COLD SPRING HARBOR SYMPOSIA ON QUANTITATIVE BIOLOGY

VOLUME LV

COLD SPRING HARBOR SYMPOSIA ON QUANTITATIVE BIOLOGY

VOLUME LV

The Brain

COLD SPRING HARBOR LABORATORY PRESS
1990

COLD SPRING HARBOR SYMPOSIA ON QUANTITATIVE BIOLOGY
VOLUME LV

© 1990 by The Cold Spring Harbor Laboratory Press
International Standard Book Number 0-87969-059-3 (cloth)
International Standard Book Number 0-87969-060-7 (paper)
International Standard Serial Number 0091-7451
Library of Congress Catalog Card Number 34-8174

COLD SPRING HARBOR SYMPOSIA ON QUANTITATIVE BIOLOGY

Founded in 1933 by
REGINALD G. HARRIS
Director of the Biological Laboratory 1924 to 1936

Previous Symposia Volumes

I (1933) Surface Phenomena
II (1934) Aspects of Growth
III (1935) Photochemical Reactions
IV (1936) Excitation Phenomena
V (1937) Internal Secretions
VI (1938) Protein Chemistry
VII (1939) Biological Oxidations
VIII (1940) Permeability and the Nature of Cell Membranes
IX (1941) Genes and Chromosomes: Structure and Organization
X (1942) The Relation of Hormones to Development
XI (1946) Heredity and Variation in Microorganisms
XII (1947) Nucleic Acids and Nucleoproteins
XIII (1948) Biological Applications of Tracer Elements
XIV (1949) Amino Acids and Proteins
XV (1950) Origin and Evolution of Man
XVI (1951) Genes and Mutations
XVII (1952) The Neuron
XVIII (1953) Viruses
XIX (1954) The Mammalian Fetus: Physiological Aspects of Development
XX (1955) Population Genetics: The Nature and Causes of Genetic Variability in Population
XXI (1956) Genetic Mechanisms: Structure and Function
XXII (1957) Population Studies: Animal Ecology and Demography
XXIII (1958) Exchange of Genetic Material: Mechanism and Consequences
XXIV (1959) Genetics and Twentieth Century Darwinism
XXV (1960) Biological Clocks

XXVI (1961) Cellular Regulatory Mechanisms
XXVII (1962) Basic Mechanisms in Animal Virus Biology
XXVIII (1963) Synthesis and Structure of Macromolecules
XXIX (1964) Human Genetics
XXX (1965) Sensory Receptors
XXXI (1966) The Genetic Code
XXXII (1967) Antibodies
XXXIII (1968) Replication of DNA in Microorganisms
XXXIV (1969) The Mechanism of Protein Synthesis
XXXV (1970) Transcription of Genetic Material
XXXVI (1971) Structure and Function of Proteins at the Three-dimensional Level
XXXVII (1972) The Mechanism of Muscle Contraction
XXXVIII (1973) Chromosome Structure and Function
XXXIX (1974) Tumor Viruses
XL (1975) The Synapse
XLI (1976) Origins of Lymphocyte Diversity
XLII (1977) Chromatin
XLIII (1978) DNA: Replication and Recombination
XLIV (1979) Viral Oncogenes
XLV (1980) Movable Genetic Elements
XLVI (1981) Organization of the Cytoplasm
XLVII (1982) Structures of DNA
XLVIII (1983) Molecular Neurobiology
XLIX (1984) Recombination at the DNA Level
L (1985) Molecular Biology of Development
LI (1986) Molecular Biology of *Homo sapiens*
LII (1987) Evolution of Catalytic Function
LIII (1988) Molecular Biology of Signal Transduction
LIV (1989) Immunological Recognition

All Cold Spring Harbor Laboratory Press publications may be ordered directly from Cold Spring Harbor Laboratory Press, 10 Skyline Drive, Plainview, New York 11803. Phone: 1-800-843-4388. In New York (516)349-1930. FAX: (516)349-1946.

Symposium Participants

ABELIOVICH, ASA, Dept. of Biology, Massachusetts Institute of Technology, Cambridge

ADAMS, PAUL, Dept. of Neurobiology and Behavior, Howard Hughes Medical Institute, State University of New York, Stony Brook

ADEREM, ALAN, Dept. of Cellular Physiology and Immunology, Rockefeller University, New York, New York

AGOSTON, DENES, Laboratory of Cell Biology and National Institute of Mental Health, National Institutes of Health, Bethesda, Maryland

ALBERINI, CRISTINA, Instituto di Chimica, Faculty of Medicine, University of Brescia, Italy

ALDRICH, RICHARD, Dept. of Neurobiology, Stanford University School of Medicine, California

ALLMAN, JOHN, Dept. of Biology, California Institute of Technology, Pasadena

ALTMAN, JENNIFER, Saunders Scientific Publications, London, England

ANDERSEN, PER, Institute of Neurophysiology, University of Oslo, Norway

ANDERSEN, RICHARD, Dept. of Brain and Cognitive Sciences, Massachusetts Institute of Technology, Cambridge

ANDERSON, DAVID, Dept. of Biology, California Institute of Technology, Pasadena

AXEL, RICHARD, Institute of Cancer Research, Columbia University College of Physicians & Surgeons, New York, New York

BADING, HILMAR, Dept. of Neurobiology and Molecular Genetics, Harvard Medical School, Boston, Massachusetts

BARABAN, JAY, Dept. of Neuroscience, Johns Hopkins University School of Medicine, Baltimore, Maryland

BARGMANN, CORI, Dept. of Biology, Massachusetts Institute of Technology, Cambridge

BARINAGA, MARCIA, *Science*, Berkeley, California

BAYLOR, DENIS, Dept. of Neurobiology, Stanford University School of Medicine, California

BEGEMANN, MARTIN, Dept. of Molecular and Developmental Biology, Rockefeller University, New York, New York

BEKKERS, JOHN, Dept. of Molecular Neurobiology, Salk Institute, La Jolla, San Diego, California

BENZER, SEYMOUR, Dept. of Biology, California Institute of Technology, Pasadena

BERG, HOWARD, Dept. of Cellular and Developmental Biology, Harvard University, Cambridge

BHUSHAN, VIKAS, University of California School of Medicine, San Francisco

BIZZI, EMILIO, Dept. of Brain and Cognitive Sciences, Massachusetts of Technology, Cambridge

BLAKEMORE, COLIN, Dept. of Physiology, University of Oxford, England

BLISS, TIMOTHY, Dept. of Neurophysiology and Neuropharmacology, National Institute for Medical Research, London, England

BONHOEFFER, FRIEDRICH, Abteilung Physikalische Biologie, Max-Planck Institut, Tubingen, Federal Republic of Germany

BONHOEFFER, TOBIAS, Neurobiology Laboratory, Rockefeller University, New York, New York

BOWER, JAMES, Dept. of Biology, California Institute of Technology, Pasadena

BRANDWEIN, HARVEY, Pall Corporation, Glen Cove, New York

BREFORT, GEORGES, Research Directorate, Rhone-Poulenc/Sante, Antony, France

BUCK, LINDA, Howard Hughes Medical Institute, Columbia University College of Physicians & Surgeons, New York, New York

BUELL, GARY, Pharmacia Genetics, La Jolla, California

BURROUS, MARY, Dept. of Neurobiology, Rockefeller University, New York, New York

BUSCH, CHRISTOPHER, Dept. of Medical Research, Max-Planck Institut, Heidelberg, Federal Republic of Germany

BUTMAN, JOHN, Dept. of Biology, Washington University, St. Louis, Missouri

BYRNE, JOHN, Dept. of Neurobiology and Anatomy, University of Texas Medical School, Houston

CADD, GARY, Dept. of Pharmacology, Howard Hughes Medical Institute, University of Washington, Seattle

CAPORALE, LYNN, Dept. of Industrial and Academic Relations, Merck Sharp & Dohme Research Laboratories, West Point, Pennsylvania

CARDOZO, DAVID, Dept. of Neurobiology, Harvard Medical School, Boston, Massachusetts

CATE, JOHN, Depts. of Pathology and Laboratory Medicine, Medical University of South Carolina, Charleston

CEPKO, CONSTANCE, Dept. of Genetics, Harvard Medical School, Boston, Massachusetts

CHANDA, PRANAB, Depts. of Microbiology and Biotechnology, Wyeth-Ayerst Laboratories, Philadelphia, Pennsylvania

CHANGEUX, JEAN-PIERRE, Dept. of Molecular Neurobiology, Institut Pasteur, Paris, France

CHAVEZ-NORIEGA, LAURA, Salk Institute, La Jolla, San Diego, California

CHEN, JOSEPH, Depts. of Physiology and Biophysics, New York University Medical Center, New York

CHU, HUNG-MING, Neuroscience Program, Harvard University, Boston, Massachusetts

CHUN, JEROLD, Whitehead Institute, Cambridge, Massachusetts

CLOTHIAUX, EUGENE, Center of Neuroscience and Physics, Brown University, Providence, Rhode Island

COHEN-CORY, SUSANA, Dept. of Neurobiology, Rockefeller University, New York, New York

COLBY, CAROL, Laboratory for Sensorimotor Research, National Eye Institute, National Institutes of Health, Bethesda, Maryland

CONSTANTINE-PATON, MARTHA, Neuroscience Program, Dept. of Biology, Yale University, New Haven, Connecticut

COREY, DAVID, Dept. of Neurology, Massachusetts General Hospital, Boston

COWAN, WILLIAM, Howard Hughes Medical Institute, National Institutes of Health, Bethesda, Maryland

CRICK, FRANCIS, Salk Institute, La Jolla, San Diego, California

CURRAN, THOMAS, Dept. of Molecular Oncology and Virology, Roche Institute of Molecular Biology, Nutley, New Jersey

DAMASIO, ANTONIO, Dept. of Neurology, University of Iowa Hospital and Clinics, Iowa City

DAMASIO, HANNA, Dept. of Neurology, University of Iowa College of Medicine, Iowa City

DARNELL, ROBERT, Dept. of Neurology, Cornell University Medical College, New York, New York

DATTA, MILTON, Dept. of Biochemistry and Biophysics, Columbia University, New York

DE CHARMS, CHRISTOPHER, Dept. of Physiology, University of California, San Francisco

DESIMONE, ROBERT, Dept. of Neuropsychology, National Institute of Mental Health, Bethesda, Maryland

DIAMOND, JEFF, Dept. of Ophthalmology, University of California, San Francisco

DOWMAN, JOHN, Dept. of Neurosciences, Medical Research Council, London, England

DUFFY, CHARLES, Laboratory for Sensorimotor Research, National Eye Institute, National Institutes of Health, Bethesda, Maryland

DUHAMEL, JEAN-RENE, National Eye Institute, National Institutes of Health, Bethesda, Maryland

EDELMAN, GERALD, Neurosciences Research Program, Rockefeller University Neurosciences Institute, New York, New York

ERKMAN, LINDA, Dept. of Biochemistry, Sciences II, The University, Geneva, Switzerland

ESSEN, LARS-OLIVER, Institute of Neurobiology, University of Heidelberg, Federal Republic of Germany

FAGG, GRAHAM, Ciba-Geigy Ltd., Basel, Switzerland

FEKETE, DONNA, Dept. of Genetics, Harvard Medical School, Boston, Massachusetts

FINGER, WOLFGANG, Universitat Tubingen, Federal Republic of Germany

FISCHBACH, GERALD, Depts. of Anatomy and Neurobiology, Washington University School of Medicine, St. Louis, Missouri

FRIEDBERG, MARC, Dept. of Neurobiology, Brown University, Providence, Rhode Island

FURTH, MARK, Dept. of Molecular and Cell Biology, Regeneron Pharmaceuticals, Inc., Tarrytown, New York

GARDNER, DANIEL, Dept. of Physiology, Cornell University Medical College, New York, New York

GASIC, GREGORY, Molecular Neurobiology Laboratory, Salk Institute, La Jolla, San Diego, California

GAUL, ULRIKE, Dept. of Cell and Molecular Biology, Howard Hughes Medical Institute, University of California, Berkeley

GEORGOPOULOS, APOSTOLOS, Dept. of Neuroscience, Johns Hopkins University School of Medicine, Baltimore, Maryland

GHEZ, CLAUDE, Dept. of Neurobiology and Behavior, Research Foundation for Mental Hygiene, Inc., New York, New York

GILBERT, CHARLES, Dept. of Neurobiology, Rockefeller University, New York, New York

GLASER, DONALD, Dept. of Physics and Neurobiology, University of California, Berkeley

GOLDBERG, MICHAEL, National Eye Institute, National Institutes of Health, Bethesda, Maryland

GOLDMAN, STEVEN, Dept. of Neurology, Cornell University Medical College, New York, New York

GOLDMAN-RAKIC, PATRICIA, Dept. of Neuroanatomy, Yale University School of Medicine, New Haven, Connecticut

GOODMAN, COREY, Dept. of Molecular and Cell Biology, Howard Hughes Medical Institute, University of California, Berkeley

GRANT, SETH, Center for Neurobiology and Behavior, Howard Hughes Medical Institute, Columbia University, New York, New York

GREENGARD, PAUL, Dept. of Molecular and Cellular Neuroscience, Rockefeller University, New York, New York

GREGA, DEBRA, Dept. of Research and Development, Boehringer Mannheim Corporation, Indianapolis, Indiana

GRILLNER, STEN, Nobel Institute for Neurophysiology, Karolinska Institutet, Stockholm, Sweden

GRUMET, MARTIN, Dept. of Developmental and Molecular Biology, Rockefeller University, New York, New York

HATTA, KOHEI, Institute of Neuroscience, University of Oregon, Eugene

HEGDE, ASHOK, Centre for Cellular and Molecular Biology, Hyderabad, India

HEINEMANN, STEPHEN, Dept. of Molecular Neurobiology, Salk Institute, La Jolla, San Diego, California

HEN, RENE, LGME de Centre National de la Recherche Scientifique, Strasbourg, France

HILDAGO, ANDREA, Dept. of Neurology, Cornell University Medical College, New York, New York

HIRANO, ARLENE, Dept. of Neurobiology, Rockefeller University, New York, New York

HIRSCH, JUDITH, Dept. of Neurobiology, Rockefeller, University, New York, New York

HOCKFIELD, SUSAN, Dept. of Neuroanatomy, Yale University School of Medicine, New Haven, Connecticut

HOGAN, NEVILLE, Dept. of Mechanical Engineering, Massachusetts Institute of Technology, Cambridge, Massachusetts

HOMONOFF, MARC, New York, New York

HOOK, VIVIAN, Uniformed Services University Health Sciences, Bethesda, Maryland

HOPKINS, NANCY, Center for Cancer Research, Massachusetts Institute of Technology, Cambridge

HORVITZ, H. ROBERT, Dept. of Biology, Howard Hughes Medical Institute, Massachusetts Institute of Technology, Cambridge

HUBEL, DAVID, Dept. of Neurobiology, Harvard Medical School, Boston, Massachusetts

HUDSPETH, JAMES, Dept. of Cell Biology and Neuroscience, University of Texas Southwestern Medical Center, Dallas, Texas

IINO, YUICHI, Center for Neurobiology and Behavior, Columbia University, New York, New York

IZUMO, SEIGO, Dept. of Molecular Medicine, Beth Israel Hospital, Boston, Massachusetts

JACEWICZ, MICHAEL, Dept. of Neurology and Neuroscience, Cornell University Medical Center, New York, New York

JACK, JULIAN, University Laboratory of Physiology, Physiological Society, Oxford, England

JALONEN, TUULA, Dept. of Biomedical Sciences, University of Tampere, Finland

JAN, LILY, Howard Hughes Medical Institute, University of California, San Francisco

JAN, YUH NUNG, Dept. of Physiology, University of California, San Francisco

JEN, JOANNA, Dept. of Molecular Neurobiology, Salk Institute, La Jolla, San Diego, California

JESSELL, THOMAS, Depts. of Biochemistry and Molecular Biophysics, Columbia University College of Physicians & Surgeons, New York, New York

JOHNSON, KENNETH, Dept. of Neuroscience, Johns Hopkins University School of Medicine, Baltimore, Maryland

JONES, EDWARD, Depts. of Anatomy and Neurobiology, University of California College of Medicine, Irvine

JONES, KEVIN, Dept. of Physiology, Howard Hughes Medical Institute, University of California, San Francisco

JORGENSEN, ERIK, Dept. of Biology, Massachusetts Institute of Technology, Cambridge

JULESZ, BELA, Laboratory of Vision Research, California Institute of Technology and Rutgers University, New Brunswick, New Jersey

KANDEL, ERIC, Center for Neurobiology and Behavior, Columbia University College of Physicians & Surgeons, New York, New York

KAPLAN, JOSHUA, Dept. of Biology, Massachusetts Institute of Technology, Cambridge

KATER, STANLEY, Depts. of Neuronal Growth and Development, Anatomy and Neurobiology,

Colorado State University, Fort Collins, Colorado

KAY, ALAN, Dept. of Biophysics, AT&T Bell Laboratories, Murray Hill, New Jersey

KELNER, KATRINA, *Science Magazine*, Washington, D.C.

KENNEDY, MARY, Dept. of Biology, California Institute of Technology, Pasadena, California

KIMMEL, BRUCE, Dept. of Molecular and Cell Biology, University of California, Berkeley

KIMURA, FUMITAKA, Dept. of Neurophysiology, Biomedical Research Center, Osaka University Medical School, Japan

KLINZ, STEPHAN, ETH Institute of Neurobiology, Zurich, Switzerland

KOCH, CHRISTOF, Dept. of Computational and Neural Systems, California Institute of Technology, Pasadena

KOCH, MICHEL, European Molecular Biology Laboratory, Outstation Hamburg, Federal Republic of Germany

KONISHI, MARK, Dept. of Biology, California Institute of Technology, Pasadena

KOTRLA, KATHRYN, Dept. of Psychiatry, Baylor College of Medicine, Houston, Texas

KUBO, TAI, Dept. of Neurobiology and Behavior, Columbia University College of Physicians & Surgeons, New York, New York

KURODA, YOICHIRO, Dept. of Neurochemistry, Tokyo Metropolitan Institute for Neuroscience, Japan

KUROKAWA, TAISUKE, Dept. of Physiology, Fukui Medical School, Japan

LA MANTIA, ANTHONY, Depts. of Anatomy and Neurobiology, Washington University School of Medicine, St. Louis, Missouri

LEHR, ANNE, Dept. of Cell Biology, National Institute of Mental Health, National Institutes of Health, Bethesda, Maryland

LI, CONGYI, Cell and Molecular Biology Program, University of Wisconsin, Madison

LILLIEN, LAURA, Dept. of Genetics, Harvard Medical School, Boston, Massachusetts

LISBERGER, STEPHEN, Dept. of Physiology, University of California, San Francisco

LIVINGSTONE, MARGARET, Dept. of Neurobiology, Harvard Medical School, Boston, Massachusetts

LLINAS, RONDOLFO, Depts. of Physiology and Biophysics, New York University School of Medicine, New York

LO, MATTHEW, ICI Americas, Wilmington, Delaware

LOEB, GERALD, Dept. of Physiology, Queen's University, Kingston, Canada

LU, BAI, Dept. of Molecular Neuroscience, Rockefeller University, New York, New York

MAC LEISH, PETER, Dept. of Neurobiology, Rockefeller University, New York, New York

MAHAN, LAWRENCE, Dept. of Cell Biology, National Institute of Mental Health, National Institutes of Health, Bethesda, Maryland

MARGOLSKEE, ROBERT, Dept. of Neurosciences, Roche Institute of Molecular Biology, Nutley, New Jersey

MARICQ, ANDREA, Dept. of Pharmacology, University of California, San Francisco

MARONEY, ANNA, Dept. of Microbiology, Howard Hughes Medical Institute, University of Pennsylvania, Philadelphia

MAROTEAUX, LUC, Institut de Chimie Biologique, Centre National Recherche Scientifique, LGME, Strasbourg, France

MARRION, NEIL, Depts. of Neurobiology and Behavior, Howard Hughes Medical Research Laboratory, State University of New York, Stony Brook

MARTIN, KEVAN, Dept. of Pharmacology, Medical Research Council, Oxford, England

McALLISTER, GEORGE, Neuroscience Research Centre, Merck Sharp & Dohme Research Laboratories, Essex, England

McCARTHY, BRIAN, Depts. of Neurobiology and Behavior, State University of New York, Stony Brook

McCLENDON, EVELYN, Depts. of Neurobiology and Anatomy, University of Texas Health Science Center, Houston

McKAY, RONALD, Depts. of Brain and Cognitive Sciences, and Biology, Massachusetts Institute of Technology, Cambridge

McMAHAN, UEL JACK, Dept. of Neurobiology, Stanford University School of Medicine, California

MERZENICH, MICHAEL, Coleman Memorial Laboratory, University of California, San Francisco

MIAKE-LYE, RYN, *Cell Magazine*, Cambridge, Massachusetts

MIKLOS, GEORGE, Molecular Neurobiology Group, Australian National University, Canberra

MILNER, BRENDA, Montreal Neurological Institute, McGill University, Canada

MOLNAR, ZOLTAN, Physiology Laboratory, University of Oxford, England

MONTAGUE, P. READ, Neurosciences Institute, New York, New York

MORIGIWA, KATSUKO, Dept. of Physiology, Osaka University Medical School, Japan

MORRIS, RICHARD, Dept. of Pharmacology, University of Edinburgh Medical School, Scotland

MOUNTCASTLE, VERNON, Bard Laboratories, Department of Neuroscience, Johns Hopkins University School of Medicine, Baltimore, Maryland

MOVSHON, J. ANTHONY, Center for Neural Science, New York University, New York

MURAKOSHI, TAKAYUKI, Neurobiology Laboratory, Rockefeller University, New York, New York

MURASE, KAZUYUKI, Dept. of Information Science, Fukui University, Japan

NAIRN, ANGUS, Dept. of Molecular and Cellular Neuroscience, Rockefeller University, New York, New York

NAKANISHI, NOBUKI, Howard Hughes Medical Institute, Columbia University College of Physicians & Surgeons, New York, New York

NAKAYAMA, KEN, Smith-Kettlewell Eye Research Institute, San Francisco, California

NATHANS, JEREMY, Dept. of Molecular Biology and Genetics, Howard Hughes Medical Institute, Johns Hopkins School of Medicine, Baltimore, Maryland

NAVE, KLAUS-ARMIN, Dept. of Molecular Neurobiology, Salk Institute, La Jolla, San Diego, California

NEWSOME, WILLIAM, Dept. of Neurobiology, Stanford University School of Medicine, California

NICOLL, ROGER, Dept. of Pharmacology, University of California, San Francisco

NIKOLICS, KAROLY, Dept. of Developmental Biology, Genentech, Inc., South San Francisco, California

NINIO, JACQUES, Institut Jacques Monod, Paris, France

NIRENBERG, SHEILA, Dept. of Genetics, Harvard Medical School, Boston, New York

NODA, TERUMI, Dept. of Physiology, Fukui Medical School, Japan

NUMA, SHOSAKU, Depts. of Medical Chemistry and Molecular Genetics, Kyoto University Faculty of Medicine, Japan

O'CONNOR, WILLIAM, Dept. of Pharmacology, Karolinska Institute, Stockholm, Sweden

O'LEARY, DENNIS, Depts. of Anatomy and Neurobiology, Washington University School of Medicine, St. Louis, Missouri

OBERDORFER, MICHAEL, National Eye Institute, National Institutes of Health, Bethesda, Maryland

OVERBEEK, PAUL, Dept. of Cell Biology, Howard Hughes Medical Institute, Baylor College of Medicine, Houston, Texas

PATTERSON, PAUL, Dept. of Biology, California Institute of Technology, Pasadena

PEINADO, ALEX, Dept. of Neurobiology, Rockefeller University, New York, New York

POGGIO, GIAN, Dept. of Neuroscience, Bard Laboratories, Johns Hopkins University School of Medicine, Baltimore, Maryland

POGGIO, TOMASCO, Artificial Intelligence Laboratory, Massachusetts Institute of Technology, Cambridge and IRST, Trento, Italy

PRIETO, ANNE, Dept. of Molecular and Developmental Biology, Rockefeller University, New York, New York

PULSINELLI, WILLIAM, Dept. of Neurology, Cornell University Medical College, New York, New York

PURVES, DALE, Depts of Anatomy and Neurobiology, Washington University School of Medicine, St. Louis, Missouri

QUINN, WILLIAM, Depts. of Brain and Cognitive Sciences, and Biology, Massachusetts Institute of Technology, Cambridge

RAFF, MARTIN, Dept. of Biology, University College, London, England

RAICHLE, MARCUS, Dept. of Radiation Sciences, Washington University Medical Center, St. Louis, Missouri

RAKIC, PASKO, Section of Neuroanatomy, Yale University School of Medicine, New Haven, Connecticut

RAMIREZ, ROSAURA, Dept. of Biology, University of Puerto Rico, Rio Piedras

RAO, YI, Dept. of Physiology, University of California, San Francisco

REICHARDT, LOUIS, Dept. of Physiology, Howard Hughes Medical Institute, University of California, San Francisco

REINAGEL, PAMELA, Harvard University, Boston, Massachusetts

ROBINSON, DAVID, Dept. of Opthamology, Johns Hopkins University, Baltimore, Maryland

ROLLS, EDMUND, Dept. of Experimental Psychology, University of Oxford, England

RONNETT, GABRIELE, Dept. of Neurology and Neuroscience, Johns Hopkins University, Baltimore, Maryland

ROUTTENBERG, ARYEH, Cresap Neuroscience Laboratory, Northwestern University, Evanston, Illinois

RUBIN, MICHAEL, Dept. of Molecular and Cellular Neuroscience, Rockefeller University, New York, New York

RUVKUN, GARY, Dept. of Molecular Biology, Massachusetts General Hospital, Boston

SAKMANN, BERT, Abteilung Zellphysiologie, Max-Planck Institut, Heidelberg, Federal Republic of Germany

SANES, JOSHUA, Dept. of Anatomy and Neurobiology, Washington University School of Medicine, St. Louis, Missouri

SARON, CLIFFORD, Dept. of Neuroscience, Albert Einstein College of Medicine, Bronx, New York

SAWIN, ELIZABETH, Dept. of Biology, Massachusetts Institute of Technology, Cambridge

SCHAEFFER, ERIC, Dept. of Molecular and Cellular Neuroscience, Rockefeller University, New York, New York

SCHELLER, RICHARD, Herrin Laboratory, Dept. of Biological Sciences, Stanford University, California

SCHWARTZ, JAMES, Howard Hughes Medical Institute, Columbia College of Physicians & Surgeons, New York, New York

SCHWARZ, ULI, Dept. of Biochemistry, Max-Planck Institut, Tubingen, Federal Republic of Germany

SEEBURG, PETER, Zentrum fur Molekulare Biologie, University of Heidelberg, ZMBH, Federal Republic of Germany

SEJNOWSKI, TERRENCE, Salk Institute and University of California, San Deigo

SHATZ, CARLA, Dept. of Neurobiology, Stanford University School of Medicine, California

SHNEIDER, NEIL, Howard Hughes Medical Institute, Columbia University, New York, New York

SHOOLMAN, HARVEY, Blackwell Scientific Publications Ltd., Oxford, England

SIGUENZA, JUAN ALBERTO, Departamento de Morfologia/Medicina, Universidad Autonoma de Madrid, Spain

SILVA, ALCINO, Center for Cancer Research, Massachusetts Institute of Technology, Cambridge

SINGER, WOLF, Dept. of Neurophysiology, Brain Research, Max-Planck Institut, Frankfurt, Federal Republic of Germany

SMITH, MARTIN, Dept. of Chemical and Biological Screening, Upjohn Company, Kalamazoo, Michigan

SPARKS, DAVID, Dept. of Psychology, University of Pennsylvania, Philadelphia

SQUIRE, LARRY, University of California, and Veterans' Administration Medical Center, San Diego

STARK, RACHEL, Dept. of Audiology and Speech Sciences, Purdue University, West Lafayette, Indiana

STEINMETZ, MICHAEL, Dept. of Neuroscience, Johns Hopkins University School of Medicine, Baltimore, Maryland

STEVENS, CHARLES, Dept. of Molecular Neurobiology, Salk Institute, La Jolla, San Diego, California

STRYKER, MICHAEL, Dept. of Physiology and Neuroscience, University of California, San Francisco

SUBRAMANIAN, ALAP, Max-Planck Institut for Molekulare Genetik, Berlin, Federal Republic of Germany

SUGA, NUBUO, Dept. of Biology, Washington University, St. Louis, Missouri

SZAPIEL, SUSAN, Dept. of Neurobiology, Rockefeller University, New York, New York

TAKEICHI, MASATOSHI, Dept. of Biophysics, Faculty of Science, Kyoto University, Japan

TANK, DAVID, Computational Neuroscience Group, Bell Laboratories, Murray Hill, New Jersey

TOMICH, PAUL, Dept. of Chemical and Biological Screening, Upjohn Company, Kalamazoo, Michigan

TORRE, VINCENT, Dept. of Physics, Universita di Genova, Italy

TSAO, FRITZ, Dept. of Psychology, Hillsdale College, Michigan

TSIEN, RICHARD, Dept. of Molecular and Cellular Physiology, Stanford University Medical Center, California

TSIEN, ROGER, Howard Hughes Medical Institute, University of California, San Diego

TULLY, TIM, Dept. of Biology, Brandeis University, Waltham, Massachusetts

ULLMAN, SHIMON, Artificial Intelligence Laboratory, Massachusetts Institute of Technology, Cambridge

UNNIKRISHNAN, K.P., Dept. of Computer Science, General Motors Research Laboratories, Warren, Michigan

VALENZUELA, DARIO, Dept. of Developmental Biology, Howard Hughes Medical Institute, Massachusetts General Hospital, Boston

VAN ESSEN, DAVID, Dept. of Biology, California Institute of Technology, Pasadena

VAN VACTOR, DAVID, Dept. of Biological Chemistry, University of California, Los Angeles

VANDENBERG, ROBERT, Garvan Institute of Medical Research, St. Vincent's Hospital, Sydney, Australia

VETTER, MONICA, Dept. of Physiology, University of California, San Francisco

VIVEROS, HUMBERTO, Division of Medicinal Biochemistry, Burroughs Wellcome Company, Research Triangle Park, North Carolina

VOYVODIC, JAMES, Dept. of Biology, University College, London, England

WAGNER, JOHN, Dana-Farber Cancer Institute, Boston, Massachusetts

WALTER, GERNOT, Dept. of Pathology, University of California, San Diego

WATSON, JAMES, Cold Spring Harbor Laboratory, Cold Spring Harbor, New York

WESTHEIMER, GERALD, Dept. of Molecular and Cell Biology, University of California, Berkeley

WHITE, W. FROST, Dept. of Neuroscience, Pfizer Central Research, Groton, Connecticut

WIESEL, TORSTEN, Dept. of Neurobiology, Rockefeller University, New York, New York

WILLIAMS, JOHN, Dept. of Neurophysiology and Neuropharmacy, National Institute for Medical Research, London, England

WILLIAMSON, DAVID, Dept. of Developmental and Molecular Biology, Rockefeller University, New York, New York

WITUNSKI, MICHAEL, Kiawah Island, South Carolina

WOOD, JOHN, Dept. of Molecular Genetics, Lilly Research Laboratories, Indianapolis, Indiana

WORLEY, PAUL, Dept. of Neuroscience, Johns Hopkins University School of Medicine, Baltimore, Maryland

WURTZ, ROBERT, Laboratory for Sensorimotor Research, National Eye Institute, National Institutes of Health, Bethesda, Maryland

YAMAMORI, TETSUO, Dept. of Biology, California Institute of Technology, Pasadena

YAMANE, T., Dept. of Biophysics, AT&T Bell Laboratories, Murray Hill, New Jersey

YAMASAKI, SONNY, Laboratory for Sensorimotor Research, National Eye Institute, National Institutes of Health, Bethesda, Maryland

YANCOPOULOS, GEORGE, Regeneron Pharmaceuticals, Inc., Tarrytown, New York

YANG, XIANJIE, Dept. of Genetics, Harvard Medical School, Boston, Massachusetts

YIN, JERRY, Dept. of Brain and Cognitive Sciences, Massachusetts Institute of Technology, Cambridge

YU, VICTOR, Eukaryotic Regulatory Biology Program, University of California, San Diego

YUSTE, RAFAEL, Dept. of Neurobiology, Rockefeller University, New York, New York

ZEKI, SEMIR, Dept. of Anatomy and Developmental Biology, University College, London, England

ZHAO, BIAO, Dept. of Neurobiology and Behavior, Columbia University, New York, New York

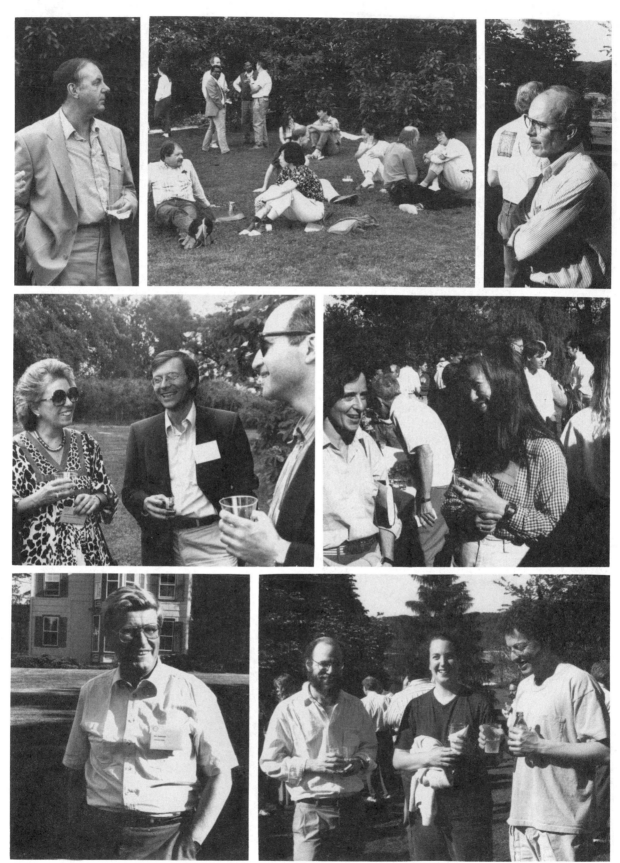

First row: J.J.B. Jack; Wine and Cheese Party; D. Baylor
Second row: H. Damasio, T. Sejnowski, C. Gilbert; S. Hockfield, L. Jan
Third row: P. Andersen; H. Horvitz, B. Sawin, A. Abeliovich

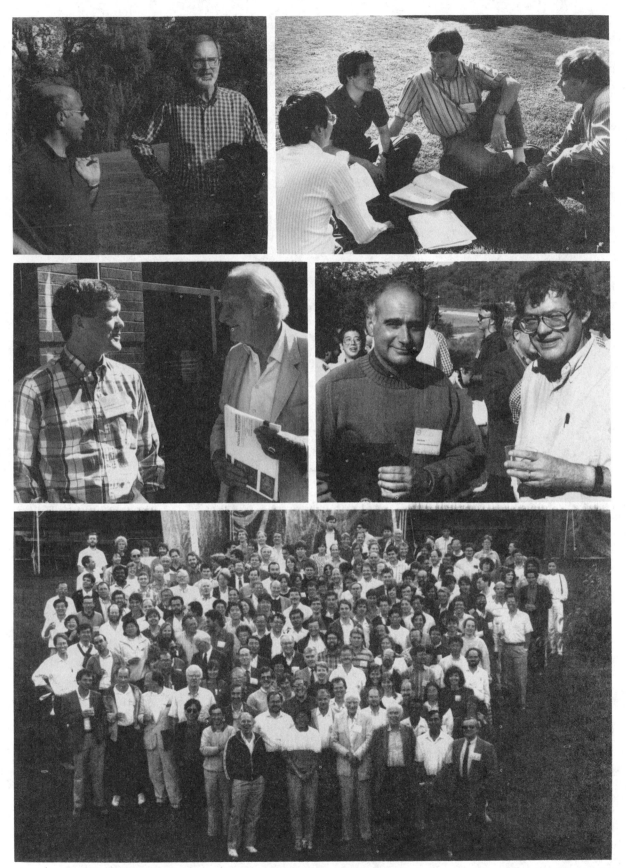

First row: S. Zeki, M. Raichle; R. Tsien, R.Tsien, T. Bonhoeffer, F. Bonhoeffer
Second row: J. Witkowski, F. Crick; J. Byrne, C.F. Stevens

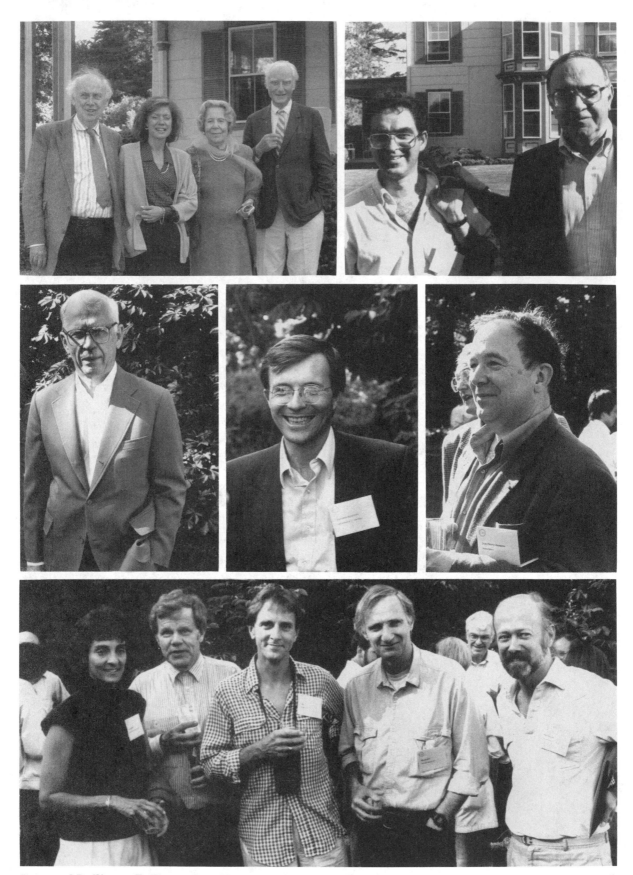

First row: J.D. Watson, E. Watson, L.A. Hazen, F. Crick; T. Poggio, G.F. Poggio
Second row: V.B. Mountcastle; T. Sejnowski; J.-P. Changeux
Third row: C. Shatz, F. Bonhoeffer, C. Blakemore, M.C. Raff, P.H. Patterson

Foreword

The brain will be to the next century what the gene has been to the 20th century. At the start of this century, we knew that genes were on chromosomes, but what they were chemically or how they functioned was a total mystery. Now, of course, much, much more is known about the brain. This has been far from a sleepy century for brain research, and an extraordinary accumulation of anatomical data is now being complemented by experiments localizing definite tasks to specific collections of nerve cells. But compared to the gene, the brain, at least in today's ignorance, seems an infinitely more daunting objective. No one has any precise ideas about how complex perceptions are stored in our brains, much less retrieved when our memories work as we wish.

How we will reach these objectives is far from clear, except for the virtual truism that we should diversify our approaches and at least for the present not divert too many of our resources toward any one approach. We must also see to it that the theorists learn the facts of the experimentalists and that the experimentalists also begin seriously to learn what the neural modelers are up to. It was with this objective that we decided to hold the 1990 Symposium (our 55th) on The Brain. This was to be our sixth symposium that focused on nerve cells. In 1936, we focused on Excitation Phenomena; in 1952, on The Neuron; in 1966, on Sensory Perception; in 1975, on The Synapse; and in 1983, on Molecular Neurobiology. The intervals between neurobiology-oriented meetings have steadily shortened and will likely continue to do so given the increasing number of talented young scientists who now see the brain as the ultimate challenge for biology.

In choosing the speakers, I needed much advice, and in particular, I thank Max Cowan, Francis Crick, Tom Jessell, Eric Kandel, Charles Stevens, and Terry Sejnowski. Later in organizing the final program and in selecting the order in which the symposium papers appear in these volumes, I particularly thank Eric Kandel, whose advice has been invaluable to me since the start of our neurobiology summer teaching program in 1971. The final program contained 105 presentations given over a one-week-long period before an audience that totaled 320. On opening night, there were splendid introductory talks by Shosaku Numa, Martin Raff, Sten Grillner, William Newsome, and Marcus Raichle. The summary, artfully given, was by Michael Stryker. The final result was a wonderful, although intellectually exhausting, experience that more than justified the money and time needed for its organization and execution.

Financial support for such a large meeting as the Symposium comes from many sources. We gratefully acknowledge the National Institute of Mental Health (an Institute of the Alcohol, Drug Abuse, and Mental Health Administration); the National Cancer Institute, the National Institute of Child Health and Human Development, the National Institute of Neurological Disorders and Stroke (divisions of the National Institutes of Health); the U.S. Department of Energy; and the National Science Foundation. Essential funds also came from our Corporate Sponsors: Alafi Capital Company; American Cyanamid Company; AMGen Inc.; Applied Biosystems, Inc.; Becton Dickinson and Company; Boehringer Mannheim Corporation; Bristol-Meyers Squibb Company; Ciba-Geigy Corporation/Ciba-Geigy Limited; Diagnostic Products Corporation; E.I. du Pont de Nemours & Company; Eastman Kodak Company; Genentech, Inc.; Genetics Institute; Hoffmann-La Roche Inc.; Johnson & Johnson; Life Technologies, Inc.; Eli Lilly and Company; Millipore Corporation; Monsanto Company; Pall Corporation; Perkin-Elmer Cetus Instruments; Pfizer Inc.; Pharmacia Inc.; Schering-Plough Corporation; The Upjohn Company; The Wellcome Research Laboratories, Burroughs Wellcome Co.; and Wyeth-Ayerst Research.

Registration and housing for the participants were organized with care and courtesy by the staff of the Meetings Office: Maureen Berejka, Barbara Ward, Karen Otto, Diane Tighe, Michela McBride, and Marge Stellabotte. Jim Hope and his staff provided admirable catering, and once again Herb Parsons and his assistants delivered a flawless audiovisual service. These books were edited by Dorothy Brown, Patricia Barker, and Ralph Battey, assisted by Joan Ebert, Mary Cozza, and Inez Sialiano, and their production was overseen by Nancy Ford.

James D. Watson
January 31, 1990

Contents

Neural Development

Cognitive Neuroscience

COLD SPRING HARBOR SYMPOSIA ON QUANTITATIVE BIOLOGY

VOLUME LV

Molecular Insights into Excitation-Contraction Coupling

S. Numa, T. Tanabe, H. Takeshima, A. Mikami, T. Niidome,
S. Nishimura, B.A. Adams,* and K.G. Beam*

Departments of Medical Chemistry and Molecular Genetics, Kyoto University Faculty of Medicine, Kyoto 606, Japan;
*Department of Physiology, College of Veterinary Medicine and Biomedical Sciences, Colorado State University,
Fort Collins, Colorado 80523

Excitation-contraction (E-C) coupling represents an essential feature of muscle function. In skeletal muscle, depolarization of transverse tubules (T tubules), infoldings of the cell-surface membrane, causes Ca^{++} to be released from the sarcoplasmic reticulum (SR) without requiring entry of extracellular Ca^{++} (Armstrong et al. 1972); the Ca^{++} released from the SR triggers contraction. One hypothesis for how skeletal muscle E-C coupling occurs is that a "voltage sensor" located in the T-tubular membrane is responsible for controlling the release of Ca^{++} from the SR (Schneider and Chandler 1973). Specifically, T-tubular depolarization induces a molecular rearrangement of the voltage sensor, which is postulated to gate calcium flow across the SR. Consistent with this hypothesis is the presence in skeletal muscle of voltage-dependent intramembrane charge movement (Schneider and Chandler 1973). The mechanism of depolarization-contraction coupling in cardiac muscle differs from that in skeletal muscle in that Ca^{++} influx across the sarcolemma is required for contraction. The dihydropyridine (DHP)-sensitive L-type calcium channel represents a major pathway for entry of extracellular Ca^{++} in cardiac cells (for review, see Bean 1989), and this entry triggers the subsequent large release of Ca^{++} from the SR (Fabiato 1985; Beuckelmann and Wier 1988; Näbauer et al. 1989).

In an attempt to understand the molecular basis of E-C coupling, we have investigated the DHP receptor as a potential T-tubular voltage sensor (and/or calcium channel) and the ryanodine receptor as a calcium release channel in the SR. The primary structure of the DHP receptor, deduced by cloning and sequencing the cDNA (Tanabe et al. 1987), has revealed that this receptor is homologous with the voltage-gated sodium channel (for review, see Numa and Noda 1986), comprising four repeating units of homology. Each of the four internal repeats contains the characteristic, highly conserved segment S4 with clustered, regularly spaced, positively charged amino acid residues, which probably serve to sense voltage (Noda et al. 1984, 1986; Stühmer et al. 1989). The structural similarity to the voltage-gated sodium channel has suggested that the DHP receptor in skeletal muscle T tubules may have a dual function, acting both as the voltage sensor for E-C coupling and as a calcium channel (Tanabe et al. 1987). An involvement of the T-tubular DHP receptor in E-C coupling has also been suggested on the basis of observed effects of DHP on intramembrane charge move-

ment and myoplasmic calcium transients (Rios and Brum 1987). However, there has not yet been a direct demonstration that the DHP receptor functions as the voltage sensor for E-C coupling. To address this issue, we have used mice with muscular dysgenesis, a fatal autosomal recessive mutation (Gluecksohn-Waelsch 1963) that is expressed in skeletal muscle as a failure of E-C coupling (Powell and Fambrough 1973; Klaus et al. 1983) and absence of the slow DHP-sensitive L-type calcium current (Beam et al. 1986; Rieger et al. 1987). The results obtained are described below. Molecular characteristics of the ryanodine receptor from the skeletal muscle SR, revealed by cloning and sequencing the cDNA, are also discussed.

Dual Role of the Skeletal Muscle DHP Receptor

Myotubes from dysgenic mice were subjected to microinjection into nuclei of an expression plasmid carrying the cDNA encoding the rabbit skeletal muscle (pCAC6) or cardiac (pCARD1) DHP receptor (Tanabe et al. 1988, 1990a). Both pCAC6-injected and pCARD1-injected dysgenic myotubes displayed contractions spontaneously or in response to electrical stimulation. Approximately 180 myotubes survived injection with pCAC6 and 68 of these exhibited E-C coupling, 17 contracting spontaneously and 51 in response to electrical stimulation. Of approximately 530 myotubes that survived injection with pCARD1, depolarization-contraction coupling was produced in 89 cases (10 spontaneous and 79 electrically evoked). None of the dysgenic myotubes injected with the vector plasmid as a control (~200 myotubes survived) were observed to contract either spontaneously or in response to electrical stimulation.

Although the injection of either pCAC6 or pCARD1 produced depolarization-contraction coupling in dysgenic myotubes, the nature of this coupling was different for the two kinds of DHP receptor. Dysgenic myotubes injected with pCAC6 underwent electrically evoked contractions in normal rodent Ringer's solution (Fig. 1A, a and d), in the absence of extracellular Ca^{++} (Fig. 1A, b), and in the presence of Cd^{++}, a calcium channel blocker (Fig. 1A, e). In contrast, pCARD1-injected dysgenic myotubes displayed electrically evoked contractions in normal rodent Ringer's solution (Fig. 1B, a and d), but not in Ca^{++}-free (Fig. 1B, b) or

A   **B**

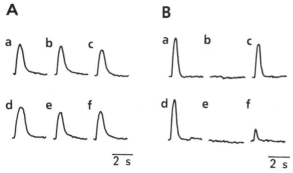

diac-type" E-C coupling, which does require entry of extracellular Ca^{++}.

The muscular dysgenesis mutation selectively eliminates slow L-type calcium current (I_{slow}) without affecting transient T-type calcium current (I_{fast}) (Beam et al. 1986; Rieger et al. 1987). Dysgenic myotubes that had been injected with pCAC6 or pCARD1 and observed to contract exhibited L-type calcium currents (Fig. 2). However, the kinetics and voltage dependence of the L-type currents produced were different between pCAC6- and pCARD1-injected myotubes. In pCAC6-injected myotubes, the rate of activation was slow (Fig. 2A), being similar to that observed in normal skeletal muscle (Sanchez and Stefani 1978; Donaldson and Beam 1983). In contrast, the L-type calcium current in pCARD1-injected myotubes was activated more rapidly (Fig. 2B), like the L-type current in cardiac muscle (Isenberg and Klöckner 1982; Lee and Tsien 1982). The function of the DHP receptors as L-type calcium channels is supported by the finding that functional DHP-sensitive calcium channels result from the expression of the cardiac DHP receptor cDNA in *Xenopus* oocytes (Mikami et al. 1989), as well as from the expression of the skeletal muscle DHP receptor in murine L cells (Perez-Reyes et al. 1989).

The finding that both E-C coupling and L-type calcium current missing in dysgenic muscle can be restored by injection of pCAC6 indicates that the skeletal muscle DHP receptor has a dual functional role, acting both as an essential component of E-C coupling and as an L-type calcium channel. On the other hand, the cardiac DHP receptor expressed in skeletal muscle is able to function as an L-type calcium channel, but cannot directly control release of Ca^{++} from the SR. The behaviors of the expressed DHP receptors mirror the physiological situations in skeletal and cardiac mus-

Figure 1. Comparison of electrically evoked contractions in dysgenic myotubes injected with the expression plasmid pCAC6 for the skeletal muscle DHP receptor (*A*) or with pCARD1 for the cardiac DHP receptor (*B*). Cells were first bathed in normal rodent Ringer's solution (*a,d*), next exposed to either Ca^{++}-free (*b*) or 0.5 mM Cd^{++}-containing (*e*) Ringer, and finally returned to normal Ringer (*c,f*). Recovery of electrically evoked contraction in the pCARD1-injected cell after exposure to Cd^{++} was incomplete during the ~5-min wash with normal Cd^{++}-free Ringer. However, after being returned to culture medium and maintained for ~30 min in the tissue-culture incubator, the cell regained the ability to contract vigorously. The blockade of contraction in pCARD1-injected myotubes by brief exposures to lower concentrations of Cd^{++} was readily reversible. For the methods of electrical stimulation and optical recording of contraction, see Tanabe et al. (1988). The normal rodent Ringer contained (in mM) 146 NaCl, 5 KCl, 2 CaCl$_2$, 1 MgCl$_2$, and 10 HEPES (pH 7.4 with NaOH). The Ca^{++}-free Ringer was made by equimolar substitution of Mg^{++} for Ca^{++} in the normal rodent Ringer. (Horizontal calibration: 2 sec. Vertical scale: arbitrary units.) (Reprinted, with permission, from Tanabe et al. 1990a.)

Cd^{++}-containing (Fig. 1B, e) Ringer's solution. Thus, injection of pCAC6 restores E-C coupling that resembles normal skeletal muscle E-C coupling ("skeletal-type"), which does not require entry of extracellular Ca^{++}, whereas injection of pCARD1 produces "car-

A   **B**

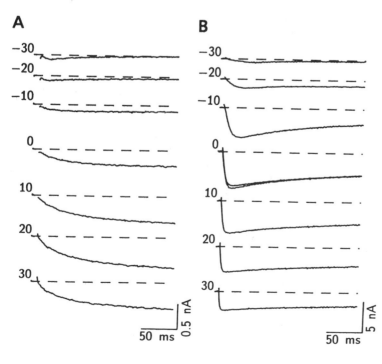

Figure 2. Comparison of calcium currents in dysgenic myotubes injected with pCAC6 (*A*) or pCARD1 (*B*). Calcium currents were measured using the whole-cell variant of the patch-clamp technique (Hamill et al. 1981). The test potential (in mV) is indicated next to each current trace. For both the cells shown, only a small amount of I_{fast} was present. The contribution of I_{fast} to the total current in the pCARD1-injected cell can be seen by comparing the two current traces for the 0-mV test potential. The larger current trace was obtained from the standard holding potential (−80 mV for all the data reported here). The smaller current trace was obtained for an identical 0-mV test pulse that was preceded by a 1-sec step to −40 mV, which selectively inactivates I_{fast}. The average maximum L-type current (normalized by linear cell capacitance) was 4.4 ± 2.7 pA/pF (mean ± s.d., range 1.0–12.4 pA/pF, $n = 26$) in pCAC6-injected myotubes and 28.0 ± 10.0 pA/pF (range 12.5–56.1 pA/pF, $n = 31$) in pCARD1-injected myotubes. (Reprinted, with permission, from Tanabe et al. 1990a.)

cle. The restoration of the functional defects in dysgenic muscle, together with blot hybridization analysis of genomic DNA and skeletal muscle RNA, suggests that the muscular dysgenesis mutation alters the skeletal muscle DHP receptor gene (Tanabe et al. 1988).

Regions of the DHP Receptor Determining Skeletal-type Excitation-Contraction Coupling

An attempt was next made to identify the regions responsible for the functional differences observed between the skeletal muscle and cardiac DHP receptors (Tanabe et al. 1990b). The major differences in primary structure between the two DHP receptors (Tanabe et al. 1987; Mikami et al. 1989) reside in the large, putative cytoplasmic regions, i.e., the amino- and carboxy-terminal regions as well as the regions linking repeats I and II (I-II loop) and repeats II and III (II-III loop). To test whether these regions of the skeletal muscle DHP receptor are required for skeletal-type E-C coupling, we constructed five different expression plasmids carrying chimeric DHP receptor cDNAs (pCSk7 and pCSk1-4), as illustrated schematically in Figure 3A. These constructions used the cardiac DHP receptor as the basic structure in which the large, putative cytoplasmic regions were replaced by the corresponding regions of the skeletal muscle DHP receptor.

Dysgenic myotubes injected with each of the five chimeric plasmids did indeed display electrically evoked contractions; the number of responsive myotubes relative to the number of tested myotubes was comparable to that for pCAC6- or pCARD1-injected myotubes (see above). Although not systematically monitored, spontaneous contractions were also observed in some myotubes injected with each of the chimeric plasmids. Myotubes that had been injected with a chimeric plasmid and observed to contract all showed L-type calcium currents. The L-type currents induced by the chimeric plasmids displayed a rapid rate of activation, which was very similar to that in pCARD1-injected myotubes (see Fig. 2B) and much faster than that in pCAC6-injected myotubes (see Fig. 2A). Thus, this property characteristic of the cardiac L-type calcium channel is maintained even when its major putative cytoplasmic regions are replaced by their skeletal muscle counterparts.

Examination of electrically evoked contractions showed that dysgenic myotubes expressing pCSk7, which encodes the chimeric DHP receptor with all the major putative cytoplasmic regions replaced by their skeletal muscle counterparts (Fig. 3A, c), exhibited E-C coupling (Fig. 3B, c) similar to that produced by pCAC6 (Fig. 3B, a). Thus, switching these regions of the DHP receptor from cardiac to skeletal muscle changed the character of E-C coupling from cardiac-type (Fig. 3B, b) to skeletal-type (Fig. 3B, a).

We next examined whether replacement of a single putative cytoplasmic region is sufficient to produce this change. Dysgenic myotubes expressing either pCSk1, which encodes the chimera with only the amino-terminal region replaced (Fig. 3A, d), or pCSk4, which encodes the chimera with only the carboxy-terminal region replaced (Fig. 3A, g), displayed cardiac-type E-C coupling (Fig. 3B, d and g). In contrast, myotubes expressing pCSk3, which encodes the chimera with only the II-III loop replaced (Fig. 3A, f), showed skeletal-type E-C coupling (Fig. 3B, f). Altogether, 42 myotubes expressing pCSk3 and 20 expressing pCSk7 were tested and all were found to display skeletal-type E-C coupling. The fact that myotubes expressing pCSk3 or pCSk7 exhibited weaker contraction in Ca^{++}-free or Cd^{++}-containing Ringer's solution than in normal Ringer's solution (Fig. 3B, c and f) can be accounted for by entry of extracellular Ca^{++} contributing to the contraction of these myotubes in normal Ringer's solution. When tested under identical conditions (extracellularly applied stimulus with a duration of 5 msec), myotubes expressing pCSk2, which encodes the chimera with only the I-II loop replaced (Fig. 3A, e), showed cardiac-type E-C coupling. When the stimulus duration was increased to 20 msec, however, weak contractions were observed in some myotubes expressing pCSk2 both in Ca^{++}-free (9 of 23 tested) and in Cd^{++}-containing (14 of 20 tested) Ringer's solution. These weak contractions, barely resolvable by the contraction-monitoring apparatus, are evident as a brief, small, upward deflection at the beginning of the trace (Fig. 3B, e, traces 2 and 3). Even with the longer stimulus of 20-msec duration, myotubes expressing pCSk1 ($n = 15$), pCSk4 ($n = 13$), or pCARD1 ($n = 15$) never showed contractions in Ca^{++}-free or Cd^{++}-containing Ringer's solution. In conclusion, pCSk3 produces effective skeletal-type E-C coupling. pCSk2 is also able to produce skeletal-type E-C coupling, although the efficiency is so low that the amount of Ca^{++} released from the SR exceeds the threshold for contraction in only a fraction of cells.

The above results indicate that the II-III loop of the skeletal muscle DHP receptor is a major determinant site for skeletal-type E-C coupling, that the I-II loop is possibly less important, and that the amino- and carboxy-terminal regions are probably unimportant. Alternatively, the weaker skeletal-type E-C coupling observed with pCSk2 than with pCSk3 may mean that the I-II loop and the II-III loop are both critical, but that the I-II loop is more functionally interchangeable between the cardiac and skeletal muscle DHP receptors than is the II-III loop. Similarly, it is possible that the putative cytoplasmic region linking repeats III and IV, which is highly conserved between the two DHP receptors, is also important in skeletal-type E-C coupling. The finding that expression of pCSk3 and pCSk7 produces skeletal-type E-C coupling but rapidly activating, cardiac-type calcium current shows that the slow activation of the skeletal muscle L-type channel is not an obligatory consequence of the DHP receptor serving as the voltage sensor for E-C coupling. This finding also suggests that the putative membrane-spanning and

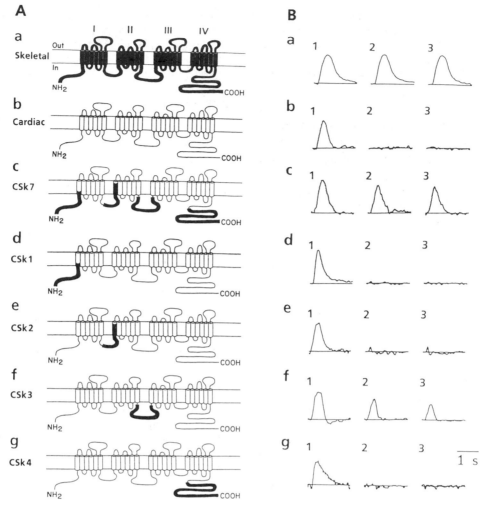

Figure 3. (*A*) Schematic representation of the structures of the skeletal muscle (*a*), cardiac (*b*), and chimeric DHP receptors (*c–g*). For each DHP receptor, the four units of homology (repeats I–IV) are displayed linearly and the six putative transmembrane segments (S1–S6 from left to right) in each repeat are shown by cylinders. The darkly shaded areas indicate regions of the skeletal muscle DHP receptor. Note that the junctional sequences common to the skeletal muscle and cardiac DHP receptors are not darkly shaded and that the exchanged portion of segment S1 of repeat II is very similar in amino acid sequence between the two DHP receptors (see below). The compositions of the individual chimeric DHP receptors are as follows (C and Sk denote the cardiac and the skeletal muscle DHP receptor, respectively, and the numbers in parentheses indicate amino acid numbers; the junctional sequences common to the two DHP receptors are represented by amino acid numbers of the cardiac DHP receptor). CSk7: Sk (1–55), C (159–464), Sk (364–448), C (571–787), Sk (666–791), C (923–1634), and Sk (1510–1873). CSk1: Sk (1–55) and C (159–2171). CSk2: C (1–464), Sk (364–448), and C (571–2171). CSk3: C (1–787), Sk (666–791), and C (923–2171). CSk4: C (1–1634) and Sk (1510–1873). (*B*) Comparison of electrically evoked contractions in dysgenic myotubes injected with pCAC6 (*a*), pCARD1 (*b*), pCSk7 (*c*), pCSk1 (*d*), pCSk2 (*e*), pCSk3 (*f*), or pCSk4 (*g*). Contractions were recorded initially in normal rodent Ringer's solution (trace 1) and subsequently in a test solution that was either Ca^{++}-free (trace 2) or 0.5 mM Cd^{++}-containing (trace 3) Ringer's solution. A period in normal Ringer sufficient for full recovery was interspersed between exposures to the two test solutions. The stimulus duration was 5 msec for all the traces, except 20 msec for *e*, traces 2 and 3. (Horizontal calibration: 1 sec. Vertical scale: arbitrary units.) (Reprinted, with permission, from Tanabe et al. 1990b.)

adjacent regions of the DHP receptor, forming the channel and its entrances, are important in determining the properties of L-type calcium current.

DHP Receptor as the Voltage Sensor for Skeletal Muscle Excitation-Contraction Coupling

To test the hypothesis that the DHP receptor represents the voltage sensor for skeletal muscle E-C coupling, we measured intramembrane charge movement in dysgenic myotubes before and after injection with

expression plasmids carrying the skeletal muscle, cardiac, or chimeric DHP receptors (Adams et al. 1990). Using a standard pulse protocol in which depolarizing test pulses were administered directly from a holding potential of −80 mV, we found that the maximum quantity of mobile charge (Q_{max}; normalized by linear cell capacitance) in dysgenic myotubes (7.6 ± 3.2 nC/μF; mean ± S.D., $n = 15$) was smaller than, but still a surprisingly large fraction of, that in normal myotubes (12.2 ± 2.9 nC/μF, $n = 12$). We then designed a "prepulse" protocol (modified from Bean and Rios 1989), which consisted of a 1-second prepulse to -30 mV and a subsequent 20–40-msec repolarization to a pedestal potential (-50 mV), followed by depolarization to varying test potentials. This procedure led to complete inactivation of both sodium current and I_{fast} calcium current without affecting the L-type calcium current I_{slow}. Additionally, with the prepulse protocol, part of the charge movement in both normal and dysgenic myotubes was immobilized. Compared to the standard protocol, Q_{max} measured with the prepulse protocol was reduced by an average of 4.8 nC/μF (normal) and 5.4 nC/μF (dysgenic), the remaining immobilization-resistant charge being 7.4 ± 1.7 nC/μF ($n = 12$) and 2.2 ± 0.6 nC/μF ($n = 15$), respectively, in normal and dysgenic myotubes (see Fig. 4, inset). The comparable reduction of charge movement in normal and dysgenic myotubes is consistent with the idea that the immobilized charge arises from gating of sodium and I_{fast} calcium channels and that these are present at comparable levels in the two kinds of myotubes.

We next examined whether the immobilization-resistant charge movement deficient in dysgenic myotubes could be restored by injecting them with the expression plasmid pCAC6 encoding the skeletal muscle DHP receptor, pCARD1 encoding the cardiac DHP receptor, or pCSk1-4 and pCSk7 encoding chimeric DHP receptors. All of these expression plasmids were indeed found to restore immobilization-resistant charge movements (Fig. 4; for the chimeras, only data for pCSk7 are shown). The kinetics and voltage dependence of the restored immobilization-resistant charge were similar for the skeletal muscle, cardiac, and five different chimeric cDNAs.

By expressing cDNAs in dysgenic myotubes, we have shown that the skeletal muscle DHP receptor is responsible for the bulk of intramembrane charge movement

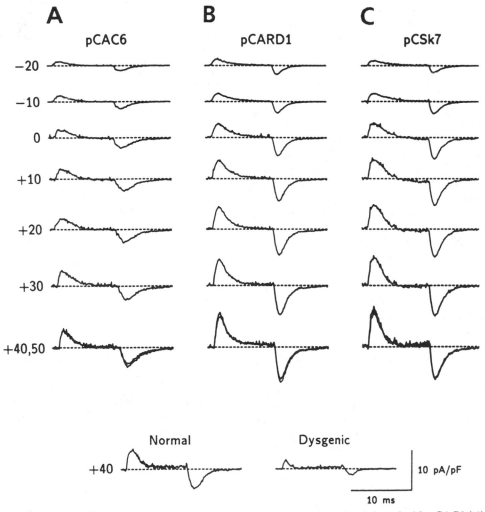

Figure 4. Restoration of immobilization-resistant charge movement in dysgenic myotubes injected with pCAC6 (*A*), pCARD1 (*B*), or pCSk7 (*C*). Injection of pCSk1-4 resulted in charge movements similar to those illustrated here for pCAC6, pCARD1, and pCSk7. (*Inset*) Representative immobilization-resistant charge movements measured from a normal myotube (*left*) and a noninjected dysgenic myotube (*right*). Immobilization-resistant charge movements were measured for the indicated test potentials using the prepulse protocol described in the text. (Reprinted, with permission, from Adams et al. 1990.)

in normal skeletal muscle. This result, together with the finding that expression of the skeletal muscle DHP receptor cDNA restores E-C coupling in dysgenic myotubes, provides evidence that the skeletal muscle DHP receptor functions as the voltage sensor for E-C coupling. Skeletal muscle, cardiac, and chimeric DHP receptor constructs all restore charge movements with very similar voltage-dependent behavior, independent of the nature of the L-type current (slowly or rapidly activating) or E-C coupling (skeletal- or cardiac-type) produced by them. This similarity in voltage dependence seems reasonable given that the S4 segments, which probably represent voltage-sensing regions (Noda et al. 1984, 1986; Stühmer et al. 1989), are highly conserved between the skeletal muscle and cardiac DHP receptors.

Structural Characteristics of the Ryanodine Receptor

Another component required for E-C coupling is the calcium release channel in the SR. This channel has been purified as the ryanodine receptor, which has been morphologically identified with the "foot" structure spanning the junctional gap between the SR and T-tubule membranes (Imagawa et al. 1987; Inui et al. 1987; Block et al. 1988; Lai et al. 1988). We deduced the complete amino acid sequence (5037 residues) of the ryanodine receptor from rabbit skeletal muscle SR by cloning and sequencing the cDNA (Takeshima et al. 1989). Expression of the ryanodine receptor cDNA in Chinese hamster ovary cells produces calcium release channel activity (Penner et al. 1989). The predicted structure of the ryanodine receptor is schematically shown in Figure 5. The carboxy-terminal tenth of the receptor protein contains four putative transmembrane segments. In view of the proposed homotetrameric structure of the ryanodine receptor (Lai et al. 1988; Wagenknecht et al. 1989), it seems likely that the putative transmembrane segments in the carboxy-terminal region, contributed by each of the four monomeric units, surround a central pore to form the calcium release channel. Interestingly, the putative cytoplasmic region preceding and close to segment M1 of the ryanodine receptor contains candidates for binding sites for modulators of the calcium release channel, such as Ca^{++} and ATP (for review, see Endo 1977). These observations suggest that the ryanodine receptor molecule consists of two main parts. The carboxy-terminal portion, which includes both the channel-forming region and the modulator-binding sites, is responsible for the calcium release channel activity, whereas the preceding large cytoplasmic region corresponds to the foot structure. The proposed architecture of the ryanodine receptor molecule is consistent with the electron microscopic observations reported previously (Lai et al. 1988; Wagenknecht et al. 1989).

Another way of releasing Ca^{++} from an intracellular store involves the inositol-1,4,5-trisphosphate-gated calcium channel (for review, see Berridge 1987; Ferris

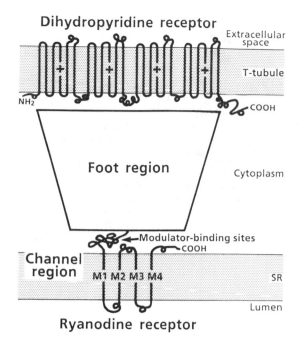

Figure 5. Structural features of the ryanodine receptor, together with the DHP receptor, in the triad junction of skeletal muscle. The carboxy-terminal channel region, including the putative transmembrane segments M1–M4 and the putative modulator-binding sites, and the large cytoplasmic region, corresponding to the foot structure, of the ryanodine receptor are shown schematically. The putative transmembrane segments of the T-tubular DHP receptor (see Fig. 3A) are also shown, and the probable voltage-sensing segment S4 of each repeat is indicated by a plus sign. (Reprinted, with permission, from Takeshima et al. 1989.)

et al. 1989). This channel protein has recently been found to be similar in amino acid sequence to the ryanodine receptor, particularly in the carboxy-terminal region (Furuichi et al. 1989).

CONCLUSIONS

Using skeletal muscle myotubes from dysgenic mice, in which both E-C coupling and L-type calcium current are missing, we have investigated the molecular mechanism of E-C coupling. The results obtained provide evidence that the skeletal muscle DHP receptor has a dual role, functioning both as the voltage sensor for E-C coupling and as the L-type calcium channel. They also identify regions of the DHP receptor critical for skeletal muscle E-C coupling. It is an attractive hypothesis that these regions of the DHP receptor interact directly with the foot region of the ryanodine receptor to gate the calcium release channel present in the latter receptor.

REFERENCES

Adams, B.A., T. Tanabe, A. Mikami, S. Numa, and K.G. Beam. 1990. Intramembrane charge movement restored in dysgenic skeletal muscle by injection of dihydropyridine receptor cDNAs. *Nature* **346:** 569.

Armstrong, C.M., F.M. Bezanilla, and P. Horowicz. 1972.

Twitches in the presence of ethylene glycol bis(β -amino-ethyl ether)-N,N′-tetraacetic acid. *Biochim. Biophys. Acta* **267**: 605.

Beam, K.G., C.M. Knudson, and J.A. Powell. 1986. A lethal mutation in mice eliminates the slow calcium current in skeletal muscle cells. *Nature* **320**: 168.

Bean, B.P. 1989. Classes of calcium channels in vertebrate cells. *Annu. Rev. Physiol.* **51**: 367.

Bean, B.P. and E. Rios. 1989. Nonlinear charge movement in mammalian cardiac ventricular cells. Components from Na and Ca channel gating. *J. Gen. Physiol.* **94**: 65.

Berridge, M.J. 1987. Inositol trisphosphate and diacyl-glycerol: Two interacting second messengers. *Annu. Rev. Biochem.* **56**: 159.

Beuckelmann, D.J. and W.G. Wier. 1988. Mechanism of release of calcium from sarcoplasmic reticulum of guinea-pig cardiac cells. *J. Physiol.* **405**: 233.

Block, B.A., T. Imagawa, K.P. Campbell, and C. Franzini-Armstrong. 1988. Structural evidence for direct interaction between the molecular components of the transverse tubule/sarcoplasmic reticulum junction in skeletal muscle. *J. Cell Biol.* **107**: 2587.

Donaldson, P.L. and K.G. Beam. 1983. Calcium currents in a fast-twitch skeletal muscle of the rat. *J. Gen. Physiol.* **82**: 449.

Endo, M. 1977. Calcium release from the sarcoplasmic reticulum. *Physiol. Rev.* **57**: 71.

Fabiato, A. 1985. Simulated calcium current can both cause calcium loading in and trigger calcium release from the sarcoplasmic reticulum of a skinned canine cardiac Purkinje cell. *J. Gen. Physiol.* **85**: 291.

Ferris, C.D., R.L. Huganir, S. Supattapone, and S. H. Snyder. 1989. Purified inositol 1,4,5-trisphosphate receptor mediates calcium flux in reconstituted lipid vesicles. *Nature* **342**: 87.

Furuichi, T., S. Yoshikawa, A. Miyawaki, K. Wada, N. Maeda, and K. Mikoshiba. 1989. Primary structure and functional expression of the inositol 1,4,5-trisphosphate-binding protein P_{400}. *Nature* **342**: 32.

Glueckschn-Waelsch, S. 1963. Lethal genes and analysis of differentiation. In higher organisms lethal genes serve as tools for studies of cell differentiation and cell genetics. *Science* **142**: 1269.

Hamill, O.P., A. Marty, E. Neher, B. Sakmann, and F.J. Sigworth. 1981. Improved patch-clamp techniques for high-resolution current recording from cells and cell-free membrane patches. *Pfluegers Arch. Eur. J. Physiol.* **391**: 85.

Imagawa, T., J.S. Smith, R. Coronado, and K.P. Campbell. 1987. Purified ryanodine receptor from skeletal muscle sarcoplasmic reticulum is the Ca^{2+}-permeable pore of the calcium release channel. *J. Biol. Chem.* **262**: 16636.

Inui, M., A. Saito, and S. Fleischer. 1987. Purification of the ryanodine receptor and identity with feet structures of junctional terminal cisternae of sarcoplasmic reticulum from fast skeletal muscle. *J. Biol. Chem.* **262**: 1740.

Isenberg, G. and U. Klöckner. 1982. Calcium currents of isolated bovine ventricular myocytes are fast and of large amplitude. *Pfluegers Arch. Eur. J. Physiol.* **395**: 30.

Klaus, M.M., S.P. Scordilis, J.M. Rapalus, R.T. Briggs, and J.A. Powell. 1983. Evidence for dysfunction in the regulation of cytosolic Ca^{2+} in excitation-contraction uncoupled dysgenic muscle. *Dev. Biol.* **99**: 152.

Lai, F.A., H.P. Erickson, E. Rousseau, Q.-Y. Liu, and G. Meissner. 1988. Purification and reconstitution of the calcium release channel from skeletal muscle. *Nature* **331**: 315.

Lee, K.S. and R.W. Tsien. 1982. Reversal of current through calcium channels in dialysed single heart cells. *Nature* **297**: 498.

Mikami, A., K. Imoto, T. Tanabe, T. Niidome, Y. Mori, H. Takeshima, S. Narumiya, and S. Numa. 1989. Primary structure and functional expression of the cardiac dihydropyridine-sensitive calcium channel. *Nature* **340**: 230.

Näbauer, M., G. Callewaert, L. Cleemann, and M. Morad. 1989. Regulation of calcium release is gated by calcium current, not gating charge, in cardiac myocytes. *Science* **244**: 800.

Noda, M., T. Ikeda, T. Kayano, H. Suzuki, H. Takeshima, M. Kurasaki, H. Takahashi, and S. Numa. 1986. Existence of distinct sodium channel messenger RNAs in rat brain. *Nature* **320**: 188.

Noda, M., S. Shimizu, T. Tanabe, T. Takai, T. Kayano, T. Ikeda, H. Takahashi, H. Nakayama, Y. Kanaoka, N. Minamino, K. Kangawa, H. Matsuo, M.A. Raftery, T. Hirose, S. Inayama, H. Hayashida, T. Miyata, and S. Numa. 1984. Primary structure of *Electrophorus electricus* sodium channel deduced from cDNA sequence. *Nature* **312**: 121.

Numa, S. and M. Noda. 1986. Molecular structure of sodium channels. *Ann. N.Y. Acad. Sci.* **479**: 338.

Penner, R., E. Neher, H. Takeshima, S. Nishimura, and S. Numa. 1989. Functional expression of the calcium release channel from skeletal muscle ryanodine receptor cDNA. *FEBS Lett.* **259**: 217.

Perez-Reyes, E., H.S. Kim, A.E. Lacerda, W. Horne, X. Wei, D. Rampe, K.P. Campbell, A.M. Brown, and L. Birnbaumer. 1989. Induction of calcium currents by the expression of the α_1-subunit of the dihydropyridine receptor from skeletal muscle. *Nature* **340**: 233.

Powell, J.A. and D.M. Fambrough. 1973. Electrical properties of normal and dysgenic mouse skeletal muscle in culture. *J. Cell. Physiol.* **82**: 21.

Rieger, F., R. Bournaud, T. Shimahara, L. Garcia, M. Pinon-Raymond, G. Romey, and M. Lazdunski. 1987. Restoration of dysgenic muscle contraction and calcium channel function by co-culture with normal spinal cord neurons. *Nature* **330**: 563.

Rios, E. and G. Brum. 1987. Involvement of dihydropyridine receptors in excitation-contraction coupling in skeletal muscle. *Nature* **325**: 717.

Sanchez, J.A. and E. Stefani. 1978. Inward calcium current in twitch muscle fibres of the frog. *J. Physiol.* **283**: 197.

Schneider, M.F. and W.K. Chandler. 1973. Voltage dependent charge movement in skeletal muscle: A possible step in excitation-contraction coupling. *Nature* **242**: 244.

Stühmer, W., F. Conti, H. Suzuki, X. Wang, M. Noda, N. Yahagi, H. Kubo, and S. Numa. 1989. Structural parts involved in activation and inactivation of the sodium channel. *Nature* **339**: 597.

Takeshima, H., S. Nishimura, T. Matsumoto, H. Ishida, K. Kangawa, N. Minamino, H. Matsuo, M. Ueda, M. Hanaoka, T. Hirose, and S. Numa. 1989. Primary structure and expression from complementary DNA of skeletal muscle ryanodine receptor. *Nature* **339**: 439.

Tanabe, T., K.G. Beam, J.A. Powell, and S. Numa. 1988. Restoration of excitation-contraction coupling and slow calcium current in dysgenic muscle by dihydropyridine receptor complementary DNA. *Nature* **336**: 134.

Tanabe, T., A. Mikami, S. Numa, and K.G. Beam. 1990a. Cardiac-type excitation-contraction coupling in dysgenic skeletal muscle injected with cardiac dihydropyridine receptor cDNA. *Nature* **344**: 451.

Tanabe, T., K.G. Beam, B.A. Adams, T. Niidome, and S. Numa. 1990b. Regions of the skeletal muscle dihydropyridine receptor critical for excitation-contraction coupling. *Nature* **346**: 567.

Tanabe, T., H. Takeshima, A. Mikami, V. Flockerzi, H. Takahashi, K. Kangawa, M. Kojima, H. Matsuo, T. Hirose, and S. Numa. 1987. Primary structure of the receptor for calcium channel blockers from skeletal muscle. *Nature* **328**: 313.

Wagenknecht, T., R. Grassucci, J. Frank, A. Saito, M. Inui, and S. Fleischer. 1989. Three-dimensional architecture of the calcium channel/foot structure of sarcoplasmic reticulum. *Nature* **338**: 167.

Molecular Studies of Voltage-gated Potassium Channels

E. Isacoff, D. Papazian,* L. Timpe, Y.-N. Jan, and L.-Y. Jan

*The Howard Hughes Medical Institute and the Departments of Physiology and Biochemistry, University of California, San Francisco, California 94143; *Department of Physiology, University of California, Los Angeles, California 90072*

Excitability and synaptic efficacy in the nervous system are regulated by a variety of potassium channels. Transmitter-induced alterations in the behavior of these channels are capable of effecting the short- and long-term modulation of synaptic transmission that may underlie some forms of memory and learning. These potassium channels are diverse pharmacologically and can be broken down into several subgroups on the basis of whether they are activated by voltage or second messengers and on whether they inactivate. The differences in gating among channels with similar ion selectivity suggest that there exist certain common pore-forming domains in diverse potassium channels that otherwise possess specialized regions specific for gating. Studies of the molecular nature of potassium channels have been made possible by the cloning of the voltage-activated *Shaker* potassium channel in *Drosophila* and of related genes in invertebrates and vertebrates.

The *Shaker* Phenotype

Shaker mutations were first isolated decades ago on the basis of the leg-shaking phenotype induced under ether anesthesia (Catsch 1944; Kaplan and Trout 1969). The first indication of a potassium channel defect emerged in a study of neuromuscular transmission in *Shaker* mutant larvae (Jan et al. 1977). Abnormally large and prolonged postsynaptic potentials were recorded in these larval muscles that could be accounted for by prolonged transmitter release from the nerve terminals (Jan et al. 1977). Since the mutant phenotype could be mimicked by treating the wild-type larval preparation with a potassium channel blocker, 4-aminopyridine (4-AP), it appeared likely that *Shaker* mutations affected a 4-AP-sensitive potassium channel. Subsequent voltage-clamp and single-channel analyses have shown that *Shaker* mutations affect a rapidly inactivating voltage-gated potassium channel, the A channel, in larval and pupal muscles (Salkoff 1983; Wu and Haugland 1985; Solc et al. 1987; Timpe and Jan 1987). A similar defect in the central neurons has also been reported (Baker and Salkoff 1990). This defect in potassium channel function is likely responsible for the prolonged transmitter release from the larval nerve terminals, since it also prolongs the axonal action potential recorded intracellularly from the cervical giant fibers of adult *Shaker* mutant flies (Tanouye et al. 1981).

EXPERIMENTAL PROCEDURES

The molecular and electrophysiological methods employed in the studies reported here have been described previously (Timpe et al. 1988a,b; Isacoff et al. 1990). Briefly, *Xenopus* oocytes were injected with transcripts of *Shaker* cDNAs. A two-electrode voltage clamp was used to record macroscopic currents (11°C), and patch clamping in the outside-out configuration was done to record single-channel activity (22°C).

RESULTS

The *Shaker* Gene Gives Rise to Different A Channel Subtypes by Alternative Splicing

The cloning of the *Shaker* gene (Baumann et al. 1987; Kamb et al. 1987; Papazian et al. 1987; Tempel et al. 1987) revealed that it is alternatively spliced, giving rise to a number of different protein-coding sequences (Papazian et al. 1987; Tempel et al. 1987; Kamb et al. 1988; Pongs et al. 1988; Schwarz et al. 1988). Each of the five full-length *Shaker* cDNAs resembles one quarter of the α subunit of sodium and calcium channels (Fig. 1). *Shaker* transcripts produce functional inactivating potassium channels when expressed in *Xenopus* oocytes (Iverson et al. 1988; Timpe et al. 1988a,b). These *Shaker* variants have a potassium selectivity, voltage dependence, and 4-AP sensitivity that are similar not only to each other, but also to the *Shaker* channels recorded in *Drosophila* muscles. The different *Shaker* products differ, however, in their inactivation kinetics.

Macroscopic inactivation of *Shaker* currents has both fast and slow components (Fig. 2). The alternatively spliced products differ in the time constants of both components and in the magnitude of the slower component. With large depolarization, the channels open briefly and synchronously, soon after the membrane potential is stepped to the depolarized level, producing the fast component of macroscopic inactivation (Figs. 2 and 3) (Solc et al. 1987). The slower component is due to reopenings later in the step (Zagotta et al. 1989; Zagotta and Aldrich 1989), which progressively decrease in frequency with time (Fig. 3).

A comparison of channels induced by naturally occurring, chimeric, and mutant *Shaker* variants that differ only at their amino- or carboxy-terminal regions (Figs. 2, 3, and 4) indicates the importance that these

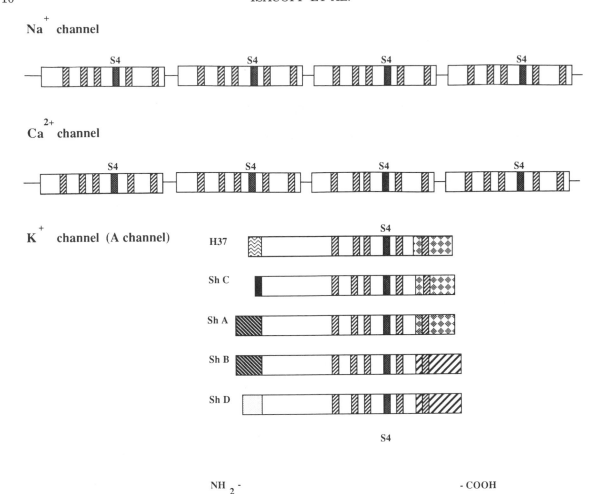

Figure 1. Schematic representation of the primary structure of voltage-sensitive ion channels. The α subunits of sodium and calcium channels are large and are composed of four internally homologous domains. Each of the five alternatively spliced products of the *Shaker* potassium channel gene that have been isolated resembles a single one of these four domains. Each domain of the sodium and calcium channels, and each alternatively spliced *Shaker* product, contains multiple stretches of 19 or more predominantly hydrophobic residues that are potentially membrane spanning (crosshatched) and one S4 segment (labeled above) that has a basic residue at every third position. (Adapted from Jan and Jan 1989.)

alternative ends have in determining inactivation gating. Variants containing the carboxy-terminal region of ShA inactivate to completion rapidly (Fig. 2, left panels), whereas those containing the carboxy-terminal region of ShB require considerably longer to decay to baseline (Fig. 2, right panels); this decay time is 40–50 times longer for ShB and ShB(Δ17–25) than for ShA and ShA(Δ17–25), respectively. These differences in macroscopic currents are due to differences in the probability of reopening between variants containing the two carboxy-terminal regions. For example, whereas ShB channels reopen several times during the depolarization, ShA channels open at the beginning of the step but reopen rarely and only early in the step (Fig. 3). In addition to inactivating rapidly, channels containing the carboxy-terminal region of ShA recover from inactivation much more slowly (e.g., ShA requires 30–60 times longer to recover than ShB (Fig. 4) (Timpe et al. 1988b). These observations suggest that there are two

inactive states that *Shaker* channels enter: a first inactivated state from which they recover rapidly, even during sustained depolarization, and a second, more stable inactive state from which they recover only during repolarization. Apparently, channels encoded by *Shaker* products containing the carboxy-terminal region of ShA rapidly enter a very stable inactive state, whereas those encoded by products containing the carboxy-terminal region of ShB enter the stable inactive state far more slowly.

The amino-terminal region also appears to play a critical role in inactivation. Constructs differing in the amino-terminal region produce channels that inactivate and recover from inactivation at different rates (Figs. 2 and 4). Comprehensive mutagenesis of the alternative amino-terminal region common to ShA and ShB has shown directly that it plays an important role in inactivation gating, with deletions in the first 20 amino acids strongly slowing inactivation of ShB (Hoshi et al. 1989;

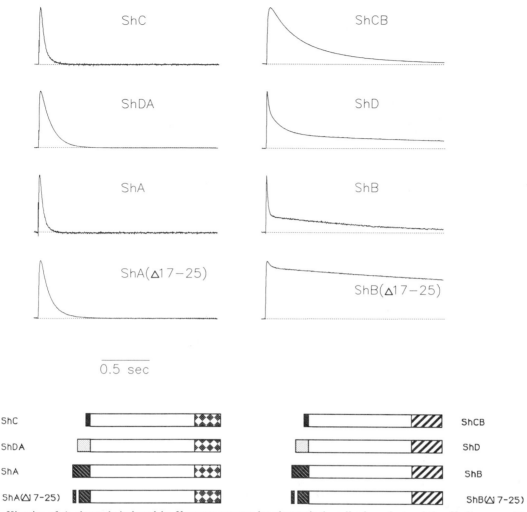

Figure 2. Kinetics of A channels induced in *Xenopus* oocytes by alternatively spliced products of the *Shaker* gene. Both the amino- and carboxy-terminal regions play a role in determining the rate of the fast component of inactivation and the magnitude of the slow component of inactivation. The role of the amino terminus can be seen by comparing the kinetics of channels encoded by variants displayed in the left panels as a group (ShC, ShDA, ShA, and ShA[Δ17–25]) and by comparing those in the right panels as a group (ShCB, ShD, ShB, and ShB[Δ17–25]). The role of the carboxy-terminal region can be seen by examining horizontal pairs. ShCB and ShDA are chimeric cDNA constructs (E. Isacoff, unpubl.) that have not been found in flies. Note the slowing of inactivation in the mutants ShB(Δ17–25) (Isacoff et al. 1990) and ShA(Δ17–25) (E. Isacoff, unpubl.) in which amino acids 17–25 were deleted from the amino terminus common to ShB and ShA. Currents were evoked by 2-sec depolarizations from −100 mV to +40 mV.

Aldrich et al., this volume). When a nine-amino-acid deletion mutation (of residues 17-25) is made in the amino-terminal region common to ShA and ShB, inactivation is slowed by about threefold for both the fast and slow components of ShB (Isacoff et al. 1990) and for the fast component of ShA (Fig. 2). The prolongation of the macroscopic currents in these mutants is partly due to a prolongation of single-channel burst duration, as shown in the ShB background in Figure 3; i.e., this is due to a slowed rate of transition into the first inactive state.

Aldrich and colleagues (this volume) suggest that the amino-terminal region forms a ball that has a net positive charge and produces inactivation by binding to a negatively charged region at the cytoplasmic mouth of the pore and plugging the permeation pathway. In this model, which is similar to one proposed by Armstrong

and Bezanilla (1977) for sodium channels (Bezanilla and Armstrong 1977), *Shaker* products with different amino-terminal regions produce plugs with different on and off rates. The three positively charged residues deleted in ShB(Δ17–25) and ShA(Δ17–25) (amino acids 17, 18, and 19) may form part of the plug, but they cannot account for all of the interaction between the plug and the negatively charged region, since a slowed inactivation still takes place in these mutants (Fig. 3). Two other alternative amino-terminal regions contain some positively charged amino acids (Kamb et al. 1988; Schwarz et al. 1988). In contrast, the amino-terminal region specific to ShC consists of entirely hydrophobic residues (Schwarz et al. 1988) but ShC channels nevertheless inactivate as rapidly as ShA (Fig. 2) (Timpe et al. 1988a), suggesting that other portions of the protein also contribute to plug formation.

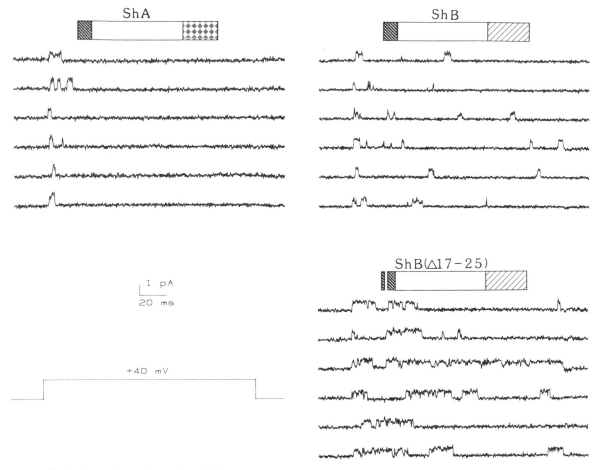

Figure 3. Single-channel recordings from *Shaker* products with different amino- and carboxy-terminal regions. In all three variants, depolarization to +40 mV evokes openings early in the step. ShA channels reopen rarely, whereas ShB channels reopen several times, with decreasing frequency, later in the step. This suggests that ShA channels enter a stable inactive state more rapidly than ShB channels. ShB(Δ17–25) channels reopen frequently, as do ShB channels, but have longer bursts, indicating a slowing of the transition into the first inactive state in the mutant. Steps were given to outside-out patches from a holding potential of −100 mV at 4-sec intervals for ShB and ShB(Δ17--25) and from a holding potential of −120 mV at 10-sec intervals for ShA.

Beyond these general observations about the kinetic properties peculiar to variant amino- or carboxy-terminal regions, it is also evident that the combination of amino and carboxyl termini is critical in determining how a channel behaves. For example, although ShC and ShA are very similar in inactivation onset, when these two amino-terminal regions are placed in the context of the carboxy-terminal region of ShB—as ShCB and ShB—their kinetics are remarkably different (Fig. 2). Similarly, the inactivation kinetics of ShDA and ShA(Δ17–25) are very similar, whereas those of ShD and ShB(Δ17–25) differ greatly (Fig. 2). These observations suggest that the amino- and carboxy-terminal regions interact in inactivation gating, a possibility addressed below.

In summary, a comparison of the *Shaker* alternative splicing products indicates that the voltage sensor and pore are likely encoded by the common core of the protein, which includes the S4 and other proposed transmembrane segments (with the exception of H6,

which is, nevertheless, almost completely conserved), whereas inactivation is at least partly controlled by the alternative amino- and carboxy-terminal regions (Figs. 2, 3, and 4) (Iverson et al. 1988; Timpe et al. 1988a,b).

The differences in inactivation kinetics of the alternative splicing products may be of physiological significance because these products are differentially distributed in the central nervous system of *Drosophila*. Whereas a widespread, although nonuniform, distribution is revealed by antibodies against the core region of the protein sequence shared by different *Shaker* products, antibodies against the amino-terminal region of a subset of the *Shaker* products show a much more restricted staining pattern (Schwarz et al. 1990). These observations suggest that different *Shaker* products may, in fact, generate distinct kinetic subtypes of A channels in different neurons. These channels may enhance synaptic transmission by undergoing cumulative inactivation during trains of activity. The type of activity required to produce such an event would be expected

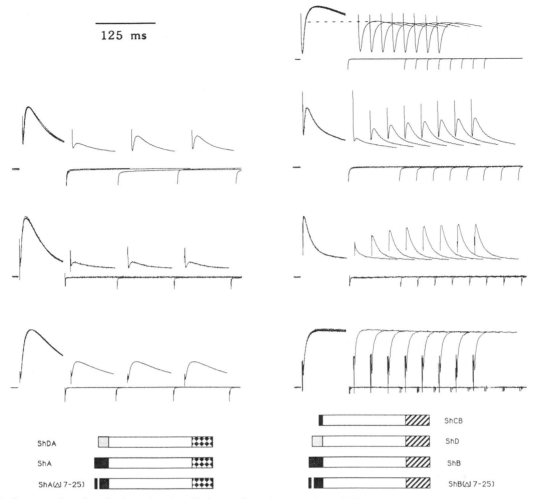

125 ms

ShDA
ShA
ShA(∆ 7-25)

ShCB
ShD
ShB
ShB(∆ 7-25)

Figure 4. Recovery from inactivation of variant *Shaker* products. Recovery is rapid (complete within seconds) for *Shaker* variants containing the carboxy-terminal region of ShB (with the exception of the chimera ShCB) and very slow (requiring many minutes) for variants containing carboxy-terminal region of ShA. Cells were held at −100 mV, and a pair of 100-msec-long pulses to +40 mV, separated by varying intervals, were given once every 20–60 sec.

to depend on the inactivation kinetics of the variants encoding the relevant channels, with more slowly recovering variants affected at lower frequencies of activity.

Multiple Genes Coding for Different Potassium Channel Polypeptides Are Found in Vertebrates and Invertebrates

Clearly, alternative splicing of a potassium channel gene accounts for only part of channel diversity in *Drosophila*. Deletions of most of the *Shaker* locus from the genome have no effect on other potassium currents, including a neuronal A current that activates at considerably more hyperpolarized potentials than *Shaker* (Salkoff 1983; Solc et al. 1987). Some of these potassium currents have been shown to be affected by mutations of other genes (Ganetzky and Wu 1986). It appears that potassium channels that differ in voltage dependence, calcium sensitivity, and pharmacology derive from a number of distinct potassium channel genes. Several potassium channel genes have already

been isolated from both *Drosophila* and mammals (cf. Jan and Jan 1990b). They encode potassium channel polypeptides that are structurally related to the *Shaker* products. Interestingly, for the closest mammalian homologs to *Shaker*, diversity appears to be generated by the existence of a family of separate genes encoded by single exons, rather than by alternative splicing of a single gene (Chandy et al. 1990).

The predicted *Shaker* potassium channel polypeptides, and their homologs in *Drosophila* and mammals, resemble each other, as well as one of the four internally homologous domains of sodium and calcium channel α subunits, in predicted transmembrane topology, including the presence of one putative transmembrane segment rich in positively charged amino acids called the S4 (Fig. 1). These homologies between voltage-activated channels have led to the suggestion that potassium channels may form into multisubunit channels by assembly of several identical polypeptides and that each subunit of a potassium channel, or pseudo-subunit of the sodium and calcium channels, possesses in its S4 segment its own voltage sensor.

Heteromultimeric Potassium Channels Expressed in *Xenopus* Oocytes Have Distinct Properties

Although detailed biochemical and structural analyses of potassium channels have not yet been carried out, electrophysiological studies have been used to test the hypothesis that the channels are composed of several like subunits. When two different species of *Shaker* mRNAs (ShA and ShB, or ShA and the slowly inactivating amino-terminal deletion mutant ShB(Δ17–25)) are mixed and coinjected into oocytes, they generate currents that cannot be fit by the arithmetic sum of the currents that each mRNA induces individually (Fig. 5A,B) (Isacoff et al. 1990); i.e., they cannot be accounted for by the independent expression of the two different populations of channels. Instead, most of the channels that are made in the coinjected oocytes inactivate (Fig. 5A) and recover from inactivation (Fig. 5C) with complex intermediate kinetics. This finding is taken to indicate that polypeptides encoded by the two mRNAs coassemble into heteromultimeric channels. Similar conclusions have also been reached by studies in which two species of mRNAs coding for different rat brain potassium channel polypeptides were coinjected (Christie et al. 1990; Ruppersberg et al. 1990).

The multisubunit character of the channel implies that there may be as many inactivation gates as there are subunits or, alternatively, that one joint gate may exist to which each polypeptide contributes its own amino- and carboxy-terminal regions. It also opens the possibility that the interaction in inactivation gating

between the amino- and carboxy-terminal regions, discussed above, may occur between subunits as well as within a subunit. The idea that interaction between subunits plays a role in inactivation gating seems reasonable by analogy with sodium channels in which the junction of the carboxyl terminus of the third and the amino terminus of the fourth internally homologous domains (Fig. 1) appears to be critical for inactivation (Vassilev et al. 1988). Related evidence has been obtained for potassium channels by the construction of tandem dimers of *Shaker* (Isacoff et al. 1990), in which two subunits are encoded by a single mRNA with the carboxyl terminus of the first copy tethered to the amino terminus of the second. These tandem constructs produce functional channels with relatively normal inactivation kinetics, both when the channels are homomultimers (Fig. 6A) and when they are heteromultimers (Fig. 6B).

The finding that tandem dimers produce functional channels indicates that, like sodium channels, *Shaker* channels likely have both amino and carboxyl termini on the same side of the membrane and that they are composed of an even number of similar subunits. The apparent absence in coinjection experiments of a current component with rates equal to those of the homomultimers (most obvious for ShB(Δ17–25; Fig. 5) suggests that either heteromultimer formation is favored over homomultimerization or that assembly is random but that the number of subunits is sufficiently large (≥ 4) so that the contribution by homomultimers to the overall current ($\leq 1/16$) is too small to detect.

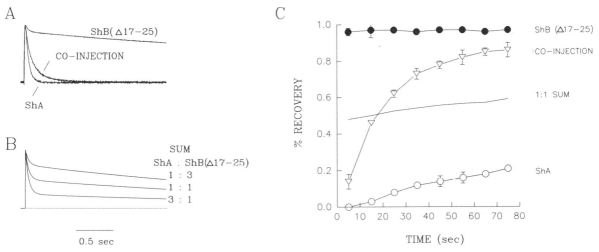

Figure 5. Potassium channels are formed by coassembly of several like subunits. (*A*) Normalized and superimposed currents from oocytes injected with mRNA from ShA and ShB(Δ17–25) or coinjected with equal amounts of the two show that the coinjected oocytes express channels with kinetics that differ from those expressed in oocytes injected with either mRNA alone. (*B*) Arithmetic sums of average time constants of ShA and ShB(Δ17–25) currents in ratios of 1:3, 1:1, and 3:1 predict macroscopic currents that would be produced by the expression in coinjected oocytes if the two variant *Shaker* mRNAs produced two independent populations of channels. These predictions clearly do not resemble the actual currents measured in coinjected oocytes as shown in panel *A*. (*C*) Recovery from inactivation following a 400-msec depolarization to +40 mV is very fast for ShB(Δ17–25), very slow for ShA, and intermediate for the coinjected oocytes. The kinetics of recovery in the coinjected oocytes cannot be accounted for by the arithmetic sum of independent populations of ShA and ShB(Δ17–25) channels as shown for the predicted 1:1 sum of the individual kinetics of ShA and ShB(Δ17–25). These results indicate that the channels formed in the coinjected oocytes are likely mixed subunit channels formed by coassembly of ShA and ShB(Δ17–25) polypeptides. (Adapted from Isacoff et al. 1990.)

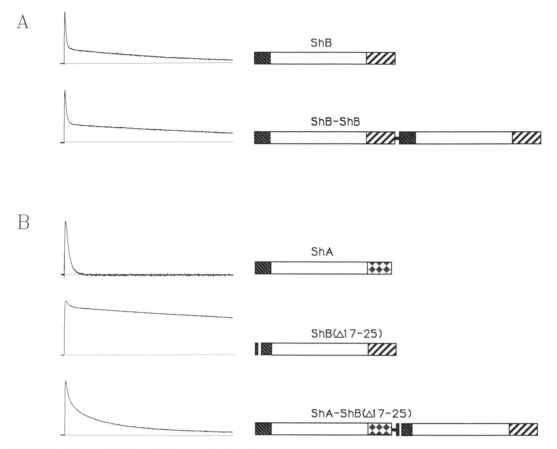

Figure 6. Tandem dimers of *Shaker* cDNAs encode functional channels. (Tandem dimers were made by fusing the 3′ end of the first copy, via a ten-glutamine linker, to the codon encoding the sixth amino acid of the second copy.) (*A*) Inactivation of the tandem dimer ShB–ShB resembles that of the wild-type ShB but has a slightly slower and larger second component. (*B*) As for the production of heteromultimeric channels in oocytes coinjected with two separate *Shaker* mRNA variants, tandem dimers containing two variants produce channels with kinetics that are distinct from those of channels produced by either variant on its own. These results indicate that *Shaker* potassium channels are likely composed of an even number of subunits and that both the amino and carboxyl termini are likely to be on the same side of the membrane. (Adapted from Isacoff et al. 1990.)

Coassembly also occurs between potassium channel polypeptides from the rat (RCK1) and fly (ShB) (Isacoff et al. 1990), indicating that the tertiary structure of channel polypeptides that have diverged evolutionarily can be similar enough to allow for functional interaction, despite the fact that they are only 75% identical in the conserved core at the level of amino acid sequence. The compatibility of divergent channel polypeptides suggests that the capacity for coassembly is as relevant for the functional grouping of potassium channel genes as is sequence homology. It remains to be determined whether heteromultimeric channels form in vivo. If so, the coassembly of different combinations of potassium channel polypeptides provides an additional parameter for the generation of functional diversity.

Structural Similarity between Voltage-gated and Second-messenger-gated Channels

Although a number of voltage-gated potassium channel sequences have been found to be related, it remains an open question as to whether other potassium chan-

nels, e.g., 4-AP-insensitive channels and channels that are gated chemically by substances such as calcium or ATP, also share structural similarity with *Shaker*. A significant sequence similarity has been found between known voltage-gated cation channels and a cGMP-gated cation channel, indicating that the superfamily of voltage-gated cation channels also includes a channel that is gated by a second messenger (Jan and Jan 1990a). This similarity, however, is restricted to a small set of highly conserved residues located in the proposed transmembrane segments. Therefore, although this superfamily may include other channels that are gated by second messengers, and although these channel genes may in several other instances encode a single subunit of a multimeric channel, the overall primary sequence similarity will probably prove to be extremely low.

Involvement of the S4 Sequence in Voltage-dependent Activation of the Channel

Voltage-gated potassium channels contain a charged intrinsic voltage sensor (the gating charge) that detects

Table 1. Midpoints of Conductance-Voltage Curves of S4 Mutants

Position	R362	R365	R368	R371	K374	R377	K380
Basic							
Substitution	+12	0	0	+64	0	+29[a]	0
Neutralization	+20	−12	+53[a]	−16	null	null	0

Values (in millivolts) are expressed relative to the midpoint of wild-type ShB (−10 mV) so that + and − indicate depolarizing and hyperpolarizing shifts, respectively, and 0 indicates similarity to ShB.

[a] Accompanied by a decrease in slope.

changes in potential across the membrane, responds to these changes by a movement of charges in the membrane electric field, and presumably triggers the conformational change leading to channel opening. The S4 segment has been proposed to function as the voltage sensor because it contains a basic residue at every third or fourth position, with mainly hydrophobic residues at the intervening positions. These positively charged residues have been proposed to constitute the channel's gating charge and their displacement (toward the extracellular face of the membrane during depolarization and toward the cytoplasmic face during hyperpolarization) to produce the channel's gating current.

To test the S4 model, we have substituted each of the seven basic residues in the S4 sequence of ShB individually with the other basic residue (replacing arginine with lysine and vice versa) or with the uncharged residue glutamine (D.M. Papazian et al., in prep.). These mutations do not affect the channel's potassium selectivity, as reflected by the reversal potentials at 1 mM and 40 mM external potassium, or the rate of inactivation. A large fraction of these mutations, however, affected the voltage dependence of channel activation, as determined from normalized conductance-voltage (g-v) curves. The g-v curves were fit to Boltzmann distributions, and the midpoints (Table 1) and slopes were measured. In addition to shifts in midpoints that occurred with little or no change in slope, two mutations greatly reduced the slope of the voltage dependence curve. The specificity of the effects of these S4 mutations on the channel's voltage dependence suggests that the S4 sequence is involved in the voltage-dependent activation of this potassium channel. Similar conclusions have been reached for the sodium channel (Stuhmer et al. 1989). The quantitative effects of individual S4 mutations in *Shaker*, however, are not predicted by simple considerations of the electrostatic interaction between charged residues and the membrane electric field. Rather, interactions between the S4 sequence and other parts of the channel molecule are likely to be important in determining the ease of transitions between closed and open states, the stability of the various states, and, possibly, the extent of cooperativity between subunits during the transitions.

SUMMARY

The cloning and characterization of the voltage-activated *Shaker* potassium channel gene in *Drosophila*

have led to the identification of structural elements involved in potassium channel gating. As found for the voltage-activated sodium channel, the S4 segment, located in the conserved core of the protein, plays a central role in voltage-dependent activation. Potassium channels appear to be formed by the assembly of several polypeptides into multisubunit channels. This is directly analogous to the proposed folding of the four internally homologous pseudosubunits of sodium and calcium channels. The amino- and carboxy-terminal regions of *Shaker* channels are specialized for, and appear to interact in, inactivation gating. This interaction probably includes interaction between subunits, as may be said for the role in inactivation gating of the junction between the carboxyl terminus of the third domain and amino terminus of the fourth domain of sodium channel (Vassilev et al. 1988). The capacity for coassembly in potassium channels extends not only to the alternatively spliced products of the same gene, but also to the products of different genes. Heteromultimeric channels that are formed in this way have kinetic and pharmacological properties that differ from homomultimers of their constituents and, as such, broaden the functional diversity of channels that can be produced by any given number of compatible potassium channel genes.

ACKNOWLEDGMENTS

The authors thank D. Muhlrad, K. Bornschlegel, and R. Tuma for technical assistance and K. Prewitt for help with the preparation of the manuscript. E.Y.I. is an MDA postdoctoral fellow. Y.N.J and L.Y.J are Howard Hughes investigators.

REFERENCES

Armstrong, C.M. and F. Bezanilla. 1977. Inactivation of the sodium channel. II. Gating current experiments. *J. Gen. Physiol.* **70**: 567.

Baker, K. and L. Salkoff. 1990. The *Drosophila Shaker* gene codes for a unique K$^+$ current in a subset of neurons. *Neuron* **4**: 129.

Baumann, A., I. Krah-Jentzens, R. Mueller, F. Mueller-Holtkamp, R. Seidel, N. Kecskemethy, J. Casal, A. Ferrus, and O. Pongs. 1987. Molecular organization of the maternal effect region of the *Shaker* complex of *Drosophila*: Characterization of an I$_A$ channel transcript with homology to vertebrate Na$^+$ channel. *EMBO J.* **6**: 3419.

Bezanilla, F. and C.M. Armstrong. 1977. Inactivation of the sodium channels. I. Sodium current experiments. *J. Gen. Physiol.* **70**: 549.

Catsch, A. 1944. Eine erbliche Storung des Bewegungsmechanismus bei *Drosophila melanogaster*. *Z. Indukt. Abstammungs Vererbungsl.* **82:** 64.

Chandy, K.G., C.B. Williams, R.H. Spencer, B.A. Aguilar, S. Ghanshari, B.L. Tempel, and G.A. Gutman. 1990. A family of three mouse potassium channel genes with intronless coding regions. *Science* **247:** 973.

Christie, M.J., R.A. North, P.B. Osborn, J. Douglass, and J.P. Adelman. 1990. Heteropolymeric potassium channels expressed in *Xenopus* oocytes form cloned subunits. *Neuron* **2:** 405.

Ganetzky, B. and C.F. Wu. 1986. Neurogenetics of membrane excitability in *Drosophila*. *Annu. Rev. Genet.* **20:** 13.

Hoshi, T., W.N. Zagotta, and R.W. Aldrich. 1989. Mutations in the amino terminal variable domain alter inactivation of *Shaker B* potassium channels in *Xenopus* oocytes. *Abstr. Soc. Neurosci.* **15:** 338.

Isacoff, E.Y., Y.N. Jan, and L.Y. Jan. 1990. Evidence for the formation of heteromultimeric potassium channels in *Xenopus* oocytes. *Nature* **345:** 530.

Iverson, L.E., M.A. Tanouye, H.A. Lester, N. Davidson, and B. Rudy. 1988. Expression of A-type potassium channels from *Shaker* cDNAs. *Proc. Natl. Acad. Sci.* **85:** 5723.

Jan, L.Y. and Y.N. Jan. 1989. Voltage-sensitive ion channels. *Cell* **56:** 13.

―――. 1990a. A superfamily of ion channels. *Nature* **345:** 672.

―――. 1990b. How might the diversity of potassium channels be generated? *Trends Neurosci.* **13:** (in press).

Jan, Y.N., L.Y. Jan, and J.J. Dennis. 1977. Two mutations of synaptic transmission in *Drosophila*. *Proc. R. Soc. Lond. B Biol. Sci.* **198:** 87.

Kamb, A., L.E. Iverson, and M.A. Tanouye. 1987. Molecular characterization of *Shaker*, a *Drosophila* gene that encodes a potassium channel. *Cell* **50:** 405.

Kamb, A., J. Tseng-Crank, and M.A. Tanouye. 1988. Multiple products of the *Drosophila Shaker* gene may contribute to potassium channel diversity. *Neuron* **1:** 421.

Kaplan, W.D. and W.E. Trout. 1969. The behavior of four neurological mutants of *Drosophila*. *Genetics* **61:** 399.

Papazian, D.M., T.L. Schwarz, B.L. Tempel, Y.N. Jan, and L.Y. Jan. 1987. Cloning of genomic and complementary DNA from *Shaker*, a putative potassium channel gene from *Drosophila*. *Science* **237:** 749.

Pongs, O., N. Kecskemethy, R. Mueller, I. Krah-Jentzens, A. Baumann, H.H. Kiltz, I. Canal, S. Llamazares, and A. Ferrus. 1988. *Shaker* encodes a family of putative potassium channel proteins in the nervous system of *Drosophila*. *EMBO J.* **7:** 1087.

Ruppersberg, J.P., K.H. Schroter, B. Sakmann, M. Stocker, S. Sewing, and O. Pongs. 1990. Heteromultimeric channels formed by rat brain potassium channel proteins. *Nature* **345:** 535.

Salkoff, L.B. 1983. Genetic and voltage-clamp analysis of a *Drosophila* potassium channel. *Cold Spring Harbor Symp. Quant. Biol.* **48:** 221.

Schwarz, T.L., B.L. Tempel, D.M. Papazian, Y.N. Jan, and L.Y. Jan. 1988. Multiple potassium channel components are produced by alternative splicing at the *Shaker* locus in *Drosophila*. *Nature* **331:** 137.

Schwarz, T.L., D.M. Papazian, R.C. Carretto, Y.N. Jan, and L.Y. Jan. 1990. Immunological characterization of K^+ channel components from the *Shaker* locus and differential distribution of splicing variants in *Drosophila*. *Neuron* **4:** 119.

Solc, C.K., W.N. Zagotta, and R.W. Aldrich. 1987. Single-channel and genetic analyses reveal two distinct A-type potassium channels in *Drosophila*. *Science* **236:** 1084.

Stuhmer, W., F. Conti, H. Suzuki, X.D. Wong, M. Noda, N. Yahagi, H. Kubo, and S. Numa. 1989. Structural parts involved in activation and inactivation of the sodium channel. *Nature* **339:** 597.

Tanouye, M.A., A. Ferrus, and S.C. Fujita. 1981. Abnormal action potentials associated with the *Shaker* complex locus of *Drosophila*. *Proc. Natl. Acad. Sci.* **78:** 6548.

Tempel, B.L., D.M. Papazian, T.L. Schwarz, Y.N. Jan, and L.Y. Jan. 1987. Sequence of a probable potassium channel component encoded at the *Shaker* locus of *Drosophila*. *Science* **237:** 770.

Timpe, L.C. and L.Y. Jan. 1987. Gene dosage and complementation analysis of the *Shaker* locus in *Drosophila*. *J. Neurosci.* **7:** 1307.

Timpe, L.C., Y.N. Jan, and L.Y. Jan. 1988a. Four cDNA clones from the *Shaker* locus of *Drosophila* induce kinetically distinct A-type potassium currents in *Xenopus* oocytes. *Neuron* **1:** 659.

Timpe, L.C., T.L. Schwarz, B.L. Tempel, D.M. Papazian, Y.N. Jan, and L.Y. Jan. 1988b. Expression of functional potassium channel from *Shaker* cDNA in *Xenopus* oocytes. *Nature* **331:** 143.

Vassilev, P.M., T. Scheuer, and W.A. Catterall. 1988. Identification of an intracellular peptide segment involved in sodium channel inactivation. *Science* **241:** 1658.

Wu, C.-F. and F.N. Haugland. 1985. Voltage clamp analysis of membrane currents in larval muscle fibers of *Drosophila* alteration of potassium currents in *Shaker* mutants. *J. Neurosci.* **5:** 2626.

Zagotta, W.N. and R.W. Aldrich. 1989. Voltage-dependent gating of *Shaker* A-type potassium channels in *Drosophila* muscle. *J. Gen. Physiol.* **95:** 29.

Zagotta, W.N., T. Hoshi, and R.W. Aldrich. 1989a. Gating of single *Shaker* potassium channels in *Drosophila* muscle and in *Xenopus* oocytes injected with *Shaker* mRNA. *Proc. Natl. Acad. Sci.* **86:** 7243.

Zagotta, W.N., S. Germeraad, S.S. Garber, T. Hoshi, and R.W. Aldrich. 1989b. Properties of ShB A-type K^+ channels expressed in *Shaker* mutant *Drosophila* by germline transformation. *Neuron* **3:** 773.

Differences in Gating among Amino-terminal Variants of *Shaker* Potassium Channels

R.W. Aldrich, T. Hoshi, and W.N. Zagotta

Department of Neurobiology, Stanford University School of Medicine, Stanford, California 94305

Voltage-dependent potassium channels are key molecular elements in the control of membrane excitability and signaling in the nervous system. They play critical roles in the pacemaker activity of endogenously active neurons and are important in the modulation of synaptic function. Potassium channels have been shown to play a central role in the control and modulation of neurotransmitter release. Alterations in potassium channels in presynaptic terminals of *Shaker Drosophila* mutants lead to delayed action potential repolarization and hyperexcitability at the neuromuscular junction. These effects underlie the behavioral defects in the mutant flies.

The *Shaker* voltage-dependent potassium channel gene was isolated and sequenced from *Drosophila* (Baumann et al. 1987; Kamb et al. 1987; Tempel et al. 1987). It is a member of a class of voltage-dependent potassium channels whose members have been also found in mammalian brain (Baumann et al. 1988; Tempel et al. 1988; Christie et al. 1989; Frech et al. 1989; McKinnon 1989; Stühmer et al. 1989). A hydropathy analysis of the deduced protein sequence suggested that the *Shaker* protein spans the membrane six times, with both the amino and carboxyl termini facing the intracellular side (Pongs et al. 1988). The *Shaker* gene gives rise to a large family of transcripts by alternative mRNA splicing (Kamb et al. 1988; Pongs et al. 1988; Schwarz et al. 1988). Generally, these alternatively spliced variants of *Shaker* share the same core region containing putative membrane-spanning regions, but they differ in the amino- and carboxy-terminal regions that are thought to face the intracellular side. Many of these RNAs individually produce macroscopic potassium currents when injected into *Xenopus* oocytes (Iverson et al. 1988; Timpe et al. 1988a,b).

An extensive analysis of gating kinetics of single *Shaker* potassium channels in cultured embryonic *Drosophila* myotubes revealed that inactivation is strongly coupled to activation and has very little, if any, intrinsic voltage dependence (Zagotta and Aldrich 1990). The lack of voltage dependence of inactivation implies no movement of charged particles through the membrane electrical field during the inactivation transition and suggests the involvement of nonmembrane-spanning domains in inactivation. The involvement of cytoplasmic domains in inactivation is further supported by the finding that channels in patches treated with internal trypsin lose the ability to inactivate, whereas external trypsin has no effect on inactivation (T. Hoshi et al., in prep.).

Previous studies have shown that ShB and ShD channels differ in the time course of inactivation of macroscopic currents, as measured by the two-electrode voltage-clamp method in *Xenopus* oocytes (Timpe et al. 1988a,b). We have investigated further the role of the amino-terminal region of the *Shaker* protein in the inactivation process of the channel. We have examined the gating of single channels expressed in *Xenopus* oocytes of three *Shaker* variants that differ only in the amino-terminal variable regions.

METHODS

RNA and oocyte preparation. ShB, ShD, and ShC cDNAs, cloned into the *Eco*RI site of the plasmid expression vector pSP72 (Promega, Madison, Wisconsin), were obtained from the laboratory of L.Y. Jan and Y.N. Jan (University of California, San Francisco). The ShB and ShD inserts utilized the T7 promoter of this vector, whereas the ShC insert utilized the SP6 promoter. In addition, the ShC construct had been modified by removing a *Sac*I fragment from the 5'-untranslated region to improve translation efficiency. The ShC/B construct was prepared by replacing the *Eco*RI-*Bsm*I fragment containing the 3' end of ShC with the same fragment from ShB. The pSP72 plasmids with *Shaker* inserts were linearized with a restriction enzyme that cuts at the 3' end of the insert and were used as templates for runoff transcription. Transcription reactions were conducted with 5–10 μg of template DNA, 500 μM NTPs, 500 μM m^{7}G(5')ppp(5')G (a cap analog), 160 units of RNasin (Promega), and 40 units of T7 or SP6 RNA polymerase in a standard transcription buffer. The template DNA was removed with DNase (RQ1 DNase, Promega), and RNA was purified by extracting with 1:1 phenol:chloroform and chloroform, precipitated with ethanol, and resuspended in 10 μl of DEPC-treated water. Oocytes were injected with mRNA in a manner similar to that described previously (Zagotta et al. 1989). Female *Xenopus laevis* were obtained from Xenopus I (Ann Arbor, Michigan) and maintained at room temperature (20–22°C). The frogs were anesthetized by immersing them in 0.1–0.2% ethyl-*m*-aminobenzoate (MS222; Sigma). A small incision was made on the abdomen, and the ovarian lobes were removed. The follicular cell layer was then removed by digestion with collagenase (2 mg/ml; Type IA, Sigma) in OR2 solution (in mM: 82.5 NaCl, 2.5 KCl, 1 MgCl$_2$, 5 HEPES, pH 7.6 with NaOH) for 2–3 hours. The large oocytes (>1 mm) were thcn transferred to ND96 solution (in mM: 96 NaCl, 2 KCl, 1.8 CaCl$_2$, 1 MgCl$_2$, 5 HEPES, pH 7.6 with NaOH) and pressure-injected with mRNA. Typically, each oocyte received 40 nl of mRNA solution. Injected oocytes were maintained in ND96 solution supplemented with 2.5 mM Na pyruvate, 100 units/ml penicillin, and 100 μg/ml streptomycin at 18°C. Oocytes were suitable for patch-clamp experiments starting 36 hours after the injection and for up to 7 days. The incubation medium was changed daily. Immediately before patch-clamp experiments, the oocytes were incubated in a hypertonic "stripping" medium (in mM: 220 N-methyl-glucamine [NMG], 220 aspartic acid, 2 MgCl$_2$, 10 EGTA, 10 HEPES, pH 7.2 with NMG) for 5–10 minutes, and the vitelline membrane was mechanically removed with fine forceps.

Electrophysiology and data analysis. Unitary currents were recorded using cell-attached, inside-out and outside-out configurations of the patch-clamp method (Hamill et al. 1981). Because stretch-activated chan-nels, which are endogenously present in *Xenopus* oo-cytes, tend not to open in the outside-out configuration, the outside-out configuration was used most frequently. In cell-free patch configurations, the external solution typically contained (in mM) 140 NaCl, 2 KCl, 6 MgCl$_2$, 10 HEPES, pH 7.1 with NaOH. The cytoplasmic solution typically contained (in mM) 140 KCl, 2 MgCl$_2$, 1 CaCl$_2$, 11 EGTA, 10 HEPES, 10 nM free Ca^{++}, pH 7.2 with NMG. Occasionally, 70 mM KCl was replaced with 70 mM KF. For the cell-attached configuration, the bath solution contained (in mM) 140 KCl, 2 MgCl$_2$, 11 EGTA, 10 HEPES, pH 7.1 with NMG for the myotube and 98 KCl, 3 MgCl$_2$, 1 EGTA, 10 HEPES, pH 7.2 with NMG for oocytes. Experiments were performed at 20°C. Single-channel data were analyzed as described previously (Hoshi and Aldrich 1988a,b; Zagotta et al. 1989).

RESULTS

Previous studies have shown that ShB and ShD chan-nels differ in the time course of inactivation of macro-scopic currents, as measured by two-electrode voltage-clamp in *Xenopus* oocytes (Timpe et al. 1988a,b). These differences in gating between channel variants

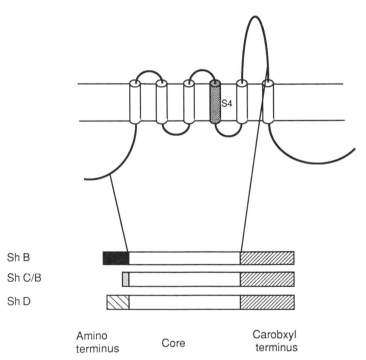

Amino Terminal Amino Acid Sequences

MAAVAGLYGLGEDRQHRKKQQQQQQHQKEQLEQKEEQKKIAERKLQLREQQLQRNSLDGYG **ShB**

MTMWQSGGMGGHGSQNNPWMKLMGIVHKERRHTGNVQSQSGSNERNLNQ **ShD**

MQMILVAGG **ShC**

Figure 1. Structural organization of ShB, ShC/B, and ShD channels. Identical shadings mean identical amino acid sequences. The amino-terminal amino acid sequences of the three variants are shown below.

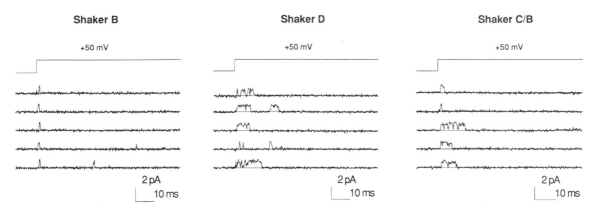

Figure 2. Representative single-channel records obtained from *Xenopus* oocytes injected with ShB, ShD, and ShC/B RNAs in inside-out patches. In each group, the single-channel openings were obtained in response to voltage steps to +50 mV from the holding voltage of −100 mV. Upward transitions are opening transitions.

with relatively small structural differences are valuable in providing preliminary identification of structural domains involved in gating. Figure 1 shows the differences in amino acid sequences among ShB, ShD, and ShC/B, along with a possible folding pattern of the *Shaker* polypeptide through the membrane. Because there is no signal sequence, the amino terminus is thought to reside on the cytoplasmic side of the membrane. By analogy with sodium and calcium channels, an even number of membrane-spanning regions have been proposed. Below the structural diagram is a schematic representation of three *Shaker* variants that vary only in their amino-terminal variable regions, a region consisting of less than 10% of the total amino acid residues. ShB and ShD were isolated from cDNA libraries (Schwarz et al. 1988); ShC/B is a chimera made of the amino-terminal region of ShC and the carboxy-terminal variable region of ShB. We expressed ShB, ShC/B, and ShD channels in *Xenopus* oocytes and recorded and analyzed their respective single-channel currents. Figure 2 shows five representative single-channel records from each of the three different variants. Channels

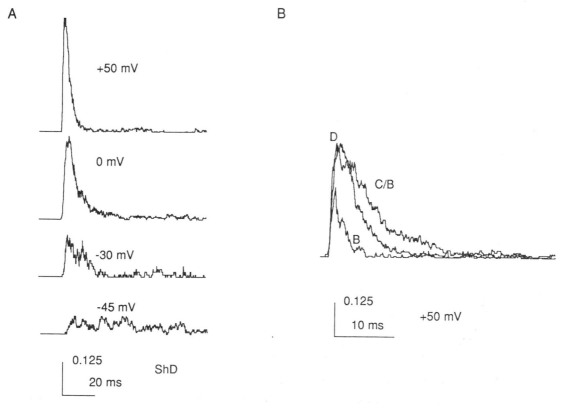

Figure 3. Time course of the probability of channels being open after a voltage step. (*A*) Ensemble averages from a patch containing a few ShD channels. The averages were converted to probabilities ($P[t]$) by dividing the average current by the single-channel current amplitude and the number of channels in the patch. (*B*) Superimposed averages from patches containing either ShB, ShD, or ShC/B channels during steps to +50 mV.

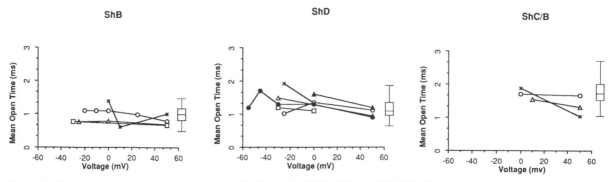

Figure 4. Mean open durations as a function of voltage for ShB, ShD, and ShC/B. No appreciable or consistent voltage dependence is seen in the mean open durations. Box plots of mean open durations from a number of patches with channels from each variant are located to the right of each graph. Mean open durations are long in ShC/B, short in ShB, and intermediate in ShD.

from all three variants had conductances of approximately 10 pSiemans in our recording solutions. Openings of all three types of channels tended to occur in bursts separated by long-lasting closures. ShB bursts usually consisted of only single or double openings, whereas both ShD and ShC/B channels had on the average more openings in their bursts. In some records,

especially in ShB and ShD, more than one burst could be observed during a voltage pulse.

The gating of *Shaker* potassium channels is strongly voltage-dependent. Figure 3A shows ensemble averages constructed from a large number of single-channel records like the ones shown in Figure 2 recorded after steps to different voltages. These averages show the

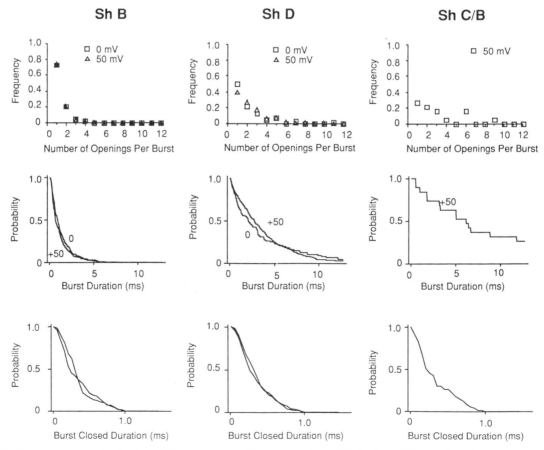

Figure 5. Burst parameters for the three different variants. The top row shows distributions of the number of openings in a burst, the middle row shows burst duration distributions, and the bottom row shows distributions of closed durations during a burst. For ShB and ShD, none of these distributions change significantly between 0 mV and +50 mV. It was difficult to obtain enough data from ShC/B channels to compare distributions from different voltages because of their slow recovery from inactivation. The burst durations are significantly longer in ShD and ShC/B relative to ShB.

probability of the channel being open versus time after a step in the membrane voltage ($P[t]$). After steps to -45 mV, $P(t)$ rises and declines slowly. As the voltage is made more positive, $P(t)$ increases and becomes more transient. This high degree of voltage dependence in the channel gating implies a significant rearrangement of charged particles in the membrane electrical field during at least some of the conformational transitions among closed, open, and inactivated states. The differences in gating among the different variants are shown in Figure 3B. ShB channels decay faster and reach a lower peak probability of being open than do ShD channels or ShC/B channels. For *Shaker* channels (Zagotta et al. 1989; Zagotta and Aldrich 1990), as well as for voltage-gated sodium channels (Aldrich et al. 1983; Aldrich and Stevens 1987), activation and inactivation are coupled, and inactivation of open channels is not very voltage-dependent. The voltage dependence in the ensemble averages shown in Figure 3A comes from voltage-dependent opening transitions. These differences in $P(t)$ values arise from differences in transition rates between various states, which cause differences in the average amount of time a channel stays open, the average number of openings during a burst of openings, or the interval between bursts. How long and frequently the channel stays open is negatively correlated with the inactivation rate of the channel (Zagotta and Aldrich 1990). The more frequently the channel opens, and the longer it stays open, the less the inactivation rate. Multiple bursts reflect returns from an inactivated state to the open state, with the interburst interval determined by the rate of return. We have examined the statistical properties of bursts of channel openings to determine the relative differences in opening, closing, and inactivation rates.

The open durations are not appreciably dependent on voltage. Figure 4 shows mean open durations from several patches of each variant at a number of voltages. The mean open durations show no significant or appreciable voltage dependence. Box plots at the right of each graph show distributions of mean open times from a number of patches for each variant, including patches where data were obtained only for a single voltage. ShC/B channels had significantly longer mean open durations than ShB or ShD variants.

The properties of bursts of channel openings are shown in Figure 5 for the three variants. Consistent with the slower decay of the ensemble averages (Fig. 3), the burst durations of ShD and ShC/B are much longer than those of ShB. For ShB and ShD, the number of openings per burst, the burst duration, and the closed durations within a burst did not show any appreciable voltage dependence between 0 mV and +50 mV. ShC/B recovered from inactivation so slowly that it was difficult to record data at both 0 mV and +50 mV (see below).

In addition to its longer open durations and higher average number of openings per burst, ShC/B exhibits another type of gating behavior that contributes to its slow decay in $P(t)$. The ShC/B channel can exist in two

different gating modes. Figure 6 shows a series of records recorded from a patch containing a few ShC/B channels. During a few of the traces, one of the channels does not inactivate with the typical time course, but continues to open and close for a long time, often until the end of the pulse. When in the slow mode, the channels behave as if they cannot inactivate. Although the channels enter the slow mode fairly often, they do not reside in it for more than a few records. In a population of ShC/B channels, only a few will be in the slow mode at any time, but those that are will contribute to the slow decay in the probability of being open. Similar shifts between high-probability and low-probability gating modes have been reported for other potassium channels (Cooper and Shrier 1989), calcium channels (Hess et al. 1984), and sodium channels (Moorman et al. 1990). Slow gating modes were not seen in either ShB or ShD.

ShC/B also differed from the other two variants in its slow recovery from inactivation. In contrast to ShB and ShD, additional bursts rarely occurred after termination of the first burst. This implies that the rate for returning from the inactivated state back to the open state is much slower for ShC/B than for the other

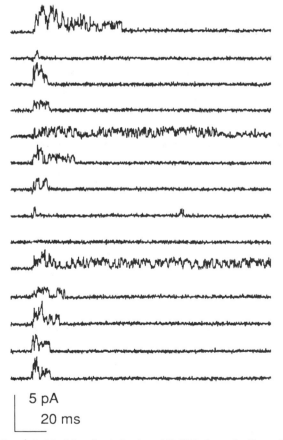

Figure 6. Modal gating behavior of ShC/B channels. Records from a patch containing a few ShC/B channels show an alternation between the usual short bursts of openings and a mode where a channel continues opening and closing for a long period of time. The voltage was +50 mV.

variants. In fact, ShC/B channels could remain in inactivated states for a number of subsequent voltage steps. Figure 7 shows a series of records recorded from ShB channels every 5 seconds. Occasional stretches of two blank records are evident, but the channels open during most traces. ShC/B channels, on the other hand, open rarely when voltage pulses are repeated every 5 or 10 seconds. Only when records are taken once every 20 seconds do the channels open with higher probability. At least two channels were present in this patch. The slow recovery of ShC/B channels from inactivation is reminiscent of the slow recovery seen with ShC and ShA, which share a carboxy-terminal domain different from ShB and ShD. The slow recovery in ShC/B demonstrates that the ShC amino-terminal variable region also contributes to slow recovery.

The contribution of burst openings and multiple bursts to the overall probability of a channel being open after a voltage step can be seen by comparing ensemble averages of single-channel records, distributions of open durations, and distributions of the probability of

channels being open at times after first opening. Figure 8 shows ensemble averages of records taken during steps to +50 mV from patches with ShB, ShD, and ShC/B channels. As described in Figure 3, the probability of ShB channels being open after the voltage step decays much more rapidly than that of either ShD or ShC/B channels. The curves on the right demonstrate the relative contributions of first and later openings to the ensemble averages for the three variants. We have previously made use of a conditional probability function $m(t)$ that describes the probability of a channel being open as a function of time after the first opening (Zagotta et al. 1989). This function can be measured by synchronizing an ensemble of records from a single-channel patch, such as those shown in Figure 2, at the time of the first channel opening and averaging them.

The $m(t)$ function has contributions from openings in the first burst and from openings in subsequent bursts, but not from transitions among closed states before the first opening. For native *Shaker* channels in *Drosophila*

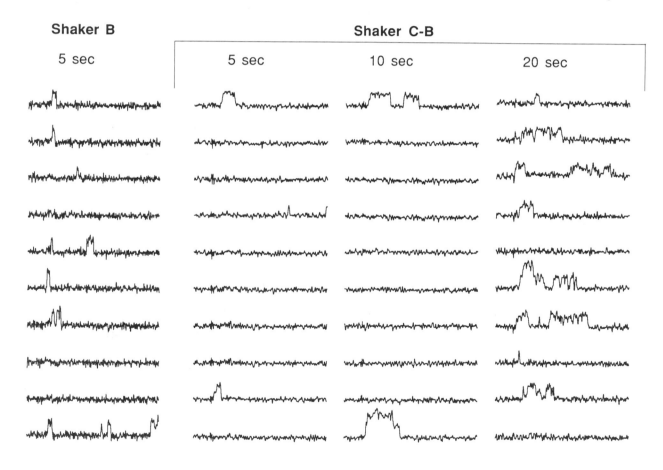

Figure 7. Slow recovery of ShC/B channels. When patches containing ShC/B channels were pulsed with a repetition interval of 5 sec, openings were rare and followed by long runs of records without openings. Patches containing ShB channels open much more readily at this interpulse interval. ShC/B channels opened much more frequently when the interpulse interval was increased to 20 sec. This patch had at least two channels. The voltage was +50 mV.

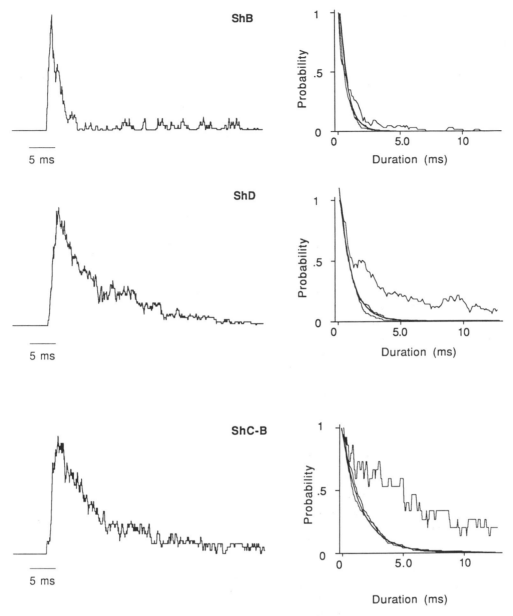

Figure 8. Contribution of first and subsequent openings to $P(t)$. The left column shows ensemble averages from the three variants recorded at +50 mV. The amplitudes are scaled to allow better comparison of the time courses. The right column shows open-duration durations from the same patches as the averages obtained at both 0 mV and +50 mV. These distributions are superimposed with single exponential functions. The slower-decaying functions in each of the panels are $m(t)$, the conditional probability of the channel being open at times after the initial opening, recorded at +50 mV. The differences between the open duration distributions and the $m(t)$ distributions reflect burst openings after the initial opening and bursts after the initial burst. ShB has little contribution from these additional openings, whereas ShC/B has a large contribution. ShD is intermediate.

muscle, and for ShB and ShD in oocytes, $m(t)$ does not depend on voltage, indicating that all of the gating transitions after the first opening, including the closings within the burst and inactivation, do not involve movement of charge through the membrane and that the voltage dependence in macroscopic current kinetics arises from transitions in the activation pathway (Zagotta et al. 1989). The right-hand column of Figure 3 shows $m(t)$ functions for ShB, ShD, and ShC/B, overlaid in each case with open duration distributions from records at 0 mV and +50 mV. The open-duration distributions

can be adequately fitted with single exponential functions, suggesting a single open state. The contribution of first openings to $m(t)$ can be assessed by comparing $m(t)$ (the slower-decaying traces) with the open-duration distributions. ShB channels have shorter open-durations and little contribution from later openings. ShC/B channels, on the other hand, have much longer open durations and considerable contribution from later openings. ShD channels behave intermediate between ShB and ShC/B in open duration and contribution of later openings.

DISCUSSION

The results obtained from the alternatively spliced variants are consistent with the hypothesis that the amino-terminal region of the channel is involved in inactivation. Channel bursts can be interpreted in terms of a simple-state diagram (Zagotta et al. 1989; Zagotta and Aldrich 1990);

$$\text{Closed} \underset{k_{OC}}{\overset{k_{CO}}{\rightleftharpoons}} \text{Open} \underset{k_{IO}}{\overset{k_{OI}}{\rightleftharpoons}} \text{Inactivated}$$

This is a simplified diagram that considers only open and closed states within a burst and the inactivated state that channels occupy upon termination of a burst. A burst consists of transitions between the closed and open states. Each burst is terminated by the channel making a transition to the inactivated state. The mean amount of time a channel resides in the open state is equal to the reciprocal of the transition rates leaving the open state, $1/(k_{OC} + k_{OI})$. The mean number of openings in a burst is equal to $(k_{OC} + k_{OI})/k_{OI}$ and is determined by the relative probabilities of continuing the burst, $k_{OC}/(k_{OC} + k_{OI})$, and terminating the burst, $k_{OI}/k_{OC} + k_{OI})$. The lack of voltage dependence in both the mean open duration and the mean number of openings per burst means that both k_{OI} and k_{OC} are not voltage-dependent, and therefore charge does not move through the membrane during these transitions. The longer mean open duration and greater mean number of openings per burst indicate a slower inactivation rate in ShC/B and ShD relative to ShB. The results show that inactivation is fastest in ShB, intermediate in ShD, and slowest in ShC/B. The mean closed duration during the burst is equal to $1/k_{CO}$. The lack of voltage dependence in the mean burst closed duration indicates that the opening step is also voltage-independent. The similarity of the burst closed duration distributions among the different channel variants suggests that the molecular rearrangements that underlie this transition are not different between the different variants. After termination of a burst by a transition to the inactivated state, a channel may return to the open state and enter another burst. The mean time between bursts is equal to $1/k_{IO}$. The slow recovery of ShC/B from inactivation indicates a small k_{IO} and therefore an inactivated state that is energetically much more stable than the inactivated states of ShB and ShD.

Our results show that variations in amino acid sequence in a fairly small region of the *Shaker* protein near the amino terminus can cause changes in channel inactivation rates. It is interesting that ShB, with the fastest inactivation rate, has the longest and most hydrophilic amino-terminal variable region. On the other hand, ShC/B inactivates the slowest and has the shortest and most hydrophobic amino-terminal sequence. ShD is intermediate in length, hydrophobicity, and inactivation rate. This trend could be explored further by using site-directed mutagenesis to make changes in

length and hydrophobicity in individual variants and determining the effects on inactivation.

ACKNOWLEDGMENTS

This work was supported by U.S. Public Health Service grant NS-23924, by an American Heart Association California Affiliate postdoctoral fellowship to T.H., and by training grant NS-07158 to W.Z.

REFERENCES

Aldrich, R. and S. Stevens. 1987. Voltage-dependent gating of single sodium channels from mammalian neuroblastoma cells. *J. Neurosci.* **7:** 418.

Aldrich, R., D. Corey, and C. Stevens. 1983. A reinterpretation of mammalian sodium channel gating based on single channel recording. *Nature* **306:** 436.

Baumann, A., A. Grupe, A. Ackermann, and O. Pongs. 1988. Structure of the voltage-dependent potassium channel is highly conserved from *Drosophila* to vertebrate central nervous systems. *EMBO J.* **7:** 2457.

Baumann, A., I. Krah-Jentgens, R. Muller, F. Muller-Holtkamp, R. Seidel, N. Kecskemethy, J. Casal, A. Rerrus, and O. Pongs. 1987. Molecular organization of the maternal effect region of the *Shaker* complex of *Drosophila*: Characterization of an IA channel transcript with homology to vertebrate Na$^+$ channel. *EMBO J.* **6:** 3419.

Christie, M.J., J.P. Adelman, J. Douglass, and R.A. North. 1989. Expression of a cloned rat brain potassium channel in *Xenopus* oocytes. *Science* **244:** 221.

Cooper, E. and A. Shrier. 1989. Inactivation of A currents and A channels on rat nodose neurons in culture. *J. Gen. Physiol.* **94:** 881.

Frech, G.C., A.M.J. VanDongen, G. Schuster, A.M. Brown, and R.H. Joho. 1989. A novel potassium channel with delayed rectifier properties isolated from rat brain by expression cloning. *Nature* **340:** 642.

Hamill, O.P., A. Marty, E. Neher, B. Sakmann, and F.J. Sigworth. 1981. Improved patch clamp techniques for high-resolution current recording from cells and cell-free membrane patches. *Pfluegers Arch. Eur. J. Physiol.* **391:** 85.

Hess, P., J.B. Lansman, and R.W. Tsien. 1984. Different modes of Ca channel gating behaviour favored by dihydropyridine Ca agonists and antagonists. *Nature* **311:** 538.

Hoshi, T. and R.W. Aldrich. 1988a. Voltage-dependent K$^+$ currents and underlying single K$^+$ channels in pheochromocytoma cells. *J. Gen. Physiol.* **91:** 73.

———. 1988b. Gating kinetics of four classes of voltage-dependent K$^+$ channels in pheochromocytoma cells. *J. Gen. Physiol.* **91:** 107.

Iverson, L.E., M.A. Tanouye, H.A. Lester, N. Davidson, and B. Rudy. 1988. A-type potassium channels expressed from *Shaker* locus cDNA. *Proc. Natl. Acad. Sci.* **85:** 5723.

Kamb, A., L.E. Iverson, and M.A. Tanouye. 1988. Molecular characterization of *Shaker*, a *Drosophila* gene that encodes a potassium channel. *Cell* **50:** 405.

Kamb, A., J. Tseng-Crank, and M.A. Tanouye. 1988. Multiple products of the *Drosophila Shaker* gene may contribute to potassium channel diversity. *Neuron* **1:** 421.

McKinnon, D. 1989. Isolation of a cDNA clone coding for a putative second potassium channel indicates the existence of a gene family. *J. Biol. Chem.* **264:** 8230.

Moorman, J.R., G.E. Kirsch, A.M.J. VanDongen, R.H. Joho, and A.M. Brown. 1990. Fast and slow gating of sodium channels encoded by a single mRNA. *Neuron* **4:** 243.

Pongs, O., N. Kecskemethy, R. Muller, I. Kreh-Jentgens, A. Baumann, H.H. Kiltz, I. Canal, S. Llamazares, and A. Ferrus. 1988. *Shaker* encodes a family of putative potassium channel proteins in the nervous system of *Drosophila. EMBO J.* **7:** 1087.

Schwarz, T.L., B.L. Tempel, D.M. Papazian, Y.N. Jan, and L.Y. Jan. 1988. Multiple potassium-channel components are produced by alternative spicing at the *Shaker* locus of *Drosophila. Nature* **331:** 137.

Stühmer, W., J.P. Ruppersberg, K.H. Schroter, B. Sakmann, M. Stocker, K.P. Giese, A. Perschke, A. Baumann, and O. Pongs. 1989. Molecular basis of functional diversity of voltage-gated potassium channels in mammalian brain. *EMBO J.* **8:** 3235.

Tempel, B.L., Y.N. Jan, and L.Y. Jan. 1988. Cloning of a probable potassium channel gene from mouse brain. *Nature* **332:** 837.

Tempel, B.L., D.M. Papazian, T.L. Schwarz, Y.N. Jan, and L.Y. Jan. 1987. Sequence of a probable potassium channel component encoded at *Shaker* locus of *Drosophila. Science* **237:** 770.

Timpe, L.C., Y.N. Jan, and L.Y. Jan. 1988a. Four cDNA clones from the *Shaker* locus of *Drosophila* induce kinetically distinct A-type potassium currents in *Xenopus* oocytes. *Neuron* **I:** 659.

Timpe, L.C., T.L. Schwarz, B.L. Tempel, D.M. Papazian, Y.N. Jan, and L.Y. Jan. 1988b. Expression of functional potassium channels from *Shaker* cDNA in *Xenopus* oocytes. *Nature* **331:** 143.

Zagotta, W.N. and R.W. Aldrich. 1990. Voltage-dependent gating of *Shaker* A-type potassium channels in *Drosophila* muscle. *J. Gen. Physiol.* **95:** 29.

Zagotta, W.N., T. Hoshi, and R.W. Aldrich. 1989. Gating of single *Shaker* K$^+$ channels in *Drosophila* muscle and in *Xenopus* oocytes injected with *Shaker* mRNA. *Proc Natl. Acad. Sci.* **86:** 7243.

The GABA_A Receptor Family: Molecular and Functional Diversity

P.H. Seeburg, W. Wisden, T.A. Verdoorn,* D.B. Pritchett, P. Werner,
A. Herb, H. Lüddens, R. Sprengel, and B. Sakmann*

*Laboratory of Molecular Neuroendocrinology, Center for Molecular Biology, University of Heidelberg;
Abteilung Zellphysiologie, Max-Planck-Institut für Medizinische Forschung, Heidelberg, Federal Republic of Germany

Fast excitatory and inhibitory signal transmission in the central nervous system (CNS) is mediated, in large part, by ion channels gated by amino acids and their derivatives (Dingledine et al. 1988). Many of these channels are built to a common design (Unwin 1989) of which the prototype is the nicotinic acetylcholine receptor (Changeux et al. 1984). The receptors/channels are assembled from several homologous subunits to form allosterically interacting transmembrane glycoprotein complexes. The main inhibitory channel is constituted by the GABA_A receptor, which occurs in virtually every neuron in the brain; it is estimated that approximately one third of all synapses in the CNS are GABAergic (Bloom and Iversen 1971). Notably, the GABA_A receptor (Olsen and Venter 1986; Stephenson 1988; Olsen and Tobin 1990) is the site of action of anxiolytics, anticonvulsants, hypnotics, anesthetics, and muscle relaxants, and hence knowledge of its structural and functional diversity is of pivotal interest to both neuroscientists and clinicians.

To study the molecular and functional diversity of GABA_A receptors in the brain, we have developed an integrated approach consisting of the molecular cloning of receptor subunits, the visualization of their distribution in the neuraxis, the recombinant expression of these receptor constituents, and the functional analysis of expressed receptors by electrophysiology and ligand-binding studies. Although these studies are ongoing, it is evident that the mammalian brain recruits for GABAergic signaling an array of GABA-gated channels, which differ in molecular composition in different neuronal populations and display distinct kinetic and modulatory properties.

METHODS

Molecular cloning. A cDNA library (10^6 recombinant phage) constructed in λgt10 from polyadenylated rat forebrain RNA was repeatedly screened with a 96-fold degenerate ^{32}P-labeled 23-mer oligonucleotide encoding a conserved octameric peptide sequence in TMII of GABA_A receptor subunits: 5'-AC(A,C)AC (A,T)GT(G,T)CT (A,C,G)AC(A,C)ATGAC(A,C) AC-3'. Only indicated third-position choices were included. Cloned cDNAs hybridizing to the 23-mer were sequenced in λgt10 or after subcloning into M13 vectors. Sequencing reactions using the 23-mer oligonu-

cleotide were performed with the 0.5 μM primer, and reactions were carried out at 55°C when recombinant λ DNA was used as template. Full-length clones were often obtained by rescreening the library using identified cDNA segments as probes.

In situ hybridization. In situ hybridization was performed as described previously (Wisden et al. 1988) using as probes subunit-specific oligonucleotides extended at their 3' termini by [^{35}S]dAMP. Hybridization of the probe (1 pg/μl; 1000 dpm/μl) was done overnight at 42°C in a buffer containing 50% formamide/ 4 × SSC/10% dextransulfate. Sections were washed at 60°C in 1 × SSC. Exposure time was 1 week on Kodak XAR-5 film. Brain structures were identified using the atlas of Paxinos and Watson (1986). Parallel sections hybridized with 20-fold excess of unlabeled oligonucleotides in addition to the labeled probe resulted in the absence of signal (not shown).

Recombinant expression. Transformed human embryonic kidney 293 cells (ATCC CRL 1573) were grown in minimum essential medium (MEM; GIBCO) supplemented with 10% fetal bovine serum containing 100 units of penicillin (GIBCO) and 100 units of streptomycin (GIBCO) per milliliter in a 6% CO_2/94% air incubator. Exponentially growing cells were trypsinized and seeded at 2×10^5 per 35-mm dish in 2 ml of growth medium. The transfection was performed by using the calcium phosphate precipitation technique (Chen and Okayama 1987). The cloned cDNAs of human GABA_A receptor subunits α_1, β_1, and γ_2 (Schofield et al. 1987; Pritchett et al. 1989b), inserted singly or together into the eukaryotic expression vector pCIS2 (Gorman et al. 1990), were used to perform the transfection. The cells were incubated in the presence (3 μg per 35-mm dish) of one or two supercoiled plasmids for 12–16 hours at 37°C under 3% CO_2/97% air. The medium was removed, and the cells were rinsed twice with growth medium, refed, and incubated in the same medium for 24 hours at 37°C under 6% CO_2/94% air before electrophysiological studies.

Ligand binding. Human embryonic kidney 293 cells transfected with expression vectors (10 plates, 10 cm each; 4×10^6 cells and 20 μg of DNA per plate) were washed twice with phosphate-buffered saline (PBS) and scraped into 10 ml of PBS. The cell pellet (500 mg) was homogenized in a Polytron tissue homogenizer (Brinkmann) in 10 ml of 10 mM potassium phosphate (pH 7.4) and centrifuged (50,000g, 20 min). This procedure was repeated three times, and the final pellet was resuspended in potassium phosphate buffer (pH 7.4) containing 100 mM KCl. For each concentration of displacing ligand, duplicate samples, each equivalent to 10^6 cells (100 μg protein) were incubated (4°C, 60 min) in 1 ml containing 4 pmoles of [^{3}H]Ro 15-1788 (75 Ci/mole). Nonspecific binding was determined by competition in the presence of 1 μM clonazepam. Filtered samples were washed twice with 5 ml of homogenization buffer, and filter-retained radioactivity was determined by liquid scintillation counting.

Electrophysiology. Transfected 293 cells grown on coverslips were transferred to the stage of an inverted microscope and bathed in normal Ringer's solution (NRR) containing (in mM) 135 NaCl, 5.4 KCl, 1.0 MgCl$_2$, 1.8 CaCl$_2$, 5 HEPES at pH 7.2. Patch-clamp techniques were used to measure GABA-activated currents in the whole-cell and outside-out configuration (Hamill et al. 1981) using a List EPC-7 amplifier (Darmstadt, Federal Republic of Germany). The pipet solution contained (in mM) 140 CsCl, 1.0 MgCl$_2$, 11 EGTA, and 10 HEPES at pH 7.3. Confluent clusters of these kidney cells are electrically coupled (Pritchett et al. 1988). Therefore, signals recorded from one cell in such cluster may arise from events occurring in one or more of its neighbors. We used the amplitude of GABA-activated currents in electrically coupled cell clusters to determine the overall effectiveness of the transfection. For quantitative measurements of whole-cell currents, only cells that did not contact other cells upon visual inspection were used. GABA (Research Biochemicals Inc.) was dissolved in NRR and applied by U-tube to allow rapid application of known concentrations. The use of this fast application system greatly improved the measurement of time course and amplitude of the response.

RESULTS

Subunits of GABA$_A$ Receptors

The mammalian brain synthesizes an array of GABA$_A$ receptor subunits, whose existence was uncovered by molecular biological studies (Schofield et al. 1987; Levitan et al. 1988; Pritchett et al. 1989b; Shivers et al. 1989; Ymer et al. 1989a,b, 1990; Lüddens et al. 1990; Pritchett and Seeburg 1990). The subunits share the same architectural design (Fig. 1) and can be grouped into different classes according to their sequence (Table 1). They are similar in size ($\sim$450–550 amino acid residues) and contain four putative membrane-spanning segments (TMI to TMIV), of which three are located approximately in the middle of the molecule and a fourth segment is at or near the carboxyl terminus. As predicted from the cDNA sequences, all subunits are biosynthesized in a preform containing a signal sequence attached to the mature amino ter-

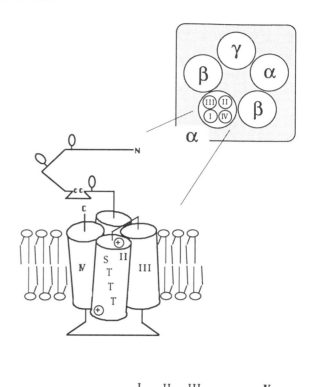

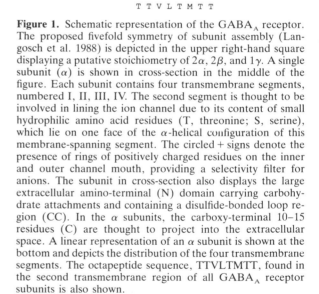

Figure 1. Schematic representation of the GABA$_A$ receptor. The proposed fivefold symmetry of subunit assembly (Langosch et al. 1988) is depicted in the upper right-hand square displaying a putative stoichiometry of 2α, 2β, and 1γ. A single subunit (α) is shown in cross-section in the middle of the figure. Each subunit contains four transmembrane segments, numbered I, II, III, IV. The second segment is thought to be involved in lining the ion channel due to its content of small hydrophilic amino acid residues (T, threonine; S, serine), which lie on one face of the α-helical configuration of this membrane-spanning segment. The circled + signs denote the presence of rings of positively charged residues on the inner and outer channel mouth, providing a selectivity filter for anions. The subunit in cross-section also displays the large extracellular amino-terminal (N) domain carrying carbohydrate attachments and containing a disulfide-bonded loop region (CC). In the α subunits, the carboxy-terminal 10–15 residues (C) are thought to project into the extracellular space. A linear representation of an α subunit is shown at the bottom and depicts the distribution of the four transmembrane segments. The octapeptide sequence, TTVLTMTT, found in the second transmembrane region of all GABA$_A$ receptor subunits is also shown.

minus, and hence the amino-terminal half of each subunit that precedes the first transmembrane segment is predicted to be extracellularly located. This large extracellular domain ($\sim$220 residues) contains several N-linked glycosylation sites, in keeping with the glycosylated nature of natural GABA$_A$ receptors (Stephenson 1988).

In all subunits, the extracellular domain features a 15-residue disulfide-bonded β-structural loop, which is also found in the closely related subunits of the strychnine-sensitive glycine receptor (Grenningloh et al.

Table 1. GABA$_A$ Receptor Subunits

Subunit classes (30–40%)	α	β	γ	δ
Variants (60–75%)	α_1	β_1	γ_1	δ_1
	α_2	β_2	γ_2	
	α_3	β_3		
	α_4			
	α_5			
	α_6			

Listed are cloned GABA$_A$ receptor subunits characterized by sequence analysis and recombinant expression. The α class contains numerous variants, and the δ class is represented by only one member.

1987, 1990a,b) and in all subunits of the nicotinic acetylcholine receptor (Noda et al. 1983). The transmembrane segments TMI through TMIV show the highest sequence conservation among the GABA$_A$ receptor subunits, reflecting their special function in channel formation (Finer-Moore and Stroud 1984). In particular, TMII contains an octapeptide sequence, TTVLTMTT, conserved also in the ligand-binding subunits of the glycine receptor (Grenningloh et al. 1987, 1990b). The presence of this conserved sequence facilitated the isolation of a variety of subunit cDNAs (Pritchett et al. 1989b; Shivers et al. 1989; Ymer et al.

```
       α1                                   QPSQDELKDNTTVFT   R  D        L ERV E K D F    47
       α2                                   NIQEDEAKNNITIFT   R  D        L DSI E F N Y    47
       α3         QGESRRQEPGDFVKQDIGGLSPKHAPDIPDDSTDNITIFT   R  D        L DAV E K D Y    72
       α4                                   QNSKDEKLCPEIFT   S  D        F GPV E K D Y    46
       α5                        HFGFSQMPTSSVQDETNDNITIFT   G  D        L ERI Q R D Y    56
       α6                                   QAQLEDEGNFYSENVS   N  E        F GAV E K D Y    48
CONSENSUS          ..................................RILD.LL.GYDNRLRPG.G...T.V.T.I.VT

   HD    I     SWK E  KFK  MTV R   LMAS I     H    VA    M    L ITED  L     TVR E   H ED   147
   TD    I     KWK E  KFK  MNI R   LMAS I     H    VA    M    L IQDD  L     TVQ E   H ED   147
   TD    I     TWH E  KFD  MKI P   LLAS I     H    MA    T    L LVDN  L     TIH E   H ED   172
   VE    M     TWI K  KYD  IEI R   MMVT V     R    VS    A    F IMRN  I     TIS E   R VD   146
   TE    I     SWK E  RFK  MQR P   LLAS I     H    IA    T    L LEDD  L     MIS E   Q ED   156
   VE    M     TRT E  KFK  AEI S   LMVS I     R    IA    T    F LMHN  I     TIN D   R VN   148
SFGPVSD..MEYT.DVFFRQ...D.RL...GP...L.LNN....K.WTPDTFF.NGKKS..HNMT.PNKL.R....GT.LYTMRL...A.CPM.L..FPM
                                                               •

                                                                     TM1
A A       TRA VV E TREPAR  V AEDG R N  D L QTVDSGIVQSS   VV  TH   K  I  |V  T L          L|  247
A S       TTS VT I TYNASD  Q APDG R N  D L QSIGKETIKSS   TV  AH   K  I  |V  T L          L|  247
V A       TKA VI S TLGKNK  E AQDG R N  D L HVVGTEIIRSS   VV  TH   K  I  |V  T L          L|  272
G A       PKS MI T TKGPEK  E PKES S V  D I QTVSSETIKSI   IV  VY   R  M  |M  T I          I|  246
A A       PNS VV V TNGSTK  V AEDG R N  H M QTVGTENISTS   TI  AH   K  I  |V  T L          L|  256
G A       PKS II T KKGPLY  E PEES S L  D I QTVSSETIKSN   VI  VY   Q  M  |M  I T          I|  248
D.H.CPLKFGSYAY...E..Y.W......SV.V....S.L.QY.L.G..........TGEY..MT..FHL.RK.GYR.IQ.Y.PCIMTVILSQVSFW.N

        TM2                              TM3
R |     V          S| N    A    |  I   Y        T  | KRGYAWDGKSV...VPEKPKKVKDPLIKKNNTYAPTA    344
R |     V          S| N    A    |  I   Y        T  | KRGWAWDGKSV...VNDKKKEKG.SVMIQNNAYAVAV    343
R |     V          T| N    A    |  M   Y        T  | KRSWAWEGKKVPEALEMKKKTPAAPTKKTSTTFNIVG    372
K |     I          S| H    S    |  I   F        A  | NIQMQKAKKKISKPPPEVPAAPVLKEKHTETSLQNTH    346
R |     V          S| N    A    |  I   Y        T  | KRGWAWDGKKALEAAKIKKKERELILNKSTNAFTTGK    356
K |     I          S| H    S    |  I   F        A  | NLQSQKAERQAQTAAKPPVAKSKTTESLEAEIVVHSD    348
.ESVPARTVFG.TTVLTMTTLSI.AR.SLPKV.YATAMDWF.AVC.AFVFSALIEFA.VNYFT.................................

TSYTPNLARGD............................................PGLATIAKSAT..........IEPKEVKPETKPPEPKKTF...   385
ANYAPNL.SKP............................................DVLSTISKSAT..........TPEPNKKPENKPAEAKKTF...   383
TTYPINL.AKD............................................TEFSTISKAAAAPSASSTPTVIASPKTTYVQDSPAETKKTY...   422
ANLNMRKRTNALVHSESDVNSRTEVGNHSSKTTAAQESSETTPKAHLASSPNPFSRANAAETISAAARGLSSAASPSPHGTLQPAPLRSASARPAFGARL   446
LTHPPNIPKEQL...........................................PGGTGNAVGT............ASIRASEEKTSESKKTYN...   396
SKYHLKKRISSL...........................................TLPIVPSSEA.....SKVLSRTPILPSTPVTPPLLLPAIG...   395
.....................................................................................................

                                      TM4
...........................NSV   I |RLS  A   LL GI   L   AT| LNREPQLKAPTPHQ            428
...........................NSV   I |RMS  V   VL GT   L   AT| LNREPVLGVSP               423
...........................NSV   V |KIS  I   VL AI   L   AT| VNRESAIKGMIRKQ            465
GRIKTTVNTTGVPGNVSATPPPSAPPPSGSGT   I |KYA  L   VT GA   M   VV| LSKDTMEKSESLM             517
.............................SI   I |KMS  V   IL GT   L   AT| LNREPVIKGATSPK            438
.............................GT   I |QYS  L   VA AG   L   IV| LSKDTMEVSSTVE             437
..............................SK.D.|..RI.FP..F..FN.VYW..Y|.............
```

Figure 2. Polypeptide sequences of six variants of the rat GABA$_A$ receptor a subunit class. Sequences are without signal peptides, are presented in the single-letter code, and are individually numbered at the right. A consensus sequence highlights the short stretches of amino acids conserved in all variants. Pairwise comparisons between α variants show a range of overall sequence identity of 60–75%.

1990). As illustrated by the octapeptide sequence, TMII contains several small hydrophilic residues whose existence in this transmembrane region is in keeping with the proposed function of TMII in lining the ion channel (Sakmann et al. 1985; Giraudat et al. 1986; Hucho et al. 1986; Imoto et al. 1988). Since the channel intrinsic to the GABA$_A$ receptor conducts chloride ions, it comes as no surprise that positively charged residues are clustered in the vicinity of the transmembrane segments and presumably serve to provide a selectivity filter for anions at the inner- and outerchannel mouth. The importance of charged residues on channel properties has been elegantly demonstrated for the nicotinic acetylcholine receptor (Imoto et al. 1988).

As summarized in Table 1, the α, β, and γ subunit classes comprise variants. This fact is particularly evident for the α subunit class, where six variants characterized to date display approximately 70% sequence identity in pairwise combinations. Our studies suggest that these variants define different GABA$_A$ receptor subtypes in the brain. To illustrate the distribution of sequence differences among such variants, Figure 2 compares the primary structures of the six α variants from rat. Interestingly, the region between the β-structural loop and TMI contains a segment in which the sequence conservation among the α variants is low. This region is probably accessible to allosteric ligands and may contribute to the disparate pharmacological properties of GABA$_A$ receptor subtypes. The comparison also indicates that the large intracellular domain between TMIII and TMIV shows no homology between the variants.

Patterns of Subunit mRNA Expression in the Rat Brain

A particularly powerful method for analyzing the expression of different GABA$_A$ receptor subunits is to visualize by in situ hybridization (Young et al. 1986) the synthesis of the cognate mRNAs in sections of brain. Due to the often abundant expression of these mRNAs in the neuraxis, ^{35}S-labeled oligonucleotides constructed to subunit-specific sequences yield valuable information about possible subunit partners of natural GABA$_A$ receptors (Séquier et al. 1988; Wisden et al. 1988; 1989a,b; Lolait et al. 1989; Shivers et al. 1989). Although there is as yet no systematic comparison of the distribution of all GABA$_A$ receptor subunit mRNAs, the available data serve to indicate the hitherto unappreciated complexity of GABAergic signal transmission in the CNS.

Figure 3 shows the differential distribution of α_1, α_2, and α_3 mRNAs in horizontal sections of the rat brain. Strikingly, α_1 mRNA is expressed fairly ubiquitously throughout the neuraxis. Highest levels of α_1 mRNA are seen in mitral cells of the olfactory bulb, in the hippocampal formation, in the cerebellum, and in the inferior colliculi (Figs. 3A and 4A). Lowest levels of this RNA are observed in the caudate nucleus (Fig. 4A). The α_2 mRNA is very highly expressed in the hippocampus (Fig. 3B), whereas α_3 mRNA is hardly expressed at all in this structure but is prominent in all cortical layers and in the superior colliculi (Fig. 3C). Both α_2 and α_3 mRNAs are rare in the cerebellum.

The distribution of β_1, β_2, and β_3 mRNAs is shown in

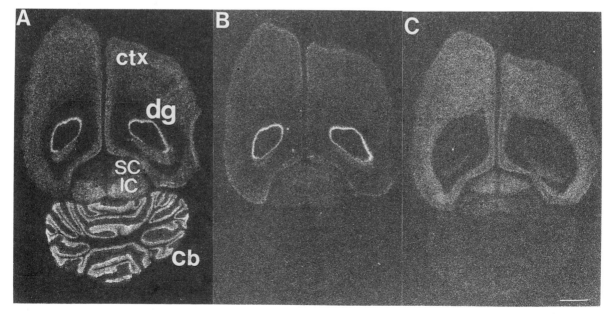

Figure 3. Differential distribution of α_1 (A), α_2 (B), and α_3 (C) mRNAs in horizontal sections of rat brain. (Cb) Cerebellum; (ctx) cortex; (dg) dentate gyrus; (IC) inferior colliculus; (SC) superior colliculus. Bar, 2.25 mm.

Figures 4 and 5, where these RNAs are also compared to α_1 mRNA. As judged from these pictures, the β_1 mRNA appears to be the rarest β subunit, and highest levels of this RNA are found in the cortex, hippocampus, and the mitral cells of the olfactory bulb (Figs. 4B and 5B). In contrast to β_2 and β_3 mRNAs, β_1 mRNA is absent from cerebellum. The β_2 mRNA is prominently localized in most of the areas also expressing the α_1 mRNA. Both β_2 and β_3 mRNAs are synthesized in the olfactory bulb, cortex, hippocampus, and cerebellum. In the olfactory bulb, β_2 mRNA is found in mitral cells, glomeruli, and the external plexiform layer, whereas β_3 is found in mitral cells, glomeruli, and granule cells. The most pronounced difference between β_2 and β_3

mRNAs is the high expression of β_3 mRNA in the caudate putamen, and the conspicuous absence of this mRNA in thalamus (Fig. 5C,D).

The distribution in brain of the γ variants is shown in Figure 6. Both mRNAs are widely expressed in the brain but show differential synthesis in certain areas. The γ_1 mRNA is highly enriched in the septum, and the γ_2 mRNA is prominently synthesized in the cerebellum, inferior colliculi, and hippocampus (Shivers et al. 1989; Ymer et al. 1990). Figure 6 also shows the distribution of α_6 mRNA, which appears to be confined completely to the granule cells of the cerebellum (Lüddens et al. 1990). No expression can be detected in the rest of the brain. Thus, the α_6 mRNA displays the most

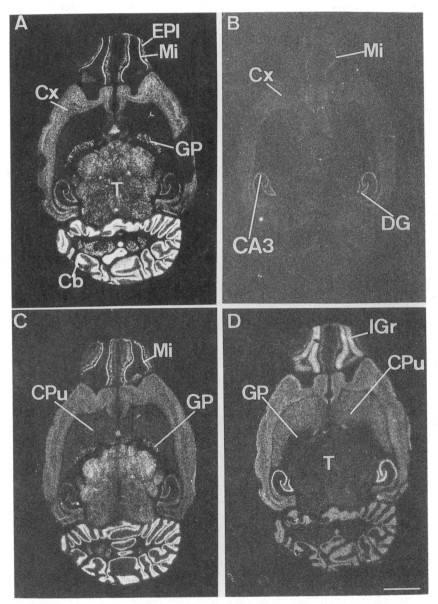

Figure 4. Different distribution of α_1 (A), β_1 (B), β_2 (C), and β_3 (D) mRNAs in horizontal sections of rat brains. (Cb) Cerebellum; (CPu) caudate putamen; (Cx) Cortex; (DG) dentate gyrus; (EPI) external plexiform layer; (GP) globus pallidus; (Mi) mitral cell layer; (IGr) internal granule cell layer of olfactory bulb; (T) thalamus. Bar, 5 mm.

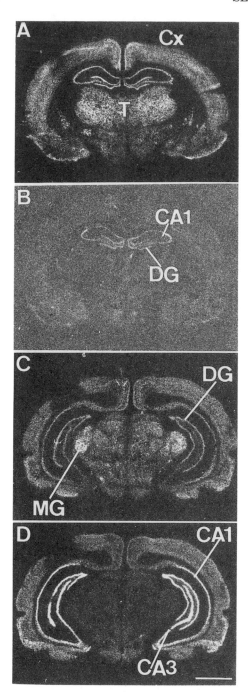

Figure 5. Different distribution of α_1 (A), β_1 (B), β_2 (C), and β_3 (D) mRNAs in thalamus of hippocampus (coronal sections). (Cx) Cortex; (DG) dentate gyrus; (MG) medial geniculate. Bar, 5 mm.

restricted expression pattern of any $GABA_A$ receptor subunit gene to date, indicating a specialized function for receptors containing this subunit.

The available data suggest likely subunit partners in natural $GABA_A$ receptors. Thus, in many areas of the brain, α_1, β_2, and γ_2 mRNAs are seen to colocalize, indicating that receptors assembled from these subunits constitute a major receptor population. Indeed, recombinant coexpression of these subunits recreates a ben-

zodiazepine-binding site displaying the properties of the $GABA_A$/benzodiazepine type I receptor (Pritchett et al. 1989a). Other subtypes may include receptors containing α_2 and β_3 subunits as the cognate mRNAs colocalize throughout most of the CNS, with the exception of the cerebellum.

Although the data obtained by in situ hybridization are suggestive of possible subunit partners for defined receptor subtypes, a detailed analysis of distinct neuronal populations paints a more complex picture. Mitral cells of the olfactory bulb express at least α_1, β_1, β_2, β_3, and γ_2 subunits (Shivers et al. 1989; Wisden et al. 1989b). Hippocampal dentate granule cells synthesize every subunit (except possibly α_6), and cerebellar granule cells express at a minimum α_1, α_6, β_2, β_3, γ_2, and δ subunits. The cases listed serve to illustrate that particular neuronal populations in different parts of the neuraxis seem to elaborate more subunits than can be assembled into one receptor type. Hence, these subunits might assemble in a promiscuous manner to generate an array of receptor subtypes. Alternatively, a cellular sorting mechanism could lead to preferred assemblies in distinct neuronal structures, e.g., dendritic synapses. The development of subunit-specific antibodies (Ewert et al. 1990) should address this important issue.

Pharmacological Properties of Recombinant $GABA_A$/Benzodiazepine Receptors

The complexity of $GABA_A$ receptors can be studied by the recombinant expression of diverse combinations of subunits and the subsequent analysis of the receptors generated. We chose a transient mammalian cell expression system, originally developed by C. Gorman (Gorman et al. 1990), to permit the efficient expression of one, two, or three different receptor subunits. To evaluate the properties of recombinant receptors, cells were analyzed by ligand binding and ligand competition studies. Importantly, these experiments led to an understanding of the molecular requirements in modeling a high-affinity benzodiazepine-binding site (Pritchett et al. 1989b).

Such a site was manifest solely upon coexpression of α, β, and γ subunits, whereas dual combinations of α, β, and γ subunits showed only high-affinity sites for [^{3}H]muscimol. Interestingly, benzodiazepine-binding sites with disparate affinities could be built by substituting different α variants, suggesting that, indeed, these α variants participate in the formation of different $GABA_A$ receptor subtypes (Pritchett et al. 1989a; Puia et al. 1989; Pritchett and Seeburg 1990). That the pharmacological properties of recombinant receptors match and extend those of natural receptors is illustrated in Table 2, which lists the affinities of several ligands binding to allosteric sites of recombinantly expressed receptors. Receptors containing the α_1 variant display the known properties of benzodiazepine type I receptors (Squires et al. 1979; Nielsen and Braestrup 1980; Olsen and Venter 1986), an abundant receptor

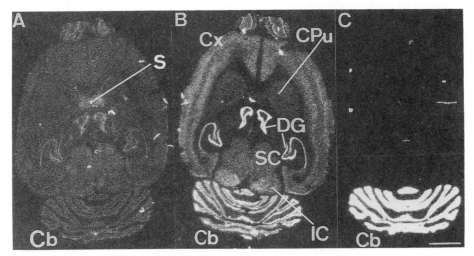

Figure 6. Distribution of γ_1 (A), γ_2 (B), and α_6 (C) mRNAs in horizontal sections of rat brain. (DG) Dentate gyrus; (Cx) cortex; (CPu) caudate putamen; (Cb) cerebellum; (IC) inferior colliculus; (SC) superior colliculus. Bar, 2.5 mm.

population in brain and the main site in the cerebellum (Young et al. 1981; Niddam et al. 1987).

Receptors containing the α_2, α_3, or α_5 variants have much in common with the GABA$_A$/benzodiazepine type II receptors described by ligand-binding studies in brain membranes. However, distinct differences are apparent among these three recombinant receptors (Blankenfeld et al. 1990; Pritchett and Seeburg 1990), suggesting the molecular heterogeneity of classically defined type II receptors. In particular, the affinity of α_5-subunit-containing receptors toward CL218872 is higher than at type II receptors, whereas zolpidem, a hypnotic imidazopyridine compound (Arbilla et al. 1986), acting at the benzodiazepine-recognition site of certain GABA$_A$ receptors, displays no measurable affinity at α_5 receptors.

Equally important is the observation that the γ variants (besides being necessary constituents in forming the benzodiazepine-recognition site) modulate the pharmacology of this site (Ymer et al. 1990). This finding may reflect the fact that the γ subunits are closest in sequence to the α subunits (sequence similarity is ~40%). It is curious in this respect that photoaffinity labeling of GABA$_A$ receptors by [^{3}H]benzodiazepine ligands occur via the α subunits (Fuchs et al. 1988, 1990). Hence, the γ subunits seem to induce a particular conformation in the α subunits conducive to forming the benzodiazepine-recognition site.

Electrophysiological Properties of Recombinant GABA$_A$ Receptors

The analysis of channel properties of simple recombinant GABA$_A$ receptors provides an excellent means in assigning specific contributions of individual subunits to the overall channel characteristics, e.g., gating and desensitization behavior, conductance, and rectification properties. In a series of experiments, cultured mammalian cells engineered for the transient expression of GABA$_A$ receptors composed of α_1, β_2; α_1, γ_2 and α_1, β_2, and γ_2 subunits were studied using patch-clamp techniques (Verdoorn et al. 1990). Importantly, these subunit combinations showed GABA-activated currents having distinctly different properties. GABA$_A$ receptors formed of α_1 and β_2 subunits desensitized more rapidly, showed greater outward rectification, and displayed smaller single-channel conductances than GABA$_A$ receptors assembled from α_1 and γ_2 subunits (see Fig. 7 and Table 3). Hence, the γ_2 subunit functionally contributes to the formation of larger channels. This is also evident with receptors composed of α_1, β_2,

Table 2. Pharmacological Properties of Recombinant GABA$_A$ Receptor Subtypes

Compounds	Receptors			
	$\alpha_1\beta_3\gamma_2$	$\alpha_2\beta_3\gamma_2$	$\alpha_3\beta_3\gamma_2$	$\alpha_5\beta_3\gamma_2$
CL218872	120 ± 18	1800 ± 600	1500 ± 200	490 ± 120
2-Oxoquazepam	16 ± 2	225 ± 12	201 ± 18	190 ± 15
Zolpidem	19 ± 3.5	450 ± 21	400 ± 43	>15,000
Ro 15-1788	0.7 ± 0.1	1.0 ± 0.1	0.6 ± 0.2	0.5 ± 0.1
β-CCM	0.8 ± 0.2	3.4 ± 0.35	4.1 ± 0.6	27 ± 5

Data were obtained from washed membranes of transiently expressing cultured 293 cells and represent K_i values (mean ± S.E.M.). These values were determined by displacement of [^{3}H]Ro 15-1788 binding and were calculated according to the equation of Cheng and Prusoff (1973). (β-CCM) Methyl-β-carboline-3-carboxylate.

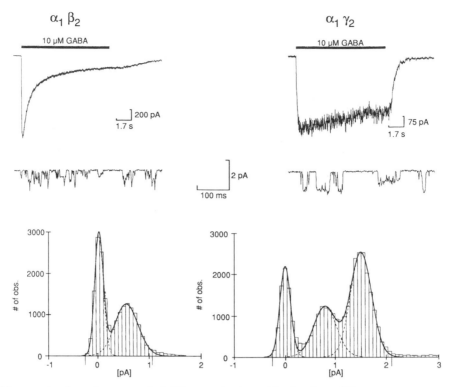

Figure 7. GABA$_A$ receptor channels composed of different subunit combinations have different electrophysiological properties. The currents are evoked by GABA measured in whole-cell (−60 mV, top traces) and outside-out (−50 mV, middle traces) recording configurations. (*Left*) Currents mediated by $\alpha_1\beta_2$ GABA$_A$ receptors; (*right*) currents caused by activation of $\alpha_1\gamma_2$ GABA$_A$ receptors. (*Bottom*) "All points" histograms compiled from the single-channel recordings. The histograms are fitted with the sum of two or three gaussians. Besides a peak at 0 pA representing the baseline current, a single peak at 0.55 pA is seen in patches containing $\alpha_1\beta_2$ GABA$_A$ receptors. In contrast, two single-channel current amplitudes of 0.78 and 1.5 pA are apparent in $\alpha_1\gamma_2$ GABA$_A$ receptors.

and γ_2 subunits. These, different from the dual-subunit combinations, show a significantly steeper slope in the concentration-response curve. This trait, combined with a large channel conductance and high outward rectification, constitutes a unique set of properties of the triple-subunit receptor (Table 3). The triple-subunit combination is also the simplest receptor to show high-affinity benzodiazepine binding (see above).

Curiously, the analysis of single-channel events of the subunit combinations tested, although showing different channel conductances for β or γ subunit-containing receptors, failed to produce evidence for the several subconductance states seen in natural GABA-gated channels (Bormann and Clapham 1985; Smith et al. 1989). This may indicate the presence of different receptor populations in the analyzed membrane patches.

Table 3. Electrophysiological Properties of Recombinant GABA$_A$ Receptors

Properties	Receptors		
	$\alpha_1\beta_2$	$\alpha_1\gamma_2$	$\alpha_1\beta_2\gamma_2$
Conc/Resp Slope	1.18 ± 0.08 (n = 5)	1.46 ± 0.10 (n = 8)	2.12 ± 0.12[a] (n = 9)
Rectification Ratio[b]	2.87 ± 0.46 (n = 7)	1.47 ± 0.29 (n = 7)	2.84 ± 0.36 (n = 5)
Main single channel Conductance (pS)[c]	11.3 ± 0.23 (n = 6)	30.8 ± 1.0 (n = 7)	32.0 ± 0.8 (n = 4)

[a] Indicated value is significantly different from values obtained with the other subunit combinations ($p <0.05$, two-tailed t-test).

[b] Estimated from the current-voltage relationship by dividing the cord conductance at 100 mV by the cord conductance at −100 mV.

[c] Measured in outside-out patches.

Recombinant and Synaptic GABA_A Receptors

Functional comparisons between GABA_A channels reconstituted in transfected cells and those that mediate synaptic transmission may be useful to elucidate the subunit composition of native GABA receptors. Recent measurements on rat hippocampal slices (Edwards et al. 1990) of the size and time course of GABA-mediated quantal inhibitory postsynaptic currents (IPSCs) in granule cell synapses (Fig. 8A) were used to numerically reconstruct the shape of IPSCs (Busch and Sakmann, this volume) as illustrated in Figure 8B. The decay time course of IPSCs largely reflects the closure of GABA_A channels, assuming that GABA concentration in the synaptic cleft falls rapidly following release from a vesicle. To compare the gating properties of GABA_A receptors in granule cell synapses with those of GABA_A receptors reconstituted from different subunits, we compared the relaxation times of measured GABA-induced current fluctuations with those predicted for synaptic GABA_A receptors calculated from the shape of the quantal IPSC. Figure 8C shows the power-density spectrum (Neher and Stevens 1977) of GABA-activated currents recorded from 293 cells transiently expressing the α, β, and γ subunits of the rat GABA_A receptor (Verdoorn et al. 1990). This spectrum of current fluctuations characterizing the recombinant channels closely resembles that calculated for the reaction scheme used to reconstruct the shape of the IPSC (Fig. 8D). The result is not inconsistent with the idea that granule cell IPSCs (shown in Fig. 8A) are mediated by a GABA_A receptor composed of α, β, and γ subunits.

Obviously, a comparison of gating properties of synaptic and reconstituted GABA_A receptors is only a first step in identifying the subunit composition of synaptic receptors in various brain regions. One way to obtain more direct evidence for the presence of a particular subunit or combination of subunits would be to compare the effects of pharmacological agents on IPSCs and on currents mediated by GABA-gated chan-

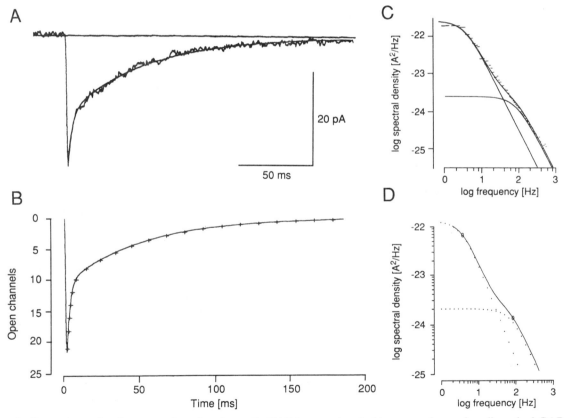

Figure 8. Comparison of gating properties of postsynaptic GABA_A receptors in hippocampal granule cells and of GABA_A receptors reconstituted from α, β, and γ subunits in 293 cells. (*A*) Record of averaged quantal IPSCs showing fast rise time and slower, doubly exponential decay time course, with time constants of 2.5 msec and 56 msec, respectively. −50 mV membrane potential, 22°C. (Modified from Edwards et al. 1990.) (*B*) Numerically reconstructed IPSC in response to the release of a quantum of GABA, assuming fast rise and decay of GABA in the synaptic cleft. Decay time constants are 2.5 msec and 52 msec, respectively. The reaction scheme assumes opening of GABA_A channels from singly and doubly liganded states. (*C*) Power density spectrum of GABA (10 μM)-activated whole-cell currents recorded from 293 cells transiently expressing $\alpha_1\beta_2$ and γ_2 subunits. −50 mV membrane potential and comparable ionic conditions are the same as those in *A*. Relaxation times are 2.1 msec and 36 msec, respectively. Single-channel conductance is 32 pS. (Modified from Verdoorn et al. 1990.) (*D*) Power density spectrum calculated for hypothetical currents induced by 10 μM GABA on synaptic GABA_A channels using the same reaction scheme as used for the reconstruction of the IPSC shown in *A* and *B*.

nels reconstituted from various subunits. A complication that may arise regarding such an approach may be the fact that GABA$_A$ receptor subunits are promiscuous in their assembly and hence could form a mosaic of receptor subtypes that are colocalized in the postsynaptic membrane.

SUMMARY AND OUTLOOK

The GABA$_A$ receptor constitutes an excellent example for the concept that diversity of signaling in the CNS is achieved by relatively few types of neurotransmitters, each targeting different receptors and receptor subtypes (Schofield et al. 1990). Often, these receptors are members of two superfamilies, the G-protein-coupled receptors and the ligand-gated ion channels. The GABAergic system exemplifies this phenomenon: GABA binds to and activates the G-protein-linked GABA$_B$ receptor (Bowery 1989) and the ligand-gated anion channel, the GABA$_A$ receptor. GABA has been clearly shown to activate the two classes of receptors simultaneously on the same cell (Dutar and Nicoll 1988). The GABA$_A$ receptor is composed of several homologous subunits, each the product of a distinct gene. Preliminary evidence suggests that some of the subunit-encoding genes are clustered, allowing for a concerted gene regulation in neuronal populations (Buckle et al. 1989).

As of now, 12 GABA$_A$ receptor subunits are characterized by structure and functional expression. Although these subunits can be grouped into distinct sequence classes (α, β, γ, δ), upon recombinant expression, each subunit seems to form oligohomomeric receptor/channels that can be gated by GABA, potentiated by barbiturates (Pritchett et al. 1988; Shivers et al. 1989) and neurosteroids (Puia et al. 1990), and show sensitivity to bicuculline, a competitive GABA antagonist, as well as to the channel blocker picrotoxin (Pritchett et al. 1988). A similar propensity to form functional homo-oligomeric receptors has been observed with the ligand-binding subunit of the strychnine-sensitive glycine receptor (Sontheimer et al. 1989). This property of single subunits suggests a functional correlate to the conserved structural properties of the subunits. However, certain allosteric interactions known to occur in natural GABA$_A$ receptors cannot be mimicked by homo-oligomeric subunit assemblies. Rather, two different subunits need to coassemble, preferably an α and γ subunit, to permit benzodiazepine-mediated potentiation of GABA-elicited currents. High-affinity binding sites for [^{3}H]benzodiazepines have only been observed with receptors composed of α, β, and γ subunits (Pritchett et al. 1989b).

Although channel properties and pharmacological characterization of simple subunit combinations prove invaluable to study the contribution of individual subunits to GABA$_A$ receptors, there has been no extensive correlation to natural receptors. The number of synthetic GABA$_A$ receptors that could be recombinantly expressed in cell lines from cloned cDNAs is immense. Thus, to narrow down these combinations of subunits, the results of in situ hybridization and immunocytochemical studies (Ewert et al. 1990) are important. Since through technical advances it now seems possible to perform patch-clamping on individual neurons in slices (Edwards et al. 1989), it may prove feasible to correlate in vivo GABA$_A$ responses on defined parts of a cell with those obtained from synthetic combinations of subunits, and thus infer the composition of the receptor. Hence, an important future task will be the elucidation of natural receptors regarding subunit composition and exact cellular localization.

It is, however, becoming increasingly clear that some neurons synthesize more subunits than can be assembled into a single receptor subtype. For fine tuning of GABAergic signaling, one would anticipate that neurons have developed ways of sorting different subtypes to different subcellular locations. Thus, it may be advantageous for efficient signal transmission to insert GABA$_A$ receptors having long channel open times and/or larger conductances into more distally located synapses and to incorporate other subtype(s) into proximal synapses. However, these considerations are highly speculative and need experimental corroboration. Several laboratories are presently developing subunit-specific antibodies that could be recruited for immuno-electron microscopy to investigate the existence of disparate GABA$_A$ receptor subtypes in different synapses of the same neuron. Until such a subtype arrangement is shown, the random assembly of subunits to generate a multitude of receptor subtypes remains a possible, although less attractive, option of how neurons handle diversity of subunit expression.

ACKNOWLEDGMENTS

We extend our gratitude to our former colleagues, Brenda D. Shivers, Sanie Ymer, and Peter R. Schofield, whose contributions were germane to our present understanding of GABA$_A$ receptor heterogeneity. We thank our colleagues Iris Killisch, Hannah Monyer, Andreas Draguhn, Markus Ewert, Kari Keinänen, Martin Köhler, and Bernd Sommer for their creative input into various aspects of this work and Sabine Grünewald, Annette Herold, and Gillian Muncke for excellent technical support. Additionally, W.W. thanks Andrew Gundlach for kindly providing some of the rat brain sections and Stephen P. Hunt and Brian J. Morris for their initial guidance with regard to mRNA localization. We acknowledge Ina Baro and Jutta Rami for their efficient help in photography and manuscript preparation. W.W. and T.A.V. gratefully acknowledge the support of EMBO and von Humboldt fellowships, respectively. This work was funded by the Max-Planck-Society to B.S. and by grants from the Deutsche Forschungsgemeinschaft and the German Ministry of Research and Technology (BMFT) to P.H.S.

REFERENCES

Arbilla, S., J. Allen, A. Wick, and S.Z. Langer. 1986. High affinity [^{3}H]zolpidem binding in rat brain: An imidazopyridine with agonist properties at central benzodiazepine receptors. *Eur. J. Pharmacol.* **130:** 257.

Blankenfeld, G., S. Ymer, D.B.Pritchett, H.Sontheimer, M. Ewert, P.H. Seeburg, and H. Kettenmann. 1990. Differential benzodiazepine pharmacology of recombinant GABA$_A$ receptors. *Neurosci. Lett.* (in press).

Bloom, F.E. and L.L. Iversen. 1971. Localizing [^{3}H]GABA in nerve terminals of rat cerebral cortex by electron microscopic autoradiography. *Nature* **229:** 628.

Bormann, J. and D.E. Clapham. 1985. γ-Aminobutyric acid receptor channels in adrenal chromaffin cells: A patch clamp study. *Proc. Natl. Acad. Sci.* **82:** 2168.

Bowery, N.G. 1989. GABA$_A$ receptors and their significance in mammalian pharmacology. *Trends Pharmacol. Sci.* **10:** 401.

Buckle, V.J., N. Fujita, A.S. Ryder-Cook, J.M.J. Derry, R.V. Lebo, P.R. Schofield, P.H. Seeburg, A.N. Bateson, M.G. Darlison, and E.A. Barnard. 1989. Chromosomal localization of GABA$_A$ receptor subunit genes: Relationship to human genetic disease. *Neuron* **3:** 647.

Changeux, J.-P., A. Devillers-Thiery, and P. Chemouilli. 1984. Acetylcholine receptor: An allosteric protein. *Science* **225:** 1335.

Chen, C. and H. Okayama. 1987. High efficiency transformation of mammalian cells by plasmid DNA. *Mol. Cell. Biol.* **7:** 2745.

Cheng, Y.C. and W.H. Prusoff. 1973. Relationship between the inhibition constant (K_i) and the concentration of inhibitor which causes 50 per cent inhibition (IC$_{50}$) of an enzymatic reaction. *Biochem. Pharmacol.* **22:** 3099.

Dingledine, R., I.M. Boland, N.I. Chamberlin, K. Kawasaki, N.W. Kleckner, S.F. Traynelis, and T.A. Verdoorn. 1988. Amino acid receptors and uptake systems in the mammalian central nervous system. *CRC Crit. Rev. Neurobiol.* **4:** 1.

Dutar, P. and R.A. Nicoll. 1988. A physiological role for GABA$_B$ receptors in the central nervous system. *Nature* **322:** 156.

Edwards, F.A., A. Konnerth, and B. Sakmann. 1990. Quantal analysis of inhibitory synaptic transmission in the dentate gyrus of rat hippocampal slices: A patch clamp study. *J. Physiol.* (in press).

Edwards, F.A., A. Konnerth, B. Sakmann, and T. Takahashi. 1989. A thin slice preparation for patch clamp recordings from neurones of the mammalian central nervous system. *Pfluegers Arch. Eur. J. Physiol.* **414:** 600.

Ewert, M., B.D. Shivers, H. Lüddens, H. Möhler, and P.H. Seeburg. 1990. Subunit selectivity and epitope characterization of monoclonal antibodies directed against the GABA$_A$/benzodiazepine receptor. *J. Cell Biol.* **110:** 2043.

Finer-Moore, J. and R.M. Stroud. 1984. Amphipathic analysis and possible formation of ion channel in an acetylcholine receptor. *Proc. Natl. Acad. Sci.* **81:** 155.

Fuchs, K., D. Adamiker, and W. Sieghart. 1990. Identification of α_2- and α_3-subunits of the GABA$_A$-benzodiazepine receptor complex purified from the brains of young rats. *FEBS Lett.* **261:** 52.

Fuchs, K., H. Möhler, and W. Sieghart. 1988. Various proteins from rat brain, specifically and irreversibly labeled by [^{3}H]flunitrazepam, are distinct α-subunits of the GABA$_A$-benzodiazepine receptor complex. *Neurosci. Lett.* **90:** 314.

Giraudat, J., M. Dennis, T. Heidmann, J.-Y. Chang, and J.P. Changeux. 1986. Structure of the high-affinity binding site for non-competitive blockers of the acetylcholine receptor: Serine-262 of the δ subunit is labeled by [^{3}H]chlorpromazine. *Proc. Natl. Acad. Sci.* **83:** 2719.

Gorman, C.M., D.R. Gies, and G. MacCray. 1990. Transient production of proteins using an adenovirus transformed cell line. *DNA Protein Eng. Techniq.* **2:** 3.

Grenningloh, G., I. Pribilla, P. Prior, G. Multhaup, K. Beyreuther, O. Taleb, and H. Betz. 1990a. Cloning and expression of the 58 kd β subunit of the inhibitory glycine receptor. *Neuron* **4:** 963.

Grenningloh, G., A. Rienitz, O. Schmitt, C. Methfessel, M. Zensen, K. Beyreuther, E.D. Gundelfinger, and H. Betz. 1987. The strychnine-binding subunit of the glycine receptor shows homology with nicotinic acetylcholine receptors. *Nature* **328:** 215.

Grenningloh, G., V. Schmieden, P.R. Schofield, P.H. Seeburg, T. Siddique, T.K. Mohandas, C.M. Becker, and H. Betz. 1990b. Alpha subunit variants of the human glycine receptor: Primary structures, functional expression and chromosomal localization of the corresponding genes. *EMBO J.* **9:** 771.

Hamill, O.P., A. Marty, E. Neher, B. Sakmann, and F.J. Sigworth. 1981. Improved patch-clamp techniques for high-resolution current recording from cells and cell-free membrane patches. *Pfluegers Arch. Eur. J. Physiol.* **391:** 85.

Hucho, F., W. Oberthur, and F. Lottspeich. 1986. The ion channel of the nicotinic acetylcholine receptor is formed by the homologous helices MII of the receptor subunits. *FEBS Lett.* **205:** 137.

Imoto, K., C. Busch, B. Sakmann, M. Mishina, T. Konno, J. Nakai, H. Bujo, Y. Mori, K. Fukuda, and S. Numa. 1988. Rings of negatively charged amino acids determine the acetylcholine receptor channel conductance. *Nature* **335:** 645.

Langosch, D., L. Thomas, and H. Betz. 1988. Conserved quaternary structure of ligand-gated ion channels; the postsynaptic glycine receptor is a pentamer. *Proc. Natl. Acad. Sci.* **85:** 7394.

Levitan, E.S., P.R. Schofield, D.R. Burt, L.M. Rhee, W. Wisden, M. Köhler, H. Rodriguez, F.A. Stephenson, M.G. Darlison, E.A. Barnard, and P.H. Seeburg. 1988. Structural and functional basis for GABA$_A$ receptor heterogeneity. *Nature* **335:** 76.

Lolait, S.J., A.M. O'Carroll, K. Kusano, and L.C. Mahan. 1989. Pharmacological characterization and region-specific expression in brain of β_2- and β_3-subunits of the rat GABA$_A$ receptor. *FEBS Lett.* **258:** 17.

Lüddens, H., D.B. Pritchett, M. Köhler, I. Killisch, K. Keinänen, H. Monyer, R. Sprengel, and P.H. Seeburg. 1990. A cerebellar GABA$_A$ receptor selective for a behavioural alcohol antagonist. *Nature* **346:** 648.

Neher, E. and C.F. Stevens. 1977. Conductance fluctuations and ionic pores in membranes. *Annu. Rev. Biophys. Bioeng.* **6:** 345.

Niddam, R., A. Dubois, B. Scatton, S. Arbilla, and S.Z. Langer. 1987. Autoradiographic localization of [^{3}H]zolpidem binding sites in the rat CNS: Comparison with the distribution of [^{3}H]flunitrazepam binding sites. *J. Neurochem.* **49:** 890.

Nielsen, M. and C. Braestrup. 1980. Ethyl β-carboline-3-carboxylate shows differential benzodiazepine receptor interaction. *Nature* **286:** 606.

Noda, M., H. Takahashi, T. Tanabe, M. Toyosato, S. Kikyotani, Y. Furutani, T. Hirose, H. Takashima, S. Inayama, T. Miyata, and S. Numa. 1983. Structural homology of *Torpedo californica* acetylcholine receptor subunits. *Nature* **302:** 528.

Olsen, R.W. and A.J. Tobin. 1990. Molecular biology of GABA$_A$ receptors. *FASEB J.* **4:** 1469.

Olsen, R. and C.J. Venter. 1986. Benzodiazepine/GABA$_A$ receptors and chloride channels: Structural and functional properties. A.R. Liss, New York.

Paxinos, I.G. and C. Watson. 1986. *The rat brain in stereotaxic coordinates*, 2nd edition. Academic Press, Sydney.

Pritchett, D.B. and P.H. Seeburg. 1990. GABA$_A$ receptor α_5 subunit creates novel type II benzodiazepine receptor pharmacology. *J. Neurochem.* **54:** 1802.

Pritchett, D.B., H. Lüddens, and P.H. Seeburg. 1989a. Type I and type II GABA$_A$/benzodiazepine receptors produced in transfected cells. *Science* **245:** 1389.

Pritchett, D.B., H. Sontheimer, C.M. Gorman, H. Kettenmann, P.H. Seeburg, and P.R. Schofield. 1988. Ligand-gating and allosteric potentiation of human GABA$_A$ receptor subunits in a transient mammalian cell expression system. *Science* **242:** 1306.

Pritchett, D.B., H. Sontheimer, B.D. Shivers, S. Ymer, H. Kettenmann, P.R. Schofield, and P.H. Seeburg. 1989b. A novel GABA$_A$ receptor subunit is important for benzodiazepine pharmacology. *Nature* **338:** 582.

Puia, G., M.R. Santi, D.B. Pritchett, P.H. Seeburg, and E. Costa. 1989. Negative allosteric modulation of native and reconstituted GABA$_A$ receptors. *Proc. Natl. Acad. Sci.* **86:** 7275.

Puia, G., M.R. Santi, S. Vicini, D.B. Pritchett, R.H. Purdy, S.M. Paul, P.H. Seeburg, and E. Costa. 1990. Neurosteroids act on recombinant human GABA$_A$ receptors. *Neuron* **4:** 759.

Sakmann, B., C. Methfessel, M. Mishina, T. Takahashi, T. Takai, M. Kurasaki, K. Fukuda, and S. Numa. 1985. Role of acetylcholine receptor subunits in gating of the channel. *Nature* **318:** 538.

Schofield, P.R., B.D. Shivers, and P.H. Seeburg. 1990. The role of receptor subtype diversity in the CNS. *Trends Neurosci.* **13:** 8.

Schofield, P.R., M.G. Darlison, N. Fujita, H. Rodriguez, D.R. Burt, F.A. Stephenson, I.M. Rhee, J. Ramachandran, T.A. Glencorse, V. Reale, P.H. Seeburg, and E.A. Barnard. 1987. The brain GABA$_A$ receptor: Cloning and functional expression of the cDNAs encoding its subunits. *Nature* **328:** 221.

Séquier, J.M., J.G. Richards, P. Malherbe, G.W. Price, S. Mathews, and H. Möhler. 1988. Mapping of brain areas containing RNA homologous to cDNAs encoding the α and β subunits of the rat GABA$_A$ γ-aminobutyric receptor. *Proc. Natl. Acad. Sci.* **85:** 7815.

Shivers, B.D., I. Killisch, R. Sprengel, H. Sontheimer, M. Köhler, P.R. Schofield, and P.H. Seeburg. 1989. Two novel GABA$_A$ receptor subunits exist in distinct neuronal subpopulations. *Neuron* **3:** 327.

Smith, S.M., R. Zoree, and R.N. McBurney. 1989. Conductance states activated by glycine and GABA in rat cultured spinal neurones. *J. Membr. Biol.* **180:** 45.

Sontheimer, H., C.M. Becker, D.B. Pritchett, P.R. Schofield, G. Grenningloh, H. Kettenmann, H. Betz, and P.H. Seeburg. 1989. Functional chloride channels by mammalian cell expression of rat glycine receptor subunit. *Neuron* **2:** 1491.

Stephenson, F.A. 1988. Understanding the GABA$_A$ receptor: A chemically gated ion channel. *Biochem. J.* **249:** 21.

Squires, R.F., D.I. Benson, C. Braestrup. J. Coupet, C.A. Klepner, V. Myers, and B. Beer. 1979. Some properties of brain specific benzodiazepine receptors: New evidence for multiple receptors. *Pharmacol Biochem. Behav.* **10:** 825.

Unwin, N. 1989. The structure of ion channels in membranes of excitable cells. *Neuron* **3:** 665.

Verdoorn, T.A., A. Draguhn, S. Ymer, P.H. Seeburg, and B. Sakmann. 1990. Functional properties of recombinant GABA$_A$ receptors depend on subunit composition. *Neuron* **4:** 919.

Wisden, W., L.A. McNaughton, M.G. Darlison, S.P. Hunt, and E.A. Barnard. 1989a. Differential distribution of GABA$_A$ receptor mRNAs in bovine cerebellum—Localization of α_2 mRNA in Bergmann glia layer. *Neurosci. Lett.* **106:** 7.

Wisden, W., B.J. Morris, M.G. Darlison, S.P. Hunt, and E.A. Barnard. 1988. Distinct GABA$_A$ receptor α subunit mRNAs show differential patterns of expression in bovine brain. *Neuron* **1:** 937.

———. 1989b. Localization of GABA$_A$ receptor α-subunit mRNAs in relation to receptor subtypes. *Mol. Brain Res.* **5:** 305.

Ymer, S., A. Draguhn, M. Köhler, P.R. Schofield, and P.H. Seeburg. 1989a. Sequence and expression of novel GABA$_A$ receptor α subunit. *FEBS Lett.* **258:** 119.

Ymer, S., P.R. Schofield, A. Draguhn, P. Werner, M. Köhler, and P.H. Seeburg. 1989b. GABA$_A$ receptor β subunit heterogeneity: Functional expression of cloned cDNAs. *EMBO J.* **8:** 1665.

Ymer, S., A. Draguhn, W. Wisden, P. Werner, K. Keinänen, P.R. Schofield, D.B. Pritchett, and P.H. Seeburg. 1990. Structural and functional characterization of the γ_1 subunit of GABA$_A$/benzodiazepine receptors. *EMBO J.* **9:** 3261.

Young, W.S., III, E. Mezey, and R.W. Siegel. 1986. Quantitative in situ hybridization histochemistry reveals increased levels of corticotrophin-releasing factor mRNA after adrenalectomy in rats. *Neurosci. Lett.* **70:** 198.

Young, W.S., III, D. Niehoff, M.J. Kuhar, B. Beer, and A.S. Lippa. 1981. Multiple benzodiazepine receptor localization by light microscopic radiochemistry. *J. Pharmacol. Exp. Ther.* **216:** 425.

Glutamate Receptor GluR-K1: Structure, Function, and Expression in the Brain

M. Hollmann,* S.W. Rogers,* A. O'Shea-Greenfield,* E.S. Deneris,*‡
T.E. Hughes,§ G.P. Gasic,*† and S. Heinemann*

*Molecular Neurobiology Laboratory, The Salk Institute for Biological Studies, †The Howard Hughes Medical
Institute, La Jolla, California 92037; §Department of Neuroscience, University of California,
San Diego, California 92093

The excitatory action of L-glutamate (GLU) on neurons, discovered more than 35 years ago (Hayashi 1954), has become the focus of considerable research interest. Although initially controversial, it is now generally accepted that excitatory amino acids (EAA) serve as neurotransmitters at the majority of all excitatory synapses in the brain (Monaghan et al. 1989). At least five pharmacologically different glutamate receptor subtypes have been recognized on the basis of their differential sensitivities to a variety of antagonists. These subtypes have been named NMDA (N-methyl-D-aspartate), KA (kainate), AMPA (α-amino-3-hydroxy-5-methyl-isooxazol-4-propionate), AP4 (L-2-amino-4-phosphono butyrate), and ACPD (1-aminocyclopentyl-1,3-dicarboxylate), with the names derived from the most active agonists that have been discovered for each subtype (Monaghan et al. 1989). The first four of these receptor subtypes are referred to as ionotropic or type I receptors (Strange 1988) because they contain integral, ligand-gated ion channels. The AMPA subtype formerly was called the QA (quisqualate) receptor. The fifth subtype, the ACPD receptor, is a metabotropic or type II receptor, which is linked to a second-messenger system that utilizes inositol triphosphate as its effector (Sugiyama et al. 1987).

The current interest in glutamate receptors has been sparked by two important discoveries. First, the finding that glutamate receptors are involved in phenomena underlying synaptic plasticity suggested a role for glutamate receptors in higher brain functions. The importance of NMDA receptors in developmental plasticity has been shown in the visual cortex (Bear and Singer 1986; Constantine-Paton et al. 1990) and in the olfactory system (Woo et al. 1987). Even more attention, however, was attracted by the crucial role NMDA receptors play in the phenomenon of long-term potentiation (LTP) (Collingridge et al. 1983). LTP, a long-lasting increase in postsynaptic responses after a brief presynaptic high-frequency stimulation, might be an electrophysiological correlate of memory formation (Eccles 1983).

The second discovery was that glutamate receptors might be involved in a number of neurological disorders such as Huntington's disease, Alzheimer's disease, and epilepsy. These receptors may also be involved in causing massive neuronal death during periods of hypoglycemia or ischemia (for an overview, see Olney 1989). In all these cases, the NMDA receptor is the prime suspect thought to mediate the detrimental effects of glutamate.

To better understand the role of glutamate receptors in the aforementioned phenomena, the receptors themselves have to be characterized at the molecular level. Ideally, this requires isolation of the receptor protein and/or cloning of the genes coding for the different subtypes. Despite numerous attempts during the past 15 years, however, no protein has yet been purified to homogeneity that has the properties of glutamate receptors, i.e., that functions as a ligand-gated ion channel or second-messenger-linked receptor in reconstituted systems. The proteins that have been isolated to date bind KA (Gregor et al. 1988; Hampson and Wenthold 1988; Klein et al. 1988) or GLU (Brose et al. 1989; Chen et al. 1989), but their functional properties remain unclear.

Since all attempts to isolate glutamate receptors by protein biochemical methods have failed, we chose a molecular cloning approach. We selected a cloning strategy that did not require any structural knowledge of the receptor to be isolated: expression in Xenopus oocytes. Several workers had succeeded in expressing glutamate receptors in oocytes injected with total brain poly(A)$^+$ RNA and fractions thereof (Gundersen et al. 1984; Sumikawa et al. 1984; Sugiyama et al. 1987; Verdoorn et al. 1987; Fong et al. 1988; Kushner et al. 1988). However, the absolute prerequisite for this cloning strategy, which is functional expression of a glutamate receptor from transcripts made in vitro from a cDNA library template DNA, had not been achieved.

We succeeded in constructing a cDNA library that contained functional glutamate receptor clones as assayed in Xenopus oocytes and in isolating a single cDNA that, upon transcription in vitro and injection into Xenopus oocytes, expressed a functional glutamate receptor (Hollmann et al. 1989). This receptor displays electrophysiological and pharmacological properties

---

‡Present address: Department of Neuroscience, Case Western Reserve, Cleveland, Ohio 44106.

compatible with those reported for the KA receptor subtype; hence, we named the receptor GluR-K1, where K1 indicates a receptor subunit of the KA type. The cDNA sequence and the deduced amino acid sequence were analyzed for sequence or structural homologies with other known ligand-gated ion channel proteins, as well as with the concurrently reported sequences of KA-binding proteins (Gregor et al. 1989; Wada et al. 1989). The electrophysiological and pharmacological properties of GluR-K1 expressed in *Xenopus* oocytes were compared with published data for KA receptors obtained in more complex systems, and the regional distribution of GluR-K1 mRNA in the brain was mapped by in situ hybridization. Patterns of GluR-K1 RNA distribution were compared with GluR-K1 protein distribution as revealed immunohistochemically by antisera raised against GluR-K1/bacterial *trp*E fusion proteins.

METHODS

RNA was isolated by the guanidine isothiocyanate method (Chirgwin et al. 1979), and poly(A)$^+$ was selected (Aviv and Leder 1972). Library construction followed the protocol of Stratagene (La Jolla, California), supplied with the company's Uni-ZAP™XR cloning kit. Transcripts were made in vitro using Stratagene's RNA transcription kit.

Sequencing was performed using the dideoxynucleotide chain-termination method (Sanger et al. 1977) on deleted, overlapping subclones generated from both strands in the bacteriophage vector M13mp19, using the Cyclone™ kit of United States Biochemical. Northern blots were carried out as described previously (Hollmann et al. 1989), and in situ hybridization followed the protocol of Deneris et al. (1988).

Xenopus oocytes were prepared, injected with RNA, and maintained in Barth's saline as described previously (Hollmann et al. 1989). Voltage recording and voltage clamp recording were performed as described previously (Hollmann et al. 1989).

Antibodies to a portion of the putative extracellular domain of GluR-K1 (residues 185–449) were made using fusion proteins generated by the *trp*E bacterial overexpression system (Dieckmann and Tzagoloff 1975). Immunohistochemical localization of GluR-K1 was performed as described previously (Hughes et al. 1989).

RESULTS

Isolation of the Functional KA-gated Ion Channel cDNA GluR-K1

As the starting material for our expression cloning approach, we used poly(A)$^+$ RNA isolated from rat forebrain. *Xenopus* oocytes were injected with 75 ng of this RNA and were analyzed 2 days after injection by voltage recording for responses to bath-applied subtype-specific glutamate receptor agonists. Figure 1,

which summarizes our expression cloning strategy, shows the responses obtained from a single oocyte. We were able to detect four of the five subtypes of glutamate receptors: the NMDA, KA, AMPA, and the ACPD receptor. The fifth type, the AP4 receptor, was never seen in any injected oocyte. In addition, when we used poly(A)$^+$ RNA isolated from certain brain regions such as cerebellum, hippocampus, and brain stem, we never found a response to AP4. The responses to NMDA and KA showed the smooth characteristics that are indicative of the activation of ligand-gated ion channels. QA and GLU, however, yielded compound responses consisting of a smooth component of fast onset (the ligand-gated ion channel activation) and an oscillatory component of slow onset, which can be attributed to activation of the second-messenger-linked metabotropic ACPD receptor (Hirono et al. 1988). Not every oocyte examined showed the ACPD receptor response, whereas all other responses were seen in every oocyte checked.

We used the poly(A)$^+$ mRNA to construct a directional cDNA library, using the commercially available Uni-ZAP™ XR kit (Stratagene, La Jolla, California). The phage vector λZAPII (see Fig. 1) accommodates cDNA inserts between a T3 and a T7 RNA polymerase promoter in a directional fashion. This results in the 5' ends of all cDNA inserts being located downstream from the T3 promoter, which thus can be used to obtain "sense" transcripts in vitro, whereas the T7 promoter is useful to obtain "antisense" control transcripts. The library constructed had an average insert size of ~2 kbp and contained ~850,000 independent clones that were amplified in 18 separate batches of 47,000 clones each (18 "sublibraries"). These 18 sublibraries were used to generate template DNA, which in turn was employed to synthesize RNA transcripts in vitro.

To determine whether any functional glutamate receptor messages were represented in the library, aliquots from the 18 batches of RNA transcripts were pooled, and the mixture was injected into *Xenopus* oocytes. No responses were seen 3, 5, 7, and 9 days after injection, but on day 10, the only surviving oocyte from a batch of 20 gave a small 1–2-mV response to 100 μM KA, and to the KA receptor agonist domoic acid (DOM) tested at 10 μM (Fig. 1). Those small responses were reproducible, showed fast onset, and were immediately reversible when agonist superfusion was switched to standard frog Ringer superfusion. The observation that a second agonist, DOM at a tenfold lower concentration, gave the same responses, whereas other neurotransmitter receptor agonists like γ-amino butyric acid (GABA) and glycine (both tested at 100 μM) elicited no responses, indicated that the small responses seen were not artifactual. No other glutamate receptor agonist produced a response. This, however, does not prove that functional clones are absent from the library. It could merely reflect the detection limit of the method. As seen in Figure 1, the response to KA in the original poly(A)$^+$ RNA had been considerably larger than the responses to any other agonist

Isolation of rat forebrain poly(A)⁺ RNA

$\downarrow$

Injection of RNA into *Xenopus* oocytes, and voltage recording of oocyte responses to glutamate receptor agonists

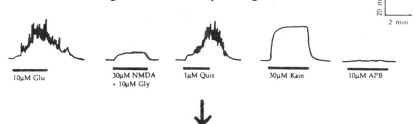

$\downarrow$

Construction of a directional cDNA expression library from the rat forebrain poly(A)⁺ RNA, using the phage vector λZAP
18 individually amplified sublibraries of ~47,000 clones each were established, comprising a total of ~850,000 independent clones

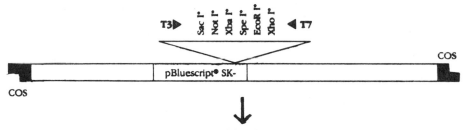

$\downarrow$

In vitro synthesis of RNA from each individual sublibrary, and test in oocytes of the pool of these transcripts, with agonists for all subtypes of glutamate receptors

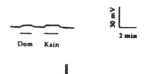

$\downarrow$

Test in oocytes of all individual sublibrary transcripts

$\downarrow$

Subdivision of the pool of ~47,000 clones from sublibrary testing positive for kainate receptor into 100 pools of ~470 independent clones

$\downarrow$

Plating of phages in positive pool at low density to allow picking of individual phage clones

$\downarrow$

Identification of a single clone coding for a kainate receptor

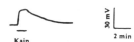

Figure 1. Strategy followed for the isolation of the glutamate receptor cDNA clone GluR-K1. All traces shown represent voltage recordings. (*Top traces*) 75 ng of poly(A)⁺ RNA, 2 days after injection; (*middle traces*) 25 ng of pooled library transcripts, 10 days after injection; (*lower traces*) 25 ng of GluR-K1 phage transcript, 3 days after injection. (Traces from Hollmann et al. 1989.)

tested; if the same ratio of response sizes was represented in the library, the KA response would be the only one detectable.

After obtaining the initial KA response, we tested oocytes injected with transcripts made from the different sublibraries for KA-evoked depolarizations. Three sublibraries gave KA responses that were slightly larger than the ones initially seen with the total library transcripts. The sublibrary with the largest signal was selected for further subdivision. Successively smaller pools of clones (4000, 400, 40) were analyzed, and in each case, the pool with the strongest signal was pursued. Finally, after having recorded from a total of ~1000 oocytes, we were able to isolate a single clone that upon transcription in vitro and injection into oocytes, elicited a KA response (see Fig. 1, bottom). This finding meant that a single cDNA encoding a single protein was sufficient to form a functional receptor. However, the response elicited by the purified clone was clearly smaller than the one initially seen with the poly(A)$^+$ RNA. This indicated that the receptor in vivo probably contains additional subunits that are not absolutely required for channel function but which increase the efficiency of the channel.

Molecular Structure of GluR-K1

Nucleotide and deduced amino acid sequence. The 3-kb cDNA insert of the phage clone encoding GluR-K1 was subcloned into the vector M13 and sequenced (Fig. 2). The cDNA of 2992 bp contained an open reading frame of 2712 bp, coding for 907 amino acids. No long poly(A) tail was found at the 3' end of the clone, and a polyadenylation signal was absent from the sequence. The deduced amino acid sequence revealed the presence of a signal peptide (predicted to be 18 amino acids long), thus putting the mature receptor protein at a total length of 889 amino acids, equivalent to a native molecular mass of 99,769 daltons.

The presence of a signal peptide suggests that the amino terminus is located extracellularly. There are six potential N-glycosylation sites in the extracellular portion of the receptor between the amino terminus and the first predicted transmembrane domain (Hollmann et al. 1989). No cAMP-dependent phosphorylation sites are predicted in GluR-K1. Since modulation of KA receptors by cAMP-dependent phosphorylation has been reported (Liman et al. 1989), this finding adds another piece of evidence to the notion that GluR-K1 probably is just one subunit of a multisubunit complex.

Transmembrane domain structure. To make a prediction for the transmembrane structure for GluR-K1, we analyzed hydropathy plots of the amino acid sequence. Two different algorithms (Kyte and Doolittle

1982; Rao and Argos 1986) predicted that there is a cluster of possible transmembrane domains (TMDs) in the region between amino acids 460 and 620 and another single TMD near the carboxyl terminus of the protein (Figs. 3A and 8A). This general pattern of putative TMD arrangement is typical for ligand-gated ion channel subunits and has been found in all nicotinic acetylcholine receptor (nAChR) subunits (Deneris et al. 1989; Boulter et al. 1990), GABA$_A$ receptor (GABA$_A$R) subunits (Schofield et al. 1987; Shivers et al. 1989), and glycine receptor (GlyR) subunits (Grenningloh et al. 1987, 1990). In the TMD "cluster" area, there are four regions that meet the minimal requirements for TMDs. In Figure 3A, these regions have been marked and numbered I, II, IIa, and III. Regions II and III are solidly hydrophobic, and it can be safely assumed that these two regions represent TMDs. Regions I and IIa, however, are both weakly hydrophobic, and it is not clear whether either of them should be assigned putative TMD status. Strictly on the basis of hydropathy, one would probably tend to disregard both regions; but in light of what is known about the structure of other ligand-gated ion channels, it is tempting to anticipate a cluster of three TMDs.

Figure 3B illustrates the two models of TMD arrangement possible assuming that three TMDs are present in the cluster region. In model I, hydrophobic regions I, II, and III are considered to be actual TMDs, whereas in model II, hydrophobic regions II, IIa, and III form the cluster. From these two models, certain predictions can be made: The amino acid loop between hydrophobic regions I and II is either intracellular (model I) or extracellular (model II), and conversely, the amino acid loop between hydrophobic regions II and IIa is either extracellular (model I) or intracellular (model II). Thus, peptide antibodies directed against these amino acid loop regions should enable us to differentiate between the two models. These experiments are currently in progress.

Sequence homologies with nicotinic acetylcholine receptors. When the amino acid sequence of GluR-K1 is compared to the sequences of nAChRs (Deneris et al. 1989), GABA$_A$Rs (Schofield et al. 1987), and the GlyR (Grenningloh et al. 1987), little overall homology is found. This might explain why low-stringency screening for glutamate receptors using nAChR or GABA$_A$R probes proved unsuccessful. To identify possible localized sequence homologies, we concentrated on two key regions in ligand-gated ion channels: (1) the proposed "signature" for neurotransmitter receptor-channel complexes (Barnard et al. 1987), the so-called "cysteine loop" or "disulfide loop," which is located close to the amino terminus of the protein in the extracellular domain of all ligand-gated ion channels, and (2) the

Figure 2. Nucleotide and deduced amino-acid sequence of clone GluR-K1. Numbering starts at first nucleotide of the codon for the predicted amino-terminal amino acid of the mature protein. Nucleotides upstream of 5'-terminal base carry negative numbers. Nucleotides −1 to −54 code for putative signal peptide. (*) Predicted glycosylation sites, (▼) cysteine loop region. Predicted transmembrane domains are boxed. (Reprinted, with permission, from Hollmann et al. 1989.)

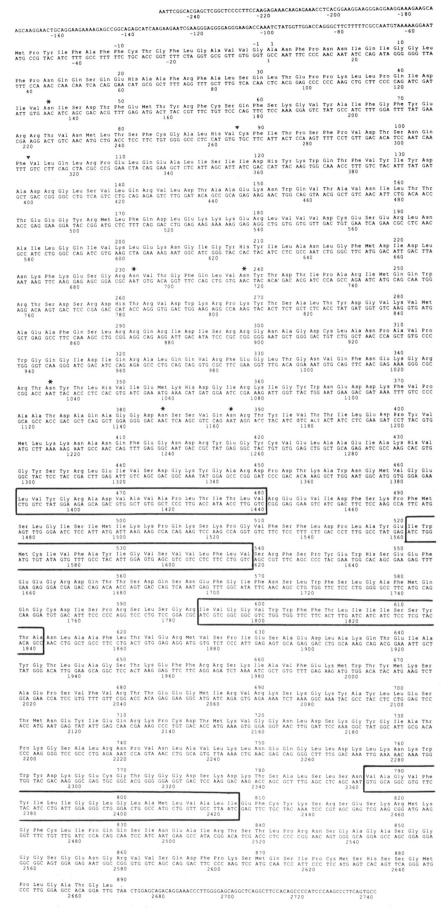

Figure 2. (*See facing page for legend.*)

45

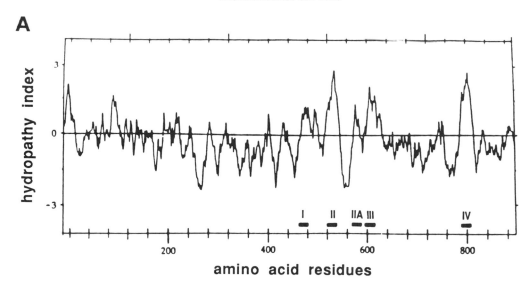

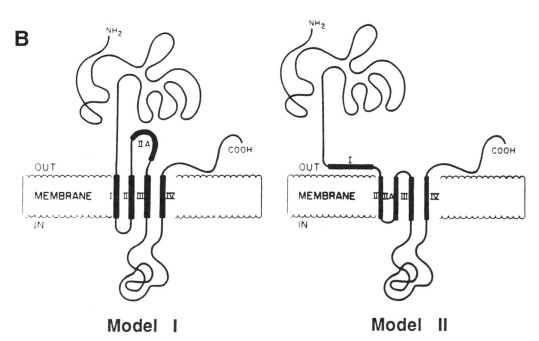

Figure 3. (*A*) Hydropathy plot of GluR-K1 (residues −18 to 889), using the algorithm of Kyte and Doolittle (1982) at a window setting of 15. Bars mark hydrophobic regions discussed in the text. (Modified from Hollmann et al. 1989.) (*B*) Two models of possible TMD arrangement in GluR-K1.

second putative TMD that is believed to line the ion channel.

A sequence with some homology with the cysteine loop was found, indeed, in the predicted amino-terminal extracellular domain of GluR-K1 (Fig. 4A). A "core structure" of the amino acid sequence F-P-X-D-X-X-N was found to be conserved. The cysteine loop in GluR-K1, however, lacks one of the key features of this structure, namely its second cysteine residue, which is supposed to be present 14 amino acids carboxy-terminal from the first cysteine residue (Barnard et al. 1987). Since the function of the cysteine loop in ligand-gated ion channels is unknown, one can only speculate as to whether it should be conserved in glutamate receptors.

TMD II is thought to be the ion-channel-lining domain in the nAChR (Hucho and Hilgenfeld 1989), and the same has been suggested for the GABA$_A$R (Barnard et al. 1987) and the GlyR (Betz and Becker 1988). Since glutamate receptors flux cations much like nAChRs, the amino acid sequences lining their channels might be expected to share similarities, but to be quite different from the respective sequences of the anion-fluxing GABA$_A$Rs and GlyRs. Indeed, when comparing the putative TMD II sequences (Fig. 4B,C), GluR-K1 appears to be more closely related to nAChRs than to either GABA$_A$R or GlyR. In Figure 4B, the hydrophobic region II of GluR-K1 (TMD II of our model I) has been selected for comparison, where-

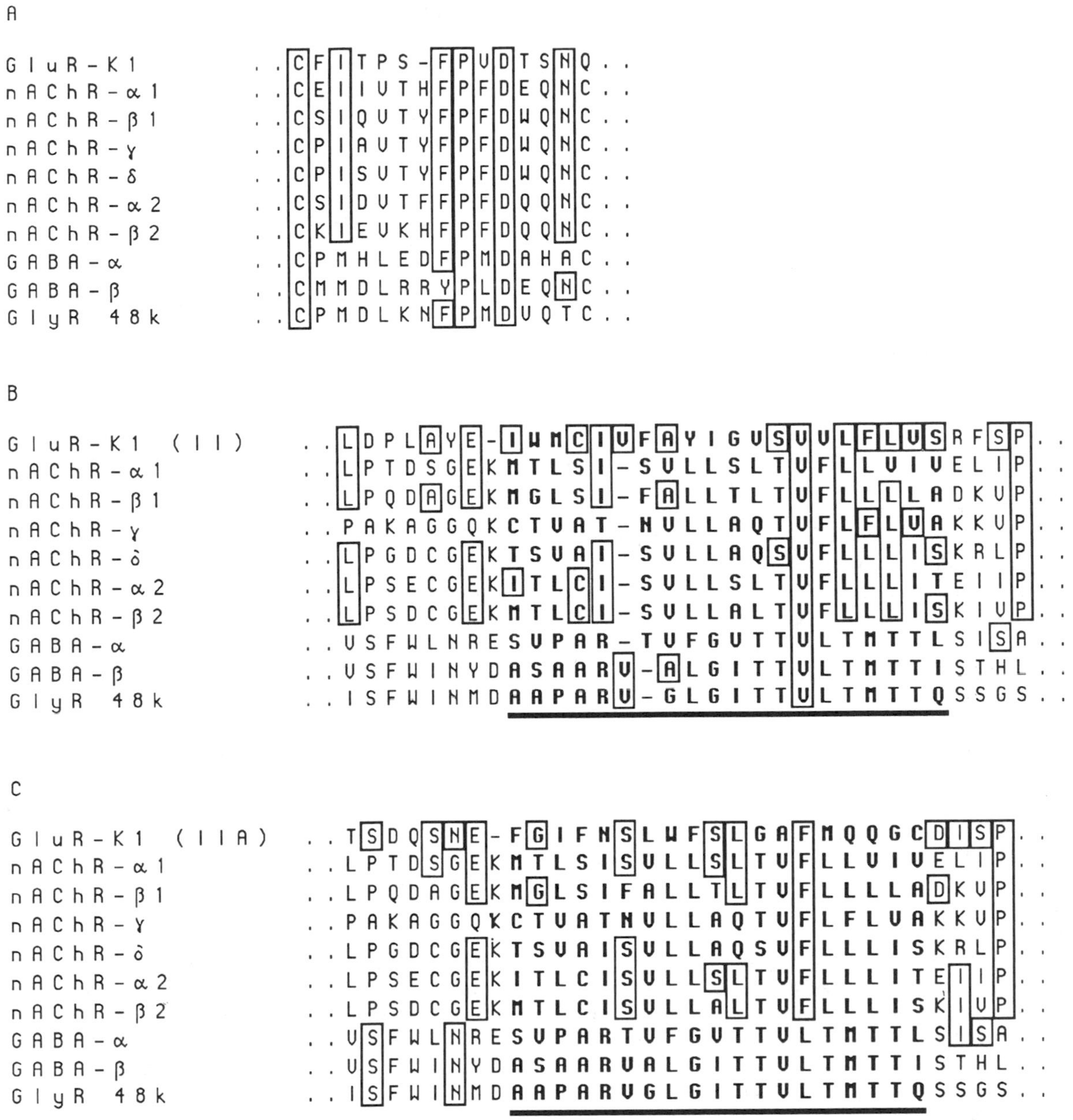

A

```
GluR-K1      . . C F I T P S - F P V D T S N Q . .
nAChR-α1     . . C E I I V T H F P F D E Q N C . .
nAChR-β1     . . C S I Q V T Y F P F D W Q N C . .
nAChR-γ      . . C P I A V T Y F P F D W Q N C . .
nAChR-δ      . . C P I S V T Y F P F D W Q N C . .
nAChR-α2     . . C S I D V T F F P F D Q Q N C . .
nAChR-β2     . . C K I E V K H F P F D Q Q N C . .
GABA-α       . . C P M H L E D F P M D A H A C . .
GABA-β       . . C M M D L R R Y P L D E Q N C . .
GlyR 48k     . . C P M D L K N F P M D V Q T C . .
```

B

```
GluR-K1 (II)  . . L D P L A Y E - I W M C I V F A Y I G V S V V L F L V S R F S P . .
nAChR-α1      . . L P T D S G E K M T L S I - S V L L S L T V F L L V I V E L I P . .
nAChR-β1      . . L P Q D A G E K M G L S I - F A L L T L T V F L L L L A D K V P . .
nAChR-γ       . . P A K A G G Q K C T V A T - N V L L A Q T V F L F L V A K K V P . .
nAChR-δ       . . L P G D C G E K T S V A I - S V L L A Q S V F L L L I S K R L P . .
nAChR-α2      . . L P S E C G E K I T L C I - S V L L S L T V F L L L I T E I I P . .
nAChR-β2      . . L P S D C G E K M T L C I - S V L L A L T V F L L L I S K I V P . .
GABA-α        . . V S F W L N R E S V P A R - T V F G V T T V L T M T T L S I S A . .
GABA-β        . . V S F W I N Y D A S A A R V - A L G I T T V L T M T T I S T H L . .
GlyR 48k      . . I S F W I N M D A A P A R V - G L G I T T V L T M T T Q S S G S . .
```

C

```
GluR-K1 (IIA)  . . T S D Q S N E - F G I F N S L W F S L G A F M Q Q G C D I S P . .
nAChR-α1       . . L P T D S G E K M T L S I S V L L S L T V F L L V I V E L I P . .
nAChR-β1       . . L P Q D A G E K M G L S I F A L L T L T V F L L L L A D K V P . .
nAChR-γ        . . P A K A G G Q K C T V A T N V L L A Q T V F L F L V A K K V P . .
nAChR-δ        . . L P G D C G E K T S V A I S V L L A Q S V F L L L I S K R L P . .
nAChR-α2       . . L P S E C G E K I T L C I S V L L S L T V F L L L I T E I I P . .
nAChR-β2       . . L P S D C G E K M T L C I S V L L A L T V F L L L I S K I V P . .
GABA-α         . . V S F W L N R E S V P A R T V F G V T T V L T M T T L S I S A . .
GABA-β         . . V S F W I N Y D A S A A R V A L G I T T V L T M T T I S T H L . .
GlyR 48k       . . I S F W I N M D A A P A R V G L G I T T V L T M T T Q S S G S . .
```

Figure 4. Sequence comparison between GluR-K1 and mouse muscle nAChR subunits α1, β1, γ, δ (Heinemann et al. 1986), rat brain nAChR subunits α2 and β2 (Deneris et al. 1989), bovine brain GABA$_A$R subunits α and β (Barnard et al. 1987), and rat brain GlyR 48-kD subunit (Grenningloh et al. 1987). Boxed residues are found at identical positions in GluR-K1 as well as in at least one other sequence. One gap has been introduced arbitrarily. (A) Cysteine loop regions; (B) predicted hydrophobic region II of GluR-K1, and TMD II regions of other sequences (underlined, plus flanking sequences); (C) predicted hydrophobic region IIa of GluR-K1, and predicted TMD II regions of other sequences (underlined, plus flanking sequences). (Modified from Hollmann et al. 1989.)

as in Figure 4C, a similar comparison is made using hydrophobic region IIa (TMD II of model II). The hydrophobic region IIa shows significantly less homology, leading us to favor model I over model II. Supporting evidence for model I is also furnished by the fact that only this model features a proline residue at position 12 in TMD I, a conserved feature in all ligand-gated ion channel subunits (Barnard et al. 1987).

Functional Analysis of GluR-K1

General observations. When transcripts made in vitro from clone GluR-K1 are injected into *Xenopus* oocytes, KA-evoked depolarizations can be recorded 2–3 days after injection. The size of the response is dependent on the amount of RNA injected. As little as 10 pg of RNA yields measurable depolarizations, and responses increase up to at least 10 ng. When a particular oocyte is monitored over a period of several days, it shows a steady increase in the size of the response. This indicates that (1) the RNA injected is not degraded rapidly and (2) the receptor proteins synthesized are stable in the oocyte. It was probably the combination of these two features that allowed us to detect the initial KA response from our library in an exceptionally long-surviving oocyte (see above).

Antisense transcripts of GluR-K1 were injected as a control for the specificity of the responses. Such transcripts did not elicit responses to glutamate receptor agonists or to other neurotransmitter receptor agonists such as GABA, glycine, or nicotine. However, during these control experiments, we observed a very small response (1–4 mV under voltage recording) to glycine that was strychnine-insensitive. This response could also be seen in uninjected or water-injected oocytes and thus represented a response endogenous to the oocyte. However, we did not see this response in every oocyte. This property of *Xenopus* oocytes did not cause any problems in our experiments, but it could possibly interfere when measurements of NMDA receptors expressed from poly(A)$^+$ RNA are attempted.

Pharmacology of GluR-K1. Our designation of GluR-K1 as a KA receptor subunit was prompted by the fact that KA and DOM, a known KA receptor agonist, were the most potent agonists. This was illustrated by the fact that during the initial expression cloning steps, when pools of clones were measured, no other agonists, including GLU and QA, elicited responses. GLU, in fact, is known to be only a poor agonist at KA receptors (Monaghan et al. 1989). The response to KA did not desensitize significantly, even during constant KA superfusion for 10 minutes. This is a property exclusive to KA receptors among the members of the glutamate receptor family (Verdoorn and Dingledine 1988). KA and DOM dose-response curves (Fig. 5A) yielded EC$_{50}$ values close to those reported in the literature for KA receptors expressed from poly(A)$^+$ RNA (Hirono et al. 1988). Notably, DOM (EC$_{50}$ = 1.8 μM) had a 20-fold higher affinity for the receptor than KA (EC$_{50}$ = 39 μM). Inhibition curves recorded for several glutamate receptor antagonists also support the classification of GluR-K1 as a KA receptor subunit (Fig. 5B). CNQX (6-cyano-7-nitro-quinoxaline-2,3-dione), an inhibitor of non-NMDA receptors (Monaghan et al. 1989), was the most efficacious of these compounds, inhibiting GluR-K1 responses to 100 μM KA with an IC$_{50}$ of ~ 1.5 μM. Kynurenic acid (KYN), a nonselective glutamate receptor antagonist, inhibited responses to KA with an IC$_{50}$ of ~ 300 μM; and GDEE (glutamate diethylester), a weak QA receptor antagonist (Monaghan et al. 1989), showed no inhibition (IC$_{50}$ $\geq$ 5 mM). However, a possible inhibitory effect might have been obscured by the weak agonist properties this antagonist has on GluR-K1 (Hollmann et al. 1989). The competitive NMDA receptor antagonist APV (D-(-)2-amino-5-phos-

phonovaleric acid) showed no significant inhibition (IC$_{50}$ $\geq$ 3 mM). Several other antagonists reported to act on glutamate receptors (Foster and Fagg 1984; Fagg 1985; Monaghan et al. 1989) were tested at 1 mM for their ability to inhibit responses to 30 μM KA (Fig. 5C). γ-D-Glutamylglycine (DGG), which inhibits KA as well as NMDA receptors, showed some inhibitory potency, as did γ-D-glutamylaminomethylsulfonic acid (GAMS), a known KA and QA receptor antagonist. 2,3-*cis*-Piperidine dicarboxylic acid (PDA), which is believed to block all subtypes of glutamate receptors, had a potency comparable to DGG and GAMS. Two NMDA channel blockers, 3-(2-carboxypiperazin-4-yl)-propyl-1-phosphate (CPP) and dibenzocyclohepteneimine (MK-801) had only weak antagonist properties. The same was true for D,L-threo-β-hydroxyaspartic acid (OH-ASP), a glutamate transport inhibitor.

When oocytes injected with large amounts (10 ng) of RNA were analyzed, QA as well as AMPA (α-amino-3-hydroxy-5-methyl-isoxazole-4-propionic acid) and GLU elicited small responses. These responses usually were seen more clearly in oocytes that had survived for 4 or 5 days after injection, probably due to the above-mentioned constant increase in responses with time. Figure 5D shows dose-response curves for KA and QA. Both curves have been recorded from a single oocyte and are presented without normalization to maximal responses. It is evident that QA has a much higher affinity than KA for GluR-K1 but has a very low efficacy for opening the ion channel. In contrast, KA, having a lower affinity, is much more efficient in fluxing ions. QA competes with KA for the same binding site on the GluR-K1 protein, as is revealed by blocking experiments (Fig. 5E). Very small concentrations of QA are sufficient to block the KA response completely: We found an IC$_{50}$ of ~ 1 μM for the competition. Thus, the blocking action of QA occurs with an IC$_{50}$ comparable to the EC$_{50}$ of its agonist action for opening the channel. AMPA and GLU were less effective, but they also inhibited KA responses (data not shown).

Current/voltage relationship of responses. Oocytes injected with brain poly(A)$^+$ RNA display linear I/V curves for their responses to KA and QA (Verdoorn and Dingledine 1988). Similarly, KA-gated currents measured in retinal horizontal cells (Liman et al. 1989) have linear, nonrectifying I/V relationships. The KA responses of GluR-K1-injected oocytes, however, display a strongly rectifying I/V curve (Fig. 5F, filled squares), indicating that GluR-K1 receptors behave differently from the KA receptor(s) in vivo. Oocytes injected with rat hippocampal poly(A)$^+$ RNA for comparison yielded a linear I/V curve as expected (Fig. 5F, open squares). This finding provides further evidence that GluR-K1 most probably is a KA-receptor subunit that functions as a part of a heterooligomeric receptor-channel complex in vivo. In support of this idea, we were able to isolate several additional cDNA clones that share extensive sequence identities with GluR-K1.

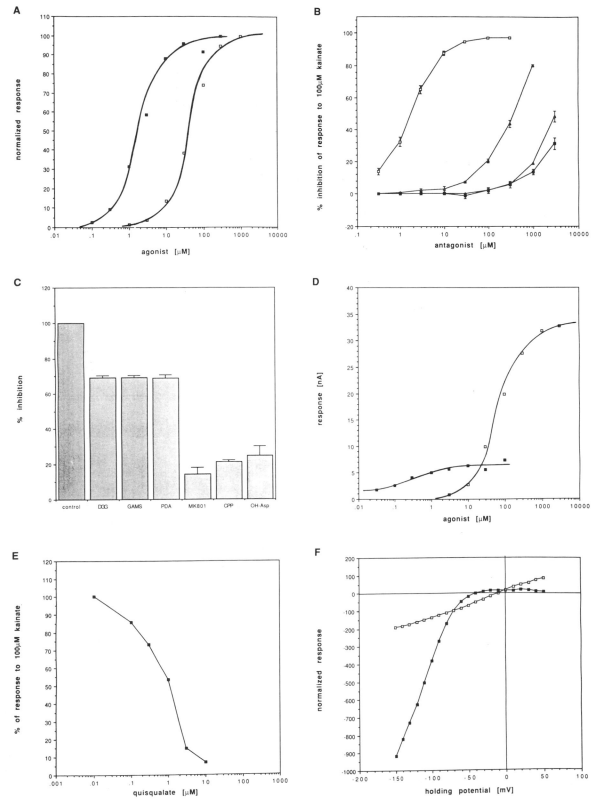

Figure 5. Pharmacological and electrophysiological properties of GluR-K1. Oocytes injected with GluR-K1 transcript (*A* and *C*: 1.25 ng, *B* and *F*: 2 ng, *D* and *E*: 10 ng) were recorded under voltage clamp 2–3 days after injection. Holding potential was -70 mV, except for *B* (-100 mV). (*A*) Dose-response curves (average values, $n = 3$) for KA ($\square$) and DOM ($\blacksquare$). Curves drawn free-hand. (*B*) Inhibition curves of CNQX ($\square$), KYN ($\blacktriangle$), GDEE ($\blacksquare$), and APV ($\triangle$). Average values $\pm$s.e.m. ($n = 3$). (*C*) Inhibition of responses to 100 μM KA by various antagonists. Average values $\pm$s.e.m. ($n = 3$). (*D*) Dose-response curves for QA ($\blacksquare$) and KA ($\square$), measured in the same oocyte. Curves drawn free-hand. (*E*) Dose-response curve of QA inhibition of responses to 100 μM KA. (*F*) Current-voltage relationships (I/V curves) of responses to 100 μM KA of GluR-K1 ($\blacksquare$) and rat hippocampal poly(A)$^+$ RNA (HipA$^+$, 25 ng) ($\square$). Average values, $n = 3$ and 2 for GluR-K1 and HipA$^+$, respectively. Currents normalized to responses recorded at -70 mV.

These clones, upon coexpression with GluR-K1 in *Xenopus* oocytes, modify the electrophysiological and pharmacological properties of GluR-K1 (J. Boulter et al., in prep.).

Regional Tissue Distribution of mRNA and Receptor Protein

Northern blot analysis. The GluR-K1 cDNA was used as a probe on Northern blots under high-stringency conditions to analyze the size and distribution of GluR-K1 mRNA in the brain and in control tissues (Fig. 6). The strongest hybridization signals were found in hippocampus and cerebellum, whereas the signals were less intense in cortex and barely visible in brain stem. No hybridization was found in lung or liver poly(A)$^+$ RNA. Three different RNAs were observed, with sizes of 3.2, 3.9, and 5.2 kb. The 5.2-kb band showed the strongest signal. The different size classes seen are all large enough to represent transcripts of full-length cDNAs, and they may either be splice variants or reflect utilization of different polyadenylation sites.

In situ hybridization analysis. To obtain additional information on the distribution of GluR-K1 message in

the brain, we used ^{35}S-labeled antisense riboprobes transcribed from GluR-K1 for in situ hybridization on coronal rat brain sections (Fig. 7A,C). The message distribution seen confirmed the results obtained with the Northern blot technique: The strongest label was found in the hippocampal formation, over the pyramidal cell layer in Ammon's horn, and in the polymorph and granule cell layers of the dentate gyrus (DG). To a somewhat lesser degree, but still very strong, was the labeling of Purkinje cell layers (PUR) in the cerebellum (Fig. 7C). Cortex (COR) showed an intermediate level of staining with some areas being very prominent, such as the piriform cortex (PC). The layers of the cortex appeared to be differentially labeled. Other areas of dense labeling included the medial habenula (MH), the central nucleus of the amygdala (CNA), and the ventral medial hypothalamus (VMH). Brain stem (BS) was almost devoid of any signal. To confirm the staining pattern described, we used two additional antisense probes, which were specific for the untranslated regions at the 3' end and the 5' end of GluR-K1, respectively. These probes gave staining patterns identical to those obtained with the full-length probe. A detailed analysis of GluR-K1 message distribution is in preparation (E.S. Deneris et al., in prep.).

Immunohistochemical localization of GluR-K1 receptors. To analyze the regional distribution of GluR-K1 protein in rat brain, we prepared antibodies against a fusion protein of bacterial *trp*E protein with an extracellular portion (amino acids 185–449) of GluR-K1. This antiserum recognizes a 105-kD protein on Western blots of brain tissue homogenates, which is compatible with the size of 99.8 kD calculated from the deduced amino acid sequence of GluR-K1, if one allows for some secondary modification like glycosylation. Indeed, after treatment with endoglycosidases H and F, the molecular mass of the immunoreactive species dropped from 105 kD to 97 kD, which is well within the error range of the predicted value.

Using this antiserum for immunohistochemical analysis of rat brain coronal sections (Fig. 7B), we found staining to be similar to the in situ hybridization labeling pattern. All regions labeled for GluR-K1 message were stained with the antibody, with the notable exception of the medial habenula, which, despite a very strong in situ hybridization signal, showed no immunoreactivity. Immunostaining for the receptor protein, however, does not necessarily have to coincide with the mRNA distribution. It is possible that (1) the RNA is not translated or (2) it is translated in the somata of efferent cells within the medial habenula, whereupon the receptor protein is rapidly transported anterogradely to the interpeduncular nucleus, the synaptic target of the medial habenula. The finding that the antibody staining pattern is very similar to the labeling pattern found by in situ hybridization suggests that the antiserum indeed recognizes the GluR-K1 protein. This antiserum will be used to purify the GluR-K1 protein and to screen for immunologically related proteins.

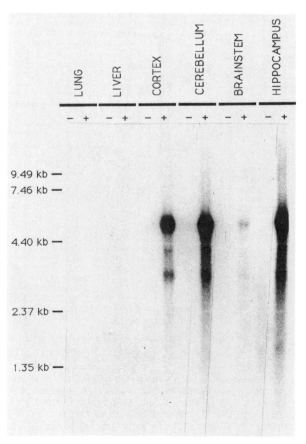

Figure 6. Northern blot analysis for GluR-K1 message, of poly(A)$^+$ RNA (3 μg) and poly(A)$^-$ control RNA (6 μg) prepared from different rat tissues. (Reprinted, with permission, from Hollmann et al. 1989.)

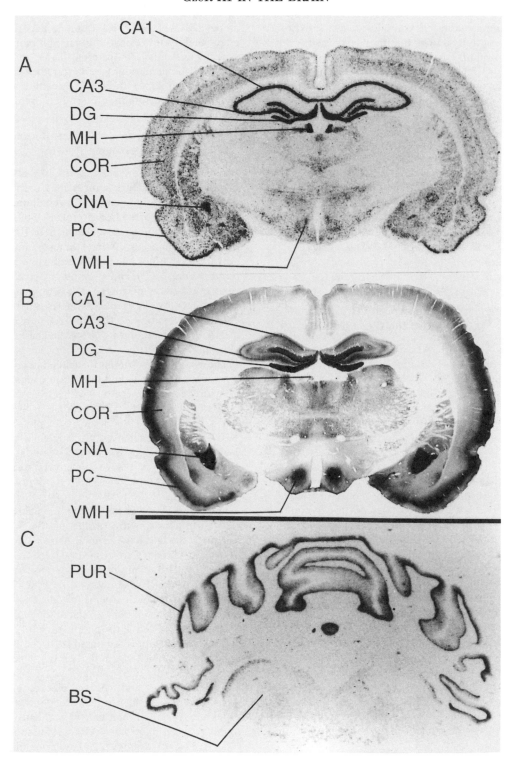

Figure 7. (*A*,*C*) Coronal rat brain sections probed with full-length ^{35}S-labeled antisense riboprobes of GluR-K1. (*B*) Coronal rat brain section of the same area shown in *A*, immunostained with antiserum prepared against the extracellular domain of GluR-K1. (BS) Brain stem; (CA1, CA3) hippocampal pyramidal cell layers in Ammon's horn; (CNA) central nucleus of the amygdala; (COR) cortex; (DG) dentate gyrus; (MH) medial habenula; (PC) piriform cortex; (PUR) Purkinje cells; (VMH) ventral medial hypothalamus.

The immunohistochemical staining pattern observed does not completely match the KA-binding sites mapped in ligand-binding studies. Most notably, the strong immunoreactivity of the pyramidal cells throughout Ammon's horn is quite different from the binding of KA, which was predominantly seen in the stratum lucidum of CA3 and, to a lesser extent, in the dentate gyrus, leaving the CA1 region nearly devoid of any staining (Monaghan and Cotman 1982; Unnerstall and Wamsley 1983; Patel et al. 1986). However, KA ligand-binding studies are complicated by the existence of both low-affinity and high-affinity binding sites. Most studies do not differentiate between the two sites (Patel et al. 1986). Interestingly, when these two sites are analyzed separately (Patel et al. 1986), the distribution of the low-affinity binding sites matches much better the immunostaining seen for GluR-K1. It has been suggested that the low-affinity KA-binding sites are identical to QA-binding sites (Honore et al. 1986). Therefore, it is noteworthy that the GluR-K1 immunostaining looks very similar to staining patterns reported for the binding of AMPA, a QA receptor agonist (Olsen et al. 1987). These observations are consistent with our findings that QA binds to GluR-K1 and suggest that GluR-K1 might represent the low-affinity KA-binding sites as seen in ligand-binding studies.

DISCUSSION

GluR-K1 and the Superfamily Hypothesis of Ligand-gated Ion Channels

The cloning of the $GABA_A$ receptor (Schofield et al. 1987) and the 48-kD subunit of the glycine receptor (Grenningloh et al. 1987) revealed structural similarities and localized sequence identities both between these receptors and to nAChR subunits. This led to the hypothesis of a "superfamily" of evolutionarily related ligand-gated ion channels (Barnard et al. 1987; Schofield et al. 1987). It was also suggested that this superfamily would include the glutamate receptors, which at that time were structurally uncharacterized. The cloning of the first glutamate receptor (Hollmann et al. 1989) allows us to reexamine this hypothesis. GlyR and $GABA_A$R share greater sequence identities with each other (34% and 39% for $GABA_A\alpha$ and $GABA_A\beta$, respectively) than with nAChRs (15–19%). This was explained by the fact that $GABA_A$R and GlyR mediate inhibition, whereas nAChRs mediate excitation. From this it would follow that glutamate receptors should share higher sequence identity with nAChRs than with either $GABA_A$Rs or GlyRs. However, as noted previously, no significant sequence identity was detected between GluR-K1 and either of these ligand-gated ion channels, except in the region of the cysteine loop and the putative channel-lining TMD II region. Nevertheless, these few identities were indeed more pronounced between GluR-K1 and the nAChRs than between GluR-K1 and the inhibitory receptors.

GluR-K1 also reveals differences in the general structure of the protein. First, it is about twice as big as all other ligand-gated ion channel subunits, and second, the TMDs are much more widely spaced apart, although they exhibit the same conspicuous "cluster of 3 + 1" TMD pattern. These differences, along with the weak sequence identity, raise doubt as to the applicability of the superfamily hypothesis to all ligand-gated ion channels. This concept might be valid only for $GABA_A$Rs and GlyRs. The conserved TMD pattern and the sequence identities in the putative channel-lining TMD of GluR-K1 (and in nAChRs as well) might merely reflect evolutionary pressure to form a functional channel for cations. Thus, these common structural features might be better explained by convergent evolution of unrelated genes than by divergent evolution of a common ancestral receptor.

Structural Comparison of GluR-K1 and Cloned KA-binding Proteins

Concurrent with the cloning of GluR-K1, the cDNA sequences of two high-affinity KA-binding proteins (KBPs) from frog and chicken cerebellum, respectively, have been reported (Gregor et al. 1989; Wada et al. 1989). It has been suggested that these KBPs are KA-gated ion channels or subunits thereof. However, channel function has not been reported for the chicken KBP (Gregor et al. 1989), and attempts to express functional channels from the frog KBP cDNA in *Xenopus* oocytes have failed (Wada et al. 1989). Nevertheless, high-affinity KA binding of the frog KBP expressed from cDNA transfected into COS cells has been shown (Wada et al. 1989).

The KBPs from frog and chicken share some structural features with ligand-gated ion channel subunits. They are similar in size to nAChRs, $GABA_A$Rs, and GlyRs (49.0 kD and 51.8 kD for the frog and chicken KBPs, respectively), and hydropathy plots suggest four TMDs in a "cluster of 3 + 1" arrangement (Fig. 8B,C). The KBPs share approximately 53% sequence identity with each other and have some very weak localized sequence identities with nAChRs, most notably in their TMDs (Wada et al. 1989). Comparison of the KBPs with GluR-K1 reveals that the amino acid sequence as well as the hydropathy profile of the KBPs is very similar to the carboxy-terminal half of GluR-K1 (Fig. 8), as if the KBPs were truncated versions of a GluR-K1-like protein. The predicted transmembrane domains in the KBPs (Gregor et al. 1989; Wada et al. 1989) match with our model II for GluR-K1. Since both KBPs lack a hydrophobic stretch in the region where in GluR-K1 we predict hydrophobic region I, our model I of TMD assignment is not possible for the KBPs. In the region where GluR-K1 and KBP sequences overlap, there is 34% and 35% amino acid sequence identity between GluR-K1 and frog and chicken KBP, respectively, and 27% of the residues are identical in all three proteins. A similar amount of sequence identity is found between different $GABA_A$R subunits (Barnard et al. 1987), for example, and suggests that GluR-K1 and the KBPs belong to the same family of proteins, which have evolved from a common ancestral protein. Whether the KBPs are subunits of KA-gated ion channels or through evolution have acquired a different function remains to be established.

It is tempting to speculate that the KBPs serve a quite different purpose than GluR-K1, since they display high-affinity KA binding and are localized preferentially at extrajunctional sites (Dechesne et al. 1990) and on glial cells (Somogyi et al. 1990). GluR-K1, in contrast, responds to KA only with low affinity,

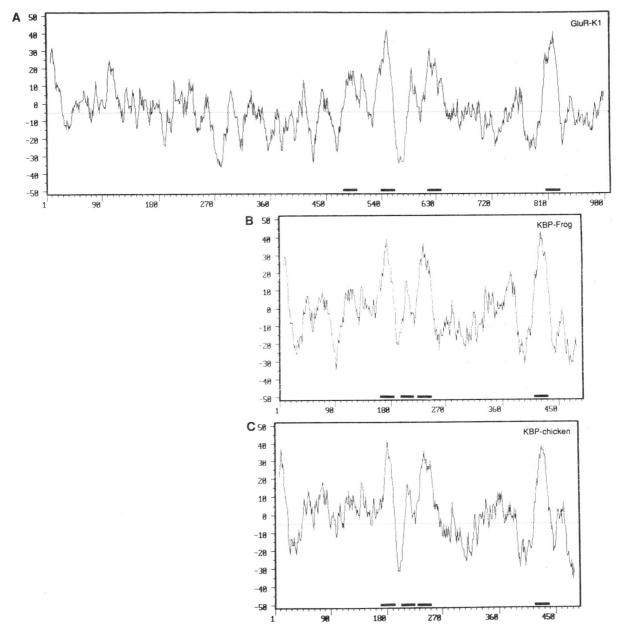

Figure 8. Comparison of hydropathy plots of GluR-K1 (*A*), the frog KBP (*B*) (sequence data from Wada et al. 1989), and the chicken KBP (*C*) (sequence data from Gregor et al. 1989). The algorithm of Kyte and Doolittle (1982) was used at a window setting of 15. All TMD assignments as proposed in the original publications. For the comparison, TMD I of the KBPs were lined up with the TMD II of GluR-K1.

is localized on neurons, and is enriched in postsynaptic densities (S.W. Rogers et al., in prep.), suggesting a postsynaptic role for this protein. Thus, it is possible that the KBPs represent the high-affinity binding sites seen in ligand-binding studies (Patel et al. 1986), whereas GluR-K1 probably represents the low-affinity sites (see above).

KA and QA Receptors: Are They Separate Molecular Entities?

Recent debate has focused on the question of whether KA and QA activate separate receptors or act at the same receptor complex, frequently called the "non-NMDA" receptor. Our findings that QA can activate GluR-K1, although less efficaciously than KA, lend support to the hypothesis that KA receptors and QA receptors are identical proteins. This is further strengthened by our observation that QA competitively blocks the action of KA at GluR-K1 expressed in oocytes. This blocking of KA responses by QA has been observed in poly(A)$^+$ RNA-injected oocytes as well as in isolated neurons, and it has been interpreted as evidence for the existence of a single receptor for KA and QA (Ishida and Neyton 1985; Verdoorn and Dingledine 1988; Kiskin et al. 1990). However, given the complexity of the systems analyzed, alternative explanations involving complicated models of allosteric interactions of different proteins or coactivation of several independent receptors could not be ruled out (Perouansky and Grantyn 1989).

The experiments reported here demonstrate that both agonists can act on the same protein. It appears that, at least in GluR-K1, both KA and QA bind to the same ligand binding site, and activate the same ion channel, but with different efficacies. It is possible, however, that other non-NMDA receptors exist which may be selectively activated by either KA or QA. The relative efficacy of KA or QA at non-NMDA receptors may depend on the subunit composition of the receptor complex. As discussed earlier, it is likely that GluR-K1 combines with one or more other subunits to form a channel in vivo (J. Boulter et al., in prep.). These additional subunits might regulate the relative channel opening efficacies of KA and QA, and/or regulate the channel open time or desensitization properties. Thus, combinations of different subunits might account for the agonist-dependent variations in non-NMDA receptor/channel properties observed (Perouansky and Grantyn 1989; Tang et al. 1989).

ACKNOWLEDGMENTS

This work was supported by a postdoctoral fellowship of the Deutsche Forschungsgemeinschaft to M.H., National Institutes of Health postdoctoral fellowships to S.W.R. and E.D., National Eye Institute grant EY-08362-01 to T.E.H., a Howard Hughes Medical Institute postdoctoral fellowship to G.P.G., the Fritz B. Burns foundation (S.H.), a National Institute of Neurological and Communicative Disorders and Stroke grant to S.H.

REFERENCES

Aviv, H. and P. Leder. 1972. Purification of biologically active globin messenger RNA by chromatography on oligothymidylic acid-cellulose. *Proc. Natl. Acad. Sci.* **69:** 1408.

Barnard, E., M.G. Darlison, and P. Seeburg. 1987. Molecular biology of the GABA_A receptor: The receptor/channel superfamily. *Trends Neurosci.* **10:** 502.

Bear, M.F. and W. Singer. 1986. Involvement of excitatory amino acid receptors in the experience-dependent development of visual cortex. *Nature* **320:** 172.

Betz, H. and C.-M. Becker. 1988. The mammalian glycine receptor—Biology and structure of a neuronal chloride channel protein. *Neurochem. Int.* **13:** 137.

Boulter, J., A. O'Shea-Greenfield, R.M. Duvoisin, J.G. Connolly, E. Wada, A. Jensen, P.D. Gardner, M. Ballivet, E.S. Deneris, D. McKinnon, S. Heinemann, and J. Patrick. 1990. α3, α5, and β4: Three members of the rat neuronal nicotinic acetylcholine receptor-related gene family form of gene cluster. *J. Biol. Chem.* **265:** 4472.

Brose, N., S. Halpain, C. Suchanek, and R. Jahn. 1989. Characterization and partial purification of a chloride- and calcium-dependent glutamate-binding protein from rat brain. *J. Biol. Chem.* **264:** 9619.

Chen, J-W., M.D. Cunningham, N. Galton, and E.K. Michaelis. 1989. Immune labeling and purification of a 71-kDa glutamate-binding protein from brain synaptic membranes. *J. Biol. Chem.* **263:** 417.

Chirgwin, J.M., A.E. Przybyla, R.J. MacDonald, and W.J. Rutter. 1979. Isolation of biologically active ribonucleic acid from sources enriched in ribonuclease. *Biochemistry* **18:** 5294.

Collingridge, G.L., S.J. Kehl, and H. McLennan. 1983. Excitatory amino acids in synaptic transmission in the Schaffer collateral-commissural pathway of the rat hippocampus. *J. Physiol.* **334:** 132.

Constantine-Paton, M., H.T. Cline, and E. Debski. 1990. Patterned activity, synaptic convergence and the NMDA receptor in developing visual pathways. *Annu. Rev. Neurosci.* **13:** 129.

Dechesne, C.J., M.D. Oberdorfer, D.R. Hampson, K.D. Wheaton, A.J. Nazarali, G. Coping, and R.J. Wenthold. 1990. Distribution of a putative kainic acid receptor in the frog central nervous system determined with monoclonal and polyclonal antibodies: Evidence for synaptic and extrasynaptic localization. *J. Neurosci.* **10:** 479.

Deneris, E.S., J. Boulter, L.W. Swanson, J. Patrick, and S. Heinemann. 1989. β3: A new member of nicotinic acetylcholine receptor gene family is expressed in brain. *J. Biol. Chem.* **264:** 6268.

Deneris, E.S., J. Connolly, J. Boulter, E. Wada, K. Wada, L.W. Swanson, J. Patrick, and S. Heinemann. 1988. Primary structure and expression of β2: A novel subunit of neuronal nicotinic acetylcholine receptors. *Neuron* **1:** 45.

Dieckmann, C.L. and A. Tzagoloff. 1975. Assembly of the mitochondrial membrane system. *J. Biol. Chem.* **260:** 1513.

Eccles, J.C. 1983. Calcium in long-term potentiation as a model for memory. *Neuroscience* **10:** 1071.

Fagg, G.E. 1985. L-glutamate, excitatory amino acid receptors and brain function. *Trends Neurosci.* **8:** 207.

Fong, T.M., N. Davidson, and H.A. Lester. 1988. Properties of two classes of rat brain acidic amino acid receptors induced by distinct mRNA populations in *Xenopus* oocytes. *Synapse* **2:** 657.

Foster, A.C. and G.E. Fagg. 1984. Acidic amino acid binding sites in mammalian neuronal membranes: Their characteristics and relationship to synaptic receptors. *Brain Res. Rev.* **7:** 103.

Gregor, P., N. Eshhar, A. Ortega, and V.I. Teichberg. 1988. Isolation, immunochemical characterization and localization of the kainate sub-class of glutamate receptor from chick cerebellum. *EMBO J.* **7:** 2673.

Gregor, P., I. Mano, I. Maoz, M. McKeown, and V.I. Teichberg. 1989. Molecular structure of the chick cerebellar kainate-binding subunit of a putative glutamate receptor. *Nature* **342:** 689.

Grenningloh, G., A. Rienitz, B. Schmitt, C. Methfessel, M. Zensen, K. Beyreuther, E.D. Gundelfinger, and H. Betz. 1987. The strychnine-binding subunit of the glycine receptor shows homology with nicotinic acetylcholine receptors. *Nature* **328:** 215.

Grenningloh, G., V. Schmieden, P.R. Schofield, P.H. Seeburg, T. Siddique, T.K. Mohandas, C.-M. Becker, and H. Betz. 1990. Alpha subunit variants of the human glycine receptor: Primary structures, functional expression and chromosomal localization of the corresponding genes. *EMBO J.* **9:** 771.

Gundersen, C.B., R. Miledi, and I. Parker. 1984. Glutamate and kainate receptors induced by rat brain messenger RNA in *Xenopus* oocytes. *Proc. R. Soc. Lond. B Biol. Sci.* **221:** 127.

Hayashi, T. 1954. Effects of sodium glutamate on the nervous system. *Keio J. Med.* **3:** 183.

Hampson, D.R. and R.J. Wenthold. 1988. A kainic acid receptor from frog brain purified using domoic acid affinity chromatography. *J. Biol. Chem.* **263:** 2500.

Heinemann, S., G. Asouline, M. Ballivet, J. Boulter, J. Connolly, E. Deneris, K. Evans, S. Evans, J. Forrest, P. Gardner, D. Goldman, A. Kochhar, W. Luyten, P. Mason, D. Treco, K. Wada, and J. Patrick. 1986. Molecular biology of the neural and muscle acetylcholine receptors. In *Molecular neurobiology* (ed. J. Patrick and S. Heinemann), p. 45. Plenum Press, New York.

Hirono, C., I. Ito, S. Yamagishi, and H. Sugiyama. 1988. Characterization of glutamate receptors induced in *Xenopus* oocytes after injection of rat brain mRNA. *Neurosci. Res.* **6**: 106.

Hollmann, M., A. O'Shea-Greenfield, S.W. Rogers, and S. Heinemann. 1989. Cloning by functional expression of a member of the glutamate receptor family. *Nature* **342**: 643.

Honore, T., J. Drejer, and M. Nielsen. 1986. Calcium discriminates two [^{3}H]kainate binding sites with different molecular target sizes in rat cortex. *Neurosci. Lett.* **65**: 47.

Hucho, F. and R. Hilgenfeld. 1989. The selectivity filter of a ligand-gated ion channel. The helix-M2 model of the ion channel of the nicotinic acetylcholine receptor. *FEBS Lett.* **257**: 17.

Hughes, T.E., R.G. Carey, J. Victoria, A.L. de Blas, and H.J. Karten. 1989. Immunohistochemical localization of GABA$_A$ receptors in the retina of the primate *Saimiri sciureus*. *Vis. Neurosci.* **2**: 565.

Ishida, A.T. and J. Neyton. 1985. Quisqualate and L-glutamate inhibit retinal horizontal-cell response to kainate. *Proc. Natl. Acad. Sci.* **82**: 1837.

Kiskin, N.I., O.A. Krishtal, and A.Y. Tsyndrenko. 1990. Cross-desensitization reveals pharmacological specificity of excitatory amino acid receptors in isolated hippocampal neurons. *Eur. J. Neurosci.* **2**: 461.

Klein, A.U., B. Niederoest, K.H. Winterhalter, M. Cuenod, and P. Streit. 1988. A kainate binding protein in pigeon cerebellum: Purification and localization by monoclonal antibody. *Neurosci. Lett.* **95**: 359.

Kushner, L., J. Lerma, R.S. Zukin, and M.V.L. Bennett. 1988. Coexpression of *N*-methyl-D-aspartate and phencyclidine receptors in *Xenopus* oocytes injected with rat brain mRNA. *Proc. Natl. Acad. Sci.* **85**: 3250.

Kyte, J. and R.F. Doolittle. 1982. A simple method for displaying the hydropathic character of a protein. *J. Mol. Biol.* **157**: 105.

Liman, E.R., A.G. Knapp, and J.E. Dowling. 1989. Enhancement of kainate-gated currents in retinal horizontal cells by cyclic AMP-dependent protein kinase. *Brain Res.* **481**: 399.

Monaghan, D.T. and C.W. Cotman. 1982. The distribution of [^{3}H]kainic acid binding sites in rat CNS as determined by autoradiography. *Brain Res.* **252**: 91.

Monaghan, D.T., R.J Bridges, and C.W. Cotman. 1989. The excitatory amino acid receptors: Their classes, pharmacology, and distinct properties in the function of the central nervous system. *Annu. Rev. Pharmacol. Toxicol.* **29**: 365.

Olney, J.W. 1989. Excitotoxicity and *N*-methyl-D-aspartate receptors. *Drug Dev. Res.* **17**: 299.

Olsen, R.W., O. Szamraj, and C.R. Houser. 1987. [^{3}H]AMPA binding to glutamate receptor subpopulations in rat brain. *Brain Res.* **402**: 243.

Patel, S., B.S. Meldrum, and J.F. Collins. 1986. Distribution of [^{3}H]kainic acid and binding sites in the rat brain: *In vivo* and *in vitro* receptor autoradiography. *Neurosci. Lett.* **70**: 301.

Perouansky, M. and R. Grantyn. 1989. Separation of quisqualate- and kainate-selective glutamate receptors in cultured neurons from the rat superior colliculus. *Neurosci.* **9**: 70.

Rao, J.K.M. and P. Argos. 1986. A conformational preference parameter to predict helices in integral membrane proteins. *Biochim. Biophys. Acta* **869**: 197.

Sanger, F., S. Nicklen, and A.R. Coulson. 1977. DNA sequencing with chain-terminating inhibitors. *Proc. Natl. Acad. Sci.* **74**: 5463.

Schofield, P.R., M.G. Darlison, N. Fujita, D.R. Burt, F.A. Stephenson, H. Rodriguez, L.M. Rhee, J. Ramachandran, V. Reale, T.A. Glencorse, P.H. Seeburg, and E.A. Barnard. 1987. Sequence and functional expression of the GABA$_A$ receptor shows a ligand-gated receptor superfamily. *Nature* **328**: 221.

Shivers, B.D., I. Killisch, R. Sprengel, H. Sontheimer, M. Köhler, P.R. Schofield, and P.H. Seeburg. 1989. Two novel GABA$_A$ receptor subunits exist in distinct neuronal subpopulations. *Neuron* **3**: 327.

Somogyi, P., N. Eshhar, V.I. Teichberg, and J.D.B. Roberts. 1990. Subcellular localization of a putative kainate receptor in Bergmann glial cells using a monoclonal antibody in the chick and fish cerebellar cortex. *Neuroscience* **35**: 9.

Strange, P.G. 1988. The structure and mechanism of neurotransmitter receptors. *Biochem. J.* **249**: 309.

Sugiyama, H., I. Ito, and C. Hirono. 1987. A new type of glutamate receptor linked to inositol phospholipid metabolism. *Nature* **325**: 531.

Sumikawa, K., I. Parker, and R. Miledi. 1984. Partial purification and functional expression of brain mRNAs coding for neurotransmitter receptors and voltage-operated channels. *Proc. Natl. Acad. Sci.* **81**: 7994.

Tang, C.-M., M. Dichter, and M. Morad. 1989. Quisqualate activates a rapidly inactivating high conductance ionic channel in hippocampal neurons. *Science* **243**: 1474.

Unnerstall, J.R. and J.K. Wamsley. 1983. Autoradiographic localization of high-affinity [^{3}H]kainic acid binding sites in the rat forebrain. *Eur. J. Pharmacol.* **86**: 361.

Verdoorn, T.A. and R. Dingledine. 1988. Excitatory amino acid receptors expressed in *Xenopus* oocytes: Agonist pharmacology. *Mol. Pharmacol.* **34**: 298.

Verdoorn, T.A., N.W. Kleckner, and R. Dingledine. 1987. Rat brain *N*-methyl-D-aspartate receptors expressed in *Xenopus* oocytes. *Science* **238**: 1114.

Wada, K., C.J. Dechesne, S. Shimasaki, R.G. King, K. Kusano, A. Buonanno, D.R. Hampson, C. Banner, R.J. Wenthold, and Y. Nakatani. 1989. Sequence and expression of a frog brain complementary DNA encoding a kainate-binding protein. *Nature* **342**: 684.

Woo, C.C., R. Coopersmith, and M. Leon. 1987. Localized changes in olfactory bulb morphology associated with early olfactory learning. *J. Comp. Neurol.* **263**: 113.

Quantal Analysis of Excitatory Synaptic Mechanisms in the Mammalian Central Nervous System

J.J.B. Jack, D.M. Kullmann, A.U. Larkman, G. Major, and K.J. Stratford
Laboratory of Physiology, Oxford University, Oxford OX1 3PT, England

The quantal hypothesis of transmitter release has as its essential feature that transmitter is released in multimolecular packets and that normal release consists of an integral number of these units. The experimental evidence for this account comes from studies of the postjunctional effect (postjunctional potential or current) and was first obtained at the vertebrate neuromuscular junction (Fatt and Katz 1952; del Castillo and Katz 1954; Boyd and Martin 1956). Subsequently, the same description has been given for a variety of other junctions. This work has been admirably reviewed previously (see, e.g., Martin 1977; Redman 1990), and the present paper has a more limited aim. We highlight the main features of the description of quantal mechanisms in the mammalian central nervous system and the way in which this has been found to differ from the description at the neuromuscular junction. Most of the results obtained so far have come from studies in the spinal cord, so this work will be reviewed first before we briefly turn to studies in the hippocampus. Our own hippocampal work, although still at an early stage, has highlighted some additional complexities that were not apparent in the spinal cord studies. Our results to date are therefore summarized, and their possible implications for quantal analysis at other synapses are discussed in the final section of the paper.

Analyses of quantal release in central nerve cells are complicated by the difficulty that spontaneously recorded synaptic potentials, which might be analogous to spontaneous miniature end-plate potentials, could arise from synaptic sites other than those being activated. This prevents an independent measure of the unit quantal amplitude, which would provide a guide to the expected levels of the evoked synaptic potential. Furthermore, the presence of so many synaptic sites, contributing spontaneous synaptic activity, greatly increases the total background noise so that resolution of the amplitudes of the evoked potential is extremely difficult. These problems led Edwards et al. (1976a,b) to devise an alternative approach, in which the contaminating noise is measured separately and then an optimization method is used to estimate the most likely form of the synaptic potential amplitude fluctuations. In these earlier studies (Edwards et al. 1976a,b; Jack et al. 1981), the statistical criterion used was to minimize the sum of squared differences, but Ling and Tolhurst (1983) showed that a better approach was to maximize the likelihood estimator (MLE) (see also Everitt and Hand 1981; Titterington et al. 1985; Kullmann 1989).

QUANTAL STUDIES IN THE MAMMALIAN SPINAL CORD

Most of the studies in the mammalian central nervous system using these techniques have analyzed the fluctuations in amplitude of excitatory synaptic potentials (EPSPs) evoked by group 1a spindle afferent fibers in either motoneurons or cells of the dorsal spinocerebellar tract (DSCT). If one assumes that the studies using these techniques have obtained reliable results, then there are some striking differences, as well as similarities, between the results obtained in the mammalian spinal cord and the neuromuscular junction. There are four main features of the description in the spinal cord: (1) The estimated peak amplitude levels show equal spacing, i.e., the EPSP fluctuates in peak amplitude between integral multiples of a unit size, known as the quantal amplitude; (2) there is no detectable variance associated with each component peak amplitude level; (3) the probability density function describing the proportion of trials at each component amplitude level is, in general, not fitted well by either a Poisson or a simple binomial distribution but is compatible with a compound binomial distribution; and (4) in the motoneuron, it has been possible to estimate the quantal amplitude for synaptic potentials generated at different electrotonic distances from the recording site at the soma. These quantal amplitudes do not show the electrotonic attenuation expected if the same amount of charge was injected at each site, implying that the total inward charge movement associated with a single quantum varies systematically, being up to five or ten times greater in the distal dendrites than near the soma. Each of these four features is considered in more detail below.

Component Amplitudes Are Equally Spaced

This first feature, which is identical to the description at the neuromuscular junction, seems on the face of it to be unproblematic. Most of the analyses in spinal cord neurons have been performed on single group 1a fiber inputs, but Figure 1 shows an example of two functionally different monosynaptic excitatory inputs to a single motoneuron. If the synaptic terminals associated with a single input were aggregated at similar electrotonic locations, each quantal effect recorded at the soma would have a similar time course and suffer similar delay and amplitude attenuation. Against this

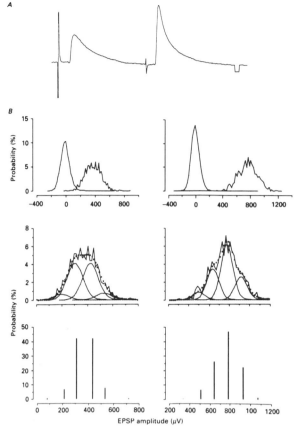

Figure 1. (*A*) The average time course of 850 intracellular records of two EPSPs evoked in a motoneuron by stimulation of group 1a spindle afferent and descending tract (ventral quadrant; VQ) fibers. Both inputs generate a monosynaptic excitation. At the end of the trace, there is a 100 μV 1 msec calibration pulse. (*B*) An illustration of the analysis procedure for the 1a (*left*) and VQ (*right*) EPSPs. The top row shows the frequency histograms for the independently recorded noise (the left of each pair of histograms) and for the EPSP peak amplitudes. The histogram bin widths were 15 μV (1a) and 20 μV (VQ). The noise histograms represent 12,000 independent samples compared with the 850 making up the EPSP histogram. Note the suggestion of peaks in the EPSP histogram for the VQ (*right*). The middle row shows the EPSP histograms again, with the maximum likelihood estimates of the underlying distributions. The dotted lines, obtained by summing these distributions, are in good agreement with the observed amplitude histograms. The bottom row shows the resolved discrete distributions with the noise removed. Both EPSPs fluctuate between four main peak amplitudes with roughly equal spacing of ~ 100 μV. (Reprinted, with permission, from Harrison et al. 1989.)

simple suggestion is the histological observation that the synaptic boutons of a single group 1a fiber are not always closely aggregated, although they may be for some fibers (Burke et al. 1979; Brown and Fyffe 1981; Redman and Walmsley 1983). It would therefore be expected that unequal spacing between amplitude levels should be detected. There may be two explanations for the fact that unequal spacing is not commonly observed. First, there is suggestive evidence, presented by Henneman et al. (1984), that different boutons of a

single fiber may be active or nonreleasing and that the nonreleasing boutons may be at a separate location from those usually active. Thus, in one motoneuron, they reported that the average time courses of all ten single-fiber EPSPs recorded were explicable by assuming a single electrical model of the cell and a single time course of the synaptic current (see Fig. 3 in Henneman et al. 1984). It is unlikely that such a result could be obtained if each of the single-fiber EPSPs were generated by groups of boutons that were electrotonically dispersed (see Walmsley and Stuklis 1989). Furthermore, the time courses of some of the EPSPs subsequently changed in such a way that the additional component of the EPSP must have arisen from a different region of the motoneuron (see Fig. 4 in Henneman et al. 1984). In some circumstances, the composite origin of an EPSP may be discerned from the time courses of its components, and a few examples of this kind have been analyzed (see e.g., Figs. 2 and 3 in Edwards et al. 1976b and Fig. 9 in Jack et al. 1981). In only one case was unequal spacing evident, whereas in the other two examples the quantal amplitude of the slower time course component was comparable to that of the faster component. This may be the second explanation for the relative consistency in the observation of equal spacing: Providing the peaks of the components of the EPSP arising from different electrotonic regions are roughly aligned, the observation that their quantal amplitudes are similar will lead to equal spacing. Harrison et al. (1989) also observed that the quantal amplitudes generated by different excitatory inputs to the same motoneuron (1a EPSPs vs. descending fiber EPSPs) were of roughly equal size, whatever their electrotonic location (see Fig. 6 in Harrison et al. 1989).

Variance of Each Component Amplitude Is Low

Edwards et al. (1976a) reported that over a third of the single-fiber 1a EPSPs they recorded showed no statistical fluctuation in amplitude other than that contributed by background noise. This was one observation that led them to suggest the "all or nothing" hypothesis for synaptic action at a single synaptic terminal, in contrast with the conventional quantal mechanism—as at the neuromuscular junction—where considerable variance is associated with each quantal amplitude (coefficient of variation, $CV = 30\%$). The lack of variance associated with single amplitude EPSPs was explored further by Harrison et al. (1989), and they reported that over 20% of their small amplitude EPSPs (< 150 μV peak voltage) showed no more fluctuation than could be accounted for by the background noise. Both of these studies therefore described a proportion of the EPSPs as showing no detectable amplitude fluctuation. Since the average amplitude of these EPSPs was comparable to the quantal amplitude in those EPSPs that did show amplitude fluctuations, it is reasonable to assume that they represent the release of single quanta and that the difference from the neuromuscular junction lies simply in the fact that there is minimal variance associated with repeated release of single quanta.

This analysis was also taken further by Jack et al. (1981) (see Fig. 2) and Walmsley et al. (1988). In both of these studies, a careful analysis was performed of the amount of possible variance associated with each com-

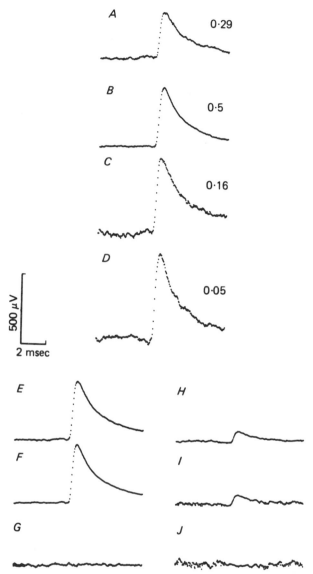

Figure 2. (A, B, C, D) The time course of the four components of a group 1a EPSP recorded in a motoneuron. The figures on the right of each EPSP time course indicate the probability with which they occur. The peak amplitudes of these components are 302, 406, 505, and 607 μV, respectively; thus, on a quantal account, they are assumed to represent the effect of the release of 3, 4, 5, and 6 quanta, respectively. (E,H) The reconstructed time courses of the mean and s.d. of the EPSP, obtained by combining the time courses of each component, weighted by their probability. (F,I) The measured time course of the mean and s.d. of the EPSP. (G,J) The differences E and F and H and I, respectively, plotted at twice the gain of the other records. Notice that there is no residual mean or s.d. time course to be accounted for, implying that there is no significant additional variance associated with each of the four components. (Reprinted, with permission, from Jack et al. 1981.)

ponent amplitude of a fluctuating EPSP. In both, it was concluded that the CV for each component amplitude was less than 5%. This is an even more striking conclusion than the lack of variance associated with repeated release of quanta from a single release site, since a particular component amplitude may represent quantal release from *alternative* release sites. For example, if there were two sites, each releasing intermittently and the quanta associated with them were 80 and 100 μV, respectively (each being invariant in amplitude), the amplitude fluctuation pattern would be 0, 80, 100, and 180 μV; if this were resolved into an amplitude fluctuation pattern of 0, 90, and 180 μV, there would be some additional variance associated with the 90 μV component.

These results, both for single-amplitude EPSPs and for EPSPs that fluctuate in amplitude, are quite different from the results for the neuromuscular junction, where the CV associated with a single quantum is 30%. The CV increases in proportion to the square root of the number of quanta (such as Fig. 2B) released, so that the independent sum of four quanta would show a CV of 60%. Walmsley et al. (1988) considered the quantal variance for an EPSP composed of up to 15 quanta and found that assuming a CV of as little as 6% for each quantum gave a less satisfactory fit to the histogram than assuming zero quantal variance.

Although there is more than one possible explanation for these results, the interpretation offered by Jack et al. (1981) was that there is a relatively small number of receptors in the subsynaptic membrane that are saturated by the release of a much larger number of transmitter molecules associated with each quantum. This possibility is taken up again below.

Release Probabilities Are Nonuniform

In their classical study of the quantal components of the end-plate potential, del Castillo and Katz (1954) pointed out that ". . . a Poisson distribution would be obtained even from a nonuniform population." They gave as an example a synaptic population consisting of, say, 500 units, where on average one quantum is released per trial, ". . . then the average chance of any unit responding to one impulse would be 1/500, but individual probabilities may be considerably higher for some and much smaller for many other members of the population." Recent experimental work at the frog neuromuscular junction (see Robitaille and Tremblay 1987) has confirmed the existence of nonuniform release probabilities; one reason why this has been difficult to establish clearly is that, as first pointed out by Brown et al. (1976), it is often very difficult to distinguish between binomial distributions where the probabilities are all equal (simple case) or where they are nonuniform (compound distribution). The possibility that statistical fluctuations at the group 1a excitatory synapse may be best represented by a compound binomial distribution was first raised by Jack et al. (1981), but a convincing demonstration of nonuniform release probabilities was first provided by Walmsley and his colleagues for group 1a excitation of the DSCT cells (see Walmsley et al. 1987, 1988).

Given that the probability of release may be nonuniform, it is of interest to consider whether all synaptic junctions are comparable in the maximum number of quanta released (N) and the distribution of the release probabilities (p). There does appear to be a qualitative difference between single-group 1a fiber excitation of DSCT cells compared with motoneurons. In DSCT cells, the value of N reported by Walmsley et al. (1987) ranged from 3 to 30, whereas the motoneuron data provide N values ranging between 1 and 10. Underlying these differences in N, there may also be a difference in the distribution of probabilities, which is most readily illustrated by considering the ratio of $p = 1$ to those where $0 < p < 1$. A higher proportion of the active release sites on the DSCT cell have unit probabilities (e.g., 23 out of 30, 8 out of 15, and so on, with an *average* probability of 0.76), whereas the active sites on the motoneuron show a generally smaller proportion with $p = 1$ (maximum reported by Edwards et al. [1989] in their Fig. 5 is 4, with an $N = 10$). These apparent differences may be matched to the different functional operation of these two types of synapses, as well as to their underlying structural differences. Although there are still only fragmentary data (see Lüscher 1990; Redman 1990), the evidence strongly suggests that for the group 1a synapse on the motoneuron, a large proportion of the release sites (assuming at least one release site per bouton) are inactive ($p = 0$) under the conditions of the experiment but that many can be brought to release by factors that enhance synaptic efficacy. A high proportion of release sites with $p < 1$ may provide greater scope for presynaptic increase in the efficacy of a connection. This will be referred to again in the section on hippocampal synaptic action.

Quantal Charge Varies Systematically with Synaptic Location

This last feature (see Fig. 3) is not relevant to the vertebrate neuromuscular junction, where the junctional area occupies a single location with a total electrotonic spread of a fraction of a space constant. It would not therefore be expected that the peak amplitude of quantal end-plate potentials would suffer much variation because of the exact site at which transmitter was released. Variations in quantal size are more likely to be due to variations in the number of transmitter molecules available to activate the postjunctional receptors. Under normal circumstances, there are ample numbers of receptors available to respond to the amount of transmitter released (Hartzell et al. 1975). The receptors are thus not saturated, and individual quantal amplitudes will be set by the number of molecules released and their diffusional efficiency in reaching receptors before destruction by acetylcholinesterase. The observation by Fatt and Katz (1952) that at a particular junction there is a relatively high coefficient

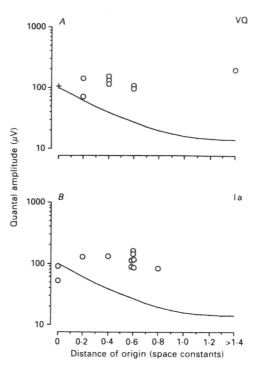

Figure 3. Symbols show the relationship between quantal amplitude, recorded at the soma, and the estimated electrotonic location at which the synaptic potential was generated. Quantal amplitude was estimated from the mean interval between discrete amplitudes in the MLE solutions. Electrotonic distance was estimated from the normalized rise time and half width of each EPSP, using the method of Jack et al. (1971). (*A*) Descending fiber EPSPs; (*B*) group 1a EPSPs. The continuous line in each graph represents the expected distribution of peak amplitudes if each quantal amplitude was generated by the same charge transfer, assuming a standard model of the motoneuron and the synaptic current time course. (Reprinted, with permission, from Harrison et al. 1989.)

of variation (30%) in the peak amplitude of quantal potentials is presumably attributable to these factors. Quantitative studies indicate that, on average, a quantum represents the effect of 3000 molecules of acetylcholine (ACh) opening 1500 ACh receptor ionophores (see Kuffler et al. 1984).

In contrast, an estimate may be made of the number of activated channels associated with a single excitatory quantum on the motoneuron. Finkel and Redman (1983), in a voltage-clamp study, found that the average peak conductance needed to generate a somatic EPSP with a peak amplitude of 100 μV was 5 nS. If one assumes that the single channel conductance is about 30–60 pS at 37°C (estimates, using a Q_{10} of 1.3 from the room temperature values of 18 pS and 35 pS made by Trussell and Fischbach [1989] and Tang et al. [1989] in chick spinal neurons and rat hippocampal neurons, respectively), the number of channels opened is of the order of 75–150, one order of magnitude less than at the end-plate. As with the ACh receptor, dose-response studies suggest that two molecules of transmitter are required to achieve opening of the ionophore (Tang et al. 1989; Trussell and Fischbach 1989), so this calculation suggests that between 150 and 300 glutamate molecules are effective in this case. If the average number of glutamate molecules released per quantum is roughly 5000 (in line with cholinergic synapses), this would be entirely consistent with the suggestion that the observed low quantal variance is the result of saturation of the subsynaptic receptors. On the other hand, quanta generated at remote dendritic locations may have up to ten times as much charge transferred, implying that up to 750–1500 channels are opened and 1500–3000 molecules of glutamate are effective. These values are closer to the likely number of transmitter molecules associated with a quantum and mean that incomplete saturation of the receptors, and hence greater quantal variance, is more likely to occur at distal synapses. These calculations have been presented because they both address the issue of lack of quantal variability and offer a possible functional explanation for this otherwise curious design. The systematic variation of postsynaptic receptor density might be an appropriate mechanism for ensuring that the efficacy of excitatory synapses on the motoneuron was largely independent of their location on the cell. Such a design would only succeed if there were sufficient transmitter molecules in a quantum to saturate the receptors at all but possibly the most distal synapses. The derived data presented above are entirely consistent with this suggestion.

CRITIQUE OF THE ABOVE CONCLUSIONS

Reliability of the Optimization Method

Edwards et al. (1976a) and subsequent investigators were forced into the use of optimization methods to extract the underlying amplitude fluctuation pattern of the EPSP because the signal-to-noise ratio was so unfavorable. These optimization methods are notoriously ill-conditioned, and it is possible that some of the published results, especially in the earlier papers by Edwards et al. (1976a,b) and to some extent in Jack et al. (1981) are potentially unreliable. The major difficulty is whether the correct number of component amplitudes is found; as pointed out by Redman (1990), if the signal-to-noise ratio is poor and the sample size small, the optimization procedure is likely to give a smaller number of components than is correct. If the opposite error occurs and spurious extra components are introduced, there is less likely to be a problem because the apparent signal-to-noise ratio (judged by the ratio of the average separation of the components to the noise standard deviation) will not be as good, and more caution will be exercised in accepting the result.

Jack et al. (1981) demonstrated that the background noise was so substantially dominated by low-frequency components that the signal-to-noise ratio was improved by using peak amplitude rather than the area of the synaptic potential as a measure of its size (see Fig. 12 in Jack et al. 1981). Furthermore, the closer together in time the baseline and peak regions are, the better the

signal-to-noise ratio. One obvious corollary to this is that synaptic potentials with a rapid rise time provide, other things being equal, a better opportunity to make a reliable resolution of their amplitude fluctuations. Put another way, synaptic potentials arising well out in the dendritic tree, with slower rise times, will tend to have a poorer signal-to-noise ratio. It will not therefore be surprising that most of the convincing experimental evidence for the conclusions listed above comes from EPSPs generated in the proximal part of the dendritic tree.

How would the conclusions be modified if the estimates of amplitude fluctuations in the more distal EPSPs were unreliable? At first sight, the most obvious feature for skepticism is the last, since distal EPSPs might have been resolved into a smaller number of components than they actually have and so have yielded erroneously large quantal amplitudes. Inspection of Figure 3 shows that there is only a very limited sample of distal EPSPs whose quantal amplitude has been judged reliable. Nevertheless, this figure illustrates that the main part of the expected attenuation occurs in the initial propagation of the synaptic potential; the assumed electrical model shows that the relative increase in rise time is much less than the relative reduction in peak amplitude (see also Figs. 3.12 to 3.14 in Jack et al. 1983). Thus, it should be possible to obtain reliable resolution of EPSP amplitude fluctuations in the proximal half of the dendritic tree, and the conclusion that there is more quantal charge transfer at distal locations should still be valid.

The first three conclusions have been largely derived from studies of EPSPs arising in the proximal half of the dendritic tree, and it is therefore an open question whether they apply also to the more distal EPSP. In particular, there is very little good evidence published that the most distal EPSPs have a very low coefficient of variation. If the calculations given above about quantal charge and synaptic location are roughly correct, there is certainly more likelihood that additional variance is associated with distal EPSPs, as the estimated number of postsynaptic receptors opened more closely approaches the likely number of transmitter molecules in a quantum.

Independence of Noise and Signal

Apart from the reliability of the method used, there is one major premise of the method that needs discussion. In the methods adopted by Edwards et al. (1976a) and subsequently followed in all the literature so far (see, however, Solodkin et al. 1987), it is assumed that the background noise is *independent* of the signal and that it *adds linearly* with the signal. Some test of the latter assumption was made implicitly by Jack et al. (1981) when they extracted the time course of a component amplitude from different sets of sweeps where the noise biased the peak amplitude in one direction or another (see Figs. 2 and 6 in Jack et al. 1981). Although these tests are not decisive, they suggest that there is little difference in the amplitude of the components for different types of noise bias. The simplest interpretation is that there was linear addition of the two signals.

The question of independence of the signal and the noise is more difficult to address. It has already been indicated that a major part of the background noise has a low frequency, and this certainly represents, in large part, spontaneous synaptic potentials. Among the release sites that could, in principle, be contributing to the background noise are therefore the release sites from which signal is being evoked. To take a simple example, imagine a postsynaptic cell in which there is only one release site active, both spontaneously and in response to a stimulus. If the release site behaved in an "all or nothing" manner and, furthermore, showed a period of refractoriness after release (either spontaneous or evoked), it would be expected that the background noise when release was successfully evoked would be different from noise measured at an entirely separate time. The noise measured independently would consist of instrumental noise plus the occasional spontaneous synaptic potential, whereas the noise occurring when release was evoked might be purely instrumental (depending on the relative durations of refractoriness and of the synaptic potential). Thus, a lower noise standard deviation (S.D.) would be associated with evoked release. It is difficult to estimate how important this effect might be, but it is likely to be much more prominent under circumstances where effort has been made to reduce synaptic activity in the majority of terminals. It would also be more important if the input from which the signal is evoked is one that as a result of regular stimulation shows a well-developed mechanism of delayed release (i.e., enhanced "spontaneous" release, as a result of stimulation; see Magleby 1987).

If this possibility had occurred in the spinal cord studies, it would weaken the conclusion that there is a low coefficient of variation for each quantum. To the degree that the background noise is an overestimate of the noise associated with release of a quantum, the variability of the quantum can be increased.

Problems of Stationarity

To extract the amplitude fluctuation pattern from the background noise successfully, it is important to accumulate a large number of trials. This reduces the error to which the optimization method is prone as a result of finite sampling. Unfortunately, the larger the number of trials collected, the less likely it is that the preparation remains in a completely stationary state.

Recent work by Trussell and Fischbach (1989), Tang et al. (1989), and Mayer and Vyclicky (1989) raises a particular issue that may contribute to nonstationarity: levels of extracellular glutamate. The conventional estimate for extracellular glutamate in the brain is of the order of 2–4 μM. The above investigators have all demonstrated that the kinetically fast α-amino-3-hydroxy-5 methyl-isoxazole-4-propionic acid (AMPA)

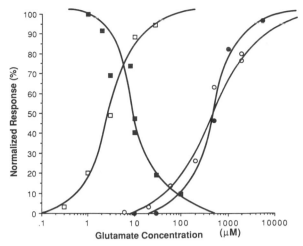

Figure 4. Concentration-response curves for the activation and desensitization of AMPA and NMDA receptors by glutamate. The curve drawn through the open squares shows the activation of NMDA receptors (Mayer 1989), whereas the closed squares show the reduction of the response by AMPA receptors following desensitization by a conditioning pulse of glutamate at the indicated concentration (Trussell and Fischbach 1989). Note that both curves span a similar range of glutamate concentrations. To the right are shown concentration-activation curves for AMPA receptors as determined by Mayer (1989) ($\bigcirc$) and Trussell and Fischbach (1989) ($\bullet$). Redrawn from Mayer (1989) and Trussell and Fischbach (1989).

(or quisqualate) receptor, which is the responding receptor for fast glutamatergic EPSPs, can be desensitized by surprisingly low levels of extracellular glutamate ($K_d = 10$ μM), whereas activation of the same receptor requires very much larger amounts of glutamate (see Fig. 4; $K_d = 300$–500 μM). It therefore seems likely that ambient extracellular glutamate levels could produce desensitization of a proportion of the AMPA receptors. Mayer (1989) has shown that the dose-response curve for N-methyl-D-aspartate (NMDA) receptor activation by glutamate spans a similar range of glutamate concentration as for the desensitization of the AMPA receptor (Fig. 4). Sah et al. (1989) have shown that there is activation of NMDA receptors in the resting hippocampal slice preparation, suggesting that the glutamate level, in this situation at least, is in the range for AMPA desensitization.

The issue therefore raised by these data is whether, either as a result of spontaneous variations in activity levels or as a result of stimulation, changes in the extracellular glutamate level can alter the proportion of nondesensitized AMPA receptors over time. If, as seems likely, this is a real possibility, then it would be a mechanism for producing quantal variability even if there was always saturation of all available postsynaptic receptors by a quantum of released glutamate.

QUANTAL ANALYSIS OF EXCITATION IN THE HIPPOCAMPUS

Redman and his colleagues have already devoted considerable effort to performing a quantal analysis of the CA3 to CA1 excitatory action in the hippocampus (Sayer et al. 1989, 1990). In their most elegant experiments, they evoked single-fiber EPSPs in CA1 neurons by intracellular stimulation of CA3 cells. A total of 76 such EPSPs was obtained, and a large number of trials were recorded for many of these. However, the levels of contaminating noise, measured in the prestimulus baseline period, were high compared with spinal cord studies (S.D. of the noise distribution, 127–459 μV), and reliable quantal analysis could only be performed for one EPSP, which gave a mean quantal amplitude of 278 μV. In other experiments, they evoked EPSPs by minimal extracellular stimulation and were able to achieve lower noise levels (70–138 μV S.D.; Sayer et al. 1989). Two further EPSPs were found that could be analyzed reliably and gave mean quantal amplitudes of 193 and 224 μV. They stressed that these values were likely to represent upper bounds. Smaller values might have been obtained had lower noise levels permitted their resolution, and they suggested that the quantal amplitude usually must have been smaller than 200 μV.

With these results in mind, we undertook a series of experiments to perform quantal analysis of excitatory inputs to hippocampal CA1 cells in slices, with the reduction of the background noise as a first priority. Picrotoxin and APV were used to block γ-aminobutyric acid (GABA$_A$) and NMDA responses, and the divalent cation concentrations in the bathing medium were elevated to reduce spontaneous spiking and synaptic activity. Minimal extracellular stimulation was used to evoke EPSPs, and recordings were made using relatively low-resistance microelectrodes (usually 15–50 MΩ). Lower noise levels were achieved, and we were able to record 16 EPSPs with noise S.D. between 47 and 80 μV and a further 16 with less than 150 μV. Using fairly high stimulation rates (1–5 Hz; usually 3–5 Hz), very large numbers of trials were recorded in most cases (1000–12000; often > 5000). Despite these apparent technical achievements, however, further difficulties emerged. This was perhaps to have been expected, given the comment of Sayer et al. (1989) that with their noise levels, they should have been able to resolve quantal amplitudes as small as 110 μV in some cases.

Nonstationarity

With the relatively high stimulation rates we employed, the mean EPSP peak amplitude usually decreased with time, often in an approximately exponential manner (Fig. 5). The averages of successive 100-trial epochs also showed smaller, apparently random changes and occasional larger jumps. When amplitude histograms were prepared from very large numbers of trials, they were either smooth or showed bizarre patterns of peaks, leading us to suspect that some selection of more stable periods of data would be necessary. Initially, we selected epochs of data for which the 100-trial averages of the EPSP mean and S.D. and the noise S.D. showed no trend or obvious jumps. In several

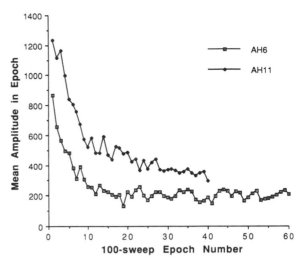

Figure 5. Graphs showing the changes in mean peak amplitude of EPSPs evoked in hippocampal CA1 pyramidal cells during repetitive stimulation. Successive 100-trial average peak amplitudes are shown for EPSPs in two cells, both stimulated at 5 Hz, over 4000 trials (*upper line*) or 6000 trials (*lower line*). The EPSPs show a progressive decline in amplitude with an approximately exponential time course, but the 100-trial averages also show both minor variations and occasional larger jumps in amplitude.

cases, such regions yielded amplitude histograms with clear, regularly spaced peaks. However, it was soon apparent that similar histograms could sometimes be obtained from periods when the EPSP mean amplitude showed a downward trend. The final procedure adopted was that the data were combed for epochs of 400 or more trials that yielded amplitude histograms with clear peaks whose positions remained unchanged when the epoch was subdivided (Fig. 6). These did not generally include the first 100–200 trials, when the mean was decreasing rapidly or periods showing obvious jumps in the 100-trial average, but otherwise their occurrence was difficult to predict. These relatively stable epochs were usually separated by periods when the histograms were smooth or showed peaks that were not evenly spaced and whose positions invariably changed dramatically when the epoch was subdivided. Epochs of 400–1800 trials meeting our criteria for stability were obtained for 38 out of 60 EPSPs examined. Many EPSPs showed several such epochs, but often only one was analyzed fully.

Several reasons for the apparent instability of the amplitude fluctuation pattern can be proposed: (1) *Changes in the quality of the impalement during the recording session.* Changes in resting potential or the leak around the recording microelectrode might alter the amplitude and time course of the EPSP and hence obscure the underlying fluctuation pattern. Any obvious changes were noted at the time of the experiment, but such occurrences did not correlate well with changes in the fluctuation pattern. Smaller changes could, of course, have gone unnoticed. (2) *Changes in the extracellular field potential.* Some EPSPs had an

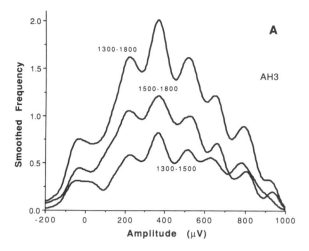

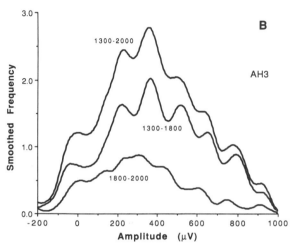

Figure 6. (*A*) Upper graph shows an amplitude histogram for 500 consecutive trials (trial nos. 1300–1800 of a longer run of data) of a hippocampal EPSP, binned finely (5 μV), and smoothed using a moving Gaussian filter. The histogram shows clear, approximately equally spaced peaks and satisfied our criterion for stability in that when the epoch of data was subdivided into two parts (middle and lower graphs, with unequal numbers of trials to avoid excessive overlap and confusion of the lines), both histograms showed peaks at similar locations. (*B*) Upper graph shows an amplitude histogram for the same EPSP as in *A* but for 700 trials nos. 1300–2000. The addition into the data set of trials 1800–2000 has resulted in a histogram with less clear peaks than for trials 1300–1800 (middle graph; same as upper graph in *A*). The histogram for the additional 200 trials (lower graph) shows rudimentary peaks, but most are not aligned with the peaks in the previous 500 trials. It seems likely that some change in the recorded fluctuation pattern occurred after trial 1800, and the inclusion of additional trials after that time tends to obscure the previous pattern.

associated field potential that may have changed in amplitude during the recording session, possibly as a result of synaptic depression during prolonged stimulation. This would cause the absolute locations of peaks in the amplitude histogram to drift with time, although their relative positions might be unaffected. Evidence for this behavior was obtained for several EPSPs. (3) *Changes in the magnitude of the charge transfer associ-*

ated with the release of a quantum of transmitter. Hippocampal synapses are eminently modifiable and "physiological" changes in efficacy could occur during the recording period. Similar changes could also result from changes in the degree of receptor desensitization caused by changes in extracellular glutamate concentration, as discussed above. Increases in glutamate levels might result from stimulation of the synapses producing the EPSP being recorded or others in the vicinity or following spontaneous activity within the slice. Glutamate levels may be particularly prone to variation in the in vitro slice preparation, where degenerating neuronal elements may release relatively large amounts of transmitter and potassium ions and where glial uptake may also be compromised (Sarantis and Attwell 1990).

Interaction between Signal and Noise

Epochs of data showing relative stability usually yielded amplitude histograms with clear, evenly spaced peaks. The heights and locations of the peaks were measured using a simple visual fitting routine. Additionally, the histograms were then analyzed using a variant of the MLE procedure described above. Most histogram peaks appeared sharper than would be predicted from the measured baseline noise. The optimization procedure was therefore repeated several times using a range of variance levels, and the solution that gave the best fit to the recorded amplitude histogram was determined using χ^2 statistics. Because the peaks within a given histogram were generally of similar sharpness, the algorithm was constrained to use the same variance for each component amplitude. For most EPSPs (25 out of 38) the optimal MLE solution gave a pattern of component amplitudes that corresponded closely to the positions and heights of the histogram peaks as measured visually (Fig. 7). The mean quantal amplitudes for these EPSPs ranged between 84 and 198 μV, with a mean of 133 μV. The spacing of the component amplitudes was fairly equal, with a mean coefficient of variation of 15%. However, the variances that gave the optimum MLE solutions were, almost without exception, lower than the variances of the corresponding measured baseline noise distributions. The mean of the measured noise s.d. values was 96 ± 39 μV, whereas the mean of the s.d. values giving optimal MLE solutions was 53 ± 17 μV. For the remaining 13 EPSPs, the optimal MLE result contained additional component amplitudes that did not match visible peaks in the amplitude histogram. In each case, one of the variance levels used did produce a solution that matched the peak locations, but a better fit to the data was obtained by using a lower variance level and including one or more additional component amplitudes. These were often of lower probability than either of their neighboring components, and usually resulted in highly unequal spacing. For these EPSPs also, the s.d. used for the optimal MLE result was lower than that of the baseline noise.

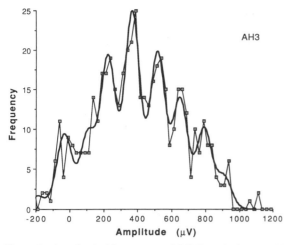

AH3

Figure 7. Amplitude histogram and MLE analysis result for the 500 trials (nos. 1300–1800) of the EPSP in Fig. 6. The square symbols show the amplitude histogram unfiltered and with a bin width of 25 μV. The mean separation between the component amplitudes of the optimal MLE solution was 137 ± 13 μV. This optimal solution was obtained assuming a S.D. of 45 μV for the distributions associated with each component amplitude, and the sum of these distributions is shown by the continuous line. The distribution of the independently measured baseline noise, however, had a S.D. of 76 μV, indicating a possible nonindependence of EPSP and noise.

These results suggest that the assumption used in the spinal cord studies that the EPSP and the baseline noise are independent cannot be made for the hippocampal EPSPs considered here. That there should be some mismatch between the noise measured in the baseline period and apparent in the amplitude histogram is perhaps not surprising, since the epochs of data used to construct the histograms were selected partly for the clarity of their pattern of peaks. The inclusion of additional trials, from either before or after the epoch selected, would result in less sharp peaks and so would require the use of a higher variance to obtain an optimal fit to the data. However, the magnitude of the mismatch in most cases argues for the operation of an additional mechanism. A possible explanation is the phenomenon of delayed or enhanced spontaneous release, as discussed above. It seems likely that such a mechanism could operate here, especially given our observation that baseline noise levels tend to increase during repetitive synaptic stimulation and decline again afterwards. The issue is whether delayed release from the small number of synapses undergoing stimulation (<20) could exert a significant effect, given the very large number of synapses potentially available to contribute to the noise (~20,000). By analyzing and simulating the recorded baseline noise, we found that the low-frequency component of the noise could arise from surprisingly low rates of spontaneous release of quanta, so that enhanced release from a small number of synapses would make a substantial difference to the overall noise level. This might only apply in cases where the level of spontaneous transmitter release had been reduced, as was done here.

Quantal Variance

The shapes of the amplitude histograms we obtained argued against the variance associated with the repeated release of quanta from a given site being high. In general, peaks corresponding to the release of several quanta were as sharp as those corresponding to the release of only one or two. Also, most histograms were fitted better using variance levels lower than the prestimulus baseline noise distribution. Nevertheless, we tried to explore the effect of including quantal variance in the analysis. The variance used for the MLE analysis was split into two components. One was constant for all discrete amplitudes, representing the contaminating noise. The other component was scaled linearly with the number of quanta associated with each discrete amplitude, representing the quantal variance. MLE optimizations were then performed for each EPSP using a range of quantal variances for each of a range of overall variances. For those EPSPs tested where the original MLE result had matched the visible histogram peaks, the optimal solutions were obtained with zero or very low levels of quantal variance (contrasting with the findings of Bekkers and Stevens [1989], for cultured hippocampal cells). However, the goodness of the fits obtained was much less sensitive to the level of quantal variance than to the overall variance level. Thus, the inclusion of some quantal variance in overall variance levels close to the optimal resulted in only slightly inferior fits. In the case of one EPSP for which the original MLE optimization result had not lined up with the visible histogram peaks, the inclusion of some quantal variance resulted in an improved fit to the data and a solution that closely matched the peaks. Thus, although the level of quantal variance in our EPSPs was generally low, the precise level may be difficult to determine and may vary between EPSPs. Our preliminary calculations indicate that the number of glutamate receptors activated by a single quantum of transmitter in the hippocampus is even lower than for the motoneuron (see above), in line with the calculations of Bekkers and Stevens (1989).

Statistical Description of Quantal Release

The use of extracellular stimulation to evoke the EPSPs in this study is not ideal. More than one fiber could have been stimulated, and the stimulation may not always have been reliable. The in vitro slice is not a perfect physiological preparation because it contains a proportion of unhealthy tissue, which makes problems such as action potential propagation failure more likely than in an intact animal. In view of these uncertainties, caution will need to be exercised in deciding whether the release probability densities for these EPSPs conformed to Poisson, simple, or compound binomial distributions. There was, however, one striking qualitative difference between the amplitude histograms we obtained as compared with the data from the spinal cord. At the frequencies of stimulation employed in this study, the smallest amplitude of the EPSPs was usually near zero, even if the mean amplitude was as much as 1 mV. Qualitatively, this means that there are few if any release sites with $p = 1$. Since the N values in this study are usually greater than 6, this would imply that, if the statistical description does prove to be of a binomial form (simple or compound), the average value of probability associated with each release site is lower than in the 1a synapse at either the motoneuron or DSCT cells. Thus, the hippocampal synapses are "set" in such a way that a greater presynaptic enhancement of synaptic efficacy could be produced by an increase in the average probability of release.

Quantal Charge and Synaptic Location

As yet, we have not systematically explored the relationship between electrotonic location of the input and the magnitude of the quantal amplitude as recorded at the soma for hippocampal neurons. Such an analysis requires an adequate electrical model of the dendritic structure of the neuron. Turner and his colleagues have made substantial progress in this area (see Turner 1988). However, given the difficulties we encountered in modeling pyramidal neurons of the visual cortex (see Jack et al. 1989; Stratford et al. 1989), it is likely that further modeling effort will be required before the quantitative allocation of electrotonic location can be performed reliably.

CONCLUDING REMARKS

The study of excitatory action in the hippocampus, although still at a very preliminary stage, has raised problems that were unexpected on the basis of studies in the spinal cord. The two major features, which had not been detected in the spinal cord studies, are the apparent lack of independence of noise and evoked EPSP (see, however, Solodkin et al. 1987, for the special case of spike-triggered averaging from intact spindle afferents) and the problem of stationarity. These problems may be particular to the in vitro slice preparation and/or to the hippocampus, but it is worth considering how they would affect the interpretation of the studies of excitation in the spinal cord. As already pointed out, the main consequence would be that (for those solutions that were found to be acceptable statistically) the quantal variance might not be negligible. The other three features of the quantal analysis of excitation in the spinal cord are unlikely to be affected. Thus, the suggestion remains that quantal charge is, in some manner, adjusted to synaptic location. It is premature to speculate whether this phenomenon will be more general, since it has only been observed for two different inputs on a single class of cell (the motoneuron). It is possible that this linear mechanism for boosting the amplitude of distally generated EPSPs will only be found in cells where the dendrites do not have significant nonlinear boosting mechanisms such as dendritic action potentials.

The other notable feature of the spinal cord studies that also needs to be explored for synapses in the brain is the statistical description of transmitter release: The evidence that neither a Poisson or simple binomial description applies for spinal cord synapses seems compelling. Although it may not be surprising that individual release sites are not all set to exactly the same probability value, this more complicated description does have an awkward implication for experimenters wishing to perform a simplified form of quantal analysis, without resolution of each component amplitude, to determine the locus of an induced change in synaptic efficacy. Experimental measures, such as the concurrent changes in the mean and variance of a distribution, do not provide sufficient information to make more than a qualitative conclusion about the nature of such changes, in particular, whether the change is due to variation in the quantal size, the average number of quanta released, or both. It therefore remains a matter of considerable importance to obtain a complete and reliable quantal analysis, taking account of the possible difficulties outlined in this paper and others that technical improvements may reveal in the future. In this way, a secure assessment of the relative, quantitative importance of pre- and postsynaptic factors contributing to changes such as long-term potentiation and depression will be made possible.

REFERENCES

Bekkers, J.S. and C.F. Stevens. 1989. NMDA and non-NMDA receptors are co-localized at individual excitatory synapses in cultured rat hippocampus. *Nature* **341**: 230.

Boyd, I.A. and A.R. Martin. 1956. The end-plate potential in mammalian muscle. *J. Physiol.* **132**: 74.

Brown, A.G. and R.E.W. Fyffe. 1981. Direct observations on the contacts made between 1a afferent fibres and alpha-motoneurones in the cat's lumbosacral spinal cord. *J. Physiol.* **313**: 121.

Brown, T.H., D.H. Perkel, and M.W. Feldman. 1976. Evoked neurotransmitter release: Statistical effects of nonuniformity and nonstationarity. *Proc. Natl. Acad. Sci.* **73**: 2913.

Burke, R.E., B. Walmsley, and J.A. Hodgson. 1979. HRP anatomy of group 1a afferent contacts on alpha motoneurones. *Brain. Res.* **160**: 347.

del Castillo, J. and B. Katz. 1954. Quantal components of the end plate potential. *J. Physiol.* **124**: 560.

Edwards, F.R., S.J. Redman, and B. Walmsley. 1976a. Statistical fluctuations in charge transfer at 1a synapses on spinal motoneurones. *J. Physiol.* **259**: 665.

———. 1976b. Non-quantal fluctuations and transmission failures in charge transfer at 1a synapses on spinal motoneurones. *J. Physiol.* **259**: 689.

Edwards, F.R., P.J. Harrison, J.J.B. Jack, and D.M. Kullmann. 1989. Reduction by baclofen of monosynaptic EPSPs in lumbosacral motoneurones of the anaesthetized cat. *J. Physiol.* **416**: 539.

Everitt, B.S. and D.J. Hand. 1981. *Finite mixture distributions*. Chapman and Hall, London.

Fatt, P. and B. Katz. 1952. Spontaneous subthreshold activity at motor nerve endings. *J. Physiol.* **117**: 109.

Finkel, A.S. and S.J. Redman. 1983. The synaptic current evoked in cat spinal motoneurones by impulses in single group 1a axons. *J. Physiol.* **342**: 615.

Harrison, P.J., J.J.B. Jack, and D.M. Kullmann. 1989. Monosynaptic EPSPs in cat lumbosacral motoneurones from group 1a afferents and fibres descending in the spinal cord. *J. Physiol.* **412:** 43.

Hartzell, H.C., S.W. Kuffler, and D. Yoshikami. 1975. Postsynaptic potentiation: Interaction between quanta of acetylcholine at the skeletal neuromuscular synapse. *J. Physiol.* **251:** 427.

Henneman, E., H.-R. Lüscher, and J. Mathis. 1984. Simultaneously active and inactive synapses of single 1a fibres on cat spinal motoneurones. *J. Physiol.* **352:** 147.

Jack, J.J.B., D. Noble, and R.W. Tsien. 1983. *Electrical current flow in excitable cells.* Clarendon Press, Oxford.

Jack, J.J.B., S.J. Redman, and K. Wong. 1981. The components of synaptic potentials evoked in cat spinal motoneurones by impulses in single group 1a afferents. *J. Physiol.* **321:** 65.

Jack, J.J.B., S. Miller, R. Porter, and S.J. Redman. 1971. The time course of minimal excitatory post-synaptic potentials evoked in spinal motoneurones by group 1a afferent fibres. *J. Physiol.* **215:** 353.

Jack, J.J.B., A.U. Larkman, G. Major, A.J.R. Mason, and K.J. Stratford. 1989. Simplified representations and compartmental modelling of cortical pyramidal neurones. *J. Physiol.* **417:** 3P.

Kuffler, S.W., J.G. Nichols, and A.R. Martin. 1984. Microphysiology of chemical transmission. In *From neuron to brain,* p.263. Sinauer, Sunderland, Massachusetts.

Kullmann, D.M. 1989. Applications of the expectation-maximization algorithm to quantal analysis of postsynaptic potentials. *J. Neurosci. Methods* **30:** 231.

Ling, L. and D.J. Tolhurst. 1983. Recovering the parameters of finite mixtures of normal distributions from a noisy record: An empirical comparison of different estimating procedures. *J. Neurosci. Methods* **8:** 309.

Lüscher, H.-R. 1990. Transmission failure and its relief in the spinal monosynaptic reflex arc. In *The segmental motor system* (ed. M.D. Binder and L.M. Mendell), p. 328. Oxford University Press, New York.

Magleby, K.L. 1987. Short-term changes in synaptic efficacy. In *Synaptic function* (ed. G.M. Edelman et al.), p. 21. Wiley, New York.

Martin, A.R. 1977. Junctional transmission. II. Presynaptic mechanisms. In *Handbook of physiology*, Section I: *The nervous system* (ed. E.R. Kandel), p. 329. American Physiological Society, Bethesda.

Mayer, M.L. 1989. Activation and desensitization of glutamate receptors in mammalian CNS. In *Ion transport* (ed. D. Keeling and C. Benham), p. 183. Academic Press, London.

Mayer, M.L. and L. Vyklicky. 1989. Concanavalin A selectively reduces desensitization of mammalian neuronal quisqualate receptors. *Proc. Natl. Acad. Sci.* **86:** 1411.

Redman, S. 1990. Quantal analysis of synaptic potentials in neurons of the central nervous system. *Physiol. Rev.* **70:** 165.

Redman, S. and B. Walmsley. 1983. The time course of synaptic potentials evoked in cat spinal motoneurones at identified group 1a synapses. *J. Physiol.* **343:** 117.

Robitaille, R. and J.P. Tremblay. 1987. Non-uniform release at the frog neuromuscular junction: Evidence of morphological and physiological plasticity. *Brain Res. Rev.* **12:** 95.

Sah, P., S. Hestrin, and R.A. Nicoll. 1989. Tonic activation of NMDA receptors by ambient glutamate enhances excitability of neurons. *Science* **246:** 815.

Sarantis, M. and D. Attwell. 1990. Glutamate uptake in mammalian retinal glia is voltage- and potassium-dependent. *Brain Res.* **516:** 322.

Sayer, R.J., M.J. Friedlander, and S.J. Redman. 1990. The time course and amplitude of EPSPs evoked at synapses between pairs of CA3/CA1 neurons in the hippocampal slice. *J. Neurosci.* **10:** 826.

Sayer, R.J., S.J. Redman, and P. Andersen. 1989. Amplitude fluctuations in small EPSPs recorded from CA1 pyramidal cells in the guinea pig hippocampal slice. *J. Neurosci.* **9:** 840.

Solodkin, M., O. Ruiz De Leon, L. Zamora, I. Jimenez, W.F. Collins III, L.M. Mendell, and P. Rudomin. 1987. Non-linear interactions between background noise and 1a single fibre EPSPs evoked in spinal motoneurones. *Soc. Neurosci. Abstr.* **13:** 1697.

Stratford, K., A. Mason, A. Larkman, G. Major, and J. Jack. 1989. The modelling of pyramidal neurones in the visual cortex. In *The computing neurone* (ed. R. Durbin et al.), p. 296. Addison-Wesley, Wokingham, England.

Tang, C.-M., M. Dichter, and M. Morad. 1989. Quisqualate activates a rapidly inactivating high conductance ionic channel in hippocampal neurons. *Science* **243:** 1474.

Titterington, D.M., A.F.M. Smith, and U.E. Makov. 1985. *Statistical analysis of finite mixture distributions.* Wiley, Chichester, England.

Trussell, L.O. and G.D. Fischbach. 1989. Glutamate receptor desensitization and its role in synaptic transmission. *Neuron* **3:** 209.

Turner, D.A. 1988. Waveform and amplitude characteristics of evoked responses to dendritic stimulation of CA1 guinea-pig pyramidal cells. *J. Physiol.* **395:** 419.

Walmsley, B. and R. Stuklis. 1989. Effects of spatial and temporal dispersion of synaptic input on the time course of synaptic potentials. *J. Neurophysiol.* **61:** 681.

Walmsley, B., F.R. Edwards, and D.J. Tracey. 1987. The probabilistic nature of synaptic transmission at a mammalian excitatory central synapse. *J. Neurosci.* **7:** 1037.

———. 1988. Nonuniform release probabilities underlie quantal synaptic transmission at a mammalian excitatory central synapse. *J. Neurophysiol.* **60:** 889.

Synaptic Transmission in Hippocampal Neurons: Numerical Reconstruction of Quantal IPSCs

C. BUSCH AND B. SAKMANN

Max-Planck-Institut für Medizinische Forschung Abteilung Zellphysiologie, D-6900 Heidelberg, Federal Republic of Germany

Most of what is known about transmission at chemical synapses derives from experiments on the peripheral synapses. The mechanism of transmitter release, as defined by the quantum hypothesis, has been discovered at the neuromuscular junction (Katz 1969). Briefly, this hypothesis states that evoked synaptic currents consist of integral multiples of a quantal current due to the liberation of transmitter in multimolecular packets containing several thousand acetylcholine (ACh) molecules. The experimental basis is the observation that end-plate potentials (EPPs) fluctuate in a quantal fashion. Fluctuation analysis and single-channel recording of ACh-activated currents subsequently have indicated that one quantum of transmitter opens about 1000–2000 postsynaptic ion channels (Katz and Miledi 1972; Anderson and Stevens 1973; Neher and Sakmann 1976). The number of channels activated by a packet transmitter is determined by the number of transmitter molecules reaching the postsynaptic receptors (Hartzell et al. 1975). The shape of the postsynaptic current generated by a quantum of ACh is mostly governed by the gating kinetics of the end-plate channels assuming that the transmitter concentration in the cleft, following the release of ACh, rises and falls in a pulse-like fashion (Magleby and Stevens 1972; Wathey et al. 1979).

In the mammalian central nervous system (CNS), experimental evidence for what determines the size and shape of quantal currents is more sparse. In most reports, clear quantal fluctuation of postsynaptic potentials or currents is not easily detectable (for review, see Redman 1990). The estimated number of channels activated by one quantum differs over several orders of magnitude. The factors determining the size, rise, and decay time of quantal synaptic currents in CNS synapses are unknown mostly because of poor amplitude resolution. This lack of resolution is largely due to the use of high-resistance intracellular pipettes and to the small size of quantal currents (see, e.g., Collingridge et al. 1984).

The resolution is greatly increased by making use of a recently developed preparation: slices of brain tissue with locally exposed neuronal somata that allow the application of patch-clamp techniques (Edwards et al. 1989). The higher resolution offered by this technique permits a more accurate measurement of size and time course of quantal events in CNS neurons in their normal environment. Granule cells in the rat hippocampus have the inhibitory synapses located on or close to their soma (Lübbers and Frotscher 1987), and the evoked inhibitory postsynaptic currents (IPSCs) can be elicited by stimulating single presynaptic neurons via a fine-tipped extracellular pipette (Sakmann et al. 1989). This preparation has provided data on size and shape of inhibitory quantal currents that is more quantitative than previously possible (Edwards et al. 1990). We have attempted here to model the postsynaptic conductance change in hippocampal granule cells when a quantum of γ-aminobutyric acid (GABA) is liberated. We have used assumptions on diffusion of GABA in the cleft and the gating mechanism of the $GABA_A$ receptor ($GABA_A R$) channel. These calculations were performed to select between different mechanisms that might govern the activation of the rather small number of postsynaptic $GABA_A R$ channels activated by a single quantum of transmitter (Sakmann et al. 1989; Edwards et al. 1990).

MEASUREMENT OF QUANTAL IPSCs IN CNS SYNAPSES

Quantal IPSCs in Hippocampal Neurons

The key for being able to resolve quantal contributions of IPSCs is the higher resolution of currents provided by using patch pipettes for the whole-cell current recording. This offers the possibility of a considerably lower access resistance to the cell interior as compared with the much higher resistance provided by conventional intracellular recording pipettes (Hamill et al. 1981). For the patch pipette technique to be applicable to CNS neurons, it was necessary to gain free access to the soma of neurons in brain slices. The relatively simple procedure that is used for the localized cleaning of somata of individual neurons in brain slices is shown schematically in Figure 1A. Cell debris and neuropil on the surface of the slice are removed mechanically by blowing extracellular solution against the surface of the slice and removing the debris by slight suction, thus exposing the soma of single neurons in the deeper layers and allowing a tight contact to be established between soma membrane and the measuring patch pipette (Fig. 1B).

A further requirement for quantal analysis of IPSCs is to stimulate a single presynaptic neuron. This is easily achieved in thin slices of hippocampal tissue (150–400 μm thickness), which allows the visualization of both

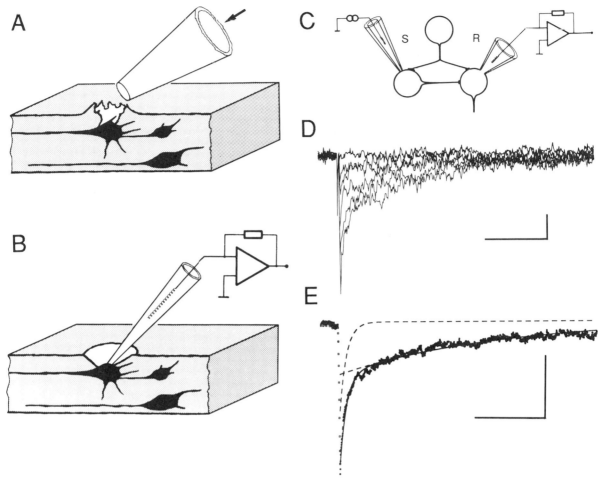

Figure 1. Measurement of quantal IPSCs in brain slices. Schematic illustration of the method of localized cleaning of brain slices (*A*) to expose neuronal somata for whole-cell recording (*B*) with patch pipettes. (*C*) Schematic diagram of the arrangement of stimulation (S) and recording (R) pipettes for measurement of stimulus-evoked IPSCs in rat hippocampal slices. Stimulus excites either the soma of a presynaptic neuron, or stimulation is via axon collaterals of another neuron. (*D*) Fluctuating peak amplitudes of successive stimulus-evoked IPSCs. (Reprinted, with permission, from Sakmann et al. 1989.) (*E*) Size and time course of quantal IPSC. Average of 40 spontaneously occurring miniature IPSCs. (From an experiment done by F. Edwards, pers. comm.) Bars: (*D*) 25 pA, 50 msec; (*E*) 10 pA, 50 msec.

the neuron recorded from and those lying nearby in the surrounding area. Neighboring neurons can be electrically stimulated via a second extracellular pipette, the tip of which is placed onto the cell soma (Fig. 1C). In many cases, unitary IPSCs were recorded that fluctuated in amplitude when the presynaptic neuron was stimulated with constant stimulus (Fig. 1D).

Size and Time Course of Quantal Currents

When the amplitude of a large number of such stimulus-evoked IPSCs was measured, amplitude histograms in 8 of 12 experiments show peaks that are equally spaced when fitted with sums of Gaussian distributions. The average peak distance in these experiments was rather small, varying between 7 and 21 pA (at -50 mV) in different experiments (Edwards et al. 1990). These experiments suggest that the release of GABA at these synapses is quantal in nature with a quantal event of relatively small size. Single-channel

recording of GABA-activated currents in patches isolated from the soma of granule cell indicated that under similar conditions, single-channel current amplitudes fall into two broad classes of about 0.7 pA and 1.2 pA average size (Edwards et al. 1990). Assuming that sub- and perisynaptic channels have the same conductance, the average sizes of the quantal event would indicate that at the peak of quantal IPSCs, about 10–30 $GABA_A R$ channels are open. This is a surprisingly small number when compared with the number of channels activated by a quantum of transmitter at the neuromuscular synapse or in the CNS of lamprey or gold fish (Gold and Martin 1983; Korn and Faber 1987). The quantal IPSCs show a characteristic time course, a fast rise to the peak with rise times smaller than 1 msec, followed by a slower double exponential decay. Figure 1E shows the average of spontaneously occurring quantal IPSCs together with two exponentials fitted to the decay time course. In summary, the experiments indicate that the quantal IPSC size is rather small, involving the opening of about 10–30 channels, has a small variability of the peak amplitude in terms of open channels, and is characterized by a fast rise time and a slower double-exponential decay time course (Edwards et al. 1990).

RECONSTRUCTION OF QUANTAL IPSCs

We have attempted to reconstruct numerically the shape and size of the quantal IPSC making use of the models proposed earlier for the reconstruction of quantal events at the neuromuscular junction (Wathey et al. 1979) but modifying them with respect to these newly described features of IPSCs and the morphology of CNS synapses. The model should simulate the fast rise time course, the small number of channels open at the peak, and the double exponential decay of quantal IPSCs. To reconstruct the quantal IPSCs, we have made several assumptions on the release process, the geometry of granule cell synapses, and the properties of $GABA_AR$ channels. In brief, the equation for diffusion of GABA from a quasi-point source into a flat open cylinder representing the synaptic cleft (Eccles and Jaeger 1958; Wathey et al. 1979) was combined with the equations describing the gating of $GABA_AR$ channels in the postsynaptic membrane by GABA.

Assumptions on the Diffusion of Transmitter

Following the considerations of Eccles and Jaeger (1958) on diffusion of transmitter out of the synaptic cleft, we assumed that GABA acts briefly by reversibly binding to $GABA_ARs$. GABA is cleared out of the synaptic cleft by delayed diffusional loss, as proposed by Wathey et al. (1979) in their reconstruction of the quantal event at the neuromuscular synapse. The diffusion coefficient for GABA was set to $3 \times 10^{-6} cm^2 sec^{-1}$ for all simulations. The following assumptions concerning the release, diffusion processes, and receptors were made in all cases: (1) The release of GABA is simulated by the instantaneous appearance of a bell-shaped transmitter cloud (initial diameter 50 nm) at the center of the cleft. (2) This cloud spreads by diffusion over the synaptic cleft (Fig. 2A,B). The number of free GABA molecules in the cleft is reduced by diffusional loss at the edge of the cleft and by binding to receptors. The interaction with the receptors "buffers" the diffusion, i.e., the diffusional loss depends on the assumptions on the receptor density and the reaction scheme for channel gating. (3) Diffusion of GABA away from the cleft occurs so rapidly that the concentration outside the cleft is zero. (4) Radial symmetry with respect to the release site and an instantaneous distribution of the transmitter over the height of the cleft is assumed; the calculations can thus be carried out in one dimension along the radius of the cleft. (5) $GABA_ARs$ are distributed homogeneously on the postsynaptic surface of the synaptic cleft, except in one type of simulation in which an inhomogeneous receptor distribution was assumed.

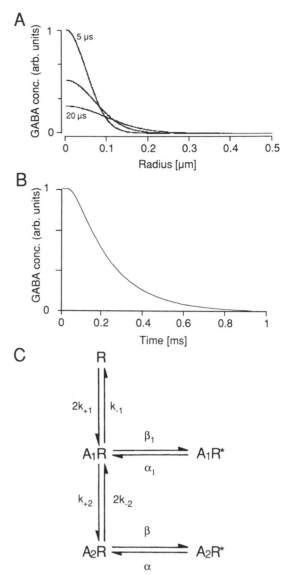

Figure 2. Diffusion of GABA in the synaptic cleft and reaction scheme describing activation of $GABA_AR$ channels. (A) Spatial density of free GABA in the synaptic cleft 5, 10, and 20 μsec after the release. The X-axis indicates distance from the release site (assumed to be at the cleft center). The concentration near the cleft center decreases rapidly as the transmitter cloud spreads over the cleft. (B) Change in amount of free GABA in the entire synaptic cleft during the first millisecond after release. (C) Reaction scheme describing interaction of GABA with $GABA_ARs$ and channel opening and closing. A represents a GABA molecule, R represents the resting $GABA_AR$, and A_1R and A_2R represent single- and double-liganded receptors. The open states of the channel are indicated by an asterisk. The conductance of the channel in the two open states is the same.

Assumptions on the Gating of $GABA_AR$ Channels

The time course of IPSC decay displays at least two time constants. This could indicate that the $GABA_ARs$ that mediate IPSCs can adopt multiple open states. We assumed that IPSCs are generated by the activation of a single class of $GABA_AR$ channels having a reaction mechanism involving three closed and two open states of the receptor. Each open state has the same conductance of 10 pS and arises from single- or double-liganded GABA$_A$Rs, respectively (Fig. 2C). For simplicity, we also assumed for all simulations that the two binding sites are independent and equivalent, that the binding step is diffusion-limited, and that the microscopic dissociation constant K_D at each site is 30 μM. The channel closing rates α and α_1 are essentially determined by the two observed IPSC decay time constants, and depending on the assumed amount of GABA in a vesicle, we have varied the channel opening rates β and β_1 such that the fast and the slow decay components have similar amplitudes (Table 1).

Numerical Methods for Reconstruction

To couple the diffusion of GABA molecules to the gating of GABA$_A$R channels, the distribution of GABA in the cleft volume was calculated for each time step. Concentrations are converted into surface densities by projecting them onto the cleft surface; the cleft height (0.05 μm for all simulations) is the scaling factor for this projection. The cleft radius (0.5 μm for most simulations) determines the scaling factor between the surface densities and the number of GABA or GABA$_A$R molecules in the cleft. With the assumed geometry, 25,000 GABA molecules in the cleft correspond to an average concentration of 1 mM and a surface density of 32,000 molecules/μm^2. Following the method of Wathey et al. (1979), the differential equations that relate diffusion, binding and channel opening are solved simultaneously by a finite-difference method on a mainframe (Convex) computer. For each time step, the densities of free and bound transmitter and of the receptor's channels in each of the five possible states were calculated using the Q-matrix method of Colquhoun and Hawkes (1977). The spatial integral of the density of open channels, multiplied by the transmembrane voltage and the single-channel conductance, yields the instantaneous current.

NUMBER OF GABA MOLECULES AND GABA$_A$Rs

At the neuromuscular junction, both the number of neurotransmitter molecules released and the number of receptors in a quantal area (Land et al. 1980) are roughly on the order of 10,000. The number of channels activated by a quantum of transmitter (1000–2000) is about 100 times higher than in the synapses we simulate here. To simulate the much smaller response, one possibility is to assume that the number of GABA molecules and the number of GABA$_A$Rs found are both reduced by a similar factor. We will refer to this model as the matched GABA/GABAR case. How large must this reduction be for the model to predict a peak response of about 20 open channels? It turned out that 400 GABA molecules (the corresponding vesicular GABA concentration is 81 mM with a vesicle diameter of 25 nm) released in a cleft with 400 receptors/μm^2 (314 receptors in the postsynaptic membrane) simulated the quantal IPSC well (Fig. 3A), but of course these values are not unique. The peak of the IPSC represents the opening of both single- and double-liganded GABA$_A$Rs. The fast IPSC decay component is caused by the faster closure of singly occupied channels, whereas the long-lasting decay component is caused by the closure of double-liganded channels (Fig. 3A). The number of free GABA molecules in the cleft decreases rapidly during the first millisecond mostly through diffusion of GABA out of the cleft (Fig. 3B). At the peak of the IPSC, the density of open channels is highest at the center of the knob opposite the release site, as expected. Predominantly, these are double-liganded channels (Fig. 3C). Even at the cleft center, i.e., opposite a release site, only about half of the available channels are opened at the peak.

With the assumption of a "matched" ratio of GABA/GABAR, the peak amplitude of a quantal IPSC varies strongly as a function of both the number of GABA molecules released and the number of

Table 1. Comparison of the Assumptions Made for the Different Numerical Reconstructions of Quantal IPCSs

Model	Low $\dfrac{\text{[GABA]}}{\text{[GABAR]}}$	Matched $\dfrac{\text{[GABA]}}{\text{[GABAR]}}$	High $\dfrac{\text{[GABA]}}{\text{[GABAR]}}$	
GABAR distribution	homogeneous	homogeneous	homogeneous	aggregated
No. GABA molecules	120 (5.1 μM)	400 (17 μM)	12,000 (0.5 mM)	2,000 (85 μM)
No. GABA$_A$R	3,927	314	25	30
k_{+1} (M^{-1} s^{-1})	10^8	10^8	10^8	10^8
k_{+2} (M^{-1} s^{-1})	10^8	10^8	10^8	10^8
k_{-1} (s^{-1})	3,000	3,000	3,000	3,000
k_{-2} (s^{-1})	3,000	3,000	3,000	3,000
β (s^{-1})	10,000	2,500	2,500	2,000
β_1 (s^{-1})	700	400	12,000	2,500
α (s^{-1})	55	30	28	30
α_1 (s^{-1})	4,000	600	2,800	700

The GABA concentrations indicated in brackets would result if the assumed number of released GABA molecules in a vesicle were distributed evenly in the cleft space that is represented by an open cylinder with a radius of 0.5 μm and 0.05 μm height. Rate constants refer to the reaction scheme shown in Fig. 2C.

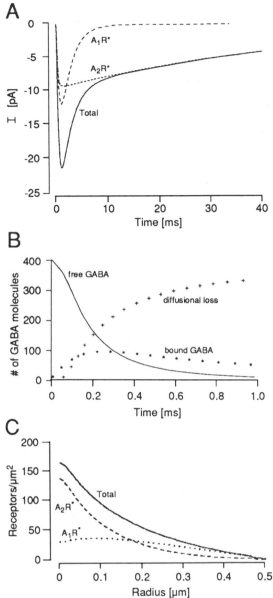

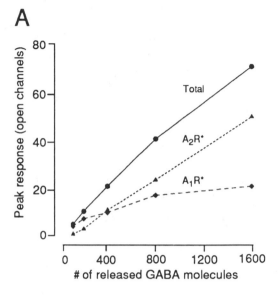

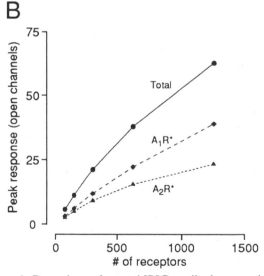

GABA$_A$Rs in the knob, and small variations in both variables have drastic effects on quantal size (Fig. 4A,B). For example, increasing the number of GABA molecules in a vesicle from 400 to 480 would increase the number of open channels from 21 to 25. Similarly, increasing the number of GABA$_A$Rs in the postsynaptic membrane from 314 to 400 would increase the number of channels open at the IPSC peak from 21 to 26.

Figure 3. Simulation of rise and decay time course of a quantal IPSC with the matched GABA/GABAR assumption. (*A*) Reconstruction of the fast rise, peak amplitude, and double exponential decay of quantal IPSC. Continuous curve represents the total current. The time from 20% to 80% of the peak response is 0.36 msec. The decay time course is fitted by the sum of two exponential components with time constants of 2.1 and 47 msec. Current mediated by single-liganded (labeled A_1R^*) and double-liganded (A_2R^*) open channels have similar amplitudes (broken lines). Model parameters are listed in Table 1. (*B*) Buffered diffusion of GABA out of the cleft. Assuming a vesicle diameter of 25 nm, the vesicular GABA concentration in this simulation is 81 mM. Continuous curve represents the change with time of the number of free GABA molecules in the cleft. Symbols indicate the change with time of GABA bound to GABA$_A$Rs (asterisk) or GABA lost by diffusion (plus). (*C*) Spatial distribution of open channels at the peak of the IPSC. The density of open channels at the peak of the response varies with the distance from the cleft center for single occupied open channels (dotted curve), double occupied open channels (dashed curve), and their sum (continuous curve). Note that double-liganded open channels are concentrated near the center of the cleft.

Figure 4. Dependence of quantal IPSC amplitude on number of GABA molecules released from a vesicle and GABA$_A$Rs in the postsynaptic membrane. Same simulation as in Fig. 3. (*A*) Dependence of the IPSC peak response on the number of released GABA molecules. This number (standard value used for the simulation shown in Fig. 3 is 400) was varied between 100 and 1600. The peak response (continuous curve) and the number of double-liganded open channels at the peak (▲) are nearly proportional to the amount of GABA, whereas the single-occupied open channels (◆) show a much weaker dependence. (*B*) Number of GABA$_A$Rs is altered by varying their density in the postsynaptic membrane between 79 and 1256/μm^2 (standard value used in the simulation shown in Fig. 3 is 314). The peak amplitude is roughly proportional to the number of receptors in the knob.

Thus, the peak amplitude of quantal IPSCs would be very sensitive to small variations of pre- and postsynaptic factors like vesicle and knob size.

Experimentally determined values for the number of GABA molecules in a vesicle or the number of $GABA_A Rs$ in the "quantal area" are not available yet for CNS synapses, and we have assumed much smaller values than those determined for peripheral cholinergic synapses to account for the much smaller size of quantal IPSCs. It seems, however, possible that only one of these variables is much smaller in the CNS synapses, and either a small number of GABA molecules could be released on a larger number of densely packed $GABA_A Rs$ (low GABA/GABAR case) or alternatively a large number of GABA molecules could be released on relatively fewer $GABA_A Rs$ (high GABA/GABAR case). We have therefore investigated whether with these assumptions, quantal IPSCs also could be reconstructed.

Small Number of GABA Molecules Released on Larger Number of $GABA_A Rs$

In this case, it was assumed that $GABA_A R$ density is $5000/\mu m^2$ corresponding to 3927 receptors in the synaptic membrane of a single knob. It was asked what is the minimal number of GABA molecules per vesicle that reproduces the observed fast rise, peak response, and time course of the IPSCs? The minimal number of GABA molecules per vesicle for which we could simulate the IPSC with a reasonable set of rate constants (see Table 1) was 120 molecules (the corresponding vesicular GABA concentration is 24 mM). As in the previous simulation, both single- and double-liganded channels are open at the peak, and the fast and slow decays are due to closure of single- and double-liganded channels (Fig. 5A, Table 1). The number of free GABA molecules in the cleft decreases rapidly due to binding to receptors, and after 0.1 msec, already 107 of the 120 released GABA molecules are bound. Binding traps GABA opposite the release site and prevents GABA molecules from leaving the cleft by diffusion (Fig. 5B). For example, after 1 msec, only 17 GABA molecules have left the cleft. Because of the high receptor density and the fact that nearly all receptors are free to bind GABA, the rebinding probability for a dissociated GABA molecule is relatively high in this model. The open channels are concentrated opposite the release site, and most of them are located within a distance of 0.1 μm from the center of the cleft (Fig. 5C). This domain comprises only 4% of the total postsynaptic area. Even at the cleft center, fewer than 20% of the available channels are open.

Large Number of GABA Molecules Released on a Smaller Number of GABARs

In this simulation, it was assumed that 12,000 GABA molecules are released per vesicle (vesicular concentration is 2.4 M), and it was investigated what would be the minimal number of postsynaptic $GABA_A Rs$ that allows reproduction of the observed IPSCs. The minimal number of $GABA_A Rs$ turned out to be 25 per knob. The two IPSC decay components reflect closure of single- and double-liganded $GABA_A Rs$ (Fig. 5D, Table 1), as in the other simulations. There is no significant reduction in GABA concentration by binding, and the transmitter is lost rapidly by diffusion out of the cleft (Fig. 5E). For example, the number of GABA molecules in the cleft is reduced to 25% of its initial value 0.34 msec after release. Figure 5F shows the spatial distribution of open channels at the peak; they are almost evenly distributed over the entire postsynaptic membrane, and their density falls off sharply at the cleft edge. In this simulation, nearly all $GABA_A Rs$ in the synaptic knob are opened with the double-liganded channels being concentrated at the center and the single-liganded channels being concentrated at the edges.

Factors Affecting Variability in Size of Quantal IPSCs

The numerical reconstructions of quantal IPSCs described above could isolate the sources of variability in quantal IPSC amplitudes. Model calculations on the detectability of quantal peaks in amplitude histograms of stimulus-evoked IPSCs have indicated that the coefficient of variation of quantal IPSC amplitudes should not exceed 15%, corresponding to a variation of only three to six channels for a quantal event, depending on the $GABA_A R$ subtype in the synaptic membrane (Edwards et al. 1990). In principle, variability of quantal IPSC peak amplitudes could arise from the release and diffusion of GABA in the cleft, the number and density of $GABA_A Rs$ in the postsynaptic membrane, and the gating mechanism itself. In the matched GABA/GABAR simulation, variability is due to both pre- and postsynaptic factors (Fig. 4A,B), whereas in the two other simulations, variability is limited to one or the other.

Amount of GABA in a Vesicle

If in the low or matched GABA/GABAR assumptions the amount of GABA in a vesicle is varied in the range from 25% to 400% of the assumed standard values (120 and 400 molecules, respectively), the change in peak amplitude is nearly proportional to the change in the number of GABA molecules. For example, in the low GABA/GABAR simulation, a difference of only 20 GABA molecules in a vesicle would change the peak amplitude by four channels. Thus, if these assumptions were true, the experimentally observed small variability of IPSCs would require that vesicle size and filling are kept constant within a very narrow range. In contrast, in the case of the high GABA/GABAR assumption, the quantal IPSC amplitude varies much less with the amount of released GABA. A 50% reduction of the amount of GABA in a

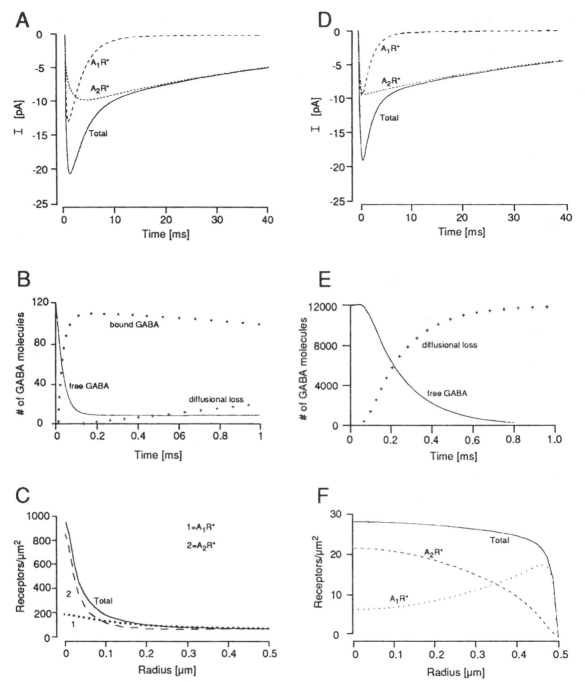

Figure 5. Comparison of simulations with "low" and "high" GABA/GABAR assumptions. The left column shows simulations with low GABA/GABAR assumption. (*A*) Reconstructed time course of quantal IPSC (continuous curve) and the time course of channels opening from single- and double-liganded receptors (broken lines). Model parameters are given in Table 1. (*B*) Slow diffusion of GABA. Vesicular GABA concentration is 21 mM. The amount of free (continuous curve) and bound (asterisk) GABA changes initially very rapidly. Because of the nearly complete binding of GABA to $GABA_A Rs$ (more than 100 of the 120 molecules are bound after 0.1 msec), the diffusional loss of GABA (plus) is slow. After 1 msec, only about 20 GABA molecules have left the cleft by diffusion. (*C*) Disk of open channels at the peak of the IPSC. The open channels (continuous curve) concentrate within a distance of 0.1 μm from the cleft center opposite the release site. This domain comprises only 4% of the cleft area. Note differences in the densities of single-liganded (dots) and double-liganded (dashes) open channels. Right column shows simulations with high GABA/GABAR assumption. (*D*) Reconstruction of quantal IPSC (continuous curve) and the change in time of open single- and double-liganded channels (broken lines). Model parameters are given in Table 1. (*E*) Time course of the change in GABA concentration in the cleft. Vesicular GABA concentration is 2.4 M. GABA is lost rapidly from the cleft by diffusion, and no significant buffering of the diffusional loss by binding to receptors occurs, since the number of GABA molecules is 500 times higher than the number of $GABA_A Rs$. After 1 msec, nearly all GABA molecules have left the cleft (plus). (*F*) Saturated knob of open channels. At the peak of the IPSC, nearly all channels in the postsynaptic membrane are open; the single-liganded (dots) and double-liganded (dashes) open channels, however, are distributed unevenly in the postsynaptic area, with the single-liganded channels predominating at the edge of the cleft.

vesicle amounting to a difference of several thousand molecules reduces the peak response by less than 10% (Fig. 6A). Thus, with the high GABA/GABAR assumption, the peak IPSC amplitude would be more or less independent of vesicle size and filling over a relatively large range.

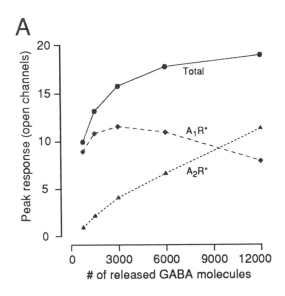

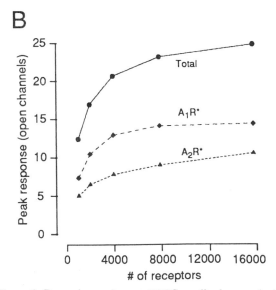

Figure 6. Dependence of quantal IPSC amplitude on vesicular GABA amount and postsynaptic GABA$_A$R channel density. (*A*) Weak dependence of quantal size on the amount of released GABA in the high GABA/GABAR simulation. 12,000 GABA molecules are released per quantum. A reduction of 50% (6000 GABA molecules) has only little effect on the peak of the IPSC; the number of single-liganded (♦) and double-liganded (▲) open channels, however, varies significantly with the amount of GABA. (*B*) Weak dependence of quantal size on receptor number in the low GABA/GABAR assumption. A 50% reduction of the receptor density (standard case assumes 5000/μm^2) reduces the peak response only by 15%.

Number of GABA$_A$Rs in a Synaptic Knob

It could also be assumed that the number of GABA$_A$Rs in the postsynaptic membrane is variable because of different GABA$_A$R densities or different knob sizes. As expected, the size of the IPSC peak amplitude varies almost linearly with the number of receptors in the high or matched GABA/GABAR assumption, and small differences in the receptor number between different knobs would cause large variations in IPSC amplitudes. The narrow distribution of IPSC peak amplitudes would then indicate a small variation in size and receptor density of different knobs. Conversely, receptor number and knob size would not be critical with the low GABA/GABAR assumption. For example, increasing the density of receptors from 5000 to 10,000/μm^2, which would double the receptor number in the quantal area, increases the number of open channels at the peak only from 20 to 23 (Fig. 6B).

AGGREGATION OF GABA$_A$Rs

The implausible features of the models described above are that the IPSC peak response depends very critically on the released amount of GABA, the number of GABA$_A$Rs, and hence the cleft radius or even both. It seems that additional assumptions are necessary. A further model that reconstructs IPSCs and in which the peak amplitude is not so critically dependent on vesicular GABA content or synapse geometry assumed that a small number of GABA$_A$Rs are concentrated in the postsynaptic area opposite the release site, in contrast with the other models that assume an even distribution of GABA$_A$Rs in the entire postsynaptic membrane. A constant and small number of clustered GABA$_A$Rs could be achieved, for example, by association of GABA$_A$Rs with cytoskeletal elements. The appearance of synapses in the electron microscope supports this assumption, since in many CNS synapses, postsynaptic densities, which could constitute receptor aggregates, are concentrated in a small area of 0.1–0.3-μm diameter opposite the presynaptic grid. For simplicity, we assume that the receptor density described is a radial-symmetrical Gaussian-shaped bell, the parameters being the number of receptors in the cluster and the standard deviation of the Gaussian. We assumed that 2000 GABA molecules are released into a standard cleft of 0.5-μm radius with an aggregate of 30 GABA$_A$Rs in the postsynaptic membrane. The profile of receptor density is bell shaped with a standard deviation of 0.1 μm (see Fig. 7B, inset). The highest receptor density (opposite the release site) is 480/μm^2 and is close to zero at a distance of 0.25 μm away from the release site. The simulated IPSC is mediated by single- and double-liganded receptors as in the other simulations (Fig. 7A). The profile of the open channels at the peak (Fig. 7B) indicates that over the whole cleft, about 70% of the available channels are opened. As expected, the dependence of the peak amplitude on the number of released GABA molecules is weak (Fig.

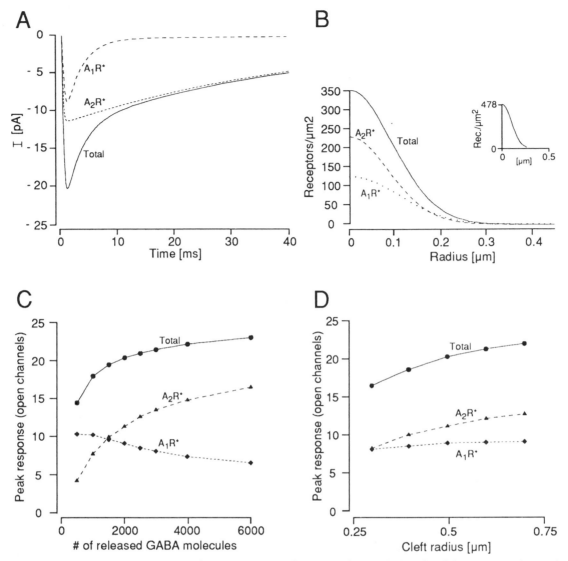

Figure 7. Simulation of quantal IPSCs assuming aggregation of GABA$_A$Rs in a small domain of the postsynaptic membrane (geometry of receptor aggregate is shown schematically in the inset of panel *B*). (*A*) Reconstruction of the time course of simulated IPSC (continuous line). As in the other models, the two IPSC decay components reflect the closure of single- and double-liganded channels (broken lines). (*B*) Distribution of open channels in the postsynaptic membrane at the peak of the IPSC. The insert shows the profile of the assumed receptor density in the GABA$_A$R aggregate opposite a release site. The X-axis of the inset indicates the distance from the cleft center. Size and structure of the GABA$_A$R aggregate do not depend on the cleft radius. At the peak of the IPSC, about 70% of the available channels are open (continuous curve). In the central domain, there are more double-liganded (A_2R^*, dashed line) channels than single-liganded ones (A_1R^*, dotted line); more than 0.1 μm away from the center, densities of single- and double-occupied open channels are similar. (*C*) Dependence of the IPSC peak response on the number of released GABA molecules. If the standard value (2000 molecules, corresponding to a vesicular GABA concentration of about 0.4 M) is halved or doubled, only slight changes in the peak response are expected. The number of single- and double-liganded channels open at the peak (labeled A_1R^* and A_2R^*, respectively) varies strongly with the amount of GABA. The peak amplitude varies little over a large range of GABA molecules. It varies strongly only if the number of GABA molecules is reduced by more than 50% of the standard value. (*D*) The dependence of the quantal IPSC peak on the cleft radius. Varying the cleft radius between 0.25 and 0.75 μm has only a relatively weak effect on the size of a quantal IPSC.

7C), and varying the number of released GABA molecules from 1000 to 4000 increases the peak response only from 18 to 22 channels. The IPSC peak amplitude is also only weakly dependent on the radius of the synaptic cleft (Fig. 7D). The small predicted dependence is mainly due to the diffusion process, since a larger cleft keeps the GABA molecules for a longer time in the cleft space because diffusion out of the receptor domain is slowed down. Hence, according to

this model, the variation of vesicle sizes as well as that of the knob sizes is not as critical as in the other three simulations to explain the small variation of the quantal IPSC peak amplitudes.

DISCUSSION

The aim of the quantal IPSC reconstructions presented here was to investigate whether the size and

time course of quantal IPSCs, as measured in hippocampal granule cells, could be simulated using simple assumptions on the diffusion of GABA in the
synaptic cleft and the gating scheme describing the
interaction of GABA with postsynaptic GABA$_A$Rs.
These reconstructions rely heavily on previous models
described for the reconstruction of a quantal event at
the neuromuscular junction (Wathey et al. 1979). It
turned out that the time course of a quantal IPSC could
be readily reconstructed using the diffusion model of
Eccles and Jaeger (1958) and a gating scheme for the
GABA$_A$R, which assumes that the channel can adopt
two open states. The small number of channels mediating quantal IPSCs prompted us to investigate, by simulations, the dependence of the size of IPSCs on the
number of GABA molecules released from a vesicle
and the number of GABA$_A$R channels in the postsynaptic membrane, since so far neither the number of
GABA molecules in a vesicle nor the density of postsynaptic GABA$_A$Rs is experimentally determined.

Determinants of IPSC Time Course

The rise time of simulated IPSCs can be reconstructed by the sequential binding of GABA to the
GABA$_A$R at two binding sites activating two open
states from the single- and double-liganded state, respectively. The double exponential decay time course
in the simulated IPSCs reflects the closing of the
GABA$_A$R channel from the two open states.

If the reaction scheme of Figure 2C applies and if the
size and variability of the IPSCs would be determined
predominantly by the amount of GABA contained in
vesicles, a larger peak amplitude of the quantal IPSCs,
caused by an increase in the number of released GABA
molecules, should occur together with an increased
relative amplitude of the slower decay component.
Thus, A_s and A_f are the amplitudes of the slow and fast
component, and the peak amplitude A_p is the sum of
the two components, a positive correlation between A_p
and A_s/A_f (see, for example, Fig. 4, matched GABA/
GABAR assumption) is expected because at the bifur-
cation $A_1R \rightarrow A_1R^*$ or $A_1R \rightarrow A_2R$, only the second
pathway is dependent on GABA concentration. If the
size and variation in the amplitude of the IPSCs are,
however, caused predominantly by variations in knob
size, the ratio A_s/A_f should vary differently with peak
amplitudes. Changing the radius of the postsynaptic
disk in the matched GABA/GABAR case from 0.4 to
0.6 μm without altering receptor density would change
the average peak amplitude changes from 15 to 28 open
channels and A_s/A_f from 1.19 to 1.0. Thus, an inverse
relation between the peak amplitude A_p and the ratio
A_s/A_f of quantal events arising from knobs with different sizes is expected. This is because of the assumption
that when the transmitter cloud reaches the edge of the
cleft, the GABA concentration is very low compared
with the central area. The larger response that a larger
knob produces is caused primarily by openings of the
single-liganded receptors, which mediate the fast decay

component. Obviously, these relations also depend on
the rate constants of the reaction scheme and would be
hardly detectable in the model assuming receptor aggregation.

Determinants of Quantal Size and Variability

The simulation assuming matched number of GABA
and GABA$_A$Rs seems unrealistic, since the peak amplitude of quantal IPSCs depends so critically on both
the GABA content of vesicles and postsynaptic geometry of synaptic knobs (Fig. 4). We therefore investigated two limiting cases in which the peak amplitude is
dependent only on either vesicle content or size of
postsynaptic area. An interesting feature of the IPSCs
reconstructed with the low GABA/GABAR assumption is that the open channels are concentrated in a disk
opposite the release site in a quantal area (Land et al.
1980) that is very small compared with the total area of
the postsynaptic membrane. Little lateral spread of
transmitter occurs during the rise time of the IPSC,
since all GABA molecules are trapped on GABA$_A$Rs
in the quantal area. It could be imagined, using this
model, that several release sites in a knob would
mediate independent quantal events if release sites
were separated by more than 0.2 μm. The finding of a
grid of release sites separated from each other by 0.08
μm in the presynaptic membrane (Akert and Pfenninger 1969) would be consistent with several release sites
per synaptic knob which, depending on their separation, would be interacting or noninteracting. The unrealistic feature of this model is, however, that the size
of quantal IPSCs is so steeply dependent on the vesicular content of GABA and hence on the vesicle diameter. For an average diameter of 25 nm, the assumed
vesicular concentration is 24 mM. The experimentally
observed variation in the peak responses would imply
that the vesicle diameter would be constant within
about 1 nm. For example, assuming 15% more GABA
molecules in a vesicle (138 molecules instead of 120)
increases the response from 20 to 24 open channels.
Under the assumption of a constant vesicular concentration, this increase in the amount of released GABA
corresponds to a difference in vesicle diameter of only
1.2 nm, i.e., less than the thickness of the vesicular
membrane.

The appealing feature of the IPSCs reconstructed
with the high GABA/GABAR assumption is that large
variations in the number of GABA molecules contained in a vesicle would not drastically affect the size
of quantal IPSCs and consequently the variability of
IPSC amplitudes because of differences in vesicle size
or filling would be low. Differences of GABA of several thousand molecules in a vesicle that could be caused
by different vesicle sizes would change the peak amplitude of quantal IPSCs by only a few channels. The
quantal size would, however, be critically dependent on
the area of the postsynaptic membrane of knobs. Assuming that GABA$_A$Rs are homogeneously distributed
and that their density is similar in different knobs, the

postsynaptic quantal area in different knobs should not differ by more than 15%, i.e., the diameter should be the same within less than 0.1 μm. In addition, it would have to be postulated that receptor density decreases abruptly at the edge of the synaptic cleft and that the perisynaptic membrane does not contain GABA$_A$Rs. This also seems an unrealistic assumption given the observation that GABA-activated currents can be recorded from patches of perisynaptic soma membrane.

The high GABA/GABAR model making the additional assumption of clustering of GABA$_A$R channels in the postsynaptic membrane can correctly reproduce the time course of quantal IPSCs, and their size is much less dependent on the geometry of vesicles and on synaptic geometry than in the other models. For example, assuming a constant vesicular concentration and a vesicle diameter of 25 nm per 2000 GABA molecules, 1000 and 4000 GABA molecules correspond, respectively, to vesicle diameters of 19.8 and 31.5 nm, i.e., a difference of nearly half the diameter of the standard vesicle. Also, a threefold increase in the radius of the synaptic knob, from 0.25 to 0.75 μm, changes the number of channels open at the peak only by four channels. At present, it seems to be the most plausible one to explain the size and variability of quantal IPSCs in hippocampal granule cell synapses. The main question remaining, however, would be how the clustering of a small and relatively constant number of GABA$_A$Rs in different synaptic knobs is achieved.

OUTLOOK

A problem of the numerical reconstructions of IPSCs is that the gating scheme for the opening of GABA$_A$R channels is, at present, not sufficiently resolved. If, however, the molecular identity of synaptic GABA$_A$Rs were known, their gating properties could be determined, for example, by using recombinant GABA$_A$Rs expressed in a host cell, and this would drastically reduce the number of assumptions to be made for IPSC reconstructions. One way to identify the molecular composition of synaptic GABA$_A$Rs would be to map the functional and pharmacological properties of recombinant GABA$_A$R subtypes in host cells (Verdoorn et al. 1990) and to investigate which of their properties can be observed in recordings of IPSCs in brain slice preparations.

In the reconstructions described above, it was also assumed that a homogeneous class of GABA$_A$Rs is present in the synaptic knobs. However, recordings of GABA-activated, single-channel currents in tissue-cultured neurons, hippocampal granule cells, as well as in transfected host cells, have also shown that GABA$_A$R channels fall into several functional subclasses. Therefore, an alternative explanation for the complex shape of IPSCs may be that it reflects the superposition of single-channel currents generated by simultaneous activation of different GABA$_A$R subtypes. In cholinergic synapses where synaptic currents with double exponential decay time courses were ob-

served (Sakmann and Brenner 1978; Fischbach and Schuetze 1980; Henderson and Brehm 1989), this indicated the presence of a mosaic of AChR channel subtypes of different molecular structure (Mishina et al. 1986). By analogy, coactivation of GABA$_A$R subtypes in the postsynaptic membrane by nerve-released GABA also could account for the double exponential decay of quantal IPSCs.

Whatever the exact determinants of size and time course of quantal IPSCs turn out to be, the small number of channels activated by a quantum of transmitter may represent a matching of synaptic input to the low conductance of the granule cell (Sakmann et al. 1989) and thus allowing a fine tuning of inhibition. The weight of a particular synaptic knob could be significantly changed, for example, by insertion of a different GABA$_A$R subtype. The small size of quantal events in hippocampal neurons seems to be ideally suited to compute, with high precision, specific patterns of electrical activity from somatic and dendritic inputs arising from only few presynaptic neurons.

REFERENCES

Akert, K. and K. Pfenninger. 1969. Synaptic fine structure and neural dynamics. *Symp. Soc. Cell Biol.* **8:** 245.

Anderson, C.R. and C.F. Stevens. 1973. Voltage clamp analysis of acetylcholine produced end-plate current fluctuations at frog neuromuscular junction. *J. Physiol.* **235:** 655.

Collingridge, G.L., P.W. Gage, and B. Robertson. 1984. Inhibitory post-synaptic currents in rat hippocampal CA1 neurones. *J. Physiol.* **356:** 551.

Colquhoun, D. and A.G. Hawkes. 1977. Relaxation and fluctuations of membrane currents that flow through drug-operated channels. *Proc. R. Soc. Lond. B Biol. Sci.* **199:** 231.

Eccles, J.C. and J.C. Jaeger. 1958. The relationship between the mode of operation and the dimensions of the junctional regions at synapses and motor end-organs. *Proc. R. Soc. Lond. B. Biol. Sci.* **148:** 38.

Edwards, F.A., A. Konnerth, and B. Sakmann. 1990. Quantal synaptic transmission in the central nervous system: A patch clamp study of IPSCs in rat hippocampal slices. (With an appendix by C. Busch). *J. Physiol.* **430:** (in press).

Edwards, F.A., A. Konnerth, B. Sakmann, and T. Takahashi. 1989. A thin slice preparation for patch clamp recordings from neurones of the mammalian central nervous system. *Pfluegers Arch. Eur. J. Physiol.* **414:** 600.

Fischbach, G.D. and S.M. Schuetze. 1980. A post-natal decrease in acetylcholine channel open time at rat end-plates. *J. Physiol.* **303:** 125.

Gold, M.R. and A.R. Martin. 1983. Characteristics of inhibitory post-synaptic currents in brain-stem neurones of the lamprey. *J. Physiol.* **312:** 85.

Hamill, O.P., A. Marty, E. Neher, B. Sakmann, and F.J. Sigworth. 1981. Improved patch clamp techniques for high-resolution current recordings from cells and cell-free patches. *Pfluegers Arch Eur. J. Physiol.* **391:** 85.

Hartzell, H.C., S.W. Kuffler, and D. Yoshikami. 1975. Postsynaptic potentiation: Interaction between quanta of acetylcholine at the skeletal neuromuscular synapse. *J. Physiol.* **251:** 427.

Henderson, L.P. and P. Brehm. 1989. The single-channel basis for the slow kinetics of synaptic currents in vertebrate slow muscle fibers. *Neuron* **2:** 1399.

Katz, B. 1969. *The release of neural transmitter substances.* Liverpool University Press, England.

Katz, B. and R. Miledi. 1972. The statistical nature of the acetylcholine potential and its molecular components. *J. Physiol.* **224:** 665.

Korn, H. and D.S. Faber. 1987. Regulation and significance of probabilistic release mechanisms at central synapses. In *Synaptic function* (ed. G. Edelman et al.), p. 57. Wiley, New York.

Land, B.R., E.E. Salpeter, and M.M. Salpeter. 1980. Acetylcholine receptor site density affects the rising phase of miniature endplate currents. *Proc. Natl. Acad. Sci.* **77:** 3736.

Lübbers, K. and M. Frotscher. 1987. Fine structure and synaptic connections of identified neurons in the rat *Fascia dentata. Anat. Embryol.* **177:** 1.

Magleby, K.L. and C.F. Stevens. 1972. A quantitative description of end-plate currents. *J. Physiol.* **223:** 173.

Mishina, M., T. Takai, K. Imoto, M. Nodi, T. Takahashi, S. Numa, C. Methfessel, and B. Sakmann. 1986. Molecular distinction between fetal and adult forms of muscle acetylcholine receptor. *Nature* **321:** 406.

Neher, E. and B. Sakmann. 1976. Single channel currents recorded from membrane of denervated frog muscle fibers. *Nature* **260:** 779.

Redman, S. 1990. Quantal analysis of synaptic potentials in neurones of the central nervous system. *Physiol. Rev.* **70:** 165.

Sakmann, B. and H.R. Brenner. 1978. Change in synaptic channel gating during neuromuscular development. *Nature* **276:** 401.

Sakmann, B., F.A. Edwards, A. Konnerth, and T. Takahashi. 1989. Patch clamp techniques used for studying synaptic transmission in slices of mammalian brain. *Q. J. Exp. Physiol.* **74:** 1107.

Verdoorn, T.A., A. Draguhn, S. Ymer, P. Seeburg, and B. Sakmann. 1990. Functional properties of recombinant rat $GABA_A$Rs depend on subunit composition. *Neuron* **4:** 919.

Wathey, J.C., M.M. Nass, and H.A. Lester. 1979. Numerical reconstruction of the quantal event at nicotinic synapses. *Biophys. J.* **27:** 145.

Excitatory Synaptic Integration in Hippocampal Pyramids and Dentate Granule Cells

P. ANDERSEN, M. RAASTAD, AND J.F. STORM

Institute of Neurophysiology, University of Oslo, Norway

Excitatory synapses on hippocampal pyramids are exclusively located to dendritic spines, usually in a 1:1 proportion. The number of spines indicates a convergence of as many as 12,000 excitatory boutons per CA1 pyramidal cell in rats. Activation of a single afferent fiber produces a unitary excitatory postsynaptic potential (EPSP) of about 150 μV, probably produced by a single quantum of transmitter. Surprisingly, in view of the large synaptic convergence, these microelectrode experiments suggest that only 100–300 synchronously active excitatory synapses are necessary to make the cell discharge. Even more astounding, whole-cell patch recording gave single fiber EPSPs of 1–4 mV, suggesting that only about ten coactive presynaptic cells are required to discharge a young CA1 cell.

The release probability is normally low but may be increased by facilitatory processes. On average, each afferent fiber has few boutons (mostly one but up to five) in contact with a given CA1 pyramid. Synapses in various parts of the dendritic tree are nearly equipotent. Excitatory postsynaptic potentials produced by neighboring synapses sum linearly, both with each other and with hyperpolarizing inhibitory potentials. Cable theoretical considerations suggest that the sum will be greater for synapses contacting the same secondary dendrite than for more distributed dendritic contacts.

Three types of inhibitory neurons provide different classes of interference. The chandelier cells terminate on the initial axons of a large number of pyramidal cells, thus capable of producing a widespread and effective inhibition. By hyperpolarizing the soma of a smaller number of cells, basket cells counteract all excitatory inputs with these cells, irrespective of synaptic location. In contrast with these two forms of global inhibition, stellate cells may cause a shunting form of inhibition at specific dendritic sites. Such local inhibition effectively removes the influence of synapses lying further distally on the same dendritic branch, whereas it has either no effect or even a certain facilitatory influence on more centrally placed inputs. After-hyperpolarization also reduces the efficiency of an excitatory synaptic drive but only for discharging neurons.

Finally, synaptic efficiency, and thereby integration, depends heavily on several activity-dependent plastic changes: facilitation, augmentation, posttetanic potentiation, and long-term potentiation, listed in order of increasing duration. The large number of factors that influence the synaptic interplay makes an individual pyramidal cell into a quite complicated calculating machine that is far more intricate than a simple switching device.

PROPERTIES OF EXCITATORY SYNAPSES IN THE HIPPOCAMPAL FORMATION

Pyramidal cells receive a large convergence of excitatory synapses, suggesting that a major task of these cells is to integrate signals coming from a variety of sources. It is often tacitly assumed that a substantial fraction of the total synaptic population must be activated to discharge the neurons. In this paper, we reexamine this question in the light of recently acquired information.

Important knowledge in this context is not only the types and number of excitatory synapses that are available for recruitment, but also the rules for their interaction and the many modulatory processes imposed on these cells, as well as their active and passive membrane properties.

The wealth of data that recently has accumulated in this area has made it evident that a single cortical pyramid is a far more complex unit than we thought a few years ago. For this reason, it may be of interest to discuss some of the factors that influence the excitatory synaptic integration in a single cortical neuron. Because so much work has been aimed at the hippocampal formation, synapses on dentate granule cells and on CA1 pyramidal cells are the topics of this paper.

Spine Synapses

Both on dentate granule cells and on hippocampal pyramidal cells, virtually all excitatory contacts are found on spines (Andersen et al. 1966). Most spines are contacted by a single bouton only (Westrum and Blackstad 1962; Harris and Stevens 1988), although some spines on dentate granule cells carry two boutons. West and Andersen (1980) estimated that each granule cell receives about 10,000 synapses, most of which are excitatory. Amaral et al. (1990) give a somewhat lower estimate: 5600 in the outer blade and 3600 for granule cells in the lower blade. On the basis of a three-dimensional reconstruction of two Golgi-impregnated guinea pig CA1 cells, Blackstad (1985) calculated the total length of the dendrites to 11,130 and 10,170 μm, respectively. If the conservative estimate of 1 spine per μm dendritic length (Wenzel et al. 1973; Andersen et al. 1987) is used, the number of spines on one cell will also be just over 10,000. An estimate of 11,000 spines was given by Amaral et al. (1990). A similar number (between 10,500 and 13,200 spines) was found by counting the number of dendritic spines in a representative sample of rat CA1 pyramidal cells filled with horseradish peroxidase (HRP) (P. Andersen, unpubl.). Consequently, hippocampal pyramidal cells probably receive the same number of boutons. In all cases, the use of sections along the dendritic segments may have caused an underestimation of the spine number because spines running transversely to the plane of section are difficult to find.

Number of Boutons per Fiber

A single fiber need not have the same probability of transmitter release at each of its en passage boutons. An open question is also how many contacts a fiber makes with an individual target cell. After filling radiatum fibers in rat hippocampal slices with HRP, the average distance between boutons in the CA1 area was measured (P. Andersen, unpubl.). Assuming a fixation shrinkage of 15%, the average interbouton distance was $7.8 + 1.8 \mu m$ (s.d., $n = 620$). There was no significant difference at different somatofugal levels of the CA1 dendritic field. For an assessment of the number of contacts per cell, the double conical dendritic tree of each CA1 pyramidal cell was imagined to be collapsed into a thin cylinder in a unicellular palisade structure. The diameter of one of these cylinders represents the width of the "private" territory of a single CA1 pyramid for its exclusive reception of afferent fibers.

Taking the average soma diameter to be $20 \mu m$ and four layers of equally sized ellipsoid somata in the pyramidal layer, the average diameter of a cylinder into which all dendritic branches of a CA1 cell could be fit would measure $20/4^{1/2} = 10 \mu m$. Thus, on average, the most likely number of contacts between a single radiatum fiber and a CA1 cell is $10/7.8 = 1.3$. For the granule cells, the diameter of the equivalent dendritic cylinder measures $5.6 \mu m$ (West and Andersen 1980), but no data exist on the interbouton distance of the perforant path fibers.

A complicating factor is the presence of multiple axons on hippocampal cells (Finch and Babb 1981; Tamamaki et al. 1984), opening the possibility for a higher number of contacts between a single cell and a target neuron than the figure given above. Unfortunately, no detailed information is available on this point.

Summation of EPSPs

Because of the large synaptic convergence on CA1 pyramidal cells, nonlinear interaction might be thought to occur. However, when spatially restricted synaptic inputs were activated simultaneously, EPSPs up to 2.5 mV summed perfectly linearly (Langmoen and Andersen 1983). The apparent deficit in the summed re-

cords that was observed with larger EPSPs could be explained by an addition of inhibitory potentials. However, for reasons of occlusion, only inputs more than 75 μm apart could be tested, leaving the possibility that nonlinear summation occurs for more closely spaced synapses. Naturally, nonlinear summation is more likely to occur when the coactivated synapses contact neighboring spines on the same secondary dendrite than when they contact different dendritic branches.

Contribution from a Single Afferent Fiber

An estimation of the amplitude of the depolarization produced in single CA1 pyramidal cell by an impulse in a single afferent fiber is not easily obtained. The main difficulty is the large amplitude of the background noise that drowns the small unitary EPSPs. An estimate of this unit size was made by constant strength stimulation of a small number of afferent fibers with intracellular recording of the resulting EPSPs. After a large number of trials, a deconvolution of the resulting amplitude histogram gave a value of about $160 \mu V$ for the unitary EPSP (Sayer et al. 1989). This value has the same order of magnitude as an earlier estimate of single fiber EPSPs in dentate granule cells ($\sim 100 \mu V$), based on amplitude variability and minimal amplitude steps (McNaughton et al. 1981).

A higher estimate ($286 \mu V$) was made by Hess et al. (1987). However, the latter investigators used a relatively small sample to construct their amplitude histograms. In addition, because of the high background noise level in the CA1 cells under standard recording conditions, there is great difficulty attached to the application of the methods of failures and variance. In combination, these factors make the latter estimation somewhat uncertain.

Recently, Sayer (1988) succeeded in measuring the amplitude of a single fiber EPSP by impaling pairs of connected CA3 and CA1 cells in slices from guinea pig hippocampus. By stimulating the CA3 neuron with intracellular pulses and by recording a large number of responses from the CA1 neuron, the average unitary EPSP was found to be $131 \mu V$ (range $30-665 \mu V$) in a sample of seven cells.

Whole-cell Patch Recording

Using a recently available technique for whole-cell patch recording in brain slices (Edwards et al. 1989), we have recorded spontaneous and electrically induced excitatory postsynaptic currents (EPSCs) from CA1 hippocampal neurons in young rats (5–20 days). Inhibitory currents were blocked by 5–10 μM bicuculline chloride.

Without stimulation, voltage clamp recordings showed apparently randomly occurring, spontaneous, inward currents superimposed on the background noise. The spontaneous currents had amplitudes of up to 20 pA, rise times of 2–16 msec, and half decay times of 15–50 msec. Since they were blocked by 10 μM tetrodotoxin (TTX) or by 10 μM CNQX, they are probably synaptic currents generated by spontaneously discharging presynaptic neurons.

Inward currents of the same time course and amplitude (2–20 pA) could also be elicited by electrical stimulation of afferent fibers (Fig. 1). At specific positions and certain critical stimulation strengths, they sometimes appeared in an all-or-none fashion. More often, the response jumped between the baseline level (failures) and a set of current values, suggesting that a small number of afferent fibers were stimulated intermittently (Fig. 1). The individual responses differed in both latency and amplitude, but the rise times were similar. Because these evoked elementary currents had the same range of amplitude, rise time, and half decay time as the spontaneous currents, we interpret each of them as being due to the synaptic effect of a single afferent fiber.

Regarding the considerable variability of the observed elementary currents, there are several possibilities (Fig. 2). On the presynaptic side, there are three possible explanations for the observed variability: (1) Apart from a number of failures, the stimuli may randomly excite one member at a time of a small number of equally excitable fibers (Fig. 2C: fiber 1, 2, and 3);

(2) alternatively, a single, regularly excited fiber may have several contacts on the same target cell (Fig. 2A, a, b, and c), each with its own release probability; and (3) a third possibility is that the regularly excited single fiber with a single bouton (Fig. 2B) releases a variable amount of transmitter per trial. In addition, several postsynaptic factors may influence the variability of the synaptic currents.

Further evidence that a single or a small number of fibers were stimulated under these conditions was obtained when a stimulating electrode was moved in regular steps at right angles to the fiber direction. Points from which no response could be elicited were flanked by positions from which elementary synaptic currents were elicited. The transition was often abrupt, occurring by a movement of 5–10 μm only.

Large Elementary Synaptic Potentials with Patch Recording in Young Rats

To test the potency of single excitatory synapses, we initially elicited elementary excitatory currents in CA1 and dentate granule cells under voltage clamp with just threshold stimulation as described above. With identical stimulation parameters, but under current clamp

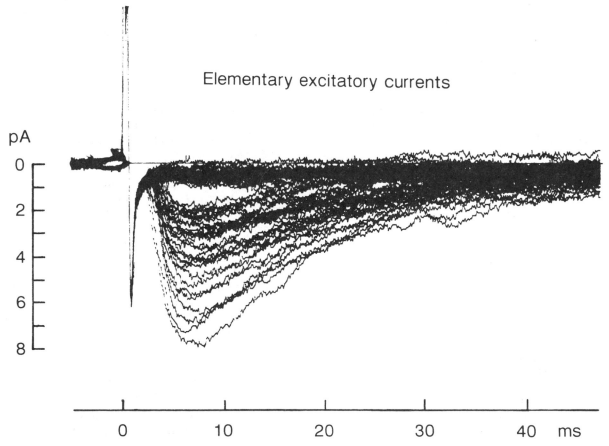

Figure 1. Excitatory synaptic currents recorded from a dentate granule cell in response to a weak but constant strength stimulation of medial perforant path fibers. In addition to a large number of failures, there are a number of discrete responses that have similar rise times but varying amplitudes and start latencies.

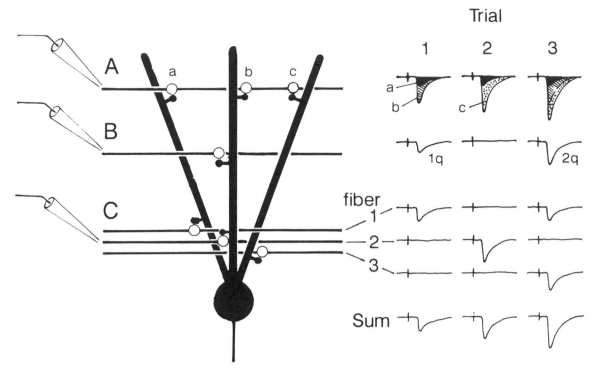

Figure 2. Diagram of possible mechanisms for the variability of the elementary excitatory currents evoked by weak stimulation of afferent fibers to a dentate or hippocampal neuron. The left half gives three possible synaptic arrangements, whereas the right side illustrates possible corresponding responses to three sequential stimuli (1–3). (*A*) A single fiber may have several contacts (a, b, c) with individual probabilities of transmitter release. To the right, the contribution from the various boutons are indicated by different shadings. (*B*) A fiber may have a single contact that releases a variable number of transmitter quanta, in sequence: 1, 0, 2. (*C*) The stimulating electrode may excite a small bundle of fibers so that either a few or none of them is excited. Fiber 1 is excited in trials 1 and 3, fiber 2 is only excited in trial 2, and fiber 3 is excited only in trial 3. The variability of the summed postsynaptic response seen below is due to the number of stimulated fibers and to the amplitude of the individual excitatory currents.

conditions, the elementary synaptic potentials in both cell types typically contributed from 1 to 4 mV and had a duration of about 200 msec in cells from 5–20-day-old rats.

When a short tetanic stimulation (3–10 stimuli at 100 Hz) was delivered at threshold strength for a single excitatory event, the build-up of the summated EPSPs often triggered an action potential, usually after 3–6 stimuli. This was seen both at moderately depolarized conditions and, in nearly half the cases, when the cell was maintained at a normal resting potential. The amplitude growth was due partly to summation of the long-lasting EPSPs and partly to facilitation of the participating EPSPs. Thus, a short tetanic activation at a strength that activates a small number of afferent fibers is able to bring the cell to discharge. In fact, it appears as a possibility that a single fiber should be able to do the same, provided the elementary EPSC elicited by that fiber belongs to the larger of the range in question, i.e., measuring 10–20 pA.

The remarkable effectiveness of a single fiber input indicated by these results seems to depend on the high input resistance of cells recorded with the patch technique. Thus, whole-cell patch recording gave considerably higher input resistance and membrane time constant than penetrating microelectrodes normally show.

For CA1 pyramidal cells and patch electrodes, the mean value of the R_{in} was from 0.5 to 1 GΩ and for the membrane time constant 60–100 msec. The corresponding values for the dentate granule cells were 0.7–2 GΩ and 50–140 msec. These values are about ten times larger than those usually obtained with penetrating microelectrodes. Consequently, the EPSPs were much larger and more prolonged than seen with conventional recordings.

Although the reason for the different input resistance obtained with the two recording techniques is not fully understood (Storm 1990), we believe that the patch clamp data are reliable, partly because the high R_{in} could be recorded within 100 msec of establishing the whole-cell configuration and also because it remained unchanged for the duration of the recording (usually 30–60 minutes).

How Many Synapses Are Needed to Discharge a Pyramidal Cell?

Two methods have been used to calculate the degree of synaptic convergence necessary to discharge the neuron: (1) estimation of the number of functional fibers in an intact fiber strand left by a near-total deafferentation, which by stimulation is able to discharge most pyramidal cells in the target area and (2) calculation of the ratio between the amplitude of an EPSP at spike threshold and the amplitude of a single fiber EPSP.

After progressively larger lesions of afferent fibers in stratum radiatum were made in hippocampal slices in guinea pigs, the smallest remaining tissue bridge that gave effective activation of all cells when stimulated was about 30–35 μm thick (Andersen et al. 1980; Sayer et al. 1989). The combined thicknesses of stratum radiatum and oriens, where the excitatory synapses are found, measure about 750 μm. Assuming evenly distributed fibers, the strand originally contained about 4% of the total amount of afferent fibers to CA1. A good deal of the fibers in the strand were probably damaged by the shearing forces of the razor blade chips used for making the microlesion; thus, an estimate was made that only about half of the fibers originally present were functionally active. In this case, the required number of activated synapses should lie around 2% of the total or about 240.

A second method starts with the average amplitude of an EPSP at the threshold for action potential generation (discharge probability of 0.5). From a large number of cells in rat hippocampal slices, the threshold EPSP value lies around 12–15 mV. Because this potential is the sum of EPSPs produced by individual fibers, the number of the latter can be found if we know the average amplitude of single fiber EPSPs. If we assume a mean value of 150 μV (Sayer 1988; Sayer et al. 1989), a minimal number of 15/0.15 = 100 synchronously active afferent fibers seem to be required to drive a CA1 pyramidal cell synaptically. Thus, these two methods give estimates of 100–240 synapses, which is only 1–2% of the total number of excitatory synapses.

An Estimate of the Smallest Effective Synaptic Convergence

The findings with whole-cell patch recording represent a down-regulation of the afferent fibers thought necessary to bring about cell discharge from a normal membrane potential. After the estimates referred to above, the revision suggested by the patch recording experiments is surprising. Given single fiber EPSPs of 1–4 mV, a reasonable estimate may be around 10 in these young cells. Although only a few afferent fibers seem necessary to drive one of the cells in question under the experimental circumstances, the input resistance may be lower in older preparations because of the conductances activated by the heavier synaptic bombardment.

The small degree of synaptic recruitment needed invites speculation about the consequences of the large synaptic convergence found on cortical neurons and, in fact, the need for this convergence. Assuming 10 as the minimal number of synchronously active fibers to cause a cell discharge and 100 as a usual figure, logically, the cell could be described as a set of AND gates, each with 10–100 input lines. Because each such assemblage of coactive fibers is able to drive the cell, the 10,000 afferents may be organized as 100–1000 AND gates feeding into a single OR gate. However, to bring about a cell discharge does not require that the same fibers are active each time. In fact, the high input resistance of some cells makes them more electrotonically compact than earlier estimates. Hence, the cable attenuation due to dendritic location of the synapses will be smaller than hitherto thought (Turner 1984, 1988). Thus, any congregation of 10–100 synchronously active fibers would do, thereby relaxing the requirement for synchrony of the CA3 neurons in order to drive the target CA1 cells.

Another scenario is that the recorded currents represent the larger events of a wide distribution and that the vast majority of excitatory synapses are either silent or produce currents so small that they drown in the background noise. A further conjecture is that such silent synapses may be in a dormant state to be brought into a more efficient state during learning and other types of activity-dependent modulation.

ACKNOWLEDGMENTS

We thank our colleagues Drs. Theodor Blackstad, Hu Guo-Yuan, Øivind Hvalby, Iver Langmoen, Stephen Redman, Rodney Sayer, and Mari Trommald for their collaboration, on which much of our review is based. The work was supported by the Norwegian Medical Research Council (RMF/NAVF) grant 326.88.007.

REFERENCES

Amaral, D.G., N. Ishizuka, and B. Claiborne. 1990. Neurons, numbers and the hippocampal network: Understanding the brain through the hippocampus. *Prog. Brain Res.* **83:** 1.

Andersen, P., T.W. Blackstad, and T. Lømo. 1966. Location and identification of excitatory synapses on hippocampal pyramidal cells. *Exp. Brain Res.* **1:** 236.

Andersen, P., T. Blackstad, G. Hulleberg, J.L. Vaaland, and M. Trommald. 1987. Dimensions of dendritic spines of rat dentate granule cells during long-term potentiation (LTP). *J. Physiol.* **390:** 264P.

Andersen, P., H. Silfvenius, S.H. Sundberg, and O. Sveen. 1980. A comparison of distal and proximal dendritic synapses on CA1 pyramids in guinea-pig hippocampal slices *in vitro*. *J. Physiol.* **307:** 273.

Blackstad, T.W. 1985. Laminar specificity of dendritic morphology: Examples from the guinea pig hippocampal region. In *Quantitative neuroanatomy in transmitter research* (ed. L.F. Agnati and K. Fuxe), p. 55. Macmillan, London.

Edwards, F.A., A. Konnerth, B. Sakmann, and T. Takahasi. 1989. A thin slice preparation for patch clamp recordings from neurones of the mammalian central nervous system. *Pfluegers Arch. Eur. J. Physiol.* **414:** 600.

Finch, D.M. and T.L. Babb. 1981. Demonstration of caudally directed hippocampal efferents in the rat by intracellular injection of horseradish peroxidase. *Brain Res.* **214:** 405.

Harris, K.M. and J.K. Stevens. 1988. Study of dendritic spines by serial electron microscopy and three-dimensional reconstructions. In *Intrinsic determinants of neuronal form and function* (ed. R.J. Lasek and M.M. Black), p. 179. A.R. Liss, New York.

Hess, G., U. Kuhnt, and L.L. Voronin. 1987. Quantal analysis of paired-pulse facilitation in guinea pig hippocampal slices. *Neurosci. Lett.* **77**: 187.

Langmoen, I.A. and P. Andersen. 1983. Summation of excitatory postsynaptic potentials in hippocampal pyramidal cells. *J. Neurophysiol.* **50**: 1320.

McNaughton, B.L., C.A. Barnes, and P. Andersen. 1981. Synaptic efficacy and EPSP summation in granule cells of rat fascia dentate studies in vitro. *J. Neurophysiol.* **46**: 952.

Sayer, R.J. 1988. "Synaptic transmission between CA3 and CA1 neurones in the guinea pig hippocampal slice." Ph.D. thesis, Australian National University, Canberra.

Sayer, R.J., S.J. Redman, and P. Andersen. 1989. Amplitude fluctuations in small EPSPs recorded from CA1 pyramidal cells in the guinea pig hippocampal slice. *J. Neurosci.* **9**: 840.

Storm, J.F. 1990. Why is the input conductance of hippocampal neurons impaled with microelectrodes so much higher than when giga-seal patch pipettes are used? *Soc. Neurosci. Abstr.* **15**: (in press).

Tamamaki, N., K. Watanabe, and Y. Nojko. 1984. A whole image of the hippocampal pyramidal neuron revealed by intracellular pressure-injection of horseradish peroxidase. *Brain Res.* **307**: 336.

Turner, D.A. 1984. Conductance transients onto dendritic spines in a segmental cable model of hippocampal neurons. *Biophys. J.* **46**: 85.

———. 1988. Waveform and amplitude characteristics of evoked responses to dendritic stimulation of CA1 guinea-pig pyramidal cells. *J. Physiol.* **395**: 419.

Wenzel, J., W. Kirsche, G. Kunz, H. Neumann, M. Wenzel, and E. Winkelmann. 1973. Licht- und elektronenmikroskopische Untersuchungen uber die Dendritenspines an Pyramiden-Neuronen des Hippocampus (CA1) bei der Ratte. *J. Hirnforsch.* **13**: 387.

West, M.J. and A.H. Andersen. 1980. An allometric study of the area dentata in the rat and mouse. *Brain Res. Rev.* **2**: 317.

Westrum, L.E. and T.W. Blackstad. 1962. An electron microscopic study of the stratum radiatum of the rat hippocampus (regio superior, CA_1) with particular emphasis on synaptology. *J. Comp. Neurol.* **119**: 281.

Physiological Properties of Excitatory Synaptic Transmission in the Central Nervous System

S. HESTRIN,* D.J. PERKEL,* P. SAH,† T. MANABE,† P. RENNER,† AND R.A. NICOLL*†

*Departments of *Physiology and †Pharmacology, University of California, San Francisco, California 94143-0450*

Excitatory synapses are the most common type of synapse in the brain. Although it had long been suspected that glutamate might be the transmitter at these synapses, it is only recently with the development of selective glutamate receptor antagonists that this issue has been clearly settled. Electophysiological analysis of excitatory synapses has been difficult for a number of reasons: (1) The reversal potential is far removed from the resting potential, (2) the synapses are located on dendrites at various electrotonic distances from the recording site, and (3) the synaptic potentials are often voltage-dependent. The introduction of whole-cell recording techniques to brain slices (Barnes and Werblin 1986; Blanton et al. 1989; Coleman and Miller 1989; Edwards et al. 1989) offers considerable advantages to the analysis of excitatory synaptic action. In this paper, we summarize some of our results obtained by applying this technique to excitatory synapses recorded in the hippocampus and cerebellum.

EXPERIMENTAL PROCEDURES

The experimental procedures used in this work have been described in detail elsewhere (Barnes and Werblin 1986; Edwards et al. 1989; Hestrin et al. 1990b; Perkel et al. 1990).

RESULTS AND DISCUSSION

Dual Component EPSC Recorded in Hippocampal Pyramidal Neurons

We have studied the pharmacological and biophysical properties of the excitatory postsynaptic current (EPSC) in the CA1 region of the rat hippocampus. In these studies, we have used the whole-cell patch clamp technique to record from pyramidal neurons in thin ($\sim$ 100–250 μm) slices (Hestrin et al. 1990b). The purpose of these studies was to show that the whole-cell recording technique preserves synaptic physiology and to obtain a rigorous characterization of the time course and voltage dependence of the N-methyl-D-aspartate (NMDA) and non-NMDA receptor-mediated EPSC evoked by stimulating Schaffer collateral-commissural afferents in stratum radiatum. Another purpose of these studies was to test the adequacy of the voltage-clamp to control the synaptic membrane potential in pyramidal neurons with extended dendritic structure.

The input impedance of the cells from which we recorded was in the range of 200–900 MOhms. Under voltage clamp, small voltage steps produced capacitative transients that could be fitted with the sum of two exponential functions as expected for a cell with an extended dendritic structure. EPSCs could be evoked by stimulating the Schaffer collateral-commissural fibers. These EPSCs were graded in size with respect to stimulus strength ranging from about ten to several hundred pA, depending on the stimulus strength. The noise level of this recording technique allows the detection of EPSCs as small as about 5 pA.

EPSCs recorded over a range of membrane potentials are illustrated in Figure 1. When the cell is clamped at −100 mV, the EPSC decays with a single fast-time constant. However, at more depolarized membrane potentials, a second, slow component measured at the peak of the response is linear (Fig. 1B), whereas the slow component measured 25 msec after the peak has a region of negative slope (Fig. 1B).

The effect of the selective NMDA antagonist D,L-2-amino-5-phosphonovalerate (APV) is illustrated in Figure 2A. At a holding potential of −80 mV, APV had little effect, whereas at more depolarized potentials, it blocked the slow component of the EPSC. Conversely, application of the selective non-NMDA antagonist 6-cyano-7-nitroquinoxaline-2,3-dione (CNQX) blocked the EPSC at a holding potential of −80 mV while removing the fast component without effect on the slow component at more depolarized potentials (Fig. 2B).

These results show that the whole-cell recording technique can be used to analyze the properties of the EPSC in pyramidal neurons. However, since the synaptic contact is known to be on dendritic spines, which could be electrically remote from the soma, it is important to determine to what extent the synaptic membrane could be controlled. We found that the adequacy of the voltage clamp depends on the distance of the synapse from the soma. In Figure 3B, the non-NMDA EPSCs from 61 different synapses, located at different distances from the somata, are plotted. We found that, for "near" EPCs that exhibited a rapid rising phase, the decay time constant of the non-NMDA EPSC could be measured accurately. In contrast with "far" synapses, which exhibited a slow rising phase, the decay of the EPSC reflects the electrotonic filtering effect of the dendrites. We have tested the adequacy of the voltage control in near synapses in several ways: (1) We

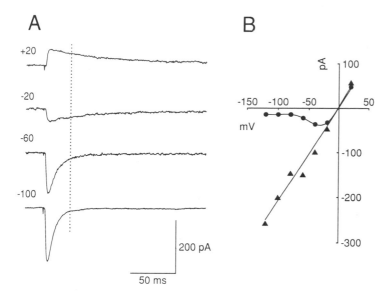

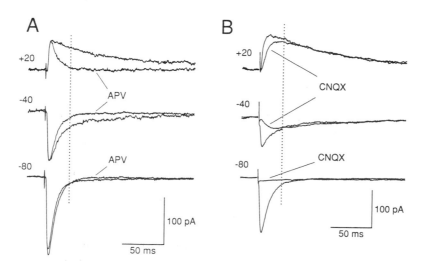

Figure 1. Voltage-dependent properties of the hippocampal EPSC. (*A*) The EPSC was recorded at the indicated membrane potentials. (*B*) The currents measured at the peak of the EPSC (▲) and at 25 msec after the peak (●, dotted line in *A*) are plotted in relation to the membrane potential. (Reprinted, with permission, from Hestrin et al. 1990b.)

showed that the reversal potential for both components and the shape of the I/V relation of the NMDA component corresponds to those expected from single-channel measurements, and (2) we showed that if we change the membrane potential during the decay phase of the EPSC, the response to the voltage step is faster than the EPSC decay, indicating that the synaptic membrane is under dynamic control (see Hestrin et al. 1990b).

Using paired recording in the spinal cord of *Xenopus* embryos, Dale and Roberts (1985) showed that NMDA and non-NMDA components could be segregated. However, in cultured hippocampal neurons, approximately 70% of miniature EPSCs were found to have both NMDA and non-NMDA components, indicating that in this system, the release of a single quantum of transmitter has access to both types of receptors (Bekkers and Stevens 1989). The situation in

the adult hippocampus is unclear. It is conceivable, for instance, that entirely segregated fiber tracts, or interneurons, could preferentially activate one set of receptors. To address the issue of colocalization of receptors, we have compared the relative contribution of NMDA and non-NMDA components with EPSCs evoked with just suprathreshold stimulation to EPSCs evoked with considerably stronger stimulation. If a substantial fraction of synapses had only one receptor subtype present, one would expect differences in the relative contributions with different stimulus strengths. However, EPSCs obtained at different stimulus strengths maintained the same relative contributions of the NMDA and non-NMDA components (Fig. 4A). This result is consistent with colocalization of receptors at a substantial number of synaptic boutons. Moreover, we found that the miniature EPSCs recorded in the

Figure 2. Pharmacological separation of two components to the EPSC. (*A*) The effect of APV. The EPSC was recorded before and during the application of 50 μM DL-APV at the indicated membrane potentials. (*B*) The effect of CNQX. The EPSC was recorded before and during the application of 10 μM CNQX at the indicated membrane potentials. (Reprinted, with permission, from Hestrin et al. 1990b.)

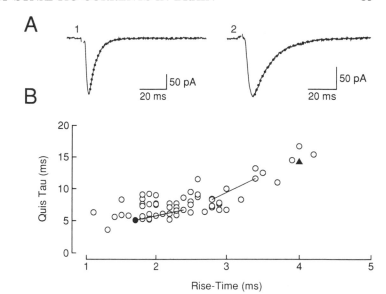

Figure 3. Kinetics of the quisqualate components. (*A*) EPSCs recorded from two neurons at −90 mV. The rise times (10–90%) were 1.7 msec (*A1*) and 4.0 msec (*A2*). The dotted lines were single-exponential fits with time constants of 5 (*A1*) and 14 msec (*A2*). (*B*) The rise times are plotted against the decay time constants of the quisqualate components measured from 61 synapses. (●, ▲) The EPSCs shown in A1 and A2, respectively. The continuous lines in *B* indicate values obtained from the same cells at near and far synapses. (Reprinted, with permission, from Hestrin et al. 1990b.)

absence of added Mg^{++} were composed of both an APV-sensitive and an APV-insensitive component (Fig. 4B). Thus, our data suggest that in CA1 pyramidal cells, both evoked and spontaneous EPSCs are mediated by colocalized receptor subtypes.

Given the marked difference in time course for the NMDA and non-NMDA components of the EPSC, one might expect them to behave quite differently during repetitive stimulation. When pyramidal neurons were held at −100 mV and the afferents were stimulated at a rate of 25 Hz, the resulting EPSCs exhibited little summation or change in amplitude (Fig. 5, top). How-

ever, at a holding potential of −40 mV, the EPSCs summated dramatically and exhibited significant depression (Fig. 5, bottom). Since the EPSCs recorded at −100 mV, which are mediated by non-NMDA receptors, do not exhibit summation or depression, these properties observed at −40 mV must be mediated postsynaptically by the NMDA receptors. The marked summation of the NMDA component will have at least two consequences. In the unclamped cell, repetitive stimulation will quickly depolarize the cell and unblock the NMDA receptors, and if the NMDA receptors are not saturated at a single bouton, more NMDA re-

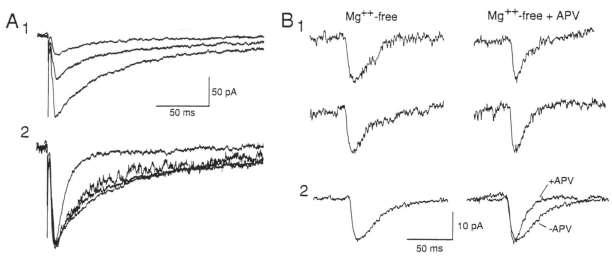

Figure 4. Colocalization of NMDA and non-NMDA receptors. (*A*) Comparison of the relative contribution of NMDA- and non-NMDA-mediated components to the EPSC at different stimulus strengths. The cell was held at −40 mV, and in *A1,* EPSCs evoked at three different stimulus strengths were recorded. Each record is an average of 40 trials. In *A2,* the three records have all been scaled to the peak of the response. In addition, the EPSC evoked at −80 mV, which results entirely from the activation of non-NMDA receptors, is superimposed. It can be seen that the slow NMDA components of the EPSCs are virtually superimposable (S. Hestrin et al., unpubl.). (*B*) Comparison of decay of sucrose-evoked miniature EPSCs recorded in Mg^{++}-free solution with and without APV. *B1* shows two representative examples, and *B2* is the average of five events. For comparison, the trace in APV also has superimposed the trace obtained in the absence of APV (T. Manabe et al., unpubl.).

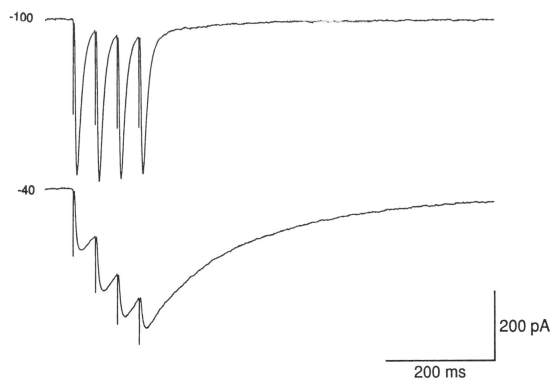

Figure 5. Effect of repetitive stimulation on the NMDA and non-NMDA components of the EPSC. The cell was initially held at −100 mV and stimulated repetitively. The cell was then held at −40 mV, and the stimuli were repeated (S. Hestrin et al., unpubl.).

ceptors on the spine will be activated. Both of these effects would explain why repetitive stimulation is so effective in inducing long-term potentiation (LTP).

EPSC Recorded in Hippocampal Interneurons

Apart from the pyramidal neurons, several types of interneurons are known to be present in the CA1 region of the hippocampus (Cajal 1911; Lorenté de Nó 1934). Whereas the synapses made by the Schaffer collateral-commissural afferents are on the dendritic spines of pyramidal neurons, synapses of the same afferents onto interneurons are made directly onto the dendritic shaft, which is aspiny (Seress and Ribak 1985). Thus, this system can be used to ask whether the structure of the dendritic spines plays a role in the physiological properties of the EPSC (Sah et al. 1990).

We have identified interneurons, as such, by their location outside the cell layer, their nonpyramidal somata, their lack of a main apical dendrite, and their morphology as seen with Lucifer Yellow epifluorescence. We found that the EPSC onto interneurons consists of an NMDA and non-NMDA components, which are quantitatively very similar to those recorded from pyramidal neurons in the same region. These data suggest that the local geometry of the synapse and the dendritic spine in particular do not play an important role in shaping the EPSC. These results also corroborated our previous conclusion that, for synapses within a short distance from the soma, the recorded EPSC

decay reflects the conductance change at the synapse and is not appreciably filtered by the spine or the dendritic cable.

A Single-component EPSC Recorded in Purkinje Cells

The dual-component EPSC found in the hippocampal CA1 region is generally similar to the EPSC found in other central nervous system regions (for review, see Collingridge and Lester 1989; Nicoll et al. 1990). Purkinje cells receive two types of excitatory inputs: one from inferior olivary climbing fibers and the other from parallel fibers originating from cerebellar granule cells (Eccles et al. 1967; Ito 1984). It has been reported that both EPSCs might be mediated by a single, non-NMDA receptor type (Hirano and Hagiwara 1988; Kano et al. 1988; Garthwaite and Beaumont 1989; Konnerth et al. 1990). However, the receptor type(s) mediating these EPSCs remains uncertain, and it has been suggested that NMDA receptors might mediate the climbing fiber EPSC (Kimura et al. 1985).

We have addressed the question of receptor type using the whole-cell recording technique in combination with the selective NMDA receptor antagonist APV and the selective non-NMDA receptor antagonist CNQX (Perkel et al. 1990). To improve the detectability of a possible NMDA receptor-mediated component, we perfused the cerebellar slices with nominally Mg^{++}-free Ringer's solution and examined the EPSC at a

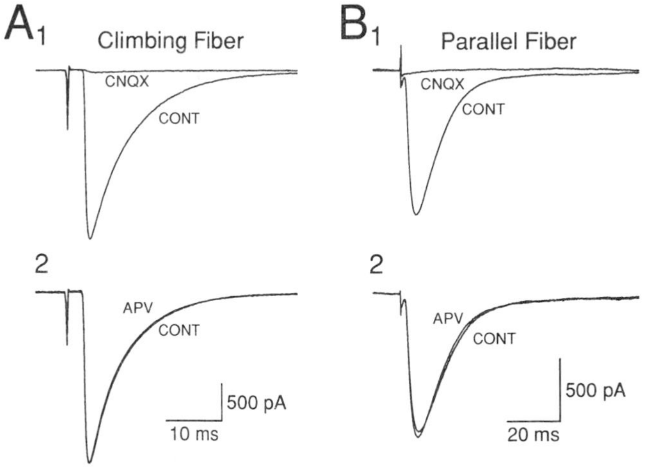

Figure 6. Pharmacological properties of synaptic currents evoked by climbing-fiber and parallel-fiber stimulation in the cerebellum. (*A*) The climbing-fiber EPSC was blocked by CNQX (*A1*) and was not affected by APV (*A2*). *A1* shows superimposed responses in control solution (CONT) and in solution containing 10 μM CNQX. *A2* illustrates superimposed EPSCs in the same cell in control solution (CONT) and in solution containing 50 μM DL-APV. (*B*) Effects of CNQX (*B1*) and APV (*B2*) on parallel-fiber EPSCs in a different Purkinje cell. Same conventions and concentrations as in *A*. (Reprinted, with permission, from Perkel et al. 1990.)

range of membrane potentials. Under these conditions, we found that the application of 10 μM CNQX reduced the climbing fiber EPSC by more than 95% and completely blocked the parallel fiber EPSC (Fig. 6A1,B1). In contrast, perfusion of the slices with DL-APV (50 μM) had no effect on the synaptic currents of either type (Fig. 6A1,B1).

Although these results indicate that synaptically released transmitter does not have access to NMDA receptors, they do not rule out the possibility that extrasynaptic NMDA receptors may be present on Purkinje cells. We have examined this question by applying NMDA (10–100 μM) to the bath while Purkinje cells were held at −40 mV or bathed in Ringer's solution containing no added Mg^{++}. Under these conditions, we did not observe any NMDA-evoked current. On the other hand, bath application of glutamate or aspartate did result in the generation of a large current. However, this current was essentially blocked by CNQX. From these results, we have concluded that both parallel-fiber and climbing-fiber EPSCs are mediated by non-NMDA-type receptors and that NMDA receptors are not present on Purkinje cells at synaptic or extrasynaptic sites.

Mechanisms Generating the Time Course of the Dual-component EPSC

In the pyramidal neurons of the hippocampal CA1 region, the non-NMDA component of the EPSC lasts for only a few milliseconds, whereas the NMDA component requires several milliseconds to reach the peak and lasts for more than 100 msec (Collingridge et al. 1988a; Forsythe and Westbrook 1988; Hestrin et al. 1990b). The slow time course of the NMDA component is surprising given that both receptor types are activated by transmitter release from the same nerve terminal (see Fig. 4B) (Bekkers and Stevens 1989). We considered two models to explain the time course of the NMDA component: (1) Effective transmitter concentration rises and falls slowly; and (2) transmitter concentration increase is brief, but NMDA channel activa-

tion-deactivation is slow. We have examined these possibilities using whole-cell recording from hippocampal pyramidal neurons in 200–300-μm thick slices (Hestrin et al. 1990a).

The two components of the EPSC could be isolated using their known pharmacological properties and voltage dependence (Hestrin et al. 1990b). The NMDA component could be recorded in isolation by applying CNQX and holding the cell at −40 mV membrane potential. The non-NMDA component could be isolated by holding the cell at membrane potentials more negative than −80 mV or by applying the NMDA antagonist APV.

Superimposing the NMDA and non-NMDA components (Fig. 7A) shows the remarkably slow time course of the NMDA component and demonstrates that the non-NMDA component actually decays before the NMDA component peaked. It has been reported that the sensitivity of the NMDA receptors to glutamate is considerably higher than that of the non-NMDA receptors (Mayer 1989). Thus, if these receptors are colocalized (Bekkers and Stevens 1989; see above) and if the released glutamate has equal access to both receptor types, the slow rise of the NMDA component could reflect a slow opening rate of the NMDA channels compared with the non-NMDA channels or that the NMDA receptors are located at some distance from the site of glutamate release and thus depend on diffusion for this activation.

If the rate-limiting step in the rise or decay of the EPSC reflects diffusion of transmitter, one would expect that the EPSC time course would show little temperature sensitivity (Magleby and Stevens 1972). However, we found that the rising phase of the NMDA component, as well as the decay phase of both components, shows high-temperature sensitivity (Fig. 7B; Q_{10} for these processes was 2.5–3.3). The high-temperature sensitivity of these processes indicates that free diffusion does not limit their time course. In addition, we found that partial blockade of the NMDA receptors by a slowly dissociating antagonist CPP (Benveniste and Mayer 1990) does not speed the decay of the NMDA

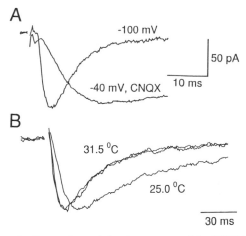

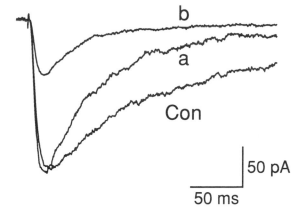

Figure 7. Comparison of the time course of the NMDA and non-NMDA receptor components of the EPSC and the temperature sensitivity of the NMDA receptor component. (*A*) The non-NMDA component of the EPSC recorded at −100 mV rose faster than the NMDA component observed after application of CNQX at a holding potential of −40 mV. Note that the NMDA component actually continues to rise during the falling phase of the non-NMDA-mediated synaptic current. (*B*) Temperature effects on the time course of the NMDA-mediated component. Synaptic current measured at a holding potential of −40 mV in the presence of 10 μM CNQX. A reduction of 6.5°C in the bath reversibly reduced the rate of decay, as well as the rate of rise of the EPSC. The peak current has been normalized. (Reprinted, with permission, from Hestrin et al. 1990a.)

Figure 8. Effect of 40 μM MK-801 on the NMDA-mediated EPSC. The cell was held at −40 mV membrane potential in the presence of CNQX. Repeated stimulation resulted in a decrease of amplitude. Trace *a* is an average of the first five responses after application. Trace *b* is an average of the response to stimulation 20–24. (Reprinted, with permission, from Hestrin et al. 1990a.)

component, indicating that buffered diffusion, known to occur at the neuromuscular junction (Katz and Miledi 1973; Magleby and Terrar 1975), is not involved in the slow decay phase of the NMDA EPSC.

We next considered the possibility that a temperature-sensitive glutamate uptake from synaptic regions controls the decay of the EPSC. Uptake of transmitter does not appear to be rate limiting, since we found that known blockers of glutamate uptake (dihydrokainate and threo-3-hydroxyl-D,L-asparate), although greatly potentiating responses to exogenous glutamate, had no effect on the EPSC decay (Hestrin et al. 1990a).

Given that our experiments have failed to provide evidence that diffusion or uptake affects the time course of the NMDA EPSC, we considered the role of NMDA channel kinetics in determining the EPSC decay. At the neuromuscular junction, the rise of acetylcholine (ACh) concentration is brief, and the decay of the EPSC reflects the closure of ACh receptor channels. Drugs that block open ACh channels accelerate the EPSC decay by modifying channel kinetics (Adams 1976). Thus, we tested the effects of MK-801 and ketamine, which have been shown to block open NMDA channels (MacDonald et al. 1987; Huettner and Bean 1988).

In these experiments, baseline data were collected for at least 10 minutes before application of the drug (Fig. 8, Con). Stimulation was then stopped, and MK-801 (10–80 μM) was applied. (Because these drugs primarily block open NMDA channels, this would ensure that the drugs were present at the receptor channel but that, at the time of the first stimulus, had not

blocked the channels.) After 7–10 minutes of drug application, stimulation was resumed. The amplitude of the initial response recorded in MK-801 was on average only slightly reduced. The time constant of the decay, however, was reduced to 46% of control by 40 μM MK-801 and to 67% of control by 80 μM MK-801. Similar results were obtained with ketamine (50 μM), which is also an open channel blocker of the NMDA channel. Further stimulation resulted in gradual decline in the EPSC amplitude with no significant change in the EPSC decay. The gradual decline of the amplitude suggested that only a small fraction of the available NMDA channels are activated during each EPSC.

Our data suggest that diffusion or uptake of transmitter does not determine the decay of the NMDA EPSC. On the other hand, drugs known to affect channel kinetics markedly affected the EPSC time course. Thus, our results are more compatible with a model in which decay of the NMDA EPSC is determined by intrinsically slow channel kinetics.

CONCLUDING REMARKS

The detailed properties of synaptic transmission and the mechanisms underlying EPSCs in the central nervous system are difficult to study with standard recording techniques. In particular, the excitatory currents, which can be voltage-dependent, are faster than the time constant of most neurons. We have shown in this paper that the application of whole-cell recording to brain slices allowing visual identification of cells can be used to study the physiology and the mechanisms underlying excitatory synaptic currents. Using these techniques, we studied four EPSCs: the Schaffer collateral-commissural to CA1 pyramidal and nonpyramidal neurons and the climbing fiber and parallel fiber input to cerebellar Purkinje cells. The hippocampal EPSCs are mediated by NMDA and non-NMDA receptors, whereas the EPSCs onto Purkinje cells are mediated by a non-NMDA receptor type. Further subdivision of the non-NMDA receptors cannot be excluded; thus, the receptors mediating transmission in the cerebellum could be different from those mediating non-NMDA EPSC in the hippocampus. We have provided evidence that the tenfold difference in the kinetics of the dual components mediating the EPSCs reflects differences in postsynaptic channel properties. The striking kinetic differences of the NMDA and the non-NMDA-mediated synaptic currents play a crucial role in the induction of LTP. During low-frequency stimulation, the fast decay of the non-NMDA EPSC coupled with disynaptic inhibition (Collingridge et al. 1988a) results in only brief membrane depolarization preventing the activation of the NMDA conductance. However, during high-frequency stimulation, the slowly deactivating NMDA EPSCs result in its nearly maximal activation concomitant with non-NMDA-dependent depolarization, aided by use-dependent depression of the synaptic inhibition (Collingridge et al. 1988b; Davies et al. 1990). Thus, the time course and short-term plasticity of these three synaptic currents prevent induction of LTP by low-frequency stimuli, although greatly facilitating its induction by high-frequency stimuli.

REFERENCES

Adams, P.R. 1976. Drug blockade of open end-plate channels. *J. Physiol.* **260**: 531.

Barnes, S. and F. Werblin. 1986. Gated currents generate single spike activity in amacrine cells of the tiger salamander retina. *Proc. Natl. Acad. Sci.* **83**: 1509.

Bekkers, J.M. and C.F. Stevens. 1989. NMDA and non-NMDA receptors are co-localized at individual excitatory synapses in cultured rat hippocampus. *Nature* **341**: 230.

Benveniste, M. and M.L. Mayer. 1990. Kinetic experiments with competitive NMDA receptor antagonists. *Biophys. J.* **55**: 121a.

Blanton, M.G., J.J. LoTurco, and A.R. Kriegstein. 1989. Whole-cell recording from neurons in slices of reptilian and mammalian cerebral cortex. *J. Neurosci. Methods* **30**: 203.

Cajal, S.R. 1911. *Histologie du systeme nerveux de l'homme et des vertebrés.* Maloine, Paris.

Coleman, P.A. and R.F. Miller. 1989. Measurements of passive membrane parameters with whole-cell recording from neurons in the intact amphibian retina. *J. Neurophysiol.* **61**: 218.

Collingridge, G.L. and R.A.J. Lester. 1989. Excitatory amino acid receptors in the vertebrate central nervous system. *Pharmacol. Rev.* **40**: 143.

Collingridge, G.L., C.E. Herron, and R.A.J. Lester. 1988a. Synaptic activation of N-methyl-D-aspartate receptors in the Schaffer collateral-commissural pathway of rat hippocampus. *J. Physiol.* **399**: 283.

———. 1988b. Frequency-dependent N-methyl-D-aspartate receptor-mediated synaptic transmission in rat hippocampus. *J. Physiol.* **399**: 301.

Dale, N. and A. Roberts. 1985. Dual-component amino-acid-mediated synaptic potentials: Excitatory drive for swimming in Xenopus embryos. *J. Physiol.* **363**: 35.

Davies, C.H., S.N. Davies, and G.L. Collingridge. 1990. Paired-pulse depression of monosynaptic GABA-mediated inhibitory postsynaptic responses in rat hippocampus. *J. Physiol.* **424**: 513.

Eccles, J.C., M. Ito, and J. Szentagothai. 1967. *The cerebellum as a neuronal machine.* Springer-Verlag, New York.

Edwards, F.A., A. Konnerth, B. Sakmann, and T. Takahashi. 1989. A thin slice preparation for patch clamp recordings from neurones of the mammalian central nervous system. *Pfluegers Arch. Eur. J. Physiol.* **414**: 600.

Forsythe, I.D. and G.L. Westbrook. 1988. Slow excitatory postsynaptic currents mediated by N-methyl-D-aspartate receptors on cultured mouse central neurons. *J. Physiol.* **396**: 515.

Garthwaite, J. and P.S. Beaumont. 1989. Excitatory amino acid receptors in the parallel fibre pathway in rat cerebellar slices. *Neurosci. Lett.* **107**: 151.

Hestrin, S., P. Sah, and R.A. Nicoll. 1990a. Mechanisms generating the time course of dual component excitatory synaptic currents recorded in hippocampal slices. *Neuron* **5**: 247.

Hestrin, S., R.A. Nicoll, D.J. Perkel, and P. Sah. 1990b. Analysis of excitatory synaptic action in the rat hippocampus using whole-cell recording from thin slices. *J. Physiol.* **422**: 203.

Hirano, T. and S. Hagiwara. 1988. Synaptic transmission between rat cerebellar granule and Purkinje cells in dissociated culture: Effects of excitatory-amino acid transmitter antagonists. *Proc. Natl. Acad. Sci.* **85**: 934.

Huettner, J.E. and B.P. Bean. 1988. Block of N-methyl-D-aspartate-activated current by the anticonvulsant MK-801: Selective binding to open channels. *Proc. Natl. Acad. Sci.* **85**: 1307.

Ito, M. 1984. *The cerebellum and neural control.* Raven Press, New York.

Kano, M., M. Kato, and H.S. Chang. 1988. The glutamate receptor subtype mediating parallel fibre-Purkinje cell transmission in rabbit cerebellar cortex. *Neurosci. Res.* **5**: 325.

Katz, B. and R. Miledi. 1973. The binding of acetylcholine to receptors and its removal from the synaptic cleft. *J. Physiol.* **231**: 549.

Kimura, H., K. Okamoto, and Y. Sakai. 1985. Pharmacological evidence for L-aspartate as the neurotransmitter of cerebellar climbing fibres in the guinea-pig. *J. Physiol.* **365**: 103.

Konnerth, A., I. Llano, and C.M. Armstrong. 1990. Synaptic currents in cerebellar Purkinje cells. *Proc. Natl. Acad. Sci.* **87**: 2662.

Lorenté de Nó, R. 1934. Studies on the structure of the cerebral cortex. II. Continuation of the study of the ammonic system. *J. Psychol. Neurol.* **46**: 113.

MacDonald, J.F., Z. Miljkovic, and P. Pennefather. 1987. Use-dependent block of excitatory amino acid currents in cultured neurons by ketamine. *J. Neurophysiol.* **58**: 251.

Magleby, K.L. and C.F. Stevens. 1972. The effect of voltage on the time course of end-plate currents. *J. Physiol.* **223**: 151.

Magleby, K.L. and D.A. Terrar. 1975. Factors affecting the time course of decay of end-plate currents: A possible cooperative action of acetylcholine on receptors at the frog neuromuscular junction. *J. Physiol.* **244**: 467.

Mayer, M.L. 1989. Activation and desensitization of glutamate receptors in mammalian CNS. In *Ion transport* (ed. C.D. Benham and D.J. Keeling), p. 183. Academic Press, London.

Nicoll, R.A., R.C. Malenka, and J.A. Kauer. 1990. Functional comparison of neurotransmitter receptor subtypes in mammalian central nervous system. *Physiol. Rev.* **70**: 513.

Perkel, D.J., S. Hestrin, P. Sah, and R.A. Nicoll. 1990. Excitatory synaptic currents in cerebellar Purkinje cells. *Proc. R. Soc. Lond. B Biol. Sci.* **241**: 116.

Sah, P., S. Hestrin, and R.A. Nicoll. 1990. Properties of excitatory postsynaptic currents recorded in vitro from rat hippocampal interneurons. *J. Physiol.* **430**: 605.

Seress, L. and C.E. Ribak. 1985. A combined Golgi-electron microscopic study of non-pyramidal neurons in the CA1 area of hippocampus. *J. Neurocytol.* **14**: 717.

Short-term Electrophysiological Actions of Insulin on *Aplysia* Neurons: Identification of a Possible Novel Modulatory Second-messenger Mechanism

J.H. Schwartz,* E. Shapiro,* S.D. Brown,† and A.R. Saltiel‡
*Howard Hughes Medical Institute, Center for Neurobiology and Behavior and †Department of Pharmacology,
Columbia University, New York, New York 10032; ‡Rockefeller University, New York, New York 10021

At several identified *Aplysia* synapses, transmitter release is enhanced through the action of the cAMP-dependent protein kinase as well as by protein kinase C (Braha et al. 1990; Sacktor and Schwartz 1990). Release is diminished by 12-lipoxygenase metabolites of arachidonic acid (Piomelli et al. 1987a,b, 1989). The cAMP-dependent kinase and protein kinase C are thought to produce presynaptic facilitation by phosphorylating different protein substrates: cAMP, the K_s^+ channel and protein kinase C, possibly cytoskeleton-associated proteins analogous to vertebrate synapsin that affect synaptic vesicle mobilization (P. Greengard pers. comm.). The 12-lipoxygenase metabolites reverse the effects of cAMP on the K_s^+ channel.

All of the electrophysiological evidence available thus far suggests that hydroperoxyeicosatetrenoic acid (12-HPETE) or its metabolite 8-hydroxy-11,12-epoxy-eicosatrienoic acid (8-HEpETE) operates directly on the K_s^+ channel in the membrane (Belardetti et al. 1989; Buttner et al. 1989). Nevertheless, a redundant molecular second-messenger pathway, for example, activation of cytoplasmic protein phosphatases, has not yet been ruled out.

In search of a second-messenger pathway for activating protein phosphatases, we discovered a possible novel inhibitory mechanism. Although this mechanism might be the first signal-transduction pathway that modulates synaptic activity in the short term by phosphorylation with a tyrosine-specific protein kinase, as we shall see, it does not appear to modulate K^+ channels specifically.

A year after Banting and Best (1922) identified insulin as the hypoglycemic hormone in vertebrates, Collip (1923) provided evidence for an insulin-like activity in the gut of a mollusc. In the intervening years, similar peptides have been found in most metazoan phyla that possess nervous systems, invertebrate and vertebrate, from coelenterates to humans (Blundell and Wood 1975; Thorpe and Duve 1984). Many of these peptides have primary structures similar to insulin; this similarity has been convincingly proved by recombinant DNA technology (Steiner et al. 1985; Adachi et al. 1989; Smit 1990).

In invertebrates, insulin-like peptides have been convincingly localized to neurons and, in several instances, have been shown to fulfill some of the classical criteria expected of neurotransmitters. In addition to being present and pharmacologically active when applied exogenously, they can be synthesized in neurons and released synaptically (Thorpe and Duve 1984; LeRoith

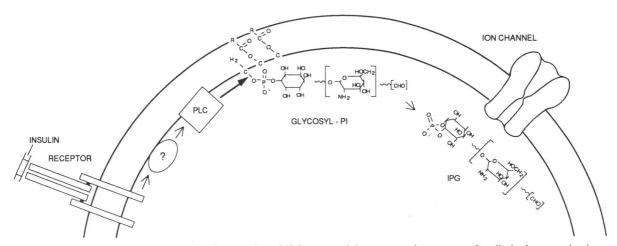

Figure 1. Scheme for the receptor-mediated generation of IPG as a modulatory second messenger. Insulin is shown activating a conventional tyrosine-kinase-type of receptor leading to the hydrolysis of glycosyl phosphatidylinositol (GLYCOSYL-PI) in the inner leaflet of the plasma membrane by a phospholipase C (PLC). Products of this reaction are phosphorylated forms of inositol glycans (IPG). Activation of the phospholipase may involve a transducing protein (?). IPG directly or indirectly modulates the functioning of an ion channel. (Adapted from Saltiel et al. 1986.)

et al. 1986). In contrast, the status of insulin and insulin-related peptides as neurotransmitters in vertebrate brain is much less secure (LeRoith et al. 1986; Baskin et al. 1987, 1988; Adamo et al. 1989).

The presence of insulin in nervous systems of diverse species as well as its actions on neurons led us to examine the electrophysiological effects of the mammalian hormone on neurons of the marine gastropod mollusc, *Aplysia californica*. Saltiel and Cuatrecasas (1986) showed that some of the metabolic effects of insulin in vertebrate liver, fat, and muscle cells are mediated by the intracellular generation of an inositol phosphate glycan (IPG) enzyme modulator (Fig. 1) (Saltiel et al. 1986; Saltiel 1987). IPG is a complex oligosaccharide that is released from the plasma membrane by hydrolysis of a glycosyl-phosphatidylinositol (PI) precursor through the activation of a specific PI-phospholipase C and that has been shown to affect the state of protein phosphorylation in vertebrate cells (Saltiel 1987).

RESULTS

Injection of IPG

To test its possible role as an intracellular mediator, we injected IPG purified from rat liver plasma membranes into L14 and L10. We chose these identified *Aplysia* neurons because they both show prominent inhibition produced by the action of 12-lipoxygenase metabolites on K_S^+-like channels. Intracellular injection of IPG caused a rapid onset hyperpolarization of L14 (Fig. 2, top). The hyperpolarization was associated

with a decrease in membrane conductance and was not a result of delayed rectification (Fig. 2, bottom). The hyperpolarization produced by injecting IPG lasts 10–30 minutes and frequently occurred as soon as the cell was impaled. In nine experiments, six with L14 and three with L10, injection of IPG hyperpolarized the cells by -8.6 mV ± 2.9 mV (S.E.M.). In control experiments, injection of the column elution buffer used to purify IPG (1 ml of 0.5 M TEA-formate lyophilized and diluted in water) had no effect on membrane potential or membrane input conductance (mean hyperpolarization: -0.8 mV ± 0.5 mV, $n = 4$).

The hyperpolarizing increase in membrane resistance observed is not consistent with the interaction of IPG with either the cAMP or the arachidonic acid second-messenger pathways. As already noted, cAMP causes a depolarizing decrease in K^+ conductance, and eicosanoids cause an increase in K^+ conductance. Moreover, prior injection of IPG into L14 did not prevent the changes in conductance produced by either histamine (data not shown) or cAMP, further differentiating these signal transduction pathways (Fig. 3). Injection of IPG did not affect the response of L14 to serotonin, a modulatory neurotransmitter that increases cAMP in the cell (Bernier et al. 1982).

Action of Vertebrate Insulins

It seemed reasonable next to test the effects of insulin on *Aplysia* neurons. Although four molluscan insulin-like peptide (MIP) transcripts have been cloned from the pond snail *Lymnea* by the group at the Free University in Amsterdam (Smit et al. 1988; Smit 1990),

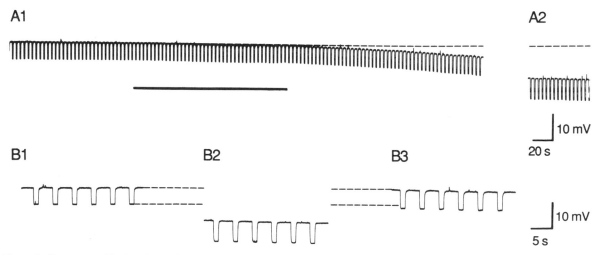

Figure 2. Response of L14 to intracellular injection of IPG. IPG was purified from rat liver membranes (Saltiel and Cuatrecasas 1986) and injected through one barrel of a double-barrelled micropipette; the other was used for recording voltage and passing current (Eisenstadt et al. 1973). Membrane potential was monitored with an independent single microelectrode. (*A1*) Injection of IPG rapidly hyperpolarized L14 at the resting potential (-50 mV). The progress of the injection (bar) was assessed visually by the movement of the air-fluid interface in the injection barrel during pressure puffs. (*A2*) At 6 min after the start of the injection, the membrane potential was hyperpolarized to -65 mV. (*B1*) The recording at a faster time-scale showed L14s membrane conductance (monitored with 1.0-sec current pulses at 0.2 Hz) before injection of IPG. (*B2*) After the injection, L14s membrane potential was hyperpolarized, and its membrane conductance decreased. L14 was hyperpolarized by -15 mV. (*B3*) After the injection, L14 was artificially depolarized back to a resting potential of -50 mV by passing current. The membrane conductance was still decreased by 10%, ruling out effects of delayed rectification. (Reprinted, with permission, from Shapiro et al. 1991.)

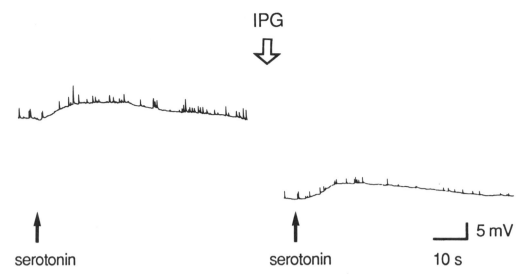

Figure 3. Response of L14 to serotonin was unaffected by IPG. Serotonin (10^{-4} M in artificial seawater) was applied to the cell body of L14 (5-sec puff delivering a 2-μl volume [arrow]) and produced a slow depolarizing response (L14 voltage, upper traces). L14's membrane potential was −62 mV. After the injection of IPG (open arrow), L14 was hyperpolarized to −74 mV (note baseline shift); nevertheless, application of serotonin (second arrow) still caused a full-sized depolarization. (Reprinted, with permission, from Shapiro et al. 1991.)

none are available for physiological testing. Nevertheless, immunocytochemical studies with antisera raised against peptides with MIP sequences indicate that MIP-like immunoreactivity is present in as yet unidentified *Aplysia* neurons in the abdominal ganglion (van Minnen and Schallig 1990). Perhaps most intriguing, insulins have been shown to be present both in neurons of the central nervous system and in the gut (Ebberink and Joosse 1985). Thus, unlike the situation in mammals where insulin in the brain has always been controversial, there is no doubt, at least in molluscs, that some insulin-like peptides are neuropeptides (Baskin et al. 1987, 1988; Adamo et al. 1989).

Application of insulin to L14 and L10 resulted in a hyperpolarization associated with decreased membrane conductances (Fig. 4A). The concentrations of insulins used (both human recombinant, Eli Lilly, Indianapolis, Indiana, and porcine, Calbiochem, San Diego, California) admittedly were quite high (up to 0.5 mg/ml) in the puff pipette, which corresponds approximately to an order of magnitude lower dose at the cell's membrane. At a normal resting potential (trace at −60 mV), a 5-second puff of porcine insulin hyperpolarized L14 and caused a decrease in the membrane conductance monitored with short current pulses. When the membrane potential of L14 was depolarized by passing current, the response to insulin was diminished and then reversed. A summary of the responses of L14 to insulin as a function of membrane voltage is shown in Figure 4B. The response to insulin is not linear with voltage, and it reversed at about −35 mV.

As with IPG, the decreased conductance produced by insulin is not consistent with modulation of a K^+ conductance alone. Further evidence that insulin does not act on a K^+ channel is that a high K^+ seawater (50 mM, replacing Na^+) produced only a small change in

the reversal potential of the response from −20 mV to −25 mV (or 5 mV), much less than the 29-mV change predicted by the Nernst equation for a pure K^+ response (data not shown).

Insulin also hyperpolarized cell L10 through a decrease in membrane conductance, but left upper quadrant cells were not affected by insulin at all, and another identified cell, R15, was depolarized (data not shown). Thus, as with other neurotransmitters, insulin does not produce the same electrophysiological action on all *Aplysia* neurons.

Production of IPG in *Aplysia* Neurons

Is there a physiological link between the effects of insulin and the action of injected IPG? To provide further evidence that insulin activates the production of IPG as a second messenger that modulates synaptic function, we next showed that IPG is actually present in *Aplysia* neurons and that the injection of IPG occludes the effects of applied insulin.

We found that a glycosyl-phosphatidylinositol lipid precursor is present in *Aplysia* neurons and is hydrolyzed in response to insulin (Table 1 and Fig. 5). Neural components from the central ganglia of ten *Aplysia* labeled with [³H]glucosamine were incubated with insulin. After 5 minutes, the nervous tissue was extracted in chloroform/methanol, and the organic and aqueous phases were separated. In control ganglia, a major [³H]glucosamine-labeled lipid was identified by thin-layer chromatography that migrated with vertebrate glycosyl phosphatidylinositol. The *Aplysia* lipid was sensitive to hydrolysis by *Bacillus thuringiensis* PI-phospholipase C. The exposure of the labeled ganglia to insulin caused a 50% decrease in the amount of label recovered in glycosyl phosphatidylinositol. Analysis of

A

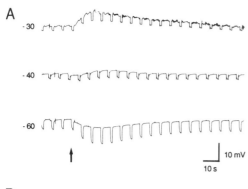

B

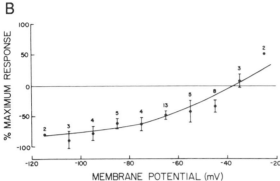

Figure 4. Response of L14 to insulin. (*A*) Experiments were performed on isolated abdominal ganglia of *Aplysia* (100–200 g) in artificial seawater (460 mM NaCl, 10 mM KCl, 11 mM CaCl₂, 55 mM MgCl₂, 10 mM Tris-HCl, pH 7.4); the connective tissue sheath was dissected away to expose the cell body of L14. Standard intracellular electrophysiological recording techniques were used to record voltage and inject current. Current was passed through an independent microelectrode as hyperpolarizing pulses to measure membrane resistance and as a constant current to control membrane potential. Insulins were prepared as stock solutions in 10 mM sodium acetate buffer, pH 6.0, and were diluted in seawater for application from a micropipette 1 mm above the ganglion. (*B*) Summary of six independent experiments showing the response of L14 to insulin as a function of membrane voltage. Responses (combined at 10-mV intervals) in each experiment were normalized to the maximal response for that preparation. Values are number of responses at each voltage ± S.E.M. (Reprinted, with permission, from Shapiro et al. 1991.)

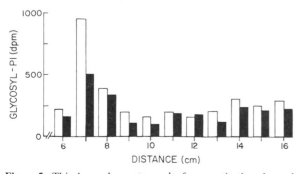

Figure 5. Thin-layer chromatography for quantitating glycosyl phosphatidylinositol from *Aplysia* neural components. See footnote to Table 1. (■) Insulin-treated; (□) control.

Table 1. Formation of iPG in *Aplysia* Neural Components

	Experiment (dpm)		Experiment (dpm)	
	glycosyl-PI	IPG	glycosyl-PI	IPG
Control	2211	477	976	501
Insulin	726	746	506	895

The connective tissue sheath was removed from abdominal and pleural-pedal ganglia, and their neural components were washed with seawater and incubated at 15°C overnight for labeling with [³H]glucosamine. The labeled neural components were exposed to porcine insulin (100 μg/ml) or to the seawater alone (control) for 5 min. The tissue was extracted with chloroform/methanol/6 N HCl and centrifuged. The supernatant was dried and extracted again with water-saturated butanol and then with water alone. The phases were separated, and the lower aqueous phase was extracted with butanol. [³H]IPG was quantitated by SAX HPLC (Saltiel et al. 1986). The butanol phases were combined, washed with water, and dried under N₂. The resulting lipids were chromatographed on thin-layer chromatography (Saltiel et al. 1986). One example of a separation by thin-layer chromatography for the quantitation of glycosyl-PI is shown in Fig. 5.

the aqueous phase by ion-exchange high-performance liquid chromatography revealed that exposure of *Aplysia* neural components to insulin caused an 80% increase of the label in IPG.

Injection of IPG occludes the action of insulin (Fig. 6). In an L14 cell hyperpolarized by the injection of IPG, application of insulin failed to elicit the response seen before the injection of IPG.

DISCUSSION

These results suggest that an endogenous *Aplysia* insulin-like neuropeptide acts as a modulatory transmitter through the release of IPG as a second messenger. Several important questions still need to be answered: (1) Is the synaptic modulation observed produced by a tyrosine-specific protein kinase (as with the known vertebrate receptors for insulin and for insulin growth factor I [IGF-I]) or through a signal transduction mechanism involving a transducing G protein (as with IGF-II) (Fernandez-Almonacid and Rosen 1987; Adamo et al. 1989; Garofalo and Rosen 1989; Okamoto et al. 1990)? The insulin superfamily is clearly distinct from the insulin-receptor family. An important, and general, question that is difficult to address experimentally is whether the evolution of a neuropeptide family occurs in step with the evolution of its receptors. Clearly, the consequences of different rates or extents of evolutionary change should bear importantly on the synaptic action mediated by the neuropeptide, and hence ultimately on its behavioral effects. From the evolutionary information now available, it would appear that multiple constraints on the evolution of the members of the insulin superfamily, as well as constraints on their receptors, did not result in coordinate change (see Blundell and Wood 1975; Steiner et al. 1985; LeRoith et al. 1986; Adamo et al. 1989; Smit 1990). Thus, it is not at all certain that the many invertebrate insulin-like peptides all use the same

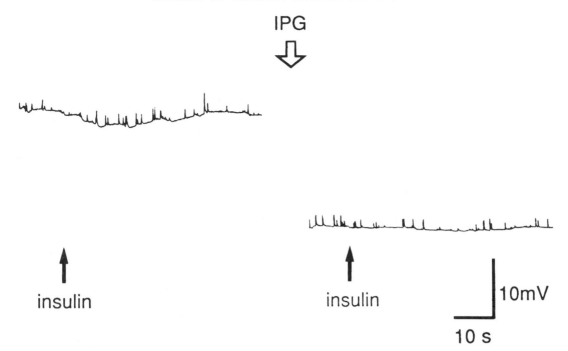

Figure 6. Injection of IPG occludes the response to insulin. (*Left*) Porcine insulin (1 μl of 0.1 mg/ml) was applied to an L14 cell with a resting potential of −62 mV and elicited a hyperpolarizing response. (*Right*) After the injection, L14's resting potential was −74 mV. Application of insulin now had no effect. For further experimental details, see Fig. 3.

receptor mechanism. (2) What is the structure of the endogenous ("true") molluscan neuropeptide whose action is mimicked by vertebrate insulin? The high concentrations of insulins needed to produce the effects observed in *Aplysia* neurons suggest that mammalian insulin is a poor homolog. (3) What are the neural circuits in which the modulated synapses occur, and what are their behavioral function? A speculative answer to this question can be offered with L14. L14 is a group of three motor neurons that produce inking, a defensive behavior with a high threshold (see Kandel 1979). The biophysical properties of L14 cells are appropriate to the all-or-none nature of the behavior they mediate. L14 cells have a lower membrane potential than most *Aplysia* neurons and are electrically coupled. Insulin, a peptide physiologically associated with feeding behavior, may also function to suppress defensive behaviors while the animal eats. The motivational balance between self-protection through the production of a cloud of ink and feeding may sometimes be tipped in favor of feeding.

The possibility that *Aplysia* neurons synthesize and release an insulin reinforces the idea that peptides of the insulin superfamily may act not only as hormones to control growth and metabolism, but also as modulatory neurotransmitters. Neuropeptides that function as hormones or growth factors to initiate longer-term metabolic, behavioral, or developmental processes also can produce short-term electrophysiological effects on neurons. Thus, bag cell peptides in *Aplysia* initiate a complex and long-lasting behavioral program (Rothman et al. 1983) but also have immediate modulatory

actions (Mayeri et al. 1985). Conversely, vasoactive intestinal peptide, regarded as a neuropeptide transmitter, has recently been shown to act as a growth factor for cultured sympathetic neuroblasts (Pincus et al. 1990). Furthermore, classical small-molecule transmitters such as serotonin and glutamate can regulate neuronal growth in tissue culture, perhaps by modulating ion channels in growth cones (Hayden et al. 1984; Mattson and Hater 1987; Mattson et al. 1988). Finally, fibroblasts transfected with a cDNA for a serotonin receptor respond to the transmitter with neoplastic growth (Julius et al. 1989). Thus, the distinction is blurred between agents involved in short-term synaptic modulation and long-term developmental programs. It is attractive to think that the immediate neurotransmitter effects of insulin and other peptide hormones constitute early steps in a longer metabolic or behavioral program. These ideas can best be examined in invertebrates where the effects on behavior can be tested, the neurons producing the behavior identified, and the specific synaptic mechanisms modulated studied directly.

ACKNOWLEDGMENTS

Dedicated to the memory of Ora M. Rosen, who died on the morning this paper was presented, with gratitude and deepest affection. We thank Dr. Irving Kupfermann for suggesting the possible behavioral role of insulin action on L14 and Jillayn Lindahl for preparing the manuscript. A.R. Saltiel is supported by National Institutes of Health grant DK-33804.

REFERENCES

Adachi, T., S. Takiya, Y. Suzuki, M. Iwami, A. Kawakami, S.Y. Takahashi, H. Ishizaki, H. Nagasawa, and A. Suzuki. 1989. cDNA structure and exression of bombyxin, an insulin-like brain secretory peptide of the silkmoth *Bombyx mori*. *J. Biol. Chem.* **264:** 7681.

Adamo, M., M.N. Raizada, and D. LeRoith. 1989. Insulin and insulin-like growth factor receptors in the nervous system. *Mol. Neurobiol.* **3:** 71.

Banting, F.C. and C.H. Best. 1922. The internal secretion of the pancreas. *J. Lab. Clin. Med.* **7:** 251.

Baskin, D.C., B.J. Wilcox, D.P. Figlewicz, and D.M. Dorsa. 1988. Insulin and insulin-like growth factors in the CNS. *Trends Neurosci.* **11:** 107.

Baskin, D.G., D.P. Figlewicz, S.C. Woods, D. Porte, Jr., and D.M. Dorsa. 1987. Insulin in the brain. *Annu. Rev. Physiol.* **49:** 335.

Belardetti, F., W.B. Campbell, J.R. Falck, G. Demontis, and M. Rosolowsky. 1989. Products of heme-catalyzed transformation of the arachidonate derivative 12-HPETE open S-type K$^+$ channels in *Aplysia*. *Neuron* **3:** 497.

Bernier, L., V.F. Castellucci, E.R. Kandel, and J.H. Schwartz. 1982. Facilitatory transmitter causes a selective and prolonged increase in adenosine 3′:5′-monophosphate in sensory neurons mediating the gill and siphon withdrawal reflex in *Aplysia*. *J. Neurosci.* **2:** 1682.

Blundell, T.L. and S.P. Wood. 1975. Is the evolution of insulin Darwinian or due to selectively neutral mutation? *Nature* **257:** 197.

Braha, O., N. Dale, B. Hochner, M. Klein, T.W. Abrams, and E.R. Kandel. 1990. Second messengers involved in the two processes of presynaptic facilitation that contribute to sensitization and dishabituation in *Aplysia* sensory neurons. *Proc. Natl. Acad. Sci.* **87:** 2040.

Buttner, N., S.A. Siegelbaum, and A. Volterra. 1989. Direct modulation of *Aplysia* S-K$^+$ channels by a 12-lipoxygenase metabolite of arachidonic acid. *Nature* **342:** 553.

Collip, J.B. 1923. The demonstration of an insulin-like substance in the tissues of the clam (*Mya arenaria*). *J. Biol. Chem.* **65:** xxxix.

Ebberink, R.H.M. and J. Joosse. 1985. Molecular properties of various snail peptides from brain and gut. *Peptides* (suppl. 3) **6:** 451.

Eisenstadt, M., J.E. Goldman, E.R. Kandel, H. Koike, J. Koester, and J.H. Schwartz. 1973. Intrasomatic injection of radioactive precursors for studying transmitter synthesis in identified neurons of *Aplysia californica*. *Proc. Natl. Acad. Sci.* **70:** 3371.

Fernandez-Almonacid, R. and O.M. Rosen. 1987. Structure and ligand specificity of the *Drosophila melanogaster* insulin receptor. *Mol. Cell Biol.* **7:** 2718.

Garofalo, R.S. and O.M. Rosen. 1989. Insulin and insulin-like growth factor 1 (IGF-1) receptors during central nervous system development: Expression of two immunologically distinct IGF-1 receptor β subunits. *Mol. Cell Biol.* **9:** 2806.

Hayden, P.G., D.P. McCobb, and S.B. Kater. 1984. Serotonin selectively inhibits growth cone motility and synaptogenesis of specific identified neurons. *Science* **226:** 561.

Julius, D., T.J. Livelli, T.M. Jessell, and R. Axel. 1989. Ectopic expression of the serotonin 1c receptor and the triggering of malignant transformation. *Science* **244:** 1057.

Kandel, E.R. 1979. *Behavioral biology of* Aplysia. W.H. Freeman, San Francisco.

LeRoith, D., G. Delahunty, G.L. Wilson, C.T. Roberts, Jr., J. Shemer, C. Hart, M.A. Lesniak, J. Shiloach, and J. Roth. 1986. Evolutionary aspects of the endocrine and nervous systems. *Recent Prog. Horm. Res.* **42:** 549.

Mattson, M.P. and S.B. Kater. 1987. Calcium regulation of neurite elongation and growth cone motility. *J. Neurosci.* **7:** 4034.

Mattson, M.P., P. Dou, and S.B. Kater. 1988. Outgrowth-regulating actions of glutamate in isolated hippocampal pyramidal neurons. *J. Neurosci.* **8:** 2087.

Mayeri, E., B.S. Rothman, P.H. Brownell, W.D. Branton, and L. Padgett. 1985. Nonsynaptic characteristics of neurotransmission mediated by egg-laying hormone in abdominal ganglion of *Aplysia*. *J. Neurosci.* **5:** 2060.

Okamoto, T., T. Katatada, Y. Murayama, M. Ui, E. Ogata, and I. Nishimoto 1990. A simple structure encodes G protein-activating function of the IGF-II mannose b-phosphate receptor. *Cell* **62:** 709.

Pincus, D.W., E.M. Di Cicco-Bloom, and I.B. Black. 1990. Vasoactive intestinal peptide regulates mitosis differentiation and survival of cultured sympathetic neuroblasts. *Nature* **343:** 564.

Piomelli, D., E. Shapiro, S.J. Feinmark, and J.H. Schwartz. 1987a. Metabolites of arachidonic acid in the nervous system of *Aplysia*: Possible mediators of synaptic modulation. *J. Neurosci.* **7:** 3675.

Piomelli, D., E. Shapiro, R. Zipkin, J.H. Schwartz, and S. Feinmark. 1989. Formation and action of 8-hydroxy-11,12-epoxy-5,9,14-icosatrienoic acid in *Aplysia*: A possible second messenger in neurons. *Proc. Natl. Acad. Sci.* **86:** 1721.

Piomelli, D., A. Volterra, N. Dale, S.A. Siegelbaum, E.R. Kandel, J.H. Schwartz, and F. Belardetti. 1987b. Lipoxygenase metabolites of arachidonic acid as second messengers for presynaptic inhibition of *Aplysia* sensory cells. *Nature* **328:** 38.

Rothman, B.S., G. Weir, and F.E. Dudek. 1983. Egg-laying hormone: Direct action on the ovotestis of *Aplysia*. *Gen. Comp. Endocrinol.* **52:** 134.

Sacktor, T.C. and J.H. Schwartz. 1990. Sensitizing stimuli cause translocation of protein kinase C in *Aplysia* sensory neurons. *Proc. Natl. Acad. Sci.* **87:** 2036.

Saltiel, A.R. 1987. Insulin generates an enzyme modulator from hepatic plasma membranes: Regulation of adenosine 3′,5′-monophosphate phosphodiesterase, pyruvate dehydroxenase and adenylate cyclase. *Endocrinology* **120:** 967.

Saltiel, A.R. and P. Cuatrecasas. 1986. Insulin stimulates the generation from hepatic plasma membranes of modulators derived from inositol glycolipid. *Proc. Natl. Acad. Sci.* **83:** 5793.

Saltiel, A.R., J. Fox, P. Sherline, and P. Cuatrecasas. 1986. Insulin-stimulated hydrolysis of a novel glycolipid generates modulators of cAMP phosphodiesterase. *Science* **233:** 967.

Shapiro, E., S.D. Brown, A.R. Saltiel, and J.H. Schwartz. 1991. Short-term action of insulin on *Aplysia* neurons: Generation of a possible novel modulator of ion channels. *J. Neurobiol.* **22:** (in press).

Smit, A.B. 1990. *The organization, neuronal expression and evolution of a family of insulin-related genes in the mollusc* Lymnaea stagnalis. Academisch Proefschrift, Vrije Universiteit te Amsterdam.

Smit, A.B., E. Vreugdenhil, R.H.M. Ebberink, W.P.M. Geraerts, J. Klootwijk, and J. Joosse. 1988. Growth-controlling molluscan neurons produce the precursor of an insulin-related peptide. *Nature* **331:** 535.

Steiner, D.F., S.J. Chan, J.M. Welsh, and S.C.M. Kwok. 1985. Structure and evolution of the insulin gene. *Annu. Rev. Genet.* **19:** 463.

Thorpe, A. and H. Duve. 1984. Insulin- and glycagon-like peptides in insects and molluscs. *Mol. Physiol.* **5:** 235.

van Minnen, J. and H. Schallig. 1990. Demonstration of insulin-related substances in the central nervous systems of pulmonates and *Aplysia californica*. *Cell Tissue Res.* **260:** 381.

Structure and Regulation of Type II Calcium/Calmodulin-dependent Protein Kinase in Central Nervous System Neurons

M.B. Kennedy, M.K. Bennett,* R.F. Bulleit,† N.E. Erondu,‡ V.R. Jennings,
S.G. Miller,§ S.S. Molloy, B.L. Patton, and L.J. Schenker

Division of Biology, California Institute of Technology, Pasadena, California 91125

In a recent talk at Caltech, David Baltimore suggested that molecular biology (the study of gene expression) and neurobiology are at similar stages. Both fields have identified many of the cast of important characters, but we still have much to learn about mechanisms and algorithms. In molecular neurobiology, the "mechanisms" are the ways that individual proteins work together to regulate release of transmitter or to modulate receptors and ion channels. The "algorithms" are the ways that these mechanisms are coordinated to allow neurons to maintain homeostasis, while at the same time adapting to changes in the external environment and storing information through molecular changes that alter the behavior of neural networks.

In the last several years, the field of molecular neurobiology has appropriately placed great emphasis on identification of the relevant "characters." By characters, we mean the proteins that make up synaptic vesicles and other synaptic organelles, transmitter receptors, ion channels, and neuronal regulatory molecules. In this paper, we describe one character that we have studied for several years, called type II $Ca^{++}/$ calmodulin-dependent protein kinase (CaM kinase II). We then discuss an interesting mechanism by which this particular protein kinase may allow neurons to store information, if only for a short time. Finally, we describe an experimental system that we hope to use to learn how the CaM kinase, together with other neuronal proteins, participates in regulatory algorithms that are important for brain function.

EXPERIMENTAL PROCEDURES

Detailed procedures for most of the experiments were presented previously (Erondu and Kennedy 1985; Miller and Kennedy 1985, 1986; Bulleit et al. 1988; Miller et al. 1988; Patton et al. 1990; S.S. Molloy and M.B. Kennedy, in prep.).

Present addresses: *Department of Biology, Stanford University, Palo Alto, California 94305; †Department of Pharmacology, University of Maryland, Baltimore, Maryland 21201; ‡Department of Biochemistry, University of Iowa, Iowa City, Iowa 52242; §Division of Cell and Developmental Biology, University of California, Berkeley, California 94720.

Immunocytochemical staining of synaptosomes. Synaptosomes were prepared from forebrains, hippocampi, and cerebelli of 8 to 12 young adult rats, by a modification of the method of Cohen et al. (1977), which is briefly summarized here. Brain regions were dissected and homogenized in a sucrose buffer. Large particles were removed by centrifugation at 1500g for 10 minutes. Crude synaptosomes and mitochondria were removed from the supernatant solution by centrifugation at 18,000g for 10 minutes and then carefully resuspended in a sucrose buffer and layered onto discontinuous sucrose density gradients. After centrifugation at 82,000g for 2 hours, an enriched synaptosome fraction was harvested from the 1.0 M:1.2 M sucrose interface. The synaptosomes were diluted fourfold with 0.32 M sucrose in bicarbonate buffer (pH 8.0) and then sedimented by centrifugation at 37,000g for 20 minutes. The pellet was gently resuspended in 1 ml or less of 0.32 M sucrose in bicarbonate buffer.

The synaptosomes were fixed and stained essentially according to the method of DeCamilli et al. (1983b). Each resuspended synaptosome pellet was fixed by slow 20-fold dilution into 4% paraformaldehyde, 0.1% glutaraldehyde, 20 mM cacodylate buffer (pH 7.4), 0.05 mM $CaCl_2$, 0.32 M sucrose at 4°C. The lightly fixed synaptosomes were recovered by centrifugation at 17,000g for 20 minutes. The pellets were gently scraped with a teflon rod into a small volume of 0.12 M phosphate (pH 7.4) and homogenized by hand in a small teflon/glass homogenizer. The resuspended pellet was passed slowly several times through a 25-gauge needle. Each suspension (100–180 μl) was placed in a tube prewarmed to 58°C. After 15 seconds, prewarmed 3% low-melting-point agarose (100–180 μl) dissolved in 5 mM phosphate (pH 7.4) was added. The mixture was stirred with a prewarmed pipette and quickly placed into warm frames constructed according to the method of DeCamilli et al. (1983b). The agarose-embedded synaptosomes were allowed to cool for 1 hour at room temperature. The resulting thin slabs were cut with a razor blade into 2 mm × 2 mm blocks. Six blocks of each sample were placed into each of several small test tubes. The blocks were first incubated for 30 minutes in 2 ml of 0.5 M Tris (pH 7.4) and then incubated for 30 minutes in 0.5 ml of Tris buffer containing 2 mg/ml sheep immunoglobulin G (IgG). Finally, they were incubated overnight at 4°C in 0.2 ml of Tris buffer containing 2 mg/ml sheep and either 40–50 μg/ml 6g9 monoclonal antibody purified from ascites fluid by chromatography on a protein A affinity column or 40 μg/ml mouse IgG. The blocks were washed at room temperature with five changes of 2 ml of solution B (20 mM phosphate [pH 7.4], 0.5 M NaCl) over 40 minutes. They were then incubated for 90 minutes in 0.15 ml of solution B containing 50 mg/ml ovalbumin, 2 mg/ml sheep IgG, and a one-fifth dilution of ferritin-conjugated sheep anti-mouse IgG antisera purchased from Janssen Life Sciences Products. The blocks were washed again with five changes of 2 ml of solution B over 40 minutes. Finally, the blocks were fixed in 2 ml of 1% glutaraldehyde, 0.12 M phosphate (pH 7.4) for 30 minutes at 4°C. The fixed blocks were washed for 20 minutes in 0.12 M phosphate (pH 7.4) at 4°C and then osmicated in ice cold 1% OsO_4 for 1 hour. After two 5-minute washes in 0.1 M phosphate (pH 7.4), the blocks were dehydrated in a graded alcohol series and embedded in epon by standard methods for sectioning. Ultrathin sections were examined and photographed with a Phillips 301 electron microscope. The number of bound ferritin grains per micrometer of postsynaptic density (PSD) was determined from photographs with the aid of a Tektronix digitizing tablet.

RESULTS AND DISCUSSION

Molecular Structure of Brain Type II CaM Kinase

Type II CaM kinase is a calmodulin-dependent protein kinase that was first purified from the brain with the use of an assay that measured its ability to phosphorylate synapsin I (Bennett et al. 1983; McGuinness et al. 1985; Miller and Kennedy 1985) or tubulin (Goldenring et al. 1983) in the presence of Ca^{++} and calmodulin. It is a large heteromultimer composed of 12 homologous subunits. The predominant holoenzyme purified from the forebrain contains, on the average, nine subunits with a molecular weight of 54,000 called α and, on the average, three subunits with molecular weights of 57,000–60,000 that are alternative products of the same gene and are called β and β'. The subunits appear to associate randomly into dodecameric holoenzymes; the ratio of subunits in holoenzymes from a particular brain region is approximately the same as the ratio of the subunit messages from that region (McGuinness et al. 1985; Miller and Kennedy 1985; Bulleit et al. 1988). This ratio varies considerably. For example, the forebrain holoenzyme contains three times as many α-subunits as β-subunits, whereas the cerebellar holoenzyme contains approximately four times as many β-subunits as α-subunits.

The α- and β-subunits are neuron-specific. The gene encoding the α-subunit is expressed at highest levels in mature forebrain neurons; whereas the gene encoding the β-subunit is expressed more uniformly in all neurons (Bulleit et al. 1988). Recently, two additional CaM kinase genes encoding γ- and δ-subunits have been isolated and sequenced (Tobimatsu et al. 1988; Tobimatsu and Fujisawa 1989). The γ- and δ-subunits are highly homologous to the α- and β-subunits but are expressed uniformly in many tissues including brain tissue.

Cellular Distribution of Type II CaM Kinase

An early finding that focused attention on the potential importance of CaM kinase II for central nervous system (CNS) function was its high concentration in the brain. The kinase is particularly highly concentrated in forebrain neurons where it comprises approximately 2% of total hippocampal protein and 1% of cortical protein (Erondu and Kennedy 1985). Within the forebrain, about half of the kinase is soluble and distributed throughout the cytosol (Kennedy et al. 1983b; Ouimet et al. 1984). The rest is associated with particulate structures (Kennedy et al. 1983b).

Association of the CaM Kinase with Postsynaptic Densities

At least one of the particulate structures that the kinase associates with is the PSD, a prominent specialization of the submembranous cytoskeleton that is attached to the postsynaptic membrane at CNS synapses (Cotman et al. 1974). The α-subunit was found to be identical to a protein that is a major constituent of highly enriched PSD fractions prepared from brain tissue (Kennedy et al. 1983a). This protein had previously been referred to as the major postsynaptic density protein (Kelly and Cotman 1978). Quantitative estimates indicate that the CaM kinase comprises 20–40% of the total protein in the PSD fraction (Miller and Kennedy 1985). Curiously, the content of CaM kinase is much reduced in PSDs isolated from the cerebellum, where the kinase is composed mainly of β-subunits. We have postulated that the α-subunit may contain a binding site for a PSD receptor protein (Miller and Kennedy 1985).

Preparation of purified PSDs from brain homogenates requires the isolation of a crude synaptosomal fraction, followed by a treatment of that fraction with detergent, either Triton X-100 (Cohen et al. 1977) or sodium lauroyl sarcosinate (Cotman et al. 1974). Finally, PSDs relatively free of membrane lipids are isolated by differential or density gradient centrifugation. Because of the necessity for detergent treatment to remove synaptosomal membranes, there has been controversy about the relationship between the composition of the PSD fraction and the true composition of PSDs in vivo. Some proteins can become denatured by detergent and may associate artifactually with the PSD fraction (Matus et al. 1980). To confirm the presence of the CaM kinase in PSDs prior to detergent treatment, we stained synaptosomes immunocytochemically with a monoclonal antibody against the CaM kinase (Fig. 1). Because these experiments were specifically designed

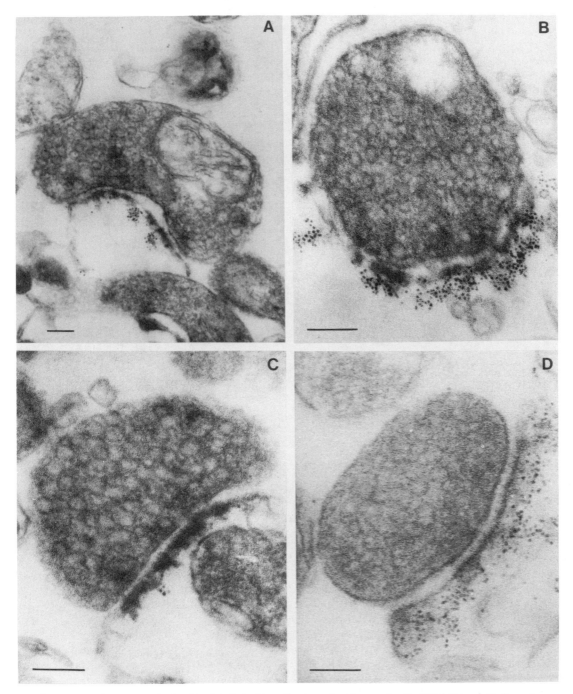

Figure 1. Synaptosomal postsynaptic densities labeled with antibody against the α-subunit of CaM kinase II. Synaptosomes were prepared, embedded in agarose, and labeled with either a specific monoclonal antibody against the α-subunit (6g9) or control mouse IgG and then with ferritin-labeled sheep anti-mouse IgG, as described in Experimental Procedures. (*A, C*) Representative synaptosomes labeled with control mouse IgG. (*B, D*) Representative synaptosomes labeled with monoclonal antibody 6g9. Bars, 100 nm.

to detect the kinase in PSDs, synaptosomes were kept intact during the incubations with antibodies. Figure 1 shows examples of forebrain synaptosomes labeled with either anti-α-subunit or control mouse antibodies and then with ferritin-labeled sheep anti-mouse IgG secondary antibodies. Figure 2A summarizes the extent of labeling with control and anti-kinase antibodies. On the average, the concentration of ferritin particles was three times higher in PSDs stained with the specific anti-α-subunit antibody. When synaptosomes from the cerebellum and from the hippocampus were labeled separately (Fig. 2B), the average density of particles in

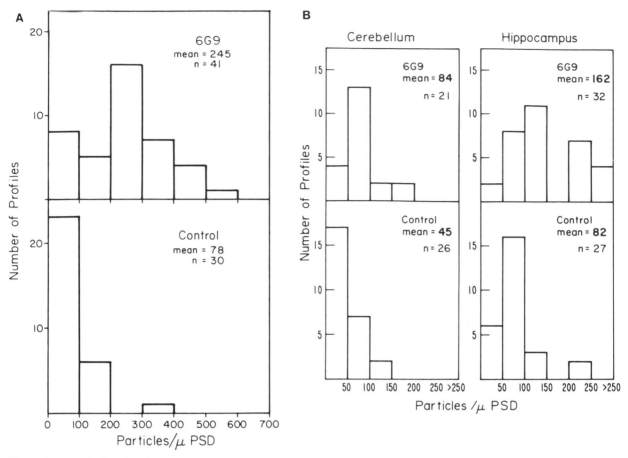

Figure 2. Quantitation of ferritin-labeling of synaptosomal postsynaptic densities. The number of ferritin grains per micrometer of PSD was determined for several synaptosomal profiles after labeling with antibodies as described in the legend to Fig. 1. (*A*) Labeling of forebrain PSDs with monoclonal antibody 6g9 or control mouse IgG. (*B*) Labeling of cerebellar and hippocampal PSDs with monoclonal antibody 6g9 or control mouse IgG.

hippocampal PSDs was approximately twice that of cerebellar PSDs. This is consistent with the earlier finding that less CaM kinase is associated with cerebellar PSDs than with forebrain PSDs; although the difference between PSDs from the two regions is greater when measured biochemically (Miller and Kennedy 1985). The results support the hypothesis that the CaM kinase is highly concentrated in PSDs in vivo. It is important to remember, however, that the kinase is not uniquely located in PSDs. About half of it is soluble and appears to be distributed throughout the neuronal cytosol (Ouimet et al. 1984; Erondu and Kennedy 1985). From the ferritin-labeling data, we estimate that the effective concentration of α-subunits in forebrain PSDs is approximately 100–400 μM. This is five to ten times higher than the concentration of α-subunits in the cytosol (19–37 μM), estimated from its abundance in forebrain homogenates (1% of total protein).

The high concentration of CaM kinase in PSDs in the hippocampus suggests that it may be an important target for the Ca^{++} current that is generated by activation of N-methyl-D-aspartate receptors. This current is necessary for induction of long-term potentiation (Malenka et al. 1988). Recent physiological studies

from the laboratories of R. Nicoll and R. Tsien indicate that inhibition of postsynaptic CaM kinase blocks induction of long-term potentiation (LTP), strengthening the hypothesis that type II CaM kinase plays a role in the generation of LTP (Malenka et al. 1989; Malinow et al. 1989).

Regulation of CaM Kinase II by Autophosphorylation

Each individual CaM kinase subunit can be autophosphorylated when the holoenzyme is activated in the presence of Ca^{++}/calmodulin (Bennett et al. 1983). This autophosphorylation is the basis of an interesting mechanism for controlling CaM kinase activity. Nonphosphorylated CaM kinase is catalytically active only in the presence of Ca^{++}/calmodulin. However, if the kinase is briefly autophosphorylated by incubating it for 5 seconds in the presence of Ca^{++}/calmodulin and ATP before it is added to assay tubes containing exogenous substrate, a new Ca^{++}-independent activity becomes apparent (Fig. 3) (Miller and Kennedy 1986). The magnitude of this activity depends on the substrate (Patton et al. 1990). With a synthetic peptide substrate,

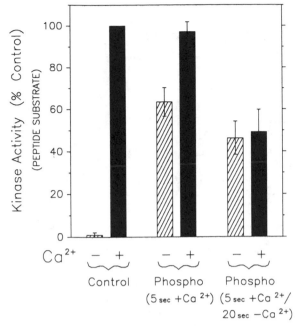

Figure 3. Effects of autophosphorylation on the kinase activity of CaM kinase II. Purified kinase was autophosphorylated and then assayed with a synthetic peptide substrate (calmodulin-dependent protein kinase substrate analog, purchased from Peninsula Laboratories) as described previously (Patton et al. 1990). Kinase was autophosphorylated for the indicated times in the presence or presence followed by absence of Ca^{++}. Control and autophosphorylated kinase was incubated in the autophosphorylation mix without Ca^{++}. Autophosphorylated kinase was then diluted into a second assay mix containing $[\gamma\text{-}^{32}P]ATP$, peptide substrate, and either EGTA or Ca^{++}/calmodulin (Patton et al. 1990). Bars represent initial rates of kinase activity expressed as a percentage of the control activity in the presence of Ca^{++}.

Second, the autophosphorylated kinase continues to phosphorylate itself as well as exogenous substrates; thus, autophosphorylation becomes Ca^{++}-independent. Third, the effects of autophosphorylation are reversible. Ca^{++}-independent activity is lost when the kinase is dephosphorylated by protein phosphatases (Lai et al. 1986; Miller and Kennedy 1986; Miller et al. 1988). Finally, autophosphorylation is restricted to individual holoenzymes. Autophosphorylated subunits within a holoenzyme can cause autophosphorylation of neighboring subunits, but one activated holoenzyme does not autophosphorylate another (Miller and Kennedy 1986).

Taken together, these properties suggest that the CaM kinase can act as a kind of switch (Fig. 4). In state 1, the kinase is completely dependent on Ca^{++} and calmodulin for activity. When sufficient autophosphorylation has occurred, the kinase is switched to state 2 in which it has a substantial Ca^{++}-independent kinase activity with exogenous substrates. Furthermore, in state 2, Ca^{++}-independent autophosphorylation can oppose dephosphorylation by cellular phosphatases, which would return the kinase to state 1. This switch mechanism may allow the CaM kinase to retain information in vivo about prior activating Ca^{++} signals. This information would be "read out" as continuing phosphorylation of functionally significant substrate proteins. The length of time that the information would be retained would depend on the balance between the rate of Ca^{++}-independent autophosphorylation and the local catalytic rate of cellular phosphatases.

Identification of Regulatory Autophosphorylation Sites

To learn more precisely how the switch mechanism operates, the specific autophosphorylation site within the CaM kinase that controls Ca^{++}-independent activity has been identified. Thr-286, located on the amino-terminal side of the calmodulin-binding domain (Fig. 5), is autophosphorylated rapidly when the kinase is activated by Ca^{++}/calmodulin (Miller et al. 1988; Schworer et al. 1988; Thiel et al. 1988). The rate of autophosphorylation and dephosphorylation of this site correlates closely with the onset and decay, respectively, of Ca^{++}-independent activity (Miller et al. 1988). The importance of Thr-286 for control of Ca^{++}-independent activity has been confirmed by experiments

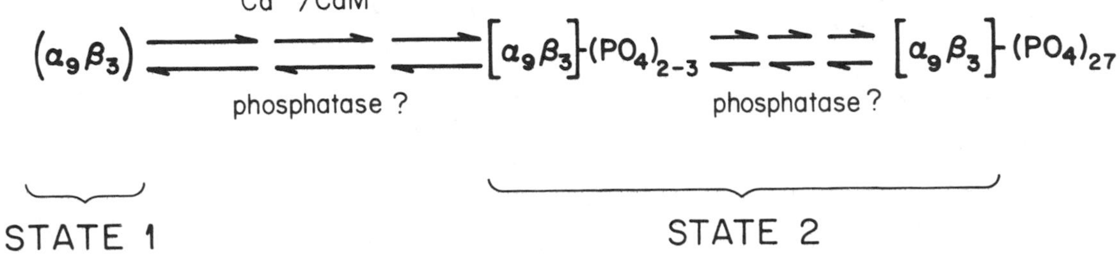

such as that used in the experiment shown in Figure 3, phosphorylation proceeds in the absence of Ca^{++} at about 60% of the rate in the presence of Ca^{++}.

This switch to a partially Ca^{++}-independent state has four important features. First, the Ca^{++}-independent activity is fully activated after addition of as little as 2–3 moles of phosphate to the CaM kinase per mole of dodecameric holoenzyme (Miller and Kennedy 1986). Therefore, the activation appears to be cooperative; autophosphorylation of one or two of the subunits in a holoenzyme produces activation of the other subunits.

$$(\alpha_9\beta_3) \underset{\text{phosphatase ?}}{\overset{Ca^{2+}/CaM}{\rightleftharpoons}} [\alpha_9\beta_3]\text{-}(PO_4)_{2-3} \underset{\text{phosphatase ?}}{\rightleftharpoons} [\alpha_9\beta_3]\text{-}(PO_4)_{27}$$

STATE 1   STATE 2

Figure 4. Hypothetical switch model of regulation of type II Ca^{++}/calmodulin-dependent protein kinase by autophosphorylation and dephosphorylation. (Modified from Miller and Kennedy 1986.)

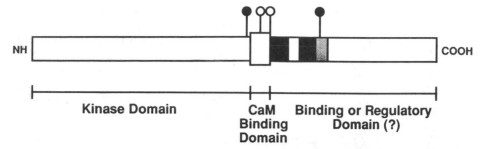

Figure 5. Location of autophosphorylation sites in the sequence of type II Ca^{++}/calmodulin-dependent protein kinase. (●) Sites that are autophosphorylated rapidly when the kinase is activated by Ca^{++}/calmodulin. The site to the left of the calmodulin-binding domain is Thr-286 in the α-subunit (287 in the β-subunit). (○) Sites that are autophosphorylated only when Ca^{++} is removed from the reaction after autophosphorylation of Thr-286. The site in the middle of the calmodulin-binding domain is Thr-305 in the α-subunit (Thr-306 in the β-subunit). The site to the right of the calmodulin-binding domain is Ser-314 in the α-subunit (Ser-315 in the β-subunit). The regions marked by dark bars or stippled bars are present only in the sequence of the β-subunit. The region marked by the stippled bar is spliced out of the β'-subunit. (Modified from Patton et al. 1990.)

in which Thr-286 was changed to leucine by in vitro mutagenesis (Hanson et al. 1989). The mutated kinase does not show Ca^{++}-independent activity upon auto-phosphorylation. The location of Thr-286 suggests a model in which its autophosphorylation partially mimics binding of calmodulin and prevents refolding of the kinase into an inactive conformation (Fig. 6).

When Ca^{++} is removed from the autophosphorylation reaction after the kinase is in state 2, a new site becomes autophosphorylated and the kinase is now insensitive to further stimulation by Ca^{++}/calmodulin (Fig. 3) (Hashimoto et al. 1987). We have identified two additional sites that are rapidly autophosphorylated only after Ca^{++} is removed from an ongoing autophosphorylation reaction. One of these, Thr-305 (Fig. 5) (Patton et al. 1990), is located in the middle of

the calmodulin-binding domain in a sequence of five amino acids that is required for high-affinity binding of calmodulin (Payne et al. 1988). The other site, Ser-314, is located at the carboxy-terminal end of the cal-modulin-binding domain. Inhibition of sensitivity to calmodulin and reversal of this inhibition correlate well with autophosphorylation and dephosphorylation of Thr-305, respectively. Autophosphorylation of Ser-314 causes only a twofold reduction in affinity for cal-modulin (Patton et al. 1990). Curiously, phosphoserine 314 is resistant to dephosphorylation by protein phos-phatases.

The sequence of regulatory events governing activity of one subunit of the CaM kinase is summarized in Figure 6. Inactive kinase is shown in Figure 6A. In the presence of Ca^{++}, calmodulin binds to a specific se-quence, resulting in a conformational change that opens the active site and allows phosphorylation of exogenous substrates (Fig. 6B). At the same time, Thr-286, next to the calmodulin-binding domain, is rapidly autophosphorylated. When Ca^{++} is removed from the reaction, calmodulin is released from the kinase (Fig. 6C). However, the phosphate group on Thr-286 prevents complete refolding of the kinase. In this state, the kinase is still active although at a some-what reduced rate. An additional site, Thr-305, located in the middle of the calmodulin-binding domain, is now autophosphorylated. In the state depicted in Figure 6C, the kinase has a substantial Ca^{++}-independent activity but cannot be further stimulated by Ca^{++}/calmodulin. It is returned to the inactive state A by dephosphoryla-tion by cellular phosphatases. This model depicts the cycle for one subunit and does not illustrate the cooperative activation of subunits within a holoen-zyme. Cooperative activation may occur by either of two mechanisms. Autophosphorylated subunits may activate adjacent subunits through allosteric conforma-tional changes transmitted through subunit-subunit in-teractions. Alternatively, autophosphorylated subunits may be able to phosphorylate neighboring subunits directly within the holoenzyme.

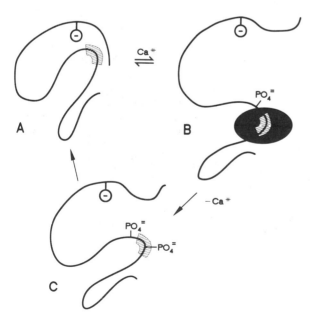

Figure 6. Schematic model of regulation of a subunit of type II Ca^{++}/calmodulin-dependent protein kinase by autophos-phorylation. See text for explanation and discussion.

Organotypic Cultures of Hippocampal Neurons

We are interested in studying how the CaM kinase functions in situ within hippocampal neurons, where it is expressed at a high concentration and has been implicated in the initiation of LTP. Physiologists have successfully studied synaptic transmission between hip-

pocampal neurons in slices prepared acutely from adult brain tissue (Nicoll 1988). However, this system may not be ideal for biochemical studies because damaged tissue at the surface of the slice cannot be separated from intact neurons at the center of the slice. Dissociated cultures of hippocampal neurons are healthy, but synapses are made randomly within the cultures

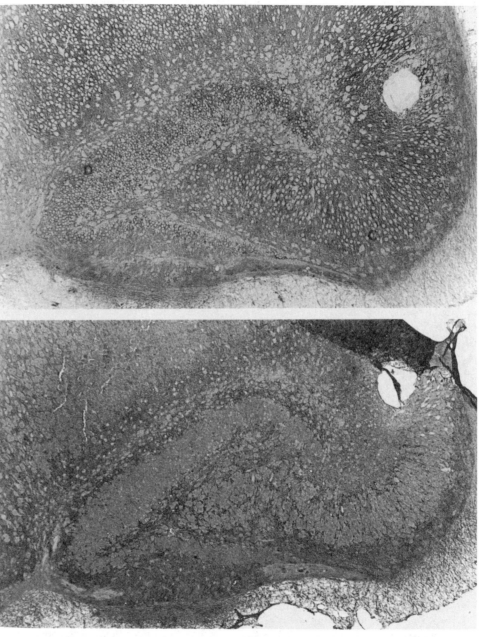

Figure 7. Immunocytochemical staining of organotypic cultures of hippocampus for the α-subunit of CaM kinase II and synapsin I. Organotypic cultures were fixed, embedded in plastic, and cut into 2-μm sections as described previously (DeCamilli et al. 1983a; S.S. Molloy and M.B. Kennedy, in prep.). The sections were etched with peroxide and then incubated with anti-α-subunit monoclonal antibody 6g9 (*top*) or rabbit antisera against synapsin I (*bottom*). The sections were then incubated with appropriate secondary antibodies coupled to horseradish peroxidase. Antibodies were visualized by reaction with diaminobenzidine, and then the sections were photographed with an Olympus Vanox microscope (S.S. Molloy and M.B. Kennedy, in prep.). The preservation of the dentate gyrus (D) and the CA pyramidal fields (C) in the cultures is evident. Cell bodies in both of these areas have spread out as the cultures flattened. Note the dark staining of cytosol and dendrites for CaM kinase (*top*). Also note the large punctate mossy fiber terminals in CA3 stained for synapsin I (*bottom*). At higher magnification, smaller punctate structures stained for synapsin I can be visualized throughout the molecular layers. Magnification, 55 $\times$.

and at relatively low density (Bartlett and Banker 1984). We have explored the use of a third preparation, organotypic cultures of hippocampal slices. This preparation was first developed by Gahwiler (1988) in Switzerland, and we have modified it slightly for our purposes (S.S. Molloy and M.B. Kennedy, in prep.). To prepare the cultures, hippocampi are dissected from 4- to 6-day-old rats and cut into 400-μm slices. The slices are fastened onto collagen-coated coverslips with a drop of liquid collagen. When the collagen has polymerized, the coverslips are placed into test tubes in 1 ml of liquid medium (Gahwiler 1984; S.S. Molloy and M.B. Kennedy, in prep.) and incubated on a roller so that the cultures are exposed periodically to air. On the fourth day, the cultures are treated with mitotic inhibitors to reduce the division of glial cells. After about 2 weeks, the cultures have shed dead tissue and flattened to a thickness of 2–3 cells (50–80 μm). They retain many anatomical characteristics of the hippocampus in vivo, including a mossy fiber projection from dentate granule cells to area CA3 and a Schaffer collateral pathway from CA3 to CA1 neurons (Gahwiler 1988). The neurons contain CaM kinase at a concentration similar to that in vivo. Immunocytochemical staining of the cultures for the α-subunit of CaM kinase (Fig. 7; top) or for the synaptic-vesicle-associated protein synapsin I (Fig. 7; bottom) produces patterns of staining similar to those in fixed tissue from adult brain (De-Camilli et al. 1983a; Ouimet et al. 1984). CaM kinase staining is dense in dendrites and cytosol with dark patches along dendrites that may represent concentrations of kinase at postsynaptic densities (S.S. Molloy and M.B. Kennedy, in prep.). Synapsin I staining is concentrated in small punctate structures that may represent presynaptic terminals. Our goal is to use these cultures to answer several specific questions. How is the CaM kinase regulated in situ? Is the switch mechanism described above used in situ? What are the substrate proteins for the CaM kinase in specific parts of the neurons. Finally, what functions does the CaM kinase regulate.

Autophosphorylation of CaM Kinase II In Situ

We attempted to determine whether Thr-286, the site that controls Ca^{++}-independent activity in vitro, could be labeled with [^{32}P]phosphate in situ (Fig. 8) (S.S. Molloy and M.B. Kennedy, in prep.). Several cultures were incubated overnight in a medium containing $^{32}PO_4$ to label ATP pools and phosphorylated proteins. The cultures were homogenized in a buffer that suppresses the activity of protein phosphatases. The CaM kinase was immunoprecipitated with specific anti-kinase monoclonal antibodies. After separation of the subunits by SDS-polyacrylamide gel electrophoresis, the α-subunit was digested with trypsin, and the labeled tryptic phosphopeptides were fractionated by high-performance liquid chromatography (HPLC) to generate a peptide map. Comparison of this map to similar maps of purified CaM kinase autophosphory-

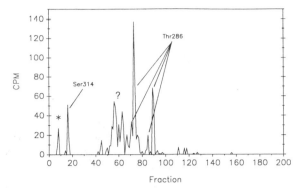

Figure 8. Phosphotryptic peptide map of the α-subunit of type II Ca^{++}/calmodulin-dependent protein kinase from cultures labeled with $^{32}PO_4$ in situ. Organotypic hippocampal cultures were incubated overnight in medium containing $^{32}PO_4$ and then homogenized. CaM kinase was immunoprecipitated from the homogenate, its subunits were separated, and phosphotryptic peptides were prepared as described previously (Miller et al. 1988; Patton et al. 1990; S.S. Molloy and M.B. Kennedy, in prep.). The peptides were fractionated by reverse-phase HPLC, and radioactivity in the fractions was counted. The four peptides marked threonine-286 were identified as phosphotryptic peptides containing phosphothreonine-286 by comparison to similar maps of the α-subunit of purified CaM kinase (Miller et al. 1988). The peptide identified as containing Ser-314 is also marked. The asterisk marks the void volume, and the question mark indicates unidentified peptides that are occasionally present in maps prepared from both purified kinase and kinase labeled in situ. They may be chemically altered forms of peptides containing Thr-305 (Patton et al. 1990; S.S. Molloy and M.B. Kennedy, in prep.).

lated in vitro (Miller et al. 1988; Patton et al. 1990) permitted identification of the most prominent site labeled with $^{32}PO_4$ in situ as Thr-286 (Fig. 8) (S.S. Molloy and M.B. Kennedy, in prep.). Thus, kinase molecules can be autophosphorylated at this site in situ, even in the absence of exogenous stimulation.

To determine the extent of autophosphorylation of Thr-286 in situ, we measured the proportion of CaM kinase in the Ca^{++}-independent state in culture homogenates. We first maximally autophosphorylated the CaM kinase in a set of homogenates by incubating them with ATP in the presence of Ca^{++}. We then determined that, in these homogenates with synapsin I as substrate, CaM kinase activity in the absence of Ca^{++} was 27% of the full activity in the presence of Ca^{++}. Synapsin I was used as substrate in these experiments because, unlike synthetic peptides, its phosphorylation in the absence of Ca^{++} in culture homogenates is catalyzed entirely by CaM kinase II (S.S. Molloy and M.B. Kennedy, in prep.). We next determined kinase activity in the absence and presence of Ca^{++} in homogenates prepared under conditions designed to preserve the state of autophosphorylation in vivo. The value was $8.4 \pm 0.4\%$, indicating that approximately 31% of the kinase in culture homogenates is in the Ca^{++}-independent state. This percentage was not reduced by extended treatment of the cultures with a variety of glutamate receptor antagonists before homogenization. Thus, the high proportion of autophosphorylated kinase in the cultures does not depend on spontaneous electrical activity. The proportion was reduced, however, by treatment of the cultures with H7, a general protein kinase inhibitor that crosses cellular membranes, or by reduction of the concentration of external Ca^{++} in the culture medium. When Ca^{++} was removed from the medium, the proportion of kinase in the Ca^{++}-independent state decreased to approximately 5% in 25–30 minutes (S.S. Molloy and M.B. Kennedy, in prep.). Therefore, both Ca^{++} and continuing kinase activity are required to maintain the autophosphorylated state in vivo.

A high percentage of CaM kinase II is in the Ca^{++}-independent state in hippocampi from intact rats. Forebrains and hippocampi were dissected from rats of increasing age and homogenized according to the method described for hippocampal cultures. The percentage of kinase in the Ca^{++}-independent state in these homogenates was 23 ± 0.9 for rats of 6 to approximately 24 days of age, and 13 ± 0.7 for rats older than 25 days, suggesting a developmental change around day 25 postnatal (S.S. Molloy and M.B. Kennedy, in prep.).

The functional significance of this high proportion of Ca^{++}-independent CaM kinase activity is at present unknown. It will be important to determine the subcellular location of the autophosphorylated kinase, as well as the identity of substrate proteins of the kinase in situ. However, the experiments with hippocampal cultures have demonstrated unequivocally that the autophosphorylation switch mechanism is used in situ. It seems likely that organotypic cultures of defined brain regions will be used extensively in the future to study the biochemistry of neuronal plasticity. They provide a system in which new methods can be developed to follow modulatory reactions through time and at particular sites within neurons.

ACKNOWLEDGMENTS

This work was supported by National Institutes of Health grants NS-17660 and training grant NS-07251, the Epilepsy Foundation of America, the McKnight Foundation, the Joseph W. Drown Foundation, the Irvine Foundation, the Gustavus and Louise Pfeiffer Research Foundation, and the Beckman Institute. We are grateful to Jean-Paul Revel and Pat Koen for help with the experiments involving electron microscopy.

REFERENCES

Bartlett, W.P. and G.A. Banker. 1984. An electron microscopic study of the development of axons and dendrites by hippocampal neurons in culture. II. Synaptic relationships. *J. Neurosci.* 4: 1954.

Bennett, M.K., N.E. Erondu, and M.B. Kennedy. 1983. Purification and characterization of a calmodulin-dependent protein kinase that is highly concentrated in brain. *J. Biol. Chem.* 258: 12735.

Bulleit, R.F., M.K. Bennett, S.S. Molloy, J.B. Hurley, and M.B. Kennedy. 1988. Conserved and variable regions in the subunits of brain type II Ca^{2+}/calmodulin-dependent protein kinase. *Neuron* 1: 63.

Cohen, R.S., F. Blomberg, K. Berzins, and P. Siekevitz. 1977. Structure of postsynaptic densities isolated from dog cerebral cortex. I. Overall morphology and protein composition. *J. Cell Biol.* 74: 181.

Cotman, C.W., G. Banker, L. Churchill, and D. Taylor. 1974. Isolation of postsynaptic densities from rat brain. *J. Cell Biol.* 63: 441.

DeCamilli, P., R. Cameron, and P. Greengard. 1983a. Synapsin I (Protein I), a nerve terminal-specific phosphoprotein. I. Its general distribution in synapses of the central and peripheral nervous system demonstrated by immunofluorescence in frozen and plastic sections. *J. Cell Biol.* 96: 1337.

DeCamilli, P., S.M. Harris, Jr., W.B. Huttner, and P. Greengard. 1983b. Synapsin I (Protein I), a nerve terminal-specific phosphoprotein. II. Its specific association with synaptic vesicles demonstrated by immunocytochemistry in agarose-embedded synaptosomes. *J. Cell Biol.* 96: 1355.

Erondu, N.E. and M.B. Kennedy. 1985. Regional distribution of type II Ca^{2+}/calmodulin-dependent protein kinase in rat brain. *J. Neurosci.* 5: 3270.

Gahwiler, B.H. 1984. Slice cultures of cerebellar, hippocampal and hypothalamic tissue. *Experientia* 40: 235.

———. 1988. Organotypic cultures of neural tissue. *Trends Neurosci.* 11: 484.

Goldenring, J.R., B. Gonzalez, J.S. McGuire, Jr., and R.J. DeLorenzo. 1983. Purification and characterization of a calmodulin-dependent kinase from rat brain cytosol able to phosphorylate tubulin and microtubule-associated protein. *J. Biol. Chem.* 258: 12632.

Hanson, P.I., M.S. Kapiloff, L.L. Lou, M.G. Rosenfeld, and H. Schulman. 1989. Expression of a multifunctional Ca^{2+}/calmodulin-dependent protein kinase and mutational analysis of its autoregulation. *Neuron* 3: 59.

Hashimoto, Y., C.M. Schworer, R.J. Colbran, and T.R. Soderling. 1987. Autophosphorylation of Ca^{2+}/calmodulin-dependent protein kinase II. Effects on total and Ca^{2+}-independent activities and kinetic parameters. *J. Biol. Chem.* 262: 8051.

Kelly, P.T. and C.W. Cotman. 1978. Synaptic proteins. Characterization of tubulin and actin and identification of a distinct postsynaptic density polypeptide. *J. Cell Biol.* 79: 173.

Kennedy, M.B., M.K. Bennett, and N.E. Erondu. 1983a. Biochemical and immunochemical evidence that the "major postsynaptic density protein" is a subunit of a calmodulin-dependent protein kinase. *Proc. Natl. Acad. Sci.* 80: 7357.

Kennedy, M.B., T.L. McGuinness, and P. Greengard. 1983b. A calcium/calmodulin-dependent protein kinase from mammalian brain that phosphorylates synapsin I. Partial purification and characterization. *J. Neurosci.* 3: 818.

Lai, Y., A.C. Nairn, and P. Greengard. 1986. Autophosphorylation reversibly regulates the Ca^{2+}/calmodulin-dependence of Ca^{2+}/calmodulin-dependent protein kinase II. *Proc. Natl. Acad. Sci.* 83: 4253.

Malenka, R.C., J.A. Kauer, R.S. Zucker, and R.A. Nicoll. 1988. Postsynaptic calcium is sufficient for potentiation of hippocampal synaptic transmission. *Science* 242: 81.

Malenka, R.C., J.A. Kauer, D.J. Perkel, M.D. Mauk, P.T. Kelly, R.A. Nicoll, and M.N. Waxham. 1989. An essential role for postsynaptic calmodulin and protein kinase activity in long-term potentiation. *Nature* 340: 554.

Malinow, R., H. Schulman, and R.W. Tsien. 1989. Inhibition of postsynaptic PKC or CaMKII blocks induction but not expression of LTP. *Science* 245: 862.

Matus, A., G. Pehling, M. Ackermann, and J. Maeder. 1980. Brain postsynaptic densities: Their relationship to glial and neuronal filaments. *J. Cell Biol.* 87: 346.

McGuinness, T.L., Y. Lai, and P. Greengard. 1985. Ca^{2+}/calmodulin-dependent protein kinase II. Isozymic forms from rat forebrain and cerebellum. *J. Biol. Chem.* **260:** 1696.

Miller, S.G. and M.B. Kennedy. 1985. Distinct forebrain and cerebellar isozymes of type II Ca^{2+}/calmodulin-dependent protein kinase associate differently with the postsynaptic density fraction. *J. Biol. Chem.* **260:** 9039.

——. 1986. Regulation of brain type II Ca^{2+}/calmodulin-dependent protein kinase by autophosphorylation: A Ca^{2+}-triggered molecular switch. *Cell* **44:** 861.

Miller, S.G., B.L Patton, and M.B. Kennedy. 1988. Sequences of autophosphorylation sites in neuronal type II CaM kinase that control Ca^{2+}-independent activity. *Neuron* **1:** 593.

Nicoll, R.A. 1988. The coupling of neurotransmitter receptors to ion channels in the brain. *Science* **241:** 545.

Ouimet, C.C., T.L. McGuinness, and P. Greengard. 1984. Immunocytochemical localization of calcium/calmodulin-dependent protein kinase II in rat brain. *Proc. Natl. Acad. Sci.* **81:** 5604.

Patton, B.L., S.G. Miller, and M.B. Kennedy. 1990. Activation of type II Ca^{2+}/calmodulin dependent protein kinase by Ca^{2+}/calmodulin is inhibited by autophosphorylation of threonine within the calmodulin-binding domain. *J. Biol. Chem.* **265:** 11204.

Payne, M.E., Y.-L. Fong, T. Ono, R.J. Colbran, B.E. Kemp, T.R. Soderling, and A.R. Means. 1988. Calcium/calmodulin-dependent protein kinase II. Characterization of distinct calmodulin binding and inhibitory domains. *J. Biol. Chem.* **263:** 7190.

Schworer, C.M., R.J. Colbran, J.R. Keefer, and T.R. Soderling. 1988. Ca^{2+}/calmodulin-dependent protein kinase II. Identification of a regulatory autophosphorylation site adjacent to the inhibitory calmodulin-binding domains. *J. Biol. Chem.* **263:** 13486.

Thiel, G., A.J. Czernik, F. Gorelick, A.C. Nairn, and P. Greengard. 1988. Ca^{2+}/calmodulin-dependent protein kinase II: Identification of threonine-286 as the autophosphorylation site in the α subunit associated with the generation of Ca^{2+}-independent activity. *Proc. Natl. Acad. Sci.* **85:** 6337.

Tobimatsu, T. and H. Fujisawa. 1989. Tissue-specific expression of four types of rat calmodulin-dependent protein kinase II mRNAs. *J. Biol. Chem.* **264:** 17907.

Tobimatsu, T., I. Kameshita, and H. Fujisawa. 1988. Molecular cloning of the cDNA encoding the third polypeptide (γ) of brain calmodulin-dependent protein kinase II. *J. Biol. Chem.* **263:** 16082.

Molecular Analysis of Proteins Associated with the Synaptic Vesicle Membrane

J.K. Ngsee, W.S. Trimble, L.A. Elferink, B. Wendland, K. Miller,
N. Calakos, and R.H. Scheller

Department of Biological Sciences, Stanford University, Stanford, California 94305-5020

Neurons communicate with their targets through the quantal release of chemical transmitters. The central organelle involved in this process is the synaptic vesicle that stores the transmitters and, upon the appropriate signals, releases its contents into the synaptic cleft. The modulation of transmitter release in response to experience is likely to be a cellular mechanism of learning and memory. Thus, an understanding of the factors regulating the morphogenesis and release of synaptic vesicles is fundamental to our understanding of brain function. Synaptic vesicle proteins are synthesized in the cell body and transported to the nerve terminal via microtubule-based fast axonal transport. On arrival at the nerve terminal, vesicles are sequestered at the active zone and await the arrival of a fusogenic signal. Fusion with the presynaptic membrane and subsequent release of the luminal content is dependent on a number of factors, most notably a rise in intracellular Ca^{++}. Proteins and lipids are then recycled from the presynaptic membrane by endocytosis, and the empty vesicles are replenished with chemical transmitter by an uptake system. The precise mechanisms underlying these processes have not been characterized.

In addition to synaptic vesicles containing classical neurotransmitters, neurons often contain biologically active neuropeptides that are packaged in a separate class of large dense cored vesicles (DCV). In contrast with classical neurotransmitter-containing vesicles, the neuropeptides are synthesized solely in the cell body. Thus, the fate of the DCV membranes at the nerve terminal is not clear. Furthermore, there is a continual need to replenish proteins and lipids in the presynaptic plasma membrane. These molecules are most likely inserted into the synapse constitutively by the fusion of small transport vesicles with the plasma membrane. In light of the existence of many different vesicle classes with varying membrane proteins and luminal contents, there must exist an efficient mechanism to sort and target proteins to the different membrane compartments and to deliver the different classes of vesicles to their appropriate sites. It is likely that there also exists an efficient salvage mechanism, whereby certain protein and lipid components are retrieved from the presynaptic membrane and recycled, either within the synaptic terminal or after retrograde transport to the cell soma.

It is our hypothesis that many of the proteins regulating vesicular function either are an integral component of synaptic vesicle membrane or are associated with the synaptic vesicle membrane. Assuming similarities in some of the basic mechanisms of vesicular transport, certain proteins are likely to be common to a number of different vesicles. However, different vesicle classes must also possess specific surface molecules that are recognized by the transport apparatus, thus allowing for differential targeting. Moreover, synaptic vesicles are likely to contain additional proteins involved in triggering the rapid exocytotic event in response to an incoming stimulus. To address the underlying mechanism of vesicular trafficking and regulated exocytosis, we and several other laboratories have embarked on a biochemical and molecular characterization of the proteins associated with synaptic vesicles. In this paper, we describe three types of proteins associated with synaptic vesicles: vesicle-associated membrane protein (VAMP), synaptophysin, and a family of low-molecular-weight GTP-binding proteins.

Isolation of Cholinergic Synaptic Vesicles

One useful model for studies of the synapse is the electromotor system of the marine elasmobranchs. The electric organ contains an ordered array of electrocytes innervated by electromotor neurons whose cell bodies are located in the electric lobe. This system has been used extensively as an enriched source of cholinergic synaptic vesicles. Each vesicle has been estimated to contain approximately 50,000 molecules of acetylcholine and 15,000 molecules of ATP (Wagner et al. 1978; Whittaker and Stadler 1980). These synaptic vesicles can be purified readily by differential centrifugation, followed by sucrose density gradient flotation and controlled pore glass 3000 (CPG-3000) column chromatography (Carlson et al. 1978). Electron microscopy analysis of the membranous material following CPG-3000 chromatography is shown in Figure 1. The excluded fraction contains a collection of irregularly shaped vesicles ranging from 140 to 300 nm in size. Large multilamellar structures, probably representing disrupted plasma membrane or membranes from intracellular organelles such as mitochondria, are often seen in this fraction. In contrast, the cholinergic synaptic vesicles eluted in the later fractions are virtually free of these contaminating membrane structures. The vesicles in this fraction appear electron luscent with an average diameter of 86 ± 3 nm. This is identical in size

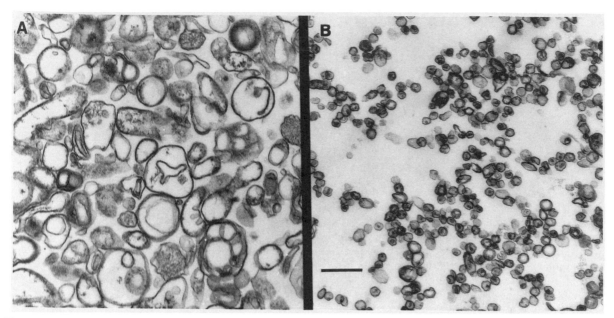

Figure 1. Electron micrograph of the membrane vesicles following CPG-3000 column chromatography as exemplified in Fig. 5. Membranes from the excluded fraction (*A*) and the synaptic vesicle fraction (*B*) were collected by centrifugation at 100,000*g* and fixed in a phosphate-buffered isotonic solution of sucrose and glutaraldehyde prior to Epon embedding and sectioning. Bar, 400 nm.

to synaptic vesicles present in the electric organ in situ. This homogeneous population of cholinergic synaptic vesicles presents a simple protein profile for biochemical and molecular analysis. Different molecular genetic approaches were undertaken in the isolation and characterization of the synaptic vesicle proteins: immunological screening of an expression library with an antiserum against purified synaptic vesicles, screening with homologous cDNA probes, and characterization of related proteins containing a defined functional domain or biological activity, such as GTP-binding.

VAMP Is a Synaptic-vesicle-associated Integral Membrane Protein

Expression screening of a *Torpedo californica* λgt11 cDNA library using a polyclonal antiserum raised against purified synaptic vesicles (Carlson and Kelly 1980) resulted in the isolation of a clone encoding a 120-amino-acid synaptic VAMP (Trimble et al. 1988). Two highly related genes, VAMP-1 and VAMP-2, were subsequently identified in the rat (Elferink et al. 1989). An 18-kD integral membrane protein in bovine synaptic vesicles (called synaptobrevin) was found to be almost identical to rat VAMP-2, and a homologous protein has also been found in *Drosophila* (Südhof et al. 1989). Comparison of the amino acid sequences of the various VAMP proteins indicates a universal structural motif. As exemplified by the two rat VAMP proteins illustrated in Figure 2, the molecules consist of four defined structural domains: (1) a proline-rich amino-terminal domain of 26–30 amino acids, (2) a highly conserved hydrophilic core of 70 amino acids, (3) a conserved hydrophobic membrane spanning domain of approximately 20 amino acids, and (4) a potential short luminal carboxy-terminal extension in the vertebrates

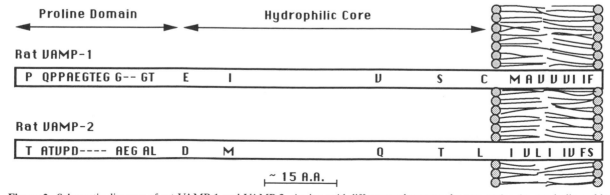

Figure 2. Schematic diagram of rat VAMP-1 and VAMP-2. Amino acid differences between the two molecules are indicated by the single amino acid code. Gaps introduced to maximize alignment between the two sequences are indicated by dashes.

and a longer 20-amino-acid stretch in *Drosophila* (Trimble et al. 1988; Südhof et al. 1989). Protease protection experiments indicate that the amino terminus extends into the cytoplasm (Trimble et al. 1988). This topology is functionally compatible with a protein involved in mediating interactions between synaptic vesicles and cytoplasmic factors or intracellular domains of membrane proteins. The lack of a well-defined signal sequence, together with the presence of a hydrophobic carboxy-terminal membrane anchor, suggests that the VAMP proteins are inserted posttranslationally into the membrane. The highly specific vesicle localization suggests that the proteins contain a domain for specific targeting to the synaptic vesicle membrane (see below). In the rat, in situ hybridization experiments reveal that the two VAMP genes are differentially expressed by neurons within the brain and spinal cord (Trimble et al. 1990). VAMP-2 expression appears to be widespread but predominates in nuclei responsible for autonomic and neuroendocrine functions, whereas VAMP-1 mRNA is found predominantly in motoneurons and in a subset of neurons that innervate them. The significance of this distribution is unknown, but it suggests that the two VAMPs have discrete functional roles.

Molecular Analysis of Synaptophysin

Synaptophysin (also known as p38) is a major integral glycoprotein in the synaptic vesicle membrane (Jahn et al. 1985; Wiedenmann and Franke 1985; Navone et al. 1986). Several groups have cloned the cDNAs encoding synaptophysin from mammalian species (Buckley et al. 1987; Leube et al. 1987; Südhof et al. 1987) and from the marine ray (Cowan et al. 1990). On the basis of the deduced amino acid sequence and biochemical analysis, the protein is predicted to span the membrane four times with both amino and carboxyl termini extending into the cytoplasm. The protein contains one N-linked glycosylation site located on the first intravesicular loop. Sequence comparison of the three mammalian synaptophysin proteins indicates that most of the nonconserved substitutions are localized to the two intravesicular loops (Fig. 3). However, comparison of the amino acid sequence of the mammalian and *Torpedo* synaptophysin shows that the highest frequency of substitutions occurs in the cytoplasmic carboxy-terminal tail. This region of the protein contains a large number of tyrosine, proline, and glutamine residues, with the tyrosines possibly serving as sites for phosphorylation (Pang et al. 1988). Despite the low similarity at the primary sequence level, there appears to exist strong functional pressures to maintain the composition of this carboxy-terminal domain. The carboxy-terminal tail has also been proposed to bind Ca^{++} (Rehm et al. 1986) despite the lack of any resemblance to the known structural motifs for Ca^{++} binding. This property is in need of confirmation using purified recombinant protein, and it has yet to be determined whether this potential Ca^{++} binding property has any correlation with the level of protein phosphorylation.

On the basis of cross-linking experiments, synaptophysin is believed to associate into a homo-hexameric complex (Thomas et al. 1988). On reconstitution into planar lipid bilayers, the protein is capable of forming a transmembrane channel with a large unit conductance, about 150 pS, and a long open time. Moreover, the properties of this channel can be altered by the addition of a synaptophysin-specific monoclonal antibody. However, it is not clear whether this channel can be mod-

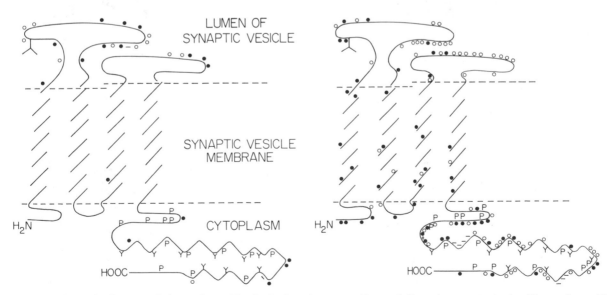

Figure 3. Schematic diagram of the amino acid substitutions in mammalian and *Torpedo* synaptophysin. The amino acid substitutions among the three mammalian species: rat, bovine, and human (*left*); the substitutions between the *Torpedo* and rat sequences (*right*). (●) Conserved substitutions; (○) nonconserved changes. The proline (P) and tyrosine (Y) residues in the carboxy-terminal cytoplasmic domain are indicated. (⅄) Glycosylation site in the first intravesicular domain. A + symbol indicates an additional amino acid, and a − symbol indicates a deleted amino acid in order to obtain maximal sequence alignment.

ulated by, or correlated with, the presumptive Ca^{++} binding property of the protein. Interestingly, this channel shows some similarity to the potassium-preferring P channel found in cholinergic synaptic vesicles (Rahamimoff et al. 1988). It remains to be seen whether the properties of the P channel can be altered by a synaptophysin-specific antibody.

A number of studies have used synaptophysin as a marker in the transport and recycling of proteins from the presynaptic membrane. In the resting neuromuscular junction, synaptophysin immunoreactivity is localized to synaptic vesicle membranes (Valtorta et al. 1988; Torri-Tarelli et al. 1990). After treatment with

α-latrotoxin in a Ca^{++}-free solution, which causes massive depletion of synaptic vesicles and prevents membrane recycling, synaptophysin is selectively associated with the plasma membrane. When membrane recycling is allowed to occur in the presence of Ca^{++} in the external medium, synaptophysin is efficiently reinserted into synaptic vesicle membranes. The properties and cellular localization of synaptophysin has also been investigated in the fibroblastic Chinese hamster ovary and neuroendocrine PC12 cells (Johnston et al. 1989; Leube et al. 1989). When the synaptophysin gene or mRNA is introduced into these cells, the expressed protein is specifically associated with the membrane of

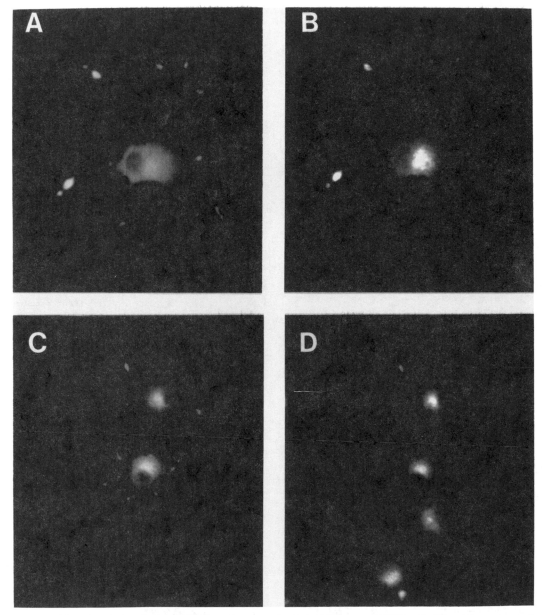

Figure 4. Immunohistochemical analysis of VAMP and synaptophysin in NGF-treated PC12 cells. The cells are treated with the primary antibodies, and the bound antibodies are detected with either fluorescein- or rhodamine-labeled secondary antibodies. (*A*) The endogenously expressed VAMP. (*B*) The same cells stained with antibodies against synaptophysin. (*C*) The expression of a transfected *Torpedo* VAMP gene in PC12 cells. (*D*) The endogenously expressed synaptophysin in these cells. Only two of the four cells in *D* are expressing the transfected *Torpedo* VAMP gene.

small diameter cytoplasmic vesicles. Moreover, a sub-population of these synaptophysin-labeled vesicles co-localizes with endocytic markers, such as transferrin receptor or internalized horseradish peroxidase, suggesting association of the protein with recycling membrane vesicles.

To gain more insights into the sorting process and to determine whether this process is applicable to all synaptic vesicle proteins, the colocalization of another synaptic vesicle protein, VAMP, with synaptophysin was examined. As shown in Figure 4, both the endogenously expressed VAMP (Fig. 4A) and synaptophysin (Fig. 4B) are selectively localized to the tips of neurite processes of nerve growth factor (NGF)-treated PC12 cells. There are, however, subtle differences in the distribution of the two proteins in the cell body. The endogenous VAMP exhibits a diffused network-like distribution, whereas synaptophysin shows a strong preference for the perinuclear Golgi complex. Protein expressed by a transfected *Torpedo* VAMP gene (Fig. 4C,D) appears adequately recognized by the transport apparatus and retains its colocalization with synaptophysin in the tips of the neurite processes. In the cell soma, the *Torpedo* VAMP is preferentially associated with the Golgi complex. Combined with earlier studies, the cellular colocalization of VAMP and synaptophysin suggests that the two proteins are derived initially from the Golgi complex, transported in synaptic vesicles or in similarly sized transport vesicles to the presynaptic terminal, and recycled after fusion with the plasma membrane.

GTP-binding Proteins Associated with the Synaptic Vesicle Membranes

The underlying mechanisms for intracellular signaling and correct targeting of vesicles may involve two families of GTP-binding proteins: the heterotrimeric forms often found coupled to receptors containing seven transmembrane domains (Stryer 1986; Gilman 1987; Neer and Clapham 1988) and the smaller Ras-like family with an apparent molecular mass between 20 and 29 kD. In the heterotrimeric G proteins, the complex is usually localized to the inner surface of the plasma membrane. However, they have also been detected on chromaffin granules (Tanaka et al. 1987; Brocklehurst and Pollard 1988) and synaptic vesicle membranes (Toutant et al. 1987; Ngsee et al. 1990). The α-subunit possesses an intrinsic GTPase activity that hydrolyzes the bound GTP, leading to regeneration of the inactive complex. In contrast, Ras and perhaps all of the low-molecular-weight GTP-binding proteins have a relatively low intrinsic GTPase activity that can be dramatically enhanced by a cytosolic GTPase-activating protein termed GAP (Trahey and McCormick 1987).

Several biological functions have been attributed to the low-molecular-weight GTP-binding proteins. By analogy with the α-subunit and the localization of the Ras protein to the inner surface of the plasma membrane, they are implicated to play a role in signal transduction. Thus, with the large number of Ras-like proteins described in recent years, it would appear that the cell possesses an elaborate system to control the intricate balance of intracellular levels of second messengers. In addition, the low-molecular-weight GTP-binding proteins have been proposed to serve as molecular switches in regulating the vectorial transport of intracellular vesicles (Bourne 1988). This is supported by the ability of the nonhydrolyzable GTP analog, GTPγS, to block the fusion of vesicles derived from the Golgi complex (Melançon et al. 1987) and the disruption of the constitutive secretory process in yeast by mutations in either the *YPT1* (Schmitt et al. 1986; Wagner et al. 1987; Segev et al. 1988; Bacon et al. 1989) or *SEC4* locus (Salminen and Novick 1987; Goud et al. 1988; Walworth et al. 1989), both of which encode Ras-like GTP-binding proteins.

As a prerequisite to mediating critical aspects of signal transduction, synaptic transmission, or in regulating the vectorial transport of secretory vesicles, it is essential that the GTP-binding proteins involved be localized near the synapse or associated with synaptic vesicles. The GTP-binding proteins associated with purified cholinergic synaptic vesicles from the electric ray were examined using the $[\alpha\text{-}^{32}\text{P}]$GTP overlay technique (McGrath et al. 1984; Lapetina and Reep 1987). As shown in Figure 5, two different size classes of GTP-binding proteins are associated with the synaptic vesicle membranes: one or more with molecular masses between 37 and 41 kD and at least three to five with molecular masses between 20 and 29 kD. Since the larger GTP-binding proteins are ADP-ribosylated with pertussis toxin, they are considered more closely related to G_o or G_i (Ngsee et al. 1990). Conversely, two or more of the low-molecular-weight GTP-binding proteins are modified by ADP-ribosylation with botulinum toxin C3. Although this is not directly related to the inhibition of neurotransmitter release by botulinum A, C1, and D toxins, ADP-ribosylation of a low-molecular-weight GTP-binding protein, RhoC, has been shown to cause disruption of the cytoskeletal network (Chardin et al. 1989). These studies suggest that Rho and perhaps other low-molecular-weight GTP-binding proteins are involved in the control of microfilament assembly and cellular morphogenesis.

The presence of multiple GTP-binding proteins associated with synaptic vesicles raises a number of interesting questions, foremost of which is the identity of these GTP-binding proteins. It is also not clear what type of receptor, if any, is coupled to these GTP-binding proteins. It will also be interesting to determine whether the different GTP-binding proteins are uniformly distributed among all of the vesicles or differentially associated with a subpopulation of vesicles. Recently, a low-molecular-weight GTP-binding protein, Rab3, has been shown to be tightly associated with synaptic vesicles (Mollard et al. 1990) suggesting a possible role in synaptic vesicle function.

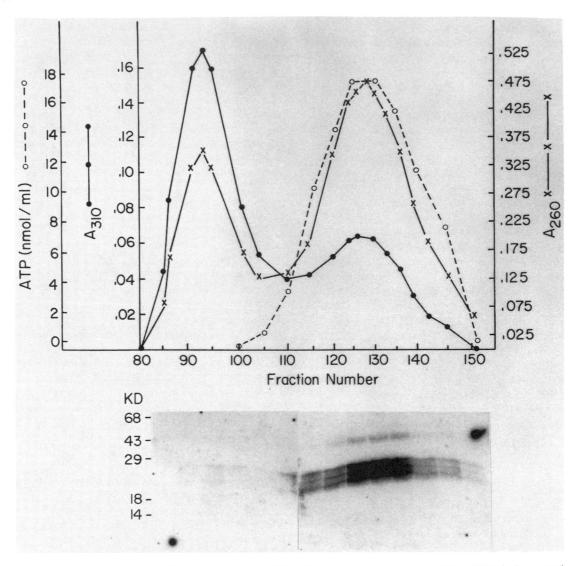

Figure 5. Size fractionation of membrane vesicles on a CPG-3000 column and association of the GTP-binding proteins with synaptic vesicle membranes. The ATP-containing fractions following flotation sucrose density gradient centrifugation were pooled and fractionated on a CPG-3000 column (2.5 × 220 cm) equilibrated in 10 mM HEPES-NaOH pH 7.0, 10 mM EGTA, 0.2 M sucrose, and 0.3 M NaCl. The fractions (5 ml) were analyzed for ATP content, A_{310}, A_{260}, and $[\alpha\text{-}^{32}P]$GTP binding. Membranes from the excluded and included peaks are shown in Fig. 1.

FUTURE PERSPECTIVES

As stated earlier, one of the goals in studying the proteins associated with synaptic vesicles is to understand the mechanism underlying membrane flow and vesicular trafficking at the nerve terminal. The localization and topology of VAMP support a possible role in some aspect of vesicle function. Its structural motif also offers opportunities for molecular characterization of the domains required for specific localization and function in synaptic vesicles. These questions are also pertinent to synaptophysin. In addition, synaptophysin is the most likely candidate identified to date for the potassium-preferring P channel activity observed in cholinergic synaptic vesicles. Although it is not clear whether phosphorylation of synaptophysin has any ef-

fect on its biological properties, it does provide the cell with a rapid means to modulate the activity of the molecule.

By analogy with cardiac myocytes, the heterotrimeric G_o- or G_i-like proteins may also be coupled to ion channels, thus exerting a strong influence on the intracellular level of Ca^{++}. The identities of these G proteins and their respective receptors await molecular characterization. Functionally, the low-molecular-weight GTP-binding proteins may be divided into three classes. Those containing the putative Ras effector domain are likely to play a role in transducing stimuli, such as those signaling axonal growth and remodeling. These processes involve the reorganization of the cytoskeletal network and may require a second set of low-molecular-weight GTP-binding proteins, such as Rho.

Finally, transport, targeting, and recycling of membrane vesicles in the nerve terminal may require the presence of a third set of low-molecular-weight GTP-binding proteins to ensure fidelity and unidirectionality. The low-molecular-weight GTP-binding proteins exhibiting the putative SEC4/YPT1 effector domain are the most prominent candidates for this role. To maintain the complexity of membrane trafficking at the nerve terminal, it is likely that each low-molecular-weight GTP-binding protein is localized to a limited number of membrane compartments. This view is consistent with the existence of a large family of low-molecular-weight GTP-binding proteins. Further subcellular localization and functional analysis will provide a greater understanding of the role of these proteins in controlling endocytosis and exocytosis.

It is an eventual goal of molecular neurobiology to develop a complete understanding of the events that underlie transmitter metabolism in the nerve terminal. The proteins associated with synaptic vesicles discussed above represent a small sample of the molecules found in the nerve terminal, but they provide an excellent focus for these studies. The ultimate challenge lies in elucidating the molecular mechanisms of learning and memory. Understanding the synaptic modulation of transmitter metabolism in response to neuronal activity is a critical step in this endeavor.

ACKNOWLEDGMENTS

J.K.N. is supported by a postdoctoral fellowship from the Medical Research Council of Canada. W.S.T. is a recipient of a Centennial Fellowship from the Medical Research Council of Canada. R.H.S. is a Presidential Young Investigator and Pew scholar. This work is supported by a grant from the National Institute of Mental Health.

REFERENCES

Bacon, R.A., A. Salminen, H. Ruohola, P. Novick, and S. Ferro-Novick. 1989. The GTP-binding protein YPT1 is required for transport *in vitro*: The Golgi apparatus is defective in ypt1 mutants. *J. Cell Biol.* **109:** 1015.

Bourne, H.R. 1988. Do GTPases direct membrane traffic in secretion? *Cell* **53:** 669.

Brocklehurst, K.W. and H.B. Pollard. 1988. Pertussis toxin stimulates delayed-onset, Ca^{2+}-dependent catecholamine release and the ADP-ribosylation of a 40 kDa protein in bovine adrenal chromaffin cells. *FEBS Lett.* **234:** 439.

Buckley, K.M., E. Floor, and R.B. Kelly. 1987. Cloning and sequence analysis of cDNA encoding p38, a major synaptic vesicle protein. *J. Cell Biol.* **105:** 2447.

Carlson, S.S. and R.B. Kelly. 1980. An antiserum specific for cholinergic synaptic vesicles from electric ray. *J. Cell Biol.* **87:** 98.

Carlson, S.S., J.A. Wagner, and R.B. Kelly. 1978. Purification of synaptic vesicles from elasmobranch electric organ and the use of biophysical criteria to demonstrate purity. *Biochemistry* **17:** 1188.

Chardin, P., P. Boquet, P. Madaule, M.R. Popoff, E.J. Rubin, and D.M. Gill. 1989. The mammalian G protein rhoC is ADP-ribosylated by *Clostridium botulinum* exoenzyme C3 and affects actin microfilaments in Vero cells. *EMBO J.* **8:** 1087.

Cowan, D.M., M. Linial, and R.H. Scheller. 1990. *Torpedo* synaptophysin: Evolution of a synaptic vesicle protein. *Brain Res.* **509:** 1.

Elferink, L.A., W.S. Trimble, and R.H. Scheller. 1989. Two vesicle-associated membrane protein genes are differentially expressed in the rat central nervous system. *J. Biol. Chem.* **264:** 11061.

Gilman, A.G. 1987. G proteins: Transducers of receptor-generated signals. *Annu. Rev. Biochem.* **56:** 615.

Goud, B., A. Salminen, N.C. Walworth, and P.J. Novick. 1988. A GTP-binding protein required for secretion rapidly associates with secretory vesicles and plasma membrane in yeast. *Cell* **53:** 753.

Jahn, R., W. Schiebler, C. Ouimet, and P. Greengard. 1985. A 38,000-Dalton membrane protein (p38) present in synaptic vesicles. *Proc. Natl. Acad. Sci.* **82:** 4137.

Johnston, P.A., P.L. Cameron, H. Stukenbrok, R. Jahn, P.D. Camilli, and T.C. Südhof. 1989. Synaptophysin is targeted to similar microvesicles in PC12 and CHO cells. *EMBO J.* **8:** 2863.

Lapetina, E.G. and B.R. Reep. 1987. Specific binding of $[\alpha^{-32}P]GTP$ to cytosolic and membrane-bound proteins of human platelets correlates with the activation of phospholipase C. *Proc. Natl. Acad. Sci.* **84:** 2261.

Leube, R.E., B. Wiedenmann, and W.W. Franke. 1989. Topogenesis and sorting of synaptophysin: Synthesis of a synaptic vesicle protein from a gene transfected into non-neuroendocrine cells. *Cell* **59:** 433.

Leube, R.E., P. Kaiser, A. Seiter, R. Zimbelmann, W.W. Franke, H. Rehm, P. Knaus, P. Prior, H. Betz, H. Reinke, K. Beyreuther, and B. Wiedenmann. 1987. Synaptophysin: Molecular organization and mRNA expression as determined from cloned cDNA. *EMBO J.* **2:** 1265.

McGrath, J.P., D.J. Capon, D.V. Goeddel, and A.D. Levinson. 1984. Comparative biochemical properties of normal and activated human ras p21 protein. *Nature* **310:** 644.

Melançon, P., T. Serafini, M.L. Gleason, L. Orci, and J.E. Rothman. 1987. Involvement of GTP-binding "G" proteins in transport through the Golgi stack. *Cell* **51:** 1053.

Mollard, F.G.V., G.A. Mignery, M. Baumert, M.S. Perin, T.J. Hanson, P.M. Burger, R. Jahn, and T.C. Südhof. 1990. rab3 is a small GTP-binding protein exclusively localized to synaptic vesicles. *Proc. Natl. Acad. Sci.* **87:** 1988.

Navone, F., R. Jahn, G. DiGioia, H. Stukenbrok, P. Greengard, and P.D. Camilli. 1986. Protein p38: An integral membrane protein specific for small vesicles of neurons and neuroendocrine cells. *J. Cell Biol.* **103:** 2511.

Neer, E.J., and D.E. Clapham. 1988. Roles of G protein subunits in transmembrane signalling. *Nature* **333:** 129.

Ngsee, J.K., K. Miller, B. Wendland, and R.H. Scheller. 1990. Multiple GTP-binding proteins from cholinergic synaptic vesicles. *J. Neurosci.* **10:** 317.

Pang, D.T., J.K.T. Wang, F. Valtorta, F. Benfenati, and P. Greengard. 1988. Protein tyrosine phosphorylation in synaptic vesicles. *Proc. Natl. Acad. Sci.* **85:** 762.

Rahamimoff, R., S.A. DeReimer, B. Sakmann, H. Stadler, and N. Yakir. 1988. Ion channels in synaptic vesicles from *Torpedo* electric organ. *Proc. Natl. Acad. Sci.* **85:** 5310.

Rehm, H., B. Wiedenmann, and H. Betz. 1986. Molecular characterization of synaptophysin, a major calcium-binding protein of the synaptic vesicle membrane. *EMBO J.* **5:** 535.

Salminen, A., and P.J. Novick. 1987. A ras-like protein is required for a post-Golgi event in yeast secretion. *Cell* **49:** 527.

Schmitt, H.D., P. Wagner, E. Pfaff, and D. Gallwitz. 1986. The ras-related YPT1 gene product in yeast: A GTP-binding protein that might be involved in microtubule organization. *Cell* **47:** 401.

Segev, N., I. Mulholland, and D. Botstein. 1988. The yeast

GTP-binding YPT1 protein and a mammalian counterpart are associated with the secretory machinery. *Cell* **52:** 915.

Stryer, L. 1986. G proteins: A family of signal transducers. *Annu. Rev. Cell Biol.* **2:** 391.

Südhof, T.C., M. Baumert, M.S. Perin, and R. Jahn. 1989. A synaptic vesicle membrane protein is conserved from mammals to *Drosophila. Neuron* **2:** 1475.

Südhof, T.C., F. Lottspeich, P. Greengard, E. Mehl, and R. Jahn. 1987. A synaptic vesicle protein with a novel cytoplasmic domain and four transmembrane regions. *Science* **238:** 1142.

Tanaka, T., H. Yokohama, M. Negishi, H. Hayashi, S. Ito, and O. Hayaishi. 1987. Pertussis toxin facilitates secretogogue-induced catecholamine release from cultured bovine adrenal chromaffin cells. *Biochem. Biophys. Res. Comm.* **144:** 907.

Thomas, L., K. Hartung, D. Langosch, H. Rehm, E. Bamberg, W.W. Franke, and H. Betz. 1988. Identification of synaptophysin as a hexameric channel protein of the synaptic vesicle membrane. *Science* **242:** 1050.

Torri-Tarelli, F., A. Villa, F. Valtorta, P.D. Camilli, P. Greengard, and B. Ceccarelli. 1990. Redistribution of synaptophysin and synapsin I during α-latrotoxin-induced release of neurotransmitter at the neuromuscular junction. *J. Cell Biol.* **110:** 449.

Toutant, M., J. Bockaert, V. Homburger, and B. Rouot. 1987. G-proteins in *Torpedo marmorata* electric organ. Differential distribution in pre- and post-synaptic membranes and synaptic vesicles. *FEBS Lett.* **222:** 51.

Trahey, M. and F. McCormick. 1987. A cytoplasmic protein stimulates normal N-ras p21 GTPase, but does not affect oncogenic mutants. *Science* **238:** 542.

Trimble, W.S., D.M. Cowan, and R.H. Scheller. 1988. VAMP-1: A synaptic vesicle-associated integral membrane protein. *Proc. Natl. Acad. Sci.* **85:** 4538.

Trimble, W.S., T.S. Gray, L.A. Elferink, M.C. Wilson, and R.H. Scheller. 1990. Distinct patterns of expression of two VAMP genes within the rat brain. *J. Neurosci.* **10:** 1380.

Valtorta, F., R. Jahn, R. Fesce, P. Greengard, and B. Cecarelli. 1988. Synaptophysin (p38) at the frog neuromuscular junction: Its incorporation into the axolemma and recycling after intense quantal secretion. *J. Cell Biol.* **107:** 2717.

Wagner, J.A., S.S. Carlson, and R.B. Kelly. 1978. Chemical and physical characterization of cholinergic synaptic vesicles. *Biochemistry* **17:** 1199.

Wagner, P., C.M.T. Molenaar, A.J.G. Rauh, R. Brokel, H.D. Schmitt, and D. Gallwitz. 1987. Biochemical properties of the ras-related YPT protein in yeast: A mutational analysis. *EMBO J.* **6 :** 2373.

Walworth, N.C., B. Goud, A.K. Kabcenell, and P.J. Novick. 1989. Mutational analysis of SEC4 suggests a cyclical mechanism for the regulation of vesicular traffic. *EMBO J.* **8:** 1685.

Whittiker, V.P. and H. Stadler. 1980. The structure and function of cholinergic synaptic vesicles. In *Proteins of the nervous system* (ed. R.A. Bradshaw and D.M. Schnieder), p. 231. Raven, New York.

Wiedenmann, B. and W. W. Franke. 1985. Identification and localization of synaptophysin, an integral membrane protein of M_r 38,000 characteristic of presynaptic vesicles. *Cell* **41:** 1017.

Presynaptic Mechanisms in Hippocampal Long-term Potentiation

T.V.P. Bliss, M.L. Errington, M.A. Lynch, and J.H. Williams

Division of Neurophysiology and Neuropharmacology, National Institute for Medical Research, London NW7 1AA

Long-term potentiation (LTP) is the name given to the sustained enhancement of synaptic transmission that is produced in certain cortical synapses and, in particular, in those of the principal excitatory hippocampal pathways, by brief episodes of tetanic stimulation (Bliss and Lømo 1973; for review, see Teyler and DiScenna 1987; Bliss and Lynch 1988). The ease with which LTP can be elicited, its prolonged duration, its properties of associativity and pathway specificity, and its presence in the hippocampus, a cortical structure essential for the formation of new memories in humans, are among the features that have helped foster the widespread assumption that LTP provides the synaptic basis of at least some aspects of memory in vertebrates. A highly satisfying account, based on the voltage-dependent properties of the N-methyl-D-aspartate (NMDA) subtype of glutamate receptor, can be given for the events leading up to the induction of LTP in the perforant path and Schaffer-collateral projections (Gustafsson and Wigström 1988; Collingridge and Singer 1990). Different and less well-understood mechanisms apply to LTP in the mossy fiber projection that links granule cells to CA3 pyramidal cells (Harris and Cotman 1986; Jaffe and Johnston 1990; Zalutsky and Nicoll 1990). In contrast to the consensus that exists regarding the induction of LTP, the mechanisms underlying the maintenance of the effect have remained the subject of lively disagreement for the best part of a decade. Early debates on the locus of LTP tended to assume that all the cellular machinery necessary to produce an increase in synaptic efficacy was in place in the presynaptic terminal or, alternatively, in the postsynaptic spine. Post-tetanic potentiation, a presynaptic model for synaptic plasticity, had long been studied at the neuromuscular junction (Brown and von Euler 1938), in sympathetic ganglia (Cannon and Rosenblueth 1937; Bronk 1939), and in monosynaptic spinal reflexes (Lloyd 1949), while changes in receptor density at the neuromuscular junction after denervation provided a model for a postsynaptic mechanism (Cannon and Rosenblueth 1949). Once the role of the postsynaptic cell in the induction of LTP became firmly established (Lynch et al. 1983; Kelso et al. 1986; Sastry et al. 1986; Wigström et al. 1986; Hvalby et al. 1987), a case could no longer be made for a purely presynaptic mechanism, at least in those pathways in which induction was dependent on the NMDA receptor. This does not, however, exclude a role for the presynaptic terminal in the expression or maintenance of LTP. In this paper, we consider in vivo and in vitro evidence that LTP is associated with a sustained increase in the concentration of glutamate in hippocampal perfusates. The simplest, although not the only, interpretation of these results is that there is an increase in the release of the putative transmitter glutamate from potentiated terminals and that, consequently, LTP is at least partly accounted for by an increase in transmitter release. If LTP is associated with a sustained increase in transmitter release, the question arises as to the nature of the signal that carries information across the synapse from the postsynaptic site of induction. We describe experiments to investigate the hypothesis that a membrane lipid, arachidonic acid, acts as a retrograde transynaptic messenger in LTP.

METHODS

Push-pull perfusion experiments in anesthetized rats. Experiments were performed on adult rats (Sprague-Dawley, 200–300 g) anesthetized with urethane (1.5 ml/kg). The concentration of extracellular glutamate or of arachidonic acid and its metabolites was monitored by perfusing the desired region (molecular layer of the dentate gyrus or stratum radiatum of area CA1) with artificial cerebrospinal fluid (ACSF; 3 mM KCl, 120 mM NaCl, 1.2 mM $MgCl_2$, 1.5 mM $CaCl_2$, 1.2 mM NaH_2PO_4, 23 mM $NaHCO_3$, 11 mM D-glucose, continuously gassed with 95% O_2 and 5% CO_2) at 6.5 μl/min through a push-pull cannula using a dual peristaltic pump (Fig. 1). Perfusates were collected over dry ice in a fraction collector and stored at $-70°C$ for subsequent analysis.

Recording electrodes of insulated stainless steel wire were attached to the cannula, as described previously (Errington et al. 1983), and field potentials were sampled from synaptic and cell body regions. For experiments in the dentate gyrus, a stimulating electrode was placed in the angular bundle to activate fibers of the ipsilateral perforant path, and for experiments in area CA1, the Schaffer-commissural system was activated with an electrode positioned in the fimbria of the contralateral hippocampus close to the midline. Test shocks were delivered throughout the experiment at 30-second intervals. LTP was induced by three trains (250 Hz for 200 msec) at the same intensity as the test stimulus in the case of CA1 experiments, or twice the intensity in the case of dentate experiments, and with an interval of 1 minute between each train.

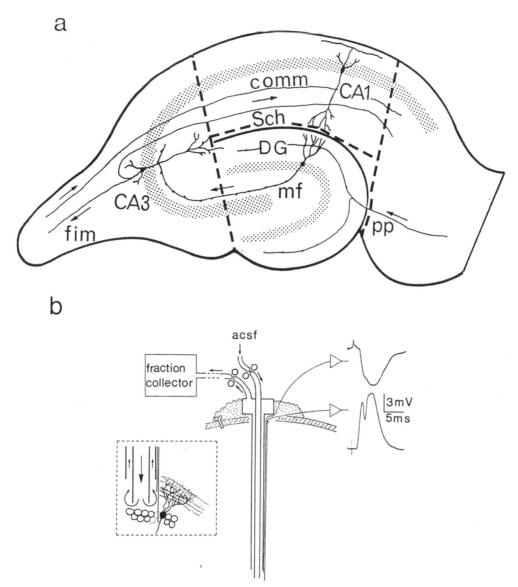

Figure 1. (*a*) Diagram of principal excitatory pathways in the hippocampus. The dashed lines indicate where cuts are made to obtain minislices from area CA1 and dentate gyrus. (*b*) Diagram of push-pull cannula in dentate gyrus (*inset*) with field potentials recorded from the molecular layer (upper trace) and granule cell layer (lower trace). (ACSF) Artificial cerebrospinal fluid; (CA1, CA3) pyramidal cell fields of areas CA1 and CA3; (DG) dentate gyrus; (fim) fimbria; (mf) mossy fibers; (pp) perforant path; (Sch, comm) Schaffer-collateral and commissural fibers.

In vitro experiments. Complete transverse slices or minislices comprising the dentate gyrus or area CA1 (Lynch et al. 1982) were maintained in a modified interface chamber at a temperature of 29–30°C. Slices were perfused at 100 μl/min with ACSF having the same composition as that used for in vivo perfusion, except in the case of dentate minislices in which, to obtain reliable LTP, the concentration of MgCl$_2$ was reduced to 75 μM. Samples were collected every 2 minutes and stored as above. Test stimuli were delivered at 30-second intervals to the perforant path or to the Schaffer-collateral system, and population excitatory postsynaptic potentials (EPSPs) were recorded from the molecular layer of the dentate gyrus or stratum radiatum of area CA1, respectively. LTP was induced by four trains of ten pulses at 100 Hz, at 1.5 times test intensity, and with 1.5 seconds between trains.

Separation and detection of glutamate, arachidonic acid and its 12-lipoxygenase derivatives, and other fatty acids. To measure glutamate, samples of perfusate were thawed, derivatized with an equal volume of *o*-phthalaldehyde/mercaptopropionic acid, separated by reverse-phase high-performance liquid chromatography (HPLC), and estimated fluorometrically (Bliss et al. 1986b).

Arachidonic acid and other fatty acids were assayed as follows. Samples of perfusate (20 μl) were added to chloroform:methanol (2:1, 800 μl) containing 1 μl margaric acid (internal standard) and shaken for 10 minutes to extract fatty acids into the organic phase. After centrifugation and evaporation of the chloroform phase to dryness, the samples were resuspended in ethanol for analysis. Fatty acids were derivatized to 2-nitrophenylhydrazides, separated by reverse-phase HPLC, and detected by UV spectroscopy at 230 nm (Miwa et al. 1986). Concentrations were calculated by the internal standard method. The 12-lipoxygenase metabolites, 12-hydroperoxyeicosatetraenoic acid (12-HPETE) and 12-hydroxyeicosatetraenoic acid (12-HETE) (Cascade Biochem Ltd, University of Reading, United Kingdom), were extracted as above and separated by reverse-phase HPLC and detected by UV spectroscopy at 230 nm. Concentrations were calculated with reference to standard curves.

Preparation of fatty acids for perfusion. Arachidonic or other fatty acids were dissolved in ethanol by sonication. Aliquots (1 mM in ACSF containing ascorbic acid) were stored at −70°C. For perfusion, aliquots were thawed 15–20 minutes before use, diluted in ACSF to give a final concentration of 50 μM fatty acid, 25 μM ascorbic acid, and 0.25% ethanol.

RESULTS

Glutamate Release: In Vivo Experiments

In a number of previous studies in the anesthetized rat, we have examined the correlation between LTP in the dentate gyrus and the concentration of glutamate and other amino acids in push-pull perfusates (Dolphin et al. 1982; Bliss et al. 1986b; Errington et al. 1987; Lynch et al. 1989a) and have consistently found that LTP is accompanied by a sustained increase in the release of glutamate. In the present experiments, we have extended this study to area CA1. We began by establishing that glutamate release in this region is partly stimulus-dependent, as we had previously shown to be the case in the dentate gyrus (Bliss et al. 1986b). In Figure 2, mean glutamate content for three successive 15-minute collection intervals is displayed for the dentate gyrus and for area CA1; samples in the first and third intervals were collected during 1/30-Hz stimulation of the perforant path and Schaffer-commissural projection, respectively. During the second 15-minute period, the stimulus frequency was increased to 1 Hz. In both areas, release during the period of enhanced activity was significantly greater than during the two periods at 1/30 Hz.

We next investigated the relationship between LTP and glutamate release in CA1. In contrast to a report by Aniksztejn et al. (1989), we find that in this region also there is an increase in glutamate release after the induction of LTP. Glutamate concentrations in successive 15-minute perfusates from stratum radiatum of area CA1 are shown in Figure 3 for six animals in which LTP was induced by tetanic stimulation of the Schaffer-commissural projection. The profile of glutamate release in these animals may be compared with a control

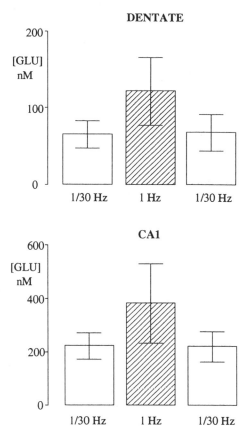

Figure 2. Stimulus-dependent release of glutamate from the hippocampus of the anesthetized rat. Mean concentration of glutamate in push-pull perfusates from dentate gyrus (*top*) and area CA1 (*bottom*) are displayed for consecutive 15-min periods during which stimuli were given at 1/30 Hz, 1 Hz, and 1/30 Hz to the perforant path or commissural projection to CA1, respectively. $n = 6$ for dentate gyrus and $n = 8$ for CA1. In both regions, release during stimulation at 1 Hz is significantly higher than for the preceding and following periods at 1/30 Hz ($p < 0.05$, Wilcoxin test for paired differences).

series in which the tetanus given to the experimental group was replaced by a regime in which the same total number of stimuli was given, but at a lower frequency which did not induce LTP (Fig. 3). Despite the considerable variability both between animals and between samples, the induction of LTP was followed by an increase in glutamate concentration, which was sustained in five of the six animals for periods ranging from 45 to 120 minutes. No such change occurred in the control group. For comparison, the results of a similar and previously reported experiment in the dentate gyrus are also shown in Figure 3 (Lynch et al. 1989a).

Glutamate Release: In Vitro Experiments

The first account of increased transmitter release after tetanic stimulation in the hippocampus (Skrede and Malthe-Sørenssen 1981) was based on the use of ^{3}H-labeled D-aspartate as a marker for glutamate release in the transverse hippocampal slice. Can a similar increase be detected in the release of endogenous gluta-

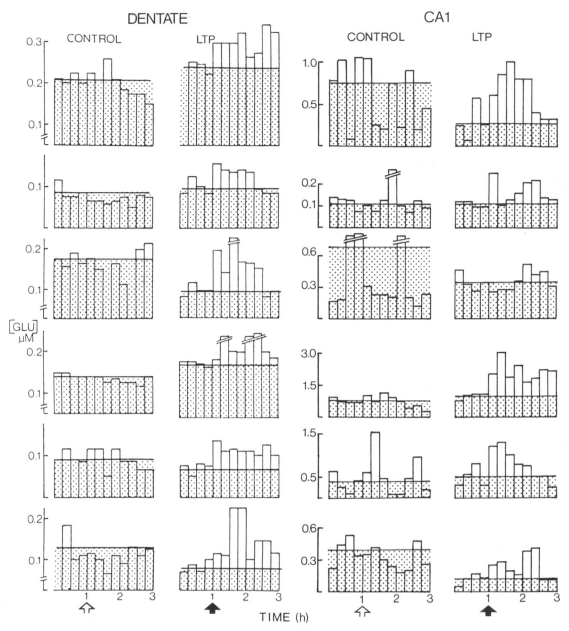

Figure 3. Relationship between LTP and release of endogenous glutamate from dentate gyrus and area CA1 in the anesthetized rat. The concentration of glutamate in consecutive 15-min samples is shown for each animal in control and LTP groups. For all animals, test stimuli were given throughout at a frequency of 1/30 Hz. LTP was induced by high-frequency stimulation (closed arrows); control animals received the same total number of extra stimuli in a low-frequency regime, which did not produce LTP (open arrows; see Methods). The mean concentration of glutamate in the first hour is indicated by stippling. Occasional failures in HPLC analysis are indicated by blank entries. Off-scale values, reading from top to bottom, left to right, are 0.29 μM, 0.25 μM, 0.28 μM, 0.31 μM (dentate) and 0.42 μM, 1.13 μM, 1.48 μM, and 1.10 μM (CA1). (Data for dentate gyrus are from Lynch et al. 1989a.)

mate in vitro? Our first attempt to answer this question was designed to maximize both the concentration of glutamate released into the perfusate and the number of potentiated synapses. Eight transverse slices were maintained in the chamber, and potentiation was induced by brief exposure to an elevated concentration of calcium (5 mM for 15 min). This procedure induces a stimulus-independent, long-term enhancement of synaptic transmission in excitatory hippocampal pathways (Turner et al. 1982; Higashima and Yamamoto

1985; Bliss et al. 1986a; Reymann et al. 1986). It may therefore be presumed that by exposing slices to high calcium, a substantial proportion of excitatory synapses in each slice will be potentiated. To monitor potentiation, one slice from the eight in the bath was chosen at random, and electrodes were placed to record evoked potentials in dentate gyrus and area CA1. As shown in Figure 4, a sustained increase in glutamate release was detected in the potentiated group, whereas in the control group, there was a slow downward drift in gluta-

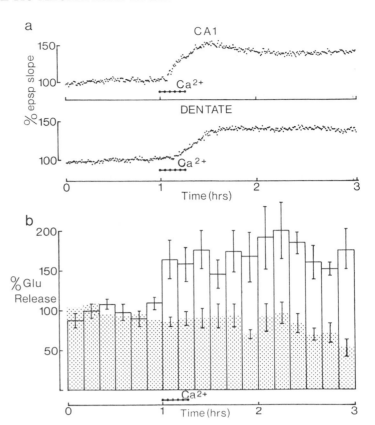

Figure 4. Calcium-induced LTP in vitro is accompanied by an increase in glutamate release. (*a*) Mean slope of the population EPSP (normalized with respect to the mean value in the first hour) in area CA1 and in the dentate gyrus in response to test shocks given at 1/30 Hz to the Schaffer-commissural and perforant path projections, respectively ($n = 11$). After 1 hr, slices were perfused with a medium containing 5 mM $CaCl_2$ for 15 min (dotted bar). (*b*) Concentration of glutamate (mean ± S.E.M.) in consecutive 10 min samples of perfusate from the experimental group (open histograms, $n = 11$) and from a control group that was perfused with normal medium throughout the experiment (stippled histograms, $n = 11$). For clarity, error bars are omitted from the control group for the first hour.

mate concentration. Although we cannot tell from this experiment whether all three hippocampal subfields contribute to the increase, it is likely to derive at least in part from the dentate gyrus because calcium-induced potentiation in that region is accompanied by increased glutamate release in vivo (Bliss et al. 1986a).

More recently, we have turned our attention to tetanus-induced LTP in hippocampal minislices. With this technique (Lynch et al. 1982), LTP can be studied in isolated regions, and the source of glutamate can thus be assigned to a particular subfield without ambiguity. Because LTP is difficult to induce in the dentate gyrus in normal ACSF (Wigström and Gustafsson 1983), dentate minislices were exposed to a lower concentration of Mg^{++} (see Methods). Early results from this continuing series of experiments are presented in Figure 5. The histograms show the mean glutamate concentrations in 4-minute samples collected at intervals before and after the induction of LTP (arrow) during test stimulation at 1/30 Hz. There is a clear and sustained increase in glutamate concentration after the induction of LTP. The two hatched histograms indicate the glutamate concentrations during two periods of stimulation at 1 Hz. In both cases, before and after the induction of LTP, there is a stimulus-dependent increase in transmitter release.

Experiments on the Role of Arachidonic Acid

In 1987, arachidonic acid or its 12-lipoxygenase metabolites were shown to act as intracellular second

messengers in *Aplysia* sensory neurons by Piomelli et al. (1987), who suggested that these small lipid-soluble molecules would be good candidates for intercellular messengers in LTP. This idea received early support when it was found that the lipoxygenase and phospholipase A_2 inhibitor, nordihydroguaiaretic acid (NDGA), blocks the induction of both calcium-induced potentiation and tetanus-induced LTP (Williams and Bliss 1988, 1989; Lynch et al. 1989a; Okada et al. 1989) and that bath-applied NMDA stimulates the release of free arachidonic acid from striatal (Dumuis et al. 1988), cerebellar (Lazarewicz et al. 1988), and hippocampal (Sanfeliu et al. 1990) neurons in culture. We also reported that LTP is associated with a sustained increase in the release of a compound that we identified as arachidonic acid (Lynch et al. 1989a) but which we now believe to be an autooxidative metabolite of arachidonic acid. Using a derivatization method (see Methods), we have repeated these measurements on push-pull perfusates from the dentate gyrus obtained by Dr. Clive Bramham at the University of Bergen and have confirmed that there is an increase in the release of free arachidonic acid in LTP (Fig. 6). In the same perfusates, we found a similar LTP-related increase in the concentration of the lipoxygenase metabolites 12-HPETE and 12-HETE. Unlike the increase in arachidonic acid and 12-HETE, which persisted for the duration of the experiment, the concentration of 12-HPETE declined to baseline in the second hour after induction of LTP (Fig. 6). We have also measured the concentration of other membrane-associ-

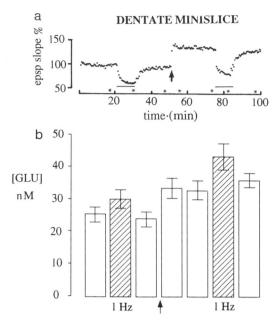

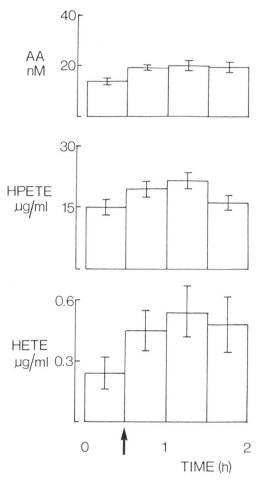

Figure 5. Relationship between glutamate release, stimulus frequency, and LTP in the dentate minislice. (*a*) Mean slope of the population EPSP (normalized with respect to the first 20 min) evoked in the molecular layer by test stimuli delivered at 1/30 Hz. The plot is the mean of data from 16 slices (recordings were made and perfusate was collected from pairs of slices in eight experiments). LTP was induced by tetanic stimulation at the time indicated by the arrow (see Methods). Bars indicate two 10-min periods of stimulation at 1 Hz, one before and the other after the induction of LTP. Note the rapid habituation of the evoked response in each case. (*b*) Mean glutamate content (mean ± S.E.M., $n = 8$) in 4-min samples of perfusate collected at the times marked by the asterisks in *a*. Note the transient increase in release during the periods of stimulation at 1 Hz compared with preceding value at 1/30 Hz (for both 1-Hz periods, $p < 0.01$, Wilcoxin test for paired differences) and the sustained increase associated with LTP.

Figure 6. LTP is accompanied by increases in the concentration of arachidonic acid and its lipoxygenase metabolites in perfusates from the dentate gyrus of the anesthetized rat. Histograms show the mean concentration (mean ± S.E.M.) of arachidonic acid, HPETE, and HETE in successive 1/2-hr periods before and after tetanic stimulation was delivered to induce LTP (↑). In all cases, with the exception of HPETE in the third interval after the tetanus, values after induction of LTP were significantly higher than the corresponding value before the tetanus ($p < 0.05$, Wilcoxin test for paired differences).

ated unsaturated and saturated fatty acids of similar chain length: oleic acid (which along with arachidonic acid has been shown to prolong LTP in the dentate gyrus [Linden et al. 1987]), linoleic, linolenic, palmitic, and stearic acids. No statistically significant changes in the concentration of any of these fatty acids were found in perfusates from the dentate gyrus following the induction of LTP.

If arachidonic acid is an extracellular messenger, linking the postsynaptic site of induction of LTP with the presynaptic terminal to produce a long-term modulation of transmitter release, it might be predicted that arachidonic acid itself would affect synaptic transmission and transmitter release. Although arachidonic acid blocks glutamate uptake into cultured glial cells (Barbour et al. 1989), it produces little effect on synaptic potentials or on glutamate content of hippocampal perfusates in the dentate gyrus (Williams et al. 1989), although it does enhance K^+-stimulated release of [^{3}H]glutamate from hippocampal synaptosomes (Lynch and Voss 1990). However, when combined with

a transient period of enhanced synaptic activity, arachidonic acid leads both in vivo and in vitro (Fig. 7) to a delayed but persistent potentiation in the dentate gyrus and in area CA1 (Williams et al. 1989). This effect, which we have called (forgive us) delayed arachidonic-acid-induced activity-dependent potentiation, is not elicited by a range of other fatty acids (Fig. 8) (Bliss and Williams 1990). It thus appears, first, that the LTP-associated increase in the release of arachidonic acid into the extracellular compartment is specific to arachidonic acid and, second, that the delayed potentiation produced by arachidonic acid is unlikely to reflect an increase in membrane fluidity, since other unsaturated fatty acids failed to produce the effect.

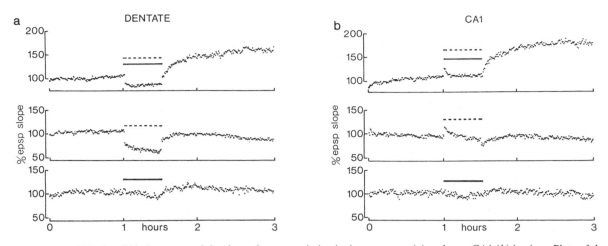

Figure 7. Arachidonic acid induces an activity-dependent potentiation in dentate gyrus (*a*) and area CA1 (*b*) in vitro. Plots of the mean slope of the population EPSP evoked by test stimuli delivered at 1/30 Hz to the perforant path or Schaffer-commissural fibers, respectively, are normalized with respect to the mean value in the first hour. Recordings were made from CA1 and dentate gyrus in the same slice (*n* = 6). Results from three protocols are presented. (*Top*) Arachidonic acid (50 μM) was added to the perfusion medium for 30 min at the time indicated by the solid line, and for the same period, the frequency of stimulation was increased from 1/30 Hz to 1/4 Hz (dashed line). Note the delayed and persistent increase in the slope of the population EPSP. Increased stimulation alone (*middle*) or arachidonic acid alone (*bottom*) produced no long-term increase in synaptic efficacy. (Data for dentate gyrus from Williams et al. 1989.)

DISCUSSION

Two separate but related issues have been addressed in these experiments and will be discussed in turn: first, the relationship between transmitter release and the expression of LTP, and second, the role of arachidonic acid as a putative extracellular messenger in LTP.

Extracellular Glutamate and LTP

Analysis of the glutamate content of hippocampal perfusates from two hippocampal areas, CA1 and dentate gyrus, points to an increase in the concentration of extracellular glutamate, lasting for an hour or more (Fig. 3). In the dentate gyrus, this increase does not occur when the induction of LTP is blocked by the NMDA receptor antagonist D(-)amino-5-phosphonovalerate (APV) or by a variety of pharmacological or physiological maneuvers (Bliss et al. 1986b; Errington et al. 1987; Lynch et al. 1989a). We have observed a similar block in area CA1 with APV (M.L. Errington et al. unpubl.), although in this region, the increase in glutamate release with LTP is less reliable and less persistent than in the dentate gyrus (Fig. 3) and is not always observed with the in vivo push-pull technique (Aniksztejn et al. 1989). Other experimental techniques have also yielded results that indicate a presynaptic involvement in the expression of LTP. In a number of ex vivo studies, we have measured the ability of hippocampal slices or synaptosomes to release radiolabeled glutamate and aspartate in response to a depolarizing stimulus (40 mM K$^+$). Tissue was prepared from area CA1 or dentate gyrus in which LTP had been induced in vivo. In both regions, we found an enhanced K$^+$-stimulated release of glutamate and/or aspartate in potentiated tissue relative to control tissue (Bliss and Lynch 1988). The increase was invariably restricted to the Ca^{++}-dependent component of release. Moreover, the capacity of the high-affinity Na$^+$-coupled glutamate uptake carrier was not affected. On this evidence, the potentiation of K$^+$-induced release reflects a change in the Ca^{++}-dependent, exocytotic component of the release process, rather than a decrease in uptake. In general, an increase in Ca^{++}-dependent release could be expressed as an increase in spontaneous quantal release and/or an increase in activity-dependent release. Major new evidence in favor of an activity-dependent increase has come from quantal analysis of LTP using the whole-cell patch clamp technique (Bekkers and Stevens 1990; Malinow and Tsien 1990; for a dissenting view, see Foster and McNaughton 1991). The statistical changes observed, including a reduction in the number of failures at presumptive single synapses, are most easily interpreted in terms of an increase in the probability of release after the invasion of a terminal by an action potential. Stimulation of a population of potentiated synapses would therefore result in the release of more transmitter per stimulus.

Our perfusion experiments, on the other hand, suggest that there is in addition an increase in the activity-independent release of endogenous glutamate. The stimulus-dependent increase that occurs both in vivo (Fig. 2) and in vitro (Fig. 5) is surprisingly modest, given the 30-fold increase in the rate of stimulation. It is not likely, particularly in the hippocampal slice, that spontaneous cell firing contributes significantly to background release, and it is reasonable to conclude that a substantial proportion of the glutamate in hippocampal perfusates derives from an activity-independent pool.

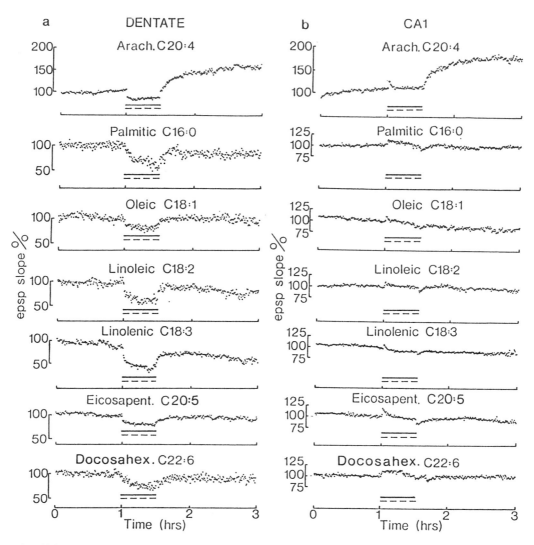

Figure 8. Specificity of activity-dependent, arachidonate-induced potentiation in dentate gyrus (*a*) and area CA1 (*b*). The conjunction protocol described in Fig. 7 was repeated for a range of endogenous saturated and unsaturated fatty acids of a similar chain length to arachidonic acid. Only arachidonate (*top*, same data as in Fig. 7) produced a persistent potentiation of synaptic transmission (*n* = 6 for arachidonic acid and *n* = 3 for the other fatty acids). (Eicosapent.) Eicosapentanoic acid; (Docosahex.) docosahexanoic acid.

Preliminary measurements of glutamate release from slices bathed in medium containing tetrodotoxin or low Ca^{++} are consistent with this assumption (J.H. Williams et al., unpubl.). The conclusion that increased glutamate release in LTP derives at least in part from activity-independent sources is hard to escape. Further experiments, e.g., of the kind illustrated in Figure 5, will be required to establish the relative contributions of activity-dependent and activity-independent sources to the increase in extracellular glutamate in LTP and to reconcile the apparent discrepancy in this regard between endogenous release and release of radiolabeled markers.

The Ca^{++}-independent movement of glutamate across the membrane is regulated by the reversible Na^{+}-coupled uptake carrier (Nicolls 1989), which is present in glia and nerve terminals and probably also in dendrites. There are therefore several potential sources for

an increase in extracellular concentration of glutamate in LTP. Whatever the source(s), a change in the tonic level of extracellular glutamate can be expected to modulate certain aspects of synaptic function in vivo. The dissociation constant for the binding of glutamate to the NMDA receptor is near the estimated concentration for extracellular glutamate, and there is evidence that the excitability of hippocampal neurons is affected by the level of tonic activation of the NMDA receptor (Sah et al. 1989), which at physiological levels of glycine is likely to be substantially nondesensitizing (Vyklicky et al. 1990). Persistent changes in the concentration of extracellular glutamate may thus promote long-term changes in the postsynaptic excitability of the cell.

In summary, there appear to be two components of the increased release in glutamate associated with LTP: a component resulting from enhanced exocytosis at presynaptic terminals and a component reflecting a change in calcium-independent handling of glutamate. The first component accounts, at least in part, for the sustained enhancement of the EPSP; it is possible that the second component plays a role in generating the long-term changes in excitability associated with LTP (Bliss and Lømo 1973; Andersen et al. 1980).

Is Arachidonic Acid a Retrograde Messenger?

Evidence consistent with the proposition that arachidonic acid or one of its lipoxygenase metabolites is a retrograde messenger in LTP includes the following: The lipoxygenase and phospholipase A_2 inhibitor, NDGA blocks the induction of LTP in vivo (Lynch et al. 1989a) and in vitro (Williams and Bliss 1989). Arachidonic acid but not a range of other fatty acids tested induces a delayed, activity-dependent potentiation of synaptic transmission (Figs. 7 and 8), which occludes with tetanus-induced LTP in vivo (Williams et al. 1989) and in vitro (Bliss and Williams 1990). LTP in the dentate gyrus is accompanied by an increase in the extracellular release of arachidonic acid and of its lipoxygenase metabolites, 12-HPETE and 12-HETE. Experiments in which the concentration of free arachidonic acid was measured in membrane fractions prepared from control and potentiated hippocampus suggest that the postsynaptic cell, rather than glia or presynaptic terminals, is the source of the increased efflux of arachidonic acid, 12-HETE, and 12-HPETE (Lynch et al. l989b). Although these observations are broadly consistent with a retrograde messenger role for arachidonic acid or its lipoxygenase metabolites, many questions remain to be answered. For instance, the experiments illustrated in Figure 7 demonstrate that transient exposure to arachidonic acid in conjunction with increased activity produces a persistent potentiation. What then is the function of the sustained increase in the release of arachidonate? Again, it is apparent that arachidonic acid or its metabolites acting alone cannot explain the early phase of LTP. Is there another messenger, possibly acting in synergy with rapidly released arachidonic acid, that mediates this early phase? One candidate is nitric oxide (NO), a molecule that acts as an intercellular messenger in peripheral tissue and that is released from cerebellar cells in culture by NMDA (Garthwaite et al. 1988). However, N_ω-nitro-L-arginine, an inhibitor of NO synthase, does not block the induction of LTP in vitro (T.V.P. Bliss et al. unpubl.).

Finally, how might arachidonic acid induce an increase in transmitter release? Arachidonic acid, 12-HPETE, and 12-HETE all significantly increase K^+-stimulated release of labeled glutamate from synaptosomes prepared from dentate gyrus (Lynch and Voss 1990). Some insight into how this could be achieved is gained from the parallel finding that phosphoinositide turnover in the same preparation is stimulated by arachidonic acid, 12-HPETE, and 12-HETE. The two second messengers produced by hydrolysis of phos-

phoinositide bisphosphate, diacylglycerol and inositol trisphosphate (IP_3), stimulate transmitter release in a variety of preparations, the former by the activation of protein kinase C and the latter by releasing calcium from nonmitochondrial intracellular stores (see Lynch 1989). Consistent with this scheme are two further observations: Arachidonic acid stimulates an increase in synaptosomal calcium, and the concentration of calcium in synaptosomes prepared from potentiated dentate gyrus 45 minutes after the induction of LTP is significantly higher than in control tissues (Lynch and Voss 1991). These effects of arachidonic acid may be secondary to phosphoinositide turnover, since arachidonic acid and IP_3 induce dose-dependent and nonadditive increases in synaptosomal calcium concentration (Lynch and Voss 1991).

In summary, our evidence suggests that one route by which arachidonic acid can influence transmitter release is by stimulating phosphoinositide turnover; an additional route is by direct activation of protein kinase C (Murikami and Routtenberg 1985; Sekiguchi et al. 1987; Linden and Routtenberg 1989). The immediate challenge is to establish causal links between these effects and the calcium-dependent and calcium-independent components of enhanced transmitter release in LTP.

REFERENCES

Andersen, P., S.H. Sundberg, O. Sveen, and H. Wigström. 1980. Possible mechanisms for long-lasting potentiation of synaptic transmission in hippocampal slices from guinea pigs. J. Physiol. 302: 463.

Aniksztejn, L., M.P. Roisin, R. Amsellem, and Y. Ben-Ari. 1989. Long-term potentiation in the hippocampus of the anaesthetized rat is not associated with a sustained enhanced release of endogenous excitatory amino acids. Neuroscience 28: 187.

Barbour, B., M. Szatkowski, N. Ingledew and D. Attwell. 1989. Arachidonic acid induces a prolonged inhibition of glutamate uptake into glial cells. Nature 342: 918.

Bekkers, J.M. and C.F. Stevens. 1990. Presynaptic mechanisms for long-term potentiation in the hippocampus. Nature 346: 724.

Bliss, T.V.P. and T. Lømo. 1973. Long-lasting potentiation of synaptic transmission in the dentate area of the anaesthetized rabbit following stimulation of the perforant path. J. Physiol. 232: 331.

Bliss, T.V.P. and M.A. Lynch. 1988. Long-term potentiation of synaptic transmission in the hippocampus: Properties and mechanisms. In Long-term potentiation: From biophysics to behavior (ed. P.W. Landfield and S.A. Deadwyler), p. 3. A.R. Liss, New York.

Bliss, T.V.P. and J.H. Williams. 1990. Arachidonic acid-induced, activity-dependent potentiation of synaptic transmission in the hippocampus. Soc. Neurosci. Abstr. 16: 145.

Bliss, T.V.P., M.L. Errington, and M.A. Lynch. 1986a. Calcium-induced long-term potentiation in the dentate gyrus is accompanied by a sustained increase in transmitter release. In Excitatory amino acid transmitters (ed. T.P. Hicks and D. Lodge), p. 337. A.R. Liss, New York.

Bliss, T.V.P., R.M. Douglas, M.L. Errington, and M.A. Lynch. 1986b. Correlation between long-term potentiation and release of endogenous amino acids from dentate gyrus of anaesthetized rats. J. Physiol. 377: 391.

Bronk, D.W. 1939. Synaptic mechanisms in sympathetic ganglia. J. Neurophysiol. 2: 380.

Brown, G.L. and U.S. von Euler. 1938. The after-effects of a tetanus on mammalian muscle. *J. Physiol.* **93**: 39.

Cannon, W.B. and A. Rosenblueth. 1937. The transmission of impulses through a sympathetic ganglion. *Am. J. Physiol.* **119**: 221.

———. 1949. *The supersensitivity of denervated structures: A law of denervation.* MacMillan, New York.

Collingridge, G.L. and W. Singer. 1990. Excitatory amino acid receptors and synaptic plasticity. *Trends Pharmacol. Sci.* **11**: 290.

Dolphin, A.C., M.L. Errington, and T.V.P. Bliss. 1982. Long-term potentiation of the perforant path in vivo is associated with increased glutamate release. *Nature* **297**: 496.

Dumuis, A., M. Sebben, L. Haynes, J.-P. Pin, and J. Bockaert. 1988. NMDA receptors activate the arachidonic acid cascade system in striatal neurones. *Nature* **336**: 68.

Errington, M.L., A.C. Dolphin, and T.V.P. Bliss. 1983. A method for combining field potential recording with local perfusion in the hippocampus of the anaesthetized rat. *J. Neurosci. Methods* **7**: 353.

Errington, M.L., M.A. Lynch, and T.V.P. Bliss. 1987. Long-term potentiation in the dentate gyrus: Induction and increased glutamate release are blocked by D(-)aminophosphonovalerate. *Neuroscience* **20**: 279.

Foster, T.C. and B.L. McNaughton. 1991. Long-term enhancement of CA1 synaptic transmission is due to increased quantal size, not quantal content. *Hippocampus* **1**: (in press).

Garthwaite, J., S.L. Charles, and R. Chess-Williams. 1988. Endothelium-derived relaxing factor release on activation of NMDA receptors suggests role as intercellular messenger in the brain. *Nature* **336**: 385.

Gustafsson B. and H. Wigström. 1988. Physiological mechanisms underlying long-term potentiation. *Trends Neurosci.* **11**: 156.

Harris, E.W. and C.W. Cotman. 1986. Long-term potentiation of guinea-pig mossy fiber responses is not blocked by *N*-methyl-D-aspartate receptors. *Neurosci. Lett.* **70**: 132.

Higashima, M. and C. Yamamoto. 1985. Two components of long-term potentiation in mossy fibre-induced excitation in hippocampus. *Exp. Neurol.* **90**: 529.

Hvalby, Ø., J.-C. Lacaille, P. Andersen, and G.-Y. Hu. 1987. Postsynaptic long-term potentiation follows coupling of dendritic glutamate application and synaptic activation. *Experientia* **43**: 599.

Jaffe, D. and D. Johnston. 1990. Induction of long-term potentiation at hippocampal mossy-fiber synapses follows a Hebbian rule. *J. Neurophysiol.* **64**: 948.

Kelso, S.R., A.H. Ganong, and T.H. Brown. 1986. Hebbian synapses in hippocampus. *Proc. Natl. Acad. Sci.* **84**: 5326.

Lazarewicz, J.W., J.T. Wroblewski, M.E. Palmer, and E. Costa. 1988. Activation of *N*-methyl-D-aspartate-sensitive glutamate receptors stimulates arachidonic acid release in primary cultures of cerebellar granule cells. *Neuropharmacology* **27**: 765.

Linden, D.J. and A. Routtenberg. 1989. The role of protein kinase C in long-term potentiation: A testable model. *Brain Res. Rev.* **14**: 296.

Linden, D.J., F.-S. Sheu, K. Murakami, and A. Routtenberg. 1987. Enhancement of long-term potentiation by *cis*-unsaturated fatty acid: Relation to protein kinase C and phospholipase A_2. *J. Neurosci.* **7**: 3783.

Lloyd, D.P.C. 1949. Post-tetanic potentiation of response in monosynaptic reflex pathways of the spinal cord. *J. Gen. Physiol.* **33**: 147.

Lynch, G., S. Halpain, and M. Baudry. 1982. Effects of high-frequency stimulation on glutamate binding studied with a modified *in vitro* hippocampal slice preparation. *Brain Res.* **244**: 101.

Lynch, G., J. Larson, S. Kelso, G. Barrionuevo, and F. Schottler. 1983. Intracellular injections of EGTA block induction of hippocampal long-term potentiation. *Nature* **305**: 719.

Lynch, M.A. 1989. Mechanisms underlying induction and maintenance of long-term potentiation in the hippocampus. *BioEssays* **10**: 85.

Lynch, M.A. and K. Voss. 1990. Arachidonic acid increases inositol phospholipid metabolism and glutamate release in synaptosomes prepared from hippocampal tissue. *J. Neurochem.* **55**: 215.

———. 1991. Presynaptic changes in long-term potentiation: Elevated synaptosomal calcium concentration and basal phosphoinositide in dentate gyrus. *J. Neurochem.* (in press).

Lynch, M.A., M.L. Errington, and T.V.P. Bliss. 1989a. Nordihydroguaiaretic acid blocks the synaptic component of long-term potentiation and the associated increases in release of glutamate and arachidonate: An *in vivo* study in the dentate gyrus of the rat. *Neuroscience* **30**: 693.

Lynch, M.A., M.P. Clements, K.L. Voss, and T.V.P. Bliss. 1989b. Increased postsynaptic release and presynaptic actions of arachidonic acid suggest a retrograde messenger role in long-term potentiation. *Soc. Neurosci. Abstr.* **15**: 86.

Malinow, R. and R.W. Tsien. 1990. Presynaptic enhancement shown by whole-cell recordings of long-term potentiation in hippocampal slices. *Nature* **346**: 177.

Miwa, H., M. Yamamoto, and T. Nishida. 1986. Assay of free and total fatty acids (as 2-nitrophenylhydrazines) by high performance liquid chromatography. *Clin. Chim. Acta* **155**: 95.

Murikami, K. and A. Routtenberg. 1985. Direct activation of purified protein kinase C by unsaturated fatty acids (oleate and arachidonate) in the absence of phospholipids and Ca^{2+}. *FEBS Lett.* **192**: 189.

Nicolls, D.C. 1989. Release of glutamate, aspartate, and γ-aminobutyric acid from isolated nerve terminals. *J. Neurochem.* **52**: 331.

Okada, D., S. Yamagishi, and H. Sugiyama. 1989. Differential effects of phospholipase inhibitors in long-term potentiation in the rat hippocampal mossy fibre synapses and Schaffer-commissural synapses. *Neurosci. Lett.* **100**: 141.

Piomelli, D., A. Volterra, N. Dale, S.A. Siegelbaum, E.R. Kandel, J.H. Schwartz, and F. Belardetti. 1987. Lipoxygenase metabolites of arachidonic acid as second messengers for presynaptic inhibition of *Aplysia* sensory cells. *Nature* **328**: 38.

Reymann, K.G., H.K. Matthies, U. Frey, V.S. Vorobyev, and H. Matthies. 1986. Calcium-induced long-term potentiation in the hippocampal slice: Characterization of the time course and conditions. *Brain Res. Bull.* **17**: 291.

Sah, P., S. Hestrin, and R.A. Nicoll. 1989. Tonic activation of NMDA receptors by ambient glutamate enhances excitability of neurons. *Science* **246**: 815.

Sanfeliu, C., A. Hunt, and A.J. Patel. 1990. Exposure of *N*-methyl-D-aspartate increases release of arachidonic acid in primary cultures of rat hippocampal neurons and not in astrocytes. *Brain Res.* **526**: 241.

Sastry, B.R., J.W. Goh, and A. Auyeung. 1986. Associative induction of posttetanic and long-term potentiation in CA1 neurons of rat hippocampus. *Science* **232**: 988.

Sekiguchi, K., M. Tsukuda, K. Ogita, U. Kiddawa, and Y. Nishizuka. 1987. Three distinct forms of rat brain protein kinase C: Differential response to unsaturated fatty acids. *Biochem. Biophys. Res. Commun.* **145**: 797.

Skrede, K.K. and D. Malthe-Sørenssen. 1981. Increased resting and evoked release of transmitter following repetitive electrical tetanization in hippocampus: A biochemical correlate to long-lasting potentiation. *Brain. Res.* **208**: 436.

Teyler, T.J. and P. DiScenna. 1987. Long-term potentiation. *Annu. Rev. Neurosci.* **10**: 131.

Turner R.W., K.G. Baimbridge, and J.J. Miller. 1982. Calcium-induced long-term potentiation in the hippocampus. *Neuroscience* **7**: 1411.

Vyklicky, L., Jr., M. Benveniste, and M.L. Mayer. 1990. Modulation of *N*-methyl-D-aspartic acid desensitization by glycine in mouse cultured hippocampal neurones. *J. Physiol.* **428**: 313.

Wigström, H. and B. Gustafsson. 1983. Facilitated induction of hippocampal long-lasting potentiation during blockade of inhibition. *Nature* **301**: 603.

Wigström, H., B. Gustafsson, Y.-Y. Huang, and W.C. Abraham. 1986. Hippocampal long-lasting potentiation is induced by pairing single afferent volleys with intracellularly injected depolarizing current pulses. *Acta Physiol. Scand.* **126**: 317.

Williams, J.H. and T.V.P. Bliss. 1988. Induction but not maintenance of calcium-induced long-term potentiation in dentate gyrus and area CA1 of the hippocampal slice is blocked by nordihydroguaiaretic acid. *Neurosci. Lett.* **88**: 81.

————. 1989. An *in vitro* study of the effect of lipoxygenase and cyclo-oxygenase inhibitors of arachidonic acid on the induction and maintenance of long-term potentiation in the hippocampus. *Neurosci. Lett.* **107**: 301.

Williams, J.H., M.L. Errington, M.A. Lynch, and T.V.P. Bliss. 1989. Arachidonic acid induces a long-term activity-dependent enhancement of synaptic transmission in the hippocampus. *Nature* **341**: 739.

Zalutsky, R.A. and R.A. Nicoll. 1990. Comparison of two forms of long-term potentiation in single hippocampal neurons. *Science* **248**: 1618.

Computational Implications of NMDA Receptor Channels

J.M. Bekkers and C.F. Stevens
The Salk Institute, Howard Hughes Medical Institute, La Jolla, California 92037

Of the various types of glutamate receptors abundantly present in the brain, the one that selectively binds the glutamate analog *N*-methyl-D-aspartate (NMDA) has recently attracted considerable attention. Here, we describe the properties of NMDA receptor channels and explore some of the implications these properties might have for neural computational mechanisms.

A recently identified family of glutamate receptors (Hollmann et al., this volume) has emphasized the diversity of excitatory amino acid receptor types that are found in the brain. One convenient way to define family membership is by pharmacological classification: Receptors belong either to the NMDA class—those activated specifically by this agonist—or to the non-NMDA class. The non-NMDA class of channels can be further subdivided into receptors activated by either of the two glutamate analogs: kainic acid and α-amino-3-hydroxy-5-methyl-isoxazole-4-propionic acid (AMPA). As a shorthand, we shall refer to non-NMDA receptors as AMPA receptors. Although the key role of NMDA receptors in the phenomenon of long-term potentiation (LTP) has been recognized since 1983 (Collingridge et al. 1983), the widespread participation of these receptors in neuronal computations has been appreciated only in the last few years. In the following sections, we review the role of NMDA receptors in the functioning of neuronal circuits, describe special properties of the NMDA receptor channel, and consider some possible uses that receptor properties might have for performing computations.

Participation of NMDA Receptors in Synaptic Transmission

Until relatively recently, NMDA receptors were thought not to participate in "normal" synaptic transmission. The basis for this belief was the observation that the specific NMDA receptor antagonist APV had no effect on synaptic potentials evoked by electrical stimulation of afferents. Salt (1986) discovered, however, that the response to natural sensory stimulation was blocked by APV, whereas the responses to electrical stimulation of the sensory afferents were unaffected by this drug. This paradoxical result is a consequence of special properties of NMDA receptor channels to be considered in the next section. During the past several years, a number of investigators have demonstrated

that NMDA receptors play a prominent role in the normal synaptic response of numerous systems (see Collingridge and Lester 1989). More recently, interest has focused on determining which attributes of a cell's response are mediated by NMDA class receptors and which are mediated by the AMPA class. We give a few examples here.

The first special role for NMDA receptors in neuronal computations was elucidated by Grillner and collaborators, who showed that NMDA induces oscillatory activity in lamprey spinal neurons involved in pattern formation for locomotion (Wallen and Grillner 1985, 1987; Moore et al. 1987), and they suggested that the voltage dependence of NMDA receptor activation and the calcium influx through these channels (Hill et al. 1989) are key for the generation of these oscillations. The current status of this work is discussed by Grillner et al. (this volume). Foutz et al. (1989) have described the participation of NMDA receptors in the generation of respiratory rhythms in mammals. These authors find that NMDA receptors are responsible for activating the inspiratory "off-switch." This function is, by an independent pathway, also provided by vagal afferents that report on the lung's extent of inflation. Vagotimized animals treated with APV do not terminate the discharge of their inspiratory neurons and thus are locked in a state of maintained inspiration.

Certain weakly electric fish use electric fields generated by their electric organs both for navigation and for communication with other fish of the same species. The frequency of the electric organ discharge is determined by a pacemaker nucleus, and their "song" has different spectral characteristics according to whether the fish are communicating with one another or are navigating in waters populated by other fish. When one fish enters the electric field generated by another, it shifts the frequency of its own electric organ discharge to avoid having its navigational field distorted by the other fish's field: This frequency shift is called the jamming avoidance response. When communicating, the fish produce a rapid rise in the frequency of electric organ discharge, a "chirp." Dye et al. (1989) have determined that chirps depend on AMPA receptors, but that the jamming avoidance response is mediated by NMDA receptors.

Neurons of area 17 use NMDA receptors in processing normal input. Fox et al. (1990) have identified what appears to be at least one of the special functions of

NMDA receptors in the processing of visual information: APV causes a decrease in contrast sensitivity without completely blocking the neuronal response to visual stimulation. Although the details of how NMDA receptor properties relate to the special computations performed by neurons have not been elucidated in any of these examples, the experiments provide convincing evidence that NMDA receptors are used for a separate computational mode. We turn now to a description of some of the special NMDA receptor properties.

Properties of the NMDA Receptor Channel

Agonist binding. The NMDA receptor possesses the unusual, and possibly unique, property of requiring the binding of two distinct neurotransmitters, both glutamate and glycine, for activation (Johnson and Ascher 1987). The "usual" transmitter is glutamate, but the application of this transmitter is ineffective unless glycine is also present. Glutamate and glycine bind to distinct sites, and the glycine site is saturated at concentrations of about 1 μM. Glutamate is released by presynaptic terminals, but the source of glycine is, as yet, unknown. An elucidation of this glycine regulatory action is a prerequisite for a full understanding of NMDA receptor function.

Patneau and Mayer (1990) determined the dose-response relation for the NMDA receptor and found that the binding of two glutamate molecules is required for receptor activation; the dissociation constant for the binding sites is close to 1 μM, a value almost an order of magnitude lower than that for the AMPA receptors. The fraction of activated receptors $f(A)$ is given by

$$f(A) = A^2/(1 + 2A + A^2)$$

where A is the glutamate concentration divided by the dissociation constant equal to 1.1 μM.

Glutamate receptor channels desensitize in the maintained presence of glutamate, but this important process has not yet been characterized in full detail. The dose-response relations described above may have been influenced by desensitization; the seriousness of this possible artifact is unknown.

Permeation and selectivity. NMDA receptor channels permit the flux of all alkali metal cations, with essentially the same permeability (Ascher et al. 1988). The receptor's pore is also highly permeable to calcium but not at all to magnesium (Jahr and Stevens 1987). Because calcium preemptively occupies the pore for a relatively long time as it passes through, increasing the calcium concentration produces a decrease in the single channel conductance (C.E. Jahr and C.F. Stevens, unpubl.). Specifically, conductance h (in pS) is given by

$$h = (H + 5a)/(1 + 0.42a)$$

where a is the calcium ion activity and $H = 53$ pS is the limiting single-channel conductance in the absence of calcium ions; note that H depends on the monovalent ion concentration (here assumed to be 165 mM). The calcium ion activity a under these circumstances is approximately (calcium concentration)/4 over the physiological range. That portion of the single channel conductance arising from the calcium flux is $5a/(1 + 0.42a)$, and this expression can be used, together with information about membrane potential, to calculate the quantity of calcium ions that flow through the channels. The "block" of these channels by calcium is not voltage-dependent.

Because calcium ions permeate the NMDA receptor pore, the reversal potential for this channel depends on the calcium concentration. The following equation gives the approximate change in reversal potential V_o when the external calcium concentration is increased from zero to C, assuming the intracellular calcium concentration is close to zero.

$$V_o = (50.8\,[57C + 4m]\,[\ln\{0.167[57C + 4m]\} - \ln\{0.667m\}])/(171C + 8m)$$

where C is the calcium concentration and m is the monovalent ion concentration; V_o is in millivolts and concentrations are in millimolars (C.E. Jahr and C.F. Stevens, unpubl.). When the intracellular and extracellular monovalent cation concentrations are equal, V_o gives the absolute reversal potential.

Gating. Jahr and Stevens (1990a) described the gating of NMDA receptor channels. They found that the channel behavior in the range of physiological magnesium concentrations can be described by assuming the channel can occupy three distinct states: open, closed, and blocked. The transitions are permitted from the open and blocked states to closed. According to this analysis, a channel opens and then makes a number of transitions into the blocked state before finally closing. The mean time for remaining in the activated state is about 10 msec, and this activated state is, after agonist binding, reentered from the closed state repeatedly for about 150 msec (at room temperature) before the channel finally closes and dissociates its bound glutamate. An important feature of this channel revealed by this analysis is that the channel can close even when a magnesium ion is blocking its pore.

The analysis (Jahr and Stevens 1990b) also provides a confirmation of the conclusion, first made by Nowak et al. (1984) and Mayer et al. (1984), that the magnesium ion must move through part of the membrane field to reach its blocking site. This position of the blocking site gives a voltage dependence to the block that endows the channel with what is, in effect, gating determined by the neuron's membrane potential. As a result of this "gating," the fraction of time the channel remains open in the presence of a given concentration of glutamate depends on voltage according to the equation

$$g(V) = 1/(1 + \exp[-0.062V][C_{Mg}/3.57])$$

where $g(V)$ is the fraction of the available NMDA receptor channel conductance expressed at voltage V(mV) and C_{Mg} is the extracellular magnesium concentration (mM).

Bekkers and Stevens (1989b) have shown that the same quantum of glutamate activates both the AMPA and NMDA receptor channels at hippocampal synapses; thus, transmission can be dual functional at a single synapse. The AMPA component is rapid and behaves much like the synaptic transmission familiar at the neuromuscular junction, but the NMDA receptor channel, by virtue of the properties described above, is quite different. Whereas the AMPA component of synaptic conductance rises rapidly and declines to zero in a few milliseconds, the NMDA component rises slowly to its peak value—it increases with about the same time course as the AMPA component decays—and then decays with a time constant of about 150 msec (at room temperature). This slow rise and very slow decay are consequences of the channel gating kinetics noted above. According to the analysis cited earlier, the channel closes at the same rate whether the magnesium-blocking site is occupied or not. This means that the time course of the channel activation proceeds in the same way independent of voltage. That is, at negative voltages, even if essentially no current flows through the channel because its magnesium-blocking site is occupied virtually all of the time, the channel still remains in its activated state for the usual several hundred milliseconds duration. If the neuron's voltage becomes sufficiently positive during this time, the magnesium block will be relieved and ions will flow through the channel. This situation gives rise to the concept of *occult conductance:* Once the NMDA receptors are briefly occupied, any depolarization will reveal the activated state of the channels. In this way, the activation of other of the neuron's synapses can alter the strength of a synapse.

When multiple boutons are activated, these occult conductances can all add linearly (Bekkers and Stevens 1989a). This means that the activity of some synapses can "read out" the prior activity of other synapses. We return to the properties of this occult conductance later.

Computational Implications of NMDA Receptor Channels

As described above, the NMDA receptors have four properties that distinguish them from other ligand gated channels in the brain. First, they require the presence of a cotransmitter, glycine, for their activation. Second, they are strongly permeable to calcium ions and can permit a significant influx of this ion. Third, voltage and glutamate (and glycine) control their opening probability. Finally, they endow synapses with a relatively long memory by remaining in the "activated" state for several hundreds of milliseconds (at room temperature), even when they are in their occult state. Each of these special properties can potentially

be used computationally. We consider them in turn. The concept of *synaptic strength* is central to understanding computation in neural circuits. As we will note, various properties of NMDA receptor channels relate specifically to the control of synaptic strength.

The fact that glycine is required as a cotransmitter provides the possibility of a mechanism through which the strength of the NMDA receptor component of synaptic transmission could be regulated; speculations about how this mechanism could be used computationally, however, are premature given the limited amount of information currently available. The problem is that glycine has not been established to be the molecule actually used in regulation—some peptide or peptide fragment might be the functional cotransmitter—and the mechanism by which glycine levels (or the levels of the putative other cotransmitter) are regulated are unknown. Even the sign of the regulatory process is unknown. For example, a real regulatory molecule might act by blocking an ongoing cotransmitter effect of glycine. One possibility that attracts us is that glycine is the natural regulatory molecule and that its levels are controlled by the uptake mechanisms in glial cells. On this theory, glia would integrate metabolic information together with regulatory signals from neurotransmitters and then modulate in some appropriate way the synaptic strength contributed by the neuron's NMDA receptors.

Calcium influx through NMDA receptor channels provides a possibly effective computational mechanism. Grillner et al. (this volume) have discussed the possibility that calcium ions entering through NMDA receptor channels can open calcium-activated potassium channels and thus participate in pattern generating voltages. Bekkers and Stevens (1989a) have previously shown that the amount of calcium that enters dendritic spines is related to the extent to which that synapse's activity is correlated with the activation of other synapses on the neuron; the NMDA receptor channels can thus be used to calculate a cross-correlation function. According to this analysis, calcium could represent the degree of correlation in activity that is used to increase synaptic strength in LTP. In both of these instances, the computation being carried out by neurons is represented by the amount of calcium that enters through NMDA receptor channels.

Because NMDA receptor channels are blocked by magnesium ions at voltages near the resting potential, one might expect that applications of NMDA would not depolarize neurons. This would be true under certain circumstances, for example, at sufficiently high magnesium concentrations, but at physiological levels of magnesium and with typical resting conductances of neurons, NMDA can quite potently depolarize neurons. This phenomenon is illustrated by the following typical example. A hippocampal pyramidal neuron has a resting input conductance of about 10 nS and receives on the order of 10^4 synapses. If each synapse has an NMDA component with a peak conductance of 0.2 nS (Bekkers and Stevens 1989b), then the depolarization

V caused by simultaneous activation n synapses (in the presence of 6-cyano-7-nitroquinoxaline-2,3-dione so that only the NMDA component is revealed) would be given by the equation

$$V = -70(0.01)/(0.01 + g[V,n])$$

where the resting potential is assumed to be -70 mV and the NMDA contribution $g(V,n)$ is, for magnesium concentration C_{Mg} mM,

$$g(V,n) = 0.2n/(1 + \exp[-0.062V][C_{Mg}/3.57])$$

The depolarization that would result is plotted in Figure 1. The simultaneous activation of only 400 synapses (4% of those the neuron receives) is thus sufficient to produce a peak depolarization of about 40 mV through NMDA receptors alone. As is apparent from Figure 1, the relation between depolarization and number of activated synapses is highly nonlinear; the activity of 100 synapses would produce only about a 10-mV peak depolarization.

The voltage dependence of NMDA receptor channels provides a special way in which synaptic strength is regulated. Typically, the strength of a synapse is a well-defined quantity that reflects the history of use, extracellular ion concentrations, adenosine levels, and a host of other factors. When NMDA receptors are activated, however, an occult conductance develops, and the extent to which this conductance is expressed depends on the neuron's membrane potential, which in turn is set by the activity of other synapses and the activation of various voltage-gated channels. Synaptic strength in this circumstance is determined in part by the sum total of the neuron's synaptic input.

The example cited above assumed the simultaneous activation of synapses, but the fourth special property of NMDA receptor, their long duration of activation from a single, brief glutamate application, together with the fact that their closing rate is independent of whether or not they happen to be conducting current, means that temporal summation can quite effectively build a considerable occult conductance. These properties explain Salt's (1986) observation that natural activation of synapses is so much more effective in depolarizing a neuron than is single-shock stimulation of afferents. When single shocks are used, the NMDA component of the conductance is almost entirely occult, and the responses are entirely mediated by the AMPA component of the conductance. However, with repetitive (or natural) stimulation, the NMDA components are temporally summed and the potential conductance reaches sufficient levels to produce significant depolarization as is clear from Figure 1. The responses to natural stimulation are thus altered when the NMDA component is removed by APV.

SUMMARY

We have summarized the quantitative relations developed so far for the description of NMDA receptor function. One of the most important gaps in our knowledge relates to desensitization. A full quantitative treatment of computational uses of NMDA receptor channels must await a formalization of this process and also a more detailed examination of the occupation of closed states of the receptor whose binding sites are occupied. As this information becomes available and the role of NMDA receptors in the function of brain circuits is further explored, we should be able to define accurately this second computational mode.

ACKNOWLEDGMENTS

This work was supported by the Howard Hughes Medical Institute and grant NS-12961 from the National Institutes of Health to C.F.S.

REFERENCES

Ascher, P., P. Bregestovski, and L. Nowak. 1988. *N*-methyl-D-aspartate-activated channels of mouse central neurones in magnesium-free solutions. *J. Physiol.* **339:** 207.

Bekkers, J.M. and C.F. Stevens. 1989a. Dual modes of excitatory synaptic transmission in the brain. In *Proceedings of the 1st NIMH Conference* (ed. S. Zaleman and R. Scheller), p. 39. U.S. Department of Health and Human Services, Rockville, Maryland.

———. 1989b. NMDA and non-NMDA receptors are co-localized at individual excitatory synapses in cultured rat hippocampus. *Nature* **341:** 230.

Collingridge, G.L. and R.A.J. Lester. 1989. Excitatory amino acid receptors in the vertebrate central nervous system. *Pharmacol. Rev.* **40:** 143.

Collingridge, G.L., S.J. Kehl, and H. McLennan. 1983. Excitatory amino acids in synaptic transmission in the Schaffer collateral-commissural pathway of the rat hippocampus. *J. Physiol.* **334:** 33.

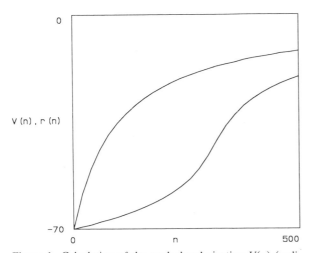

Figure 1. Calculation of the peak depolarization $V(n)$ (ordinate) produced by the NMDA component when n (abscissa) synapses are activated simultaneously on a hippocampal neuron (S-shaped curve). The top curve, $r(n)$, shows what the depolarization response would have been had the NMDA receptor channels not been voltage-dependent. The difference between the top and bottom curves is a reflection of the extent to which the NMDA receptor conductance is occult.

Dye, J., W. Heiligenberg, C.H. Keller, and M. Kawasaki. 1989. Different classes of glutamate receptors mediate distinct behaviors in a single brainstem nucleus. *Proc. Natl. Acad. Sci.* **86**: 8993.

Foutz, A.S., J. Champagnat, and M. Denavit-Saubie. 1989. Involvement of *N*-methyl-D-aspartate (NMDA) receptors in respiratory rhythmogenesis. *Brain Res.* **500**: 199.

Fox, K., H. Sato, and N. Daw. 1990. The effect of varying stimulus intensity on NMDA-receptor activity in cat visual cortex. *J. Neurophysiol.* (in press).

Hill, R.H., L. Brodin, and S. Grillner. 1989. Activation of *N*-methyl-D-aspartate (NMDA) receptors augments repolarizing responses in lamprey spinal neurons. *Brain Res.* **499**: 388.

Jahr, C.E. and C.F. Stevens. 1987. Glutamate activates multiple single channel conductances in hippocampal neurons. *Nature* **325**: 522.

———. 1990a. A quantitative description of NMDA receptor-channel kinetic behavior. *J. Neurosci.* **10**: 1830.

———. 1990b. Voltage dependence of NMDA-activated macroscopic conductances predicted by single-channel kinetics. *Neuroscience* **10**: 3178.

Johnson, J.W. and P. Ascher. 1987. Glycine potentiates the NMDA response in cultured mouse brain neurons. *Nature* **325**: 529.

Mayer, M.L., G.L. Westbrook, and P.B. Guthrie. 1984. Voltage-dependent block by Mg^{2+} of NMDA responses in spinal cord neurones. *Nature* **309**: 261.

Moore, L.E., R.H. Hill, and S. Grillner. 1987. Voltage clamp analysis of lamprey neurons—Role of *N*-methyl-D-aspartate receptors in fictive locomotion. *Brain Res.* **419**: 397.

Nowak, L. P. Bregestovski, P. Ascher, A. Herbert, and Z. Prochiantz. 1984. Magnesium gates glutamate-activated channels in mouse central neurones. *Nature* **307**: 462.

Patneau, D.K. and M.L. Mayer. 1990. Structure-activity relationships for amino acid transmitter candidates acting at *N*-methyl-D-aspartate and quisqualate receptors. *J. Neurosci.* **10**: 2385.

Salt, T.E. 1986. Mediation of thalamic sensory input by both NMDA receptors and non-NMDA receptors. *Nature* **322**: 263.

Wallen, P. and S. Grillner. 1985. The effect of current passage on *N*-methyl-D-aspartate-induced, tetrodoxin-resistant membrane potential oscillations in lamprey neurons active during locomotion. *Neurosci. Lett.* **56**: 87.

———. 1987. *N*-methyl-D-aspartate receptor-induced, inherent oscillatory activity in neurons active during fictive locomotion in the lamprey. *J. Neurosci.* **7**: 2745.

Modified Hebbian Rule for Synaptic Enhancement in the Hippocampus and the Visual Cortex

T. BONHOEFFER,*‡§ A. KOSSEL,† J. BOLZ,† AND A. AERTSEN‡

*The Rockefeller University, Neurobiology Laboratory, New York, New York 10021;
†Friedrich-Miescher-Laboratorium der Max-Planck-Gesellschaft and ‡Max-Planck-Institut für biologische Kybernetik, 7400 Tübingen, Federal Republic of Germany

Ramón y Cajal (1909, 1911) was the first to suggest that synapses might be the locations at which memory is laid down in the brain. Some 50 years later, Donald Hebb proposed the physiological condition under which this might happen (Hebb 1949). He invoked the notion of "synaptic plasticity": Activity occurring simultaneously at the neurons pre- and postsynaptic to a particular synapse would lead to an increase in the efficacy of that synapse. This postulate later became known as the Hebb rule and was widely adopted by both experimentors and theoreticians. Hebb's model of synaptic plasticity provided a natural explanation for many experimental observations on learning, memory, and development.

Despite the intuitive appeal of Hebb's idea and its wide acceptance, it took quite some time before its validity could be established by direct experimental evidence. Wigström, Gustafsson, and co-workers (Wigström et al. 1986; Gustafsson et al. 1987) showed

that simultaneous activation of pre- and postsynaptic neurons in a hippocampal slice can enhance a synapse. Once this result had been obtained, it was an obvious question whether this enhancement was confined to only those synapses that had actually received the concurrent stimulation or whether it was a more global phenomenon that also extended to other synapses. At first sight, it would seem advantageous if the enhancement occurred as locally as possible. This caused many people to assume, at least implicitly, that the biological mechanism underlying the strengthening of synapses should also follow this rule. It was shown that synaptic enhancement shows postsynaptic specificity: If a synapse (Fig. 1, synapse A) on a postsynaptic neuron is enhanced, a neighboring synapse on the same cell but receiving input from a different afferent fiber (Fig. 1, synapse B) will not be affected (Gustafsson et al. 1987).

In our experiments, we set out to investigate whether this spatial confinement also holds along the presynaptic fiber. To this end, we stimulated a set of afferent fibers with one stimulating electrode (conditioning stimulus) and recorded intracellularly from two postsynaptic neurons (cf. Fig. 1). Potentiation was induced

§ Present address: Max-Planck Institute for Brian Research, Deutschordenstrasse 46, D-6000 Frankfurt/Main 71, Federal Republic of Germany.

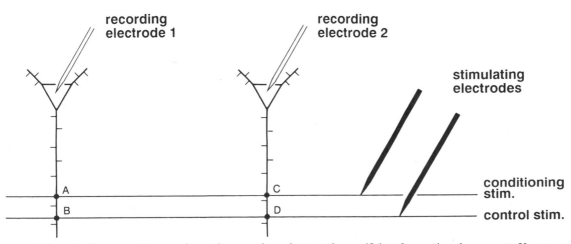

paired cell   **unpaired cell**

Figure 1. Schematic diagram of the experimental approach used to test the specificity of synaptic enhancement. If synapse A is enhanced by simultaneous stimulation with the conditioning stimulus and intracellular current injection into the paired cell, would synapses on a nearby cell (C) also be affected?

by pairing the "conditioning stimuli" with postsynaptic depolarization in one cell (paired cell) but not in the other (unpaired cell). The question was whether the enhancement that was induced in synapse A would spread to the neighboring synapse C. We chose to investigate this question in two different systems: slice cultures of the hippocampus and conventional slices of the visual cortex.

METHODS

Slice cultures. Hippocampal slice cultures were prepared following the method of Gähwiler (Gähwiler 1981, 1984; Gähwiler and Brown 1985). Three- to seven-day-old rats were decapitated, and their hippocampi were removed. The tissue was cut into 350-μm-thick sections using a McIlwain tissue chopper. They were glued onto glass coverslips with 15 μl of plasma (Difco TC chicken plasma) coagulated by 15 μl of a thrombin solution. After the plasma clot hardened, the coverslips were transferred into culture test tubes (Nunclon) containing 750 μl of culture medium and put into a roller drum incubator at 34°C. Within 1–2 weeks, the slices flattened to monolayer thickness and were suitable for our experiments. We were able to maintain these cultures viable for up to 6 months.

For electrophysiological recordings, we placed the coverslip with a slice culture into the recording chamber that was perfused at 30 ml/hr with a modified Hanks' balanced salt solution (HBSS + 2 mM $CaCl_2$). The temperature of the solution was kept at 33 ± 1°C with a conventional temperature-controlling system. The chamber itself was mounted on an inverted microscope, which allowed easy access with stimulating and recording electrodes from above without obstructing the view of the preparation. For more details regarding the recording setup, see Bonhoeffer and Staiger (1988).

Acute slices. Two- to four-week-old rats were anesthetized with ether and decapitated, and their brains were removed. After storing the brain in ice-cold artificial cerebrospinal fluid, a block of 5×5 mm^2 of the visual cortex was prepared and cut into 350-μm-thick slices using the egg-slicer technique (Katz 1987). For storage and recording from the slices, we used an interface chamber.

Pairing experiment. In the hippocampus, stimulating electrodes were placed in the Schaffer-collaterals of the CA3 or CA1 region (cf. Fig. 4, top). For intracellular recordings, we impaled neurons in the pyramidal layer of the CA1 region (intracellular electrodes were filled with 3 M KCl [resistance 60–100 MΩ] or 3 M K-acetate [resistance 100–220 MΩ]). In the cortex, two stimulating electrodes (distance ~1.5 mm) were positioned in the white matter of the slice. We recorded intracellularly from two closely neighboring cells (distance <200 μm).

The strength of the test stimulus (a single pulse with duration of 50 μsec; interstimulus interval [ISI] 4 sec) to the presynaptic fibers was set so that we could record a stable, subthreshold excitatory postsynaptic potential (EPSP) in the postsynaptic neurons or that the neurons fired only occasionally. After the responses to the test stimulus were stable, we applied a pairing paradigm similar to the one developed by Gustafsson et al. (1987): Concurrent to the presynaptic stimulus, we depolarized one of the intracellularly recorded neurons by injecting a 0.5–5-nA current pulse with a duration of 100 msec, starting 10 msec prior to the test stimulus. The other neuron did not receive any depolarizing current injection. In fact, our intracellular recordings from the second neuron allowed us to make sure that there was not even an artifactual depolarization in this neuron. In some cases, we used a second stimulating electrode as a control. In this case, we alternated between the two presynaptic stimuli, which we called control and conditioning stimuli. During the pairing, we applied postsynaptic stimulation only concurrently with the conditioning stimulus.

After 30–60 such pairings (ISI 4 sec), we stopped applying the depolarizing current pulse and recorded again the response of the neurons to the test stimulus only. In a few experiments, we used a modified pairing procedure: We alternated presynaptic stimuli paired with current injection and presynaptic stimuli alone (thereby doubling the inter-pairing interval) to monitor the progress of synaptic enhancement.

Optical recording. Voltage-sensitive dyes were used to monitor the evoked responses of neurons surrounding the postsynaptically stimulated one before and after the pairing (for details regarding the optical recording technique, see Bonhoeffer and Staiger 1988). The slice culture was viewed with an inverted microscope (Zeiss IM 35) equipped with a rhodamine epifluorescence filter set. The slice culture was illuminated by a mercury lamp with a stabilized power supply. The image of the slice culture was projected with a microscope objective (Zeiss 63 × /1.25 oil immersion) onto a 12 × 12 photodiode array (Centronics M144-5) mounted on the microscope. The signals from the photodiodes were amplified and recorded with a microcomputer (DEC LSI 11/73). The data were transferred to a VAX 750 for further signal processing.

We used the styryl dyes RH 237 (Grinvald et al. 1982) and RH 414 (Grinvald et al. 1984) for our experiments. The medium in the chamber was exchanged for 1–1.5 ml of the voltage-sensitive dye, and perfusion was stopped for 30 minutes. After recommencing perfusion, we waited 10–20 minutes to ensure that the dye that had not bound to cell membranes was washed out. To minimize photodynamic damage, we only recorded fluorescence signals every 30 seconds. Only on every third sweep was a stimulus delivered (i.e., ISI 90 sec), and the remaining two sweeps were used for signal correction purposes (Bonhoeffer and Staiger 1988).

RESULTS

Figure 2 shows how synaptic strengthening can be induced in hippocampal slice cultures. We stimulated the Schaffer-collaterals in a hippocampal slice culture and recorded intracellularly from a neuron in the CA1 region. After collecting a baseline response (Fig. 2A, before) from the neuron, we applied the pairing procedure. The presynaptic stimuli were presented concurrently with postsynaptic current injection of 0.6 nA, which caused the neuron to fire. After this procedure, the responses of the neuron were clearly different from before (Fig. 2A, after). Three main features could indicate that the synapses between the fibers and the neuron were potentiated: (1) The initial slope of the EPSP values was much steeper after a successful pairing than before; (2) if spikes occurred in response to the stimulus, they did so with a much shorter latency than before the pairing; and (3) if the postsynaptic neuron did not generate spikes, an increased amplitude of the EPSP was an indication of successful enhancement. In the case shown in Figure 2, criteria 1 and 2 were met. Although condition 3 also seems to have been fulfilled, it was not of great value since the occurrence of a spike before the maximum of the EPSP was reached distorted the shape of the EPSP.

Since in this experiment pairing and test stimuli were alternated, we were in a position to examine the temporal development of synaptic enhancement. To illustrate the temporal aspects, we chose a different way of displaying the data (Fig. 2B). Membrane potentials are now coded in gray levels, with a higher value corresponding to a darker gray. Each single response corresponds to a horizontal line in the display, with the gray value variation along this line portraying the time course of the membrane potential. Successive responses are plotted above each other; consequently, the vertical axis represents time as it proceeds from trial to trial throughout the experiment. This allows one not only to look at selected responses (as in Fig. 2A), but also to show every single response of the intracellularly recorded neuron during the entire experiment within one picture, thereby making changes in the responses over time readily detectable. In Figure 2B, one can observe how during the pairing phase (the horizontal band between 2 and 7 min), the latencies of the action potentials (which manifest themselves as dark spots) elicited by the intervening test stimuli gradually declined until a stable minimum was reached. In addition, one observes a decrease in the variation of horizontal position of the dark spots as time proceeds. This indicates that, because of the pairing, spikes occurred earlier not only with respect to the stimulus, but also in a more reliable fashion. Summarizing, these data show that in slice cultures of the hippocampus, synaptic enhancement can be induced by simultaneously stimulating pre- and postsynaptic neurons.

The goal of our experiments was to test whether this potentiation is well restricted spatially on the presynaptic axons. To this end, we placed an extracellular stimulating electrode in the Schaffer-collaterals and impaled a postsynaptic neuron in the CA1 region of the hippocampal slice culture. To record simultaneously the responses from different postsynaptic neurons, we recorded optically with voltage-sensitive dyes. We utilized a 12×12 photodiode array to measure optically the responses of all the neurons in a field of 280×280 μm^2. Before synaptic enhancement, the responses of all of these neurons to the presynaptic stimulus were measured. We then induced the enhancement exactly as described above, by pairing postsynaptic stimuli to one neuron with single presynaptic stimuli to the Schaffer-collaterals. After this procedure, the responses from all of the neurons were tested again.

The data from such an experiment are displayed in Figure 3. The thin curves in the figure show averaged responses of the neurons before potentiation of the synapses and the thick curves show the responses after potentiation of the synapses. The position of the postsynaptically stimulated neuron is marked with an asterisk. Despite the local postsynaptic stimulus, not only the response of this one neuron, but also those of neighboring neurons were enhanced. It should be emphasized that this spread cannot be attributed to poor spatial resolution: We have shown elsewhere (Bonhoeffer and Staiger 1988) that the optical recording procedure permits "single-cell resolution" in hippocampal slice cultures. We thus conclude from these data that not only the synapses that actually received the paired stimulation, but also other synapses connecting from the stimulated fibers to different postsynaptic neurons were enhanced.

We performed 26 of these experiments, in 11 of which potentiation could be induced and measured optically. In each of these 11 cases, we found a spread of the effect which amounted to at least some 150 μm around the depolarized neuron.

To corroborate this finding obtained with optical methods by conventional electrophysiology, we also performed double intracellular recordings. The stimulating electrode was again placed in the Schaffer-collaterals near the CA3 region. In this case, however, we impaled two pyramidal cells lying close together (distance <60 μm) in the CA1 region of the hippocampus (cf. Fig. 4, top). After testing the responses of both cells to the test stimulus (Fig. 4a,f), we depolarized cell 1 strongly during the presynaptic stimulus (Fig. 4b), whereas no current was injected into cell 2 (Fig. 4g). Recording from both cells simultaneously enabled us to always make sure that the depolarization of cell 1 had no effect on the membrane potential of cell 2. After 30 pairings of the pre- and postsynaptic stimuli, we tested both cells again with the original test stimulus. Again, the responses of *both* cells were potentiated (Fig. 4c,h): The initial slopes of the EPSPs in both cells are steeper, in turn causing the action potentials to occur more reliably and earlier with respect to the stimulus. The effect was rather long-lasting: After 10 minutes (Fig. 4d,i) and even after 30 minutes (Fig. 4e,j), enhancement was still clearly visible in both cells.

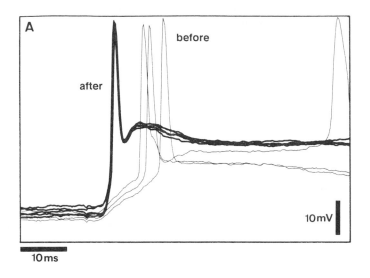

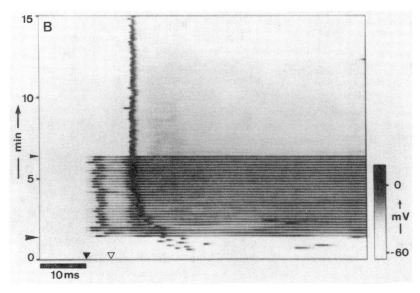

Figure 2. Enhancement of synapses by paired stimulation. The stimulating electrode was situated in the Schaffer-collaterals. An intracellular electrode recorded from a pyramidal neuron in the CA1 region. (*A*) Some responses of the neuron to single test stimuli before pairing are displayed as thin curves. The initial slope of the EPSPs was very gentle. This caused the action potentials to occur (if at all) very late after the test stimulus. After 30 simultaneous presentations of an intracellular depolarizing current pulse and the extracellular single stimulus to the Schaffer-collaterals (ISI 4 sec), the response of the neuron was enhanced. This is shown in the thick curves: After pairing, every test stimulus elicited an action potential that occurred with a much shorter latency than before the pairing. Amplitude and initial slope of the EPSPs also showed a substantial increase. (*B*) The data from the same experiment as in *A* are displayed with emphasis on the temporal development of the enhancement. In this experiment, we applied a test stimulus (at the time indicated by the open triangle on the horizontal axis) to the Schaffer-collaterals after each individual pairing. Thus, one can observe the temporal development of the synaptic enhancement. The data are displayed as a matrix composed of 180 single horizontal lines (corresponding to 180 recorded sweeps, covering a total of 15 min). Each line represents the intracellularly recorded membrane potential, the values being coded according to the gray scale in the right-hand part of the figure. Black spots in the figure thus correspond to high values of the membrane potential (i.e., spikes). One can discern three horizontal bands in the figure, each corresponding to a particular phase of the experiment. The lower band (the first 2 min; between 0 and the large arrowhead on the vertical axis) shows the responses of the neuron to the test stimulus before pairing. One can see that a spike does not occur in every trace, but when it does, it occurs irregularly and quite late. The middle band (the following 5 min; between the large and the small arrowhead on the vertical axis) is composed of 30 responses measured during the paired stimulation (note the early spike pair elicited by the depolarizing current, which was applied between the triangles on the horizontal axis), alternating with 30 responses to the presynaptic stimulus alone. One can clearly observe that the latency of the spikes invoked by the test-stimulus gradually declined and settled after some 20 pairings. The upper band (the final 8 min, above the small arrowhead on the vertical axis) shows the responses after pairing: Each trace contained a spike and their occurrences remained as regular and early as in the late stage of the pairing. The postsynaptic depolarizing current was 0.6 nA in this experiment.

140

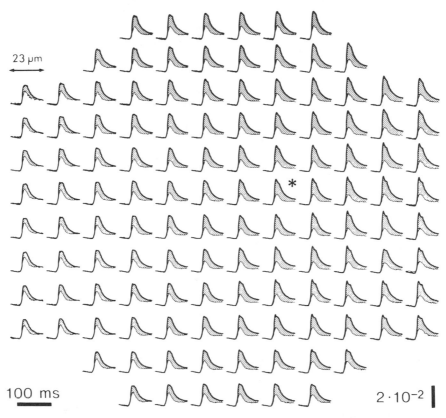

Figure 3. Optically recorded responses of CA1 neurons before and after synaptic enhancement by concurrent pre- and postsynaptic stimulation. We used the voltage-sensitive dye RH 237. Every element of the 12×12 photodiode array recorded from an area of 23×23 μm^2. The vertical scale bar denotes the relative fluorescence change $\Delta F/F$, which is a measure for membrane potential changes of the neurons. The thin traces are averages of two responses (ISI 90 sec) of the neurons before pairing. Synaptic enhancement was induced as described in the text, by pairing stimulation to the afferent fibers with local depolarization of only one neuron. This neuron was located under the photodiode marked with an asterisk. After this procedure, the neurons were tested again. Their responses are displayed in the thick traces, which represent an average of 10 traces (corresponding to 15 min) after the enhancement. The difference between the responses before and after the pairing is hatched. One clearly sees that not only the responses of the one postsynaptically depolarized neuron, but the responses of many of the surrounding neurons are also enhanced.

We performed nine experiments similar to the one of Figure 4 in which we could record from both neurons over a long enough period of time (> 30 min); in six of these, we could induce statistically significant enhancement ($p < 0.01$, taking the spike latency as a measure; for the exact statistics, see Bonhoeffer et al. 1989). In all six cases where we observed potentiation of the response of cell 1, it was accompanied by a significantly increased response in cell 2. In other words, whenever synaptic enhancement could be induced (which was not always the case), we observed enhanced responses in both cells.

These data suggest that in hippocampal slice cultures, synaptic enhancement is not strictly localized on the presynaptic fibers. If a synapse is strengthened by concurrent pre- and postsynaptic stimulation, neighboring synapses, despite not having received the postsynaptic stimulus, also enhance their efficacy.

To assess the functional significance of the observed spread of synaptic enhancement, it is crucial to know whether one can observe this phenomenon in other brain regions as well. Since much work has been done

on plasticity in the visual cortex, this seemed the appropriate preparation for testing whether the modification of Hebb's mechanism has to be extended to the neocortex or whether it is a peculiarity of the hippocampus.

To investigate whether the spread of enhancement could also be observed in the visual cortex, we prepared acute slices from this brain region and performed an experiment very similar to the one described above for the hippocampus. We recorded from two cortical cells lying very close together (distance < 200 μm) and stimulated two sets of afferent fibers with stimulating electrodes in the white matter. The synapses were again enhanced by pairing one of the presynaptic stimuli (the conditioning stimulus) with depolarization of one postsynaptic neuron (the "paired cell").

Figure 5 illustrates the result of such an experiment: The thin traces show averaged responses of two cells recorded simultaneously before initiating synaptic enhancement by pairing the conditioning stimulus with a depolarizing current pulse into one of the two cells, the paired cell. The thick traces show the averaged responses 15 minutes after the pairing. One can observe a

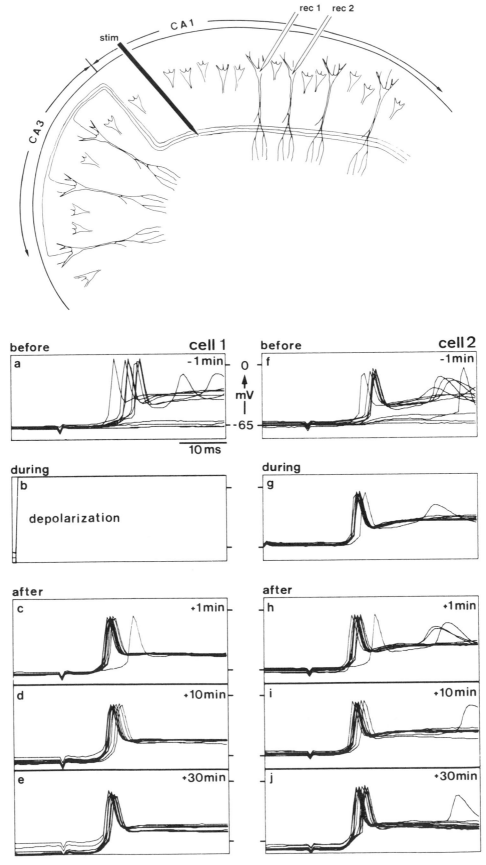

Figure 4. (*See facing page for legend.*)

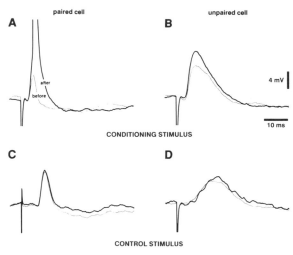

Figure 5. Double intracellular recording of two cortical cells. Although a depolarization of 2 nA in only one of the cells was paired with the conditioning stimulus, both cells showed an increased response to the stimulus following the pairing paradigm and an unchanged response to the control stimulus. (*A*) Averaged EPSPs of cell 1 (paired cell) in response to the conditioning stimulus. The thin trace displays the averaged response of the cell taken at the beginning of the recording (6 trials), the thick trace shows the averaged response 15 min after the pairing (4 trials). A marked increase in the response could be observed. It manifested itself in a bigger and steeper EPSP that reached the firing threshold of the cell. This increase lasted for more than 60 min (data not shown). (*B*) The responses of the simultaneously recorded second (unpaired) cell were also increased 15 min after the pairing, although this cell did not receive any current injection. (*C, D*) The cells' responses to the control stimulus, which was not given during pairing, remained unchanged for the observed period for the paired cell (*C, see footnote at bottom of page*), as well as for the unpaired cell (*D*).

marked potentiation of the synaptic response in the cell that had received the current injection (Fig. 5A). This result is similar to earlier reports showing synaptic strengthening after simultaneous pre- and postsynaptic stimulation in cortical slices (Bindman et al. 1988). However, an enhanced response was also observed in an adjacent cell that had not received current injections (Fig. 5B, unpaired cell). The increased response of the

---

In the original data of Fig. 5C were a few responses in which a spike occurred before pairing. For the averaging, we discarded these trials. We assert that this is legitimate, since action potentials only occurred before pairing. Thus, if there was a change in synaptic efficacy before as opposed to after the pairing at all, synaptic strength would have decreased in this control.

unpaired cell was only obtained after the paired cell was potentiated; repeated application to the conditioning stimulus or current injections alone did not lead to an enhanced response of either cell. Moreover, the response to a control stimulus that was presented before and after but not during the postsynaptic current injections remained unchanged (Fig. 5C,D). The latter result indicates that synaptic enhancement was selective to the paired input fibers and therefore spatially restricted on the postsynaptic site, the cells' dendrites. In contrast, the effect was *not* well confined at the presynaptic site: The response to the conditioning stimulus increased in both the paired and unpaired cell. We were able to initiate synaptic enhancement in 4 out of 15 double cell recordings. This relatively low success rate had to be expected from earlier reports of synaptic enhancement in the neocortex using a similar experimental procedure (Bindman et al. 1988). In every case in which we could obtain an enhanced response of the paired cell, the unpaired cell showed a comparable increase in its synaptic response (Kossel et al. 1990). Thus, in all cases of successful pairing, the strengthening of the paired cell went along with an increased response in the unpaired cell. The enhancement persisted in the paired and unpaired cells for up to 100 minutes after the end of the pairing procedure.

DISCUSSION

Our results show that enhancement is not restricted to the synapses that actually receive paired pre- and postsynaptic stimulation, but rather it extends to neighboring synapses as well. It had been shown previously that in the hippocampus and in the neocortex, synaptic enhancement is input-specific (Gustafsson et al. 1987; Bindman et al. 1988), i.e., if some synapses on a dendrite are enhanced, neighboring synapses on the same dendrite are not. This finding, however, is not at variance with our observations, which show that the mechanism performing the enhancement seems unable to restrict such strengthening to a single site on the presynaptic axons (cf. Fig. 1).

There are several mechanisms that could account for such a spread. Although the induction of long-term potentiation (LTP) is mediated by the postsynaptic entry of Ca^{++} ions through channels gated by the N-methyl-D-aspartate (NMDA) receptor (Collingridge et al. 1983; Nowak et al. 1984), several studies suggest that its maintenance requires a retrograde messenger that leads to presynaptic changes (Dolphin et al. 1982; Davies et al. 1989; Williams et al. 1989). If this process

---

Figure 4. Double intracellular recording during synaptic enhancement. The upper part of the figure shows the experimental situation: A stimulation electrode was placed in the Schaffer-collaterals. Two intracellular electrodes recorded the membrane potentials of two pyramidal cells lying close together (30 μm) in the CA1 region of a hippocampal slice culture; 1 min after the responses to the test stimulus were recorded (*a, f*), the synapses were enhanced by simultaneous depolarization of cell 1 and extracellular stimulation (*b*). The current injection (5 nA) into cell 1 had no effect on cell 2 (*g*); neither electric nor synaptic coupling between the two cells could be seen. Nevertheless, 1 min (*c, h*), 10 min (*d, i*), and 30 min (*e, j*) later, one could observe a long-lasting enhancement of the synapses of both cells: The initial slope of their EPSPs was considerably steeper. This in turn caused their action potentials to occur much more reliably and much earlier with respect to the stimulus.

of strengthening were mediated by a second messenger system within the presynaptic fiber, this second messenger might well travel over substantial distances within the fiber and thus cause enhancement to occur at more than one terminal. Alternatively, retrograde messengers might diffuse from the postsynaptic cell and directly influence nearby cells. If these fibers were to react to such a diffusible substance only if they had been active shortly before, one would observe the described effect: Enhancement would spread along the presynaptic fibers but remain input-specific.

Arachidonic acid and its metabolites have been proposed as key candidates for such a retrograde messenger (Bevan and Wood 1987; Piomelli et al. 1987; Williams et al. 1989). Arachidonic acid is released from cells after induction of LTP, and this release is triggered by activation of the NMDA receptors (Dumuis et al. 1988; Lazarewicz et al. 1988). In the hippocampus, stimulation of the perforant path in the presence of arachidonic acid leads to an increase in synaptic transmission (Williams et al. 1989). Such an activity-dependent potentiation by a retrograde messenger could explain our finding that the response to the conditioning stimulus was potentiated, whereas the response to the unpaired control stimulus was not affected.

An interesting observation, which might be related to our results, was made in recent experiments of Sastry et al. (1988). These investigators show that depolarization of a glial cell concurrent with afferent stimulation of the Schaffer-collaterals (but not depolarization alone) leads to potentiation of the field EPSP of neighboring neurons. This observation is similar to the results presented here. Yet, Sastry et al. depolarized a glial cell, whereas we injected current into a postsynaptic neuron. In view of their finding, one might argue that our postsynaptic depolarization was so strong that it spread to neighboring glial cells, in turn causing an enhancement similar to the result described above (Sastry et al. 1988). One should keep in mind, though, that recordings from *neurons* close to the depolarized neuron (as close as 20 μm) never showed such crosstalk.

Apart from electrical, artifactual crosstalk, there might, however, be a "physiological crosstalk." Very strong activity of a neuron (in our case caused by current injection) will lead to a substantially increased potassium level in the immediate vicinity of the active cell. This elevated potassium level will cause adjacent glial cells to depolarize (much more than an adjacent neuron [Baylor and Nicholls 1969]), which could create a situation similar to the one induced by Sastry et al. artificially. Lacking simultaneous recordings from neighboring glial cells, we were, however, unable to determine whether this depolarization is substantial enough to explain our result by an effect similar to the one described above.

Another possible explanation of our results is that the two neurons in which we observed enhancement were synaptically connected. We therefore ensured before and after every experiment that firing one neuron

by current injection did not induce an EPSP in the other cell. The few cases in which we found the two cells interconnected were not included in the present data.

We performed all of these tests at resting potential, assuming that synaptic connections would manifest themselves at the resting state of the membrane. If there were, however, synapses in the hippocampus or in the neocortex that purely relied on NMDA receptors for synaptic transmission, this assumption would not hold true. These synaptic connections would become apparent and thus effective only in a depolarized neuron. It is not clear whether pure NMDA synapses exist. Although for the neocortex such synapses have been described previously (Thomson 1986), subsequent reports failed to find these synapses (Jones and Baughman 1988; Sutor and Hablitz 1989). Thus, if pure NMDA synapses exist, they are apparently not a very widespread phenomenon. We therefore consider it unlikely that they provide an explanation for all the experiments we report here.

Whatever the mechanism for the spread of enhancement, it is of functional relevance that strong firing of one or a few neurons paired with presynaptic stimulation can induce synaptic strengthening in a substantial number of neighboring neurons. This observation indicates that in the neocortex and in the hippocampus of young animals, the Hebbian rule in its usual interpretation is not strictly valid. Although coincident activity at some synapse is required to alter synaptic strength, other synapses on the presynaptically activated fibers for which this simultaneity did not apply also show enhanced efficacy. At first sight, such a modified Hebbian mechanism might seem to have great disadvantages. When synaptic changes are not strictly localized, a great deal of the specificity inherent in Hebb's rule is lost. On the other hand, one can also conceive of advantageous consequences of such "synaptic recruitment." It might enable the nervous system to form reliable connections without requiring too many coincident firings; thereby, it might profitably serve as an amplification mechanism, causing coincidences between a few neurons to be sufficient to enhance connections reliably within a larger group of neurons.

Another consequence of the presynaptic spread of enhancement might be envisaged in a developmental context: the formation of functionally interconnected groups of nerve cells (e.g., the ocular dominance columns) in the developing central nervous system. The described spread of synaptic strengthening would tend to induce a correlation between the anatomical proximity of neurons and the similarity of their functional properties. In other words, it would cause functionally related neurons to be clustered in space, as indeed they are (e.g., in the visual [Hubel and Wiesel 1968] and somatosensory [Kaas et al. 1979] cortex).

Most theories dealing with map formation in the developing neocortex have to postulate an interaction between the cortical neurons, which has a bell-shaped profile. Such interaction, together with the classical

Hebbian rule, yields reliable formation of ocular dominance (Miller et al. 1989) and orientation (Durbin and Mitchison 1990) columns. Similar local cooperativity rules have also been applied in the context of map formation in artificial neuronal networks (Kohonen 1982; Saarinen and Kohonen 1985). Our experimental data prompted us and other investigators (Gally et al. 1990) to hypothesize (a detailed theoretical study is currently in progress in our laboratory [H. Preissl et al., in prep.]) that the observed spread of enhancement, in particular in the neocortex, could play the role of the theoretically postulated bell-shaped interaction. It might introduce the desired positive correlation between neighboring neurons and thereby make any assumptions about intracortical neuronal interactions superfluous.

We thus propose that the mechanism described here could be responsible for the formation of cortical maps. It might give rise to what seems to be a general principle of organization in the cortex: Stimulus parameters are represented in an orderly fashion across the cortical surface, and neurons with similar properties are clustered in space.

ACKNOWLEDGMENTS

We thank Volker Staiger for his excellent assistance in many of the experiments and Ed Callaway and Richard Morris for valuable comments on the manuscript. Shirley Würth helped improve the English.

REFERENCES

Baylor, D.A. and J.G. Nicholls. 1969. Changes in extracellular potassium concentration produced by neuronal activity in the central nervous system of the leech. *J. Physiol.* **203:** 555.

Bevan, S. and J.N. Wood. 1987. Arachidonic-acid metabolites as second messengers. *Nature* **328:** 20.

Bindman, L.J., K.P.S.J. Murphy, and S. Pockett. 1988. Postsynaptic control of the induction of long-term changes in efficacy of transmission at neocortical synapses in slices of rat brain. *J. Neurophysiol.* **60:** 1053.

Bonhoeffer, T. and V. Staiger. 1988. Optical recording with single cell resolution from monolayered slice cultures of rat hippocampus. *Neurosci. Lett.* **92:** 259.

Bonhoeffer, T., V. Staiger, and A. Aertsen. 1989. Synaptic plasticity in rat hippocampal slice cultures: Local "Hebbian"conjunction of pre- and postsynaptic stimulation leads to distributed synaptic enhancement. *Proc. Natl. Acad. Sci.* **86:** 8113.

Collingridge, G.L., S.J. Kehl, and H. McLennan. 1983. Excitatory amino acids in synaptic transmission in the Schaffer collateral-comissural pathway of the rat hippocampus. *J. Physiol.* **334:** 33.

Davies, S.N., R.A.J. Lester, K.G. Reymann, and G.L. Collingridge. 1989. Temporally distinct pre- and postsynaptic mechanisms maintain long-term potentiation. *Nature* **338:** 500.

Dolphin, A.C., M.L. Errington, and T.V.P. Bliss. 1982. Long-term potentiation of the perforant path in vivo is associated with increased glutamate release. *Nature* **297:** 496.

Dumuis, A., M. Sebben, L. Haynes, J.P. Pin, and J. Bock-aert. 1988. NMDA receptors activate the arachidonic acid cascade system in striatal neurons. *Nature* **336:** 68.

Durbin, R. and G. Mitchison. 1990. A dimension reduction framework for understanding cortical maps. *Nature* **343:** 644.

Gähwiler, B.H. 1981. Organotypic monolayer cultures of nervous tissue. *J. Neurosci. Methods* **4:** 329.

———. 1984. Development of the hippocampus in vitro: Cell types, synapses and receptors. *Neuroscience* **11:** 751.

Gähwiler, B.H. and D.A. Brown. 1985. Functional innervation of cultured hippocampal neurones by cholinergic afferents from co-cultured septal explants. *Nature* **313:** 577.

Gally, J.A., P.R. Montague, G.N. Reeke, and G.M. Edelman. 1990. The NO hypothesis: Possible effects of a short-lived, rapidly diffusible signal in the development and function of the nervous system. *Proc. Natl. Acad. Sci.* **87:** 3547.

Grinvald, A., R. Hildesheim, I.C. Farber, and L. Anglister. 1982. Improved fluorescence probes for the measurement of rapid changes in membrane potential. *Biophys. J.* **39:** 301.

Grinvald, A., L. Anglister, J.A. Freeman, R. Hildesheim, and A. Manker. 1984. Real-time optical imaging of naturally evoked electrical activity in intact frog brain. *Nature* **308:** 848.

Gustafsson, B., H. Wigström, W.C. Abraham, and Y.-Y. Huang. 1987. Long term potentiation in the hippocampus using depolarizing current pulses as the conditioning stimulus to single volley synaptic potentials. *J. Neurosci.* **7:** 774.

Hebb, D.O. 1949. *The organization of behavior. A neuropsychological theory.* Wiley, New York.

Hubel, D.H. and T.N. Wiesel. 1968. Receptive fields and functional architecture of monkey striate cortex. *J. Physiol.* **195:** 215.

Jones, K.A. and R.W. Baughman. 1988. NMDA- and non-NMDA-receptor components of excitatory synaptic potentials recorded from cells in layer V of rat visual cortex. *J. Neurosci.* **8:** 3522.

Kaas, J.H., R.J. Nelson, M. Sur, C.-S. Lin, and M.M. Merzenich. 1979. Multiple representation of the body within the primary somatosensory cortex of primates. *Science* **204:** 521.

Katz, L.C. 1987. Local circuitry of identified projection neurons in cat visual cortex brain slices. *J. Neurosci.* **7:** 1223.

Kohonen, T. 1982. Self-organized formation of topologically correct feature maps. *Biol. Cybern.* **43:** 59.

Kossel, A., T. Bonhoeffer, and J. Bolz. 1990. Non-Hebbian synapses in rat visual cortex. *NeuroReport* **1:** 115.

Lazarewicz, J.W., J.T. Wroblewski, M.E. Palmer, and E. Costa. 1988. Activation of N-methyl-D-aspartate-sensitive glutamate receptors stimulates arachidonic acid release in primary cultures of cerebellar granule cells. *Neuropharmacology* **27:** 765.

Miller, K.D., J.B. Keller, and M.P. Stryker. 1989. Ocular dominance column development: Analysis and simulation. *Science* **245:** 605.

Nowak, L., P. Bregestovski, P. Ascher, A. Herbet, and A. Prochiantz. 1984. Magnesium gates glutamate-activated channels in mouse central neurones. *Nature* **307:** 462.

Piomelli, D., A. Volterra, N. Dale, S.A. Siegelbaum, E.R. Kandel, J.H. Schwartz, and F. Belardetti. 1987. Lipoxigenase metabolites of arachidonic acid as second messengers for presynaptic inhibition of *Aplysia* sensory cells. *Nature* **328:** 38.

Ramón y Cajal, S. 1909 and 1911. *Histologie du systéme nerveux de l'homme et des vertébrés*, volumes 1 and 2. Maloine, Paris.

Saarinen, J. and T. Kohonen. 1985. Self-organized formation of colour maps in a model cortex. *Perception* **14:** 711.

Sastry, B.R., J.W. Goh, P.B.Y. May, and S.S. Chirwa. 1988. The involvement of nonspiking cells in long-term potentiation of synaptic transmission in the hippocampus. *Can. J. Physiol. Pharmacol.* **66:** 841.

Sutor, B. and J.J. Hablitz. 1989. EPSPs in rat neocortical neurons in vitro. II. Involvement of *N*-methyl-D-aspartate receptors in the generation of EPSPs. *J. Neurophysiol.* **61:** 621.

Thomson, A.M. 1986. A magnesium-sensitive post-synaptic potential in rat cerebral cortex resembles neuronal responses to *N*-methylaspartate. *J. Physiol.* **370:** 531.

Wigström, H., B. Gustafsson, Y.-Y. Huang, and W.C. Abraham. 1986. Hippocampal long-term potentiation is induced by pairing single afferent volleys with intracellularly injected depolarizing current pulses. *Acta Physiol. Scand.* **126:** 317.

Williams, J.H., M.L. Errington, M.A. Lynch, and T.V. Bliss. 1989. Arachidonic acid induces a long-term activity-dependent enhancement of synaptic transmission in the hippocampus. *Nature* **341:** 739.

Long-term Potentiation: Presynaptic Enhancement following Postsynaptic Activation of Ca^{++}-dependent Protein Kinases

R.W. Tsien and R. Malinow*

Department of Molecular and Cellular Physiology, Beckman Center, Stanford University Medical Center, Stanford, California 94305

It is widely believed that long-lasting changes in synaptic function provide the cellular basis for learning and memory in both vertebrates and invertebrates (Hebb 1949; Eccles 1953; Goelet et al. 1985; Alkon and Nelson 1990). The most thoroughly characterized example of such synaptic plasticity in the mammalian nervous system is long-term potentiation (LTP). The remarkable feature of LTP is that a short burst of synaptic activity can trigger persistent enhancement of synaptic transmission lasting at least several hours and possibly weeks or longer (Bliss and Gardner-Medwin 1973). First found in the hippocampus (Lomo 1966; Bliss and Lomo 1973), this phenomenon has recently been described in areas of the mammalian central nervous system including visual cortex (Artola and Singer 1987) and motor cortex (Iriki et al. 1989). There is intense interest in understanding the cellular and molecular basis for this form of synaptic plasticity (Lynch and Baudry 1984; Collingridge and Bliss 1987; Bliss and Lynch 1988; Brown et al. 1988; Nicoll et al. 1988; Cotman et al. 1989; Kennedy 1989; Malenka et al. 1989a; Stevens 1989).

Most studies on mechanisms of LTP have focused on synaptic transmission in the CA1 field of the hippocampus, at synapses between Schaffer collaterals and CA1 pyramidal cells, an area rich in N-methyl-D-aspartate (NMDA) receptors (Cotman et al. 1989) and Ca^{++}-dependent protein kinases (Nishizuka 1988; Kennedy 1989). Induction of LTP requires a temporal conjunction of presynaptic transmitter release and postsynaptic depolarization (Malinow and Miller 1986; Collingridge and Bliss 1987; Gustafsson et al. 1987; Brown et al. 1988), a combination of events resembling that envisioned by Hebb (1949). It is generally agreed that these factors work together: glutamate to activate the NMDA receptor channel and postsynaptic depolarization to free the channel from block by extracellular Mg^{++} (Ascher and Nowak 1988; Mayer and Westbrook 1987). The NMDA receptor allows a significant Ca^{++} influx (MacDermott et al. 1986) and increases [Ca^{++}]$_i$ in postsynaptic spines (Regehr and Tank 1990); the rise in [Ca^{++}]$_i$ is necessary for LTP (Lynch et al. 1983; Malenka et al. 1988).

Many questions remain about what happens next. What is the mechanism of the long-lasting synaptic modification and its relationship to Ca^{++} signaling? Our work has been directed toward understanding the role of Ca^{++}-dependent protein kinases and elucidating the nature of the persistent change. A key question is whether synaptic transmission is strengthened by increased transmitter release or enhanced postsynaptic receptivity. There is considerable controversy about this issue. Evidence in favor of a strictly postsynaptic mechanism for the expression of LTP has come from the groups of Gary Lynch (Muller et al. 1988) and Roger Nicoll (Kauer et al. 1988). Their results indicated that the expression of LTP was associated with a selective enhancement of the response of α-amino-3-hydroxy-5-methyl-4-isoxazole proprionate (AMPA) receptors but not NMDA receptors. Thus, they concluded that the locus of expression must be postsynaptic. This conclusion is appealingly simple: If induction and expression of LTP are both localized within the postsynaptic spine, they could be linked by purely intracellular signaling mechanisms.

On the other hand, early evidence from Timothy Bliss and colleagues and other investigators has provided support for enhancement of presynaptic release. Using a push-pull cannula system in vivo, Dolphin et al. (1982) found evidence for increased release of [^{3}H]glutamate in the dentate gyrus in association with LTP and proposed that presynaptic release was elevated (see also Skrede and Malthe-Sorenssen 1981). However, Bliss et al. (1986) were careful to point out that some questions remain unanswered. Which type of cell is the source of the increase? Could the increased concentration of glutamate in the perfusate be due to decreased uptake? If presynaptic glutamate release is truly increased, is this evoked by action potentials or merely an increase in nonquantal leakage? What is the nature of the retrograde communication across the synaptic cleft that must be postulated to link postsynaptic induction and presynaptic expression? Having discussed these questions, Bliss and Lynch (1988) concluded that the available evidence provided " . . . plausible though not conclusive reasons for attributing the enhanced release to an increase in the amount of transmitter released per action potential from potentiated terminals; it is probable that only a rigorous

---

*Present address: Department of Physiology and Biophysics, University of Iowa, Iowa City, Iowa 52242.

quantal analysis, not presently available, will finally settle the issue."

This paper describes progress toward such analysis. A major obstacle to statistical analysis of synaptic variability has been the poor signal-to-noise ratio of conventional intracellular recordings (for review, see Redman 1990). We have overcome this problem by applying the whole-cell voltage clamp technique to study synaptic transmission in conventional hippocampal slices (Malinow and Tsien 1990a). We find that robust LTP can be recorded with much improved signal resolution and biochemical access to the postsynaptic cell. Prolonged dialysis of the postsynaptic cell blocks the triggering of LTP with no effect on expression of LTP. The improved signal resolution unmasks a large trial-to-trial variability reflecting the probabilistic nature of transmitter release. Changes in the synaptic variability, and a decrease in the proportion of synaptic failures during LTP provide two lines of evidence to demonstrate that transmitter release is significantly enhanced (Malinow and Tsien 1990a). These biophysical approaches are complemented by studies in which we explored mechanisms of LTP induction and expression and their localization by direct intracellular injection of protein kinase inhibitors into individual postsynaptic cells (Malinow et al. 1989).

EXPERIMENTAL STRATEGY AND METHODS

Transverse hippocampal slices (400–500 μm) were obtained from 3–5 week-old rats by standard methods (Alger and Nicoll 1982). Slices were submerged and superfused continuously with a modified Earle's solution containing NaCl (119 mM), KCl (2.5 mM), MgCl$_2$ (1.3 mM), CaCl$_2$ (2.5 mM), NaH$_2$PO$_4$ (1.0 mM), NaHCO$_3$ (26.2 mM), and glucose (11 mM), and they were gassed with 95% O$_2$/5% CO$_2$ (pH 7.4) at room temperature (22°C). Picrotoxin (20 μM) was used to block inhibitory transmission, and a cut was made between regions CA3 and CA1 to prevent epileptiform activity. Synaptic transmission was elicited with bipolar stainless steel stimulating electrodes at two locations; each electrode delivered a stimulus every 4 seconds; stimuli from the two electrodes were separated by 2 seconds. Excitatory postsynaptic currents (EPSCs) were recorded with a patch electrode (3–7 MΩ tip resistance, no fire polishing or Sylgard coating) in the whole-cell mode (Axopatch 1D). Pipette solution contained Cs-gluconate (100 mM), EGTA (0.6 mM), MgCl$_2$ (5 mM), ATP (2 mM), GTP (0.3 mM), and HEPES (40 mM, pH 7.2 with CsOH). Holding potential was kept constant at a level between −60 and −70 mV. EPSCs were amplified 50–500-fold, filtered at 1 kHz, digitized at 10 kHz, and stored. For a given experiment, EPSC amplitudes were determined by averaging the current over a 10–20 msec window at the peak response and subtracting a baseline estimate from the same record. A similar procedure was used to measure the background noise before the synaptic stimulation (Sayer et al. 1989).

RESULTS

Whole-cell Recordings from Hippocampal Slices

We were able to make whole-cell voltage clamp recordings from CA1 neurons in rat hippocampal slices without special procedures for exposing or cleaning the neurons (see also Barnes and Werblin 1987; Coleman and Miller 1989; Blanton et al. 1989). Positive pressure was applied to the recording pipette during penetration of the slice; high-resistance (1–5 GΩ) seals on cell bodies 2–3 cell diameters below the surface were then obtained by suction. After breaking into the cell, synaptic currents were elicited with bipolar stimulation electrodes placed in the stratum radiatum of CA1. Stable synaptic recordings could be maintained for as long as 10 hours. The input resistance was typically 100–200 MΩ in whole-cell recordings.

Whole-cell current recording offers better resolution than even the most favorable microelectrode recordings (Sayer et al. 1989; Redman 1990; Foster and McNaughton 1991). The low background noise of whole-cell recordings facilitated the study of small synaptic responses. In most experiments, we used minimal stimulation, only slightly stronger than the highest stimulus that gave only failures. Under these conditions, activation is thought to be restricted to a single synapse onto the monitored neuron (McNaughton et al. 1981; Foster and McNaughton 1991). (This was supported by experiments in which a single CA3 neuron was directly stimulated by an intracellular microelectrode while simultaneously recording from a CA1 neuron [Malinow and Tsien 1990b].) The resulting synaptic currents showed a large intertrial variability that was much greater than the background noise but with similar time courses (Fig. 1a,b), supporting the view that they originated from the same synapse. There were occasional clear failures (Figs. 1a and 4a,b) and sporadic spontaneous events that resembled the elicited response, ranging in amplitude from less than 1 pA up to about 10 pA (Fig. 1b, inset).

The average synaptic current for minimal stimulation was 6.7 pA in a representative series of 17 experiments. This is in reasonable agreement with estimates of synaptic current from minimal excitatory postsynaptic potentials (EPSPs) recorded with high-resistance microelectrodes if one allows for the measured input resistance in those experiments (Sayer et al. 1990; Foster and McNaughton 1991).

Whole-cell Recordings of LTP

To optimize the chances of obtaining LTP under whole-cell recording conditions, we used internal solutions with minimal Ca^{++} buffering to avoid block of LTP and with Cs$+$ as the main cation to enhance voltage control of the postsynaptic membrane. We also included ATP and GTP in the internal solution to allow activity of protein kinases or GTP-binding proteins. After a stable baseline period of 10–15 minutes, we were able to induce LTP by pairing a steady postsynap-

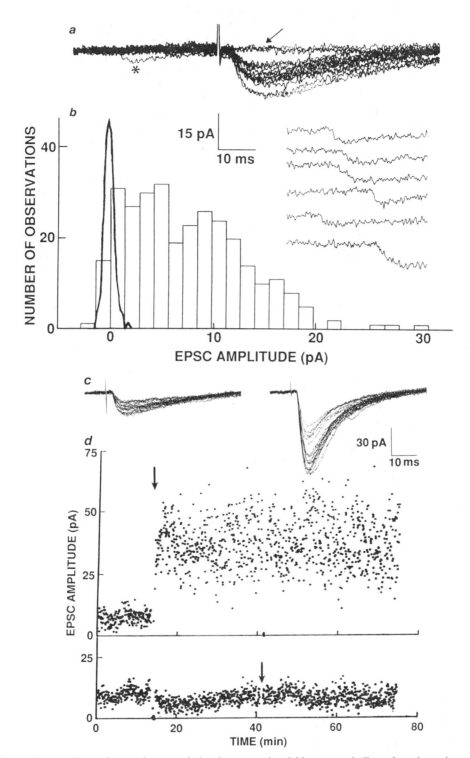

Figure 1. Whole-cell recordings of synaptic transmission in conventional hippocampal slices show large intertrial variability, synapse-specific LTP, and loss of induction but not expression with prolonged dialysis. (*a*) Shown are 16 consecutive records of synaptic currents superimposed. Note spontaneous event in baseline period (asterisk) and synaptic failures (arrows). (*b*) Amplitude distribution histograms for 200 consecutive synaptic currents (bars) and baseline noise (smooth curve). Bin sizes were 1.4 pA for EPSC and 0.14 pA for baseline noise. (*Inset*) Representative spontaneous synaptic currents. Note the variability in amplitude and time course but general similarity to evoked responses. (*c,d*) Plots of synaptic responses against time in a postsynaptic cell receiving two independent inputs. (*c*) LTP was selectively induced in one pathway by a pairing procedure 15 min following break-in (arrows); in the other pathway (*d*), the pairing procedure was applied 25 min later but failed to induce LTP, in contrast to the maintenance of LTP in *c*. In the pairing procedure, the cell was depolarized from −70 mV to ∼0 mV, whereas the paired (conditioned) pathway was stimulated 40 times at 2 Hz with no change in stimulus strength. Nonconditioned pathway received no stimuli during the postsynaptic depolarization. (*Inset*) Families of consecutive current records showing EPSCs of conditioned pathway collected before (*left*) and 30 min after (*right*) pairing. (Reprinted, with permission, from Malinow and Tsien 1990a.)

149

tic depolarization to about 0 mV with continued activation of the test pathway (40 stimuli at 2 Hz). This pairing procedure resulted in LTP in 14 of 18 experiments (Figs. 1c, 3, top, and 4c). In contrast, no potentiation was found in transmission through a simultaneously monitored control pathway that did not receive presynaptic stimuli during the postsynaptic depolarization (Figs. 1d and 3, bottom). Furthermore, synaptic stimulation at 2 Hz without postsynaptic depolarization did not give synaptic enhancement ($n = 5$). Thus, the potentiation was synapse-specific and required a combination of presynaptic activity and postsynaptic depolarization, just as seen in conventional recordings of LTP.

To investigate whether diffusible cytoplasmic factors are involved in potentiation, we attempted to trigger LTP at different times after gaining whole-cell access

(Fig. 1c,d). Pairing soon after beginning whole cell recording (~20 minutes or less) consistently resulted in LTP lasting more than 1 hour (Figs. 1, 3, and 4). However, no potentiation was found with pairing more than 30 minutes after whole-cell access (6 of 7 experiments). One possibility is that some diffusible postsynaptic component is needed to trigger LTP but not to maintain the potentiation.

Analysis of Presynaptic and Postsynaptic Factors

To understand the basis of the synaptic variability and its possible relation to fluctuations in transmitter release, we modified presynaptic or postsynaptic functions by changing the bathing medium (Fig. 2). Elevating $[Ca^{++}]_o$ to increase presynaptic release enhanced

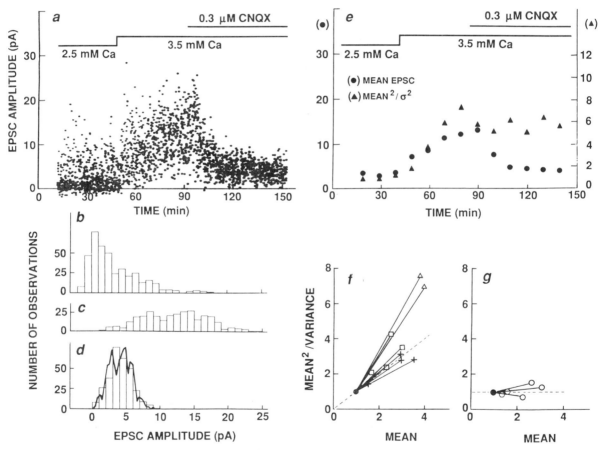

Figure 2. Selective changes in presynaptic and postsynaptic function produce expected changes in mean and variance of synaptic currents. Agents acting through presynaptic mechanisms affect shape of distribution histograms and M^2/σ^2, whereas inhibition of postsynaptic receptors does not. (a) EPSC amplitude plotted against time. Bathing calcium was elevated from 2.5 mM to 3.5 mM, and 0.3 μM CNQX was applied where shown. (b,c,d) Amplitude distribution histograms for 300 EPSCs before manipulation (b), after elevation of calcium (c), and after subsequent addition of CNQX (d). Continuous line in d shows data from c, normalized to mean EPSC amplitude in d. Note close agreement of normalized histograms. (e) Plot of mean EPSC amplitude, M (●) and M^2/σ^2 (▲) for the experiment shown in a with τ = 10 min (150 trials). (f) Plot of M^2/σ^2 against M for several presynaptic manipulations: Ca increased from 2.5 to 3.5 mM (△); Mg decreased from 1.3 to 0.65 mM in the presence of 50 μM APV (□); increased stimulus strength to recruit more fibers (+). (g) Plot of M^2/σ^2 against M for experiments in which CNQX (0.2–0.3 μM) was bath applied. For each experiment in f and g, lines connect points obtained before and after manipulation; M and M^2/σ^2 were computed for 300 trials prior to the manipulation and 300 trials at the peak of the effect, and normalized by the values corresponding to the smaller M for that experiment. Note that presynaptic manipulations that are thought to increase p affect M^2/σ^2 more than the mean, whereas increasing stimulus strength, which increases N, affects M^2/σ^2 as much as M. These findings are expected for a binomial release process (see text). (Reprinted, with permission, from Malinow and Tsien 1990a.)

the synaptic currents (Fig. 2a). The amplitude histogram changed from a highly skewed distribution (Fig. 2b) to a nearly symmetrical bell shape (Fig. 2c). In contrast, when we added low concentrations of the glutamate receptor antagonist 6-cyano-7-nitroquinoxaline-2,3-dione (CNQX) to modify postsynaptic responsiveness, the average synaptic current was dramatically reduced, but the shape of the distribution remained unchanged (Fig. 2a,e). Thus, the distributions before and after CNQX matched closely when normalized by their means (Fig. 2d). Similar results were obtained with CNQX at lower $[Ca^{++}]_o$ (not shown).

To obtain a simple and revealing index of synaptic variability, we computed $CV^{-2} = M^2\sigma^2$ where CV is the coefficient of variation, M is the mean synaptic current, and σ^2 is the variance about M for a given epoch of consecutive responses from t to $t + \tau$. This kind of analysis has been applied to synaptic transmission in other systems (see, e.g., del Castillo and Katz 1954; Martin 1977). We can compute the expected behavior of $M^2\sigma^2$ if we make assumptions regarding the mechanisms underlying synaptic transmission. In the simplified case of a binomial distribution of transmitter release, where p is the probability of release for each of N available quanta, v is the vesicular content, and z is the postsynaptic response to a fixed amount of transmitter,

$$M^2/\sigma^2 = (Npvz)^2/Np(1 - p)(vz)^2 = Np/(1 - p)$$

Thus, M^2/σ^2 is independent of changes in z and is a useful measure of some changes in presynaptic function but not all factors (e.g., v). It increases in proportion to N and at least linearly with p, as experimentally confirmed at the neuromuscular junction (del Castillo and Katz 1954). The lack of dependence of M^2/σ^2 on the postsynaptic responsiveness (z) holds for more general cases as long as z does not vary from trial to trial within a given epoch (see Malinow and Tsien 1990a).

Assuming z is constant for an epoch, the theory predicts that changes in M^2/σ^2 between epochs will result from changes in release characteristics but not postsynaptic modifications. This was tested by examining changes in M^2/σ^2 following interventions known to affect presynaptic or postsynaptic mechanisms. Figure 2e shows that raising extracellular calcium dramatically increased M^2/σ^2. This was found for all experimental maneuvers expected to affect presynaptic release: lowering magnesium, application of 4-aminopyridine (not shown), or increasing the stimulus strength to recruit more afferent fibers (see Fig. 2f, $n = 10$). In general, M^2/σ^2 increased at least as much as the mean synaptic current. In contrast, addition of CNQX produced no significant change in M^2/σ^2, despite its large effect on synaptic transmission (see Fig. 2e,g; $n = 5$).

Changes during LTP

Does M^2/σ^2 change with LTP? Figure 3 (bottom) compares M^2/σ^2 of the test pathway with that of the

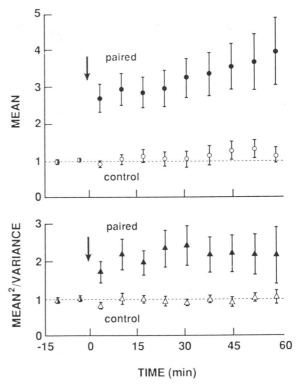

Figure 3. A synapse-specific increase in M^2/σ^2 associated with LTP. Results from the 14 of 18 experiments that showed LTP with pairing (in the other 4 experiments with no LTP, M^2/σ^2 remained unchanged, not shown). (*Top*) Ensemble averages and S.E.M. values of M for the paired pathway (●) and the control pathway (○, $n = 10$; in 4 experiments this pathway was not monitored). (↓) Time of pairing procedure (as in Fig. 1b). (*Bottom*) Ensemble averages of M^2/σ^2 for paired (▲) and nonpaired (△) pathways for the same experiments as in *a*. (Reprinted, with permission, from Malinow and Tsien 1990a.)

control (unpaired) pathway for the 14 experiments showing potentiation of mean synaptic current (Fig. 3, top). After pairing, M^2/σ^2 increased significantly in the test pathway with no change in the control pathway. The increase in M^2/σ^2 with LTP could arise from various presynaptic mechanisms: an increase in the number of available vesicles, an increase in the probability of release of some or all vesicles, or changes in nonvesicular release. It would not be expected from uniform changes in the number, sensitivity, or conductance of glutamate receptor channels, or in the effectiveness of charge transfer from spines to dendrites.

If the expression of LTP involves an increased probability of release or a greater number of available quanta, one would expect fewer failures of transmission during LTP. Figure 4 illustrates an experiment where failures and responses were clearly resolvable. The amplitude distribution histogram displayed a distinct peak at 0 amplitude, which matched the amplitude distribution of the noise (inset). The area under the 0 amplitude peak was used to estimate the percentage of failures. In this experiment, the proportion of failures was 27% prior to pairing and fell to 11% between 5 and 22 minutes after pairing. This change accompanied a

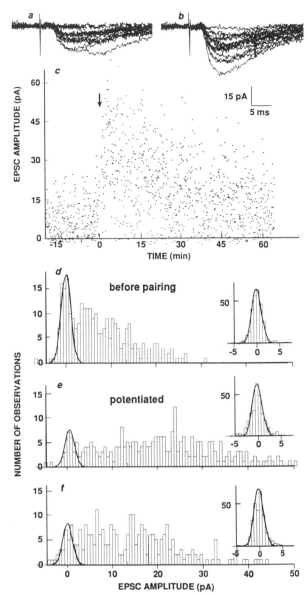

Figure 4. Decreases in the proportion of synaptic failures associated with LTP. (*a,b*) Groups of 16 consecutive EPSCs taken before (*a*) and 40 min after (*b*) a pairing procedure to induce LTP. (*c*) Amplitude of EPSCs elicited by minimal stimulation plotted against time. (↓) Pairing procedure (see Fig. 1). (*d,e*) Amplitude distribution histograms for 17 min epochs prior to pairing (*d*, from $t = -17$ to $t = 0$) and after pairing (*e* from $t = 5$ to $t = 22$ min; *f* from $t = 40$ to $t = 57$ min). Smooth curves are Gaussians whose height was adjusted to fit the first peak in the amplitude distribution. The half-width of the Gaussians, 2.5 pA, was obtained by fitting amplitude histograms of the baseline noise during the same epochs (*insets*). The proportion of failures was estimated as the area under the Gaussian curve. (Reprinted, with permission, from Malinow and Tsien 1990a.)

2.8-fold increase in mean synaptic current. During a later epoch (from $t = 40$ to $t = 57$ min), the synaptic enhancement was 2.1-fold relative to control, and the proportion of failures was 15%.

This decrease in the proportion of failures was a consistent finding. Figure 5 shows collected results from

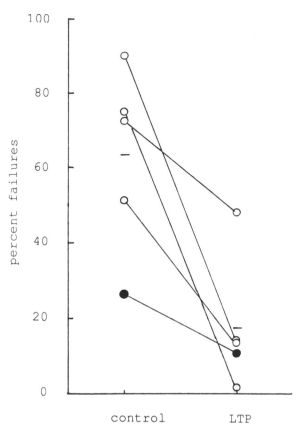

Figure 5. Consistent decrease in proportion of synaptic failures during LTP. Collected results from five experiments. Horizontal lines show mean percentage of failures (63 ± 11% in control before pairing and 17 ± 8% during LTP after pairing). (●) Results from experiment illustrated in Fig. 4. The two experiments with the highest percentage of failures in control were recordings of one-to-one transmission from presynaptic CA3 neurons stimulated with an intracellular microelectrode. (Data from Malinow and Tsien 1990a.)

five experiments where failures could be clearly resolved. Three of the recordings were obtained with minimal stimulation, and two were obtained with intracellular microelectrode stimulation of a CA3 neuron (Malinow and Tsien 1990b). The collected data from all five experiments showed a mean (± s.e.m.) decrease in failures from 63 ± 11% in control to 17 ± 8% after pairing, consistent with a greater likelihood of transmitter release during LTP. This conclusion is supported by the overall amplitude distribution, which changes from a skewed shape in control (Fig. 4d) to a bell-shape during LTP (Fig. 4e), as with increasing extracellular Ca (Fig. 2b,c).

Changes in NMDA Receptor-mediated Transmission Can Be Detected

If presynaptic transmitter release is enhanced, one might expect to find an increase in both the kainate/quisqualate (K/Q)-sensitive and NMDA-sensitive components of the EPSP. The available evidence is not consistent. On one hand, Kauer et al. (1988) and Muller and Lynch (1988) found no significant increase in the NMDA component under conditions that normally produce LTP; thus, they concluded that the expression of LTP must be purely postsynaptic. On the other hand, Bashir and Collingridge (1990) have reported a significant potentiation of NMDA-mediated transmission under very similar conditions.

We have looked for changes in the NMDA-sensitive component under conditions similar to those in our other experiments. To reveal the NMDA receptor component, the external $[Mg^{++}]_o$ was lowered to 0.65 mM, the membrane potential was held near -60 mV, and K/Q receptors were blocked by including 1–10 μM CNQX in the superfusing solutions. Figure 6 shows a representative experiment (Fig. 6A) and collected results from nine recordings, obtained in the presence of 1 μM CNQX (Fig. 6B). The results show a clear and significant increase in the NMDA component during LTP in the test pathway (Fig. 6B) but not in the control

pathways (not shown). The potentiated EPSPs were completely blocked by the NMDA receptor blocker 2-amino-5-phosphonovalerate (APV). Thus, our findings show that an enhancement of the NMDA-receptor component can be detected.

Further investigations will be needed to understand how our results and those of Bashir and Collingridge (1990) may be reconciled with the results of Kauer et al. (1988) and Muller and Lynch (1988). We find that the NMDA response is quite sensitive to membrane potential; even a few millivolts hyperpolarization (which can occur after a tetanus) can reduce the NMDA response by 50%. Thus, in all our experiments, the NMDA-mediated transmission in the control pathway was monitored and found to be unchanged. Similarly, ambient glycine concentration can affect NMDA responses (Johnsen and Ascher 1987; Thompson et al. 1989), and this action can be modulated by CNQX (Lester et al. 1989). To allow for such complications, we looked for LTP of the NMDA component under a variety of conditions: with 1 μM CNQX (Fig. 6), with 10 μM CNQX, and with 10 μM CNQX plus exogenous glycine. In all cases, there was clear and significant potentiation of an APV-sensitive EPSP. If anything, the potentiation was more pronounced with 1 μM CNQX or with 10 μM CNQX plus 300 μM glycine than with 10 μM CNQX alone, but the differences were not dramatic enough to be statistically significant.

In addition to the experimental considerations mentioned above, another possibility is that the NMDA receptor was closer to saturation in the earlier experiments. In our opinion, the possibility of NMDA saturation was not excluded by previous arguments based on the demonstration of synaptic potentiation with paired pulses (Muller and Lynch 1988) or after tetani (Kauer et al. 1988). These forms of potentiation can take place by recruitment of silent boutons and by previously active boutons, so some enhancement would be seen regardless of NMDA receptor saturation at previously active boutons. In contrast, during LTP, enhancement of transmission is thought to be restricted to previously active synapses since local transmitter release must occur to induce LTP. NMDA receptor saturation would thus impose a more stringent limitation during LTP than with paired pulse facilitation or posttetanic potentiation.

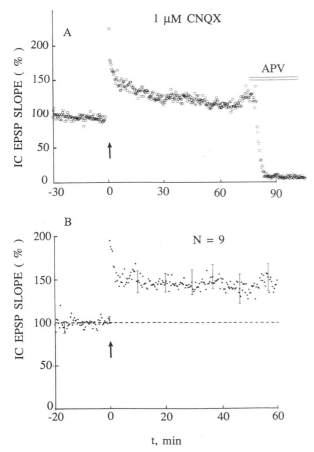

Figure 6. Enhancement of NMDA-receptor response during LTP. (*A*) Representative experiment in the presence of 1 μM CNQX to block K/Q receptors. Relative amplitude of EPSP, recorded with an intracellular microelectrode plotted against time. (↑) Tetanic stimulation. Abolition of EPSPs by 50 μM APV demonstrates that EPSP was mediated by NMDA receptors. For further experimental details, see Malinow et al. 1989. (*B*) Collected results from similar experiments in a total of nine slices. EPSP amplitudes were normalized to control values before tetanic stimulation and then the ensemble was averaged. Bars indicate S.E.M. Note significant and long-lasting potentiation of the NMDA-receptor-mediated response.

Signal Transduction between Postsynaptic Induction and Presynaptic Expression: Role of Ca^{++}-dependent Protein Kinases

A key question at this point is how a rise in postsynaptic $[Ca^{++}]_i$ can lead to a long-lasting enhancement of presynaptic function. A generic working hypothesis, favored by many investigators, is that Ca^{++} acts through a signal transduction pathway that involves a Ca^{++}-dependent protein kinase such as protein kinase C (PKC) or multifunctional Ca/calmodulin-dependent protein kinase (CaMKII) (see Malinow et al. 1988; Cotman et al. 1989; Kennedy 1989; Malenka

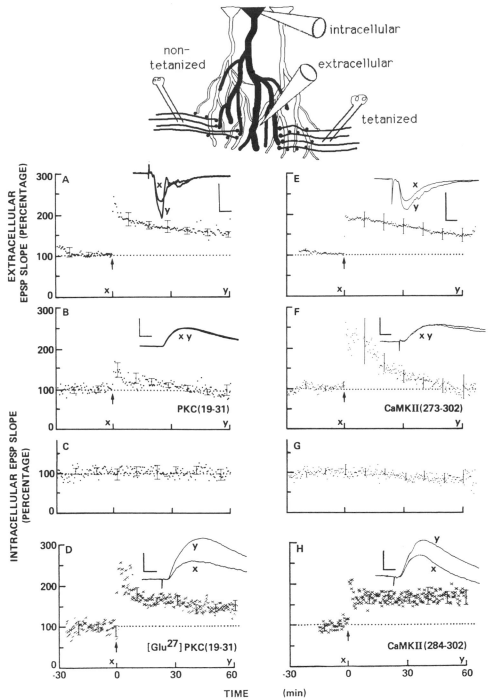

Figure 7. Selective postsynaptic block of PKC or CaMKII prevents LTP. Diagram shows stimulation and recording conditions (see text). (*A*) Extracellular recordings of transmission show persistent potentiation following a tetanus (↑). (*B*) Simultaneous monitoring of synaptic potentials using an intracellular microelectrode whose tip is filled with 3 mM PKC(19–31) (*n* = 8). Following the tetanus, there is no persistent potentiation. (*C*) Transmission in a nontetanized pathway monitored through the same PKC(19–31)-containing electrode is constant throughout the experiment, indicating no nonspecific depressant effect on basal synaptic transmission. (*D*) Transmission monitored in a different set of slices with 3 mM [Glu-27]PKC(19–31) in the intracellular electrode, shows LTP after a conditioning tetanus (*n* = 6 pathways from three slices). (*E–H*) Recordings of transmission in experiments testing the involvement of CaMKII. (*E*) Extracellular monitoring shows LTP after tetanic stimulation. (*F*) Simultaneous monitoring of synaptic potentials with intracellular electrode containing 1.1 mM CaMKII(273–302) shows no persistent potentiation after tetanic conditioning. (*G*) Transmission in a nontetanized pathway monitored with the CaMKII(273–302)-containing electrode is constant throughout the experiment. (*H*) Transmission monitored in a different set of slices, using 1.1 mM CaMKII(284–302) in the intracellular electrode, shows LTP after a tetanus (*n* = 5 pathways from three slices). Error bars indicate S.E.M. values for representative time points. (*Insets*) Average of ten consecutive potentials obtained at the times designated on time axis. Scale bars: (*A* and *E*) 0.33 mV and 12.5 msec; (*B,D,F* and *H*) 5 mV and 12.5 msec. Peptides PKC(19–31) and PKC(19–36) were generously provided by Dr. John J. Nestor, Jr., Dr. Bruce Kemp, and Dr. Tim Mietzner, respectively. (Reprinted, with permission, from Malinow et al. 1989.)

et al. 1989b). We have tested these ideas by postsynaptic intracellular injection of peptides that are potent and selective inhibitors of either PKC or CaMKII (Malinow et al. 1989). PKC(19–31) or PKC(19–36) are peptide fragments forming the pseudosubstrate region of the PKC regulatory domain (House and Kemp 1987). They are more than 600-fold more potent as blockers of PKC (IC50 ~0.1 μM) than as blockers of CaMK. In contrast, the Glu-27 derivative of PKC(19–31) is relatively inactive against either kinase and serves as a useful control against nonspecific effects.

The results of intracellular injection of peptides are illustrated in Figure 7 (left). PKC(19-31) and PKC(19-36) blocked LTP when delivered to the postsynaptic cell with the recording intracellular microelectrode. They had no significant effect on transmission to a group of neighboring cells monitored extracellularly; [Glu-27]PKC(19–31), the control peptide, failed to block LTP. These results are compatible with effects of injecting PKC (Hu et al. 1987) or PKC inhibitory peptides (Andersen et al. 1990).

To investigate the role of postsynaptic CaMKII, we used the peptide fragment CaMKII(273–302), which inhibits CaMKII at much lower concentrations than PKC. A control was provided by CaMKII(284–302), a shorter peptide that is much less effective in blocking CaMKII. When delivered to postsynaptic cells through the recording microelectrode, CaMKII(273–302) blocks LTP (Fig. 7, right), whereas CaMKII(284–302) does not. We obtained similar results with a calmodulin-blocking peptide (not shown; see also Malenka et al. 1989b). The effects of the CaMKII fragments are almost certainly not explained by block of PKC, since CaMKII(284–302) is more effective than CaMKII(273–302) in blocking PKC but much less effective in preventing LTP (Malinow et al. 1989). We thus conclude that postsynaptic PKC and CaMKII are both required for the establishment of LTP.

Persistent Signaling Outside the Postsynaptic Cell?

To determine if the postsynaptic kinases are involved in the expression of LTP, we impaled cells with microelectrodes containing protein kinase inhibitors after the high-frequency stimulation had already established potentiated transmission (Fig. 9, insets). To our surprise, we found that established LTP was not suppressed by intracellular postsynaptic H-7. Delayed introduction of a combination of PKC(19–31) and CaMKII(273–302) was similarly ineffective (Tsien et al. 1990). Control procedures showed that the agents were successfully delivered and that LTP had indeed been established before the impalement. Thus, once established, the persistent signal is inaccessible to postsynaptic injection of H-7 (or to the kinase-blocking peptides). Interestingly, established LTP remains sensitive to bath application of H-7 (Figs. 8 and 9E). The effect of bath-applied H-7 is selective for the potentiated pathway (Fig. 8). Thus, we conclude that the maintenance of LTP depends on H-7-sensitive persis-

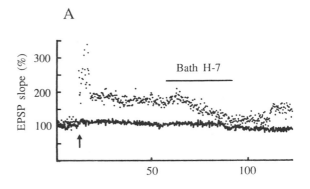

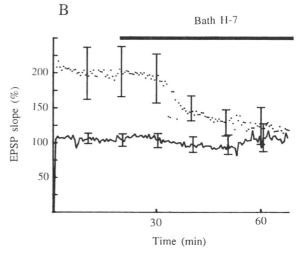

Figure 8. Expression of LTP is reversibly inhibited by bath applied H-7. (*A*) Representative experiment. (↑) Tetanic stimulation. For experimental details, see Malinow et al. 1988. (*B*) Ensemble average of EPSP amplitudes in 20 experiments plotted against time. Transmission from two different pathways is monitored with an extracellular electrode. One pathway (unconnected dots) was previously potentiated by delivery of a high-frequency stimulus, whereas the other pathway (connected dots) was not conditioned. H-7 (50–300 μM) was applied to the bath as indicated. Note that the drug acts relatively selectively in suppressing the potentiation in the conditioned pathway while leaving transmission in the control pathway essentially unaffected.

tent signaling somewhere outside the postsynaptic cell, possibly in the presynaptic terminal.

DISCUSSION AND CONCLUSIONS

The main conclusions of our studies are as follows: Whole-cell recordings can be used to study synaptic transmission in neurons well below the surface of conventional brain slices over many hours. This method allows access to deeper cells that are more likely to retain intact dendritic structures and functional properties. The approach is an alternative to methods that require cleaning of the surface of slices but provide better visibility (Edwards et al. 1989).

Whole-cell recordings offer a much better signal-to-noise ratio than conventional intracellular recordings, facilitating statistical analysis of small synaptic signals. Under favorable circumstances, quantal re-

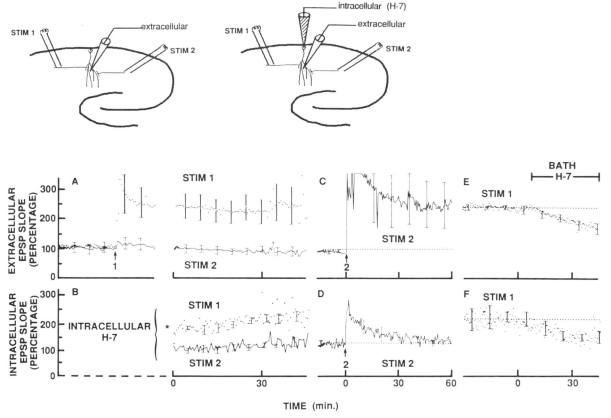

Figure 9. Expression of LTP is insensitive to postsynaptic H-7 application. (*Insets*) Recording configurations before and after delayed impalement with an H-7-containing microelectrode. (*A*) Synaptic potentials are monitored extracellularly (no microelectrode) in response to alternate stimulation of two independent pathways (unconnected points: stim 1; and connected points: stim 2). Tetanic conditioning is delivered to stim 1 (↑, 1). After the establishment of stable LTP, an intracellular recording with an H-7-containing electrode is obtained (*B*) and monitoring of synaptic potentials begins within 2 min of penetration (at $t = 0$ on lower axis). As monitored by the H-7-containing intracellular electrode, synaptic transmission from the potentiated pathway (stim 1, asterisk) does not decay during the observation period and parallels transmission from the unpotentiated pathway (stim 2) ($n = 13$). In this panel, synaptic strength in each pathway is normalized relative to average data for the first 5 min of transmission in the untetanized pathway. (*C,D*) To determine whether H-7 from the intracellular electrode has reached the synaptic zone, the previously unpotentiated pathway (stim 2) is tested for the ability to generate LTP (seven slices). Delivery of a tetanus to stim 2 results in slowly decaying potentiation but no LTP as monitored with the intracellular electrode (*D*) despite a large persistent potentiation seen with the extracellular electrode (*C*). (*E,F*) In eight slices, H-7 is subsequently bath applied, and a comparable synaptic diminution of pathway 1 is seen with both extracellular monitoring and with the H-7-filled intracellular microelectrode. Occlusion or reduction of the effect of externally applied H-7 would have been expected if postsynaptic H-7 had already inhibited the potentiated transmission. (Reprinted, with permission, from Malinow et al. 1989.)

sponses can be distinguished from synaptic failures (Figs. 1 and 4).

Experiments conform with theory in supporting M^2/σ^2 as a simple measure of changes in presynaptic function in hippocampal slices. This approach might be useful in characterizing neuroactive drugs whose locus of action is unknown.

Synapses can display LTP even after the postsynaptic cell has been accessed by a whole-cell recording pipette. This opens up the possibility of probing the postsynaptic mechanisms of LTP with a wide range of biochemical compounds that could not be reliably delivered with intracellular microelectrodes. Some obvious possibilities include large proteins or even nucleic acids.

Interestingly, the ability to undergo LTP was lost following longer periods of whole-cell recording, as if

some key cytoplasmic constituent were washed out, although LTP established earlier during the recording did not decay. This contrast supports the idea that induction and persistence of LTP involve different molecular events, possibly in different locations (Goh and Pennefather 1989; Malinow et al. 1989; Segal and Patchornik 1989).

When LTP was induced relatively soon after break-in, the degree of potentiation was large, ranging up to tenfold and averaging more than threefold. The magnitude of the enhancement is considerably greater than seen with other recording methods. The difference was not due to depressed levels of basal transmission in whole-cell recordings; the number or frequency of presynaptic action potentials (40 stimuli at 2 Hz) was certainly not excessive. One possibility is that whole-cell recordings are particularly effective in achieving strong depolarizations of postsynaptic spines (particularly with cesium as the main internal cation). Whatever the explanation, the whole-cell experiments provide a measure of the inherent power of the mechanisms underlying LTP. A large degree of persistent synaptic plasticity is of obvious interest for neural modeling (see, e.g., McNaughton and Morris 1987).

LTP of up to tenfold was seen with intracellular stimulation of single CA3 neurons (Malinow and Tsien 1990b). This provides the first direct evidence that LTP is a property of one-to-one connections between presynaptic and postsynaptic neurons, rather than an emergent property of a large number of converging presynaptic inputs (cf. Friedlander et al. 1990).

Biophysical analysis and biochemical approaches provide three complementary lines of evidence for an enhancement of presynaptic function during LTP, as suggested previously by other approaches (Skrede and Malthe-Sorenssen 1981; Dolphin et al. 1982; Routtenberg 1985; Malenka et al. 1986; Malinow et al. 1989).

The analysis of M^2/σ^2 is relatively model independent and does not require failures. M^2/σ^2 increased significantly and remained elevated during LTP; it was unchanged in pathways not undergoing potentiation (Fig. 3, bottom). LTP was associated with a clear change in M^2/σ^2, and the shape of the amplitude histogram was similar to that seen with elevated $[Ca^{++}]_o$.

An analysis based on failures gives a more direct view of presynaptic function. This method does not require that a single synapse be activated, an issue for analyses based on changes in M^2/σ^2. In all cases where unitary events were large relative to the background noise so that failures were clearly resolved, the occurrence of failures was greatly diminished; the proportion of failures fell by about threefold during LTP (e.g., Fig. 4e). In some experiments, failures were common during the control run and completely disappeared with LTP.

Although all the biophysical results support an increase in the likelihood of transmitter release, they do not exclude some change in postsynaptic responsivity. We found that M increased more than M^2/σ^2, particularly 30–60 minutes after pairing; the late change in M might reflect a delayed increase in postsynaptic responsivity as suggested by iontophoretic application of AMPA (Davies et al. 1989). This possibility might be in line with a recent report of minimal EPSPs in which an increase in quantal size but no clear change in quantal content was detected in association with a 30% potentiation (Foster and McNaughton 1991). The enhancement of transmitter release may have been more pronounced in our experiments simply because the potentiation was much larger.

A third and rather different line of evidence is based on postsynaptic injection of inhibitors of protein kinases, H-7, or peptide inhibitors of Ca^{++}-dependent kinases. After its establishment, LTP appears unresponsive to postsynaptic H-7 or to delivery of both peptides in combination, although it remains sensitive to externally applied H-7 (Fig. 8). These results suggest

that LTP is maintained by a signaling pathway not entirely contained within the postsynaptic cell. One possibility is that the pathway includes a presynaptic protein kinase such as PKC.

Our evidence supporting presynaptic changes with LTP is striking in light of previous studies showing that induction is postsynaptic (Lynch et al. 1983; Kelso et al. 1986; Malinow and Miller 1986; Sastry et al. 1986; Wigstrom et al. 1986; Malenka et al. 1988; Malinow et al. 1989). The combination of results makes it difficult to escape the conclusion that a retrograde message must travel from the conditioned postsynaptic cell to modify presynaptic function (see Bliss and Lynch 1988). Since the proportion of failures decreases and M^2/σ^2 increases soon after pairing, the retrograde signaling must occur promptly.

A retrograde message might act jointly with a presynaptic signal (e.g., elevated $[Ca^{++}]_i$). This would constitute a presynaptic AND function somewhat similar to the AND operation of glutamate plus depolarization at the postsynaptic NMDA receptor. In principle, the retrograde signal could spread laterally along the postsynaptic afferent to modify synaptic boutons onto other postsynaptic cells (Bonhoeffer et al. 1989).

An enhancement of presynaptic function effectively increases the signal-to-noise ratio of evoked synaptic release relative to "background noise" produced by the ambient level of glutamate within brain tissue. For signal processing, this is a more robust and efficient mechanism than an elevated postsynaptic receptivity, which would increase both signal and noise together.

ACKNOWLEDGMENTS

We are grateful to Dr. Daniel Madison for contributing some of the H-7 experiments illustrated in Figure 8. We thank Drs. D.D. Friel, J.A. Kauer, D.V. Madison, and R.S. Zucker for helpful discussion. This work was supported by Javits Investigator award NS-24067 to R.W.T.

REFERENCES

Alger, B.E. and R.A. Nicoll. 1982. Feed-forward dendritic inhibition of rat hippocampal pyramidal cells studied *in vitro*. *J. Physiol.* **328:** 105.

Alkon, D.L. and T.J. Nelson. 1990. Specificity of molecular changes in neurons involved in memory storage. *FASEB J.* **4:** 1567.

Andersen, P., J.M. Godfraind, P. Greengard, O. Hvalby, A. Nairn, M. Raastad, and J.F. Storm. 1990. Injection of a peptide inhibitor of protein kinase C blocks the induction of long-term potentiation in rat hippocampal cells *in vitro*. *J. Physiol.* **429:** 25P.

Artola, A. and W. Singer. 1987. Long-term potentiation and NMDA receptors in rat visual cortex. *Nature* **330:** 649.

Ascher, P. and L. Nowak. 1988. Electrophysiological studies of NMDA receptors. *Trends Neurosci.* **10:** 284.

Barnes, S. and F. Werblin. 1987. Gated currents generate single spike activity in amacrine cells of the tiger salamander retina. *Proc. Natl. Acad. Sci.* **83:** 1509.

Bashir, Z.I. and G.L. Collingridge. 1990. Potentiation of an

NMDA receptor-mediated EPSP in rat hippocampal slices *in vitro*. *J. Physiol.* **425:** 23P.

Blanton, M.G., J.J. Lo Turco, and A.R. Kriegstein. 1989. Whole cell recording from neurons in slices of reptilian and mammalian cerebral cortex. *J. Neurosci. Methods* **30:** 203.

Bliss, T.V.P. and A. Gardner-Medwin. 1973. Long-lasting potentiation of synaptic transmission in the dentate area of the unanaesthetized rabbit following stimulation of the perforant path. *J. Physiol.* **232:** 357.

Bliss, T.V.P. and T. Lomo. 1973. Long-lasting potentiation of synaptic transmission in the dentate area of the anaesthetized rabbit following stimulation of the perforant path. *J. Physiol* **232:** 331.

Bliss, T.V.P. and M. Lynch. 1988. Long-term potentiation of synaptic transmission in the hippocampus: Properties and mechanisms. In *Long-term potentiation: From biophysics to behavior* (ed. P.W. Landfield and S.A. Deadwyler), p. 3. A.R. Liss, New York.

Bliss, T.V.P., R.M. Douglas, M.L. Errington, and M.A. Lynch. 1986. Correlation between long-term potentiation and release of endogenous amino acids from dentate gyrus of anaesthetized rats. *J. Physiol.* **377:** 391.

Bonhoeffer, T., V. Staiger, A. Aertsen. 1989. Synaptic plasticity in rat hippocampal slice cultures: Local "Hebbian" conjunction of pre- and postsynaptic stimulation leads to distributed synaptic enhancement. *Proc. Natl. Acad. Sci.* **86:** 8113.

Brown, T.H., P.F. Chapman, E.W. Kairiss, and C.L. Keenan. 1988. Long-term synaptic potentiation. *Science* **242:** 724.

Coleman, P.A. and R.F. Miller. 1989. Measurement of passive membrane parameters with whole-cell recordings from neurons in the intact amphibian retina. *J. Neurophysiol.* **61:** 218.

Collingridge, G.L. and T.V.P. Bliss. 1987. NMDA receptors— Their role in long-term potentiation. *Trends Neurosci.* **10:** 288.

Cotman, C.W., R.J. Bridges, J.S. Taube, A.S. Clark, J.W. Geddes, and D.T. Monaghan. 1989. The role of the NMDA receptor in central nervous system plasticity and pathology. *J. Natl. Inst. Health Res.* **1:** 65.

Davies, S.N., R.A.J. Lester, K.G. Reymann, and G.L. Collingridge. 1989. Temporally distinct pre- and post-synaptic mechanisms maintain long-term potentiation. *Nature* **330:** 500.

del Castillo, J. and B. Katz. 1954. Quantal components of the end-plate potential. *J. Physiol.* **124:** 560.

Dolphin, A.C., M.L. Errington, and T.V.P. Bliss. 1982. Long-term potentiation of the perforant path *in vivo* is associated with increased glutamate release. *Nature* **297:** 496.

Eccles, J.C. 1953. *The neurophysiological basis of mind.* Clarendon Press, Oxford.

Edwards F.A., A. Konnerth, and T. Sakmann. 1989. A thin slice preparation for patch clamp recordings from synaptically connected neurones of the mammalian central nervous system. *Pfluegers Arch. Eur. J. Physiol.* **414:** 600.

Foster, T.C. and B.L. McNaughton. 1991. Long-term synaptic enhancement in CA1 is due to increased quantal size, not quantal content. *Hippocampus* (in press).

Friedlander, J.J., R.J. Sayer, and S.J. Redman. 1990. Evaluation of long-term potentiation of small compound and unitary EPSPs at the hippocampal CA3-CA1 synapse. *J. Neurosci.* **10:** 814.

Goelet, P., V.F. Castellucci, S. Schacher, and E.R. Kandel. 1985. The long and short of long-term memory—A molecular framework. *Nature* **322:** 419.

Goh, J.W. and P.A. Pennefather. 1989. Pertussis toxin-sensitive G protein in hippocampal long-term potentiation. *Science* **244:** 980.

Gustafsson, B., H. Wigstrom, W.C. Abraham, and Y.Y. Huang. 1987. Long-term potentiation in the hippocampus using depolarizing current pulses as the conditioning stimulus to single volley synaptic potentials. *J. Neurosci.* **7:** 774.

Hebb, D.O. 1949. *The organization of behavior.* Wiley, New York.

House, C. and B.E. Kemp. 1987. Protein kinase C contains a pseudosubstrate prototope in its regulatory domain. *Science* **238:** 1726.

Hu, G.Y., O. Hvalby, S.I. Walaas, K.A. Albert, P. Skjelfo, P. Andersen, and P. Greengard. 1987. Protein kinase C injection into hippocampal pyramidal cells elicits features of long-term potentiation. *Nature* **328:** 426.

Iriki, A., C. Pavlides, A. Keller, and H. Asanuma. 1989. Long-term potentiation in the motor cortex. *Science* **246:** 1385.

Johnson, J.W. and P. Ascher. 1987. Glycine potentiates the NMDA response in cultured mouse brain neurons. *Nature* **325:** 529.

Kauer, J.A., R.C. Malenka, and R.A. Nicoll. 1988. A persistent postsynaptic modification mediates long-term potentiation in the hippocampus. *Neuron* **1:** 911.

Kelso, S.R., A.H. Ganong, and T.H. Brown. 1986. Hebbian synapses in hippocampus. *Proc. Natl. Acad. Sci.* **83:** 5326.

Kennedy, M.B. 1989. Regulation of synaptic transmission in the central nervous system: Long-term potentiation. *Cell* **59:** 777.

Lester, A.J.R, M.L. Quarum, J.D. Parker, E. Weber, and C.E. Jahr. 1989. Interaction of 6-cyano-7-nitroquinoxaline-2,3-dione with the N-methyl-D-aspartate receptor-associated glycine binding site. *Mol. Pharmacol.* **35:** 565.

Lomo, T. 1966. Frequency potentiation of excitatory synaptic activity in the dentate area of the hippocampal formation. *Acta Physiol. Scand. (suppl.)* **277:** 128.

Lynch, G. and M. Baudry. 1984. The biochemistry of memory: A new and specific hypothesis. *Science* **224:** 1057.

Lynch, G., J. Larson, S. Kelso, G, Barrionuevo, and F. Schottler. 1983. Intracellular injections of EGTA block induction of hippocampal long-term potentiation. *Nature* **305:** 719.

MacDermott, A.B., M.L. Mayer, G.L. Westbrook, S.J. Smith, and J.L. Barker. 1986. NMDA-receptor activation increases cytoplasmic calcium concentration in cultured spinal cord neurones. *Nature* **321:** 519.

Malenka, R.C., D.V. Madison, and R.A. Nicoll. 1986. Potentiation of synaptic transmission in the hippocampus by phorbol esters. *Nature* **321:** 695.

Malenka, R.C., J.A. Kauer, D.J. Perkel, and R.A. Nicoll. 1989a. The impact of postsynaptic calcium on synaptic transmission—Its role in long-term potentiation. *Trends Neurosci.* **12:** 444.

Malenka, R.C., J.A. Kauer, R.S. Zucker, and R.A. Nicoll. 1988. Postsynaptic calcium is sufficient for potentiation of hippocampal synaptic transmission. *Science* **242:** 81.

Malenka, R.C., J.A. Kauer, D.J. Perkel, M.D. Mauk, P.T. Kelly, R.A. Nicoll, and M.N. Waxham. 1989b. An essential role for postsynaptic calmodulin and protein kinase activity in long-term potentiation. *Nature* **340:** 554.

Malinow, R. and J.P. Miller. 1986. Postsynaptic hyperpolarization during conditioning reversibly blocks induction of long-term potentiaton. *Nature* **321:** 529.

Malinow, R. and R.W. Tsien. 1990a. Presynaptic enhancement revealed by whole cell recordings of long-term potentiation in hippocampal slices. *Nature* **346:** 177.

———. 1990b. Long-term potentiation of synaptic transmission between individual CA3 and CA1 neurons in rat hippocampal slices. *Soc. Neurosci. Abstr.* **16:** 145.

Malinow, R., D.V. Madison, and R.W. Tsien. 1988. Persistent protein kinase activity underlying long-term potentiation. *Nature* **335:** 820.

Malinow, R., H. Schulman, and R.W. Tsien. 1989. Inhibition of postsynaptic PKC or CaMKII blocks induction but not expression of LTP. *Science* **245:** 862.

Martin, A.R. 1977. Junctional transmission. II. Presynaptic mechanisms. In *Handbook of physiology: The nervous system* (ed. E.R. Kandel), p. 329. American Physiological Society, Bethesda, Maryland.

Mayer, M.L., and G.L. Westbrook. 1987. The physiology of excitatory amino acids in the vertebrate central nervous system. *Prog. Neurobiol.* **28:** 197.

McNaughton, B.L. and R.G.M. Morris. 1987. Hippocampal synaptic enhancement and information storage within a distributed memory system. *Trends Neurosci.* **10:** 408.

McNaughton, B.L., C.A. Barnes, and P. Andersen. 1981. Synaptic efficacy and EPSP summation in granule cells of rat fascia dentat studied in vitro. *J. Neurophysiol.* **46:** 952.

Muller, D. and G. Lynch. 1988. Long-term potentation differentially affects two components of synaptic responses in hippocampus. *Proc. Natl. Acad. Sci.* **85:** 9346.

Muller, D., M. Joly, and G. Lynch. 1988. Contributions of quisqualate and NMDA receptors to the induction and expression of LTP. *Science* **242:** 1694.

Nicoll, R.A., J.A. Kauer, and R.C. Malenka. 1988. The current excitement in long-term potentiation. *Neuron* **1:** 97.

Nishizuka, Y. 1988. The molecular heterogeneity of protein kinase C and its implications for cellular regulation. *Nature* **334:** 661.

Redman, S.J. 1990. Quantal analysis of synaptic potentials in neurons of the central nervous system. *Physiol. Rev.* **70:** 165.

Regehr, W.G. and D.W. Tank. 1990. Postsynaptic NMDA-receptor mediated calcium accumulation in hippocampal CA1 pyramidal cell dendrites. *Nature* **345:** 807.

Routtenberg, A. 1985. Protein kinase C activation leading to protein F1 phosphorylation may regulate synaptic plasticity by presynaptic terminal growth. *Behav. Neural Biol.* **44:** 186.

Sastry, B.R., J.W. Goh, and A. Auyeung. 1986. Associative induction of posttetanic and long-term potentiation in CA1 neurons of rat hippocampus. *Science* **232:** 988.

Sayer, R.J., M.J. Friedlander, and S.J. Redman. 1990. The time course and amplitude of EPSPs evoked at synapses between pairs of CA3/CA1 neurons in the hippocampal slice. *J. Neurosci.* **10:** 826.

Sayer, R.J., S.J. Redman, and P. Andersen. 1990. Amplitude fluctuations in small EPSPs recorded from CA1 pyramidal cells in the guinea-pig hippocampal slice. *J. Neurosci.* **9:** 840.

Segal, M. and A. Patchornik. 1989. Modulation of $(Ca)_1$ by a caged EGTA affects neuronal plasticity in the rat hippocampus. *Soc. Neurosci. Abstr.* **15:** 166.

Skrede, K.K. and D. Malthe-Sorenssen. 1981. Increased resting and evoked release of transmitter following repetitive electrical tetanization in hippocampus: A biochemical correlate to long-lasting synaptic potentiation. *Brain Res.* **208:** 436.

Stevens, C.F. 1989. Strengthening the synapses. *Nature* **338:** 460.

Thompson, A.M., V.E. Walker, and D.M. Flynn. 1989. Glycerine enhances NMDA-receptor mediated synaptic potentials in neocortical slices. *Nature* **338:** 422.

Tsien, R.W., H. Schulman, and R. Malinow. 1990. Peptide inhibitors of PKC and CaMK block induction but not expression of long-term potentiation. *Adv. Second Messenger Phosphoprotein Res.* **24:** 101.

Wigstrom, H., B. Gustafsson, Y.Y. Huang, and W.C. Abraham. 1986. Hippocampal long-term potentiation is induced by pairing single afferent volleys with intracellularly injected depolarizing pulses. *Acta Physiol. Scand.* **126:** 317.

Toward a Representational Hypothesis of the Role of Hippocampal Synaptic Plasticity in Spatial and Other Forms of Learning

R.G.M. MORRIS

Department of Pharmacology, University of Edinburgh Medical School, Edinburgh EH8 9JZ, Scotland

One reason for the current interest in the neural mechanisms of activity-dependent synaptic plasticity, particularly those involved in hippocampal long-term potentiation (LTP), is the idea that these same mechanisms may overlap with those actually used by the nervous system in certain kinds of learning. Several different theoretical and experimental approaches have been taken to investigate this possibility (Laroche and Bloch 1982; McNaughton 1983; Lynch 1986; Teyler and Discenna 1986; Barnes 1988; Berger and Sclabassi 1988; Morris et al. 1990a; Singer 1990), but this paper focuses on a hitherto neglected aspect of the problem: the interface between the properties and mechanisms of LTP, on the one hand, and recent neuropsychological theories about the organization of memory, on the other. Aspects of a "representational" hypothesis concerning the role LTP could play in storing information about the relationship between events are then outlined and evaluated against available evidence.

Properties and Mechanisms of LTP Relevant to a Role in Learning

LTP is a sustained enhancement of communication between afferent fibers and their target cells consisting of increases in both synaptic efficacy (synaptic LTP) and the ease with which spike activity is generated by summated excitatory postsynaptic potentials. It was first reported in detail by Bliss and Lomo (1973) and has since been intensively investigated at many different levels of analysis (for review, see Landfield and Deadwyler 1988). Certain properties of hippocampal LTP have seemed particularly relevant to its possible role in memory. These include that it can be induced by brief physiologically realistic patterns of stimulation (Larson and Lynch 1986; Rose and Dunwiddie 1986) not dissimilar to those that have been recorded from single cells in hippocampus (O'Keefe 1979; Fox et al. 1986; McNaughton 1989; T. Otto et al., in prep.). Furthermore, as in many forms of learning, the induction of LTP obeys an associative principle in requiring the conjunction of two events, presynaptic stimulation and postsynaptic depolarization, and thus shows a measure of postsynaptic specificity (Kelso et al. 1986; Wigstrom et al. 1986; cf. Bonhoeffer et al., this volume). It

develops rapidly after induction (McNaughton 1983; Gustafsson et al. 1989), and like many forms of memory, it can last for extended periods of time (Bliss and Gardner-Medwin 1973; Barnes 1979; Racine et al. 1983). LTP does not last indefinitely but decays according to three separate time courses, suggesting that it may consist of several overlapping components (Abraham and Otani 1990).

Work on its underlying mechanisms has established that activation of a dual voltage- and ligand-gated receptor that detects the conjunction of presynaptic activity and postsynaptic depolarization (the N-methyl-D-aspartate [NMDA] receptor) is an essential step in the induction of most forms of LTP. Its prominence in hippocampus is thus partly due to the high density of NMDA receptors found in subregions of this structure (Monaghan and Cotman 1985) and partly due to the prevailing balance of excitation and inhibition. The occurrence of LTP elsewhere (e.g., neocortex) is now well-documented, but it has usually proved necessary to block inhibition with γ-aminobutyric acid antagonists to see the phenomenon reliably (see, e.g., Artola and Singer 1987). Blocking NMDA receptors with selective antagonists such as 2-amino-5-phosphonopentanoic acid (APV) provides a convenient and reliable way of preventing the induction of LTP in a dose-dependent manner (Collingridge et al. 1983; Harris et al. 1984), albeit a method that can have other effects on physiological function (Kleinschmidt et al. 1987; Dale 1989; Fox et al. 1989; Sillito et al. 1990). However, because hippocampal NMDA receptors participate minimally in fast synaptic transmission, it is possible to block the slower but longer-lasting currents associated with NMDA receptor activation selectively (see Hestrin et al., this volume). Achieving such selectivity in vivo for the purposes of behavioral studies requires both careful titration of dose and direct administration to the brain (because APV penetrates the blood-brain barrier very poorly). The mechanisms of expression of LTP are less well understood, including whether it is predominantly a pre- or postsynaptic phenomenon (see chapters by Bliss et al.; Bekkers and Stevens; Tsien and Manilow; all this volume), but specific agents that interfere with its expression and maintenance may eventually become available for use in behavioral studies also.

Aspects of the Neuropsychology of Memory Relevant to the Possible Role of Hippocampal LTP

If hippocampal LTP is involved in learning and memory, it is reasonable to expect (1) that it will be involved in the types of learning dependent on the integrity of the hippocampus, (2) that its induction will only occur during certain modes of hippocampal information processing, and thus (3) that it will only be involved in a subset of hippocampal-dependent types of learning. It follows that we must have some idea of the types of information processing carried out by the hippocampus before any specific hypothesis of what hippocampal LTP may be doing can be outlined.

Work on the psychological processes involved in learning and memory in animals has established that these are organized into a number of neuropsychologically dissociable systems. Certain tasks apparently acquired in a strictly dispositional manner, such as the learning of simple brightness and pattern discriminations, motor skills, and some aspects of classical and instrumental conditioning, are unaffected by damage to structures in the medial temporal lobe. In these, behavioral dispositions to respond in a particular way are acquired over the course of training, but animals neither need nor develop flexible access to the information causally responsible for the learned behavior. Other tasks, such as object discrimination learning, delayed matching- or nonmatching-to-sample, place discrimination, and object-place conditional learning, are sometimes (although not always) affected by medial temporal lobe damage (Mishkin 1982; see also Squire et al.; Rolls; both this volume). Unfortunately, these latter tasks do not fall naturally into any obvious category. Despite many years of ingenious experimentation guided by a variety of theoretical formulations, there remains considerable disagreement about both the psychological organization of the memory systems dependent on the integrity of the medial temporal lobe and exactly what role(s) the various structures within it (e.g., hippocampus, amygdala, entorhinal cortex, and parahippocampal gyrus) might be performing. Faced with this uncertainty at the "process" level, the task of building a neurobiological theory of learning and memory, in which hippocampal LTP may or may not play a role, must seem forlorn. However, an emerging consensus is that the hippocampus processes information for transfer into long-term memory in the neocortex in a manner that enables episodic or declarative memory, or what I call here a "representational" form of memory. It may also be involved in information retrieval.

One distinctive psychological feature of representational processing is that information both about the nature of the logical relationship between stimuli and about the stimuli themselves is processed and then stored in long-term memory. Subsequent presentation of a stimulus will then evoke not only the memory representation of the event, action, or stimulus with which it was associated, but also information about the nature of the relationship between them. The associated cue might be a simple stimulus that predicted the event, an action on the part of the animal that brings about some consequence or contextual information indicating where or when the event occurred. Why animals have this separate memory system and why it evolved remain unclear, but various features of the system are becoming apparent. One is that access to factual information, independent of behavior, is an essential prerequisite of reasoning. Thus, retrieval from memory of two independent associations may enable further information to be inferred. In a similar vein, encoding contextual information helps resolve ambiguities concerning memory for similar events occurring in different contexts and provides additional recall cues for the retrieval of information from long-term memory. Representational processing is clearly associative, but it differs from the associative processes involved in the acquisition of dispositional skills in ways that are not yet fully understood. Clearly, it involves processing information about both the events themselves and the nature of the relationship between them. Thus, the content of what is learned differs from dispositional memory where tendencies to behave in a particular way are acquired, but the reason why such behavior is appropriate may not be accessible to the animal's memory. However, the conditions under which these two types of learning take place need not differ. Thus, the arrangement of a simple pairing of one stimulus or action (A) with another (B) may, depending on the pairing arrangement, result in the acquisition of knowledge that A predicts B (causal knowledge), is near to B (spatial knowledge), or even that A means B (semantic knowledge); or it may proceed dispositionally such that A merely acquires value and/or nothing more than the capacity to evoke a response (assuming that B is a biologically significant event). This overlap of the conditions required for acquisition makes the task of designing behavioral experiments to dissociate the two processes very difficult (see Dickinson 1980). In contemporary studies of animal learning, some types of representational coding have been identified by procedures such as reinforcer devaluation in which an animal's desire for a predicted object (B) is experimentally reduced without reexposing the animal to the cue (A) that predicts that object. If subsequent presentation of cue A now fails to evoke anticipatory behavior of the type it used to evoke prior to reinforcer (B) devaluation, it may be inferred that the animal has stored not only memory representations of cues A and B, but also the relationship between them (Rescorla 1988). However, such procedures have not yet been explored in neuropsychological or neuropharmacological studies.

A relevant albeit limited illustration of the difference between representational and dispositional learning is the comparison between allocentric spatial learning and visual discrimination learning. Spatial learning involves learning the location of an object and, some have argued, forming either a "map" of space (O'Keefe and Nadel 1978) or remembering the "whole scene" (Gaffan and Harrison 1989). Either process would require building a rich representation of the relative locations of numerous cues and storing these in long-term memory in a manner that would later enable an animal to search accurately for a target from any direction or to distinguish two scenes consisting of identical objects. Visual discrimination learning, on the other hand, need involve no more than associating one cue with reward and another with nonreward. The former type of learning is impaired by lesions of the hippocampus in the rat, and the latter is not (O'Keefe and Nadel 1978; Morris et al. 1986a). Although this represents only a single dissociation and is thus a weak foundation upon which to base any claim of functional specificity,[1] some of the

experimental work discussed below uses these two types of tasks to investigate whether blocking LTP affects either or both types of memory.

It is worth noting in passing that there has recently been some uncertainty concerning the hitherto well-established notion that lesions of the hippocampus cause deficits in allocentric spatial learning. Jarrard (1986) recently showed that ibotenate lesions of the hippocampus may not always prevent the relearning of either reference or working-memory components of performance in versions of Olton and Samuelson's (1976) radial-maze task. Accordingly, in a joint study with L.E. Jarrard and F. Schenk (Morris et al. 1990b), the effects of such lesions on the acquisition of place-navigation spatial reference memory in a water-maze task (Morris 1981) have been reexamined. Selective lesions of hippocampus (HPC), subiculum (SUB), or hippocampus plus subiculum (HPC + SUB) were made

---

[1] The importance and pitfalls of establishing functional dissociation in experimental neuropsychology have been discussed in detail by Weiskrantz (1968) and Shallice (1989).

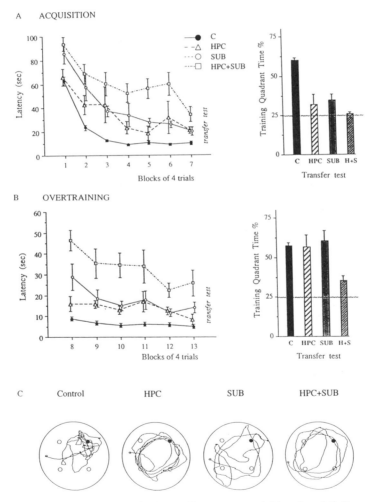

Figure 1. Ibotenate hippocampal lesions impair but do not totally prevent spatial learning. (*A*) Escape latency (sec ± 1 S.E.M.) and transfer test performance (% training quadrant time ± 1 S.E.M. with platform absent) of control, HPC-, SUB-, and HPC + SUB-lesioned rats trained postoperatively on a simple place-navigation water escape task. Note impairment in all lesioned groups that also, in the transfer test, perform at or only just above chance levels. (*B*) Escape latencies during, and transfer test performance after, a series of overtraining trials. The HPC and SUB groups were still impaired but, by the end of overtraining, showed as good a spatial bias to the training quadrant as controls. (*C*) Paths taken by typical animals of each group during the first transfer test. Note "circling" strategy in HPC-lesioned rat and its absence in the SUB-lesioned rat.

by infusing small volumes of the neurotoxin into multiple sites within each structure. The behavioral findings indicated that, although both the HPC and SUB lesions caused impairments in the initial postoperative acquisition of place-navigation (Fig. 1A), they did not prevent eventual learning, except by the HPC + SUB-lesion group, to levels of performance almost as effective as those of controls (Fig. 1B). Interestingly, qualitative observations of the paths taken to find the hidden platform indicated that, at an intermediate stage of training, different types of paths were shown by the different groups (Fig. 1C). The improvements in performance with overtraining indicate that the long-term storage of spatial information is unlikely to be in hippocampus and, for various reasons including the difference in paths shown by the HPC and SUB groups, point to hippocampal cell loss causing a dual deficit: a slower rate of place-learning and a separate navigational impairment. An intriguing possibility is that these deficits reflect distinct modes of processing in hippocampus: a storage and retrieval mode.

A Representational Hypothesis

The above discussion summarizes the essential background for a more specific hypothesis about the role of hippocampal LTP over and beyond the very general statement of an "involvement" in learning alluded to above. Specifically, I propose that hippocampal LTP participates in the mechanisms responsible for ensuring that the logical relationships that underlie associative representational memory are stored in long-term memory in the neocortex along with information about the stimulus events themselves.

The essence of this hypothesis is the recognition of a fundamental distinction between detecting that two events are associated and representing the nature of their association in memory. Clearly, the induction of LTP entails no more than the associative conjunction of presynaptic activity with postsynaptic depolarization and thus on its own cannot be more than a mechanism for detecting associations. In this respect, it shares with activity-dependent modulation of presynaptic facilitation (Kandel and Schwartz 1982) the property of being a mechanism of plasticity rather than of learning per se (see Morris 1990). However, embedded into appropriate circuitry, an LTP mechanism could potentially play a very important role in ensuring that stimuli and the associative relationships into which they enter in any given task or context are stored together. In realizing this possibility, it would be necessary for information computed or passing through the hippocampus to include not only concrete information about the identity of objects or events, but also information of a more abstract nature, such as the fact that one event occurred before another, that one object was near another, or could be seen when near another, and so on. The fact the locus of control for LTP induction is postsynaptic is very important for it enormously expands the scope for interaction between spatially dispersed patterns of

neural activity representing both concrete and more abstract information. Clearly, the core idea of this hypothesis is a matter of speculation and a full statement of it would involve details of how information is represented within the hippocampal matrix, of the processing to which it is subject in the different subfields of dentate gyrus, CA3 and CA1, and of how the hippocampus interacts with cortex in laying down long-term memory traces. McNaughton and Morris (1987) have sketched out, in a strictly qualitative way, how certain aspects of its anatomical organization (e.g., topographic vs. nontopographic projections from entorhinal cortex, the lamella organization of the mossy fiber projections, and the extensive longitudinal connections of the outputs of CA3) may enable certain simple types of representational processing. For example, we showed how, if information is represented as a spatially distributed pattern of activation, an LTP-like mechanism of synaptic change could enable one cue to evoke a memory representation of another using known hippocampal circuitry. This process is very different from the modulation of an existing reflex (or even a cryptic one) and captures better the spirit of modern work in animal learning. However, the McNaughton and Morris (1987) paper was limited not only by the lack of quantitative modeling (cf. Hawkins 1989), but also because it failed to explain how different kinds of associative relations could be computed or identify whether hippocampal circuitry is specifically organized to deal with spatial but not other types of associative relationship (and if so why). A claim for associative specificity is sometimes made on the basis that hippocampal lesions fail to affect classical conditioning. However, such a claim should be treated with caution for precisely the reason given earlier: Many conditioning procedures engage both dispositional and representational learning processes. The failure to see lesion-induced conditioning impairments may be because dispositional processes are spared rather than because the hippocampus is only involved in some types of representational memory processing but not others.

In any event, in even this skeletal form, the representational hypothesis makes three predictions: (1) The neural mechanisms underlying hippocampal LTP are required for some forms of learning but not others,[2] (2) LTP-like changes induced in the course of learning may prove difficult to detect; and (3) LTP should not be required for retrieval. These predictions are limited but may be sufficient to distinguish the validity of the representational hypothesis from certain others, notably from the ideas that LTP is involved in many kinds of learning without regard to their neuropsychological status (see, e.g., Laroche and Bloch 1982), that it plays a role in indexing memory locations in cortex (Teyler

---

[2]Of course, no one believes that the physiological phenomenon of LTP itself is involved in memory. The shorthand "role of LTP in learning" (used hereafter) is intended to capture the more exact idea that some subset of the neural mechanisms underlying LTP are activated during and required for certain kinds of learning.

and Discenna 1986), or finally that it plays no special role in memory processing at all. As summarized below, the available evidence provides support for each of these predictions, but there are both gaps in our understanding and conflicting evidence on each point.

Prediction I: The neural mechanisms underlying hippocampal LTP are required for some forms of learning but not others. The idea that LTP mechanisms are required for representational learning has now been examined in a number of experiments of increasing precision. A first step was the finding that blocking LTP in either of two different ways was sufficient to cause a selective impairment in such learning. A second step has been to establish that this impairment is seen across exactly the range of conditions at which LTP in vivo is itself impaired.

Following observations that the decay time course of LTP is correlated with the learning rate (Barnes 1979), McNaughton et al. (1986) showed that saturation of LTP ("enhancement") causes an anterograde spatial learning impairment. Rats were prepared with bilateral stimulating (perforant path) and recording electrodes (dentate hilus) and then trained in the Barnes circle-maze task. Once all animals were escaping relatively rapidly with minimal errors to a dark escape tunnel at one location on the maze, they were subject to several days of either high-frequency (HF) LTP-inducing electrical stimulation or low-frequency (LF) stimulation (groups HF and LF, respectively). The effects of the HF stimulation were to saturate LTP so that no further changes in synaptic efficacy could be achieved. The animals were then returned to the maze and required to

learn a new tunnel location. Two results of interest were that (1) group HF failed to learn the new tunnel location but (2) both it and group LF continued to approach the old tunnel location preferentially at the start of retraining. Other experiments in the same series established (3) that saturation also impaired spatial memory when given posttrial within a few minutes of each daily training trial and (4) was without effect on a short-term memory radial-maze task. In a complimentary set of experiments, Morris et al. (1986b) explored a different way of blocking LTP: the use of chronic intraventricular infusion of APV at an infusion concentration shown to be sufficient to block LTP in vivo. Separate groups of rats were trained in two different tasks. One was a spatial localization task involving escape from water onto a platform hidden at a particular location in space, and the other was a two-platform discrimination task in which the animals had to learn to distinguish a gray object from a black-and-white striped one of roughly equivalent luminosity. The results showed a selective impairment of spatial learning without effect on visual discrimination (Fig. 2). Taken together, these experiments indicate that two radically different ways of blocking LTP have the equivalent effect of causing an impairment of spatial learning. The McNaughton et al. (1986) experiment adds the important information that saturation of LTP has no effect on information stored in long-term memory prior to the HF stimulation, whereas the selective profile of impairment in the Morris et al. (1986b) study indicates that the drug-induced impairment of spatial learning was not due to a gross disturbance of vision, movement, or incentive to learn.

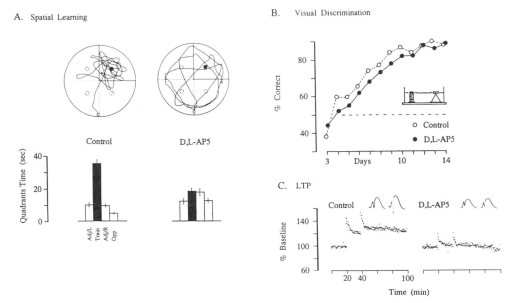

Figure 2. Intraventricular infusion of APV causes a selective impairment of learning. (*A*) Performance during a posttraining transfer test by typical animals from the control and APV (AP5) groups. Times (sec ± 1 S.E.M.) spent in each of the four quadrants of the pool during the 60-sec test (training quadrant = black) are shown below. (*B*) Lack of impairment in learning a dispositional visual discrimination task involving a choice between two discriminable objects. (*C*) Induction of hippocampal LTP under urethane anesthesia in control but not in APV-treated rats. *Y* axis is mean early rising slope values of dentate hilus field potentials.

There is, however, a logical weakness to both sets of experiments. Both point to a correlation between the ability to learn certain tasks and the capacity for LTP, but neither establishes a definitive causal relation. The logical point is that in each experiment, both the blockade of LTP and the spatial learning impairment are each dependent consequences of an independent treatment. It is clearly logically fallacious to presume, in the absence of further evidence, that one dependent consequence (e.g., the blockade of LTP) is the cause of the other (the spatial learning impairment). Both McNaughton's group and my own have attempted to address this problem in various ways. In one ingenious experiment, Castro et al. (1989) reasoned that if HF stimulation was indeed causing the learning impairment by saturating LTP, rats for whom a period of several days was allowed to elapse after LTP induction before retraining commenced might not show such an impairment if the LTP had by then decayed to baseline. This prediction was fulfilled. My own efforts to address the problem have involved attempting to identify whether APV is causing its impairment by blocking LTP or via "side-effects" (for a critical perspective, see Mondadori et al. 1989; Keith and Rudy 1990). Relevant experiments include comparing visual and olfactory discrimination control tasks of varying task difficulty (Morris 1989, expt. 2; Reid and Morris 1990), measuring drug diffusion from the intraventricular cannula through the brain (S.P. Butcher et al., in prep.), examining the effects of local infusion of APV into hippocampus (Morris et al. 1989), measuring and controlling sensorimotor side-effects (Morris 1989, expt. 3) and finally, examining the detailed dose-response profile of APV on both spatial learning and LTP in vivo (S. Davis et al., in prep.). Morris et al. (1990a) discuss these and related issues in detail. We recognized that pharmacological experiments concerned with behavior are fraught with interpretative difficulties and that APV clearly has a variety of effects on physiological function beyond effects on LTP (including effects on excitability [Abraham and Kairiss 1988], the hippocampal θ-rhythm [Leung and Desborough 1988], and sensory transduction in the geniculo-striate pathway [Daw et al. 1990; Sillito et al. 1990]). Great care must therefore be exercised in designing and executing behavioral experiments that use a pharmacological method of examining the functional role of LTP.

Of these efforts to explore specificity, the dose-response analysis (S. Davis et al., in prep.) is arguably the most important. The Morris et al. (1986b) experiment established that an infusion concentration of APV sufficient to block LTP in vivo was sufficient to impair spatial learning. This finding leaves open the possibility that a drug concentration could be found at which LTP is blocked completely but spatial learning proceeds normally. Such a finding would severely compromise if

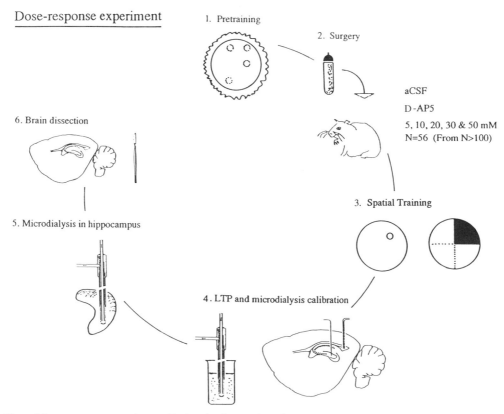

Figure 3. Plan of dose-response experiment. Each animal was taken through each phase, and usable data were obtained from 56 rats. These were later assigned to groups on the basis of APV content in the hippocampal whole tissue dissected during the final phase.

not even disprove the representational LTP hypothesis. The general plan of the dose-response experiment is shown in Figure 3. The behavioral protocol began with 3 days of nonspatial pretraining (which helps to reduce sensorimotor side-effects). The rats were then given surgery for implanting minipumps containing either artificial cerebrospinal fluid (aCSF) or various concentrations of APV or given a sham operation (i.e., no minipump). Beginning 3 days later, all rats were given 5 days of spatial training followed on the last day by a transfer test. On the next day or any of the succeeding 3 days, an attempt was made to induce LTP in vivo under urethane anesthesia. After this and while still under anesthesia, the extracellular fluid in hippocampus was sampled for 2 hours using microdialysis probes. Finally, each animal was sacrificed, their brains were removed, and various brain regions were dissected for whole-tissue measurements of APV and endogenous amino acids using high-performance liquid chromatography.

It proved convenient to divide the 56 rats who completed all phases of this experiment into groups on the basis of their APV concentration in hippocampal whole tissue. This was done in an arbitrary way by assigning rats with no APV to a control group and assigning rats with between 0.01 and 0.10, 0.11 and 0.20, 0.21 and 0.30, and above 0.31 nmole/mg wet weight to separate groups. This sorting process enabled us to establish that the minipumps per se had no effect on learning (i.e., the aCSF and sham rats performed equivalently) and to identify certain rats who had shown sensorimotor abnormalities during training as the very rats with extremely high whole-tissue APV concentrations (well above 0.31 nmole/mg). Analysis of the remaining animals showed that there was a parallel dose-related impairment of both spatial learning and LTP in vivo (Fig. 4). Mean escape latency increased as a function of whole-tissue content, whereas the amount of LTP that could be evoked (measured 30 min posttetanus) declined.

A more subtle feature of the results, however, emerged from the microdialysis measurements. These established that the extracellular concentration of APV in hippocampus was some 30 times lower than the whole-tissue content. At first, we were puzzled by this finding, wondering if there had been some mistake in the calibration measurements, but careful reworking of values failed to reveal any source of error. Whole-tissue measurements do not, of course, establish in which of several compartments the drug is located (neurons, glia, or extracellular space). Thus, a mismatch between these two indices of drug content was not unexpected; it was the scale of the mismatch that was puzzling. Biochemical experiments conducted in collaboration with M. Kessler (University of California, Irvine) and R. Griffiths (University of St. Andrews) established that APV does not inhibit the uptake of L-[^{3}H]glutamate on the high-affinity glutamate uptake carrier, nor is D-[^{3}H]APV itself taken up. However, a clue to the fate of the infused APV that remains in the brain came when, following a suggestion from J. Watkins (University of Bristol), we added 20 mM EGTA to the infusion medium of the microdialysis probes (switching to a calcium-free buffer for this part of the experiment only) and found a dramatic eightfold increase in APV concentration in the perfusate lasting at least 40 minutes (Fig. 5). This finding suggests that a significant proportion of the whole-tissue APV may be "trapped" in extracellular space by a calcium-dependent mechanism (N.B. Bear et al. [1990], who observed a similar trapping phenomenon in visual cortex slices). Whatever the mechanism, the finding gave us greater confidence in our measurements of extracellular APV concentration enabling an examination of whether the impairments of both spatial learning and

A. Relation to Whole Tissue   B. EGTA

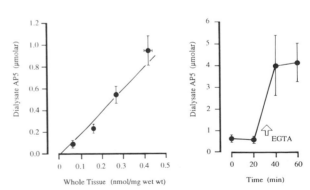

Figure 5. Dose-response study. (*A*) Relationship between true dialysate concentration (μM) and whole-tissue APV content (nmole/mg). The calibrated recovery rate for the microdialysis probes was 6.1%, which yields a ratio of (circa) 30:1 between whole-tissue levels and effective interstitial concentration. (*B*) Massive release of APV in the dialysate upon switching to a continuous infusion of 20 mM EGTA in a Ca^{++} buffer. The capacity to release APV into the dialysate provides independent validation of the discrepancy between the whole-tissue and extracellular concentrations.

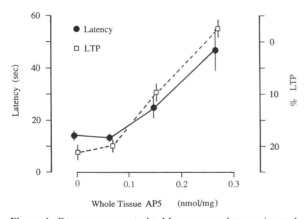

Figure 4. Dose-response study. Mean escape latency (sec ± 1 S.E.M.) and LTP (percentage above baseline 30 min posttetanus) as a function of APV levels in hippocampal whole tissue. Note parallel dose-response functions but the apparently high whole-tissue levels of APV required to block LTP completely.

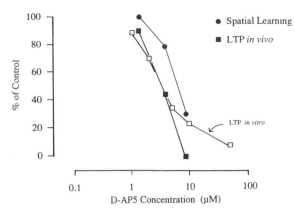

Figure 6. Dose-response study. Comparison of dose-response profile of spatial learning and LTP in vivo (this study) with published data on LTP in vitro. X axis is bath concentration of APV (D-AP5) in the Harris et al. (1984) hippocampal slice experiment and our estimates of effective interstitial APV concentration in hippocampus in vivo across groups.

LTP in vivo occurred across an equivalent dose range to that required to block NMDA receptors in vitro. Such a comparison required that the data be normalized, and this was done for the behavioral data by comparing the savings in escape latencies across spatial training relative to the baseline level shown by each group at the end of nonspatial pretraining. For the LTP in vivo data, the normalization was in relation to the LTP shown by controls. Plotting the results in this way points to a remarkable parallel: The impairments in spatial learning and LTP in vivo are not only parallel, but occur across exactly the same dose range as the APV-induced blockade of LTP in vitro (Fig. 6). Although this finding by no means exhausts the possibilities for alternative interpretations, it does provide striking support for the hypothesis that one type of representational learning dependent on normal hippocampal function requires activation of hippocampal NMDA receptors in vivo.

Prediction 2: LTP-like changes induced in the course of learning may prove difficult to detect. The prediction that LTP-like changes might prove difficult to detect after even the types of learning believed to require it may seem paradoxical but follows from the property of synapse specificity. The prediction is an unfortunate one because behaviorally induced LTP would, were it easy to obtain, be a straightforward way to investigate the functional significance of LTP. Animals would be implanted with electrodes, and recordings of field-potentials would be taken before and after a learning experience. An increase in the field-potential slope could indicate that an LTP mechanism had been activated during that particular type of learning. Unfortunately, although increases in neuronal excitability (Weisz et al. 1984; Sharp et al. 1985) in transmitter release (Laroche et al. 1987) and/or second messengers implicated in LTP (Laroche et al. 1990) have each been observed, little or no long-lasting changes in the early rising slope of extracellularly recorded field

potentials have been found (Sharp et al. 1985). Where slope changes have been seen, they have sometimes been traced to modulation by behavioral state (Hargreaves et al. 1990). However, an exploration-induced, behavior-independent, short-lasting change in evoked-potential slope has been reported recently (Sharp et al. 1989), and this, despite its duration, may be dependent on an LTP-like mechanism (Green et al. 1990).

LTP-like changes might be difficult to detect after learning for two reasons: (1) because of the link between synapse specificity and storage capacity and (2) the possibility that LTP is accompanied by long-term depression. Suppose, first, that the hippocampus functions as an associative matrix of roughly the kind whose implementation in hippocampus was discussed by McNaughton and Morris (1987). Associative synaptic conjunctions that could trigger long-term increases in synaptic efficacy would, if the matrix were operating at near optimal signal-to-noise levels of efficiency (Willshaw and Dayan 1990), occur in proportion to the product of the probability of activity on afferent fibers (p) and the probability of sustained depolarization (activity) of their target cells (r). Assuming that discrete events are represented as spatiotemporal patterns of activity and inactivity and that a relatively sparse distributed code is used to maximize storage capacity (i.e., p is small), the proportion of synapses that will increase following an individual learning experience will likely be very small (proportional to $p \times r$). It follows that changes in population measures, such as field potentials, will prove difficult to detect. This experimental problem is also implicit in Marr's (1971) theory of hippocampus as a "simple-memory" because he arbitrarily assumes that the number of events that it can store is equal to the number of seconds in a day (about 10^5; see Willshaw and Buckingham 1990), and we should cautiously assume that an individual learning experience would be but a fraction of these. One way to get around these problems might be to record from individual cells, selecting only those responsive to relevant events at the outset of training, and to look for changes in the probability of cell firing after learning (see Rolls, this volume). This has the advantage that the magnitude of the change sought is now no longer the product of two small probabilities, but it suffers from the difficulty that changes in cell-firing can arise for reasons other than alterations in synaptic efficacy on a subset of excitatory afferents. The second reason why LTP-like changes may prove difficult to detect is that it is sometimes associated with heterosynaptic depression of synapses presynaptically inactive at the time of induction (Lynch et al. 1977; Levy and Steward 1979) or associative (homosynaptic) depression of afferents active out-of-phase with the conditioning tetani (Stanton and Sejnowski 1988). If either type of depression were also to occur during learning, it is likely that of the larger number (N) of afferents stimulated physiologically when probing for behavioral LTP, one subset ($n1$) would be potentiated, whereas another subset ($n2$) would be depressed. Long-term depression could effectively serve a normalizing function ensuring that

$$\sum_{i=1}^{N} w_i = \text{constant}$$

across successive learning episodes (where w_i is the synaptic weight of the ith terminal of a neuron with N terminals). Accordingly, like a microphone hung in the center of a crowded football stadium attempting to record individual conversations in the crowd, recordings of field potentials in vivo would fail to detect the rapidly shifting undercurrents of synaptic change that are going on as patterns of activity occur successively within the hippocampal matrix. Unit recordings may here prove more helpful because an LTP-induced increase in the capacity of the $n1$ connections to drive a single cell would be unaffected by down-regulation of the $n2$ connections.

Prediction 3: LTP should not be required for retrieval. Seeking whether LTP is involved in encoding, retrieval, or any other psychological process involved in memory is important for several reasons. First, Teyler and Discenna's (1986) hippocampal indexing theory seems to predict that saturation of LTP would impair retrieval of long-term memories held in the neocortex (because saturating LTP should disrupt the index of information in the hippocampus about the cortical loci of the long-term memories). Second, an involvement in encoding is central to the representational hypothesis because it provides the mechanism with which concrete stimuli and abstract associative relationships are linked. Third, blocking LTP pharmacologically may have different retrograde effects on spatial memory from those induced by ibotenate hippocampal lesions.

We have already seen that McNaughton et al. (1986) showed that rats given HF stimulation sufficient to

saturate LTP were as accurate as LF-stimulated rats in returning (during retraining) to the tunnel location used in pretraining. These findings are inconsistent with Teyler and Discenna's (1986) theory. However, blocking LTP by saturating synaptic weights may have different effects on hippocampal electrophysiology from the pharmacological blockade at baseline. Accordingly, a complimentary but more extensive study using APV has recently been conducted in my laboratory.

The effect of a drug on retrieval is usually investigated by training animals in its absence but later testing them without changing the behavioral procedure in its presence. This design suffers from the weakness that the lack of an effect on retrieval is revealed solely as a null result. The design may be extended by including other groups which, as in the McNaughton et al. (1986) study, are required to learn a reversal of the task trained initially. This extended design permits more rigorous comparison of encoding versus retrieval processes by providing both a second index of retrieval and confirmation that the same drug concentration is sufficient to impair new learning. Our implementation of this extended design involved giving rats initial training in the water maze until they were performing well at one trial per day (i.e., performance being dependent on retrieval from long-term memory). They were then implanted with minipumps containing either aCSF or 30 mM APV and divided into four groups, two of which had the hidden escape platform at the same location it had occupied during pretraining (Groups Same) and two of which had it in the opposite location (Groups Different, i.e., in NE if it had previously occupied SW or vice versa).

The crucial observations were what happened on the first trial of retraining and the immediately succeeding trials. As shown qualitatively in Figure 7, rats in

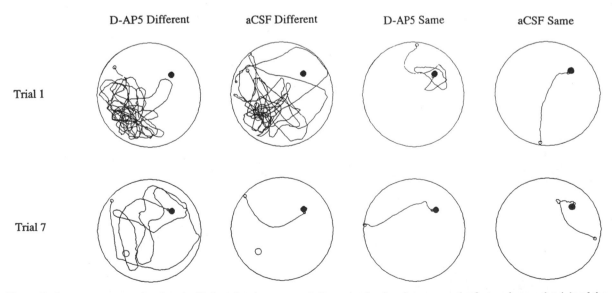

Figure 7. Storage versus retrieval study. Paths taken by representative animals of each group on the first and seventh trials of the drug phase. The escape platform was in SW during pretraining for the two Groups Different and in NE throughout the experiment for the Groups Same.

Groups Different swam persistently in the former location of the platform on the first trial of retraining, and their mean escape latency was consequently very high (82 ± 10 sec; no trial was allowed to exceed 120 sec). Importantly, the APV Different rats were as persistent in searching in the formerly correct location as the aCSF-Different rats. Rats in Groups Same swam directly to the platform on this trial, but there was some hint of inaccuracy by the APV-treated rats on this first trial as they approached the platform. By trial 7 of retraining, all groups were swimming accurately to the platform, except from Group APV Different. Its failure to learn the new platform location indicates that the drug concentration was indeed sufficient to impair new learning. Thus, as in the McNaughton et al. (1986) saturation study, the very same group of animals who failed to show a retrieval impairment (on trial 1 of retraining) did show a learning impairment as retraining proceeded. More formal analyses of both escape latency (Fig. 8) and spatial bias (data not shown) bear out these qualitative observations. For example, a quantitative index of spatial bias measuring the relative tendency of animals to visit the old (pretraining) platform location versus their tendency to visit the opposite one (i.e., new one for Groups Different) showed that all groups were equally biased to the old platform location on trial 1.

Once again, two radically different treatments, whose only obvious common consequence is to block LTP, each cause new learning impairments without impairing retrieval. This finding points to LTP being at least one of the mechanisms used by the hippocampus for building associative representations and storing information in long-term memory in cortex. It also has wider ramifications. Although earlier control studies ruled out the possibility of a gross disturbance of vision on the basis of the successful learning of a visual discrimination task by drug-treated rats (cf. Fox et al. 1989; Sillito et al. 1990), the present results render less likely the possibility of an even more subtle sensorimotor disturbance, such as an inability to see distal cues. APV-treated rats were just as likely as controls to approach the correct general vicinity of the pool on their first trial (i.e., prior to the effects of any retraining) and failed to show any disturbance when retraining was conducted with the platform in the same location as it had occupied in pretraining.

It is noteworthy that if the same type of experiment is conducted using ibotenate hippocampal lesioned rats, a very different result prevails (J.J. Bolhuis et al., in prep.). Specifically, even when the escape platform remains in the same location as it occupied during pretraining, lesioned rats show a severe impairment on the first postlesion trial, which continues (but lessens) throughout up to 24 trials of retraining (Fig. 9). Although this result is consistent with the idea that some long-term information storage could be in hippocampus, a closer analysis reveals that at least part of the deficit shown by hippocampal rats is due to their navigational (i.e., retrieval) deficit.

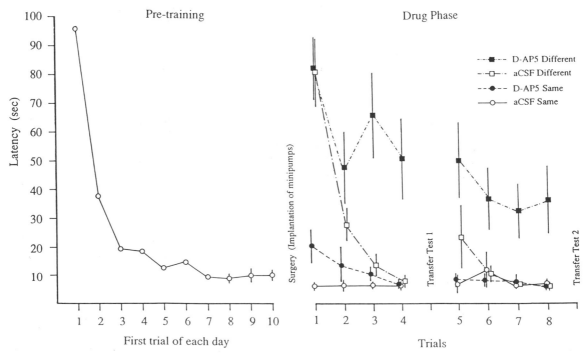

Figure 8. Storage versus retrieval study. Escape latency (sec $\pm$ 1 S.E.M.) during pretraining and drug phases. Note absence of deficit in the Group APV Same but the failure to learn a new platform location in Group APV Different.

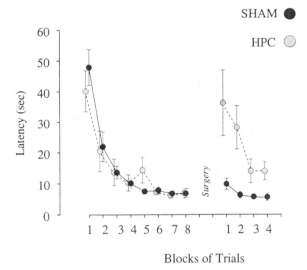

Figure 9. Ibotenate hippocampal lesions cause disruption of the retrieval of spatial information. After extensive spatial pretraining (8 blocks of 6 trials), sham-lesion and HPC groups were retrained to the same platform location. HPC-lesioned rats showed an initial impairment that ameliorated over trials.

CONCLUSION

In considering the idea that LTP could be involved in learning, it should not be overlooked that the hypothesis might have fallen at the first hurdle. It could have turned out that blocking LTP, whether pharmacologically or by physiological saturation to asymptote, would have failed to impair any type of learning. Alternatively, as proponents of the view that LTP has no special status in relationship to memory processing could equally argue, blocking LTP might impair learning but also impair a wide variety of other psychological processes. This latter assertion is harder to disprove, but evidence summarized above is barely consistent with such a position. Animals in whom LTP has been blocked in either of two ways can see, attend, move around in a coordinated way, and learn some but not other tasks. They can also retrieve information from long-term memory relevant for the performance of tasks that they can no longer learn. This profile of impairment is reasonably selective. Furthermore, it should be noted that several of the objections often raised to the idea that LTP could play a role in learning have been undermined by recent neurobiological research. To take one example, the apparent need for long trains of high-frequency afferent stimulation to induce LTP (which seems most unphysiological) is now recognized as a convenience rather than a necessity, following the discovery that LTP can be induced by pairing single afferent volleys with postsynaptic depolarization (Wigstrom et al. 1986). Similarly, recognition of the role and mechanisms of NMDA-receptor activation in LTP has suggested a new hypothesis concerning the functional significance of the hippocampal θ-rhythm (Larson and Lynch 1986; Pavlides et al. 1988;

Morris et al. 1990a). In short and on the basis of progress in both neuropsychological and neurobiological domains, I believe the burden of proof has now shifted away from concern about whether LTP plays a role in learning to the more analytical issue of how it participates in learning.

The representational hypothesis shown in this paper has been contrasted with one theory of memory consolidation (Laroche and Bloch 1982) which, although giving relevant prominence to distinguishing between active and inactive states of memory, ignores certain important neuropsychological distinctions. There is nothing in this theory to lead one to expect that blocking LTP would impair some types of learning but not others. It has also been contrasted with an indexing theory (Teyler and Discenna 1986) that, in my view, suffers conceptually from treating the brain as if it were a digital computer in requiring "addresses" to access information rather than as a system capable of recalling information associatively in a content addressable way. LTP is precisely the kind of synaptic process that a biologically realistic, distributed, associative memory requires to store information. In addition, Teyler and Discenna's (1986) hypothesis makes the incorrect prediction that saturating synaptic weights in hippocampus should cause retrograde amnesia. However, there is clearly one aspect of the representational hypothesis that goes well beyond currently available evidence. An explicit assertion of this paper has been that there are two fundamentally different kinds of associative learning. One is a simple process wherein reflexes are modulated, cues assume value, and behavioral dispositions are acquired. The other is a much more sophisticated process through which different kinds of logical relationships can be learned, information inferred or set in context, and ambiguities resolved. The central claim is that LTP is somehow crucial for the latter type of learning but unnecessary for the former. On the basis of this framework, it would be expected that limiting the representational demands of an erstwhile representational task should, as happens with hippocampal disruption (Eichenbaum et al. 1990), reduce the requirement for LTP activation during learning; that blocking LTP should disrupt context-dependent learning and certain conditional tasks; and that it might prevent an animal from reacting appropriately to reinforcer devaluation. Nearly 20 years ago, Bliss and Lomo (1973, p355) wondered ". . .whether or not the intact animal makes use in real life of a property which has been revealed by synchronous repetitive volleys to a population of fibres." The answer seems to be yes, but we clearly need a deeper understanding of precisely the kind of associative processes in which LTP participates.

ACKNOWLEDGMENTS

I am grateful to several colleagues for permission to refer to their experimental data in this paper, notably Johan Bolhuis, Steve Butcher, Sabrina Davis, Len Jarrard, Francoise Schenk, and Caroline Stewart. The work was supported by a Medical Research Council Program grant held by R.G.M.M. and D.J. Willshaw and by grants from the Wellcome Trust and the European Economic Community.

REFERENCES

Abraham, W.C. and E.W. Kairiss. 1988. Spontaneous complex spikes of hippocampal pyramidal cells are truncated by APV in urethane anaesthetised rats. *Neurosci. Lett.* **89:** 36.

Abraham, W.C. and S. Otani. 1990. Macromolecules and the maintenance of long-term potentiation. In *Kindling and synaptic plasticity: The legacy of Graham Goddard* (ed. F. Morrell), Birkhauser, Boston. (In press.)

Artola, A. and W. Singer. 1987. Long term potentiation and NMDA receptors in rat visual cortex. *Nature* **330:** 649.

Barnes, C.A. 1979. Memory deficits associated with senescence: A neurophysiological and behavioral study in the rat. *J. Comp. Physiol. Psychol.* **93:** 74.

———. 1988. Spatial learning and memory processes: The search for their neurobiological mechanisms in the rat. *Trends Neurosci.* **11:**163.

Bear, M.F., A. Kleinschmidt, Q. Gu, and W. Singer. 1990. Disruption of experience-dependent modifications in the striate-cortex by infusion of an NMDA receptor antagonist. *J. Neurosci.* **10:** 909.

Berger, T. and R. Sclabassi. 1988. Long term potentiation and its relation to hippocampal pyramidal cell activity and behavioural learning during classical conditioning. In *Long term potentiation: From biophysics to behavior* (ed. P.W. Landfield and S.A. Deadwyler), p. 467. A.R. Liss, New York.

Bliss, T.V.P. and A.R. Gardner-Medwin. 1973. Long lasting potentiation of synaptic transmission in the dentate area of the unanaesthetized rabbit following stimulation of the perforant path. *J. Physiol.* **232:** 357.

Bliss, T.V.P. and T. Lomo. 1973. Long lasting potentiation of synaptic transmission in the dentate area of the anaesthetized rabbit following stimulation of the perforant path. *J. Physiol.* **232:** 331.

Castro, C.A., L.H. Silbert, B.L. McNaughton, and C.A. Barnes. 1989. Recovery of spatial following decay of experimental saturation of LTE at perforant path synapses. *Nature* **342:** 545.

Collingridge, G.L., S.J. Kehl, and H. McLennan. 1983. Excitatory amino acids in synaptic transmission in the Schaffer collateral-commissural pathway of the rat hippocampus. *J. Physiol.* **334:** 33.

Dale, N. 1989. The role of NMDA receptors in synaptic integration and the organisation of complex neural patterns. In *The NMDA receptor* (ed. J.C. Watkins and G.L. Collingridge), p. 93. IRL Press, Oxford.

Daw, N., K. Fox, and N. Sato. 1990. The effect of varying stimulus intensity of NMDA-receptor activity in cat visual cortex. *J. Physiol.* **420:** 46P.

Dickinson, A. 1980. *Contemporary animal learning theory.* Cambridge University Press, Cambridge, England.

Eichenbaum, H., C. Stewart, and R.G.M. Morris. 1990. Hippocampal representation in place learning: The effects of fornix transection. *J. Neurosci.* (in press).

Fox, K., H. Sato, and N. Daw. 1989. The location and function of NMDA receptors in cat and kitten visual cortex. *J. Neurosci.* **9:** 2443.

Fox, S.E., S. Wolfson, and J.B. Ranck, Jr. 1986. Hippocampal theta rhythm and the firing of neurons in walking and urethane anaesthetised rats. *Exp. Brain Res.* **62:** 495.

Gaffan, D. and S. Harrison. 1989. Place memory and scene memory: Effects of fornix transection in the monkey. *Exp. Brain Res.* **74:** 202.

Green, F.J., B.L. McNaughton, and C.A. Barnes. 1990. Exploration-dependent modulation of evoked responses in fascia dentata: Dissociation of motor, EEG and sensory factors and evidence for a synaptic efficacy change. *J. Neurosci.* **10:** 1455.

Gustafsson, B., F. Asztely, E. Hanse, and H. Wigstrom. 1989. Onset characteristics of long-term potentiation in the guinea-pig hippocampal CA1 region *in vitro*. *Eur. J. Neurosci.* **1:** 382.

Harris, E.W., A.H. Ganong, and C.W. Cotman. 1984. Long-term potentiation in the hippocampus involves activation of N-methyl-D-aspartate receptors. *Brain Res.* **323:** 132.

Hargreaves, E.L., D.P. Cain, and C.H. Vanderwolf. 1990. Learning and behavioural long-term potentiation: Importance of controlling for motor activity. *J. Neurosci.* **10:** 1472.

Hawkins, R.D. 1989. A biologically realistic neural-network model for higher-order features of classical conditioning. In *Parallel distributed processing: Implications for psychology and neurobiology* (ed. R.G.M. Morris), p. 214. Clarendon Press, Oxford.

Jarrard, L.E. 1986. Selective hippocampal lesions and behaviour: Implications for current research and theorising. In *The hippocampus* (ed. R.L. Isaacson and K.H. Pribram), vol. 4, p. 93. Plenum Press, New York.

Kandel, E.R. and J.H. Schwartz. 1982. Molecular biology of learning: Modulation of transmitter release. *Science* **218:** 433.

Keith, J.R. and J.W. Rudy. 1990. Why NMDA receptor-dependent long-term potentiation may not be a mechanism of learning and memory: Reappraisal of the NMDA receptor blockade strategy. *Psychobiology* **18:** 251.

Kelso, S.R., A.H. Ganong, and T.H. Brown. 1986. Hebbian synapses in hippocampus. *Proc. Natl. Acad. Sci.* **83:** 5326.

Kleinschmidt, A., M.F. Bear, and W. Singer. 1987. Blockade of "NMDA" receptors disrupts experience-dependent plasticity of kitten striate cortex. *Science* **238:** 355.

Landfield, P. and S.A. Deadwyler. 1988. *Long term potentiation: From biophysics to behavior.* A.R. Liss, New York.

Laroche, S. and V. Bloch. 1982. Conditioning of hippocampal cells and long-term potentiation: An approach to mechanisms of post-trial memory facilitation. In *Neuronal plasticity and memory formation* (ed. C. Ajmone-Marsen and H. Matthies), p. 575. Raven Press, New York.

Laroche, S., M.L. Errington, M.A. Lynch, and T.V.P. Bliss. 1987. Increase in [³H]-glutamate release from slices of dentate gyrus and hippocampus following classical conditioning in the rat. *Behav. Brain Res.* **25:** 23.

Laroche, S., C. Redini-del Negro, M.P. Clements, and M.A. Lynch. 1990. Long term activation of phosphonoinositide turnover is associated with increased release of amino acids in the dentate gyrus and hippocampus following classical conditioning in the rat. *Eur. J. Neurosci.* **6:** 534.

Larson, J. and G. Lynch. 1986. Induction of synaptic potentiation in hippocampus by patterned stimulation involves two events. *Science* **232:** 985.

Leung, L.-W.S. and K.A. Desborough. 1988. APV, an N-methyl-D-aspartate receptor antagonist, blocks the hippocampal theta rhythm in behaving rats. *Brain Res.* **463:** 148.

Levy, W.B., Jr. and O. Steward. 1979. Synapses as associative memory elements in the hippocampal formation. *Brain Res.* **175:** 233.

Lynch, G. 1986. *Synapses, circuits and the beginnings of memory.* Bradford Books, MIT Press, Cambridge, Massachusetts.

Lynch, G., T. Dunwiddie, and V. Gribkoff. 1977. Heterosynaptic depression: A post-synaptic correlate of long-term potentiation. *Nature* **266:** 737.

Marr, D. 1971. Simple memory: A theory of archicortex. *Philos. Trans. R. Soc. Lond. B Biol. Sci.* **262:** 23.

McNaughton, B.L. 1983. Activity-dependent modulation of hippocampal efficacy: Some implications for memory processes. In *Neurobiology of the hippocampus* (ed. W. Siefert), p. 233. Academic Press, London.

———. 1989. Neuronal mechanisms for spatial computation and information storage. In *Neural connections, mental computations* (ed. L. Nadel et al.), p. 285. Bradford Books, MIT Press, Cambridge, Massachusetts.

McNaughton, B.L. and R.G.M. Morris. 1987. Hippocampal synaptic enhancement and information storage within a distributed memory system. *Trends Neurosci.* **10:** 408.

McNaughton, B.L., C.A. Barnes, G. Rao, J. Baldwin, and M. Rasmussen. 1986. Long-term enhancement of hippocampal synaptic transmission and the acquisition of spatial information. *J. Neurosci.* **6:** 563.

Mishkin, M. 1982. A memory system in the monkey. *Philos. Trans. R. Soc. Lond. B Biol. Sci.* **298:** 85.

Monaghan, D.T. and C.W. Cotman. 1985. Distribution of *N*-methyl-*D*-aspartate sensitive L-[³H]-glutamate binding sites in rat brain. *J. Neurosci.* **5:** 2909.

Mondadori, C., L. Weiskrantz, H. Buerki, F. Petschke, and G.E. Fagg. 1989. NMDA receptor antagonists can enhance or impair learning performance in animals. *Exp. Brain Res.* **75:** 449.

Morris, R.G.M. 1981. Place navigation does not depend on the presence of local cues. *Learn. Motiv.* **12:** 239.

———. 1989. Synaptic plasticity and learning: Selective impairment of learning in rats and blockade of long term potentiation in vivo by the *N*-methyl-*D*-aspartate receptor antagonist AP5. *J. Neurosci.* **9:** 3040.

———. 1990. Synaptic plasticity, neural architecture and forms of learning. In *Brain organisation and memory: Cells, systems and circuits* (ed. J.L. McGaugh et al.). Oxford University Press, New York. (In press.)

Morris, R.G.M., S. Davis, and S.P. Butcher. 1990a. Hippocampal synaptic plasticity and NMDA receptors: A role in information storage? *Philos. Trans. R. Soc. Lond. B Biol. Sci.* **329:** 187.

Morris, R.G.M., J.J. Hagan, and J.N.P. Rawlins. 1986a. Allocentric spatial learning by hippocampectomised rats: A further attempt to dissociate the "spatial mapping" and "working memory" theories of hippocampal function. *Q. J. Exp. Psychol.* **38B:** 365.

Morris, R.G.M., R.F. Halliwell, and N. Bowery. 1989. Synaptic plasticity and learning. II. Do different kinds of plasticity underly different kinds of learning? *Neuropsychologia* **27:** 41.

Morris, R.G.M., E. Anderson, G.S. Lynch, and M. Baudry. 1986b. Selective impairment of learning and blockade of long term potentiation by an *N*-methyl-*D*-aspartate receptor antagonist, AP5. *Nature* **319:** 774.

Morris, R.G.M., F. Schenk, F. Tweedie, and L.E. Jarrard. 1990b. Dissociation between components of spatial learning following ibotenic acid lesions of hippocampus and/or subiculum. *Eur. J. Neurosci.* (in press).

O'Keefe, J. 1979. A review of the hippocampal place cells. *Prog. Neurobiol.* **13:** 419.

O'Keefe, J. and L. Nadel. 1978. *The hippocampus as a cognitive map.* Oxford University Press, Oxford.

Olton, D.S. and R.J. Samuelson. 1976. Remembrance of places passed: Spatial memory in rats. *J. Exp. Psychol. Anim. Behav. Processes* **2:** 97.

Pavlides, C., Y.J. Greenstein, M. Grudman, and J. Winson. 1988. Long-term potentiation in the dentate gyrus is induced preferentially on the positive phase of theta rhythm. *Brain Res.* **439:** 383.

Racine, R.J., N.W. Milgram, and S. Hafner. 1983. Long-term potentiation phenomena in the rat limbic forebrain. *Brain Res.* **260:** 217.

Reid, I.C. and R.G.M. Morris. 1990. NMDA receptors and learning: A framework for classifying some recent studies. *Fidia Res. Found. Symp. Ser.* (in press).

Rescorla, R.A. 1988. Behavioral studies of Pavlovian conditioning. *Annu. Rev. Neurosci.* **11:** 329.

Rose, G.M. and T.V. Dunwiddie. 1986. Induction of hippocampal long-term potentiation using physiologically patterned stimulation. *Neurosci. Lett.* **69:** 244.

Shallice, T. 1989. *From neuropsychology to mental structure.* Cambridge University Press, Cambridge, England.

Sharp, P., B.L. McNaughton, and C.A. Barnes. 1985. Enhancement of hippocampal field potentials in rats exposed to a novel complex environment. *Brain Res.* **339:** 361.

———. 1989. Exploration-dependent modulation of evoked responses in fascia dentata: Fundamental observations and time course. *Psychobiology* **17:** 257.

Sillito, A., P.C. Murphy, T.E. Salt, and C.I. Moody. 1990. The dependence of retino-geniculate transmission in the cat on NMDA receptors. *J. Neurophysiol.* **63:** 347.

Singer, W. 1990. Ontogenetic self-organization and learning. In *Brain organization and memory: Cells, systems and circuits* (ed. J.L. McGaugh et al.), p. 211. Oxford University Press, New York.

Stanton, P. and T.J. Sejnowski. 1988. Associative long term depression in the hippocampus induced by hebbian covariance. *Nature* **339:** 215.

Teyler, T.J. and P. Discenna. 1986. The hippocampal memory indexing theory. *Behav. Neurosci.* **100:** 147.

Weiskrantz, L. 1968. Some traps and pontifications. In *Analysis of behavioural change* (ed. L. Weiskrantz), p. 415. Harper and Row, New York.

Weisz, D.J., G.A. Clark, and R.F. Thompson. 1984. Increased responsivity of dentate granule cells during nictitating membrane response conditioning in rabbit. *Behav. Brain Res.* **12:** 145.

Wigstrom, H., B. Gustafsson, Y.-Y. Huang, and W.C. Abraham. 1986. Hippocampal long-lasting potentiation is induced by pairing single afferent volleys with intracellularly injected depolarising current phases. *Acta Physiol. Scand.* **126:** 317.

Willshaw, D.J. and J. Buckingham. 1990. An assessment of Marr's theory of hippocampus. *Philos. Trans. R. Soc. Lond. B Biol. Sci.* **329:** 205.

Willshaw, D.J. and P. Dayan. 1990. Optimal plasticity from matrix memories: What goes up must come down. *Neural Computat.* **2:** 85.

Neuronal and Network Determinants of Simple and Higher-order Features of Associative Learning: Experimental and Modeling Approaches

J.H. BYRNE, D.A. BAXTER, D.V. BUONOMANO, AND J.L. RAYMOND
Department of Neurobiology and Anatomy, The University of Texas Medical School, Houston, Texas 77225

One of the fundamental problems in neurobiology is to understand events occurring within individual neurons and within neural networks that contribute to learning and memory. An equally important and related problem is to discover what the mechanistic relationships are between different forms of learning. Two approaches, one empirical and the other modeling, are currently being used to examine these problems. The empirical approach involves examining a particular behavior that is modified by learning, finding the neural circuit producing the behavior, determining in what ways neurons within the circuit are modified by learning, and identifying the cellular and subcellular processes underlying the neuronal plasticity (see Byrne 1987). The modeling approach involves formulating mathematical descriptions of the proposed cellular mechanisms and neural circuits and examining whether simulations of the resultant model can account for features of the plasticity and of the behavior (see Byrne and Berry 1989; Hawkins and Bower 1989). Neither approach is exclusive of the other. Indeed, each approach benefits from insights provided by the other.

In this paper, we summarize some of our initial attempts to apply a combination of empirical and modeling approaches to extend our understanding of the mechanisms of and relationships between several forms of associative learning in *Aplysia*. The most extensive empirical studies of learning in *Aplysia* have focused on two defensive behaviors, the siphon-withdrawal and the tail-withdrawal reflexes. The synaptic connections between the sensory and motor neurons that mediate these reflexes exhibit a number of plastic properties, which in turn can be related to nonassociative and associative learning (see Kandel and Schwartz 1982; Byrne 1987). Previously, we developed a single-cell mathematical model of these sensory neurons (Gingrich and Byrne 1985, 1987; Gingrich et al. 1988). This single-cell model accurately simulates many aspects of empirically observed neuronal plasticity that contribute to simple forms of nonassociative and associative learning. In the present study, derivatives of this single-cell model are incorporated into two relatively simple neural networks, and the ability of these networks to simulate features of associative learning is examined. A three-cell network successfully simulates the features of two higher-order examples of classical conditioning, specifically, second-order conditioning and blocking. A six-cell network successfully simulates several features of operant conditioning, including sensitivity to the contingency, intensity, and delay of reinforcement, reversal learning, and extinction. These results illustrate that the same neuronal plasticity that underlies simple forms of classical conditioning can, at least in theory, also underlie higher-order features of classical conditioning and operant conditioning.

Single-cell Model for Simple Forms of Learning

Our current understanding of the various biochemical and biophysical mechanisms that contribute to plasticity within the sensory neurons of *Aplysia* has allowed the development of formal descriptions of these processes. The approach has been to transform these processes into mathematical formalisms, assign values to the parameters that agree with published data, and fit the components together to create a model of transmitter release at the sensory-to-motor synapse. The details of this single-cell model have been described previously (Gingrich and Byrne 1985, 1987; Gingrich et al. 1988; Byrne and Gingrich 1989; Byrne et al. 1989). The general features of the single-cell model are illustrated in Figure 1A and discussed below.

Release, storage, and mobilization of transmitter. The model contains differential equations describing two pools of transmitter, a readily releasable pool (P_R) and a storage pool (P_S). The releasable pool contains vesicles that are in close proximity to release sites. During a simulated action potential, an influx of Ca^{++} (I_{Ca}) through voltage-dependent Ca^{++} channels causes the release of transmitter (T_R) from this pool. Thus, the amount of transmitter released is a function of both the dynamics of Ca^{++} influx and the number of vesicles in the releasable pool. As a consequence of release, P_R is depleted. Depletion of transmitter is a cellular mechanism contributing to synaptic depression, which is a neuronal correlate of habituation (Castellucci et al. 1970; Byrne 1982). To offset depletion, transmitter is delivered (mobilized) from a storage pool to the releasable pool. Vesicles move from one pool to the other via three fluxes, one driven by diffusion (F_D), another driven by Ca^{++} (F_C), and the third driven by levels of cAMP (F_{cAMP}). The storage pool is replenished by synthesis of new vesicles (flux F_N). Mobilization of

A

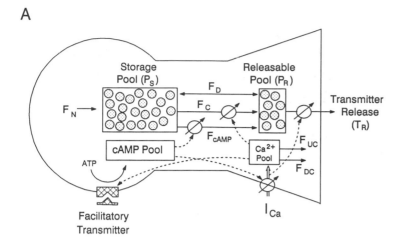

B

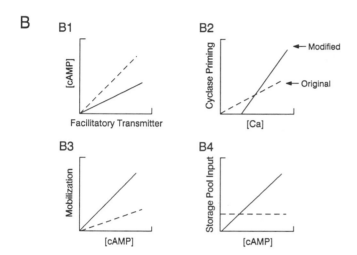

Figure 1. Single-cell model for nonassociative and associative learning. (*A*) Components of a single-cell model for learning that reflect the properties of sensory neurons in *Aplysia*. The circles with arrows through their centers represent elements of the model that are modulated positively by other variables. See text for details. (*B*) Properties of the original single-cell model were modified for simulations of second-order conditioning and blocking in the present study. See text for details. Unless otherwise noted, all equations and parameters are as described by Gingrich and Byrne (1985, 1987).

transmitter has been described as one of the cellular mechanisms contributing to presynaptic facilitation in sensory neurons (Gingrich and Byrne 1985; Hochner et al. 1986a,b; Gingrich et al. 1988; Bhara et al. 1990), which is a neuronal correlate of sensitization and dishabituation (Carew et al. 1971; Walters et al. 1983). A second mechanism contributing to presynaptic facilitation is spike broadening (see below).

Regulation of Ca^{++}. The influx of Ca^{++} during simulated action potentials leads to the release of transmitter and accumulation of intracellular Ca^{++}. The pool of intracellular Ca^{++} is contained in two volumes (not shown): the submembrane compartment, which represents a thin layer of the cytosol immediately adjacent to the membrane, and the interior compartment, which represents a larger fraction of the cytosol further away from the membrane. The Ca^{++} within the submembrane compartment regulates the release of transmitter, whereas the Ca^{++} within the interior compartment contributes to the regulation of mobilization and to the regulation of cAMP synthesis (see below). Two

fluxes remove Ca^{++} from the interior compartment; one represents active buffering of Ca^{++} by organelles (F_{UC}), and one represents diffusion of Ca^{++} into an innermost compartment that serves as a Ca^{++} sink (F_{DC}).

Regulation of cAMP. The model also includes equations describing the concentration of cAMP and its effects on the release of transmitter. Facilitatory transmitters activate adenylate cyclase (Bernier et al. 1982; Ocorr and Byrne 1985; Ocorr et al. 1985), which leads to increased synthesis of cAMP. Increased levels of cAMP contribute to an increase in the duration of the action potential (Klein et al. 1982; Baxter and Byrne 1990), which results in an increase in the influx of Ca^{++}, and hence, an increase in the release of transmitter.

Empirical results indicate that the activity of adenylate cyclase is also regulated by intracellular levels of Ca^{++} (Ocorr et al. 1985; Abrams and Kandel 1988; Eliot et al. 1989). In the model, an influx of Ca^{++} during spikes that precede the facilitatory transmitter primes the cyclase and amplifies the subsequent stimulation of cAMP synthesis by the facilitatory transmitter. Thus, convergence at adenylate cyclase of the Ca^{++} signal and the facilitatory transmitter results in an associative amplification of the synthesis of cAMP, which in turn leads to an enhancement of presynaptic facilitation. This associative form of neuronal plasticity is termed activity-dependent neuromodulation and is believed to be a neuronal correlate of classical conditioning in *Aplysia* (Hawkins et al. 1983; Walters and Byrne 1983; Buonomano and Byrne 1990).

Simulations of Higher-order Features of Classical Conditioning

Little is known about the neural mechanisms responsible for higher-order forms of classical conditioning. Hawkins and Kandel (1984), however, illustrated in a theoretical paper how the neural circuit and cellular mechanisms that underlie simple forms of nonassociative learning and classical conditioning in *Aplysia* could also account for some higher-order features of classical conditioning such as second-order conditioning and blocking. Although these two features have not been examined behaviorally in *Aplysia*, we examined the ability of the single-cell model to simulate these two higher-order features of classical conditioning when incorporated into an appropriate neural circuit.

Figure 2A illustrates a simplified schematic of the type of neural circuit that mediates the defensive withdrawal reflexes in *Aplysia* and helps to illustrate how associative plasticity in sensory neurons is related to differential classical conditioning. In a differential classical conditioning paradigm, there are two conditioned stimuli (CS1 and CS2). Initially, the two sensory neurons (SN1 and SN2), which constitute the pathways for the conditioned stimuli, make weak, subthreshold connections to a response system (e.g., a motor neuron, MN). Delivering a reinforcing or unconditioned stimulus (US) alone has two effects. First, the US activates the response system and produces the unconditioned response (UR). Second, the US activates a diffuse modulatory system (e.g., a facilitatory neuron, FN) that nonspecifically enhances the release of transmitter from all of the sensory neurons. This nonspecific presynaptic facilitation contributes to sensitization in *Aplysia* (see Kandel and Schwartz 1982). Temporal specificity, a characteristic of associative learning, occurs when there is pairing of a conditioned stimulus, spike activity in sensory neuron 1 ($CS1^+$), with the US. This pairing causes a selective amplification of the modulatory effects in that specific sensory neuron via activity-dependent neuromodulation. Unpaired activity does not amplify the effects of the US in sensory neuron 2 ($CS2^-$) because the intracellular levels of Ca^{++} are low at the time of the US. The amplification of the modulatory effects in the paired sensory neuron leads to an enhancement of the ability of sensory neuron 1 to activate the response system and produce the conditioned response (CR).

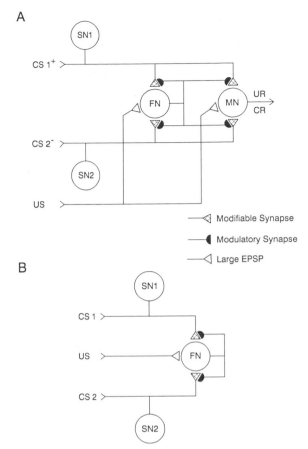

Figure 2. Simplified schematics of the type of neural circuit that mediates defensive withdrawal reflexes in *Aplysia*. (*A*) Sensory neurons (SN1 and SN2) make excitatory monosynaptic connections onto a motor neuron (MN). In addition, the sensory neurons make synaptic connections with a facilitatory neuron (FN) that feeds back onto the sensory neurons and presynaptically facilitates transmitter release from the sensory neurons. (*B*) Three-cell neural network used to simulate higher-order features of classical conditioning.

A critical feature of this circuit is that the modulatory input not only enhances the connections from the sensory neurons to the motor neuron, but also enhances the connections between the sensory neurons and the facilitatory neuron. This has two consequences, one practical and the other theoretical. First, from a practical point of view, the circuit can be simplified by eliminating the motor neuron (Fig. 2B) and using the excitatory postsynaptic potentials (EPSPs) in the facilitatory neuron as a measure of synaptic plasticity. Second, from a theoretical point of view, a sensory neuron whose EPSP is enhanced by conditioning can "take control" of the facilitatory neuron. This possibility has fundamental implications with respect to neural models of second-order conditioning and blocking.

To simulate second-order conditioning and blocking, the single-cell model has been incorporated into the three-cell network shown in Figure 2B. Two model sensory neurons (SN1 and SN2) with identical properties make synaptic contact with a facilitatory neuron (FN). Activity in the individual sensory neurons represents separate pathways for conditioned stimuli (CS1 and CS2). The transmitter released from each sensory neuron produces excitatory conductance changes in the facilitatory neuron. The facilitatory neuron feeds back onto the sensory neurons, providing modulatory output in response to either the US or suprathreshold stimulation from the sensory neurons.

Properties of the network elements. In the present study, three properties of the single-cell model are modified from those originally described by Gingrich and Byrne (1985, 1987) (Fig. 1B). First, the magnitude of associative plasticity is increased by decreasing the Ca^{++}-independent cAMP synthesis (Fig. 1B1) and increasing the Ca^{++}-dependent cAMP synthesis (Fig. 1B2). Second, a threshold is introduced that intracellular levels of Ca^{++} must surpass before Ca^{++} can prime adenylate cyclase (Fig. 1B2). Third, the cAMP-dependent mobilization is enhanced by increasing the cAMP-dependent flux of transmitter (Fig. 1B3) and by making the flux of transmitter into the storage pool sensitive to the levels of cAMP (Fig. 1B4).

Because there are few experimental data on the properties of the facilitatory neuron, it is modeled as an element that sums its synaptic inputs and initiates a burst of action potentials if that sum equals or exceeds a threshold (for specific details, see Buonomano et al.

1990). The duration of the burst is a linear function of the time period that the input to the facilitatory neuron remains above threshold. The presentation of the US always produces a strong input to the facilitatory neuron that stimulates the release of the facilitatory transmitter, which in turn activates adenylate cyclase in the sensory neuron. As suggested by Hawkins and Kandel (1984), an important assumed property of the facilitatory neuron is that its output diminishes or accommodates rapidly (within the duration of the US), and that the recovery from accommodation is relatively slow.

Simulations of second-order conditioning. The defining feature of second-order conditioning is that a conditioned stimulus (CS1) can come to function as a reinforcing stimulus for the conditioning of a second conditioned stimulus (CS2) (see Rescorla 1988). As illustrated in Figure 3A, the training paradigm for second-order conditioning proceeds in two phases. During phase I, CS1 is paired with the US at an optimal interstimulus interval (interval between the onset of the CS and onset of the US; ISI) for associative conditioning, whereas CS2 is presented unpaired with the US (the 15-sec ISI does not lead to any associative increase in the strength of CS2). During phase II, the presentation of the US is terminated, and CS2 is paired with

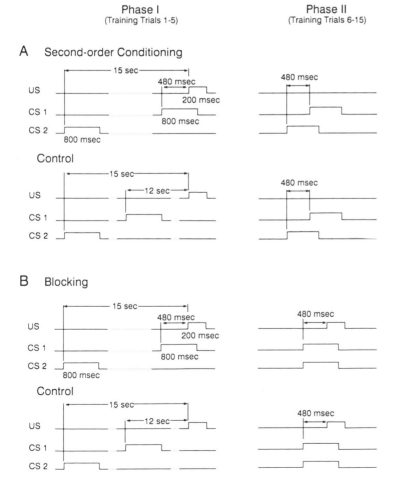

Figure 3. Stimulation paradigms for simulating second-order conditioning and blocking. (A) Second-order conditioning. During phase I of second-order conditioning, CS1 (spike activity in SN1) is temporally paired with the US, while CS2 is presented in an unpaired fashion. During phase II, CS2 is paired with CS1 in the absence of any US. The control paradigm for second-order conditioning is similar to the experimental paradigm, except that both CS1 and CS2 are presented unpaired with the US during phase I. (*B*) Blocking. During phase I of blocking, CS1 is paired with the US and CS2 is presented unpaired with the US. During phase II, both CS1 and CS2 are presented simultaneously and paired with the US. The control paradigm for blocking is similar to the experimental paradigm except that during phase I, CS1 is presented unpaired with the US. In all simulations, each CS consists of an 800-msec train of spikes at 25 Hz in the modeled sensory neurons, the US is a 200-msec, suprathreshold activation of the facilitatory neuron, and the intertrial interval is 5 min.

CS1. The critical question is whether the previously conditioned CS1 will act as a secondary reinforcer for CS2. If this is the case, then CS2 should undergo associative enhancement during phase II of second-order conditioning. In phase I of the control paradigm, both CS1 and CS2 are presented unpaired with the US, whereas in phase II, CS1 and CS2 are paired as above. Second-order conditioning should only occur if CS1 has been paired previously with the US; thus, during phase II of the control paradigm, there should be no associative enhancement of CS2.

Figure 4 illustrates a simulation of second-order conditioning. The amplitudes of the EPSPs at the sensory-to-facilitatory neuron synapses are plotted in Part A. During phase I, the synaptic strength of the CS1 cell (SN1) undergoes associative enhancement and increases dramatically. Because the CS1 cell is paired with the US during phase I, this associative enhancement represents first-order classical conditioning. In contrast, the synaptic strength of the CS2 cell (SN2), which is not paired with the US, does not change significantly. During phase II, the presentation of the US is terminated, and activity in the CS2 cell is paired with activity in the CS1 cell. The synaptic strength of

the CS2 cell is enhanced during phase II. As illustrated by the control paradigm, if activity in the CS1 cell is unpaired with the US during phase I, there is no enhancement of the CS2 cell during phase II of the control paradigm. In other words, the prior conditioning of the CS1 cell during phase I allows it to act as a secondary reinforcer and to induce an associative enhancement in the synaptic strength of the CS2 cell. Thus, the increase of the synaptic strength of the CS2 cell during phase II is a simulation of an example of second-order conditioning.

Details of how the synaptic outputs of the two sensory neurons and the facilitatory neuron change during the simulation of second-order conditioning are shown in Part B of Figure 4. At the start of training (trial 1), the facilitatory neuron is active only during the presentation of the US. Initially, the EPSPs from both the CS1 cell (EPSP 1) and the CS2 cell (EPSP 2) are too weak to activate the facilitatory neuron. However, because the CS1 cell is paired with US, the amplitude of EPSP 1 undergoes significant associative enhancement, and eventually EPSP 1 surpasses the threshold for activating the facilitatory neuron (trial 5). In subsequent trials (e.g., trials 6 and 10), the CS1 cell stimulates the

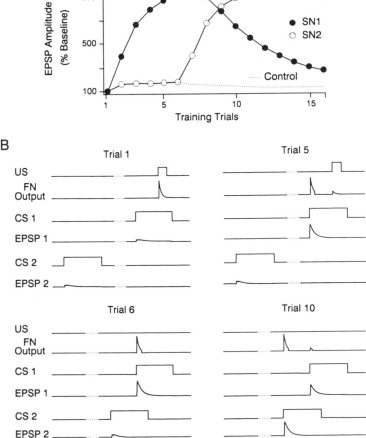

Figure 4. Simulation of second-order conditioning. (*A*) Second-order conditioning of transmitter release. The baseline values of the EPSPs produced by the CS cells are normalized to 100%. During first-order conditioning (phase I, trials 1–5), only the CS1 cell (SN1) shows a significant increase in strength. During phase II (trials 6–15), the EPSPs produced by CS2 exhibit an increase in strength due to second-order conditioning. During phase I of the control paradigm, neither CS cell exhibits an increase in strength. Phase II of the control paradigm (dotted line) illustrates that without preconditioning of CS1 no associative plasticity is observed in the CS2 cell. (*B*) Stimuli and synaptic outputs of network elements during second-order conditioning. The outputs of the sensory neurons and facilitatory neuron are plotted at various points during training. Initially, neither CS cell is strong enough to activate the facilitatory neuron, which is activated only by the US (trial 1). By the end of phase I, CS1 is able to activate the facilitatory neuron (trial 5). The CS1 cell can now function as a reinforcing stimulus for the CS2 cell by activating the facilitatory neuron (trial 6), and EPSP 2 undergoes associative enhancement (trial 10). Note that the duration of the CS outlasts the actual duration of the EPSPs. This is due to synaptic depression. In addition, the output of the facilitatory neuron decreases during the US. This is due to accommodation. The facilitatory neuron recovers from accommodation within about 30 sec.

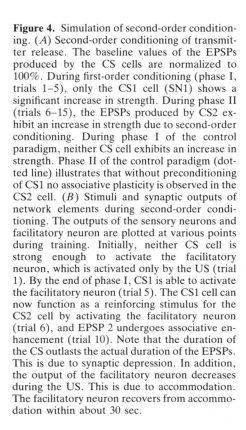

facilitatory neuron, and thus functions as a secondary reinforcer for the CS2 cell. Because of the secondary reinforcement provided by the CS1 cell, the amplitude of EPSP 2 undergoes significant associative enhancement, even though no US is explicitly presented during that phase of training. In this model, second-order conditioning results directly from the ability of a previously conditioned CS to take control of the facilitatory neuron and thus serve as a secondary reinforcer to another CS in the absence of a US.

Simulations of blocking. Blocking is a phenomenon in which previous conditioning of a conditioned stimulus (CS1) can decrease or block subsequent conditioning of a second conditioned stimulus (CS2) presented as part of the compound stimulus (CS1/CS2). A blocking paradigm consists of two phases (Fig. 3B) (see Rescorla 1988). During phase I, CS1 is paired with the US, while CS2 is presented unpaired with the US. During phase II, CS1 and CS2 are activated simultaneously, and this compound (CS1/CS2) is paired with the US. If blocking occurs, then prior conditioning of CS1 should prevent the associative enhancement of CS2 during phase II even though CS2 is paired with a

US. The expected or control level of associative enhancement of CS2 can be determined by activating both CS1 and CS2 in an unpaired fashion with the US during phase I and presenting the compound CS1/CS2 paired with the US in phase II.

Figure 5 illustrates a simulation of blocking. During phase I, the synaptic strength of the CS1 cell (SN1) increases, whereas the synaptic strength of the CS2 cell (SN2) does not change. During phase II, the compound CS1/CS2 is paired with the US. Although the CS2 cell is paired with the US during phase II, the synaptic strength of the CS2 cell does not increase. The control paradigm illustrates that enhancement of the CS2 cell (SN2) does occur if the CS1 cell (SN1) has not been paired previously with the US. Thus, the prior conditioning of the CS1 cell completely blocks associative enhancement of the CS2 cell.

Details of how the synaptic outputs of the two sensory neurons and the facilitatory neuron change during the simulation of blocking are shown in Figure 5B. Initially (trial 1), EPSP 1 and EPSP 2 are weak, and the facilitatory neuron is activated only by the US. As the CS1 cell undergoes enhancement (trial 5), EPSP 1 becomes large enough to activate the facilitatory

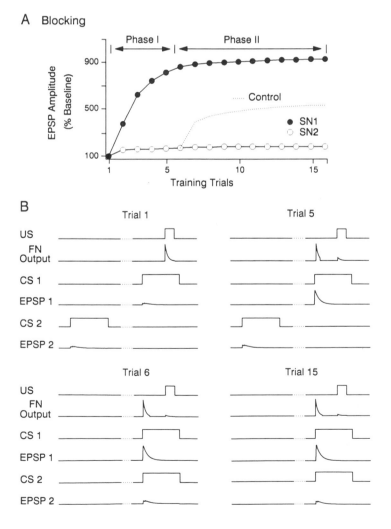

Figure 5. Simulation of blocking. (*A*) Blocking of associative enhancement of transmitter release. During phase I (trials 1–5), the CS1 cell exhibits first-order conditioning and the CS2 cell remains essentially unchanged. During phase II (trials 6–15), associative plasticity in the CS2 cell is blocked and the synaptic strength of the CS2 cell remains unchanged. (*B*) Stimuli and synaptic outputs of network elements during blocking. The output of the sensory neurons and facilitatory neuron are shown during different training trials. Initially, neither CS cell is strong enough to activate the facilitatory neuron, which is activated only by the US (trial 1). After first-order conditioning (trial 5), EPSP 1 can activate the facilitatory neuron but is not strong enough to fully accommodate it. During trial 6, both the CS1 and CS2 cells are activated simultaneously and their summed output activates the facilitatory neuron and more completely accommodates it. Thus, during the US, the output of facilitatory neuron is insignificant, and associative plasticity in the CS2 cell is completely blocked.

neuron. There are two important consequences of this CS1-induced activity in the facilitatory neuron. First, due to accommodation, the output of the facilitatory neuron in response to the actual US becomes insignificant (e.g., trials 6 and 10). Second, during the compound CS1/CS2 stimulus, the facilitatory neuron is activated almost immediately after the onset of CS2, rather than 480 msec after onset, which is the optimal ISI for associative plasticity. (The ISI function for associative plasticity in the single-cell model is directly related to the dynamics of intracellular levels of Ca^{++} [Gingrich and Byrne 1987].) An aspect of blocking for which it is difficult to account is the fact that while the CS2 cell undergoes little or no associative plasticity, associative plasticity in the CS1 cell must continue in order to prevent extinction. In our model, this property emerges because the CS1 cell has broader action potentials that permit a greater influx of Ca^{++}, which is necessary for associative plasticity. In contrast, the CS2 cell does not have enough of an influx of Ca^{++} to induce associative plasticity during the activation of the facilitatory neuron (Buonomano et al. 1990). Thus, the detailed description of subcellular processes can unmask phenomena relevant to the simulation of blocking that are not captured by less detailed models.

It is interesting to note that the single-cell model as originally described by Gingrich and Byrne (1985, 1987), when incorporated into this circuit, can simulate second-order conditioning but only partial blocking (Byrne et al. 1988; Buonomano et al. 1990). Blocking is only partial, in part, because the ISI function of the original single-cell model predicts some associative conditioning at an ISI of 0 msec (Gingrich and Byrne 1987), whereas the Ca^{++} threshold of the modified model prevents associative conditioning at an ISI of 0 msec (Buonomano et al. 1990). As an alternative to modifying the original single-cell model, complete blocking can be simulated by incorporating inhibitory neurons into the neural circuit (Buonomano et al. 1990). Experimental evidence indicates that the US stimulates not only facilitatory neurons, but also inhibitory neurons (Mackey et al. 1987; Buonomano et al. 1988), and the modeling studies suggest that this inhibition could contribute to blocking.

Simulations of Elementary Features of Operant Conditioning

Another type of associative learning that has been studied experimentally in *Aplysia* is operant conditioning. Classical conditioning and operant conditioning have been distinguished in terms of the paradigms that govern the presentation of the reinforcing stimuli (see Mackintosh 1974). In classical conditioning, presentation of the reinforcing stimulus (the US) is contingent on the presentation of another stimulus (the CS). This contingency is independent of the behavior of the animal. In contrast, during operant conditioning, presentation of the reinforcement is contingent on the performance of a particular behavior (the operant) by

the animal. Thus, during operant conditioning, the animal has the opportunity to control the delivery of reinforcement. Despite operational distinctions, it is not known whether the cellular processes underlying classical conditioning and operant conditioning are fundamentally different or whether these forms of learning may share at least some aspects of a common underlying mechanism. One method of addressing this issue is to construct computational models of neural circuits containing elements whose properties reflect the cellular mechanisms contributing to a form of associative plasticity that is believed to underlie classical conditioning, and to test whether this form of associative plasticity can, at least in theory, also underlie operant conditioning.

The most extensive empirical studies of operant conditioning in *Aplysia* have focused on head-waving behavior (Cook and Carew 1986, 1988, 1989a,b,c,d; Baxter et al. 1990). Head-waving is a naturally occurring behavior in which animals sweep their heads from side to side to probe their environment. Following operant conditioning, animals significantly increase the amount of time they spend head-waving to one side compared to their baseline performance. The analysis of operant conditioning of head-waving is being extended to the cellular level by examining operant modification of the activity of individual motor neurons that innervate the neck muscles (Cook and Carew 1988; Baxter et al. 1990). Thus, *Aplysia* are capable of expressing operant conditioning of head-waving at the level of intact behavior and at the level of individual central motor neurons.

Although the neuronal elements and circuit underlying head-waving behavior are not known, the artificial neural network shown in Figure 6A simulates an oscillatory pattern of behavior similar to the side-to-side movement of head-waving. The neural network contains three types of elements: pattern-generating elements (PGs), associative elements (AEs), and motor neurons (MNs). Two spontaneously active and mutually inhibitory neurons comprise the central pattern generator that initiates the spontaneous behavior within the network (output A or output B), which serves as the target of operant training.

The neurons of the pattern generator are modeled as having essentially four membrane currents: two types of Ca^{++} current, a voltage-gated K^+ current, and an inhibitory synaptic current. One of the Ca^{++} currents has a low threshold of activation and is activated at the resting potential. This low-threshold Ca^{++} current depolarizes the membrane potential toward threshold and thus drives spontaneous spike activity in the neurons of the pattern generator. The simulated spikes activate the voltage-gated K^+ current, which produces an afterhyperpolarization following each spike. The low-threshold Ca^{++} current undergoes Ca^{++}-dependent inactivation, such that as intracellular Ca^{++} accumulates, this Ca^{++} current decreases gradually, thereby slowing the spontaneous activity. During the spontaneous activity, the second Ca^{++} current, a voltage-

A

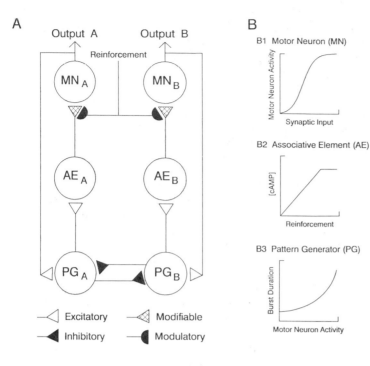

Output A   Output B

Reinforcement

MN$_A$ MN$_B$

AE$_A$ AE$_B$

PG$_A$ PG$_B$

◁— Excitatory   ◬— Modifiable

◀— Inhibitory   ◖— Modulatory

B

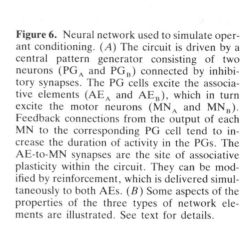

B1 Motor Neuron (MN)

Motor Neuron Activity

Synaptic Input

B2 Associative Element (AE)

[cAMP]

Reinforcement

B3 Pattern Generator (PG)

Burst Duration

Motor Neuron Activity

Figure 6. Neural network used to simulate operant conditioning. (*A*) The circuit is driven by a central pattern generator consisting of two neurons (PG$_A$ and PG$_B$) connected by inhibitory synapses. The PG cells excite the associative elements (AE$_A$ and AE$_B$), which in turn excite the motor neurons (MN$_A$ and MN$_B$). Feedback connections from the output of each MN to the corresponding PG cell tend to increase the duration of activity in the PGs. The AE-to-MN synapses are the site of associative plasticity within the circuit. They can be modified by reinforcement, which is delivered simultaneously to both AEs. (*B*) Some aspects of the properties of the three types of network elements are illustrated. See text for details.

gated Ca^{++} current, is also activated and contributes to the accumulation of intracellular Ca^{++}. Thus, the voltage-gated Ca^{++} current indirectly contributes to the slowing of spontaneous activity. The inhibitory synaptic current originates from the contralateral neuron in the pattern generator. The inhibitory synapses allow only one neuron of the pattern generator to be active at a time. Thus, when pattern-generating element A (PG$_A$) is active, it inhibits activity in pattern generator B (PG$_B$). The rate of spontaneous activity in PG$_A$ gradually slows, however, because of the accumulation of intracellular Ca^{++}, and this slowing allows PG$_B$ eventually to overcome the diminishing synaptic inhibition. When PG$_B$ recovers and becomes spontaneously active, PG$_B$ synaptically inhibits PG$_A$. Eventually, activity in PG$_B$ slows and PG$_A$ becomes active. An average burst of activity in either neuron of the pattern generator lasts about 13 seconds, and activity in these two neurons oscillates back and forth at a baseline rate of about 26 seconds for one cycle.

The neurons of the pattern generator each make an excitatory connection onto an associative element (AE). Each action potential in a pattern-generating element initiates an action potential in its respective follower associative element. The properties of these associative elements are similar to the single-cell model illustrated in Figure 1, but four properties have been modified in order to adapt these elements to the prolonged periods of activity in these simulations. First, a saturation level or "ceiling" has been added to the intracellular concentration of cAMP (Fig. 6B2). Second, Ca^{++}-independent synthesis of cAMP has been eliminated. Third, transmitter depletion has been reduced by eliminating depletion of the storage pool and by reducing the release of transmitter. The latter was accomplished by scaling down I$_{Ca}$ and the gain constant

in the function that defines T$_R$. Fourth, I$_{Ca}$ was allowed to recover from voltage-dependent inactivation faster. These associative elements are the only elements in the network that are capable of activity-dependent neuromodulation (i.e., associative enhancement of synaptic strength). The neural pathways for reinforcement impinge on both associative elements. Reinforcement, like the US in the simulations of classical conditioning, activates adenylate cyclase, which in turn facilitates the connection between the associative elements and the respective motor neurons. This synaptic facilitation is enhanced by prior activity in the associative element via the activity-dependent neuromodulation learning rule.

Activity in the motor neurons (MN$_A$ and MN$_B$) is driven by synaptic input from the associative elements (Fig. 6B1). Activity in the motor neurons serves as the measure of network behavior, and the output of the motor neurons feeds back onto the neurons in the pattern generator. This feedback from the motor neurons contributes to the maintenance of bursts of activity in the neurons of the pattern generator by reducing the conductance of the voltage-gated Ca^{++} current. The greater the feedback, the less is the accumulation of intracellular Ca^{++} and inactivation of the low-threshold Ca^{++} current, and therefore, the longer is the duration of the burst (Fig. 6B3).

The basic operant training protocol consists of a 5-minute baseline phase and one or more 40-minute training phases. During the baseline phase, no reinforcement is delivered. During training, activity in one of the motor neurons is chosen as the reinforced behavior, and reinforcement is delivered whenever activity in that motor neuron exceeds a certain criterion level. The results of one such simulation are shown in Figure 7. When reinforcement is contingent on activity in MN$_A$ (Fig. 7A), two effects are observed. There is an

A   Contingent Reinforcement

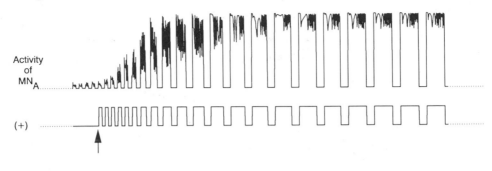

1 min

B   Random Reinforcement

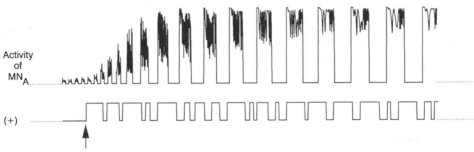

Figure 7. Network output during simulation of operant conditioning. (*A*) Simulation of contingent reinforcement. The top trace represents the activity in the motor neurons. The upward deflections represent temporally summating EPSPs, and the duration of an upward deflection represents the duration of a burst of activity in MN_A. When MN_A is silent, MN_B is active (not shown). The lower trace illustrates the delivery of reinforcement. Training begins at the arrow. When reinforcement is contingent on the expression of output A (i.e., activity in MN_A), the duration of activity in MN_A increases. (*B*) Simulation of random reinforcement. When reinforcement is random, the durations of activity in both MN_A and MN_B increase to an equal extent.

increase in the amplitude of motor neuron activity, and more to the point, there is an increase in the duration of each burst in the motor neuron. Thus, during the training phase, the network simulates the defining feature of operant conditioning, an increase in the amount of time it spends producing the reinforced behavior, i.e., output A (time A). As a control procedure, reinforcement is delivered randomly during the training phase (Fig. 7B), i.e., it is not contingent on activity in either motor neuron. When the reinforcement is random, the durations of bursts of activity in both motor neurons increase to an equal extent. Thus, there is no net change in the relative amount of time the network spends expressing either output A or B. The results of these two simulations are plotted in Figure 8A. During the baseline phase, the durations of bursts of activity are equal in each motor neuron. When reinforcement is contingent on activity in motor neuron A during the training phase, the network spends increasingly more time expressing output A. In contrast, when reinforcement is random, the network does not show any systematic preference for expressing either output A or B.

These results can be understood by referring to Figure 6A. During contingent training, reinforcement (activation of adenylate cyclase) always coincides with activity (and therefore high Ca^{++} levels) in associative element A (AE_A). Because of the mutual inhibition between the neurons of the central pattern generator, reinforcement is always delivered during a time when associative element B (AE_B) is inactive and contains only the small amount of Ca^{++} from its last burst that has not yet been buffered. Reinforcement therefore facilitates both AE-to-MN synapses, but enhances AE_A-to-MN_A to a much greater degree because of the high Ca^{++} levels in AE_A, which are necessary for associative plasticity. Consequently, enhanced activity in PG_A results (via AE_A) in greater activity in MN_A and hence greater positive feedback to PG_A, which in turn results in a longer burst on that side. In the non-reinforced motor neuron, MN_B, activity and the feedback to the central pattern generator do not change to the same extent.

During random reinforcement, the reinforcement is sometimes delivered during activity in MN_A and is sometimes delivered during activity in MN_B. Therefore, both AE-to-MN connections are facilitated to a comparable degree, the activities of both motor neurons increase, feedback to both neurons of the central pattern generator is increased, and thus, bursts in both neurons of the central pattern generator are increased. However, since, on average, both sides are facilitated equally, there is no change in the relative amount of

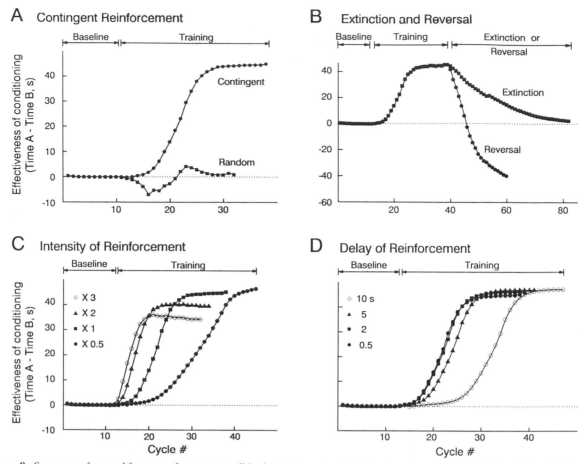

Figure 8. Summary of several features of operant conditioning that are simulated by a learning rule originally derived to simulate classical conditioning. In all plots, baseline spontaneous activity is simulated for 5 min, and training periods last for 40 min. The effectiveness of conditioning is calculated as the difference between the time spent expressing output A (time A) and the time spent expressing output B (time B) for each cycle, where a cycle is one complete oscillation of the network through a burst of activity in each motor neuron. For example, during the baseline period, the duration of activity is equal in each motor neuron, and therefore the difference between the two is plotted as 0. The number of cycles that occur during the 40-min training period depends on the duration of each cycle. Thus, the curves may not appear to be of equal length in various simulations, even though the duration of training is always 40 min. (*A*) The data from Fig. 7 are plotted. When reinforcement is contingent on output A, the network simulates operant conditioning, in that it increases the amount of time it spends expressing output. In contrast, random reinforcement does not differentially increase the duration of activity in either motor neuron. (*B*) During simulations of extinction, there is a gradual reduction in the duration of activity in motor neuron A. During simulations of reversal learning, time A rapidly decreases and time B increases. (*C*) Increasing the intensity of reinforcement increases the rate of acquisition of the operant response, whereas decreasing the intensity decreases the rate of acquisition. (*D*) Increasing the delay of reinforcement slows the acquisition of the operant response.

time the network spends expressing either output A or B.

Additional simulations illustrate that this neural network and this form of associative plasticity can simulate several other features of operant conditioning. A three-phase baseline-training-training protocol is used to examine extinction and reversal learning (Fig. 8B). During the first training phase, reinforcement is contingent on the expression of output A, and during this phase, time A increases dramatically. During simulations of extinction, no reinforcement occurs during the second 40-minute training phase, and there is a gradual reduction in the duration of activity in motor neuron A. During simulations of reversal learning, the contingency of reinforcement is reversed during the second 40-minute training period (i.e., reinforcement is now

delivered in response to activity in motor neuron B). As a result of reversal training, time A rapidly decreases and indeed, time B, which is now being reinforced, increases. The results of these simulations are very similar to the behavioral studies of extinction and reversal learning of head-waving in *Aplysia* (Cook and Carew 1986; Baxter et al. 1989, 1990).

The influence of two aspects of the presentation of reinforcement was examined also: the intensity of reinforcement and the delay of reinforcement. Behavioral studies indicate that increasing the intensity of reinforcement generally leads to faster acquisition in simple operant conditioning tasks (see Flaherty 1985). Figure 8C illustrates the simulation of this feature of operant conditioning. During the training phase, delivery of reinforcement is contingent on the expression of output

A. The intensity of the reinforcement is varied by altering the gain constant in the function that relates the reinforcement (activation of adenylate cyclase) to synthesis of cAMP (i.e., the slope of the function in Fig. 1B1). Reducing the intensity by one half ($\times 0.5$) significantly slows acquisition, whereas increasing the intensity twofold ($\times 2$) or threefold ($\times 3$) increases the rate of acquisition. It also has been well established that delaying reinforcement impedes acquisition in simple operant conditioning tasks (see Flaherty 1985). Figure 8D illustrates the simulation of this feature of operant conditioning. During previous simulations, reinforcement was delivered 0.5 second after the beginning of activity in the selected motor neuron. Increasing the delay of reinforcement beyond 2 seconds slows the rate of acquisition. The effects of intensity and delay of reinforcement on operant conditioning of head-waving in *Aplysia* have not been examined. The results of these simulations, however, are qualitatively similar to those generally reported for operant conditioning of simple tasks in vertebrates.

CONCLUDING REMARKS

In summary, previous work has shown that small neural networks similar to that shown in Figure 2B are able to simulate some higher-order features of classical conditioning (Gluck and Thompson 1987; Hawkins 1989a,b). The present study extends these observations by showing that the same holds true when the construct of the elements better reflects our understanding of real neurons. Furthermore, the present results indicate that an empirically derived model of a form of associative plasticity that is believed to underlie classical conditioning, when incorporated into an appropriate circuit, can simulate features of operant conditioning. Thus, in principle, a simple associative learning rule can be used as a "building block" to construct more complex forms of learning.

It should be emphasized that we do not know the properties of the interneurons that may be involved in second-order conditioning and blocking, nor do we know whether the basic mechanism for operant conditioning in *Aplysia* is the same as that for classical conditioning. In the near future, a major experimental question to be answered is the extent to which the mechanisms for associative learning are common both within any one animal and between different species. Although many common features are emerging, there seem to be some differences. Thus, it will be important to understand the extent to which specific mechanisms are used selectively for one type of conditioning and not another. Irrespective of the particular example of learning and memory that is analyzed, whether it be simple or complex, the results of this paper indicate that it will be important to pay attention to three major details: the details of the circuit interactions, the details of the learning rule, and the details of the intrinsic biophysical properties of the neurons within the circuit.

ACKNOWLEDGMENTS

We thank S. Patel for his assistance with computer programming and graphics. This research was supported by Air Force Office of Scientific Research grant 87-0274 and National Institute of Mental Health Award KO-2 MH-00649 to J.H.B., National Institute of Mental Health fellowship F31 MH-09895 to D.V.B., and National Science Foundation fellowship RCD-8851871 to J.L.R.

REFERENCES

Abrams, T.W. and E.R. Kandel. 1988. Is contiguity detection in classical conditioning a system or a cellular property? Learning in *Aplysia* suggests a possible molecular site. *Trends Neurosci.* **11**: 128.

Baxter, D.A. and J.H. Byrne. 1990. Differential effects of cAMP and serotonin on membrane current, action potential duration and excitability in somata of pleural sensory neurons of *Aplysia. J. Neurophysiol.* **64**: (in press).

Baxter, D.A., J.L. Raymond, D.V. Buonomano, and J.H. Byrne. 1989. Operant conditioning can be simulated by small networks of neuron-like elements. *Soc. Neurosci. Abstr.* **15**: 1263.

Baxter, D.A., D.V. Buonomano, J.L. Raymond, D.G. Cook, F.M. Kuenzi, T.J. Carew, and J.H. Byrne. 1990. Empirically derived adaptive elements and networks simulate associative learning. In *Quantitative analysis of behavior: Neural networks of conditioning and action* (ed. M. L. Commons et al.). Lawrence Erlbaum, Hillsdale, New Jersey. (In press.)

Bernier, L., V. F. Castellucci, and E. R. Kandel. 1982. Facilitatory transmitter causes a selective and prolonged increase in adenosine 3':5'-monophosphate in sensory neurons mediating the gill and siphon withdrawal reflex in *Aplysia. J. Neurosci.* **2**: 1682.

Bhara, O., N. Dale, B. Hochner, M. Klein, T.W. Abrams, and E.R. Kandel. 1990. Second messengers involved in the two processes of presynaptic facilitation that contribute to sensitization and dishabituation in *Aplysia* sensory neurons. *Proc. Natl. Acad. Sci.* **87**: 2040.

Buonomano, D.V. and J.H. Byrne. 1990. Long-term synaptic changes produced by a cellular analogue of classical conditioning in *Aplysia. Science* **249**: 420.

Buonomano, D.V., D.A. Baxter, and J.H. Byrne. 1990. Small networks of empirically derived adaptive elements simulate some higher-order features of classical conditioning. *Neural Networks* **3**: (in press).

Buonomano, D.V., L.J. Cleary, and J.H. Byrne. 1988. Inhibitory interneuron produces heterosynaptic inhibition of the sensory-motor connection mediating the tail withdrawal reflex in *Aplysia. Soc. Neurosci. Abstr.* **14**: 841.

Byrne, J.H. 1982. Analysis of the synaptic depression contributing to habituation of gill-withdrawal reflex in *Aplysia. J. Neurophysiol.* **48**: 431.

———. 1987. Cellular analysis of associative learning. *Physiol. Rev.* **67**: 329.

Byrne, J.H. and W.O. Berry, eds. 1989. *Neural models of plasticity.* Academic Press, San Diego.

Byrne, J.H. and K.J. Gingrich. 1989. Mathematical model of cellular and molecular processes contributing to associative and nonassociative learning in *Aplysia.* In *Neural model of plasticity* (ed. J.H. Byrne and W.O. Berry), p. 58. Academic Press, San Diego.

Byrne, J.H., K.J. Gingrich, and D.A. Baxter. 1989. Computational capabilities of single neurons: Relationship to simple forms of associative and nonassociative learning in *Aplysia.* In *Computational models of learning in simple systems* (ed. R.D. Hawkins and G.H. Bower), p. 31. Academic Press, San Diego.

Byrne, J.H., D. Buonomano, I. Corcos, S. Patel, and D.A. Baxter. 1988. Small networks of adaptive elements that reflect the properties of neurons in *Aplysia* exhibit higher-order features of classical conditioning. *Soc. Neurosci. Abstr.* **14:** 840.

Carew, T.J., V.F. Castellucci, and E.R. Kandel. 1971. An analysis of dishabituation and sensitization of the gill-withdrawal reflex in *Aplysia. Int. J. Neurosci.* **2:** 79.

Carew, T.J., R.D. Hawkins, and E.R. Kandel. 1983. Differential classical conditioning of a defensive withdrawal reflex in *Aplysia californica. Science* **219:** 397.

Castellucci, V.F., H. Pinsker, I. Kupfermann, and E.R. Kandel. 1970. Neuronal mechanisms of habituation and dishabituation of the gill-withdrawal in *Aplysia. Science* **167:** 1745.

Cook, D.G. and T.J. Carew. 1986. Operant conditioning of head waving in *Aplysia. Proc. Natl. Acad. Sci.* **83:** 1120.

———. 1988. Operant conditioning of identified neck muscles and individual motor neurons in *Aplysia. Soc. Neurosci. Abstr.* **14:** 607.

———. 1989a. Operant conditioning of head waving in *Aplysia* I: Identified muscles involved in the operant response. *J. Neurosci.* **9:** 3097.

———. 1989b. Operant conditioning of head waving in *Aplysia* II: Contingent modification of electromyographic activity in identified muscles. *J. Neurosci.* **9:** 3107.

———. 1989c. Operant conditioning of head waving in *Aplysia* III: Cellular analysis of possible reinforcement pathways. *J. Neurosci.* **9:** 3115.

———. 1989d. Identification of reinforcement pathways necessary for operant conditioning in *Aplysia. Soc. Neurosci. Abstr.* **15:** 1265.

Eliot, L.S., Y. Dudai, E.R. Kandel, and T.W. Abrams. 1989. Ca^{2+}/calmodulin sensitivity may be common to all forms of neural adenylate cyclase. *Proc. Natl. Acad. Sci.* **86:** 9564.

Flaherty, C.F. 1985. *Animal learning and cognition.* Alfred Knopf, New York.

Gingrich, K.J. and J.H. Byrne. 1985. Simulation of synaptic depression, posttetanic potentiation and presynaptic facilitation of synaptic potentials from sensory neurons mediating gill-withdrawal reflex in *Aplysia. J. Neurophysiol.* **53:** 652.

———. 1987. Single-cell model for associative learning. *J. Neurophysiol.* **57:** 1705.

Gingrich, K.J., D.A. Baxter, and J.H. Byrne. 1988. Mathematical model of cellular mechanisms contributing to presynaptic facilitation. *Brain Res. Bull.* **21:** 513.

Gluck, M.A. and R.F. Thompson. 1987. Modeling the neural substrate of associative learning and memory: A computational approach. *Psychol. Rev.* **94:** 176.

Hawkins, R.D. 1989a. A simple circuit model for higher-order features of classical conditioning. In *Neural models of plasticity* (ed. J.H. Byrne and W.O. Berry), p. 73. Academic Press, San Diego.

———. 1989b. A biologically based computational model for several simple forms of learning. In *Computational models of learning in simple neural systems* (ed. R.D. Hawkins and G.H. Bower), p. 65. Academic Press, San Diego.

Hawkins, R.D. and G.H. Bower, eds. 1989. *Computational models of learning in simple neural systems.* Academic Press, San Diego.

Hawkins, R.D. and E.R. Kandel. 1984. Is there a cell biological alphabet for simple forms of learning? *Psychol. Rev.* **91:** 375.

Hawkins, R.D., T.W. Abrams, T.J. Carew, and E.R. Kandel. 1983. A cellular mechanism of classical conditioning in *Aplysia*: Activity-dependent amplification of presynaptic facilitation. *Science* **219:** 400.

Hochner, B., M. Klein, S. Schacher, and E.R. Kandel. 1986a. Action potential duration and the modulation of transmitter release from the sensory neurons of *Aplysia* in presynaptic facilitation and behavioral sensitization. *Proc. Natl. Acad. Sci.* **83:** 8410.

———. 1986b. Additional component in the cellular mechanisms of presynaptic facilitation contributing to behavioral dishabituation in *Aplysia. Proc. Natl. Acad. Sci.* **83:** 8794.

Kandel, E.R. and J.H. Schwartz. 1982. Molecular biology of learning: Modulation of transmitter release. *Science* **218:** 433.

Klein, M., J. Camardo, and E.R. Kandel. 1982. Serotonin modulates a specific potassium current in sensory neurons that show presynaptic facilitation in *Aplysia. Proc. Natl. Acad. Sci.* **79:** 5713.

Mackey, S.L., D.L. Glanzman, S.A. Small, A.M. Dyke, E.R. Kandel, and R.D. Hawkins. 1987. Tail shocks produce inhibition as well as sensitization of the siphon-withdrawal reflex of *Aplysia*: Possible role for presynaptic inhibition mediated by the peptide Phe-Met-Arg-Phe-NH_2. *Proc. Natl. Acad. Sci.* **84:** 8730.

Mackintosh, N.J. 1974. *The psychology of animal learning.* Academic Press, New York.

Ocorr, K.A. and J.H. Byrne. 1985. Membrane responses and changes in cAMP levels in *Aplysia* sensory neurons produced by serotonin, tryptamine, FMRFamide and small cardioactive peptide (SCP_B). *Neurosci. Lett.* **55:** 113.

Ocorr, K.A., E.T. Walters, and J.H. Byrne. 1985. Associative conditioning analog selectively increases cAMP levels of tail sensory neurons in *Aplysia. Proc. Natl. Acad. Sci.* **82:** 2548.

Rescorla, R.A. 1988. Behavioral studies of pavlovian conditioning. *Annu. Rev. Neurosci.* **11:** 329.

Walters, E.T. and J.H. Byrne. 1983. Associative conditioning of single neurons suggests a cellular mechanism for learning. *Science* **219:** 405.

Walters, E.T., J.H. Byrne, T.J. Carew, and E.R. Kandel. 1983. Mechanoafferent neurons innervating the tail of *Aplysia*. II. Modulation by sensitizing stimulation. *J. Neurophysiol.* **50:** 1543.

Long-term Facilitation in *Aplysia:* Persistent Phosphorylation and Structural Changes

S. Schacher, D. Glanzman, A. Barzilai, P. Dash, S.G.N. Grant,
F. Keller, M. Mayford, and E.R. Kandel
*Howard Hughes Medical Institute and Center for Neurobiology and Behavior, Columbia University
College of Physicians & Surgeons, New York, New York 10032*

For most learning tasks, memory in human beings and experimental animals appears to be a single, graded, continuous process whose duration is related to the number of training trials. Repetition of a task usually increases both the strength and the duration of the memory for that task (Ebbinghaus 1885). As a result, long-term memory has often been thought to be a graded extension of short-term memory (Weiskrantz 1970; Craik and Lockhart 1972; Wickelgren 1973). Yet a variety of studies indicate that memory is probably not unitary but has at least two forms, each of which subserves a family of time courses: a short-term form that can last seconds, minutes, or hours, and a long-term form that can last days, weeks, or years (James 1890; McGaugh 1966; Atkinson and Shiffrin 1968; Davis and Squire 1984); e.g., several clinical conditions can dissociate short-term from long-term memory in humans (Russell and Nathan 1946; Barbizet 1970). A similar dissociation can be demonstrated in experimental animals using inhibitors of protein synthesis (Flexner et al. 1963; Agranoff 1967; Barondes 1970).

We have found a similar situation with short- and long-term memory for behavioral sensitization in the gill-and-siphon-withdrawal reflex of *Aplysia*. Long-term sensitization resembles a graded extension of the short-term form in both strength and duration (Pinsker et al. 1970, 1973; Frost et al. 1985). Nevertheless, the long-term behavioral process can be dissociated from the short-term form by inhibition of protein synthesis (Castellucci et al. 1989). Cellular studies of memory storage for sensitization in this reflex indicate that both the behavioral similarities and the differences can be detected in a monosynaptic pathway consisting of the sensory and motor neurons participating in this reflex (Castellucci et al. 1970; Montarolo et al. 1986). Although the long-term change in the synaptic connection between the sensory and motor neurons resembles a graded extension of the short-term change, its induction is selectively blocked by inhibitors of transcription or translation.

Since this monosynaptic pathway can be reconstituted in dissociated cell culture (Rayport and Schacher 1986), we have used this simple in vitro system as a model to examine the cellular mechanisms contributing to the similarities and differences between short- and long-term memory. In this two-cell system in culture, serotonin (5-HT), a transmitter released by sensitizing stimuli (Glanzman et al. 1989b; Mackey et al. 1989), can substitute for a shock to the tail, the reinforcing stimulus used for the intact animal (Montarolo et al. 1986). A single application of 5-HT produces short-term changes in synaptic effectiveness lasting minutes. In contrast, four or five repeated applications of 5-HT over 1.5 hours, designed to simulate four to five tail stimuli, produce long-term changes lasting more than 1 day (Montarolo et al. 1986; Dale et al. 1988; Schacher et al. 1990). As is the case with behavior, the long-term changes on the cellular level are surprisingly similar to the short-term changes. Both the long-term and the short-term changes occur at the same locus: the connections between the sensory and motor neurons. Both types of changes involve an increase in synaptic strength (Frost et al. 1985; Scholz and Byrne 1987; Dale et al. 1988, 1990). A quantal analysis has revealed that the increase in synaptic strength is due, in each case, to an enhanced release of transmitter and is accompanied in both cases by an increase in excitability of the sensory neurons attributable to a depression of the S-K$^+$ current (Castellucci and Kandel 1976; Dale et al. 1987, 1990; Scholz and Byrne 1987). Moreover, the same modulatory transmitter (5-HT) and also the same second-messenger system can produce both short- and long-term facilitation. Thus, whereas a transient exposure to cAMP causes transient facilitation, repeated or prolonged application of cAMP causes persistent facilitation (Brunelli 1976; Scholz and Byrne 1988; Schacher et al. 1988; Braha et al. 1990).

Despite these several similarities, the short-term cellular changes in *Aplysia* differ from the long-term changes in an important way. The short-term change involves only covalent modification of preexisting proteins; it is not blocked by inhibitors of transcription or translation (Schwartz et al. 1971; Montarolo et al. 1986). In contrast, these inhibitors selectively block the induction of the long-term changes (Montarolo et al. 1986; Dale et al. 1987; Schacher et al. 1988). Thus, as is the case for long-term behavioral changes (Castellucci et al. 1989), the long-term cellular changes may require the expression of genes and proteins not required for the short-term changes. What is the function of these genes and proteins? We recently have examined this set of connections on the ultrastructural and molecular levels and here summarize our studies, delineating two functional, transcriptionally dependent changes that

seem to define two molecular themes important for
long-term memory storage in the connections between
the sensory and motor neurons (Fig. 1).

First, there is in the long-term a persistent phosphorylation of the same set of substrate proteins involved in
setting up the short-term process. These physiological
and biochemical data indicate that the long-term resembles the short-term in part because the same substrate proteins are persistently phosphorylated (Sweatt
and Kandel 1989). However, whereas in the short-term

the phosphorylation requires an increase in the basal
level of cAMP and a consequent activation of the
cAMP-dependent protein kinase, in the long-term the
phosphorylation no longer requires elevated levels of
cAMP (Bernier et al. 1982) and seems to be maintained by an autonomously active kinase (Greenberg et
al. 1987; Bergold et al. 1990).

Second, in the long-term, there is a growth of additional synaptic connections (Bailey and Chen 1983,
1988a,b, 1989; Glanzman et al. 1990). This learning-

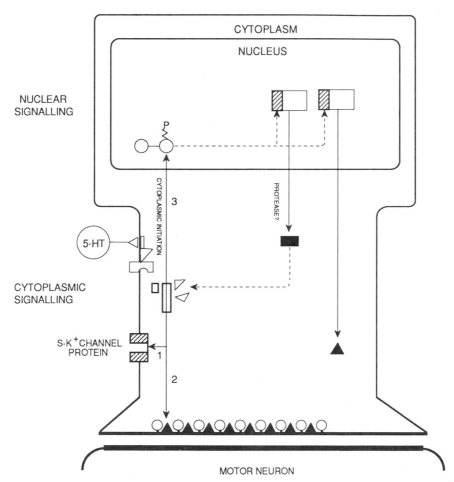

Figure 1. Schematic outline of the two major sets of changes that accompany long-term memory: persistent phosphorylation and
structural changes. We have focused on the presynaptic neuron at a synapse and consider changes in ion channels, transmitter
release mechanisms, and structural changes at active zones. Similar changes in the properties and insertion of receptors are likely
to occur in postsynaptic cells. In this model, an extracellular signal, a transmitter released by modulatory neurons, acts on a
presynaptic neuron to initiate separate memory processes with different durations. Short-term memory, which has a time course
of minutes to hours, involves covalent modification of preexisting proteins. Common components of cytoplasmic signaling
(membrane receptor, transducing proteins, amplifier enzyme, adenylyl cyclase, cytoplasmic signal, cAMP, Ca^{++}, and protein
kinases A) are used to modify target proteins: gated K^+ channels (1) transmitter mobilizing and release mechanism (2). The
duration of these modifications determines the retention of memory. For intermediate memory, this short-term memory system
can be prolonged to last hours by similar covalent modifications that are self-reinforcing, as in the case of autocatalytic
phosphorylation of a protein kinase (see Goelet et al. 1986). Unlike these covalent modification mechanisms (pathways 1 and 2),
the acquisition of long-term memory lasting more than 1 day (pathway 3) is dependent on the phosphorylation of one or more
CREB-like transcriptional activators. This phosphorylation is initiated by the second-messenger system involved in short-term
memory. The two classes of modified transacting regulators activate effector genes. It is the induced synthesis of the proteins of
these genes (black rectangle and black triangle) that is blocked by the inhibition of protein synthesis during learning. One
consequence of gene induction is a persistent phosphorylation due to the maintained activity of the same protein kinase involved
in the short-term process. In the sensory neuron, this involves a down-regulation of the regulatory subunit of the cAMP-
dependent protein kinase, which might occur by activation of a specific protease. A second consequence is the activation of genes
for proteins important for this structural change.

related growth bears some resemblance to that of synapse formation (Glanzman et al. 1989a, 1990).

These two sets of findings suggest that with repeated exposure, the modulatory transmitter acts as a growth factor to increase the synthesis of new proteins and the laying down of additional synaptic connections.

LONG-TERM FACILITATION INVOLVES PERSISTENT PHOSPHORYLATION

The initial evidence for persistent phosphorylation came from attempts to examine the mechanisms in the sensory neurons that might account for the graded similarity between short- and long-term memory (Sweatt and Kandel 1989). It was found that a single exposure to 5-HT (a transmitter released in response to behavioral sensitizing stimuli) or to cAMP (a second messenger for 5-HT), which is increased with short-term sensitization, produces short-term facilitation lasting minutes in the connections between the sensory and motor neurons (Brunelli et al. 1976; Castellucci et al. 1980, 1982; Klein et al. 1982). The action of 5-HT or cAMP leads to a short-term increase in phosphorylation of substrate proteins that is not dependent on transcription or translation. In contrast, repeated or prolonged exposure to 5-HT or cAMP, which induce long-term changes in synaptic transmission lasting one or more days (Montarolo et al. 1986; Scholz and Byrne 1988), induces long-term increases in phosphorylation of the same proteins. However, this persistent phosphorylation is dependent for its induction on both translation and transcription (Fig. 2).

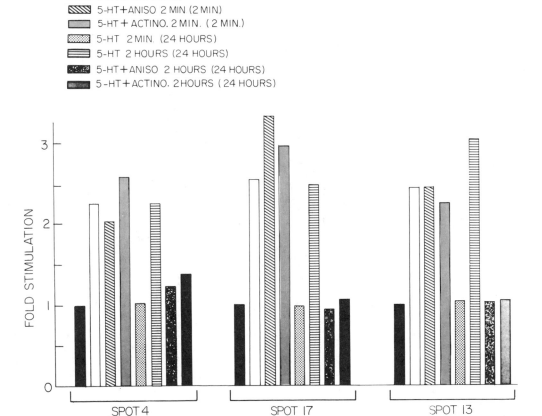

Figure 2. Persistent phosphorylation. Short- and long-term effects of 5-HT on the phosphorylation of individual proteins. Values given are the ratios of stimulated to control for ^{32}P content of three representative spots. Treatments were as follows: 5-HT 2 min (2 min), 40 μM 5-HT applied for 2 min and assayed at 2 min ($n = 6$); 5-HT + ANISO 2 min (2 min), 40 μM 5-HT applied for 2 min in the presence of 10 μM anisomycin and assayed at 2 min ($n = 1$); 5-HT + ACTINO 2 min (2 min), 40 μM 5-HT applied for 2 min in the presence of 50 μg ml^{-1} actinomycin D and assayed at 2 min ($n = 1$); 5-HT 2 min (24 hr), 40 μM 5-HT applied for 2 min, washed out, and protein phosphorylation assayed at 24 hr ($n = 3$); 5-HT 2 hr (24 hr), 40 μM 5-HT applied for 2 hr, washed out, and protein phosphorylation assayed at 24 hr ($n = 7$); 5-HT + ANISO 2 hr (24 hr), 40 μM 5-HT applied for 2 hr in the presence of 10 μM anisomycin, then both agents washed out and protein phosphorylation assayed at 24 hr ($n = 3$); 5-HT + ACTINO 2 hr (24 hr), 40 μM 5-HT applied for 2 hr in the presence of 50 μg ml^{-1} actinomycin D, then both agents washed out and protein phosphorylation assayed at 24 hr ($n = 3$). Where anisomycin or actinomycin D was applied, they were added either 30 min before stimulation (for samples incubated 2 hr with stimulus) or 2.5 hr before stimulation (for samples incubated for 2 min with stimulus) and present during stimulation. (Modified from Sweatt and Kandel 1989.)

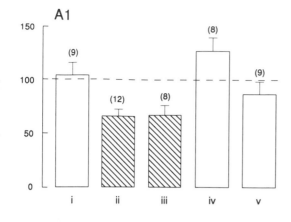

A1

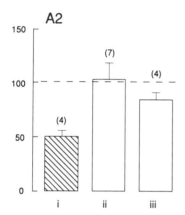

A2

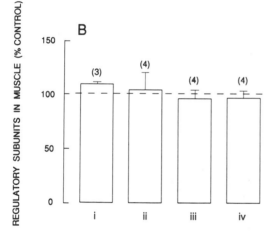

B

Figure 3. Change in the amount of regulatory subunits in sensory clusters 24 hr after induction of either short-term or long-term facilitation by 5-HT and by increased intracellular cAMP. Percent change (mean ± S.E.M.) in regulatory subunits is determined by averaging the difference between the incorporation of $[^{32}\text{P}]$8-azido-cAMP in control and experimental clusters for M_r 52,000 and 47,000 components 24 hr after beginning each treatment. The change in the muscle M_r 55,000 regulatory subunit was assayed similarly. The muscle regulatory subunits of M_r 55,000 are structurally related to the nervous system subunits in the region of cAMP binding (Dale et al. 1987; Schacher et al. 1988). The number of times each experiment was done is shown in parentheses. Treatments that induce long-term facilitation are indicated by hatching. (*A1*) Decrease in regulatory subunits after treatments with 5-HT that induce long-term facilitation has a critical period for new protein synthesis. The percent change in regulatory subunits was determined 24 hr after treatment for 5 min with 5-HT (40 μM) (bar *i*); 2 hr with 5-HT (bar *ii*); 2 hr with 5-HT followed by washing and 3 hr with anisomycin (50 μg/ml) (bar *iii*); with anisomycin added 30 min before 5-HT, after which both 5-HT and anisomycin were removed 2 hr later by washing extensively (bar *iv*); or 3 hr with anisomycin alone (bar *v*). (*A2*) Elevation of intracellular cAMP can produce the decrease in regulatory subunits. The change in regulatory subunits was determined 24 hr after a 2-hr treatment with CPT-cAMP (100 μM) with isobutyl methylxanthine (IBMX) (100 μM) (bar *i*); CPT-cAMP (bar *ii*); or IBMX alone (bar *iii*). (*B*) Elevation of intracellular cAMP by 5-HT (10 μM) or SCP$_\text{B}$ (10 μM) has no effect on the muscle regulatory subunit. The change in regulatory subunits was determined immediately after (bars *i* and *ii*) or 24 hr after (bars *iii* and *iv*) 1.5-hr treatment with either SCP$_\text{B}$ (bars *i* and *iii*) or 5-HT (bars *ii* and *iv*). (Reprinted, with permission, from Bergold et al. 1990.)

To explore possible mechanisms underlying the persistent phosphorylation, Bergold et al. (1990) next examined changes in the properties of the *Aplysia* cAMP-dependent protein kinase (A kinase), a heterodimer consisting of two regulatory subunits that inhibit two catalytic subunits. The A kinase is activated during both short-term and long-term sensitization, and the amount of the regulatory subunit is lowered, as compared to the catalytic subunit, in the sensory cells of long-term behaviorally sensitized animals (Greenberg et al. 1987). Bergold et al. (1990) found that facilitatory stimuli (5-HT or cAMP) also diminish the ratio of the regulatory to catalytic subunits in the sensory neurons and that this reduction in the regulatory subunit requires new protein synthesis (Fig. 3). Thus, one of the functions of the macromolecular synthesis required for long-term facilitation is to synthesize proteins that regulate the cAMP-dependent kinase in a long-term manner. This long-term down-regulation of the regulatory subunit makes the catalytic subunit more autonomous of cAMP, and this could account for the persistent increase in protein phosphorylation observed in long-term facilitation. We do not as yet know, however, how this reduction in the regulatory subunit comes about. It appears not to occur at the level of transcription of the regulatory subunit (Bergold et al. 1990; J.H. Schwartz and P.J. Bergold, pers. comm.) and it may involve the induction or activation of a protease that cleaves the regulatory subunit.

Because the memory for different learning processes in vertebrates and invertebrates seems similarly graded, a transcriptionally dependent persistent increase in protein phosphorylation might prove to be a general mechanism for long-term memory. Indeed, a requirement for protein synthesis has recently been found in studies of long-term potentiation in the hippocampus (Frey et al. 1988; Otani and Abraham 1989; Otani et al. 1989), a learning-related process thought to use either protein kinase C or a Ca^{++}-calmodulin-dependent kinase (Malenka et al. 1989; Malinow et al. 1989). Similarly, there is a requirement for protein synthesis in the long-term biophysical changes in the eye of *Hermissenda* (Crow and Forrester 1990), a change thought to involve protein kinase C (Farley and Auerbach 1986; Alkon et al. 1988). These several findings raise the interesting possibility that as the long-term memory processes in different learning systems persist, they do so because the relevant protein kinases—such as the cAMP-dependent kinase, protein kinase C, and the Ca^{++}-calmodulin-dependent kinase—might all be capable of a transcriptionally dependent persistent increase in activity.

INDUCTION OF LONG-TERM FACILITATION SEEMS TO REQUIRE CREB-LIKE TRANSCRIPTIONAL ACTIVATORS

Further evidence relating to the transcriptional dependence of the long-term facilitation comes from the examination of change in specific proteins induced by 5-HT. Barzilai et al. (1989) found that repeated exposure to 5-HT rapidly stimulates transcriptionally dependent changes in 15 early proteins (which change their level of expression within 15–30 min) as well as a number of later ones. Of the early proteins, 10 showed increases and 5 showed decreases in net incorporation of [^{35}S]methionine. The same 15 early proteins were also induced by cAMP. In these features—rapid induction, transcriptional dependence, and second-messenger mediation—these early proteins appear to resemble the immediate-early gene products induced in vertebrate cells by growth factors. In vertebrates, some of the immediate-early genes encode regulators; others encode effector proteins, including those that inhibit growth (Sorrentino 1989).

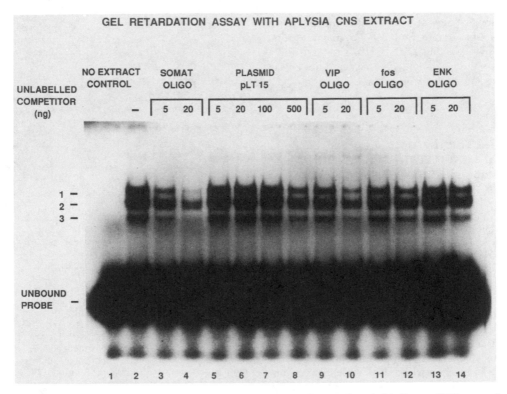

Figure 4. Specific binding of *Aplysia* CNS extract to CRE of rat somatostatin gene. Protein binding to CRE was performed by gel retardation assay. The positions of the free and of the three retarded bands are shown. The probe and the probe plus extract in the absence of competitor are in lanes *1* and *2*. The three retarded bands can be competed out specifically by nonradioactive somatostatin CRE (lanes *3* and *4*) but not by linear nonspecific plasmid DNA (lanes *5–8*). The competition by CRE sequence from VIP (−99 to −58), *fos* (−330 to −276), and enkephalin (−114 to −70) is shown in lanes *9–11*. (Reprinted, with permission, from Dash et al. 1990.)

What turns on these early proteins and triggers the long-term process? Most cAMP-inducible genes so far studied are activated by specific transcription factors that bind to an enhancer sequence TGACGTCA, called the cAMP-responsive element (CRE) (Montminy et al. 1986). The CRE binds as a dimer of 43-kD protein subunits, the enhancer binding protein called CREBP. Dash et al. (1990) therefore examined extracts of *Aplysia* sensory neurons and found that they contain proteins that specifically bind to a mammalian (somatostatin) CRE sequence (Figs. 4 and 5). One of the *Aplysia* proteins resembles in its DNA binding a mammalian CREB protein, as determined by a DNase protection assay (Fig. 5). This protein is approximately 45 kD and serves as a substrate for the A kinase (Dash et al. 1990).

To examine whether these CREB-like proteins are essential to activate the long-term process, Dash et al. (1990) injected oligonucleotides containing the CRE sequence into the nucleus of a sensory neuron. This selectively blocked the long-term increase in synaptic strength without affecting short-term facilitation (Figs. 6 and 7). Injection of control enhancer sequences fails to block the increase in synaptic strength (Fig. 7). These results indicate that one or more CREB-like transcriptional activators are required for the expression of long-term facilitation. Although these results are consistent with the finding that long-term facilitation in the sensory neurons is induced by cAMP, other second messengers may also contribute. Indeed, Dash et al. (1990) and Greenberg and his colleagues (pers. comm.) have found that CREB is a substrate for a number of kinases, including Ca^{++}/calmodulin kinase II, C kinase, and casein kinase II.

THE STRUCTURAL CHANGES ASSOCIATED WITH LONG-TERM FACILITATION RESEMBLE THOSE THAT UNDERLIE SYNAPSE FORMATION DURING DEVELOPMENT

Ever since the work of Ramón y Cajal (1911), neurobiologists have suggested that learning in vertebrates may involve the growth of new anatomical connections in the brain similar to those that occur during development (see, e.g., Bennett et al. 1964; Diamond et al. 1966; Fifkova and Van Harreveld 1977; Lee et al. 1980; Chang and Greenough 1984; Desmond and Levy 1986a,b). With regard to invertebrates, the morphological studies by Bailey and Chen (1983, 1988a, 1989) first indicated that long-term modification of *Aplysia*'s gill-and-siphon-withdrawal reflex is accompanied by long-lasting structural changes in the sensory and motor neurons. Many of these changes can now also be examined in the sensory to motor neuron connections reconstituted in dissociated cell culture (Glanzman et al. 1990). Moreover, in these studies, Glanzman et al. (1989a) have discovered a parallel between structural changes in *Aplysia* sensory neurons that occur during in vitro development of sensorimotor cul-

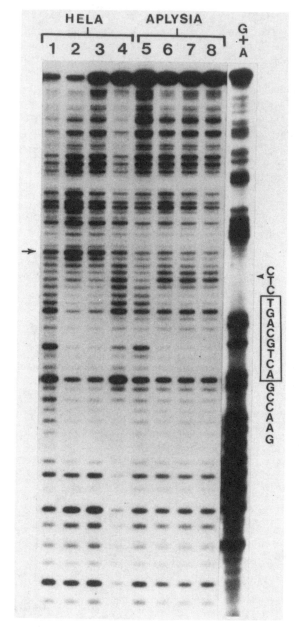

Figure 5. Analysis of the protein-DNA interaction at the CRE site. DNase I footprinting of the coding strand of the rat somatostatin CRE with HeLa nuclear and *Aplysia* CNS extract. An autoradiograph of the sequencing gel is shown. Two retarded bands were seen using HeLa nuclear extract. The footprints of the unbound (lane *1*), nonspecifically bound (lane *4*), and the two retarded bands (lanes *2* and *3*) are shown. The footprints of the unbound band (lane *5*) and three retarded bands (lanes *6—8*) with the partially purified heparin-agarose fraction of the *Aplysia* CNS extract are shown. The DNase I hypersensitive sites are shown by the arrows. The same probe was independently cleaved with piperidin (A + G ladder) for sequence alignment of the CRE motif and is shown at the right. (Reprinted, with permission, from Dash et al. 1990.)

tures and those that accompany learning-related long-term synaptic plasticity. Specifically, in both situations, the structural changes depend critically on the presence of an appropriate target motor neuron.

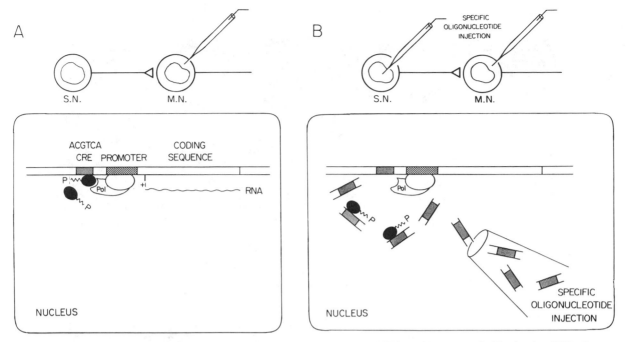

Figure 6. *Aplysia* sensorimotor neuron culture system used to study the inhibition of long-term facilitation by CRE oligonucleotide injection. A schematic representation of the experimental design before and after the injection of CRE. (*A*) Binding of CREB to the CRE of cAMP-inducible genes in the nucleus of the sensory neuron. (*B*) Consequence of injecting excess oligonucleotides that encode CRE. These compete with the normal binding of CREB to the endogenous genes. (Reprinted, with permission, from Dash et al. 1990.)

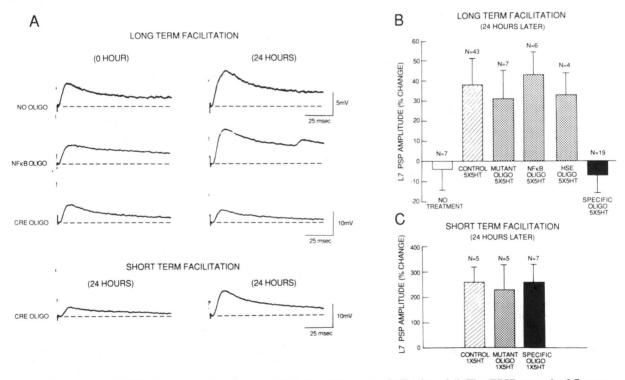

Figure 7. Injection of CRE oligonucleotides blocks 5-HT-induced long-term facilitation. (*A*) The EPSP onto the L7 motor neuron at 0 hr (before 5-HT treatment) is compared with the first EPSP 24 hr after the treatment. Injection of the control oligonucleotide does not affect the increase in the EPSP, whereas the CRE injection blocks the increase 24 hr after treatment. Short-term facilitation in the presence of 5-HT is not affected by CRE oligonucleotide injection 24 hr after the long-term training procedure. (*B*) Summary of the blockade of the 5-HT-induced increase in long-term facilitation by CRE injection. The height of each bar is the percentage change in the EPSP amplitude ± S.E.M. retested 24 hr after treatment. (A two-tailed *t*-test comparison of means indicated that the decrease in EPSP in cultures injected with CRE oligonucleotide is significantly different [$p < 0.05$] from the increase in the EPSP in the cells injected with either the mutant or NFκB oligonucleotides.) (*C*) Summary of the pooled data for short-term facilitation 24 hr after injection. In contrast to long-term facilitation, the 5-HT (5 μM) was applied after the EPSP was first depressed. Five stimuli were given with an interstimulus interval of 30 sec, and this resulted in 70–80% depression in EPSP amplitude. This 5-HT now produced an increase in EPSP amplitude by the seventh stimulus. The increase in short-term facilitation was measured by calculating the percentage increase in the seventh EPSP amplitude as compared to the fifth EPSP amplitude. Because the facilitation here was of a depressed EPSP, the percent facilitation is larger than the long-term, where only the nondepressed EPSP was examined. (Reprinted, with permission, from Dash et al. 1990.)

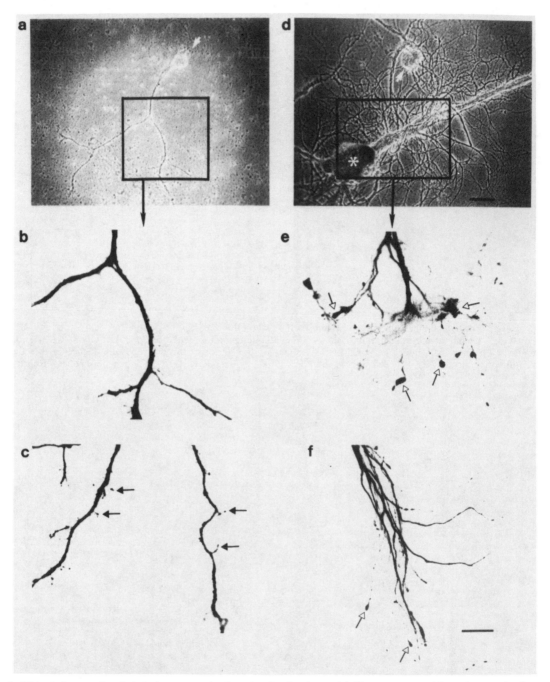

Figure 8. Video micrographs of *Aplysia* neurons in dissociated cell culture. (*a*) Phase-contrast video micrograph of a sensory neuron (white arrow) in culture alone. (*b*) Fluorescence video micrograph of the outlined region of the neuritic field of the sensory neuron shown in *a*. (*c*) Fluorescence video micrograph of a region of the neuritic field of a sensory neuron alone in culture (a different neuron from that shown in *a*. The neurites are studded with tiny spine-like protrusions (black arrows). This image was made by averaging eight video frames and contrast-enhancing the averaged image with a computer. (*d*) Phase-contrast video micrograph of a sensory neuron (white arrow) in culture together with an L7 motor neuron (cell body indicated by asterisk). The majority of outgrowth is from the L7 cell. Note the very large neurite of L7 running diagonally across the micrograph. This neurite actually consists of three separate axons, which are taken out from the abdominal ganglion along with the L7 soma during dissociation and which collapse together when the cell is plated down in the culture dish. This large neurite does not therefore represent in vitro outgrowth of L7 in culture but, instead, is composed of original axons of L7. The smaller motor neurites represent outgrowth that has occurred since L7 was placed into culture. Firing of the sensory neuron evoked a 24-mV EPSP in the L7 cell. Bar, 100 μm. (*e*) Fluorescence video micrograph of the outlined region of the neuritic field of the sensory neuron shown in *d*. The processes of the sensory neuron are shown contacting the major neurites of L7. In this region the neurites of the sensory neuron are relatively smaller and have many varicosities (some of which are indicated by open arrows) on its processes. (*f*) Fluorescence video micrograph of a region of the neuritic field of a different sensory neuron in culture with an L7 cell. The neurites are smooth and lack spine-like protrusions. Two varicosities are indicated by open arrows. This sensory cell evoked a 30-mV EPSP in L7. Average of 16 video frames, contrast-enhanced by computer. Bar, 50 μm. (Reprinted, with permission, from Glanzman et al. 1989a.)

194

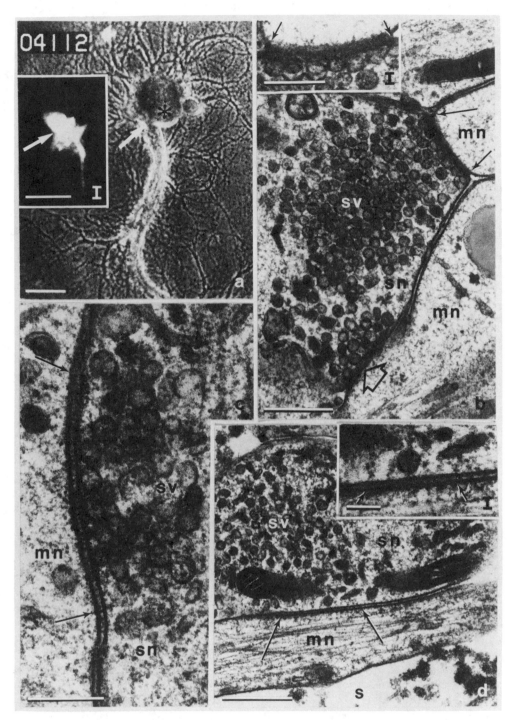

Figure 9. Correlative light/electron microscopy analyses of sensorimotor synapses. (*a*) Phase-contrast micrograph of sensorimotor culture after 5 days. White arrow indicates the large fluorescently labeled sensory neuron structure (inset I) near the motor cell body (*) and along the proximal portion of the initial segment of the motor axons. Bar, 100 μm. Bar in I, 50 μm. (*b,c*) Electron micrographs of areas within the region containing contacts between the sensory and motor cells. (*b*) One synapse has a bisynaptic configuration containing clusters of synaptic vesicles (sv) in the sensory neuron (sn) process at both junctional sites (arrows) along the motor neuron processes (mn). Variably lucent 65–90 ±5 nm and a few 100 ± 8 nm dense cored presynaptic vesicles occur next to or in contact with the specialized membrane junctional complex. Bar, 0.5 μm. Inset (I) shows higher-power view of one of the synapses (between arrows) with a junctional gap of 40–80 ± 20 nm. Linear 3–5 ± 2 nm structural elements appear to span the gap, and some extend into the cytoplasm of both processes. Bar, 0.25 μm. (*c*) Portion of another synaptic junction between the same sensory (sn) and motor (mn) cell with a more convex configuration (between arrows). Linear and other densities are present in the slightly widened gap of the active zone area. Several presynaptic dense projections with finer fibrous elements appear to extend to nearby synaptic vesicles (sv). Bar, 0.25 μm. (*d*) Portion of a sensory neuron (sn) varicosity containing a number of synapse-like vesicles (sv) adjoining a fine caliber motor neuron (mn) process and the polylysine substrate (s) in the distal neuritic outgrowth region. Intergap densities appear between the two processes (between arrows). Bar, 0.5 μm. Inset (I) is a higher-power view of this area showing that the intergap densities lack the structured, linear ordering of the densities in the synaptic clefts (*b* and *c*) and lack presynaptic specializations (dense projections and clusters of synaptic vesicles). Bar, 0.1 μm. (Reprinted, with permission, from Glanzman et al. 1989a.)

The Structure of the Presynaptic Neuron Is Modified by Contact with an Appropriate Target during Development

Glanzman et al. (1989a) initially examined the structure of sensory neurons placed into dissociated cell culture either alone or together with a target neuron, the identified gill-and-siphon-motor neuron L7. The outgrowth of sensory neurons in the absence of a motor neuron is relatively simple. These sensory neurons have neurites with relatively few branches and varicosities, and their neurites tend to be thick, consisting of bundles, or fascicles, of finer processes (Fig. 8, a–c). In contrast, sensory neurons grown together with motor neuron L7 have a more complex structure. Their outgrowth tends to consist of finer neurites, and these neurites have more branches and more varicosities (Fig. 8, d–f). In addition to inducing a structural elaboration of sensory neurons, L7 motor neurons appear to guide the sensory outgrowth. In cocultures, the neurites of sensory neurons tend to grow along the processes of L7 and are particularly attracted to the initial segment of L7's original axons.

Interestingly, the enhanced structural complexity induced in sensory neurons by the motor cell appears to depend on the ability of the sensory neuron to form chemical synaptic connections with L7 cells. Sensory neurons grown in cell culture together with an inappropriate target—a motor cell with which they do not normally form chemical synapses in the ganglion—have significantly less complex structures than do cocultures of sensory neurons grown together with an appropriate target. Indeed, sensory neurons grown with inappropriate target cells appear much like sensory neurons grown alone. Thus, the enhanced structural complexity induced in sensory neurons by L7 motor neurons in vitro is not simply due to the presence of another neuron but is related to synapse formation. Moreover, the number of varicosities on a sensory neuron's processes is significantly correlated with the strength of its synaptic connection to the motor neuron, as indicated by the sensorimotor excitatory postsynaptic potential (EPSP). Correlative fluorescence and electron microscopy reveal that many of these sensory varicosities contain active zones (Fig. 9).

The regulation of the structural complexity of Aplysia sensory neurons by the appropriate target cell during in vitro development appears to be due to a local interaction with the postsynaptic cell. Different regions of the outgrowth of the same sensory neuron may be relatively simple or complex depending on whether they contact an L7 cell. Moreover, the guidance of the sensory outgrowth by the postsynaptic cell indicates that the motor neuron's surface is an attractive substrate for the growing sensory processes. These interactions between the sensory and the motor neuron may depend on a constituent of L7's surface membrane (Sperry 1963; Walter et al. 1987) or a diffusible factor released locally from L7 (Davies et al. 1987; Levi-Montalcini 1987; Tessier-Lavigne et al. 1988).

Long-term Morphological Changes in Aplysia Sensory Neurons In Vitro Due to 5-HT Are Also Regulated by the Postsynaptic Motor Neuron

Bailey and Chen (1983, 1988a, 1989) found that behavioral training that produced long-term sensitization of the gill-and-siphon-withdrawal reflex also produced long-lasting morphological changes in siphon sensory neurons in the Aplysia abdominal ganglion. Using horseradish peroxidase to visualize the terminals of the sensory neurons, Bailey and Chen analyzed the changes in the number, size, and extent of the active zones and in the number and distribution of the synaptic vesicles, the likely storage sites of transmitter quanta. They found two sorts of changes. First, the sensory neurons of sensitized animals had more varicose expansions than controls (30% increase after 1 day of training; 100% increase after 4 days of training). Second, a larger percentage of varicosities had an active zone. The mean ratio of active zones to varicosities increased from 41% in control animals to 65% in animals sensitized with 4 days of training.

To study these learning-related presynaptic morphological changes more directly, and to relate them to long-term synaptic changes, Glanzman et al. (1990) performed experiments on in vitro Aplysia sensorimotor synapses. Using low-light-level video microscopy, Glanzman et al. were able to image the sensory neuron in vitro before and after it had been treated with five repeated applications of 5-HT. They found that 24 hours after 5-HT treatment, there was a significant increase in the number of presynaptic varicosities in sensory-L7 cocultures (Figs. 10 and 11). Moreover, the increase in varicosity number was correlated with the long-term synaptic enhancement (Fig. 11). Interestingly, this morphological effect of 5-HT again depended on the presence of an appropriate target cell. Sensory neurons alone in cell culture did not exhibit long-term morphological changes when treated with repeated applications of 5-HT.

These findings and those of Bailey and Chen suggest that long-term sensitization of the Aplysia withdrawal reflex is mediated in part by structural changes in presynaptic sensory neurons, which require a postsynaptic target for their expression. At present, we do not know the nature of the postsynaptic cell's contribution to the presynaptic changes. It might be a constituent of the motor cell's membrane or, conversely, it might be a diffusible factor released from the motor cell's processes.

Irrespective of the specific mechanisms for interaction, the 5-HT-induced long-term in vitro growth resembles in two ways the in vitro development of the sensory neurons (the growth that occurs during the first 5 days in cell culture): (1) The growth of the sensory neuron induced by 5-HT also requires the postsynaptic motor neuron. (2) The growth induced by 5-HT appears to be guided by the motor neuron in that it is not cell-wide but restricted to those sensory neurites in contact with L7.

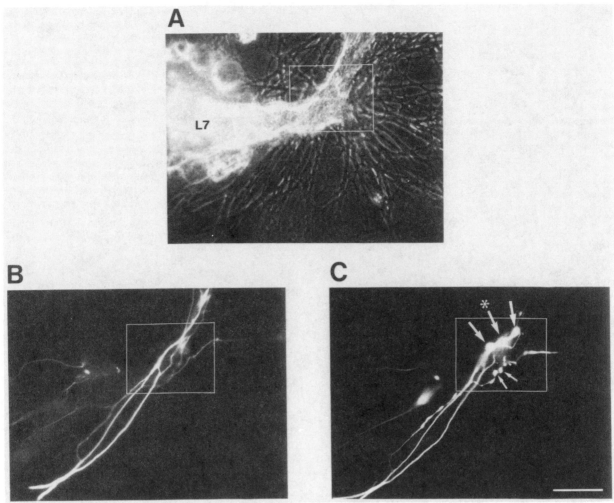

Figure 10. Phase-contrast (*A*) and fluorescence (*B* and *C*) video micrographs of a 5-HT-treated coculture. The same region of the coculture is shown in all three micrographs, so that the relation between presynaptic and postsynaptic structures can be seen. All of the neurites visible in *A* belong to the motor neuron L7. The sensory processes are finer and run along the motor neurites. They are therefore not apparent in the phase-contrast micrograph. Note in *A* a portion of L7's soma and the large initial segment of the major motor axon, which in this coculture has an elbow-like shape. This neurite actually represents three separate motor axons that collapse together when the cell is taken out of the abdominal ganglion and placed into cell culture. (*B*) Fluorescence micrograph of the processes of a single, dye-labeled sensory neuron before 5-HT treatment. By comparing *A* and *B*, one can see where the sensory neuron contacts the initial segment of L7. Note that in the outlined region there are no sensory varicosities. (*C*) Fluorescence micrograph of the same sensory neuron approximately 24 hr after 5-HT treatment. Note the presence of several new varicosities in the outlined region (arrows). This same coculture was fixed after reimaging the sensory neuron and prepared for electron microscopy (see Fig. 11). Bar, 50 μm. (Reprinted, with permission, from Glanzman et al. 1990.)

Structural Changes Accompanying Long-term Facilitation May Involve the Regulation of Expression of a Group of Developmentally Regulated Cell Adhesion Molecules

What molecular mechanisms contribute to synaptic growth? To begin to explore the roles of the early proteins in the induction of the structural change accompanying long-term facilitation, Mayford et al. (1990) focused on four proteins, D_1–D_4, which decrease their expression in a transcriptionally dependent manner following application of 5-HT or cAMP. These proteins have molecular masses that range from 100 kD to 140 kD. Peptide mapping indicates that they are related. These four proteins cross-react selectively and specifically with two monoclonal antibodies raised by Keller and Schacher (1990) against proteins in the neuropil region of *Aplysia* neurons. Their biochemical characterization indicates that they have characteristics of cell adhesion molecules. They are intrinsic membrane proteins that are glycosylated. They are specific to the nervous system and are especially enriched in the processes of neurons and in their synaptic terminals, and they promote neurite fasciculation.

Mayford et al. (1990) have cloned a cDNA coding for one of the molecular species by screening a λgt11 cDNA expression library from *Aplysia* CNS with the monoclonal antibodies. The deduced amino acid sequence shows that the proteins are members of the immunoglobulin superfamily of adhesion molecules,

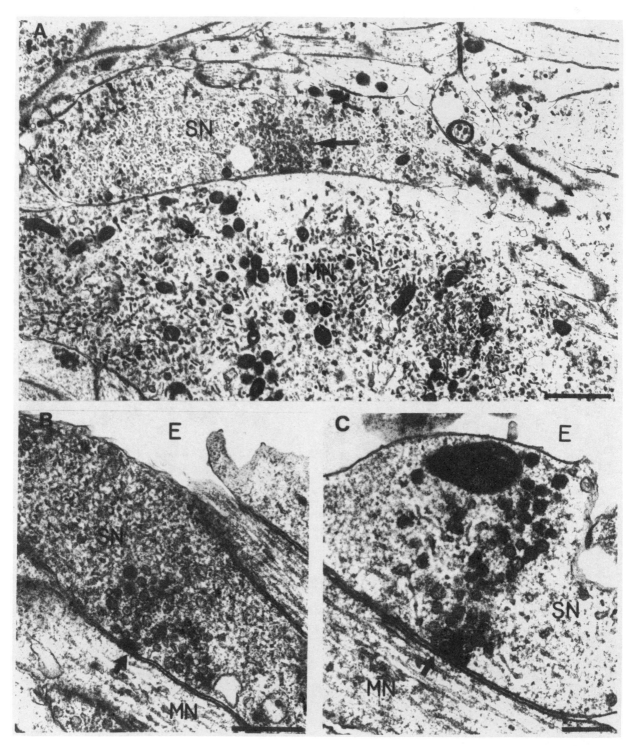

Figure 11. Electron micrographs made of the coculture shown in Fig. 10 following 5-HT treatment and reimaging of the sensory neuron. Because of the distinctive elbow-like shape of the initial segment of L7 in this coculture, it was possible to identify the new varicosities that appear in Fig. 10C in the thin sections cut through this region of the coculture. (*A*) Electron micrograph of a region of one of the three larger varicosities (indicated by the asterisk) shown in Fig. 10C. An active zone (arrow) can be seen. (SN) Sensory neuron; (MN) motor neuron. Bar, 1 μm. (*B*) Electron micrograph of a region of one of the smaller varicosities indicated by the small arrows in Fig. 10C. An active zone is indicated by the arrow. (E) Extracellular space. Bar, 0.50 μm. (*C*) Electron micrograph of a region of another of the smaller varicosities indicated by the small arrows in 10C. The arrow here indicates an active zone. Note the relation of E, the extracellular space, to the sensory neuron structures in *B* and *C* and compare to the positions of the smaller varicosities (small arrows) in 10C. Bar, 0.25 μm.

which includes N-CAM and fasciclin II. Consistent with their role as cell adhesion molecules, monoclonal antibodies against the proteins perturb axon fasciculation in the sensory neurons and increase the number of fine diameter neurites in cultures of sensory neurons. Because long-term facilitation is associated with structural changes in sensorimotor synapses, the down-regulation of adhesion molecules may be one step in a growth program activated by 5-HT.

In contrast to their localization in the adult, these proteins are found widely expressed in pregastrulation embryos (Fig. 12). S.G.N. Grant et al. (in prep.) have found that the D proteins can be detected as early as the two-cell embryo (day 1) on the cell surface at the junction between blastomeres. Throughout the blastula and gastrula stages, the D proteins are present on all cells and are enriched at points of cell-cell contact. With development of the segmentation cavity (day 3) and establishment of longitudinal polarity, expression becomes restricted first to the ectoderm and then to the posterior pole of the animal, where the ectoderm is proliferating and differentiating (days 4–5). Within this posterior ectoderm, which gives rise to many structures, D-protein expression appears to localize to an ectoderm bud invaginating into the segmentation cavity. As the animals hatch to form free-swimming larvae, the D proteins are seen in the first neurons of the cerebral ganglia and now are lost from all other ectodermal structures (day 10). Throughout all the subsequent premetamorphic and postmetamorphic stages of juvenile development, D expression is neuron-specific.

This embryological pattern in the expression of proteins D_1–D_4 also is similar to that of the N-CAM cell adhesion molecules in vertebrate development (Levi et al. 1987) and suggests that the *Aplysia* CAM may have a comparable role in morphogenic events during embryogenesis. These studies therefore suggest that proteins D_1–D_4, which play a role in early embryogenesis, are reutilized in the adult, specifically in the nervous system, where they are modulated during synaptic plasticity (Fig. 13). These results support the idea that development of neurons and their connections, as well

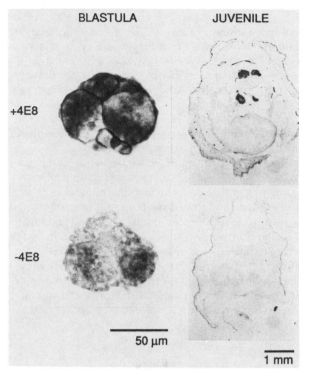

Figure 12. Expression of D proteins during *Aplysia* embryogenesis, detected by immunostaining with monoclonal antibody 4E8. Cryostat sections of blastula (*left* panels) and stage 11 juvenile animals (*right* panels) were reacted with (*upper* panels) or without (*lower* panels) the 4E8 antibody. Expression of D proteins is on the surface of all blastomeres at the blastula stage and is restricted to neurons in juvenile animals.

as the plasticity at mature synapses, may depend on the expression and regulation of a common set of molecules.

OVERALL VIEW

Our studies suggest an interesting relationship between aspects of development and long-term memory storage. This relationship is based on several features.

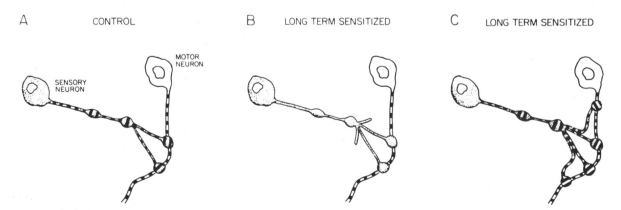

Figure 13. *Aplysia* cell adhesion molecules (indicated in stripes) are transiently decreased in expression following exposure to 5-HT and prior to process outgrowth. (*A*) Control. (*B*) One hour following training. (*C*) After outgrowth.

First, in initiating the long-term process, 5-HT, a modulatory transmitter, and cAMP, a second messenger, important for long-term synaptic plasticity, stimulate protein synthesis (Barzilai et al. 1989), much as do NGF and other growth factors important in development (Garrels and Schubert 1979; for review, see Schneider and Johnson 1989). Second, in addition to an overall stimulation, 5-HT and cAMP activate a specific set of proteins that bears at least a partial resemblance to the immediate-early proteins evident in quiescent cells activated to enter the cell cycle by serum and growth factors. Third, the long-term synaptic plasticity involves a growth of synaptic connections. Fourth, as is the case for synapse formation, the learning-related growth requires the presence of an appropriate target. Finally, the learning-related growth is associated with reorganization of immunoglobulin-related cell adhesion molecules present during early embryogenesis. These data suggest that synapse formation during development and learning-related growth changes may share certain common molecular regulatory mechanisms.

REFERENCES

Agranoff, B.W. 1967. Agents that block memory. In *The neurosciences: A study program* (ed. G.C. Quarton et al.), p. 756. Rockefeller University Press, New York.

Alkon, D.L., S. Naito, M. Kubota, C. Chen, B. Bank, J. Smallwood, P. Gollant, and H. Rasmussen. 1988. Regulation of *Hermissenda* K$^+$ channels by cytoplasmic and membrane associated C-kinase. *J. Neurochem.* **51:** 903.

Atkinson, R.C. and R.M. Shiffrin. 1968. Human memory: A proposed system and its control processes. In *The psychology of learning and motivation* (ed. K.W. Spence and J.T. Spence), vol. 2, p. 89. Academic Press, New York.

Barbizet, J. 1970. *Human memory and its pathology.* Freeman Press, San Francisco.

Barondes, S.H. 1970. Multiple steps in the biology of memory. In *The neurosciences: Second study program* (ed. F.O. Schmitt et al.), p. 272. Rockefeller University Press, New York.

Bailey, C.H. and M. Chen. 1983. Morphological basis of long-term habituation and sensitization in *Aplysia. Science* **220:** 91.

———. 1988a. Long-term memory in *Aplysia* modulates the total varicosities of single identified sensory neurons. *Proc. Natl. Acad. Sci.* **85:** 2373.

———. 1988b. Long-term sensitization in *Aplysia* increases the number of presynaptic contacts onto the identified gill motor neuron L7. *Proc. Natl. Acad. Sci.* **85:** 9356.

———. 1989. Time course of structural changes at identified sensory neuron synapses during long-term sensitization in *Aplysia. J. Neurosci.* **9:** 1774.

Barzilai, A., T.E. Kennedy, J.D. Sweatt, and E.R. Kandel. 1989. 5-HT modulates protein synthesis and the expression of specific proteins during long-term facilitation in *Aplysia* sensory neurons. *Neuron* **2:** 1577.

Bennett, E.L., M.C. Diamond, D. Krech, and M.R. Rosenzweig. 1964. Chemical and anatomical plasticity of the brain. *Science* **146:** 610.

Bergold, P.J., J.D. Sweatt, I. Winicov, K.R. Weiss, E.R. Kandel, and J.H. Schwartz. 1990. Protein synthesis during acquisition of long-term facilitation is needed for the persistent loss of regulatory subunits of the *Aplysia* cAMP-dependent protein kinase. *Proc. Natl. Acad. Sci.* **87:** 3788.

Bernier, L., V.F. Castellucci, E.R. Kandel, and J.H.

Schwartz. 1982. Facilitatory transmitter causes a selective and prolonged increase in cAMP in sensory neurons mediating the gill- and siphon-withdrawal reflex in *Aplysia. J. Neurosci.* **2:** 1682.

Braha, O., N. Dale, B. Hochner, M. Klein, T.W. Abrams, and E.R. Kandel. 1990. Second messengers involved in the two processes of presynaptic facilitation that contribute to sensitization and dishabituation in *Aplysia* sensory neurons. *Proc. Natl. Acad. Sci.* **87:** 2040.

Brunelli, M., V.F. Castellucci, and E.R. Kandel. 1976. Synaptic facilitation and behavioral sensitization in *Aplysia*: Possible role of serotonin and cyclic AMP. *Science* **194:** 1178.

Cajal, S.R. 1911. *Histologie du Système Nerveux de l'Homme & des Vertébrés,* vol. 2. (translated by L. Azoulay). Instituto Ramón y Cajal, 1955, Madrid.

Castellucci, V.F. and E.R. Kandel. 1976. Presynaptic facilitation as a mechanism for behavioral sensitization in *Aplysia. Science* **194:** 1176.

Castellucci, V.F., H. Blumenfeld, P. Goelet, and E.R. Kandel. 1989. Inhibitor of protein synthesis blocks long-term behavioral sensitization in the isolated gill-withdrawal reflex of *Aplysia. J. Neurobiol.* **20:** 1.

Castellucci, V.F., H.M. Pinsker, I. Kupfermann, and E.R. Kandel. 1970. Neuronal mechanisms of habituation and dishabituation of the gill-withdrawal reflex in *Aplysia. Science* **167:** 1745.

Castellucci, V.F., A.C. Nairn, P. Greengard, J.H. Schwartz, and E.R. Kandel. 1982. Inhibitor of cAMP-dependent protein kinase blocks presynaptic facilitation in *Aplysia. J. Neurosci.* **2:** 1673.

Castellucci, V.F., E.R. Kandel, J.H. Schwartz, F.D. Wilson, A.C. Nairn, and P. Greengard. 1980. Intracellular injection of the catalytic subunit of cAMP-dependent protein kinase stimulates facilitation of transmitter release underlying behavioral sensitization in *Aplysia. Proc. Natl. Acad. Sci.* **77:** 7492.

Chang, F.-L.F. and W.T. Greenough. 1984. Transient and enduring morphological correlates of synaptic activity and efficacy change in rat hippocampal slice. *Brain. Res.* **309:** 35.

Craik, F.I.M. and R.S. Lockhart. 1972. Levels of processing: A framework for memory research. *J. Verb. Learn. Verb. Behav.* **11:** 671.

Crow, T. and J. Forrester. 1990. Inhibition of protein synthesis blocks long-term enhancement of generator potentials produced by one-trial *in vivo* conditioning in *Hermissenda. Proc. Natl. Acad. Sci.* **87:** 4490.

Dale, N. and E.R. Kandel. 1990. Facilitatory and inhibitory transmitters modulate spontaneous transmitter release at cultured *Aplysia* sensorimotor synapses. *J. Physiol.* **421:** 203.

Dale, N., E.R. Kandel, and S. Schacher. 1987. Serotonin produces long-term changes in the excitability of *Aplysia* sensory neurons in culture that depends on new protein synthesis. *J. Neurosci.* **7:** 2232.

Dale, N., S. Schacher, and E.R. Kandel. 1988. Long-term facilitation in *Aplysia* involves increase in transmitter release. *Science* **239:** 282.

Dash, P., B. Hochner, and E.R. Kandel. 1990. Injection of the cAMP-responsive element into the nucleus of *Aplysia* sensory neurons blocks long-term facilitation. *Nature* **345:** 718.

Davis, H.P. and L.R. Squire. 1984. Protein synthesis and memory: A review. *Psychol. Bull.* **96:** 518.

Davies, A.M., C. Bandtlow, R. Heumann, S. Korsching, H. Rohrer, and H. Thoenen. 1987. Timing and site of nerve growth factor synthesis in developing skin in relation to innervation and expression of the receptor. *Nature* **326:** 353.

Desmond, N.L. and W.B. Levy. 1986a. Changes in the numerical density of synaptic contacts with long-term potentiation in the hippocampal dentate gyrus. *J. Comp. Neurol.* **253:** 466.

————. 1986b. Changes in the postsynaptic density with long-term potentiation in the dentate gyrus. *J. Comp. Neurol.* **253:** 476.

Diamond, M.C., F. Law, H. Rhodes, B. Linder, M.R. Rosenzweig, D. Krech, and E.L. Bennett. 1966. Increases in cortical depth and glia numbers in rats subjected to enriched environment. *J. Comp. Neurol.* **128:** 117.

Ebbinghaus, H. 1885. *Memory: A contribution to experimental psychology.* (Reprinted.) Dover, New York.

Farley, J. and S. Auerbach. 1986. Protein kinase C activation induces conductance changes in *Hermissenda* photoreceptors like those seen in associative learning. *Nature* **319:** 220.

Fifkova, E. and A. Van Harreveld. 1977. Long-lasting morphological changes in dendritic spines of dentate granular cells following stimulation of the entorhinal area. *J. Neurocytol.* **6:** 211.

Flexner, J.B., L.B. Flexner, and E. Stellar. 1963. Memory in mice as affected by intracerebral puromycin. *Science* **141:** 567.

Frey, U., M. Krug, K.G. Reymann, and H. Matthies. 1988. Anisomycin, an inhibitor of protein synthesis, blocks late phases of LTP phenomena in the hippocampal CA1 region *in vitro. Brain Res.* **452:** 57.

Frost, W.N., V.G. Castellucci, R.D. Hawkins, and E.R. Kandel. 1985. The monosynaptic connections made by the sensory neurons of the gill- and siphon-withdrawal reflex participate in the storage of long-term memory for sensitization. *Proc. Natl. Acad. Sci.* **82:** 8266.

Garrels, J.I. and D. Schubert. 1979. Modulation of protein synthesis by nerve growth factor. *J. Biol. Chem.* **254:** 7978.

Glanzman, D.L., E.R. Kandel, and S. Schacher. 1989a. Identified target motor neuron regulates neurite outgrowth and synaptic formation of *Aplysia* sensory neurons *in vitro. Neuron* **3:** 441.

————. 1990. Target-dependent structural changes accompanying long-term synaptic facilitation in *Aplysia* neurons. *Science* **249:** 799.

Glanzman, D.L., S.L. Mackey, R.D. Hawkins, A.M. Dyke, P.E. Lloyd, and E.R. Kandel. 1989b. Depletion of serotonin in the nervous system of *Aplysia* reduces the behavioral enhancement of gill-withdrawal as well as the heterosynaptic facilitation produced by tail shock. *J. Neurosci.* **9:** 4200.

Goelet, P., V.F. Castellucci, S. Schacher, and E.R. Kandel. 1986. The long and short of long-term memory—A molecular framework. *Nature* **322:** 419.

Greenberg, S.M., V.F. Castellucci, H. Bayley, and J.H. Schwartz. 1987. A molecular mechanism for long-term sensitization in *Aplysia. Nature* **329:** 62.

James, W. 1890. *The principles of psychology,* 2 vols. Holt, New York.

Keller, F. and S. Schacher. 1990. Neuron-specific membrane glycoproteins promoting neurite fasciculation in *Aplysia californica. J. Cell Biol.* (in press).

Klein, M., J. Camardo, and E.R. Kandel. 1982. Serotonin modulates a specific potassium current in the sensory neurons that show presynaptic facilitation in *Aplysia. Proc. Natl. Acad. Sci.* **79:** 5713.

Lee, K.S., F. Schotler, M. Oliver, and G. Lynch. 1980. Brief bursts of high-frequency stimulation produce two types of structural change in rat hippocampus. *J. Neurophysiol.* **2:** 247.

Levi, G., K.L. Crossin, and G.M. Edelman. 1987. Expression sequences and distribution of two primary cell adhesion molecules during embryonic development of *Xenopus laevis. J. Cell Biol.* **105:** 2359.

Levi-Montalcini, R. 1987. The nerve growth factor 35 years later. *Science* **237:** 1154.

Mackey, S.L., E.R. Kandel, and R.D. Hawkins. 1989. Identified serotonergic neurons LCB1 and RCB1 in the cerebral ganglia of *Aplysia* produce presynaptic facilitation of siphon sensory neurons. *J. Neurosci.* **9:** 4227.

Malenka, R.C., J.A. Kauer, D.J. Perkel, M.D. Mark, P.T. Kelly, R.A. Nicoll, and N.N. Waxham. 1989. An essential role for postsynaptic calmodulin and protein kinase activity in long-term potentiation. *Nature* **340:** 554.

Malinow, R., H. Schulman, and R.N. Tsien. 1989. Inhibition of postsynaptic PKC or CaMKII blocks induction but not expression of LTPD. *Science* **245:** 862.

Mayford, M., F. Keller, A. Barzilai, S. Schacher, and E.R. Kandel. 1990. Cloning of a neural cell adhesion molecule from *Aplysia* that is modulated in the sensory neurons in response to 5-HT. *Soc. Neurosci. Abstr.* **16:** 627.

McGaugh, J.L. 1966. Time-dependent processes in memory storage. *Science* **153:** 1351.

Montarolo, P.G., P. Goelet, V.F. Castellucci, J. Morgan, E.R. Kandel, and S. Schacher. 1986. A critical period for macromolecular synthesis in long-term heterosynaptic facilitation in *Aplysia. Science* **234:** 1249.

Montminy, M.R., K.R. Sevarino, J.A. Wagner, G. Mondel, and R.H. Goodman. 1986. Identification of a cyclic AMP responsive element within the rat somastatin gene. *Proc. Natl. Acad. Sci.* **86:** 6682.

Otani, S. and W.C. Abraham. 1989. Inhibition of protein synthesis in the dentate gyrus, but not the entorhinal cortex, blocks maintenance of long-term potentiation. *Neurosci. Lett.* **106:** 175.

Otani, S., C.J. Marshall, W.P. Tate, G.V. Goddard, and W.C. Abraham. 1989. Maintenance of long-term potentiation in rat dentate gyrus requires protein synthesis but not messenger RNA synthesis immediately post-teranization. *Neuroscience* **28:** 519.

Pinsker, H.M., W.A. Hening, T.J. Carew, and E.R. Kandel. 1973. Long-term sensitization of a defensive withdrawal reflex in *Aplysia. Science* **182:** 1039.

Pinsker, H.M., I. Kupfermann, V.F. Castellucci, and E.R. Kandel. 1970. Habituation and dishabituation of the gill-withdrawal reflex in *Aplysia. Science* **167:** 1740.

Ramón y Cajal, S. 1911. *Histologie du Systéme Nerveux de l'Homme et des Vertébrés,* vol. 2. A Maloine, Paris. (Reprinted by Consejo Superior de Investigationes Cientificas, Instituto Ramón Y Cajal, Madrid, 1955.)

Rayport, S.G. and S. Schacher. 1986. Synaptic plasticity *in vitro:* Cell culture of identified *Aplysia* neurons mediating short-term habituation and sensitization. *J. Neurosci.* **6:** 759.

Russell, W.R. and P.W. Nathan. 1946. Traumatic amnesia. *Brain* **69:** 280.

Schacher, S., V.F. Castellucci, and E.R. Kandel. 1988. cAMP evokes long-term facilitation in *Aplysia* sensory neurons that requires new protein synthesis. *Science* **240:** 1667.

Schacher, S., P.G. Montarolo, and E.R. Kandel. 1990. Selective short- and long-term effects of serotonin, small cardioactive peptide, and tetanic stimulation on sensorimotor synapses in *Aplysia* in culture. *J. Neurosci.* (in press).

Schneider, W.D. and E.M. Johnson, Jr. 1989. Neurotrophic molecules. *Ann. Neurol.* **26:** 489.

Scholz, K.P. and J.H. Byrne. 1987. Long-term sensitization in *Aplysia:* Biophysical correlates in tail sensory neurons. *Science* **235:** 685.

————. 1988. Intercellular injection of cyclic AMP induces a long-term reduction of neuronal potassium current. *Science* **240:** 1664.

Schwartz, J.H., V.F. Castellucci, and E.R. Kandel. 1971. Functioning of identified neurons and synapses in abdominal ganglion of *Aplysia* in the absence of protein synthesis. *J. Neurophysiol.* **34:** 939.

Sorrentino, V. 1989. Growth factors, growth inhibitors and cell cycle control. *Anticancer Res.* **9:** 1925.

Sperry, R.W. 1963. Chemoaffinity in the orderly growth of nerve fiber patterns and connections. *Proc. Natl. Acad. Sci.* **78:** 703.

Sweatt, J.D. and E.R. Kandel. 1989. Persistent and transcriptionally-dependent increase in protein phosphorylation in long-term facilitation of *Aplysia* sensory neurons. *Nature* **339:** 51.

Tessier-Lavigne, M., M. Placzek, A.G.S. Lumsden, J. Dodd, and T.M. Jessell. 1988. Chemotropic guidance of developing axons in the mammalian central nervous system. *Nature* **336:** 775.

Walter, J., B. Kern-Veits, J. Huf, B. Stoltze, and F. Bonhoeffer. 1987. Recognition of position-specific properties of tectal cell membranes by retinal axons *in vitro*. *Development* **101:** 85.

Weiskrantz, L. 1970. A long-term view of short-term memory in psychology. In *Short-term changes in neural activity and behaviour* (ed. G. Horn and R.A. Hinde), p. 63. Cambridge University Press, England.

Wickelgren, W.A. 1973. The long and the short of memory. *Psychol. Bull.* **80:** 425.

Genetic Dissection of Memory Formation in *Drosophila melanogaster*

T. TULLY,* S. BOYNTON,* C. BRANDES,* J.M. DURA,†
R. MIHALEK,* T. PREAT,* AND A. VILLELLA*

*Department of Biology, Brandeis University, Waltham, Massachusetts 02254; †Centre de Génétique
Moléculaire du C.N.R.S., 91190 Gif-sur-Yvette, France

Over a decade ago, the last mutagenesis to generate mutations affecting associative learning in *Drosophila* ended. In all, about 3500 strains, mutagenized with ethylmethane sulfonate (EMS), were screened first in S. Benzer's laboratory at CalTech and then in W.G. Quinn's laboratory at Princeton (for review, see Aceves-Pina et al. 1983). Associative learning was assayed with an olfactory shock-avoidance conditioning procedure specifically designed to produce an average learning index for a population of flies, which were trained and tested en masse (Quinn et al. 1974). The conditioning procedure employed two conditioned stimuli (CSs): Flies received electric shock (US) if they approached one odor (CS+), but not if they approached a second odor (CS−). In a subsequent test trial, one could conclude that associative learning occurred only if more flies avoided the CS+ than the CS−, and only in this case would the learning index be greater than zero (for more details, see Tully 1984). Significantly, this discriminative, group conditioning procedure precluded the time-consuming process of assaying learning in individuals, thereby increasing the efficiency of screening thousands of mutant strains (see also Tully 1986).

When the mutagenic dust had settled, six mutant strains showed no shock-avoidance conditioning but normal olfactory acuity and shock reactivity. Initial genetic complementation tests suggested that five genes on the X chromosome were mutated. Two EMS-induced alleles of the *dunce* gene were isolated by D. Byers in Benzer's laboratory (Dudai et al. 1976; Byers et al. 1981), while P. Sziber in Quinn's laboratory isolated one mutant allele for each of the *rutabaga, cabbage, turnip,* and *radish* genes (Aceves-Pina and Quinn 1979; Duerr and Quinn 1982; Aceves-Pina et al. 1983). P. Sziber also identified a sixth X-linked gene, *amnesiac*, by conditioning flies from mutant strains with a modified shock-avoidance procedure in which conditioned responses were assayed 45 minutes after training. Under these conditions, *amnesiac* mutants learned normally but showed abnormally rapid memory loss (Quinn et al. 1979). Flies from each of these six mutant strains subsequently were shown to perform poorly in several other behavioral tasks thought to involve some aspect of learning (Siegel and Hall 1979; Booker and Quinn 1981; Duerr and Quinn 1982; Folkers 1982;

Gailey et al. 1982, 1984; Tempel et al. 1983; Kyriacou and Hall 1984).

A fundamental genetic issue that arises from such mutagenesis is whether the aberrant phenotype of a mutant strain is produced by one or more than one mutation. The EMS procedure employed was designed to produce one lethal mutation in about 30% of X chromosomes (Lewis and Bacher 1968). Two or more viable mutations on the same chromosome can be produced, however. Moreover, mutagenized flies already may carry spontaneous mutations, which then might be isolated in the phenotypic screen. Evidence for two (complementing) mutations on the same chromosome frequently has been documented in mutagenesis for other traits. Sometimes the mutations affected unrelated phenotypes (Johnson et al. 1981); sometimes they affected similar phenotypes (Baker and Carpenter 1972; Kulkarni and Hall 1987).

Examples of each outcome also exist for the learning mutants. The *dunce* gene now is known to be involved with both associative learning and female fertility. Unlike *dunce²* mutants, however, *dunce¹* flies were not sterile. Subsequent genetic analyses later revealed that *dunce¹* flies carried a second mutation, a dominant suppressor of sterility, in another X-linked gene (Saltz et al. 1982); *rutabaga* flies also carry a second, X-linked mutation that produces "blistered" wings (T. Tully, unpubl.). Mutant *turnip* flies appear to be even more complicated genetically: The *turnip* X chromosome carries a lethal mutation and a suppressor of lethality, both of which map distal to the *turnip* locus (R.F. Smith et al., unpubl.), and a third mutation that affects protein kinase C (PKC) activity (Smith et al. 1986). The PKC-disrupting mutation most likely is not solely responsible for abnormal learning in *turnip* flies. This phenotype may result from an interaction between the "PKC" mutation and at least one other autosomal gene (Tully 1986). Given such caveats, it is important to note that genetic analyses only with *dunce, rutabaga,* and *amnesiac* flies have provided clear evidence that their mutant behaviors result from single-gene mutations (Byers 1980; Byers et al. 1981; Livingstone et al. 1984; Dudai et al. 1985; Livingstone 1985; Tully and Gergen 1986). Convincing evidence for the *cabbage, radish,* and *turnip* strains still is lacking.

Of the three bona fide single-gene learning/memory

mutations, biochemical abnormalities have been identified for two (for reviews, see Kiger and Saltz 1985; Heisenberg 1989). The *dunce* mutations disrupt a cAMP-specific phosphodiesterase (Byers et al. 1981; Kiger et al. 1981; Kauvar 1982; Shotwell 1983), and the *rutabaga* mutation disrupts several biochemical properties of adenylate cyclase (Livingstone et al. 1984; Dudai et al. 1985; Livingstone 1985). Davis and Davidson (1984) capitalized on the aberrant phosphodiesterase activity of *dunce* mutants to obtain DNA clones from the *dunce* region via linkage analyses with restriction site polymorphisms. Subsequent DNA sequence analysis has confirmed that the *dunce* gene encodes a phosphodiesterase (Chen et al. 1986).

Although these biochemical discoveries, implicating the cAMP cell-signaling pathway with associative learning in *Drosophila*, are impressive, one can argue that little progress toward a molecular understanding of the phenotype has been made. Compared to analyses of many other phenotypes in fruit flies, in fact, this behavior-genetic analysis has proceeded at glacial speed. In hindsight, however, we can attribute such slow progress to two technical problems:

1. Measuring differences among individuals (or genotypes) for behavioral phenotypes is time-consuming. Learning and memory, in particular, require excessive time to assay. Furthermore, since behavioral responses are ephemeral in design, many environmental factors conspire to make individual scores vary, thereby demanding larger sample sizes to obtain accurate estimates of genotypic effects. Thus, routine genetic experiments to generate new mutations or to map single-gene effects require such an investment of time as to make even the most resolute hesitate.

2. In addition to frequently isolating more than one mutation per chromosome, EMS mutageneses also usually produce single base-pair substitutions or small deletions, which are difficult to detect at the DNA level with existing molecular techniques. Therefore, further genetic experiments are required to isolate (molecularly visible) chromosomal breakpoints in or near the gene of interest. Even then, a tedious chromosomal walk often is necessary to clone the relevant stretch of genomic DNA. Importantly, identification of a second, pleiotropic phenotype that is easier to assay than the behavioral one can speed up genetic experiments. In fact, such was the case for the *dunce* and *rutabaga* genes. Usually, however, looking for pleiotropic effects is akin to looking for a needle in a haystack. A case in point is work on the *amnesiac* gene. Extensive biochemical experiments have detected no pleiotropic effects, and a chromosomal walk is mired in repetitive DNA (C. Brandes and T. Tully, unpubl.).

To remedy this situation, we at Brandeis have begun a mutagenesis in *Drosophila* to isolate new mutations affecting associative learning and memory. Our mutagens are genetically engineered P-element transposons

(see Bier et al. 1989), which first can be mobilized to jump randomly into genes, thereby disrupting them. Then, further transposition can be stabilized. Significantly, these P-element mutators represent molecular "tags," which are used to identify adjacent DNA sequence from the disrupted gene, thereby expediting its cloning. In addition, these mutators contain functional DNA sequences from other *Drosophila* genes, which encode products involved with eye pigmentation. Thus, in an appropriate genetic background, the mutator provides a "pleiotropic" morphological tag, which greatly facilitates subsequent genetic analyses of the behavioral phenotype. We describe behavioral and genetic work on the first P-element insertion mutant we have isolated.

To interpret the phenotype of our new mutant properly, we first describe behavioral experiments on normal (wild-type) and *amnesiac* flies. We have focused our attention on memory formation after an olfactory classical conditioning procedure (Tully and Quinn 1985). Our results suggest that three behaviorally distinct phases, or components, of memory underlie normal memory retention during the first 7 hours after training. Moreover, the *amnesiac* mutation may disrupt one of these components. We also introduce a new training procedure that substantially improves 24-hour memory in wild-type flies.

METHODS

Subjects. *Drosophila melanogaster* were of the wild-type Canton-S (Can-S) strain, a *white^{1118}* strain, and the *amnesiac* memory mutant strain (Quinn et al. 1979). Over the years, we have observed that the abnormal behavioral phenotypes of many of the extant learning/memory mutants become more normal with time. Presumably, flies carrying the mutant phenotype are less fit than wild-type flies, and natural selection over generations produces an accumulation of phenotype-ameliorating modifying alleles in the genetic background of mutant flies. To minimize this effect, we (1) replaced the second and third chromosomes in the original *amnesiac* strain, using the double balancer strain *y; Pm/CyO; Sb/TM6*, (2) maintained the *amnesiac* X chromosome over the *FM7a* X-chromosome balancer, which itself was outcrossed repeatedly to the Can-S strain to "cantonize" the autosomes, (3) only bred heterozygous *amn/FM7a* females (*amn* is recessive to the *amn⁺* allele in *FM7a* flies) to *FM7a* males every generation, and (4) bred homozygous *amn* flies every few months to use in behavioral experiments.

The mutant *latheo (lat)* was generated in our laboratory from an ongoing P-element insertional mutagenesis, the general details of which have been published elsewhere (Cooley et al. 1988; Tully 1990). We used a "mutator" strain, *w,9.3*, which contained a single, genetically engineered P-element transposon on the X chromosome (D. Coen and D. Anxolabehare, in prep.) in conjunction with the *SbΔ2-3, ry/TM6* "transposase donor" strain (Robertson et al. 1988). Independent transposition events were isolated first in heterozygous form, and then strains homozygous for each single P-element insertion were bred. Mutant *latheo* flies were the first to satisfy our behavioral and genetic criteria (see below). The appropriate control strain for behavioral comparisons with *latheo* was *white[1118]* [w(H)], which was cantonized by 4 generations of outcrossing to Can-S flies. Heterozygous, *w, lat/w, +* flies were outcrossed to *white* flies each generation to minimize any possible accumulation of genetic modifiers. Homozygous *w, lat/w, lat* flies then were bred regularly from the heterozygous strain for use in behavioral experiments.

Classical conditioning. Tully and Quinn (1985) modified the T-maze chamber of Dudai et al. (1976) so that carefully controlled currents of air could be drawn through it (Fig. 1). In this manner, the instrumental shock-avoidance conditioning procedure of Quinn et al. (1974) was adapted to a classical conditioning procedure, in which flies always received negative reinforcement in the presence of the CS[+]. About 100 flies were sequestered in a closed chamber and were trained by exposing them sequentially to two odors (either 3-octanol [OCT] or 4-methylcyclohexanol [MCH]) delivered in air currents. In the standard procedure, flies received a 60-second presentation of the first odor (CS[+]) along with 12 1.25-second 60-V (DC) pulses of electric shock every 5 seconds (US), a 30-second rest, a 60-second presentation of the second odor (CS[-]) without shock, and finally another 30-second rest.

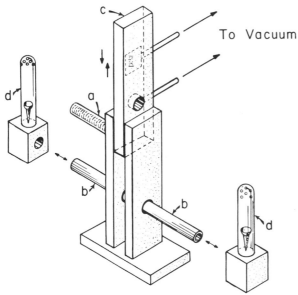

Figure 1. Classical conditioning apparatus of Tully and Quinn (1985). A group of about 100 flies are sequestered in the training chamber (*a*) and exposed sequentially to two different odors (contained in *d*)—one presented alone and the other presented along with electric shock. After training, flies are transferred via a miniature elevator (*c*) to the choice point of a T-maze, where they are exposed to the same two odors simultaneously in converging currents of air. After the test trial, flies are trapped in the arms of the T-maze (*b*), anesthetized, and counted (see text for more details).

To test for conditioned avoidance, flies were tapped gently into an elevator-like sliding compartment and were transported to the T-maze choice point of the teaching machine, between converging currents of OCT and MCH. After 120 seconds, the center compartment was slid up, trapping flies in the arms of the T-maze. Typically, 90% of wild-type (Can-S) flies avoided the CS[+], 5% avoided the CS[-], and 5% remained at the choice point.

After conclusion of the test trial, flies were anesthetized and counted. A "half lambda" was calculated as the fraction of flies avoiding the CS[+] (they ran toward CS[-]) minus the fraction of flies avoiding the CS[-] (they ran toward CS[+]). Flies remaining at the choice point were included in the total used to compute fractions. A second group of flies then was trained and tested as above using reciprocal odors for CS[+] and CS[-] (i.e., if OCT was CS[+] for the first group, then MCH was CS[+] for the second). A half lambda was calculated for the second group of flies, and then the two half lambdas were averaged to yield one learning index. In this manner, nonassociative changes in odor avoidance and any slight odor biases were eliminated arithmetically from the learning index. Concentrations of OCT and MCH were adjusted so that naive flies distributed themselves 50:50 in the T-maze during the test trial. Thus, if no associative learning occurred, then the learning index would be zero. Conversely, if all flies learned perfectly to associate a specific odor with electric shock, then all flies would avoid the CS[+] and the learning index would be one. Typically, wild-type flies yielded an average learning index of 0.85 (for more details, see Tully and Quinn 1985).

Memory retention. Groups of flies were trained as above, except that the CS[-] was presented first, followed by the CS[+]. Within 90 seconds after training, the flies were removed from the training chamber and stored at 25°C in the dark for 10, 15, 20, 30, 60, 120, or 180 minutes in plastic test tubes (Falcon no. 2017) containing pieces of filter paper soaked in 4% sucrose solution. Flies were aspirated from the test tubes to the choice point of the T-maze 70 seconds before the usual 120-second test trial. At retention time 0 in Figure 2, flies were transferred from the training chamber to the T-maze choice point 120 seconds after the shock stimulus ended. In memory retention experiments with *latheo* flies, equal numbers of mutant and *w(H)* control flies were mixed and then were trained, stored in glass shell vials with food, and tested together. Afterward, learning indices for each strain were obtained by separating the two genotypes according to eye color (*latheo* flies were red-eyed; *w(H)* flies were white-eyed).

Retrograde amnesia. Groups of flies were transferred 0, 10, 20, 30, 60, or 120 minutes after training (second odor shocked as above) to a 3.5 × 1.2-cm glass test tube, and the test tube was submerged in salted ice water (0°C) for 2 minutes. Flies stopped moving and fell to the bottom of the test tube within 30 seconds

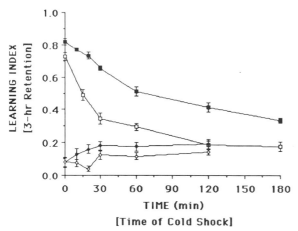

Figure 2. Memory retention and anesthesia-resistant memory in wild-type (Canton-S) and *amnesiac* flies. Retention was determined by training flies in the standard classical conditioning procedure and then by assaying conditioned avoidance responses (LEARNING INDEX) at various intervals (TIME) afterward. Memory decays with time in wild-type flies (■) but decays more quickly in *amnesiac* flies (□). Anesthesia-resistant memory was inferred from retrograde amnesia experiments, in which 3-hr retention was assayed in flies that received cold-shock anesthesia at various intervals (Time of Cold Shock) after training. Flies showed progressively higher 3-hr memory scores as the interval of time between training and cold-shock anesthesia increased. This result implies that an anesthesia-resistant phase of memory begins to form during training and reaches maximal levels 1–2 hr later. Interestingly, anesthesia-resistant memory levels were similar in wild-type (◆) and *amnesiac* (◇) flies. *n* = 18 and 8 learning indices at each memory retention interval for wild-type and *amnesiac* flies, respectively. *n* = 8 and 12 learning indices at each cold-shock interval for wild-type and *amnesiac* flies, respectively.

after being placed in ice water. Flies recovered from this "cold-shock" within 30 seconds after being removed to 25°C. Three-hour retention was assayed for each of these posttraining cold-shock groups, as well as for a pretraining control group that was cold-shocked 60 minutes before training. During the time intervals between training and cold-shock, and between cold-shock and testing, flies were stored in plastic test tubes containing a strip of filter paper soaked with 4% sucrose.

Reversal learning. After one training cycle, during which the second odor was paired with shock, groups of flies were retrained 0, 10, 20, 30, 60, or 180 minutes later by pairing the reciprocal odor with shock, i.e., if OCT was CS$^+$ in cycle 1, then MCH was CS$^+$ in cycle 2. Conditioned avoidance responses were measured immediately after cycle 2 training by transferring the flies to the T-maze for 120 seconds. To calculate a learning index, "CS$^+$" was the CS$^+$ of cycle 2. During the time intervals between cycle 1 and cycle 2 training, flies were stored in glass shell vials containing their usual food medium.

Long-term memory. Groups of flies received ten, instead of one, training cycles, with a 15-minute intercycle interval. Odor concentrations were a 10^{-3} dilu-

tion in mineral oil. Conditioned avoidance responses were tested 24 hours after training in the usual manner. During the retention interval, flies were stored in glass shell vials with food. They then were transferred to the T-maze choice point 90 seconds before the 120-second test trial began.

RESULTS

Memory Retention and Retrograde Amnesia in Wild-type and *amnesiac* Flies

Figure 2 compares memory retention curves between wild-type (Can-S) and *amnesiac* flies. As originally reported by Tully and Quinn (1985), *amnesiac* flies showed near-normal learning followed by a more rapid memory decay during the first hour after training. Thereafter, the *amnesiac* memory decay rate was similar to that of wild-type flies, suggesting that the *amnesiac* mutation interfered with early memory formation.

Results from retrograde amnesia experiments seem to support this notion. Cold-shock anesthesia administered to wild-type flies immediately after training served to diminish 3-hour retention levels. This amnestic effect was less severe, however, when cold-shock was administered at later intervals after training (see Fig. 2; cf. Quinn and Dudai 1976; Tempel et al. 1983; Tully 1988). Interestingly, the effect of retrograde amnesia in *amnesiac* flies was similar to that in wild-type flies.

Traditionally, retrograde amnestic effects have been interpreted to indicate that an anesthesia-resistant phase of memory begins to form during training, or immediately thereafter, reaching maximal levels within a few hours (cf. Andrew 1980). Thus, memory formation after classical conditioning in *Drosophila* appears to be composed of anesthesia-sensitive and anesthesia-resistant components. This idea is visualized in Figure 2 by plotting results from the retrograde amnesia experiments along with the memory retention curves of wild-type (Can-S) and *amnesiac* flies. Comparisons of memory retention curves with the anesthesia-resistant memory (ARM) curves suggest that a cold-shock-sensitive phase of memory still is present 2 hours after training in wild-type flies. In contrast, no such memory phase is detectable 2 hours after training in *amnesiac* flies. In other words, ARM can account entirely for memory levels 2 (or more) hours after training in *amnesiac* flies but not in wild-type flies. So what is the nature of the cold-shock-sensitive phase of memory in wild-type flies?

Components of Memory

One approach to answering the question above is to decompose the wild-type memory retention curve into additive components. First, the ARM curve (wild-type and *amn* data combined) can be subtracted from the *amnesiac* retention curve to reveal a short-term component presumably present in both wild-type and *amnesiac* flies. Second, the *amnesiac* retention curve can be subtracted from the wild-type retention curve to reveal another component presumably present in wild-type flies but missing in *amnesiac* flies. Thus, Figure 3 shows the three resulting hypothetical components of memory, which we refer to as short-term memory (STM), middle-term memory (MTM), and anesthesia-resistant memory (ARM). The kinetics of these three memory components are surprisingly similar to a model of memory formation proposed earlier (Tully 1988) and to results from pharmacological experiments on memory formation in chicks and on long-term potentiation (Gibbs and Ng 1976; Patterson et al. 1986; Matthies 1989).

At this stage of model building, we must emphasize two important points: (1) The components of memory that we have derived are based on the assumptions that memory phases act additively to produce overall memory retention and that the *amnesiac* mutation eliminates a specific component. (2) Although we empirically can distinguish the ARM component from earlier components (STM and MTM), we have not yet provided experimental evidence for the existence of separate STM and MTM components. These memory components exist only by assuming that the *amnesiac* mutation disrupts MTM specifically. An alternative hypothesis is that classical conditioning produces only one early (cold-shock-sensitive) phase of memory and therefore the *amnesiac* mutation produces a quantitative effect on this early phase (STM), rather than eliminating a qualitatively different component (MTM). Interpretation of results from the next experiment begins to shed light on these two alternative hypotheses.

Reversal Learning in Wild-type and *amnesiac* Flies

Although reversal learning per se has been done before with olfactory conditioning in *Drosophila*

(Quinn et al. 1974, 1979; Dudai 1983; Tully and Quinn 1985), we extended the experiment to determine the interaction of reversal learning (but not memory induced by it) with memory present at *several* retention intervals after cycle 1 training (see Methods). Much to our surprise, the resulting "reversal retention" curves of wild-type and *amnesiac* flies were not significantly different (Fig. 4). One way to interpret these results is that an environmental manipulation (reversal learning) has eliminated the phenotypic difference in (cycle 1) memory between wild-type and *amnesiac* flies (compare Figs. 2 and 4).

More detailed analysis of results from the reversal learning experiment also supports the hypothesis that STM and MTM are functionally distinct phases of memory. Figure 5 plots the observed reversal retention curve for wild-type and *amnesiac* flies combined (open diamonds connected by solid line), along with other "retention" curves representing hypothetical outcomes of the experiment. First, if reversal learning had no effect whatsoever, then the lowest curve in Figure 5 would represent memory retention induced by cycle 1 training. The learning indices are negative because of the way they are calculated in the reversal learning experiment (see Methods). Second, if reversal learning always was of the same magnitude (represented by arrows in Fig. 5) and *interacted additively* with cycle 1 memory at all retention intervals, then one expected reversal retention curve would resemble the curve at the top of the arrows in Figure 5. It follows that the difference between the observed reversal retention curve and this expected reversal retention curve (hatched area in Fig. 5) represents the *non*additive interaction of reversal learning with cycle 1 memory. Finally, if reversal learning completely disrupted cycle

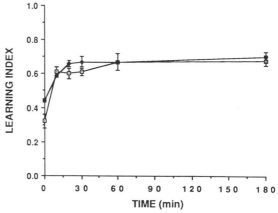

Figure 4. "Reversal retention" in wild-type (□) and *amnesiac* (◆) flies. Groups of flies were trained in the standard classical conditioning procedure in cycle 1. At various time intervals after cycle 1 training, the flies then were retrained (cycle 2) to the reciprocal odor combination, i.e., the odor that was CS⁺ in cycle 1 was CS⁻ in cycle 2 and vice versa (reversal learning). Conditioned avoidance responses (learning index) were assayed immediately after cycle 2 (re)training. The resulting reversal retention curves were similar for wild-type and *amnesiac* flies. $n = 4$ at 0, 10, 20, 30, and 60 retention intervals for wild-type and *amnesiac* flies. $n = 2$ for both genotypes at the 180-min interval.

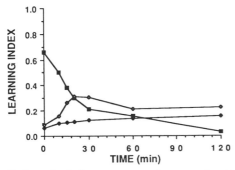

Figure 3. Hypothetical components of memory in wild-type flies. Anesthesia-resistant memory (ARM) component (◆), the average of wild-type and *amnesiac* data, was derived empirically from retrograde amnesia experiments. The short-term memory (STM) component (■) was obtained by subtracting ARM from the *amnesiac* retention curve in Fig. 2. The middle-term memory (MTM) component (◇) was obtained by subtracting the *amnesiac* retention curve from the wild-type retention curve. See text for more details.

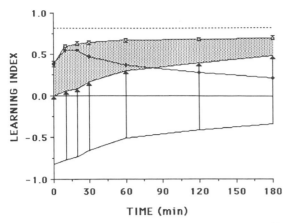

Figure 5. Reversal retention (for wild-type and *amnesiac* flies combined) in relation to hypothetical outcomes. If reversal learning did not occur, then the lowest line would be expected. If, however, reversal learning (*arrows*) interacted additively with memory of cycle 1 training, then the line on top of the arrows would be expected. The difference (*hatched area*) between this line and the observed reversal retention curve (◇) represents the nonadditive interaction of reversal learning with cycle 1 memory. This nonadditive effect (◆) can be considered a component of cycle 1 memory that is disrupted or "erased" by reversal learning and is similar to the hypothetical MTM component in Fig. 3. If reversal learning completely disrupted cycle 1 memory, then the dotted line would be expected. The difference between this line and the observed reversal retention curve represents cycle 1 memory that is not disrupted by reversal learning. Interestingly, this reversal-resistant memory appears to be composed of two components, perhaps corresponding to STM and ARM (see Fig. 3).

1 memory at all retention intervals, then a second expected reversal retention curve would be the dotted line in Figure 5.

A more meaningful interpretation of this analysis is that reversal learning disrupts or "erases" a component of cycle-1-induced memory. The kinetics of this phase of memory (solid diamonds connected by solid line in Fig. 5) are strikingly similar to those of the MTM component in Figure 3. These observations suggest that MTM in wild-type flies may be disrupted by reversal learning. Moreover, the existence of such a reversal learning-sensitive (MTM) phase in wild-type flies supports the hypothesis that the *amnesiac* mutation completely disrupts the same component of memory.

One final observation is that the difference between the second expected reversal retention curve (dotted line) and the observed reversal retention curve (open diamonds connected by solid line) represents reversal learning-resistant memory, which appears to be composed of two components—an early one lasting about 30 minutes and a later one lasting at least 180 minutes. These kinetics are similar to that of STM and ARM, suggesting that STM may be reversal learning-resistant, whereas MTM is reversal learning-sensitive (i.e., the two phases are functionally distinct). Taken together with the observation that the *amnesiac* mutation appears primarily to disrupt MTM, these data also suggest that STM, MTM, and ARM are genetically distinct components.

Long-term Memory

Traditional views of memory consolidation would postulate that ARM (see Figs. 2 and 3) in *Drosophila* is a form of long-term memory. In fact, ARM levels in wild-type flies can account for overall retention levels 7 hours after classical conditioning (S. Boynton and T. Tully, data not shown), and ARM still is detectable 24 hours after similar training (Dudai et al. 1988). Moreover, memory retention in *amnesiac* flies can last 24 hours (Tully and Quinn 1985), and we have shown that ARM can account for overall retention levels in this mutant strain within 3 hours after training (see Fig. 2).

We have been perplexed, however, over the low levels of 24-hour memory displayed by wild-type flies. At best, our standard classical conditioning procedure yields 24-hour memory scores of 0.16 ± 0.03. Past attempts to increase 24-hour memory via extended training procedures failed, whether such training was massed or distributed (T. Tully and S. Boynton, unpubl.; cf. Woodworth and Schlosberg 1954). Recently, however, we have produced 24-hour memory scores of 0.44 ± 0.01 (a threefold improvement) by using a distributed training procedure with diluted odor concentrations (see Methods). In addition, conditioned avoidance responses still can be detected at least 4 days after such training (T. Preat and T. Tully, in prep.). Taken together, these data clearly demonstrate the existence in *Drosophila* of long-term memory with behavioral properties similar to long-term memories in other species (also see Tully and Quinn 1985 for additional behavioral properties of classical conditioned olfactory avoidance responses).

Behavioral and Genetic Characterization of a New Mutant *latheo*

For the last 3 years, we have been generating autosomal mutations via a P-element insertional mutagenesis (see Methods). The breeding scheme was designed so that random transposition events were isolated on autosomes, and strains were made homozygous for each independent P-element insertion. Groups of flies from each of these mutant strains then were classically conditioned and tested 3 hours after training. Any strain that produced a mean 3-hour memory score reliably and significantly lower than that of control *w(H)* flies was subjected to further behavioral and genetic analyses. To date, we have screened over 2000 mutant strains, have identified one new mutant (described below), and still are "chasing" nine other putative mutants.

In Figure 6, we compare memory retention during the first 180 minutes after training in *latheo* flies with that in *lat+* control flies. In these experiments, the appropriate control strain was *w(H)*, instead of Can-S, since the P-element transpositions were induced in a *w(H)* genetic background (see Methods). As shown, memory retention in *latheo* flies was significantly lower than that in wild-type flies at every retention interval,

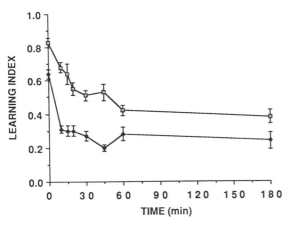

Figure 6. Memory retention in control *w(H)* (□) and mutant *latheo* (◆) flies, which were trained and tested together (see text). Mutant flies show less memory at all retention intervals. In addition, memory in *latheo* flies decays more rapidly during the first 15 min after training. $n = 6,4,4,4,8,4,8$, and 6 learning indices for retention intervals 0,10,15,20,30,45,60, and 180, respectively, for both genotypes.

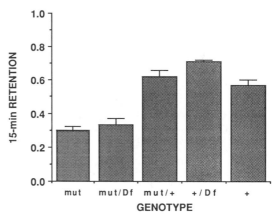

Figure 7. Cytological mapping of the mutant *latheo* phenotype. Flies from a strain carrying a small chromosomal deficiency (Df) of the *latheo* region were mated with *latheo* flies (mut), or with *w(H)* flies (+) to produce the genotypes shown here. Heterozygous mut/+ flies produce normal scores, indicating that the *latheo* mutation is recessive to its wild-type allele. More importantly, mut/Df flies produce mutant scores, and +/Df flies produce normal scores, indicating that the mutant phenotype maps to the region containing the P-element insertion. $n = 2$ learning indices for each genotype.

including 180 minutes. More interestingly, *latheo* memory decayed more rapidly during the first 15 minutes after training (this effect appeared as a significant interaction between TIME and STRAIN in a 2-way ANOVA). Importantly, olfactory avoidance responses to OCT versus Air or to MCH versus Air over a wide range of odor concentrations (a test of olfactory acuity) and escape responses to electric shock from 0 to 60 V (a test of shock reactivity), were normal in naive (untrained) *latheo* flies (S. Boynton and T. Tully, data not shown). Thus, the observed performance deficit in *latheo* flies most likely does not result from abnormal function of sensory or motor systems underlying conditioned avoidance responses.

Corroborative results from two sets of genetic experiments confirm that the mutant phenotype of *latheo* flies was produced by a single-gene mutation associated with a P-element insertion. In the first set of experiments, the cytological location of the autosomal P-element insert was mapped in situ using chromosome squashes from *latheo* flies and DNA sequence from the P-element mutator as a probe. Next, a strain carrying a chromosomal deficiency (Df) of the *latheo* region was obtained from the *Drosophila* stock center in Bloomington, Indiana, and these flies were mated with either *latheo* (mut) or *w(H)* (+) flies to produce mut/Df, +/Df, or mut/+ heterozygous offspring. Finally, 15-minute memory retention was assayed in these heterozygotes, as well as in mut/mut and +/+ homozygotes. Figure 7 shows that mut/Df flies yielded a mutant memory score, whereas mut/+ and Df/+ flies yielded wild-type memory scores. These results indicate that the mutation responsible for the *latheo* phenotype maps to a region close to the P-element insertion and that the *lat* mutant allele is recessive to its wild-type counterpart.

In a second set of experiments, a breeding scheme was designed to produce excisions of the P-element insert in *latheo* flies. To date, nine independent excision events, visualized by loss of rcd eyes in some *latheo* progeny, have been isolated, and strains homozygous for each excision allele have been bred. Fifteen-minute retention scores produced by two of these excision strains were similar to those of *w(H)* flies (S. Boynton and T. Tully, data not shown). The appearance of wild-type "revertant" flies is expected only if the (previously disrupted) gene containing a P-element insertion actually is responsible for the mutant phenotype of *latheo* flies.

DISCUSSION

We are encouraged by results from behavioral experiments on wild-type and *amnesiac* flies suggesting that memory formation after classical conditioning is composed of three distinct phases (STM, MTM, and ARM) with distinct properties. STM and ARM appear to be reversal learning-resistant, MTM is not; ARM is cold-shock anesthesia-resistant, MTM is not (we do not yet know if STM is cold-shock-sensitive). Most importantly, the *amnesiac* mutation specifically may disrupt MTM, leaving STM and ARM substantially intact. If this "components of memory" hypothesis withstands further behavioral and genetic scrutiny, then we will be able to conclude two important facts: (1) These memory phases are genetically distinct and (2) ARM, and possibly LTM, can be induced by STM in the absence of MTM. This latter conclusion would establish the notion that memory formation proceeds in a parallel rather than, or in addition to, a sequential fashion.

The behavioral experiments reported here, however, were neither perfect nor perfectly designed. Consequently, it is important to stress that our component model of memory formation must be considered preliminary. More behavioral and genetic work must be done, in particular, to determine whether ARM is completely normal in *amnesiac* flies (see Fig. 2), to establish a functional distinction between STM and MTM, and to assay each of these memory phases independently in *amnesiac* and other learning/memory mutants. Finally, we only have begun to study the relation of our distributed training-induced LTM to the other memory phases in normal and mutant flies. On the behavioral level alone, the next decade promises to be intriguing.

Memory retention in mutant *latheo* flies resembles that of *amnesiac* flies, suggesting that both genes are involved with MTM. We may confirm this notion by studying memory formation in *amnesiac, latheo* double mutants. Many such "phenogenetic" analyses of different genotypic combinations will be possible as additional P-element mutants are identified, contributing in yet another way to our understanding of the molecular basis of associative memory.

Molecular genetic analysis of our new P-element insertional mutants also holds great promise. These mutations contain both a morphological and a molecular "tag," which will expedite molecular cloning of these new learning/memory genes. In this manner, we can gain experimental access to gene products without making any assumptions about, or doing needle-in-haystack searches for, underlying biochemical, physiological, or structural mechanisms of memory formation. With the gene products in hand, we will be able to ask whether similar genes and protein are involved with learning and memory in other species.

ACKNOWLEDGMENTS

This work was supported by grants from the National Institutes of Health (GM-33205 and NS-25621) and the McKnight Foundation, and by a John Merck Scholarship in the Biology of Developmental Disabilities in Children. We thank W. Engels, E. Bier, and D. Coen for sending us fly stocks for the mutagenesis and M. Del Vecchio for generating mutant strains.

REFERENCES

Aceves-Pina, E.O. and W.G. Quinn. 1979. Learning in normal and mutant *Drosophila* larvae. *Science* **206:** 93.

Aceves-Pina, E.O., R. Booker, J.S. Duerr, M.S. Livingstone, W.G. Quinn, R.F. Smith, P.P. Sziber, B.L. Tempel, and T.P. Tully. 1983. Learning and memory in *Drosophila*, studied with mutants. *Cold Spring Harbor Symp. Quant. Biol.* **48:** 831.

Andrew, R.J. 1980. The functional organization of phases of memory consolidation. In *Advances in the study of behavior* (ed. R.A. Rosenblatt et al.), vol. 11, p. 337. Academic Press, New York.

Baker, B.S. and A.T.C. Carpenter. 1972. Genetic analysis of sex chromosomal meiotic mutants in *Drosophila melanogaster. Genetics* **71:** 255.

Bier, E., H. Vaessin, S. Shepherd, K. Lee, K. McCall, S. Barbel, L. Ackermann, R. Carretto, T. Uemura, E. Grell, L.Y. Jan, and Y.N. Jan. 1989. Searching for pattern and mutation in the *Drosophila* genome with a P-*lacZ* vector. *Genes Dev.* **3:** 1273.

Booker, R. and W.G. Quinn. 1981. Conditioning of leg position in normal and mutant *Drosophila. Proc. Natl. Acad. Sci.* **78:** 3940.

Byers, D. 1980. "Studies on learning and cyclic AMP phosphodiesterase of the *dunce* mutant of *Drosophila melanogaster.*" Ph.D. thesis, California Institute of Technology, Pasadena.

Byers, D., R.L. Davis, and J.A Kiger. 1981. Defect in cyclic AMP phosphodiesterase due to the *dunce* mutation of learning in *Drosophila melanogaster. Nature* **289:** 79.

Chen, C.-N., S. Denomen, and R.L. Davis. 1986. Molecular analysis of cDNA clones and the corresponding genomic coding sequences of the *Drosophila dunce*[+] gene, the structural gene for cAMP-dependent phosphodiesterase. *Proc. Natl. Acad. Sci.* **83:** 9313.

Cooley, L. C. Berg, and A. Spradling. 1988. Controlling P element insertional mutagenesis. *Trends Genet.* **4:** 254.

Davis, R.L. and N. Davidson. 1984. Isolation of *Drosophila melanogaster* dunce chromosomal region and recombinational mapping of dunce sequences with restriction site polymorphisms as genetic markers. *Mol. Cell. Biol.* **4:** 358.

Dudai, Y. 1983. Mutations affect storage and use of memory differentially in *Drosophila. Proc. Natl. Acad. Sci.* **80:** 5445.

Dudai, Y., G. Corfas, and S. Hazvi. 1988. What is the possible contribution of Ca^{2+}-stimulated adenylate cyclase to acquisition, consolidation and retention of an associative olfactory memory in *Drosophila? J. Comp. Physiol. A* **162:** 101.

Dudai, Y., B. Sher, D. Segal, and Y. Yovell. 1985. Defective responsiveness of adenylate cyclase to forskolin in the *Drosophila* memory mutant *rutabaga. J. Neurogenet.* **2:** 365.

Dudai, Y., Y.N. Jan, D. Byers, W.G. Quinn, and S. Benzer. 1976. *dunce*, a mutant of *Drosophila* deficient in learning. *Proc. Natl. Acad. Sci.* **73:** 1684.

Duerr, J.S. and W.G. Quinn. 1982. Three *Drosophila* mutations that block associative learning also affect habituation and sensitization. *Proc. Natl. Acad. Sci.* **79:** 3646.

Folkers, E. 1982. Visual learning and memory of *Drosophila melanogaster* wild-type CS and the mutants *dunce, amnesiac, turnip* and *rutabaga. J. Insect. Physiol.* **28:** 535.

Gailey, D.A., F.R. Jackson, and R.W. Siegel. 1982. Male courtship in *Drosophila*: The conditioned response to immature males and its genetic control. *Genetics* **102:** 771.

———. 1984. Conditioning mutations in *Drosophila melanogaster* affect an experience-dependent behavioral modification in courting males. *Genetics* **106:** 613.

Gibbs, M.E. and K.T. Ng. 1976. Memory formation: A new three-phase model. *Neurosci. Lett.* **2:** 165.

Heisenberg, M. 1989. Genetic approach to learning and memory (mnemogenetics) in *Drosophila melanogaster*. In *Fundamentals of memory formation: Neuronal plasticity and brain function* (ed. H. Rahmann), p. 3. Gustav Fischer Verlag, Stuttgart.

Johnson, C.D., J.G. Duckett, J.G. Culotti, R.K. Herman, P.M. Meneely, and R.L. Russell. 1981. An acetylcholinesterase-deficient mutant of the nematode *Caenorhabditis elegans. Genetics* **97:** 261.

Kauvar, L.M. 1982. Defective cyclic adenosine 3'5' monophosphate phosphodiesterase in the *Drosophila* memory mutant *dunce. J. Neurosci.* **3:** 1347.

Kiger, J.A. and H.K. Saltz. 1985. Cyclic nucleotide metabolism and physiology of the fruit fly *Drosophila melanogaster. Adv. Insect Physiol.* **18:** 141.

Kiger, J.A., R.L. Davis, H.K. Saltz, T. Fletcher, and M. Bowling. 1981. Genetic analysis of cyclic nucleotide phosphodiesterase in *Drosophila melanogaster. Adv. Cyclic Nucleotide Res.* **14:** 273.

Kulkarni, S.J. and J.C. Hall. 1987. Behavioral and cytogenetic analysis of the *cacophony* courtship song mutant and interacting genetic variants in *Drosophila melanogaster.* *Genetics* **115**: 461.

Kyriacou, C.P. and J.C. Hall. 1984. Learning and memory mutations impair acoustic priming of mating behavior in *Drosophila. Nature* **308**: 62.

Lewis, E.B. and F. Bacher. 1968. Method of feeding ethyl methane sulfonate to *Drosophila* males. *Drosophila Inf. Service* **43**: 193.

Livingstone, M.S. 1985. Genetic dissection of *Drosophila* adenylate cyclase. *Proc. Natl. Acad. Sci.* **82**: 5992.

Livingstone, M.S., P.P. Sziber, and W.G. Quinn. 1984. Loss of calcium/calmodulin responsiveness in adenylate cyclase of *rutabaga,* a *Drosophila* learning mutant. *Cell* **37**: 205.

Matthies, H.J. 1989. In search of cellular mechanisms of memory. *Prog. Neurobiol.* **32**: 277.

Patterson, T.A., M.C. Alvarado, I.T. Warner, E.L. Bennett, and M.R. Rosenzweig. 1986. Memory stages and brain asymmetry in chick learning. *Behav. Neurosci.* **100**: 856.

Quinn, W.G. and Y. Dudai. 1976. Memory phases in *Drosophila. Nature* **262**: 576.

Quinn, W.G., W.A. Harris, and S. Benzer. 1974. Conditioned behavior in *Drosophila melanogaster. Proc. Natl. Acad. Sci.* **71**: 708.

Quinn, W.G., P.P. Sziber, and R. Booker. 1979. The *Drosophila* memory mutant *amnesiac. Nature* **277**: 212.

Robertson, H.M., C.R. Preston, R.W. Phillis, D.M. Johnson-Schlitz, W.K. Benz, and W.R. Engels. 1988. A stable genomic source of *P* element transposase in *Drosophila melanogaster. Genetics* **118**: 461.

Saltz, H.K., R.L. Davis, and J.A. Kiger. 1982. Genetic analysis of chromosome 3D4 in *Drosophila melanogaster,* the *dunce* gene and *sperm-amotile* genes. *Genetics* **100**: 587.

Shotwell, S.L. 1983. Cyclic adenosine 3′:5′-monophosphate phosphodiesterase and its role in learning in *Drosophila. J. Neurosci.* **3**: 739.

Siegel, R.W. and J.C. Hall. 1979. Conditioned responses in courtship behavior of normal and mutant *Drosophila. Proc. Natl. Acad. Sci.* **76**: 3430.

Smith, R.F., K.-W. Choi, T. Tully, and W.G. Quinn. 1986. Deficient protein kinase C activity in *turnip,* a *Drosophila* learning mutant. *Soc. Neurosci. Abstr.* **12**: 399.

Tempel, B.L., N. Bonini, D.R. Dawson, and W.G. Quinn. 1983. Reward learning in normal and mutant *Drosophila. Proc. Natl. Acad. Sci.* **80**: 1482.

Tully. T. 1984. *Drosophila* learning: Behavior and biochemistry. *Behav. Genet.* **14**: 527.

———. 1986. Measuring learning in individual flies is not necessary to study the effects of single-gene mutations in *Drosophila:* A reply to Holliday and Hirsch. *Behav. Genet.* **16**: 449.

———. 1988. On the road to a better understanding of learning and memory in *Drosophila melanogaster.* In *Modulation of synaptic transmission and plasticity in nervous systems* (ed. G. Hertting and H.Ch. Spatz), p. 401. Springer-Verlag, Berlin.

———. 1990. *Drosophila*'s role in identifying the building blocks of associative learning and memory. In *Perspectives in cognitive neuroscience* (ed. R.G. Lister and H.J. Weingartner). Oxford University Press, New York. (In press.)

Tully, T. and J.P. Gergen. 1986. Deletion mapping of the *Drosophila* memory mutant *amnesiac. J. Neurogenet.* **3**: 33.

Tully, T. and W.G. Quinn. 1985. Classical conditioning and retention in normal and mutant *Drosophila melanogaster. J. Comp. Physiol.* **157**: 263.

Woodworth, R.S. and H. Schlosberg. 1954. *Experimental psychology,* p. 786. Holt, Rinehart and Winston, New York.

Synaptic Regulation of Immediate-Early Genes in Brain

P.F. Worley,*† A.J. Cole,*† T.H. Murphy,* B.A. Christy,‡¶
Y. Nakabeppu,‡¶ and J.M. Baraban*§

*Departments of *Neuroscience, †Neurology, ‡Molecular Genetics, §Psychiatry and Behavioral Sciences, and
¶Howard Hughes Medical Institute, Johns Hopkins University School of Medicine, Baltimore, Maryland 21205*

Rapid genomic responses to neuronal stimulation may play a critical role in long-term synaptic plasticity. This concept emerged from behavioral studies indicating that new protein synthesis shortly after training is required for long-term memory of a learned task (Agranoff 1981). Recent work in invertebrate preparations has strengthened this idea by demonstrating that neurotransmitter-induced long-term synaptic plasticity requires RNA and protein synthesis during a critical time window immediately following stimulation (Montarolo et al. 1986). These studies prompted the suggestion that genes, like c-*fos*, that are rapidly induced by cell-surface-receptor stimulation by either growth factors or neurotransmitters (Greenberg et al. 1985, 1986) might be involved in the early genomic response underlying long-term synaptic plasticity (Berridge 1986; Goelet et al. 1986).

c-*fos* is a member of a group of genes, referred to as cellular immediate-early genes (IEGs), that are rapidly and transiently activated in quiescent fibroblasts by growth factors (see Cochran et al. 1983; Linzer and Nathans 1983; Greenberg and Ziff 1984; Lau and Nathans 1987). Activation of IEGs occurs by increased transcription and is thought to represent the primary genomic response to growth factor stimulation, since it does not require protein synthesis. Several IEGs code for transcription factors. These include members of the *fos* and *jun* families, which dimerize to form the transcription regulatory complex AP1 (Halazonetis et al. 1988; Nakabeppu et al. 1988; Rauscher et al. 1988), as well as *nur/77* (Hazel et al. 1988; also termed NGFI-B [Milbrandt 1988]), which belongs to the steroid receptor superfamily of transcription factors, *zif/268* (Christy et al. 1988; also termed egr-1 [Sukhatme et al. 1988], Krox 24 [Lemaire et al. 1988], and NGFI-A [Milbrandt 1987]), and *Krox-20* (Chavrier et al. 1989), which are members of a family of proteins characterized by zinc-finger motifs in their DNA-binding domains.

Several lines of evidence indicate that these IEGs play a key role in growth factor action. For example, blockade of c-*fos* induction interrupts the growth-factor-induced cell-cycle transition of quiescent fibroblasts (Nishikura and Murray 1987; Riabowol et al. 1988). Abundant evidence has accumulated that c-*fos*, as well as several other IEGs that encode transcription factors, is activated by neuronal stimulation both in

vitro and in vivo (for review, see Sheng and Greenberg 1990). Accordingly, a rapid genomic response similar to that involved in growth factor action may play a key role in neuronal plasticity.

To examine the hypothesized role of the IEG response in synaptic plasticity, we studied the regulation of several IEGs in the long-term potentiation (LTP) paradigm, a well-characterized model of synaptic plasticity. In this paradigm, brief high-frequency stimulation of perforant path afferents to dentate granule cells elicits a long-lasting increase in synaptic responses to subsequent volleys. We found that the IEG *zif/268* is induced in dentate neurons by LTP stimulation (Cole et al. 1989). Moreover, the pharmacology of *zif/268* mRNA induction appears similar to that of LTP, since both require *N*-methyl-D-aspartate (NMDA)-type glutamate receptor activation (Nicoll et al. 1988).

Because the LTP studies involved artificial, synchronous electrical stimulation of a major afferent pathway, they raise concern that transcription factor induction might require severe or artificial stimuli and thus may not be relevant to processes underlying normal neuronal plasticity thought to underlie learning and memory. Initial characterization of *zif/268* mRNA levels in brain had demonstrated prominent basal levels in adult neocortex (Milbrandt 1987; Christy et al. 1988; Lemaire et al. 1988; Sukhatme et al. 1988). Accordingly, we have sought to understand the neural mechanisms regulating basal expression of *zif/268*, as well as other IEGs, on the premise that these basal levels reflect induction by physiological stimuli. In particular, we have focused on the visual cortex, since this brain area has been well characterized and its afferent activity can be manipulated readily. Our studies indicate that physiological visual stimulation is sufficient to elicit a robust IEG response in cortical neurons that may be mediated by NMDA receptor activation. Similar synaptic regulation of transcription factors is displayed by primary cortical neuronal cultures, providing an in vitro preparation to examine intracellular pathways regulating IEGs in brain neurons.

METHODS

Animal preparation. Sprague-Dawley rats or BALB/c mice were used in all experiments. For intra-

ocular injections of tetrodotoxin (TTX), animals were

ocular injections of tetrodotoxin (TTX), animals were briefly anesthetized with water-saturated diethyl ether, and 2 μl of 1 mM TTX in saline was injected with a microsyringe into the vitreal space. In experiments examining effects of dark-rearing, midterm pregnant female rats and subsequent litters were housed in complete darkness until time of sacrifice (12 days to 6 weeks). Dark-adaptation was performed by placing normally reared adult rats in complete darkness for 1 day to 3 weeks. All animals were sacrificed by guillotine decapitation.

In situ hybridization and Northern analysis. These procedures were performed as described previously (Saffen et al. 1988; Cole et al. 1989, 1990).

Gel-shift assays. Nuclear extracts from cortex and hippocampus were prepared according to the method of Dignam et al. (1983). Gel-shift assays were performed as described previously (Nakabeppu et al. 1988; Christy and Nathans 1989).

Immunohistochemistry. Cryostat sections (10 μm) were fixed in 2% paraformaldehyde, and immunoreactivity was detected by the ABC immunoperoxidase method (Vector Labs). Immunostaining of primary cortical cultures was performed in a similar fashion. Affinity-purified rabbit polyclonal antisera selective for Jun-B, c-Jun, and Zif/268 were used. Characterization of these antisera is described by Y. Nakabeppu et al. (in prep.). Omission of primary antibody resulted in complete loss of nuclear staining.

Cell culture. Cell cultures were prepared from day-17 gestation Sprague-Dawley rat fetal cerebral cortex, using a papain dissociation method (Huettner and Baughman 1986). The dissociated cells were resuspended at a density of 1×10^6 cells/ml in minimal essential medium (MEM) supplemented with 5.5 g/liter glucose, 2 mM glutamine, 10% fetal calf serum, 5% heat-inactivated horse serum, 100 units/ml penicillin, and 0.1 mg/ml streptomycin, plated onto polylysine-coated (10 μg/ml) 24-well culture dishes in 0.5 ml of medium, and placed in a 37°C CO_2-buffered incubator. The cultures were fed by addition of MEM with 5.5 g/liter glucose, 5% heat-inactivated horse serum, and 2 mM glutamine, after 4–6, 12–14, and 19–21 days in culture, by removal and replacement of approximately 60% of the medium. To avoid mechanical stimulation associated with changing medium, cells were fed at least 24 hours before fixation for immunostaining. In addition, compounds were diluted directly into culture medium without removal of medium from the cells.

RESULTS

NMDA Receptor Antagonists Selectively Reduce Basal Levels of *zif/268* in Cortex

In situ hybridization studies demonstrate a prominent laminar distribution of *zif/268* mRNA in adult rat or mouse cortex (Fig. 1). Northern analysis of cortical RNA confirms that *zif/268* mRNA is easily detectable in control cortex. Since we had found in previous studies that synaptic NMDA receptor activation increases *zif/268* mRNA in the dentate gyrus, we wondered if the high basal level expression of *zif/268*

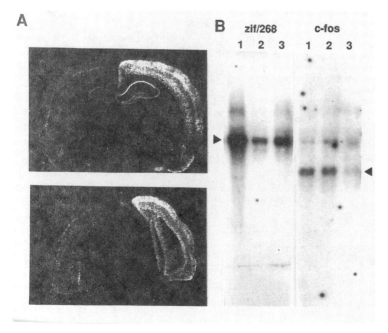

Figure 1. NMDA receptor antagonists reduce basal level of *zif/268* mRNA in rat forebrain. (*A*) *zif/268* in situ autoradiogram. The right half brain of each autoradiogram is from a control animal and the left half brain is from an animal treated with MK-801 (3 mg/kg, i.p.) 4 hr prior to sacrifice. Top autoradiogram demonstrates that MK-801 reduces levels of *zif/268* mRNA in neocortex, pyriform cortex, and hippocampus. Bottom autoradiogram demonstrates reductions in visual cortex. Reductions in *zif/268* mRNA, as assayed by in situ hybridization, are produced by MK-801 doses as low as 0.3 mg/kg and are also produced by CGS-19755 (10 mg/kg, i.p.). (*B*) Northern analysis of rat cortex RNA. Lane *1* is from a control animal. Lanes *2* and *3* are from animals treated with MK-801 (3 mg/kg, i.p.) for 4 hr and 20 hr, respectively.

mRNA in cortex might reflect tonic activation of NMDA-type glutamate receptors. Administration of MK-801 (0.1–3 mg/kg, i.p.) or CGS-19755 (10 mg/kg), agents that block NMDA responses in vivo (Wong et al. 1986; Abraham and Mason 1988; Lodge et al. 1988; Murphy et al. 1988), markedly reduces *zif/268* mRNA levels in cortex (Fig. 1). Reduction of *zif/268* mRNA is detected within 1 hour of administering MK-801 (3 mg/kg), and levels remain reduced for 20 hours, consistent with the long half-life of MK-801 (Abraham and Mason 1988). These reductions are most prominent in regions expressing highest basal levels, including neocortex and pyriform cortex. In contrast, basal levels of c-*fos* mRNA in cortex appear lower than those of *zif/268* and are not rapidly reduced by MK-801. However, a delayed reduction is evident 20 hours after MK-801 administration (Fig. 1).

To examine the effect of NMDA receptor antagonists on transcription factor proteins, we monitored sequence-specific DNA-binding activity in nuclear extracts from cortex. Binding activity to the consensus sequence for *zif/268* is enriched in control cortex relative to hippocampus and is markedly reduced within 4 hours of MK-801 (3 mg/kg) administration (Fig. 2). AP1-binding activity in cortex is unchanged 4 hours after MK-801 and is only moderately reduced after 20 hours. To examine further the specificity of this reduction in binding to the *zif/268* consensus sequence by MK-801, we also assayed DNA-binding activity to two other consensus sequences: one for Sp1, a DNA-binding protein, that, like Zif/268, contains a zinc finger

DNA-binding domain (Kadonaga et al. 1987) and the other, referred to as the serum response element (SRE), recognized by a structurally distinct DNA-binding protein (Treisman 1987). Binding activity to the Sp1 and SRE consensus sequences is not affected by MK-801 treatment (Fig. 2). Accordingly, *zif/268* appears to be particularly responsive to NMDA receptor blockade.

To further characterize the regulation of Zif/268 by NMDA receptor blockade, we monitored Zif/268 immunohistochemically. In the neocortex, Zif/268-like immunoreactivity displays a marked laminar pattern with staining observed predominantly in nuclei of neurons (see Fig. 4). The laminar pattern fits well with that observed with in situ hybridization studies of *zif/268* mRNA. Likewise, Zif/268 immunoreactivity is markedly reduced 4 hours after administration of MK-801 (3 mg/kg, i.p.).

Visual Activity Modulates Basal Expression of *zif/268* in Visual Cortex

Since NMDA receptor antagonists reduce levels of *zif/268* mRNA, sequence-specific DNA-binding activity, and immunoreactivity in cortex, we examined the possibility that NMDA receptor activation associated with normal levels of synaptic transmission provides the physiological stimulus for persistent activation of *zif/268*. In the visual cortex, excitatory synaptic responses to visual stimuli include a prominent NMDA receptor-mediated component (Tsumoto et al. 1987; Hagahara

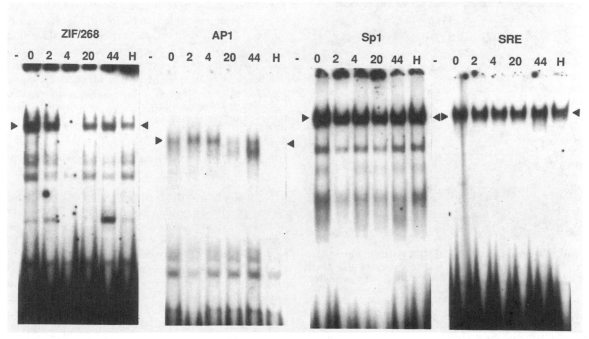

Figure 2. NMDA receptor antagonist rapidly and selectively reduces *zif/268* sequence-specific DNA binding. Nuclear extracts were prepared from rat control cortex (lane *0*), control hippocampus (lane *H*), and from cortex of animals 2, 4, 20, and 44 hr after MK-801 (3 mg/kg, i.p.) administration and used for gel-shift assays (Nakabeppu et al. 1988; Christy and Nathans 1989). Arrowheads indicate bands reflecting specific DNA-binding activity.

et al. 1988; Jones and Baughman 1988; Fox et al. 1989; Miller et al. 1989). Accordingly, we blocked retinal output with intraocular injections of TTX and monitored *zif/268* mRNA and immunoreactivity in visual cortex. In rats and mice, visual pathways from the optic nerve to primary visual cortex are nearly completely crossed (Zilles et al. 1984). Within 1 hour of monocular intravitreal injection of TTX, *zif/268* mRNA levels are markedly reduced in the contralateral primary visual cortex (Fig. 3). Reductions are selective for the primary visual cortex, since levels of *zif/268* mRNA in adjacent cingulate or visual association cortex (Paxinos and Watson 1982; Miller and Vogt 1984; Zilles et al. 1984) are not affected by this treatment. Within the visual cortex, dramatic reductions in *zif/268* immunostaining are seen in layers II–IV and VI, which contain highest basal levels. These results suggest that retinal activity drives *zif/268* expression in all of these layers. Similar effects of monocular TTX injection on *zif/268*

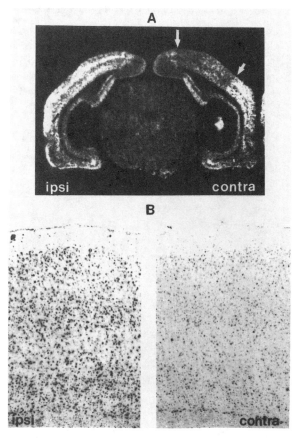

Figure 3. Monocular injection of TTX results in rapid reductions in *zif/268* mRNA in the contralateral visual cortex of adult rat. TTX (2 μl of 1 mM solution in saline) was injected into the vitreous, and 2 hr later the animal was sacrificed. (*A*) Low power (3 ×) in situ autoradiogram demonstrating reductions in *zif/268* mRNA in the contralateral primary visual cortex (arrows). (*B*) *zif/268* mRNA is localized with digoxigenin-labeled riboprobe (Genius Kit; Boehringer Mannheim) in visual cortex ipsilateral and contralateral to TTX injection. Magnification, 30 ×. Laminar pattern of neuronal labeling is seen in ipsilateral cortex with marked reductions of labeling in contralateral cortex.

mRNA were seen in both rats and mice. In contrast to the rapid and dramatic reductions in *zif/268* mRNA following intraocular TTX injections, in situ hybridization signals for mRNAs of several other transcription regulatory factors, c-*fos*, c-*jun*, *jun-B*, or *Krox-20*, are unaffected.

To determine whether TTX treatments also produce the expected decrease in Zif/268 protein, we performed immunohistochemistry on adjacent tissue sections. Within 4 hours of monocular TTX injection, Zif/268 immunoreactivity is reduced in nuclei of neurons in all layers of the contralateral primary visual cortex (Fig. 4). Reductions are most dramatic in layer IV neurons, which express highest levels in control cortex. In contrast to reductions in Zif/268, immunostaining with antisera selective for c-*jun* or *jun-B* shows little change after TTX injection.

Intraocular TTX injection is likely to totally block activity of retinal ganglion cells. Since retinal ganglion cell activity is not totally suppressed under dark conditions, we wanted to determine whether the critical retinal activity that regulates *zif/268* in the visual cortex is light-dependent. Accordingly, we monitored *zif/268* expression in visual cortex of rats that were maintained in the dark for 1 day to 3 weeks (dark-adaptation). *zif/268* mRNA and immunostaining are reduced in visual cortex of dark-adapted animals compared to levels in visual cortex of control animals maintained in normal diurnal lighting conditions. These reductions in *zif/268* mRNA and immunostaining appear to be less marked than those due to TTX injection, but are anatomically more widespread, involving both primary visual cortex and adjacent association cortex (Paxinos and Watson 1983; Miller and Vogt 1984; Zilles et al. 1984). Moreover, reductions in *zif/268* are observed after 4 days of dark-adaptation but not 1 day, in contrast to the very rapid reduction induced by intraocular TTX. As expected, reexposure of dark-adapted rats to ambient laboratory light results in rapid increases in *zif/268* mRNA (Fig. 5) and immunoreactivity. Levels of *zif/268* mRNA and immunoreactivity return to control levels within 1 hour of light exposure.

Regulation of Transcription Factors during Postnatal Development: Role of Activity

Rat pups do not open their eyes until the second week of life (day 14). Accordingly, we wondered whether the appearance of *zif/268* displays a similar developmental delay in visual cortex. Examination of *zif/268* mRNA (Fig. 6) and immunoreactivity reveals a delayed rise in *zif/268* expression throughout the cortex, beginning between postnatal days 11 and 16 and reaching peak levels by day 21. Gel-shift assays of *zif/268* and AP1-binding activity demonstrate a similar delayed developmental profile. In contrast, Sp1-binding activity does not change significantly during postnatal development.

To examine the role of activity in the developmental regulation of *zif/268*, we compared *zif/268* mRNA

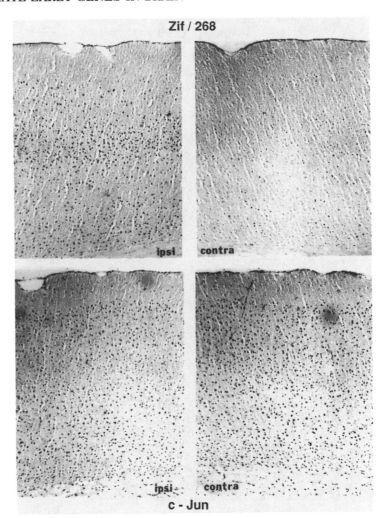

Figure 4. Monocular injection of TTX rapidly reduces immunostaining for Zif/268 but not c-Jun in contralateral visual cortex. Adult mice were prepared as in Fig. 3 and sacrificed 5 hr after TTX administration. Immunoreactivity is visualized with the ABC immunoperoxidase method. Photomicrographs (magnification, 43 ×) show the full thickness of the visual cortex ipsilateral and contralateral to TTX administration.

levels and immunostaining in visual cortex of animals that were either raised under normal diurnal lighting conditions or in complete darkness from birth. In the visual cortex of postnatal day-12 animals, levels of *zif/268* mRNA and immunostaining are nearly identical in dark-reared and normally reared animals. However, by postnatal day 21, *zif/268* mRNA (Fig. 7) and immunostaining are markedly less in dark-reared animals. The lower levels of *zif/268* mRNA in dark-reared animals appear to be due to reduced visual stimulation, since returning dark-reared animals to a normally illuminated cage results in rapid (within 30 minutes of light exposure) increases in *zif/268* mRNA and immunostaining. NMDA receptors appear to be involved in the light-induced increase in *zif/268*, since it is blocked by pretreatment with MK-801 (3 mg/kg; Fig. 7).

In comparing the IEG response to light exposure in dark-adapted (normally reared adult animals placed in dark for several days) and dark-reared animals (3-week-old animals raised in dark from birth), several differences are apparent. Dark-reared animals display a more robust *zif/268* response to light. Moreover, increases in c-*fos* and *jun-B* mRNA are noted following light exposure in dark-reared animals, whereas in dark-adapted animals, these other transcription factors are not markedly altered by light exposure. In addition, the anatomic distribution of the *zif/268* response to light exposure in dark-reared animals is more widespread than in dark-adapted animals. Specifically, *zif/268* increases are observed in both visual cortex and entorhinal cortex following light exposure in dark-reared animals, whereas increases are limited to primary visual and association cortex in dark-adapted animals (Fig. 5). The neuroanatomic basis for light-induced activation of *zif/268* in the entorhinal cortex is unknown but may involve developmentally restricted corticocortical projections from the visual cortex (Innocenti 1981). Taken together, these data indicate qualitative differences in activity-dependent transcription factor regulation in adult and developing brain.

Developmental and Activity-dependent Regulation of Transcription Factors in Primary Cortical Cell Cultures

The in vivo studies described above demonstrate marked developmental and activity-dependent regula-

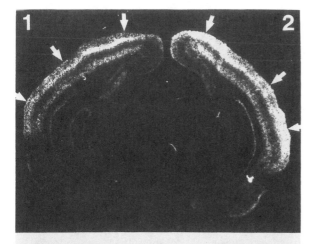

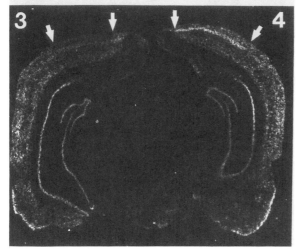

Figure 5. Light induces increases in *zif/268* mRNA in visual cortex of dark-adapted rats. Adult rats were housed in complete darkness for 4 days (dark-adapted) and sacrificed in the dark (hemibrains 1 and 3) or returned to normal laboratory light conditions (hemibrains 2 and 4) for 30 min prior to sacrifice. Autoradiograms of *zif/268* in situ hybridization demonstrate light-dependent induction of *zif/268* mRNA in superficial layers of primary and association visual cortex (top autoradiogram; compare 1 and 2). In more rostral areas (bottom autoradiogram), light induces *zif/268* in layer IV of visual cortex (compare 3 and 4 between arrows).

tion of *zif/268* and other IEGs in cortical neurons. With the ultimate goal of defining the intracellular pathways mediating these responses, we have examined whether primary cortical neuronal cultures display similar IEG responses and therefore might be suitable for further studies of synaptic regulation of IEGs. In initial studies, we monitored the developmental profile of c-Jun, Jun-B, and Zif/268 in primary cortical cultures. The proportion of c-Jun and Jun-B immunoreactive neurons increases markedly over the course of 3 weeks in culture. Antisera selective for either c-Jun or Jun-B stain approximately one fourth of neurons in 21-day cultures. Basal Jun-B immunostaining appears to be associated primarily with the nuclei of neurons, whereas c-Jun immunostaining is associated with nuclei of both neurons and glia. *zif/268* immunostaining also appears

to increase during this period in culture; however, staining is less robust than that of c-Jun and Jun-B.

In preliminary studies, we have examined the possibility that basal expression of these transcription factors is regulated by synaptic activity. Addition of the sodium channel blocker TTX (10 μM) to the culture medium markedly reduces the number of Jun-B immunoreactive neurons after 4–6 hours. In contrast, c-Jun immunoreactivity is unaffected by TTX. Similar results were obtained when NMDA receptor antagonists MK-801 (10 μM; Fig. 8) or AP-5 (30 μM) are added to cultures. In contrast, 10 μM atropine, a muscarinic receptor antagonist, fails to reduce levels of Jun-B immunostaining. The differential response of Jun-B and c-Jun is likely to represent differences in synaptic regulatory mechanisms rather than differences in protein turnover rates, since the time course of reduction in c-Jun immunostaining after cycloheximide (10 μg/ml) is similar to that of Jun-B, since immunostaining for both proteins is markedly reduced after 4–6 hours of cycloheximide treatment (Fig. 8). Accordingly, basal levels of both c-Jun and Jun-B immunostaining require ongoing protein synthesis; however, only Jun-B appears to be sensitive to NMDA receptor blockade.

DISCUSSION

Our central observation is that *zif/268* is regulated in brain by natural stimuli. Previously, we reported that *zif/268* mRNA is selectively induced by electrically evoked synaptic stimuli that result in long-term potentiation (LTP; Cole et al. 1989). The present study extends these observations by demonstrating that basal levels of *zif/268* mRNA, sequence-specific DNA-binding activity, and immunoreactivity are regulated throughout the forebrain by mechanisms that involve NMDA receptors. In the visual cortex, where the major excitatory input can be easily manipulated, blockade of afferent activity by intraocular injection of TTX results in pronounced reductions of *zif/268* mRNA and immunoreactivity. Additionally, reducing visual activity by placing animals in the dark decreases levels of *zif/268* mRNA and immunoreactivity, and upon reexposure to light, these markers rapidly return to control levels. Accordingly, light-dependent retinal activity appears to be important for *zif/268* regulation in visual cortex.

In systems where IEG induction has been characterized (for review, see Lau and Nathans 1990), responses are typically rapid and transient. Following stimulation of fibroblasts (Lau and Nathans 1987) or PC-12 cells (Greenberg et al. 1985), transcription factor mRNA levels increase rapidly, peak within 30–60 minutes, and return to basal levels typically within 2 hours. A similar time course occurs in brain after seizures (Morgan et al. 1987; Saffen et al. 1988). Transcription factor proteins are also rapidly and transiently induced after stimulation both in cell-culture systems (Kruijer et al. 1984) and in brain (Morgan et al. 1987; Sonnenberg et al. 1989; Y. Nakabeppu et al., in prep.). The relatively

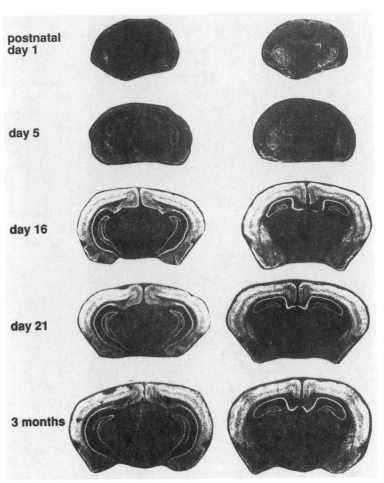

Figure 6. Developmental regulation of *zif/268* mRNA in rat forebrain. Autoradiograms of *zif/268* in situ hybridization at indicated postnatal day. Left column is at level of visual cortex; right column is at levels of dorsal hippocampus and somatosensory cortex.

high basal levels of *zif/268* mRNA, sequence-specific DNA-binding activity, and immunoreactivity present in control brain might appear to represent an exception to previous studies demonstrating transient expression of IEG transcription factors. However, the rapid reduction in *zif/268* markers following intraocular TTX or NMDA receptor antagonists suggests a short half-life of *zif/268* mRNA and protein under basal conditions. Additionally, in dark-adapted or dark-reared animals, light exposure causes rapid increases in *zif/268* mRNA and immunostaining. Accordingly, basal levels are likely to represent tonic production of short-lived *zif/268* mRNA and protein in response to normal synaptic activity. Similarly, in primary neuronal cultures, basal levels of Jun-B immunoreactivity are rapidly reduced by agents that block NMDA-dependent synaptic transmission and by protein synthesis inhibition, suggesting that these levels are driven by spontaneous synaptic activity.

A notable feature of the transcription factor response to activity, both in vivo and in primary cortical cell cultures, is the specificity of the response. In contrast to the rapid, marked suppression of *zif/268* in the adult brain by NMDA antagonists or blockade of retinal activity, several other IEGs are relatively unaffected by these treatments. A similar response specificity occurs in hippocampal granule cells following LTP-inducing stimuli that reproducibly induce *zif/268* mRNA but inconsistently induce c-*fos*, c-*jun*, and *jun-B* (Cole et al. 1989). In the primary cortical culture system, *jun-B* but not c-*jun* immunostaining is rapidly reduced in neurons by agents that suppress synaptic transmission. Similar differential activation of transcription factors has been demonstrated in PC-12 cells (Bartel et al. 1989). Therefore, it appears likely that activation of distinct sets of transcription factors may contribute to differences in neuronal responses to stimulation.

Although systemic administration of NMDA receptor antagonists blocks activation of *zif/268* in vivo, we cannot conclude that synaptic activation of NMDA receptors is the stimulus directly linked to regulation of *zif/268* under physiological conditions. Recent evidence suggests that NMDA receptors, under certain conditions, may function as voltage-sensitive ion channels due to ambient extracellular glutamate concentrations that are sufficient to partially occupy NMDA receptors (Sah et al. 1989). Under these conditions, NMDA receptor stimulation may exert a permissive influence, whereas excitatory effects of other transmitter receptors may provide the stimulus for indirect activation of the NMDA receptor ion channels. Another factor which needs to be emphasized is that

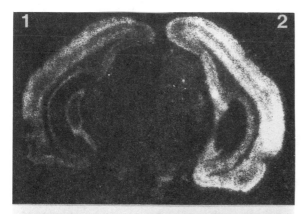

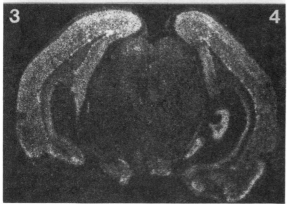

Figure 7. NMDA receptor antagonist blocks light-induced increases in *zif/268* mRNA in cortex of dark-reared animals. Rats were housed in complete darkness until postnatal day 21. Animals were then either sacrificed in the dark (hemibrain 1) or exposed to normal laboratory lighting for 30 min prior to sacrifice (hemibrain 2). Other dark-reared animals received MK-801 (3 mg/kg, i.p.) 60 min prior to sacrifice in the dark (hemibrain 4) or 30 min prior to light exposure (30 min) and subsequent sacrifice (hemibrain 3).

systemically administered NMDA receptor antagonists produce behavioral sedation, indicating widespread reduction in neuronal activity. Accordingly, the reduction in *zif/268* mRNA, DNA-binding activity, and immunostaining in the forebrain by NMDA receptor antagonists cannot be taken as compelling evidence that *zif/268* is regulated exclusively or directly by synaptic NMDA receptor activity under physiological conditions. Nevertheless, it is interesting to note that light-induced excitatory potentials in both adult (Hagihara et al. 1988; Miller et al. 1989) and developing (Tsumoto et al. 1987; Fox et al. 1989) visual cortex contain a significant NMDA receptor-mediated component. Moreover, basal levels of *zif/268* mRNA, sequence-specific DNA-binding activity, and immunoreactivity are enriched in cortex relative to hippocampus, a structure with low levels of normal spontaneous activity (Mizumori et al. 1989). Furthermore, the ability of NMDA receptor antagonists to block activation of *zif/268* in hippocampal granule cells by perforant path stimulation indicates that this receptor may be closely linked to *zif/268* activation.

In the cortical culture preparation, mechanisms of activation are more accessible for study. Synaptically released neurotransmitters appear to regulate *jun-B*, since TTX and NMDA receptor antagonists (AP-5, MK-801) reduce Jun-B immunostaining. These data support a major role for NMDA-dependent synaptic mechanisms in regulating Jun-B. Current models suggest that rises in intracellular calcium may couple membrane events to gene activation (Sheng and Greenberg 1990). This in vitro system should be useful in future studies to examine more precisely how NMDA receptors regulate transcription factor expression.

The present observations strongly suggest that transcription factors play a key role in neuronal physiology, since they appear to be continuously activated by natural stimuli. In the visual cortex, there is compelling evidence for activity-dependent neural plasticity both in adult and in developing animals. Our data indicate that manipulations that induce plasticity are associated with altered expression of *zif/268*. In adult animals, monocular deprivation induces changes in levels within the visual cortex of cytochrome oxidase (Hendrickson et al. 1981; Wong-Riley and Carroll 1984) and calcium and calmodulin-dependent protein kinase (Hendry and Kennedy 1986), as well as changes in neurotransmitter phenotype (Hendry and Jones 1986; Hendry et al. 1988). Recent data indicate that the retinotopic cortical map is reorganized after retinal lesions (Kaas et al. 1990), providing electrophysiological evidence of plasticity in the adult visual cortex. In contrast to these biochemical and electrophysiological changes that require days or weeks of visual deprivation, changes in *zif/268* expression occur within minutes to hours, consistent with its proposed regulatory role in orchestrating alterations in gene expression underlying neuronal plasticity.

In the developing brain, synaptic connectivity of neurons in the visual cortex is critically dependent on the activity of visual afferents during a period of development referred to as the critical period (Hubel and Wiesel 1970; Hubel et al. 1977; LeVay et al. 1980). Temporary monocular occlusion during the critical period, but not during adulthood, results in marked and permanent alterations in synaptic connectivity. The critical period has been most extensively examined in cats and monkeys; however, there is evidence that visual development in rodents is also activity-dependent (Cragg 1967; Valverde 1971; Gabbott et al. 1986; Gabbott and Stewart 1987). The critical period typically coincides with eye opening and extends for an interval thereafter that is species-specific. Remarkably, the critical period can be extended into adulthood by rearing animals in complete darkness (Cynader and Mitchell 1980). Exposure of dark-reared animals to light results in rapid and dramatic changes in protein phosphorylation (Aoki and Siekevitz 1985) and protein synthesis (Rose 1967; Richardson and Rose 1972) in the visual cortex, thought to underlie cortical plasticity. Taken together, these observations suggest that determinants of developmental plasticity operative during

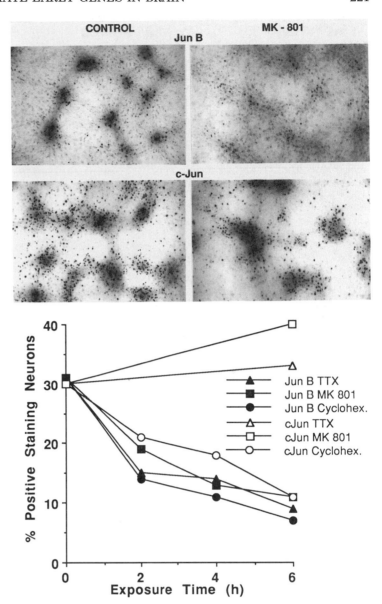

Figure 8. TTX and MK-801 reduce Jun-B but not c-Jun immunostaining in neurons of primary cortical cultures. Primary cultures of E17 rat fetuses were prepared as described in Methods and maintained 22–24 days in vitro. Final concentrations of drugs were TTX, 10 μM; MK-801, 10μM; cycloheximide, 10 μg/ml. Photomicrographs (bright field magnification, 68×) of Jun-B and c-Jun immunostaining in control cultures and 6 hr after addition of MK-801. Dark punctate immunostaining is associated with nuclei. Immunoreactive neurons were counted in random microscopic fields and expressed as the percentage of total neurons.

the normal critical period may be evoked and studied in dark-reared animals during the interval following first light exposure and emphasize differences in the degree of plasticity of developing and adult brain. As noted, dark-rearing appears to block the normal developmental increase in expression of several transcription factors, whereas subsequent light exposure triggers their rapid induction. As compared with the adult, transcription factor responses in developing animals are more robust, more extensive anatomically, and appear to affect a broader range of transcription factors. Moreover, NMDA receptors, thought to be involved in plasticity in both adult (Artola and Singer 1987) and developing (Kleinschmidt et al. 1987) visual cortex, appear to play a key role in regulating transcription factor activation in both adult and developing animals.

In summary, the induction of *zif/268* by artificial electrically induced synaptic stimulation in the LTP paradigm suggests that a rapid genomic response, similar to that induced by growth factors, may play a key role in orchestrating a program of gene expression underlying long-term synaptic plasticity. Studies described above examining the regulation of *zif/268* and other transcription factors in visual cortex suggest that these IEGs may well play a similar role in the synaptic plasticity induced by natural stimulation in both developing and adult cortical neurons.

ACKNOWLEDGMENTS

We are grateful to D. Nathans for advice and encouragement in conducting these studies and to D. Saffen and A. Lanahan for helpful comments and technical assistance. This research was supported by grants from the Esther and Joseph A. Klingenstein Fund (P.F.W.), Lucille P. Markey Charitable Trust (J.M.B.), Joseph P. Kennedy Foundation (J.M.B.), U.S. Public Health Service grant DA-00266 (J.M.B.), National Research

Service Award training grant (T.H.M.), Clinical Investigator Development Award K08-NS01360 (A.J.C.), and an American Academy of Neurology research fellowship (A.J.C.). J.M.B. is a Lucille P. Markey Scholar. We thank D. Lawrence for expert secretarial assistance.

REFERENCES

Abraham, W.C. and S.E. Mason. 1988. Effects of the NMDA receptor/channel antagonists CPP and MK801 on hippocampal field potentials and long-term potentiation in anesthetized rats. *Brain Res.* **462:** 40.

Agranoff, B.W. 1981. Learning and memory: Biochemical approaches. In *Basic neurochemistry,* 3rd edition (ed. G.J. Siegel et al.), p. 801. Little Brown and Company, Boston.

Aoki, C. and P. Siekevitz. 1985. Ontogenetic changes in the cyclic adenosine 3′, 5′-monophosphate-stimulatable phosphorylation of cat visual cortex proteins, particularly of microtubule-associated protein 2 (MAP 2): Effects of normal and dark rearing and the exposure to light. *J. Neurosci.* **5:** 2465.

Artola, A. and W. Singer. 1987. Long-term potentiation and NMDA receptors in rat visual cortex. *Nature* **330:** 649.

Bartel, D.P., M. Sheng, L.F. Lau, and M.E. Greenberg. 1989. Growth factors and membrane depolarization activate distinct program of early response gene expression: Dissociation of *fos* and *jun* induction. *Genes Dev.* **3:** 304.

Berridge, M. 1986. Second messenger dualism in neuromodulation and memory. *Nature* **323:** 294.

Chavrier, P., U. Janssen-Timmen, M.-G. Mattei, M. Zerial, R. Bravo, and P. Charnay. 1989. Structure, chromosome location, and expression of the mouse zinc finger gene *Krox-20*: Multiple gene products and coregulation with the proto-oncogene c-*fos. Mol. Cell. Biol.* **9:** 787.

Christy, B. and D. Nathans. 1989. DNA binding site of the growth factor-inducible protein Zif268. *Proc. Natl. Acad. Sci.* **86:** 8737.

Christy, B.A., L.F. Lau, and D. Nathans. 1988. A gene activated in mouse 3T3 cells by serum growth factors encodes a protein with "zinc finger" sequences. *Proc. Natl. Acad. Sci.* **85:** 7857.

Cochran, B.H., A.C. Reffel, and C.D. Stiles. 1983. Molecular cloning of gene sequences regulated by platelet-derived growth factor. *Cell* **33:** 939.

Cole, A.J., D.W. Saffen, J.M. Baraban, and P.F. Worley. 1989. Rapid increase of an immediate early gene messenger RNA in hippocampal neurons by synaptic NMDA receptor activation. *Nature* **340:** 474.

Cole, A.J., S. Abu-Shakra, D.W. Saffen, J.M. Baraban, and P.F. Worley. 1990. Rapid rise in transcription factor messenger RNAs in rat brain after electroshock induced seizures. *J. Neurochem.* (in press).

Cragg, B.G. 1967. Changes in visual cortex on first exposure of rats to light. *Nature* **215:** 251.

Cynader, M. and D.E. Mitchell. 1980. Prolonged sensitivity to monocular deprivation in dark-reared cats. *J. Neurophysiol.* **43:** 1026.

Dignam, J.D., R.M. Lebowitz, and R.G. Roeder. 1983. Accurate transcription initiation by RNA polymerase II in a soluble extract from isolated mammalian nuclei. *Nucleic Acids Res.* **11:** 1475.

Fox, K., H. Sato, and N. Daw. 1989. The location and function of NMDA receptors in cat and kitten visual cortex. *J. Neurosci.* **9:** 2443.

Gabbott, P.L.A. and M.G. Stewart. 1987. Quantitative morphological effects of dark-rearing and light exposure on the synaptic connectivity of layer 4 in the rat visual cortex (area 17). *Exp. Brain Res.* **68:** 103.

Gabbott, P.L.A., M.G. Stewart, and S.P.R. Rose. 1986. The quantitative effects of dark-rearing and light exposure on the laminary composition and depth distribution of neurons and glia in the visual cortex (area 17) of the rat. *Exp. Brain Res.* **64:** 225.

Goelet, P., V.F. Castellucci, S. Schacher, and E.R. Kandel. 1986. The long and the short of long-term memory—A molecular framework. *Nature* **322:** 419.

Greenberg, M.E. and E.B. Ziff. 1984. Stimulation of 3T3 cells induces transcription of the c-*fos* proto-oncogene. *Nature* **311:** 433.

Greenberg, M.E., L.A. Greene, and E.B. Ziff. 1985. Nerve growth factor and epidermal growth factor induce rapid transient changes in proto-oncogene transcription in PC12 cells. *J. Biol. Chem.* **260:** 14101.

Greenberg, M.E., E.B. Ziff, and L.A. Greene. 1986. Stimulation of neuronal acetylcholine receptor induces rapid gene transcription. *Science* **234:** 80.

Hagihara, K., T. Tsumoto, H. Sato, and Y. Hata. 1988. Actions of excitatory amino acid antagonists on geniculocortical transmission in the cat's visual cortex. *Exp. Brain Res.* **69:** 407.

Halazonetis, T.D., K. Georgopoulos, M.E. Greenberg, and P. Leder. 1988. c-Jun dimerizes with itself and with c-Fos, forming complexes of different DNA binding affinities. *Cell* **55:** 917.

Hazel, T.G., D. Nathans, and L.F. Lau. 1988. A gene inducible by serum growth factors encodes a member of the steroid and thyroid hormone receptor superfamily. *Proc. Natl. Acad. Sci.* **85:** 8444.

Hendrickson, A.E., S.P. Hunt, and J.-Y. Wu. 1981. Immunocytochemical localization of glutamic acid decarboxylase in monkey striate cortex. *Nature* **292:** 506.

Hendry, S.H.C. and E.G. Jones. 1986. Reduction in number of immunostained GABAergic neurones in deprived-eye dominance columns of monkey area 17. *Nature* **320:** 750.

Hendry, S.H.C. and M.B. Kennedy. 1986. Immunoreactivity for a calmodulin-dependent protein kinase is selectively increased in macaque striate cortex after monocular deprivation. *Proc. Natl. Acad. Sci.* **83:** 1536.

Hendry, S.H.C., E.G. Jones, and N. Burstein. 1988. Activity-dependent regulation of tachykinin-like immunoreactivity in neurons of monkey visual cortex. *J. Neurosci.* **8:** 1225.

Hubel, D.H. and T.N. Wiesel. 1970. The period of susceptibility to the physiological effects of unilateral eye closure in kittens. *J. Physiol.* **206:** 419.

Hubel, D.H., T.N. Wiesel, and S. LeVay. 1977. Plasticity of ocular dominance columns in monkey striate cortex. *Philos. Trans. R. Soc. Lond. B. Biol. Sci.* **278:** 377.

Huettner, J.E. and R.W. Baughman. 1986. Primary culture of identified neurons from the visual cortex of postnatal rats. *J. Neurosci.* **6:** 3044.

Innocenti, G.M. 1981. Growth and reshaping of axons in the establishment of visual callosal connections. *Science* **212:** 825.

Jones, K.A. and R.W. Baughman. 1988. NMDA- and non-NMDA-receptor components of excitatory synaptic potentials recorded from cells in layer V of rat visual cortex. *J. Neurosci.* **8:** 3522.

Kaas, J.H., L.A. Krubitzer, Y.M. Chino, A.L. Langston, E.H. Polley, and N. Blair. 1990. Reorganization of retinotopic cortical maps in adult mammals after lesions of the retina. *Science* **248:** 229.

Kadonaga, J.T., K.R. Carner, F.R. Masiarz, and R. Tjian. 1987. Isolation of cDNA encoding transcription factor Sp1 and functional analysis of the DNA binding domain. *Cell* **51:** 1079.

Kleinschmidt, A., M.F. Bear, and W. Singer. 1987. Blockade of "NMDA" receptors disrupts experience-dependent plasticity of kitten striate cortex. *Science* **238:** 355.

Kruijer, W., J. Cooper, T. Hunter, and I.M. Verma. 1984. Platelet-derived growth factor induces rapid but transient expression of the c-*fos* gene and protein. *Nature* **312:** 711.

Lau, L.F. and D. Nathans. 1987. Expression of a set of growth-related immediate early genes in BALB/c 3T3 cells: Coordinate regulation with *c-fos* or *c-myc*. *Proc. Natl. Acad. Sci.* **84**: 1182.

———. 1990. Genes induced by serum growth factors. In *Hormonal control of gene transcription. Molecular aspects of cell regulation* (ed. G. Foulkes and P. Cohen), vol. 6. Elsevier Biomedical, New York. (In press.)

Lemaire, P., O. Revelant, R. Bravo, and P. Charnay. 1988. Two mouse genes encoding potential transcription factors with identical DNA-binding domains are activated by growth factors in cultured cells. *Proc. Natl. Acad. Sci.* **85**: 4691.

LeVay, S.T.N., T.N. Wiesel, and D.H. Hubel. 1980. The development of ocular dominance columns in normal and visually deprived monkeys. *J. Comp. Neurol.* **191**: 1.

Linzer, D.L.H. and D. Nathans. 1983. Growth-related changes in specific mRNAs of cultured mouse cells. *Proc. Natl. Acad. Sci.* 80: 4271.

Lodge, D., S.N. Davies, M.G. Jones, J. Millar, and D.T. Manallack. 1988. A comparison between the *in vivo* and *in vitro* activity of five potent and competitive NMDA antagonists. *Br. J. Pharmacol.* **95**: 957.

Milbrandt, J. 1987. A nerve growth factor-induced gene encodes a possible transcriptional regulatory factor. *Science* **238**: 797.

———. 1988. Nerve growth factor induces a gene homologous to the glucocorticoid receptor gene. *Neuron* **1**: 183.

Miller, K.D., B. Chapman, and M.P. Stryker. 1989. Visual responses in adult cat visual cortex depend on N-methyl-D-aspartate receptors. *Proc. Natl. Acad. Sci.* **86**: 5183.

Miller, M.W. and B.A. Vogt. 1984. Direct connections of rat visual cortex with sensory, motor, and association cortices. *J. Comp. Neurol.* **226**: 184.

Mizumori, S.J.Y., B.L. McNaughton, and C.A Barnes. 1989. A comparison of supramammillary and medial septal influences on hippocampal field potentials and single-unit activity. *J. Neurophysiol.* **61**: 15.

Montarolo, P.G., P. Goelet, V.F. Catelluci, J. Morgan, E.R. Kandel, and S. Schacher. 1986. A critical period for macromolecular synthesis in long-term heterosynaptic facilitation in *Aplysia*. *Science* **234**: 1249.

Morgan, J.I., D.R. Cohen, J.L. Hempstead, and T. Curran. 1987. Mapping patterns of *c-fos* expression in the central nervous system after seizure. *Science* **237**: 192.

Murphy, D.E., A.J. Hutchison, S.D. Hurt, M. Williams, and M.A. Sills. 1988. Characterization of the binding of [³H]-CGS 19755: A novel N-methyl-D-aspartate antagonist with nanomolar affinity in rat brain. *Br. J. Pharmacol.* **95**: 932.

Nakabeppu, Y., K. Ryder, and D. Nathans. 1988. DNA binding activities of three murine Jun proteins: Stimulation by Fos. *Cell* **55**: 907.

Nicoll, R.A., J.A. Kauer, and R.C. Malenka. 1988. The current excitement in long-term potentiation. *Neuron* **1**: 97.

Nishikura, K. and J.M. Murray. 1987. Antisense RNA or protooncogene *c-fos* blocks renewed growth or quiescent 3T3 cells. *Mol. Cell. Biol.* **7**: 639.

Paxinos, G. and C. Watson. 1982. The rat brain in sterotaxic coordinates. In *The rat brain*. Academic Press, New York.

Rauscher, F.J., P.J. Voulalas, B.R. Franza, Jr., and T. Curran. 1988. Fos and Jun bind cooperatively to the AP-1 site: Reconstruction *in vitro*. *Genes Dev.* **2**: 1687.

Riabowol, K.T., R.J. Vosatka, E.B. Ziff, N.J. Lamb, and J.R. Feramisco. 1988. Microinjection of *fos*-specific antibodies blocks DNA synthesis in fibroblast cells. *Mol. Cell. Biol.* **8**: 1670.

Richardson, K. and S.P.R. Rose. 1972. Changes in [³H]lysine incorporation following first exposure to light. *Brain Res.* **44**: 299.

Rose, S.P.R. 1967. Changes in visual cortex on first exposure of rats to light. *Nature* **215**: 253.

Saffen, D.W., A.J. Cole, P.F. Worley, B.A. Christy, K. Ryder, and J.M. Baraban. 1988. Convulsant-induced increase in transcription factor messenger RNAs in rat brain. *Proc. Natl. Acad. Sci.* **85**: 7795.

Sah, P., S. Hestrin, and R.A. Nicoll. 1989. Tonic activation of NMDA receptors by ambient glutamate enhances excitability of neurons. *Science* **246**: 815.

Sheng, M. and M.E. Greenberg. 1990. The regulation and function of c-*fos* and other immediate early genes in the nervous system. *Neuron* **4**: 477.

Sonnenberg, J.L., P.F. MacGregor-Leon, T. Curran, and J.I. Morgan. 1989. Dynamic alterations occur in the levels and composition of transcription factor AP-1 complexes after seizure. *Neuron* **3**: 359.

Sukhatme, V.P., X. Cao, L.C. Chang, C.-H. Tsai-Morris, D. Stamenkovich, P.C.P. Ferreira, D.R. Cohen, S.A. Edwards, T.B. Shows, T. Curran, M.M. Le Beau, and E.D. Adamson. 1988. A zinc finger-encoding gene coregulated with c-*fos* during growth and differentiation, and after cellular depolarization. *Cell* **53**: 37.

Treisman, R. 1987. Identification and purification of a polypeptide that binds to the c-*fos* serum response element. *EMBO J.* **6**: 2711.

Tsumoto, T., K. Hagihara, H. Sato, and Y. Hata. 1987. NMDA receptors in the visual cortex of young kittens are more effective than those of adult cats. *Nature* **327**: 513.

Valverde, F. 1971. Rate and extent of recovery from dark rearing in the visual cortex of the mouse. *Brain Res.* **33**: 1.

Wong, E.H.F., J.A. Kemp, T. Priestley, A.R. Knight, G.N. Woodruff, and L.L. Iversen. 1986. The anticonvulsant MK-801 is a potent N-methyl-D-aspartate antagonist. *Proc. Natl. Acad. Sci.* **83**: 7104.

Wong-Riley, M. and E.W. Carroll. 1984. Effect of impulse blockade on cytochrome oxidase activity in monkey visual system. *Nature* **307**: 572.

Zilles, K., A. Wree, A. Schleicher, and I. Divac. 1984. The monocular and binocular subfields of the rat's primary visual cortex: A quantitative morphological approach. *J. Comp. Neurol.* **226**: 391.

Inducible Proto-oncogene Transcription Factors: Third Messengers in the Brain?

T. Curran,* C. Abate,* D.R. Cohen,* P.F. MacGregor,* F.J. Rauscher III,*
J.L. Sonnenberg,* J.A. Connor,† and J.I. Morgan†
*Department of Molecular Oncology and Virology, †Department of Neurosciences,
Roche Institute of Molecular Biology, Roche Research Center, Nutley, New Jersey 07110

Neglected for several years, the nucleus is now undergoing a renaissance in neurobiology. Although it has long been appreciated that the diversity of the nervous system must have its basis in the selective regulation of gene expression and there have been many indications that altered gene expression contributes to processes that underlie neural plasticity, it is only recently that the specific molecular probes for studying such phenomena have become available (see, e.g., Vaessin et al.; Jones et al.; Schacher et al.; Worley et al.; all this volume). A great deal of effort is now being directed toward understanding the molecular events that occur in the nucleus to orchestrate cell-type-specific and stimulus-evoked alterations in gene regulation. Although the neuron has many unique properties, it is becoming increasingly clear that its behavior is governed by many of the same signaling molecules that operate in other cell types. We have borrowed concepts and reagents from the field of oncogene research and applied these to the study of the nervous system. Here, we describe the several steps that have led us to suggest that the very same transcription factors that have been implicated in the regulation of cell growth, and that are capable of causing oncogenic transformation, also play a role as inducible transcription factors in stimulus-response coupling in the nervous system.

fos and *jun*: Inducible Proto-oncogene Transcription Factors

The oncogenes *fos* and *jun* were first described as the transforming genes carried by the FBJ murine sarcoma virus (Curran and Teich 1982) and avian sarcoma virus 17 (Maki et al. 1987), respectively. Their normal cellular homologs, c-*fos* and c-*jun*, are expressed at relatively low levels in the majority of cell types. However, they are induced transiently to very high levels by a great variety of extracellular stimuli (for reviews, see Curran 1988; Cohen and Curran 1989). Although initial studies on the regulation of c-*fos* and c-*jun* expression were concerned primarily with mitogenic stimuli, it has become clear that these genes function as components of a relatively common signal transduction cascade (Fig. 1). Both c-*fos* and c-*jun* are members of the set of genes known as cellular immediate-early genes (Curran and Morgan 1987; Lau and Nathans 1987).

This gene set has been defined operationally by the fact that expression is induced rapidly by a range of extracellular stimuli, even in the presence of protein synthesis inhibitors. This is a feature shared with the immediate-early genes of several viruses. Cellular immediate-early genes have been proposed to function in coupling short-term stimuli to long-term changes in cellular phenotype. This hypothesis was strengthened by the discovery that both c-*fos* and c-*jun* encode proteins (Fos and Jun, respectively) that function in transcriptional regulation. Indeed, Fos and Jun form a heterodimeric complex that interacts with the regulatory element known as the transcription factor AP-1 (activator protein-1) binding site (for review, see Curran and Franza 1988). Interestingly, Jun was previously identified as the Fos-associated protein p39 (Rauscher et al. 1988b). Thus, two independently isolated oncogenes encode proteins that function cooperatively as a bimolecular complex to regulate target gene expression in response to cell stimulation.

The situation has been made more complex by the discovery that both *fos* and *jun* are members of gene families. The other family members are also induced by extracellular stimuli, and they are all capable of forming heterodimeric and homodimeric complexes with similar, although not identical, DNA-binding specificities (Cohen and Curran 1988; Ryder et al. 1988, 1989; Cohen et al. 1989; Zerial et al. 1989). All of the Jun family members can form homodimeric and heterodimeric complexes with each other, whereas the Fos family members only form heterodimeric complexes with Jun-related proteins (Nakabeppu et al. 1988; Rauscher et al. 1988a; Cohen et al. 1989; Zerial et al. 1989). Although all of these homodimers and heterodimers are considered to be AP-1 complexes with specificities for so-called *TPA*-responsive elements (TRE, consensus sequence TGACTCA), it is clear that they can also interact with *cAMP*-responsive elements (CRE, consensus sequence TGACGTCA) (Fig. 1). Furthermore, one of the CRE-binding proteins (CRE-BP1) forms heterodimers with Jun that have a high degree of specificity for CRE sites (Macgregor et al. 1990).

The terms TRE and CRE are quite narrow and perhaps now misleading. These DNA sequence motifs are present in many regulatory elements, and they

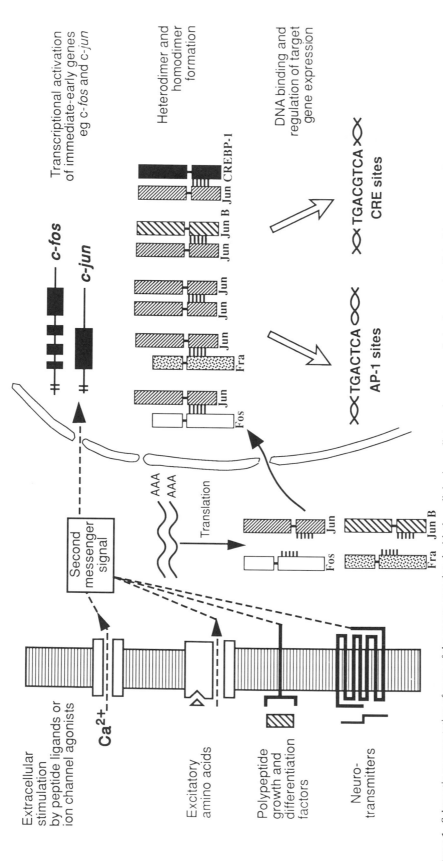

Figure 1. Schematic representation of some of the events associated with the cellular immediate-early response. Induction can be elicited by an array of extracellular stimuli acting on several second-messenger systems. The mechanism whereby the signal reaches the nucleus and activates immediate-early gene transcription is not yet clear. The result of activation is the transient elevation of mRNA levels and increased synthesis of immediate-early proteins. The Fos and Jun family members are rapidly transported to the nucleus, where they form heterodimeric and homodimeric protein complexes. The Jun proteins can also form heterodimeric complexes with CRE-BP1, a CRE-binding protein, which is expressed at high basal levels in the brain. The dimeric complexes have varying affinities for a range of regulatory elements containing AP-1 and CRE sites. Although not shown here, it is likely that other protein-protein interactions and posttranslational modifications influence the selection of DNA-binding sites on target genes.

contribute both negatively and positively to basal and regulated rates of transcription. In a general sense, the proteins encoded by the *fos* and *jun* gene families function as "intermediary transcription factors" that are responsive to a variety of second-messenger signals in many situations. The question that is often provoked by illustrations like Figure 1 is, "Wherein lies the specificity?" If similar DNA-binding proteins are induced by mitogenic, differentiation-inducing, and depolarizing stimuli, how can they mediate distinct phenotypic responses? The short answer is that no one really knows. However, there are many variables in the cellular immediate-early response that, in combination, likely contribute to the recognition of specific target genes in each situation.

1. Different subsets of immediate-early genes are induced by distinct stimuli.
2. The proteins encoded by these genes interact with different resident proteins whose presence is dictated by the phenotype of the stimulated cell. For example, CRE-BP1 (which forms heterodimers with Jun) is not usually inducible but is expressed at particularly high levels in brain (Maekawa et al. 1989; Macgregor et al. 1990).
3. Both Fos and Jun undergo extensive posttranslational modification. The degree of modification of Fos, primarily phosphorylation, depends on the nature of the inducing stimulus (Fig. 3).
4. Although consensus AP-1 and CRE sites are illustrated in Figure 1, there are many variations of these sites. Thus, particular variations of these DNA sequences may be preferentially recognized by specific dimeric complexes.
5. Only certain regulatory sites may be available in each differentiated cell type. This specificity could be mediated by nuclear or chromatin organization or by the presence of proteins that mask certain binding sites.
6. AP-1 and CRE sites are usually present in complex regulatory elements and are surrounded by binding sites for other transcription factors. Thus, the recognition of target genes may rely as much on protein-protein contacts with these other factors as on protein-DNA interactions. Therefore, target genes may be selected by a "key-in-lock" mechanism that is specified by other inducible or resident transcription factors.
7. We have recently identified a novel reduction/oxidation mechanism that regulates the DNA-binding activity of Fos and Jun (Abate et al. 1990a). This may provide an additional layer of regulation of the Fos, Jun, and CREB proteins.

The nucleus can be viewed as a complex arena in which multiple signal transduction pathways converge. We are only beginning to scrape the surface of the molecular interactions among transcriptional regulatory molecules that are required to mediate biological responses in individual cell types to environmental cues.

Structure/Function Relationships in Fos and Jun

There have been several investigations of the structural basis of dimerization and DNA binding in Fos and Jun (Kouzarides and Ziff 1988; Gentz et al. 1989; O'Shea et al. 1989; Ransone et al. 1989; Schuermann et al. 1989; Turner and Tjian 1989). These studies were prompted by the proposal of a model, termed the leucine zipper, suggesting that dimerization was mediated by a zipper-like interaction between a heptad repeat of five leucines arranged as an α helix in each protein (Landschulz et al. 1988). The model has now been refined, and it appears that the leucine zipper is more akin to the coiled-coil structure. It involves a parallel interaction of α helices in the zipper region (Gentz et al. 1989; O'Shea et al. 1989) that bring into juxtaposition regions of each protein rich in basic amino acids. The basic regions of Fos and Jun each contact both strands of DNA in a bipartite DNA-binding domain (Abate et al. 1990b). A schematic representation of the Fos-Jun heterodimer is presented in Figure 2. The zipper and basic regions are highly conserved among the *fos* and *jun* family members. The regions of each protein that function in transcriptional activation in vitro (an acidic region in Fos and a proline-glutamine-rich region in Jun) are indicated (Bohmann and Tjian 1989; Abate et al. 1990c). Fos also contains a domain that acts independently of the leucine zipper and basic regions as a transcriptional repressor in cotransfection assays (Gius et al. 1990). This region has an indirect effect on the *serum response element* (SRE) and it may function to turn off the immediate-early response. Although the leucine zipper is the primary dimerization domain, and the basic region is the primary DNA-binding domain in Fos and Jun, it should be kept in mind that the whole

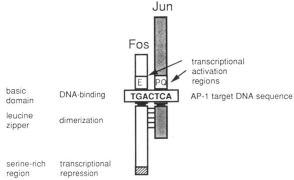

Figure 2. Functional domains in the Fos-Jun heterodimer. Several functional regions in Fos and Jun have been defined in mutagenesis and biochemical studies. The leucine zipper is the primary region associated with dimerization (illustrated by parallel lines) and the basic region (shown in contact with the AP-1 site) is the primary region involved in DNA binding. However, other parts of the proteins influence these functions (Cohen and Curran 1990). Glutamic acid-rich (E) and proline-glutamine-rich (P-Q) regions associated with transcriptional activation in vitro (Bohmann and Tjian 1989; Abate et al. 1990c) and a repression region identified in cotransfection assays (Gius et al. 1990) have also been defined.

228 CURRAN ET AL.

proteins interact and amino acids outside of these motifs also contribute to dimerization and DNA binding (Cohen and Curran 1990).

Induction of Fos in PC-12 Cells

The first indication of a possible association between c-*fos* and neuronal cells was the observation that c-*fos* could be induced in PC-12 pheochromocytoma cells by treatment with nerve growth factor (NGF) (Curran and Morgan 1985; Greenberg et al. 1985; Kruijer et al. 1985). An example of the induction of Fos by NGF is shown in Figure 3. This was an important demonstration of the fact that induction of cellular immediate-early genes is not only associated with mitogenic signaling. The discovery that voltage-gated calcium influxes (Morgan and Curran 1986), such as those elicited by depolarization, and stimulation of the acetylcholine receptor (Greenberg et al. 1986) could also induce c-*fos* expression cemented the connection between the immediate-early response and neuronal stimuli. As shown in Figure 3, Fos is induced by depolarization with 50 mM potassium chloride (KCl). This action is calcium-channel-dependent and is blocked by calcium channel antagonists such as nisoldipine (Morgan and Curran 1986). In addition, barium ions (1 mM) in the external saline that enter the cell through the voltage-gated calcium channel (Hagiwara et al. 1974) also trigger the induction of c-*fos* expression. Experiments using the calcium indicator fura-2 have demonstrated that depolarizing levels of KCl provoke a rapid increase in intracellular free calcium (Fig. 4). These increases were largely eliminated by calcium channel antagonists (Fig. 4). Peak concentrations of free calcium observed with potassium depolarizations were in the range of 0.6–1 µM. This establishes a link between intracellular free calcium levels and induction of c-*fos* expression. The exact mechanism whereby calcium and, indeed, barium inside the cell elicit c-*fos* induction remains unclear.

The majority of the c-*fos* protein induced by KCl and barium has a lower apparent molecular weight, which is

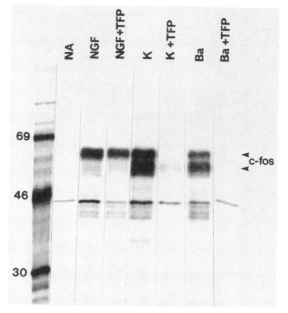

Figure 3. Induction of Fos in PC-12 cells. Cultures of PC-12 cells were incubated in DMEM with no additions (NA), nerve growth factor (NGF) at 200 ng/ml⁻¹, NGF at 200 ng/ml⁻¹ plus 15 µM trifluoperazine (TFP), 50 mM potassium chloride (K), 50 mM potassium chloride plus 15 µM trifluoperazine, 1 mM barium chloride (Ba), or 1 mM barium chloride plus 15 µM trifluoperazine for 30 min before labeling with [³⁵S]methionine. Cells were lysed, and Fos was immuno-precipitated from solubilized extracts using anti-Fos antibodies. Proteins were analyzed by electrophoresis on SDS polyacrylamide gels and were visualized by autoradiography. The numbers on the left indicate the molecular weights of [¹⁴C]methyl-labeled marker proteins (Amersham). Arrows indicate the positions of the c-*fos* proteins. (Reprinted, with permission, from Curran and Morgan 1986.)

a result of a decreased posttranslational modification, compared to that obtained with NGF (Fig. 3). The lack of modification is not absolute; rather, the modification process is slower in KCl- or barium-treated cells. The effect can be abolished by adding NGF to KCl-treated cultures as little as 5 minutes before lysing the cells.

Figure 4. Calcium levels in stimulated PC-12 cells. Freshly dispersed PC-12 cells were suspended in serum-free DMEM containing 4 µM fura-2/AM and allowed to settle onto a polylysine-coated glass coverslip (#1) mounted in the imaging chamber. Incubation times of 15–25 min at 30°C were sufficient to allow the cells to load with indicator and stick to the coverslip, after which the cells were rinsed with HEPES-buffered Krebs saline, removing the extracellular fura-2/AM. Relatively flat clusters of cells were selected for experimentation (lower right detail of figure shows fluorescence excited by 380 nm light). Details of the ratiometric determination of free calcium levels are given elsewhere (Connor 1986; Connor et al. 1987). The left-hand column shows calcium changes elicited by 50 mM K saline (Na substituted). Color coding of levels is given in the upper right portion. Measurements are shown at 20 sec after the exchange of saline, approximately the peak of the response, and at 2 min in high K, when levels had decayed to an intermediate plateau. The diversity in calcium response shown here was typical of all groups of cells examined. Normal resting levels of calcium were restored within 2 min in 4.7 mM K saline, and subsequent responses to high K challenges were approximately the same as the one shown. The right-hand column shows the response of the same cells given the same K challenge but in nifedipine (10 µM) saline. Both the peak and plateau responses were greatly attenuated; in nifedipine the peak responses never reached levels greater than 200 nM, whereas plateau levels were generally only slightly above the unstimulated values. Similar results were obtained in PC-12 cells cultured on the glass coverslips for several days before experimentation.

Figure 6. Induction of Fos immunoreactivity in the dentate gyrus by Metrazole. Three hours after administration of Metrazole, tissues were prepared for immunocytochemistry by fixation with paraformaldehyde. A coronal section through the dentate gyrus was stained with anti-Fos antibodies. Bound antibody was detected with an avidin-biotin-peroxidase complex. (dg) Dentate gyrus; (hc) hippocampus.

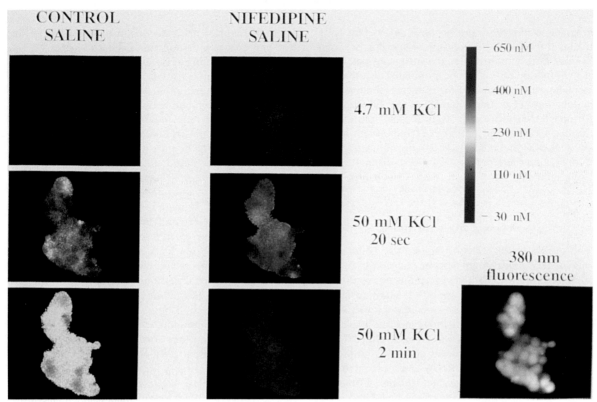

CONTROL
SALINE

NIFEDIPINE
SALINE

4.7 mM KCl

650 nM

400 nM

230 nM

110 nM

30 nM

50 mM KCl
20 sec

50 mM KCl
2 min

380 nm
fluorescence

Figure 4. (*See facing page for legend.*)

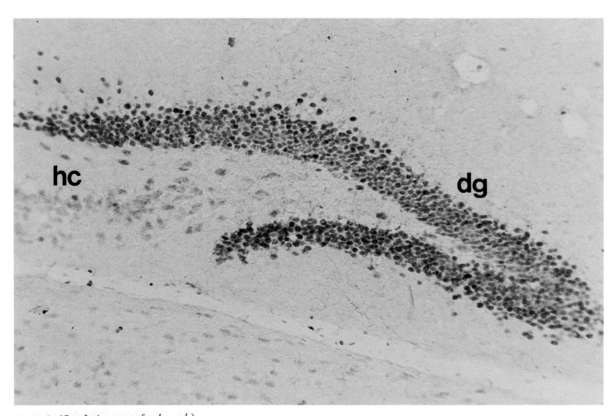

hc

dg

Figure 6. (*See facing page for legend.*)

The simplest interpretation of these data is that NGF activates the kinases that phosphorylate Fos, whereas KCl does not. This provides the intriguing possibility that the function of Fos can be modulated differentially depending on the nature of the inducing stimulus. The signaling pathways that mediate c-*fos* induction by NGF and KCl are distinct; NGF does not require extracellular calcium and, unlike KCl and barium induction, it is not affected by the calmodulin antagonist trifluoperazine (TFP) (Fig. 3). Indeed, distinct 5′ regulatory elements in c-*fos* mediate NGF- and KCl-induced expression (Sheng et al. 1988).

Induction of *fos* in the Brain

The studies on PC-12 cells implied that cellular immediate-early genes might also be induced by neuromodulators in vivo. To investigate this possibility, we examined the effects of a range of pharmacological agents on the levels of expression of c-*fos* mRNA in mouse brain. All agents were inoculated intraperitoneally, and whole-brain RNA was isolated after 90 minutes, as described by Morgan et al. (1987). Although modest increases in c-*fos* mRNA levels were detected with isoproteronol, reserpine, and codeine, a dramatic increase was obtained with the convulsant pentylenetetrazole (Metrazole) (Fig. 5). Induction of c-*fos* by Metrazole is dose-dependent and is blocked by anticonvulsants such as Diazepam (Morgan et al. 1987). The cells that express c-*fos* were identified as neurons by double-labeling immunocytochemistry (Morgan et al. 1987). This was accomplished using a rabbit antibody raised against Fos amino acids 127–152 (Curran et al. 1985) and a monoclonal antibody specific for

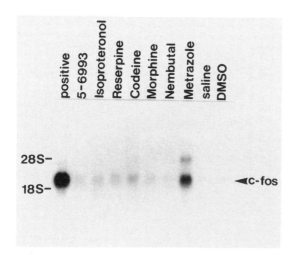

Figure 5. Induction of Fos mRNA in brain. Mice were injected intraperitoneally with the compounds listed. After 90 min, whole-brain RNA was isolated as described previously (Morgan et al. 1987). Aliquots (10 μg) were analyzed by electrophoresis on an agarose-formaldehyde gel. RNA was transferred onto nitrocellulose and hybridized with a *fos*-specific probe. The positive control is RNA extracted from PC-12 cells after treatment with barium.

neurofilaments. This technique also allowed us to map the neuronal populations that exhibited increased Fos-like immunostaining at different times after seizure. In untreated mice, positive neurons were detected sporadically throughout the brain but particularly in the pyriform and cingulate cortices, anterior olfactory nucleus, dentate gyrus, and hippocampus. However, 3 hours after administration of Metrazole, all of the granule cells in the dentate gyrus stained strongly positive (Fig. 6). Increased staining of the dentate gyrus was first evident after 30 minutes and was maximal after 60 minutes. There was an increase in both the number and intensity of stained neurons in defined cortical regions between 60 and 90 minutes. Subsequently, staining of further cortical layers and regions became evident. By 4 hours after treatment, essentially all neurons in the cortex and limbic system were labeled. Although occasional neurons were labeled in the hippocampus up to 90 minutes, the entire structure became Fos-positive by 3 hours. At 90 minutes after drug administration, immunoreactivity was also observed in the amygdala, septum, and olfactory bulb. Fos was conspicuously absent from some areas of brain at all times examined, notably the superior and inferior colliculi, the geniculate bodies, central gray, substantia nigra, and cerebellar cortex. Thus, after seizure, there ensues a successive recruitment of specific cohorts of neurons expressing c-*fos* throughout the cerebral cortex and limbic system.

A Complex Immediate-Early Response in Neurons

We investigated the regulation of expression of a range of cellular immediate-early genes in the seizure model system. As shown in Figure 7, increases were detected in the levels of c-*fos*, c-*jun*, *jun*B, and *egr*-1 in whole-brain and hippocampal RNAs. *egr*-1 encodes a zinc-finger-containing protein that is thought to function in transcriptional regulation (Sukhatme et al. 1988). Increases were also detected in proenkephalin mRNA levels, as reported previously in other seizure model systems (Iadarola et al. 1986; White and Gall 1987). Both *jun*B and *egr*-1 showed similar temporal patterns of induction as c-*fos*, with maximal stimulation occurring in the hippocampus at 30–60 minutes after treatment and returning to basal levels by 2–4 hours. The time course of proenkephalin mRNA induction was slightly delayed compared to that of the immediate-early gene mRNAs. One hour after injection of Metrazole, proenkephalin mRNA in the hippocampus was increased compared to control animals and remained elevated for at least 6 hours, consistent with the long half-life of this mRNA. Thus, the level of proenkephalin mRNA increased in the hippocampus after elevation of c-*fos* and c-*jun* mRNAs. The basal level of proenkephalin mRNA in whole-brain samples was high, and no increase was observed after seizure. These data suggested that the proenkephalin gene might be a target for regulation by immediate-early genes in the hippocampus but not in other regions of the central

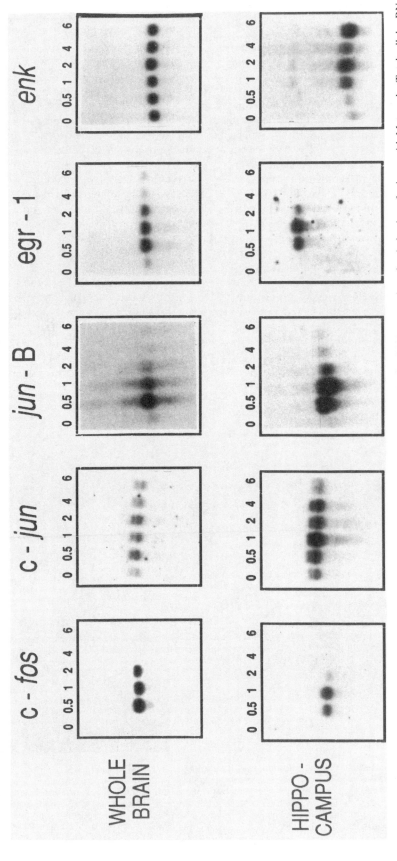

Figure 7. Induction of immediate-early genes in the brain. Time-course of immediate-early gene and *enk* mRNA expression after induction of seizure with Metrazole. Total cellular RNA was extracted from whole mouse brain and dissected rat hippocampus at the indicated times (in hours) after induction of seizure by intraperitoneal injection of Metrazole (45 mg/kg^{-1}). Each RNA (2 μg) was analyzed by electrophoresis on 0.8% agarose gels in the presence of 2.2 M formaldehyde. The total RNA content of each lane was monitored by staining with ethidium bromide. RNAs were transferred onto nitrocellulose and hybridized with *c-fos*, *c-jun*, *jun*B, *egr*-1, and *enk* probes. The nitrocellulose membrane was washed with 2 × standard sodium citrate plus 0.1% SDS for 90 min at 55°C prior to autoradiography. (Reprinted, with permission, from Sonnenberg et al. 1989b.)

231

nervous system. Indeed, we demonstrated subsequently that Fos and Jun bind cooperatively to the ENK-2 sequence in the 5' control region of proenkephalin (Sonnenberg et al. 1989b). The ENK-2 site has been shown to contribute to the regulation of proenkephalin following stimulation of cells by phorbol esters and cAMP analogs (Comb et al. 1988). Furthermore, co-transfection of c-*fos* and c-*jun* stimulated expression from the proenkephalin promoter in F9 cells (Sonnenberg et al. 1989b). However, it should be noted that many transcription factors can interact with the proenkephalin regulatory region, and it is likely that several proteins contribute to the regulation of proenkephalin transcription in response to physiological stimuli.

We were rather surprised to discover that the Fos-related gene *fra*-1 was not induced by seizure-provoking stimuli (Cohen and Curran 1988). However, the induction of several Fos-related proteins was detected by Western blot analysis in several seizure paradigms (Sonnenberg et al. 1989a,c). Induction of Fos and several Fra are illustrated in Figure 8A following injection of *N*-methyl-D-aspartate (NMDA), an agonist of a subclass of excitatory glutamate receptors. In addition to Fos, at least two inducible Fos-related antigens (46K and 35K) were detected by immunoblot analysis. The 46K Fra was induced to high levels later than Fos,

between 2 and 4 hours after seizure, and declined thereafter, reaching basal levels by 8 hours. The 35K Fra was sometimes the most abundant protein recognized by anti-Fos antibodies in control samples. Despite variability in basal levels, 35K Fra increased after seizure, attaining maximal levels after 4 hours. It is possible that the many bands detected on the gel in the 46K and 35K regions represent either distinct proteins or multiple modified forms of the same protein. All of the Fra detected by Western analysis apparently contribute to increased levels of AP-1 DNA-binding activity in the brain after seizure. As shown in Figure 8B, elevated levels of AP-1 gel-shift activity are detected 8 hours after induction of seizure by Metrazole. This is a much longer time course than Fos expression, which has returned to basal values by 4 hours. Thus, there is a complex interplay among several inducible Fos- and Jun-related proteins that leads to prolonged (at least 8 hr) increases in transcription factor AP-1 levels in neurons after stimulation. These changes can be triggered by a relatively brief (15 min) period of seizure (Sonnenberg et al. 1989a). Thus, neuronal stimuli elicit a programmed series of alterations in the levels and composition of transcription factor AP-1. After induction, there often ensues a refractory period for reinduction by the same stimuli. This period of refractoriness is

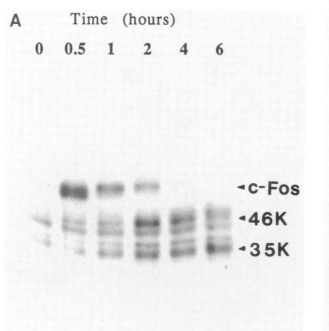

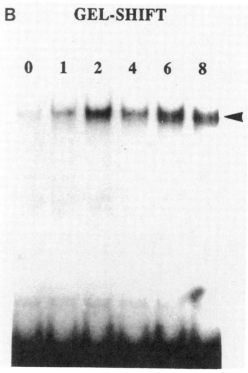

Figure 8. Induction of Fra and AP-1 activity in brain. (*A*) Time-course of Fos and Fra induction following NMDA treatment. Immunoblot analysis was performed using brain nuclear extracts prepared at the indicated times after administration of NMDA. The positions of Fos and Fra are indicated by arrowheads. (Reprinted, with permission, from Sonnenberg et al. 1989c.) (*B*) Time-course of induction of AP-1-binding activity after seizure. Male Sprague-Dawley rats were injected intraperitoneally with Metrazole (50 mg/kg^{-1}). At the indicated times following Metrazole administration, rat hippocampal tissue was used to prepare brain nuclear extracts for gel-shift assays. Gel-shift assays were carried out using an oligonucleotide corresponding to the AP-1 site from the human metallothionein$_A$ gene as described previously (Rauscher et al. 1988a). The position of AP-1-binding activity is indicated by an arrowhead. (Reprinted, with permission, from Sonnenberg et al. 1989a.)

coincident with the time-course of Fra expression. We have shown that at least *fra*-1 and c-*fos* are capable of repressing immediate-early gene expression in cotransfection assays (Gius et al. 1991). These results suggest that there is a higher order of organization of the neuronal immediate-early response that could be a common feature of nuclear signal transduction processes in many cell types.

What Does It All Mean?

The seizure model system has allowed us to characterize the molecular details of the cellular immediate-early response in the central nervous system. Seizure provokes a massive and relatively synchronized neuronal activation event in defined subsets of neurons. Using pharmacological agonists and antagonists of excitatory and inhibitory amino acid receptors, we have shown that several receptor types contribute to the response. The identification of occasional Fos-positive neurons in control mice suggested that the immediate-early response might be triggered transiently by physiological stimuli. There have now been many studies using electrical and physiological stimuli, e.g., water deprivation, light, or pain, that demonstrate induction in specific neuronal targets in the nervous system (for review, see Morgan and Curran 1991). In these situations, the signal that triggers the immediate-early response in individual cell types has not yet been defined. However, it is likely that an integration of several stimuli is required. The most difficult question to answer is, "What comes next?" Although proenkephalin has been identified as a potential target gene of Fos and Jun in the nervous system (Sonnenberg et al. 1989b), it is clear that many other transcription factors contribute to its regulation. Studies on fibroblasts in culture have shown that induction of immediate-early genes is not sufficient in itself to signal mitogenesis. Other signal transduction pathways operating in concert are required. Thus, the immediate-early response cannot be considered in isolation; it must be integrated into the particular context of the stimulated cell. The questions that must be answered in the future are, "What are the available target genes in specific cells?" "What are the cooperating basal or inducible transcription factors?" "What are the other important signals, e.g., activated kinases, ion fluxes?" "How does regulation of target genes influence the long-term phenotype of a stimulated neuron?"

REFERENCES

Abate, C., L. Patel, F.J. Rauscher III, and T. Curran. 1990a. Redox regulation of Fos and Jun DNA-binding activity *in vitro*. *Science* 249: 1157.

Abate, C., F.J. Rauscher III, R. Gentz, and T. Curran. 1990b. Expression and purification of the leucine zipper and the DNA-binding domains of Fos and Jun: both Fos and Jun directly contact DNA. *Proc. Natl. Acad. Sci.* 87: 1032.

Abate, C., D. Luk, E. Gagne, R.G. Roeder, and T. Curran.

1990c. Fos and Jun cooperate in transcriptional regulation via heterologous activation domains. *Mol. Cell. Biol.* 10: 5532.

Bohmann, D. and R. Tjian. 1989. Biochemical analysis of transcriptional activation by Jun: differential activity of c- and v-Jun. *Cell* 59: 709.

Cohen, D.R. and T. Curran. 1988. *fra*-1: A serum inducible, cellular immediate-early gene that encodes a Fos-related antigen. *Mol. Cell. Biol.* 8: 2063.

———. 1989. The structure and function of the *fos* proto-oncogene. *Crit. Rev. Oncogen.* 1: 65.

———. 1990. Analysis of DNA-binding functions in Fos and Jun by domain-swapping: Involvement of residues outside the leucine zipper/basic region. *Oncogene* 5: 929.

Cohen, D.R., P.C.P. Ferreira, R. Gentz, B.R. Franza, Jr. and T. Curran. 1989. The product of a Fos-related gene, *fra*-1, binds cooperatively to the AP-1 site with Jun: Transcription factor AP-1 is comprised of multiple protein complexes. *Genes Dev.* 3: 173.

Comb, M., N. Mermod, S.E. Hyman, J. Pearlberg, M.E. Ross, and H.M. Goodman. 1988. Proteins bound at adjacent DNA elements act synergistically to regulate human proenkephalin cAMP inducible transcription. *EMBO J.* 7: 3793.

Connor, J.A. 1986. Digital imaging of free calcium changes and of spatial gradients in growing processes in single, mammalian central nervous system cells. *Proc. Natl. Acad. Sci.* 83: 6179.

Connor, J.A., M.C. Cornwall, and G.H. Williams. 1987. Spatially resolved cytosolic calcium response to angiotensin II and potassium in rat glomerulosa cells measured by digital imaging techniques. *J. Biol. Chem.* 62: 2919.

Curran, T. 1988. The *fos* oncogene. In *The oncogene handbook* (ed. E.P. Reddy et al.), p. 307. Elsevier, Amsterdam.

Curran, T. and B.R. Franza, Jr. 1988. Fos and Jun: The AP-1 connection. *Cell* 55: 395.

Curran, T. and J.I. Morgan. 1985. Superinduction of *fos* by nerve growth factor in the presence of peripherally active benzodiazepines. *Science* 229: 1265.

———. 1986. Barium modulates c-*fos* expression and post-translational modification. *Proc. Natl. Acad. Sci.* 83: 8521.

———. 1987. Memories of *fos*. *BioEssays* 7: 255.

Curran, T. and N.M. Teich. 1982. Candidate product of the FBJ murine osteosarcoma virus oncogene: Characterization of a 55,000 dalton phosphoprotein. *J. Virol.* 42: 114.

Curran, T., C. van Beveren, N. Ling, and I.M. Verma. 1985. Viral and cellular *fos* proteins are complexed with a 39,000 dalton cellular protein. *Mol. Cell. Biol.* 5: 167.

Gentz, R., F.J. Rauscher III, C. Abate, and T. Curran. 1989. Parallel association of Fos and Jun leucine zippers juxtaposes DNA binding domains. *Science* 243: 1695.

Gius, D., X. Cao, F.J. Rauscher III, D.R. Cohen, T. Curran, and V.P. Sukhatme. 1990. Transcriptional activation and repression by Fos are independent functions: The C-terminus represses immediate-early gene expression via CArG elements. *Mol. Cell. Biol.* 10: 4243.

Greenberg, M., L.A. Greene, and E.B. Ziff. 1985. Nerve growth factor and epidermal growth factor induce rapid transient changes in proto-oncogene transcription in PC12. *J. Biol. Chem.* 260: 14101.

Greenberg, M.E., E.B. Ziff, and L.A. Greene. 1986. Stimulation of neuronal acetylcholine receptors induces rapid gene transcription. *Science* 234: 80.

Hagiwara, S., H. Fukuda, and D.C. Eaton. 1974. Membrane currents carried by Ca, Sr, and Ba in barnacle muscle fiber during voltage clamp. *J. Gen. Physiol.* 63: 564.

Iadarola, M.J., C. Shin, J.O. McNamara, and H.-Y. Yang. 1986. Changes in dynorphin, enkephalin and cholecystokinin content of hippocampus and substantia nigra after amygdala kindling. *Brain Res.* 365: 1985.

Kouzarides, T. and E. Ziff. 1988. The role of the leucine zipper in the *fos*-*jun* interaction. *Nature* 336: 646.

Kruijer, W., D. Schubert, and I.M. Verma. 1985. Induction of the proto-oncogene fos by nerve growth factor. *Proc. Natl. Acad. Sci.* **82:** 7330.

Landschulz, W.H., P.F. Johnson, and S.L. McKnight. 1988. The leucine zipper: A hypothetical structure common to a new class of DNA binding proteins. *Science* **240:** 1759.

Lau, L.F. and D. Nathans. 1987. Expression of a set of growth-related immediate-early genes in BALB/c 3T3 cells: Coordinate regulation with c-*fos* or c-*myc*. *Proc. Natl. Acad. Sci.* **84:** 1182.

Macgregor, P.F., C. Abate, and T. Curran. 1990. Direct cloning of leucine zipper proteins: Jun binds cooperatively to the CRE with CRE-BP1. *Oncogene* **5:** 451.

Maekawa, T., H. Sakura, C. Kanei-Ishii, T. Sudo, T. Yoshimura, J. Fujisawa, M. Yoshida, and R. Ishii. 1989. Leucine zipper structure of the protein CRE-BP1 binding to the cAMP response element in brain. *EMBO J.* **8:** 2023.

Maki, Y., T.J. Bos, C. Davis, M. Starbuck, and P.K. Vogt. 1987. Avian sarcoma virus 17 carries a new oncogene, *jun*. *Proc. Natl. Acad. Sci.* **84:** 2848.

Morgan, J.I. and T. Curran. 1986. The role of ion flux in the control of c-*fos* expression. *Nature* **322:** 552.

―――. 1990. Stimulus-transcription coupling in the nervous system: Involvement of the inducible proto-oncogenes *fos* and *jun*. *Annu. Rev. Neurosci.* (in press).

Morgan, J.I., D.R. Cohen, J.L. Hempstead, and T. Curran. 1987. Mapping patterns of c-*fos* expression in the central nervous system after seizure. *Science* **237:** 192.

Nakabeppu, Y., K. Ryder, and D. Nathans. 1988. DNA binding activities of three murine *jun* proteins: Stimulation by Fos. *Cell* **55:** 907.

O'Shea, E.K., R. Rutlowski, W.F. Stafford III, and P.S. Kim. 1989. Preferential heterodimer formation by isolated leucine zippers from Fos and Jun. *Science* **245:** 646.

Ransone, L.J., J. Visvader, P. Sassone-Corsi, and I.M. Verma. 1989. Fos-Jun interaction: Mutational analysis of the leucine zipper domain of both proteins. *Genes Dev.* **3:** 770.

Rauscher, F.J. III, P.J. Voulalas, B.R. Franza, Jr., and T. Curran. 1988a. Fos and Jun bind cooperatively to the AP-1 site: Reconstitution *in vitro*. *Genes Dev.* **2:** 1687.

Rauscher, F.J. III, D.R. Cohen, T. Curran, T.J. Bos, P.K. Vogt, D. Bohmann, R. Tjian, and B.R. Franza, Jr. 1988b. Fos-associated protein p39 is the product of the *jun* proto-oncogene. *Science* **240:** 1010

Ryder, K., L.F. Lau, and D. Nathans. 1988. A gene activated by growth factors is related to the oncogene v-*jun*. *Proc. Natl. Acad. Sci.* **85:** 1487.

Ryder, K., A. Lanahan, E. Perez-Albuerne, and D. Nathans. 1989. Jun-D: A third member of the Jun gene family. *Proc. Natl. Acad. Sci.* **86:** 1500.

Schuermann, M., M. Neuberg, J.B. Hunter, T. Jenuwein, R.P. Ryseck, R. Bravo, and R. Muller. 1989. The leucine repeat motif in *fos* protein mediates complex formation with Jun/AP-1 and is required for transformation. *Cell* **56:** 507.

Sheng, M., S.T. Dougan, G. McFadden, and M. Greenberg. 1988. Calcium and growth factor pathways of c-*fos* transcriptional activation require distinct upstream regulatory sequences. *Mol. Cell. Biol.* **8:** 2787.

Sonnenberg, J.L., P.F. Macgregor-Leon, T. Curran, and J.I. Morgan. 1989a. Dynamic alterations occur in the levels and composition of transcription factor AP-1 complexes after seizure. *Neuron* **3:** 359.

Sonnenberg, J.L., F.J. Rauscher III, J.I. Morgan, and T. Curran. 1989b. Regulation of proenkephalin by proto-oncogenes *fos* and *jun*. *Science* **246:** 1622.

Sonnenberg, J.L., C. Mitchelmore, P.F. Macgregor-Leon, J. Hempstead, J.I. Morgan, and T. Curran. 1989c. Glutamate receptor agonists increase the expression of Fos, Fra and AP-1 DNA binding activity in the mammalian brain. *J. Neurosci. Res.* **24:** 72.

Sukhatme, V.P., X. Cao, L.C. Chang, C. Tsai-Morris, D. Stamenkovich, P.C. Ferre, D.R. Cohen, S.A. Edwards, T.B. Shows, T. Curran, M.M. LeBeau, and E.D. Adamson. 1988. A zinc finger-encoding gene coregulated with c-*fos* during growth and differentiation, and after cellular depolarization. *Cell* **53:** 37.

Turner, R. and R. Tjian. 1989. Leucine repeats and an adjacent DNA-binding domain mediate the formation of functional cFos-cJun heterodimers. *Science* **243:** 1689.

White, J.D. and C.M. Gall. 1987. Differential regulation of neuropeptide and proto-oncogene mRNA content in the hippocampus following recurrent seizures. *Mol. Brain Res.* **3:** 21.

Zerial, M., L. Toschi, R.P. Ryseck, M. Schuermann, R. Müller, and R. Bravo. 1989. The product of a novel growth factor activated gene, *fos*B, interacts with Jun proteins enhancing their DNA binding activity. *EMBO J.* **8:** 805.

An Analysis of the Cell-Cell Interactions That Control the Proliferation and Differentiation of a Bipotential Glial Progenitor Cell in Culture

M.C. RAFF, I.K. HART, W.D. RICHARDSON, AND L.E. LILLIEN

Biology Department, Medawar Building, University College London, London WC1E 6BT, England

The neurons and macroglial cells of the mammalian central nervous system (CNS) develop from neuroepithelial cells that initially all look alike. To begin to analyze the mechanisms that underlie this cell-diversification process, we have studied the differentiation of macroglial cells in dissociated cell cultures of the developing rat optic nerve. This experimental system is attractive because the process of glial cell diversification can be studied in the absence of neurons, and the cellular and molecular environment of the cultures can be readily manipulated.

In optic nerve cultures, three types of differentiated macroglial cells can be distinguished by their morphology and antigenic phenotype: oligodendrocytes and two types of astrocytes (Raff et al. 1983b). Studies in vitro have established that type-1 astrocytes develop from one type of precursor cell, whereas type-2 astrocytes and oligodendrocytes develop from a common bipotential precursor, called an O-2A progenitor cell (Raff et al. 1983a, 1984a). Cells with the characteristic antigenic phenotype of each of the three types of differentiated glial cells present in optic nerve cultures can be found in cell suspensions prepared from the developing optic nerve or brain. Studies of such cell suspensions suggest that type-1 astrocytes first appear at embryonic day 15–16 (E15–16), oligodendrocytes appear around the day of birth, and type-2 astrocytes appear in the second postnatal week (Abney et al. 1981; Miller et al. 1985; Williams et al. 1985). Remarkably, these glial cells develop on the same schedule in cultures of embryonic brain cells (Abney et al. 1981; Williams et al. 1985; Lillien et al. 1988), suggesting that the mechanisms that control the timing and direction of glial differentiation operate in vitro and therefore can be analyzed in culture.

The complexity of brain cell cultures, however, makes such an analysis difficult. In simpler optic nerve cell cultures, O-2A progenitor cells do not develop on their normal schedule but instead differentiate prematurely: In serum-free medium, they differentiate within 2–3 days into oligodendrocytes, whereas in the presence of 10% fetal calf serum (FCS), they differentiate within 2–3 days into type-2 astrocytes (Raff et al. 1983a, 1984b). These findings indicate that environmental factors can dramatically influence both the timing and direction of O-2A progenitor cell differentiation and that the environment in optic nerve cell cultures is different from that in either brain cultures or the developing optic nerve. By manipulating the environment in optic nerve cell cultures so that the development of O-2A progenitor cells more closely resembles their development in brain cell cultures and in vivo, we have uncovered a number of cell-cell interactions that apparently control this development and have begun to identify some of the signaling molecules involved.

Oligodendrocyte Development Occurs by Default

If a single O-2A progenitor cell is cultured alone in a microwell in serum-free medium, it prematurely stops dividing and differentiates into an oligodendrocyte (Temple and Raff 1985), suggesting that oligodendrocyte development is the default pathway that O-2A progenitor cells follow when they are deprived of signals from their neighbors. Type-1 astrocytes, the first glial cells to develop in the optic nerve, seem to be responsible for keeping O-2A progenitor cells proliferating in vivo (Noble and Murray 1984): When embryonic optic nerve cells are cultured in serum-free medium, the O-2A progenitor cells stop dividing and differentiate into oligodendrocytes prematurely, just as in single-cell cultures; however, if the optic nerve cells are cultured on monolayers of type-1 astrocytes, or in medium conditioned by such cultures, the progenitor cells continue to proliferate and differentiate into oligodendrocytes on the same schedule as they do in vivo (Raff et al. 1985).

Several lines of evidence indicate that platelet-derived growth factor (PDGF) plays an important part in mediating the interaction between type-1 astrocytes and O-2A progenitor cells in vitro: (1) PDGF is a potent mitogen for O-2A progenitor cells in vitro (Noble et al. 1988). (2) If added to embryonic optic nerve cell cultures, PDGF reconstitutes the normal timing of oligodendrocyte development; the O-2A progenitor cells continue to proliferate and oligodendrocytes begin to develop on the equivalent of the day of birth, just as in vivo (Raff et al. 1988). (3) Type-1 astrocytes synthesize and secrete PDGF in vitro; they make mRNA that encodes the PDGF A chain but not the B chain, suggesting that they make the AA homodimer form of PDGF (Richardson et al. 1988). (4) The mitogenic activity for O-2A progenitor cells in type-1 astrocyte-conditioned medium cofractionates on gel-filtration columns with iodinated PDGF (Richardson et al. 1988). (5) Treatment of type-1 astrocyte-conditioned medium with anti-PDGF antibodies neutralizes both its mitogenic activity for O-2A progenitor cells (Richardson et al. 1988) and its ability to reconstitute the normal timing of oligodendrocyte development in embryonic optic nerve cell cultures (Raff et al. 1988). As both PDGF (Raff et al. 1988) and PDGF A-chain mRNA (Pringle et al. 1989) are present in the developing optic nerve, it seems likely that PDGF also plays a role in stimulating O-2A progenitor cell proliferation in vivo.

No matter how much PDGF is added to embryonic optic nerve cell cultures, however, O-2A progenitor cells do not proliferate indefinitely (Raff et al. 1988). They seem to have an intrinsic timing mechanism that limits either the number of times that they can divide or the length of time that they can proliferate in response to PDGF (Temple and Raff 1986; Raff et al. 1988); when the limit is reached, the cells stop dividing and differentiate by default into oligodendrocytes. If this view of oligodendrocyte development is correct, then the key to understanding the timing mechanism that controls the onset of oligodendrocyte differentiation is to determine why O-2A progenitor cells become mitotically unresponsive to PDGF. Studies of newly formed oligodendrocytes have shown that although these cells no longer divide in response to PDGF, they still have large numbers of (α-type) PDGF receptors on their surface (Hart et al. 1989b) and show an increase in cytosolic Ca^{++} in response to PDGF (Hart et al. 1989a). Moreover, O-2A progenitor cells are stimulated to proliferate if they are treated with both a Ca^{++} ionophore (to increase cytosolic Ca^{++}) and a phorbol ester (to activate protein kinase C), but newly formed oligodendrocytes are not; interestingly, O-2A progenitor cells treated in this way stop dividing and differentiate into oligodendrocytes on the same schedule as they do when they are stimulated to proliferate by PDGF (Hart et al. 1989a). Taken together, these findings suggest that the timing mechanism that controls the onset of mitotic unresponsiveness to PDGF depends on a change in the progenitor cell that, in part at least, lies downstream from the PDGF receptors and the early events that they activate. We have found that PDGF stimulates an increase in the expression of the immediate-early genes c-*fos* and c-*jun* in newly formed oligodendrocytes (I.K. Hart et al., in prep.), indicating that at least one signaling pathway from the PDGF receptors to the nucleus still operates in these cells, even though the cells are no longer mitotically responsive to PDGF.

Type-2 Astrocyte Development Depends on Both Diffusible and Nondiffusible Signals Produced by Non-O-2A Lineage Cells

Unlike oligodendrocyte development, type-2 astrocyte development in serum-free cultures requires in-ducing signals from other cells. When newborn optic nerve cells are cultured in the absence of serum, but in the presence of added PDGF to keep the O-2A progenitor cells proliferating, oligodendrocytes begin to develop immediately, whereas type-2 astrocytes only begin to develop after 7–10 days (Lillien and Raff 1990). If postnatal day 8 (P8) optic nerve cells are cultured under the same conditions, type-2 astrocytes develop sooner (within 4 days), as might be expected if the timing in culture reflects a timing mechanism that operates in vivo. If P8 cells are cultured at low density under the same conditions, however, oligodendrocytes develop, but type-2 astrocytes do not, even after several weeks. Type-2 astrocyte development can be reconstituted in such low-density P8 cultures if non-O-2A lineage cells (mainly type-1 astrocytes, meningeal cells, macrophages, and endothelial cells) from newborn optic nerve are added to the cultures; the timing of type-2 astrocyte development in these mixed-age cultures reflects the age of the non-O-2A lineage cells, rather than the age of the O-2A progenitor cells (Lillien and Raff 1990). Thus, non-O-2A lineage cells are required for type-2 astrocyte development and seem to be responsible for timing this development.

The type-2 astrocyte-inducing signal produced by non-O-2A lineage cells is complex and consists of both diffusible and nondiffusible signaling molecules (Lillien et al. 1990). Evidence for a diffusible signaling molecule comes from the findings that low-salt extracts of 3-week-old rat optic nerve (Hughes and Raff 1987), as well as supernatants and extracts of serum-free brain cultures in which type-2 astrocytes are developing (Lillien et al. 1988), contain an activity that induces O-2A progenitor cells to express the astrocyte-specific marker glial fibrillary acidic protein (GFAP) within 24 hours in serum-free optic nerve cell cultures. In both cases, the amount of activity greatly increases around the time that type-2 astrocytes are developing in the nerve or in culture. The type-2 astrocyte-inducing activity in these extracts seems to be due to ciliary neurotrophic factor (CNTF), a 23-kD protein that was initially defined as a survival factor for chick ciliary neurons (Manthorpe et al. 1986; Lin et al. 1989; Stöckli et al. 1989): Not only does purified CNTF have the same GFAP-inducing activity as the extracts (Hughes et al. 1988; Lillien et al. 1988), but the activity in extracts cofractionates by SDS-PAGE with purified CNTF (Hughes et al. 1988), and antibodies made against a synthetic peptide corresponding to the carboxyl terminus of CNTF remove more than 95% of the GFAP-inducing activity from optic nerve extracts (M. Sendtner et al., unpubl.). There is evidence that type-1 astrocytes are the main producers of CNTF both in vitro (Lillien et al. 1988) and in vivo (M. Sendtner, pers. comm.).

CNTF or low-salt extracts of optic nerve or brain cultures, however, are, on their own, not enough to induce O-2A progenitor cells to differentiate into stable type-2 astrocytes in culture (Hughes and Raff 1987; Hughes et al. 1988; Lillien et al. 1988). No matter how much CNTF or extract is added, the progenitor cells are induced to express GFAP only transiently and then go on to develop into oligodendrocytes (Lillien and Raff 1990). These findings suggest that additional signals are required for type-2 astrocyte development; these signals seem not to be diffusible, as they are not present in supernatants or low-salt extracts of brain cultures in which stable type-2 astrocytes are developing (Lillien et al. 1988). The missing signals are apparently bound to the extracellular matrix (ECM). When O-2A progenitor cells are cultured in the presence of CNTF on ECM prepared from 1–2-week-old cultures of newborn optic nerve cells, they rapidly develop into stable type-2 astrocytes (Lillien et al. 1990). Both CNTF and the ECM are required for stable type-2 astrocyte development, and single-cell experiments indicate that both act directly on O-2A progenitor cells (Lillien et al. 1990). The ECM can be shown to have at least two actions on the progenitor cells: It inhibits their differentiation into oligodendrocytes, and it collaborates with CNTF to induce them to differentiate into type-2 astrocytes (Lillien et al. 1990); although it is clear that inhibition of the default pathway (to oligodendrocyte) is not sufficient to induce type-2 astrocyte differentiation, it is uncertain whether this inhibition is required for type-2 astrocyte development. Both activities can be removed by washing the ECM with 2 M NaCl. Treatment of such a salt-washed ECM with a 2 M NaCl extract of 3-week-old optic nerve reconstitutes both activities, suggesting that both are present in the developing optic nerve (Lillien et al. 1990). Preliminary evidence suggests that the two activities are mediated by different ECM-associated molecules and that the molecules that inhibit oligodendrocyte differentiation might be similar to basic fibroblast growth factor (bFGF), whereas the molecules that collaborate with CNTF to induce type-2 astrocyte development might not be (Lillien et al. 1990). As ECM produced by cultures of endothelial cells or meningeal cells (which contain endothelial cells) has both activities, whereas ECM produced by cultures of type-1 astrocytes or O-2A lineage cells has neither, it seems likely that the ECM-associated signals are produced by mesenchymal cells rather than by glial cells (Lillien et al. 1990).

CONCLUSIONS

O-2A progenitor cells can develop into either oligodendrocytes or type-2 astrocytes in vitro. Oligodendrocyte development seems to occur by default when progenitor cells become mitotically unresponsive to PDGF, which is secreted by type-1 astrocytes. In contrast, type-2 astrocyte development is induced by a combination of CNTF, which is also secreted by type-1 astrocytes, and ECM-associated molecules, which are secreted by mesenchymal cells. Whereas the timing of oligodendrocyte development seems to depend on an intrinsic mechanism in the O-2A progenitor cell, the timing of type-2 astrocyte development seems to depend on the timed production of the inducing signals.

Although it is reassuring that PDGF, CNTF, and the ECM-associated activities are present in the developing optic nerve, there is a pressing need to determine whether O-2A progenitor cells develop into type-2 astrocytes in vivo and whether the same mechanisms that control the timing and direction of O-2A progenitor cell differentiation in vitro also do so in vivo.

ACKNOWLEDGMENTS

I.K.H. was supported by a Medical Research Council training fellowship and L.E.L. was supported by a fellowship from the National Multiple Sclerosis Society of the United States and by a grant from the Wellcome Trust. The work reviewed here was supported by the Medical Research Council.

REFERENCES

Abney, E., P.F. Bartlett, and M.C. Raff. 1981. Astrocytes, ependymal cells and oligodendrocytes develop on schedule in dissociated cell cultures of embryonic rat brain. *Dev. Biol.* **83:** 301.
Hart, I.K., W.D. Richardson, S.R. Bolsover, and M.C. Raff. 1989a. PDGF and intracellular signaling in the timing of oligodendrocyte differentiation. *J. Cell Biol.* **109:** 3411.
Hart, I.K., W.D. Richardson, C.H. Heldin, B. Westermark, and M.C. Raff. 1989b. PDGF receptors on cells of the oligodendrocyte-type-2 astrocyte (O-2A) cell lineage. *Development* **105:** 595.
Hughes, S.M. and M.C. Raff. 1987. An inducer protein may control the timing of fate switching in a bipotential glial progenitor cell in rat optic nerve. *Development* **101:** 157.
Hughes, S.M., L.E. Lillien, M.C. Raff, H. Rohrer, and M. Sendtner. 1988. Ciliary neurotrophic factor induces type-2 astrocyte differentiation in culture. *Nature* **335:** 70.
Lillien, L.E. and M.C. Raff. 1990. Analysis of the cell-cell interactions that control type-2 astrocyte development in vitro. *Neuron* **4:** 525.
Lillien, L.E., M. Sendtner, and M.C. Raff. 1990. Extracellular-matrix-associated molecules collaborate with ciliary neurotrophic factor to induce type-2 astrocyte development. *J. Cell Biol.* **111:** 685.
Lillien, L.E., M. Sendtner, H. Rohrer, S. Hughes, and M.C. Raff. 1988. Type-2 astrocyte development in rat brain cultures is initiated by a CNTF-like protein produced by type-1 astrocytes. *Neuron* **1:** 485.
Lin, L.F.H., D. Mismer, J.D. Lile, L.G. Armes, E.T. Butler, J.L. Vannice, and F. Collins. 1989. Purification, cloning, and expression of ciliary neurotrophic factor (CNTF). *Science* **246:** 1023.
Manthorpe, M., S.D. Skaper, L.R. Williams, and S. Varon. 1986. Purification of adult rat sciatic nerve ciliary neurotrophic factor. *Brain Res.* **367:** 282.
Miller, R.H., S. David, R. Patel, E.R. Abney, and M.C. Raff. 1985. A quantitative immunohistochemical study of macroglial cell development in the rat optic nerve: In vivo evidence for two distinct astrocyte lineages. *Dev. Biol.* **111:** 35.
Noble, M. and K. Murray. 1984. Purified astrocytes promote the in vitro division of a bipotential glial progenitor cell. *EMBO J.* **3:** 2243.
Noble, M., K. Murray, P. Stroobant, M.D. Waterfield, and P. Riddle. 1988. Platelet-derived growth factor promotes division and motility and inhibits premature differentiation of the oligodendrocyte/type-2 astrocyte progenitor cell. *Nature* **333:** 560.
Pringle, N., E.J. Collarini, M.J. Mosley, C.H. Heldin, B. Westermark, and W.D. Richardson. 1989. PDGF A-chain

homodimers drive proliferation of bipotential (O 2A) glial progenitor cells in the developing rat optic nerve. *EMBO J.* **8:** 1049.

Raff, M.C., E.R. Abney, and J. Fok-Seang. 1985. Reconstitution of a developmental clock in vitro: A critical role for astrocytes in the timing of oligodendrocyte differentiation. *Cell* **42:** 61.

Raff, M.C., E.R. Abney, and R.H. Miller. 1984a. Two glial cell lineages diverge prenatally in rat optic nerve. *Dev. Biol.* **106:** 53.

Raff, M.C., R.H. Miller, and M. Noble. 1983a. A glial progenitor cell that develops *in vitro* into an astrocyte or an oligodendrocyte depending on the culture medium. *Nature* **303:** 390.

Raff, M.C., B.P. Williams, and R.H. Miller. 1984b. The *in vitro* differentiation of a bipotential glial progenitor cell. *EMBO J.* **3:** 1857.

Raff, M.C., E.R. Abney, J. Cohen, R. Lindsay, and M. Noble. 1983b. Two types of astrocytes in cultures of developing rat white matter: Differences in morphology, surface gangliosides, and growth characteristics. *J. Neurosci.* **3:** 1289.

Raff, M.C., L.E. Lillien, W.D. Richardson, J.F. Burne, and M.D. Noble. 1988. Platelet-derived growth factor from astrocytes drives the clock that times oligodendrocyte development in culture. *Nature* **333:** 562.

Richardson, W.D., N. Pringle, M.J. Mosley, B. Westermark, and M. Dubois-Dalcq. 1988. A role for platelet-derived growth factor in normal gliogenesis in the central nervous system. *Cell* **53:** 309.

Stöckli, K.A., F. Lottspeich, M. Sendtner, P. Masiakowski, P. Carroll, R. Gotz, D. Lindholm, and H. Thoenen. 1989. Molecular cloning, expression and regional distribution of ciliary neurotrophic factor. *Nature* **342:** 920.

Temple, S. and M.C. Raff. 1985. Differentiation of a bipotential glial progenitor cell in single cell microculture. *Nature* **313:** 223.

———. 1986. Clonal analysis of oligodendrocyte development in culture: Evidence for a developmental clock that counts cell divisions. *Cell* **44:** 773.

Williams, B.P., E.R. Abney, and M.C. Raff. 1985. Macroglial cell development in embryonic rat brain: Studies using monoclonal antibodies, fluorescence activated cell sorting, and cell culture. *Dev. Biol.* **112:** 126.

Role of Helix-Loop-Helix Proteins in *Drosophila* Neurogenesis

H. VAESSIN, M. CAUDY,* E. BIER,† L.-Y. JAN, AND Y.-N. JAN
Howard Hughes Medical Institute and Departments of Physiology and Biochemistry, University of California, San Francisco, California 94143

The development of the nervous system in invertebrate and vertebrate systems is initiated by the determination of a subset of neuroectodermal cells to become neuronal precursor cells. In this process, neuroectodermal cells choose between two principal developmental pathways and subsequently differentiate into either neuronal or epidermal precursors. In the early developmental processes of spatial subdivision and segmentation in *Drosophila* (and to some degree in vertebrate systems), DNA-binding proteins containing either the homeobox or zinc finger domain are instrumental. These classes of transcription factors have not been found to be regulators of the initial steps of neurogenesis. In contrast, several members of a recently defined class of DNA-binding proteins containing the so-called helix-loop-helix (HLH) domain play an important role in the choice between neurogenesis and epidermogenesis in *Drosophila* (Ghysen and Dambly-Chaudiere 1989; Knust and Campos-Ortega 1989). Other HLH-domain-containing proteins also appear to control cell fate, such as mesoderm formation (Thisse et al. 1988) and muscle determination (Davis et al. 1987) in invertebrates as well as vertebrates. The HLH-domain-containing proteins form homo- or heterodimeric protein complexes and bind DNA in a sequence-specific way (Murre et al. 1989a). The involvement of multiple HLH-domain-containing proteins in the same developmental process therefore raises the possibility that a large number of different DNA-binding protein complexes can be formed by combining different HLH proteins.

In *Drosophila*, at least ten HLH-protein-encoding transcription units from five different genomic loci are involved in the regulation of neuronal versus epidermal precursor formation (Alonso and Cabrera 1988; Caudy et al. 1988b; Klämbt et al. 1989; Rushlow et al. 1989; Ellis et al. 1990; Garrell and Modolell 1990). Here, we present a brief overview of the early events in neurogenesis and discuss the role of several HLH proteins in this process.

Proneural and Neurogenic Genes Are Required for *Drosophila* Neurogenesis

In *Drosophila melanogaster*, the process of neuronal precursor determination can be subdivided into two major steps (Fig. 1). In the first step, cells acquire the capacity to choose between two developmental pathways, namely, neurogenesis versus epidermogenesis. This decision is dependent on the expression of the "proneural" genes (Ghysen and Dambly-Chaudiere 1989). In a subsequent step, cells that have initiated neurogenic differentiation actively suppress the neurogenic potential of neighboring cells influencing them into the epidermogenic pathway. The underlying mechanism appears to be mediated through lateral inhibition, a type of cell-cell communication process. The function of the "neurogenic" genes is essential for this

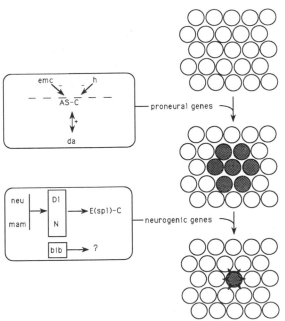

Figure 1. Main steps in the determination of neuronal precursor cells in *Drosophila*. Genomic loci known to be functional in these two steps are indicated. *emc* and *h* are separated by a dashed line from the other proneural genes, as these two loci are only known to function in the development of the adult nervous system.

Present address: *Department of Cell Biology and Anatomy, Cornell University Medical College, New York, New York 10021; †Department of Biology, University of California, San Diego, La Jolla, California 92093.

VAESSIN ET AL.

interaction between the neuronal precursor and its neighbors (for reviews, see Artavanis-Tsakonas 1988; Campos-Ortega 1988; Ghysen and Dambly-Chaudiere 1989; Knust and Campos-Ortega 1989; Jan and Jan 1990; Campos-Ortega and Jan 1991).

The known proneural genes, *daughterless* (*da*) and four genes forming the *achaete-scute complex* (*AS-C*), encode HLH-domain-containing proteins. Loss of various proneural gene functions results in the absence of some or all of the neuronal precursor cells of the larval peripheral nervous system (PNS) (Fig. 2B) (Dambly-Chaudiere and Ghysen 1987; Caudy et al. 1988a). The

da and *AS-C* genes are also essential for the proper development of the larval central nervous system (CNS) (Jimenez and Campos-Ortega 1987). Whether the functions of these genes in the CNS are similar to those in the PNS is not yet known. For the development of the adult PNS, two loci, *extramacrochaetae* (*emc*) and *hairy* (*h*), behave genetically as negative regulators of the two *AS-C* genes *T4* and *T5*, respectively (Moscoso del Prado and Garcia-Bellido 1984). Both of these loci also encode protein products containing the HLH motif (Ellis et al. 1990; Garrel and Modolell 1990).

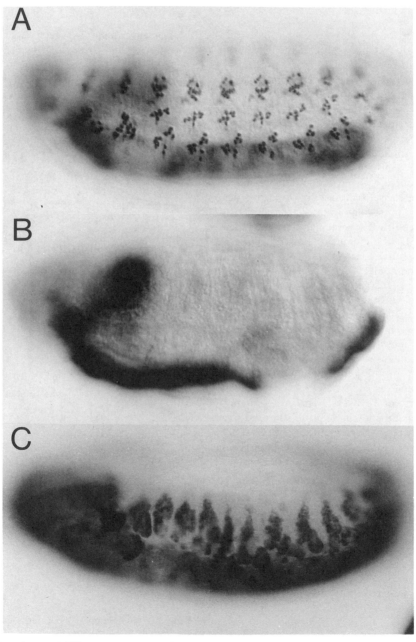

Figure 2. *Drosophila* embryos of different genotypes stained with the neuronal nuclei-specific monoclonal antibody *44C11* (Bier et al. 1988). (*A*) Wild-type embryo. Peripheral neurons are visible in the focal plane. In the background, a developed CNS is visible. (*B*) Mutant embryo homozygous for a loss of function mutation of the proneural gene *da*. In the periphery, no neurons can be detected. In the background, interruptions in the ventral cord of the CNS are apparent. (*C*) Embryo homozygous for *Df(3R)E(spl)*[RA7.1], a partial deletion of the *E(spl)* complex (Knust et al. 1987). Hyperplasia of both the CNS and PNS is evident.

The neurogenic genes appear to be involved in the lateral inhibition and include at least six zygotically expressed genes. Loss of function of any of the neurogenic genes causes most or all cells in the ectoderm to differentiate as neuronal precursors, resulting in a hyperplasia of the nervous system at the expense of epidermal development (Campos-Ortega 1988). Three of the neurogenic genes, *Notch*, *Delta*, and *big brain*, encode membrane proteins and may directly mediate the communication process between neighboring cells (Wharton et al. 1985; Kidd et al. 1986; Vaessin et al. 1987; Kopczynski et al. 1988; Rao et al. 1990). There are also neurogenic genes that encode presumably nuclear proteins. In particular, the *m5*, *m7*, and *m8* genes of the *Enhancer of split (E[spl])* complex (Knust et al. 1987) encode highly related HLH proteins (Klämbt et al. 1989). These proteins are thought to be involved in the transduction of signals transmitted from one cell to another; they may control the cell fate by regulating transcription (Brand and Campos-Ortega 1988).

Genetic interactions have been observed between proneural and neurogenic genes, as well as between members of each group. Of specific interest here are interactions observed between *da* and *AS-C* (Dambly-Chandiere et al. 1988), between *AS-C T4* and *emc*, between *AS-C T5* and *h* (Moscoso del Prado and Garcia-Bellido 1984), and between either *da* or the *AS-C* and the neurogenic *E(spl))* complex (Brand and Campos-Ortega 1988). Moreover, those HLH proteins that have similar functions share sequence similarities beyond the HLH domain and form subfamilies (Table 1). Although the observation of genetic interaction per se does not allow one to draw conclusions on the underlying molecular basis of this interaction, the functional properties of the HLH domain common to the protein products of these loci suggest a number of mechanistic possibilities.

Combinatorial Use of HLH Proteins Can Generate a Large Array of Regulatory Functions

HLH proteins normally function as dimers and may act as transcriptional regulators. The intrinsic functional features of the HLH domain provide a basis for a wide array of potential regulatory mechanisms. Originally

defined in the human enhancer binding proteins E12 and E47, the HLH domain is characterized by an array of amino acids that have been hypothesized to form two amphipathic helices (Murre et al. 1989a). In this model, helices I and II are separated by a much less conserved loop structure of variable length. In addition, the first helix is preceded by a basic domain containing clusters of basic amino acids (Fig. 3).

Murre et al. (1989a) have shown for E12 and E47 that the HLH region has two principal properties: It binds DNA as dimeric protein complexes in a sequence-specific manner, and it mediates homo- and heterodimer formation between HLH proteins. Studies of *MyoD* by Davis et al. (1990) and *da* (H. Vaessin et al., in prep.) indicate that these two functions are located in different parts of this domain. Specific point mutations in the basic domain of *MyoD* or deletion of the basic domain in *da* abolishes the capacity of the HLH domain to bind to the target sequence. These mutations, however, do not seem to interfere with the capacity of the respective proteins to form homo- or heterodimeric protein complexes. Thus, the HLH region appears to be essential for the formation of the protein complexes, whereas the basic domain is required for DNA binding (Davis et al. 1990). A similar arrangement of adjacent DNA-binding domains and dimerization domains has been found in leucine zipper proteins, which form another major class of eukaryotic DNA-binding proteins and include the Jun/Fos or AP1 family of transcription factors (Schuermann et al. 1989). In the HLH protein TFE3, a transcriptional activation region has also been mapped (Beckmann et al. 1990), indicating that this particular HLH protein can act as a transcriptional activator.

Different homodimers and heterodimers of HLH proteins bind preferentially to different binding sites. For a DNA-binding protein to control directly the transcriptional activity of a gene, there must be binding sites in the regulatory region of that gene. Potential binding sites for the products of *da* and the *AS-C* have been identified in the regulatory regions of several transcription units of the *AS-C* and the *E(spl)* complex (H. Vaessin et al., in prep.). These loci have been shown in genetic studies to interact with each other, as well as

Table 1. Grouping of *Drosophila* HLH Proteins Involved in Neurogenesis into Subfamilies

Global expression		Spaciotemporal-specific expression			
basic domain absent			basic domain present		
				carboxy terminus = WRPW	
		AS-C subfamily	*E(spl)* subfamily	*h/44c* subfamily	
emc (*Id*)	*da* (*E12/E47*)	AS-C T3 AS-C T4 AS-C T5 AS-C T8 (*mash1/mash2*)	*E(spl) m5* *E(spl) m7* *E(spl) m8* — —	*h* *44C* — —	

Vertebrate proteins with high similarity in the HLH regions are indicated in parenthesis below the corresponding *Drosophila* proteins.

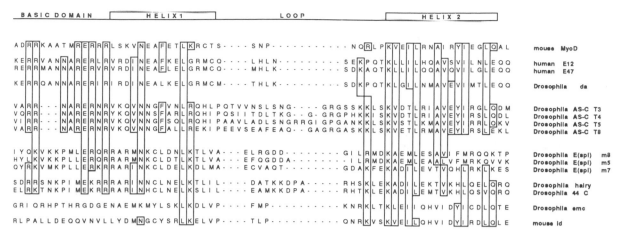

Figure 3. Alignment of the HLH domain and the adjacent basic domain of HLH proteins involved in *Drosophila* neurogenesis. For comparison, the vertebrate HLH proteins *E12*, *E47*, *Id*, and *MyoD1* are shown. The presumed extent of the basic domain, helix 1, loop, and helix 2, is marked (Murre et al. 1989a; Davis et al. 1990).

with the *da* locus (Brand and Campos-Ortega 1988; Dambly-Chaudiere et al. 1988). The identified binding sites have in common the presence of a core sequence that shows variable degrees of similarity to the *kE2* motif (GGCAGGTGG), which functions as a tissue-specific enhancer for the expression of the immunoglobulin *κ* light chain. This sequence is recognized by a variety of HLH proteins including heterodimers of *da* and *AS-C T3* and heterodimers of the human enhancer binding proteins E12 and MyoD. Under the same experimental conditions, homodimeric complexes bind only weakly if at all, suggesting that heterodimers bind better than homodimers to at least some binding sites (Murre et al. 1989b). Indeed, for myoblast induction by *MyoD*, the availability of *E12/E47* protein is essential (Benezra et al. 1990). Flanking sequences also affect binding of HLH proteins. We found that different combinations of *Drosophila* HLH proteins show different properties of binding to sites that are embedded within their normal sequence context in the regulatory regions of *Drosophila* genes encoding HLH proteins. Besides heterodimeric protein complexes of *da* and *AS-C*, homodimers of the respective proteins also bind some of these binding sites. Moreover, these dimers bind the different sites differently. For example, one site in the *AS-C* is recognized specifically by the homodimeric *AS-C T3* protein but is not recognized by either heterodimers of *da* and *AS-C T3* or by homodimers of the *da* protein (H. Vaessin et al., in prep.). These studies demonstrate the potential of the combinatorial use of HLH proteins in autoregulation, as well as in controlling the expression of other genes. It remains to be determined in vivo whether different combinations of the homodimers and heterodimers bind to different DNA sequences and regulate transcription of specific genes.

Certain HLH proteins can function as negative regulators. The separate DNA-binding (the basic domain) and dimerization (HLH domain) functions of the HLH proteins (Davis et al. 1990; H. Vaessin et al., in prep.) suggest a possible mechanism of negative regulation. An HLH protein with either no basic domain or a basic domain that is incompatible with DNA binding may combine with an HLH protein with a functional basic domain and form a heterodimer that cannot bind DNA, thereby inhibiting the binding of the HLH proteins with functional basic domains to their target sequences. This notion is strongly supported by the recent identification of two HLH proteins (*emc* and *Id*) that lack a basic domain (Benezra et al. 1990; Ellis et al. 1990; Garrell and Modolell 1990). The *Id* protein inhibits myoblast induction by *MyoD*, apparently by forming heterodimeric complexes that do not bind to DNA. In vitro binding assays demonstrate that the *Id* protein inhibits DNA binding by heterodimers of *MyoD* and *E12* (Benezra et al. 1990). The high degree of sequence similarity between *Id* and *emc* proteins in the HLH region suggests that the *emc* protein may act in a similar way in the regulation of *AS-C* activity and/or *da* activity. In this scenario, the *emc* protein would compete with other HLH proteins, such as *da* or *AS-C* proteins, in their formation of homodimers or heterodimers capable of binding DNA. This could account for the genetically defined role of *emc* as a negative regulator of *AS-C* functions.

When proline replaces an alanine in the basic domain of *MyoD*, the mutant *MyoD* protein inhibits DNA binding by other HLH proteins (Davis et al. 1990). Because this alanine is immediately adjacent to where a proline residue is found in all three *E(spl)* HLH proteins and in the *h* protein product, this has led to the hypothesis that the *E(spl)* and *h* gene products act as inhibitors, similar to the functions proposed for the *Id* and *emc* proteins. Other modes of action of these gene products, however, remain possible. The *E(spl)* and *h* proteins have basic domains that show significant sequence similarity with the basic domains of other HLH proteins that are known to bind DNA. It is possible that the conservation of these basic domains is due to an unknown function of these basic domains. However, it is perhaps more likely that the *E(spl)* and *h* proteins bind to DNA. These putative targets would presumably differ in sequence from the binding sites of *da* and *AS-C*. In the case of the *E(spl)* HLH proteins, sites of this type could be crucial in the activation of the epidermal differentiation program in the epidermoblasts.

In summary, the specific features of the HLH domain suggest the potential for a variety of regulatory activities. The ability of HLH proteins to form homodimers, as well as heterodimeric protein complexes, the large number of known HLH proteins involved in neurogenesis, and the different binding preferences of these different protein complexes for specific target sites allow the possibility of complex combinatorial signaling in the specification of cell fate and the formation of the highly heterogeneous nervous system.

Regulatory Network or Cascade?

It is possible that the determination of neuronal precursor cells involves a regulatory cascade, with the proneural genes acting before the neurogenic genes. Such a view, however, appears simplistic in light of the complex expression patterns of these genes (Cabrera et al. 1987; Knust et al. 1987; Romani et al. 1987). Although the proneural genes are largely responsible for imparting certain blastoderm cells with the basic potential to differentiate as neuronal precursors, the subsequent steps are likely to involve cross-regulatory interactions between proneural genes and neurogenic genes. In this later stage, the expression of the *AS-C* becomes restricted to cells that actually become neuronal precursors (Cabrera et al. 1987; Romani et al. 1987), whereas *E(spl)* transcripts become limited to the epidermal precursors (Knust et al. 1987). Prior to neuroblast formation, the patterns of expression of these genes appear to overlap extensively. From the mutant analysis, it is not clear what function, if any, is mediated by the early expression. The presence of potential binding sites in the control regions of both gene complexes suggests that the HLH proteins encoded by these loci may be directly involved in restricting their expression to specific cell types and that such cross-regulatory interactions could take place before neuroblast formation.

HLH proteins are also expressed during later steps of neurogenesis. By using the enhancer trap method (Bier et al. 1989), we have isolated a gene with neuron-specific expression at the chromosomal location 44C. This gene also encodes an HLH protein (Fig. 3), which can be detected after the neuronal precursor cells have delaminated from the neuroectoderm (E. Bier et al., unpubl.). The expression of this HLH protein is therefore later than the time of action of the HLH proteins encoded by the proneural and neurogenic genes.

Functional Redundancy among HLH Proteins

Of the ten genes that encode HLH proteins and are involved in *Drosophila* neuronal precursor determination, seven are from two gene complexes, the *AS-C* and the *E(spl)* complexes. The products of the different transcription units within each complex share a significantly higher degree of sequence similarity. This is true for the two helix regions, the loop, as well as for the basic domain (Alonso and Cabrera 1988; Klämbt et al. 1989). Interestingly, both gene complexes appear to contain genes with redundant functions. For example, only the loss of several transcription units of the *E(spl)* complex results in a strong mutant phenotype; loss of individual transcription units results only in very weak or no mutant phenotypes at all (Campos-Ortega 1988; Ziemer et al. 1988; Knust and Campos-Ortega 1989). It remains to be seen whether redundancies are also inherent to other subgroups of HLH proteins. In the case of the muscle differentiation, several HLH proteins have been demonstrated to have the same fundamental capacity to induce muscle differentiation on their own in cell lines (Wright et al. 1989). The examples of the *AS-C* and the *E(spl)* gene complex emphasize the possibility of redundant functions of similar HLH proteins with overlapping expression patterns.

CONCLUSIONS

Genes encoding HLH proteins play a crucial role in the initial steps of neurogenesis in *D. melanogaster*. At least ten different HLH proteins are involved. They most likely function as transcriptional regulators to control target gene expression. The known properties of HLH domains suggest a wide range of possible molecular mechanisms (see Fig. 4). The binding of homodimers or heterodimers to a given regulatory sequence may have different effects on transcription (Fig. 4A,B). There could be competition between different homo- or heterodimers for different target sites (Fig. 4C). The formation of DNA-binding protein complexes may be inhibited by the formation of non-DNA-binding complexes. There may also be competition at the level of dimerization to give rise to protein complexes with very different binding specificities (Fig. 4D). The range of mechanistic possibilities inherent in the structure of the HLH protein could provide the necessary complexity needed in the regulation of nervous system development.

Because functional redundancy is a possible feature of HLH proteins, classical genetic mutation analysis may not be sufficient to identify all of the relevant loci. It may be necessary to take other approaches, such as reverse genetic methods that start with the isolation of novel HLH-protein-coding genes, followed by mutational analysis, or mutant screening schemes based on genetic interaction. The use of the enhancer trap method has led to the identification of the 44C locus, which encodes an HLH protein and is likely to act in later steps of neuronal differentiation.

A

B

C

D

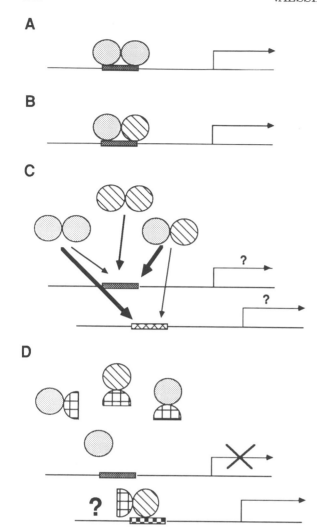

Figure 4. Possible mechanisms of function of proteins containing the HLH domain in the transcriptional regulation of downstream genes (see text).

Whether HLH proteins are also involved in neurogenesis of the vertebrate nervous system is not yet known. This seems likely, however, because other developmental processes, like mesoderm formation or muscle differentiation, involve highly conserved HLH proteins in *Drosophila*, as well as in vertebrates (Hopwood et al. 1989; Benezra et al. 1990). HLH proteins with high degrees of similarities in the HLH domain have been identified from fairly distant species, e.g., *twist* in *Drosophila* and *Xtwi* in *Xenopus* (Thisse et al. 1988; Hopwood et al. 1989), the homolog of mouse *MyoD* in *Caenorhabditis elegans* (Benezra et al. 1990), and the mouse homolog of *AS-C* (*mash1*/*mash2*; see Mori et al., this volume). The observation that these related proteins have comparable tissue distributions and developmental profiles provides support for the idea that HLH proteins in vertebrates may also be found to control the early events of neuronal precursor formation.

ACKNOWLEDGMENTS

H.V. was partially supported by a postdoctoral fellowship from the Deutsche Forschungsgemeinschaft. L.Y.J. and Y.N.J. are Howard Hughes Investigators.

REFERENCES

Artavanis-Tsakonas, S. 1988. The molecular biology of the *Notch* locus and the fine tuning of differentiation in *Drosophila*. *Trends Genet.* **4:** 95.

Alonso, M.C. and C.V. Cabrera. 1988. The *achaete-scute complex* of *Drosophila melanogaster* comprises four homologous genes. *EMBO J.* **7:** 2585.

Beckmann, H., L.K. Su, and T. Kadesch. 1990. TFE3: A helix-loop-helix protein that activates transcription through the immunoglobulin enhancer uE3 motif. *Genes Dev.* **4:** 167.

Benezra, R., R.L. Davis, D. Lockshon, D.L. Turner, and H. Weintraub. 1990. The protein Id: A negative regulator of helix-loop-helix DNA binding proteins. *Cell* **61:** 49.

Bier, E., L. Ackermann, S. Barbel, L.Y. Jan, and Y.N. Jan. 1988. Identification and characterization of a neuron-specific nuclear antigen in *Drosophila*. *Science* **240:** 913.

Bier, E., H. Vaessin, S. Shepherd, K. Lee, K. McCall, S. Barbel, L. Ackermann, R. Carretto, T. Uemura, E. Grell, L.Y. Jan, and Y.N. Jan. 1989. Searching for pattern and mutation in the *Drosophila* genome with a P-*lacZ* vector. *Genes Dev.* **3:** 1273.

Brand, M. and J.A. Campos-Ortega. 1988. Two groups of interrelated genes regulate early neurogenesis in *Drosophila melanogaster*. *Roux's Arch. Dev. Biol.* **197:** 457.

Cabrera, C.V., A. Martinez-Arias, and M. Bate. 1987. The expression of three members of the *achaete-scute* gene complex correlates with neuroblast segregation in *Drosophila*. *Cell* **50:** 425.

Campos-Ortega, J.A. 1988. Cellular interactions during early neurogenesis of *Drosophila melanogaster*. *Trends Neurosci.* **11:** 400.

Campos-Ortega, J.A. and Y.N. Jan. 1991. Genetic and molecular basis of neurogenesis in *Drosophila melanogaster*. *Annu. Rev. Neurosci.* (in press).

Caudy, M., E.H. Grell, C. Dambly-Chaudiere, A. Ghysen, L.Y. Jan, and Y.N. Jan. 1988a. The maternal sex determination gene *daughterless* has zygotic activity necessary for the formation of peripheral neurons in *Drosophila*. *Genes Dev.* **2:** 843.

Caudy, M., H. Vaessin, M. Brand, R. Tuma, L.Y. Jan, and Y.N. Jan. 1988b. *daughterless*, a gene essential for both neurogenesis and sex determination in *Drosophila*, has sequence similarities to *myc* and the *achaete-scute* complex. *Cell* **55:** 1061.

Dambly-Chaudiere, C. and A. Ghysen. 1987. Independent subpatterns of sense organs require independent genes of the *achaete-scute complex* in *Drosophila* larvae. *Genes Dev.* **1:** 297.

Dambly-Chaudiere, C., A. Ghysen, L.Y. Jan, and Y.N. Jan. 1988. The determination of sense organs in *Drosophila*: Interaction of *scute* with *daughterless*. *Roux's Arch. Dev. Biol.* **197:** 419.

Davis, R.L., H. Weintraub, and A.B. Lassar. 1987. Expression of a single transfected cDNA converts fibroblasts to myoblasts. *Cell* **51:** 987.

Davis, R.L., P.-F. Cheng, A.B. Lassar, and H. Weintraub. 1990. The MyoD DNA binding domain contains a recognition code for muscle-specific gene activation. *Cell* **60:** 733.

Ellis, H.M., D.R. Spann, and J.W. Posakony. 1990. *extramacrochaetae*, a negative regulator of sensory organ development in *Drosophila*, defines a new class of helix-loop-helix proteins. *Cell* **61:** 27.

Garrell, J. and J. Modolell. 1990. The *Drosophila extramacrochaetae* locus, and antagonist of proneural genes that, like these genes, encodes a helix-loop-helix protein. *Cell* **61:** 39.

Ghysen, A. and C. Dambly-Chaudiere. 1989. Genesis of the *Drosophila* peripheral nervous system. *Trends Genet.* **5:** 251.

Hopwood, N.D., A. Pluck, and J.B. Gurdon. 1989. A *Xenopus* mRNA related to *Drosophila twist* is expressed in response to induction in the mesoderm and the neural crest. *Cell* **59:** 893.

Jan, Y.N. and L.Y. Jan. 1990. Genes required for specifying cell fates in *Drosophila* embryonic nervous system. *Trends Neurosci.* (in press).

Jimenez, F. and J.A. Campos-Ortega. 1987. Genes in subdivision 1B of the *Drosophila melanogaster* X-chromosome and their influence on neural development. *J. Neurogenet.* **4:** 179.

Kidd, S., M.R. Kelley, and M.W. Young. 1986. Sequence of the *Notch* locus of *Drosophila melanogaster*: Relationship of the encoded protein to mammalian clotting and growth factors. *Mol. Cell. Biol.* **6:** 3094.

Klämbt, C., E. Kunst, K. Tietze, and J.A. Campos-Ortega. 1989. Closely related transcripts encoded by the neurogenic gene complex *Enhancer of split* of *Drosophila melanogaster*. *EMBO J.* **8:** 203.

Knust, E. and J.A. Campos-Ortega. 1989. The molecular genetics of early neurogenesis in *Drosophila melanogaster*. *BioEssays* **11:** 95.

Knust, E., K. Tietze and J.A. Campos-Ortega. 1987. Molecular analysis of the neurogenic locus *Enhancer of split* of *Drosophila melanogaster*. *EMBO J.* **6:** 4413.

Kopczynski, C.C., A.K. Alton, K. Fechtel, P.J. Kooh, and M.A.T. Muskavitch. 1988. *Delta*, a *Drosophila* neurogenic gene, is transcriptionally complex and encodes a protein related to blood coagulation factors and epidermal growth factor of vertebrates. *Genes Dev.* **2:** 1723.

Moscoso del Prado, J. and A. Garcia-Bellido. 1984. Genetic regulation of the *achaete-scute complex* of *Drosophila melanogaster*. *Roux's Arch. Dev. Biol.* **193:** 242.

Murre, C., P. Schonleber-McCaw, and D. Baltimore. 1989a. A new DNA binding and dimerization motif in immunoglobulin enhancer binding, *daughterless*, *MyoD*, and *myc* proteins. *Cell* **56:** 777.

Murre, C., P. Schonleber-McCaw, H. Vaessin, M. Caudy, L.Y. Jan, Y.N. Jan, C.V. Cabrera, J.N. Buskin, S.D. Hauschka, A.B. Lassar, H. Weintraub, and D. Baltimore. 1989b. Interactions between heterologous helix-loop-helix proteins generate complexes that bind specifically to a common DNA sequence. *Cell* **58:** 537.

Rao, Y., L.Y. Jan, and Y.N. Jan. 1990. Similarity of the product of the *Drosophila* neurogenic gene *big brain* to transmembrane channel proteins. *Nature* **345:** 163.

Romani, S., S. Campuzano, and J. Modolell. 1987. The *achaete-scute complex* is expressed in neurogenic regions of *Drosophila* embryos. *EMBO J.* **6:** 2085.

Rushlow, C.A., A. Hogan, S.M. Pinchin, K.M. Howe, M. Lardelli, and D. Ish-Horowicz. 1989. The *Drosophila hairy* protein acts in both segmentation and bristle patterning and shows homology to N-myc. *EMBO J.* **8:** 3095.

Schuermann, M., M. Neuberg, J.B. Hunter, T. Jenuwein, R.-P. Ryseck, R. Bravo, and R. Mueller. 1989. The leucine repeat motif in fos protein mediates complex formation with Jun/AP-1 and is required for transformation. *Cell* **56:** 507.

Thisse, B., C. Stoetzel, C. Gorostiza-Thisse, and F. Perrin-Schmitt. 1988. Sequence of the *twist* gene and nuclear localization of its protein in endomesodermal cells of early *Drosophila* embryos. *EMBO J.* **7:** 2175.

Vaessin, H., K.A. Bremer, E. Kunst, and J.A. Campos-Ortega. 1987. The neurogenic locus *Delta* of *Drosophila melanogaster* is expressed in neurogenic territories and encodes a putative transmembrane protein with EGF-like repeats. *EMBO J.* **6:** 3431.

Wharton, K.A., K.M. Johansen, T. Xu, and S. Artavanis-Tsakonas. 1985. Nucleotide sequence from the neurogenic locus *Notch* implies a gene product that shares homology with proteins containing EGF-like repeats. *Cell* **43:** 567.

Wright, W.E., D.A. Sassoon, and V.K. Lin. 1989. Myogenin, a factor regulating myogenesis, has a domain homologous to MyoD. *Cell* **56:** 607.

Ziemer, A., K. Tietze, and J.A. Campos-Ortega. 1988. Genetic analysis of *Enhancer of split*, a locus involved in neurogenesis in *Drosophila melanogaster*. *Genetics* **119:** 63.

Generation of Neuronal Diversity: Analogies and Homologies with Hematopoiesis

H. Nawa,* T. Yamamori, T. Le,† and P.H. Patterson
Biology Division, California Institute of Technology, Pasadena, California 91125

The immense variety of neuronal phenotypes in the vertebrate nervous system is apparent in considering just the process of chemical transmission. There are approximately 12 known classical neurotransmitters and more than 30 neuropeptides thus far identified, and individual neurons simultaneously synthesize, store, and secrete one or more classical transmitters in addition to three or more neuropeptides. The transmitters and peptides are expressed in an exceedingly large number of different combinations in different parts of the nervous system. Although there are useful generalizations as to the frequency of certain transmitter-peptide combinations, there are innumerable exceptions to these rules. How the particular combinations produced in each neuron are specified during development is a challenging question. The magnitude of this problem becomes clear if one calculates the number of possible combinations if a neuron is to produce 2 transmitters out of a possible 12 and 3 peptides out of a possible 30. There are 267,960 different potential phenotypes in this example.

It has become increasingly clear that such phenotypic decisions are not made solely on the basis of a cell's lineage history. Clonal analysis in both the central and peripheral vertebrate nervous systems in situ has demonstrated that multipotential precursor cells can, right up to their final division, give rise to a variety of neurons and, in some cases, glia (Turner and Cepko 1987; Holt et al. 1988; Price and Thurlow 1988; Wetts and Fraser 1988; Bronner-Fraser and Fraser 1989; Galileo et al. 1990). This suggests that the precursor cells (and their immediate daughter cells) are not committed to a single fate (see also Tomlinson 1988; Anderson 1989). That postmitotic neurons can be influenced in their phenotypic choices by environmental signals has been convincingly shown for cells of both peripheral and central origin in vitro (see, e.g., Patterson 1978; Kessler et al. 1984; Iacovitti et al. 1989; Adler and Hatlee 1989; Schoenen et al. 1989). Moreover, a variety of manipulations of cell position in vivo have indicated that the identity of a neuron's target can influence transmitter and peptide choices (McMahon and Gibson 1987; Schotzinger and Landis 1988; Wall and Taghert 1989). Many of these choices are revers-

ible, and changes in transmitter and peptide phenotype can be part of normal development in situ, as growing neurons encounter new environments, in both vertebrate and invertebrate systems (Hayashi et al. 1983; Landis and Keefe 1983; Gesser and Larsson 1985; Happola et al. 1986; Koizumi and Bode 1986; Tublitz and Sylwester 1990).

What are the intercellular signals that control these phenotypic decisions? Using primary neuronal cultures as assay systems, it has been possible to identify a number of these signals and to characterize their biological activities and their biochemical properties (Fukada 1985; Wong and Kessler 1987; Adler et al. 1989; Lin et al. 1989; McManaman et al. 1989; Saadat et al. 1989; Stockli et al. 1989; Yamamori et al. 1989; Rao et al. 1990a). An early generalization that is arising from this work is that although these neuronal differentiation factors have distinct effects on a target neuron population, their effects can be partially overlapping or redundant. For instance, several factors with discrete biochemical properties can induce acetylcholine (ACh) production in cultured striatal and sympathetic neurons, but their effects on the expression of other transmitters and neuropeptides are distinct (Kessler 1986; Nawa and Patterson 1990). This emerging picture has a striking parallel in the control of phenotypic decisions in the hematopoietic system. Here too, biochemically diverse proteins produce distinct differentiation responses, but their effects can be partially overlapping (Metcalf 1989). Thus, although four hematopoietic regulators, with no sequence identity, elicit different arrays of derivatives from multipotential stem cell precursors, all four promote granulocyte and/or macrophage differentiation. In fact, this analogy between the nervous and hematopoietic systems has recently been carried a step further with the demonstration that the same protein can influence differentiation in both systems (Yamamori et al. 1989).

In this paper, we further examine the effects of this recombinant protein, known as leukemia inhibitory factor (LIF) and cholinergic differentiation factor (CDF), on cultured neurons. We present the dose-dependence of its effects on the expression of various transmitters and neuropeptides in sympathetic neurons, and we show that it can act on another type of neuron eliciting somewhat different effects. The developmental profile of the onset of neuropeptide induction is also presented, and the reversibility of these

Present addresses: *Institute of Immunology, Kyoto University, Kyoto, Japan; †University of California Medical School, San Francisco, California 94143.

effects is described. The conclusions are that CDF/LIF can act on several different types of neurons, that the response in each neuron is probably influenced by its lineage history, and that the factor must be continually present to maintain its effects on neuropeptide gene expression.

METHODS

Cell cultures. Sympathetic neuron cultures were prepared from neonatal rat superior cervical ganglia (SCG) using enzymatic dissociation and growth in L15-CO_2 medium plus 5% rat serum and nerve growth factor (NGF), according to the methods of Hawrot and Patterson (1979). Sensory neuron cultures were also prepared from dorsal root ganglia (DRG) of neonatal rats in the same way and grown in F-12 medium containing the N2 medium nutrient supplement and NGF (Lindsay 1988). Serum-free, heart-cell-conditioned medium (CM) was prepared according to the method of Fukada (1980).

Transmitter and neuropeptide assays. After 14–16 days in culture, the intact sympathetic and sensory neurons were assayed for ACh and catecholamine (CA) synthesis from radioactive precursors, according to the methods of Mains and Patterson (1973). Sister neuronal cultures containing 1–6000 neurons were also extracted, and their neuropeptide contents were assayed by radioimmunoassay, according to the methods of Nawa and Sah (1990). The authenticity of these peptides was previously determined by high-performance liquid chromatography (Nawa and Sah 1990). The data are expressed as fmoles transmitter or peptide per 1000 neurons assayed.

Materials. Recombinant mouse and human CDF/LIF produced by *Escherichia coli* (Gearing et al. 1989) was the kind gift from Dr. D. Metcalf and associates at the Walter and Eliza Hall Institute in Melbourne. NGF was produced by J. Carnahan. All other materials were produced according to the methods of Hawrot and Patterson (1979) and Nawa and Patterson (1990).

RESULTS

Induction of Neuropeptides by Recombinant CDF/LIF

It was shown previously that heart cell CM can induce the synthesis of several neuropeptides and their mRNAs, as well as ACh in cultured sympathetic neurons (Nawa and Sah 1990). Moreover, these neurons can respond to recombinant CDF/LIF by the induction of ACh synthesis and the reduction of CA synthesis (Yamamori et al. 1989). Therefore, we sought to determine whether the peptide inductions by CM were also due to CDF/LIF (see also Nawa and Patterson 1990). Using recombinant CDF/LIF, we find that this protein does increase neuronal substance P (SP) and somatostatin (SOM), whereas it reduces neuropeptide

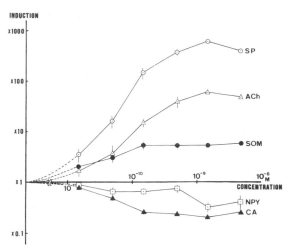

Figure 1. Dose dependence of recombinant CDF/LIF effects on neurotransmitter and neuropeptide choice. Recombinant mouse CDF/LIF was added at various concentrations (abcissa) to cultured sympathetic neurons for 12 days. Transmitter synthesis and peptide content were measured as described in Methods. The values are normalized to neuron number by counting neurons, and the data are calculated as the mean ± S.E.M. The ratio to the control (no CDF/LIF) value is shown on the ordinate. The control values were SP = 0.07 ± 0.03, SOM = 34.0 ± 2.0, and NPY = 1100.0 ± 200.0 fmoles/1000 neurons, and ACh = 170.0 ± 2.0, and CA = 3600.0 ± 500.0 fmoles/1000 neurons/hour. The cultures contained the following numbers of neurons: control = 8448 ± 1260, 17 pM = 6971 ± 774, 50 pM = 6507 ± 788, 170 pM = 5016 ± 1027, 500 pM = 2760 ± 270, 1.7 nM = 1582 ± 224, 5 nM = 1020 ± 39. The lower number of surviving neurons at the higher CDF/LIF concentrations is not yet explained. Since such an effect was not observed for purified CDF (Fukada 1985; Nawa and Patterson 1990), it is possible that the recombinant preparation contains a toxic contaminant. It is clear, however, that differential survival of various populations of predetermined neurons is not the explanation for the effects on transmitter/peptide phenotype (Patterson 1978; Potter et al. 1986; Nawa and Sah 1990).

Y (NPY) (Fig. 1). The inductions of ACh, SP, and SOM were observed at CDF/LIF concentrations well below 0.1 nM, with approximately 2 nM required for maximal induction of SP and ACh. The reductions in CA and NPY were less marked but required protein concentrations similar to those for the positive inductions. These effects are all consistent with previous results obtained using the protein purified from CM. The NPY suppression was not obvious when crude heart cell CM was added to the neurons (Nawa and Sah 1990; see also Marek and Mains 1989). The lack of effect with CM could be due to a lower concentration of CDF/LIF in the medium than was added with the recombinant protein or to the presence of a factor in the medium that acted to counter the effect of CDF/LIF.

Time Course of Peptide Induction and Its Reversibility

The induction of ACh synthesis in cultured sympathetic neurons by heart cell CM is slow, requiring several weeks for the major increase to occur (Patterson and Chun 1977; see also Johnson et al. 1976). Given that the same protein can induce the production of several neuropeptides, it was of interest to determine whether the peptide changes followed a time course similar to that of ACh. When sympathetic neurons are grown in a 100% volume equivalent of heart cell CM, the developmental profiles of SP and SOM induction (Fig. 2) are both very similar to that observed previously for ACh. The major induction of vasoactive intestinal polypeptide (VIP), however, is considerably slower, with the major increase occurring after 12 days and still rising at 24 days. Thus, there appear to be two phases in the VIP induction, the second of which does not correspond in time to those of ACh, SP, and SOM.

These changes in phenotype in postmitotic neurons raise the question of reversibility and age dependence. The culture paradigm offers an excellent opportunity to ask whether the neuropeptide changes induced by CM are reversible. When CM was withdrawn from the sympathetic neurons on day 12, a dramatic decline in SP, SOM, and VIP levels was observed (Fig. 2). The apparent rise in VIP seen at day 24 in the absence of CM is unexplained at present. Overall then, not only the induction of these peptides, but their maintenance appears to be completely dependent on the continued presence of CM.

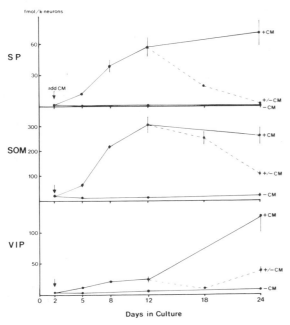

Figure 2. Time course of neuropeptide induction and its reversibility. Sympathetic neurons were grown in 100% volume equivalent of heart cell CM from day 2. On days 5, 8, 12, and 24, total peptides were extracted from three sister cultures, and radioimmunoassays were carried out for SP, SOM, and VIP (solid lines). On day 12, CM was withdrawn from some of the CM cultures to assess the reversibility of its effects (dashed lines). The culture medium was changed every 2 days, and 10 μm cytosine arabinoside was added on days 0, 2, 5, 10, and 16 to suppress nonneuronal cell proliferation. Neuronal numbers did not differ significantly among the various groups of cultures.

Neuronal Specificity of CDF/LIF

The dramatic changes in gene expression elicited in sympathetic neurons by CDF/LIF raises the question as to whether this factor is specific for these neurons or whether it can act in a widespread fashion in the nervous system. If it can act on other neurons, does it induce the same set of transmitters and peptides that it does in sympathetic neurons? Since a similar cholinergic factor from skeletal muscle can induce ACh synthesis in cultured sensory neurons from nodose ganglia (Mathieu et al. 1984), we tested recombinant CDF/LIF on sensory neurons, in this case from DRG. The results of such an experiment are given in Table 1. The most significant changes induced by CDF/LIF in the DRG neurons are 13-fold increases in ACh synthesis and VIP content. There is also a small reduction in SP. Therefore, CDF/LIF does alter the phenotype of sensory neurons, and it induces several of the same changes that it does in sympathetic neurons, namely, ACh and VIP induction. The effects on the DRG neurons are, however, not identical to those with sympathetic neurons, since SP and SOM are not increased in the sensory neurons. A reduction in CA synthesis is also not apparent, but the control levels of CA synthesis are too low to be sure if a CA suppression effect could be seen. Similarly, the large errors in the NPY measurements mitigated against drawing firm conclusions about a lowering of the level of this peptide. These results support the idea that a neuron's lineage history can influence its particular response to a given differentiation factor.

DISCUSSION

Hematopoietic Analogy

There are several parallels in the generation of cell diversity in the neural crest lineage and in the hematopoietic system: Both systems appear to arise from multipotent stem cells that give rise to progenitor cells committed to particular sublineages, and in both systems, extracellular signals can influence which differentiation pathways are taken (Anderson 1989). It is the last point concerning phenotypic instructive factors to which the present work relates. It was previously shown that the CDF from heart cells can alter neuropeptide as well as neurotransmitter expression in cultured sympathetic neurons (Nawa and Patterson 1990), and we here demonstrate that recombinant CDF/LIF duplicates these various activities (see also Yamamori et al. 1989). That this protein also influences the proliferation and differentiation of a myeloid cell line (Gearing et al. 1987) draws the two systems together at the molecular level as well. It should be noted, however, that it is not yet known how or when LIF acts in the hematopoietic lineage (Metcalf and Gearing 1989). Recent evidence implicates CDF/LIF in the control of cell proliferation and differentiation in many different tissues, from the earliest embryo through adulthood (Gough and Williams 1989). These findings suggest

Table 1. Effect of CDF/LIF on Neurotransmitter and Neuropeptide Choices in Sympathetic and Sensory Neurons

Neuron	CDF/LIF	ACh	CA	SP	SOM	VIP	NPY
SCG	+	4400 ± 400	730 ± 180	59 ± 6.0	48 ± 5	9.7 ± 0.6	
	−	330 ± 50	3200 ± 300	0.4 ± 0.0	4 ± 2	1.1 ± 0.4	
DRG	+	53 ± 5	0.4 ± 0.2	2.1 ± 0.2	2.5 ± 1.3	2.7 ± 0.4	66 ± 28
	−	4 ± 4	0.6 ± 0.4	5.0 ± 0.9	3.5 ± 1.6	0.2 ± 0.2	75 ± 21

Sympathetic neurons from the SCG were cultured in serum-containing medium with or without 1 nM recombinant human CDF/LIF for 12 days. Sensory neurons from the DRG were grown in defined medium as described in Methods. To suppress nonneuronal cell growth, 10 μM cytosine arabinoside was added during the first 7 days (SCG) or between 24 and 48 hours (DRG). The number of neurons did not differ significantly between the various groups of cultures, and nonneuronal cells were not observed in the SCG cultures. Some nonneuronal cells were observed in the DRG cultures, numbering <10% of the total cell population. Transmitters and peptides were assayed as described in Methods. ACh and CA values are expressed as fmoles/1000 neurons/hour, and the peptides are expressed as fmoles/1000 neurons.

that it may be rewarding to study the effects of other cytokines and hematopoietic regulators on neuronal phenotypic choices, as well as to investigate whether neuronal factors can influence hematopoietic decisions.

Role of CDF/LIF In Situ

To understand the role of CDF/LIF in neuronal development in the intact organism, it will be necessary to localize the factor in situ, describe which cells have receptors for it, and to perform appropriate perturbation experiments. Although such data are not yet available, one can ask if the effects of CDF/LIF on cultured neurons mimic any of the phenotypes known from descriptive studies of normal neurons. The present experiments and those of Nawa and Patterson (1990) show that CDF/LIF can each induce the expression of ACh and VIP while causing a corresponding reduction in CA and NPY. The striking aspect of these results is that these are precisely the pairs of transmitters and peptides that are generally colocalized together in cholinergic (ACh + VIP) and noradrenergic (CA + NPY) peripheral neurons; these pairings have been termed one of the organizational principles of the sympathetic nervous system (Lundberg et al. 1982). Thus, we would expect that the natural neuronal differentiation signal operating in the sweat glands of the rat foot pad, for instance, where the noradrenergic-to-cholinergic switch in phenotype is observed during normal development (Landis and Keefe 1983), would regulate these pairs of transmitters and peptides coordinately, as does CDF/LIF. The simplest picture would then involve a unique neuronal differentiation signal for each distinct combination of transmitters and peptides.

There are, however, a great many exceptions to the general rules of transmitter/peptide pairings. NPY is sometimes found in cholinergic neurons, for instance, and VIP in noncholinergic neurons (cf. Leblanc and Landis 1988). To take these exceptions into account, simple models might include separate differentiation factors for each transmitter and peptide or factors that both suppress and induce single or combinations of transmitters and peptides. Although it is clearly too

early to draw firm conclusions, the data that are available support both alternatives. That is, some purified neuronal differentiation factors, such as CDF/LIF, ciliary neurotrophic factor, and membrane-associated neurotransmitter stimulating factor, can each induce the expression of several transmitters and peptides as well as suppress others (Wong and Kessler 1987; Ernsberger et al. 1989; Nawa and Patterson 1990; Rao et al. 1990a), whereas several newly described factors appear to have more narrow effects on neuronal gene expression (Nawa and Patterson 1990).

In the particular case of the sympathetic innervation of the sweat gland in the rat, a combination of factors may be required to explain the observed transmitter/peptide phenotype. These axons switch from a CA phenotype to an ACh-VIP-CGRP (calcitonin-gene-related peptide) phenotype on arrival at this target (Landis et al. 1988; Schotzinger and Landis 1988). It is particularly noteworthy that SP has not been detected in these neurons because all three cholinergic factors known to act on cultured sympathetic neurons do induce SP (Wong and Kessler 1987; Nawa and Sah 1990; Rao et al. 1990b and unpubl.). Three hypotheses that can reconcile these results are as follows: (1) In none of these proteins is the factor acting normally in the sweat gland, (2) the sympathetic neurons do not show an SP response to CDF (for instance) in vivo, and (3) the SP part of the response to CDF (for example) is counterbalanced by another factor in the sweat gland that acts to suppress SP expression. In this regard, it is interesting that soluble extracts of rat foot pads (including sweat glands) contain a factor(s) that mimics the action of the known cholinergic factors on cultured sympathetic neurons, including the induction of SP (Rao et al. 1990b and unpubl.).

Neuronal Targets for CDF/LIF

Another aspect of the role of CDF/LIF concerns how many types of neurons respond to it. That is, does the protein act only on the sympathetic neurons that were used as the assay for its purification, or can it act on other neurons that are normally cholinergic? Can it induce cholinergic properties in neurons that do not normally display such a phenotype? The investigations of Weber et al. (1985) demonstrated that skeletal muscle CM contains a cholinergic neuronal differentiation factor that very closely resembles CDF/LIF. The skeletal muscle protein can enhance cholinergic differentiation in cultures of partially purified rat motor neurons and nodose ganglion sensory neurons without altering neuronal survival (Mathieu et al. 1984; Martinou et al. 1989). These findings suggest a potentially widespread role for this factor. We assayed recombinant CDF/LIF on another population of neurons, DRG sensory neurons, that are not known to produce ACh normally in situ. CDF/LIF does enhance ACh synthesis in these neurons, as well as VIP expression. Quantitatively, the observed increases are not as great as those seen with sympathetic neurons, but we have not yet attempted to optimize this effect by testing higher concentrations of factor or by testing DRG neurons from different developmental stages.

What does the apparently widespread distribution of putative receptors for CDF/LIF mean for its biological role? One possibility is that normally, in vivo, most neurons are not responsive to this factor. That is, the response observed here represents a derepression of the receptor in culture (or some other aspect of the response pathway); normally, expression of the CDF/LIF receptor is closely regulated and restricted in developmental time and location. It is also possible that many neurons do have the capacity to respond to this factor in situ but that expression of CDF/LIF itself is closely regulated and restricted in developmental time and location. Yet another possibility is that many neurons do express the CDF/LIF receptor and do encounter the factor in situ, but they are prevented from responding to it by another factor in their environment. Such factors might include glial cells (Spiegel et al. 1990) and neuronal activity (Walicke et al. 1977), both of which have been shown to inhibit the response of cultured sympathetic neurons to cholinergic or peptidergic factors.

Reversibility of the CDF/LIF Effects

How permanent are the effects of CDF/LIF? Put another way, if the early decision to become catecholaminergic is reversible, is the subsequent decision to become cholinergic similarly plastic? Vidal et al. (1987) found that removal of skeletal muscle CM from sympathetic neurons at later times in culture resulted in a leveling off of the rise in choline acetyltransferase activity and a concomitant induction of tyrosine hydroxylase activity. Reversibility in cholinergic development was observed by Patterson and Chun (1977), but they found that such changes became quantitatively less with neuronal age in culture. Similarly, although mature sympathetic neurons taken from adult rats can become cholinergic when exposed to the appropriate environment in culture, they do so at a lower frequency or with a slower time course (Wakshull et al. 1979; Johnson et

al. 1980; Potter et al. 1986; see also Lindsay et al. 1989). In an entirely in vivo paradigm, Coulombe and Bronner-Fraser (1986) showed that cholinergic, parasympathetic neurons could store catecholamines when transplanted to the appropriate environment.

The present experiments extend the reversibility phenomenon to neuropeptide expression. These findings, taken with those reviewed above (and McMahon and Gibson 1987), imply that the transmitter and peptide phenotypes observed in mature neurons in the adult organism are being actively maintained by the appropriate differentiation factors. This idea is consistent with the adult vertebrate nervous system being in a state of dynamic equilibrium. In this view, rather than being static or fixed, maturity actually represents a balance between regression of processes and connections, and sprouting of new processes and the formation of novel connections (Patterson and Purves 1982; Purves and Lichtman 1985). It may be that this continual remodeling of the system could also involve the chemical identity of the neurons, an extreme form of synaptic plasticity.

ACKNOWLEDGMENTS

We are grateful to Dr. Donald Metcalf and colleagues of the Walter and Eliza Hall Institute for Medical Research in Melbourne for recombinant LIF. We thank D. McDowell for help with the preparation of tissue culture materials and J. Carnahan for preparation of NGF. This work was supported by the National Institute of Neurological Disorders and Stroke (Javits Neuroscience Investigator Award) and a McKnight Foundation Neuroscience Research Project Award (P.H.P.); by the Muscular Dystrophy Association, the Del Webb Foundation and the Japanese Ministry of Education, Science, and Culture (H.N.); by a Caltech Summer Undergraduate Research Fellowship (T.L.); and by the Alzheimer's Disease and Related Disorders Association (T.Y.).

REFERENCES

Adler, R. and M. Hatlee. 1989. Plasticity and differentiation of embryonic retinal cells after terminal mitosis. *Science* **243:** 391.

Adler, J.E., L.S. Schleifer, and L.B. Black. 1989. Partial purification and characterization of a membrane-derived factor regulating neurotransmitter phenotypic expression. *Proc. Natl. Acad. Sci.* **86:** 1080.

Anderson, D.J. 1989. The neural crest cell lineage problem: Neuropoiesis? *Neuron* **3:** 1.

Bronner-Fraser, M. and S. Fraser. 1989. Developmental potential of avian trunk neural crest cells in situ. *Neuron* **3:** 755.

Coulombe, J.N. and M. Bronner-Fraser. 1986. Cholinergic neurones acquire adrenergic neurotransmitters when transplanted into an embryo. *Nature* **324:** 569.

Ernsberger, U., M. Sendtner, and H. Rohrer. 1989. Proliferation and differentiation of embryonic chick sympathetic neurons: Effects of ciliary neurotrophic factor. *Neuron* **2:** 1275.

Fukada, K. 1980. Hormonal control of neurotransmitter choice in sympathetic neuron cultures. *Nature* **287:** 553.

———. 1985. Purification and partial characterization of a cholinergic differentiation factor. *Proc. Natl. Acad. Sci.* **82:** 8795.

Galileo, D.S., G.E. Gray, G.C. Owens, J. Majors, and J.R. Sanes. 1990. Neurons and glia arise from a common progenitor in chicken optic tectum: Demonstration with two retroviruses and cell type-specific antibodies. *Proc. Natl. Acad. Sci.* **87:** 458.

Gearing, D.P., N.A. Nicola, D. Metcalf, S. Foote, T.A. Willson, N.M. Gough, and R.L. Williams. 1989. Production of leukemia inhibitory factor (LIF) in *Escherichia coli* by a novel procedure and its use in maintaining embryonic stem (EC) cells in culture. *Biotechnology* **7:** 1157.

Gearing, D.P., N.M. Gough, J.A. King, D.J. Hilton, N.A. Nicola, R.J. Simpson, E.C. Nice, A. Kelso, and D. Metcalf. 1987. Molecular cloning and expression of cDNA encoding a murine myeloid leukaemia inhibitory factor (LIF). *EMBO J.* **6:** 3395.

Gesser, B.P. and L.I. Larsson. 1985. Changes from enkephalin-like to gastrin/cholecystokinin-like immunoreactivity in snail neurons. *J. Neurosci.* **5:** 1412.

Gough, N.M. and R.L. Williams. 1989. The pleiotropic actions of leukemia inhibitory factor. *Cancer Cells* **1:** 77.

Happola, O., H. Paivarinta, S. Soinila, and H. Steinbusch. 1986. Pre- and postnatal development of 5-hydroxytryptamine-immunoreactive cells in the superior cervical ganglion of the rat. *J. Auton. Nerv. Syst.* **15:** 21.

Hawrot, E. and P.H. Patterson. 1979. Long-term culture of dissociated sympathetic neurons. *Methods Enzymol.* **53:** 574.

Hayashi, M., D. Edgar, and H. Thoenen. 1983. The development of substance P, somatostatin and vasoactive intestinal polypeptide in sympathetic and spinal sensory ganglia of the chick embryo. *Neuroscience* **10:** 31.

Holt, C.E., T.W. Bertsch, H.M. Ellis, and W.A. Harris. 1988. Cellular determination in the *Xenopus* retina is independent of lineage and birth date. *Neuron* **1:** 15.

Iacovitti, L., M.J. Evinger, T.H. Joh, and D.J. Reis. 1989. A muscle-derived factor(s) induces expression of a catecholamine phenotype neurons in neurons of cultured rat cerebral cortex. *J. Neurosci.* **9:** 3529.

Johnson, M., C.D. Ross, and R.P. Bunge. 1980. Morphological and biochemical studies on the development of cholinergic properties in cultured sympathetic neurons. II. Dependence on postnatal age. *J. Cell Biol.* **84:** 692.

Johnson, M., D. Ross, M. Meyers, R. Rees, R. Bunge, E. Wakshull, and H. Burton. 1976. Synaptic vesicle cytochemistry changes when cultured sympathetic neurones develop cholinergic interactions. *Nature* **262:** 308.

Kessler, J.A. 1986. Differential regulation of cholinergic and peptidergic development in the rat striatum in culture. *Dev. Biol.* **113:** 77.

Kessler, J.A., J.E. Adler, G.M. Jonakait, and I.B. Black. 1984. Target organ regulation of substance P in sympathetic neurons in culture. *Dev. Biol.* **103:** 71.

Koizumi, O. and H.R. Bode. 1986. Plasticity in the nervous system of adult hydra. I. The position-dependent expression of MRFamide-like immunoreactivity. *Dev. Biol.* **116:** 407.

Landis, S.C. and D. Keefe. 1983. Evidence for neurotransmitter plasticity in vivo: Developmental changes in the properties of cholinergic sympathetic neurons. *Dev. Biol.* **98:** 349.

Landis, S.C., M. Schwab, and R.E. Siegel. 1988. Evidence for neurotransmitter plasticity in vivo. II. Immunocytochemical studies of rat sweat gland innervation. *Dev. Biol.* **126:** 129.

Leblanc, G. and S.C. Landis. 1988. Target specificity of neuropeptide Y-immunoreactive cranial parasympathetic neurons. *J. Neurosci.* **8:** 146.

Lindsay, R. 1988. Nerve growth factors (NGF, BDNF) en-

hance axonal regeneration but are not required for survival of adult sensory neurons. *J. Neurosci.* **8:** 2394.

Lindsay, R., C. Lockett, J. Sternberg, and J. Winter. 1989. Neuropeptide expression in cultures of adult sensory neurons — Modulation of substance-P and calcitonin gene-related peptide levels by nerve growth-factor. *Neuroscience* **33:** 53.

Lin, L.-F.H., D. Mismer, J.D. Lile, L.G. Armes, E.T. Butler, J.L. Vannice, and F. Collins. 1989. Purification, cloning and expression of ciliary neurotrophic factor (CNTF). *Science* **246:** 1023.

Lundberg, J.M., T. Hokfelt, A. Anggard, L. Terenius, R. Elde, K. Markey, M. Goldstein, and J. Kimmel. 1982. Organizational principles in the peripheral sympathetic nervous system: Subdivision by coexisting peptides (somatostatin-, avian pancreatic polypeptide-, and vasoactive intestinal polypeptide-like immunoreactive materials). *Proc. Natl. Acad. Sci.* **79:** 1303.

Mains, R.E. and P.H. Patterson. 1973. Primary cultures of dissociated sympathetic neurons. I. Establishment of long-term growth in culture and studies of differentiated properties. *J. Cell Biol.* **59:** 329.

Marek, K.L. and R.E. Mains. 1989. Biosynthesis, development and regulation of neuropeptide Y in superior cervical ganglion culture. *J. Neurochem.* **52:** 1807.

Martinou, J.C., A.L.V. Thai, G. Cassar, F. Roubinet, and M.J. Weber. 1989. Characterization of two factors enhancing choline acetyltransferase activity in cultures of purified rat motoneurons. *J. Neurosci.* **9:** 3645.

Mathieu, C., A. Moisand, and M.J. Weber. 1984. Acetylcholine metabolism by cultured neurons from rat nodose ganglia: Regulation by a macromolecule from muscle-conditioned medium. *Neuroscience* **13:** 1373.

McMahon, S.B. and S. Gibson. 1987. Peptide expression is altered when afferent nerves reinnervate inappropriate tissue. *Neurosci. Lett.* **73:** 9.

McManaman, J., F. Crawford, R. Clark, J. Richker, and F. Fuller. 1989. Multiple factors from skeletal muscle: Demonstration of effects of basic neurotrophic fibroblast growth factor and comparisons with the 22-kilodalton choline acetyltransferase development factor. *J. Neurochem.* **53:** 1763.

Metcalf, D. 1989. The molecular control of cell division, differentiation commitment and maturation in haemopoietic cells. *Nature* **339:** 27.

Metcalf, D. and D.P. Gearing. 1989. Fatal syndrome in mice engrafted with cells producing high levels of the leukemia inhibitory factor. *Proc. Natl. Acad. Sci.* **86:** 5948.

Nawa, H. and P.H. Patterson. 1990. Separation and partial characterization of neuropeptide-inducing factors in heart cell conditioned medium. *Neuron* **4:** 269.

Nawa, H. and D.W.Y. Sah. 1990. Different biological activities in conditioned media control the expression of a variety of neuropeptides in cultured sympathetic neurons. *Neuron* **4:** 279.

Patterson, P.H. 1978. Environmental determination of autonomic neurotransmitter functions. *Annu. Rev. Neurosci.* **1:** 1.

Patterson, P.H. and L.L.Y. Chun. 1977. The induction of acetylcholine synthesis in primary cultures of dissociated rat sympathetic neurons. II. Developmental aspects. *Dev. Biol.* **60:** 473.

Patterson, P.H. and D. Purves. 1982. *Readings in developmental neurobiology.* Cold Spring Harbor Laboratory, Cold Spring Harbor, New York.

Potter, D.D., S.C. Landis, S.G. Matsumoto, and E.J. Furshpan. 1986. Synaptic functions in rat sympathetic neurons in microcultures. II. Adrenergic/cholinergic dual status and plasticity. *J. Neurosci.* **6:** 1080.

Price, J. and L. Thurlow. 1988. Cell lineage in the rat cerebral cortex. A study using retroviral-mediated gene-transfer. *Development* **104:** 473.

Purves, D. and J.W. Lichtman. 1985. *Principles of neural*

development. Sinauer Associates, Sunderland, Massachusetts.

Rao, M.S., S.C. Landis, and P.H. Patterson. 1990a. The cholinergic neuronal differentiation factor from heart cell conditioned medium is different from the cholinergic factors in sciatic nerve and spinal cord. *Dev. Biol.* **139:** 65.

Rao, M.S., P.H. Patterson, and S.C. Landis. 1990b. Characterization of a target derived cholinergic differentiation factor present in rat sweat glands. *Soc. Neurosci. Abstr.* **16:** (in press).

Saadat, S., M. Sendtner, and H. Rohrer. 1989. Ciliary neurotrophic factor induces cholinergic differentiation of rat sympathetic neurons in culture. *J. Cell Biol.* **108:** 1807.

Schoenen, J., P. Delree, P. Leprince, and G. Moonen. 1989. Neurotransmitter phenotype plasticity in cultured dissociated adult rat dorsal root ganglia: An immunochemical study. *J. Neurosci. Res.* **22:** 473.

Schotzinger, R.J. and S.C. Landis. 1988. Cholinergic phenotype developed by noradrenergic sympathetic neurons after innervation of a novel cholinergic target *in vivo*. *Nature* **335:** 637.

Spiegel, K., V. Wong, and J.A. Kessler. 1990. Translational regulation of somatostatin in cultured sympathetic neurons. *Neuron* **4:** 303.

Stockli, K.A., F. Lottspeich, M. Sendtner, P. Masiakowski, P. Caroll, R. Gotz, D. Lindholm, and H. Thoenen. 1989. Molecular cloning, expression and regional distribution of rat ciliary neurotrophic factor. *Nature* **342:** 920.

Tomlinson, A. 1988. Cellular interactions in the developing *Drosophila* eye. *Development* **104:** 183.

Tublitz, N.J. and A.W. Sylwester. 1990. Postembryonic alteration of transmitter phenotype in individually identified peptidergic neurons. *J. Neurosci.* **10:** 161.

Turner, D. and C.L. Cepko. 1987. A common progenitor for neurons and glia persists in rat retina late in development. *Nature* **328:** 131.

Vidal, S., B. Raynaud, D. Clarous, and M.J. Weber. 1987. Neurotransmitter plasticity of cultured sympathetic neurones. Are the effects of muscle-conditioned medium reversible? *Development* **101:** 617.

Wakshull, E., M.I. Johnson, and H. Burton. 1979. Postnatal rat sympathetic neurons in culture. II. Synaptic transmission by postnatal neurons. *J. Neurophysiol.* **42:** 1426.

Walicke, P.A., R.B. Campenot, and P.H. Patterson. 1977. Determination of transmitter function by neuronal activity. *Proc. Natl. Acad. Sci.* **74:** 5767.

Wall, J.B. and P.H. Taghert. 1989. Regulation of neuropeptide phenotypes in identified neurons of *Manduca* embryos. *Soc. Neurosci. Abstr.* **15:** 448.

Weber, M.J., B. Raynaud, and C. Delteil. 1985. Molecular properties of a cholinergic differentiation factor from muscle-conditioned medium. *J. Neurochem.* **45:** 1541.

Wetts, R. and S.E. Fraser. 1988. Multipotent precursors can give rise to all major cell types of the frog retina. *Science* **239:** 1142.

Wong, V. and J.A. Kessler. 1987. Solubilization of a membrane factor that stimulates levels of substance P and choline acetyltransferase in sympathetic neurons. *Proc. Natl. Acad. Sci.* **84:** 8726.

Yamamori, T., K. Fukada, R. Aebersold, S. Korsching, M.-J. Fann, and P.H. Patterson. 1989. The cholinergic neuronal differentiation factor from heart cells is identical to leukemia inhibitory factor. *Science* **246:** 1412.

Contributions of Cell-extrinsic and Cell-intrinsic Factors to the Differentiation of a Neural-crest-derived Neuroendocrine Progenitor Cell

N. Mori,† S.J. Birren,* R. Stein,‡ D. Stemple,* D.J. Vandenbergh,*
C.W. Wuenschell,† and D.J. Anderson†

*Division of Biology 216-76 and †Howard Hughes Medical Institute, California Institute of Technology, Pasadena,
California 91125; ‡Department of Biochemistry, Tel Aviv University, Tel Aviv, Israel

A central question in developmental neurobiology concerns the mechanisms that generate cellular diversity in the vertebrate nervous system. Cell lineage analyses have established that many progenitor cells in the developing nervous system are multipotent (Turner and Cepko 1987; Holt et al. 1988; Wetts and Fraser 1988). However, the mechanisms that control the differentiation of such progenitor cells are poorly understood. It is assumed that both the developmental history of a progenitor cell and its interactions with its local environment influence its final choice of developmental fate. Few experimental systems are available, however, in which it has been possible to dissect the relative contributions of these two factors to the differentiation program. In the vertebrate nervous system, only two well-defined multipotential progenitor cells have been isolated and studied in detail. These are the O2A progenitor, which gives rise to two types of glial cells in the central nervous system (Raff 1989), and the sympathoadrenal progenitor (Doupe et al. 1985b; Anderson and Axel 1986), which generates either the sympathetic neurons or adrenal medullary chromaffin cells of the peripheral nervous system.

The Sympathoadrenal Progenitor Has a Restricted Repertoire of Developmental Fates

Sympathoadrenal progenitors derive from a population of neural crest cells that detach from the top of the neural tube and migrate throughout the embryo. Lineage tracing studies, performed both in vitro (Sieber-Blum and Cohen 1980; Baroffio et al. 1988) and in vivo (Bronner-Fraser and Fraser 1989), have indicated that single cells in the premigratory crest are initially multipotent and are able to generate most or all crest derivatives. These include not only sympathetic neurons and chromaffin cells, but other neuronal populations such as sensory and parasympathetic, as well as nonneuronal cell types including glia and melanocytes. As neural crest cells migrate and localize in the periphery, however, they appear to become developmentally restricted, perhaps analogous to the gradual narrowing of the developmental potential observed in

hematopoiesis (Anderson 1989). The sympathoadrenal progenitor appears to represent one such developmentally restricted progenitor cell. These progenitors are first detectable concomitant with the aggregation of crest cells to form the sympathetic ganglion primordia (Fig. 1). They can be visualized using several antigenic markers including tyrosine hydroxylase (TH), the rate-limiting enzyme in catecholamine biosynthesis (Cochard et al. 1979). After this initial aggregation, some of the cells in this population remain in the ganglion primordia and differentiate into sympathetic neurons, whereas others continue migrating ventrally to invade the mesodermally derived adrenal primordium (Fig. 1). The latter proliferate and differentiate into chromaffin cells, which ultimately form the medullary zone of the adrenal gland.

Experiments in primary cell culture originally suggested that environmental factors determine the ultimate fate of progenitors in this sublineage. It was shown that postnatal (Unsicker et al. 1978) or even adult (Doupe

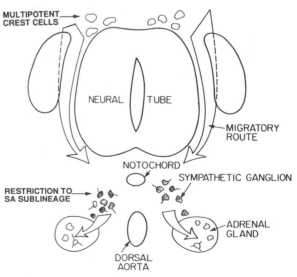

Figure 1. Schematic indicating the migratory route taken by cells in the sympathoadrenal lineage. A cross section through the spinal cord in the thoraco-lumbar region is shown.

et al. 1985a) chromaffin cells could be induced to transdifferentiate into sympathetic neuron-like cells by
nerve growth factor (NGF). This transdifferentiation
could be slowed or blocked by glucocorticoid (GC),
suggesting that the high local concentration of these
steroids in the surrounding adrenal cortex could similarly inhibit the neuronal differentiation of chromaffin
precursors in vivo (Unsicker et al. 1978). The idea that
the microenvironment of sympathoadrenal lineage cells
is important in controlling their differentiation in vivo is
supported by the observation that TH$^+$ cells in the
sympathetic ganglion and the adrenal gland acquire
distinct antigenic phenotypes only a few days after
migration has ended (Fig. 2).

To determine whether individual sympathoadrenal
progenitors are bipotential, we have isolated these cells
from fetal rat adrenal glands, using cell-surface monoclonal antibodies and fluorescence-activated cell sorting

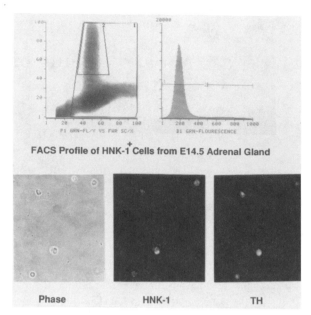

FACS Profile of HNK-1$^+$ Cells from E14.5 Adrenal Gland

Phase   HNK-1   TH

Figure 3. Isolation of sympathoadrenal progenitor cells from
E14.5 rat adrenal gland by FACS using monoclonal antibody
HNK-1. (*Top, left*) Forward light scatter (abscissa) versus
fluorescence intensity (ordinate). Gated region 2 delimits cell
population isolated. (*Top, right*) Histogram of fluorescence
intensity versus cell number. The HNK-1$^+$ cells represent
approximately 10% of the adrenal population. (*Bottom*)
FACS-isolated progenitors several hours after plating. The
same field is shown photographed with phase contrast optics
(*left*), fluorescein-HNK-1 (*middle*), or rhodamine-TH (*right*).
Note that all the HNK-1$^+$ cells are also TH$^+$.

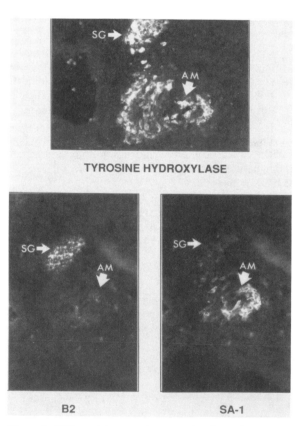

TYROSINE HYDROXYLASE

B2   SA-1

Figure 2. Differential expression of antigenic markers by embryonic sympathoadrenal cells in the ganglion and adrenal
primordia in vivo. Shown are sections through the caudal
thoracic region of an E15.5 rat embryo. Cells in both the
sympathetic ganglion (SG) and adrenal medulla (AM) stain
with an antibody to TH (*top*). Note the individual cells between the SG and AM, which may be migrating to the adrenal. (*Bottom*) Fluorescence photomicrographs of the same
section double-labeled with monoclonal antibody B2 (*left*),
which selectively labels primitive sympathetic neurons (Anderson and Axel 1986) and SA-1 (*right*), which selectively
labels adrenal chromaffin cells. (J. Carnahan and P.H. Patterson, unpubl.).

(FACS) (Anderson and Axel 1986; Anderson 1988)
(Fig. 3). In culture, the differentiation of such progenitors into chromaffin cells (Fig. 4) is absolutely
dependent on the addition of exogenous GC to the
culture medium (Anderson and Axel 1986; Seidl and
Unsicker 1989; A. Michelsohn and D.J. Anderson, unpubl.). In the absence of GC, these progenitors initiate
neuronal differentiation (Fig. 4), a process that can be
promoted by specific growth factors (see below). Quantitative analysis of cell populations and serial observations of single cells strongly suggest that individual
progenitors in these cultures are indeed bipotential
(Anderson and Axe 1986). Similar observations have
been made for progenitors isolated from postnatal
(Doupe et al. 1985b) and, more recently, fetal superior
cervical sympathetic ganglia (J. Carnahan and P.H.
Patterson, pers. comm.). This conclusion is supported
by recent in vivo observations showing that, in the
ganglion primordia, chromaffin-specific and neuron-
specific markers are transiently coexpressed by individual progenitor cells (D.J. Anderson et al.,
unpubl.). Taken together, these data suggest that a
common, developmentally restricted progenitor cell
initially populates both the sympathetic ganglia and the
adrenal gland and then differentiates into either sympathetic neurons or chromaffin cells under the influence
of factors differentially distributed in these alternative
sites of migratory arrest.

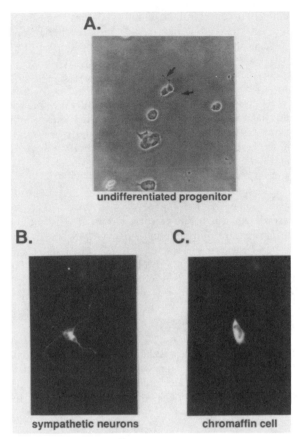

Figure 4. FACS-isolated progenitors develop into sympathetic neurons or chromaffin cells, in vitro. (A) Phase-contrast micrograph of progenitor cells after 24 hours in culture. (→) Note the short cytoplasmic extensions characteristic of such cells. (B) Progenitors after 2–3 days in serum-containing medium. Under these conditions, the cells begin to differentiate into neurons, extending short neurites, but they eventually die. Neurite extension is enhanced by addition of FGF (not shown). (C) Progenitors after 2–3 days in 5 μM dexamethasone. Note the difference in morphology from the cells in B. Cells in both B and C are labeled with an anti-TH antibody. However, cells such as those in B also express neurofilaments, whereas those in C express the chromaffin marker PNMT (not shown).

Neuronal Differentiation of Sympathoadrenal Progenitors May Be Controlled by Polypeptide Factors Acting in a Cascade

The requirement of GC for chromaffin cell differentiation in vitro is consistent with the fact that in vivo these cells normally develop within the adrenal gland, the major site of GC synthesis. In contrast, the identification of factors promoting neuronal differentiation and their relationship to molecules present in vivo has been more difficult to establish. As NGF converts both chromaffin cells (Unsicker et al. 1978) and PC12 cells (Greene and Tischler 1976) into sympathetic neuron-like cells, this molecule initially seemed like a reasonable candidate for the factor that promotes neuronal differentiation of sympathetic neuroblasts in vivo. However, subsequent studies of the timing and location

of NGF synthesis in the embryo indicated that NGF is unlikely to be playing such a role. NGF is initially produced in the targets of sympathetic innervation, not in the ganglia, and is not made until the neurons have already grown their axons to these targets (Davies et al. 1987; Korsching and Thoenen 1988). Moreover, freshly isolated sympathoadrenal progenitor cells are initially unresponsive to NGF in vitro (Anderson and Axel 1986; Ernsberger et al. 1989). Such findings have led to the search for other factors that might promote neuronal differentiation in this system.

One such factor may be fibroblast growth factor (FGF). FGF is the only factor other than NGF able to induce the expression of neuron-specific mRNAs in PC12 cells (Leonard et al. 1987; Stein et al. 1988a). Moreover, both basic (Stemple et al. 1988) and acidic (Claude et al. 1988) FGF can promote the transdifferentiation of postnatal chromaffin cells into neurons. However, FGF cannot act subsequently as a survival factor for the sympathetic neurons generated from chromaffin cells. Rather, FGF induces an NGF dependence in these cells (Stemple et al. 1988). Taken to-

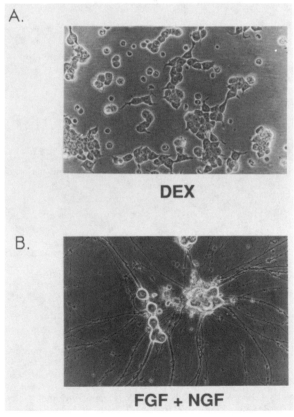

Figure 5. Immortalized sympathoadrenal progenitor cells can differentiate into stable, postmitotic neurons. (A) MAH cells maintained in 5 μM dexamethasone. Note the morphologic similarity to the primary cells shown in Fig. 4A. (B) A small proportion (<0.1%) of MAH cells develop into neurons in the presence of bFGF (10 ng/ml) + NGF (50 ng/ml). The cells shown had been maintained for approximately 4 weeks in culture at the time this photograph was taken. The magnification in A is twice that in B.

gether, these results suggested a potential role for FGF in the initial stages of neuronal differentiation in the sympathoadrenal lineage.

To address this question, we first generated immortal cell lines from sympathoadrenal progenitors by retroviral transduction of the v-*myc* oncogene (Fig. 5A). These lines appear to have retained many of the morphologic and antigenic properties of their normal (i.e., nonimmortalized) counterparts (Birren and Anderson 1990). Such cell lines facilitate cell biological and molecular experiments by providing large numbers of easily available cells. We have named these cell lines MAH cells, for *myc*-infected, *a*drenal-derived, *H*NK-1-positive cells (Birren and Anderson 1990). MAH cells represent the first case where a well-defined neuronal progenitor population has been first isolated and then immortalized.

A striking feature of MAH cells is that they respond to basic FGF (bFGF) by extending long neurites, but they do not do so in response to NGF. This is because these cells do not express the NGF receptor (NGFR), as determined by hybridization of MAH cell mRNA with cloned NGFR cDNA probes (Birren and Anderson 1990). Like normal chromaffin cells, MAH cells

induced to differentiate with FGF alone die several days after extending neurites. In the presence of both FGF and NGF, however, a small proportion of MAH cells become postmitotic neurons that are stable for many weeks in culture if supplied with NGF (Fig. 5B). In the presence of a blocking anti-NGF antibody, however, these MAH-derived neurons rapidly die, indicating that they are now dependent on the neurotrophic factor for survival. Northern blot analysis has confirmed that treatment of MAH cells with FGF induces the de novo expression of NGFR mRNA (Birren and Anderson 1990).

Taken together, these data suggest that neuronal development in this lineage may involve a relay, or cascade, in which one factor (perhaps FGF) initiates differentiation and simultaneously primes the cell to respond to a second factor (NGF), which then subserves further maturation and survival (Fig. 6). The extent to which FGF exerts such an effect on normal progenitors is now under investigation. Interestingly, when cultured at high density, such progenitors appear to initiate neuronal differentiation spontaneously. Such an effect could be due to an autocrine action of FGF or an FGF-like molecule. Whatever the case, the data suggest that the initial stages of neuronal differentiation in this lineage occur independently of NGF (Coughlin and Collins 1985) but involve an induction of the NGFR. As NGF appears able to up-regulate expres-

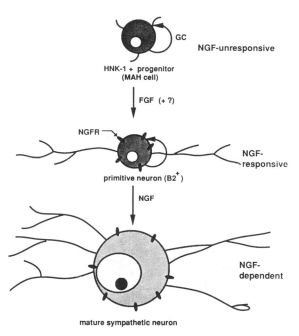

Figure 6. Stages of neuronal differentiation in the sympathoadrenal lineage. The sympathoadrenal progenitors represented by MAH cells (*top*) extend neurites in response to FGF but do not yet express NGF receptors. In the presence of glucocorticoid, these cells divide (*circular arrow*) but do not differentiate. Following treatment with FGF, a primitive neuron can be observed that bears processes and is still dividing. This cell type has been described in primary cultures previously (Anderson and Axel 1986; Anderson 1988). At least a subpopulation of these primitive neurons begins to express the NGF receptor. In the presence of NGF, these cells mature into postmitotic neurons with large cell bodies, prominent nucleoli, and extensive networks of neurites. Such neurons are then dependent on NGF for survival. (Reprinted, with permission, from Birren and Anderson 1990.)

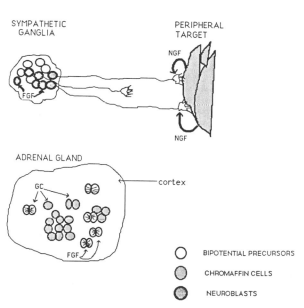

Figure 7. A two-stage model for sympathetic neuron development. (*Top*) FGF (or a different factor with similar biological activity) induces progenitor proliferation and neuronal differentiation locally in the sympathetic ganglion primordia. These differentiating cells extend processes toward their targets. The appearance of NGF in targets coincides with the arrival of the sympathetic afferent fibers. At or near the target, neurons acquire responsiveness to and dependence on NGF, which thereby supports their survival and further maturation. (*Bottom*) In the adrenal gland, GC permits FGF to mitotically expand the developing endocrine population but prevents the factor from inducing neuronal differentiation.

sion of its own receptor (at least in PC12 cells; Doherty et al. 1988), it may be that the initiating factor simply provides sufficient NGFR to establish an NGF autoregulatory loop that is in turn primarily responsible for the induction of full NGF-responsiveness and NGF-dependence.

This "two-factor" model would fit well with the fact that, in vivo, neuronal differentiation is initiated at a site (the ganglia) distant from that where NGF is eventually synthesized (Korsching and Thoenen 1988) (Fig. 7). According to this view, FGF (or a molecule with similar biological activity) would act locally in the ganglia to trigger initial neurite outgrowth. At the same time, the induction of NGFR expression would ensure that by the time the growing axons arrived at the periphery, they would have acquired competence to be supported by target-derived NGF. Moreover, the induction of an absolute NGF dependence in these growing neurons would ensure the death of any cells that failed to grow to an appropriate target. Studies are now in progress to determine whether mRNAs encoding FGF or related members of the FGF gene family (Hébert et al. 1990) are indeed present in embryonic sympathetic ganglia at the stage when neuronal differentiation normally occurs. Recent immunocyto-

chemical evidence suggests that bFGF, at least, is present in embryonic chick sympathetic neurons (Kalcheim and Neufeld 1990).

Derepression of Neural-specific Genes May Be a Developmental Prerequisite for Their Regulation by Environmental Factors

The foregoing data indicate that the development of sympathoadrenal derivatives occurs through the action of diffusible factors on a progenitor cell with a restricted repertoire of developmental fates. Studies of gene expression in PC12 cells indicate that, at the molecular level, these factors act by up- and down-regulating terminal-differentiation genes specific to the neuronal and chromaffin phenotypes, respectively (Leonard et al. 1987; Stein et al. 1988a). In other words, NGF and FGF induce neuron-specific genes and suppress chromaffin-specific genes, and vice versa for GC. The "repertoire of fates" in a committed sympathoadrenal progenitor cell is therefore reflected molecularly in batteries of neuron-specific and chromaffin-specific genes that can be activated or repressed by FGF/NGF and GC. The question thus is how this repertoire first becomes established in the pro-

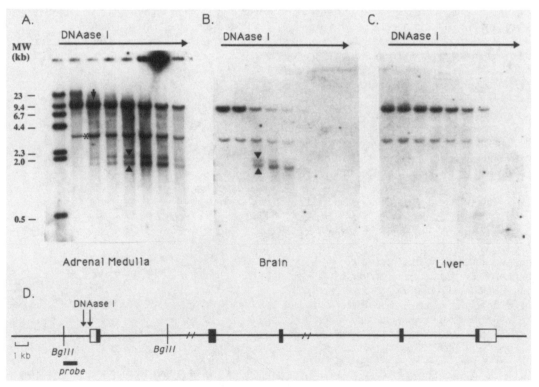

Figure 8. Identification of two DNase 1 HSS in the SCG10 gene that are lineage-specific. (*A*, *B*, *C*) Southern blots of DNase-1-digested, *Bgl*II-restricted genomic DNA from adult AM (*A*), E18 brain (*B*), and liver (*C*). The two HSS are indicated by the presence of the two subbands running at 1.8 and 2 kb (*A* and *B*, arrowheads). The arrow pointing down indicates the 8-kb *Bgl*II parent band (*A*). The faint band at ~3 kb (asterisk) represents cross-hybridization of the probe to the immediately upstream *Bgl*II fragment, due to a repeat sequence. (*D*) Schematic illustrating the location of the sites in the SCG10 gene. (■) Coding exons; (□) noncoding exons. The complete intron-exon organization of this gene has not been determined. Vertical lines demarcate the 8-kb *Bgl*II parent band containing the HSS. The size and location of the probe are indicated. (Reprinted, with permission, from Vandenbergh et al. 1989.)

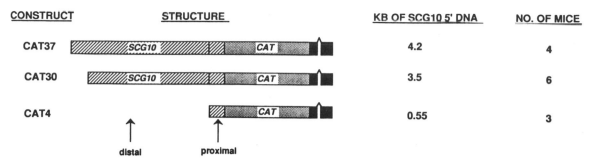

CONSTRUCT	STRUCTURE	KB OF SCG10 5' DNA	NO. OF MICE
CAT37		4.2	4
CAT30		3.5	6
CAT4		0.55	3

Figure 9. Schematic illustrating SCG10-CAT gene fusion constructs used to generate transgenic mice. The "proximal" region in CAT4 extends from a *Pvu*II site in the 5'-untranslated region of the mRNA to an *Eco*RI site ~0.5 kb upstream. The distal region in CAT37 contains an additional 3.7 kb of 5'-flanking DNA. CAT30 is 0.7 kb shorter than CAT37 at its 5' end. The number of independent integrants generated for each construct is indicated. For each integrant, between 1 and 30 copies of the gene were present. (Reprinted, with permission, from Wuenschell et al. 1990.)

genitor cell. The determination of this repertoire is presumably closely related to the commitment of early neural crest cells to the sympathoadrenal sublineage.

Both FGF and GC are factors that exert a broad range of effects on cells of different lineages through the activation of transcription factors. In the case of GC, the receptor itself is a transcription factor (Chandler et al. 1983); in the case of FGF (and NGF), the receptors activate transcription factors indirectly via second messenger pathways (Sheng and Greenberg 1990). The specificity of action of these factors on cells of a given lineage must therefore be determined, at least in part, by the set of target genes that their corresponding transcription factors can activate or repress. One mechanism that has been proposed to account for the selectivity of target gene activation is the accessibility of such genes to transcription factors in chromatin (Robins et al. 1982; Burch and Weintraub 1983). According to this view, the repertoire of fates available to a sympathoadrenal progenitor cell would be established as a set of genes maintained in a chromatin configuration accessible to transcription factors activated by FGF and/or GC (Anderson and Axel 1985).

As an initial test of this hypothesis, we examined the chromatin structure of a neuron-specific gene that can be induced by FGF or NGF in sympathoadrenal cells. This gene, SCG10, encodes a 22-kD vesicle-associated protein that accumulates in the growth cones of developing and regenerating neurons (Stein et al. 1988b). We examined SCG10 chromatin structure in adult adrenal chromaffin cells because these cells retain the capacity to transdifferentiate into neurons in response to FGF or NGF, and because SCG10 is induced during this transdifferentiation (Anderson and Axel 1985). As an index of an accessible or "open" chromatin structure, we used the well-established criterion of sensitivity to digestion by DNase I (Gross and Garrard 1988).

We found that SCG10 exhibits a specific pattern of DNase I hypersensitivity in the nuclei of adult chromaffin cells (Vandenbergh et al. 1989). This pattern, marked by two cleavage sites in the promoter region of the gene (Fig. 8A), is also found in neurons expressing high levels of SCG10 (Fig. 8B) but not in nonneuronal

cells (Fig. 8C). Thus, these hypersensitive sites appear to define a state of the SCG10 gene that is characteristic of both neurons and chromaffin cells and is therefore independent of whether or not the gene is expressed at high levels. We anticipate but have not yet proven that these sites appear in ontogeny at the time that neural crest cells initially commit to the sympathoadrenal lineage, since this is the earliest time that the SCG10 gene is detectably transcribed (Anderson and Axel 1986). The persistence of this DNase-sensitive chromatin structure in adult chromaffin cells, moreover, could in part account for the phenotypic plasticity exhibited by these cells (Vandenbergh et al. 1989).

To gain further insight into the mechanisms controlling the assembly of this state of the SCG10 gene, we

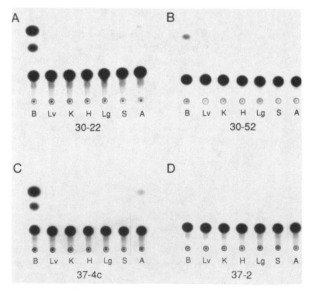

Figure 10. Neuron-specific expression of CAT37 and CAT30 in transgenic mice. Two representative integrants for CAT30 (*A, B*) and CAT37 (*C, D*) are shown. CAT enzymatic activity was assayed using 50 μg of protein from the indicated adult tissues: (B) brain; (Lv) liver; (K) kidney; (H) heart; (Lg) lung; (S) spleen; (A) adrenal gland. (*A, B*) 40 μg of adrenal gland protein was used. Note that in the two lines expressing the highest levels of CAT in brain (*A, C*) a low level of expression is also detected in the adrenal gland. (Reprinted, with permission, from Wuenschell et al. 1990.)

have examined the formation of the hypersensitive sites in transgenic mice (Wuenschell et al. 1990). We generated several mice containing varying lengths of SCG10 5'-flanking DNA fused to the heterologous reporter gene CAT (bacterial chloramphenicol acetyltransferase) (Fig. 9). All of these gene fusion constructs contained the proximal region of the SCG10 promoter to which the DNase-I-hypersensitive sites map in the endogenous gene. However, these constructs varied in the amount of SCG10 DNA lying upstream of this region (Fig. 9).

We found that 3.5 kb of SCG10 5'-flanking DNA appeared sufficient to reconstitute correctly the pattern of endogenous SCG10 gene expression, at least at the gross tissue level (Wuenschell et al. 1990). A high level of transcription was detected in brain tissue, a very low level in adrenal gland tissue, and no expression in various nonneuronal tissues (Fig. 10). Importantly, in these mice, the two DNase-hypersensitive sites formed in their characteristic position in the transgene in a neuron-specific manner (Fig. 11C,D) (Vandenbergh et al. 1989). Surprisingly, deletion of the distal region of the SCG10 5'-flanking DNA (Fig. 9, CAT4) resulted in deregulated expression of the transgene (Fig. 12A–C). In these mice, moreover, the hypersensitive sites formed in their characteristic position in liver, an inappropriate tissue, as well as in brain tissue (Fig. 11A,B).

These results suggested that the two hypersensitive sites reflect a state of the SCG10 gene that can, in principle, form in any cell type. The formation of this state is apparently blocked in nonneuronal cells by sequences lying upstream of the proximal hypersensitive region. In an independent set of transient expression experiments (Mori et al. 1990), we showed that this upstream region has the properties of a silencer, which strongly suppresses transcription from the SCG10 promoter in nonneuronal, but not in neuronal-cell lines (Fig. 13). This silencer, moreover, can act in an orientation-independent and relatively position-insensitive manner to suppress transcription from a heterologous promoter as well (Fig. 14).

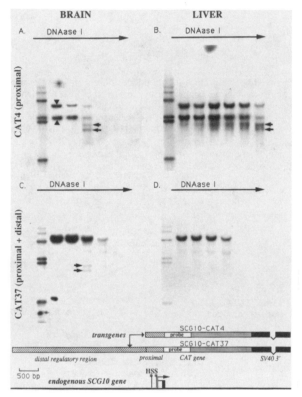

Figure 11. Formation of the HSS in transgenic mice containing SCG10-CAT gene fusion constructs. The HSS were assayed in the brains (A, C) and livers (B, D) of two transgenic mice expressing either the transgene SCG10-CAT4 (A, B) or SCG10-CAT37 (C, D). The structure of these two gene fusion constructs relative to the endogenous SCG10 gene is illustrated below the Southern blots. Note that the twin HSS map within the proximal regulatory region contained within both transgene constructs. CAT4 (A, B), which contains only the 450-bp proximal regulatory region, contains the HSS in both tissues (A, B, horizontal arrows). CAT37 (C, D), which contains the entire 4-kb 5' region of SCG10, is expressed in brain nuclei but not liver nuclei and contains the HSS only in brain nuclei (C, horizontal arrows). The band at ~3 kb reflects a weak HSS that is also present in the endogenous gene but is not tissue-specific (data not shown). The probe used (schematic) contains only CAT coding DNA and therefore detects only the transgene on these Southern blots. Two parent bands are detected in the CAT4 mouse (A, B, arrowheads) due to the tandem ligation of two copies of the transgene. A single band is detected for the CAT37 mouse. (Reprinted, with permission, from Vandenbergh et al. 1990.)

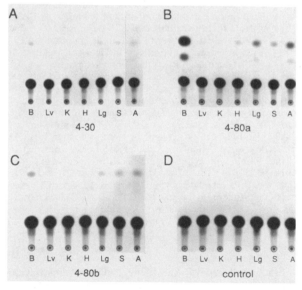

Figure 12. SCG10-CAT constructs lacking the distal silencer region exhibit deregulated expression in transgenic mice. Shown are CAT assays from three different integrants harboring the CAT4 construct in A, B, and C, respectively. In D, a nontransgenic control is shown. Tissue abbreviations are the same as those in Fig. 10. Note that varying levels of CAT activity can be detected in some or all nonneuronal tissues in all three transgenic mice. Quantitative analysis of such assays indicates that despite their loss of tight tissue specificity, the relative level of CAT activity is always highest in brain tissue for each mouse (Wuenschell et al. 1990).

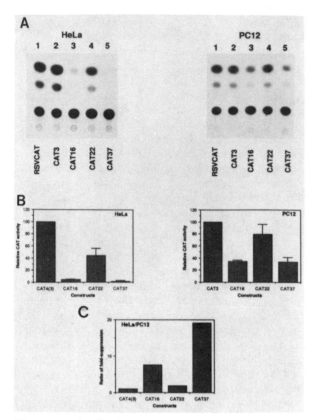

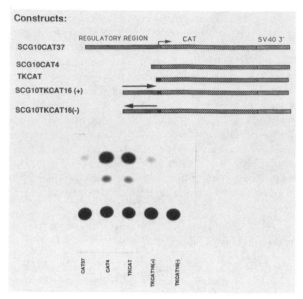

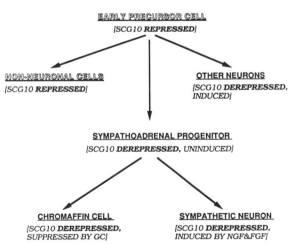

Figure 13. Identification of a constitutive enhancer in the proximal region and of a cell-preferred silencer in the distal region. (*A*) Representative CAT enzymatic activity assays from an experiment in which the indicated constructs were transfected into HeLa and PC12 cells, in parallel. CAT3 contains the promoter-proximal region and is similar to CAT4 (Fig. 9). Note that the activity of CAT3 is comparable to that of RSV-CAT in both HeLa and PC12 cells, and that CAT37 and CAT16 are strongly suppressed in HeLa cells relative to CAT3. (*B*) Quantification of the suppression activity. CAT activity was normalized to that of the cotransfected internal control plasmid, pRSV*lacZ*. The activity of CAT3 (or CAT4) was set at 100%, and the fractional activity shown by the other constructs was calculated. The data shown are the mean ± range of two independent experiments. (*C*) Suppression by CAT37 and CAT16 is stronger in HeLa cells than in PC12 cells. Fold suppression was calculated for each construct in each cell line as the reciprocal of the activity relative to CAT3 (from *B* above). The ratio of this value for HeLa and PC12 cells was then calculated. Thus, for example, CAT37 is suppressed 55-fold in HeLa cells and 2.8-fold in PC12 cells (relative to CAT3), so the ratio of fold suppression is 19.4. (Reprinted, with permission, from Mori et al. 1990.)

Figure 14. Orientation-independent inhibition of transcription from a heterologous promoter by the SCG10 silencer element. The constructs shown were assayed by transient transfection in HeLa cells. TKCAT contains the HSV TK promoter to position −109 (McKnight and Kingsbury 1982). SCG10CAT 16(+) contains 1.6 kb of SCG10 DNA located immediately upstream of the proximal promoter-enhancer region contained in CAT4 (for details, see Mori et al. 1990). Note that in either orientation, this DNA suppresses transcription from the TK promoter.

Figure 15. Model to suggest the role of the silencer element during neuronal lineage diversification. Early neuroepithelial precursor cells maintain the SCG10 gene in a repressed state. With the appearance of committed sympathoadrenal progenitor cells, the gene becomes derepressed as a result of functional inactivation of the silencer. Such a derepression also occurs in other neuronal lineages. In nonneuronal lineages, SCG10 remains in a repressed state. Later in sympathoadrenal development, the gene is either further induced by FGF and NGF in sympathetic neurons or suppressed by GC in adrenal chromaffin cells. This induction or suppression is superimposed on the derepressed state of the gene. Note that cells indicated in white letters are those in which the silencer is active; those indicated in black are cells in which the silencer is inactive. (Reprinted, with permission, from Mori et al. 1990.)

Since deletion of the silencer permits an SCG10 transgene to assume an accessible chromatin configuration in an inappropriate tissue, it is reasonable to conclude that the endogenous gene acquires this configuration during normal development because of the loss or inactivation of proteins that interact with the silencer. Thus, the open state of the SCG10 gene in sympathoadrenal progenitors may reflect the fact that this gene has undergone a specific derepression event (Fig. 15). It is not clear whether this derepression occurs by an actual "opening" of chromatin or simply by the relief from a repression imposed by sequence-specific silencer-binding factors. Whatever the case, we imagine that such a derepression is a prerequisite for the subsequent modulation (Stein et al. 1988a) of SCG10 expression by FGF/NGF and GC. It is likely, however, that the acquisition of such a derepressed state is insufficient to confer full regulatability on these genes. Progenitor cells must also acquire receptors for FGF and NGF, as well as signal-transduction components and transcription factors that specifically interact with the SCG10 gene in its derepressed state. Nevertheless, we believe that the derepression of SCG10 may define an important developmental step, in which an apparently cell-intrinsic mechanism affects the genomic response of a progenitor cell to a set of specific environmental influences. An understanding of the mechanism of SCG10 derepression may therefore yield insights into the molecular basis for the segregation of neural crest cells into the sympathoadrenal and other neuronal sublineages.

ACKNOWLEDGMENTS

Some of the work described in this paper was supported by National Institutes of Health (NIH) grant NS-23476, Searle Scholars and National Science Foundation Presidential Young Awards to D.J.A., and a U.S.-Israeli Binational Science Foundation grant to R.S. We thank LiChing Lo and Steven Padilla for technical assistance and Helen Walsh for preparation of the manuscript. We are also grateful to our colleagues Paul Patterson and Barbara Wold for frequent helpful discussions. S.J.B. was supported by a Damon Runyon-Walter Winchell postdoctoral fellowship and D.J.V. and C.W.W. by NIH fellowships.

REFERENCES

Anderson, D.J. 1988. Cell fate and gene expression in the developing neural crest. *NATO ASI Ser. H* **22:** 188.
———. 1989. The neural crest cell lineage problem: Neuropoiesis? *Neuron* **3:** 1.
Anderson, D.J. and R. Axel. 1985. Molecular probes for the development and plasticity of neural crest derivatives. *Cell* **42:** 649.
Anderson, D.J. and R. Axel. 1986. A bipotential neuroendocrine precursor whose choice of cell fate is determined by NGF and glucocorticoid. *Cell* **47:** 1079.
Baroffio, A., E. Dupin, and N.M. Le Douarin. 1988. Clone-forming ability and differentiation potential of migratory neural crest cells. *Proc. Natl. Acad. Sci.* **85:** 5325.
Birren, S.J. and D.J. Anderson. 1990. A v-*myc*-immortalized sympathoadrenal progenitor cell line in which neuronal differentiation is initiated by FGF but not NGF. *Neuron* **4:** 189.
Bronner-Fraser, M. and S. Fraser. 1989. Developmental potential of avian trunk neural crest cells in situ. *Neuron* **3:** 755.
Burch, J.B.E. and H. Weintraub. 1983. Temporal order of chromatin structure changes associated with activation of the major chicken vitellogenin gene. *Cell* **33:** 65.
Chandler, V.L., B.A. Maler, and K.R. Yamomoto. 1983. DNA sequences bound specifically by glucocorticoid receptor in vitro render a heterologous promoter hormone responsive in vivo. *Cell* **33:** 489.
Claude, P., I.M. Parada, K.A. Gordon, P.A. D'Amore, and J.A. Wagner. 1988. Acidic fibroblast growth factor stimulates adrenal chromaffin cells to proliferate and to extend neurites, but is not a long-term survival factor. *Neuron* **1:** 783.
Cochard, P., M. Goldstein, and I. Black. 1979. Initial development of the noradrenergic phenotype in automatic neuroblasts of the rat embryo in vivo. *Dev. Biol.* **71:** 100.
Coughlin, M.D. and M.D. Collins. 1985. Nerve growth factor-independent development of embryonic mouse sympathetic neurons in dissociated cell culture. *Dev. Biol.* **110:** 392.
Davies, A.M., C. Bandtlow, R. Heumann, S. Korsching, H. Rohrer, and H. Thoenen. 1987. The site and timing of nerve growth factor (NGF) synthesis in developing skin in relation to its innervation by sensory neurons and their expression of NGF receptors. *Nature* **326:** 353.
Doherty, P., P. Seaton, T. Flanigan, and F.S. Walsh. 1988. Factors controlling the expression of the NGF receptor in PC12 cells. *Neurosci. Lett.* **92:** 222.
Doupe, A.J., S.C. Landis, and P.H. Patterson. 1985a. Environmental influences in the development of neural crest derivatives: Glucocorticoids, growth factors and chromaffin cell plasticity. *J. Neurosci.* **5:** 2119.
Doupe, A.J., P.H. Patterson, and S.C. Landis. 1985b. Small intensely fluorescent (SIF) cells in culture: Role of glucocorticoids and growth factors in their development and phenotypic interconversions with other neural crest derivatives. *J. Neurosci.* **5:** 2143.
Ernsberger, U., D. Edgar, and H. Rohner. 1989. The survival of early chick sympathetic neurons in vitro is dependent on a suitable substrate but independent of NGF. *Dev. Biol.* **135:** 250.
Greene, L.A. and A.S. Tischler. 1976. Establishment of a noradrenergic clonal line of rat adrenal phaeochromocytoma cells which respond to nerve growth factor. *Proc. Natl. Acad. Sci.* **73:** 2424.
Gross, D.S. and W.T. Garrard. 1988. Nuclear hypersensitive sites in chromatin. *Annu. Rev. Biochem.* **57:** 159.
Hébert, J.M., C. Basilico, M. Goldfarb, O. Haub, and G.R. Martin. 1990. Isolation of cDNAs encoding four mouse FGF family members and characterization of their expression patterns during embryogenesis. *Dev. Biol.* (in press).
Holt, C.E., T.W. Bertsch, H.M. Ellis, and W.A. Harris. 1988. Cellular determination in the *Xenopus* retina is independent of lineage and birth date. *Neuron* **1:** 15.
Kalcheim, C. and G. Neufeld. 1990. Expression of basic fibroblast growth factor in the nervous system of early avian embryos. *Development* **109:** 203.
Korsching, S. and H. Thoenen. 1988. Developmental changes of nerve growth factor levels in sympathetic ganglia and their target organs. *Dev. Biol.* **126:** 40.
Leonard, D.G.B., E.B. Ziff, and L.A. Greene. 1987. Identification and characterization of mRNAs regulated by nerve growth factor in PC12 cells. *Mol. Cell. Biol.* **7:** 3156.
McKnight, S.L. and R. Kingsbury. 1982. Transcriptional control signals of a eukaryotic protein-coding gene. *Science* **217:** 316.
Mori, N., R. Stein, O. Sigmund, and D.J. Anderson. 1990. A cell type-preferred silencer element that controls the neural-specific expression of the SCG10 gene. *Neuron* **4:** 583.
Raff, M. C. 1989. Glial cell diversification in the rat optic nerve. *Science* **243:** 1450.
Robins, D.M., I. Paek, P.H. Seeburg, and R. Axel. 1982. Regulated expression of human growth hormone genes in mouse cells. *Cell* **29:** 623.
Seidl, K. and K. Unsicker. 1989. The determination of the adrenal medullary cell fate during embryogenesis. *Dev. Biol.* **136:** 481.
Sheng, M. and M.E. Greenberg. 1990. The regulation and

function of c-*fos* and other immediate early genes in the nervous system. *Neuron* **4:** 477.

Sieber-Blum, M. and A.M. Cohen. 1980. Clonal analysis of quail neural crest cells: They are pluripotent and differentiate *in vitro* in the absence of non crest cells. *Dev. Biol.* **80:** 96.

Stein, R., O. Sigmund, and D.J. Anderson. 1988a. The induction of a neural-specific gene, SCG10, by nerve growth factor in PC12 cells is transcriptional, protein synthesis dependent, and glucocorticoid inhibitable. *Dev. Biol.* **127:** 316.

Stein, R., N. Mori, K. Matthews, L.-C. Lo, and D.J. Anderson. 1988. The NGF-inducible SCG10 mRNA encodes a novel membrane-bound protein present in growth cones and abundant in developing neurons. *Neuron* **1:** 463.

Stemple, D.L., N.K. Mahanthappa, and D.J. Anderson. 1988. Basic FGF induces neuronal differentiation, cell division, and NGF dependence in chromaffin cells: A sequence of events in sympathetic development. *Neuron* **1:** 517.

Turner, D.H. and C. Cepko. 1987. A common progenitor for neurons and glia persists in rat retina late in development. *Nature* **328:** 131.

Unsicker, K., B. Drisch, J. Otten, and H. Thoenen. 1978. Nerve growth factor-induced fiber outgrowth from isolated rat adrenal chromaffin cells: Impairment by glucocorticoids. *Proc. Natl. Acad. Sci.* **75:** 3498.

Vandenbergh, D.J., C.W. Wuenschell, N. Mori, and D.J. Anderson. 1989. Chromatin structure as a molecular marker of cell lineage and developmental potential in neural crest-derived chromaffin cells. *Neuron* **3:** 507.

Wetts, R. and S.E. Fraser. 1988. Multipotent precursors can give rise to all major cell types of the frog retina. *Science* **239:** 1142.

Wuenschell, C.W., N. Mori, and D.J. Anderson. 1990. Analysis of SCG10 gene expression in transgenic mice reveals that neural specificity is achieved through selective derepression. *Neuron* **4:** 595.

Studies of Cortical Development Using Retrovirus Vectors

C.L. CEPKO,* C.P. AUSTIN,*† C. WALSH,*† E.F. RYDER,*
A. HALLIDAY,*‡ AND S. FIELDS-BERRY*

*Harvard Medical School, Department of Genetics, Boston, Massachusetts 02115; †Department of Neurology, and ‡Department of Neurosurgery, Massachusetts General Hospital, Boston, Massachusetts 02114

Precise descriptions of patterns of cell division, migration, and differentiation provide a logical foundation for understanding the molecular genetics of these processes. Model systems such as *Caenorhabditis elegans* and *Drosophila melanogaster* have illustrated this concept regarding the developing nervous system. Isolation and characterization of genes that mediate cellular determination have been greatly facilitated by detailed knowledge of cell behavior during development of invertebrates. To characterize analogous genes in vertebrates, equally precise descriptions of neural development are needed.

Progress has been made in describing patterns of neural cell division and cell lineage in some vertebrate systems in recent years. Methods that allow the labeling of neural progenitor cells directly, such as dye microinjection (Wetts and Fraser 1988) and retrovirus-mediated gene transfer (for discussion, see Price 1987; Cepko 1988; Sanes 1989) have shown that neural progenitors in the retina (Turner and Cepko 1987; Holt et al. 1988; Wetts and Fraser 1988; Turner et al. 1990) and tectum (Gray et al. 1988; Galileo et al. 1990) are multipotential: Many types of neurons, as well as glial cells, can be produced from single progenitor cells even at late stages of neurogenesis. This suggests that lineage itself does not determine cell fate and that fate may reflect environmental interactions that remain as yet poorly understood. These same studies have shown that the migratory patterns of retinal and tectal neurons are remarkably constrained: With few exceptions, clonally related cells remain adjacent or follow carefully orchestrated migratory paths. Similar studies in the mammalian cerebral cortex, on the other hand, have suggested slightly different developmental rules and have pushed the limits of present labeling methods. This paper discusses our understanding of the data obtained to date using retroviral vectors to investigate cortical development, and it illustrates the impetus for further refining our tools.

Like the retina and the tectum, the cerebral cortex forms a fairly uniform sheet that is highly structured in two orthogonal planes. Parallel to the pial surface are six laminae; cells in each lamina share similar morphology, transmitter characteristics, and afferent and efferent connections. Perpendicular to the six laminae, the cortex is organized on functional grounds. Columns of neurons share responsiveness to stimuli in precise regions of the body surface, auditory space, or visual space (for examples, see Hubel and Weisel 1962; Mountcastle 1979). Arrays of columns form spatially distinct areas of the cortex that subserve particular functions. Each of these areas tends to show a characteristic specialization in the laminar pattern of neurons; these local variations make up the "cytoarchitectonic" map of the cortex (Brodmann 1909; Caviness 1975).

Unlike several other brain regions, neurons in the developing cortex are not produced in their adult locations but migrate across several cell layers which anticipate the laminae of the mature cortex (Boulder Committee 1970). Cortical neurons, generated primarily in the ventricular zone (VZ), migrate via radial glial fibers through the intermediate zone (IZ), an area composed of afferent and efferent processes and migrating cells. Ultimately, most cells arrest migration in one of two laminae composed of densely packed cells, the subplate (SP) or cortical plate (CP), whereas a final uppermost layer, the marginal zone (MZ), contains few cells at all stages of development. Whereas the SP is a transient structure thought to provide a scaffold for cortical development (Shatz et al. 1988 and this volume), the CP progressively enlarges to form most of the adult cortex.

The long migration of cortical neurons along radial glial fibers raises several possibilities concerning the generation of cortical organization relative to this migration. One possibility is that the cytoarchitectonic map of the cortex derives from a "proto-map" among cortical progenitors within the VZ (Reznikov et al. 1984; Rakic 1988; Leise 1990). The translation of this proto-map onto the developing CP could occur via migration of related cells along tightly circumscribed paths described by juxtaposed radial glial cells. Another possibility is that neurons remain fairly uncommitted until reaching their final destination, with commitment being the result of environmental interactions within the IZ and/or CP.

Experiments designed to test such hypotheses directly, in which newly postmitotic cells were challenged with a change in their environment, have suggested that cellular commitment is a complex, multistage process. Commitment to a laminar fate appears to occur near the time that a cell becomes postmitotic (McConnell 1988, 1991). On the other hand, commitment to particular functional domains and cytoarchitectonic areas appears to be a later process, dependent on interactions with environmental components, perhaps including thalamic afferents or other cortical cells (O'Leary and Stanfield 1989; Schlagger and O'Leary 1988; O'Leary 1989; Shatz et al., this volume). Experiments using a different approach, in which tetraparental mice were used to examine mixing of progenitor cells during the formation of cortical structures, have similarly led to the suggestion that a considerable amount of mixing occurs during the formation of these structures (Goldowitz 1987; Crandall and Herrup 1990).

A careful description of cell interactions during neurogenesis and neuronal migration in the cortex, using marking techniques that label cortical progenitors and their progeny, can provide important insights into these processes. One marking technique successfully used in the vertebrate central nervous system (CNS) employs a replication-incompetent retroviral vector, discussed in several recent reviews (Price 1987; Cepko 1988; Sanes 1989). Retroviral vectors can stably and genetically tag cells via integration of an easily assayable histochemical marker gene. Whereas lineage studies in several parts of the CNS provided fairly simple and reproducible patterns of label, which were straightforward to interpret, the rodent cerebral cortex has been harder to analyze presumably because of the complexity of cortical cell generation, migration, and specification. Some investigators have emphasized that clonally related cortical neurons remain radially arrayed, even in the adult animal (Luskin et al. 1988), whereas others have reported variable degrees of spatial dispersion (Price and Thurlow 1988; Walsh and Cepko 1988; Austin and Cepko 1990). Reconciliation of these differing results has been difficult because of utilization of different experimental animals, vectors, timing of infection and harvest, and methods of analysis of labeled cells in the cortex.

We are pursuing analysis of cortical lineage using retroviruses in several different ways. One approach is to use the current technology as systematically and quantitatively as possible to study the migration patterns and spatial relationships of retrovirally labeled cells in the developing mouse cerebral cortex. A large number of animals have been infected at an early point in neocortical histogenesis and have been harvested at 2, 3, 4, and 6 days postinfection. Quantitative analysis and computer-assisted three-dimensional reconstruction of all labeled cells in the developing cortex at multiple early time points have been carried out (Austin and Cepko 1990).

Two other approaches are being pursued. One is the development of retroviral vectors that encode distinct histochemical marker genes. We anticipate that this strategy will yield two to four distinguishable histochemical tags that can be used simultaneously. This will enable determination of clonal boundaries where the degree of migration is fairly moderate. In situations where the degree of migration is extensive, the number of distinct viral tags will need to be fairly large (e.g., > 4) in order to make definitive clonal boundary assign-

ments. To this end, we are developing a library of lacZ-encoding retrovirus vectors carrying inserts of 10–400 bp. Each member of this library will be identified using the polymerase chain reaction (PCR). Together, these approaches should enable an understanding of the migration patterns and lineal relationships among cortical cells.

EXPERIMENTAL PROCEDURES

The general approach is to infect progenitor cells with a replication-incompetent retrovirus vector that encodes a gene whose product can be assayed histochemically in infected tissue. The BAG retrovirus has proven to be quite useful in this regard (Price et al. 1987). BAG encodes and expresses two genes, the *Escherichia coli lacZ* gene and the Tn5 *neo* gene. *lacZ* encodes β-galactosidase (β-Gal), an enzyme that has been widely used to tag cells. Its popularity is due to several features. A substrate, 5-bromo-4-chloro-3-indolyl-β-D-galactosidase (X-Gal), which can be applied to whole mounts or tissue sections, forms a blue precipitate upon hydrolysis in situ. In addition, β-Gal does not seem to affect development or activity of cells, even though it is often expressed at a high level.

BAG virus is produced by transfection of the BAG plasmid into murine fibroblasts that encode all of the genes necessary for production of a virus capsid (for methodological details, see Cepko 1989). Supernatants of such "packaging cells" contain infectious BAG virions, which are quantitated by infection of mouse fibroblasts in vitro. Virions are then concentrated by centrifugation, retitered, and tested for the presence of replication-competent helper viruses. Stocks of appropriate titer (e.g., $> 10^6$ cfu/ml) that are free of helper virus are stored indefinitely at $-80°C$.

Infection of cortical progenitors is accomplished by introduction of the virus into the lateral ventricles of midgestation mouse or rat embryos. Viral inoculum, approximately 1 μl, is introduced via insertion of a drawn glass pipette through the uterine wall and into the ventricular system. Pressure is applied and the ventricles can be seen to fill with a dye (e.g., fast green or trypan blue) that is added to the viral inoculum. Animals are sacrificed at intervals beginning at 2 days postinfection and continuing into the adult period. The animal is perfused with paraformaldehyde and either intact brains or cryostat sections are exposed to X-Gal. In certain cases, serial reconstruction of the entire brain has been carried out. CARP software (Biographics, Dallas, Texas) was used to reconstruct the surface of the brain and lateral ventricles and to plot the location of all labeled cells.

RESULTS AND DISCUSSION

Initial Observations of Rat Cortical Cells

Our first series of experiments was performed on midgestation rat embryos (Walsh and Cepko 1988).

The patterns of distribution of labeled cells within the cortex were evaluated after short (3–5 days) and long (>5 days) survival times. It was noted that labeled cells were fairly tightly clustered if examination was performed within several days of infection. However, after long survival times, the labeled cells were separated by variable distances, often >200 μm (Fig. 1). Patterns of label after both short and long survival periods were observed to vary in a regionally specific manner with more radial patterns of migration noted in the medial and dorsal areas relative to the lateral areas.

To determine whether dispersion was an artifact created by selective expression of *lacZ*, which was driven by the long terminal repeat (LTR) promoter of Moloney murine leukemia virus in BAG, alternative constructs were made in which *lacZ* was expressed from cellular promoters (Turner et al. 1990; C. Walsh et al., unpubl.). The rat β-actin promoter and the human histone 4 promoter have been proposed to act as constitutive promoters and were thus chosen for these constructs. In addition, the SV40 early promoter, another promoter observed to have activity in a wide variety of cells, was used. Infection with the constructs containing the cellular promoters resulted in the same overall patterns of labeled cells as seen with BAG (Fig. 1b,c). The SV40 promoter produced the lowest level of label and was difficult to interpret (data not shown).

We also addressed the issue of whether replication-competent "helper" virus, which is capable of promoting horizontal spread of the vectors, could be the cause of the dispersed pattern of label. Stocks were examined for the presence of helper virus using an assay capable of detecting very few (1–10) wild-type particles within the injected inoculum and were found to be negative. Moreover, the virus encoding the histone promoter was crippled in such a way as to prohibit transmission after the first round of infection (Cone et al. 1987). This vector thus could not be spread even if wild-type virus had been present. As mentioned above and shown in Figure 1c, the vector encoding the histone promoter yielded the same pattern of label as the other vectors.

It was of interest to determine which cell types were distributed in the various patterns observed after both short and long survival periods. In embryonic material, cells do not exhibit morphologies indicative of their eventual fate. However, in neonatal and adult material, many cells exhibited "Golgi-like" labeling, allowing distinct cell types to be identified. The most dispersed cells frequently appeared to be neurons (Fig. 2a–c). However, a rather curious lack of uniformity was noted regarding the filling of processes. As shown in Figure 2b, cells with well-filled processes could be seen quite close to cells with no staining of their processes. This may reflect a cell-type restriction in transport of β-Gal

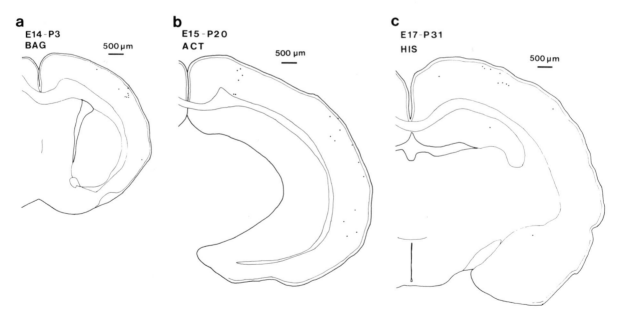

Figure 1. Camera lucida drawings representing cells labeled by expression of β-Gal from different promoters. All plotted cells were identified as presumptive neurons. Each drawing represents a superimposition of up to 11 consecutive coronal sections, each 90-μm thick and covering about 1 mm rostrocaudally. Groups were chosen for illustration because they were well separated from other labeled cells. Age of infection and harvest are as indicated in each panel. (*a*) Cells in the brain of a rat infected with BAG virus (Price et al. 1987) in which the viral LTR directs expression of β-Gal. Some labeled cells are single, whereas others form a loosely organized cluster covering 500 μm mediolaterally and about the same distance rostrocaudally. (*b*) Cells from a rat infected with the ACT virus (Turner et al. 1990) in which the rat β-actin promoter directs expression of β-Gal. A group of cells in the dorsomedial cortex forms a radial array covering about 200 μm—unusually close spacing in our material. Most labeled neurons are more widely separated from one another, as seen in more lateral parts of this cortex. (*c*) Cells from a brain infected with the HIS virus (Turner et al. 1990) in which the human histone 4 promoter is used to express the β-Gal. Labeled cells tend to be more superficial in the cortex following these later injections. Using this vector, labeled cortical cells were also usually single or arranged in groups that cover hundreds of microns.

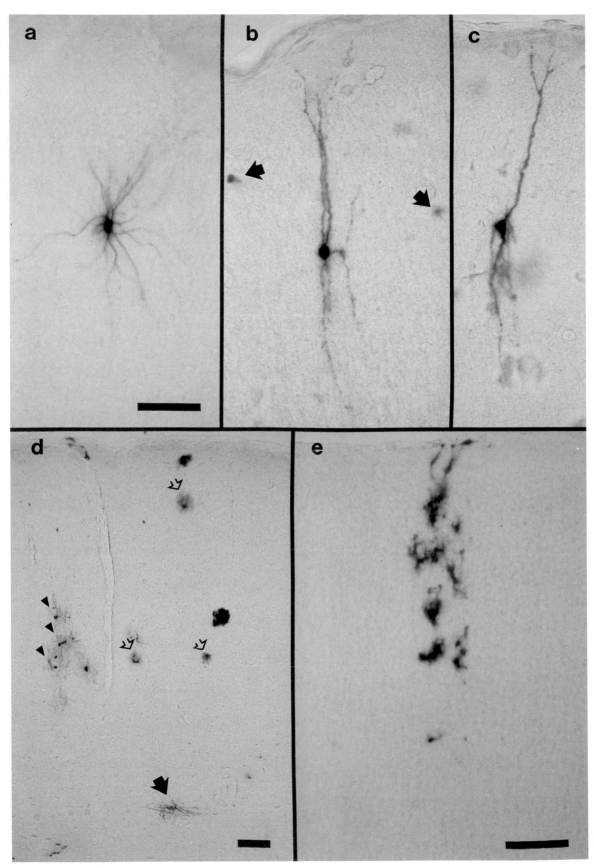

Figure 2. (*See facing page for legend.*)

to processes, but additional factors may come into play as well. Deeply stained cell soma, with no process filling, were especially common when any of the alternative, non-LTR, promoters were used, and may reflect some aspect of the mRNA structure. In contrast, glial processes were observed to stain regardless of the promoter used.

Whereas cells with neuronal morphology were often quite dispersed, cells exhibiting glial morphology were fairly tightly clustered and, as expected, were not identifiable until the postnatal period (Fig. 2d,e). The putative glial clusters, observed within gray or white matter, were often quite extensive and contained cells of varied morphologies (Ryder et al. 1988). Occasionally, a single, extensive group was seen in both gray and white matter. When in the white matter, clusters with glial morphology were sometimes distributed in patterns oriented along the axes of the white matter tract. Such patterns were seen in animals injected postnatally and in animals injected with extremely low doses of virus. Since the retrovirus can only integrate and express in cells that are mitotic, the observation of labeled cells from postnatal inoculation also suggests that these cells were glia; neuronal birthdays are complete by the end of gestation, and thus their progenitors cannot be infected postnatally.

The above observations led us to propose that neurons did not follow tightly circumscribed paths to the CP. The extent of the dispersion also made the hypothesis that there was a lineage basis for the allocation of cells to discrete cytoarchitectonic domains untenable, since cells were not found grouped in restricted domains of 30–380 μm, the range reported for cytoarchitectonic domains in rodents (for summary, see Liese 1990). This led us to propose that lineage was not an underlying mechanism for the development of discrete functional domains in the cortex. However, since there was so much dispersion, we were unable to assign clonal boundaries and report the precise location of clonally related cells within the CP or the exact nature of the final lineal relationships among neurons or between neurons and glia.

Quantitative Analysis of Mouse Cortical Cells

As the initial studies of rat cortex suggested that migration patterns varied in a regionally specific manner, we initiated a systematic and quantitative study of the migration patterns of cortical cells (Austin and Cepko 1990). Mice were used since their brains are approximately one half the size of rat brains and thus comprise fewer sections.

The lateral ventricles of embryonic day 12 (E12) mice were infected with a constant amount of BAG virus. Animals were then sacrificed at E14 ($n = 11$), E15 ($n = 11$), E16 ($n = 12$), E18 ($n = 15$), postnatal day 3 (P3; $n = 7$), P11 ($n = 2$), and P35 ($n = 2$). Coronal cryostat sections (90 μm) of the brain were stained with X-Gal, and all blue cortical cells ($n > 5000$) were recorded.

To provide some framework for a quantitative analysis of the large number of labeled cells, an algorithm for grouping cells was developed. Although the algorithm leads to an oversimplification of the continuum of patterns that were observed, it provides a rough description of reproducible patterns and their frequency. For purposes of categorization of cellular location, the developing cerebral wall was divided into four mediolateral areas ("domains") using easily identifiable and reproducible landmarks (Fig. 3). Since sections were not counterstained and most of the tissue was from embryos, no attempt was made to correlate these four domains with the more limited and rigorously defined cytoarchitectonic areas present in the adult (Caviness 1975). Inventory was then taken of all cells in the neocortex, as defined by Caviness (1975). An algorithm for grouping cells was designed on the basis of these preliminary observations.

Cells were designated as a "group" using the following criteria: (1) The cells were on the same or adjacent sections; (2) they were in the same or adjacent of the four mediolateral cortical domains; and (3) not more than one source in the VZ from which the cells emanated could be identified. This third criterion was made after it was noted that there did not appear to be lateral displacement of VZ cells, i.e., all labeled VZ cells in close proximity to other labeled VZ cells were either radially aligned or immediately adjacent. If clusters of cells that met the first two criteria were in the vicinity of spatially distinct labeled VZ cells, they were assigned to separate groups, based on which area of the VZ was most likely responsible for their origin. This situation occurred infrequently at all time points, and almost never at E18, since there were few labeled cells in the VZ by this harvest date. Note was made of the number of sections and which mediolateral areas each group occupied.

Statistical analysis of the grouping algorithm. A number of statistical methods were used to determine whether groups of cells were clonally related (for a complete description, see Austin and Cepko 1990). Using the series of mice described above, where infection was at E12 and harvests were at E14–E18, the

---

Figure 2. Photomicrographs illustrating rat neural cells labeled with the BAG virus (Price et al. 1987), taken either from rats injected at E17 and processed as adults (*a,d,e*) or injected at E16 and processed at P10 (*b,c*). (*a*) A stellate cell in layer IV shows Golgi-like filling of its dendrites. Similar staining is seen in immature pyramidal cells in layer III in *b* and *c*. Two other cells in *b* show little or no staining of cell processes (arrows), making identification of cell type impossible. (*d*) A group of labeled glial cells. A wide variety of glial morphologies is represented here, including presumptive oligodendrocytes at the junction of gray and white matter (closed arrow), presumptive astrocytes of the gray matter (open arrows), and presumptive oligodendrocytes in the gray matter (arrowheads). Other cell types are not as darkly stained or are obscured by very dense reaction product. (*e*) A tightly radial cluster of glial cells is seen to be widely separated from other labeled cells. Bars: (*a,b,c*) 50 μm; (*d,e*) 100 μm.

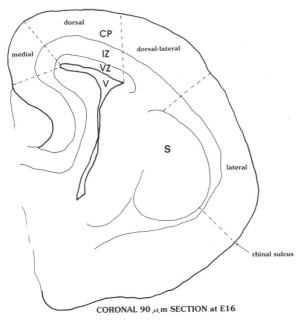

CORONAL 90 μm SECTION at E16

Figure 3. Designations of medial-lateral domains for grouping of labeled cells. Four "domains" of the developing cerebral wall were defined, using easily identifiable and reproducible landmarks. The medial domain extended from the border between the cingulate field and hippocampal formation to a line connecting the medial corner of the ventricle with the apex of the interhemispheric fissure. The dorsal domain extended to a line drawn perpendicular to the pial surface from the lateral corner of the ventricle. The dorsolateral domain extended to a line drawn at a 45° angle between the dorsal surface of the striatum and the pial surface. The lateral domain extended to the rhinal fissure. This example is taken from an E16 brain in coronal section at the level of the striatum. (S) Striatum; (V) ventricle; (VZ) ventricular zone; (IZ) intermediate zone; (CP) cortical plate. (Reprinted, with permission, from Austin and Cepko 1990).

number of cells per group over time and the number of groups over time were quantitated. The number of groups over time was found to be the same, approximately 17 groups per cortex, with no statistical difference among harvest dates, whereas the number of cells per group was observed to increase over time. The means of the number of cells per group were 2.1 (range 1–6) at E14, 3.9 (range 1–11) at E15, 4.1 (range 1–17) at E16, and 6.3 (range 1–35) at E18. Since there are no data that describe the patterns of proliferation of cortical progenitors throughout the period of histogenesis examined here, it is impossible to determine whether these values of group sizes are in agreement with those expected of clonal proliferation. However, one would expect clone size to increase with survival time and clone number to remain the same regardless of survival time. It is interesting to note that the range of group size was fairly broad, much as was observed in the retina (Turner et al. 1990), where the range was 1–234 cells per clone.

Further evidence that most groups were clones was provided by a dilution analysis. An additional 21 animals were injected with serial threefold dilutions of

virus at E12 and were harvested at E16. The number of groups relative to the viral dilution and the number of cells per group at different dilutions were quantitated. These analyses revealed that although the distribution in the number of cells per group was fairly broad, it was independent of virus dose. Moreover, there was a linear relationship between the number of groups and the virus dose.

The quantitative analysis described above can be used to indicate that the majority of group assignments accurately reflect clonal boundaries. An individual group, or rare categories of groups, may or may not represent clones, since the statistical analysis only applies to the majority. The type of analysis used here probably represents the limit of use of a single marker virus for determining clonal boundaries of cortical cells. Further confidence in the identification of clonal boundaries of individual clones, especially those that are rarely observed, will await further advances in the methodology, as described above.

Three-dimensional reconstructions of all neocortical cells.

The locations of all labeled neocortical cells were plotted for three-dimensional reconstruction to appreciate the distribution of labeled cells within the cortex. These reconstructions (not shown because of lack of space, see Austin and Cepko 1990) illustrated several points: (1) Groups were distributed widely throughout both hemispheres, and there was no identifiable injection point; (2) individual groups were easily distinguishable at E14, but the explicit criteria designed to define groups were needed to identify individual groups at later time points; and (3) cells initially appeared to migrate radially out of the ventricular zone, but with increasing time after injection, they became increasingly dispersed in both mediolateral and anteroposterior dimensions, as previously observed in the rat cortex (Walsh and Cepko 1988). Anteroposterior dispersion was greatest at the frontal and occipital poles. Increased anterior-posterior dispersion at the poles is presumably due to the fact that the lateral ventricle, which does not extend to the very rostral and caudal extremes of the cortex, must nonetheless supply cells destined for these areas.

Distribution and morphology of labeled cells.

Characteristic migration patterns could be identified in each cortical area, as demonstrated by camera lucida reconstructions of a small number of sections (Fig. 4). Cellular leading and/or trailing processes provided information as to the probable direction of migration of the cells (Figs. 5 and 6). Migration was inferred from this static material from the cells' appearance, their alignment with respect to the pial and ventricular surfaces, and their distribution further from the ventricle with increasing survival times. A summary of the observed patterns is given below.

In the medial domain, groups were strikingly radial after survival times of 2 and 3 days (Fig. 4a) and in some cases up to 6 days. However, tangential dispersion within the IZ, and to a lesser extent within the CP,

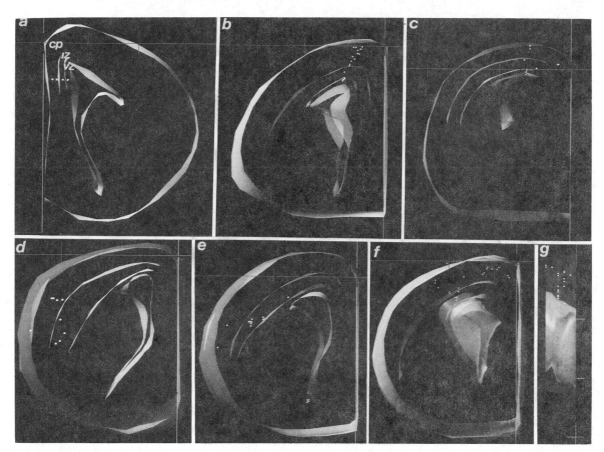

Figure 4. Camera lucida reconstructions of groups in several domains. Animals were infected with BAG at E12 and harvested at the times indicated below. The brain outline, (CP/SP)-IZ border, IZ-(SVZ/VZ) border, and lateral ventricle were traced into the CARP database and reconstructed in three dimensions. These structures are labeled in *a* for reference. In all reconstructions, the dorsoventral and mediolateral axes (appearing as ordinate and abscissa, respectively) with 1-mm hatch marks are displayed for spatial orientation and scale. (*a*) Medial domain; E15 harvest; cells were strictly radially arrayed and restricted to the medial domain. (*b*) Dorsal domain; E18 harvest; cells migrated radially through the VZ and IZ and dispersed approximately 100 μm within the CP. (*c*) Dorsal domain; E16 harvest; after migrating strictly radially through the VZ, cells appear to bifurcate in the IZ to reach different medial-lateral domains of the CP. (*d*) Lateral domain; E15 harvest; two separate paths of migration are evident, leading to wide separation in the CP. (*e*) Lateral domain; E16 harvest; cells migrated tangentially in the IZ but diverged to reach points separated by 300 μm in the CP. (*f,g*) A widely dispersed group occupying medial, dorsal, and dorsolateral domains; E18 harvest; *f* and *g* show coronal and side views, respectively, of all cells in the group; both illustrate that the initial migration out of the VZ was radial and was followed by dispersion of cells in the IZ to allow delivery of cells to widely separated points in the CP. A photograph of a portion of this group is shown in Figure 6f. (Reprinted, with permission, from Austin and Cepko 1990.)

was seen with increasing survival time. By E18, cells in medial domain groups were separated by up to 300 μm in the CP, and only 43% of groups occupying the medial area were restricted to that area alone.

In the dorsal domain, radially aligned cells were also seen here (Figs. 4b and 5a–c), but again they were most common after short survival times. By 4 days after infection (E16), migration parallel to the pial surface (Fig. 5c) and often bifurcation of groups in the IZ (Fig. 4c), and continued more limited spread (of up to 100 μm) in the CP, made nonradial groups increasingly common. By 6 days after infection, cells in the CP were separated by up to 500 μm within the dorsal domain alone, and only 30% of all groups occupying the dorsal area were restricted to this domain.

In the dorsolateral domain, radial migration from the VZ to CP was only occasionally observed. More com-

monly, cells migrated roughly radially, often in single file, only through the dorsolateral VZ, after which they moved laterally in the IZ for a variable distance before turning orthogonal to the pial surface again, to migrate radially through the dorsolateral SP and CP (Fig. 5d). Cells within groups demonstrated great variability in the extent of their lateral migration and consequently arrived in the CP separated by a variety of distances. Spread of cells to other areas was most common in the dorsolateral cortex, with only 21% of groups occupying the dorsolateral areas being restricted to their area of origin by 6 days after infection.

In the lateral domain, there were more cells than in any other single area or combination of areas at every time point beyond E14 because of the large extent of neocortical surface subserved by this designation. Both the distance between the generative region in the dorsal

VZ and the lateral domain and the presence of sub-cortical structures caused labeled cells to follow circuitous and variable paths to their final positions (Fig. 4d,e). Cells typically migrated through the VZ roughly perpendicular to the ventricular surface. In the subventricular zone (SVZ) or IZ, they turned and migrated parallel to the pial surface for up to 500 μm (Fig. 5f), thereafter turning orthogonally to the pial surface once again at the level of the IZ-SP border to migrate radially to the CP. Migration of a group of cells along a single path to the CP was seen only rarely (Fig. 4e). As in the dorsolateral domain, cells much more commonly turned orthogonally at different points over the lateral convexity of the cerebrum to take up positions within the CP that separated by variable distances (Figs. 4d and 5e); 38% of the groups were restricted to the lateral area only by 6 days after infection.

In the combinations of domains, cells within groups sometimes occupied more than one mediolateral area (Fig. 4f,g). Inference of the routes of migration taken by widely dispersed cells was difficult given data from E18 animals alone, but examination of patterns from earlier harvests showed that cells in a group may bifurcate into subgroups in the IZ or become widely separated within the IZ. No evidence for tangential translation of cells within the VZ was seen, and separation in the CP itself was limited to approximately 100 μm.

Quantitation of dispersion. With increasing survival time after infection, the number of groups restricted to a single medial-lateral domain decreased, and the number of groups occupying two, three, or all four domains increased in a stepwise fashion. At E14, 94% of the groups were restricted to one medial-lateral domain; at E16, 73% were restricted; and by E18, 52% were restricted to one domain. By E18, approximately 10% of the groups occupied each of the combinations of two domains, and another 10% occupied the three domains dorsal, dorsolateral, and lateral. Fewer groups occupied the medial domain in combinations with other areas. Groups that contained cells in all four domains were uncommon even at E18 and appeared most frequently at the frontal poles.

Anteroposterior dispersion of cells also increased with survival time but was generally less extensive than dispersion in the mediolateral dimension. At E14, 72% of the groups occupied only one 90 μm section; at E16 and E18, this figure was 46% and 35%, respectively. Although groups occupying a single section remained most common at every time point, by 6 days after injection, more than 15% of groups occupied five or more sections, corresponding to an anteroposterior dispersion of greater than 450 μm.

Relationship of migration patterns to the radial glial system. A great deal of evidence has suggested that radial glia provide support for neuronal migration (Rakic 1972, 1978, 1981; Rakic et al. 1974; for review, see Hatten 1990). The majority of these data have been collected in primates using reagents that have not been effective in defining radial glia in mice. The recent availability of monoclonal antibodies that stain murine radial glial fibers sensitively and specifically has allowed a precise description of these fibers in mice. The relationship of migration patterns observed after retroviral infection and the morphology of the radial glial system can now be addressed. Caviness and colleagues (Gaddiseux et al. 1989, 1990a,b) have shown a regional variation in the path of murine radial glial fibers that corresponds with the patterns of migration described above. Moreover, a correspondence was demonstrated directly by reacting BAG-infected, X-Gal-stained tissue with RC2, a radial glial-specific monoclonal antibody (Misson et al. 1989). In these preparations, the majority of X-Gal$^+$ cells that exhibited an axis of elongation had the same orientation as radial glial fibers within their immediate environment.

The timing of commitment to functional domains. Although the observations discussed above from studies using both mice and rats suggest that the radial glial system provides support for migration, it appears that the radial glial system does not always constrain the migration of sibling cells to a narrow path that leads to strictly circumscribed final locations. The wide variation in migration patterns, and the variable amount of dispersion among sibling cells, suggests that commitment to a particular cytoarchitectonic area or functional domain does not occur within cells of the VZ, an interpretation in agreement with previous results using transplants.

O'Leary and colleagues used heterotopic transplantation of embryonic cortical domains to investigate the timing of commitment to a particular functional domain (for review, see O'Leary 1989; McConnell 1991). When small pieces of presumptive visual cortex were engrafted into the motor cortical area, layer 5 cells exhibited a pattern of connections that they normally lose during development in the visual area (Stanfield and O'Leary 1985; O'Leary and Stanfield 1989). A similar plasticity was noted when the converse transplantation was performed (O'Leary and Stanfield 1989). The patterning of groups of cortical cells also appears to be plastic. When visual cortex was transplanted to the somatosensory area, the graft organized into barrels—the characteristic pattern of layer 4 cells of the somatosensory cortex (Schlagger and O'Leary 1988). The cells within all of these grafts were postmitotic and in many cases postmigratory, arguing for a lack of commitment in progenitor (VZ) cells for these cortical areas.

The timing of commitment to a particular functional domain or cytoarchitectonic area may vary among cortical cells. Although the experiments of O'Leary and colleagues suggest that commitment occurs after migration, migrating cells presumably destined for the limbic system express an antigen, LAMP, specific for cells of that system (Horton and Levitt 1988). Since similar markers are not available for other cortical areas, it is difficult to predict whether the early commitment of cells of the limbic system is unique. However, the fact that commitment to somatosensory and motor cortical areas is not stable until after migration, whereas commitment to a limbic system fate appears to occur when cells begin to migrate, suggests that timing of commitment is variable and may involve multiple steps.

It is worth considering the impact of variation in the timing of commitment on migration patterns. Sibling cells that are committed to an area when they leave the VZ probably follow a particular fascicle or juxtaposed fascicles of radial glia to their final, common destination. Examination of migration patterns reveals that the regions in which this is most likely to occur would be in the dorsal and medial cortex. However, the variability in patterns in these areas indicates that migration of sibling cells to a tightly restricted area does not always occur. Alternatively, sibling cells that become postmitotic and leave the VZ without commitment to an area may distribute in a random manner along the radial glial fibers most accessible to them. In the latter scenario, commitment to an area may occur as cells are

migrating, and it is conceivable that sibling cells become committed at different points during migration. The events leading to commitment may be somewhat stochastic in their timing, so that a cell could become committed to an area as it begins migration, whereas its sibling may become committed after it randomly distributes to an available site within the CP. This difference in timing could result in sibling cells becoming committed to different areas, leading to variable amounts of separation of sibling cells within the CP. It is interesting to speculate that commitment before or during migration may lead a cell to follow a particular path to its destination. Recognition of such a path may entail recognition of specific cues on radial glial cells, although there is presently no evidence that radial glia possess such cues (Hatten 1990). Cells presumably would become interactive with such cues after, but not before, commitment to a particular area.

The lack of precise delivery of sibling cells to fairly limited areas of the CP does not rule out lineage as an

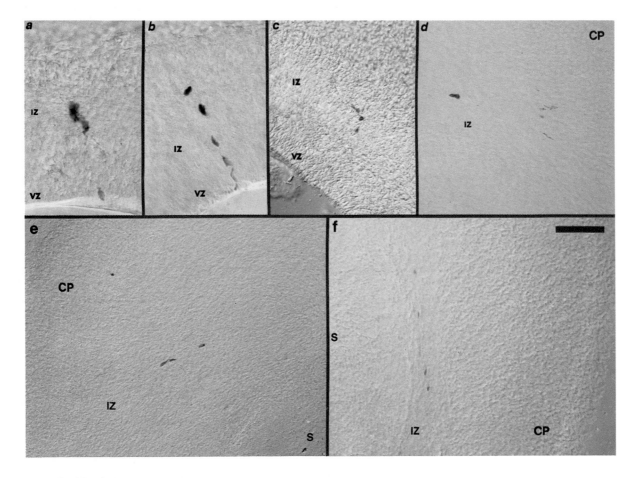

Figure 5. Morphology of migrating cells. Mice were infected at E12 with BAG and harvested at the indicated times. (*a*) E14; dorsal domain; a cell within the VZ and two newly postmitotic cells migrating radially in the IZ are shown. (*b*) E15; dorsal domain; a cell with a ventricular process and three radially migrating cells are shown. (*c*) E16; dorsal domain; three cells are shown migrating within the IZ. The leading cell has a process that is aligned along fibers that run parallel to the pial surface. (*d*) E16; border between dorsolateral and lateral domains; cells can be seen leaving the IZ and entering the CP. (5d Reprinted, with permission, from Austin and Cepko 1990.) (*e*) E15; lateral domain; cells can be seen migrating within the IZ with one cell having left the IZ and having entered the CP earlier than the others. (*f*) E16; lateral domain; migration of four cells within the lateral IZ. Bar: (*a,b*) 50 μm; (*c,d,e,f*) 100 μm.

influence on the development of cortical organization. It appears that functional domains and cytoarchitectonic areas, as they are currently defined, do not develop from a precise proto-map within VZ cells. However, there may be lineage-determined "compartments" that are arrayed along the anterior-posterior axis. This suggestion can be made as there was minor dispersion along this axis compared with that within the medial-lateral plane. Patterns reported in chimeric mice (Goldowitz 1987; Crandall and Herrup 1990) similarly suggest that mixing is not extensive along the anterior-posterior axis. These findings are intriguing in light of recent reports that homeobox and zinc-finger genes in the mouse neural tube appear to be expressed within domains with fairly sharp anterior, and in some cases, posterior borders (Holland and Hogan 1988; Wilkinson et al. 1989). The observed lack of dispersion along the anterior-posterior axis may, on the other hand, simply reflect the array of radial glial fibers (Gadisseux et al. 1989). However, it does appear that cells can switch radial glial fibers during migration (Rakic et al. 1974), and thus there is a possibility for migration along the anterior-posterior axis. Further transplantation experiments will be necessary to determine whether lineage does influence development via the establishment of domains of a different sort than are currently defined on the basis of anatomy and physiology.

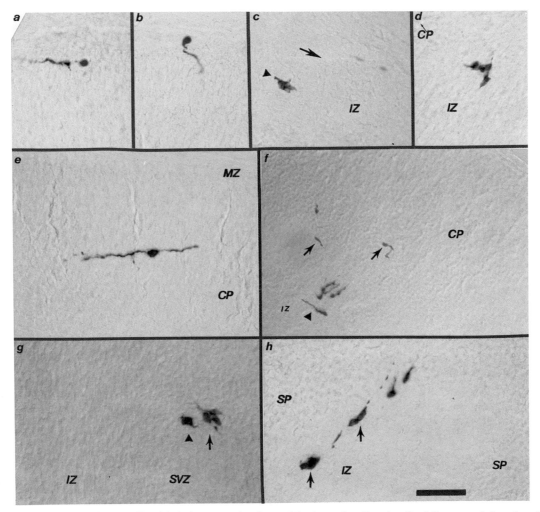

Figure 6. Morphology of MZ cells, tightly juxtaposed cells, and horizontally aligned cells. Mice were infected at E12 and harvested at the indicated times. (*a,b*) E18; dorsolateral domain; MZ cells with the morphology of Cajal-Retzius cells are shown. (*c*) E16; lateral domain; a cluster of five cells (arrowhead) and two well-separated cells are shown in the lateral IZ. An arrow indicates the direction of inferred migration. (*d*) E15; lateral domain; a cluster of four cells within the lateral IZ is shown. The CP is off the photograph in the direction indicated by the arrow. (*e*) E18; dorsal domain; a cell with horizontal processes in the middle of the CP is shown. (*f*) A portion of a group (see camera lucida in Fig. 4f,g) that spans the medial, dorsal, and dorsolateral domain. Several cells are aligned counter to the direction of the radial glial system (arrows) with one cell demonstrating morphology suggestive of a subplate cell (arrowhead). (6f, Reprinted, with permission, from Austin and Cepko 1990.) (*g*) E15; lateral domain (posterior region); a triplet (arrow) and doublet (arrowhead) of cells are shown. (*h*) E18; medial and dorsal domains; a group of cells within the IZ, including two doublets (arrows), migrating along the dorsal-medial border are shown. Bar: (*a–e,g,h*) 50 μm; (*f*) 100 μm.

Analysis of postnatal brains. Seven mouse brains were analyzed after harvest at P3, two were analyzed after harvest at P11, and two were analyzed after harvest at P35. These brains were not included in the quantitative analysis because increased spread of labeled cells, as well as the appearance of large numbers of labeled astrocytes (making up greater than 30% of labeled cells after P11) and oligodendrocytes (appearing at P35 and later) made impossible designations of groups in the manner described. However, it can be concluded from these findings that progenitors for glial cells must be mitotically active at E12, since retroviral integration requires that cells undergo an S phase. It has been shown that radial glial cells, which are mitotically active during this period, undergo a transformation into astrocytes late in embryogenesis and during the neonatal period (Voigt 1989). As described further below, only two cells out of the over 5000 cells observed in mouse embryonic cortex had the morphology of radial glia. Similarly, when RC2- and X-Gal-stained sections were examined, double-stained cells were found to be rare, indicating that the lack of detection of blue radial glia was not simply due to lack of process-filling by β-Gal in these cells. Thus, the majority of glia observed in the postnatal brains were probably not derived from radial glial cells. This observation does not conflict with the fact that radial glia transform into astrocytes; it rather suggests that all astrocytes do not derive from radial glia. However, other explanations, such as inactivity of the promoters within radial glial cells, could also explain the lack of staining of radial glial cells with X-Gal.

Morphology of unusual classes of cells. Although the majority of cells exhibited the morphology of migrating neural cells with leading and trailing processes aligned along the radial glia, several other types of cells were observed as well and are described below.

Clusters of cells closely apposed to each other were commonly seen, usually composed of from two to three cells but up to five cells (Fig. 6c,d,g,h). At each time point, such clusters were evenly distributed throughout each mediolateral domain and were most prevalent in the upper VZ, SVZ, and IZ. These cells probably do not represent transfer of β-Gal or X-Gal among infected and uninfected cells, since cells within each cluster were always equally blue. Moreover, in cases where cells are known to be connected by gap junctions (e.g., rod photoreceptors), single-labeled cells are a very frequent occurrence (Turner and Cepko 1987).

Clusters may be due to an incomplete separation of sibling cells that result from a terminal mitosis in the VZ wherein both daughter cells become postmitotic. Although this may account for some of the two-cell clusters, it cannot be the explanation for all clusters. One group contained four two-cell clusters, and several groups contained greater than two cells. An alternative hypothesis is that they result from cell division outside of the VZ. Cells that incorporate [3H]thymidine in the SVZ (Boulder Committee 1970), as well as IZ and CP

of rat embryos of E20 and older (Altman and Bayer 1990a,b) have been reported. Altman and Bayer (1990a,b) interpret replication in the IZ and CP as that of locally replicating glial cells. The clusters reported here in embryonic mouse tissue may be glial cells or their progenitors, with some mitotic activity occurring earlier in mouse than in rat. However, since clusters contain cells that exhibit a variety of morphologies (Fig. 6c,g,h), no conclusion regarding their eventual fate can be drawn; they may sometimes contain cells that are neurons or their progenitors, whereas at other times they may contain glia or glial progenitors.

In cells within the MZ, cells had either astrocytic morphology or possessed a single, long process that descended tangentially within the MZ or into layer 2 (Fig. 6a,b). These cells were not seen at all at E14, rarely at E15 and E16, and commonly at E18. They were usually part of larger groups that spanned other cortical layers. Neurons found in the MZ, the Cajal-Retzius cells, are reported to be among the earliest-born neocortical cells. The exact timing of their appearance as differentiated cells within the mouse superficial zone has not been reported, and thus it is difficult to determine whether the time of appearance of X-Gal$^+$ MZ cells conforms to that of Cajal-Retzius cells. In the rat neocortex, large, horizontal, differentiated cells appear in the superficial region beginning at E16, and they appear to have their birthdays beginning at E15 (Bayer and Altman 1990). Small-to-medium cells of the superficial zone appear slightly later and reside below the large, earlier-generated cells. Since the cells observed here have a morphology reminiscent of that reported for Cajal-Retzius cells (Marin-Padilla and Marin-Padilla 1982) and appear as differentiated cells relatively early, they most likely belong to this class.

Cells that could be described as "horizontal," either because they had horizontal processes and/or because their cell bodies were horizontally aligned, were occasionally seen within the CP or the IZ. The CP horizontal cells were bipolar, with long, unbranching processes quite reminiscent of those of neurons (Fig. 6e). The identity of these cells is not clear. Those closest to the IZ may be SP cells, although most were not observed in close proximity to the IZ; rather, they were seen at varied depths within the CP. They may represent a transient class and/or a class of neurons that differentiates quite early. Quantitative studies of adult tissue will be necessary to compare their frequency within mature tissue.

Within the IZ, there was a minority of cells ($< 10\%$) that were horizontally aligned, counter to the orientation of fibers of the radial glial system within their immediate environment. As discussed above, the majority of cells exhibited an axis of elongation that was the same as the known direction of radial glial fibers within that locale. Examples of anomalously aligned cells are shown in Figure 6f (also see Fig. 1F in Walsh and Cepko 1988 and Fig. 13E in Austin and Cepko 1990). Such cells were often within close proximity to cells oriented in the more standard fashion, suggestive of alignment along radial glia and with CP cells. Some of these cells are candidates for "subplate" cells, which can reside within the IZ. Others may be of the type described by Altman and Bayer (1990b), which are horizontal cells aligned at either the outer or inner margin of the IZ. They used [³H]thymidine-labeling protocols to suggest that these cells were progenitors of neurons. Our present studies cannot address the ultimate fate of these cells, but they may suggest an interesting exception to the rule of radial-glial-directed migration.

Possible Lineal Relationships among Neurons and Glia

Lineage analyses of rodent retina and chick optic tectum have demonstrated that neurons and glia can have a common progenitor (Turner and Cepko 1987; Wetts and Fraser 1988; Holt et al. 1988; Galileo et al. 1990). In retina, even two-cell clones could contain both a neuron and a Müller glial cell. Moreover, the only clones that contained >1 Müller cell were large clones containing primarily neurons, and these were only observed when infection was early in retinal histogenesis. These observations strongly suggest that there is not a distinct mitotic glial progenitor during normal development of the retina.

Within the cortex, the lineal relationship of neurons and glia has been addressed in studies of progenitors in vitro and in vivo. Cultures of individual, embryonic rat septal cells give rise to both neurons and glia 22% of the time (Temple 1989). Primary cultures of embryonic cortical progenitors have yielded differing results for different groups. One group observed that almost all (99%) clones contained only neurons or only glia (Luskin et al. 1988), whereas another group observed mixtures of several morphological types at a high frequency (Price et al. 1987). Cell lines established from neonatal rodent olfactory bulbs and cerebellum, where neurogenesis and gliogenesis occur during the first few postnatal weeks, are multipotent and produce cells of neuronal and glial phenotype (Frederiksen et al. 1988; Ryder et al. 1990). Interestingly, lines established from neonatal cortex were neither multipotent nor capable of producing neurons but produced only glia (Ryder et al. 1990). Cortex similarly produces only glia during the neonatal period, which was the period from which the lines were established.

When in situ lineage analysis was attempted, the extensive migration of cortical cells made it difficult to define clonal boundaries in adult animals when neuronal and glial morphologies are distinct. However, many examples of neurons and glia that were very closely juxtaposed within adult tissue were observed after infections in the early to mid-period of cortical neurogenesis. Within embryonic tissue, at times when dispersion is not very extensive, occasionally cells with the morphology of radial glia were very close to cells that appeared within the CP or migrating toward the CP (Fig. 7). In such cases, where there is a very low density

of labeled cells throughout the cortex, it is tempting to speculate that the putative radial glial cells and neurons share a common progenitor at E12. Alternatively, since radial glia are mitotic (Levitt et al. 1981; Misson et al. 1988), they may produce neurons during this period of neurogenesis.

Although a definitive resolution of clonal boundaries will be required to determine the relationships among neurons and glia, we favor the following speculative hypothesis. During the embryonic period, progenitors are multipotent (much as suggested by Schaper 1897a,b) and produce primarily postmitotic neurons, presumably because of environmental influences. At a lower rate, they produce glial progenitors that migrate throughout the tissue, including the CP. These committed glial progenitors are envisioned to be almost entirely nonmitotic during the embryonic period but may occasionally divide outside of the VZ. Such infrequent mitoses may account for some of the tightly juxtaposed cells that we observed outside of the VZ. During the postnatal period, a mitotic signal(s) would activate the glial progenitors, causing them to divide

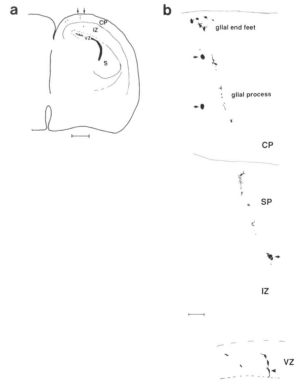

Figure 7. Camera lucida of a group in the dorsal domain of an E16 mouse infected at E12 with BAG virus. Two 90-μm coronal sections from approximately midway through the cortex were superimposed. Section contours are shown at low magnification in *a*. The portion of *a* indicated by arrows is shown at higher magnification in *b*. Cells of varied morphology, suggestive of radial glia (arrowhead indicates the most likely cell body for the radial glial cell), and migrating or postmigratory neurons (arrows) are shown. Four additional cell bodies were observed within the VZ (including the SVZ). Glial-like processes were seen coursing through the sections and terminate in glial end feet within the pial surface and MZ. Bars: (*a*) 400 μm; (*b*) 200 μm.

throughout the tissue and produce the relatively clustered glia that we observed. We thus propose that a committed progenitor that gives rise only to neurons is not present within the VZ, but that the progenitor that gives rise to neurons can also give rise to glia, much as was observed within the retina. A difference between the committed glial progenitor within the cortex and the glial cell within the retina is that the cortical glial progenitor is mitotic during normal development, but the retinal glial cell is mitotic only after injury. This hypothesis is congruent with the observations of cell lines and could explain some of the confusion in interpretation of various experiments.

CONCLUSIONS

Use of the retroviral marking method has allowed an illustration of the complexity of migration patterns of rodent cortical cells. The architecture of the radial glial system appears to provide a basis for the patterns reported here. This system is envisioned to provide a scaffolding for migration, as opposed to an active role in constraining dispersion of sibling cells, since the data strongly suggest that lineage does not play a dominant role in the allocation of cells to narrowly defined functional domains.

REFERENCES

Altman, J. and S.A. Bayer. 1990a. Vertical compartmentation and cellular transformations in the germinal matrices of the embryonic rat cerebral cortex. *Exp. Neurol.* **107:** 23.

———. 1990b. Horizontal compartmentation in the germinal matrices and intermediate zone of the embryonic rat cerebral cortex. *Exp. Neurol.* **107:** 36.

Austin, C.P. and C.L. Cepko. 1990. Cellular migration patterns in the developing mouse cerebral cortex. *Development* **110:** 713.

Bayer, S.A. and J. Altman. 1990. Development of layer I and the subplate in the rat neocortex. *Exp. Neurol.* **107:** 48.

Boulder Committee. 1970. Embryonic vertebrate central nervous system: Revised terminology. *Anat. Rec.* **166:** 257.

Brodmann, K. 1909. *Vergleichende Lokalisationslehre der Grosshirnrinde in ihren Prinzipien dargestellt auf Grund des Zellenbaues.* J.A. Barth, Leipzig.

Caviness, V.S., Jr. 1975. Architectonic map of neocortex of the normal mouse. *J. Comp. Neurol.* **164:** 247.

Cepko, C. 1988. Retrovirus vectors and their applications in neurobiology. *Neuron* **1:** 345.

———. 1989. Lineage analysis in the vertebrate nervous system by retrovirus-mediated gene transfer. *Methods Neurosci.* **1:** 367.

Cone, R.D., A. Weber-Benarous, D. Baorto, and R. Mulligan. 1987. Regulated expression of a complete human β-globin gene encoded by a transmissible retrovirus vector. *Mol. Cell. Biol.* **7:** 887.

Crandall, J.E. and K. Herrup. 1990. Patterns of cell lineage in the cerebral cortex reveal evidence for developmental boundaries. *Exp. Neurol.* **109:** 131.

Frederiksen, K., P.S. Jat, N. Valz, D. Levy, and R. McKay. 1988. Immortalization of precursor cells from the mammalian CNS. *Neuron* **1:** 439.

Gadisseux, J.F., P. Evrard, J.P. Misson, and V.A. Caviness, Jr. 1989. Dynamic structure of the radial glial fiber system of the developing murine cerebral wall. An immunocytochemical analysis. *Dev. Brain. Res.* **50:** 55.

———. 1990a. Dynamic changes in the density of radial glial fibers of the developing murine cerebral wall: A quantitative immunohistological analysis. *J. Comp. Neurol.* (in press).

Gadisseux, J.F., H.J. Kadhim, P. Van de Bosch de Aguilar, V.S. Caviness, Jr., and P. Evrard. 1990b. Neuron migration within the radial glial system of the developing murine cerebrum: An electron microscopic and autoradiographic analysis. *Dev. Brain Res.* **52:** 39.

Galileo, D.S., G.E. Gray, G.C. Owens, J. Majors, and J.R. Sanes. 1990. Neurons and glia arise from a common progenitor in chick optic tectum: Demonstration with two retroviruses and cell type-specific antibodies. *Proc. Natl. Acad. Sci.* **87:** 458.

Goldowitz, D. 1987. Cell partitioning and mixing in the formation of the CNS: Analysis of the cortical somatosensory barrels in chimeric mice. *Dev. Brain Res.* **35:** 1.

Gray, G.E., J.C. Glover, J. Majors, and J.R. Sanes. 1988. Radial arrangement of clonally related cells in the chicken optic tectum: Lineage analysis with a recombinant retrovirus. *Proc. Natl. Acad. Sci.* **85:** 7356.

Hatten, M.E. 1990. Riding the glial monorail: A common mechanism for glial-guided neuronal migration in different regions of the developing mammalian brain. *Trends Neurosci.* **13:** 179.

Holland, P.W.H. and B.L.M. Hogan. 1988. Expression of homeobox genes during mouse development: A review. *Genes Dev.* **2:** 773.

Holt, C.E., T.W. Bertsch, H.M. Ellis, and W.A. Harris. 1988. Cellular determination in the *Xenopus* retina is independent of lineage and birth date. *Neuron* **1:** 15.

Horton, H.L. and P. Levitt. 1988. A unique membrane protein is expressed on early developing limbic system axons and cortical targets. *J. Neurosci.* **8:** 4653.

Hubel, D.H. and T.N. Weisel. 1962. Receptive fields, binocular interaction and functional architecture in the cat's visual cortex. *J. Physiol.* **160:** 106.

Leise, E.M. 1990. Modular construction of nervous system: A basic principle of design for invertebrates and vertebrates. *Brain Res. Rev.* **15:** 1.

Levitt, P., M.L. Cooper, and P. Rakic. 1981. Coexistence of neuronal and glial precursor cells in the cerebral ventricular zone of the fetal monkey: An ultrastructural immunoperoxidase analysis. *J. Neurosci.* **1:** 27.

Luskin, M.B., A.L. Pearlman, and J.R. Sanes. 1988. Cell lineage in the cerebral cortex of the mouse studied in vivo and in vitro with a recombinant retrovirus. *Neuron* **1:** 635.

Marin-Padilla, M. and T.M. Marin-Padilla. 1982. Origin, prenatal development and structural organization of layer I of the human cerebral (motor) cortex: A Golgi study. *Anat. Embryol.* **164:** 161.

McConnell, S.K. 1988. Fates of visual cortical neurons in the ferret after isochronic and heterochronic transplantation. *J. Neurosci.* **8:** 945.

———. 1991. The generation of neuronal diversity in the central nervous system. *Annu. Rev. Neurosci.* **14:** (in press).

Misson, J.-P., M.A. Edwards, M. Yamamoto, and V.S. Caviness, Jr. 1988. Identification of radial glial cells within the developing murine central nervous system: Studies based upon a new immunohistochemical marker. *Dev. Brain Res.* **44:** 95.

Misson, J.-P., C.P. Austin, C. Takahashi, C. Cepko, and V.S. Caviness, Jr. 1989. Migrating neurons of the murine cerebrum ascend in parallel to radial glial fibers: Analysis based upon double-labeling of migrating neurons and radial fibers. *Soc. Neurosci. Abstr.* **15:** 599.

Mountcastle, V.B. 1979. An organizing principle for cerebral function: The unit module and the distributed system. In *The neurosciences: Fourth study program* (ed. F.O. Schmitt and F.G. Worden), p. 21. MIT Press, Cambridge, Massachusetts.

O'Leary, D.D.M. 1989. Do cortical areas emerge from a protocortex? *Trends Neurosci.* **12:** 400.

O'Leary, D.D.M. and B.B. Stanfield. 1989. Selective elimination of axons extended by developing cortical neurons is dependent on regional locale: Experiments utilizing cortical transplants. *J. Neurosci.* **9:** 2230.

Price, J. 1987. Retroviruses and the study of cell lineage. *Development* **101:** 409.

Price, J. and L. Thurlow. 1988. Cell lineage in the rat cerebral cortex: A study using retroviral-mediated gene transfer. *Development* **104:** 473.

Price, J., D. Turner, and C. Cepko. 1987. Lineage analysis in the vertebrate nervous system by retrovirus-mediated gene transfer. *Proc. Natl. Acad. Sci.* **84:** 154.

Rakic, P. 1972. Mode of cell migration to the superficial layers of fetal monkey neocortex. *J. Comp. Neurol.* **145:** 61.

———. 1978. Neuronal migration and contact guidance in primate telencephalon. *Postgrad. Med. J.* **54:** 25.

———. 1981. Developmental events leading to laminar and areal organization of the neocortex. In *The organization of the cerebral cortex* (ed. F.O. Schmitt et al.), p. 7. MIT Press, Cambridge, Massachusetts.

———. 1988. Specification of cerebral cortical areas. *Science* **241:** 170.

Rakic, P., L. Stensaas, E.P. Sayre, and R.L. Sidman. 1974. Computer-aided three-dimensional reconstruction and quantitative analysis of cells from serial electron microscopic montages of foetal monkey brain. *Nature* **250:** 31.

Reznikov, K.Y., Z. Fulop, and F. Hajos. 1984. Mosaicism of the ventricular layer as the developmental basis of neocortical columnar organization. *Anat. Embryol.* **170:** 99.

Ryder, E.F., E.Y. Snyder, and C.L. Cepko. 1990. Establishment and characterization of multipotent neural cell lines using retrovirus vector-mediated oncogene transfer. *J. Neurobiol.* **21:** 356.

Ryder, E.F., C. Walsh, and C.L. Cepko. 1988. A common precursor for astrocytes and oligodendrocytes. *Soc. Neurosci. Abstr.* **14:** 892.

Sanes, J.R. 1989. Analysing cell lineage with a recombinant retrovirus. *Trends. Neurosci.* **12:** 21.

Schaper, A. 1987a. Die fruhesten Differenzierungsvorganger im Centralnervensystem. *Arch. Entwicklungsmech. Org.* **5:** 81.

———. 1987b. The earliest differentiation in the central nervous system of vertebrates. *Science* **5:** 430.

Schlaggar, B.L., and D.D.M. O'Leary. 1988. Fetal visual cortex transplanted to somatosensory region of newborn rats develops barrel-like features. *Soc. Neurosci. Abstr.* **14:** 475.

Shatz, C.J., J.J. Chun, and M.B. Luskin. 1988. The role of the subplate in the development of the mammalian telencephalon. In *Cerebral cortex* (ed. A. Peters and E.G. Jones), p. 35. Plenum Press, New York.

Stanfield, B.B. and D.D.M. O'Leary. 1985. Fetal occipital cortical neurons transplanted to the rostral cortex can extend and maintain a pyramidal tract axon. *Nature* **313:** 135.

Temple, S. 1989. Division and differentiation of isolated CNS blast cells in microculture. *Nature* **340:** 471.

Turner, D.L. and C.P. Cepko. 1987. A common progenitor for neurons and glia persists in rat retina late in development. *Nature* **328:** 131.

Turner, D.L., E.Y. Snyder, and C.L. Cepko. 1990. Lineage-independent determination of cell type in the embryonic mouse retina. *Neuron* **4:** 833.

Voigt, T. 1989. Development of glial cells in the cerebral wall of ferrets: Direct tracing of their transformation from radial glia into astrocytes. *J. Comp. Neurol.* **289:** 74.

Walsh, C. and C.L. Cepko. 1988. Clonally related cortical cells show several migration patterns. *Science* **241:** 1342.

Wetts, R. and S.E. Fraser. 1988. Multipotent precursors can give rise to all major cell types of the frog retina. *Science* **239:** 1142.

Wilkinson, D.G., S. Bhatt, R. Chavrier, R. Bravo, and P. Charnay. 1989. Segment-specific expression of zinc-finger gene in the developing nervous system of the mouse. *Nature* **337:** 461.

Guidance of Developing Axons by Diffusible Chemoattractants

M. Placzek,* M. Tessier-Lavigne,† T. Yamada,† J. Dodd,* and T.M. Jessell†
*Center for Neurobiology and Behavior and †Howard Hughes Medical Institute, Columbia University,
New York, New York 10032

One of the first steps in the formation of specific neuronal connections is the projection of axons to their targets through diverse and changing environments. The selection of pathways by neuronal growth cones occurs with a high degree of precision and appears to be under the control of locally acting guidance cues that direct growth cones to a succession of intermediate targets (Dodd and Jessell 1988; Harrelson and Goodman 1988). Many of the molecules that regulate growth cone extension and navigation are expressed in the extracellular matrix or on the surface of cells along the pathways taken by developing axons. Some of these molecules, such as laminin, are present in restricted regions of the developing nervous system and may influence the pathway choice of axons (Cohen et al. 1986; Riggott and Moody 1987; Tomaselli and Reichart 1989). Others, such as neural cell adhesion molecules N-CAM and N-cadherin, appear to act as adhesive substrates that promote growth cone extension (Edelman 1988; Jessell 1988; Takeichi 1988).

In addition to the recognition of cues provided by cells along the pathway of developing axons, it is possible that growth cones are oriented by gradients of chemoattractant molecules that are released selectively by intermediate or final cellular targets. Although chemotropism has been invoked on repeated occasions (Ramón y Cajal 1909; Trinkaus 1985), the evidence in favor of this mechanism of axon guidance has remained equivocal. A local source of the trophic molecule nerve growth factor (NGF) can reorient regenerating sensory axons in vitro (Letourneau 1978; Gundersen and Barrett 1979) and appears to attract sympathetic axons in vivo (Menesini-Chen et al. 1978). However, it is unclear whether NGF normally exerts a tropic action in the guidance of axons within the developing embryo (see Davies 1987). More recent studies suggest that developing axons may be guided by chemotropic factors other than NGF. Trigeminal sensory neurons extend axons in vitro in response to a diffusible factor distinct from NGF that is secreted by one of their normal target tissues, the maxillary epithelium (Lumsden and Davies 1983, 1986). A similar in vitro analysis has suggested that the axons of corticospinal projection neurons extend collateral branches toward one of their final targets, the basilar pons, in response to a diffusible factor secreted by pontine tissue (Heffner et al. 1990).

We have been examining the cues responsible for the guidance of axons of commissural neurons in the embryonic rat spinal cord (see Fig. 1). Commissural neurons differentiate in the dorsal spinal cord and extend axons ventrally, close to the lateral edge of the spinal cord (Holley 1982; Altman and Bayer 1984; Wentworth 1984; Dodd et al. 1988). When commissural axons reach a point just dorsal to the motor column, they alter their trajectory and project through the motoneuron column toward the floor plate, a specialized group of epithelial cells located at the ventral midline of the spinal cord (Jessell et al. 1989). The directed growth of commissural axons to the ventral midline raises the possibility that they are guided by a chemotropic factor secreted by the floor plate.

In this paper, we discuss evidence that supports the idea that commissural axons are guided by a floor-plate-specific chemotropic factor (Tessier-Lavigne et al. 1988; Placzek et al. 1990a). Our studies show that floor plate cells secrete a diffusible factor(s) that influences the orientation of commissural axon growth in vitro without affecting other embryonic spinal cord axons. We also provide preliminary evidence that the floor plate can orient the growth of commissural axons in the developing chick embryo in vivo. The floor plate factor can diffuse considerable distances through the neural epithelium and can override intrinsic polarity cues within the epithelium to reorient essentially all commissural axons. The orienting effect of the floor plate occurs in the absence of any detectable effect on the survival or differentiation of commissural neurons or on the rate of axon growth. These findings provide support for the hypothesis that gradients of chemotropic factors guide developing axons to their targets in the vertebrate nervous system.

EXPERIMENTAL PROCEDURES

Culture. For explant cultures, one- to four-segment long pieces of dorsal spinal cord and floor plate from 24–27 somite stage rat embryos (E11–E11.5) were dissected and embedded in three-dimensional collagen gels (Fig. 1c) and cultured in supplemented Ham's F12 medium (Tessier-Lavigne et al. 1988) at 37°C in a 5% CO_2 environment. To generate conditioned medium, floor plates dissected from E11 and E13 rat embryos or the dorsal part of the E11 spinal cord were collected in L15 medium and plated in tissue culture dishes. After overnight incubation in supplemented Ham's F12 containing 5% horse serum, tissues were cultured in

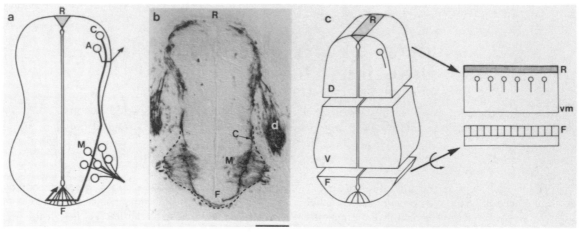

Figure 1. (*a*, *b*) Trajectory of commissural axons in the embryonic rat spinal cord. (*a*) Schematic diagram of a transverse section of an E12 rat spinal cord showing the location of the first three classes of differentiated neurons and their prospective axonal trajectories. Motoneurons (M) differentiate in the ventral region of the spinal cord from E10.5 and extend axons to their target muscles. Commissural (C) and association (A) neurons differentiate from E11 in the dorsal region of the spinal cord, adjacent to the roof plate (R). Association axons project laterally to join the ipsilateral lateral funiculus (→). Commissural axons grow ventrally along the lateral margin of the spinal cord to the motor column, then alter their trajectory and course directly through the nascent motor column to the floor plate (F). After crossing the midline of the spinal cord at the floor plate, commissural axons turn by 90° to form longitudinal projections in the contralateral ventrolateral funiculus (→). (*b*) Transverse section of E12 rat spinal cord at the cervical level, labeled with a monoclonal antibody to the TAG-1 antigen. Motor and commissural axons but not association axons express TAG-1. Commissural axons project toward the floor plate. TAG-1⁺ neurons in the dorsal root ganglia (d) can also be seen. Note that the spinal cord shown here is at a more advanced stage of development than those used for explant cultures (see below). (*c*) Schematic diagram of the main experimental protocol. Each section of E11 spinal cord (see below) was dissected into three portions: a dorsal explant (D) comprising the dorsal third or half, a floor plate explant (F) comprising the ventral-most fifth, and the remaining ventral explant without floor plate (V), which contained most of the motoneurons. Explants were then embedded in three-dimensional collagen matrices in appropriate orientations. Calibration: 100 μm. (Reprinted, with permission, from Tessier-Lavigne et al. 1988.)

serum-free supplemented Ham's F12 for a further 48–60 hours. Tissues dissected from 100 E11 or 40 E13 embryos were used to condition 1 ml of medium. Floor-plate-conditioned medium could be frozen at −20°C for periods up to a month without detectable loss of activity. Before use, conditioned medium was diluted with an equal volume of fresh supplemented Ham's F12 medium containing 10% horse serum.

Immunocytochemistry and dye labeling. Explants cultured in collagen gels and sections of whole embryos were processed for immunocytochemistry as described previously (Dodd et al. 1988; Tessier-Lavigne et al. 1988). TAG-1, an axonal glycoprotein, was detected using monoclonal antibody 4D7 (Yamamoto et al. 1986) or with rabbit anti-TAG-1 antibodies (Dodd et al. 1988). Cellular retinoic acid binding protein (CRABP) was detected using affinity-purified turkey anti-CRABP antibodies (a gift from W. Blaner, Columbia University).

Retrograde or anterograde labeling of commissural neurons in explant culture was performed with DiI (1,1′-dioctadecyl-3,3,3′,3′-tetramethylindocarbocyanine perchlorate, molecular probes; 2.5 mg/ml in dimethylformamide) (see Honig and Hume 1986; Godement ct al. 1987; Placzek et al. 1990). Explants were fixed in 4% paraformaldehyde in 0.12 M phosphate buffer (pH 7.4) for 24–48 hours and washed extensively in phosphate-buffered saline (PBS). The top layer of collagen above the region to be injected was removed

and 5–30 nl of DiI was injected into the tissue using a glass microcapillary. DiI was allowed to diffuse at 4°C for 1–5 days, and explants were then examined under a Zeiss Axioplan with epifluorescence optics.

Chick embryo grafts. The vitelline membrane above the area to be operated was removed. An incision was made through ectoderm and mesoderm, leaving endoderm intact. An incision was made adjacent to the closing neural tube at nonsegmented levels. Grafts of chick or rat floor plate were positioned within the cut and embryos were allowed to develop for a further 40–48 hours at 38°C before analysis.

Assays of defined growth factors and cell-conditioned media. A panel of growth factors and media conditioned by primary cells or cell lines were tested for their ability to mimic the effect of the floor plate in evoking commissural axon outgrowth. Factors and conditioned media were added to E11 dorsal spinal cord explants grown alone in a collagen gel matrix. Axon outgrowth was assayed after 40 hours. The following factors and media did not mimic the effect of the floor plate. Factors: ciliary neurotrophic factor (rat) 10–100 ng/ml; brain-derived neurotrophic factor (porcine) 10–100 ng/ml; NGF (murine) 10–100 ng/ml; basic fibroblast growth factor (bFGF) (bovine rec. ± heparin) 1–100 ng/ml; aFGF (bovine rec. ± heparin) 10 ng/ml; transforming growth factor-α (TGF-α) (human rec.) 1–100 ng/ml; TGF-β1 (porcine rec.) 1–

100 ng/ml; TGF-β2 (porcine rec.) 1–100 ng/ml; platelet-derived growth factor (PDGF) (porcine rec.) 3 ng/ml; epidermal growth factor (EGF) (murine) 1–100 ng/ml; insulin-like growth factor (IGF-1) (human rec.) 10–100 ng/ml; IGF-II (human rec.) 10–100 ng/ml; interleukin-1 (IL-1) (human rec.) 1–10 ng/ml; IL-2(B) (human rec.) 0.1–1 units/ml; IL-3 (human rec.) 10^{-2} to 10^{-3} units; IL-4 (human rec.) 10^{-2} to 10^{-3} units; IL-6 (human rec.) 1–10 ng/ml; IL-3 (murine rec.) $\sim$1:1000 stock; IL-5 (murine rec.) $\sim$1:1000 stock; IL-6 (murine rec.) 1:1000 stock; G-colony-stimulating factor (G-CSF) (human rec.) 0.1–1 ng/ml; M-CSF (human rec.) 10^{-2} to 10^{-3} stock; GM-CSF (human rec.) 10^{-2} to 10^{-3} stock; tumor necrosis factor-α (TNF-α) (human rec.) 10^{-2} to 10^{-3} stock; TNF-β (human rec.) 10^{-2} to 10^{-3} stock; interferon α-D (human rec.) 8–80 IU/ml; interferon α-2b (human rec.) 17–170 IU/ml; interferon γ (human; leukocyte) 3–30 IU/ml; interferon (human; fibroblast) 10–100 IU/ml; leukemia inhibitory factor (murine rec.) $\sim$1:1000 stock; retinoic acid 10^{-7} to 10^{-5} M; scatter factor (murine) $\sim$1:1000 stock; laminin (EHS sarcoma) (1–100 μg/ml); fibronectin (human) 1–100 μg/ml. Combinations of bFGF/TGF-β1; TGF-β1/TGF-β2/PDGF/EGF; TGF-β1/TGF-β2/PDGF/EGF/bFGF/IGF-I/IGF-II were also tested without effect. In all cases, factors were tested at concentrations necessary to reveal their primary activities. (rec. = recombinant-DNA-derived proteins). Cell-conditioned media: 10T-1/2; COS, 3T3, XTC, P19, PC12, P388D1, MRC5, C6, RD, primary astrocyte, spleen, thymus, bone marrow, and macrophage (all rat).

RESULTS

Evidence for a Floor-plate-derived Chemoattractant

The existence of a floor-plate-derived chemoattractant was established initially by examining the effect of the floor plate on axon outgrowth from explants of dorsal spinal cord cultured in three-dimensional collagen gels. Dorsal explants were taken from rat embryos at embryonic day (E) 11, the age at which commissural neurons begin to differentiate and extend processes. Dorsal explants cultured alone for 39–44 hours show little or no axon outgrowth (Fig. 2a). In contrast, dorsal explants cultured with an E11 floor plate explant placed 100–400 μm from their ventral-most edge show axon outgrowth within 20–24 hours. After 40–44 hours, a characteristic pattern of outgrowth is observed from all of these explants, with most axons projecting

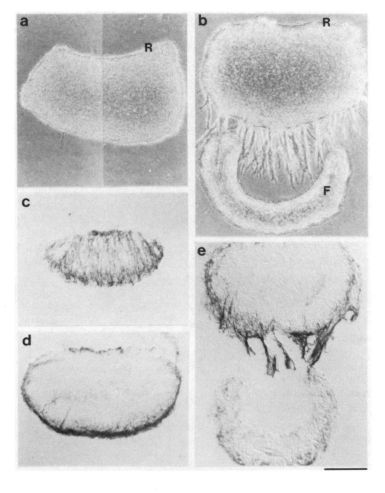

Figure 2. The floor plate promotes commissural axon outgrowth from dorsal spinal cord explants. All explants were taken from E11 rat embyros and cultured in collagen gels, as described in Fig. 1c. (*a–e*) The dorsal-ventral axis of dorsal explants is oriented vertically with the ventral downward. (*a*) Little axon outgrowth is observed from a dorsal spinal cord explant cultured alone for 44 hr. Abbreviations as in Fig. 1. (*b*) Extensive axon outgrowth is apparent from a dorsal explant cultured for 44 hr with a floor plate explant. (*c, d*) TAG-1 expression observed by immunoperoxidase labeling in cryostat sections through two different levels of a dorsal explant cultured without a floor plate for 44 hr. Extensive growth of TAG-1$^+$ axons, presumably from commissural neurons, is observed along a dorsal-ventral trajectory (*c*). These axons then extend along the inside perimeter of the explant (*d*) and do not project into the collagen gel. (*e*) TAG-1 expression observed in a cryostat section of a dorsal explant cultured with floor plate for 40 hr. TAG-1$^+$ axons are oriented along a dorsal-ventral trajectory (not shown) and project into the collagen gel. Note that the floor plate explant contains a few TAG-1$^+$ motor axons. R and F as in Fig. 1. Calibrations: (*a, b*) 150 μm; (*c, d*) 135 μm. (Reprinted, with permission, from Tessier-Lavigne et al. 1988.)

in thick fascicles from the ventral-most edge to the floor plate (Fig. 2b). Axons that project into the collagen gel are not preceded or accompanied by migrating cells, as assessed by staining with nuclear dyes (Tessier-Lavigne et al. 1988). Marked outgrowth is also observed from dorsal explants cultured alone but exposed to medium conditioned by E11 or E13 floor plate; however, under these conditions, axons emerge from all edges of the explant (Fig. 3). These experiments suggest that the floor plate secretes a diffusible factor that promotes axon outgrowth from dorsal spinal cord explants. All of the axons that project from dorsal explants in the presence of floor plate appear to derive from commissural neurons as assessed by expression of the TAG-1 glycoprotein. Studies both in vivo and in vitro indicate

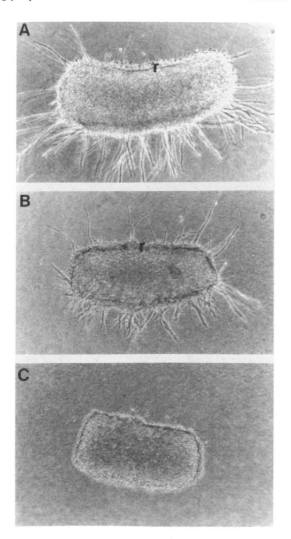

Figure 3. Medium conditioned by the floor plate evokes commissural axon outgrowth from E11 dorsal spinal cord explants. (*A*) After 40 hr in culture in the presence of floor-plate-conditioned medium, fasciculated axons emerge from the lateral- and the ventral-most edges of the dorsal explant. (*B*) Occasionally, axons also emerge from the roof plate (r) of the dorsal explant. (*C*) No outgrowth is seen from dorsal explants cultured for 40 hr in the presence of medium conditioned by dorsal spinal cord. Calibrations: (*A*, *B*, *C*) 170 μm. (Reprinted, with permission, from Placzek et al. 1990a.)

that TAG-1 is selectively expressed by commissural neurons in the dorsal spinal cord of E11 rat embryos (Figs. 1b and 2e) (Dodd et al. 1988; Furley et al. 1990).

TAG-1-labeled axons are observed within control explants at a density equal to that in explants cocultured with the floor plate. These axons are oriented along the original dorsal-ventral axis of the explants (Fig. 2c,d). Instead of projecting into the collagen gel at the ventral most edge of the explant, however, these axons remain confined to the explants, extending along its inside perimeter (Fig. 2d). This suggests that the floor-plate-derived factor promotes commissural axon outgrowth from the neural epithelium into the collagen gel. Quantitative analysis of TAG-1-labeled neurons shows that the number and length of commissural axons are similar in dorsal explants cultured alone or with a floor plate (Placzek et al. 1990a). Thus, the floor-plate-derived factor does not appear to affect the survival or differentiation of commissural neurons or the rate of growth of commissural neurons.

The effect of the floor plate on axon outgrowth appears to be selective for commissural neurons (Table 1). Axons that do not express TAG-1 and that presumably derive from association neurons are also present within dorsal explants cultured for 40–44 hours with floor plate (Placzek et al. 1990a) but are not observed projecting from the explants toward the floor plate. In addition, motor axons extend into the collagen gel from ventral explants grown alone, but the extent and pattern of axon outgrowth is not altered when ventral explants are cultured with floor plate (Table 1) (Tessier-Lavigne et al. 1988).

The specificity of expression of this chemotropic factor in embryonic rat tissues was examined at different stages of development. Expression of the chemotropic factor is largely confined to the floor plate, over its entire rostrocaudal length, during the period in which commissural axons project to the ventral midline in vivo (E11–E14) (Table 2) (Tessier-Lavigne et al. 1988). Explants of E13-PO floor plate have the same effect as E11 floor plate in evoking outgrowth of TAG-1[+] axons from dorsal explants, although lower activity is detected in floor plate explants from older embryos (Table 2). This effect is not mimicked by explants of E11–E14 dorsal spinal cord nor E11 ventral spinal cord (Table 2). However, E13 ventral spinal cord evokes the outgrowth of a small number of TAG-1-labeled axons. It is possible that ventral spinal cord cells at this age secrete low amounts of a factor that affects commissural axon outgrowth. Alternatively, the factor secreted by the floor plate may bind to the ventral spinal cord in vivo and be released slowly by the ventral explant in vitro. If the deviation in trajectory observed as commissural axons reach the dorsal aspect of the motor column indicates the point at which commissural axons first respond to the chemotropic factor, then the ventral spinal cord should contain activity detectable in the in vitro assay. It is clear though that the chemotropic activity of the floor plate always greatly exceeds that of adjacent ventral tissue. Thus, it is likely that at all

Table 1. Specifity of Neuronal Response to Floor Plate Explants

Neurons tested	Age	No. of explants	Response
Dorsal spinal cord	E11	>200	directed outgrowth of commissural axons
Ventral spinal cord	E11	10	spontaneous axon outgrowth; not increased or oriented by the floor plate
Dorsal root ganglion	E13	11	no axon outgrowth
Trigeminal ganglion	E11, E13	4	no axon outgrowth
Superior cervical ganglion	PO	3	no axon outgrowth
Retina	E14, E17	5	sparse axon outgrowth; not increased or oriented by the floor plate

Neuronal explants were cocultured in the presence or absence of a piece of E11 floor plate in a collagen gel matrix, and the pattern of axon outgrowth was examined after 40 hr. Dorsal root, trigeminal and superior cervical ganglion explants were cultured in the absence of NGF. Spontaneous axon outgrowth, presumably from motoneurons, was observed from E11 ventral spinal cord explants, but the extent and orientation of axon growth were not affected by the presence of a nearby floor plate explant.

relevant developmental stages, there is a concentration gradient of the factor in the spinal cord with its high point in or near the floor plate.

A large number of nonneural tissues, defined growth factors, and media conditioned by cultured cells fail to mimic the effect of the floor plate (Table 2, see also Experimental Procedures). Sparse outgrowth of commissural axons is, however, observed when dorsal spinal cord explants are cocultured with Rathke's pouch, embryonic limb bud mesenchyme, and dermomyotome (Table 2). It is not clear whether these tissues synthesize the floor plate chemoattractant or an unrelated activity that can also promote neurite outgrowth. Pre-liminary biochemical studies indicate that the floor plate chemoattractant is in a protein with a molecular weight of about 70,000 (M. Tessier-Lavigne et al. unpubl.).

Orientation of Commissural Axons

The findings described in the previous section show that the floor plate can promote commissural axon outgrowth into a collagen matrix but do not reveal whether the floor plate has an orienting effect on axon growth. To provide information on the orientation of commissural axons in relation to a source of floor plate

Table 2. Ability of Embryonic Rat Tissue Explants to Evoke Commissural Axon Outgrowth

Tissue	Age	No. explants tested	Dorsal explants exhibiting axon outgrowth (%)	Average no. of axon bundles/ positive explant
Floor plate: spinal cord	E11	>200	100	24
	E13	13	100	31
	E14–17	28	89	12.5
	E18–PO	48	52	5
	P6	8	0	0
Floor plate: hindbrain	E11	2	100	21
	E13	4	100	34
Floor plate: midbrain	E11	2	100	19.5
	E13	6	100	28.5
Ventral spinal cord	E11	22	0	0
	E13	21	38	3
Dorsal spinal cord	E11	22	0	0
	E13	4	0	0
Ventral midline: forebrain	E11	2	0	0
	E13	4	0	0
Rathke's pouch	E13, E14	26	30	8.5
Limb bud	E11	60	33	10 (some TAG-1⁻)
Sclerotome	E11	27	0	0
Dermomyotome	E11	30	95	5
Notochord	E10, E11	9	0	0
	E13	6	0	0

Tissues were tested for their ability to promote outgrowth of commissural axons from an E11 dorsal explant. Explants were cultured 200–400 μm from the ventral-most edge of a dorsal explant, and their effect was examined after 40 hr. In addition to the tissues shown in the table, explants of the following tissues were found not to promote commissural axon outgrowth: P9 skeletal muscle, E11 maxillary process, E11 mandibular process, E11 heart, E14 lung, E14 gut, E14 retina, E18 adrenal gland, E19 skin, P4 pituitary gland, adult choroid plexus, adult salivary gland, and adult testis.

factor, we examined the angle of emergence of axons from the ventral edge of dorsal explants under two conditions: (1) with a uniform concentration of the factor (in the form of conditioned medium) and (2) with a local source of the floor plate factor (achieved by placing a floor plate explant opposite or lateral to the ventral edge).

In the presence of conditioned medium, axons emerge from all edges of the explant (Fig. 3A,B). Axons emerge from the ventral edge of these explants with a mean angle of 5.4° ± 28.6°, where 0° indicates an angle of emergence perpendicular to the cut edge of the explant (Fig. 4A). The range of angles is broad but exhibits an approximately Gaussian distribution centered around the perpendicular. The clustering of emerging axons around the perpendicular probably reflects the existence of intrinsic cues that direct axons along a dorsal-ventral trajectory within the explant (see below).

We also examined the extent to which the angle of axon emergence is altered when outgrowth is evoked by a localized floor plate explant (Fig. 4B). With a floor plate placed opposite the ventral edge of the dorsal explant, the mean angle of emergence is 0° ± 18.2°. The angles of emergence are more sharply clustered around the perpendicular, with about half (50.4%) of the bundles emerging within ±10° of the perpendicular, compared with 27.5% in the presence of conditioned medium. Thus, cues intrinsic to the dorsal explant direct commissural axons along a dorsal-ventral trajectory within the explant, but a localized source of floor plate factor with its high point opposite the ventral edge of the explant can sharpen the distribution of angles at which the axons emerge.

The ability of the floor plate to orient commissural axons is most obvious when the floor plate explant is positioned 200–400 μm from one of the lateral edges of the dorsal explant (Fig. 4C). Under these conditions, most (91.2%) of the bundles that emerge from the ventral edge are oriented toward the floor plate (Fig. 3C), with a mean angle of emergence of 27.0° ± 21.2°. Once in the collagen gel, axons do not markedly reorient their growth (Tessier-Lavigne et al. 1988). This contrasts with the behavior of individual trigeminal sensory and corticospinal axons, which reorient as they grow through a similar matrix in response to chemoattractants (Lumsden and Davies 1983; Heffner et al. 1990). The reason why commissural axons fail to reorient in the collagen gel is unclear but could result from their growth in thick fascicles.

Because axons extend through the collagen gel in fascicles, it is possible that only a subpopulation of commissural axons respond to the floor plate and that others follow these pioneers. To avoid problems of interpretation caused by the fasciculation of axons, we examined the effect of the floor plate on commissural axonal trajectories within the dorsal neural epithelium (Placzek et al. 1990a). A floor plate explant was apposed to one end of a long dorsal explant (Fig. 5A,B), and the complete trajectory of commissural axons was assessed by injecting DiI into the region of the neural

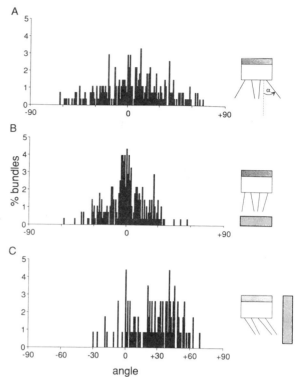

Figure 4. The floor plate orients the growth of commissural axons. Histograms of the angles of emergence of commissural axon bundles from the ventral-most edge of E11 dorsal spinal cord explants cultured either with E11 floor-plate-conditioned medium (A) with a two-segment piece of floor plate explant placed 200–400 μm from the ventral-most edge of the dorsal explant or with a long (700–1000 μm) floor plate explant placed at right angles to the roof plate of the dorsal explant at a distance of 200–400 μm (C). Schematic of the experimental protocol in each case, illustrating typical results after 40 hr in culture, is shown alongside each histogram. (A–C) Percentage of bundles emerging at each angle. (A) Angles of emergence from explants cultured in the presence of floor-plate-conditioned medium (271 bundles; 10 explants). The variance of this distribution is significantly smaller than in A (p < 0.001, F test) (B) Angles of emergence from explants cultured with a floor plate explant placed opposite the ventral-most edge (274 bundles; 10 explants). (C) Angles of emergence from explants cultured with a floor plate explant to one side (113 bundles; 10 explants). The mean angle of emergence is significantly different from that in A and B; p < 0.0001; t test. (C) Fewer fascicles extended from the ventral edge because (1) fascicles also emerged from the lateral edge (these bundles were not included in this analysis) and (2) these dorsal explants were only one segment in length, compared with the two segment stretches used in A and B. Part of the ventral spinal cord, which has no activity in isolation, was left attached to each floor plate explant to prevent the floor plate from curling. The angle at which each fascicle emerged from the ventral-most edge was measured from photographs (see diagram in A). Since the ventral-most edge of the explant tended to be convex, angles were measured from the tangent to the edge at each point. Axon bundles emerging to the left of the ordinate axis were ascribed values between 0° and −90°; those emerging to the right were given values between 0° and +90°. (Reprinted, with permission, from Placzek et al. 1990a.)

epithelium in and adjacent to the roof plate. The initial growth of DiI-labelled axons originating from this region is along the dorsal-ventral axis. Axons located close to the floor plate deviate from their dorsal-ventral trajectory and reorient toward the floor plate (Fig. 5C).

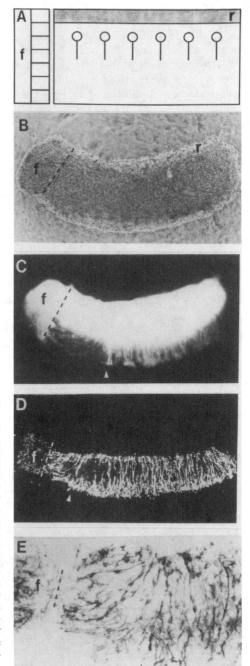

Figure 5. The floor plate reorients the growth of commissural axons within the dorsal neuroepithelium. (*A*) Diagram of the experimental protocol. A small E11 floor plate explant (f) was cultured directly apposed to the lateral edge of an 800-μm strip of E11 dorsal explant. (*B*) Phase-contrast micrograph taken after 40 hr showing that no axons have emerged from the dorsal explant. The dotted line in *B–E* indicates the point of contact between the floor plate and the dorsal explant. (*C*) Anterograde transport of DiI injected into the roof plate region reveals that axons within 300 μm of the floor plate (indicated by arrowhead) deviate from their initial dorsal-ventral trajectory and reorient toward the floor plate within the dorsal neural epithelium. (*D*) Dark-field micrograph of TAG-1 immunoperoxidase-labeled axons in a cryostat section from a similar explant to that shown in *B*. Nonfasciculated TAG-1$^+$ axons at various dorsal-ventral positions are oriented toward the floor plate. In this example, reoriented growth is apparent at a distance of 185 μm (indicated by arrowhead). Serial sections through 14 explants cultured in this manner were immunostained with TAG-1, and the distance at which turning occurred was measured from photographs of each section. The maximum distance at which TAG-1$^+$ axons reoriented their growth in each explant was used to calculate a mean distance for reorientation. (*E*) Higher-power Nomarski image of TAG-1 immunoperoxidase-labeled axons in similar dorsal explants. (*E*, *D*) Some motor axons within the floor plate explant are also TAG-1$^+$. Calibrations: (*B*, *C*) 170 μm; (*D*) 210 μm; (*E*) 70 μm. (Reprinted, with permission, from Placzek et al. 1990a.)

The distance from the floor plate over which axons turn ranges from 155 μm to 375 μm for different explants, with a mean of 243 ± 54 μm (s.d.; $n = 15$ explants). Within this range, all labeled axons reorient their growth so that they are directed toward the floor plate explant. At greater distances, axons fail to reorient toward the floor plate and continue to project along their normal dorsal-ventral route, until they reach the cut ventral edge (Fig. 5C). To determine whether the floor plate also affects commissural axons that originate from neurons located more ventrally, similar explants were sectioned and labeled with anti-TAG-1 antibodies. The pattern of TAG-1$^+$ axons throughout the neu-

ral epithelium is consistent with that of DiI-labeled axons (Fig. 5D,E), indicating that the axons of neurons located ventrally within the explants respond to the floor plate in the same way as dorsal axons. TAG-1-labeled axons reorient their growth when they are within 195 ± 47 μm (s.d.; $n = 14$ explants) of the floor plate. Thus, the floor plate can override the intrinsic dorsal-ventral polarity cues within the dorsal neural epithelium and appears to reorient all commissural axons.

It is possible that the floor plate factor diffuses within the neural epithelium for only a short distance with more distant axons reorienting their growth by fasciculating on axons closer to the floor plate, resulting in a contact-dependent cascade of fasciculation. This seems unlikely, since TAG-1$^+$ axons appear unfasciculated within the dorsal spinal cord explant (see also Holley et al. 1982; Holley and Silver 1987). However, this issue can be addressed directly by interposing a piece of E11 ventral spinal cord between the floor plate and the dorsal spinal cord. Commissural axons reorient toward the floor plate under conditions in which the nearest axons are separated from the floor plate by an interposed piece of ventral spinal cord 150–220 μm long (Placzek et al. 1990a). These results suggest that the floor plate factor can diffuse long distances through ventral neural epithelium to reorient the growth of commissural axons. The diffusion through ventral neural epithelium is pertinent, since this is the normal environment through which the factor would have to diffuse in the developing embryo. The distance at which reoriented axons are observed in these experiments could represent the maximum range of action of the factor or simply be the distance over which the factor can diffuse within the time of the experiment. Nevertheless, the point in vivo at which commissural axons break away from their initial trajectory in the dorsal spinal cord and grow to the floor plate is about 100–200 μm from the ventral midline, well within the range of action of the factor defined in vitro.

We do not know whether the orienting and outgrowth promoting actions of the floor plate are mediated by the same molecule(s). Because of this, the ability of different regions of the spinal cord to reorient commissural axon growth within neural epithelium was also tested (Placzek et al. 1990a). Commissural axons turn toward E11 and E13 floor plate. In contrast, axons do not deviate from their dorsal-ventral trajectory toward E11 dorsal or ventral spinal cord explants. Thus, at E11 only the floor plate appears to release the chemoattractant. Reorientation was not observed toward E13 dorsal spinal cord. However, TAG-1-labeled axons did reorient toward E13 ventral spinal cord from which the floor plate had been removed, but reorientation occurred only within about 10 μm of the ventral tissue and not within the remainder of the dorsal neuroepithelium (not shown). Thus, within the E11–E13 spinal cord, the regional expression of orienting activity parallels that of outgrowth promoting activity.

The results described above demonstrate that a localized source of factor, in the form of a tissue explant, can compete effectively with the intrinsic polarity cues within the dorsal explant. However, in the presence of floor-plate-conditioned medium, the pattern of TAG-1$^+$ axons within dorsal explants is not detectably different from that in explants cultured alone (Placzek et al. 1990a). Thus, a uniform concentration of factor (in the form of conditioned medium) does not prevent axons from responding to the polarity cues within the neural epithelium. Yet, floor-plate-conditioned medium promotes the extension of axons located near the dorsal or lateral edges into the collagen gel. It is possible that a gradient of the factor is established at the border be-

tween the dorsal explant and the collagen gel. For example, the factor may be degraded or otherwise inactivated by neural tissue, creating a local concentration difference that may be sufficient to direct axon outgrowth from the explant into the collagen gel. Alternatively, the factor may have growth-promoting activity even when it is not presented in a concentration gradient with the consequence that axons respond to a uniform concentration of the factor by growing into collagen. At present, we cannot exclude that the outgrowth promoting and orienting effects of the floor plate are mediated by distinct molecules. However, the specificity of expression reported above indicates that if there are distinct factors they must be restricted to the floor plate in E11 embryos.

Chemotrophic Guidance of Commissural Axons In Vivo

To provide a further test of the role of the floor-plate-derived chemoattractant in axon guidance, we have examined whether commissural axons orient their growth toward an ectopically located floor plate in vivo. Small segments of E13 rat or stage 17 chick floor plate were grafted adjacent to the neural tube of stage 10 chick embryos. Embryos were incubated for a further 40–48 hours before examination of commissural axon trajectories. Since the chick homolog of TAG-1 has not yet been identified, we used antibodies against the CRABP as a marker of chick commissural axons (Maden et al. 1989). The location of the grafted tissue was determined using monoclonal antibody (MAb) 2E7 (Dodd and Jessell 1988) to identify rat floor plate and MAb SC1 (Tanaka and Obata 1984) to identify chick floor plate.

With a grafted floor plate located near to the lateral region of the spinal cord, commissural axons could be observed to deviate from their normal ventral trajectory at a point dorsal to the motoneuron column and to emerge from the neural tube toward the ectopic floor plate (Fig. 6). CRABP immunoreactive axons on the contralateral side of the spinal cord followed their usual path and projected medially through the motor column toward the floor plate (Fig. 6). Grafts of other regions of the neural tube did not result in the deflection of commissural axons (not shown), suggesting that this effect is specific to the floor plate. These results provide preliminary evidence that the floor plate is capable of orienting commissural axons in vivo as well as in vitro.

DISCUSSION

The movement of many cell types is directed by gradients of soluble molecules emanating from a point source. For example, cellular slime molds orient their growth by chemotaxis up a gradient of cAMP, and polymorphonuclear leukocytes are attracted to leukotrienes and complement peptides (Devreotes and Zigmond 1988). The directed migration of growth cones and the ability of axons to reach their targets via aber-

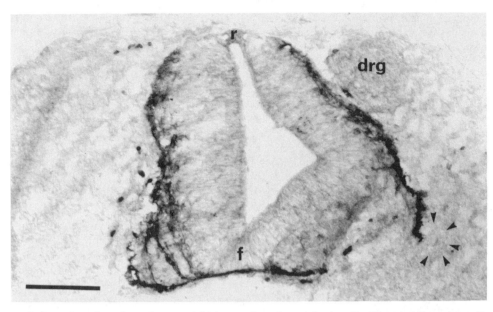

Figure 6. An ectopic floor plate alters the trajectory of chick commissural axons in vivo. Grafting a rat floor plate adjacent to the neural tube of a chick embryo causes the deviation of commissural axons from their normal trajectory. Commissural axons were identified by their expression of CRABP immunoreactivity. On the side of the spinal cord contralateral to the graft, commissural axons project ventromedially to the floor plate, but on the side adjacent to the floor plate graft no medially directed CRABP$^+$ immunoreactive axons are present in the ventral spinal cord. Axons emerge from the spinal cord and project to the region of the ectopic floor plate graft (arrowheads). Similar results were obtained with chick floor plate grafts. (r) Roof plate; (f) floor plate; (drg) dorsal root ganglion. Bar: 200 μm.

rant routes raises the possibility that growth cones can be guided by gradients of chemoattractant molecules diffusing from restricted cell populations within their targets.

A chemotropic factor should have three major characteristics. First, it should be secreted by cells present in the target region of the growing axon. Second, it should diffuse through the environment of growing axons, setting up a concentration gradient that can reorient axons at a distance from the target. Third, it should reorient axons by a direct action on the growth cones or axons of responsive neurons. Our results show that the floor plate secretes a factor that is capable of diffusing through the neural epithelium of the developing spinal cord and which can effectively reorient the growth of commissural axons. This conclusion is based primarily on two sets of observations: (1) the orientation of commissural axons growing into a collagen matrix in the presence of the floor plate factor and (2) the reorientation of commissural axons within the neural epithelium under the influence of a floor plate explant. The floor plate also appears to orient the growth of chick commissural axons in vivo.

The contribution of the floor-plate-derived chemoattractant to the guidance of commissural axons in vivo remains to be established. At one extreme, the presence and graded distribution of the factor might be an absolute requirement for the maintained ventral growth of commissural axons after they have reached the motor column. Alternatively, commissural axons may be capable of growing ventrally beyond the motor column even in the absence of floor-plate-derived fac-

tor. The role of the factor might then be to provide a cue that ensures that commissural axons project directly through the motor column to the ventral midline, rather than fasciculate with motor axons extending out of the spinal cord. Identification of the floor-plate-derived chemotropic factor will be necessary to determine in more detail the contribution of chemotropism to the guidance of commissural axons in vivo. In recent studies (Placzek et al., 1990b), we have found that expression of floor-plate-specific chemotropic activity in cells of the neural plate and neural tube can be induced by the notochord. Moreover, removal of the notochord at early stages of neural tube development prevents the expression of this chemoattractant by cells at the ventral midline. These findings indicate that chemotropic activity and probably other specialized properties of the floor plate are induced by local signals that derive from axial mesodermal cells of the notochord.

Chemotropism is likely to be only one of several guidance mechanisms that operate successively or coordinately to define the trajectory of commissural axons in vivo. The initial ventral trajectory of these axons through the dorsal spinal cord may be determined by extracellular matrix cues, in particular laminin (D. Karagogeos et al., in prep.). Moreover, once commissural growth cones arrive at the midline, their subsequent guidance appears to be regulated by contact-dependent interactions with floor plate cells (Dodd et al. 1988; Bovolenta et al. 1988; Bovolenta and Dodd 1990; Kuwada et al. 1990; Yaginuma et al. 1990).

There is evidence for the existence of target-derived

diffusible factors capable of orienting developing axons in two other neural systems. The analysis of developing mouse trigeminal sensory axons has shown that one of their peripheral targets, the maxillary arch, secretes a factor that is capable of directing their growth. When trigeminal ganglia from E10–E12 embryos are confronted with age-matched maxillary processes and limb buds (an inappropriate target), there is directed axonal growth to the maxillary process (Lumsden and Davies 1983, 1986). NGF itself has no effect on axon outgrowth from E10 trigeminal ganglia cultured on two-dimensional substrates and axon outgrowth is unaffected by antibodies to NGF. Moreover, NGF is not detected in the maxillary process until E11 (Davies 1987). These observations indicate that the E10 maxillary process secretes a diffusible factor(s), distinct from NGF, that evokes outgrowth of trigeminal sensory axons.

A diffusible factor has also been implicated in directing the growth of axons of developing corticopontine neurons (Heffner et al. 1990). In this system, evidence for chemotropism was again obtained by confronting explanted cortical tissue with pontine tissue in collagen matrices. Neurons extend axons along an apparently normal dorsal-ventral trajectory within explants of cortical tissue but project into the collagen matrix when they reach the ventral ventricular surface (Heffner et al. 1990; see also O'Leary et al., this volume). This pattern of growth is dramatically altered by explants of pontine tissue. Axons that emerge from the ventral edge of the explant reorient their growth within the collagen matrix to project toward the target. In addition, axons appear to give off collateral branches that project directly to the pontine target. These experiments provide evidence that diffusible chemoattractants can both reorient growth cones and evoke directional branching of axons. As in the other two systems discussed above, the identity of the chemotropic factor released by the pontine target tissue is not known.

Collectively, the findings discussed in this paper suggest that chemotropism plays a more prominent role in the guidance of central and peripheral neurons than appreciated previously. At present, NGF is the only defined molecule for which a chemotropic action has been demonstrated, and it remains possible that NGF has a tropic function in vivo, in addition to its well-established neurotrophic role. In vertebrate neural tissues, chemotropic factors appear to guide axons over a distance of up to 300 μm, which is well within the theoretical limit of action of diffusible signals in embryonic tissues and consistent with the range over which diffusible factors have been proposed to influence cell patterning in other organisms (Wolpert 1969; Crick 1970). The sensitivity of growth cones in detecting diffusible gradients has not yet been determined. However, other vertebrate cells, for example leukocytes, can orient in response to soluble gradients of chemotactic factors that generate only 1% differences in concentration across the diameter of the cell (Zigmond 1977). It would not be surprising if growth

cones exhibited a similar sensitivity in their ability to recognize cell-surface and diffusible guidance cues.

ACKNOWLEDGMENTS

We thank Drs. D.S. Goodman and W. Blaner for providing anti-CRABP antibodies, many colleagues for providing growth factors and cell lines, Eric Hubel and Ira Schieren for assistance with figures, and Karen Liebert for preparing the manuscript. Supported by grants to J.D. from the National Institutes of Health (NS-22993), the McKnight Endowment Fund for Neuroscience, the Joseph P. and Esther A. Klingenstein Foundation, and the Irma T. Hirschl Foundation. M.P. was supported by a fellowship from the European Molecular Biology Organization. M.T.-L. is a Lucille P. Markey Scholar and was supported in part by a grant from the Lucille P. Markey Charitable Trust. T.M.J. is an Investigator of the Howard Hughes Medical Institute.

REFERENCES

Altman, J. and S.A. Bayer. 1984. The development of the rat spinal cord. *Adv. Anat. Embryol. Cell Biol.* **85:** 1.

Bovolenta, P. and J. Dodd. 1990. Guidance of commissural growth cones at the floor plate in embryonic rat spinal cord. *Development* **109:** 435.

Bovolenta, P., T.M. Jessell, and J. Dodd. 1988. Disruption of commissural axon guidance in the absence of the midline floor plate. *Soc. Neurosci. Abstr.* **14:** 271.

Cohen, J., J.F. Burne, J. Winter, and P. Bartlett. 1986. Retinal ganglion cells lose response to laminin with maturation. *Nature* **322:** 465.

Crick, F.H.C. 1970. Diffusion in embryogenesis. *Nature* **225:** 420.

Davies, A.M. 1987. Molecular and cellular aspects of patterning sensory neurone connections in the vertebrate nervous system. *Development* **101:** 185.

Devreotes, P.N. and S.H. Zigmond. 1988. Chemotaxis in eukaryotic cells: A focus on leukocytes and *Dictyostelium*. *Annu. Rev. Cell Biol.* **4:** 649.

Dodd, J. and T.M. Jessell. 1988. Axon guidance and the patterning of neural projections in vertebrates. *Science* **242:** 692.

Dodd, J., S.B. Morton, D. Karagogeos, M. Yamamoto, and T.M. Jessell. 1988. Spatial regulation of axonal glycoprotein expression of subsets of embryonic spinal neurons. *Neuron* **1:** 105.

Edelman, G.M. 1988. Morphoregulatory molecules. *Biochemistry* **21:** 3573.

Furley,, A.J., S.B. Morton, D. Manalo, D. Karagogeos, J. Dodd, and T.M. Jessell. 1990. The axonal glycoprotein TAG-1 is an immunoglobulin superfamily member with neurite outgrowth promoting activity. *Cell* **61:** 157.

Godement, P., J. Vanselow, S. Thanos, and F. Bonhoeffer. 1987. A study in developing visual systems with a new method of staining neurons and their processes in fixed tissue. *Development* **101:** 697.

Gundersen, R.W. and J.N. Barrett. 1979. Neuronal chemotaxis: Chick dorsal-root axons turn toward high concentrations of nerve growth factor. *Science* **206:** 1079.

Harrelson, A. and C.S. Goodman. 1988. Growth cone guidance in insects: Fasciclin II is a member of the immunoglobulin superfamily. *Science* **242:** 700.

Heffner, C., A. Lumsden, and D. O'Leary. 1990. Target

control of collateral extension and directional axon growth in the mammalian brain. *Science* **247:** 217.

Holley, J.A. 1982. Early development of the circumferential axonal pathway in mouse and chick spinal cord. *J. Comp. Neurol.* **205:** 371.

Holley, J. and J. Silver. 1987. Growth pattern of pioneering chick spinal cord axons. *Dev. Biol.* **123:** 375.

Holley, J.A., H.O. Nornes, and M. Morita. 1982. Guidance of neurite growth in the transverse plane of embryonic mouse spinal cord. *J. Comp. Neurol.* **205:** 360.

Honig, M.G. and R.I. Hume. 1986. Fluorescent carbocyanine dyes allow living neurons of identified origin to be studies in long-term cultures. *J. Cell Biol.* **103:** 171.

Jessell, T.M. 1988. Adhesion molecules and the hierarchy of neuronal development. *Neuron* **1:** 3.

Jessell, T.M., P. Bovolenta, M. Placzek, M. Tessier-Lavigne, and J. Dodd. 1989. Polarity and patterning in the neural tube: The origin and function of the floor plate. *Ciba Found. Symp.* **144:** 255.

Kuwada, J.Y., R.R. Bernhardt, and A.B. Chitnis. 1990. Pathfinding by identified growth cones in the spinal cord of zebrafish embryos. *J. Neurosci.* **10:** 1299.

Letourneau, P.C. 1978. Chemotactic response of nerve fiber elongation to nerve growth factor. *Dev. Biol.* **66:** 183.

Lumsden, A. and A. Davies. 1983. Earliest sensory nerve fibers are guided to peripheral targets by attractants other than nerve growth factor. *Nature* **306:** 786.

―――. 1986. Chemotrophic effect of special target epithelium in development of the mammalian nervous system. *Nature* **323:** 538.

Maden, M., D.E. Ong, D. Summerbell, F. Chytil, and E.A. Hirst. 1989. Cellular retinoic-acid binding protein and the role of retinoic acid in the development of the chick embryo. *Dev. Biol.* **135:** 124.

Menesini-Chem, M.G., J.S. Chen, and R. Levi-Montalcini. 1978. Sympathetic nerve fiber ingrowth in the central nervous system of neonatal rodents upon intracerebral NGF injections. *Arch. Ital. Biol.* **116:** 53.

Placzek, M., M. Tessier-Lavigne, T.M. Jessell, and J. Dodd. 1990a. Orientation of commissural axons *in vitro* in response to a floor plate-derived chemoattractant. *Development* **110:** 19.

Placzek, M., M. Tessier-Levigne, T. Yanada, T. Jessell, and J. Dodd. 1990b. Mesodermal control of neural cell identity: Floor plate induction by the notochord. *Science* (in press).

Ramón y Cajal, S. 1990. *Histologie du système nerveux de l'homme et des vertébrés,* vol. 1, p. 657. Consejo Superior de Investigaciones Cientificas, Madrid.

Riggott, M.J. and S.A. Moody. 1987. Distribution of laminin and fibronectin along peripheral axon pathways in the developing chick. *J. Comp. Neurol.* **258:** 580.

Takeichi, M. 1988. The cadherins: Cell-cell adhesion molecules controlling animal morphogenesis. *Development* **102:** 639.

Tanaka, H. and K. Obata. 1984. Developmental changes in unique cell surface antigens of chick embryo spinal motonerurons and ganglion cells. *Dev. Biol.* **106:** 26.

Tessier-Lavigne, M., M. Placzek, A. Lumsden, J. Dodd, and T. Jessell. 1988. Chemotropic guidance of developing axons in the mammalian central nervous system. *Nature* **336:** 775.

Tomaselli, K.J. and L.F. Reichardt. 1989. Integrins, cadherins, and cell adhesion molecules of the immunoglobulin supefamily: Neuronal receptors that regulate axon growth and guidance. In *The assembly of the nervous system* (ed. L.T. Landmesser), p. 81. A.R. Liss, New York.

Trinkaus, J.P. 1985. Further thoughts on directional cell movement during morphogenesis. *J. Neurosci. Res.* **13:** 1.

Wentworth, L.E. 1984. The development of the cervical spinal cord of the mouse embryo. II. A Golgi analysis of sensory, commissural and association cell differentiation. *J. Comp. Neurol.* **222:** 96.

Wolpert, L. 1969. Positional information and the spatial pattern of cellular differentiation. *J. Theor. Biol.* **25:** 1.

Yaginuma, H., T. Shiga, S. Homma, R. Ishihara, and R.W. Oppenheim. 1990. Identification of early developing axon projections form spinal interneurons in the chick embryo with a neuron-specific β-tubulin antibody: Evidence for a new "pioneer" pathway in the spinal cord. *Development* **108:** 705.

Yamamoto, M., A.M. Boyer, J.E. Crandall, M. Edwards, and H. Tanaka. 1986. Distribution of stage-specific neurite-associated proteins in the developing murine nervous system recognized by a monoclonal antibody. *J. Neurosci.* **6:** 3576.

Zigmond, S.H. 1977. The ability of polymorphonuclear leukocytes to orient in gradients of chemotactic factors. *J. Cell Biol.* **75:** 606.

Mechanisms Regulating Cell Number and Type in the Mammalian Central Nervous System

R. McKay, N. Valtz, M. Cunningham, and T. Hayes

Department of Brain and Cognitive Science, Department of Biology, Massachusetts Institute of Technology
Cambridge, Massachusetts 02139

In the last decade, it has become clear that molecular biological methods will contribute in an important way to our understanding of the high-level integrative properties of the central nervous system (CNS). Some of the first evidence for this conclusion came from the use of hybridoma technology, which showed that neurons were an extraordinarily diverse group of cells and that the expression of individual antigens correlated with specific physiological features of the invertebrate and vertebrate brain (Zipser and McKay 1981; McKay and Hockfield 1982). Other recent evidence using several different techniques reinforces the conclusion that brain function is a consequence of the differentiation of large numbers of molecularly distinct neuronal types (for review, see McKay 1988).

This finding, like the time-honored joke, leads to good news and bad news. The good news is that the tools of molecular biology will give profound insight into subtle features of brain function. The bad news is that the extreme molecular complexity of the brain does not map in a simple way onto high-level brain functions. One of the challenging questions posed by these results is the embryonic origin of the molecular diversity of neurons. Spurred by this challenge, we are developing new tools to analyze the mechanisms that generate the complex arrays of neurons found in the mammalian brain.

Although very large numbers of neurons are present in the mammalian central nervous system, they are postmitotic cells, which are all generated during embryonic and postnatal development. There is good evidence that in many brain regions, distinct neurons are derived from a multipotential stem cell (for review, see McKay 1989). It follows then that neuroepithelial stem cells are crucial in regulating the appropriate numbers and types of neurons in the brain. This paper reviews some of our experiments, which analyze the proliferation and differentiation of these neuroepithelial stem cells, with particular emphasis on the cerebellum.

First, we showed that neuronal precursors can be identified by their specific pattern of gene expression. Second, we have now shown that neuronal precursor cells can proliferate and differentiate under defined conditions in primary cultures derived from the embryonic brain. This technology has allowed us to identify directly growth factors that regulate differentiation of specific neuronal precursor cells. Third, we show that immortal precursor cell lines can differentiate into neurons in response to signals generated by the developing nervous system, both in vitro and in the animal. These cell lines will allow us to take advantage of powerful molecular genetic tools to analyze the differentiation mechanisms of the neuroepithelium.

MATERIALS AND METHODS

Primary cerebellar cultures. Primary cultures were prepared from 2–4-day postnatal Sprague Dawley rats (Taconic Inc., New York). The cerebellum was dissected and treated for 3 minutes with 0.1% trypsin (Worthington Biochemicals LS3703) and 0.01% DNase (Worthington Biochemicals LS2139) in calcium-free phosphate-buffered saline (PBS). Cells were dissociated by trituration through 16-, 18-, 20-, and 22-gauge needles in the presence of 0.005% DNase in calcium- and magnesium-free PBS. The cell suspension was plated onto polyornithine-coated glass coverslips (15 μm/ml, Sigma) in 10% horse serum and 10% fetal bovine serum in Dulbecco's modified Eagle's medium (DMEM) at 1.8×10^5 cell/ml. Cerebellar cells were also grown under serum-free conditions in N2 medium (Bottenstein and Sato 1979) without insulin containing 5 ng/ml each of insulin-like growth factor-1 (IGF-1), basic fibroblast growth factor (bFGF), and nerve growth factor (NGF).

A lacZ-labeled immortal cerebellar cell line. A subclone of the ST15A cell line (Frederiksen et al. 1988) expressing the *Escherichia coli lacZ* gene product was generated by calcium-phosphate-mediated transfection of two plasmids: pBAM-Hygro conferring hygromycin resistance and pβ-AP-βGal expressing the *lacZ* gene under the control of a fragment of the human β-actin promoter. Transfected cultures were selected in 100 μg/ml hygromycin and then screened for colonies expressing high levels of β-galactosidase (β-Gal) activity.

Retroviral infection of primary cultures. Retroviruses transducing the *E. coli lacZ* were obtained from psi2 producer cell lines (Price et al. 1987; Galileo et al. 1990). Retrovirus was harvested from Bag 7 cells at 60% confluence grown overnight in 10% fetal bovine serum in DMEM. Each pool of supernatant was titered on primary cerebellar cultures. A titer was chosen that gave approximately five infected colonies per 10 mm² culture. Primary cultures were infected with Bag 7 supernatant for 2 hours at 39°C and rinsed twice with DMEM. After retroviral infection, primary cultures for clonal analysis were shifted into the N2-serum-free medium of Bottenstein and Sato (1979) without insulin, supplemented with 5 ng/ml IGF-1 (Amgen), 5 ng/ml bFGF (Amgen), and 5 ng/ml NGF (Collaborative). Cultures were fed every other day.

β-Gal histochemistry. To detect cells labeled with β-Gal, cultures were rinsed once with PBS and fixed for 15 minutes with 0.2% gluteraldehyde and 2 mM MgCl₂ in PBS (pH 7.2). Fixed cells were rinsed once with 2 mM MgCl₂ and 0.1% Triton X-100 in PBS (MTP) and incubated for 30 minutes with MTP to permeabilize cells. X-Gal (5-bromo, 4-chloro, 3-indolyl-β-D-galactopyranoside, Bachem) was prepared as a 40 mg/ml dimethylsulfoxide (DMSO) stock solution. Cells were incubated overnight at 37°C in the enzyme substrate; 5 mM potassium ferrocyanide, 5 mM potassium ferricyanide, 2 mM MgCl₂, 0.1% Triton X-100, and 1 mg/ml X-Gal in PBS (pH 7.2).

Production of anti-β-Gal antisera. An antiserum against the bacterial enzyme β-Gal was raised in New Zealand white rabbits (Hazelton), according to the immunization scheme: on day 0, a total of 1 mg of β-Gal (Sigma) emulsified in complete Freund's adjuvant was injected in three subcutaneous sites. On day 29, 1 mg of β-Gal in incomplete Freund's adjuvant was injected; this boost was repeated every 4 weeks, with bleeds collected an average of every 2 weeks after boosting.

Anti-β-Gal immunohistochemistry. The anti-β-Gal antisera described above exhibits minor cross-reactivity with an epitope transiently expressed on glial cells in primary cerebellar cultures (although this staining is significantly less than that seen with every commercially available antisera tested), requiring further purification of the serum. The antiserum was affinity-purified over a column of β-Gal enzyme (Sigma) coupled to Affigel 10 (Biorad). Affinity-purified antibody was absorbed against fixed cerebellar tissue 1 day before staining cells.

Transplants. To permit accurate and reproducible brain implants, we constructed a scaled-down stereotaxic device for neonates. Animals were anesthetized hypothermically and then placed on a device that is mounted on a copper block with a circulatory cooling system so that the hypothermic anesthesia could be maintained reliably for long periods of time. Cells were labeled with carbocyanine dye by diluting a stock solution of the dye 1:200 directly into complete media in the tissue culture dish. The cells were incubated in the dye solution for 2 hours in darkness at room temperature. The cells were then washed with three changes of PBS and incubated in complete culture medium for 12 hours. Before implantation the cells were washed again, trypsinized, and spun out of suspension before resuspension in Hank's medium. The carbocyanine dye (Molecular Probes) stock solutions were 1 mg of 1,1'-dioctadecyl-3,3,3',3'-tetramethylindocarbocyanine perchlorate (DiI) or DiO dissolved in 1 ml of ethanol or DMSO, respectively.

Cells were radiolabeled by incubating plates with tritiated thymidine ([³H]thymidine; New England Nuclear) diluted to 0.2 μCi/ml of complete culture medium. Fresh thymidine was added to the plates three times at 8-hour intervals over 24 hours. The cells to be implanted were washed three times with Hank's medium, freed from the culture plates with trypsin, and quenched with 10% fetal calf serum (FCS). Prior to implantation, the cells were washed with Hank's medium and resuspended in Hank's at a density of $10^5 \pm 10^4$ cells/μl. The cell suspension was loaded into a glass pipette (I.D., 0.5 mm; O.D., 1.0 mm) with a gently tapered tip (shank length 6 mm) with a final internal diameter of 100 μm.

Each animal was anesthetized and positioned in the aforementioned stereotaxic device. An incision was made in the skin, and a 0.5-mm diameter piece of the skull was removed over the right cerebellar hemisphere with a low-speed drill (coordinates: 1 mm lateral to the midline and 1 mm caudal to the parietal-occipital fissure). The dura was reflected, and the pipette tip was lowered perpendicular to the surface of the brain, 0.6 mm below the dura using a manual microdrive. A picospritzer (General Valve Corp.) was used to slowly pressure inject 1 μl of cell suspension over 1 minute in 4-msec pulses at a pressure of 10 psi. The pipette was slowly removed (over 1 min) to minimize the loss of cells from the injection site. At the appropriate age, the cell distribution was analyzed using standard methods.

Gene expression in ST15A cells. ST15A cells were passaged in DMEM supplemented with 10% FCS at 33°C, the permissive temperature for the temperature-sensitive T antigen. Confluent cells were rinsed with PBS, fed with DMEM containing 10% horse serum or 10% FCS, and grown at 33°C or 39°C for up to 7 days. Total RNA was prepared by scraping the cells into guanidine and pelleting through CsCl. RNA was electrophoresed on a 1% agarose gel containing 2.2 M formaldehyde and transferred to nitrocellulose. Filters were hybridized in 50% formamide, 5× SSC, 5× Denhardt's solution, 0.1% SDS, and 0.1 mg/ml salmon sperm DNA at 42°C. The same filter was stripped and reprobed with each of the following probes: mouse MPF cDNA, rat p53 cDNA, mouse retinoblastoma (RB) cDNA, human β-actin cDNA, and SV40 T antigen.

RESULTS AND DISCUSSION

A New Intermediate Filament Protein in CNS Stem Cells

To identify the precursor cells of the mammalian brain, we have defined a gene that is specifically expressed in neuronal stem cells and not in the differentiated cells of the mammalian CNS (see Fig. 1) (Fre-

A

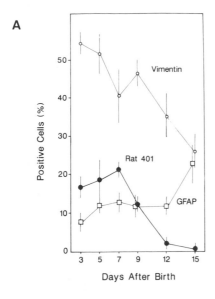

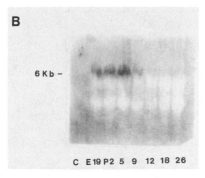

Figure 1. Nestin is expressed transiently during cerebellar development. (*A*) Cerebellar cells were dissociated on different days after birth, and the proportion of cells reacting with antibodies against different intermediate filament markers was measured. The Rat 401 antigen is an epitope on a gene that encodes nestin, a new intermediate filament protein. (This panel reprinted, with permission, from Frederiksen et al. 1988.) (*B*) The expression of the nestin gene was measured by Northern blot analysis. RNA was prepared from cerebella dissected from animals at different developmental stages from embryonic day 19 (E19) to postnatal day 26 (P26). The expression of the mRNA correlates closely with the number of Rat 401-positive cells found in the cerebellum. (This panel reprinted, with permission, from Lendahl et al. 1990.)

deriksen and McKay 1988; Lendahl et al. 1990). Both in vivo and in vitro data are described below, which show that this gene, nestin, is expressed in the immediate precursor to neurons. The nestin gene codes for a protein, which is the first example of a new class of intermediate filament protein. The function of intermediate filament proteins is not clear for any cell, but it is clear that different intermediate filament proteins are induced in cells at major developmental transitions. This feature of intermediate filament proteins makes them particularly useful as markers of cell type. Most relevant here is the fact that specific intermediate filaments are found in neurons and glial cells. For the present, the most significant feature of nestin expression is that this protein is specifically and widely ex-

pressed in the neuronal and glial precursor cells of the CNS. One other cell that has been identified to express nestin is the precursor to certain classes of muscle cell (Hockfield and McKay 1985).

Defined Growth Factors Regulate the Proliferation and Differentiation of Neuronal Precursor Cells in Primary Culture

Primary culture has been a crucial tool in our understanding of the origin of neuronal type in the peripheral nervous system (Patterson and Chun 1975; Yamamori et al. 1989). In the CNS, primary culture experiments have been important in defining the mechanisms that regulate the differentiation of glial cells (Raff 1989). Studies of CNS neuronal differentiation have been slower because it has been difficult to establish culture conditions that allow dissociated neuronal precursor cells to divide and differentiate into neurons. Some recent success has been achieved using complex culture conditions, including feeder layers or aggregate culture in the presence of serum (Reh and Kljavin 1989; Temple 1989; Watanabe and Raff 1990).

We have shown that proliferating neuronal precursors from the striatum can differentiate in dissociated culture with fully defined serum-free media (Cattaneo and McKay 1990). Defining these serum-free culture conditions is an important step to understanding the mechanisms that regulate cell number in the brain. In cultures of E14 striatum nestin-positive (Nes$^+$) cells, cells proliferate in the presence of specific growth factors; when these growth factors are removed, the cells differentiate. NGF and bFGF are two signals that control the progression of these events. In combination with FGF or after transient exposure to FGF, NGF stimulates the proliferation of Nes$^+$ striatal cells. Following NGF withdrawal, these cells become Nes$^-$, gain expression of neurofilaments, and adopt a neuronal morphology. The proliferative response to NGF is also found when E14 substantia nigra and E16 hippocampal cells were placed in culture. The interaction between NGF and FGF may occur at the level of NGF receptors: FGF induction of NGF receptors occurs during neuronal differentiation of a rat sympathoadrenal precursor cell line (Birren and Anderson 1990). Our results suggest that NGF, in addition to its well-known role in synapse formation, has an additional function controlling neuronal precursor cell number.

The analysis of differentiation of striatal neuronal precursors was possible because the majority of cells express the same responses. In many cases, several different precursor cells may be present in a single culture. Fate-mapping techniques allow the differentiation of single precursor cells to be measured. Clonal analysis has been used in several in vivo systems to define the time when cells become committed to a particular fate. Retroviruses expressing the *E. coli* β-Gal gene have been used extensively for clonal analysis in avian and mammalian systems (Turner and Cepko 1987; Luskin et al. 1988). In these in vivo studies, cell

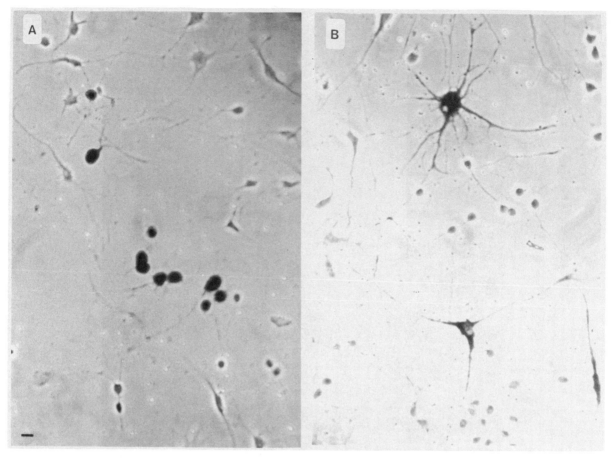

Figure 2. Neuronal precursor cells proliferate in cultures of postnatal rat cerebellum. Primary cultures were plated from the postnatal rat cerebellum and infected at limiting dilution with a β-Gal-transducing retrovirus after 1 day in vitro. After 9 DIV, the cultures were fixed and analyzed for β-Gal activity by reaction with the X-Gal substrate, which yields a blue product upon cleavage by the β-Gal enzyme. The blue cells in A and B are the progeny of two distinct cells that were infected after 1 day in culture. The clone in A are cells with the morphology of neurons. The clone in B has the morphology of astrocytes. These cells were grown in serum-free medium containing 5 ng/ml IGF-1, NGF, and bFGF. Bar, 5 μm.

morphology has been used to define the types of cell in the clone. Retrovirus infection can also be used for clonal analysis in tissue culture where signals altering cell fate can be studied. A key question here is, Can the members of a clone be detected with a method that is compatible with defining cell type? Immunohistochemistry with cell-type-specific markers is the best method for defining cell type in tissue culture. To permit clonal analysis, we have developed high-titer antisera against $E.$ $coli$ β-Gal. We have used double-label immunohistochemistry with anti-β-Gal antibodies and cell-type-specific antibodies to identify the cell type of the progeny of labeled cells in primary culture in serum-free medium.

Cells from the postnatal day-2 rat cerebellum were placed in serum-free culture, infected with the BAG 7 retrovirus after 1 day in vitro (DIV) and analyzed at 9 DIV. Cell fate of the infected clones was assessed by the morphology of X-Gal reactive cells or double-label immunohistochemistry with antibodies against β-Gal and cell-type-specific markers. By both criteria, clones of cells with neuronal properties were seen in these

cultures (see Figs. 2 and 3). Neuronal clones contained up to ten neurons, and most clones containing neurons had no other cell types present. These results show that serum-free, dissociated cultures of neuronal precursors can be used to define signals that regulate the differentiation of neurons in different regions of the brain.

Nestin-positive Cell Lines Differentiate in Coculture

The neuroepithelium is a fine-grained mosaic of precursors that give rise to the different neurons found in distinct regions of the brain. Many of these precursor populations are present in very small numbers. The small numbers of these precursors and their transient presence in the developing brain makes them hard to study. Cell lines that represent these precursor states offer two advantages: They capture the transient cell state and they allow genetic manipulation. Cell lines that represent many of the different cell types in the brain have been useful for a wide-range of experiments (see Lendahl and McKay 1990). Our group has focused

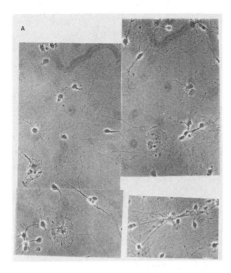

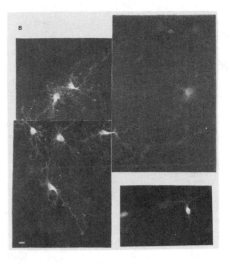

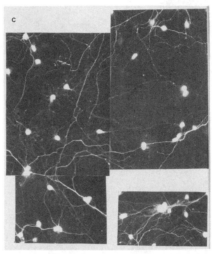

Figure 3. Neuronal precursor cells proliferate in vitro. When cultures of postnatal cerebellum were infected with a β-Gal-transducing retrovirus after 1 day in culture and analyzed 8 days later, large clones of neurons were seen. More than 12 cell bodies are seen under phase optics in *A*. Of these cells, 8 are recognized by an anti-β-Gal antiserum in *B*, indicating that they are the progeny of a single cell. The same cells are stained with an antineurofilament antibody, identifying these cells as neurons that have divided in culture. Bar: (B) 5 μm.

on CNS precursors. A critical feature of the strategy has been to use a conditional oncogene as an immortalizing agent because this allows the cells to be released from the influence of the oncogene and revert to normal control mechanisms. We have applied this strategy to many regions of the neuroepithelium to generate cell lines that express precursor markers and retain the ability to differentiate. In this paper, we specifically focus on one of these cell lines, ST15A.

The ST15A cell line was immortalized from a primary culture of postnatal day-2 cerebellum by SV40 T antigen carrying a temperature-conditional mutation. This mutation produces a protein that is stable at 33°C but rapidly degraded at 39°C. The ST15A cell line has been previously shown to express nestin and acquire some of the properties expected of either neurons or astrocytes (Frederiksen et al. 1988). However, in clonal culture, these cells do not differentiate fully. There is strong evidence that cell-cell interactions play a cen-

tral role in the differentiation of CNS neurons from their stem cells (see McKay 1989). To explore further the cell-cell signals that regulate differentiation, we exposed ST15A cells to cerebellar cells under two circumstances: by coculture with primary cerebellar cells and by transplantation into developing cerebellum. Cocultures were grown at 39°C (at this temperature, the primary cells differentiated normally). Since the body temperature of a rat is also 39°C, transplantation automatically leads to instability of the oncogenic protein in the cell line.

To allow the identification of ST15A cells in a heterogeneous cellular environment, whether in coculture or in vivo, we have used several cell-labeling methods. To follow ST15A cells in coculture, a subclone (B6) of ST15A cells expressing the bacterial enzyme β-Gal was used. In transplant experiments, we have used the β-Gal marker, lipid soluble dyes, and [3H]thymidine to follow the ST15A cells.

When B6 cells were cocultured with primary cerebellar cells, the B6 cells could be distinguished by the X-Gal reaction product for up to 10 days at the nonpermissive temperature for T antigen. When grown alone at 39°C, all the ST15A cells expressed an unremarkable flat morphology and stained blue (Fig. 4A). Under the same staining conditions, primary cerebellar cells never generated the blue product of X-Gal (Fig. 4B). In coculture, a subset of blue cells showed a dramatically different morphology from the input ST15A cells. In Figure 4C, two types of blue cells can be seen: flat cells with large nuclei similar to astrocytes and small round cells the same size as primary neurons. Figure 4C shows two clusters of small cells with morphology typical of primary neurons, and one of these clusters is clearly β-Gal-positive.

Figure 4 (D,E,F) show β-Gal-positive ST15A cells at higher magnification. In Figure 4 (D,E), both the flat cells and the small round cells can be seen. There is a striking similarity of the small blue cells to primary neurons. Figure 4F shows a third morphological class of blue cell seen in coculture. These cells were very large and elongated. This morphology is similar to the Bergman glial cell, a type of astrocyte that has been well studied in the cerebellum. The Bergman glial cell acts as a guide for the migration of differentiating granule neurons (Hatten 1990).

Under coculture conditions, the immortal cells adopt three morphologies that are similar to the morphology of neurons, astrocytes, and Bergman glial cells found in primary cultures. The presence of X-Gal-labeled small cells in the coculture is particularly striking because these small cells are morphologically similar to primary neurons. The intense blue reaction product is restricted to the cell bodies. This is the expected distribution for the X-Gal reaction product because the bacterial enzyme is not transported down the axons of mature granule neurons, as best demonstrated in transgenic mice carrying the *E. coli lacZ* gene (S. Forss-Petter et al., in prep.). The morphological differentiation of ST15A cells suggests that they can respond to signals from other cerebellar cells by differentiating into neurons and astrocytes. Double-label immunocytochemistry with antibodies to neurofilament (NF) and glial filament acidic protein (GFAP) is necessary to extend the conclusions derived from cell morphology.

Reconstructing the Brain from Immortal Cell Lines

The coculture results suggest that ST15A cells differentiate at the nonpermissive temperature for T antigen. The body temperature of rodents is nonpermissive for the temperature-sensitive A58 mutant form of T antigen. This raises the interesting question of whether ST15A cells will differentiate when they are transplanted into the developing cerebellum. ST15A cells and a control fibroblast cell line, Rat 2, were labeled with the lipid soluble dyes DiI and DiO. Then, 100,000 cells were transplanted into the cerebellum of

postnatal day-2 rats using a stereotaxic frame and a glass micropipette. The cells were delivered by control pressure pulses delivered by a picospritzer. This transplantation method was highly reproducible as shown by the distribution of transplanted cells 1–2 days after transplantation. At these short times after surgery, the transplanted cells were found clustered around the site of the transplant (Fig. 5A,B). This localization was the same for either ST15A cells or the control Rat 2 cell line. Labeled cells were found at sites distant from the original transplant 1 week after transplantation. The cells were now integrated into the host tissue (Fig. 5C,D). However, the B6 subline of ST15A cells downregulated β-Gal expression in vivo. Beyond 4 days after transplantation, only a few blue cells were seen, but here again these cells were often found in the granular layer (Fig. 5C). The integration of ST15A cells into the host tissue was also seen when transplanted ST15A cells were localized by labeling with the lipid soluble dye DiO (Fig. 5D). Rat 2 fibroblasts were also found 1 week after transplantation integrated into the host tissue often associated with blood vessels (Fig. 6). These results show that transplanted cells can migrate extensively in the developing brain. The different distributions of the ST15A cells and the Rat 2 cells suggest that the labeled cells are the transplanted cells.

When animals carrying transplants for 2 weeks were analyzed, labeled cells were not distributed uniformly in the cerebellum. A striking difference in the concentration of labeled cells was often seen at the boundary of the granule and molecular layers of the cerebellum. Figure 7 shows the distribution of ST15A cells labeled with [3H]thymidine 2 weeks after transplantation. The thymidine-labeled cell bodies were often found specifically associated with the cell bodies of the granule neurons in the granule layer (Fig. 7). The localization of the cell bodies of transplanted ST15A cells suggests that a subset of the immortalized cells are responding like granule neurons to the signals that define the structural organization of the cerebellum.

When the lipid soluble dye DiI was used to label the B6 cells, two distinct morphologies were seen. First, processes morphologically indistinguishable from those of the axons of the intrinsic granule neurons that synapse with the dendrites of Purkinje cells were found (Fig. 8A). Second, DiI-labeled cells with the morphology of Bergman glial cells were also seen (Fig. 8B). Cell morphologies of either kind were not seen when Rat 2 cells were transplanted. The autoradiographic data also show that the transplanted cell bodies can behave like granule neurons, and this supports the interpretation that immortalized cells can differentiate into granule neurons after transplantation.

Although the majority of ST15A cells cannot be followed at present by techniques that allow cell-type identification, the results we report here are based on significant technical developments in immortalization, precursor cell identification, and transplantation. Taken together, the coculture and transplant data suggest that ST15A cells can differentiate into either

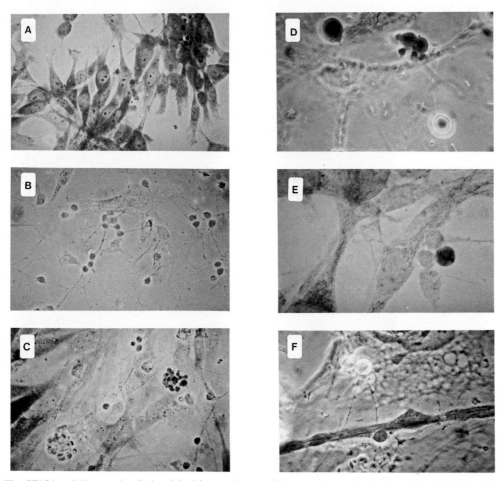

Figure 4. The ST15A cell line can be distinguished from primary cells in cocultures. A subclone of the ST15A cell line expresses the bacterial β-Gal enzyme in virtually every cell. (*A*) A clonal population of ST15A was fixed and reacted with X-Gal, a substrate for the β-Gal enzyme that yields an insoluble blue product. (*B*) Primary cerebellar cultures processed identically do not react with the X-Gal substrate. Cocultures of ST15A and primary cerebellar cells were grown for 9 days at the nonpermissive temperature for the immortalizing oncogene SV40 large T antigen. ST15A cells were distinguished by their expression of the bacterial enzyme β-Gal, which produces a blue reaction product in the presence of the substrate X-Gal. Under these conditions, the ST15A cells cease proliferating. As seen in *C*, there is a striking morphological transformation induced in a subpopulation of ST15A cells by coculture. *A, B,* and *C* were all photographed at the same magnification. Comparison of *A* and *B* shows that primary cells are significantly smaller than ST15A cells. In *C*, a cluster of ST15A cells has lost the flat morphology seen when the cells are grown alone and acquired the small round cell body size typical of primary neurons; a similar cluster of primary neurons is seen on the left side of this field. (*D,E*) Additional examples of small round ST15A cells with a similar morphology to primary cerebellar neurons are shown. In addition, larger flat ST15A cells can be seen in the same cultures. In *F*, a highly elongate blue cell is shown, and a small cell can be seen associated with a large blue ST15A cell.

neurons or glial cells. Perhaps the most extraordinary feature of these results is that precursor cell types that are only transiently present in the developing animal can be arrested in that state by T antigen and differentiate when T antigen is switched off many months or years later. The stability of the differentiated state of these cell lines makes them ideal tools in defining the mechanisms that regulate differentiation. In particular, cell lines capable of expressing different phenotypes will allow the signals that control the differentiation of these cells to be studied.

A Model for Terminal Differentiation

The strategy of using a conditional oncogene to generate cell lines capable of differentiating is based on the simple idea that a precursor cell can proliferate under one set of conditions and differentiate when these conditions are changed. We have used both SV40 T antigen and v-*myc* to generate immortal precursor cells from the cerebellum. Cell lines made with both oncogenes were capable of differentiating into neurons (Frederiksen et al. 1988). Neurons are postmitotic terminally differentiated cells. The fact that transplanted ST15A cells can be followed with a radioactive marker in their DNA suggests that these cells do not proliferate in vivo, and the differentiation of these cells suggests that they may be a model system for terminal differentiation.

There is growing understanding of the molecular mechanisms that regulate progress through the cell cycle. The protein kinase known as cdc2 in *Schizosac-*

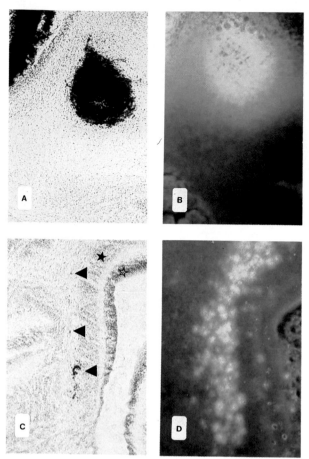

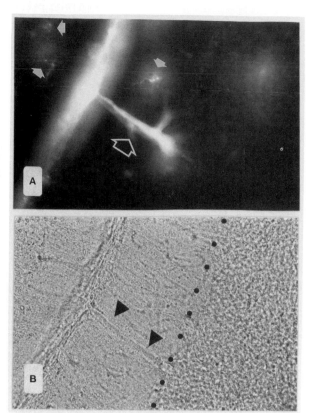

Figure 5. Transplanted conditionally immortalized cerebellar cells. The localization-labeled ST15A cells 1 day (*A,B*) and 1 week (*C,D*) after transplantation of 10^5 cells into the P2 cerebellum. (*A,C*) Tissue reacted for X-Gal histochemistry. (*B,D*) Fluorescence micrographs of adjacent sections to *A* and *C* revealing the distribution of cells labeled with the lipid soluble dye DiO. The arrow heads in *C* show the location of the few blue cells seen in the X-Gal reaction after 1 week in vivo. The open star shows the proliferative external granular layer that is still present. The solid star shows the granular layer that contains the cell bodies of mature granule neurons. The DiO-labeled cell bodies in *D* are located both in the granular layer and in the deeper white matter.

Figure 6. Transplanted fibroblasts. (*A*) Fluorescence micrograph of DiO-labeled Rat 2 cells. These cells were predominantly localized in the molecular layer, which contains the axons of granule neurons and lies above the granular layer. The boundary between the molecular layer and the granular layer is indicated by the dotted line in the phase micrograph shown in *B*. Many Rat 2 cells are seen associated with blood vessels that run perpendicular to both the surface of the cerebellum and the molecular/granular layer interface (open arrow in *A* and closed arrowheads in *B*). Single Rat 2 cells with the morphology of fibroblasts are seen in the molecular layer (closed white arrows in *A*).

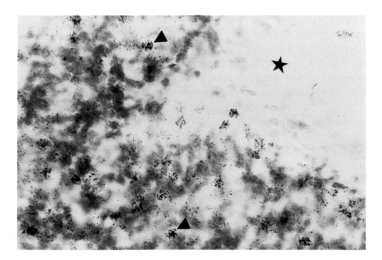

Figure 7. Thymidine autoradiographic localization of transplanted ST15A cells. ST15A cells were labeled with [^{3}H]thymidine while growing in tissue culture. These labeled cells were transplanted into the P2 cerebellum, and after 2 weeks, the tissue was fixed, sectioned, and covered with photographic emulsion. The distribution of the transplanted cells was determined by autoradiography. Many labeled nuclei were found in the granular layer. Two groups of photographic grains indicating a radiolabeled nucleus are indicated by closed arrowheads. The granular layer was revealed by Nissl staining. The overlying molecular layer (solid star) lacked radiolabeled nuclei.

charomyces pombe, CDC28 in *Saccharomyces cerevisiae,* or MPF elsewhere, plays a critical role in cell proliferation (Nurse 1990). p53 and retinoblastoma (RB) are two other genes that play a critical role in cell proliferation (Huang et al. 1988; Whyte et al. 1988; Finlay et al. 1989; Lane and Benchimol 1990), at least partly through their interactions with cdc2 (Buchkovich et al. 1989; Chen et al. 1989; Cooper and Whyte 1989; DeCaprio et al. 1989). Both the RB protein and the p53 protein bind SV40 T antigen (Lane and Crawford 1979; Linzer and Levine 1979; DeCaprio et al. 1988; Finlay et al. 1989). Northern blot analysis shows high levels of MPF mRNA in ST15A cells at the nonpermissive temperature but lower levels at the permissive temperature (Fig. 9). mRNA transcribed from the p53 gene was also reduced at the nonpermissive temperature but less rapidly than MPF. In contrast, mRNA encoded by the RB gene was not immediately altered by shifting the cells to the nonpermissive temperature. T-antigen protein levels in ST15A cells are strikingly reduced after 24 hours at the nonpermissive temperature. This result suggests that MPF mRNA levels are tightly linked to functional T-antigen expression in the ST15A cell line. These results suggest that ST15A cells may be a good model for the molecular events that occur on terminal differentiation of neurons. Downregulation of MPF expression during cerebellar and cerebral development in vivo supports the view that

transcriptional control of MPF is a key step in terminal differentiation (T. Hayes et al., unpubl.).

From Yeast to Humans

It was reported that the MAP2 kinase cDNA sequence is similar to the kinases encoded by the yeast genes *fus3* and *kss1* (Boulton et al. 1990). The *cdc2/CDC28* genes have sequence homology with the *fus3/kss1*/MAP2-kinase genes. Interestingly, when yeast cells switch from the proliferative to the conjugation cycle in response to the peptide mating factor, they also switch from dependence on the *cdc2/CDC28* kinase to *fus3* (Elion et al. 1990). The *kss1* gene is required for recovery from conjugation (Courchesne et al. 1989).

The MAP2 kinase was named because in vitro this kinase phosphorylates microtubule-associated proteins. The activity of this protein kinase is stimulated in PC12 cells within 2 minutes of NGF treatment (Miyasake et al. 1990). NGF acts to differentiate PC12 cells. We have shown that NGF can also act to stimulate the proliferation of striatal neuronal precursor cells. One model that would reconcile these two distinct roles for NGF is that NGF can interact with both the MPF and MAP2 classes of kinases. In PC12 cells, NGF might promote a switch from the MPF kinase to the related MAP2 kinase. In striatal cells, NGF might act in a converse manner to maintain the MPF activity and the

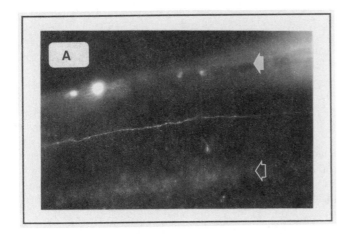

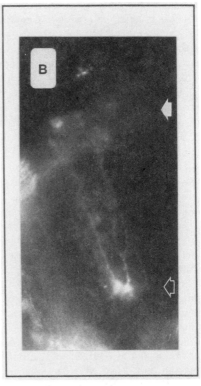

Figure 8. DiI-labeled ST15A cells transplanted into the P2 cerebellum. (*A,B*) The outer surface of the cerebellum is indicated by a closed white arrow, and the interface between the molecular and granular layers is indicated by the open white arrow. A DiI-labeled process with the morphology of a granule neuron axon can be seen in *A*. In *B*, DiI-labeled Bergman glial cells are present.

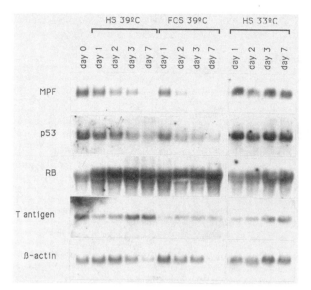

Figure 9. Expression of MPF, RB, and p53 mRNAs in differentiating ST15A cells. ST15A cells were grown to confluence in 10% FCS at 33°C (day 0). The medium and temperature were changed as indicated. Total RNA was isolated from the cells at the times shown and analyzed on Northern blots probed for the indicated sequences.

proliferating neuronal precursor state. This simple model is appealing because it implies conservation of mechanism from yeast mating to mammalian CNS differentiation. The development of new and powerful molecular genetic methods is critical if we are going to understand the origins and consequences of the molecular diversity of the nervous system. We have developed immortal cell lines because they provide the opportunity to apply recent advances in gene manipulation to the study of the mammalian nervous system. In this paper, we present data that suggest that the ST15A cell line will be useful in defining the molecular basis of neuroepithelial stem cell differentiation.

Another cell line generated in this lab, HT4, can express morphological and biochemical characteristics of neurons (G. Almazan et al., unpubl.) and N-methyl-D-aspartate receptors (Morimoto and Koshland 1990). These cells also synthesize the mRNA for NGF under the regulation of the interleukin-1 receptor (E. Cattaneo and R. McKay, unpubl.). The regulation of NGF gene expression in a neuronal context takes on added significance because HT4 cells may be an important model system for Alzheimer's disease. To determine whether HT4 cells were able to prevent cell death in vivo, they were transplanted into fimbria/fornix-lesioned rats. This work was carried out in collaboration with Dr. S. Whittemore at the University of Miami (Whittemore et al. 1990). The cholinergic basal forebrain neurons that project to the hippocampus are lost when their axons, projecting through the fimbria/fornix, are cut. However, they can be rescued when cells synthesizing NGF are placed at the lesion site. This experiment has been carried out using fibroblasts expressing a transfected NGF gene (Rosenberg et al. 1988). Both kind of cells rescue cholinergic forebrain

neurons, but the experiments are interestingly different. The HT4 cells express NGF from the normal promoter sequences and provide a model for studying the regulation of NGF transcription in the context of control pathways normally found in brain cells. Cells that synthesize and secrete NGF from the normal gene offer an alternative to engineered fibroblasts as a method of delivering NGF to the injured brain. Transplants of cell lines that differentiate may also have important implications for brain repair.

Because rodent cells can be readily handled in the laboratory, they are the focus of much of the current interest in mammalian molecular genetics. However, many of the fundamental problems in neuroscience would be better addressed in other mammalian species. Conditional immortalization of cell lines from carnivores and primates will allow these outstanding questions to be addressed at the molecular genetic level.

SUMMARY

In the developing brain, neurons are derived from multipotential precursor cells in a precise sequence, where the time when a neuron becomes postmitotic is closely linked to the differentiated function of the neuron. Work from our group (1) identifies the Nes[+] neuronal precursor state, (2) defines growth factors that regulate the proliferation of Nes[+] precursor cells and their differentiation into neurons, and (3) establishes immortal cell lines that may be useful models for the terminal differentiation of Nes[+] cells into neurons and astrocytes.

These results suggest that the basic technical requirements are now in place to define the signals that control the transition from a precursor cell to a postmitotic neuron in the mammalian CNS. Control of this terminal differentiation is a key step in generating the large numbers and types of cells in the CNS.

ACKNOWLEDGMENTS

We thank Moses Chao and Larry Zipursky for their contributions to the ideas presented here. We also thank other members of this laboratory for their criticisms of this manuscript. We are grateful to the following for providing cDNA probes: (MPF) Jeff Corden, (RB) Robert Weinberg, (p53) Helmut Zarbl, and (retroviruses) Josh Sanes and Guillermina Almazan. This work was supported by the National Institute of Health and the Pew Charitable Trust. R.M. is a scholar of the Rita Allen Foundation.

REFERENCES

Birren, S.J. and D.J. Anderson. 1990. A v-*myc*-immortalized sympathoadrenal progenitor cell line in which neuronal differentiation is initiated by FGF but not NGF. *Neuron* **4:** 189.

Bottenstein, I. and G. Sato. 1979. Growth of a rat neuroblastoma line in serum free supplemented medium. *Proc. Natl. Acad. Sci.* **76:** 514.

Boulton, T.G., G.D. Yancopoulos, J.S. Gregory, C. Slaughter, C. Moomaw, J. Hsu, and M.H. Cobb. 1990. An insulin stimulated protein kinase similar to yeast kinases involved in cell cycle control. *Science* **249:** 64.

Buchkovich, K., L.A. Duffy, and E. Harlow. 1989. The retinoblastoma protein is phosphorylated during specific phases of the cell cycle. *Cell* **58:** 1097.

Cattaneo, E. and R.D.G. McKay. 1990. Proliferation and differentiation of neuronal stem cells regulated by nerve growth factor. *Nature* **347:** 762.

Chen, P.-L., P. Scully, I.-Y. Shew, I.Y.I. Wang, and W.-H. Lee. 1989. Phosphorylation of the retinoblastoma gene product is modulated during the cell cycle and cellular differentiation. *Cell* **58:** 1193.

Cooper, I.A. and P. Whyte. 1989. RB and the cell cycle: Entrance or exit? *Cell* **58:**1009.

Courchesne, W.E., R. Kunisawa, and I. Thorner. 1989. A putative protein kinase overcomes pheromone-induced arrest of cell cycling in *S. cerevisiae. Cell* **58:** 1107.

DeCaprio, I.A., I.W. Ludlow, D. Lynch, Y. Furukawa, I. Griffin, H. Piwnica-Worms, C.-M. Huang, and D.M. Livingston. 1989. The product of the retinoblastoma susceptibility gene has properties of a cell cycle regulatory element. *Cell* **58:** 1085.

DeCaprio, I.A., I.W. Ludlow, I. Figge, I.-Y. Shew, C.-M.Huang, W.-H. Lee, E. Marsillo, E. Paucha, and D.M. Livingstone. 1988. SV40 large tumor antigen forms a specific complex with the product of the retinoblastoma susceptibility gene. *Cell* **54:** 275.

Elion, E.A., P.L. Grisafi, and G.R. Fink. 1990. FUS3 encodes a cdc2$^+$/CDC28-related kinase required for the transition from mitosis to conjugation. *Cell* **60:** 649.

Finlay, C.A., P.W. Hinds, and A.I. Levine. 1989. The p53 proto-oncogene can act as a suppressor of transformation. *Cell* **57:** 1083.

Frederiksen, K. and R. McKay. 1988. Proliferation and differentiation of rat neuroepithelial precursor cells in vivo. *J. Neurosci.* **8:** 1144.

Frederiksen, K., P.S. Jat, N. Valtz, D. Levy, and R. McKay. 1988. Immortalization of precursor cells from the mammalian CNS. *Neuron* **1:** 439.

Galileo, D.S., G.E. Gray, G.C. Owens, I. Majors, and J.R. Sanes. 1990. Neurons and glia arise from a common progenitor in chick optic tectum: Demonstration with two retroviruses and cell type specific antibodies. *Proc. Natl. Acad. Sci.* **87:** 458.

Hatten, M.E. 1990. Riding the glial monorail: A common mechanism for glial guided migration in different regions of the developing brain. *Trends Neurosci.* **13:** 179.

Hockfield, S. and R. McKay. 1985. Identification of major cell classes in the developing mammalian nervous system. *J. Neurosci.* **5:** 3310.

Huang, H.-K.S., I.-K. Yee, Y.-I. Shew, P.-L. Chen, R. Bookstein, T. Friedman, E.Y.-H.P. Lee, and W.-H. Lee. 1988. Suppression of the neoplastic phenotype by replacement of the RB gene in human cancer cells. *Science* **242:** 1563.

Lane, D.P. and S. Benchimol. 1990. p53: Oncogene or antioncogene? *Genes Dev.* **4:** 1.

Lane, D.P. and L.V. Crawford. 1979. T-antigen is bound to host protein in SV40-transformed cells. *Nature* **278:** 261.

Lendahl, U. and R.D.G. McKay. 1990. The use of cell lines in neurobiology. *Trends Neurosci.* **13:** 132.

Lendahl, U., L. Zimmerman, and R.D.G. McKay. 1990. CNS stem cells express a new intermediate filament protein. *Cell* **60:** 585.

Linzer, D.I.H. and A.I. Levine. 1979. Characterization of a 54K dalton cellular SV40 tumor antigen present in SV40 transformed cells and in uninfected embryonal carcinoma cells. *Cell* **17:** 43.

Luskin, M.B., A.L. Pearlman, and J.R. Sanes. 1988. Cell lineage in the cerebral cortex of the mouse studied in vivo and in vitro with a recombinant retrovirus. *Neuron* **1:** 635.

McKay, R.D.G. 1988. Molecular diversity of neurons. *Encyclopedia of neuroscience* (ed. G. Adelman). Burkhauser, Boston.

———. 1989. The origins of cellular diversity in the mammalian central nervous system. *Cell* **58:** 815.

McKay, R.D.G. and S.I. Hockfield. 1982. Monoclonal antibodies distinguish antigentically discrete neuronal types in the vertebrate central nervous system. *Proc. Natl. Acad. Sci.* **79:** 6747.

Miyasaka, T., M.V. Chao, P. Sherline, and A.R. Saltiel. 1990. Nerve growth factor stimulates a protein kinase in PC-12 cells that phosphorylates microtubule associated protein-2. *J. Biol. Chem.* **265:** 4730.

Morimoto, B. and D. Koshland. 1990. Excitatory amino acid uptake and *N*-methyl-D-aspartate-mediated secretion in aneural cell line. *Proc. Natl. Acad. Sci.* **87:** 3518.

Nurse, P. 1990. Universal control mechanism regulating onset of M-phase. *Nature* **344:** 503.

Patterson, P. and L.L.Y. Chun. 1975. The induction of acetyl choline synthesis in primary cultures of dissociated rat sympathetic neurons. *Dev. Biol.* **56:** 263.

Price, I., D. Turner, and C. Cepko. 1987. Lineage analysis in the vertebrate nervous system by retrovirus mediated gene transfer. *Proc. Natl. Acad. Sci.* **84:** 156.

Raff, M.C. 1989. Glial cell diversification in the rat optic nerve. *Science* **243:** 1450.

Reh, T.A. and I.I. Kljavin. 1989. Age of differentiation determines rat retinal germinal cell phenotype: Induction of differentiation by dissociation. *J. Neurosci.* **9:** 4179.

Rosenberg, M.B., T. Friedmann, R.C. Robertson, M. Tuszynski, J.A. Wolff, X.O. Breakefield, and F.H. Gage. 1988. Grafting genetically modified cells to the damaged brain: Restorative effects of NGF expression. *Science* **242:** 1575.

Temple, S. 1989. Division and differentiation of isolated CNS blast cells in microculture. *Nature* **340:** 471.

Turner, D.L. and C.L. Cepko. 1987. A common progenitor for neurons and glia persists in rat retina late in development. *Nature* **238:** 131.

Watanabe, T. and M.C. Raff. 1990. Rod photoreceptor development in vitro: Intrinsic properties of proliferating neuroepithelial cells change as development proceeds in the rat retina. *Neuron* **2:** 461.

Whittemore, S.R., V.R. Holets, R.W. Keane, D.J. Levy, and R.D.G. McKay. 1990. Transplantation of a temperature sensitive, nerve growth factor secreting, neuroblastoma cell line into adult rats with fimbria-fornix lesions rescues cholinergic septal neurons. *J. Neurosci. Res.* (in press).

Whyte, P., K. Buchovich, I. Horowitz, S. Friend, M. Raybuck, R. Weinberg, and E. Harlow. 1988. Association between an oncogene and anti-oncogene; the adenovirus E1A proteins bind to the retinoblastoma gene product. *Nature* **334:** 124.

Yamamori, T., K. Fukada, R. Abersold, S. Korsching, M.-I. Fann, and P. Patterson. 1989. The cholinergic neuronal differentiation factor from heart cells is identical to the leukemia inhibitory factor. *Science* **246:** 1412.

Zipser, B. and R.D.G. McKay. 1981. Monoclonal antibodies distinguish identifiable neurons in the leech. *Nature* **289:** 549.

Place-dependent Cell Adhesion, Process Retraction, and Spatial Signaling in Neural Morphogenesis

G.M. Edelman and B.A. Cunningham
The Rockefeller University, New York, New York 10021

The establishment of a functioning neuroanatomy during development is obviously a multistage process. In its early stages, it calls upon cellular driving forces, neurite extension and retraction, and various interactions with cell adhesion molecules (CAMs) and substrate adhesion molecules (SAMs). These early events result in the formation of particular neuroanatomical structures (Edelman 1986, 1987a). Later, during synapse formation and the establishment of refined neural maps, activity-dependent effects of correlated signals drive the formation of specific synaptic contacts (Constantine-Paton et al. 1990). The combined results of early and late events is an intricate but specifically mapped neural structure able to respond appropriately to different inputs.

Evidence is now mounting to support the idea that neural interactions involve a complex set of mutual cooperative or antagonistic effects of cell and substrate adhesion events. These interactions result in cell contacts or migration, neurite fasciculation or defasciculation, and finally the formation of metastable but specific synaptic patterns. Signaling events that lead to CAM and SAM expression in a place-dependent fashion (Edelman 1986) are of critical significance. The particular combinations of CAMs and SAMs that ensue contribute to various modulations of cell patterns. These patterns can result directly from adhesion (the case for all CAMs and most SAMs) but also from the deflection of cell growth cone migration and the induction of neurite retraction, as seen for certain SAMs such as cytotactin and its neural ligand CTB proteoglycan (Friedlander et al. 1988; Crossin et al. 1990).

In this paper, we consider the roles of some CAMs and SAMs in the early stages of neural morphogenesis. The thrust is on experimental data indicating that expression of these morphoregulatory molecules is controlled by elaborate signal loops. We first briefly consider the structure and genetic specification of some CAMs as a basis for reviewing their molecular binding mechanism and their effects on intercellular communication. Next, we discuss cytotactin as an example of a molecule with complex modulating functions, one of which is the induction of cell rounding and neurite retraction. We then describe the effects of perturbation of the functions of such CAMs and SAMs, providing evidence for the existence of signal loops that depend on cell-cell and tissue-tissue interactions. At the end of

the paper, we briefly consider some theoretical issues concerned with the possibility that short-lived diffusible signals of a different type may be important in the establishment of specific synaptic patterns underlying specific neural maps. The two subjects are related in the sense that place-dependent signals of various kinds are a common theme in both early and late neural morphogenesis. To emphasize that CAM and SAM action must be coordinated with the effects of signaling during synaptogenesis, we describe a specific model in which spatial signaling by a hypothesized postsynaptically released diffusible substance plays a key role.

CAMs: The N-CAM and L-CAM Families

The first CAM to be isolated and definitively identified in terms of function was the neural cell adhesion molecule, N-CAM (Brackenbury et al. 1977; Thiery et al. 1977). Since that time, a number of molecules related to N-CAM have been described (Table 1, Fig. 1A). A striking feature of these molecules is their structural homology with immunoglobulins and other members of the immunoglobulin superfamily (Hemperly et al. 1986; Cunningham et al. 1987; Edelman 1987b). Shortly after the analysis of N-CAM, L-CAM (a calcium-dependent CAM) was found to mediate epithelial adhesion (Bertolotti et al. 1980; Hyafil et al. 1981; Gallin et al. 1983; Ogou et al. 1983), and a series of related molecules, the cadherins (see Takeichi 1988), were described (see Table 1 and Fig. 1B). N-CAM and L-CAM are primary cell adhesion molecules, being found as early as the 2-cell stage of embryogenesis and on tissues of all germ layers (Levi et al. 1987). Thus, although N-CAM is found in the nervous system, it is seen elsewhere, as is N-cadherin, which is also found in many of the same neural locations as N-CAM (Hatta and Takeichi 1986; Volk and Geiger 1986). Many of the molecules structurally related to N-CAM (Fig. 1A) are located mainly in the nervous system and are secondary CAMs that appear only later in development. Some of these CAMs (as well as certain SAMs, see below) have important roles in the fasciculation of neurites. N-CAM-like molecules outside the nervous system have a variety of activities. One such molecule, C-CAM (Aurivillius et al. 1990), has ecto-ATPase activity (Lin and Guidotti 1989) and is probably equivalent to the biliary glycoprotein BGP1 (Hinoda et al. 1988). Although it is

Table 1. Cell-adhesion Molecules and Related Proteins

N-CAM superfamily (calcium independent)

Neural	Immune	Miscellaneous	Insects
N-CAM[a]	I-CAM-1[a]	CEA[a]	fascilin II[a]
Ng-CAM[a]/G4	I-CAM-2	NCA	amalgam
L1 (NILE)[a]	CD4	C-CAM[a] (BGP-I)	neuroglian
Nr-CAM	LAR	V-CAM	DLAR
Contactin/F11		PECAM-1/endo CAM	DPTP
F3		poliovirus receptor	
TAG-1[a]		OB-CAM	
MAG[a]		PDGF R	
P$_0$[a]		MUC 18	
		DCC	

Calcium-dependent CAMs

L-CAM[a] (uvomorulin, E-cadherin, cell CAM 120/80, ARC1)
N-cadherin/A-CAM[a]
P-cadherin[a]
T-cadherin
V-cadherin

For references to articles describing most of these molecules, see the reviews by Crossin (1990) and Takeichi (1988). For molecules not listed in these references, descriptions can be found in specific papers for C-CAM (Aurivillius et al. 1990), V-CAM (Osborn et al. 1989), PECAM-1 (Newman et al. 1990), and endo CAM (Albelda et al. 1990).

[a]Molecules with demonstrated adhesion activity.

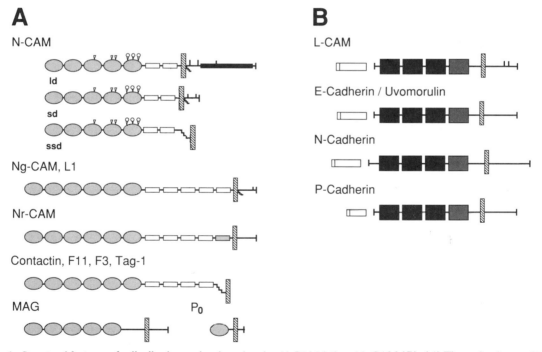

Figure 1. Structural features of cell adhesion molecules related to N-CAM (*A*) and L-CAM (*B*). (*A*) The major forms of N-CAM differ in their mode of attachment to the membrane and the size of their cytoplasmic domains. Their immunoglobulin-like domains (ovals) and fibronectin-like repeats (open rectangles) are otherwise identical. Other closely related neural CAMs resemble N-CAM in that they contain both immunoglobulin-like segments and fibronectin-like repeats that are about 20–30% identical to those in N-CAM. Of these, Ng-CAM (M. Burgoon et al., unpubl.), resembles L1 (Moos et al. 1988) and Nr-CAM (Grumet et al. 1989 and unpubl.) and contactin (Ranscht 1988) (F11; Brummendorf et al. 1989) resembles F3 (Gennarini et al. 1989) and TAG-1 (Furley et al. 1990) more closely than either resembles N-CAM. Other molecules, such as MAG (Arquint et al. 1987) and P$_0$ (Lemke and Axel 1985), have immunoglobulin-like segments only. The large stairstep symbol denotes a phosphatidylinositol link to the membrane, whereas the small symbol denotes other lipids. Arrowheads on N-CAM indicate N-linked oligosaccharides and open circles indicate polysialic acid. (*B*) Calcium-dependent CAMs are all 50% or greater in identity. They contain internal repeats (large stippled rectangles) of ~100 amino acids but do not resemble immunoglobulin; the first three repeats (closed boxes) are most closely related to one another. The number of apparent repeats may vary from three to five depending on the alignments and the criteria chosen for similarity. L-CAM (Gallin et al. 1987) and E-cadherin/uvomorulin (Nagafuchi et al. 1987; Ringwald et al. 1987) are thought to be comparable molecules in chicken and mouse. All molecules have typical signal sequences (thin open rectangles). N-cadherin (Hatta et al. 1988) is slightly larger than the others, whereas P-cadherin (Nose et al. 1987) has a substantially shorter precursor sequence (stippled thin rectangles). In both *A* and *B*, the hatched vertical bars denote the cell membrane, and the short vertical lines denote phosphoserine and phosphothreonine.

not our direct concern here, a pattern is emerging indicating that CAMs are involved in various diseases (Crossin 1990). Given the important role of these molecules in establishing cell-cell interactions to yield a normal histology, this is perhaps no surprise.

The structures of some major N-CAM forms and related molecules in the vertebrate nervous system as well as of L-CAM and related cadherins are compared in Figure 1. The key points to be emphasized are that (1) there are multiple N-CAM forms arising as products of a single gene by alternative RNA splicing, (2) N-CAM contains an unusual carbohydrate, α-2,8 polysialic acid, which can indirectly affect its binding (Hoffman and Edelman 1983) and the amount of which is developmentally regulated (Edelman and Chuong 1982; Rothbard et al. 1982), (3) L-CAM and the cadherins show no evidence of such extensive splicing or unusual carbohydrates, but as with N-CAM (Owens et al. 1987), each is the product of a single gene (Sorkin et al. 1988; Takeichi 1988), (4) N-CAM and L-CAM families show no homologies at the level of DNA or protein, and (5) certain forms in each family have a transmembrane segment, but others are associated with the cell membrane by phosphatidylinositol linkage (He et al. 1986; Hemperly et al. 1986).

Genes for L-CAM (Sorkin et al. 1988) and N-CAM (Owens et al. 1987) are present in single copies (Fig. 2). The gene for L-CAM (Fig. 2A) is much smaller than that of N-CAM; so far, no evidence of alternative splicing of the L-CAM mRNA has been seen. Comparison of the genomic DNA encoding N-CAM (Owens et al. 1987) with the protein sequences indicates the pattern of mRNA splicing that gives rise to some of the main forms of the polypeptide (Fig. 2B). Additional splicing events yield a variety of other forms, particularly in striated (Dickson et al. 1987) and cardiac (Prediger et al. 1988) muscle. Recently, a series of upstream regulatory elements have been defined previously for mouse N-CAM (Hirsch et al. 1990).

Binding by CAMs: Extracellular and Intracellular Determinants

Much remains to be done to define the exact mechanisms of CAM binding, but enough is known to provide a provisional picture that explains many of the observed phenomena. The most egregious lacuna in our knowledge concerns the specific amino acids involved in binding and the three-dimensional structure of the binding interactions as assessed by X-ray crystallography. At present, we are left only with general impressions and with some data on binding rates for N-CAM that are suggestive.

Most known CAMs bind homophilically: Each CAM on a cell specifically binds trans to its own kind on an apposing cell. Electron microscopy analysis of molecular shape by rotary shadowing of purified preparations (Becker et al. 1989) suggests that N-CAM and L-CAM have a hinged structure with their binding regions

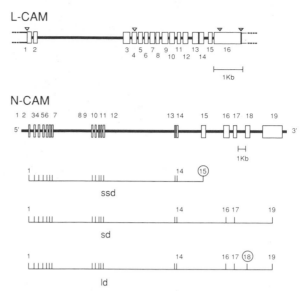

Figure 2. Organization of the genes for L-CAM and N-CAM in chicken. Open vertical rectangles denote exons that are numbered in each gene. Open triangles above the L-CAM gene are exons specifying the signal and precursor sequences; closed triangles denote the 3' untranslated segment. The N-CAM gene (Owens et al. 1987) spans more than 50 kb and includes more than 19 exons that are alternatively spliced as shown to give the large cytoplasmic domain (ld), small cytoplasmic domain (sd), and small surface domain (ssd) forms of N-CAM. Vertical lines denote exons used to encode each N-CAM polypeptide. Sequences encoded by exons 1–14 are in all forms. Exons unique to the ssd form (15) and the ld form (18) are circled. The L-CAM gene (Sorkin et al. 1988) is smaller ($\sim$ 10 kb); although it includes at least 16 exons, there is no evidence for alternative splicing.

amino-terminal to the hinge (Fig. 3A,B). A series of rate studies of the binding of synthetic vesicles containing various forms and amounts of N-CAM (Hoffman and Edelman 1983) suggest that the homophilic binding (Fig. 3C) is nonlinear (Fig. 3D). Increasing the surface density of N-CAM by a factor of 2 increases the rate of binding by a factor of 30. Decreasing the amount of α-2,8 polysialic acid (which is linked near the hinge) increases the rate of binding as well. Such decreases are seen in vivo when N-CAM is converted from a sialic-acid-rich embryonic (E) form to an adult (A) form with less sialic acid. This effect of the polysaccharide, which is itself not directly involved in binding, may result from its net negative charge, its large excluded volume, and its alteration of the various hinge angles that may be required to form multiple homophilic attachments between cells with flexible membranes.

The existence of multiply spliced forms mainly in regions outside the binding regions (Murray et al. 1986a,b; Cunningham et al. 1987; Prediger et al. 1988; Santoni et al. 1989; Thompson et al. 1989) may alter the ways in which these hinged molecules interact with each other. Whatever the case, different CAMs do not bind to each other, not even homologous molecules such as N-CAM and Ng-CAM or E-, P-, and N-cadherins. A given cell has on its surface multiple CAMs, and obviously these must rearrange in the plane

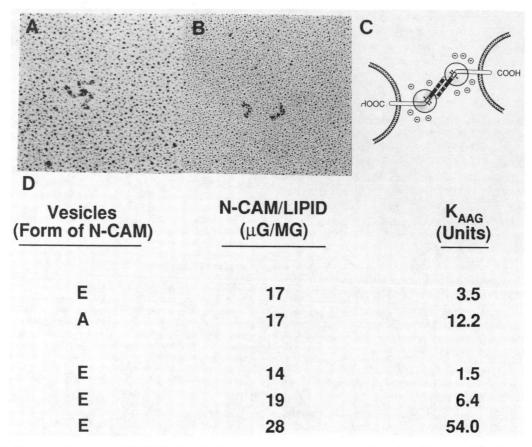

Vesicles (Form of N-CAM)	N-CAM/LIPID (μG/MG)	K_{AAG} (Units)
E	17	3.5
A	17	12.2
E	14	1.5
E	19	6.4
E	28	54.0

Figure 3. Electron micrographs of N-CAM sd and ld forms after detergent extraction from the cell surface (*A*) and the ssd form after enzymatic release (*B*) indicate that the molecule is extended with a flexible hinge, allowing for N-CAM:N-CAM interactions (*C*). Binding (*D*) is dependent on the amount of sialic acid, which is greatest on embryonic (E) forms than on adult (A) forms of N-CAM but even more so on the concentration of N-CAM in the membrane. (Adapted from Becker et al. 1989 and Hoffman and Edelman 1983.)

of the membrane to form appropriate specific homophilic attachments. Moreover, control of different combinations of CAMs of different specificity could obviously alter overall cell-binding specificity. The mobility of N-CAM in the plane of the membrane (Gall and Edelman 1981; Pollerberg et al. 1986) is consistent with this possibility; other CAMs are likely to be equally mobile, but may be modulated by particular cytoskeletal attachments.

CAM Binding and the Establishment of Intercellular Junctions

The binding properties of CAMs are consistent with the proposal (Edelman 1988a) that CAM-CAM binding is necessary for the establishment of higher-order junctions (adherens junctions, tight junctions, and desmosomes), as well as of intercellular communication via gap junctions. This has been shown to be the case in at least one in vitro experiment. S180 cells were transfected with cDNA for L-CAM (Mege et al. 1988) or N-cadherin or both (Matsuzaki et al. 1990). At confluence, the transfected cells were linked into an "epithelioid" sheet, showing a change from spindle to poly-

gonal shape, and expressed functional gap junctions as well as adherens junctions (Table 2). The two homologous CAMs acted independently and jointly to cause this change in doubly transfected cells (Matsuzaki et al. 1990). Addition of the appropriate specific antibodies dissociated the cells, which then reassumed the spindle phenotype. This treatment also reduced the gap junctions to control levels (Table 2). This formation and disruption of gap junctions correlates with specific phosphorylation of the connection that makes up the junction (Musil et al. 1990). Although not yet clearly demonstrated for neural cells, it is highly likely that the establishment and maintenance of functioning gap junctions in the nervous system will depend on CAM-CAM interactions.

Intracellular Basis of Modulation Events

The picture of CAM binding we have shown above suggests that interactions of multiple CAM arrays with the cytoskeleton must play a key role in cell adhesion. This notion, suggested over a dozen years ago (Edelman 1976), seems to be borne out by the results of a series of experiments on the cytoplasmic domain of

Table 2. Formation of Junctions in Epithelial Sheets of S180 Cells Transfected with L-CAM cDNA (S180 cells) or N-cadherin cDNA (S180cadN cells)

Cells	Total membrane measured (μm)	Percentage of membrane apposed[a]	Adherens junctions[b]	Gap junctions[c]
S180	1720	6.8	2.3	0.3
S180L	975	19.8	31.2	38.4
S180L + Fab′ anti-L-CAM	2300	6.6	5.2	4.2
S180cadN	1602	29.8	9.2	9.4
S180cadN + anti-N-cadherin	1046	23.0	3.0	0.1

Adapted from Mege et al. (1988) and Matsuzaki et al. (1990).

[a]Microns of membrane adjacent to membrane of another cell per 100 μm of total surface membrane.

[b]Number of junctions with 10- to 20-nm spacing and dense cytoplasmic inclusions per 100 μm of apposed membrane.

[c]Microns of apposed membranes with no gap per 100 μm of apposed membrane.

CAMs (Nagafuchi and Takeichi 1988, 1989; Jaffe et al. 1990). In this analysis, the ability to transfect cells lacking a given CAM with complete or mutated cDNAs for a given CAM has been particularly useful.

The largest (ld) form of N-CAM interacts with fodrin (Pollerberg et al. 1986), and L-CAM binding is affected by treatment with cytochalasin D, which dissociates actin filaments (Mege et al. 1988; Matsuzaki et al. 1990; Jaffe et al. 1990). The interaction of L-CAM with actin filaments may occur via other cytoplasmic molecules collectively termed catenins (Ozawa et al. 1989; Nagafuchi and Takeichi 1989). Transfection with cDNA modified so as to remove as few as 30 carboxy-terminal amino acids from E-cadherin or L-CAM abolishes the binding of cells (Nagafuchi and Takeichi 1988, 1989; Jaffe et al. 1990). An example is given in Table 3 for a cDNA with the bases encoding the carboxy-terminal 50 amino acids of L-CAM deleted. These findings strengthen the notion that the attachment of multiple CAM molecules to the cytoskeleton is required for cell-cell binding by CAMs.

Recently, we have carried out an experiment to explore in more detail whether specific cytoskeletal attachment would alter not only cell-cell binding, but also cell functions that are dependent on CAM adhesion, such as sorting out. Transfected cells expressing a CAM of different specificity will sort out in culture from each other, as will transfected cells expressing different amounts of the same CAM (Friedlander et al. 1989). Using this paradigm (Jaffe et al. 1990), we constructed a chimeric L/N cDNA containing bases specifying the cytoplasmic domain of the sd form of N-CAM linked to those specifying the extracellular domain of L-CAM. The behavior of cells transfected with the L/N chimeric cDNA was compared to that of cells transfected with cDNA specifying intact L-CAM.

The results (Table 3) were quite striking. Cells containing the L/N chimera and those containing L-CAM expressed each molecule to the same extent. In short-term assays, each cell type bound to itself to the same degree and the two types of transfected cells bound to each other, consistent with the fact that they expressed the same external L-CAM binding region. The different cytoplasmic domains, however, affected the behavior of these cells in cell-sorting assays. When cells expressing the L/N chimera were mixed with cells expressing L-CAM, they sorted out from each other. Moreover, in similar assays, the cells expressing the L/N chimera did not sort out from untransfected cells, whereas those expressing intact L-CAM did.

Differences in cells expressing L-CAM and those expressing the L/N chimera were also shown by specific drugs. Treatment with cytochalasin D (which dissociates actin filaments) diminished the binding of L-CAM-expressing cells but had no effect on the cells expressing the L/N chimera (Table 3). Conversely,

Table 3. Aggregation of L-cells Transfected with L-CAM cDNA (L-L cells), a Truncated L-CAM cDNA (L-L-50 cells), or an L-CAM/N-CAM Chimeric cDNA (L-L/N cells)

Treatment	Aggregation (%)[a]			
	control cells	L-L cells	L-L/N cells	L-L-50 cells
None	31 ± 2	86 ± 4	88 ± 3	26 ± 3
Fab′	34 ± 3	33 ± 4	31 ± 6	29 ± 2
Cytochalasin D	32 ± 2	44 ± 5	86 ± 3	n.d.
Nocodazole	35 ± 1	81 ± 4	66 ± 6	n.d.

Adapted from Jaffe et al. (1990).

Numbers are means ± mean deviations ($n = 2$).

[a]Percentage of aggregation after a 90-min incubation period. n.d. indicates not determined.

treatment with nocodazole (which leads to microtubule disassembly) did not alter L-CAM-expressing cells but moderately diminished binding by cells with the L/N chimera; binding by transfected cells expressing the sd form of N-CAM was decreased by nocodazole to the same extent as cells expressing the L/N chimera (not shown; see Jaffe et al. 1990).

These experiments suggest that the cytoplasmic domain of a given CAM can influence cell-cell binding and other cellular processes. Its specific and differential interactions (whether direct or indirect) with different elements of the cytoskeleton are significant in coupling adhesion events to cell migration, process extension, and sorting out. As our investigation shows, this feature of CAM binding must relate to certain interactions in the nervous system in which both CAMs and SAMs (particularly those inducing retraction) act together to affect migration and boundary formation. At this point, it is revealing to consider one such SAM, cytotactin, because it is known to affect neural migration.

Cytotactin, Cell-surface Modulation, and Neurite Retraction

Cell adhesion and migration mechanisms in morphogenesis are obviously affected by CAMs. An equally important modulating influence is provided by SAMs and molecules of the extracellular matrix (ECM). The ECM can contain as many as 50 different molecules interacting with each other in various combinations and with the cell surface by binding to surface receptors including integrins (Hynes 1987; Edelman 1988b; Ruoslahti and Giancotti 1989). In the nervous system, there is a characteristic distribution of SAMs. We discuss here one such molecule, cytotactin (Fig. 4), which has been variously named myotendinous antigen (Chiquet and Fambrough 1984), glioma-mesenchymal extracellular matrix (GMEM) (Bourdon et al. 1985), brachionectin (Erickson and Taylor 1987), J1 220/200 (Kruse et al. 1985), and tenascin (Chiquet-Ehrismann et al. 1986). This glycoprotein has a remarkable distribution in the embryo and in the brain (Grumet et al. 1985; Crossin et al. 1986; Chuong et al. 1987; Prieto et al. 1990), and it has been shown to be involved in neural cell migration (Chuong et al. 1987; Tan et al. 1987). Of particular significance is the fact that when cells are cultured in the presence of cytotactin, they remain round and show diminished ability to flatten on favorable substrates (Friedlander et al. 1988). When cultured neural cells extend neurites into a region with cytotactin present, the neurites tend to retract or be deflected (Fig. 4D,E) (Crossin et al. 1990). Cytotactin, which is made by glia and not by neurons, binds CTB proteoglycan, a molecule made by neurons (Hoffman and Edelman 1987; Hoffman et al. 1988). It also binds another SAM, fibronectin, by an independent site. The presence of fibronectin tends to neutralize cytotactin's effects on cell rounding and neurite retraction.

We have determined the sequence of the cDNA-specifying cytotactin (Jones et al. 1988, 1989) as have Spring et al. (1989). On the basis of the sequence, which includes epidermal-growth-factor-like repeats, fibronectin type III domains, and a fibrinogen-like domain (Fig. 4A), as well as experiments on binding domains (Friedlander et al. 1988) and electron microscopy (Fig. 4B), we have proposed a model (Jones et al. 1989) for the molecule (Fig. 4C). The figure is of six chains linked by their amino-terminal regions via disulfide bonds to form a so-called hexabrachion (Erickson and Iglesias 1984). A cell-binding site is in the distal portion of the arms near the fibrinogen-like domain and is near a binding region for CTB proteoglycan (Friedlander et al. 1988).

These properties of cytotactin (and its distribution and role in cell migration, discussed below) suggest that it can act as a "repulsin" or "repugnin." Preliminary experiments indicate that it also binds to cells and that it can link neurons and glia. It is not known whether this binding is via an integrin. One possible mechanism for its effects on cell shape is that it acts as a global cell-surface modulator (Edelman 1976) like the exogenous molecule, concanavalin A (Yahara and Edelman 1975). Attachment of the multivalent structure of cytotactin would affect cytoskeletal interactions and assembly, cell shape, process extension, and migration. The recent description of molecules in the nervous system that lead to growth cone collapse (Caroni and Schwab 1988; Cox et al. 1990; Davies et al. 1990; Raper and Kapfhammer 1990; Stahl et al., this volume) raises the possibility that a number of different molecular structures may act as "repulsins" and thus affect neural morphogenesis by altering neurite extension. With molecules as complex as cytotactin, however, a "repulsive" action is only one of many potential activities, and even it can be altered by interaction with other molecules in the extracellular matrix.

Local Expression of CAMs and SAMs in the Nervous System: Perturbation and Signals

Morphogenesis in the nervous system is place-dependent and must therefore depend on a complex set of signals to express CAMs and SAMs. Moreover, additional signals must be responsible for the detailed and specific synapse formation that occurs later in target sites during embryogenesis. In this section, we briefly note some facts about CAM and SAM distribution. We then consider a set of experiments showing the critical effects on neural and neuromuscular structures of perturbing CAM binding or expression.

CAMs appear in characteristic expression sequences from the time of two-cell formation until the completion of functioning neural and extraneural tissues. These sequences have been described in detail elsewhere (Crossin et al. 1985; Damjanov et al. 1986; Takeichi 1988) and will not be explicitly discussed. We only mention here certain cases that are particularly germane to the development of the nervous system. At the time of formation of the neural groove in chickens

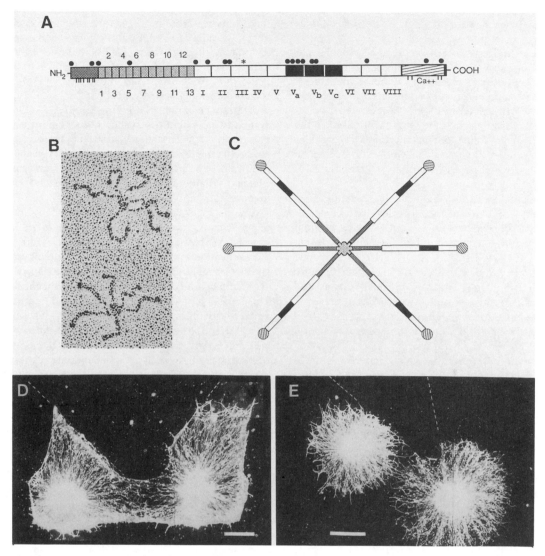

Figure 4. Structure of cytotactin (*A–C*) and its influence on neurite outgrowth (*D–E*). The linear structure (*A*) includes a cysteine rich region (dark stippling, vertical bars), 13 EGF-line repeats (1–13, light stippling), 8 to 1 fibronectin-line type III repeats (open boxes, I–VIII and closed boxes, V_a–V_c), and a fibrinogen-like unit (crosshatches). Potential glycosylation sites (closed circles) and a RGD sequence (asterisk) are indicated. Electron microscopy pictures (*B*) show hexamer units with a central hub; each arm corresponds to a single cytotactin unit as shown in *A*. A model of how each element correlates with the electron microscopy structure is given in *C*. Neurites grow out readily from dorsal root ganglia on laminin (*D*) or fibronectin (*E*) but not on combined surfaces of cytotactin and either permissive substrate (V-shaped segments indicated by white dashes). (Adapted from Jones et al. 1989 and Crossin et al. 1990.)

and the neural tube in frogs, N-CAM and N-cadherin increase, and L-CAM completely disappears in these structures (Edelman 1988a; Takeichi 1988). When neural crest cells migrate, they down-regulate N-CAM; they up-regulate its expression only after arriving at sites where they form ganglia (Thiery et al. 1985). During formation of neurites (beginning with ventral roots in the neural tube), the secondary neuron-glia CAM (Ng-CAM) appears, first on cell bodies and then almost exclusively on neurites. Subsequently, this set of events is seen at all sites of neurite fasciculation in the peripheral nervous system. Independent experiments indicate that Ng-CAM (Grumet et al. 1984) or L1 (Rathjen and Schachner 1984), its homolog in mice (Bock et al. 1985; Friedlander et al. 1986), is mainly

responsible for fasciculation of neurites in culture (Hoffman et al. 1986).

Modulation of CAMs is also important in nerve-muscle interaction. When myoblasts form myotubes by fusion, both express an isoform of N-CAM at their cell surfaces (Covault and Sanes 1985; Rieger et al. 1985). This form appears to be linked by a phosphatidylinositol moiety to the membrane (He et al. 1986; Hemperly et al. 1986). When functional synapses appear, N-CAM expression is specifically regulated and is localized at the motor endplate, leaving the surface of the myofibril essentially free of N-CAM, although an extracellular form of the molecule is found in the basal lamina.

These various examples indicate the quite specific

developmental regulation of CAM expression. A similar site-specific sequence has been found for cytotactin (Crossin et al. 1986). This molecule appears in a cephalocaudal wave of expression during gastrulation and somite formation and then appears along the sites of migration of neural crest cells (Crossin et al. 1986; Tan et al. 1987; Bronner-Fraser 1988; Mackie et al. 1988). It is also expressed at the time of tract formation in the central nervous system (CNS) and is found at particular boundaries of structures, such as whisker barrels in the somatosensory cortex (Crossin et al. 1989; Steindler et al. 1989).

It is difficult to imagine such place-dependent expression without considering that a series of local signals must specifically control CAM and SAM expression. At present, only a few candidates are known. Nerve growth factor (NGF) has been found to up-regulate Ng-CAM expression in cultured PC12 cells (McGuire et al. 1978; Friedlander et al. 1986). Thyroxine-induced metamorphosis causes a sharp switch in *Xenopus laevis* liver from L-CAM expression to N-CAM expression (Levi et al. 1990). Estradiol enhances E-cadherin (L-CAM) expression in rat granulosa cells (Blaschuk and Farookhi 1989), retinoic acid increases N-CAM expression in some embryonal carcinoma cells (Husmann et al. 1989), and transforming growth factor β enhances cytotactin expression (Pearson et al. 1988). So far, however, no in vivo signal other than thyroxine has been found, and it remains unknown whether particular neural growth factors will induce specific CAM expression. Obviously, a study of upstream positive and negative control elements for CAM and SAM transcription will prove valuable (Hirsch et al. 1990; Jones et al. 1990). In the meanwhile, a useful indicator of the function of CAMs, SAMs, and their signal loops has come from perturbation experiments.

Perturbation. Two main kinds of perturbation experiments have been employed to show how CAMs and SAMs act in vitro and in vivo. In the first, antibodies were used to block CAM binding and a search was made for ensuing morphological change. In the second, structures were removed or severed and a search was made for alterations in CAM expression. A combination of positive results from both is needed to conclude that a signal loop exists affecting CAM expression and morphogenesis.

When 6-day-old chick neural retinas were grown in organ culture for 6 more days, they formed normal-appearing retinas with well-organized plexiform layers and ganglion cells. Addition of Fab' fragments of anti-N-CAM (but not anti-Ng-CAM; Hoffman et al. 1986) at the initiation of the culture led to a mosaic and disrupted structure with altered cell spacing and invasion of the plexiform layer by ganglion cells (Buskirk et al. 1980). In in vivo experiments (Fraser et al. 1984, 1988), an agarose spike containing anti-N-CAM Fab' fragments was implanted in the tectum of *X. laevis* during development or regeneration of the retinotectal projection. After diffusion of the antibody fragments,

the retinotectal map was severely disordered, showing huge overlapping multiunit receptive fields and distorted map order. After the antibody levels declined, a more or less normal map was restored. These experiments indicate that N-CAM interactions are critical for certain morphogenetic events.

A striking example of the contribution of a CAM and SAM to the formation of neural layers is provided by perturbation of cerebellar slices with various specific antibody fragments (Hoffman et al. 1986; Chuong et al. 1987). Slices were prepared at a time when migration of external granule cells through the molecular layer to the internal granular layer was just beginning. Labeled thymidine (Moonen et al. 1982) was used to follow the migration of granular cells subsequent to their final mitosis. As shown in Figure 5, anti-Ng-CAM fragments blocked migration of cells from the external granular layer. Anti-N-CAM had little effect. In contrast, anti-cytotactin caused cells to pile up in the molecular layer. This experiment shows that a CAM made by neurons and a SAM made by glia are both required for normal layer formation. Most likely, other molecules such as CTB proteoglycan made by neurons are involved as well. These data suggest that multiple CAMs and SAMs and a coordinated regulation of their expression are likely to be the rule in neural morphogenesis and layer formation. The main conclusion from the various perturbation experiments is that the blockade of CAM or SAM function in particular places at particular times can alter morphogenesis.

Another set of experiments shows that disruption of tissue interactions alters CAM or SAM expression. The concentration of N-CAM at the motor endplate (Covault and Sanes 1985; Rieger et al. 1985) provides the opportunity to study the effects of Wallerian degeneration and regeneration after nerve crush or cut on CAM expression. Moreover, one may ask whether the signal loop altered by these maneuvers involves the same CAMs as those used in embryogenesis and whether it affects normally linked structures from the periphery to the spinal cord and back.

When the sciatic nerve was crushed or cut, N-CAM message (Covault et al. 1986) and protein (Rieger et al. 1985) reappeared in the affected muscle cells and cell surfaces, respectively. Moreover, Ng-CAM and N-CAM expression was up-regulated (Daniloff et al. 1986) in the dorsal root ganglion of the affected segment and was down-regulated in the ventral horn of the segment on the affected side (Fig. 6). Only after Wallerian regeneration occurred were the normal patterns restored. In addition, striking patterns of increased expression of N-CAM and Ng-CAM in Schwann cells at the cut or crush site were observed. The interested reader may consult the original papers for details.

This experiment is significant in showing that disruption of normal neuromuscular interaction breaks a control loop from the spinal cord to the periphery and back. Signals affecting the same CAMs used to establish embryonic morphology are then readjusted appropriately in the regeneration phase.

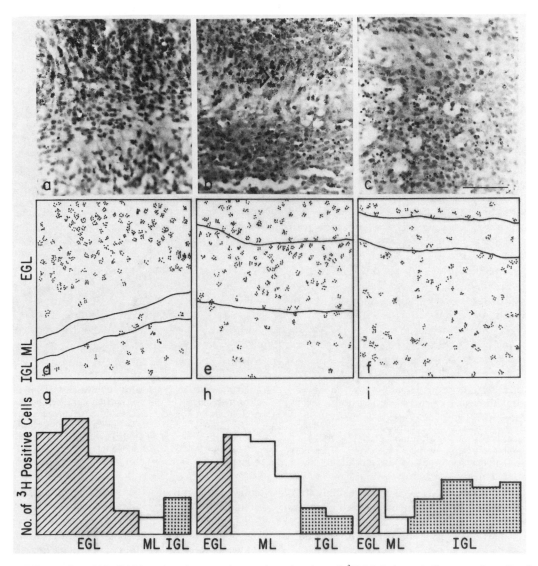

Figure 5. Effects of anti-Ng-CAM and anti-cytotactin on the migration of ^{3}H-labeled cerebellar granule cells. (*a–c*) Autoradiograms of paraffin sections of cerebellar explants that were pulse-labeled with [^{3}H]thymidine for 1 hour and cultured for 3 days in the presence of Fab′ fragments of antibodies to adhesive molecules. (*d–f*) Tracings of *a–c* highlight the silver grains and the relative thickness of the cortical layers. (*g–i*) Histograms of the number of tritiated cells versus distance along layers. (*a, d, g*) Anti-Ng-CAM; (*b, e, h*) anti-cytotactin; (*c, f, i*) nonimmune control. The arrow in *b* indicates granule cells in the molecular layer (ML), which are piled up along the Bergmann glia. Bar, 50 μm. (Reprinted, with permission, from Chuong et al. 1987.)

Signals. Such signals operate in other contexts where extracellular cues are necessary for targeting of regenerating neurites into muscle. For example, the replacement of a wedge of *X. laevis* pectoral muscle by an agarose slab containing anti-N-CAM antibodies led to a failure of neurons to target to their previous sites (Rieger et al. 1988). The floridly growing neurons branched over the muscle target, and the terminal Schwann cell sheaths were also disrupted. The presence of extracellular N-CAM in the basal lamina may in fact be the source of the necessary cues for normal retargeting of the ingrowing neurons. The function of these N-CAM forms and N-CAM on the muscle are likely to have been perturbed by the specific antibody used in this experiment.

Cytotactin expression is also modulated in the neuro-

muscular system. The molecule normally accumulates at critical sites of cell-cell interaction, specifically at the neuromuscular junction and the myotendinous junction (Daniloff et al. 1989) as well as the node of Ranvier (Rieger et al. 1986). In denervated muscle (Daniloff et al. 1989), cytotactin accumulates in interstitial spaces and near the previous synaptic sites. Its levels are elevated and remain high along the endoneurial tubes and in the perineurium until the muscle is reinnervated when levels return to normal. In dorsal root ganglia, the processes around ganglionic neurons show strong cytotactin expression after the nerve is cut and return to normal after about 30 days.

The foregoing experiments leave us with little doubt that complex dynamic signaling events underlie the effects of CAMs on morphogenesis. That the same is

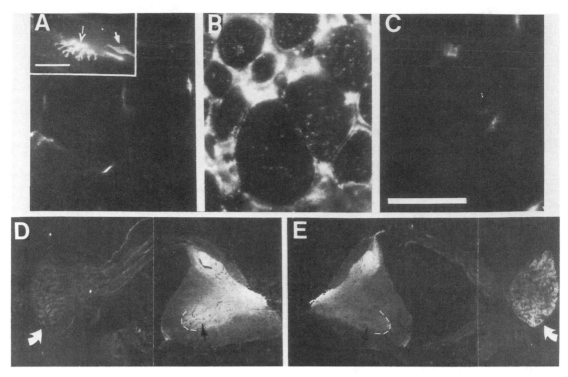

Figure 6. Changes in the expression of N-CAM in muscle (*A–C*) and Ng-CAM in spinal cord and dorsal root ganglia (*D, E*) following nerve damage. (*A*) Normal chicken gastrocnemius muscle expresses little N-CAM except at the motor end plate (inset, thin arrow) and on mononucleated cells (thick arrow). (*B*) Ten days after cutting the sciatic nerve, N-CAM expression increased dramatically but was restored to normal levels after 150 days (*C*). (*D, E*) Expression of Ng-CAM in the ventral horn (dashed line and black arrows) of the lowest lumbar section of the spinal cord and dorsal root ganglia (white arrows) is normal 20 days after cutting the sciatic nerve on the side ipsilateral to sciatic nerve lesion (*B*). Ng-CAM expression decreased in the ventral horn and increased in the ganglia on the contralateral side to the lesion. (Adapted from Daniloff et al. 1986.)

likely to be true for SAMs is revealed by the above observation and by an experiment in which cytotactin and CTB proteoglycan distributions were explored in rat whisker barrels or somatosensory cortex, before and after removal of a row of whiskers.

It is known that the formation and integrity of whisker barrels depend on sensory input from the follicle of the corresponding vibrissa (Woolsey et al. 1979). It was found (Crossin et al. 1989) that the walls of each whisker barrel expressed cytotactin (Fig. 7a) and CTB proteoglycan (not shown) soon after barrel formation. On removal of a row of whiskers (Crossin et al. 1989), the expected pattern of fusion of the corresponding row of barrels was found, and the two molecules were seen in the fused walls. In addition, the cytotactin (Fig. 7b) and proteoglycan also were expressed at low levels throughout the fused barrel structures. Whatever the role of these proteins in maintaining dendrites within each barrel (possibly encouraging their retraction upon centrifugal growth), this experiment indicates that the appropriate expression of these proteins depends on the presence of appropriate neural input signals from the afferent axons.

In view of these findings, the large number of possible alterations in signals as well as the various combinations of CAMs and SAMs under coregulation could lead to formation of a remarkable number of specific structures. This alleviates the necessity of a "place

code" for neural structure with huge numbers of CAMs acting almost at the level of individual neurons (Sperry 1963). Still, it is an interesting question to ask, for example, how many CAMs will be required to help construct the basic scaffold of neuroanatomy in a brain. This is obviously an empirical question, and it remains unanswered. One of us (Edelman 1988a) has speculated that the number of CAMs related to N-CAM would be in the dozens rather than the hundreds of thousands that would be implied by a place code. Whatever the case, the finding that N-CAM is structurally related to immunoglobulins sheds some light on how various but related CAM structures of different specificity (Table 1) may have emerged during evolution.

The N-CAM and Immunoglobulin Superfamily

As indicated in Table 1, a number of molecules with structures related to N-CAM have been discovered in neural (Fig. 1A) and nonneural tissues. Many of these have not yet been demonstrated to have functions in cell adhesion. Indeed, the finding that N-CAM is homologous to immunoglobulins and the major histocompatibility antigens indicates that many N-CAM-related structures have binding functions but are not cell adhesion molecules. This conclusion takes on even more force when one confronts the hypothesis (Edel-

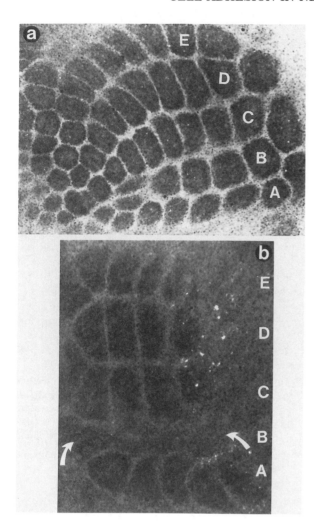

Figure 7. Localization of cytotactin in normal (*a*) and damaged (*b*) mouse whisker barrel cortex (rows A–E). (*a*) Antibodies to cytotactin stain the barrel walls but not the hollows in the P7 barrel field. (*b*) When row B of P1.5 whiskers were electrocauterized, the cytotactin at P8 was fused into a stripe in row B with no delineation between barrels. (Adapted from Crossin et al. 1989.)

man 1987b) that a precursor gene for an N-CAM-like adhesion molecule gave rise to the entire immunoglobulin superfamily and to the vertebrate system of adaptive immunity. The finding in *Drosophila* of the N-CAM-related molecules amalgam (Seeger et al. 1988), fasciclin II (Harrelson and Goodman 1988), which is a CAM, and neuroglian (Bieber et al. 1989) provides strong corroboration of this hypothesis: *Drosophila* species do not have an adaptive immune system containing major histocompatibility antigens and immunoglobulins of the kind found in vertebrate species.

We may conclude that, during evolution, the gene for such a precursor duplicated and was modified to give rise to neurally important CAMs, as well as to the molecules of adaptive immunity (Edelman 1987b). In the former class are N-CAM, Ng-CAM, the newly discovered Nr-CAM (M. Grumet et al., unpubl.), con-

tactin, TAG-1, myelin-associated glycoprotein (MAG), P_0, and the invertebrate molecules fasciclin II and neuroglian (Table 1, Fig. 1).

It remains a challenge to determine whether a specific combination of multiple different neural CAMs under control of a given set of signals can be changed by the additional place-dependent expression of a new CAM. This could occur via signaling from growth cones exploring a new region which then transfer signaling factors for that expression by retrograde transport. Models of this kind have been proposed previously (Bastiani et al. 1985; Edelman 1987a [pp. 118-119]). If CAMs are to be expressed or down-regulated in a particular fascicle at a particular place and time, such signals are likely to be transported to a cell body from a growth cone to affect transcription of a given CAM. It does not take too much imagination to see how neural branching and fasciculation events could lead to a huge variety of structures, given the combination of even several dozens of neural CAMs and the appropriate retrograde signals.

The question arises whether such signaling can also account for the specific activity-dependent establishment of synapses in neural maps. A close consideration of this problem suggests that regulation of CAM expression is necessary but not sufficient and that an additional form of place-dependent spatial signaling is required. We end this paper by a brief consideration of an hypothesis on the role of spatial signaling in converting temporally correlated activity to spatial connectivity at the level of the synapses themselves.

Back-signaling by Diffusible Substances in the Establishment of Refined Neural Mappings

However subtle CAM signaling may be and however large the CAM repertoire may be, CAMs alone cannot assure the formation of individual specific synapses that undergo activity-dependent refinement. There are many pieces of evidence suggesting that the segregation and refinement of afferent projections during development depend on correlated electrical activity and synaptic changes occurring between afferents and their target (Hubel et al. 1977; Stretavan and Shatz 1986; Stryker and Harris 1986; Cline et al. 1987; Frank 1987; Kleinschmidt et al. 1987; Schmidt 1990). The *N*-methyl-D-aspartate (NMDA) receptor and excitatory transmission have both been implicated in this activity-dependent segregation (Constantine-Paton et al. 1990). Given the remarkable specificity of such activity-driven sharpening and the wide extent of the axonal arborizations and their dendritic targets, a retrograde signal from each postsynaptic neuron only to its corresponding presynaptic neuron may be necessary but would not be sufficient to account for this sharpening. What appears to be required is a *spatial* signal that differs from those seen in NGF uptake or, for example, from those inferred from the data on CAMs.

A recent hypothesis (Gally et al. 1990) involving a rapidly diffusible substance such as nitric oxide (NO) released from a postsynaptic site suggests an alternative. Although several candidate substances remain to be ruled in or out and there may be more than one such substance, there is evidence to suggest that NO may serve as such a short-lived signal. In this hypothesis (Fig. 8), temporally correlated firing of afferents releases NO, the enzyme for which is present in the CNS. NO rapidly diffuses into the surrounding cells where it binds to the heme group of soluble guanylate cyclase, increasing cGMP synthesis. Evidence suggests that it might also stimulate ADP-ribosylase activity and this may in turn affect vesicle release. According to the hypothesis, the presence of correlated action potentials arriving at neurons in a space (regardless of their direct synaptic connectivity) would give rise to levels of NO that could facilitate growth cone branching and encourage the formation of synapses only at the terminals of active axons. This would alter the eventual location and shape of terminal arbors. Any growth cones far from dendritic targets (as in eventual white matter) or in dendritic areas releasing a diffusible signal that is not in phase with correlated electrical activity would tend not to form local branches or synapses but rather would continue to explore a target space.

This hypothesis is consistent with reports that NMDA blocking agents disrupt the formation and refinement of appropriately mapped synapses (Cline and Constantine-Paton 1990). The NO synthase is a Ca^{++}-dependent enzyme, and it has been shown that NO release is stimulated by glutamate and blocked by agents that block glutamatergic transmission (Garthwaite et al. 1988, 1989a,b). It is important to notice that the postulated return signal would act rapidly in an extended neuronal volume and that it can act epigenetically on both the postsynaptic and presynaptic sites in that space. In this way, it would naturally lead to formation of neuronal groups (Edelman 1987a). Furthermore, since NO is essential to formation of the endothelial relaxing factor, its release would contribute to the evoked vascular changes in functioning regions of the CNS that underlie changes in positron emission tomography scans.

It has not yet been shown that NO is in fact able to act in the fashion hypothesized; but, whatever the case, a variety of other signals that act in similar fashion (albeit with a lower diffusion constant) would still remain viable candidates. Among these, arachidonic acid is a notable candidate, particularly inasmuch as it has been implicated in causing long-term potentiation (Lazarewicz et al. 1988; Williams et al. 1989).

One of our main purposes in describing this notion of rapidly diffusible short-lived signals is to underscore the need for several levels of signaling during neural morphogenesis. Growth cone exploration and specific synapse formation depend in a variety of ways on molecules mediating adhesion or promoting neurite retraction. Clearly, should spatial signaling be involved in the activity-dependent synaptogenesis that occurs during

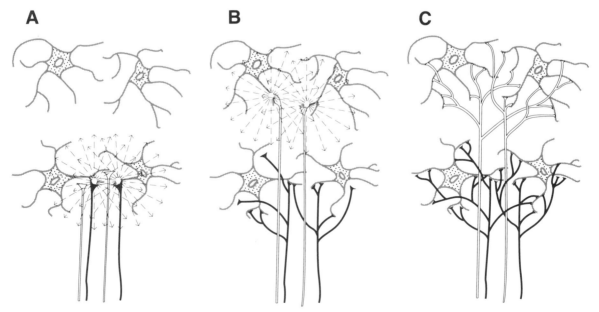

A **B** **C**

Figure 8. Schematic illustration of the mechanisms by which the formation of a short-lived, rapidly diffusing substance at active synapses might use patterns of correlated neural input to guide the segregation of terminal axonal arbors within dendritic fields. (A) Solid lines denote axons that are active at a particular instance during the period when axonal growth cones first invade dendritic fields. These axons generate the diffusive signal indicated by the dashed arrows. Axonal terminals active within the space filled by this signal are induced to form and strengthen synapses and to branch to form new growth cones. Axonal terminals not active at this instant (stippled lines) tend to weaken or break synapses and to grow out of this space. (B) At a later time during development, at an instant when the other axons (stippled lines) are active, the diffusive signal fills a space at which all axonal terminals simultaneously active tend to form synapses and branch. (C) In the adult neuroanatomy, axonal terminal arbors are segregated from one another as a result of their history of input neural activity.

formation of refined mappings, concurrent alterations in signals for CAM and SAM expression must be at least permissive, if not actively coregulated. A delicate balance of cellular driving forces, the action of morphoregulatory molecules, and several different types of signaling must be responsible for establishing functioning neuroanatomy. Identifying the different types of signaling events in terms of electrical activity, neurotransmitter action, and CAM and SAM expression and function remains one of the most challenging tasks in developmental neurobiology.

REFERENCES

Albelda, S.M., P.D. Oliver, L.H. Romer, and C.A. Buck. 1990. EndoCAM: A novel endothelial cell-cell adhesion molecule. *J. Cell Biol.* **110:** 1227.

Arquint, M., S. Roder, L.S. Chia, J. Down, D. Wilkinson, H. Bayley, P. Braun, and R. Dunn. 1987. Molecular cloning and primary structure of myelin-associated glycoprotein. *Proc. Natl. Acad. Sci.* **84:** 600.

Aurivillius, M., O.C. Hansen, M.B.S. Lazrek, E. Bock, and B. Obrink. 1990. The cell adhesion molecule Cell-CAM 105 is an ecto-ATPase and a member of the immunoglobulin superfamily. *FEBS Lett.* **264:** 267.

Bastiani, M.J., G.S. du Lac, and C.S. Goodman. 1985. *The first neuronal growth cones in insect embryos: Model systems for studying the development of neuronal specificity.* Plenum Press, New York.

Becker, J.W., H.P. Erickson, S. Hoffman, B.A. Cunningham, and G.M. Edelman. 1989. Topology of cell adhesion molecules. *Proc. Natl. Acad. Sci.* **86:** 1088.

Bertolotti, R., U. Rutishauser, and G.M. Edelman. 1980. A cell surface molecule involved in aggregation of embryonic liver cells. *Proc. Natl. Acad. Sci.* **77:** 4831.

Bieber, A.J., P.M. Snow, M. Hortsch, N.H. Patel, J.R. Jacobs, Z.R. Traquina, J. Schilling, and C.S. Goodman. 1989. *Drosophila* neuroglian: A member of the immunoglobulin superfamily with extensive homology to the vertebrate neural adhesion molecule L1. *Cell* **59:** 447.

Blaschuk, O.W. and R. Farookhi. 1989. Estradiol stimulates cadherin expression in rat granulosa cells. *Dev. Biol.* **136:** 564.

Bock, E., C. Richter-Landsberg, A. Faissner, and M. Schachner. 1985. Demonstration of immunochemical identity between the nerve growth factor-inducible large external (NILE) glycoprotein and the cell adhesion molecule-L1. *EMBO J.* **4:** 2765.

Bourdon, M.A., T.J. Matthews, S.V. Pizzo, and D.D. Bigner. 1985. Immunochemical and biochemical characterization of a glioma-associated extracellular matrix glycoprotein. *J. Cell. Biochem.* **28:** 183.

Brackenbury, R., J.-P. Thiery, U. Rutishauser, and G.M. Edelman. 1977. Adhesion among neural cells of the chick embryo. I. An immunological assay for molecules involved in cell-cell binding. *J. Biol. Chem.* **252:** 6835.

Bronner-Fraser, M. 1988. Distribution and function of tenascin during cranial neural crest development in the chick. *J. Neurosci. Res.* **21:** 135.

Brummendorf, T., J.M. Wolff, R. Frank, and F.G. Rathjen 1989. Neural cell recognition molecule F11: Homology with fibronectin type III and immunoglobulin type C domains. *Neuron* **2:** 1351.

Buskirk, D.R., J.-P. Thiery, U. Rutishauser, and G.M. Edelman. 1980. Antibodies to a neural cell adhesion molecule disrupt histogenesis in cultured chick retinae. *Nature* **285:** 488.

Caroni, P. and M.E. Schwab. 1988. Antibody against myelin-associated inhibitor of neurite growth neutralizes nonper-

missive substrate properties of CNS white matter. *Neuron* **1:** 85.

Chiquet, M. and D.M. Fambrough. 1984. Chick myotendinous antigen. I. A monoclonal antibody as a marker for tendon and muscle morphogenesis. *J. Cell Biol.* **98:** 1926.

Chiquet-Ehrismann, R., E.J. Mackie, C.A. Pearson, and T. Sakakura. 1986. Tenascin: An extracellular matrix protein involved in tissue interactions during fetal development and oncogenesis. *Cell* **47:** 131.

Chuong, C.-M., K.L. Crossin, and G.M. Edelman. 1987. Sequential expression and differential function of multiple adhesion molecules during the formation of cerebellar cortical layers. *J. Cell Biol.* **104:** 331.

Cline, H.T. and M. Constantine-Paton. 1990. NMDA receptor agonist and antagonists alter retinal ganglion cell arbor structure in the developing frog retinotectal projection. *J. Neurosci.* **10(4):** 1197.

Cline, H.T., E.A. Debski, and M. Constantine-Paton. 1987. *N*-methyl-D-aspartate receptor antagonist desegregates eye-specific stripes. *Proc. Natl. Acad. Sci.* **84:** 4342.

Constantine-Paton, M., H.T. Cline, and E. Debski. 1990. Patterned activity, synaptic convergence, and the NMDA receptor in developing visual pathways. *Annu. Rev. Neurosci.* **13:** 129.

Covault, J. and J.R. Sanes. 1985. Neural cell adhesion molecule (N-CAM) accumulates in denervated and paralyzed skeletal muscles. *Proc. Natl. Acad. Sci.* **82:** 4544.

Covault, J., J.P. Merlie, C. Goridis, and J.R. Sanes. 1986. Molecular forms of N-CAM and its RNA in developing and denervated skeletal muscle. *J. Cell Biol.* **102:** 731.

Cox, E.C., B. Muller, and F. Bonhoeffer. 1990. Axonal guidance in the chick visual system: Posterior tectal membranes induce collapse of growth cones from the temporal retina. *Neuron* **2:** 31.

Crossin, K.L. 1990. Cell adhesion molecules in embryogenesis and disease. *Ann. N.Y. Acad. Sci.* (in press).

Crossin, K.L., C.-M. Chuong, and G.M. Edelman. 1985. Expression sequences of cell adhesion molecules. *Proc. Natl. Acad. Sci.* **82:** 6942.

Crossin, K.L., S. Hoffman, S.-S. Tan, and G.M. Edelman. 1989. Cytotactin and its proteoglycan ligand mark structural and functional boundaries in somatosensory cortex of the early postnatal mouse. *Dev. Biol.* **136:** 381.

Crossin, K.L., S. Hoffman, M. Grumet, J.-P. Thiery, and G.M. Edelman. 1986. Site-restricted expression of cytotactin during development of the chicken embryo. *J. Cell Biol.* **102:** 1917.

Crossin, K.L., A.L. Prieto, S. Hoffman, F.S. Jones, and D.R. Friedlander. 1990. Expression of adhesion molecules and the establishment of boundaries during embryonic and neural development. *Exp. Neurol.* (in press).

Cunningham, B.A., J.J. Hemperly, B.A. Murray, E.A. Prediger, R. Brackenbury, and G.M. Edelman. 1987. Neural cell adhesion molecule: Structure, immunoglobulin-like domains, cell surface modulation, and alternative RNA splicing. *Science* **236:** 799.

Damjanov, I., A. Damjanov, and C.H. Damsky. 1986. Developmentally regulated expression of the cell-cell adhesion glycoprotein cell-CAM 120/80 in peri-implantation mouse embryos and extraembryonic membranes. *Dev. Biol.* **116:** 194.

Daniloff, J.K., G. Levi, M. Grumet, F. Rieger, and G.M. Edelman. 1986. Altered expression of neuronal cell adhesion molecules induced by nerve injury and repair. *J. Cell Biol.* **103:** 929.

Daniloff, J.K., K.L. Crossin, M. Pinçon-Raymond, M. Murawsky, F. Rieger, and G.M. Edelman. 1989. Expression of cytotactin in the normal and regenerating neuromuscular system. *J. Cell Biol.* **108:** 625.

Davies, J.A., G.M.W. Cook, C.D. Stern, and R.J. Keynes. 1990. Isolation from chick somites of a glycoprotein fraction that causes collapse of dorsal root ganglion growth cones. *Neuron* **2:** 11.

Dickson, G., H.J. Gower, C.H. Barton, II.M. Prentice, V.L. Elsom, S.E. Moore, R.D. Cox, C. Quinn, W. Putt, and F.S. Walsh. 1987. Human muscle neural cell adhesion molecule (N-CAM)—Identification of a muscle specific sequence in the extracellular domain. *Cell* **50:** 1119.

Edelman, G.M. 1976. Surface modulation in cell recognition and cell growth. *Science* **192:** 218.

———. 1986. Cell adhesion molecules in the regulation of animal form and tissue pattern. *Annu. Rev. Cell Biol.* **2:** 81.

———. 1987a. *Neural Darwinism: The theory of neuronal group selection.* Basic Books, New York.

———. 1987b. CAMs and Igs: Cell adhesion and the evolutionary origins of immunity. *Immunol. Rev.* **100:** 11.

———. 1988a. Morphoregulatory molecules. *Biochemistry* **27:** 3533.

———. 1988b. *Topobiology: An introduction to molecular embryology.* Basic Books, New York.

Edelman, G.M. and C.-M. Chuong. 1982. Embryonic to adult conversion of neural cell adhesion molecules in normal and staggerer mice. *Proc. Natl. Acad. Sci.* **79:** 7036.

Erickson, H.P. and J.L. Iglesias. 1984. A six-armed oligomer isolated from cell surface fibronectin preparations. *Nature* **311:** 267.

Erickson, H.P. and H.C. Taylor. 1987. Hexabrachion proteins in embryonic chicken tissues and human tumors. *J. Cell Biol.* **105:** 1387.

Frank, E. 1987. The influence of neuronal activity on patterns of synaptic connections. *Trends Neurosci.* **10:** 188.

Fraser, S.E., B.A. Murray, C.-M. Chuong, and G.M. Edelman. 1984. Alteration of the retinotectal map in *Xenopus* by antibodies to neural cell adhesion molecules. *Proc. Natl. Acad. Sci.* **81:** 4222.

Fraser, S.E., M.S. Carhart, B.A. Murray, C.-M. Chuong, and G.M. Edelman. 1988. Alterations in the *Xenopus* retinotectal projection by antibodies to *Xenopus* N-CAM. *Dev. Biol.* **129:** 217.

Friedlander, D.R., M. Grumet, and G.M. Edelman. 1986. Nerve growth factor enhances expression of neuron-glia cell adhesion molecule in PC12 cells. *J. Cell Biol.* **102:** 413.

Friedlander, D.R., S. Hoffman, and G.M. Edelman. 1988. Functional mapping of cytotactin: Proteolytic fragments active in cell-substrate adhesion. *J. Cell Biol.* **107:** 2329.

Friedlander, D.R., R.-M. Mege, B.A. Cunningham, and G.M. Edelman. 1989. Cell sorting-out is modulated by both the specificity and amount of different cell adhesion molecules (CAMs) expressed on cell surfaces. *Proc. Natl. Acad. Sci.* **86:** 7043.

Furley, A.J., S.B. Morton, D. Manalo, D. Karagogeos, J. Dodd, and T.M. Jessel. 1990. The axonal glycoprotein TAG-1 is an immunoglobulin superfamily member with neurite-promoting activity. *Cell* **61:** 157.

Gall, W.E. and G.M. Edelman. 1981. Lateral diffusion of surface molecules in animal cells and tissues. *Science* **213:** 903.

Gallin, W.J., G.M. Edelman, and B.A. Cunningham. 1983. Characterization of L-CAM, a major cell adhesion molecule from embryonic liver cells. *Proc. Natl. Acad. Sci.* **80:** 1038.

Gallin, W.J., B.C. Sorkin, G.M. Edelman, and B.A. Cunningham. 1987. Sequence analysis of a cDNA clone encoding the liver cell adhesion molecule, L-CAM. *Proc. Natl. Acad. Sci.* **84:** 2808.

Gally, J.A., P.R. Montague, G.N. Reeke, Jr., and G.M. Edelman. 1990. The NO hypothesis: Possible effects of a short-lived, rapidly diffusible signal in the development and function of the nervous system. *Proc. Natl. Acad. Sci.* **87:** 3547.

Garthwaite, J., S.L. Charles, and R. Chess-Williams. 1988. Endothelium-derived relaxing factor release on activation of NMDA receptors suggests role as intercellular messenger in the brain. *Nature* **336:** 385.

Garthwaite, J., E. Southam, and M. Anderton. 1989a. A kainate receptor linked to nitric oxide synthesis from arginine. *J. Neurochem.* **53:** 1952.

Garthwaite, J., G. Garthwaite, R.M.J. Palmer, and S. Moncada. 1989b. NMDA receptor activation induces nitric oxide synthesis from arginine in rat brain slices. *Eur. J. Pharmacol.* **172:** 413.

Gennarini, G., G. Cibelli, G. Rougon, M.-G. Mattei, and C. Goridis. 1989. The mouse neuronal cell surface protein F3: A phosphatidylinositol-anchored member of the immunoglobulin superfamily related to chicken contractin. *J. Cell Biol.* **109:** 775.

Grumet, M., S. Hoffman, and G.M. Edelman. 1984. Two antigenically related neuronal cell adhesion molecules of different specificities mediate neuron-neuron and neuron-glia adhesion. *Proc. Natl. Acad. Sci.* **81:** 267.

Grumet, M., S. Hoffman, K.L. Crossin, and G.M. Edelman. 1985. Cytotactin, an extracellular matrix protein of neural and non-neural tissues that mediates glia-neuron interaction. *Proc. Natl. Acad. Sci.* **82:** 8075.

Grumet, M., M.P. Burgoon, V. Mauro, G.M. Edelman, and B.A. Cunningham. 1989. Structure and characterization of Ng-CAM and a closely-related molecule. *J. Neurosci.* **15:** 568a.

Harrelson, A.L. and C.S. Goodman. 1988. Growth cone guidance in insects—Fasciclin II is a member of the immunoglobulin superfamily. *Science* **242:** 700.

Hatta, K. and M. Takeichi. 1986. Expression of N-cadherin adhesion molecules associated with early morphogenetic events in chick development. *Nature* **320:** 447.

Hatta, K., A. Nose, A. Nagafuchi, and M. Takeichi. 1988. Cloning and expression of cDNA encoding a neural calcium-dependent cell adhesion molecule—Its identity in the cadherin gene family. *J. Cell Biol.* **106:** 873.

He, H.T., J. Barbet, J.C. Chaix, and C. Goridis. 1986. Phosphatidylinositol is involved in the membrane attachment of NCAM-120, the smallest component of the neural cell adhesion molecule. *EMBO J.* **5:** 2489.

Hemperly, J.J., G.M. Edelman, and B.A. Cunningham. 1986. cDNA clones of N-CAM lacking a membrane-spanning region consistent with evidence for membrane attachment via a phosphatidylinositol intermediate. *Proc. Natl. Acad. Sci.* **83:** 9822.

Hinoda, Y., M. Neumaier, S.A. Hefta, Z. Drzeniek, C. Wagener, L. Shively, L.J.G. Hefta, J.E. Shively, and R.J. Paxton. 1988. Molecular cloning of a cDNA coding biliary glycoprotein. I. Primary structure of a glycoprotein immunologically crossreactive with carcinoembryonic antigen. *Proc. Natl. Acad. Sci.* **85:** 6959.

Hirsch, M.-R., L. Gaugler, H. Deagostini-Bazin, L. Bally-Cuif, and C. Goridis. 1990. Identification of positive and negative regulatory elements governing cell-type-specific expression of the neural cell adhesion molecule gene. *Mol. Cell. Biol.* **10:** 1959.

Hoffman, S. and G.M. Edelman. 1983. Kinetics of homophilic binding by E and A forms of the neural cell adhesion molecule. *Proc. Natl. Acad. Sci.* **80:** 5762.

———. 1987. A proteoglycan with HNK-1 antigenic determinants is a neuron-associated ligand for cytotactin. *Proc. Natl. Acad. Sci.* **84:** 2523.

Hoffman, S., K.L. Crossin, and G.M. Edelman. 1988. Molecular forms, binding functions, and developmental expression patterns of cytotactin and cytotactin-binding proteoglycan, an interactive pair of extracellular matrix molecules. *J. Cell Biol.* **106:** 519.

Hoffman, S., D.R. Friedlander, C.-M. Chuong, M. Grumet, and G.M. Edelman. 1986. Differential contributions of Ng-CAM and N-CAM to cell adhesion in different neural regions. *J. Cell Biol.* **103:** 145.

Hubel, D.H., T.N. Weisel, and S. LeVay. 1977. Plasticity of ocular dominance columns in monkey striate cortex. *Philos. Trans. R. Soc. London B Biol. Sci.* **278:** 377.

Husmann, M., I. Gorgen, C. Weisgerber, and D. Bitter-Suermann. 1989. Up-regulation of embryonic NCAM in an EC cell line by retinoic acid. *Dev. Biol.* **136:** 194.

Hyafil, F., C. Babinet, and F. Jacob. 1981. Cell-cell interactions in early embryogenesis: A molecular approach to the role of calcium. *Cell* **26:** 447.

Hynes, R.O. 1987. Integrins: A family of cell surface receptors. *Cell* **48:** 549.

Jaffe, S.H., D.R. Friedlander, F. Matsuzaki, K.L. Crossin, B.A. Cunningham, and G.M. Edelman. 1990. Differential effects of the cytoplasmic domains of cell adhesion molecules on cell aggregation and cell sorting. *Proc. Natl. Acad. Sci.* **87:** 3589.

Jones, F.S., K.L. Crossin, B.A. Cunningham, and G.M. Edelman. 1990. Identification and characterization of the promoter for the cytotactin gene. *Proc. Natl. Acad. Sci.* (in press).

Jones, F.S., S. Hoffman, B.A. Cunningham, and G.M. Edelman. 1989. A detailed structural model of cytotactin: Protein homologies, alternative RNA splicing, and binding regions. *Proc. Natl. Acad. Sci.* **86:** 1905.

Jones, F.S., M.P. Burgoon, S. Hoffman, K.L. Crossin, B.A. Cunningham, and G.M. Edelman. 1988. A cDNA clone for cytotactin contains sequences similar to epidermal growth factor-like repeats and segments of fibronectin and fibrinogen. *Proc. Natl. Acad. Sci.* **85:** 2186.

Kleinschmidt, A., M.F. Bear, and W. Singer. 1987. Blockade of "NMDA" receptors disrupts experience-dependent plasticity of kitten striate cortex. *Science* **238:** 355.

Kruse, J., G. Keilhauer, A. Faissner, R. Timpl, and M. Schachner. 1985. The J1 glycoprotein—A novel nervous system cell adhesion molecule of the L2/HNK-1 family. *Nature* **316:** 146.

Lazarewicz, J.W., J.T. Wroblewski, M.E. Palmer, and E. Costa. 1988. Activation of *N*-methyl-D-aspartate-sensitive glutamate receptors stimulates arachidonic acid release in primary cultures of cerebellar granule cells. *Neuropharmacology* **27:** 765.

Lemke, G. and R. Axel. 1985. Isolation and sequence of a cDNA encoding the major structural protein of peripheral myelin. *Cell* **40:** 501.

Levi, G., K.L. Crossin, and G.M. Edelman. 1987. Expression sequences and distribution of two primary cell adhesion molecules during embryonic development of *Xenopus laevis.* *J. Cell Biol.* **105:** 2359.

Levi, G., F. Broders, D. Dunon, G.M. Edelman, and J.-P. Thiery. 1990. Thyroxine-dependent modulations of the expression of the neural cell adhesion molecule N-CAM during *Xenopus laevis* metamorphosis. *Development* **109:** 681.

Lin, S. and G. Guidotti. 1989. Cloning and expression of a cDNA coding for a rat liver plasma membrane ecto-ATPase. *J. Biol. Chem.* **264:** 14408.

Mackie, E.J., R.P. Tucker, W. Halfter, R. Chiquet-Ehrismann, and H.H. Epperlein. 1988. The distribution of tenascin coincides with pathways of neural crest cell migration. *Development* **102:** 237.

Matsuzaki, F., R.-M. Mege, S.H. Jaffe, D.R. Friedlander, W.J. Gallin, J.I. Goldberg, B.A. Cunningham, and G.M. Edelman. 1990. cDNAs of cell adhesion molecules of different specificity induce changes in cell shape and border formation in cultured S180 cells. *J. Cell Biol.* **110:** 1239.

McGuire, J.C., L.A. Greene, and A.V. Furano. 1978. NGF stimulates incorporation of fucose or glucosamine into an external glycoprotein in cultured rat PC12 pheochromocytoma cells. *Cell* **15:** 357.

Mege, R.-M., F. Matsuzaki, W.J. Gallin, J.I. Goldberg, B.A. Cunningham, and G.M. Edelman. 1988. Construction of epithelioid sheets by transfection of mouse sarcoma cells with cDNAs for chicken cell adhesion molecules. *Proc. Natl. Acad. Sci.* **85:** 7274.

Moonen, G., M.P. Grau-Wagemans, and I. Selak. 1982. Plas-minogen activator-plasmin system and neuronal migration. *Nature* **298:** 753.

Moos, M., R. Tacke, H. Scherer, D. Teplow, K. Fruh, and M. Schachner. 1988. Neural adhesion molecule L1 as a member of the immunoglobulin superfamily with binding domains similar to fibronectin. *Nature* **334:** 701.

Murray, B.A., J.J. Hemperly, E.A. Prediger, G.M. Edelman, and B.A. Cunningham. 1986a. Alternatively spliced mRNAs code for different polypeptide chains of the chicken neural cell adhesion molecule (N-CAM). *J. Cell Biol.* **102:** 189.

Murray, B.A., G.C. Owens, E.A. Prediger, K.L. Crossin, B.A. Cunningham, and G.M. Edelman. 1986b. Cell surface modulation of the neural cell adhesion molecule resulting from alternative mRNA splicing in a tissue-specific developmental sequence. *J. Cell Biol.* **103:** 1431.

Musil, S.M., B.A. Cunningham, G.M. Edelman, and D.A. Goodenough.. 1990. Differences in phosphorylation of the gap junction protein connexin 43 in junctional communication-competent and -deficient cells. *J. Cell Biol.* (in press).

Nagafuchi, A. and M. Takeichi. 1988. Cell binding function of E-cadherin is regulated by the cytoplasmic domain. *EMBO J.* **7:** 3679.

———. 1989. Transmembrane control of cadherin-mediated cell adhesion: A 94 kDa protein functionally associated with a specific region of the cytoplasmic domain of E-cadherin. *Cell Regul.* **1:** 37.

Nagafuchi, A., Y. Shirayoshi, K. Okazaki, K. Yasuda, and M. Takeichi. 1987. Transformation of cell adhesion properties by exogenously introduced E-cadherin cDNA. *Nature* **329:** 341.

Newman, P.J., M.C. Berndt, J. Gorski, G.C. White II, S. Lyman, C. Paddock, and W.A. Muller. 1990. PECAM-1 (CD31) cloning and relation to adhesion molecules of the immunoglobulin gene superfamily. *Science* **247:** 1219.

Nose, A., A. Nagafuchi, and M. Takeichi. 1987. Isolation of placental cadherin cDNA—Identification of a novel gene family of cell-cell adhesion molecules. *EMBO J.* **6:** 3655.

Ogou, S.I., C. Yoshida-Noro, and M. Takeichi. 1983. Calcium-dependent cell-cell adhesion molecules common to hepatocytes and teratocarcinoma cells. *J. Cell Biol.* **97:** 944.

Osborn, L., C. Hession, R. Tizard, C. Vassallo, S. Luhowskyj, G. Chi-Rosso, and R. Lobb. 1989. Direct expression cloning of vascular cell adhesion molecule 1, a cytokine-induced endothelial protein that binds to lymphocytes. *Cell* **59:** 1203.

Owens, G.C., G.M. Edelman, and B.A. Cunningham. 1987. Organization of the neural cell adhesion molecule (N-CAM) gene: Alternative exon usage as the basis for different membrane-associated domains. *Proc. Natl. Acad. Sci.* **84:** 294.

Ozawa, M., H. Baribault, and R. Kemler. 1989. The cytoplasmic domain of the cell adhesion molecule uvomorulin associates with three independent proteins structurally related in different species. *EMBO J.* **8:** 1711.

Pearson, C.A., D. Pearson, S. Shibahara, J. Hofsteenge, and R. Chiquet-Ehrismann. 1988. Tenascin: cDNA cloning and induction by TGF-β. *EMBO J.* **7:** 2977.

Pollerberg, G.E., M. Schachner, and J. Davoust. 1986. Differentiation state-dependent surface mobilities of two forms of the neural cell adhesion molecule. *Nature* **324:** 462.

Prediger, E.A., S. Hoffman, G.M. Edelman, and B.A. Cunningham. 1988. Four exons encode a 93bp insert in three N-CAM mRNAs specific for chick heart and skeletal muscle. *Proc. Natl. Acad. Sci.* **85:** 9616.

Prieto, A.L., F.S. Jones, B.A. Cunningham, K.L. Crossin, and G.M. Edelman.. 1990. Localization during development of alternatively-spliced forms of cytotactin by *in situ* hybridization. *J. Cell Biol.* **11:** (in press).

Ranscht, B.. 1988. Sequence of contactin, 130-kD glycoprotein concentrated in areas of interneuronal contact, defines a new member of the immunoglobulin supergene family in the nervous system. *J. Cell Biol.* **107:** 1561.

Raper, J.A. and J.P. Kapfhammer. 1990. The enrichment of a neuronal growth cone collapsing activity from embryonic chick brain. *Neuron* **2:** 21.

Rathjen, F.G. and M. Schachner. 1984. Immunocytological and biochemical characterization of a new neuronal cell surface component (L1 antigen), which is involved in cell adhesion. *EMBO J.* **3:** 1.

Rieger, F., M. Grumet, and G.M. Edelman. 1985. N-CAM at the vertebrate neuromuscular junction. *J. Cell Biol.* **101:** 285.

Rieger, F., M. Nicolet, M. Pinçon-Raymond, G. Levi, and G.M. Edelman. 1988. Distribution and role in regeneration of N-CAM in basal laminae of muscle and Schwann cells. *J. Cell Biol.* **107:** 707.

Rieger, F., J.K. Daniloff, M. Pinçon-Raymond, K.L. Crossin, M. Grumet, and G.M. Edelman. 1986. Neuronal cell adhesion molecules and cytotactin are colocalized at the node of Ranvier. *J. Cell Biol.* **103:** 379.

Ringwald, M., R. Schuh, D. Vestweber, H. Eistetter, F. Lohspeich, J. Engel, R. Dotz, F. Jahnig, J. Epplen, S. Mayer, C. Muller, and R. Kemler. 1987. The structure of cell adhesion molecule uvomorulin. Insights into the molecular mechanism of Ca^{2+}-dependent cell adhesion. *EMBO J.* **6:** 3647.

Rothbard, J.B., R. Brackenbury, B.A. Cunningham, and G.M. Edelman. 1982. Differences in the carbohydrate structures of neural cell-adhesion molecules from adult and embryonic chicken brains. *J. Biol. Chem.* **257:** 11064.

Ruoslahti, E. and F.G. Giancotti. 1989. Integrins and tumor cell dissemination. *Cancer Cells Monthly Rev.* **1:** 119.

Santoni, M.J., D. Barthels, G. Vopper, A. Boned, C. Goridis, and W. Wille. 1989. Differential exon usage involving an unusual splicing mechanism generates at least eight types of NCAM cDNA in mouse brain. *EMBO J.* **8:** 385.

Schmidt, J.T.. 1990. Long-term potentiation and activity-dependent retinotopic sharpening in the regenerating retinotectal projection of goldfish: Common sensitive period and sensitivity to NMDA blockers. *J. Neurosci.* **10:** 233.

Seeger, M.A., L. Haffley, and T.C. Kaufman. 1988. Characterization of amalgam: A member of the immunoglobulin superfamily from *Drosophila. Cell* **55:** 589.

Sorkin, B.C., J.J. Hemperly, G.M. Edelman, and B.A. Cunningham. 1988. Structure of the gene for the liver cell adhesion molecule, L-CAM. *Proc. Natl. Acad. Sci.* **85:** 7617.

Sperry, R.W.. 1963. Chemoaffinity in the orderly growth of nerve fiber patterns and connections. *Proc. Natl. Acad. Sci.* **50:** 703.

Spring, J., K. Beck, and R. Chiquet-Ehrismann. 1989. Two contrary functions of tenascin: Dissection of the active sites by recombinant tenascin fragments. *Cell* **59:** 325.

Steindler, D.A., N.G.F. Cooper, A. Faissner, and M. Schachner. 1989. Boundaries defined by adhesion molecules during development of the cerebral cortex: The J1/tenascin glycoprotein in the mouse somatosensory cortical barrel field. *Dev. Biol.* **131:** 243.

Stretavan, D. and C.J. Shatz. 1986. Prenatal development of cat retinogeniculate axon arbors in the absence of binocular interactions. *J. Neurosci.* **6:** 990.

Stryker, M.P. and W.A. Harris. 1986. Binocular impulse blockade prevents the formation of ocular dominance columns in cat visual cortex. *J. Neurosci.* **6:** 2117.

Takeichi, M.. 1988. The cadherins—Cell-cell adhesion molecules controlling animal morphogenesis. *Development* **102:** 639.

Tan, S.-S., K.L. Crossin, S. Hoffman, and G.M. Edelman. 1987. Asymmetric expression in somites of cytotactin and its proteoglycan ligand is correlated with neural crest cell distribution. *Proc. Natl. Acad. Sci.* **84:** 7977.

Thiery, J.-P., G.C. Tucker, and H. Aoyama. 1985. Gangliogenesis in the avian embryo—Migration and adhesion properties of neural crest cells. In *Molecular bases of neural development* (ed. G. M. Edelman et al.), p. 181. Wiley, New York.

Thiery, J.-P., R. Brackenbury, U. Rutishauser, and G.M. Edelman. 1977. Adhesion among neural cells of the chick embryo. II. Purification and characterization of a cell adhesion molecule from neural retina. *J. Biol. Chem.* **252:** 6841.

Thompson, J., G. Dickson, S.E. Moore, H.J. Gower, W. Putt, J.G. Kenimer, C.H. Barton, and F.S. Walsh. 1989. Alternative splicing of the neural cell adhesion molecule gene generates variant extracellular domain structure in skeletal muscle and brain. *Genes Dev.* **3:** 348.

Volk, T. and B. Geiger. 1986. A-CAM—A 135 kD receptor of intercellular adherens junctions. I. Immuno-electron microscopic localization and biochemical studies. *J. Cell Biol.* **103:** 1441.

Williams, J.H., M.L. Errington, M.A. Lynch, and T.V.P. Bliss. 1989. Arachidonic acid induces a long-term activity-dependent enhancement of synaptic transmission in the hippocampus. *Nature* **341:** 739.

Woolsey, T.A., J.R. Anderson, J.R. Wann, and B.R. Stanfield. 1979. Effects of early vibrissal damage on neurons in the ventrobasal (VB) thalamus of the mouse. *J. Comp. Neurol.* **184:** 363.

Yahara, I. and G.M. Edelman. 1975. Modulation of lymphocyte receptor mobility by locally bound concanavalin A. *Proc. Natl. Acad. Sci.* **72:** 1579.

Cadherin Subclasses: Differential Expression and Their Roles in Neural Morphogenesis

M. Takeichi, H. Inuzuka, K. Shimamura, T. Fujimori, and A. Nagafuchi*

Department of Biophysics, Faculty of Science, Kyoto University, Kyoto 606, Japan

Cells are able to adhere selectively to particular cell types. This property of cells is considered to play an important role in development of the nervous system. For example, the selective adhesiveness might be essential for developing neurons to seek and bind to the particular target cells, or it might work for sorting different types of neurons and glias to establish the highly ordered stereotypic cell arrangement in neural tissues during development. In fact, it is known that disaggregated neural cells can reconstitute the original tissue-like structures when reaggregated by allocating themselves in a tissue-specific pattern (Fujisawa 1971). It is likely that such cell behaviors are regulated at least partly by the molecules involved in cell-cell adhesion, although many other factors, such as cell-matrix adhesion molecules, cell migration activators or inhibitors, chemotactic factors, and growth factors, might also be involved (Dodd and Jessel 1988).

Many classes of cell surface molecules that show cell-binding activities have been identified from neural cells, and these were classified into three molecular families: the immunoglobulin superfamily, the integrin superfamily, and the cadherin family, with some exceptions (Jessel 1988). Evidence has been accumulated that these molecules are involved in neuron-neuron, neuron-glia, or glia-glia adhesion. Although they have been operationally defined as cell adhesion molecules, their primary structures are completely different among the families, suggesting their distinct roles in cell-cell contact phenomena.

Cadherins are a group of Ca^{++}-dependent cell-cell adhesion molecules, subdivided into different members, such as E-cadherin (uvomorulin), P-cadherin, N-cadherin (A-CAM), and L-CAM (Takeichi 1988, 1990). About 50% amino acids are conserved among these molecules, and they are expressed in different cell types. Each member homophilically binds to the identical type, and, as a result, cells preferentially adhere to the cells with identical cadherins (Nose et al. 1988, 1990; Miyatani et al. 1989). Thus, cells acquire adhesive specificities by expressing different members of the cadherin family. It is therefore considered that this molecular family plays a key role in selective cell adhesion.

Expression of cadherins in embryos dynamically changes during development (Takeichi 1988). In early

neural development, the undifferentiated ectoderm expresses only E-cadherin in mammals or L-CAM in chickens. When the neural plate invaginates, it gradually loses E-cadherin or L-CAM, and instead it acquires N-cadherin (Thiery et al. 1984; Crossin et al. 1985; Hatta and Takeichi 1986; Duband et al. 1988). The neural tube whose closure has been completed strongly expresses N-cadherin, whereas the overlying ectoderm continues E-cadherin or L-CAM expression (Hatta et al. 1987). Thus, early neural epithelia express N-cadherin throughout their entire structure (Fig. 1a). Peripheral ganglia derived from neural crest cells also begin to express N-cadherin immediately after reaching their final destinations (Fig. 1b).

The pattern of expression of N-cadherin in neural tissues changes with differentiation of cells. In undifferentiated neuroepithelia, N-cadherin is almost evenly distributed (Fig. 1a). With differentiation, however, N-cadherin becomes gradually localized in particular cell layers. For example, in the spinal cord of 8-day-old chicken embryos, immunostaining intensity for N-cadherin varies with the regions of this tissue (Fig. 1b). Similarly, in the neural retina of 10-day-old chick embryos, the optic nerve fiber layer, the plexiform layers, and the outer limiting membrane express N-cadherin, but other layers do not, and thereafter this molecule gradually diminishes from most parts of the retina, except in the outer limiting membrane (Matsunaga et al. 1988a).

The role of N-cadherin in neural histogenesis has been investigated using antibodies that can inhibit the action of this molecule (Matsunaga et al. 1988a). When retinal fragments derived from early chicken embryos were incubated with such antibodies, they were dissociated into small cell clusters. Retinas from older embryos were not dissociated by the antibodies, but their histogenesis was severely affected. It was thus concluded that N-cadherin is essential for maintaining the overall structure of the undifferentiated retina, but, during development, its role becomes restricted to regulating the morphogenesis of local regions of the tissue.

It has also been shown that N-cadherin is involved in the attachment and outgrowth of axons. The retinal axons temporally express N-cadherin during development, and the neuroepithelial cells constituting the migration pathway for the axons also express this molecule. Experiments using N-cadherin-transfected cell lines demonstrated that the retinal axons use N-cadherin for their attachment to and the migration on

*Present address: Department of Information Physiology, National Institute for Physiological Sciences, Okazaki 444, Japan.

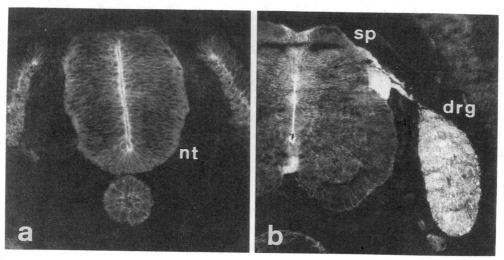

Figure 1. Immunofluorescent staining for N-cadherin in the neural tube of chicken embryos. (*a*) A transverse section of the neural tube of a 3.5-day-old embryo. (*b*) A transverse section of the spinal cord of a 8-day-old embryo. Note local differences in the staining intensity for N-cadherin in the spinal cord. The dorsal root ganglion also stained. (nt) Neural tube; (sp) spinal cord; (drg) dorsal root ganglion. Magnifications: (*a*) 232 × ; (*b*) 69 × .

the surface of other cells (Matsunaga et al. 1988b). It was also shown that N-cadherin plays a role in the attachment of axons to glial or muscle cells (Bixby et al. 1987; Tomaselli et al. 1988; Letourneau et al. 1990) and that this molecule can promote neurite outgrowth even when coated onto the surface of culture dishes (Bixby and Zhang 1990). A recent study suggested that N-cadherin is also involved in the fasciculation of retinal axons (Drazba and Lemmon 1990). From the results of these investigations, we believe that N-cadherin regulates a variety of morphogenetic events in the nervous system through its specific binding properties.

In the work presented here, we ask whether other cadherins are expressed in the nervous system, because our previous studies suggested the presence of unidentified cadherins in the neural retina (Matsunaga et al. 1988a). Since the cytoplasmic domain of cadherins is highly conserved in this molecular family (Hatta et al. 1988), antibodies raised to this domain were used to search for novel cadherins. The present work also shows that E-cadherin, which was previously thought to be an epithelial cadherin (Takeichi 1988), is expressed in some neurons. In addition, we examine whether neural development is perturbed if the pattern of expression of N-cadherin is artificially altered. Taking the results of these experiments into account, we discuss how the cadherin molecular family regulates neural morphogenesis.

EXPERIMENTAL PROCEDURES

Antibodies to the cytoplasmic domain of E-cadherin. Polyclonal antibodies against the carboxy-terminal region of E-cadherin were generated by using a protein-A fusion protein as an antigen. A *Sac*I-*Nco*I 143-bp fragment of E-cadherin cDNA, which encodes the carboxy-terminal 35-amino-acid sequence, with a short 3′ noncoding sequence following a stop codon, was blunt-

ended and inserted into the *Sma*I site of a pRIT2T vector (Pharmacia) in-frame. After transfecting N4830-1 host cells with this plasmid, the fusion protein was expressed, and then the product was affinity-purified using an IgG-Sepharose column. Rabbits were immunized with the purified fusion protein to produce antisera. The antibodies obtained were designated anti-ET35.

Microinjection of RNAs into Xenopus embryos. mRNAs were synthesized as described previously (Davanloo et al. 1984; Melton et al. 1984). Z10T6/BS, which was constructed by the insertion of chicken N-cadherin cDNA λN2 into the *Eco*RI site of a Bluescript KS+ vector (Hatta et al. 1988), was used as a template for transcription with T7 RNA polymerase (New England Biolabs). Synthesized RNAs were precipitated with ethanol, and RNA pellets were resuspended in 1.0 mM Tris–0.1 mM EDTA buffer at a final concentration of 200 μg/ml.

Eggs of *Xenopus laevis* were fertilized in vitro. One blastomere of each embryo at the 2-cell stage was microinjected with 15–30 nl of the 200 μg/ml RNA solution, and the injected embryos were allowed to develop at 23°C.

Immunostaining. Cells or tissues were fixed with 3.5% paraformaldehyde and 10 mM CaCl$_2$ in phosphate-buffered saline (PBS) at 4°C for 15–30 minutes, then postfixed with 100% methanol for 20 minutes at −20°C, and washed with 10 mM CaCl$_2$ and 0.1% Triton X-100 in PBS. The cells or cryostat sections of the tissues thus fixed were stained with antibodies to cadherins as described previously (Hatta et al. 1987).

Xenopus embryos were fixed as above, except that a saline for amphibian was used, and immunostained as whole-mount preparations according to the method of Dent et al. (1989) with some modifications. Briefly, embryos were treated with 0.3% H$_2$O$_2$ at 4°C for 3 hours and were then treated with 2% bovine serum albumin for more than 3 hours at 4°C. They then were incubated overnight at 4°C with monoclonal antibody NCD-2 to chicken N-cadherin (Hatta and Takeichi 1986) and washed. The embryos were then placed into a solution of a rabbit anti-rat immunoglobulin conjugated to horseradish peroxidase and incubated overnight at 4°C. After extensive washing, a peroxidase reaction was carried out using 0.05% diaminobenzidine, and the embryos were sectioned.

RESULTS AND DISCUSSION

Identification of a Novel Neural Cadherin

Using an antiserum raised against the cytoplasmic domain of E-cadherin (anti-ET35), we searched for novel cadherins by immunoblot analysis of the extracts of chicken embryonic neural retina. As shown in Figure 2 (left), the antibodies recognized two bands. The slowly migrating band was found to be N-cadherin, since this band reacted with antibodies to this molecule. The other band, however, reacted with none of the antibodies to identified cadherins, suggesting that it is a novel subclass of cadherin.

The expression of this novel cadherin during development of the neural retina was compared with that of N-cadherin (Fig. 2, right). The N-cadherin band was the most intense on embryonic days 5–10, and thereafter its expression decreased, as described previously

(Matsunaga et al. 1988a). In contrast, the expression of the other molecule was relatively weak on embryonic day 5, but it increased at later developmental stages and maintained the high level of expression at newly hatched stages. Thus, the temporal patterns of expression of these two molecules are complementary; N-cadherin decreases and the other one increases during embryonic development.

We then isolated cDNA clones coding for a novel cadherin using an oligonucleotide probe for the cytoplasmic domain of E-cadherin from a cDNA library derived from embryonic chicken brains and retinas (Hatta et al. 1988), and we found that the predicted amino acid sequence of this molecule is 75% identical to chicken N-cadherin but only 49% identical to L-CAM, the chicken epithelial cadherin. We designated this molecule retinal cadherin (R-cadherin).

These results demonstrated that N-cadherin is not the only cadherin in the nervous system, and they agree with the early observation that antibodies to N-cadherin cannot completely block Ca^{++}-dependent aggregation of neural retina cells (Matsunaga et al. 1988a). Antisera were raised against R-cadherin using a fusion protein of this molecule, and the preliminary results of immunostaining experiments showed that the distribution of N-cadherin and R-cadherin is indeed complementary in the neural retina of 14-day-old embryos, as expected from the immunoblot analysis. N-cadherin is localized only in the outer limiting membrane, whereas R-cadherin is detected in all other regions (data not shown).

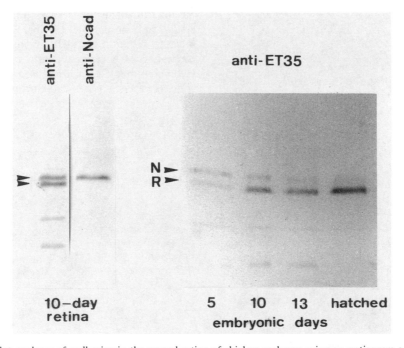

Figure 2. Immunoblot analyses of cadherins in the neural retina of chicken embryos using an antiserum against the cytoplasmic domain of E-cadherin (anti-ET35). (*Left*) Detection of the bands reacting with anti-ET35 or anti-N-cadherin (anti-Ncad) from the neural retina of 10-day-old embryos. Arrowheads indicate the cadherin bands. Bands with lower molecular weights have not been identified. (*Right*) Developmental changes in the expression of N- and the putative R-cadherin, detected with anti-ET35.

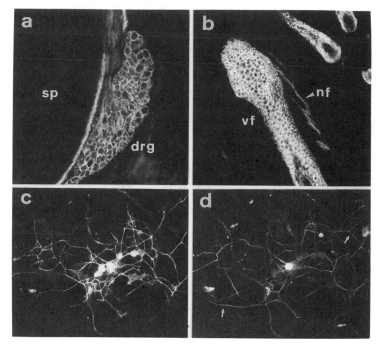

Figure 3. Immunofluorescent staining for E-cadherin expressed in the dorsal root ganglion or trigeminal ganglion cells of the mouse. (*a*) A transverse section of a dorsal root ganglion of a 15-day-old fetus. Arachnoid also expresses E-cadherin. (*b*) An oblique section of a vibrissa follicle of a newborn mouse. Note that nerve fibers reaching the follicle are stained. (*c, d*) A monolayer culture of trigeminal ganglion cells derived from a newborn mouse. This culture was double-stained for E-cadherin (*c*) and for MAP1B (*d*). The latter was stained with monoclonal antibody 1B6 (Sato-Yoshitake et al. 1989) and used as a marker for neurites. Note that some neurons express E-cadherin through their entire length. Some E-cadherin-negative neurons are indicated by arrows in *d*. Many fibroblastic cells are also positive, although weakly. (sp) Spinal cord; (vf) vibrissa follicle; (nf) nerve fibers. Magnifications: (*a, b*) 102 × ; (*c, d*) 86 × .

Expression of E-Cadherin in Sensory Neurons

E-cadherin is expressed in epithelial cells. However, immunostaining using antibodies to E-cadherin revealed that this molecule was also expressed in trigeminal ganglia (TG) and dorsal root ganglia (DRG) of fetal and newborn mice (Fig. 3a). To identify which cell types of these ganglia express E-cadherin, we disaggregated the ganglion cells and cultured them as monolayers. Immunostaining of these cultures showed that a subset of neurons expressed E-cadherin (Fig. 3c,d). In these positive neurons, the entire regions of the cells, cell body, axon, and growth cone, were stained. Other neurons, however, were completely negative.

Other cell types constituting the ganglia also stained with the antibodies to E-cadherin, although more weakly than neurons. Cells with fibroblastic morphology, probably the satellite cells, were positive (Fig. 3c). These cells generally acted as a substratum for the attachment of the neurites of E-cadherin-positive neurons in monolayer cultures. Schwann cells, identified by their spindle shape, were occasionally positive.

A target organ for trigeminal sensory fibers is hair follicles of the upper lip skin. When the vibrissa hair follicles were sectioned and stained with antibodies to E-cadherin, nerve fibers reaching the hair follicles positively reacted with the antibodies (Fig. 3b). In the central nervous system, we found that the superficial layers of the dorsal horn in the spinal cord as well as the spinal trigeminal nucleus, where many of the sensory fibers terminate, stained with E-cadherin antibodies (data not shown). These results indicate that the axons of sensory neurons express E-cadherin at their terminal regions and also suggest the possibility that their target cells express E-cadherin in both the central and peripheral terminals.

We then studied the expression of E-cadherin during development of DRG and TG. Embryonic DRG and TG express N-cadherin, as revealed previously using the chicken system (Fig. 1b) (Hatta et al. 1987). We confirmed that this was the case also in the mouse by immunoblot analysis using antisera against mouse N-cadherin (Fig. 4a). Regarding E-cadherin, early undifferentiated ganglia of mouse embryos did not express this molecule, although they had already acquired N-cadherin. The expression of E-cadherin began around embryonic day 11.5, increased during development, and continued to the adult stage, whereas the expression of N-cadherin did not increase during development but rather decreased by newborn stages (Fig. 4). Thus, only N-cadherin is expressed in early

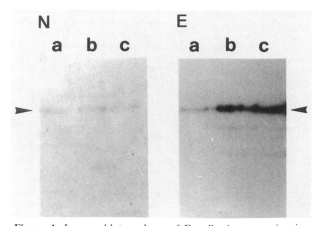

Figure 4. Immunoblot analyses of E-cadherin expression in the trigeminal ganglia in developing mice. (*a*) 13.5-day-old fetus; (*b*) 15.5-day-old fetus; and (*c*) newborn. (N) N-cadherin; (E) E-cadherin. Arrowheads indicate the positions of cadherin bands.

TG or DRG, but at later developmental stages, E-cadherin is added or substituted for N-cadherin in these ganglia at least in the mouse system.

Possible Roles of Cadherin Subclasses in Neural Histogenesis

We thus found that neural tissues express not only N-cadherin, but also R-cadherin or E-cadherin depending on the tissues. Another type of cadherin homolog that lacks the cytoplasmic domain was also identified from neural tissues (Ranscht and Dours 1989). Possibly, these are not all the cadherins expressed in the nervous system, but the total number of cadherin subclasses in the entire body remains to be studied.

Among the cadherins expressed in the nervous system, it seems that N-cadherin is the most important cell-cell adhesion molecule in maintaining the architecture of early neural tissues. All undifferentiated neuroepithelial cells express N-cadherin (Fig. 1a), and antibodies blocking this cadherin can dissociate the neuroepithelial layers into cell clusters (Matsunaga et al. 1988a). Other cadherins in the nervous system are possibly expressed at later developmental stages. In the case of E-cadherin, their expression in DRG or TG began around the stages when multiple neural cell types were differentiating, and it occurred only in a subpopulation of the ganglion cells. The expression of R-cadherin in the retina increased in more differentiated stages, although its precise localization has not yet been studied in detail. In contrast, the expression of N-cadherin tends to be depressed during development in a position-specific manner (Matsunaga et al. 1988a). These results suggest that different cell types in neural tissues acquire different sets of cadherins during development. Through this mechanism, different neural cells might acquire different adhesive specificities.

Neural tissues comprise multiple domains of functionally different cell groups. The differential expression of different cadherins in the nervous system might be associated with the formation of such domain structures. For example, in the matured neural retina, only the outer limiting membrane expresses N-cadherin. The N-cadherin-mediated adhesion could work for maintaining the cell layer with the outer limiting membrane to be separated from other regions of the retina that have no N-cadherin. An example supporting such an idea can be seen in epithelial organs that are composed of at least two domains, epithelial and mesenchymal. In these organs, epithelial cells express E-cadherin, and mesenchymal cells express N-cadherin, and this differential expression of two cadherins seems to take part in sorting of the two cell types (Nose et al. 1988). To investigate whether this kind of mechanism operates in the nervous system, however, we need more detailed information on the localization of different cadherins in neural tissues.

On the basis of homophilic interacting properties of cadherins, it can also be speculated that this molecular family might be used for the specific connection between neurons and their target cells. That is, if these cells express the same cadherins, they could automatically be connected with each other when brought into contact. It is thus noteworthy that not only the axons of sensory neurons, but also some of their peripheral target tissues, such as hair follicles, express E-cadherin (Fig. 3b). It is known that some of the sensory nerve fibers are directly connected with Merkel cells in the epidermis. It therefore should be studied in the future whether such fibers express E-cadherin and use it for their connection to the target cells. Regarding the E-cadherin staining in the dorsal horn of the spinal cord, it is not known whether this staining represents the expression of this molecule by spinal cord neurons themselves or by the terminals of sensory neurons. If the former is the case, we have to consider an interesting possibility that E-cadherin is used for the specific connections between neurons.

Perturbation of Neural Tube Formation by the Ectopic Expression of N-Cadherin

N-cadherin first appears in the nervous system at the stage of neural tube formation (Hatta et al. 1987; Duband et al. 1988). We questioned how the early morphogenesis of the neural tube was regulated by the N-cadherin expression. To answer this question, we attempted to modify the pattern of N-cadherin expression by injecting N-cadherin mRNA into *Xenopus* embryos (Fujimori et al. 1990).

Prior to such experiments, we studied the properties of *Xenopus* endogenous N-cadherin. We found that the antibodies to chicken N-cadherin reacted with *Xenopus* embryos. In immunoblot and immunostaining analyses, *Xenopus* N-cadherin became detectable at the neurula stage, in the invaginating neural tube, mesoderm, and notochord. Although the staining intensity with the antibodies was faint, the pattern of the N-cadherin expression was similar to that in the chicken. At later developmental stages, N-cadherin expression increased, maintaining a similar pattern of tissue distribution compared with chicken N-cadherin.

We also found that *Xenopus* cells expressing N-cadherin can adhere to cells expressing chicken N-cadherin, indicating that N-cadherin derived from these species can cross-bind to each other. *Xenopus* N-cadherin is thus indistinguishable from chicken N-cadherin in both functional and immunological properties.

On the basis of these data, we decided to inject chicken N-cadherin mRNA into *Xenopus* embryos to observe the consequence of its ectopic expression. Since N-cadherin is cross-reactive between both species, chicken N-cadherin expressed in *Xenopus* embryos should operate normally and can be regarded as the molecule functionally equivalent to the *Xenopus* endogenous N-cadherin.

After these preliminary experiments, one blastomere of 2-cell stage *Xenopus* embryos was injected with chicken N-cadherin mRNA and allowed to develop. Most of the injected embryos appeared to develop normally, although some embryos generated nodule-like structures or protrusions on their surface at the sites expressing ectopic N-cadherin (Fig. 5a). We then sectioned these embryos at the neurula stage and examined their internal structures. Expression of injected

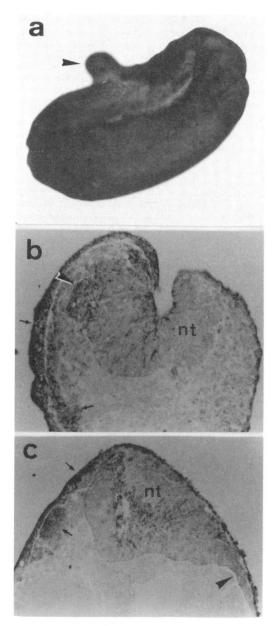

Figure 5. Effect of injection of chicken N-cadherin mRNA into *Xenopus* embryos. (*a*) A neurula-stage embryo that has a surface protrusion at the position expressing ectopic N-cadherin. The ectopic N-cadherin expression was confirmed by immunostaining for this molecule. (*b*) A transverse section of the head region of an embryo. Cells with darker outlines express ectopic N-cadherin. The regions with such cells are indicated by arrows or an arrowhead. The arrowhead indicates clumping of a fraction of neural tube cells. (*c*) A transverse section of the trunk region of an embryo. Darker regions express ectopic N-cadherin. Arrowhead indicates the fusion of the neural tube with the basal layer of the epidermis. Arrows indicate thickening of part of the epidermis and clumping of a fraction of mesodermal cells, both of which coincide with the overexpression of N-cadherin. (nt) Neural tube. Magnifications: (*a*) 26×; (*b, c*) 110×.

N-cadherin mRNA was easily detected by immunostaining of the translation products. The immunostaining for endogenous N-cadherin was not intense at this stage and therefore did not hinder the detection of the exogenous one. The ectopic N-cadherin was distributed in a mosaic pattern, and its localization varied with the embryos. In the regions with the ectopic expression of N-cadherin, various abnormal morphology of tissues was observed, and we focus below on the neural tube.

Local regions of the neural tube often expressed ectopic N-cadherin (Fig. 5b,c). Cells in such regions tended to form clumps with a clear boundary to the adjacent regions expressing only endogenous N-cadherin. In some cases, cell clumps with ectopic N-cadherin were separated from the neural tube, causing the disorganized morphology of the tube (Fig. 5b). Probably, cells acquire higher mutual adhesiveness by the ectopic N-cadherin expression and establish tighter associations to each other. Cells with weaker adhesiveness that are expressing only endogenous N-cadherin may not be able to join such cell aggregates, resulting in the separation of the two cell populations.

Another interesting effect of the ectopic N-cadherin expression was observed (Fig. 5c). In some embryos, ectopic N-cadherin occurred in the basal layer of the ectoderm, as well as in the neural tube at the dorsal region. In some of these embryos, the neural tube could not separate from the future epidermis and remained fused to the latter. In normal development, the expression of N-cadherin does not occur in the ectoderm that is separating from the neural tube. Therefore, these results can be explained by the aberrant expression of N-cadherin that prevents the separation of the epidermis and the neural tube. The surface protrusion shown in Figure 5a was associated with the high expression of exogenous N-cadherin in the epidermis and the mesoderm at the region with abnormality (data not shown).

Similar results were recently obtained by injecting *Xenopus* endogenous N-cadherin mRNA into *Xenopus* embryos (Detrick et al. 1990). These observations illustrated two important features on the morphogenetic implication of N-cadherin expression. First, the quantitative regulation of N-cadherin expression is important for the coordinated morphogenesis of tissues. The overexpression of N-cadherin induced clumping of cells, resulting in the disorganization of tissue structures. Second, the switching of cadherin expression from one type to another is indispensable for the separation of cell layers. The failure in this process led to the fusion of tissues that would otherwise be separated. The precise regulation of cadherin expression in development therefore seems essential to the normal morphogenesis of animal embryos.

SUMMARY

Cadherins homophilically bind cells. Thus, cells expressing identical cadherins adhere selectively to each other, and they do not randomly intermix with the cells expressing other types of cadherins in vitro. Neural tissues express multiple types of cadherins, and the expression of each cadherin type is spatiotemporally regulated within a tissue during development. This molecular family therefore could operate for the sorting of different cell types in the nervous system. The regulation of N-cadherin expression is also important for the early development of the neural tube. The ectopic expression of N-cadherin in *Xenopus* embryos, which was induced by mRNA injection, led to the disorganization of neural tube structures or the fusion of the neural tube to the epidermis. These results suggest that the precise regulation of cadherin expression at the quantitative as well as at the qualitative level is crucial for neural morphogenesis.

ACKNOWLEDGMENTS

The authors thank Nobutaka Hirokawa and Reiko Sato for monoclonal antibody 1B6 and Glenn Radice for his critical reading of the manuscript. This work was supported by the Ministry of Education, Science and Culture of Japan and the Science and Technology Agency of the Japanese Government.

REFERENCES

Bixby, J.L. and R. Zhang. 1990. Purified N-cadherin is a potent substrate for the rapid induction of neurite outgrowth. *J. Cell Biol.* **110:** 1253.

Bixby, J.L., J. Pratt, J. Lilien, and L. Reichardt. 1987. Neurite outgrowth on muscle cell surfaces involves extracellular matrix receptors as well Ca^{2+}-dependent and independent cell adhesion molecules. *Proc. Natl. Acad. Sci.* **84:** 2555.

Crossin, K.L., C.M. Chuong, and G.M. Edelman. 1985. Expression of sequences of cell adhesion molecules. *Proc. Natl. Acad. Sci.* **82:** 6942.

Davanloo, P., A.H. Rosenberg, J.J. Dunn, and W. Studier. 1984. Cloning and expression of the gene for bacteriophage T7 RNA polymerase. *Proc. Natl. Acad. Sci.* **81:** 2035.

Dent, J.A., A.G. Polson, and M.W. Klymkowsky. 1989. A whole-mount immunocytochemical analysis of the expression of the intermediate filament protein vimentin in *Xenopus. Development* **105:** 61.

Detrick. R.J., D. Dickey, and C.R. Kintner. 1990. The effect of N-cadherin misexpression on morphogenesis in *Xenopus* embryos. *Neuron* **4:** 493.

Dodd, J. and M.J. Jessel. 1988. Axon guidance and the patterning of neuronal projections in vertebrates. *Science* **242:** 692.

Drazba, J. and V. Lemmon. 1990. The role of cell adhesion molecules in neurite outgrowth on Muller cells. *Dev. Biol.* **138:** 82.

Duband, J.L., T. Volberg, I. Sabanay, J.P. Thiery, and B. Geiger. 1988. Spatial and temporal distribution of the adherens-junction-associated adhesion molecule A-CAM during avian embryogenesis. *Development* **103:** 325.

Fujimori, T., S. Miyatani, and M. Takeichi. 1990. Ectopic expression of N-cadherin perturbs histogenesis in *Xenopus* embryos. *Development* (in press).

Fujisawa, H. 1971. A complete reconstruction of the neural retina of chick embryo grafted onto the chorio-allantoic membrane. *Dev. Growth Differ.* **13:** 25.

Hatta, K. and M. Takeichi. 1986. Expression of N-cadherin adhesion molecules associated with early morphogenetic events in chick development. *Nature* **320:** 447.

Hatta, K., A. Nose, A. Nagafuchi, and M. Takeichi. 1988. Cloning and expression of cDNA encoding a neural calcium-dependent cell adhesion molecule: Its identity in the cadherin gene family. *J. Cell Biol.* **106:** 873.

Hatta, K., S. Takagi, H. Fujisawa, and M. Takeichi. 1987. Spatial and temporal expression pattern of N-cadherin cell adhesion molecules correlated with morphogenetic processes of chicken embryos. *Dev. Biol.* **120:** 215.

Jessel, T.M. 1988. Adhesion molecules and the hierarchy of neural development. *Neuron* **1:** 3.

Letourneau, P.C., T.A. Shattuck, F.K. Roche, M. Takeichi, and V. Lemmon. 1990. Nerve growth cone migration onto Schwann cells involves the calcium-dependent adhesion molecule, N-cadherin. *Dev. Biol.* **138:** 430.

Matsunaga, M., K. Hatta, and M. Takeichi. 1988a. Role of N-cadherin cell adhesion molecules in the histogenesis of neural retina. *Neuron* **1:** 289.

Matsunaga, M., K. Hatta, A. Nagafuchi, and M. Takeichi. 1988b. Guidance of optic nerve fibers by N-cadherin adhesion molecules. *Nature* **334:** 6177.

Melton, D.A., P.A. Krieg, M.R. Rebagliati, T. Maniatis, K. Zinn, and M.R. Green. 1984. Efficient *in vitro* synthesis of biologically active RNA and RNA hybridization probes from plasmids containing a bacteriophage SP6 promoter. *Nucleic Acids Res.* **12:** 7035.

Miyatani, S., K. Shimamura, M. Hatta, A. Nagafuchi, A. Nose, M. Matsunaga, K. Hatta, and M. Takeichi 1989. Neural cadherin: Role in selective cell-cell adhesion. *Science* **245:** 631.

Nose, A., A. Nagafuchi, and M. Takeichi. 1988. Expressed recombinant cadherins mediate cell sorting in model systems. *Cell* **54:** 993.

Nose, A., K. Tsuji, and M. Takeichi. 1990. Localization of specificity determining sites in cadherin cell adhesion molecules. *Cell* **61:** 147.

Ranscht, B. and M.T. Dours. 1989. Selective expression of a novel cadherin in the pathways of developing motor and commissural axons. *Soc. Neurosci. Abstr.* **15:** 959.

Sato-Yoshitake, R., Y. Shiomura, H. Miyasaka, and N. Hirokawa. 1989. Microtubule-associated protein 1B: Molecular structure, localization, and phosphorylation-dependent expression in developing neurons. *Neuron* **3:** 229.

Takeichi, M. 1988. The cadherins: Cell-cell adhesion molecules controlling animal morphogenesis. *Development* **102:** 639.

———. 1990. Cadherins: A molecular family important in selective cell-cell adhesion. *Annu. Rev. Biochem.* **59:** 237.

Thiery, J.P., A. Delouvee, W.J. Gallin, B.A. Cunningham, and G.M. Edelman. 1984. Ontogenetic expression of cell adhesion molecules: L-CAM is found in epithelia derived from the three primary germ layers. *Dev. Biol.* **102:** 61.

Tomaselli, K., K.M. Neugebauer, J.L. Bixby, J. Lilien, and L. Reichardt. 1988. N-cadherin and integrin: Two receptor systems that mediate neuronal process outgrowth on astrocyte surfaces. *Neuron* **1:** 33.

Molecular Genetics of Neuronal Recognition in *Drosophila*: Evolution and Function of Immunoglobulin Superfamily Cell Adhesion Molecules

G. Grenningloh, A.J. Bieber,* E.J. Rehm, P.M. Snow,† Z.R. Traquina,
M. Hortsch, N.H. Patel, and C.S. Goodman
*Howard Hughes Medical Institute, Department of Molecular and Cell Biology, University of California,
Berkeley, California 94720*

One form of neuronal recognition is the remarkable selectivity shown by neuronal growth cones in their ability to recognize and extend along specific axonal surfaces, a process called selective fasciculation. At the Cold Spring Harbor Symposium on Molecular Neurobiology in 1983, Raper, Bastiani, and Goodman (1983c) proposed on the basis of a long series of descriptive and experimental studies on the mechanisms of selective fasciculation in the grasshopper (Raper et al. 1983 a,b, 1984; Bastiani et al. 1984) that neighboring axon pathways must be differentially labeled by surface recognition molecules, which allow growth cones to distinguish among them—a notion they called the labeled pathways hypothesis. Subsequent cellular analysis from our laboratory in both the grasshopper (Bastiani et al. 1986; Doe et al. 1986; du Lac et al. 1986) and a simple vertebrate (the fish spinal cord; see Kuwada 1986) further supported this hypothesis. At about the same time, other studies from our laboratory, in collaboration with Michael Bate at Cambridge, showed that what had been learned from the large grasshopper embryo with its highly accessible identified neurons could be directly applied to the much smaller fruitfly, *Drosophila*, with its powerful genetics (Thomas et al. 1984), thus opening the door to a combined cellular, classical genetic, and molecular genetic analyses of this problem (see, e.g., Goodman et al. 1984).

Several years ago, in an attempt to identify molecules that impart specificity on the developing nervous system, our laboratory began a series of monoclonal antibody screens to identify surface glycoproteins that are differentially expressed during development on subsets of axon pathways in the insect embryo (Bastiani et al. 1987; Patel et al. 1987; Bieber et al. 1989). The long-term goal of this work was to identify and characterize the genes encoding these neuronal recognition molecules in *Drosophila*, to identify mutations in these genes, and to use these mutations as the starting point for a detailed genetic analysis of neuronal recognition.

We initially identified and subsequently cloned the genes encoding four different surface glycoproteins that are dynamically expressed on different overlapping subsets of growth cones, axon fascicles, and glia during embryonic development (Bastiani et al. 1987; Patel et al. 1987; Bieber et al. 1989). Fasciclin I and fasciclin II were initially characterized and cloned in the grasshopper (Harrelson and Goodman 1988; Snow et al. 1988; Zinn et al. 1988), and subsequently, the homologous genes were identified in *Drosophila* (Zinn et al. 1988; G. Grenningloh and E.J. Rehm, unpubl.). Fasciclin III and neuroglian, on the other hand, were initially characterized and cloned in *Drosophila* (Patel et al. 1987; Bieber et al. 1989; Snow et al. 1989), and subsequently, the neuroglian homolog was identified in the grasshopper (G. Grenningloh and E.J. Rehm, unpubl.).

One striking result from these molecular genetic studies was the finding that three of the four proteins (fasciclin II, neuroglian, and fasciclin III) are members of the same gene family: the immunoglobulin superfamily. Fasciclin II and neuroglian are highly related to a series of vertebrate neural cell adhesion molecules, including such molecules as N-CAM (Barthels et al. 1987; Cunningham et al. 1987), MAG (Arquint et al. 1987; Salzer et al. 1987), L1 (Moos et al. 1988), contactin/F11 (Ranscht 1988; Brümmendorf et al. 1989), and TAG-1 (Furley et al. 1990). Within this group, fasciclin II is related to and shares a common evolutionary ancestor with N-CAM (Harrelson and Goodman 1988); neuroglian is related to and shares a common ancestor with L1 (Bieber et al. 1989). The third of these proteins, fasciclin III, was initially described as possessing a novel structure (Snow et al. 1989). However, subsequent analyses by A. Smith in Minneapolis (University of Minnesota) and A. Williams at Oxford have indicated that fasciclin III is composed of three immunoglobulin domains that are much more divergent than those found in fasciclin II or neuroglian. The other protein uncovered by our initial immunological screen, fasciclin I, has a novel sequence and structure that is unrelated so far to any proteins described previously (Zinn et al. 1988). In vitro aggregation assays show that all four of these proteins can function as homophilic cell adhesion molecules capable of mediating cell aggregation and cell sorting (Snow et al. 1989; Elkins et al. 1990a; A.J. Bieber et al.; G. Grenningloh et al.; both unpubl.).

Present addresses: *Department of Biological Sciences, Purdue University, West Lafayette, Indiana 47907; †Department of Biological Sciences, State University of New York, Albany, New York 12222.

In this paper, we review what we have learned about the structure and function of three immunoglobulin superfamily cell adhesion molecules in *Drosophila*: fasciclin II, neuroglian, and fasciclin III. We also highlight some insights gained by comparing the sequence and expression of fasciclin II and neuroglian in two insect species that diverged some 300 million years ago (the relatively advanced *Drosophila* and the more primitive grasshopper) and by comparing them with related molecules in vertebrates. Finally, we review the discoveries of a variety of other types of immunoglobulin superfamily molecules in *Drosophila*, and we use this information to reconsider the evolution of the immunoglobulin superfamily.

Expression of Axonal Glycoproteins Can Be Dynamic and Regional

Within each neuromere of the developing insect central nervous system (CNS), there develops a scaffold of axon pathways, including a pair of bilaterally symmetric longitudinal axon tracts, a pair of commissural tracts (anterior and posterior) connecting the two sides, and a pair of nerve roots exiting the CNS on each side (the segmental and intersegmental nerve roots). Each of the major tracts is subdivided into an array of distinct axon bundles or fascicles. In the insect CNS, the first growth cones extend largely toward and along the surfaces of special glial cells (and some neurons) and in so doing establish the initial axon pathways (Bastiani and Good-

man 1986; Jacobs and Goodman 1989a,b; Jacobs et al. 1989; C. Klämbt et al., unpubl.).

As development proceeds, however, the growth cones of the bulk of later-born neurons find themselves in an environment increasingly dominated by other axons. Most of these later growth cones do not contact the glia but rather only contact the growth cones and axons of other neurons. As the scaffold of axon pathways grows larger and more complex within the CNS, these later growth cones show remarkable selectivity in their ability to recognize and extend along specific axonal surfaces, a process called selective fasciculation (Raper et al. 1983a,b). Experimental studies on the mechanisms of selective fasciculation in insects (Raper et al. 1983c, 1984; Bastiani et al. 1984, 1986; Doe et al. 1986; du Lac et al. 1986) led to the prediction (the labeled pathways hypothesis) that neighboring axon pathways are differentially labeled by surface recognition molecules, which allow growth cones to distinguish among them. This model led to the search for glycoproteins expressed on subsets of fasciculating embryonic axons.

Candidates for axonal recognition molecules were identified by generating monoclonal antibodies that recognize surface antigens expressed on subsets of axon fascicles in insect embryos. These antibodies were used to characterize, purify, and generate further antibodies against four different membrane-associated glycoproteins, fasciclin I and fasciclin II in the grasshopper (Bastiani et al. 1987) and fasciclin III and neuroglian in

Figure 1. Expression of fasciclin I and fasciclin II in the grasshopper and expression and function of neuroglian in *Drosophila*. (*A–D*) Dynamic and regional expression of the fasciclin I (black label) and fasciclin II (brown label) axonal glycoproteins in the grasshopper embryo as revealed by two rounds of anti-horseradish peroxidase (HRP) immunocytochemistry using monoclonal antibodies (MAb) and nickel enhancement for the black color. (*A*) View of the longitudinal connective on the left side between two segments in a 35% grasshopper embryo showing the first three longitudinal axon fascicles. The arrowhead marks the inside-most vMP2 fascicle, which does not express either fasciclin I or fasciclin II; the middle, brown-stained fascicle is the MP1/dMP2 fascicle, which expresses fasciclin II; and the outside, black-stained fascicle is the U fascicle, which expresses fasciclin I. Note that two different bundles of black-stained axons come together to form the U fascicle and also that many of these axons turn laterally (→) to extend out the intersegmental nerve root. (*B*) A single neuromere of a 40% grasshopper embryo showing the expression of fasciclin I (black label) on one large fascicle in the anterior commissure and one large fascicle in the posterior commissure. Many of the longitudinal bundles express fasciclin II (brown label). The arrowheads mark the choice point regions on each side where axons change from commissural pathways to longitudinal pathways and where some of these axons change from fasciclin I to fasciclin II. (*C,D*) Higher power magnification of choice point regions from two different segments where axons change from commissural to longitudinal pathways. Fasciclin I and fasciclin II are regionally expressed in that some interneurons express fasciclin I on their commissural processes and then express fasciclin II on their longitudinal axon segments after crossing the midline. Arrowheads mark the axons (as seen in this one focal plane) that have changed from the fasciclin-I-positive commissural pathway to a variety of different longitudinal pathways. After turning longitudinally, these axons still express some fasciclin I (black label) on their surface, although this protein disappears as the cells express fasciclin II (brown label) on their longitudinal axon segments. (*E,F*) The lateral cluster of sensory neurons in the A2 and A3 segments of wild-type (*E*) and *neuroglian* mutant *Drosophila* embryos (*F*) as stained with the BP104 MAb (*E*) and 22C10 MAb (*F*), respectively, showing that the null mutation in the *neuroglian* gene leads to disruption of sensory neurons. (*E*) Neuroglian is normally expressed at high levels at point of membrane apposition between sensory neurons in the *Drosophila* embryo PNS, as shown here by HRP immunocytochemistry with an anti-neuroglian monoclonal antibody (BP104; see Hortsch et al. 1990). This photo shows the normal pattern of lateral sensory neurons (including in particular the five chordotonal neurons) in a wild-type embryo. (*F*) A null lethal mutation in the *neuroglian* gene, *l(1)RA35*, leads to disruption of sensory neurons. At a gross level, the overall structure of the CNS and PNS, and in particular the peripheral nerve roots and CNS axon pathways, develop in a relatively normal way in *nrg* mutant embryos. However, although neurons do not become "unglued," there is a consistent although more subtle phenotype in *nrg* mutant embryos: The orientation and extent of contact among the normally neuroglian-positive sensory neurons in the PNS is abnormal. As shown here, the five lateral chordotonal neurons in each abdominal hemisegment normally line up in a tight row with each cell body having extensive membrane apposition with the neurons on either side of it; the chordotonal neurons are normally flattened against one another and lie in the same focal plane. In contrast, in *nrg* mutant embryos, the five chordotonal neurons are more randomly organized in a looser group with less membrane apposition, resulting in a disorganization in the alignment of their dendrites. Similar types of phenotypes are seen with other clusters of sensory neurons as well. Bar: (*A,C,D*) 10 μm; (*B*) 20 μm; (*E,F*) 6 μm.

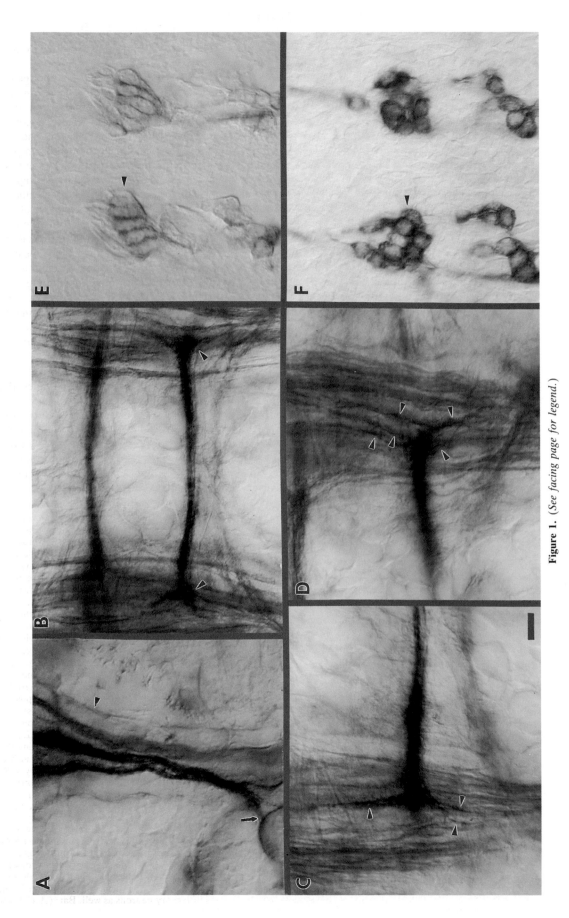

Figure 1. (*See facing page for legend.*)

329

Drosophila (Patel et al. 1987; Bieber et al. 1989). Antibodies against the fasciclin I and fasciclin II homologs in *Drosophila* were subsequently generated (fasciclin I: Zinn et al. 1988; Hortsch and Goodman 1990; fasciclin II: G. Grenningloh and E.J. Rehm., unpubl.).

The expression of these four axonal glycoproteins is consistent with their potential involvement in neuronal recognition and growth cone guidance (Fig. 1); all four proteins are dynamically expressed on subsets of growth cones and fasciculating axons and, in some cases, on the glia they extend along during the period of axon outgrowth. The pattern of expression of each protein changes during development, and in some cases, the expression of a particular protein on an individual neuron is transient during a particular stage of axon outgrowth. Each of the proteins is also expressed outside of the developing nervous system in particular patches or stripes of cells (Bastiani et al. 1987; Patel et al. 1987; Bieber et al. 1989; Hortsch et al. 1990; G. Grenningloh and E.J. Rehm; L. McAllister and K. Zinn; both unpubl.).

The four axonal glycoproteins are expressed on different but overlapping subsets of axon fascicles, neuroglian being the most widely distributed of the four, and fasciclin I, fasciclin II, and fasciclin III are expressed on more restricted subsets of axon fascicles (Fig. 1A). For example, one form of *Drosophila* neuroglian (the long form; see Hortsch et al. 1990) is expressed at high levels on all of the axons in the intersegmental nerve root, whereas the other form of neuroglian (the short form) is expressed on the glia of this nerve root along which the axons extend. All of the axons in the intersegmental nerve root also express fasciclin I, whereas only a subset of these axons express fasciclin III, and this subset stays tightly bundled within the larger nerve (J.R. Jacobs, unpubl.). In contrast, some axon pathways express only one of these four proteins, and others express none at all (Fig. 1A), leading to the suggestion that there are likely to be additional fasciclin-like proteins still awaiting future discovery.

Some features of the expression of these proteins have been remarkably conserved across many hundreds of millions of years of insect evolution. For example, fasciclin I is expressed on the surface of the aCC neuron but not on the pCC neuron in both the grasshopper and *Drosophila* (Bastiani et al. 1987; Zinn et al. 1988), and fasciclin II is expressed at high levels on the axons of the MP1/dMP2 fascicle in both the grasshopper (Harrelson and Goodman 1988) and *Drosophila* (G. Grenningloh and E.J. Rehm, unpubl.). However, some features have changed over evolution; perhaps most striking is the evolutionary change in the forms and expression of neuroglian between the grasshopper and *Drosophila* (Hortsch et al. 1990; G. Grenningloh and E.J. Rehm, unpubl.), described in a later section of this paper.

Most neurons in the insect CNS are interneurons, and many of these interneurons have long projection axons that cross the midline in one of the commissures and then extend rostrally or caudally in one of the longitudinal pathways. The growth cones of these neurons typically show no affinity for the homologous longitudinal pathway on their own (ipsilateral) side but then dramatically change as they turn and follow the same pathway on the other (contralateral) side after crossing the midline. The simplest hypothesis to explain this change in growth cone behavior after crossing the midline is to postulate that the expression of axonal recognition molecules is both dynamic and regional: Dynamic in that the molecules controlling the selective affinity for a particular longitudinal pathway are not expressed until after the growth cone crosses the midline and regional in that the molecules controlling the selective affinity for a particular commissural pathway are likely not to be expressed after the growth cone crosses the midline and turns onto a longitudinal pathway. This dynamic and regional expression of axonal glycoproteins was one of the predictions of a more detailed discussion of the labeled pathways hypothesis (see Fig. 11 in Goodman et al. 1985).

In the initial characterization of fasciclin I, fasciclin II, and fasciclin III (Bastiani et al. 1987; Patel et al. 1987), one of the key observations was that these three proteins are regionally expressed in just this predicted fashion: For example, some interneurons express fasciclin I on their commissural processes and then express fasciclin II on their longitudinal axon segments after crossing the midline (Fig. 1B–D). The discovery of the regional expression of axonal glycoproteins is not isolated to insects; similar changes have been seen in the vertebrate spinal cord, as projection interneurons express TAG-1 on their commissural processes and then express L1 on their longitudinal processes after crossing the midline (Dodd and Jessell 1988). The mechanisms that regulate this "switch" in the temporal and spatial expression of axonal glycoproteins is presently unknown.

Three of the Four Proteins Belong to the Immunoglobulin Superfamily

Monoclonal antibody affinity columns were used to purify microgram quantities of fasciclin I, fasciclin II, fasciclin III, and neuroglian proteins from kilogram quantities of lysates of grasshopper (fas I and fas II) and *Drosophila* (fas III and nrg) embryos (Bastiani et al. 1987; Patel et al. 1987; Snow et al. 1988; Bieber et al. 1989). This purified protein was used to generate serum antibodies against all four proteins (for cDNA expression cloning) and for protein microsequencing. Amino-terminal sequences were obtained for fasciclin I and neuroglian, and chemically generated fragments were microsequenced for fasciclin II and neuroglian (Snow et al. 1988; Bieber et al. 1989). Oligonucleotide probes based on protein microsequence data were used to isolate cDNA clones for fasciclin I and fasciclin II from a grasshopper embryo cDNA library (Snow et al. 1988). The serum antibody probes were used to screen a cDNA expression library to isolate cDNA clones for fasciclin III and neuroglian in *Drosophila* (Patel et al. 1987; Bieber et al. 1989). The cloning of the genes encoding three of the proteins was confirmed by comparing the deduced amino acid sequence from the cDNA clones with the protein microsequence data; the cloning of the gene encoding the fourth protein (fasciclin III) was confirmed by genetic deficiency analysis.

Full-length cDNA clones encoding fasciclin I and fasciclin II were initially isolated in grasshopper (Harrelson and Goodman 1988; Snow et al. 1988; Zinn et al. 1988). The cDNAs for the *Drosophila* homologs of both were subsequently isolated: fasciclin I using low-stringency hybridization (Zinn et al. 1988) and fasciclin II using the polymerase chain reaction (PCR) method (G. Grenningloh and E.J. Rehm, unpubl.). Fasciclin III and neuroglian, on the other hand, were initially characterized and cloned in *Drosophila* (Patel et al. 1987; Bieber et al. 1989; Snow et al. 1989). PCR was also used to clone a cDNA for the neuroglian homolog in the grasshopper (G. Grenningloh and E.J. Rehm, unpubl.).

cDNA sequence analysis reveals that three of the four proteins (fasciclin II, neuroglian, and fasciclin III) are members of the immunoglobulin superfamily (Fig. 2). What defines proteins as members of the immunoglobulin superfamily is a common domain structure (~100 amino acids), typically (but not always) with two cysteines in each domain (separated by ~50 amino acids), with many other conserved amino acids (particularly around the cysteine residues) and with a conserved deduced three-dimensional structure, called the immunoglobulin fold (see, e.g., Williams 1987; Williams and Barclay 1988). Immunoglobulin domains typically fold to form a globular structure containing two β-sheets, each consisting of three to four antiparallel β strands of five to ten amino acids each. Intrachain disulfide bonding between the conserved cysteine residues stabilizes the structure. A common characteristic of immunoglobulin-related molecules is that most of them function in some form of adhesion or recognition at the cell surface.

Three types of immunoglobulin domains have been proposed: V-, C1-, and C2-type domains (Williams and Barclay 1988). The classifications are based on the length of the domains between the conserved cysteine residues, on the predicted secondary structure of the domains, and on statistical analysis of the conserved amino acids within the domains. V-type domains are usually longer than the C-type domains, with 65–75 amino acids between the cysteine residues. The extra length of the domain allows the formation of β-sheets composed of four β strands each. The shorter C-type domains have 55–60 amino acids between the cysteine residues, giving rise to β-sheets of three and four β strands. C1 and C2 domains are distinguished on the basis of conserved sequence patterns within the domains.

Most of the immunoglobulin domains of the neural cell adhesion molecules (including N-CAM, L1, MAG, F11/contactin, TAG-1, fasciclin II, neuroglian, and

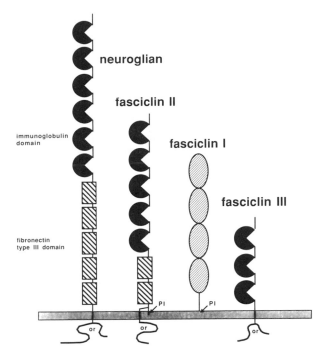

Figure 2. Schematic domain structure of the neuroglian, fasciclin II, fasciclin I, and fasciclin III axonal glycoproteins. Three of the four axon glycoproteins are members of the immunoglobulin superfamily. Two of these proteins, neuroglian and fasciclin II, have multiple immunoglobulin domains followed by multiple fibronectin type III domains; the third, fasciclin III, has more divergent immunoglobulin domains (see text). Fasciclin I has a novel structure made up of four tandem domains (Zinn et al. 1988) and is anchored to the membrane via a PI lipid membrane anchor (Hortsch and Goodman 1990). Neuroglian (Hortsch et al. 1990) and fasciclin III (P.M. Snow and Z.R. Traquina, unpubl.) have alternative cytoplasmic domains; fasciclin II also comes in different forms including one with a putative PI membrane anchor (G. Grenningloh and E.J. Rehm, unpubl.) and as a transmembrane protein with a cytoplasmic domain (Harrelson and Goodman 1988).

fasciclin III) are of the C2 type (Williams 1987). In addition to these tandem immunoglobulin domains, most of these neural cell adhesion molecules (all listed above except MAG and fasciclin III) have another type of tandem conserved repeat near to their transmembrane domains; these repeats are called fibronectin type III domains (Fig. 2) on the basis of their homology with a repeat motif first found in the extracellular matrix adhesion molecule fibronectin (Hynes 1986). Fasciclin II has five immunoglobulin C2-type domains followed by two fibronectin domains; neuroglian has six immunoglobulin C2-type domains followed by five fibronectin domains (Harrelson and Goodman 1988; Bieber et al. 1989). As described in a later section, fasciclin III has three divergent immunoglobulin domains and no fibronectin domains (Snow et al. 1989; A. Smith; A. Williams; both pers. comm.).

Fasciclin II Is Related to N-CAM

In 1988 came the discovery of the first two members of the immunoglobulin superfamily outside of the chor-

dates: amalgam in *Drosophila* (Seeger et al. 1988) and
fasciclin II in the grasshopper (Harrelson and Goodman 1988). When fasciclin II was first cloned in the
grasshopper, its extracellular portion, consisting of five
immunoglobulin C2-type domains followed by two fibronectin domains, was shown to have the greatest overall similarity with that of N-CAM (Harrelson and
Goodman 1988). Comparison of grasshopper fasciclin
II with mouse N-CAM (Barthels et al. 1987) by use of
the FAST-P alignment program (Lipman and Pearson
1985) yields an optimized score of 586; for comparison,
the score with mouse L1 (Moos et al. 1988) is 147.
Detailed analysis using the ALIGN program (Dayhoff
et al. 1983; Williams and Barclay 1988; analysis of
fasciclin II by A.F. Williams, unpubl.) indicates that
the similarity between fasciclin II and N-CAM extends
throughout the entire extracellular portion of both proteins; when fasciclin II and N-CAM domains are compared, the best match of the five immunoglobulin domains and two fibronectin type III domains of fasciclin
II is with the same seven domains of N-CAM, namely,
domain 2 with domain 2, domain 3 with domain 3, and
so on. The aligned sequences from both mouse N-CAM
and *Drosophila* fasciclin II shows that these molecules
have approximately 25–30% amino acid identity over
all seven of their extracellular domains (Fig. 3A).

The fasciclin II homolog was recently cloned in
Drosophila using PCR (G. Grenningloh and E.J.
Rehm, unpubl.). The deduced grasshopper and
Drosophila fasciclin II proteins have approximately
45% amino acid identity over most of their extracellu-

lar domains (Fig. 3A). *Drosophila*, a relatively advanced insect, and the grasshopper, a more primitive
insect, diverged some 300 million years ago. Given the
extent of amino acid identity and sequence alignment
between the *Drosophila* and grasshopper fasciclin II
proteins, it is reasonable to assume that these molecules are true homologs. Moreover, they are expressed
in a very similar way in the developing CNS; in both
insects, fasciclin II is expressed at high levels on the
MP1/dMP2 axon fascicle and on a subset of other
longitudinal axon fascicles (Harrelson and Goodman
1988; G. Grenningloh and E.J. Rehm, unpubl.).

What of the relationship between insect fasciclin II
and vertebrate N-CAM? At the molecular level, although their sequences align over all seven extracellular domains, and each appears to come in multiple
forms with different membrane attachments, they share
only about 28% amino acid identity over their extracellular domains. In addition, their patterns of expression
are quite different; fasciclin II is expressed on a restricted subset of longitudinal axon fascicles in the developing insect embryo, whereas N-CAM is more
broadly expressed on nearly all neurons throughout the
developing vertebrate CNS. This major difference in
expression, coupled with the low level of amino acid
identity, makes it difficult to assign precise molecular
homologies among these related insect and vertebrate
molecules. It may be that fasciclin II and N-CAM are
not true homologs, but rather they are related in that
they both evolved from a common ancestral molecule,
which predated the split in the two evolutionary lines
leading to the arthropods and chordates (Fig. 4). The
alignment of their sequences across all seven extracellular domains supports the notion that this common ancestor had five immunoglobulin domains and two fibronectin domains and differed from other immunoglobulin superfamily adhesion molecules that predated
the arthropod-chordate split, including, for example,
the ancestor with six immunoglobulin domains and five
fibronectin domains that gave rise to L1 and neuroglian.

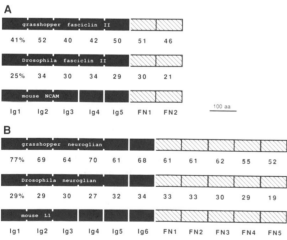

Figure 3. Summary of comparisons of *Drosophila* and grasshopper fasciclin II and mouse N-CAM and of *Drosophila* and
grasshopper neuroglian and mouse L1. Numbers shown are
percentages of amino acid identity in each domain compared
between the two species immediately above and below the
number (immunoglobulin domains are measured here as including 20 amino acids outside the two characteristic cysteine
residues; fibronectin type III domains are measured as including 20 amino acids outside the characteristic tryptophan and
tyrosine residues). Because these molecules have alternative
cytoplasmic domains and in some cases alternative membrane
linkages, all that is shown here are the extracellular regions of
each protein.

Neuroglian Is Related to L1

Neuroglian was first cloned in *Drosophila* (Bieber et
al. 1989). The initial cDNA sequence analysis revealed
that the extracellular portion of the protein consists of
six immunoglobulin C2-type domains and five fibronectin type III domains followed by a transmembrane
domain and a short cytoplasmic domain. Neuroglian
exhibits extensive structural homology with the mouse
neural adhesion molecule L1. Comparison of neuroglian with L1 using the FAST-P alignment program
yields an optimized score of 1442. Neuroglian is next
most related to contactin/F11 and TAG-1; for example, comparison of neuroglian with contactin using
FAST-P yields an optimized score of 925. The homology between neuroglian and these proteins extends
throughout most of the extracellular portion of both
molecules. The greatest similarity exists between

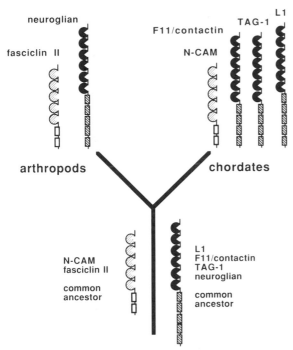

arthropods

chordates

Figure 4. Evolutionary kinship among some of the *Drosophila* and vertebrate neural cell adhesion molecules of the immunoglobulin superfamily. The present data support the notion that a number of ancestral neural cell adhesion molecules existed before the arthropod-chordate split, that these molecules had multiple immunoglobulin domains and multiple fibronectin type III domains, and that these ancestral molecules gave rise to a wide diversity of arthropod and chordate neural cell adhesion molecules. One common ancestor gave rise to fasciclin II and N-CAM, whereas another gave rise to neuroglian, L1, F11/contactin, and TAG-1. Still another must have given rise to fasciclin III, which is quite divergent from the others shown here. Moreover, the similarity of these molecules in arthropods and chordates supports the hypothesis that the mechanisms of neural adhesion and recognition are likely to have been conserved in both phyla.

neuroglian and L1, which have greater than 28% amino acid identity over the entire length of the proteins (Fig. 3B). In contrast, neuroglian has an optimized score to mouse N-CAM of only 383 and to grasshopper fasciclin II of only 182.

The neuroglian homolog was recently cloned in the grasshopper using PCR (G. Grenningloh and E.J. Rehm, unpubl.). The deduced grasshopper and *Drosophila* neuroglian proteins have approximately 65% amino acid identity over most of their extracellular domains. Over the much broader evolutionary span between *Drosophila* and the mouse, the structural similarities and the 28% amino acid identity between neuroglian and L1 suggest a common evolutionary origin. Although most related to L1, neuroglian is next most closely related to contactin/F11 and TAG-1 and then more distantly related to N-CAM, fasciclin II, and other immunoglobulin adhesion molecules. Thus, whereas fasciclin II appears to have arisen from a common ancestor of fasciclin II and N-CAM (Harrelson and Goodman 1988), neuroglian appears to have arisen

from a second common ancestor that gave rise to neuroglian, L1, contactin/F11, and TAG-1 (Fig. 4). In this subfamily of immunoglobulin neural cell adhesion molecules, neuroglian shares the greatest overall similarity with L1.

Fasciclin III Is Also a Member of the Immunoglobulin Superfamily

The sequence of a fasciclin III cDNA was initially reported as encoding a novel cell-surface protein (Snow et al. 1989). The mature protein (after cleavage of the 20-amino-acid signal sequence) consists of an extracellular domain of 326 amino acids, a transmembrane domain of 24 amino acids, and a cytoplasmic domain of 138 residues. Comparison of the sequence encoded by the cDNA with those of other proteins within the NBRF database using the FAST-P program revealed no strong sequence similarity to any known protein. However, a short sequence in the extracellular region just outside the transmembrane domain did show a relatively weak similarity to one half of an immunoglobulin domain, although it lacked the characteristic cysteine residues. Because this homology was weak and extended over only a short stretch of sequence, it was not considered significant. Thus, fasciclin III was reported as representing a novel class of cell-surface proteins (Snow et al. 1989).

Although the original sequence comparison indicated that fasciclin III did not seem to resemble any previously described protein, an independent analysis of the fasciclin III sequence by A. Smith (University of Minnesota) has revealed that fasciclin III appears to be composed of somewhat divergent immunoglobulin domains. This conclusion was initially based on alignment of the fasciclin III sequence to that of twitchin, a recently described nematode muscle protein containing 26 immunoglobulin domains, many of which lack the characteristically positioned cysteine residues (Benian et al. 1989). When the fasciclin III and twitchin sequences were analyzed using the ALIGN program of Dayhoff (Dayhoff et al. 1983; Williams and Barclay 1988), Smith concluded that the extracellular portion of fasciclin III contains three immunoglobulin-related domains, the third of which lacks the characteristic cysteine residues. The fasciclin III sequence has also been analyzed by A. Williams (Oxford), whose findings are in basic agreement with those of Smith. Williams finds three immunoglobulin-related domains, although the assignments were made with some difficulty because of the unusual sequence patterns surrounding the second cysteines. The most amino-terminal domain appears to be of the V type, whereas the second and third immunoglobulin domains are less clear; Williams suggests that they could be long C2 types but may fold as a V type. The third domain, which lacks the characteristic cysteine residues, gave the best comparison with the ALIGN program to twitchin: 17 of 26 domain comparisons gave z-scores of > 3 s.d. (usually considered a significant homology), whereas 7 of 26 gave z-scores of

>5 s.d. (a highly significant score). Thus, we conclude, with the help of A. Smith and A. Williams, that the extracellular region of fasciclin III consists of three immunoglobulin domains that are somewhat divergent from the standard C2-type domains found in many of the other neural cell adhesion molecules (Fig. 2).

All Three Immunoglobulin Superfamily Proteins Come in Multiple Forms

All three of these *Drosophila* immunoglobulin super-family axonal glycoproteins (fasciclin II, neuroglian, and fasciclin III) undergo alternative splicing to generate multiple forms of each protein having either different cytoplasmic domains or different forms of membrane attachment (Fig. 2). In none of the three cases can we detect alternative splicing in the extracellular domains. Most vertebrate genes encoding immunoglobulin superfamily molecules have introns between each immunoglobulin domain, with some like N-CAM having additional introns in the middle of each immunoglobulin domain. In contrast, fasciclin II (G. Grenningloh and E.J. Rehm, unpubl.) and neuroglian (A.J. Bieber et al., unpubl.) do not have introns between their immunoglobulin domains and, for that matter, have very few introns in the region coding their extracellular domains. Amalgam, another immunoglobulin superfamily molecule in *Drosophila* (see later section), also has no introns between its immunoglobulin domains (Seeger et al. 1988).

The initial grasshopper fasciclin II cDNA that was sequenced encodes a protein with a transmembrane domain of 25 amino acids and a cytoplasmic domain of 108 amino acids (Harrelson and Goodman 1988). A more detailed characterization of the fasciclin II gene in *Drosophila* has revealed several different mRNAs in Northern blot analysis, the most abundant of which in the embryo encodes a deduced protein that, according to cDNA sequence analysis, does not have a transmembrane domain but rather appears to have a phosphatidylinositol (PI) lipid membrane anchor (G. Grenningloh and E.J. Rehm, unpubl.). Thus, it is likely that fasciclin II comes in at least two different forms, one of which is PI linked and the other of which has a transmembrane domain. The existence of multiple forms of a neural cell adhesion molecule and, in particular, different forms of membrane attachment is reminiscent of N-CAM (Murray et al. 1986; Cunningham et al. 1987; Dickson et al. 1987; Owens et al. 1987; Barbas et al. 1988; Small et al. 1988; Santoni et al. 1989; Thompson et al. 1989), the molecule with which fasciclin II shares a common ancestor.

The neuroglian gene in *Drosophila* generates at least two different protein products by tissue-specific alternative splicing (Hortsch et al. 1990). The two protein forms differ in their cytoplasmic domains; so far, there is no evidence for a PI-linked form of neuroglian, just as there is no evidence for a PI-linked form of vertebrate L1, its closest relative. Although identical in their extracellular domains, after the transmembrane

domain, the two neuroglian protein forms share only the first 68 amino acids of their cytoplasmic domains. The short, more abundant form of the protein continues for another 17 amino acids. However, in contrast with the short form, the long form of the protein extends for another 62 amino acids. The entire cytoplasmic domain of the long form of the neuroglian protein form encompasses 148 amino acid residues compared with 85 amino acids in the cytoplasmic domain of the short form. The long form is restricted to the surface of neurons in the CNS and neurons and some support cells in the peripheral nervous system (PNS); in contrast, the short form is expressed on a wide range of other cells and tissues. Thus, whereas the mouse L1 gene appears to encode only one protein that functions largely as a neural cell adhesion molecule, its closest *Drosophila* relative, the neuroglian gene, encodes at least two protein forms that may play two different roles: one as a neural cell adhesion molecule and the other as a more general cell adhesion molecule involved in tissue and imaginal disc morphogenesis.

Some striking differences appear to have evolved in the alternative splicing of the neuroglian gene during the 300 million years of evolution that separate the more advanced insect, *Drosophila*, from the more primitive one, the grasshopper. Whereas the *Drosophila* neuroglian gene generates two different forms of the protein with different cytoplasmic domains (which are easily detectable on Western blots), the grasshopper gene appears to generate only one protein form as detected on Western blots (G. Grenningloh and E.J. Rehm, unpubl.). This single form in the grasshopper is expressed throughout many tissues of the embryo, much as is the short form of the *Drosophila* protein. Thus, although *Drosophila* does have a nervous-system-specific, alternatively spliced form of neuroglian, the more primitive grasshopper apparently does not. This conclusion is supported by the observation that the two alternatively spliced cytoplasmic domains in *Drosophila* may have recently evolved by an exon duplication. The short-form-specific exon encodes for another 17 amino acids, 11 of which are conserved in the protein sequence encoded by the long-form-specific exon (Hortsch et al. 1990). Just as with fasciclin II and neuroglian, so too *Drosophila* fasciclin III is alternatively spliced to generate at least two different protein forms with different cytoplasmic domains, each of which has a different spatial and temporal pattern of expression (P.M. Snow et al., unpubl.).

All Three Immunoglobulin Superfamily Proteins Are Homophilic Cell Adhesion Molecules

Fasciclin II is related to N-CAM, a homophilic neural cell adhesion molecule, and neuroglian is related to L1, another homophilic neural cell adhesion molecule. Moreover, fasciclin III is also a member of the immunoglobulin superfamily. Do these three *Drosophila* axonal glycoproteins function as neural cell adhesion molecules, as their structure predicts? To answer this ques-

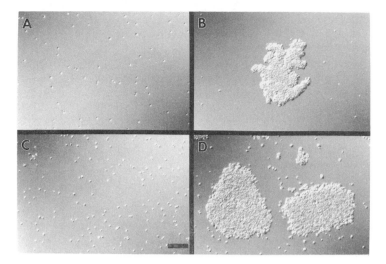

Figure 5. Homophilic aggegation of *Drosophila* S2 cells transfected with either neuroglian or fasciclin II cDNAs. *Drosophila* S2 cells normally grow in suspension without aggregating. In these studies, cDNAs encoding *Drosophila* neuroglian (*A,B*) (A.J. Bieber, unpubl.) or *Drosophila* fasciclin II (*C,D*) (G. Grenningloh and A.J. Bieber, unpubl.) were transfected into Schneider 2 (S2) cells as described previously (Snow et al. 1989). The transfected cells were heat shocked for 15–30 min and allowed to recover. In both cases, the cells aggregate in what appears to be a homophilic manner. Bar, 100 μm.

tion, we have used DNA transfection methods to test whether these proteins can confer cell aggregation in vitro in the nonadhesive *Drosophila* S2 cells, an experimental paradigm modeled after the studies on vertebrate cadherins begun by Takeichi and his colleagues (Nagafuchi et al. 1987). The first aggregation experiments using transfected *Drosophila* cDNAs and the *Drosophila* S2 cell line showed that fasciclin III can function as a homophilic cell adhesion molecule (Snow et al. 1989). In subsequent studies, we have shown that fasciclin I (the other, novel protein; Elkins et al. 1990a), neuroglian (A.J. Bieber, unpubl.), and fasciclin II (G. Grenningloh and A.J. Bieber, unpubl.) can each function as a homophilic cell adhesion molecule in vitro (Fig. 5). We have also shown that when the fasciclin-I-transfected S2 cells are heterogeneously mixed with the fasciclin-III-transfected S2 cells (Elkins et al. 1990a), the fasciclin-I-transfected S2 cells with the neuroglian-transfected S2 cells (A.J. Bieber, unpubl.), or the fasciclin-III-transfected cells with the neuroglian-transfected S2 cells (A.J. Bieber, unpubl.), they undergo cell-type-specific sorting into homogeneous aggregates. These in vitro results lead to the suggestion that these neural cell adhesion molecules (the three immunoglobulin superfamily proteins: fasciclin II, neuroglian, and fasciclin III, and the novel protein, fasciclin I) might play a similar role in cell sorting during development in vivo, particularly during axonal guidance in which they are expressed on both specific growth cones and the axon pathways they follow.

Mutations Have Been Identified in All Three Immunoglobulin Superfamily Cell Adhesion Molecules

The *Drosophila* genes encoding all three immunoglobulin superfamily cell adhesion molecules have been mapped to the polytene chromosomes and are located as follows. Neuroglian and fasciclin II are on the X chromosome, neuroglian at band 7F and fasciclin II at

band 4B, and fasciclin III is on the left arm of the second chromosome at band 36E. We have identified and/or generated mutations in all three immunoglobulin superfamily neural cell adhesion molecules, including a lethal, null mutation in the *neuroglian* gene (Bieber et al. 1989), a viable, hypomorphic P element insertion in the 5′ end of the *fasciclin II* gene (a screen for null mutations is in progress; G. Grenningloh, unpubl.), and a viable, null mutation in the *fasciclin III* gene (T. Elkins et al., unpubl.). (We have also generated a viable, null mutation in the *fasciclin I* gene [Elkins et al. 1990b].) To our knowledge, the mutations in the *fasciclin III* and *neuroglian* genes are the first known null mutations in immunoglobulin superfamily cell adhesion molecules. Of the mutations in the three immunoglobulin superfamily neural cell adhesion molecules, the one that has been analyzed in greatest detail thus far is in neuroglian.

The genetic deficiencies *Df(1)KA14* and *Df(1)RA2* delete the 7F region (which includes the *neuroglian* gene) and have breakpoints at 7F1-2;8C5 and 7D10;8A4-5, respectively. A screen for lethal point mutations in this region was undertaken previously by Lefevre and Watkins (1986), and ten lethally mutable loci were described that lie within the overlap of these two deficiencies. Antibody staining of representatives for each of these lethally mutable loci reveals that one of these loci corresponds to the *neuroglian* gene. Antibody staining experiments demonstrate that the ethylmethanesulfonate-induced mutation designated *l(1)VA142* represents a hypomorphic, lethal mutation in the *neuroglian* gene (data not shown). Mutant embryos reveal no or little expression of neuroglian in nonneuronal tissues (e.g., trachea, salivary gland, and hindgut) and reduced expression in the nervous system. However, there is still a small amount of neuroglian expression in the CNS, indicating that this is not a complete null allele of *neuroglian*.

A second lethal mutation *l(1)RA35* (Lefevre and Watkins 1986) consists of an inversion with breakpoints at 6E;7F1. Embryonic lethality is associated with the

7F1 breakpoint, and mutant embryos completely lack neuroglian expression. We have named lethal mutations in the *neuroglian* gene: *nrg*.

We have used a variety of nervous system markers for our initial analysis of the phenotype of *nrg* mutant embryos. The most striking observation is that, at a gross level, the overall structure of the CNS and PNS, and in particular the peripheral nerve roots and CNS axon pathways, develops in a relatively normal way. Clearly, normally neuroglian-positive axon pathways do not become "unglued" when this *Drosophila* L1 homolog is genetically deleted, suggesting some redundancy in overall axonal and glial adhesion systems. However, although neurons do not become "unglued," there is a consistent although more subtle phenotype in *nrg* mutant embryos: The orientation and extent of contact among the normally neuroglian-positive sensory neurons in the PNS are abnormal (Fig. 1E,F). For example, the five lateral chordotonal neurons in each abdominal hemisegment normally line up in a tight row with each cell body having extensive membrane apposition with the neurons on either side of it; the chordotonal neurons are normally flattened against one another and lie in the same focal plane. In contrast, in *nrg* mutant embryos, the five chordotonal neurons are more randomly organized in a looser group with less membrane apposition, resulting in a disorganization in the alignment of their dendrites. Similar types of phenotypes are seen with other clusters of sensory neurons as well.

Studies in vertebrates, in which antibodies were used to perturb neurite outgrowth and axon fasciculation in vitro, suggest that the systems that mediate neural cell adhesion are redundant in that perturbation of more than one system is required before major functional disruptions occur (Tomaselli et al. 1986, 1988; Bixby et al. 1987; Chang et al. 1987; Neugebauer et al. 1988); presumably, in the developing organism, these systems are not simply redundant, but rather each of the overlapping systems has a subtly different function. If such overlap of adhesion systems is at play in *Drosophila* as it appears to be in vertebrates, then multiple mutations that remove more than one cell adhesion system simultaneously may be necessary to produce gross disruptions of nervous system development. In this light, it is not so surprising that the *nrg* mutant does not lead to a grossly abnormal CNS in which axon pathways and peripheral nerve roots become unglued and highly disorganized. Rather, the *nrg* mutant does lead to a more subtle phenotype in the disruption of the precise patterning of sensory neurons, which makes us wonder if there might also be subtle abnormalities in the guidance and patterning of axons in the CNS that are not as easy to detect. It will be of interest in the future both to look for more subtle phenotypes in the behavior of individual axons in *nrg* mutant embryos and to look for more gross phenotypes in embryos mutant for *nrg* in combination with mutations in other neural cell adhesion systems, such as fasciclin II and fasciclin III.

Diversity of Immunoglobulin Superfamily Molecules in *Drosophila*

When the cloning of fasciclin II in the grasshopper (Harrelson and Goodman 1988) and amalgam in *Drosophila* (Seeger et al. 1988) was reported in 1988, it was thought that both might be neural cell adhesion molecules; indeed, fasciclin II was closely related to N-CAM and amalgam also appeared to have sequence similarity to N-CAM in its immunoglobulin domains. The next year came the cloning of *Drosophila* neuroglian, a close relative of the vertebrate neural cell adhesion molecule L1 (Bieber et al. 1989). The discovery that the first three members of the immunoglobulin superfamily outside of the chordates were found in the developing insect nervous system and that all three were thought to be candidates for neural cell adhesion molecules led to the suggestion (Harrelson and Goodman 1988; Bieber et al. 1989) that (1) the ancestral function of immunoglobulin superfamily molecules was as adhesion molecules in the developing nervous system, (2) these molecules duplicated and diverged with multiple immunoglobulin type C2 and fibronectin type III domains before the split of the arthropod and chordate lines, and (3) the molecular mechanisms of neural adhesion and recognition are likely to have been conserved in arthropods and chordates.

As more has been learned about these molecules, the second and third of these conclusions still seem valid. The present data support the notion that a number of ancestral neural cell adhesion molecules existed before the arthropod-chordate split, that these molecules had multiple immunoglobulin domains and multiple fibronectin domains, and that these ancestral molecules gave rise to a wide diversity of arthropod and chordate neural cell adhesion molecules. For example, one common ancestor gave rise to fasciclin II and N-CAM, whereas another gave rise to neuroglian, L1, F11/contactin, and TAG-1 (see Fig. 4). Still another must have given rise to fasciclin III, which is quite divergent from the others listed above. Moreover, the similarity of these molecules in arthropods and chordates supports the hypothesis that the mechanisms of neural adhesion and recognition are likely to have been conserved in both phyla.

The first conclusion on the origins of the immunoglobulin superfamily from neural cell adhesion molecules needs to be reevaluated in light of further work on amalgam and because of the discovery of a wide variety of other immunoglobulin superfamily molecules in *Drosophila* (Fig. 6). The amalgam protein has a signal sequence followed by three immunoglobulin domains (Seeger et al. 1988) but lacks either a transmembrane domain or a suitable site for a PI linkage. Recent studies have suggested that amalgam is not a cell adhesion molecule, but rather it is a secreted molecule of unknown function (M. Seeger et al., pers. comm.): First, when transfected into S2 cells, it is secreted and appears neither to mediate nor to modulate cell adhe-

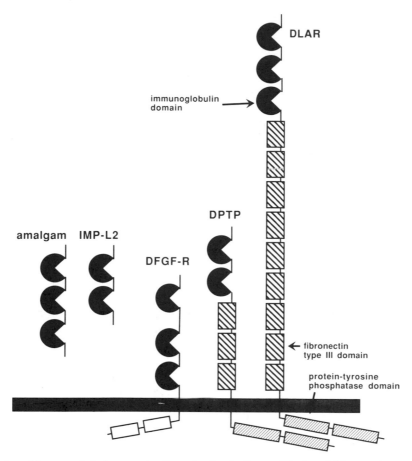

Figure 6. The diversity of immunoglobulin superfamily molecules in *Drosophila*. In addition to the three immunoglobulin superfamily neural cell adhesion molecules described in this paper (fasciclin II, neuroglian, and fasciclin III), a variety of other immunoglobulin superfamily molecules have been recently discovered in *Drosophila*. The amalgam protein has a signal sequence, followed by three immunoglobulin domains (Seeger et al. 1988) but lacks either a transmembrane domain or a suitable site for a PI linkage; recent studies suggest that amalgam is a secreted molecule of unknown function (M. Seeger et al., pers. comm.). IMP-L2 is another small, presumably secreted immunoglobulin superfamily molecule in *Drosophila* that has been discovered by J. Garbe and J. Fristrom (pers. comm.); IMP-L2 encodes a protein with a signal sequence and two immunoglobulin domains but which lacks a transmembrane domain. Two different receptor-linked protein tyrosine phosphatases (DLAR and DPTP) have been identified in *Drosophila* (Streuli et al. 1989). The extracellular regions of these proteins look very similar to the neural cell adhesion molecules in that they have multiple immunoglobulin domains followed by multiple fibronectin type III domains (DLAR has three immunoglobulin domains and nine fibronectin domains; DPTP has two immunoglobulin domains and two fibronectin domains). The cytoplasmic domains of these molecules, however, are strikingly different from fasciclin II and neuroglian: DLAR and DPTP have two tandemly repeated PTPase domains. The *Drosophila* homolog of the receptor for FGFR has been discovered by L. Glazer and B. Shilo (pers. comm.). The *Drosophila* FGFR has three immunoglobulin domains in its extracellular region, as well as a transmembrane domain and highly conserved cytoplasmic domain. Thus, the diversity of *Drosophila* proteins containing immunoglobulin domains includes three neural cell adhesion molecules (fasciclin II, neuroglian, and fasciclin III), two putative secreted molecules (amalgam and IMP-L2), two receptor-linked protein tyrosine phosphatases (DLAR and DPTP), and a growth factor receptor (DFGFR). Several of these molecules, such as fasciclin II, neuroglian, DLAR, and DFGFR, have close vertebrate relatives, if not homologs, suggesting a wide diversity of common ancestors before the arthropod-chordate split.

sion; second, in the embryo, comparison of in situ hybridization with antibody localization suggests that one set of cells secretes amalgam (the epidermis), whereas the protein binds to the surface of a different set of cells (neuronal cell bodies).

Another small, presumably secreted immunoglobulin superfamily molecule in *Drosophila* has been discovered by J. Garbe and J. Fristrom (pers. comm.). The ecdysone-inducible gene, IMP-L2, is expressed by imaginal discs and histoblasts during metamorphosis (Osterbur et al. 1988). Garbe and Fristrom have re-

cently shown that IMP-L2 encodes a protein with a signal sequence and two immunoglobulin domains but lacks a transmembrane domain. Thus, just as with amalgam, so too IMP-L2 is likely to be a secreted immunoglobulin superfamily protein.

Two different receptor-linked protein tyrosine phosphatases (DLAR and DPTP) have been identified in *Drosophila* (Streuli et al. 1989). The extracellular regions of these proteins look very similar to those of the neural cell adhesion molecules in that they have multiple immunoglobulin domains followed by multiple fibronectin type III domains (DLAR has three immuno-globulin domains and nine fibronectin domains, and DPTP has two immunoglobulin domains and two fibronectin domains). The cytoplasmic domains of these molecules, however, are strikingly different from those of fasciclin II and neuroglian: DLAR and DPTP have two tandemly repeated PTPase domains.

Finally, L. Glazer and B. Shilo (pers. comm.) have discovered the *Drosophila* homolog of the fibroblast growth factor receptor (FGFR). Just as with its vertebrate homolog, so too the *Drosophila* FGFR has three immunoglobulin domains in its extracellular region, as well as a transmembrane domain and highly conserved cytoplasmic domain. Thus, the diversity of *Drosophila* proteins containing immunoglobulin domains includes three neural cell adhesion molecules (fasciclin II, neuroglian, and fasciclin III), two putative secreted molecules (amalgam and IMP-L2), two receptor-linked protein tyrosine phosphatases (DLAR and DPTP), and a growth factor receptor (DFGFR). Several of these molecules, such as fasciclin II, neuroglian, DLAR, and DFGFR, have close vertebrate relatives, if not homologs, suggesting a wide diversity of common ancestors before the arthropod-chordate split.

These data do not support the simple hypothesis that neural cell adhesion molecules were the forerunners of the immunoglobulin superfamily at the time of the major phylogenetic branch leading to arthropods and chordates. Rather, before the split of these two lines of evolution, the proteins with immunoglobulin domains had already radiated to include a wide range of secreted and cell-surface molecules, making it difficult from these data alone to speculate on which kind of immunoglobulin molecule was the true ancestor of the whole gene family. It might have been a neural cell adhesion molecule, but then it just as easily could have been a phosphatase or a growth factor receptor. The important conclusion is that a wide diversity of immunoglobulin superfamily molecules already existed before the phyletic split. Given that *Drosophila* is an ideal organism for the genetic analysis of function, it is fortunate that so many different types of immunoglobulin superfamily molecules exist in *Drosophila*.

ACKNOWLEDGMENTS

We are indebted to Michael Bastiani, the late Tom Elkins, Allan Harrelson, Jim Schilling, and Kai Zinn for the important roles they played in the earlier studies on fasciclin II, fasciclin III, and neuroglian that laid the groundwork for the results described here. We thank Mark Seeger, Christian Klämbt, and Roger Jacobs from our own laboratory, and Thom Kaufman, Jim Garbe, Jim Fristrom, Lilly Glazer, and Benny Shilo for allowing us to refer to their unpublished results. Finally, we give a special thanks to Andrew Smith and Alan Williams for sharing with us their unpublished analysis of the structure of fasciclin III and for allowing us to refer to it here. This work was supported by postdoc-toral fellowships from the Deutsche Forschungs-gemeinschaft to G.G. and National Institutes of Health to A.B. and by grant HD-21294 to C.S.G. who is an Investigator with the Howard Hughes Medical Institute.

REFERENCES

Arquint, M., J. Roder, L.-S. Chia, J. Down, D. Wilkinson, H. Bayley, P. Braun, and R. Dunn. 1987. Molecular cloning and primary structure of myelin-associated glycoprotein. *Proc. Natl. Acad. Sci.* **84:** 600.

Barbas, J.A., J.-C. Chaix, M. Steinmetz, and C. Goridis. 1988. Differential splicing and alternative polyadenylation generates distinct NCAM transcripts and proteins in the mouse. *EMBO J.* **7:** 625.

Barthels, D., M.J. Santoni, W. Wille, C. Ruppert, J.C. Chaix, M.R. Hirsch, J.C. Fontecilla-Camps, and C. Goridis. 1987. Isolation and nucleotide sequence of mouse NCAM cDNA that codes for a M_r 79,000 polypeptide without a membrane-spanning region. *EMBO J.* **6:** 907.

Bastiani, M.J. and C.S. Goodman. 1986. Guidance of neuronal growth cones in the grasshopper embryo. III. Recognition of specific glial pathways. *J. Neurosci.* **6:** 3542.

Bastiani, M.J., S. du Lac, and C.S. Goodman. 1986. Guidance of neuronal growth cones in the grasshopper embryo. I. Recognition of a specific axonal pathway by the pCC neuron. *J. Neurosci.* **6:** 3518.

Bastiani, M.J., J.A. Raper, and C.S. Goodman. 1984. Pathfinding by neuronal growth cones in grasshopper embryos. III. Selective affinity of the G growth cone for the P cells within the A/P fascicle. *J. Neurosci.* **4:** 2311.

Bastiani, M.J., A.L. Harrelson, P.M. Snow, and C.S. Goodman. 1987. Expression of fasciclin I and II glycoproteins on subsets of axon pathways during neuronal development in the grasshopper. *Cell* **48:** 745.

Benian, G.M., J.E. Kiff, N. Necklelmann, D.G. Moerman, and R.H. Waterson. 1989. Sequence of an unusually large protein implicated in regulation of myosin activity in *C. elegans. Nature* **342:** 45.

Bieber, A.J., P.M. Snow, M. Hortsch, N. Pate, J.R. Jacobs, Z.R. Traquina, J. Schilling, and C.S. Goodman. 1989. *Drosophila* neuroglian: A member of the immunoglobulin superfamily with extensive homology to the vertebrate neural adhesion molecule L1. *Cell* **59:** 447.

Bixby, J.L., R.S. Pratt, J. Lilien, and L.F. Reichardt. 1987. Neurite outgrowth on muscle cell surfaces involves extracellular matrix receptors as well as Ca^{2+}-dependent and -independent cell adhesion molecules. *Proc. Natl. Acad. Sci.* **84:** 2555.

Brümmendorf, T., J.M. Wolff, R. Frank, and F.G. Rathjen. 1989. Neural cell recognition molecule F11: Homology with fibronectin type III and immunoglobulin type C domains. *Neuron* **2:** 1351.

Chang, S., F.G. Rathjen, and J.A. Raper. 1987. Extension of neurites on axons is impaired by antibodies against specific neural cell surface glycoproteins. *J. Cell Biol.* **104:** 355.

Cunningham, B.A., J.J. Hemperiy, B.A. Murray, E.A. Prediger, R. Brackenbury, and G.M. Edelman. 1987. Neural cell adhesion molecule: Structure, immunoglobulin-like domains, cell surface modulation and alternative RNA splicing. *Science* **236:** 799.

Dayhoff, M.O., W.C. Barker, and L.T. Hunt. 1983. Establishing homologies in protein sequences. *Methods Enzymol.* **91:** 524.

Dickson, G., H.J. Gower, C.H. Barton, H.M. Prentice, Y.L. Elsom, S.E. Moore, R.D. Cox, C. Quinn, W. Putt, and F.S. Walsh. 1987. Human muscle neural cell adhesion molecule (NCAM): Identification of a muscle-specific sequence in the extracellular domain. *Cell* **50:** 1119.

Dodd, J. and T.M. Jessell. 1988. Axon guidance and the patterning of neuronal projections in vertebrates. *Science* **242**: 692.

Doe, C.Q., M.J. Bastiani, and C.S. Goodman. 1986. Guidance of neuronal growth cones in the grasshopper embryo. IV. Temporal delay experiments. *J. Neurosci.* **6**: 3552.

du Lac, S., M.J. Bastiani, and C.S. Goodman. 1986. Guidance of neuronal growth cones in the grasshopper embryo. II. Recognition of a specific axonal pathway by the aCC neuron. *J. Neurosci.* **6**: 3532.

Elkins, T., M. Hortsch, A.J. Bieber, P.M. Snow, and C.S. Goodman. 1990a. *Drosophila* fasciclin I is a novel homophilic adhesion molecule that along with fasciclin III can mediate cell sorting. *J. Cell Biol.* **110**: 1825.

Elkins, T., K. Zinn, L. McAllister, F.M. Hoffmann, and C.S. Goodman. 1990b. Genetic analysis of a *Drosophila* neural cell adhesion molecule: Interaction of fasciclin I and Abelson tyrosine kinase mutations. *Cell* **60**: 565.

Furley, A.J., S.B. Morton, D. Manalo, D. Karagogeos, J. Dodd, and T.M. Jessell. 1990. The axonal glycoprotein TAG-1 is an immunoglobulin superfamily member with neurite outgrowth-promoting activity. *Cell* **61**: 157.

Goodman, C.S., M.J. Bastiani, J.A. Raper, and J.B.Thomas. 1985. Cell recognition during neuronal development in grasshopper and *Drosophila*. In *Molecular bases of neural development* (ed. G.M. Edelman et al.), p. 295. Neuroscience Research Foundation, Wiley, New York.

Goodman, C.S., M.J. Bastiani, C.Q. Doe, S. du Lac, S.L. Helfand, J.Y. Kuwada, and J.B. Thomas. 1984. Cell recognition during neuronal development. *Science* **225**: 1271.

Harrelson, A.L. and C.S. Goodman. 1988. Growth cone guidance in insects: Fasciclin II is a member of the immunoglobulin superfamily. *Science* **242**: 700.

Hortsch, M. and C.S. Goodman. 1990. *Drosophila* fasciclin I, a neural cell adhesion molecule, has a phosphoinositol lipid membrane anchor that is developmentally regulated. *J. Biol. Chem.* **265**: 15104.

Hortsch, M., A.J. Bieber, N.H. Patel, and C.S. Goodman. 1990. Differential splicing generates a nervous system-specific form of *Drosophila* neuroglian. *Neuron* **4**: 697.

Hynes, R.O. 1986. Molecular biology of fibronectin. *Annu. Rev. Cell Biol.* **1**: 67.

Jacobs, J.R. and C.S. Goodman. 1989a. Embryonic development of axon pathways in the Drosophila CNS: I. A glial scaffold appears before the first growth cones. *J. Neurosci.* **9**: 2402.

———. 1989b. Embryonic development of axon pathways in the *Drosophila* CNS: II. Behavior of pioneer growth cones. *J. Neurosci.* **9**: 2412.

Jacobs, J.R., Y. Hiromi, N. Patel, and C.S. Goodman. 1989. Lineage, migration, and morphogenesis of longitudinal glia in the *Drosophila* CNS as revealed by a molecular lineage marker. *Neuron* **2**: 1625.

Kuwada, J.Y. 1986. Cell recognition by neuronal growth cones in a simple vertebrate embryo. *Science* **233**: 740.

Lefevre, G. and W. Watkins. 1986. The question of the total gene number in *Drosophila melanogaster*. *Genetics* **113**: 869.

Lipman, D.J. and W.R. Pearson. 1985. Rapid and sensitive protein similarity searches. *Science* **227**: 1435.

Moos, M., R. Tacke, H. Scherer, D. Teplow, K. Früh, and M. Schachner. 1988. Neural adhesion molecule L1 is a member of the immunoglobulin superfamily with binding domains similar to fibronectin. *Nature* **334**: 701.

Murray, B.A., J.J. Hemperly, E.A. Prediger, G.M. Edelman, and B.A. Cunningham. 1986. Alternatively spliced mRNAs code for different polypeptide chains of the chicken neural cell adhesion moleculae (NCAM). *J. Cell Biol.* **102**: 189.

Nagafuchi, A., Y. Shirayoshi, K. Okazaki, K. Yasuka, and M. Takeichi. 1987. Transformation of cell adhesion properties by exogenously introduced E-cadherin cDNA. *Nature* **329**: 341.

Neugebauer, K.M., K.L. Tomaselli, J. Lilien, and L.F. Reichardt. 1988. N-cadherin, NCAM and integrins promote retinal neurite outgrowth on astrocytes in vitro. *J. Cell Biol.* **107**: 1177.

Osterbur, D.L, D.K. Fristrom, J.R. Natzle, S.J. Tojo, and J.W. Fristrom. 1988. Genes expressed during imaginal discs morphogenesis: IMP-L2, a gene expressed during imaginal disc and imaginal histoblast morphogenesis. *Dev. Biol.* **129**: 439.

Owens, G.C., G.M. Edelman, and B.A. Cunningham. 1987. Organization of the neural cell adhesion molecule (NCAM) gene: Alternative exon usage as the basis for different membrane-associated domains. *Proc. Natl. Acad. Sci.* **84**: 294.

Patel, N.H., P.M. Snow, and C.S. Goodman. 1987. Characterization and cloning of fasciclin III: A glycoprotein expressed on a subset of neurons and axon pathways in *Drosophila*. *Cell* **48**: 975.

Ranscht, B. 1988. Sequence of contactin, a 130-kD glycoprotein concentrated in areas of interneuronal contact, defines a new member of the immunoglobulin supergene family in the nervous system. *J. Cell. Biol.* **107**: 1561.

Raper, J.A., M.J. Bastiani, and C.S. Goodman. 1983a. Pathfinding by neuronal growthcones in grasshopper embryos. I. Divergent choices made by the growth cones of sibling neurons. *J. Neurosci.* **3**: 20.

———. 1983b. Pathfinding by neuronal growth cones in grasshopper embryos. II. Selective fasciculation onto specific axonal pathways. *J. Neurosci.* **3**: 31.

———. 1983c. Guidance of neuronal growth cones: selective fasciculation in the grasshopper embryo. *Cold Spring Harbor Symp. Quant. Biol.* **48**: 587.

———. 1984. Pathfinding by neuronal growth cones in grasshopper embryos. IV. The effects of ablating the A and P axons upon the behavior of the G growth cone. *J. Neurosci.* **4**: 2329.

Salzer, J.L., W.P. Holmes, and D.R. Colman. 1987. The amino acid sequences of the myelin-associated glycoproteins: Homology with the immunoglobulin gene family. *J. Cell Biol.* **104**: 957.

Santoni, M.J., D. Barthels, G. Vopper, A. Boned, C. Goridis, and W. Wille. 1989. Differential exon usage involving an unusual splicing mechanism generates at least eight types of NCAM cDNA in mouse brain. *EMBO J.* **8**: 385.

Seeger, M.A., L. Haffley, and T.C. Kaufman. 1988. Characterization of amalgam: A member of the immunoglobulin superfamily from *Drosophila*. *Cell* **55**: 589.

Small, S.J., S.L. Haines, and R.A. Akeson. 1988. Polypeptide variation in an NCAM extracellular immunoglobulin-like fold is developmentally regulated through alternative splicing. *Neuron* **1**: 1007.

Snow, P.M., A.J. Bieber, and C.S. Goodman. 1989. *Drosophila* fasciclin III: A novel homophilic adhesion molecule. *Cell* **59**: 313.

Snow, P.M., K. Zinn, A.L. Harrelson, L. McAllister, J. Schilling, M.J. Bastiani, G. Makk, and C.S. Goodman. 1988. Characterization and cloning of fasciclin I and fasciclin II glycoproteins in the grasshopper. *Proc. Natl. Acad. Sci.* **85**: 5291.

Streuli, M., N.X. Krueger, A.Y.M. Tsai, and H. Saito. 1989. A family of receptor-linked protein tyrosine phosphates in human and *Drosophila*. *Proc. Natl. Acad. Sci.* **86**: 8698.

Thomas, J.B., M.J. Bastiani, C.M. Bate, and C.S. Goodman. 1984. From grasshopper to *Drosophila*: A common plan for neuronal development. *Nature* **310**: 203.

Thompson, J., G. Dickson, S.E. Moore, N.J. Gower, W. Putt, J.G. Kenimer, C.H. Barton, and F.S. Walsh. 1989. Alternative splicing of the neural cell adhesion molecule gene generates variant extracellular domain structure in skeletal muscle and brain. *Genes Dev.* **3**: 348.

Tomaselli, K.J., L.F. Reichardt, and J.L. Bixby. 1986. Distinct molecular interactions mediate neuronal process outgrowth on non-neuronal cell surfaces and extracellular matrices. *J. Cell Biol.* **103:** 2659.

Tomaselli, K.J., K.M. Neugebauer, J.L. Bixby, J. Lilien, and L.F. Reichardt. 1988. N-cadherin and integrins: Two receptor systems that mediate neural process outgrowth on astrocyte surfaces. *Neuron* **1:** 33.

Williams, A.F. 1987. A year in the life of the immunoglobulin superfamily. *Immunol. Today* **8:** 298.

Williams, A.F. and A.N. Barclay. 1988. The immunoglobulin superfamily—Domains for cell surface recognition. *Annu. Rev. Immunol.* **6:** 381.

Zinn, K., L. McAllister, and C.S. Goodman. 1988. Sequence and expression of fasciclin I in grasshopper and *Drosophila. Cell* **53:** 577.

Neuronal Receptors That Regulate Axon Growth

L.F. Reichardt,* B. Bossy,* S. Carbonetto,† I. de Curtis,* C. Emmett,*
D.E. Hall,* M.J. Ignatius,* F. Lefcort,* E. Napolitano,* T. Large,*
K.M. Neugebauer,* and K.J. Tomaselli‡

*Howard Hughes Medical Institute, University of California, San Francisco, California 94143-0724;
†Center for Neuroscience Research, McGill University, Montreal, Quebec, Canada H3G 1A4; ‡Athena Neurosciences,
South San Francisco, California 94080

The development of neurons depends in large part on interactions with molecules in their environment. These include chemotropic and trophic factors, cell adhesion molecules (CAMs), and molecules anchored in the extracellular matrix (ECM). The number of identified proteins in each of these classes has expanded dramatically in recent years (Reichardt and Tomaselli 1991; Grenningloh et al.; Takeichi et al.; Yancopoulos et al.; all this volume). Proteins in each class have now been shown to influence major steps in neural development, including neuronal survival and differentiation, axon growth and guidance, and synapse formation. Subclasses of neurons have been shown to differ dramatically in their responses to some of these proteins, providing a potential molecular basis for determining their individual phenotypes. The same classes of molecules also regulate proliferation and differentiation of glia. Clearly, identifying these morphogenic molecules and their receptors is important for understanding neural development.

Molecules that direct the establishment of specific axonal pathways act in large part by regulating the behavior of the leading edge of the axon, the neuronal growth cone. In culture systems, soluble factors, CAMs and ECM glycoproteins have each been shown to promote and direct axon growth in the absence of other cues. In vitro assays have also identified an additional class of glycoproteins that strongly inhibits growth cone movements (see, e.g., Davies et al. 1990; Schwab 1990). Both positive and negative regulators of growth cone motility have been localized in embryos at positions appropriate for influencing neuronal behavior in vivo. Consistent with this, coculture experiments examining the growth of axons on cellular substrates suggest that the particular combination of molecules expressed on a cellular substrate and receptors expressed by a neuron regulate the extent and possibly also the orientation of axon growth in the complex molecular environment of the developing embryo.

To extend this approach, hybridoma technology has made it possible to identify and isolate the diverse cell types encountered sequentially by an individual growth cone. New methods for immortalizing cells make it possible to propagate rare cell populations. These new methodological advances make it now possible, in principle, to examine in vitro the interactions between an identified neuronal subpopulation and each of the cell types encountered by its growth cones during development in vivo. With these approaches, many of the major substrates and receptors important in regulating growth cone movements are being identified.

The Extracellular Matrix

Most nonneural cells secrete proteins and other molecules that form an ECM and constitute a major subset of the molecules with which growth cones interact during development (for review, see Sanes 1989; Reichardt and Tomaselli 1991). As shown in Figure 1, ECM glycoproteins are typically large, modular, multidomain proteins that can span several hundred nanometers. Major constituents of the ECM that stimulate neurite growth in vitro and are encountered by peripheral neurons in vivo include laminin (Ln), fibronectin (Fn), and several collagens. Recently, several additional ECM proteins able to promote neurite growth have been shown to be present at high levels during development in the central nervous system (CNS). These include tenascin, thrombospondin, and vitronectin (O'Shea and Dixit 1988; Chiquet 1989; Edelman and Cunningham, this volume; K.M. Neugebauer et al., unpubl.). As one example of an ECM molecule whose distribution has not been examined previously, the localization of vitronectin in the developing chick retina is shown in Figure 2. Prominent staining is seen in embryonic day-6 neural retina around cell bodies and in the basal lamina. In embryonic day 12, retina staining is pronounced in the inner and outer plexiform layers around ganglion cell bodies and in the fiber layer that is traversed by the axons of retinal ganglion neurons. These results suggest a role for vitronectin in differentiation of the retina.

Neuronal Receptors for the Extracellular Matrix

In the past few years, progress has been rapid in identifying receptors for the ECM. Figure 3 illustrates three general classes of ECM receptors: integrin heterodimers, the hyaluronic-acid-binding protein H-CAM (also named the Hermes antigen or CD44), and cell-surface-associated proteoglycans. Integrins are a

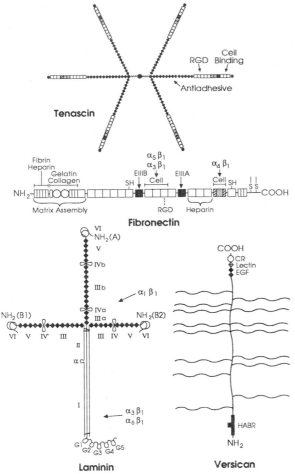

Figure 1. Examples of ECM glycoproteins and proteoglycans. Schematic structures for tenascin, Fn, and Ln, and for the proteoglycan versican are presented. Fn is a dimer, but only one subunit is shown. The positions of Fn type I (▯), Fn type II (◯), Fn type III (▢), EGF (◆), lectin (◇), complement regulatory protein (◯), and hyaluronic acid binding (━■━) domains are indicated. Approximate sites in Fn and Ln recognized by integrins are indicated (for details, see Reichardt and Tomaselli 1991).

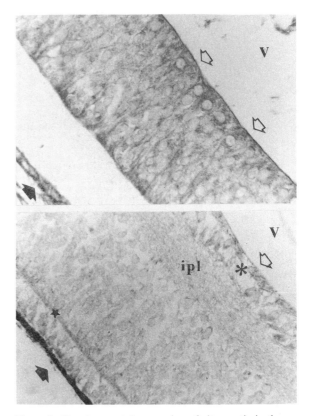

Figure 2. Developmental expression of vitronectin in the embryonic chick retina. Sections were incubated with a polyclonal rabbit antibody raised against chicken vitronectin, followed by a second antibody conjugated to horseradish peroxidase. Sections were photographed under bright-field optics so that only the reaction product and the pigment epithelium (closed arrows) are visible. The dark pigment present in the pigment epithelium layer is present in controls and does not represent vitronectin. (*Top*) Embryonic day 6. (*Bottom*) Embryonic day 12; (IPL) inner plexiform layer; (asterisk) retinal ganglion cell layer; (open arrows) optic fiber layer and basement membrane; (star) outer plexiform layer.

large family of receptors with noncovalently associated α and β subunits, each of which is a transmembrane glycoprotein. Individual integrin heterodimers, many of which are present in the nervous system, are listed with their ligands in Table 1 (cf. Hemler 1990). Their functions in the nervous system will be discussed below. H-CAM is a transmembrane receptor for hyaluronic acid (Aruffo et al. 1990). Identified originally as a lymphocyte homing receptor, H-CAM has recently been localized on both CNS glia and Schwann cells (Picker et al. 1989). Although it is not expressed by adult neurons, its functions in the developing nervous system merit attention. Syndecan is a transmembrane proteoglycan that uses glycosaminoglycan chains to bind cells to ECM glycoproteins (Saunders et al. 1989). Functions of neural receptor(s) that act similarly are described below.

Antibodies to neuronal surface proteins have been useful for identifying ECM receptors. When cell attach-

ment and neurite outgrowth are measured in quantitative assays, shown in Figure 4, the effects of such antibodies show that integrin heterodimers are the primary receptors used by neurons to attach to the vast majority of purified ECM glycoproteins. In this figure, interactions of embryonic retinal neurons with Ln, Fn, and collagen IV are virtually eliminated by function-blocking antibodies specific for the integrin β1-subunit (Hall et al. 1987). Similar results were seen using several populations of embryonic peripheral neurons (see, e.g., Bozyczko and Horwitz 1986). Interactions of retinal neurons with vitronectin are partially inhibited by antibodies to two integrin subunits, β1 and αVN, implying that more than one integrin receptor mediates interactions of retinal neurons with vitronectin (Fig. 4).

In contrast, retinal neurons appear to use proteoglycan(s) as major receptor(s) for attachment to thrombospondin. As shown in Figure 4, anti-integrin antibodies have no significant inhibitory effect on embryonic retinal neuron attachment to this protein. Instead, soluble heparin strongly inhibits attachment.

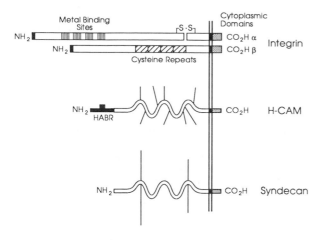

Extracellular Matrix Receptors

Figure 3. ECM receptors. Examples of three different classes of integral membrane glycoprotein receptors are shown. An integrin similar to the Fn receptor $\alpha_5\beta_1$ is shown above (see Hemler 1990). H-CAM, also named the Hermes antigen or CD44, is illustrated in the middle with a hyaluronic acid binding domain (▬▬). The positions of several carbohydrate chains are indicated by thin lines (see, e.g., Aruffo et al. 1990). The structure of sydecan, a proteoglycan that mediates binding of several cell types to several collagens and Fn, is illustrated at the bottom (Saunders et al. 1989). Positions of glycosaminoglycan chains are indicated by thin lines.

The effect of heparin appears to be specific, since it does not inhibit integrin-mediated attachment to vitronectin. Thus, retinal neurons appear to use a cell-surface proteoglycan, perhaps similar to syndecan, as a thrombospondin receptor. Since thrombospondin is expressed in the embryonic neural retina and other areas of the developing CNS (O'Shea and Dixit 1988), it is clearly important to characterize its neuronal receptors.

Using peripheral neurons, anti-integrin β_1-antibodies have been shown to virtually eliminate neurite out-

growth on two intact extracellular matrices (Tomaselli et al. 1986). Thus, integrins appear to be the major receptors used by peripheral neurons to interact with complex ECMs.

Identification of Ligands for Individual Integrin Heterodimers

Results presented above imply that integrins function as the primary receptors used by neurons to interact with a majority of proteins in the ECM. Since the integrin β_1-subunit associates with many different α subunits (see Table 1), these results needed to be extended to identify the functions of individual heterodimers. The glycoprotein Ln is particularly interesting because it has dramatic stimulatory effects not mimicked by other ECM constituents, on neuronal survival, axon outgrowth, and expression of neurotransmitters (see Reichardt and Tomaselli 1991). To determine which integrins mediate these dramatic effects, we have used neuronal cell lines to purify, characterize, and clone neuronal laminin receptors. Initially, integrins from a neuronal cell line, B50, were fractionated by Ln affinity chromatography (Ignatius and Reichardt 1988). As shown in Figure 5, a single integrin α/β_1-heterodimer with a relative molecular weight of 200K (α) and 120K (β_1) subunits was retained on Ln. An antibody was used to purify and clone the α-subunit (Ignatius et al. 1990; Tawil et al. 1990). The general structure of this α-subunit (α_1) is summarized in Table 1, which compares the major features of the different integrin α subunits known to associate with the α_1-subunit. The α_1-subunit shares major features of other integrin α subunits, including a large extracellular domain with seven repeats of an approximately 50-amino-acid motif, several potential divalent cation binding sites in the repeat region, a single transmembrane domain, and a short cytoplasmic tail. In addition, the α_1-subunit con-

Table 1. Summary of Integrin Heterodimers and their Ligands

Class	Relative molecular weight	α Subunit	Relative molecular weight	I domain	Ca/Mg sites	Cleaved	Ligands
β_1	115K	α_1	200K	+	3	−	col, Ln (E1)
		α_2	150K	+	3	−	col, Ln[a]
		α_3	150K	−	3	+	Ln (E8), Fn (RGD), col[a]
		α_4	140K	−	3	+ / −	Fn (CSI), V-CAM-1
		α_5	150K	−	4	+	Fn (RGD)
		α_6	150K	−	3	+	Ln (E8)
		α_{VN}	150K	−	4	+	Fn (RGD)[a], VN[a]
β_2	90K	α_{LFA-1}	170K	+	3	−	I-CAM-1, I-CAM-2
		α_{Mac-1}	180K	+	3	−	C3bi, Fg
		α_{p150}	150K	+	3	−	?
β_3	95K	α_{IIb}	136K	−	4	+	Fn, Vn, vWF, Fg
		α_{VN}	150K	−	4	+	Vn, Ts, vWF, Fg
β_4	205 K	α_6	150 K	−	3	+	?
β_5	90K	α_{VN}	150K	−	4	+	Vn, Fn (RGD)
β_P	95K	α_4	140K	−	3	+ / −	?

Six integrin classes, distinguished by distinct but homologous β-subunits, are shown. Each β-subunit can associate noncovalently with a subgroup of homologous α-subunits (see Hemler 1990). Abbreviations: (Col) collagen; (Fg) fibrinogen; (Fn) fibronectin; (ICAM) intercellular adhesion molecule; (Ln) laminin; (Tn) tenascin; (Ts) thrombospondin; (V-CAM) vascular cell adhesion molecule; (Vn) vitronectin; (vWF) von Willebrand factor; (RGD) RGDS site in Fn; (CS-1) CS-1 site in Fn; (E1) and (E8) elastase fragments of Ln.

[a] Indicates ligands recognized by integrins expressed in some but not all cells.

Retinal Neuron Attachment

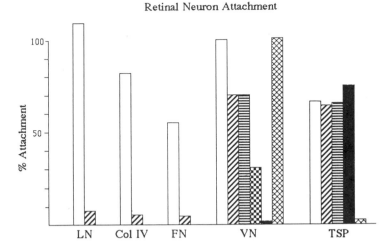

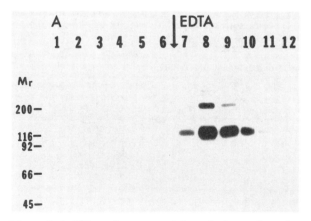

Figure 4. Effect of anti-integrin β_1-subunit-specific antibodies on cell attachment and neurite outgrowth. Cell attachment by E6 neural retinal cells was measured from left to right on laminin (LN), collagen IV (COL IV), fibronectin (FN), vitronectin (VN), and thrombospondin (TSP). Cell interactions with different matrix protein substrates were measured in control (□) or in the presence of anti-integrin β_1 [▨], anti-α_V [▤], anti-β_1, plus anti-α_V [▩], the RGDS peptide [■], or heparin [▨].

tains an insertion of an about 200-amino-acid I domain that has homology with similar domains shared by many collagen-binding proteins. This suggests that heterodimers containing the α_1-subunit may bind collagen in addition to Ln, which has been confirmed by affinity chromatography (see Hemler 1990).

In a complementary approach, we have used function-blocking α-subunit-specific antibodies to determine the ligand-binding specificities and functions of individual integrin heterodimers, including those recently shown by others to be Ln receptors (cf. Gehlsen et al. 1989; Turner et al. 1989; Sonnenberg et al. 1990). Using the JAR cell line that expresses $\alpha_1\beta_1$ and $\alpha_6\beta_1$ but not $\alpha_3\beta_1$, it was possible to show that $\alpha_1\beta_1$ and $\alpha_6\beta_1$ both function as Ln receptors, mediating binding to different domains in Ln (Hall et al. 1990; see also

Figure 5. Isolation of a neuronal integrin heterodimer by Ln-affinity chromatography. Analysis by SDS-PAGE and autoradiography of ^{125}I-labeled surface glycoproteins. ^{125}I-labeled surface, wheat-germ-agglutin-binding B50 neuroblastoma glycoproteins were applied to a Ln-affinity column in Mn^{++}/Ca^{++}. (*Lanes 1–6*) Material in the column wash fractions containing Ca^{++} and Mn^{++}. (*Lanes 7–12*) Material in fractions collected during elution with Ca^{++}-Mn^{++}-free buffer containing EDTA. The 120K subunit was shown to react with an anti-integrin β_1-subunit-specific antibody. The 200K putative integrin α-subunit was shown to be coprecipitated with the anti-integrin β_1 antibody (Ignatius and Reichardt 1988).

Sonnenberg et al. 1990). Similarly, using the rat PC12 pheochromocytoma, which expresses two major integrins, $\alpha_1\beta_1$ and $\alpha_3\beta_1$, it was possible to show that both heterodimers function as laminin receptors, again binding distinct sites on Ln (Tomaselli et al. 1990). The sites in Ln recognized by each integrin are illustrated in Figure 1. The $\alpha_1\beta_1$ heterodimer binds a site in fragment E1 near the center of Ln's cruciform structure; the $\alpha_3\beta_1$ and $\alpha_6\beta_1$ heterodimers bind sites present in fragment E8 near the foot of the long arm of Ln. Figure 6 illustrates the effects of integrin subunit-specific antibodies on neurite outgrowth by nerve-growth-factor (NGF)-primed PC12 cells on fragments of Ln. As predicted, an antibody to one α-subunit can prevent neurite outgrowth on a Ln fragment (Fig. 6), but a combination of both α-specific antibodies is needed to eliminate neurite outgrowth on intact Ln (not shown). Using the same antibodies, $\alpha_1\beta_1$ heterodimers were shown to be the only significant collagen receptor on PC12 cells (Tomaselli et al. 1990). The properties of $\alpha_3\beta_1$, described by Gehlsen et al. (1989), suggest that it mediates the weak interactions observed between PC12 cells and Fn (Tomaselli et al. 1987). A mixture of the two PC12 cell integrin heterodimers was purified and was shown to bind specifically to Ln and collagen IV after reconstitution into liposomes, mimicking the adhesive properties of the PC12 cells (Tomaselli et al. 1988a). We conclude that the interactions of PC12 cells with the ECM can be explained by the two major integrins expressed on their surfaces. In addition, neurite outgrowth by PC12 cells on Ln does not depend on the function of any one α/β integrin heterodimer.

To examine the integrins expressed by developing neurons, α- and β-subunit-specific antibodies have been used to immunoprecipitate glycoproteins expressed by sensory, sympathetic, and retinal neurons. Results summarized in Table 2 show that developing neurons express several different integrin heterodimers. Focusing on potential Ln receptors, sympathetic and sensory neurons express high levels of $\alpha_1\beta_1$ and $\alpha_3\beta_1$, each of which has been shown to function as a Ln receptor in PC12 cells (Turner et al. 1989; Tomaselli et

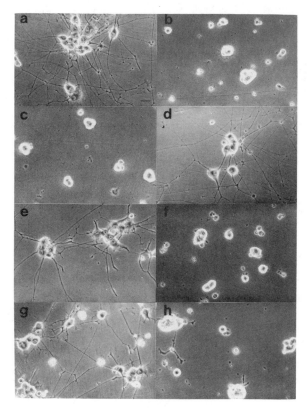

Figure 6. Neurite outgrowth by PC12 cells on Ln fragments. NGF-primed PC12 cells were cultured 16–20 hr in the presence of 50 ng/ml NGF on substrates coated with fragment E1–E4 $(a–d)$ or fragment E8 $(e–h)$ in the absence of antibodies (a,e) or in the presence of anti-β_1 (b,f), anti-α_1 (c,g), or anti-α_3 (d,h). Bar, 10 μm. (Reprinted, with permission, from Tomaselli et al. 1990.)

al. 1990). The same neurons also express one subunit of an additional Ln receptor, $\alpha_6\beta_1$, but α_6 is associated primarily in these cells with a different, large-molecular-weight β-subunit, almost certainly β_4 (see Sonnenberg et al. 1990). In contrast to $\alpha_6\beta_1$, $\alpha_6\beta_4$ does not appear to be a Ln receptor (Sonnenberg et al. 1990). Thus, the major candidates to function as Ln receptors on sympathetic and sensory neurons are $\alpha_1\beta_1$ and $\alpha_3\beta_1$. Preliminary experiments using antibodies suggest that these are the major Ln receptors mediating neurite outgrowth by embryonic sensory neurons (K.J. Tomaselli et al., unpubl.). Different results are obtained when integrin expression in embryonic E6 retinal neu-

rons is examined (Table 2). Again focusing on potential Ln receptors, the α_6-subunit is expressed at high levels, but in association with the β_1-subunit not the β_4-subunit (I. de Curtis et al., unpubl.). A comparatively low expression of the $\alpha_3\beta_1$ integrin is also seen. Although experiments are not complete, we have failed to detect in embryonic neuroretina either $\alpha_1\beta_1$ or a fourth potential Ln receptor, $\alpha_2\beta_1$ (S.T. Carbonetto and I. de Curtis, unpubl.). Thus, $\alpha_6\beta_1$ is likely to be the major Ln receptor expressed in embryonic avian retina.

Regulation of Integrin Receptor Function in Neurons

With cell adhesion and neurite outgrowth assays, it has been possible to show that the functions of selected integrins are down-regulated in neuronal subclasses at approximately the same time as these neurons innervate their targets and are reinduced by manipulations that prevent or disrupt target contact. For example, embryonic chick ciliary neurons progressively lose functional Ln receptors between embryonic days 8 and 14 (Tomaselli and Reichardt 1988). This correlates closely with the time course with which they functionally innervate the iris. These same neurons recovered substantial integrin function when explanted for 2.5 days in vitro, suggesting that target contact may regulate their integrin receptors.

In embryonic chick retinal neurons, integrin-receptor-dependent interactions with Fn and Ln diminish progressively with increasing age between embryonic days 6 and 12 (Cohen et al. 1986; Hall et al. 1987). More recently, it has been shown that ablation of the optic tectum in early embryos reduces subsequent down-regulation of integrin receptor function in retinal ganglion cells, again arguing that integrin function can be regulated by target contact (Cohen et al. 1989).

Mechanisms of integrin receptor regulation have been examined in the retina. Recently, Cohen et al. (1989) showed that a loss of Ln receptor function in retinal ganglion cells correlates with loss of receptors detected in binding assays, using ^{125}I-labeled Ln. We have prepared antibodies specific for the chick α_6-subunit and, taking advantage of the recent cloning of human α_6 (Tamura et al. 1990), have isolated and sequenced cDNAs encoding the entire chick α_6-subunit (I. de Curtis et al., unpubl.). Major structural features of this subunit, deduced from the cDNA sequence, are summarized in Table 1. Results in Table 3 show that expression of α_6 mRNA and protein is strongly downregulated between embryonic days 6 and 12 in chick retinal ganglion cells. Thus, a signal from the optic tectum seems likely to inhibit expression of the α_6 gene in retinal ganglion cells.

The function of Ln-binding integrins on the other neuronal cells in the embryonic chick retina is also down-regulated with development, but the mechanisms by which this occurs are quite different. In binding assays using ^{125}I-labeled Ln, Cohen et al. (1989) de-

Table 2. Integrins Expressed by Primary Neurons

Sensory neurons	$\alpha_1\beta_1$, $\alpha_3\beta_1$, $\alpha_5\beta_1$, $\alpha_6\beta_4$
Sympathetic neurons	$\alpha_1\beta_1$, $\alpha_3\beta_1$, $\alpha_5\beta_1$, $\alpha_6\beta_4$
Retinal neurons	$\alpha_6\beta_1$, $\alpha_3\beta_1$, $\alpha_5\beta_1$, $\alpha_{VN}\beta_1$, $\alpha_{VN}\beta_3$

Neonatal rat and mouse sensory neurons and sympathetic neurons, and embryonic E6 chick retinal neurons were labeled with ^{125}I or [3H]glucosamine. α-Subunit-specific antibodies were used in immunoprecipitations to identify individual heterodimers. Possible expression of the α_2, α_4, and α_{VN}-subunits has not been examined in peripheral neurons. The α_4-subunit is almost certainly expressed in all of these neurons because they interact with the variable domain in Fn, the domain recognized by $\alpha_4\beta_1$ but not other known integrins (for review, see Reichardt and Tomaselli 1991).

Table 3. Regulation of Integrin α_6 mRNA and Protein Levels in Retinal Neurons

	E6		E12	
	RGC	other neurons	RGC	other neurons
L1/Ng-CAM protein	+ +	+ / −	+ +	+ / −
α_6 protein	+ + +	+ + +	+ / −	+ +
α_6 mRNA	+ + +	+ +	+	+ +

Retinas were dissected from 6 (E6) and 12 (E12) day-old chick embryos. After trypsinization, the retinas were mechanically dissociated with trituration and were fractionated on a Percoll step gradient to separate retinal ganglion cells from other neurons, using a method developed by J.E. Johnson (University of Arkansas). L1/Ng-CAM was used as a marker to assess the purity of the retinal ganglion cells. L1 and the integrin α_6-subunit were quantitated on antigen blots. α_6 mRNA was quantitated on RNA blots using an α_6 cDNA probe. An actin cDNA probe was used to normalize mRNA samples.

tected a change in receptor affinity but not number in this population of neurons. Consistent with these results, we have seen continued high expression of integrin α_6 mRNA and protein in these cells as development proceeds (Table 3). Since these cells no longer bind Ln in attachment assays (Hall et al. 1987), receptor function must be lost by a posttranslational mechanism. Consistent with this model, the $\alpha_6\beta_1$ integrin has been shown to exist on the surface of unstimulated macrophages in a comparatively inactive state (Shaw et al. 1990). Activation of macrophages by interferon-γ or phorbol esters activates $\alpha_6\beta_1$-dependent adhesion to Ln. Coincident with this functional activation, the α_6-subunit is phosphorylated, and the $\alpha_6\beta_1$ heterodimer more readily associates with the cytoskeleton.

Results described above suggest that integrins can exist in more than one activity state on neuronal cell surfaces. To examine these states in more detail, we have isolated a monoclonal antibody, TASC, that binds the β_1-subunit and activates the functions of β_1-subunit-containing heterodimers (K.M. Neugebauer and L.F. Reichardt, unpubl.). Binding of TASC immunoglobulin G (IgG) or Fab fragments activates integrin β_1 heterodimers but not other adhesive mechanisms. In addition, function-blocking β_1-subunit-specific monoclonal antibodies remain able to block completely integrin function, whether or not the TASC monoclonal antibody is present. Results in Table 4 show that the TASC monoclonal antibody restores the ability of E12 chick retinal neurons to attach to Ln, providing direct evidence that they have potentially active Ln receptors on their surfaces. In the future, it should be informative to study the mechanisms by which the TASC monoclonal antibody activates the functions of these integrins.

Table 4. Activation of Ln Receptor Function by the TASC Monoclonal Antibody

Cells	Antibody	Attachment (%)
E12 retinal neurons	—	0
E12 retinal neurons	TASC	70 + / − 5
E12 retinal neurons	TASC + CSAT	0

E12 retinal neurons were incubated for 60 min on a Ln-coated substrate in the presence of the indicated monoclonal antibodies. Effects of TASC monoclonal antibody on adhesion by these neurons were detectable within 10 min (not shown).

Integrin-dependent Interactions with Cellular Substrates

As described above, the functions of integrins are required for process outgrowth by neurons on at least two different ECMs. Similarly, we demonstrated that neurite outgrowth on fibroblast monolayers is strongly dependent on β_1 integrins (Tomaselli et al. 1986). These results suggest that neurons grow on fibroblasts primarily by interacting with secreted ECM proteins assembled on the fibroblast surface. In contrast, whereas glial and muscle cells produce ECM glycoproteins in vitro, neuronal process growth on these cells is not dramatically dependent on integrin function (Tomaselli et al. 1986). Instead, neurons utilize both integrins and additional receptors to bind to multiple ligands present on nonneuronal cells. In several cases, listed in Table 5, it has been possible to identify the additional receptors and ligands. In every instance so far, they have proven to be CAMs, either a Ca^{++}-dependent cadherin or a Ca^{++}-independent adhesion molecule with an extracellular domain containing repeats of immunoglobulin and fibronectin type III domains. The general features of these molecules are described elsewhere in this volume (Takeichi et al.; Grenningloh et al.; Edelman and Cunningham). As one example of their roles in regulating axon growth, we will discuss our studies on the major cellular substrates in central nerve tracts.

Neurite Outgrowth on Astroglia

Astroglia are prominent substrates for axon growth during establishment of many central nerve tracts. Older astroglia become less able to support axon growth in vivo and in vitro (see, e.g., Smith et al. 1990). Similarly, central nerve tracts lose the ability to support extensive axon regeneration. This seems to reflect not only maturation of astroglia, but also the appearance in these tracts of proteins associated with myelin that directly inhibit axon extension (Schwab 1990). In our studies, axon growth on astroglial surfaces was shown to depend on integrin-mediated interactions with ECM constituents secreted by astroglia and on the adhesion molecules N-CAM and N-cadherin (Neugebauer et al. 1988; Tomaselli et al. 1988b). Drazba and Lemmon (1990) have demonstrated a role for L1/Ng-CAM. The

Table 5. Neuronal Receptors Involved in Axon Growth on ECM and Cellular Substrates

		Receptor			
	Substrate	β_1 integrin	N-cadherin	L1/NILE	N-CAM
Extracellular matrix	Laminin	+	−	−	−
	Fibronectin	+	n.t.	n.t.	n.t.
	Collagen	+	n.t.	n.t.	n.t.
Cell surfaces	Astrocytes	+	+	+	+
	Schwann cells	+	+	+	−
	Myotubes	+	+	n.t.	+
	Fibroblasts	+	−	−	−

This table summarizes experiments testing effects of anti-CAM or anti-integrin Fab fragments on neuronal process outgrowth on different extracellular matrix and cellular substrates. "Plus" indicates that a receptor promotes neuronal processes outgrowth. "Minus" indicates that a receptor has no detected function in promoting neuronal process outgrowth. n.t. indicates not tested. In all systems examined thus far, the individual CAMs and integrins appear to function independently as receptors to promote neuronal process outgrowth.

importance of the different receptors varies depending on the type and age of neuron. Integrins and N-cadherin appear to be the major promoters of axon growth by ciliary neurons (Tomaselli et al. 1988b); in addition to these receptors, as illustrated in Figure 7, N-CAM, L1, and additional uncharacterized molecules are also important in promoting growth cone movements by retinal neurons (Neugebauer et al. 1988; Drazba and Lemmon 1990). As described above, additional ECM constituents may well include thrombospondin and tenascin, both of which are synthesized by astroglia (cf. O'Shea and Dixit 1988; K.M. Neugebauer et al., unpubl.; Edelman and Cunningham, this volume). The importance of interactions mediated by N-CAM and integrins changes dramatically during retinal neuron development (Neugebauer et al. 1988). Since

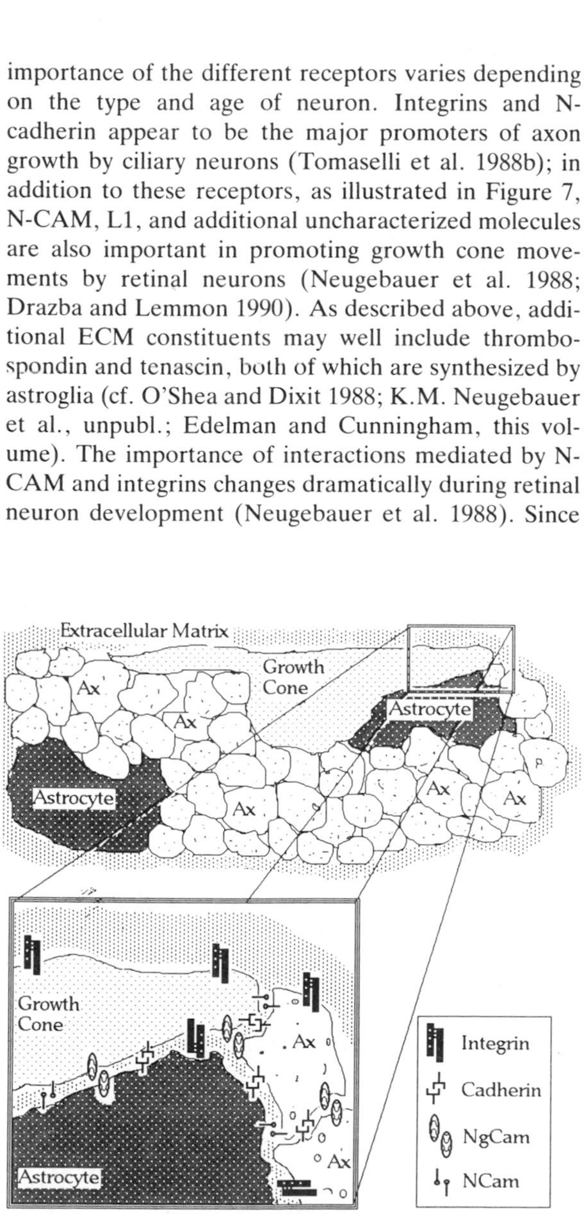

many of the CAMs described above are expressed at reduced levels in mature compared with developing central nerves (cf. Takeichi et al., this volume), it is likely that regulation of expression of these molecules in neurons and on glial substrates helps regulate the potential of these nerves to support axon growth.

Novel Adhesion Molecules

Motivated by evidence suggesting that additional adhesive interactions mediated by uncharacterized receptors and ligands promote axon growth by retinal neurons (Neugebauer et al. 1988), we have initiated efforts to identify some of these molecules. Using a molecular approach, cDNAs encoding a novel integrin α-subunit, named α_8, have been isolated (B. Bossy et al., unpubl.). Using peptides corresponding to segments of the predicted protein sequence, antibodies have been prepared and used to show that this α-subunit associates with the β_1-subunit and is strongly expressed in the developing nervous system. The ligand-binding properties of this novel integrin are being examined. Potential ligands for this receptor include both ECM constituents and cell surface proteins.

In a second approach, antibodies were prepared to peptide segments conserved in all known cadherins. These antibodies were shown to recognize each of the characterized cadherins and several additional glycoproteins that are potentially novel cadherins. Using these antibodies, we have isolated cDNAs encoding one novel cadherin, named B-cadherin, which shares the major features of each cadherin described to date (N-, E-, P-, and L-CAM), including a motif repeated five times in the extracellular domain, a single transmembrane domain, and a highly conserved cytoplasmic domain (E. Napolitano et al., unpubl.). It is distinct, however, from each of these and from the novel cadherin, R-cadherin, described by Takeichi et al. (this volume). Figure 8 documents the distribution of this cadherin in the avian optic tectum where it stains strongly ependymal cells and populations of cells, probably neurons, in layers VI and VIII. Its role in development is under investigation.

Figure 7. Model for growth cone interactions with astroglia and axons in the embryonic neuroretina. A growth cone of an embryonic day 6 retinal neuron is shown with receptors that bind independently to ECM and cell-surface proteins. (Ax) Axon. (Modified from Easter et al. 1984.)

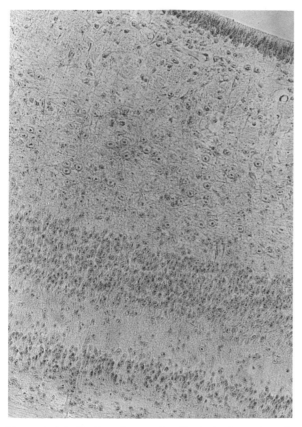

Figure 8. Distribution of a novel cadherin in the embryonic day-13 chick optic tectum. An antipeptide antibody to a primary sequence in the fifth extracellular repeat, a region with high divergence from the same region in other cadherins, was used. Note prominent staining of the ependymal cells lining the ventricle and of cells residing in layers VI and VIII of the tectum, as described by LaVail and Cowan (1971).

CONCLUSIONS

One of our objectives has been to identify the major classes of molecules that regulate growth cone movements and axon outgrowth. As a result of work from many laboratories, both ECM glycoproteins and CAMs have been shown to promote axon extension. Integrins appear to be the major but not the only class of receptors used by neurons to interact with ECM constituents. In recent investigations, the ligand specificities of individual heterodimers have been determined, and substantial progress has been made in identifying the functions of these heterodimers on the surfaces of different populations of neurons. Neurons have been shown to utilize integrins and CAMs to extend axons over cellular substrates. On different cell surfaces, different CAMs are important. The importance of individual integrins or CAMs depends on both the type and age of neurons. On most cells, multiple interactions need to be blocked to see dramatic effects on axon growth in vitro, suggesting that a combination of cues direct axon growth in vivo. Multiple cues may also exist on single-cell types in *Drosophila* (cf. Grenningloh et al., this volume). Clearly, a major future challenge is to understand the roles of the receptors and ligands described above in directing axon growth in vivo.

The integrins and CAMs share many intriguing properties. First, several are expressed most strongly during development, are down-regulated at times that correlate with target innervation, and are reexpressed after denervation. Regulation of their genes seems likely to influence axon growth during development. In PC12 cells, expression of at least two CAMs, N-CAM and L1/Ng-CAM, and one integrin subunit, α_1, are induced strongly by NGF (see, e.g., Prentice et al. 1987; Rossino et al. 1990). Collateral sprouting by sensory neurons has been shown to require NGF, which increases dramatically in denervated targets of sympathetic and sensory neurons (Diamond et al. 1987). Functionally, it is attractive to imagine that elevated NGF levels promote collateral sprouting, in part, by elevating expression of integrins and CAMs. Similarly, target contact has been shown to down-regulate integrin function in retinal neurons. As described in this paper, a major mechanism appears to be down-regulation of transcripts encoding selected integrin subunits.

Integrins, cadherins, and several Ca^{++}-independent adhesion molecules are transmembrane proteins that interact with cytoskeletal elements and are phosphorylated on their cytoplasmic domains (cf. Pollerberg et al. 1987; Shaw et al. 1990; Takeichi et al., this volume). In many cells, the activity of surface integrins can be more directly regulated by second-messenger systems that also modify their interactions with the cytoskeleton (see, e.g., Shaw et al. 1990). In addition, the function of one lymphocyte integrin is regulated by stimulated release from subplasmalemmal membrane compartments (Bainton et al. 1987). Finally, integrins have recently been shown to be inserted preferentially at leading edges of fibroblasts and to cycle rapidly between the cell surface and intracellular compartments (Bretscher 1989). Many extrinsic cues seem likely to act by regulating or directing this cycle. Each of these regulatory mechanisms is a plausible target for local factors that affect growth cone motility. Similar mechanisms may also regulate the functions of CAMs.

Finally, a major challenge is to understand what signals are transduced by binding of integrins and CAMs. Binding of these adhesive receptors to their ligands has been shown to regulate the organization of the cytoskeleton (cf. Mueller et al. 1989). In particular, they interact with the actin-based cytoskeleton, which is believed to control the behavior of the leading edge of the growth cone (cf. Mitchison and Kirschner 1988). These interactions could regulate any step in the dynamic actin cycle, which includes preferential actin polymerization at the leading edge, retrograde movement of actin filaments by an energy-dependent motor, and depolymerization of filaments in the cell interior. In addition, adhesive interactions with a cytoskeleton in motion seem likely to generate tension in the growth cone. Tension could potentially modulate dynamics of other cytoskeletal elements, such as microtubules. Intriguingly, stretch-sensitive K$^+$ channels have recently been identified in growth cones (cf. Sigurdson and Morris 1989). Regulation of these channels makes it possible, in principle, for tension to modulate membrane potential, which in turn could alter levels of cytoplasmic Ca^{++}. Changes in cytoplasmic Ca^{++} levels would be expected to have pleiotropic effects on other second messengers. In addition, cytoplasmic Ca^{++} appears to control growth cone motility directly (see, e.g., Kater and Guthrie, this volume). Thus, there are now potential mechanisms for explaining many effects of adhesive interactions on neuronal differentiation.

ACKNOWLEDGMENTS

We thank Marion Meyerson for her invaluable help in preparing the manuscript. Research has been supported by grants to L.F.R. from the National Institutes of Health and Howard Hughes Medical Institute and to S.C. from the Medical Research Foundation of Canada and the Spinal Cord Research Institute. L.F.R. is an investigator of the Howard Hughes Medical Institute. S.C. is the recipient of a Chercheur Boursier from the F.R.S.Q.

REFERENCES

Aruffo, A., I. Stamenkovic, M. Melnick, C.B. Underhill and B. Seed. 1990. CD44 is the principal cell surface receptor for hyaluronate. *Cell* **61:** 1303.

Bainton, D.F., L.J. Miller, T.K. Kishimoto, and R.A. Springer. 1987. Leukocyte adhesion receptors are stored in peroxidase-negative granules of human neutrophils. *J. Exp. Med.* **166:** 1641.

Bozyczko, D. and A. Horwitz. 1986. The participation of a putative cell surface receptor for laminin and fibronectin in peripheral neurite extension. *J. Neurosci.* **6:** 1241.

Bretscher, M.S. 1989. Endocytosis and recycling of the fibronectin receptor in CHO cells. *EMBO J.* **8:** 1341.

Chiquet, M. 1989. Tenascin/J1/cytotactin: The potential function of hexabrachion proteins in neural development. *Dev. Neurosci.* **11:** 266.

Cohen, J., J.F. Burne, J. Winter, and P. Bartlett. 1986. Retinal ganglion cells lose response to laminin with maturation. *Nature* **322:** 465.

Cohen, J., V. Nurcombe, P. Jeffrey, and D. Edgar. 1989. Developmental loss of functional laminin receptors on retinal ganglion cells is regulated by their target tissue, the optic tectum. *Development* **107:** 381.

Davies, J.A., G.M.W. Cook, C.D. Stern, and R.J. Keynes. 1990. Isolation from chick somites of a glycoprotein fraction that causes collapse of dorsal root ganglion growth cones. *Neuron* **2:** 11.

Diamond, J., M. Coughlin, L. Macintyre, M. Holmes, and B. Visheau. 1987. Evidence that endogenous β nerve growth factor is responsible for the collateral sprouting, but not the regeneration, of nociceptive axons in adult rats. *Proc. Natl. Acad. Sci.* **84:** 6596.

Drazba, J. and V. Lemmon. 1990. The role of cell adhesion molecules in neurite outgrowth on Muller cells. *Dev. Biol.* **138:** 82.

Easter, S.S., B. Bratton, and S.S. Scherer. 1984. Growth-related order of the retinal fiber layer in goldfish. *J. Neurosci.* **4:** 2173.

Gehlsen, K., K. Dickerson, W.S. Argraves, E. Engvall, and E. Ruoslahti. 1989. Subunit structure of a laminin-binding integrin and localization of its binding site on laminin. *J. Biol. Chem.* **264:** 19034.

Hall, D., K. Neugebauer, and L. Reichardt. 1987. Embryonic neural retina cell response to extracellular matrix proteins: Developmental changes and effects of the cell substratum attachment antibody, CSAT. *J. Cell Biol.* **104:** 623.

Hall, D.E., L.F. Reichardt, E. Crowley, B. Holley, H. Moezzi, A. Sonnenberg, and C.H. Damsky. 1990. The α_1/β_1 and α_6/β_1 integrin heterodimers mediate cell attachment to distinct sites on laminin. *J. Cell Biol.* **110:** 2175.

Hemler, M.E. 1990. VLA proteins in the integrin family: Structure, functions, and their role on leukocytes. *Annu. Rev. Immunol.* **8:** 365.

Ignatius, M.J. and L.F. Reichardt. 1988. Identification of a neuronal laminin receptor: An M_r 200/120 kD integrin heterodimer that binds laminin in a divalent cation-dependent manner. *Neuron* **1:** 713.

Ignatius, M.J., T.H. Large, M. Houde, J.W. Tawil, A. Barton, F. Esch, S. Carbonetto, and L.F. Reichardt. 1990. Molecular cloning of the rat integrin α_1-subunit: A receptor for laminin and collagen. *J. Cell Biol.* **111:** 709.

LaVail, J.H. and W.M. Cowan. 1971. The development of the chick optic tectum. I. Normal morphology and cytoarchitectomic development. *Brain Res.* **28:** 391.

Mitchison, T. and M. Kirschner. 1988. Cytoskeletal dynamics and nerve growth. *Neuron* **1:** 761.

Mueller, S.C., T. Kelly, M. Dai, H. Dai, and W.-T. Chen. 1989. Dynamic cytoskeleton-integrin associations induced by cell binding to immobilized fibronectin. *J. Cell Biol.* **109:** 3455.

Neugebauer, K.M., K.J. Tomaselli, J. Lilien, and L.F. Reichardt. 1988. N-cadherin, NCAM and integrins promote retinal neurite outgrowth on astrocytes in vitro. *J. Cell Biol.* **107:** 1177.

O'Shea, K.S. and V.M. Dixit. 1988. Unique distribution of the extracellular matrix component thrombospondin in the developing mouse embryo. *J. Cell Biol.* **107:** 2737.

Picker, L.J., M. Nakache, and E.C. Butcher. 1989. Monoclonal antibodies to human lymphocyte homing receptors define a novel class of adhesion molecules on diverse cell types. *J. Cell Biol.* **109:** 927.

Pollerberg, G.E., K. Burridge, K.E. Krebs, S.R. Goodman, and M. Schachner. 1987. The 180 kD component of the neural cell adhesion molecule N-CAM is involved in cell-cell contacts and cytoskeletal membrane interaction. *Cell Tissue Res.* **250:** 227.

Prentice, H.M., S.E. Moore, J.G. Dickson, P. Doherty, and F.S. Walsh. 1987. Nerve growth factor-induced changes in neural cell adhesion molecule (N-CAM) in PC12 cells. *EMBO J.* **6:** 1859.

Reichardt, L.F. and K.J. Tomaselli. 1991. Extracellular matrix molecules and their receptors: Functions in neural development. *Annu. Rev. Neurosci.* **14:** (in press).

Rossino, P., I. Gavazzi, R. Timpl, M. Aumailley, M. Abbadini, F. Giancotti, L. Silengo, P.C. Marchisio, and G. Tarone. 1990. Nerve growth factor induces increased expression of a laminin-binding integrin in rat pheochromocytoma PC12 cells. *Exp. Cell. Res.* **189:** 100.

Sanes, J.R. 1989. Extracellular matrix molecules that influence neural development. *Annu. Rev. Neurosci.* **12:** 491.

Saunders, S., M. Jalkanen, S. O'Farrell, and M. Bernfield. 1989. Molecular cloning of syndecan, an integral membrane proteoglycan. *J. Cell Biol.* **108:** 1547.

Schwab, M.E. 1990. Myelin-associated inhibitors of neurite growth. *Exp. Neurol.* **109:** 2.

Shaw, L.M., J.M. Messier, and A.M. Mercurio. 1990. The activation dependent adhesion of macrophages to laminin involves cytoskeletal anchoring and phosphorylation of the $\alpha_6\beta_1$ integrin. *J. Cell Biol.* **110:** 2167.

Sigurdson, W.J. and C.E. Morris. 1989. Stretch-activated ion channels in growth cones of snail neurons. *J. Neurosci.* **9:** 2801.

Smith, G.M., U. Rutishauser, J. Silver, and R.H. Miller. 1990. Maturation of astrocytes *in vitro* alters the extent and molecular basis of neurite outgrowth. *Dev. Biol.* **138:** 377.

Sonnenberg, A., C. Linders, P. Modderman, C. Damsky, M. Aumailley, and R. Timpl. 1990. Integrin recognition of different cell-binding fragments of laminin (P1, E3, E8) and evidence that $\alpha_6\beta_1$ but not $\alpha_6\beta_4$ functions as a major receptor for fragment E8. *J. Cell Biol.* **110:** 2145.

Tamura, R.N., C. Rozzo, L. Starr, J. Chambers, L.F. Reichardt, H.M. Cooper, and V. Quaranta. 1990. Epithelial integrin $\alpha_6\beta_4$: Complete primary structure of α_6 and variant forms of β_4. *J. Cell Biol.* **111:** 1593.

Tawil, N.J., M. Houde, R. Blacher, F. Esch, L.F. Reichardt, D.C. Turner, and S. Carbonetto. 1990. $\alpha_1\beta_1$ integrin functions as a dual laminin/collagen receptor in neural cells. *Biochemistry* **29:** 6540.

Tomaselli, K.J. and L.F. Reichardt. 1988. Peripheral motoneuron interactions with laminin and Schwann cell-derived neurite-promoting molecules: Developmental regulation of laminin receptor function. *J. Neurosci. Res.* **21:** 275.

Tomaselli, K., C. Damsky, and L. Reichardt. 1987. Interactions of a neuronal cell line (PC12) with the extracellular matrix proteins fibronectin, laminin and collagen type IV: Identification of cell surface glycoproteins involved in attachment and outgrowth. *J. Cell Biol.* **105:** 2347.

———. 1988a. Purification and characterization of mammalian integrins expressed by a rat neuronal cell line (PC12): Evidence that they function as α/β heterodimeric receptors for collagen IV and laminin. *J. Cell Biol.* **107:** 241.

Tomaselli, K.J., L.F. Reichardt, and J.L. Bixby. 1986. Distinct molecular interactions mediate neuronal process outgrowth on non-neuronal cell surfaces and extracellular matrices. *J. Cell Biol.* **103:** 2659.

Tomaselli, K.J., K.M. Neugebauer, J.L. Bixby, J. Lilien, and L.F. Reichardt. 1988b. N-cadherin and integrins: Two receptor systems that mediate neuronal process outgrowth on astrocyte surfaces. *Neuron* **1:** 33.

Tomaselli, K.J., D.E. Hall, L.A. Flier, K.R. Gehlsen, D.C. Turner, S. Carbonetto, and L.F. Reichardt. 1990. A neuronal cell line (PC12) expresses two β_1-class integrins—$\alpha_1\beta_1$ and $\alpha_3\beta_1$—that recognize different neurite outgrowth-promoting domains in laminin. *Neuron* **5:** (in press).

Turner, D.C., L.A. Flier, and S. Carbonetto. 1989. Identification of a cell-surface protein involved in PC12 cell-substratum adhesion and neurite growth on laminin and collagen. *J. Neurosci.* **9:** 3287.

Directional Cues for Retinal Axons

B. Stahl, Y. von Boxberg, B. Müller, J. Walter, U. Schwarz, and F. Bonhoeffer
Max-Planck-Institut für Entwicklungsbiologie, D-7400 Tübingen, Federal Republic of Germany

The elucidation of the mechanisms that govern the development of topographic projections in the central nervous system has been a challenge for neurobiologists for quite some time. Since the pioneering work of Sperry (1956, 1963) on the formation of neural connections in the retinotectal system of amphibia and fish, many speculations have been put forward and dismissed. One of them, which is still a tenable hypothesis, is that the axons are guided to their target site by directional cues expressed on the surface of the target organ given by the graded distribution of substances either diffusible or membrane-bound. As documented in many systems, there are in vivo directional cues for incoming axons at the target surface.

Conceptually, it is very easy to see how a gradient may determine direction. In fact, it appears almost impossible to consider directional cues without thinking of gradients. However, it is a fascinating question of how in nature axons read the gradients and how the message is converted into a directional guiding force. A major problem arises from the fact that the growth cone is very small compared with the spatial extent of the gradient in the target field. Thus, the difference in concentration of the graded component at two opposite margins of the growth cone may be as small as 1%, and this tiny difference must be sufficient to direct the growth cone. Two different mechanisms have been suggested to explain how growth cones evaluate these tiny differences. One model assumes that the gradient is amplified by autocatalysis of a locally acting activator in conjunction with inhibition by a far-reaching inhibitor (Gierer 1981, 1987). The other model, which will be briefly mentioned at the end of this paper, invokes a regulation mechanism (Walter et al. 1990a). Both models have in common that guidance is not based on gradients of adhesiveness of the substratum. Whatever the detailed mechanism by which the directional cues, i.e., the gradients, are sensed, it must be postulated that growth cones read small biochemical differences between different areas of the target organ.

In previous years, our laboratory has developed an in vitro system to test whether retinal axons recognize different tectal areas as different and whether they can be guided by tectal components. It was found that temporal retinal axons, when offered the choice between anterior and posterior tectal membranes, preferred to grow on anterior membranes. This behavior is analogous to the in vivo behavior of temporal axons that project to the anterior pole of the tectum but do not innervate the posterior tectal end. Nasal axons

showed no preference for posterior membranes. The preference of temporal axons for anterior substratum in vitro is not due to an attractive component of anterior tectum, but rather to a repellent substance in posterior tectal membranes. The biochemical characterization of a putative repellent molecule will be described in the second part of this paper.

In the first part, we briefly describe experiments showing that also nasal axons express the preference expected from the in vivo behavior, if the anterior and posterior material offered has been prefractionated by electrofocusing. They grow preferentially on membrane fractions derived from posterior tectum. This is a finding for which we have long been searching. Since it resembles the in vivo situation, it gives us more confidence in the significance of the in vitro results.

EXPERIMENTAL PROCEDURES

Retinal explants. E6 retinas were prepared as described previously (Walter et al. 1987b). In brief, 275-μm-wide strips were cut along the nasal-temporal axis. The strips were cultured on the substratum for approximately 48 hours in 2.5 ml of supplemented F12 medium at 37°C and 4% CO_2. For the stripe assay, the substratum was a membrane carpet on a nuclepore filter, the medium was supplemented with methyl cellulose to give a final concentration of 0.4% (Walter et al. 1987b). In the case of the collapse assay, laminin-coated 12-mm coverslips were used (Cox et al. 1990).

Stripe assay. Membrane stripes were prepared according to the method of Walter et al. (1987b). To produce alternating stripes of anterior and posterior membranes, a nuclepore filter (0.1 μm pore diameter) was placed onto a special silicon matrix containing many parallel channels. The first membrane suspension (150 μl) is placed onto the filter and sucked (0.03 bars, 2 min) through the channels in the silicon matrix. The membrane particles cover the filter and occlude its pores in parallel lanes. The second membranes (150 μl) are sucked (0.03 bars, 1.5 min) onto the interstitial empty lanes of the filter after replacing the silicon matrix by a fine nylon net. The membranes applied first were mixed with fluorescent beads to facilitate the identification of the stripes.

Collapse assay. The collapse assay was performed according to the method of Cox et al. (1990). In brief, membrane vesicles were added to retinal axons growing on laminin-coated coverslips. To the culture medium

(F12 medium with fetal calf serum [FCS]), 10–200 μl of membrane suspension (in culture medium with 0.4% methyl cellulose) was added slowly. After 1 hour incubation at 37°C and 4% CO_2, the axons were fixed with 1 ml of 4% paraformaldehyde in 0.33 M sucrose and phosphate-buffered saline (PBS). The next day, the coverslips were washed and mounted in glycerol/PBS. The fixed growth cones and axons were observed with an inverted microscope.

Membrane preparation. Whole tecta or brains from E9-E10 chick embryos were dissected free of pial membranes in Hank's medium. Anterior and posterior thirds were dissected and separately pooled. Pooled thirds were homogenized in 5 ml of buffer containing 4 M urea, 10 mM spermidine, protease, and neuraminidase inhibitors in PBS without Ca^{++} and Mg^{++}. Nuclei, unlysed cells, and other debris were removed by centrifugation for 30 minutes at 12,000g in a Sorvall HB4 swinging bucket rotor. The supernatant was then centrifuged 60 minutes at 125,000g. The supernatant was discarded, and the pellet was washed in F12 medium without FCS. The ultracentrifugation step was repeated, and the pellet was finally sonicated at 0°C in 0.5 ml of F12 medium.

Solubilization of membranes. Fresh membranes were solubilized in 6 M urea in 6 mM 3-[(3-cholamidopropyl)-dimethylammonio]-1-propanesulfonate (CHAPS) and PBS without Ca^{++} and Mg^{++} in a Dounce homogenizer (5 min, 0°C). Afterwards, the insoluble material was pelleted at 200,000g for 30 minutes. The pellet was discarded, and the supernatant was saved for further purification.

Column chromatography of membrane proteins and reconstitution of vesicles. Diethylaminoethyl-Sepharose (Pharmacia) was equilibrated overnight with 3 M urea in 3 mM CHAPS and PBS without Ca^{++} and Mg^{++} (~20 column volumes). Solubilized membrane proteins at a concentration of 1 mg/ml were loaded onto the column. Unbound protein was removed by washing with the above-mentioned buffer until no protein was detectable in the wash. Proteins were then eluted with 300 mM NaCl in the equilibration buffer. This step was continued until the eluted fractions were free of protein. The collapse-inducing and guiding activity was eluted with 1000 mM NaCl in equilibration buffer. Solubilized phosphatidylcholine was added to the column fractions of interest at a concentration of 1.5 mg/ml. After thorough mixing, the samples were dialyzed against PBS containing Ca^{++} and Mg^{++} (500 sample volumes) overnight. The dialysis buffer was renewed, and dialysis was continued for 6 hours. Finally, the vesicles formed were pelleted at 200,000g (30 min) and washed with F12 medium. After sonication at 0°C, these vesicles were used in the collapse assay.

Fractionation of membranes by preparative electrofocusing. Anterior and posterior membranes were homogenized in 8.5 M urea plus 2% ampholine in dis-

tilled water and subjected to preparative nonequilibrium electrofocusing in the following way: 13-cm-long glass tubes of 6-mm inner diameter were filled up to a height of 8 cm with 4.3% acrylamide solution also containing 8.5 M urea and 2% ampholine. The suspension of the membrane vesicles was loaded on top of the acrylamide and covered by 8 mm of overlay composed of 5 M urea and 2% ampholine. Electrofocusing was carried out for 6 hours at 300 mW per gel tube. Vesicle bands formed in the liquid phase of the gel system. The vesicles were collected, pelleted, and washed three times with Dulbecco's modified Eagle's medium (DMEM) plus 10% FCS.

During electrophoresis, the bulk of proteins migrate into the solid phase of the gel system, while a subpopulation of proteins stays with the lipids in the upper, liquid phase. We have evidence that proteins that are either integral membrane proteins or covalently linked to the lipids will be concentrated in these fractionated membrane vesicles. For example, the glycosyl-phosphatidylinositol-linked membrane protein F11 (Rathjen et al. 1987) is highly enriched (see Fig. 1). This assumption is supported further by the distribution of the different forms of the G4 protein (Rathjen et al. 1987) in the vesicles. It has been shown for mouse L1,

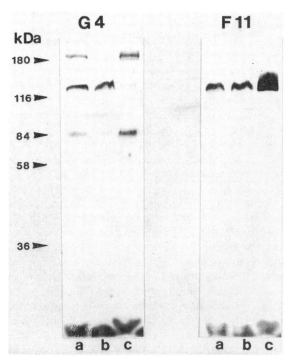

Figure 1. Enrichment of F11 and G4 protein in fractionated vesicles: Homogenates of tectum tissue E9 (lane *a*), membranes (lane *b*), and fractionated membranes (lane *c*) were separated on 7.5% acrylamide gels according to the method of Laemmli (1970) and blotted onto nitrocellulose filter. The protein concentration is the same for all three lanes. The left blot was first reacted with anti-G4 serum (gift from E. de la Rosa), and the right was reacted with anti-F11 serum (gift from M. Wolff). Then after washing, the secondary horseradish-peroxidase-coupled antibody was added, and finally the blots were developed with 4-Cl-1-naphthol.

which is closely related to the chick G4 protein, that the L1 molecule is made by the cell in a 190-kD form, which is then cleaved into a 135-kD component released from the membrane and an 80-kD integral membrane protein (Sadoul et al. 1988). In the fractionated vesicles, the intact G4 molecule (190 kD) and its membrane-anchored 80-kD part are highly enriched, whereas they are depleted of the free 135-kD form of the G4 protein (see Fig.1).

Gel electrophoresis and blotting. SDS-polyacrylamide gel electrophoresis (SDS-PAGE) was carried out on 10% polyacrylamide gels according to the method of Laemmli (1970). Nonequilibrium PH gradient gel electrophoresis, followed by SDS-PAGE in the second dimension, was performed as described previously by von Boxberg (1988). Proteins in the gels were stained with silver according to the method of Ansorge (1985).

Proteins were transferred from SDS-polyacrylamide gels to nitrocellulose (Schleicher & Schuell) according to the method of Towbin et al. (1979). Proteins on two-dimensional blots were sometimes stained with colloidal gold (Egger and Bienz 1987).

Immunization of rabbits. An antiserum was produced by subcutaneous injection of white rabbits at multiple sites with membranes from the posterior third of tecta (E9 and E10). Protein (500 μg) was injected at intervals of 2–4 weeks. Complete Freund's adjuvant was used for the first immunization, and incomplete adjuvant was used for subsequent injections. Blood was collected 5 days after the fifth immunization.

Inactivation of posterior membranes. Posterior membranes (100 μg protein/ml) were incubated with a sterile antiserum (5 volumes membrane suspension and 1 volume antiserum). During the incubation time of 3 hours at 4°C, the suspension was vigorously agitated on an Eppendorf shaker. Afterwards, the membranes were pelleted at 200,000g (30 min) and washed once in PBS. These washed membranes were used in the stripe assay.

Polyclonal antibodies and Fab fragments. Polyclonal antibodies were isolated on a column with protein A–Sepharose according to the method of Pharmacia. Fab fragments were produced from these antibodies by papain digestion (Porter 1959).

RESULTS

Guidance of Temporal and Nasal Axons on Carpets Consisting of Alternating Stripes of Anterior and Posterior Tectal Membranes

Previous experiments have shown that temporal retinal axons, when growing on a carpet of anterior and posterior tectal membranes arranged in alternating stripes, exhibit a pronounced preference for growth on anterior membranes (Fig. 2a) (Walter et al. 1987b). On the other hand, nasal retinal axons (chick, fish, and

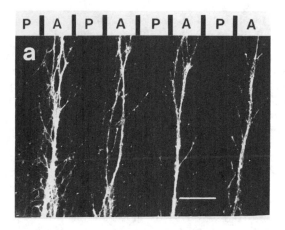

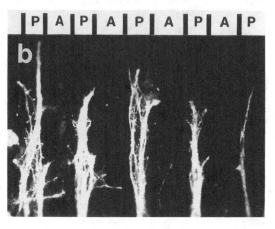

Figure 2. Guidance of temporal and nasal retinal axons on carpets consisting of alternating stripes of anterior and posterior tectal membranes. Temporal axons show a preference for anterior membranes (*a*). A preference of nasal axons for posterior tectum material is only found when the stripes are prepared from membrane vesicles prefractionated by electrofocusing (*b*). Bar, 100 μm.

mouse) show no preference for posterior over anterior stripes (Godement and Bonhoeffer 1989; Vielmetter and Stürmer 1989), although they do discriminate between tectal and retinal membranes (Bonhoeffer and Huf 1982). However, when anterior and posterior tectal membranes are subjected to an electrophoretic fractionation and reconstitution procedure, as described in Experimental Procedures, before the striped carpets are prepared, nasal axons grow preferentially on the lanes of posterior membrane preparations (Fig. 2b). The growth rate on this type of carpet is similar to the growth rate on unpurified membranes. These experiments on guidance of nasal axons by tectal membranes are still in an early phase. It is not yet known, for example, whether guidance is due to attraction by posterior or repulsion by anterior components, when the component is expressed during development or what its distribution is within the tectum. On the other hand, guidance of temporal axons in this stripe assay has been shown to be due to a repulsive or inhibitory component in posterior membranes (Walter et al. 1987a).

Identification of the Component Carrying the Guiding and the Collapse-inducing Activity

It was discovered recently that posterior tectal membranes contain a component that causes growth cones of temporal retinal axons to collapse (Cox et al. 1990). This collapse is only seen when temporal axons are exposed to posterior membranes. It is not observed when temporal axons are exposed to anterior membranes. Furthermore, nasal growth cones show little if any reaction to posterior membranes. These findings, together with the observation that guiding activity and collapse-inducing activity share some other features, for example, time of expression (B. Müller, pers. comm.) and sensitivity to phosphatidylinositol-specific phospholipase C (PI-PLC) (Walter et al. 1990b), suggested to us that both the repellent guiding activity and the collapse-inducing activity may reside in the same molecule. We therefore set out to isolate the molecule by using a guidance and a collapse assay as test.

As a first step, an antiserum against posterior tectal membranes was prepared. It recognizes and inactivates the repulsive guiding component of posterior membranes (Fig. 3), as shown by the loss of striped outgrowth upon preincubation of the posterior membranes with the serum. It also inactivates the ability of posterior membranes to induce collapse of temporal growth cones (data not shown). The serum is directed against many components of tectal membranes. When tectal membranes of anterior and posterior tectum are separated by two-dimensional electrophoresis, more than 1000 components can be detected by silver staining,

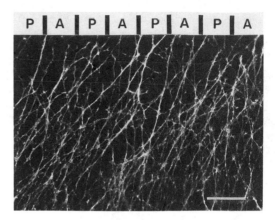

Figure 3. The guiding activity for temporal retinal axons is inactivated by antiserum. Guidance is abolished by treatment of posterior membranes with antiserum directed against posterior tectal membranes. Bar, 100 μm.

and a small percentage of the corresponding spots is recognized and stained by the antiserum. Differences between anterior and posterior membranes can be detected in the immunoblots (Fig. 4a). The most obvious difference concerns a component that is found in higher concentrations in posterior than in anterior tectum. As shown in a one-dimensional SDS gel, this component has a molecular mass of 33 kD and is probably a glycoprotein since it is detected by peanut lectin (Fig. 4b).

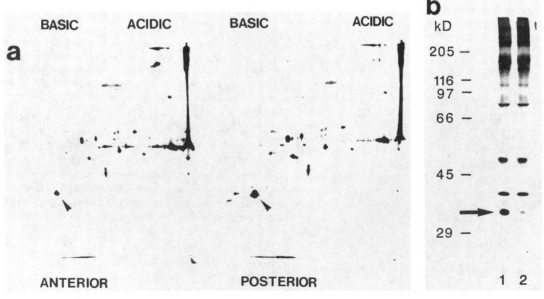

Figure 4. A 33-kD glycoprotein is found in greater amount in the posterior than in the anterior part of the optic tectum (E9). Anterior and posterior membranes were analyzed on two-dimensional blots. The blots were incubated with antibodies that prevent the decision of temporal axons in the stripe assay. Antibody binding was made visible with a peroxidase-conjugated second antibody (goat anti-rabbit). A 33-kD protein, enriched in the posterior part of the tectum is marked by an arrow (*a*). This anterior-posterior difference is also detectable on a one-dimensional blot (*b*). Posterior membranes are analyzed on lane *1*, and anterior membranes are analyzed on lane *2*. Biotinylated peanut lectin (Vector) recognizes the 33-kD protein.

Purification of the Component That Shows Guiding and Collapse-inducing Activity

To purify the 33-kD component, tissue of tecta or whole brain was homogenized in buffer containing urea and spermidine. The cell membranes (the protein composition of this crude membrane preparation is shown in Fig. 5, lane 1) were separated from cytoplasm, nuclei, and mitochondria by two centrifugation steps. They were then solubilized in buffer with urea and the detergent CHAPS, and nonsolubilized material was removed by centrifugation. The solubilized components were fractionated on DEAE-Sepharose in the presence of urea and CHAPS. Fractions were eluted with sodium chloride of stepwise increasing concentration. The composition of the first 1 M sodium chloride eluate is shown in Figure 5, lane 2. Lecithin was added to this column fraction. After mixing, the sample was dialyzed against PBS. Vesicles formed because of the removal of CHAPS.

The vesicles were purified by centrifugation and subjected to SDS gel electrophoresis. Their protein composition is shown in Figure 5, lane 3. Three protein bands are observed, but two of them are not visible in Figure 5, lane 3 (35 and 38 kD). The compound with the lowest molecular weight (33 kD) can be cleaved off the vesicles by PI-PLC (Fig. 6). Figure 6, lane 1, shows the protein composition of the vesicles before PI-PLC treatment. Figure 6, lane 2, illustrates the loss of this component upon a 60-minute PI-PLC treatment of the vesicles and its appearance in the supernatant (Fig. 6, lane 3).

The reconstituted vesicles containing all three components, when tested in the collapse and in the guiding

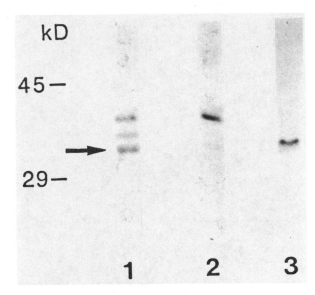

Figure 6. A 33-kD protein is released from reconstituted vesicles by treatment with the enzyme PI-PLC. A fraction containing the collapse-inducing activity was reconstituted into lecithin vesicles (lane *1*). After incubation of the reconstituted vesicles in PBS, with the enzyme PI-PLC the vesicles were pelleted and analyzed by SDS-PAGE (lane *2*). The protein pattern of the supernatant after incubation with PI-PLC is shown on lane *3*. The gels were blotted, and the blots were incubated with antibodies interfering with the decision of temporal axons in the stripe assay.

assay, have a strong collapse-inducing effect on growing temporal retinal axons (Fig. 7a; Table 1), whereas most nasal axons show no reaction (Fig. 7b; Table 1). In the guidance assay with alternating stripes from anterior membranes and a mixture of anterior membranes with vesicles, temporal axons grow exclusively on the stripes of pure anterior membranes. On these striped carpets, nasal axons often show a preference for anterior membranes. This is not unexpected, as has been discussed elsewhere (Stahl et al. 1990), and is in agreement with observations by J. Vielmetter (unpubl.).

DISCUSSION

In the initial stripe assay for retinal axons (Walter et al. 1987b), temporal axons expressed a regional selectivity with respect to the target material. They grew preferentially on material of anterior tectum (their target area), and they avoided posterior membranes (Walter et al. 1987a). However, repeated attempts to show a regional selectivity by nasal axons for their target area, the posterior tectum, failed, although nasal axons when given the choice between retinal and tectal substrate showed a clear preference for material of the target organ.

Nasal axons, like their temporal equivalents, can show regional selectivity. They have a preference for posterior membranes over anterior components when the membranes have been subjected to a fractionation

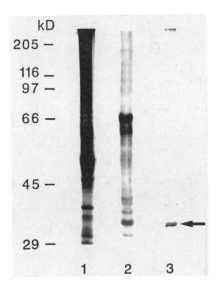

Figure 5. Protein pattern of increasingly enriched fractions of collapse-inducing activity. Samples collected during enrichment of the 33-kD component were fractionated by SDS-PAGE. Lanes from left to right show starting material (lane *1*, brain membranes), a 1 M NaCl-eluted fraction (lane *2*), and reconstituted vesicles from this fraction (lane *3*). The gel is stained with silver.

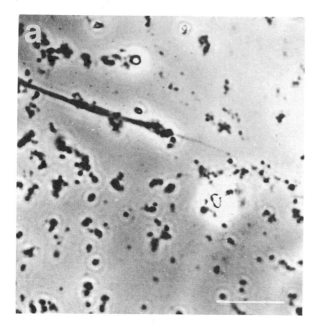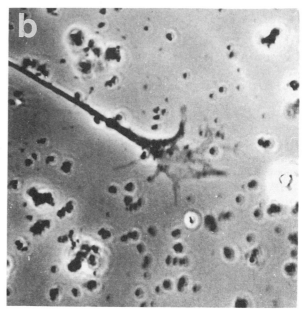

Figure 7. A fraction of reconstituted vesicles containing a 33-kD protein causes collapse of temporal retinal growth cones. Vesicles prepared from the 1 M NaCl DEAE-column fraction induce collapse of temporal retinal growth cones (*a*). Most nasal growth cones show no reaction to these vesicles (*b*). Bar, 15 μm.

and enrichment procedure before the stripe assay. This finding is consistent with the speculation that the concentration of the corresponding guiding components may be crucial in the assay. The establishment of an in vitro system in which nasal axons can be guided by position-specific cues of the tectum is the first step toward a future biochemical characterization of the guiding component(s) involved. It is not yet known whether nasal axons are attracted by posterior membranes or repelled by anterior membranes.

For the temporal axons, on the other hand, it has been shown that posterior membranes are repellent (Walter et al. 1987a) and that they can cause temporal growth cones to collapse. Since both activities, repulsion and collapse induction, show a similar age dependence (B. Müller, pers. comm.) and a similar topographic specificity (Cox et al. 1990), it has been speculated that they may be mediated by the same molecule.

During the search for the repellent and collapse-inducing molecule, we made use of an antiserum raised against tectal membranes that inhibits guidance and collapse induction (Stahl et al. 1990). The antiserum was used to detect differences in protein composition of anterior and posterior tectal membranes. Two-dimen-

sional gels reveal a conspicuous 33-kD component that is present at a higher concentration in posterior than in anterior membranes. Besides this component, which has been analyzed in detail, other reproducible differences between anterior and posterior membranes have been discovered by the use of the antiserum. The corresponding components have still to be analyzed with respect to their involvement in axonal guidance.

Besides its spatial distribution in the tectum, the 33-kD protein has two properties expected for a molecule that is repellent for temporal axons and that exhibits the collapse-inducing activity: (1) The concentration of the 33-kD component decreases with increasing developmental age at the time when the guiding activity decreases (Stahl et al. 1990); and (2) the 33-kD component is anchored in the membrane by a phosphatidylinositol anchor as documented by the PI-PLC sensitivity (Fig. 6), which corresponds to the observation that posterior membranes lose the 33-kD component and the repellent activity upon PI-PLC treatment (Walter et al. 1990b). Furthermore, reconstituted vesicles, which contain the 33-kD component, show guidance and collapse-inducing activities for temporal retinal axons. Since there are only two other components besides the 33-kD component found in these

Table 1. Collapse of Temporal Retinal Growth Cones upon Addition of Posterior Membranes or Reconstituted Vesicles Containing a 33-kD Protein

	Collapsed nasal growth cones (%)	Collapsed temporal growth cones (%)
Anterior membranes	29.2 ± 1.6	33.6 ± 7.2
Posterior membranes	32.5 ± 10.7	79.4 ± 7.3
Reconstituted vesicles	38.6 ± 8.2	85.6 ± 4.9

vesicles and since only the 33-kD component expresses the properties expected for the guiding and collapse-inducing activity, we conclude that the 33-kD glycoprotein most likely carries both the repellent and the collapse-inducing activity for temporal retinal axons. The final proof for this conclusion is still missing and will probably come from studies with functionally active monospecific antibodies.

Two different properties of tectal membranes have been discussed. Both properties have the same spatial (anterior-posterior) distribution within the tectum. They share position specificity with respect to their action on nasal and temporal retinal axons. The fact that both guidance and growth cone collapse seems to be caused by a single molecule, the 33-kD glycoprotein, suggests that these phenomena are related.

Recently, we suggested a model of axonal guidance (Walter et al. 1990a) in which it was assumed that local growth cone collapse (or paralysis) is the basis of axonal guidance. It is easy to see how, for example, temporal axons might be guided by induction of a local collapse at the sharp boundaries in the stripe assay. Wherever the temporal growth cone reaches the boundary where much of the 33-kD collapse-inducing activity is expressed, it becomes locally paralyzed and can keep growing only at that part at which it is not in contact with the 33-kD component (Walter et al. 1990a). Thus, it becomes deflected away from the boundary. However, to explain axonal guidance in a gradient field, especially at high concentration of the collapse-inducing or paralyzing activity, a further assumption is needed. In the model, it must be assumed that axons can "learn" to grow even in the presence of high concentrations of the collapse-inducing activity. They must habituate. There are, in fact, experimental indications that they may do so. Temporal axons, which are unable to invade posterior lanes at the sharp edges of the stripes (Fig. 2a), do grow quite well on or onto posterior membranes after having been exposed to the high concentration of posterior material for some time (Walter et al. 1990b; H. Baier, pers. comm.). We have recently suggested (Walter et al. 1990a) how this habituation might permit a very slight concentration difference between the two margins of a growth cone in a gradient field to be converted into a growth-cone directing force.

ACKNOWLEDGMENTS

We thank Susanne Bahde, Julita Huf, and Silvia Deiss for excellent technical assistance. We are also very grateful to Dr. Paul Whitington for reading and improving the manuscript.

REFERENCES

Ansorge, W. 1985. Fast and sensitive detection of protein and DNA bands by treatment with potassium permanganate. *J. Biochem. Biophys. Meth.* **11:** 13.

Bonhoeffer, F. and J. Huf. 1982. *In vitro* experiments on axon guidance demonstrating an anterior-posterior gradient on the tectum. *EMBO J.* **1:** 427.

Cox, E.C., B. Müller, and F. Bonhoeffer. 1990. Axonal guidance in the chick visual system: Posterior tectal membranes induce collapse of growth cones from the temporal retina. *Neuron* **4:** 31.

Egger, D. and K. Bienz. 1987. Colloidal gold staining and immunoprobing of proteins on the same nitrocellulose blot. *Anal. Biochem.* **166:** 413.

Gierer, A. 1981. Development of projections between areas of the nervous system. *Biol. Cybern.* **42:** 69.

———. 1987. Directional cues for growing axons forming the retinotectal projection. *Development* **101:** 479.

Godement, P. and F. Bonhoeffer. 1989. Cross-species recognition of tectal cues by retinal fibers in vitro. *Development* **106:** 313.

Laemmli, U.K. 1970. Cleavage of structural proteins during the assembly of the head of bacteriophage T4. *Nature* **227:** 680.

Porter, R.R. 1959. The hydrolysis of rabbit gamma-globulin and antibodies with crystalline papain. *Biochem. J.* **73:** 119.

Rathjen, F.G., M. Wolff, R. Frank, F. Bonhoeffer, and U. Rutishauser. 1987. Membrane glycoproteins involved in neurite fasciculation. *J. Cell Biol.* **104:** 343.

Sadoul, K., R. Sadoul, A. Faissner, and M. Schachner. 1988. Biochemical characterization of different molecular forms of the neural cell adhesion molecule L1. *J. Neurochem.* **50:** 510.

Sperry, R.W. 1956. The eye and the brain. *Sci. Am.* **194:** 48

———. 1963. Chemoaffinity in the orderly growth of nerve fiber patterns and connections. *Proc. Natl. Acad. Sci.* **50:** 703.

Stahl, B., B. Müller, Y. von Boxberg, E.C. Cox, and F. Bonhoeffer. 1990. Biochemical characterization of a putative axonal guidance molecule of the chick visual system. *Neuron* (in press).

Towbin, H., T. Staehelin, and J. Gordon. 1979. Electrophoretic transfer of proteins from polyacrylamide gels to nitrocellulose sheets: Procedure and some applications. *Proc. Natl. Acad. Sci.* **76:** 4350.

Vielmetter, J. and C.A.O. Stürmer. 1989. Goldfish retinal axons respond to position-specific properties of tectal cell membranes in vitro. *Neuron* **2:** 1331.

von Boxberg, Y. 1988. Protein analysis on two-dimensional polyacrylamide gels in the femtogram range: Use of a new sulfur-labeling reagent. *Anal. Biochem.* **169:** 372.

Walter, J., T. Allsopp, and F. Bonhoeffer. 1990a. A common denominator of growth cone guidance and collapse? *Trends Neurosci.* (in press).

Walter, J., S. Henke-Fahle, and F. Bonhoeffer. 1987a. Avoidance of posterior tectal membranes by temporal retinal axons. *Development* **101:** 909.

Walter, J., B. Müller, and F. Bonhoeffer. 1990b. Axonal guidance by an avoidance mechanism. *J. Physiol.* **84:** 104.

Walter, J., B. Kern-Veits, J. Huf, B. Stolze, and F. Bonhoeffer. 1987b. Recognition of position-specific properties of tectal cell membranes by retinal axons in vitro. *Development* **101:** 685.

Neuronal Growth Cone as an Integrator of Complex Environmental Information

S.B. KATER AND P.B. GUTHRIE

Program in Neuronal Growth and Development, Department of Anatomy and Neurobiology,
Colorado State University, Fort Collins, Colorado 80523

Fundamental decisions on neuronal morphology and connectivity are made at the level of the neuronal growth cone. The decision to continue outgrowth in a given direction, to turn, to branch, or to stop growing seems in many cases to depend on the many signals received and integrated by the growth cone from its external environment. The role of the growth cone may be quite different over the course of a lifetime. During early development, growth cones connect large ensembles of initially spherical neuroblasts. Interpreting the molecular terrain to be traversed at this time presents a formidable task. The growth cone also emerges as the primary organelle of pathfinding and elongation in the regenerating adult nervous system. Finally, there is compelling evidence that the growth cone is not just associated with the formation of initial connections or restoration of broken connections, but is also a tool for neural plasticity in normal mature animals (see, e.g., Purves et al. 1986). Information reaching the tips of previously stable neurites must reawaken dormant structures to restore the growth-cone-like behavior. This allows the now motile growth cone to break some connections and reform others. The spatial and temporal variables that must be considered in trying to understand the signals that alter growth cone behavior are therefore formidable.

It is possible to approach fundamental questions experimentally by analyzing processes common to most of the challenges the growth cone must meet. For instance, the process of motility itself results from displacements of cytoskeletal elements and membrane components (Kater and Letourneau 1985). Such changes are undoubtedly signaled by messengers within the cell that take their cues from information reaching the external face of the cell membrane. These cues may well be quite different at different times. On the other hand, it is reasonable to assume that at least some common strategies for pathfinding remain constant throughout the life of an organism. To address these questions, it is necessary to gather data from a variety of circumstances within the lifetime of a single organism. It is also important to compare the results obtained in one organism with those found in others. The remainder of this review examines primarily the behavior of growth cones from identified neurons of the snail *Helisoma* in cell culture. These large growth cones, with their stereotyped behavior, have proven to be a valuable model because of their high tractability and

ease of experimental manipulation. The behavior of growth cones will be examined in parallel situations from preparations including rat hippocampal neurons and mouse dorsal root ganglion cells. Taken together, we describe our present view of the growth cone as an integrator of multiple, simultaneous stimuli: some endogenous to a neuron and some from the environments through which the growth cones traverse. This paper also describes a candidate locus at which integration of several different stimuli may occur. Intracellular calcium concentrations are modifiable by many of the same agents that can modify neuronal growth cone behavior. In fact, when intracellular calcium levels are manipulated, *changes in growth cone behaviors ensue.* Accordingly, we propose that intracellular calcium may be one level at which multiple stimuli are integrated and through which decisions about growth cone behavior are ultimately determined.

Intrinsic and Extrinsic Regulators of Growth Cone Behavior

The large growth cones from different identified neurons of the snail, *Helisoma*, have allowed us to study basic decision-making processes. Although regeneration of axotomized neurons within ganglia may seem chaotic (Murphy and Kater 1980), neurons plated in culture go through a stereotypic set of behaviors (Hadley et al. 1985). These begin with the initiation of neurite outgrowth from the spherical neuronal cell bodies excised from adult ganglia. Each of these neurites is tipped by highly motile growth cones with large, broad, and flat lamellipodia and numerous filopodial extensions. The growth cones exhibit highly dynamic morphology throughout their early phases in culture. Three to five days after plating (depending on conditions and the neuron in question), a significant morphological change occurs in the growth cone that is accompanied by a cessation of outgrowth (Fig. 1A). This change is characterized by a retraction of filopodia, decrease in lamellipodial area, and a conversion to what is referred to as a "stable state" morphology. Interestingly, although each neuron undergoes this stereotyped sequence of events, specific identified neurons show distinctive differences in their final form such that neurons B5, B19, and B4, for instance, are clearly identifiable by their final morphologies in cell culture (Haydon et al. 1985). This spontaneous stabilization of

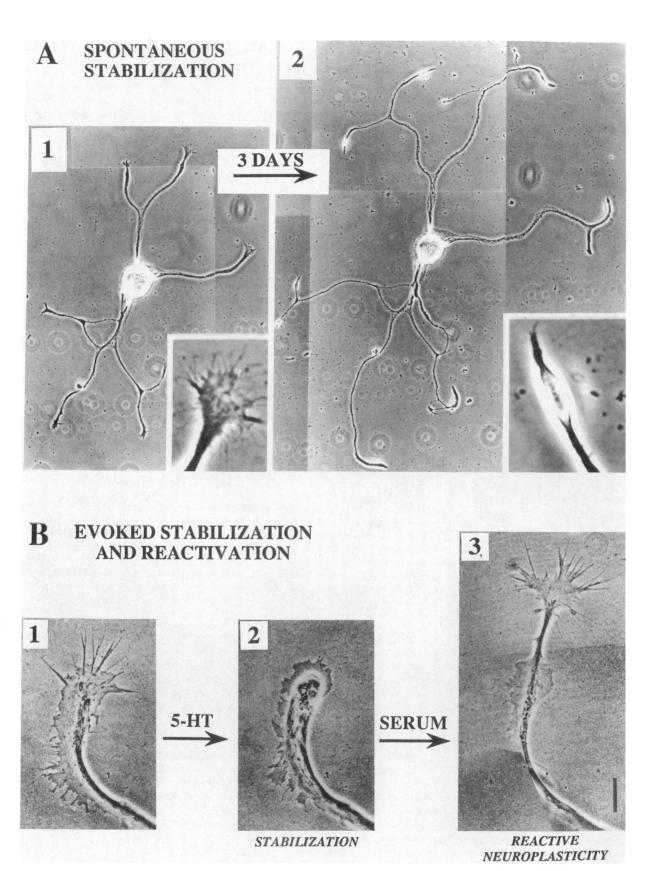

A SPONTANEOUS STABILIZATION

1

3 DAYS →

2

B EVOKED STABILIZATION AND REACTIVATION

1

5-HT →

2

SERUM →

3

STABILIZATION

REACTIVE NEUROPLASTICITY

Figure 1. (*See facing page for legend.*)

neuronal morphology appears to be an intrinsic quality characteristic of each of the neurons from *Helisoma* that we have studied. It should be emphasized that these definitive growth patterns occur even when only a single nerve cell is plated in the culture dish. What stabilizes these patterns by halting outgrowth at predefined times? It is reasonable to assume that intrinsic cues reach growth cones and significantly change them from motile to nonmotile forms. This spontaneous, intrinsically derived stabilization of growth cone activity and neuronal form is to be contrasted with a series of extrinsic cues that can impinge on growth cones and also change their behavior significantly.

Among the most interesting and perhaps somewhat unexpected extrinsic cues that we have identified as guides for neuronal growth cones are neurotransmitter molecules. These compounds, which play critical roles in intercellular communication, can also act as highly specific regulators of growth cone behavior. For example, when serotonin is applied to a neuron B19 (and other neurons of this class), growth cones abruptly go through a series of changes that closely resembles the spontaneous stabilization described earlier (Fig. 1B). Growth cone filopodia withdraw, lamellipodial surface area decreases, and the neurons cease to elongate as long as serotonin is present in the medium (Haydon et al. 1984; McCobb et al. 1988a). Such effects are highly neuron-selective. The growth cones of neuron B5 (and several other neurons belonging to this class) are unaffected by high levels (up to 10^{-4} M) of serotonin in the medium. Strikingly, it can be shown that the growth inhibitory effect of this neurotransmitter can be localized to individual growth cones. Isolation of the growth cones by transecting their neurite results in a motile organelle that can remain alive for several days. In this condition, focal application of serotonin to a neuron B19 isolated growth cone completely inhibits the motility of this structure, indicating that a single growth cone may well "read" a local environment without having a direct effect on the rest of the growth cones of this nerve cell (Haydon et al. 1984). In contrast, it should be noted that isolated growth cones never spontaneously express the stable state condition. This indicates that the stable state condition, whether environmentally evoked or occurring spontaneously, requires cues; the spontaneous ones are likely to derive from the cell body, and the others are derived from the environment.

There are several factors that can inhibit the outgrowth of nerve cells. It is important to point out, however, that factors also exist that can reawaken outgrowth from stable state growth cones (Fig. 1B). Such factors may well play critical roles in neuroplasticity, where the breaking of old connections and the formation of others implies that the stable, nongrowing neurite must be capable of conversion to an active motile form. Although not yet well characterized in *Helisoma*, one such factor(s) is derived from *Helisoma* serum. Applications of low-molecular-weight fractions (<10,000) from *Helisoma* serum reawaken dormant growth cones (Grega and Kater 1987; Kater et al. 1990). The important point lies not necessarily in the particulars of those signals that inhibit or those that will reawaken growth cones, but in the fact that growth cones are highly responsive structures that can respond to many simultaneously present environmental cues. Furthermore, such observations reinforce the idea that a fundamental property of nerve cells lies in their continued capacity for remodeling.

It is therefore clearly necessary to define sets of cues (Fig. 2) and to study both their individual and their combinatorial actions. How does the intrinsic system, timed for stabilization, interact with novel sets of environmental information? Why do different neurons differ in response to similar environmental cues? What are the common paths of integration that govern neurite outgrowth at the level of intracellular machinery?

Growth Cones as Integrators of Multiple Cues

It is clear that individual neuronal growth cones respond to a variety of cues present in their external environment. These cues almost certainly do not occur singularly but simultaneously. The growth cone must therefore be capable of integrating multiple environmental cues. In addition to external cues, information is also derived from the cell body. Such information is likely to have more global effects on all of the growth cones of a given nerve cell, whereas environmental cues may well be restricted to local effects on individual

Figure 1. Dynamic and reversible growth states underlying the generation of neuronal form. (*A*) A *Helisoma* buccal neuron B5 is plated as an individual sphere. Within 1 day after plating, new neurites have been generated, producing a simple outgrowth pattern. The neuron will continue to grow for 4–5 days, elaborating a more complex outgrowth pattern with increased neurite length and many branch points. During this period, a change has occurred in most of the growth cones of this neuron. During active outgrowth, the growth cones resemble classical cell-culture growth cones with numerous filopodia, a broadened lamellipodium, and considerable motile activity (*A1*, inset). Later in development, these growth cones undergo morphological changes that include the retraction of filopodia and lamellipodium and the cessation of further motility and outgrowth (*A2*, inset). The growth cones will remain in this nonmotile "stable state" for many days unless a new stimulus is presented. (*B*) Spontaneous stabilization can be mimicked by environmental cues. The active outgrowth of a neuron B19 growth cone is abruptly halted by the application of serotonin (5-HT, 5×10^{-7} M) (*B2*). This growth cone and all of the other growth cones not shown from this neuron would have remained in this stable state indefinitely unless presented with a novel stimulus. Low-molecular-weight *Helisoma* serum factors were added to this preparation, and significant new neurite outgrowth ensued with the production of new growth cones of characteristic form and behavior (*B3*). These two examples of growth cone behaviors illustrate the dynamic and reversible response of neuronal growth cones to both intrinsic and extrinsic cues.

DIFFERENT GROWTH CONES RESPOND DIFFERENTLY
TO THE SAME STIMULUS:

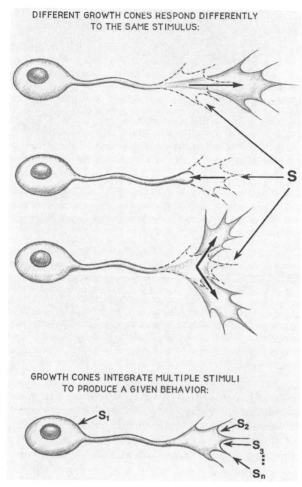

GROWTH CONES INTEGRATE MULTIPLE STIMULI
TO PRODUCE A GIVEN BEHAVIOR:

Figure 2. (*Top*) The growth cone has a discrete repertoire of behaviors that can be made in the response to a single stimulus. These behaviors include continued elongation, cessation of elongation, turning, and/or branching. Growth cones either on the same neuron or on different neurons can respond quite differently to an identical stimulus. (*Bottom*) Rarely, however, is a single stimulus encountered by a growth cone during navigation. The growth cone encounters a complex and changing environment of multiple stimuli that must be integrated, in a decision-making process, to result in the appropriate behavior. The presence of one stimulus can alter the response of the growth cone to a second cue. Whether or not a specific growth cone responds to a given stimulus may therefore involve not only the receptive capability of the growth cone, but also the presence or absence of other signals. Thus, the complex environmental information that a growth cone encounters is translated into a series of complex internal processes that bias the behavioral response of the growth cone to new environmental stimuli.

growth cones. It is noteworthy that different growth cones can respond quite differently to the same stimulus. This has already been discussed for the case of serotonin with respect to neurons B5 and B19, but it is also quite clear that the same environmental cue may differentially affect different growth cones of the same neuron. This has been most effectively demonstrated on the growth cones of embryonic hippocampal pyramidal-like neurons in cell culture (Banker and Cowan 1977, 1979). In these neurons, we have found

that neurotransmitters can have differential effects on different growth cones. For instance, glutamate can have selective effects on the dendritic growth cones of these neurons without affecting axonal growth cones (Mattson et al. 1988). Depending on glutamate concentration, dendritic growth cones stop or even regress, whereas axonal growth cones from the same neuron continue normal outgrowth. Although these results are derived from an experimental configuration for bath application of glutamate, one must consider them in the context of developing nervous systems. Within the developing nervous system, it is entirely possible that, instead of all dendritic growth cones seeing high concentrations of glutamate, only selected dendrites are exposed. Accordingly, if processes in vivo do resemble those in vitro, one might expect a highly selective sculpting of the dendritic arbor (Mattson et al. 1988). This has been mimicked in cell culture by local micropipette application to individual dendrites (Mattson et al. 1988); then local dendritic regression follows. This kind of response could have important ramifications for the fine-tuning of neuronal circuits. Not only is the dendrite in question affected, but the electrical load of synaptic input onto other areas of the neuron is changed as well.

The hippocampal pyramidal neuron also provides an example of integration of multiple environmental cues (Fig. 3). γ-Aminobutyric acid (GABA) is a key inhibitory transmitter of these neurons. Alone (or in concert with its potentiator, diazepam), it has no effect on the growth cones. However, GABA has important effects in concert with glutamate. In the presence of GABA, glutamate will no longer cause dendritic growth cones to stop or retract. Given that glutamate is a major excitatory transmitter afferent to these neurons and GABA is the major inhibitory transmitter, our present view is that outgrowth may be regulated by a balance of excitatory and inhibitory inputs to a neuron. Under conditions of excitatory imbalance (i.e., net depolarization), outgrowth would be inhibited, and, in fact, dendritic regression could ensue. Conversely, when excitatory and inhibitory inputs are balanced, dendritic out-growth will continue. This integration of two stimuli by growth cones is essentially identical to the classical synaptic integration with which we have all become so familiar. It seems reasonable that principles similar to those employed in the physiology of adult nervous systems may also be used in regulating the formation of those very same systems. An extension of this idea is illustrated by studies made of *Helisoma* growth cones, where it is possible to perform electrophysiological experiments and monitor growth cone behavior simultaneously (below).

In *Helisoma*, it has been possible to demonstrate that the inhibitory effect of serotonin on neuron B19's growth cones can be negated by the presence of acetylcholine in the same fashion that GABA negated glutamate's effect on hippocampal growth cones. Although acetylcholine in its own right has no effect on outgrowth, it does enable continued outgrowth in the pres-

Balanced Excitation and Inhibition

Excitatory Imbalance

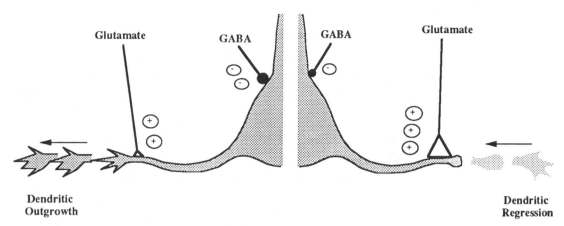

Figure 3. Experiments on embryonic hippocampal pyramidal neurons in cell culture exemplify how the response to a single stimulus can be altered by the presence of another. In the presence of high quantities of glutamate (i.e., excitatory imbalance), growth cones of dendrites cease elongation. However, in a balanced excitation-inhibition condition (i.e., glutamate in the presence of GABA) dendritic outgrowth continues. These effects are specific to the dendritic growth cones and not to axonal growth cones, indicating further the complexity of the regulation of growth cones of individual neurons. Taken together, these experiments clearly demonstrate the interactive nature of multiple stimuli on a given neuron.

ence of serotonin (McCobb et al. 1988b). The growth retarding effects of serotonin can be negated as well by experimentally imposed hyperpolarization of the cell (McCobb and Kater 1988). Again, this indicates that the growth cone is integrating a variety of signals to decide ultimately whether growth will continue or be terminated. Given that acetylcholine is the inhibitory transmitter and serotonin the excitatory transmitter, the results of membrane polarization again suggest that the mode of integration of these two stimuli may well be the same as the classical modes of synaptic integration; namely, integration may well occur at the level of membrane potential. This raises several interesting possibilities with respect to more global forms of regulation of a growth cone's behavior.

From the results just reviewed, it appears that depolarizations retard outgrowth and hyperpolarizations negate such effects, possibly, by simple membrane summation. Action potentials constitute the major depolarizations that are likely seen within developing neurons. The fact that action potentials might regulate growth cones documents a quite different form of control system. Although specific cues such as neurotransmitters or other agents could act locally on individual growth cones, action potentials may well serve to regulate the behavior of all of the growth cones on a neuron simultaneously. Given all of the caveats of branch-point failures and the need for action potential invasion of the growth cone, it seems likely that action potentials generated in the cell body could spread to most of the growth cones of the neuron. We know, in fact, that action potentials can travel quite effectively from the cell body to growth cones (Kater and Guthrie 1989). Indeed, a study of growing growth cones under

electrophysiological control has demonstrated that generation of action potentials can completely inhibit outgrowth in all neurons studied if the frequency of stimulation is high enough (Cohan and Kater 1986). It is interesting to note that this inhibition is frequency-dependent and quite different in different neurons (Cohan 1990). Thus, it is even possible to envision a specific "neural code" for the regulation of growth cone behaviors that is different for different neurons.

A striking demonstration of the integrative capability of neurons and their associated growth cones can be seen when applying multiple stimuli to *Helisoma* growth cones (McCobb 1987, McCobb et al. 1988b). When one subjects a neuron B19 growth cone to acetylcholine and serotonin simultaneously (a growth permissive condition) and then evokes action potentials, growth cone motility is abruptly terminated (Fig. 4). This case illustrates the basic thesis of this paper: Namely, the behavior of neuronal growth cones is likely determined not by unitary signals but, rather, is the result of an integration of multiple environmental and intrinsic cues. Although this is a straightforward concept, it should be emphasized that not all cues may have equal weight. For instance, in our hands, action potentials have an overwhelming growth retarding effect when fired at high frequencies. At lower frequencies, their weighting may be considerably less and their effects might well be negated by other factors. It is this view of the neuronal growth cone as an integrator of diverse environmental cues that has motivated investigations on the underlying mechanisms that integrate different kinds of stimuli and result in an effective decision-making process governing growth cone behavior.

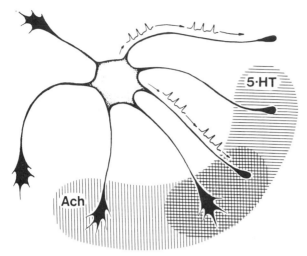

Figure 4. A schematic summary of a series of experiments on the growth cones of *Helisoma* B19 neurons (McCobb et al. 1988b). Stimuli presented individually have discrete effects on these growth cones: serotonin (5-HT) inhibits neurite elongation; acetylcholine (Ach) has no effect on neurite elongation, and action potentials rapidly inhibit neurite elongation. In the presence of acetylcholine, however, serotonin's growth-retarding effects are negated. The protective nature of Ach can be completely overridden by high-frequency bursts of action potentials. These results clearly demonstrate, again, the interactive nature of stimuli as they impinge simultaneously on the neuronal growth cone.

Intracellular Calcium as a Regulator of Growth Cone Behavior

Many of the underlying processes that may play roles in growth cone motility can be significantly affected by levels of intracellular calcium. For example, key aspects of growth cone motility, such as interactions of actin and myosin, the assembly and disassembly of microtubules, and the incorporation of membrane in the form of vesicles transported from the cell body, are thought to be regulated by the specific calcium environment. Indeed, we have found that a variety of stimuli that can affect the behavior of the neuronal growth cones do so by raising intracellular calcium (Fig. 5). Neurotransmitters, such as serotonin on *Helisoma* neurons B19 (Haydon et al. 1984, 1987; McCobb et al. 1988b) and glutamate on the dendritic growth cones of hippocampal pyramidal neurons (Mattson et al. 1988), act through rises in intracellular calcium. Both of these are dependent on influx of intracellular calcium since both can be blocked by specific calcium channel blockers. Even quite simple mechanical cues may well act through changes in intracellular calcium (Mills et al. 1988). It is also clear that other stimuli may well act through regulators other than intracellular calcium (see, e.g., Ivins and Pittman 1989). Among the important future questions is, why do individual stimuli act through different regulatory pathways? An intriguing possibility is that stimuli of one form will act through one regulatory system, whereas stimuli of a second type will act through another. For example, it may be found that stimuli, such as excitatory neu-

rotransmitters, act through intracellular calcium systems, whereas stimuli, such as surface-associated molecules, may act through other systems.

Intracellular calcium concentrations can act as a nodal point for integration of multiple, simultaneously presented environmental cues. As an example, intracellular calcium rises when serotonin is applied to a neuron B19. This rise, which could have blocked outgrowth, is negated by the experimental application of hyperpolarizing current (McCobb and Kater 1988). Alternatively, in a more physiological situation, the outgrowth-retarding effects of serotonin are negated by acetylcholine as a result of acetylcholine inhibiting the calcium rise in the growth cone (McCobb et al. 1988b). Finally, if the environment presents a complex combination of information such as serotonin, acetylcholine, and action potentials simultaneously, the growth cone integrates all of these inputs, in a weighted fashion, to determine the final calcium levels and resultant behavioral output. Some signals may well make different contributions to calcium levels than others. In fact, the generation of action potentials does result in a large rise in intracellular calcium that can override the effects of acetylcholine. This striking parallelism between calcium changes and changes in behavior reinforces the idea that calcium levels do play an important regulatory role in determining growth cone behavior. This suggests that the effects of this combination of stimuli on the behavior of the growth cone is mediated by integrating the changes in intracellular calcium produced by individual stimuli. The basic reasoning is that stimuli that would raise intracellular calcium can sum to produce even higher levels of intracellular calcium in the growth cone. Those stimuli that can negate a rise in intracellular calcium may act to balance other stimuli and thereby stabilize growth cone behavior. Taken together, these data point to intracellular calcium levels as a key nodal point of integration for many of the cues that a growth cone is likely to encounter during development.

Calcium Homeostasis

Available evidence, although limited, supports the existence of several classes of intracellular regulatory molecules that govern the behavior of growth cones. Some of these may well respond to extracellular stimuli and change cytoskeletal activity or the insertion of membrane without directly altering intracellular calcium (Forscher et al. 1987). It is clear, however, that intracellular calcium can profoundly effect the machinery of growth cone motility. Accordingly, a comprehensive understanding of the behavior of the neuronal growth cone must include an understanding of those basic mechanisms that regulate intracellular calcium.

Calcium homeostasis depends, on the one hand, on a set of mechanisms that can increase intracellular calcium and, on the other hand, on a different set of mechanisms that can decrease free calcium. A balance of the activities of these two sets of machinery results in

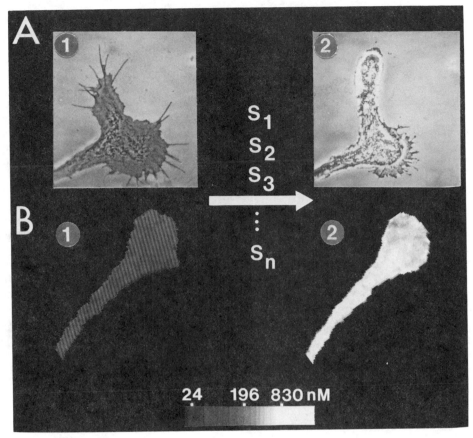

Figure 5. Many stimuli that alter the behavior of growth cones do so by increasing intracellular calcium levels. (*Top*) In the example shown, application of serotonin results, within minutes, in inhibition of the growth cone behavior. Such behavioral effects of a variety of stimuli can be negated by calcium channel blockers such as cobalt or treatments in calcium-free media. (*Bottom*) The same kind of stimulus evokes a rise in calcium that spreads throughout the growth cone. Both the behavioral response and the calcium changes can be blocked by the addition of calcium channel blockers. Calcium is indicated by grayness, with black being low concentrations (<100 nM) and white being high concentration (>1100 nM).

the apparent steady-state levels of intracellular calcium. From the variety of cell types that others have studied, we recognize multiple interactive components of the homeostasis equation (McBurney and Neeting 1987). Among those factors that can decrease intracellular calcium are the following: calcium-pumping ATPases of the endoplasmic reticulum and plasma membrane, mitochondria, and sodium/calcium exchangers. The interaction between these components is such that it is difficult to determine which specific mechanisms are playing a given role. On the other side of the equation, calcium increases can come from a variety of sources. These are classified as either transmembrane fluxes from the extracellular milieu or release from intracellular stores. The interactive nature of systems for raising intracellular calcium makes a dissection of precise causal relationships extremely difficult as well.

Many environmental stimuli evoke discrete rises in intracellular calcium followed by subsequent restoration to near base-line levels (Kater et al. 1988; Mills et al. 1988; Mills and Kater 1990; Jensen et al. 1990; Rehder et al. 1990). It would be of considerable interest to determine which subcellular components of calcium homeostasis are responsible for each phase of this

reaction. Because of the intertwined nature of these components, this represents a formidable task. By way of illustration, for many stimuli that change growth cone behavior, intracellular calcium appears to come from extracellular sources. This conclusion is drawn from the observation that rises in intracellular calcium are blocked by specific organic or inorganic calcium channel-type blockers (Cohan et al. 1987; Mattson and Kater 1987; Mattson et al. 1988). Although this indicates that increased intracellular calcium is due to an influx, it should be noted that even a small influx could equally well trigger the release of calcium from intracellular stores. Thus, attributing changes in calcium levels only to influx on the basis of channel blockers might prove spurious. Another example of the complexity of the calcium homeostatic web can be seen when attempting to inactivate individual components pharmacologically in calcium clearance systems. Within the growth cone exist a variety of mechanisms that can lower intracellular calcium in response to a massively increased influx (Jensen et al. 1990; Rehder et al. 1990). Such rises in intracellular calcium can be experimentally evoked, for example, by the addition of the calcium ionophore A23187. The growth cone, even in isolation, can compensate for these rises; despite the continued presence of A23187, intracellular calcium levels restore. In an experimental attempt to dissect which mechanism was responsible for this regulation, the sodium/calcium exchanger was blocked by lowering extracellular sodium. This does not block the ability of the growth cone to restore its intracellular calcium levels. As an alternative, FCCP (carbonyl cyanide p-trifluoromethoxyphenyl hydrazone) was employed to dissipate proton gradients to determine whether these were important for restoration in the face of a large influx induced by A23187. Again, growth cones were able to restore near normal levels. This, however, does not mean that neither mechanism is important. Indeed, the application of FCCP in concert with a low-sodium environment produces a condition where the growth cone no longer has the ability to compensate for the large influx of calcium induced by A23187 application. Clearly then, using the standard "ablative" strategies of pharmacology for determining functional roles is not satisfactory for dissecting this system. These are simple examples of the complex web of interactive mechanisms that are clearly responsible for the maintenance of intracellular calcium. Obviously, a precise dissection of the system into components may neither be possible nor likely to represent the true cellular condition. Rather, this illustrates that calcium homeostasis in the growth cone is perhaps best viewed as a complex, highly interrelated multicomponent system.

Our considerations to this point have emphasized the existence of multiple, interactive mechanisms that, in the short term, determine free calcium levels in the growth cone. It seems quite probable, however, that separate components of calcium homeostasis can be biased over longer time periods. For instance, our work revealed that glutamate, through rises in free calcium, can selectively alter dendritic growth cones of hippocampal pyramidal neurons. Long-term influences, however, can clearly modulate this effect. For example, fibroblast growth factor (FGF) can (in an RNA- and protein-synthesis-dependent fashion) antagonize the outgrowth-inhibiting actions of glutamate (Mattson et al. 1989b). Furthermore, calcium levels do not rise as dramatically when glutamate is applied following FGF incubation. This example demonstrates another temporal domain over which the responses of growth cones can be "tuned" to alter the responsiveness of a growth cone to its environment.

A final question with respect to our ability to partition calcium homeostasis within the growth cone rests with the limitations of contemporary technology. Fura-2, as a calcium indicator, reports primarily the bulk-free calcium concentrations of the cytoplasm. One must therefore be careful in interpreting results using such methods, since cycling processes, occurring near the cell membrane (Alkon and Rasmussen 1988), could produce an extremely high concentration in submembrane zones without being reported as changes in bulk calcium (Fig. 6). Foci of calcium influx close to points of calcium efflux would result in shunting of calcium,

such that high concentrations of calcium are found only in a local microenvironment. This is indicated in *Helisoma* neurons by the fact that A23187 presented continuously results in a very high rise in intracellular calcium that then appears to restore toward rest levels for the duration of an experiment, despite the continued presence of A23187 (e.g., Fig. 7). In such experiments on cell bodies (Mills and Kater 1990), one finds that the bulk levels of intracellular calcium are elevated to extremely high levels following removal of extracellular sodium. This indicates that a sodium/calcium exchange mechanism has been "handling" the large amounts of influx induced by A23187, such that changes in bulk intracellular calcium are not seen. The corollary of this condition is that local submembrane calcium cycling produces large calcium concentrations in the areas intervening between the local points of influx and efflux. Here, despite the fact that fura-2 technology fails to reveal it, high calcium levels may well have significant effects on membrane-associated, calcium-dependent molecular events. It is clear, from examples such as these, that at present we can only infer a coarse-grain picture of how calcium homeostasis and its particular subcellular components respond to environmental cues that are relevant to growth cone guidance.

Individuality of Neurons

Individual neurons express a variety of differences. Some of these may be formidable and essentially represent the "fingerprint" of that neuron, whereas others may be subtle and based primarily on the past history of one neuron as opposed to another. Figure 7 illustrates examples of straightforward differences between two neurons from *Helisoma*. Individual growth cones of B19 and B5 are quite different morphologically and behaviorally from one another. Their electrophysiological and ultrastructural properties can be quite distinctive as well (Guthrie et al. 1989). Additionally, their differential responses to environmental cues has been illustrated by their response to serotonin. There exists, however, a much more subtle, yet potentially very important, difference between these neurons in their response to environmental cues during neuronal pathfinding. This involves the basic capability of a cell to maintain its specific intracellular calcium levels.

Differences in calcium homeostatic capacity between neurons B19 and B5 appear to be quite large. These differences, undoubtedly representing intrinsic differences between these two neurons, can be demonstrated when the two neurons are challenged with the calcium ionophore A23187. Neuron B19 is unable to compensate for the new calcium influx that occurs, ultimately resulting in the death of that neuron. The same dose of A23187 applied to a neuron B5, on the other hand, neither kills that neuron nor does it alter in any significant long-term way the behavior of its growth cones. It is clear that neuron B5 shows a high compensatory capability for regulating intracellular calcium

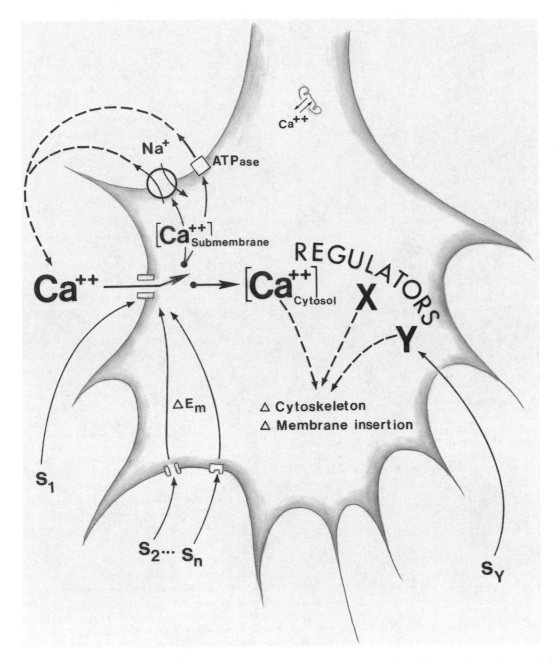

Figure 6. A summary of some of the key features of intracellular calcium and regulation of neuronal growth cone behavior. Calcium homeostasis is a complex balance of multiple processes. Some processes raise intracellular calcium, and others lower intracellular calcium. Shown here for simplicity are only three loci for affecting the influx of extracellular calcium. Stimuli can directly affect the calcium channels (S_1). Stimuli can affect other ion channels and, thus, through membrane voltage, alter voltage-dependent calcium channels (S_2). Receptors might, through other second messengers, affect calcium channels (S_n). Opening of calcium channels would result in an influx of intracellular calcium that, if it exceeded the levels of efflux of the system, would be seen as a rise in cytosolic calcium. Even visible rises in intracellular calcium, however, are often compensated for quite rapidly (Kater et al. 1988; Mills and Kater 1990) by efflux mechanisms. Given that a rise in calcium can activate and increase the efficacy of systems such as the sodium-calcium exchanger, each event that changes intracellular calcium might activate a series of interdigitating compensatory responses. The highly dynamic nature of the processes underlying calcium homeostasis seems to provide the necessary stability so that intracellular calcium changes can serve as important signals for regulating neuronal growth cone behavior. Many of these features are surmised by reading intracellular calcium levels using the fluorescent calcium indicator, fura-2. Influx sites can produce extremely high local levels of calcium. When, however, calcium efflux sites are located close to the sites of influx, local calcium shunts develop. This would maintain local high calcium levels while preventing the diffusion of calcium into the bulk cytoplasmic pool. These local calcium shunts therefore could produce extremely high local calcium levels that would often not be detectable as bulk fura-2 measurements. Nevertheless, it is clear from the very large stimuli-induced changes in cytosolic calcium that do occur that calcium does affect growth cone behavior. This cytosolic calcium likely has targets at either the cytoskeleton and/or membrane insertion. Since other stimuli are known that do not cause measurable rises in calcium but do cause changes in behavior, it is clear that other regulators (X and Y) exist that can also mediate changes in cytoskeleton and/or membrane insertion.

NEURON B 19

NEURON B 5

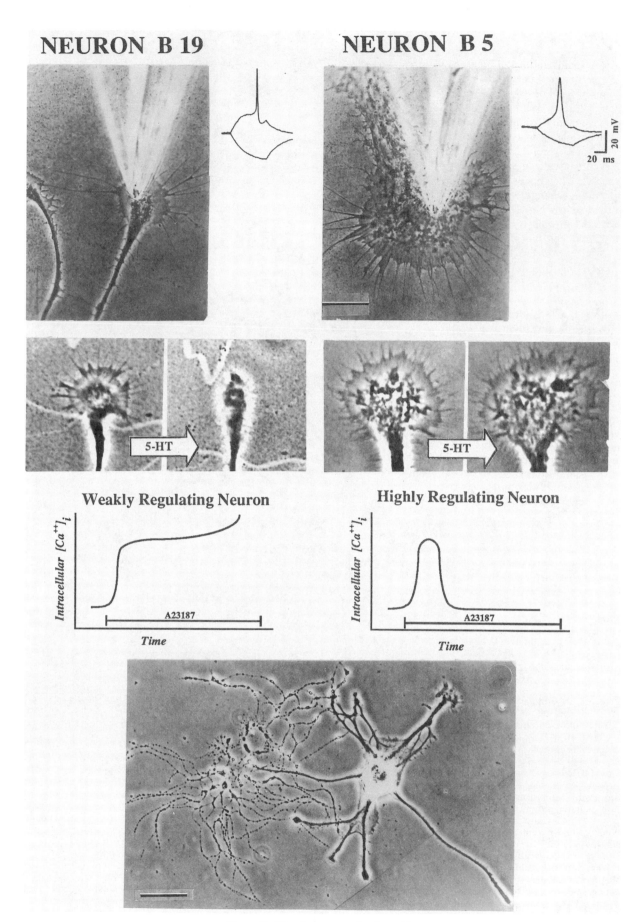

Weakly Regulating Neuron

Highly Regulating Neuron

5-HT

5-HT

20 mV

20 ms

Figure 7. (*See facing page for legend.*)

levels (Mills and Kater 1990). This is true not only for the cell body, but also for the individual growth cones (Jensen et al. 1990; Rehder et al. 1990). This means that neurons could react quite differently to a given environmental stimulus for two reasons. First, a given neuron may or may not have receptors for particular cues, and, second, its ability to handle changes in intracellular calcium may depend on the presence or absence of compensatory systems, such as the sodium/calcium exchanger. This difference in calcium-regulating capacities between different cells can be even more dramatically illustrated when comparing more widely diverging cell types.

We have plated both NCB20 cells and embryonic hippocampal pyramidal neurons in the same dish (Mattson et al. 1989a). In the face of a large dose of A23187, which results in an influx of intracellular calcium into both cell types, only hippocampal pyramidal neurons die. If, on the other hand, one performs the same experiment in the absence of external sodium, both cell types die. This indicates that NCB20 cells survive large influxes because of the presence of an active sodium/calcium exchange system. In fact, when one views intracellular calcium levels with fura-2, one finds that under normal saline conditions, A23187 causes a large rise in both cell types but that the NCB20 cells are capable of restoring themselves back to rest levels. In the absence of sodium, however, even the NCB20 cells display enormous rises in calcium for which they cannot compensate. This finding is nearly identical to those from the more closely related B19 and B5 from *Helisoma* and raises the question as to whether even more subtle differences will eventually be described. For instance, can the same neuron respond quite differently to the same environmental cues simply as a result of the past history of that neuron? As an example, a calcium rise induced by a brief mechanical stimulus to a growth cone is frequently followed by a long undershoot in intracellular levels. This undershoot appears to represent the hysteresis of the compensatory mechanisms in response to the large rise in intracellular calcium (Mills et al. 1988). Another example is from our work with Fields and Nelson (Fields et al. 1990a) on mouse dorsal root ganglion cells. Here, we have found that action potentials can inhibit outgrowth through a rise in intracellular calcium in these neuronal growth cones. However, after chronic stimulation, there is long-term modification of the calcium homeostasis in these cells.

Continued stimulation no longer inhibits outgrowth and no longer produces the large changes in intracellular calcium that were seen initially (Fields et al. 1990b). These examples point to the likelihood that calcium homeostasis could act to encode the history of the neuron and, thus, impart new specific differences between nerve cells. Two apparently identical neurons could well respond quite differently to the same environmental stimulus if one had briefly seen environmental cues to which the other had not been exposed.

CONCLUSIONS

The neuronal growth cone serves multiple roles that extend from early development and may continue to adult neuronal plasticity and even pathological neurodegeneration (Kater et al. 1989). Key to the performance of these functions is the ability to sort out and respond to the many potential influences, both intrinsic and extrinsic, that impinge on the growth cone at any given moment in time. The work reviewed emphasized the integrative capacity of growth cones, showing that the growth cone performs its behaviors through the summation of multiple, differentially weighted cues. Clearly, for many of these cues, intracellular calcium levels act as a nodal point for integration. The impressive and somewhat daunting aspect of this control system lies in the extent of interactions and modifiability of the individual components of calcium homeostasis. From this and likely other integrators, the growth cone takes its most characteristic attribute: the ability to read and interpret multiple, simultaneously impinging, environmental cues.

Clearly, the neuronal growth cone is not just the simple "battering ram" of Ramon y Cajal (1890). Rather, the growth cone emerges as a finely tuned ensemble of subcellular machinery capable of generating quite subtle aspects of neuronal form and function.

ACKNOWLEDGMENTS

We thank M. Schmidt and Drs. L. Mills, L. Davis, and M. Segal for critical input on the manuscript and D. Gidding, R. Olson, and T. Malmstrom for assistance in preparation of the manuscript and the illustrations. This work was supported by National Institutes of Health grants NS-24683, NS-26819, and NS-28323.

Figure 7. Differences in the characteristics of two identified *Helisoma* neurons and their growth cones. (*Top*) Patch recordings from isolated growth cones demonstrate that the growth cones of individual identified neurons display the distinctive signature of ionic currents characteristic of the individual neuron as a whole (Guthrie et al. 1989). (*Second Panel*) These same growth cones show quite different responses to an identical stimulus, in this case, serotonin. Serotonin completely inhibits the outgrowth of neuron B19 growth cones, whereas neuron B5 growth cones continue unaltered in their behavior. (*Third Panel*) These neurons display also quite different calcium homeostatic capacities. In the face of a challenge of increased calcium influx, experimentally evoked by the calcium ionophore A23187 being chronically applied, neurons B5 show a powerful compensatory response to the rise in intracellular calcium and eventually return toward rest levels. On the other hand, neurons B19 show no compensatory responses, and calcium concentrations can rise to toxic levels (Mills and Kater 1990). (*Bottom*) These differences in calcium homeostatic capacity are clearly demonstrated in this preparation. A neuron B5 and a neuron B19 were plated in close proximity. The addition of 0.4 μM A23187 selectively kills the neuron B19. Neuron B5 continues to grow and display all its normal characteristics. Bars: (*Top*) 10 μm; (*Bottom*) 75 μm.

REFERENCES

Alkon, D.L., and H. Rasmussen. 1988. A spatial-temporal model of cell activation. *Science* **239:** 998.

Banker, G.A., and W.M. Cowan. 1977. Rat hippocampal neurons in dispersed cell culture. *Brain Res.* **126:** 397.

———. 1979. Further observations on hippocampal neurons in dispersed cell culture. *J. Comp. Neurol.* **187:** 469.

Cohan, C.S. 1990. Frequency-dependent and cell-specific effects of electrical activity on growth cone movements of cultured *Helisoma* neurons. *J. Neurobiol.* **21:** 400.

Cohan, C.S., and S.B. Kater. 1986. Suppression of neurite elongation and growth cone motility by electrical activity. *Science* **232:** 1638.

Cohan, C.S., J.A. Connor, and S.B. Kater. 1987. Electrically and chemically mediated increases in intracellular calcium in neuronal growth cones. *J. Neurosci.* **7:** 3588.

Fields, R.D., E.A. Neale, and P.G. Nelson. 1990a. Neuronal activity inhibits growth cone motility and neurite outgrowth from mouse sensory neurons. *J. Neurosci.* (in press).

Fields, R.D., P.B. Guthrie, P.G. Nelson, and S.B. Kater. 1990b. Calcium homeostatic capacity is regulated by patterned electrical activity in growth cones of mouse DRG neurons. *Soc. Neurosci Abstr.* (in press).

Forscher, P., L.K. Kaczmarek, J. Buchanan, and S.J. Smith. 1987. Cyclic AMP induces changes in the distribution and transport of organelles within growth cones of *Aplysia* bag neurons. *J. Neurosci.* **7:** 3600.

Grega, D.S., and S.B. Kater. 1987. Reinitiation of outgrowth from dormant neurons in cell culture. *Soc. Neurosci. Abstr.* **13:** 167.

Guthrie, P.B., R.E. Lee, and S.B. Kater. 1989. A comparison of neuronal growth cone and cell body membrane: Electrophysiological and ultrastructural properties. *J. Neurosci.* **9:** 3596.

Hadley, R.D., D.A. Bodnar, and S.B. Kater. 1985. Formation of electrical synapses between isolated, cultured *Helisoma* neurons requires mutual neurite elongation. *J. Neurosci.* **5:** 3145.

Haydon, P.G., D.P. McCobb, and S.B. Kater. 1984. Serotonin selectively inhibits growth cone dynamics and synaptogenesis of specific identified neurons of *Helisoma*. *Science* **226:** 561.

———. 1987. The regulation of neurite outgrowth, growth cone motility, and electrical synaptogenesis by serotonin. *J. Neurobiol.* **18:** 197.

Haydon, P.G., C.S. Cohan, D.P. McCobb, H.R. Miller, and S.B. Kater. 1985. Neuron-specific growth cone properties as seen in identified neurons of *Helisoma*. *J. Neurosci. Res.* **13:** 135.

Ivins, J.K., and R.N. Pittman. 1989. Interactions between sympathetic growth cones *in vitro*. *Soc. Neurosci. Abstr.* **15:** 1037.

Jensen, J.R., V. Rehder, and S.B. Kater. 1990. Differences in Ca^{2+} homeostasis in growth cones and soma of an identified neuron: Na^+-dependent amplification of Ca^{2+} signals in growth cones. *Soc. Neurosci. Abstr.* **16:** (in press).

Kater, S.B. and P.B. Guthrie. 1989. The neuronal growth cone: Calcium regulation of a presecretory structure. In *Secretion and its control*. (ed. C.M. Armstrong and G.S. Oxford) p. 111. Wiley-Interscience, New York.

Kater, S.B. and P. Letourneau. 1985. *The biology of the neuronal growth cone*. A.R. Liss, New York.

Kater, S.B., P.B. Guthrie, and L.R. Mills. 1990. Integration by the neuronal growth cone: A continuum from neuroplasticity to neuropathology. In *Molecular and cellular mechanisms of neural plasticity in aging and Alzheimer's disease.* (ed. P. Coleman et al.). Elsevier, New York. (In press.)

Kater, S.B., M.P. Mattson, and P.B. Guthrie. 1989. Calcium-induced neuronal degeneration: A normal growth cone regulating signal gone awry (?). In *Calcium, membrane, aging, and Alzheimer's disease* (ed. C.W. Cottman and Lavin), vol. 568, p. 252. New York Academy of Sciences, New York. (In press.)

Kater, S.B., P.B. Guthrie, M.P. Mattson, L.R. Mills, and R.S. Zucker. 1988. Calcium homeostasis in molluscan and mammalian neurons: Dynamics of calcium regulation. *Soc. Neurosci. Abstr.* **14:** 582.

Mattson, M.P. and S.B. Kater. 1987. Calcium regulation of neurite elongation and growth cone motility. *J. Neurosci.* **7:** 4034.

Mattson, M.P., P. Dou, and S.B. Kater. 1988. Outgrowth-regulating actions of glutamate in isolated hippocampal pyramidal neurons. *J. Neurosci.* **8:** 2087.

Mattson, M.P., P.B. Guthrie, and S.B. Kater. 1989a. A role for Na^+-dependent calcium extrusion in protection against neuronal excitotoxicity. *FASEB J.* **3:** 2519.

Mattson, M.P., M. Murrain, P.B. Guthrie, and S.B. Kater. 1989b. Fibroblast growth factor and glutamate: Opposing roles in the generation and degeneration of hippocampal architecture. *J. Neurosci.* **9:** 3728.

Mattson, M.P., R.E. Lee, M.E. Adams, P.B. Guthrie, and S.B. Kater. 1988. Interactions between entorhinal axons and target hippocampal neurons: A role for glutamate in the development of hippocampal circuitry. *Neuron* **1:** 865.

McBurney, R.N. and R. Neeting. 1987. Neuronal calcium homeostasis. *Trends Neurosci.* **10:** 164.

McCobb, D.P. 1987. "Neurotransmitter regulation of outgrowth of neuronal processes." Ph.D. thesis, University of Iowa, Iowa City.

McCobb, D.P. and S.B. Kater. 1988. Membrane voltage and neurotransmitter regulation of neuronal growth cone motility. *Dev. Biol.* **130:** 599.

McCobb, D.P., P.G. Haydon, and S.B. Kater. 1988a. Dopamine and serotonin inhibition of neurite elongation of different identified neurons. *J. Neurosci. Res.* **19:** 19.

McCobb, D.P., C.S. Cohan, J.A. Connor, and S.B. Kater. 1988b. Interactive effects of serotonin and acetylcholine on neurite elongation. *Neuron* **1:** 377.

Mills, L.R. and S.B. Kater. 1990. Neuron-specific and state-specific differences in calcium homeostasis regulate the generation and degeneration on neuronal architecture. *Neuron* **2:** 149.

Mills, L.R., M. Murrain, P.B. Guthrie, and S.B. Kater. 1988. Intracellular calcium concentrations in neuronal growth cones change with induced turning and branching behavior. *Soc. Neurosci. Abstr.* **14:** 583.

Murphy, A.D. and S.B. Kater. 1980. Sprouting and functional regencration of identified neurons in *Helisoma*. *Brain Res.* **186:** 251.

Purves, D., R.D. Hadley, and J.T. Voyvodic. 1986. Dynamic changes in the dendritic morphology of individual neurons visualized over periods of up to three months in the superior cervical ganglion of living mice. *J. Neurosci.* **6:** 1051.

Ramon y Cajal, S. 1890. A quelle epoque apparaissent les expansions des cellules nerveuses de la moelle epiniere du poulet. *Anat. Anz.* **5:** 609.

Rehder, V., J.R. Jensen, P. Dou, and S.B. Kater. 1990. Calcium homeostasis in an identified neuronal growth cone. *Soc. Neurosci. Abstr.* **16:** (in press).

Neurotrophic Factors, Their Receptors, and the Signal Transduction Pathways They Activate

G.D. Yancopoulos,* P.C. Maisonpierre,* N.Y. Ip,* T.H. Aldrich,* L. Belluscio,*
T.G. Boulton,† M.H. Cobb,† S.P. Squinto,* and M.E. Furth*

*Regeneron Pharmaceuticals, Inc., Tarrytown, New York 10591-6707; †Southwestern Graduate School of Biomedical
Sciences, University of Texas, Dallas, Texas 75235-9041

The development and maintenance of the vertebrate nervous system depends on neuronal survival proteins known as neurotrophic factors (for review, see Snider and Johnson 1989). Nerve growth factor (NGF) remains the best-characterized neurotrophic factor. Understanding the role and action of NGF has been aided greatly by the apparently fortuitous discovery of a rich source of this protein in male mouse submaxillary glands, which led to the generation of NGF-neutralizing antibodies as well as the molecular cloning of NGF (Scott et al. 1983; Ullrich et al. 1983). Monoclonal antibodies to the receptor for NGF permitted the cloning of one component of this receptor (Chao et al. 1986; Radeke et al. 1987); this transmembrane protein can mediate low-affinity binding to NGF when expressed alone but can interact with other molecules to generate a high-affinity NGF-binding site (Hempstead et al. 1989). The various reagents and molecular probes for the study of NGF and its receptor have yielded a great deal of information concerning the sites and mechanisms of NGF action in cultures of primary neurons and in the animal. These studies have been complemented by work on NGF-responsive immortalized cell lines (Greene et al. 1987). Such cellular models have been used in extensive analyses of the signal transduction pathways that are triggered by NGF. Although the details of the transduction process are not yet known, increasingly strong evidence suggests that NGF can cause activation of parallel phosphorylation cascades that result in significant physiological changes within the responding cell, culminating in an altered program of gene expression (Mutoh and Guroff 1989).

Because NGF only supports a limited set of neuronal populations, the existence of additional neurotrophic factors has long been postulated. However, the extremely low abundance of such factors has impeded their molecular characterization. Nevertheless, two neurotrophic factors related to NGF, namely, brain-derived neurotrophic factor (BDNF) and neurotrophin-3 (NT-3), as well as another neurotrophic factor unrelated to the NGF/BDNF/NT-3 family called ciliary neurotrophic factor (CNTF), have recently been molecularly cloned (Leibrock et al. 1989; Lin et al. 1989; Stockli et al. 1989; Hohn et al. 1990; Maisonpierre et al. 1990a). In this paper, we describe our insights into important structural features of the NGF/NT-3/BDNF family (designated the "neurotrophin"

family) as well as the finding of an unprecedented degree of evolutionary conservation for NT-3 and BDNF. We explore the spatiotemporal distribution of NT-3 and BDNF synthesis in vivo, revealing a reciprocal relationship between the expression of these two molecules in the developing nervous system, and correlating remarkably high levels of NT-3 expression with critical events in early neural development. We also describe an "epitope tagging" method that has allowed us to define cells that bear receptors for (and display transcriptional responses to) neurotrophic factors. Finally, we describe the molecular cloning of a family of novel mammalian protein kinases, most of which are related to kinases that regulate the yeast response to pheromones, the activation of which may represent one of the earliest events triggered by NGF in responsive cells.

RESULTS AND DISCUSSION

Absolute Conservation of BDNF and NT-3 Structure in Mammals

NGF, BDNF, and NT-3 are short (~120 amino acids), basic (pI about 10) proteins that share about 50% sequence identity (Hohn et al. 1990; Maisonpierre et al. 1990a). These identities include six cysteine residues that, in active NGF, have been shown to form three disulfide bridges. Amino acids flanking these cysteine residues comprise the regions most similar among these three related proteins. All three neurotrophins seem to be initially synthesized as longer precursors that are proteolytically cleaved to release the mature neurotrophins, which essentially constitute the carboxy-terminal 120 amino acids of each precursor.

Using probes designed on the basis of the pig BDNF (Leibrock et al. 1989) and rodent NT-3 gene sequences (Hohn et al. 1990; Maisonpierre et al. 1990a), we molecularly cloned genomic DNA fragments containing the human and rat BDNF genes and the human NT-3 gene. DNA sequences obtained from the human and rat BDNF genomic clones were aligned with the known pig cDNA sequence (Fig. 1), and a sequence obtained from the human NT-3 genomic clone was similarly aligned with the mouse (Hohn et al. 1990) and rat (Maisonpierre et al. 1990) genomic NT-3 sequences (Fig. 2). Surprisingly, the predicted amino acid se-

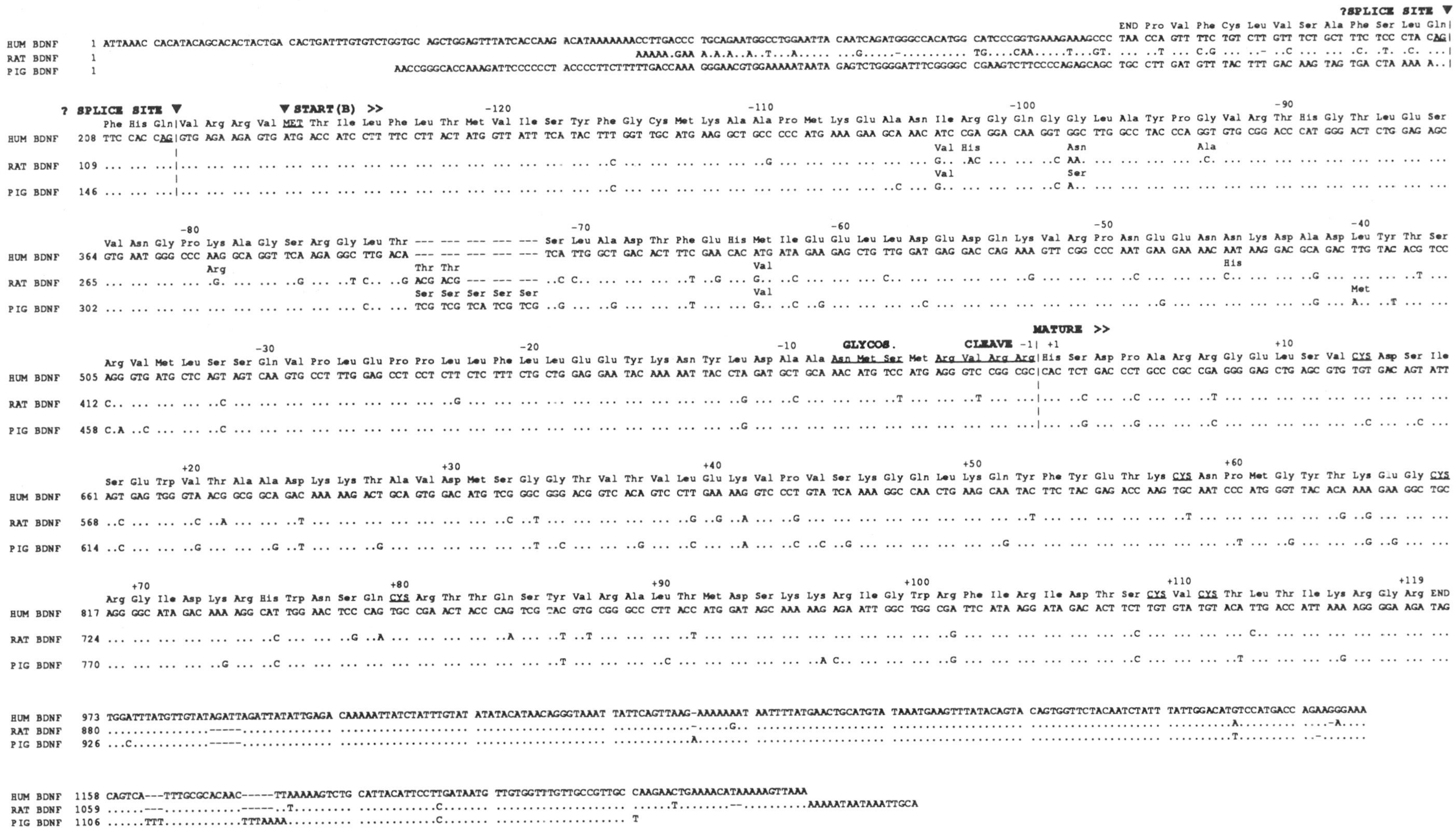

Figure 1. Comparison of human, rat, and pig BDNF nucleotide and amino acid sequences. Amino acid translation is provided above human sequence; amino acids are numbered with position +1 assigned to the first residue of mature BDNF. DNA sequence identities to the human sequence are indicated by a dot, and gaps are identified with a dash. Only amino acids differences with the human sequence are indicated for the pig and rat sequences. The potential splice acceptor sites/intron boundaries upstream of the "B start site," the B start site initiation codon, the cleavage site used to release mature BDNF, and the conserved glycosylation site just upstream of this cleavage site are indicated (significance of many of these sites discussed in Maisonpierre et al. [1990a]).

```
                                                                                                                                                              START (B) >>>
                                                                                                                         ?SPLICE |   ?SPLICE |               |                            -130
                                                        END His Arg Leu Ser Cys Gln Ser Leu Leu Leu Thr Pro Val Phe Pro --Phe Gln|Ile Leu Gln|Val Asn Lys Val|Met Ser Ile Leu Phe Tyr Val Ile Phe Leu Ala Tyr Leu Arg Gly Ile
HUM NT3     1 CCTCACAGGGCTACTCAGCC TCAGGTAGCTGGTGCCAGAA TAA CAC AGA CTC AGC TGC CAG AGC CTG CTC TTA ACA CCT GTG TTT CCT --TTT CAG|ATC TTA CAG|GTG AAC AAG GTG|ATG TCC ATC TTG TTT TAT GTG ATA TTT CTC GCT TAT CTC CGT GGC ATC
RAT NT3     1                         ••••G••••A•T•••T•• •G• •C• ••• ••- --• •T• •-- ••T •A• A•A ••• ••• •T• ••• ••• ••• TC••• •••|••• ••• •••|••• ••• ••• •••|••• ••• ••• ••• ••• ••• ••• ••• ••• ••• ••T ••• ••• ••• ••• •••
MOU NT3     1                                                                                                                                                |••• ••• ••• ••• ••• ••• ••• ••• ••• ••• ••T ••• ••• ••• ••• •••

                  -120                                    -110                                    -100                                    -90                                     -80                                     -70
              Gln Gly Asn Asn Met Asp Gln Arg Ser Leu Pro Glu Asp Ser Leu Asn Ser Leu Ile Ile Lys Leu Ile Gln Ala Asp Ile Leu Lys Asn Lys Leu Ser Lys Gln Met Val Asp Val Lys Glu Asn Tyr Gln Ser Thr Leu Pro Lys Ala Glu Ala
HUM NT3   164 CAA GGT AAC AAC ATG GAT CAA AGG AGT TTG CCA GAA GAC TCG CTC AAT TCC CTC ATT ATT AAG CTG ATC CAG GCA GAT ATT TTG AAA AAC AAG CTC TCC AAG CAG ATG GTG GAC GTT AAG GAA AAT TAC CAG AGC ACC CTG CCC AAA GCT GAG GCT

RAT NT3   139 ••• ••C ••• ••• ••• ••• ••• ••• ••• ••• ••• ••• ••• ••T ••• ••• ••• ••• ••• ••C ••• T•• ••• ••• ••G ••• ••C ••• ••• ••• ••• ••• ••• ••• ••• ••• ••A ••T ••• ••• ••• ••• ••• ••• ••• ••• ••• ••• ••• ••A ••• ••A

                          Ser
MOU NT3    49 ••• ••C ••• •G• ••• ••• ••• ••• ••• ••• ••G ••• ••• ••T ••• ••• ••• ••• ••C ••C ••• ••• ••• ••• ••G ••• ••C ••• ••• ••• ••• ••T ••• ••A ••• ••• ••• ••T ••• ••• ••• ••• ••• ••• ••• ••• ••• ••• ••• ••A ••• ••A

                                                                                                                              ?CLEAVE
                                                  -60                                     -50                                     -40                                     -30                                     -20
              Pro Arg Glu Pro Glu Gln Gly Gly Pro Arg Lys Ser Ala Phe Gln Pro Val Ile Ala Met Asp Thr Glu Leu Leu Arg Gln Gln Arg Arg Tyr Asn Ser Pro Arg Val Leu Leu Ser Asp Thr Thr Pro Leu Glu Pro Pro Pro Leu Tyr Leu Met
HUM NT3   320 CCC CGA GAG CCG GAG CAG GGA GGG CCC CGC AAG TCA GCA TTC CAG CCA GTG ATT GCA ATG GAC ACC GAA CTG CTG CGA CAA CAG AGA CGC TAC AAC TCA CCG CGG GTC CTG CTG AGC GAC ACG ACC CCC TTG GAG CCC CCG CCC TTG TAT CTC ATG

                                          Glu Ala Thr Arg     Glu             Met         Thr                                                                                  Ser
RAT NT3   295 ••• A•• ••A ••A ••• ••• ••• •A• G•• AC• •G• ••• •A• ••• ••• ••G A•• ••• ••• •CA ••• ••A ••• ••A ••A ••G ••• ••• ••• ••• ••• ••T ••• ••C ••• ••• ••• ••• ••T ••• •GC ••• ••T ••• ••• ••• ••T ••• ••A ••• ••A •••

                                          Glu Ala Thr Arg     Glu             Met         Thr                                                                                  Ser
MOU NT3   205 ••• A•G ••A ••A ••• ••• ••• •A• G•• AC• •G• ••• •AG ••• ••• ••• A•• ••• ••• •C• ••• ••A ••G ••A ••A ••G ••• ••• ••• ••• ••• ••T ••G ••C ••• ••• ••• ••• ••T ••• •GC ••• ••T ••• ••• ••• ••T ••• ••A ••C ••A •••

                                                                                          MATURE >>>
                                              -10     GLYCOS.             CLEAVE       -1| +1                                +10                                     +20                                     +30
              Glu Asp Tyr Val Gly Ser Pro Val Val Ala Asn Arg Thr Ser --- Arg Arg Lys Arg|Tyr Ala Glu His Lys Ser His Arg Gly Glu Tyr Ser Val CYS Asp Ser Glu Ser Leu Trp Val Thr Asp Lys Ser Ser Ala Ile Asp Ile Arg Gly His
HUM NT3   476 GAG GAT TAC GTG GGC AGC CCC GTG GTG GCG AAC AGA ACA TCA --- CGG CGG AAA CGG|TAC GCG GAG CAT AAG AGT CAC CGA GGG GAG TAC TCG GTA TGT GAC AGT GAG AGT CTG TGG GTG ACC GAC AAG TCA TCG GCC ATC GAC ATT CGG GGA CAC
                                                                                         |
                                  Asn             Thr                 Pro                |
RAT NT3   451 ••A ••• ••T ••• ••• •A• ••G ••• ••A A•C ••T ••• ••• ••• CCA ••• A•• ••• ••C|••T ••A ••• ••• ••• ••• ••• ••• ••A ••• ••• ••A ••G ••• ••• ••• ••• ••• ••C ••• ••• ••• ••• ••• ••C ••A ••• ••T ••• ••• ••• ••• •••
                                                                                         |
                                  Asn                                 Pro                |
MOU NT3   361 ••• ••• ••T ••• ••• •A• ••G ••• ••A ••C ••T ••• ••C ••• CCA ••• A•• ••• ••C|••T ••A ••A ••• ••• ••• ••• ••• ••A ••• ••• ••A ••G ••• ••• ••• ••• ••• ••C ••• ••• ••• ••• ••• ••C ••A ••• ••T ••• ••• ••• ••• •••

                                      +40                                     +50                                     +60                                     +70                                     +80
              Gln Val Thr Val Leu Gly Glu Ile Lys Thr Gly Asn Ser Pro Val Lys Gln Tyr Phe Tyr Glu Thr Arg CYS Lys Glu Ala Arg Pro Val Lys Asn Gly CYS Arg Gly Ile Asp Asp Lys His Trp Asn Ser Gln CYS Lys Thr Ser Gln Thr Tyr
HUM NT3   629 CAG GTC ACG GTG CTG GGG GAG ATC AAA ACG GGC AAC TCT CCC GTC AAA CAA TAT TTT TAT GAA ACG CGA TGT AAG GAA GCC AGG CCG GTC AAA AAC GGT TGC AGG GGT ATT GAT GAT AAA CAC TGG AAC TCT CAG TGC AAA ACA TCC CAA ACC TAC

RAT NT3   607 ••• ••T ••A ••• T•• ••A ••• ••• ••• ••C ••• ••• ••• ••T ••G ••• ••• ••• ••• ••• ••• ••• A•G ••• ••A ••• ••• ••• ••A ••• ••• ••• ••• ••• ••• ••G ••• ••• ••C ••• ••• ••• ••• ••• ••• ••• ••• ••G ••G ••• ••• •••

MOU NT3   517 ••• ••• ••A ••• ••• ••A ••• ••• ••• ••C ••T ••• ••• ••T ••G ••• ••• ••• ••• ••• ••• ••• A•• ••• ••A ••• ••• ••• ••• ••• ••• ••• ••• ••• ••• ••G ••• ••• ••C ••• ••• ••• ••• ••• ••• ••• ••• ••T ••G ••• ••• ••T

                              +90                                     +100                                    +110                            +119
              Val Arg Ala Leu Thr Ser Glu Asn Asn Lys Leu Val Gly Trp Arg Trp Ile Arg Ile Asp Thr Ser CYS Val CYS Ala Leu Ser Arg Lys Ile Gly Arg Thr END
HUM NT3   785 GTC CGA GCA CTG ACT TCA GAG AAC AAT AAA CTC GTG GGC TGG CGG TGG ATA CGG ATA GAC ACG TCC TGT GTG TGT GCC TTG TCG AGA AAA ATC GGA AGA ACA TGA ATTGGCATCTC TCCCCATATATAAATTATTA CTTTAAATTATATGATATGC

RAT NT3   763 ••• ••• ••• ••• ••• ••• ••A ••• ••C ••• ••• ••A ••• ••• ••C ••• ••• ••A ••• ••• ••T ••• ••• ••• ••• ••• ••• ••A ••• ••• ••• ••• ••• ••• ••• ••••••••••G ••••••C•••••••••••• ••••••••••••••••••••

MOU NT3   673 ••• ••• ••• ••• ••• ••• ••A ••• ••C ••• ••• ••A ••• ••• ••C ••• ••• ••A ••• ••• ••T ••• ••• ••• ••• ••• ••• ••• ••• ••• ••T ••• ••• ••• •••


HUM NT3   941 ATGTAGCATATAAATGTTTA TATTGTTTTTATATA-TATAA GTTGACCTTTATTTATTAAA CTTCAGCAACC-CTACAGTAT ATAAGCTT

RAT NT3   919 •••••••••••••••••••• •••••••••••••••T••••• •••••••••••••••••••• •••••••••••T•••••••••• ••••••••TTTTTTCTCAATA AAATTCGTGTGCTTGCC
```

Figure 2. Comparison of human, rat, and mouse NT-3 nucleotide and amino acid sequences. Amino acid translation is provided above the human sequence; amino acids are numbered with position +1 assigned to the first residue of mature NT-3. DNA sequence identities to the human sequence are indicated by a dot, and gaps are identified with a dash. Only amino acids differences with the human sequence are indicated for the pig and rat sequences. The potential splice acceptor sites/intron boundaries upstream of the B start site, the B start site initiation codon, a potential upstream cleavage site, as well as the cleavage site used to release mature NT-3, and the conserved glycosylation site just upstream of this latter cleavage site are indicated (significance of many of these sites discussed in Maisonpierre et al. [1990a]).

Table 1. Conservation of NGF, BDNF, and NT-3 in Mammals

	Human NGF (%)	Human BDNF (%)	Human NT-3 (%)
Cow	95 (6)	n.d.	n.d.
Pig	n.d.	100 (0)	n.d.
Rat	92 (9)	100 (0)	100 (0)
Mouse	90 (12)	100 (0)	100 (0)

The percentage of identity between the mature forms of each of the three human neurotrophins and their counterparts in other mammals is indicated. The number of amino acid differences between each compared pair is included in the parentheses. n.d. indicates not determined.

quences of the mature proteins encoded by the rat and human BDNF genes are identical to that of the porcine BDNF, whereas the mature protein predicted by the human NT-3 gene is identical to that encoded by the mouse and rat genes. This extreme degree of evolutionary conservation among the mammalian BDNF and NT-3 proteins (in each case, complete identity among three mammalian species of the 119-amino-acid mature forms) ranks both BDNF and NT-3 among the most conserved of mammalian proteins and has not been seen for any other secreted factor. The degree of evolutionary conservation of mature BDNF and NT-3 in mammals far exceeds that seen for even the relatively highly conserved NGF molecule (Table 1). The absolute conservation of these proteins in mammals implies remarkably strong evolutionary constraints on their structures.

Spatiotemporal Distribution of Neurotrophin Gene Expression

Defining neuronal populations that are dependent on particular neurotrophic factors in vivo requires detailed analyses of the availability of these factors and their receptors. Such studies with NGF have shown that this factor is synthesized in the target regions of NGF-dependent neurons in both the peripheral nervous system (PNS) and the central nervous system (CNS) (for review, see Thoenen et al. 1987). The first studies of NT-3 and BDNF mRNA expression revealed that NT-3 is broadly distributed in peripheral tissues and in the CNS (Hohn et al. 1990; Maisonpierre et al. 1990a), whereas results with BDNF were more equivocal. Initial studies with BDNF in the mouse defined a single major transcript (∼1.4 kb) for BDNF, which was seen only in the CNS (Leibrock et al. 1989); a subsequent study reported two major BDNF transcripts in the rat (1.6 and 4.0 kb), with significant expression in a limited number of peripheral tissues as well as in the CNS (Maisonpierre et al. 1990a). To explore BDNF expression further, we used rat and human BDNF probes to compare levels of BDNF mRNA in mouse, rat, and human tissues. Two major BDNF transcripts (∼1.6 and 4 kb) were seen in all three species under both high- and low-stringency hybridization conditions and using either DNA or cRNA probes. Similar tissue distributions were observed in the three species examined. In addition to substantial expression in brain, BDNF

transcripts were detectable in rat heart, lung, and muscle tissues; in mouse heart, lung, muscle, and kidney tissues; and in human lung tissue (Fig. 3A,B,C).

To obtain further insights into the potentially unique roles of each of the related neurotrophins in the CNS, we performed a more detailed comparison, by quantitative Northern blot analysis, between NT-3, BDNF, and NGF mRNA expression in developing and adult rats (Maisonpierre et al. 1990b). One striking observation is that the initial expression of all three members of the neurotrophin family occurs between the 11th and 12th day of embryonic life (E11–E12), roughly coincident with the onset of neurogenesis both in the CNS and in the PNS (Maisonpierre et al. 1990b). Furthermore, the synthesis of each factor then can be detected throughout embryonic development and is maintained in adult life. The final level of NGF, BDNF, and NT-3 mRNAs in adult rat brain is quite similar. However, the detailed pattern of expression of each neurotrophin is quite distinct with respect both to time and to regions of the CNS.

In total brain, the level of NGF mRNA remains roughly constant from about embryonic day 13 (E13), through birth, postnatal development, and in the adult (data not shown). In contrast, the expression of BDNF mRNA in the brain is relatively low in the embryo, increases significantly after birth, and is highest in the adult. Finally, the expression of NT-3 mRNA in the brain starts at much higher levels in the early embryo, peaking at about E13, remains relatively high throughout the first few weeks of postnatal development, and then decreases to the final adult level.

Because neuronal development proceeds at different rates in discrete areas of the CNS, it was important to analyze expression of the neurotrophins in specific regions. The developmental pattern of expression of NGF, BDNF, and NT-3 mRNAs in the spinal cord, cerebellum, and hippocampus is summarized in Figure 4. In these and other areas of the CNS, high levels of expression of NT-3 correlate consistently with those crucial periods in early neural development in which neurogenesis, neuronal migration, and neuronal differentiation occur. Thus, for example, NT-3 mRNA expression peaks and then decreases significantly earlier in the spinal cord (Fig. 4A) than in the cerebellum (Fig. 4B), in good accord with the timing of neuronal maturation in these regions. As in total brain, the expression pattern of BDNF in each region examined is

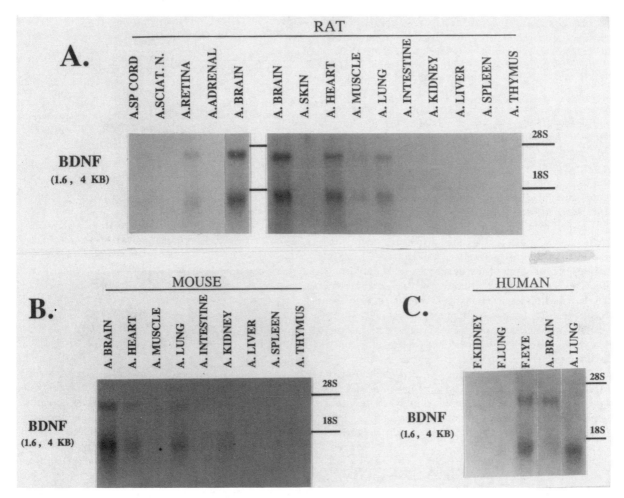

Figure 3. Expression of BDNF in indicated adult rat tissues (*A*), adult mouse tissues (*B*), and fetal and adult human tissues (*C*). Positions of 18S and 28S rRNAs are indicated on the right of each panel, whereas sizes of major BDNF transcripts are indicated in kilobases on the left. Of the total RNA, 10 μg were used in each lane; the probe prepared from rat BDNF gene was used for *A* and *B*, whereas the probe prepared from human BDNF gene was used in *C*.

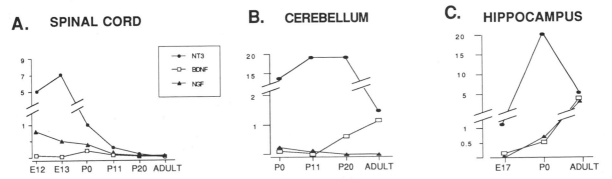

Figure 4. Developmentally regulated expression of the NT-3, BDNF, and NGF genes in the rat spinal cord (*A*), cerebellum (*B*), and hippocampus (*C*). Quantitation of neurotrophin mRNA levels in various samples was performed by comparing them with defined synthetic RNA standards. These levels were then normalized to adult brain levels to simplify comparison. The levels of all three transcripts in the adult brain are similar. Levels of NT-3, BDNF, and NGF mRNAs in total adult brain RNA are approximately 40, 45, and 30 fg/μg, respectively. In the figure, levels of all three transcripts in adult brain were arbitrarily set at 1.0 (for details, see Maisonpierre et al. 1990b).

essentially reciprocal to that of NT-3, whereas NT-3 expression decreases dramatically as neurons mature and BDNF expression increases. However, for each of the three regions shown in Figure 4, the final level of BDNF mRNA in the adult is similar to that of NT-3. Finally, the expression of NGF mRNA varies during the development of these CNS regions but not consistently; it gradually decreases from E12 through adulthood in the spinal cord, increases from E17 through adulthood in the hippocampus, and decreases from very low levels at birth to barely detectable levels in the adult cerebellum.

Because NT-3 supports the survival of at least some neurons that also can depend on NGF and/or BDNF for survival (Maisonpierre et al. 1990a) and because its expression is dramatically linked to early neural development, it is attractive to postulate that NT-3 is responsible for some of the developmentally important functions previously attributed to NGF and BDNF. NT-3 might thus act as a classical target-derived neurotrophic factor during development, the limited expression of which results in neuronal selection and pruning. However, the high levels of NT-3 expression in early development could also reflect other roles. Thus, NT-3 might be involved in regulating the proliferation or differentiation of neuronal precursors or in the guidance of migrating cells or their axons. On the other hand, BDNF may play a more important role later in development, perhaps by mediating neuronal maturation or by playing a role in neuronal maintenance. The observations that NT-3 and BDNF are reciprocally expressed during development of the CNS but achieve similar levels within the adult CNS suggest that NT-3 may act both early and late in the development of the same neuronal populations that are predominately affected late in their development by BDNF. The expression profiles of all three neurotrophins do share a similarly high level of expression in the adult hippocampus (Fig. 4C), consistent with the possibility that this region normally supplies all three neurotrophins to the basal forebrain and/or other important hippocampal afferents.

Detection of Neurotrophin Receptors Using "Ligand Tagging"

The determination of which neuronal populations respond to neurotrophic factors in vivo requires not only elucidation of the spatiotemporal distribution of factor synthesis, but also identification of the actual cells bearing receptors for these factors. In the absence of antibodies to the recently cloned neurotrophic factors or their receptors, we decided to use polymerase chain reaction (PCR) technology to engineer genetically "tagged" neurotrophic factors that could be used in binding assays to detect specifically the receptors for these ligands (S.P. Squinto et al., in prep.). In one particular example, we added a 10-amino-acid epitope derived from the human c-*myc* proto-oncogene to the carboxyl terminus of rat CNTF (Fig. 5A,B); this epitope had previously been used to tag proteins in order

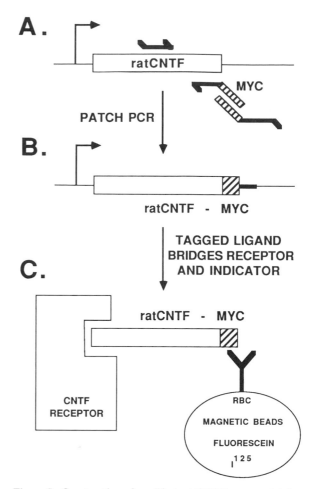

Figure 5. Construction of modified rat CNTF gene containing *myc*-epitope using three oligonucleotides and patch PCR technology (*A, B*) and use of this ligand as a bridge for identification of CNTF receptor using antibodies coupled to variety of indicators (for details, see S.P. Squinto et al., in prep.).

to follow their intracellular trafficking and their expression within embryos (Munro and Pelham 1987; McMahon and Moon 1989). A well-characterized monoclonal antibody that efficiently and specifically recognizes the "*myc* tag" (Evan et al. 1985) was coupled to a variety of reporters (e.g., red blood cells [RBC], immunobeads or magnetic beads, fluorescein or a radioisotope), allowing detection of receptors bound to the tagged ligand by rosetting, immunofluorescence, or autoradiography (Fig. 5C). Screening cell lines for rosetting using the tagged CNTF ligand revealed that receptor-positive cell lines constituted an interesting subset of all lines examined. Only neuronal cell lines were receptor-positive; although only one of the four neuroblastomas examined was rosette-positive, all three neuroepitheliomas and two of three Ewing's sarcomas (a tumor closely related to neuroepithelioma) were rosette-positive (Table 2).

A functional interaction between a protein factor and its cognate receptor results in the activation of intracellular signal transduction pathways, which can involve a number of different second messengers and protein-kinase-mediated phosphorylation cascades. These sig-

Table 2. Expression of CNTF Receptors and Responses to CNTF in a Variety of Human Neural Cell Lines

	Rosette	CNTF *fos/jun*
Neuroblastoma		
LAN-1	−	−
LAN-5	−	−
CHP-126	−	−
SY5Y	+	+
Neuroepitheliomas		
SH-EP	+	+
CHP-100	+	+
SK-N-MC	+	+
Ewing's sarcomas		
5838	+	+
EW1	+	+
RD-ES	−	−

Specific CNTF binding was assayed by red blood cell rosetting using *myc*-tagged CNTF (see text) and immediate-early gene responses (*fos/jun*) were assayed by Northern blot analysis of cells exposed to physiological levels of CNTF for 30 min (for details, see S.P. Squinto et al., in prep.).

nal transduction pathways are coordinately linked to the rapid activation of immediate-early primary response genes. Transcriptional activation of the c-*fos* and c-*jun* proto-oncogenes, which are immediate-early response genes activated by a wide variety of signals, can often serve as a useful marker of a functional interaction between a given ligand and its receptor. The presence of a functional CNTF receptor on the CNTF binding cell lines was demonstrated by a perfect correlation between the rapid induction of c-*fos* and/or c-*jun* by CNTF in these target cells and their ability to bind CNTF in the rosetting assay (Table 2). In addition to defining cell lines that might be useful for elucidating the signal transduction pathways used in the CNTF response, the "tagged ligand" strategy is also being used to define neuronal targets for CNTF, as well as other neurotrophic factors, in primary neuronal cultures and in vivo and in strategies aimed at molecularly cloning the CNTF receptor.

Molecular Cloning of Genes Encoding an NGF-induced Kinase and Its Homologs

The availability of the NGF-responsive cell line PC12 has permitted extensive analysis of the multiple intracellular signal transduction pathways triggered by the binding of NGF to its high-affinity receptor (Mutoh and Guroff 1989). One of the earliest biochemical changes detectable within NGF-activated PC12 cells is the activation of a serine-threonine protein kinase known as MAP2 kinase, thus named because *mi*crotubule-*a*ssociated *p*rotein-2 is a useful substrate for assaying its phosphorylating activity. In PC12 cells, activation of this protein kinase can be detected within 1 minute of exposure to NGF (Miyasaka et al. 1990; T.G. Boulton and M.H. Cobb, unpubl.). An identical or very similar kinase is also activated by a variety of stimuli in many other cell types, both proliferating and postmitotic (Ray and Sturgill 1987, 1988; Hoshi et al. 1988; Rossomando et al. 1989; Boulton et al. 1990a;

Ely et al. 1990). Several extracellular cues initiate signal transduction by activating protein-tyrosine kinases either intrinsic to or associated with specific cell-surface receptors; these kinases then trigger phosphorylation cascades consisting of protein serine-threonine kinases, few of which have been identified. In addition to being very rapidly activated in a variety of responses, MAP2 kinase is one of the few serine-threonine kinases known to be phosphorylated on tyrosine residues in vivo (Ray and Sturgill 1988), and it has the ability to activate at least one downstream kinase (the "S6" kinase). Thus, it has been suggested that MAP2 kinase may be a direct substrate for the protein-tyrosine kinase activity of cell-surface receptors and that it may act as a very early intermediate in a variety of phosphorylation cascades. Although the NGF receptor subunit, which has been cloned and characterized in detail, is not a protein-tyrosine kinase, it may well be associated with another subunit that has such an activity and is responsible for the rapid activation of MAP2 kinase.

We purified a MAP2 kinase based on its activation in response to insulin in fibroblasts bearing insulin receptors, obtained a partial amino acid sequence, and used this sequence to design a PCR-based strategy to clone cDNAs encoding the MAP2 kinase. This approach led to the identification of several closely related (∼80–90% identical) but distinct genes encoding novel serine-threonine kinases; one of these corresponded to the purified MAP2 kinase (Boulton et al. 1990b). We have renamed this MAP2 kinase as ERK1 (*e*xtracellular-*s*ignal *r*egulated *k*inase) and have sequentially numbered additional members of this novel family. A comparison with known protein sequences reveals that the ERK proteins are most closely related (50–55% identical) to two protein kinases, FUS3 (Elion et al. 1990) and KSS1 (Courchesne et al. 1989), involved in mediating the response to pheromones in the yeast *Saccharomyces cerevisiae* (Fig. 6). The ERK family members are significantly less related to their next closest relatives, the CDC2/CDC28 family of protein kinases (Fig. 6). The FUS3 and KSS1 kinases play antagonistic roles in regulating the cell cycle in response to mating-factor pheromones, the only peptide hormones known to mediate intercellular communication in yeast. Both kinases act by fine-tuning the activity of CDC28, a related kinase that is the indispensable regulator of the mitotic cycle. FUS3 also independently acts to trigger the onset of mating-specific functions. The ERK kinases appear to represent mammalian counterparts to the yeast kinases; they may therefore also act to regulate the cell cycle as well as the differentiated state of the cell (the latter being particularly relevant in considering their actions in postmitotic neurons) in response to extracellular signals.

The molecular cloning of a family of signal-response protein kinases, representing mammalian counterparts to the kinases used to mediate pheromone responses in unicellular organisms, should facilitate the elucidation of the roles and mechanisms of action of these enzymes in mammals. Individual members of the ERK family may mediate responses in different cell types and/or to

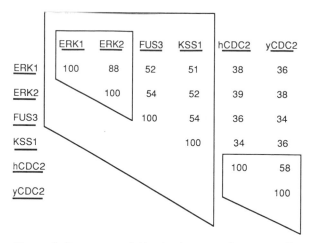

	ERK1	ERK2	FUS3	KSS1	hCDC2	yCDC2
ERK1	100	88	52	51	38	36
ERK2		100	54	52	39	38
FUS3			100	54	36	34
KSS1				100	34	36
hCDC2					100	58
yCDC2						100

Figure 6. Percentage of identity between the mammalian ERK1 and ERK2 proteins and other protein kinases. The ERK kinases comprise a mammalian family of closely related proteins (*upper left*, box), whose closest relatives are the yeast FUS3 and KSS1 kinases (larger box). These kinases are all significantly less related to their next closest relatives, the human (h) and yeast (y) CDC2 kinases, which are as related to each other (*lower right*, box) as the ERK kinases are to their putative yeast counterparts.

different stimuli. Alternatively, a growth factor may induce division in a cycling cell and a neurotrophic factor may elicit differentiation in a postmitotic neuron by triggering activation of the same initial kinase(s), with different downstream effects resulting from the presence of unique phosphorylation substrates for these kinases in the different cells.

SUMMARY

Our studies of the spatiotemporal availability of neurotrophic factors, coupled with tagged ligand binding assays that identify cells bearing receptors for these factors, should lead toward defining the physiological roles of these molecules in the animal. The use of the tagged ligands to identify factor-responsive cell lines has also provided new model systems for the examination of ligand-receptor interactions, as well as for the study of the subsequent induction of intracellular response pathways. To obtain insights into such intracellular pathways, we have molecularly cloned genes encoding a family of serine-threonine protein kinases, most closely related to kinases involved in the yeast response to pheromones. These kinases may be crucial regulators of early steps in the response of mammalian cells to neurotrophic factors as well as other extracellular signals.

ACKNOWLEDGMENTS

We thank Drs. Leonard Schleifer, Ronald Lindsay, Beth Friedman, and Stanley Weigand for enthusiastic discussions and productive scientific interactions. Our thanks to the rest of the Regeneron community, in particular to Dan Everdeen for his technical assistance and Karen Nash for superb organizational skills.

REFERENCES

Boulton, T.G., J.S. Gregory, S.M. Jong, L.H. Wang, L. Ellis, and M.H. Cobb. 1990a. Evidence for insulin-dependent activation of S6 and microtubule-associated protein-2 kinases via a human insulin receptor/v-ros hybrid. *J. Biol. Chem.* **265**(5): 2713.

Boulton, T.G., G.D. Yancopoulos, J.S. Gregory, C. Slaughter, C. Moomaw, J. Hsu, and M.H. Cobb. 1990b. An insulin-stimulated protein kinase related to yeast kinases involved in cell cycle control. *Science* **249**: 64.

Chao, M.V., M.A. Bothwell, A.H. Ross, H. Koprowski, A.A. Lanahan, C.R. Buck, and A. Sehgal. 1986. Gene transfer and molecular cloning of the human NGF receptor. *Science* **232**: 518.

Courchesne, W.E., R. Kunisawa, and J. Thorner. 1989. A putative protein kinase overcomes pheromone-induced arrest of cell cycling in *S. cerevisiae*. *Cell* **58**: 1107.

Elion, E.A., P.L. Grisafi, and G.R. Fink. 1990. FUS3 encodes a cdc2$^+$/CDC28-related kinase required for the transition from mitosis into conjugation. *Cell* **60**: 649.

Ely, C.M., K.M. Oddie, J.S. Litz, A.J. Rossomando, S.B. Kanner, T.W. Sturgill, and S.J. Parsons. 1990. A 42 kD tyrosine kinase substrate linked to chromaffin cell secretion exhibits an associated MAP kinase activity and is highly related to a 42kD mitogen-stimulated protein in fibroblasts. *J. Cell Biol.* **110**(3): 731.

Evan, G.I., G.K. Leis, G. Ramsay, and J.M. Bishop. 1985. Isolation of monoclonal antibodies specific for human c-myc proto-oncogene product. *Mol. Cell. Biol.* **12**: 3610.

Greene, L.A., J.M. Aletta, A. Rukenstein, and S.H. Green. 1987. PC12 pheochromocytoma cells: Culture, nerve growth factor treatment, and experimental exploitation. *Methods Enzymol.* **147**: 207.

Hempstead, B.L., L.S. Schleifer, and M.V. Chao. 1989. Expression of functional nerve growth factor receptors after gene transfer. *Science* **243**: 373.

Hohn, A., J. Leibrock, K. Bailey, and Y.-A. Barde. 1990. Identification and characterization of a novel member of the nerve growth factor/brain derived neurotrophic factor family. *Nature* **344**: 339.

Hoshi, M., E. Nishida, and H. Sakai. 1988. Activation of a Ca^{2+}-inhibitable protein kinase that phosphorylates microtubule-associated protein 2 in vitro by growth factors, phorbol esters, and serum in quiescent cultured human fibroblasts. *J. Biol. Chem.* **263**(11): 5396.

Leibrock, J., F. Lottspeich, A. Hohn, M. Hofer, B. Hengerer, P. Masiakowski, H. Thoenen, and Y.-A. Barde. 1989. Molecular cloning and expression of brain-derived neurotrophic factor. *Nature* **341**: 149.

Lin, L.-F.H., D. Mismer, J.D. Lile, L.G. Armes, E.T. Butler, J.L. Vannice, and F. Collins. 1989. Purification, cloning, and expression of ciliary neurotrophic factor (CNTF). *Science* **246**: 1023.

Maisonpierre, P.C., L. Belluscio, S. Squinto, N.Y. Ip, M.E. Furth, R.M. Lindsay, and G.D. Yancopoulos. 1990a. Neurotrophin-3: A neurotrophic factor related to NGF and BDNF. *Science* **247**: 1446.

Maisonpierre, P.C., L. Belluscio, B. Friedman, R.F. Alderson, S.J. Weigand, M.E. Furth, R.M. Lindsay, and G.D. Yancopoulos. 1990b. NT-3, BDNF and NGF in the developing rat nervous system: Parallel as well as reciprocal patterns of expression. *Neuron* (in press).

McMahon, A.P. and R.T. Moon. 1989. Ectopic expression of the proto-oncogene int-1 in *Xenopus* embryos leads to duplication of the embryonic axis. *Cell* **58**: 1075.

Miyasaka, T., M.-V. Chao, P. Sherline, and A.-R. Saltiel. 1990. Nerve growth factor stimulates a protein kinase in PC-12 cells that phosphorylates microtubule-associated protein-2. *J. Biol. Chem.* **265**(8): 4730.

Munro, S. and H.R.B. Pelham. 1987. A c-terminal signal prevents secretion of luminal ER proteins. *Cell* **48**: 899.

Mutoh, T. and G. Guroff. 1989. The role of phosphorylation in the action of nerve growth factor. *BioFactors* **2**: 71.

Radeke, M.J., T.P. Misko, C. Hsu, L.A. Herzenberg, and E.M. Shooter. 1987. Gene transfer and molecular cloning of the rat nerve growth factor receptor. *Nature* **325:** 593.

Ray, L.B. and T.W. Sturgill. 1987. Rapid stimulation by insulin of a serine/threonine kinase in 3T3-L1 adipocytes that phosphorylates microtubule-associated protein 2 in vitro. *Proc. Natl. Acad. Sci.* **84(6):** 1502.

———. 1988. Insulin-stimulated microtubule-associated protein kinase is phosphorylated on tyrosine and threonine in vivo. *Proc. Natl. Acad. Sci.* **85(11):** 3753.

Rossomando, A.J., D.M. Payne, M.J. Weber, and T.W. Sturgill. 1989. Evidence that pp42, a major tyrosine kinase target protein, is a mitogen-activated serine/threonine protein kinase. *Proc. Natl. Acad. Sci.* **86(18):** 6940.

Scott, J., M. Selby, M. Urdea, M. Quiroga, G.I. Bell, and W.J. Rutter. 1983. Isolation and nucleotide sequence of a cDNA encoding the precursor of mouse nerve growth factor. *Nature* **302:** 538.

Snider, W.D. and E.M. Johnson. 1989. Neurotrophic molecules. *Ann. Neurol.* **26:** 489.

Stockli, K.A., F. Lottspeich, M. Sendtner, R. Masiakowski, P. Carroll, R. Gotz, D. Lindholm, and H. Thoenen. 1989. Molecular cloning, expression and regional distribution of rat ciliary neurotrophic factor. *Nature* **342:** 920.

Thoenen, H., C. Bandtlow, and R. Heumann. 1987. The physiological function of nerve growth factor in the central nervous system: Comparison with the periphery. *Rev. Physiol. Biochem. Pharmacol.* **109:** 145.

Ullrich, A., A. Gray, C. Berman, and T.J. Dull. 1983. Human beta nerve growth factor gene sequence highly homologous to that of mouse. *Nature* **303:** 821.

Compartmentalization of Acetylcholine Receptor Gene Expression during Development of the Neuromuscular Junction

J.P. Changeux,* C. Babinet,† J.L. Bessereau,* A. Bessis,* A. Cartaud,‡
J. Cartaud,‡ P. Daubas,* A. Devillers-Thiéry,* A. Duclert,* J.A. Hill,*
B. Jasmin,‡ A. Klarsfeld,* R. Laufer,* H.O. Nghiêm,* J. Piette,*
M. Roa,* and A.M. Salmon*

*Institut Pasteur, *UA CNRS D 1284 Molecular Neurobiology and †Génétique des Mammifères, 75724 Paris Cédex 15,
France; ‡Institut Jacques Monod, CNRS and Université Paris VII, 75251 Paris Cédex 05, France*

The nicotinic acetylcholine receptor (AChR) is a membrane-bound allosteric protein engaged in intercellular communication at the cholinergic synapse. This transmembrane heterologous ($\alpha_2 \beta \gamma \delta$) pentamer operates in the millisecond time scale as an acetylcholine-gated cationic channel, and its functional architecture is actively investigated (Changeux 1981; Popot and Changeux 1984; Hucho 1986; Lindstrom et al. 1987; and this volume). In particular, the regions of the molecule that form its two main functional domains, namely, the acetylcholine-binding site and the agonist-gated ion channel, have recently been defined at the amino acid level (for review, see Changeux 1990; Galzi et al. 1990).

The AChR protein is also a dominant component of the postsynaptic membrane of the motor endplate. In the adult, the density of AChR under the motor nerve ending reaches approximately 10,000 molecules per μm^2 and drops more than 1000-fold only a few micrometers away (for review, see Salpeter and Loring 1985; Laufer and Changeux 1989b). Here, we report recent studies from this laboratory concerning the molecular mechanisms engaged in the development of this postsynaptic domain.

COMPARTMENTALIZATION OF GENE EXPRESSION AT THE ENDPLATE

Among the several mechanisms that may account for the high concentration of AChR protein under the motor nerve ending, a simple one (among others) takes into account the existence of multiple nuclei in the developing and adult muscle fiber (see Changeux 1979). The biosynthesis of AChR would take place, in a privileged manner, at nuclei that underlie the endplate. These nuclei, referred to as "fundamental" by Ranvier (1875) because of their distinct morphology, were already tentatively related to the biosynthesis of synapse-specific proteins by Couteaux (1978).

Merlie and Sanes (1985) observed by hand-dissecting the mouse diaphragm that the levels of AChR α- and δ-subunit mRNAs were higher in the subsynaptic versus extrasynaptic regions. They considered that such distribution could arise as a result of (1) directed transport of mRNA toward the synaptic regions, (2) enhanced stability of AChR mRNA near the endplates, and (3) increased transcription of AChR subunit genes by the nuclei underlying the synapse.

Compartmentalized Expression of AChR α-Subunit Gene at the Level of Endplate Nuclei Revealed by In Situ Hybridization

In a first attempt to distinguish among these possibilities, the localization of mature and unspliced mRNA transcripts coding for the α-subunit mRNA was determined in chick muscle by in situ hybridization (Fontaine et al. 1988; Fontaine and Changeux 1989). In two different muscles, the slow, multi-innervated, anterior latissimus dorsi (ALD) and the fast, singly innervated, posterior latissimus dorsi (PLD), from 15-day-old chicks, α-subunit mRNA was detected in situ at discrete regions. These domains colocalize (80% correspondence) with motor endplates identified by histochemical staining for acetylcholinesterase. At this level, the autoradiographic grains accumulate on and around the fundamental nuclei.

Initially high in early embryos, transcript levels decrease during embryonic development. In embryonic day 11 (ED11) PLD muscle, both mature and precursor mRNAs are detected all over the developing muscle fiber. Subsequently, at ED16, the total number of grains distributed along the muscle fiber decreases but several clusters of grains persist. At ED19, only one cluster is observed per muscle fiber. The distribution of mature AChR α-subunit mRNA in PLD becomes restricted to the newly formed endplate (Fontaine and Changeux 1989).

Denervation of adult ALD and PLD has been reported to increase acetylcholine sensitivity in extrajunctional areas (Bennett et al. 1973; see also Axelsson and Thesleff 1959; Miledi 1960; for review, see Salpeter and Loring 1985). Northern blot analysis of AChR α-subunit mRNA reveals substantial increases in the steady-state levels of mature mRNA in PLD and ALD 4 days after denervation of 15-day-old chicks (Fontaine

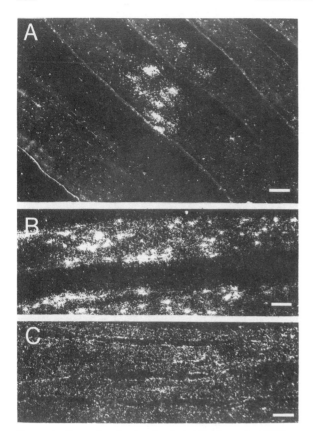

Figure 1. Detection by in situ hybridization of AChR α-subunit mRNA in posterior latissimus dorsi muscle of a 15-day-old chick. (*A*) Innervated muscle; (*B*) denervated muscle; (*C*) innervated muscle hybridized with an actin probe. (Reprinted, with permission, from Fontaine et al. 1988.)

et al. 1988) as observed in other systems (for references, see Fontaine et al. 1988; Brenner et al. 1990). In situ, clusters of grains appear at the level of about 10% of the nuclei distributed at random all along the denervated muscle fibers. A similar picture is observed using a strictly intronic probe (Fontaine and Changeux 1989), supporting the notion that the transcriptional activity (see Shieh et al. 1987; Tsay and Schmidt 1989) of individual nuclei varied under these conditions. In contrast, actin mRNA was found diffusely distributed all over muscle fibers during development and did not significantly change after denervation (see Fig. 1) (Fontaine et al. 1988; Fontaine and Changeux 1989).

These in situ results have been extended to the evolution of the other AChR subunits in the rat (Goldman and Staple 1989; Brenner et al. 1990), yet with timing differences among the diverse subunits mRNAs. Thus, nuclei in different states of AChR gene expression exist within the cytoplasm of the muscle fiber with higher transcript accumulation under the nerve endings than outside the endplate.

Spontaneous Variability of Expression of α-Subunit mRNA in Nuclei of Cultured Muscle Cells

At the adult endplate, nuclei labeled by either a mixed exonic-intronic or strictly intronic α-subunit probe are often found in the close vicinity of almost completely silent nuclei within the same cytoplasm. Interestingly, such discrete labeling can also be observed in cultured chick myotubes in the absence of nerve (Fontaine and Changeux 1989). Similar results have been reported by other groups of investigators with cultured muscle cells (Bursztajn et al. 1989; Harris et al. 1989; Horovitz et al. 1989; Berman et al. 1990). This spontaneous "mosaicism" of α-subunit mRNA accumulation appears even more striking when the overall level of α-subunit message is increased by blocking the spontaneous electrical activity of cultured chick myotubes using tetrodotoxin (TTX) (Fontaine and Changeux 1989). Thus, it was suggested that, in muscle fibers, all-or-none switches of gene expression regulate in a discrete manner the accumulation of unspliced transcripts for the α-subunit (Fontaine and Changeux 1989).

FIRST AND SECOND MESSENGERS INVOLVED IN THE COMPARTMENTALIZATION OF ACHR GENE EXPRESSION

Activity-dependent Repression of Extrajunctional AChR Biosynthesis

Chronic paralysis of the chick embryo in ovo by snake venom α-toxins or curare-like agents does not affect the initial onset of AChR biosynthesis (Giacobini et al. 1973) but prevents the elimination of extrajunctional AChR (Giacobini-Robecchi et al. 1975; Burden 1977; Bourgeois et al. 1978; Betz et al. 1980). This elimination occurs without a major change of the metabolic stability of the AChR protein and therefore represents an activity-dependent repression of AChR biosynthesis. Interestingly, a similar phenomenon can be reproduced with primary cultures of chick myotubes, which exhibit spontaneous (nonneurogenic) firing (Cohen and Fischbach 1973; Shainberg and Burstein 1976; Betz and Changeux 1979). Blocking this spontaneous electrical activity by TTX results after 24 and 48 hours of treatment in a 1.5- to 2-fold increase in surface AChR, accompanied by, respectively, a 4.5- and 13-fold increase in α-subunit mRNA level (Klarsfeld and Changeux 1985). Measurements of the steady-state levels of partially spliced forms of α-subunit mRNA show that TTX treatment significantly increases in parallel both precursor and mature mRNA levels (Klarsfeld et al. 1989; Österlund et al. 1989). Furthermore, in situ hybridization studies with strictly intronic probes (Fontaine and Changeux 1989) revealed that spontaneously contracting cultured chick myotubes display little labeling, but after 48 hours of treatment with TTX, hybridization strikingly increased. As a few examples exist of mRNA precursor stabilization without increased transcription (Leys et al. 1984; Narayan and Towle 1985), these results suggest, but do not prove, that electrical activity represses AChR biosynthesis at the level of transcription. Final proof comes from the recent finding, using nuclear run-on assays, that denervation of chick muscle enhances the transcription rates of the α-, γ- and δ-subunits (Tsay and Schmidt 1989).

Intracellular Signals Linking Electrical Activity to Gene Expression

One of the second messengers postulated to link electrical activity to the expression of AChR genes is Ca^{++} (Shainberg et al. 1976; for review, see Laufer and Changeux 1989b). On depolarization of the cell membrane, the cytoplasmic Ca^{++} concentration transiently rises. Several lines of evidence, mostly pharmacological, support the notion that a rise in intracellular Ca^{++} causes a decrease in surface AChR numbers (Shainberg et al. 1976; Birnbaum et al. 1980; Pezzementi and Schmidt 1981; McManaman et al. 1982; Smilowitz et al. 1988).

This question was further examined at the mRNA level (Klarsfeld et al. 1989). Treatment of chick myotube cultures with the Ca^{++} channel blocker verapamil was found to increase α-subunit mature messenger about 12-fold, which is in the range of the increase observed with TTX. The latter effect was completely abolished in the presence of the Ca^{++} ionophore A23187. These results support the notion that the entry of Ca^{++} through the sarcolemmal membrane during muscle depolarization contributes to the repression of α-subunit gene transcription.

The Ca^{++}-activated and phospholipid-dependent protein kinase C is an intracellular regulatory enzyme that may be activated by muscle depolarization (Vergara et al. 1985; Richter et al. 1987). Short-term exposure (up to 40 hours) of chick muscle cultures to tetradecanoyl-12,13-phorbol acetate (TPA), an activator of protein kinase C, blocks the increase in AChR α-subunit mRNA and surface AChR levels caused by TTX (Fontaine et al. 1987). When the exposure to TPA is prolonged for an extra day, probably leading to "down-regulation" of the kinase (Niedel and Blackshear 1986), surface AChR levels recover from an initial 40% decrease to reach values almost twofold above control, whereas α-subunit mRNA level increases eightfold (Klarsfeld et al. 1989).

Similar results were obtained with the protein kinase C inhibitor, staurosporine (Tamaoki et al. 1986). At concentrations (10 ng/ml) where it only marginally affects myotube morphology and does not prevent spontaneous contractions, staurosporine caused a five- to tenfold increase in surface AChR and α-subunit mRNA levels (Klarsfeld et al. 1989). Staurosporine also reversed the short-term decrease in surface AChR number elicited by TPA. Moreover, its effect on AChR expression was not additive with that of TTX, suggesting that staurosporine acts on a downstream step in the signaling pathway(s) that links membrane electrical activity to AChR biosynthesis. These results further support the suggestion (Fontaine et al. 1987) that protein kinase C contributes to the regulation of AChR α-subunit gene expression by the electrical activity of the sarcolemmal membrane. The precise relationships that may exist between the depolarization of the muscle membrane, Ca^{++} entry, and protein kinase C activation remain to be elucidated.

Subneural Regulation of AChR Gene Expression

Even after the transcriptional activity of the extrajunctional nuclei has been switched off, the biosynthesis of the AChR by the subneural nuclei persists. Soluble factors from neural tissues, which increase AChR number on cultured myotubes in vitro, have been postulated to play a role in this process (for review, see Salpeter and Loring 1985; Schuetze and Role 1987). Among them are a polypeptide of about 42 kD (ARIA) purified from chick brain (Usdin and Fischbach 1986; Falls et al., this volume) and ascorbic acid (Knaack et al. 1986).

Other potentially important compounds are the neuropeptides known to coexist (Hökfelt et al. 1986; Villar et al. 1988, 1989) with acetylcholine in spinal cord motor neurons. These include vasoactive intestinal peptide (VIP), somatostatin, and calcitonin gene-related peptide (CGRP) (Villar et al. 1988, 1989). CGRP has been localized at the level of motor nerve endings (Takami et al. 1985a,b), where it is stored within dense-core vesicles (Matteoli et al. 1988). CGRP can be released from rat neuromuscular junctions on electrical stimulation of the motor nerve (Uchida et al. 1990).

To test for a possible role of CGRP as an anterograde "trophic" factor of neural origin, primary cultures of chick myotubes were exposed to 10^{-8} to 10^{-6} M CGRP. As a result, both surface and total AChR levels increased (30–50%) without changing the AChR degradation rate (Fontaine et al. 1986; New and Mudge 1986). Moreover, CGRP elevated the steady-state level of mature α-subunit mRNA by about threefold (Fontaine et al. 1987). Under these conditions, high-molecular-weight, unspliced mRNA increased in parallel, supporting the view, with the limitations mentioned above, that CGRP stimulates the transcription of the α-subunit gene (Österlund et al. 1989).

The response to CGRP occurs independently of the rise in AChR number caused by TTX and thus does not influence the electrical activity of the muscle fiber. Moreover, under the conditions where the phorbol ester TPA abolishes the effect of TTX on AChR biosynthesis, the response to CGRP persists (Fontaine et al. 1987). Different intracellular signaling mechanisms are thus involved in the regulation of AChR gene expression by CGRP and by electrical activity (Fontaine et al. 1986, 1987; Duclert et al. 1990).

CGRP elevates intracellular levels of cAMP and activates adenylate cyclase in skeletal muscle (Takami et al. 1986; Kobayashi et al. 1987; Laufer and Changeux 1987, 1989a). Moreover, AChR biosynthesis is enhanced by membrane permeant analogs of cAMP and by compounds that activate adenylate cyclase (prostaglandin, β-adrenergic agonists, cholera toxin, forskolin) (Betz and Changeux 1979; Blosser and Appel 1980; Fontaine et al. 1987; Harris et al. 1988). Thus, cAMP may serve as one of the second messengers that mediate the action of CGRP.

Other neuropeptides, such as VIP, coexisting with acetylcholine in motoneurons also regulate cAMP levels in muscle cells (Villar et al. 1989). On the other hand, intracellular signals other than cAMP, may also contribute to the increase in subsynaptic AChR numbers. A medium conditioned for 24 hours by spinal cord cells causes, in agreement with the result of Jessell et al. (1979), an approximately twofold increase of surface ^{125}I-labeled α-bungarotoxin sites (Kirilovsky et al. 1989). This effect is additive with that of CGRP and does not involve cAMP. On the other hand, treatments by the phorbol ester TPA or by the Ca^{++} ionophore A23187 block the effects of the conditioned medium (Kirilovsky et al. 1989). These findings raise the possibility that persistence of AChR biosynthesis at the endplate may result from a direct antagonism of the electrical activity-induced repression, in addition to, or even as an alternative of, the cAMP-mediated effect of CGRP.

If, at this stage, we lack definite proof that CGRP is actually involved in the morphogenesis of the endplate and/or its maintenance, several arguments plead in favor of such a role: (1) In the chick, CGRP immunoreactive neurons are detected in the ventral horns of the spinal cord at ED6, and their number reaches a peak between ED12 and ED18 of incubation, i.e., at the moment where neuromuscular contacts become established (Villar et al. 1989). (2) Chronic paralysis of chick embryos by d-tubocurarine causes a decrease of CGRP-like immunoreactivity (Esquerda et al. 1989) and peripheral axotomy results in an increase of β- but not α-CGRP mRNA (Noguchi et al. 1990), indicating that the biosynthesis of β-CGRP in motor neurons is regulated in a "retrograde manner" by neuromuscular contacts. (3) Binding sites for CGRP are present on cultured chick myotubes (Jennings and Mudge 1989) and on embryonic muscles (Roa and Changeux 1991) in a ratio of one to ten α-bungarotoxin-binding sites. During embryonic development, the highest specific activity of CGRP-binding sites occurs between ED11 and ED14, at the moment where the number of AChR reaches a maximum (Roa and Changeux 1991). Colocalization of ^{125}I-labeled CGRP and acetylcholinesterase reaction product is detected at the level of endplates in the bulbo cavernosus muscle of the rat (Popper and Micevych 1989). CGRP appears as a *plausible* "anterograde" trophic factor that, along with others (see Falls et al.; McMahan; both this volume), may act synergistically and/or sequentially during endplate morphogenesis and maturation.

MOLECULAR MECHANISMS OF THE REGULATION OF ACHR α-SUBUNIT GENE TRANSCRIPTION

Mapping of the DNA Elements Involved in the *cis*-Regulation of Chick α-Subunit Gene Transcription in Muscle Primary Cultures

To study the regulation of AChR gene expression at the DNA level, genomic clones encoding the chicken AChR α-subunit were isolated (Klarsfeld and Changeux 1985) on the basis of the high degree of sequence identity existing between chick and *Torpedo marmorata* α-subunits (Devillers-Thiéry et al. 1983). The 5′-upstream flanking region of the AChR α-subunit gene was then cloned and sequenced. Of this upstream flanking region, 850 bp were inserted in front of the bacterial chloramphenicol acetyltransferase (CAT) gene (Klarsfeld et al. 1987), and this construct was used for transfection studies. High CAT expression was obtained in myotubes but not in cultured myoblasts nor in fibroblasts (Klarsfeld et al. 1987). Hence, the 5′-flanking region of the α-subunit gene contains DNA elements that selectively control the expression of AChR α-subunit in muscle cells during myotube differentiation. Subsequently, Wang et al. (1988) reported that the −116 to −81 region of the chicken α-subunit gene functions as an enhancer in the mouse C2C12 muscle cell line. Consistent with the latter finding, Piette et al. (1989) showed by deletion mapping that the −110 to −45 segment confers developmental control of expression in chick myotube primary cultures.

The 850-bp fragment contains a TATA and a CAAT box, an Sp1 recognition site, and the core sequence of the SV40 enhancer. An 11-bp motif found in the cardiac actin gene at position +32 (Chang et al. 1985) also occurs in this α-subunit upstream sequence at position −287 (Klarsfeld et al. 1987). Similar elements have been subsequently recognized in upstream sequences of the mouse γ-subunit gene (Gardner et al. 1987). In the δ-subunit genes from the mouse (Baldwin and Burden 1988) and chick (Wang et al. 1990), the CAAT and TATA boxes are missing, but a CANNTG motif, which characterizes the MyoD1 target sequence (Buskin and Hauschka 1989; Lassar et al. 1989), is present (Baldwin and Burden 1989; Wang et al. 1990). This element is also found in the α-subunit upstream sequence from chick (Piette et al. 1990).

Compartmentalized Expression of AChR α-Subunit Gene Conferred by an 842-bp α-Subunit Chick Promoter in Muscle of Transgenic Mice

To begin in vivo studies of the chicken α-subunit promoter, Merlie and Kornhauser (1989) introduced into the genome of mice the CAT fusion gene constructed by Klarsfeld et al. (1987). In four independently derived lines of mice, the expression of the CAT gene was found specific of skeletal muscle. Moreover, an approximately 100-fold decrease in CAT steady-state levels took place over the first 2–3 weeks after birth, and denervation reversed this effect. Thus, in the mouse, the 842 bp of the chick α-subunit promoter confers to the CAT gene the activity-dependent repression of extrajunctional AChR. Yet, as CAT is a soluble cytoplasmic enzyme, its compartmentalized expression at the endplate could not be followed.

Transgenic mice were thus generated with DNA constructs containing as a reporter gene the β-galactosidase (β-Gal) gene linked to a nuclear location signal (nls) (A. Klarsfeld et al., in prep.). Nuclei that express this reporter gene stain blue and are easily identified in situ. Among the five founder animals obtained with a −110 to +3 chick promoter fragment, none expressed β-Gal. Yet, one line derived from the progeny of one founder animal with the chick −842 to +3 promoter fragment expressed the transgene. β-Gal staining was found in the somites of embryos starting at day 9.5 of gestation and, subsequently, in the skeletal muscles (Fig. 2). A good correlation was observed with the expression of the α-subunit gene revealed by in situ hybridization. After birth, a general decline of staining takes place consistent with the repression of CAT transgene expression reported by Merlie and Kornhauser (1989).

In the diaphragm, the endplates are roughly distributed along a line running through the middle of the muscle fibers. Interestingly, at birth, when many myonuclei stain blue, a line of nuclei that react more intensely to the dye begins to be discerned. It coincides with the endplate alignment revealed on the other half of the diaphragm by the Koelle reaction for acetylcholinesterase. The staining intensity of the endplate nuclei and the contrast between junctional and extrajunctional nuclei become more striking on days 1–3, but the endplate staining subsequently fades and is no longer detected in the adult. Thus, the chick 842-bp promoter contains DNA elements that, in the mouse genetic background, suffice for the compartmentalized expression of the β-Gal reporter gene at early stages of

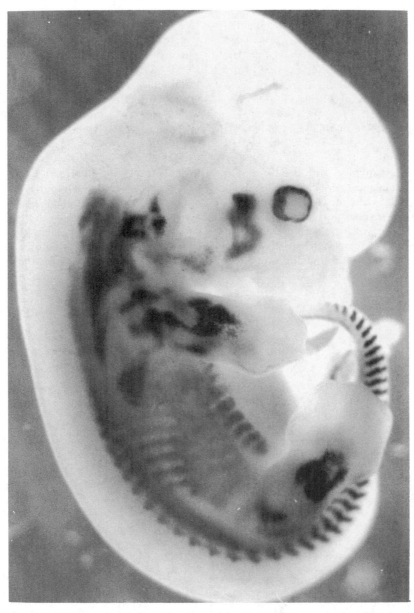

Figure 2. In toto X-Gal staining pattern of a 13-day-old embryo of the RαNLZ2 transgene line. The developing muscle masses within the limbs are clearly seen. The pattern of intercostal and paravertebral muscles is also easily recognizable. In situ hybridization with a mouse AChR α-subunit probe shows good superposition of transgene and endogenous gene expression (A. Klarsfeld et al., in prep.).

endplate morphogenesis. This differential nuclear labeling most likely reflects differential transcription of the transgene in subsynaptic versus extrasynaptic nuclei.

trans-Activating Factors Involved in the Regulation of α-Subunit Gene Transcription

A detailed analysis of the function of DNA regulatory elements present within the α-subunit upstream sequence was carried out by following the interaction of nuclear proteins with an 870-bp segment 5' to the transcription start point (Piette et al. 1989). DNase I footprinting and gel retardation experiments led to the distinction of three distinct domains of interactions ARI, ARII, and ARIII (Fig. 3). ARIII binds in addition to the ubiquitous Sp1 factor, a guanine-stretch-binding protein and a group of factors with Sp1-like specificity. The ARII domain can be further subdivided into three subdomains: ARIIa and ARIIb contain part of the enhancer sequences (Wang et al. 1988), and ARIIc contains the CAAT box motif. Each of these domains interacts with several distinct factors (see below).

During muscle differentiation, Piette et al. (1990) observed changes in the steady-state levels of several nuclear factors that interact with these DNA sequences. A factor that interacts with ARIIb and is displaced by the SV40 enhancer core element is present in differentiated myotubes and muscle fibers but is not detected in extracts of myoblasts. Other factors that interact with ARIIb are also underrepresented in myoblasts. The level of a protein binding to ARIII also varies during differentiation but in the opposite direc-

tion. In myoblasts, the guanine-stretch-binding protein appears more abundant than the Sp1 factor, whereas the opposite is true in differentiated myotubes (Piette et al. 1989).

Of particular interest is the function of two MyoD1-binding elements, one of which is adjacent to the ARIIa sequence and the other is contained within ARIIb (Piette et al. 1990). Four genes coding for proteins, which act as myogenic regulatory factors, have been identified on the basis of their ability to convert nonmuscle mesenchyme cells into myoblasts (Davis et al. 1987; Braun et al. 1989; Rhodes and Konieczny 1989; Wright et al. 1989). These proteins belong to a family characterized by a helix-loop-helix motif required for protein dimerization (Murre et al. 1989). One of these proteins, MyoD1, has been shown to trans-activate the creatine kinase gene (Lassar et al. 1989).

An eventual role of MyoD1-binding sites was investigated with the chick α-subunit promoter (Piette et al. 1990). First, it was shown that both sites bind glutathione transferase MyoD1 (Glu-MyoD) fusion protein. Moreover, cotransfection of 3T6 fibroblasts with an expression vector for either MyoD1 or myogenin trans-activates the α-subunit promoter sequences linked to the CAT gene (−842 to +20). Mutations of either MyoD1 site decrease by at least tenfold the ability of Glu-MyoD1 protein to bind to the α-subunit enhancer and inhibit the trans-activation of the α-subunit gene promoter by both MyoD1 and myogenin in 3T6 fibroblasts. In chick myotube primary cultures, any one of the two mutations reduces the activity of the 842-bp promoter by about twofold. When both sites are mutated, the activity of the pro-

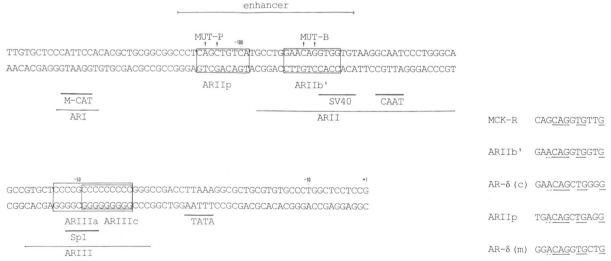

Figure 3. (*Left*) DNA-protein interactions in the 5'-upstream region of the AChR α-subunit gene. The sequence is numbered with respect to the starting point of transcription (+1). Homologies to published consensus sequences are underlined: M-CAT, SV40, CAAT, Sp1, and TATA. The three protected regions in DNase I footprinting experiments are indicated, respectively: ARI, ARII, and ARIII. The muscle-specific enhancer region is also indicated. DNA-protein interactions characterized by bandshift and methylation interference experiments are boxed: MyoD1-binding sites ARIIp and ARIIb', Sp1-binding site ARIIIa, and guanine-stretch site ARIIIc (see references in Piette et al. 1989, 1990). (*Right*) Comparison of MyoD1-binding sites in MCK gene, AChR δ-subunit gene of mouse, AChR δ-subunit gene of chicken, and AChR α-subunit gene of chicken. Conserved base pairs are underlined.

moter drops about 20-fold. The factors binding to the two MyoD1-binding sites from the α-subunit enhancer thus play a critical role in the tissue-specific expression of the α-subunit gene (Piette et al. 1990).

A direct contribution of proteins from the MyoD1 family to the activity-dependent repression of α-subunit gene transcription in extrajunctional areas remains to be established. Yet, it is noteworthy that denervation of leg muscles in postnatal day 1 (PN1) chicken causes after 4 days a general increase of transcription factors but with a marked differential effect in favor of proteins binding to the ARIIb fragment (Piette et al. 1989). Moreover, denervation of leg muscles in the mouse increases severalfold the steady-state levels of the mRNAs coding for MyoD1, myogenin, and MRF4 (A. Duclert, unpubl.). Thus, the activation of α-subunit gene transcription following denervation may result from the positive regulation of *trans*-acting factors from the MyoD1 family as a consequence of their enhanced synthesis and/or activity.

Apart from the MyoD1 family, another class of transcription factors, namely, the "early response" factors may be relevant to the control of AChR gene expression. These gene products have been implicated in the transduction of protein-kinase-C-mediated signals (for review, see Curran and Franza 1988) and in the effect of electrical activity in nerve cells (Greenberg et al. 1986; Morgan and Curran 1986; Bartel et al. 1989; Curran et al., this volume). The mRNA levels of the early response genes c-*fos* and *jun* were investigated in the mouse after denervation of lower leg muscles (Bessereau et al. 1990). As early as 1.5 hours after sciatic nerve section, c-*fos* mRNA levels reach a maximum and then return to basal levels at 6 hours, whereas c-*jun* and *jun-B* mRNA levels increase after 24 hours and remain elevated for at least 8 days. In contrast, *jun-D* mRNA levels do not change. To our knowledge, the increase of c-*fos* mRNA is the earliest gene response reported to occur in muscle after denervation and might be at the origin of a cascade of genetic events leading to the differential regulation of AChR genes.

It is thus tempting to speculate that c-*fos* and c-*jun* or *jun-B* proto-oncogene products participate in the derepression of AChR genes by muscle denervation. Yet, none of these gene products have been found to *trans*-activate the chick α-subunit promoter (J.L. Bessereau and J. Piette, unpubl.), and furthermore, c-*fos* has recently been reported to decrease the expression of the MyoD1 gene (Lassar et al. 1989). At present, the situation is unclear. Further investigations should establish whether any relationship exists between these early response genes, the genes of the MyoD1 family, and the AChR genes.

Inhibition of Protein Translation Differentially Affects the Regulation of α-Subunit mRNA Level by Electrical Activity and CGRP

The regulation of α-subunit gene expression may either involve a modulation of the "efficacy" of preex-

isting factors or require de novo synthesis of regulatory factors. To distinguish between these possibilities, primary cultures of chick myotubes were exposed to the translation inhibitors cycloheximide or anisomycin (Duclert et al. 1990). Both of these compounds blocked the increase of α-subunit mRNA caused by TTX. Under these conditions, neither the basal level of the α-subunit mRNA nor that of muscle-specific creatine phosphokinase mRNA was affected. Moreover, the high level of α-subunit mRNA caused by TTX did not persist after subsequent addition of cycloheximide. A similar requirement is found for the maintenance of a high level of α-subunit mRNA at early stages (3–4-day) of in vitro differentiation of muscle primary cultures. Thus, the continuous synthesis of a positive regulatory factor is required for the maintenance of high levels of α-subunit mRNA expression at early stages of development or following TTX treatment. The metabolic lifetime of such factor(s) appears to be rather short. On the other hand, the elevation of α-subunit mRNA level caused by CGRP does not display a requirement for constant protein synthesis, a finding consistent with the notion that electrical activity and CGRP regulate α-subunit gene expression via distinct intracellular pathways (Fontaine et al. 1987).

These data emphasize the possible role played by the metabolic turnover (rate of synthesis and/or metabolic stability) of transcription factors in controlling the expression of their target genes (Duclert et al. 1990). In this context, one may note that the turnover rate of MyoD1 is particularly fast (half-life of about 30 min) (Thayer et al. 1989).

DISCOORDINATE REGULATION OF ACHR GENES

Information available about the compartmentalization of AChR gene expression primarily concerns the gene coding for the acetylcholine-binding α-subunit in the chick. Yet, the AChR pentamer results from the assembly of four different subunits (α, β, γ, and δ). In some species (rat, calf), one of these, the γ-subunit, is replaced by a distinct subunit, named ϵ (Mishina et al. 1986) during postnatal maturation of the endplate, thereby leading to a change of single channel properties (Witzemann et al. 1987; Brenner et al. 1990). In addition, two distinct α-subunit cDNAs have been identified in *Xenopus* muscle and are coexpressed throughout muscle development (Hartman and Claudio 1990). These issues are not addressed in the following sections, which are primarily devoted to the differential expression of the four "standard" α-, β-, γ-, and δ-subunit genes.

Chromosomal Localization of AChR Genes in the Mouse

In the mouse, the genes coding for the four subunits of the AChR have been located on three chromosomes by analyzing restriction-fragment-length polymorphisms between the domestic mouse and *Mus spretus* (Robert et al. 1985). The γ- and δ-subunit genes have been found to cosegregate in this species, as in the chick (Nef et al. 1984), and are allocated to chromosome 1, whereas the β-subunit gene is located on chromosome 11 (Heidmann et al. 1986). The α-subunit gene was found closely linked to the Actc-1 gene (Heidmann et al. 1986), but the latter was incorrectly assigned to chromosome 17 by Czosnek et al. (1983). Crosby et al. (1989) have recently demonstrated that the Actc-1 gene is located on chromosome 2, thus definitively assigning the α-subunit gene to this chromosome.

The genes coding for the neuronal nicotinic AChR subunits have also been localized on mouse chromosomes (Bessis et al. 1990). The α_2-, α_3-, and β_2-subunits (for references, see Heinemann et al. 1989) have been found dispersed on chromosomes 14, 9, and 3, respectively. The α_4-subunit gene is located on chromosome 2 but not genetically linked to the α_1-subunit gene (Bessis et al. 1990). However, a cluster of α_3, α_5, β_4 genes exists on the same 60-kbp DNA fragment (Boulter et al. 1990). Nevertheless, no strict correlation can be recognized between function or organ specificity of the receptor subunits and the chromosomal localization of their genes, thus ruling out coordinate gene regulation mediated by common *cis*-acting regulatory sequences.

Differential Regulation of AChR Gene Expression in Primary Cultures of Chick Myotubes

Although the stoichiometry of the four receptor subunits is fixed in the mature receptor protein, the steady-state levels of the mRNAs coding for these subunits do not appear strictly correlated in vivo during development or after denervation in the chick (Moss et al. 1987, 1989; Shieh et al. 1988; Tsay and Schmidt 1989), in the rat (Evans et al. 1987; Goldman et al. 1988), in the mouse (Merlie et al. 1983; Buonanno and Merlie 1986; Merlie and Kornhauser 1989), or in the frog *Xenopus laevis* (Baldwin et al. 1988). It was thus suggested that during myogenesis and upon denervation "the availability of AChR subunit transcripts for translation" plays a regulatory role in surface AChR appearance (Evans et al. 1987; see also Moss et al. 1989).

In chick muscle primary cultures, a discoordinate regulation has also been reported to occur on exposure to ARIA (Harris et al. 1988). In this laboratory, using the same system, Österlund et al. (1989) and Kirilovsky et al. (1989) have compared the steady-state levels of the mRNAs coding for the α-, γ-, and δ-subunits during differentiation and in the presence of TTX and CGRP. It was found that in agreement with Harris et al. (1988), the level of α-subunit message varies to a much larger extent than those of the γ- and δ-subunit mRNAs. The levels of all these mRNAs first increase as a consequence of differentiation. Then, α-subunit mRNA level decreases drastically at the onset of spontaneous electrical activity, to rise again in the presence

of TTX or CGRP, whereas γ- and δ-subunit mRNA levels remain much more stable throughout this evolution. This situation differs somewhat from that seen in vivo, where the discoordination appears less pronounced (Moss et al. 1989).

In conclusion, the in vitro model system of chick muscle primary cultures does not strictly reproduce all the features of the developing and denervated muscle in vivo. Yet, it illustrates that (1) the level of the AChR protein in the cytoplasmic membrane may be regulated by the availability of the AChR subunit transcripts; (2) no absolute correlation exists in the expression of the several mRNAs that code for the subunits assembled in the mature proteins; and (3) the extent of coordination, which nevertheless exists between the levels of the diverse subunits mRNAs, may result from the control by common *trans*-activating factors acting on homologous DNA elements (such as MyoD1) present in the promoter of the various AChR genes dispersed, for most of them, on different chromosomes (see above).

POSTTRANSCRIPTIONAL REGULATION DURING ENDPLATE FORMATION

As discussed above, regulation at the transcription level contributes to the morphogenesis and maturation of the postsynaptic domain but may not suffice for its full development. Several additional steps of the processes of biosynthesis, degradation, and/or stabilization of the AChR proteins (Fig. 4) could be subject to posttranscriptional control.

Posttranscriptional Regulation of AChR Expression

In situ hybridization studies using either mixed exonic-intronic or strictly intronic probes for the α-subunit mRNA show that at the early stages of chick development, the evolution of precursor mRNA closely follows that of mature mRNA (Fontaine et al. 1988; Fontaine and Changeux 1989). Yet, in 15-day-old chicks, an intense hybridization was found with a mixed exonic-intronic probe, but no labeling was detected with a strictly intronic probe (Fontaine and Changeux 1989). In addition, in the transgenic mouse line, which differentially expresses the nls *lacZ* gene under the control of the 842-bp α-subunit promoter, the nuclear staining at diaphragm endplates disappears after PN10 (A. Klarsfeld et al., in prep.). These observations suggest (although they do not prove) that at late stages of endplate maturation, the transcription rate of the α-subunit gene at the level of endplate nuclei markedly decreases without a correlative decrease of mature mRNA level. In other words, a stabilization of mature mRNA (or more efficient processing of precursor mRNA) would take place at the late stages of endplate maturation.

In addition to its effect on mRNA availability, electrical activity may control the processing of AChR subunits in cultured myotubes (Carlin et al. 1986). It

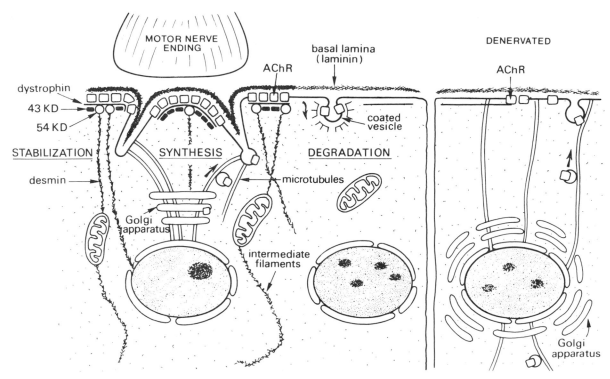

Figure 4. Diagrammatical representation of some of the elements involved in the posttranscriptional processing of the AChR in junctional and extrajunctional areas of innervated and denervated muscles. For explanation, see text.

has also been proposed that a phosphorylation-dephosphorylation reaction plays a role in the regulation of AChR subunit assembly (Ross et al. 1987). Along these lines, it was found that the activation of protein kinase C by TPA reduces the number of surface AChR without affecting α-subunit mRNA level (Fontaine et al. 1987). Such posttranscriptional regulation may account for the quantitative discrepancy systematically found between the variation of the levels of translatable α-subunit mRNA level and the changes in sarcolemmal AChR protein content (Olson et al. 1983, 1984; Klarsfeld and Changeux 1985; Evans et al. 1987; Tsay and Schmidt 1989). Thus, the processing and assembly of the receptor subunits, their transport to the postsynaptic membrane, and their stabilization/degradation may be the target of regulation by electrical activity and/or neural factors via the second messengers mentioned above.

Distribution of the Golgi Apparatus in Innervated and Denervated Chick Skeletal Muscle

The question then arises to what extent the compartmentalization revealed at the mRNA level by in situ hybridization studies persists for subsequent posttranslational processing of the receptor protein. In this context, several lines of evidence suggest that during its intracellular transport, the AChR is conveyed to the Golgi apparatus (see Merlie et al. 1983) where it becomes glycosylated (see Meunier et al. 1974; Vandlen et al. 1979). However, despite its likely involvement in

AChR processing (Fambrough and Devreotes 1978; Atsumi 1981), the precise location and organization of the Golgi apparatus in adult skeletal muscle was until now not known. These issues were investigated in PN15 chick muscle using a monoclonal antibody directed against a determinant localized to the medial compartment of the Golgi apparatus (Jasmin et al. 1989). In the ALD muscle, the Golgi apparatus appears to be restricted to areas located underneath the motor endplates. Interestingly, denervation causes a striking reorganization and expansion of the Golgi apparatus. Then, 5 days after denervation, it displays a perinuclear localization in close association with nuclei as observed in developing myotubes. Such differences in the localization of the Golgi apparatus may be related to the fact that in denervated muscle as in embryonic muscle fibers, the AChR is distributed all over the muscle fiber, whereas in the adult innervated muscle, the expression and processing of the AChR protein appears to be restricted to the subsynaptic domain (Fig. 4).

Compartmentalization of Cold Stable and Acetylated Microtubules at Chick Endplate

Microtubules, in their stable form, have been implicated in the traffic of vesicles and organelles within the cell. In chick muscle, microtubules have been identified by immunofluorescence using anti-α-tubulin antibodies following cold treatment (Jasmin et al. 1990a). Coldstable microtubules surround the subsynaptic nuclei and extend from the nuclear periphery toward the endplate. A specific antibody against acetylated α-tubulin also labels a similar subsynaptic domain. At this stage, it is not known whether the cold stable and the acetylated microtubules represent the same population. In any case, in the chick, a specialized microtubular cytoskeleton appears to be compartmentalized within the subsynaptic sarcoplasm and plausibly takes part, together with the Golgi apparatus, in the posttranslational processing and targeting of the postsynaptic membrane proteins, and in particular, of the AChR to the motor endplate (Fig. 4).

Importance of the 43K Protein in the Stability of the Postsynaptic Domain

Among the various elements that may contribute to the stability of the postsynaptic domain, one candidate is an extrinsic protein with an apparent molecular weight of 43,000 (43K protein). Initially identified in this laboratory (Sobel et al. 1977, 1978) as a major component of purified postsynaptic membranes from *T. marmorata* electric tissue, its cDNA has been cloned and sequenced from *T. californica* (Carr et al. 1987; Frail et al. 1987).

Immunocytochemical studies have shown that a protein immunologically related to the 43K protein is present at mammalian motor endplates (Froehner et al. 1981; Froehner 1984). In addition, AChR clusters arising spontaneously in cultures in the presence or in the absence of nerve cells (Burden 1985; Peng and Froehner 1985; Bloch and Froehner 1987) have been often found associated with the 43K protein.

The 43K protein is localized on the cytoplasmic side of the membrane (Elliott et al. 1980; Wennogle and Changeux 1980; St. John et al. 1982) and codistributes with the AChR (Froehner et al. 1981; Sealock 1982; Nghiêm et al. 1983; Kordeli et al. 1986, 1987a,b; Bridgman et al. 1987). Extraction of the 43K protein by mild alkaline treatment (Neubig et al. 1979) from purified *Torpedo* postsynaptic membrane fragments (Rousselet et al. 1979, 1982; Barrantes et al. 1980; Lo et al. 1980; Cartaud et al. 1981) and from myotube membranes (Bloch and Froehner 1987) increases the rotational and translational mobilities of AChR molecules within the membrane plane. After such extraction, no significant change in the permeability response to acetylcholine or of ligand binding to AChR was observed in *T. californica* AChR-rich membranes (Neubig et al. 1979). From these data, it was suggested that the 43K protein (and possibly other still unidentified peripheral components of the domain) plays a structural role contributing to the immobilization of AChR (for review, see Froehner 1986).

The developing electrocyte from *T. marmorata* represents a useful model to study early stages of AChR-43K protein interaction. Immunochemical studies were carried out at three stages of embryonic development (Kordeli et al. 1989): (1) the 45-mm (body length) embryo, before the entry of nerve endings; (2) the 80–85-mm stage, where the innervated electrocyte dis-

plays a flattened asymmetric structure; and (3) adult. At the 45-mm stage, in agreement with the earlier work of Witzemann et al. (1983), AChR was found accumulated at the ventral pole of the developing electrocyte. Double fluorescence experiments, however, failed to reveal 43K protein immunoreactivity associated with the AChR, but rather a faint, diffuse fluorescence was seen with a largely cytoplasmic distribution. On the other hand, a transient asymmetric distribution of laminin paralleling that of the AChR was seen. At the subsequent 80–85-mm stage, the AChR and the 43K protein were found codistributed on the ventral face of the cell, as in the adult electrocyte. These studies show that in the electrocyte, the AChR may cluster independently of the 43K protein and before the entry of the nerve terminals.

Two forms of the 43K proteins related to the cytoplasmic and postsynaptic membrane fractions, respectively, have been detected in *Torpedo* electrocyte. The membrane form is favored on electrocyte maturation, and this aggregation of the 43K protein at the postsynaptic membrane correlates well with the formation of the postsynaptic elements (H.O. Nghiêm et al., in prep.).

The 43K protein is phosphorylated in vivo (J.A. Hill et al., in prep.) and can be phosphorylated in vitro (Saitoh and Changeux 1980) by protein kinase A (J.A. Hill et al., in prep.); 43K protein phosphorylation, which occurs at the level of serine residues, takes place with kinetics that suggest the involvement of a reaction cascade different from that mediating AChR phosphorylation (J.A. Hill et al., in prep.). These observations raise the possibility that putative 43K protein interactions with AChR and/or cytoskeleton are regulated by 43K protein phosphorylation and thus by neural factors or electrical activity.

Presence of Dystrophin in the Subneural Domain of *Torpedo* Electroplaque

In addition to the 43K protein, several proteins have been found associated with the AChR-rich domain: the lamin-B-related 54-kD (Cartaud et al. 1989), 58-kD (Froehner 1984), 87-kD (Carr et al. 1989), and the nonspectrin 270–300-kD (Woodruff et al. 1987) proteins. With the exception of the 43K and 54-kD proteins for which respective functions of AChR stabilization and anchoring of intermediate filaments (Cartaud et al. 1989; Kordeli et al. 1987a,b) have been hypothesized, the role(s) of the other peripheral proteins is not well understood.

Recently, dystrophin (Hoffman and Kunkel 1989) has been shown to exist in *Torpedo* electrocyte (Chang et al. 1989; Jasmin et al. 1990). Detailed immunofluorescence and ultrastructural experiments performed on adult electrocytes with a polyclonal antibody directed against chick dystrophin reveal that dystrophin immunoreactivity strictly codistributes with AChR along the innervated membrane (Jasmin et al. 1990b) on its cytoplasmic face. In developing electrocytes (45-

mm stage), dystrophin is already detected at the AChR-rich ventral pole of the cells *before* the appearance of 43K protein and the entry of the nerve endings. Therefore, the interaction of dystrophin with the developing subsynaptic membrane does not seem to require the presence of the 43K protein, raising the possibility that it plays a role in the initial assembly of this membrane domain. The presence of the extracellular matrix protein, laminin (Kordeli et al. 1989), at the moment AChR molecules aggregate is consistent with the observations of Burden et al. (1979) and Sanes et al. (1978) that, at the motor endplate, the synaptic basement membrane directs both pre- and postsynaptic specializations in the course of in vivo regeneration experiments (see McMahan this volume). It also offers one explanation for our initial observation that AChR aggregates persist with a high surface density several weeks after denervation (Bourgeois et al. 1973, 1978).

CONCLUSION

Several steps in the morphogenesis and maturation of the postsynaptic domain may be subject to posttranscriptional regulation: splicing of precursor mRNA, processing and assembly of the subunits, stabilization of the postsynaptic domain through interaction with peripheral proteins (43K protein and dystrophin) and the cytoskeleton on its cytoplasmic side and with the basal lamina (see McMahan; Lehky et al.; both this volume) on its synaptic face (Fig. 4). The *T. marmorata* electrocyte has served as a useful model. Yet, the motor endplate displays features of its own (e.g., the complex folded subsynaptic apparatus and associated cytoskeleton in mammals) that may not be

shared with the innervated membrane of the electrocyte. Moreover, the exact contribution of each of these posttranscriptional processes to the targeting, immobilization, and long-term metabolic stabilization of the receptor protein remains to be elucidated (see Fischbach; Lehky et al.; McMahan; all this volume). Of particular interest is the demonstration that the increase in AChR metabolic stability takes place postnatally and is regulated by the *trans*-synaptically evoked electrical activity of the muscle fiber (Avila et al. 1989; Fumagalli et al. 1990).

A Model for Compartmentalized Gene Expression during Endplate Morphogenesis and Stabilization

In summary, during skeletal muscle development, the biosynthesis of AChR is subject to several distinct regulatory mechanisms: (1) AChR biosynthesis increases in relation with myoblast commitment, differentiation, and fusion into myotubes; (2) a compartmentalized expression of AChR genes takes place at the level of topographically distinct nuclei, under the motor nerve ending and outside the endplate; (3) this morphogenetic process results, at least in part, from activity-dependent repression of AChR gene transcription outside the endplate and persistence of AChR biosynthesis at the level of the endplate fundamental nuclei; the latter mechanism involves still unidentified anterograde neural factors released by the motor nerve endings (CGRP and ARIA are plausible candidates); (4) a discrete all-or-none switch is included in the chain of processes involved in the regulation of α-subunit gene transcription; (5) several regulations at the posttranscriptional level take place such as precursor mRNA splicing, processing and assembly of the sub-

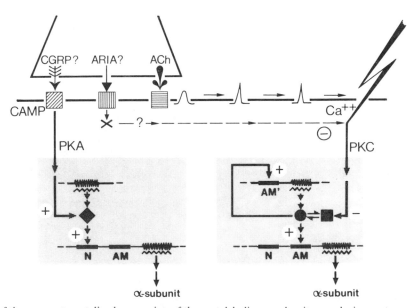

Figure 5. A model of the compartmentalized expression of the acetylcholine α-subunit gene during motor endplate formation. In this schematized diagram, the mechanisms involved in junctional and extrajunctional regulations have been drawn within distinct nuclei although they coexist in all muscle nuclei, yet with different levels of expression in the mature innervated muscle. For further explanation, see text.

units, targeting, stabilization and/or degradation of the
AChR protein in the postsynaptic membrane, and association with components of the basal lamina and/or
extrinsic membrane proteins (43K protein and dystrophin); in particular, the morphology of the cytoskeleton might be regulated by electrical activity and/
or neural factors; (6) distinct second-messenger systems are likely involved in the subneural *positive* regulation of AChR biosynthesis (e.g., cAMP and protein
kinase A) and its electrical activity-dependent *negative*
regulation outside the endplates (Ca^{++} and protein
kinase C); (7) in the case of chick α-subunit, the DNA
regulatory elements required for its compartmentalized
transcription in transgenic mice are located within the
850-bp upstream sequence; and (8) protein factors of
the MyoD1 family *trans*-activate the α-subunit gene
and may contribute, among others, to the above-mentioned regulation. Yet, the precise mechanisms of regulation of the binding activity, number, and/or turnover
of these factors by the above-mentioned second messengers remain to be elucidated.

A simple mechanism (Changeux et al. 1985, 1987;
Laufer and Changeux 1989b [with a few additions])
(see Fig. 5) that accounts for these results involves at
least three main components: (1) a defined network of
first and second messengers and of *trans*-acting regulatory proteins binding to defined *cis*-acting DNA regulatory elements; (2) a "local autocatalytic" loop, which
may be compared with the positive feedback of nuclear
factor(s) activating the promoters of their own structural genes (see Monod and Jacob 1962; Fontaine and
Changeux 1989), and (3) "long-range inhibition" of
gene expression by the electrical activity propagated
along the muscle fiber.

A computer simulation of the formalized model (M.
Kerzberg and J.P. Changeux, unpubl.) illustrates that
the mosaic adult pattern may develop from an initial
"isotropic" situation, where the genes are transcribed
in all nuclei, to a final "anisotropic" situation, where
only the subneural nuclei express AChR genes.

An important outcome of the model is that it stresses
the importance of the identification of *cis*-acting DNA
elements and *trans*-activating factors, of their interactions with the intracellular network of second and third
messengers, and of their parallel and sequential evolution in the course of endplate development. Thereby,
their study may open novel experimental approaches to
the understanding of the molecular mechanisms involved in endplate development and its epigenetic regulation.

ACKNOWLEDGMENTS

This work was supported by research grants from the
Association Française Centre les Myopathies, Collège
de France, The Université Paris VII, the Centre National de la Recherche Scientifique, the Ministère de la
Recherche, Institut National de la Santé et de la Recherche Médicale (contract 872-004), and the Direction
des Recherches Etudes et Techniques (contract 87-
211).

REFERENCES

Atsumi, S. 1981. Localization of surface and internal acetyl-choline receptors in developing fast and slow muscles of the chicken embryo. *Dev. Biol.* **86:** 22.

Avila, O.L., D.B. Drachman, and A. Pestronk. 1989. Neurotransmission regulates stability of acetylcholine receptors at the neuromuscular junction. *J. Neurosci.* **9:** 2902.

Axelsson, J. and F. Thesleff. 1959. A study of super-sensitivity in denervated mammalian skeletal muscle. *J. Physiol.* **147:** 178.

Baldwin, T.J. and S.J. Burden. 1988. Isolation and characterization of the mouse acetylcholine receptor delta subunit gene: Identification of a 148-bp *cis*-acting region that confers myotube-specific expression. *J. Cell Biol.* **107:** 2271.

———. 1989. Muscle-specific gene expression controlled by a regulatory element lacking a MyoD1-binding site. *Nature* **341:** 716.

Baldwin, T.J., C.M. Yoshihara, K. Blackmer, C.R. Kintner, and S.J. Burden. 1988. Regulation of acetylcholine receptor transcript expression during development in *Xenopus laevis*. *J. Cell Biol.* **106:** 469.

Barrantes, F.J., D.-C. Neugebauer, and H.P. Zingsheim. 1980. Peptide extraction by alkaline treatment is accompanied by rearrangement of the membrane-bound acetylcholine receptor from *Torpedo marmorata*. *FEBS Lett.* **112:** 73.

Bartel, D.P., M. Sheng, L.F. Lau, and M.E. Greenberg. 1989. Growth factors and membrane depolarization activate distinct programs of early response gene expression: Dissociation of *fos* and *jun* induction. *Genes Dev.* **3:** 304.

Bennett, M.R., A.G. Pettigrew, and R.S. Taylor. 1973. The formation of synapses in reinnervated and cross-reinnervated adult avian muscle. *J. Physiol.* **230:** 331.

Berman, S.A., S. Bursztajn, B. Bowen, and W. Gilbert. 1990. Localization of an acetylcholine receptor intron to the nuclear membrane. *Science* **247:** 212.

Bessereau, J.L., B. Fontaine, and J.P. Changeux. 1990. Denervation of mouse skeletal muscle differentially regulates the expression of the *jun* and *fos* proto-oncogenes. *New Biologist* **2:** 375.

Bessis, A., D. Simon-Chazottes, A. Devillers-Thiéry, J.L. Guénet, and J.P. Changeux. 1990. Chromosomal localization of the mouse genes coding for $\alpha2$, $\alpha3$, $\alpha4$ and $\beta2$ subunits of neuronal nicotinic acetylcholine receptor. *FEBS Lett.* **264:** 48.

Betz, H. and J.P. Changeux. 1979. Regulation of muscle acetylcholine receptor synthesis in vitro by cyclic nucleotide derivatives. *Nature* **278:** 749.

Betz, H., J.P. Bourgeois, and J.P. Changeux. 1980. Evolution of cholinergic proteins in developing slow and fast skeletal muscles from chick embryo. *J. Physiol.* **302:** 197.

Birnbaum, M., M. Reiss, and A. Shainberg. 1980. Role of calcium in the regulation of acetylcholine receptor synthesis in cultured muscle cell. *Pfluegers Arch. Eur. J. Physiol.* **385:** 37.

Bloch, R.J. and S.C. Froehner. 1987. The relationship of the postsynaptic 43K protein to acetylcholine receptors in receptor clusters isolated from cultured rat myotube. *J. Cell Biol.* **104:** 645.

Blosser, J.C. and S.H. Appel. 1980. Regulation of acetylcholine receptor by cyclic AMP. *J. Biol. Chem.* **253:** 3088.

Boulter, J., A. O'Shea-Greenfield, R.M. Duvoisin, J.G. Connolly, E. Wada, A. Jensen, P.D. Gardner, M. Ballivet, E.S. Deneris, D. McKinnon, S. Heinemann, and J. Patrick. 1990. $\alpha3$, $\alpha5$, and $\beta4$: Three members of the rat neuronal nicotinic acetylcholine receptor-related gene family form a gene cluster. *J. Biol. Chem.* **265:** 4472.

Bourgeois, J.P., J.L. Popot, and J.P. Changeux. 1973. Consequences of denervation on the distribution of the cholinergic (nicotinic) receptor sites from *Electrophorus electricus* revealed by high resolution autoradiography. *Brain Res.* **62:** 557.

Bourgeois, J.P., J.L. Popot, A. Ryter, and J.P. Changeux.

1978. Quantitative studies on the localization of the cholinergic receptor protein in the normal and denervated electroplaque from *Electrophorus electricus*. *J. Cell Biol.* **79:** 200.

Braun, T., G. Buschhausen-Denker, E. Bober, E. Tannich, and H.H. Arnold. 1989. A novel human muscle factor related to but distinct from MyoD1 induces myogenic conversion in 10T 1/2 fibroblasts. *EMBO J.* **8:** 701.

Brenner, H.R., V. Witzemann, and B. Sakmann. 1990. Imprinting of acetylcholine receptor messenger RNA accumulation in mammalian neuromuscular synapses. *Nature* **344:** 544.

Bridgman, P.C., C. Carr, S.E. Pedersen, and J.B. Cohen. 1987. Visualization of the cytoplasmic surface of *Torpedo* postsynaptic membranes by freeze-etch and immunoelectron microscopy. *J. Cell Biol.* **105:** 1829.

Burden, S. 1977. Development of the neuromuscular junction in the chick embryo: The number, distribution and stability of the acetylcholine receptors. *Dev. Biol.* **57:** 317.

———. 1985. The subsynaptic 43 KD protein is concentrated at developing nerve-muscle *in vitro*. *Proc. Natl. Acad. Sci.* **82:** 7805.

Burden, S.J., P.B. Sargent, and U.J.M. McMahan. 1979. Acetylcholine receptors in regenerating muscle accumulate at original synaptic sites in the absence of the nerve. *J. Cell Biol.* **82:** 412.

Buonanno, A. and J.P. Merlie. 1986. Transcriptional regulation of nicotinic acetylcholine receptor genes during muscle development. *J. Biol. Chem.* **261:** 11452.

Bursztajn, S., S.A. Berman, and W. Gilbert. 1989. Differential expression of acetylcholine receptor mRNA in nuclei of cultured muscle cells. *Proc. Natl. Acad. Sci.* **86:** 2928.

Buskin, J.N. and S.D. Hauschka. 1989. Identification of a myocyte nuclear factor that binds to the muscle-specific enhancer of the mouse muscle creatine kinase gene. *Mol. Cell. Biol.* **9:** 2627.

Carlin, B.E., J.C. Lawrence, Jr., J.M. Lindstrom, and J.P. Merlie. 1986. Inhibition of acetylcholine receptor assembly by activity in primary cultures of embryonic rat muscle cells. *J. Biol. Chem.* **261:** 5180.

Carr, C., G.D. Fischbach, and J.B. Cohen. 1989. A novel 87,000-M_r protein associated with acetylcholine receptors in *Torpedo* electric organ and vertebrate skeletal muscle. *J. Cell Biol.* **109:** 1753.

Carr, C., D. McCourt, and J.B. Cohen. 1987. The 43-kilodalton protein of *Torpedo* nicotinic postsynaptic membranes: Purification and determination of primary structure. *Biochemistry* **26:** 7090.

Cartaud, A., J.C. Courvalin, M.A. Ludosky, and J. Cartaud. 1989. Presence of a protein immunologically related to lamin B in the postsynaptic membrane of *Torpedo marmorata* electrocyte. *J. Cell Biol.* **109:** 1745.

Cartaud, J., A. Sobel., A. Rousselet, P.F. Devaux, and J.P. Changeux. 1981. Consequences of alkaline treatment for the ultrastructure of the acetylcholine-receptor-rich membranes from *Torpedo marmorata* electric organ. *J. Cell Biol.* **90:** 418.

Chang, H.W., E. Block, and E. Bonilla. 1989. Dystrophin in electric organ of *Torpedo californica* homologous to that in human muscle. *J. Biol. Chem.* **264:** 20831.

Chang, K.S., K.N. Rothblum, and R.J. Schwartz. 1985. The complete sequence of the chicken α-cardiac actin gene: A highly conserved vertebrate gene. *Nucleic Acids Res.* **13:** 1223.

Changeux, J.P. 1979. Molecular interactions in adult and developing neuromuscular junction. In *The Neurosciences, fourth study program* (ed. F.O. Schmitt and F.G. Worden), p.749. MIT Press, Cambridge, Massachusetts.

———. 1981. The acetylcholine receptor: An "allosteric" membrane protein. *Harvey Lect.* **75:** 85.

———. 1990. Functional architecture and dynamics of the nicotinic acetylcholine receptor: An allosteric ligand-gated ion channel. *Fidia Res. Found. Neurosci. Award Lect.* **4:** 21.

Changeux, J.P, A. Klarsfeld, and T. Heidmann. 1985. The acetylcholine receptor and molecular models for short and long term learning. In *The cellular and molecular bases of learning,* Dahlem Konferenzen, 1987 (ed. J.P. Changeux and M. Konishi) p. 31. Wiley, London.

Changeux, J.P., A. Devillers-Thiéry, J. Giraudat, M. Dennis, T. Heidmann, F. Revah, C. Mulle, O. Heidmann, A. Klarsfeld, B. Fontaine, R. Laufer, H.O. Nghiêm, E. Kordeli, and J. Cartaud. 1987. The acetylcholine receptor: Functional organisation and evolution during synapse formation. *Taniguchi Symp. Brain Sci.* **10:** 29.

Cohen, S.A. and G.D. Fischbach. 1973. Regulation of muscle acetylcholine sensitivity by muscle activity in cell culture. *Science* **181:** 76.

Couteaux, R. 1978. *Recherches morphologiques et cytochimiques sur l'organisation des tissus excitables*, p. 225. Robin and Marenge, Paris.

Crosby, J.L., S.J. Phillips, and J.H. Nadeau. 1989. The cardiac actin locus (Actc-1) is not on mouse chromosome 17 but is linked to β_2-microglobulin on chromosome 2. *Genomics* **5:** 19.

Curran, T. and B.R. Franza. 1988. Fos and Jun: The AP-1 connection. *Cell* **55:** 395.

Czosnek, H., U. Nudel, Y. Mayer, P.E. Barker, D.D. Pravtcheva, F.H. Ruddle, and D. Yaffe. 1983. The genes coding for the cardiac muscle actin, the skeletal muscle actin and the cytoplasmic β-actin are located on three different mouse chromosomes. *EMBO J.* **2:** 1977.

Davis, L., G.A. Banker, and O. Steward. 1987. Selective dendritic transport of RNA in hippocampal neurons in culture. *Nature* **330:** 477.

Devillers-Thiéry, A., J. Giraudat, M. Bentaboulet, and J.P. Changeux. 1983. Complete mRNA coding sequence of the acetylcholine binding α-subunit of *Torpedo marmorata* acetylcholine receptor: A model for the transmembrane organization of the polypeptide chain. *Proc. Natl. Acad. Sci.* **80:** 2067.

Duclert, A., J. Piette, and J.P. Changeux. 1990. Induction of acetylcholine receptor α-subunit gene expression in chicken myotubes by electrical activity blockade requires ongoing protein synthesis. *Proc. Natl. Acad. Sci.* **87:** 1391.

Elliott, J., S.G. Blanchard, W. Wu, J. Miller, C.D. Strader, P. Hartig, H.P. Moore, J. Racs, and, M.A. Raftery. 1980. Purification of *Torpedo californica* post-synaptic membranes and fractionation of their constituent proteins. *Biochem. J.* **185:** 667.

Esquerda, J.E., D. Ciutat, and J.X. Comella. 1989. Absence of histochemical immunoreactivity to calcitonin gene-related peptide (CGRP) in spinal cord motoneurons from (+)-tubocurarine-treated chick embryos. *Neurosci. Lett.* **105:** 1.

Evans, S., D. Goldman, S. Heinemann, and J. Patrick. 1987. Muscle acetylcholine receptor biosynthesis. *J. Biol. Chem.* **262:** 4911.

Fambrough, D.M. and P.N. Devreotes. 1978. Newly synthesized acetylcholine receptors are located in the Golgi apparatus. *J. Cell Biol.* **76:** 237.

Fontaine, B. and J.P. Changeux. 1989. Localization of nicotinic acetylcholine receptor α-subunit transcripts during myogenesis and motor endplate in the chick. *J. Cell Biol.* **108:** 1025.

Fontaine, B., A. Klarsfeld, and J.P. Changeux. 1987. Calcitonin-gene related peptide and muscle activity regulate acetylcholine receptor α-subunit mRNA levels by distinct intracellular pathways. *J. Cell Biol.* **105:** 1337.

Fontaine, B., A. Klarsfeld, T. Hökfelt, and J.P. Changeux. 1986. Calcitonin gene-related peptide, a peptide present in spinal cord motoneurons, increases the number of acetylcholine receptors in primary cultures of chick embryo myotubes. *Neurosci Lett.* **71:** 59.

Fontaine, B., D. Sassoon, M. Buckingham, and J.P. Changeux. 1988. Detection of the nicotinic acetylcholine receptor α-subunit mRNA by *in situ* hybridization at neuromuscular junctions of 15-day old chick striated muscles. *EMBO J.* **7:** 603.

Frail, D.E., J. Mudd, V. Shah, C. Carr, J.B. Cohen, and J.P. Merlie. 1987. cDNAs for the postsynaptic 43-kDa protein of *Torpedo* electric organ encode two proteins with different carboxyl termini. *Proc. Natl. Acad. Sci.* **84:** 6302.

Froehner, S.C. 1984. Peripheral proteins of postsynaptic membranes from *Torpedo* electric organ identified with monoclonal antibodies. *J. Cell Biol.* **99:** 88.

―――. 1986. The role of the postsynaptic cytoskeleton in AChR organization. *Trends Neurosci.* **9:** 37.

Froehner, S.C., V. Gulbrandsen, A.Y. Jeng, R.R. Neubig, and J.B. Cohen. 1981. Immunofluorescence localization at the mammalian neuromuscular junction of the M_r 43,000 protein of *Torpedo* postsynaptic membranes. *Proc. Natl. Acad. Sci.* **78:** 5230.

Fumagalli, G., S. Balbi, A. Cangiano, and T. Lømo. 1990. Regulation of turnover and number of acetylcholine receptors at neuromuscular junctions. *Neuron* **4:** 563.

Galzi, J.L., F. Revah, A. Bessis, and J.P. Changeux. 1990. Functional architecture of the nicotinic acetylcholine receptor: From the electric organ to brain. *Annu. Rev. Pharmacol. Toxicol.* (in press).

Gardner, P.D., S. Heinemann, and J. Patrick. 1987. Transcriptional regulation of nicotinic acetylcholine receptor genes: Identification of control elements of a γ-subunit gene. *Mol. Brain Res.* **3:** 69.

Giacobini, G., G. Filogamo, M. Weber, P. Boquet, and J.P. Changeux. 1973. Effect of a snake-neurotoxin on the development of innervated motor muscles in chick embryo. *Proc. Natl. Acad. Sci.* **70:** 1708.

Giacobini-Robecchi, M.G., G. Giacobini, G. Filogamo, and J.P. Changeux. 1975. Effect of the type A toxin from C. Botulinum on the development of skeletal muscles and of their innervation in chick embryo. *Brain Res.* **83:** 107.

Goldman, D. and J. Staple. 1989. Spatial and temporal expression of acetylcholine receptor RNAs in innervated and denervated rat soleus muscle. *Neuron* **3:** 219.

Goldman, D., H.R. Brenner, and S. Heinemann. 1988. Acetylcholine receptor α-, β-, γ-, and δ-subunit mRNA levels are regulated by muscle activity. *Neuron* **1:** 329.

Greenberg, M.E., E.B. Ziff, and A.G. Lloyd. 1986. Stimulation of neuronal acetylcholine receptors induces rapid gene transcription. *Science* **234:** 80.

Harris, D.A., D.L. Falls, and G.P. Fischbach. 1989. Differential activation of myotube nuclei following exposure to an acetylcholine receptor-inducing factor. *Nature* **337:** 173.

Harris, D.A., D.L. Falls, R.M. Dill-Devor, and G.D. Fischbach. 1988. Acetylcholine receptor-inducing factor from chicken brain increases the level of mRNA encoding the receptor α-subunit. *Proc. Natl. Acad. Sci.* **85:** 1983.

Hartman, D.S. and T. Claudio. 1990. Coexpression of two-distinct muscle acetylcholine receptor α-subunits during development. *Nature* **343:** 372.

Heidmann, O., A. Buonanno, B. Goeffroy, B. Robert, J.L. Guénet, J.P. Merlie, and J.P. Changeux. 1986. Chromosomal localization of the nicotinic acetylcholine receptor genes in the mouse. *Science* **234:** 866.

Heinemann, S., J. Boulter, E. Deneris, J. Connolly, P. Gardner, E. Wada, K. Wada, R. Duvoisin, M. Ballivet, L. Swanson, and J. Patrick. 1989. Brain and muscle nicotinic acetylcholine receptor: A gene family. *NATO ASI Ser. Ser. H. Cell. Biol.* **32:** 13.

Hoffman, E.P. and L.M. Kunkel. 1989. Dystrophin abnormalities in Duchenne/Becker muscular dystrophy. *Neuron* **2:** 1019.

Hökfelt, T., V.R. Holets, W. Staines, B. Meister, T. Melander, M. Schalling, M. Schultzberg, J. Freedman, H. Björklund, L. Olson, B. Lindk, L.G. Elfvin, J. Lundberg, J.A. Lindgren, B. Samuelsson, L. Terenius, C. Post, B. Everitt, and M. Goldstein. 1986. Coexistence of neuronal messengers—An overview. *Prog. Brain Res.* **68:** 33.

Horovitz, O., V. Spitsberg, and M.M. Salpeter. 1989. Regulation of acetylcholine receptor synthesis at the level of translation in rat primary muscle cells. *J. Cell Biol.* **108:** 1817.

Hucho, F. 1986. The nicotinic acetylcholine receptor and its ion channel. *Eur. J. Biochem.* **158:** 211.

Jasmin, B.J., J.P. Changeux, and J. Cartaud. 1990a. Compartmentalization of cold-stable and acetylated microtubules in the subsynaptic domain of chick skeletal muscle fibre. *Nature* **344:** 673.

Jasmin, B.J., J. Cartaud, M. Bornens, and J.P. Changeux. 1989. Golgi apparatus in chick skeletal muscle: Changes in its distribution during endplate development and after denervation. *Proc. Natl. Acad. Sci.* **86:** 7218.

Jasmin, B.J., A. Cartaud, M.A. Ludosky, J.P. Changeux, and J. Cartaud. 1990b. Asymmetric distribution of dystrophin in developing and adult *Torpedo marmorata* electrocyte: Evidence for its association with the acetylcholine receptor-rich membrane. *Proc. Natl. Acad. Sci.* **87:** 3938.

Jennings, C.G.B. and A.W. Mudge. 1989. Chick myotubes in culture express high-affinity receptors for calcitonin gene-related peptide. *Brain Res.* **504:** 199.

Jessell, T.M., R.E. Siegel, and G.D. Fischbach. 1979. Induction of acetylcholine receptors on cultured skeletal muscle by a factor extracted from brain and spinal cord. *Proc. Natl. Acad. Sci.* **76:** 5397.

Kirilovsky, J., A. Duclert, B. Fontaine, A. Devillers-Thiéry, M. Österlund, and J.P. Changeux. 1989. Acetylcholine receptor expression in primary cultures of embryonic chick myotubes. II. Comparison between the effects of spinal cord cells and calcitonin gene-related peptide. *Neuroscience* **32:** 289.

Klarsfeld, A. and J.P. Changeux. 1985. Activity regulates the level of acetylcholine receptor alpha-subunit mRNA in cultured chick myotubes. *Proc. Natl. Acad. Sci.* **82:** 4558.

Klarsfeld, A., P. Daubas, B. Bourachot, and J.P. Changeux. 1987. A 5' flanking region of the chicken acetylcholine receptor α-subunit gene confers tissue-specificity and developmental control of expression in transfected cells. *Mol. Cell. Biol.* **7:** 951.

Klarsfeld, A., R. Laufer, B. Fontaine, A. Devillers-Thiéry, C. Dubreuil, and J.P. Changeux. 1989. Regulation of muscle AChR α-subunit gene expression by electrical activity: Involvement of protein kinase C and Ca^{++}. *Neuron* **2:** 1229.

Knaack, D., I. Shen, M.M. Salpeter, and T.R. Podleski. 1986. Selective effects of ascorbic acid on acetylcholine receptor number and distribution. *J. Cell Biol.* **102:** 795.

Kobayashi, H., K. Hashimoto, S. Uchida, J. Sakuma, K. Takami, M. Tohyama, F. Izumi, and H. Yoshida. 1987. Calcitonin gene related peptide stimulates adenylate cyclase activity in rat striated muscle. *Experientia* **43:** 314.

Kordeli, E., J. Cartaud, H.O. Nghiêm, and J.P. Changeux. 1987a. *In situ* localization of soluble and filamentous actin in *Torpedo marmorata* electrocyte. *Biol. Cell* **59:** 61.

―――. 1987b. The *Torpedo* electrocyte: A model system for the study of receptor-cytoskeleton interaction. *J. Recept. Res.* **7:** 77.

Kordeli, E., J. Cartaud, H.O. Nghiêm, A. Devillers-Thiéry, and J.P. Changeux. 1989. Asynchronous assembly of the acetylcholine receptor and of the 43KD-v_1 protein in the postsynaptic membrane of developing *Torpedo marmorata* electrocyte. *J. Cell Biol.* **108:** 127.

Kordeli, E., J. Cartaud, H.O. Nghiêm, L.A. Pradel, C. Dubreuil, D. Paulin, and J.P. Changeux. 1986. Evidence for a polarity in the distribution of proteins from the cytoskeleton in *Torpedo marmorata* electrocytes. *J. Cell Biol.* **102:** 748.

Lassar, A.B., M.J. Thayer, R.W. Overell, and H. Weintraub. 1989. Transformation by activated *ras* or *fos* prevents myogenesis by inhibiting expression of MyoD1. *Cell* **58:** 659.

Laufer, R. and J.P. Changeux. 1987. Calcitonin gene-related peptide elevates cyclic AMP levels in chick skeletal muscle: Possible neurotrophic role for a coexisting neuronal messenger. *EMBO J.* **6:** 901.

―――. 1989a. Calcitonin gene-related peptide and cyclic AMP stimulate phosphoinositide turnover in skeletal muscle cells: Interaction between two second messenger systems. *J. Biol. Chem.* **264:** 2683.

————. 1989b. Activity dependent regulation of gene expression in muscle and neuronal cells. *Mol. Neurobiol.* **3:** 1.

Leys, E.J., G.F. Crouse, and R.E. Kellems. 1984. Dihydrofolate reductase gene expression in cultured mouse cells is regulated by transcript stabilization in the nucleus. *J. Cell Biol.* **99:** 180.

Lindstrom, J., R. Schoepfer, and P. Whiting. 1987. Molecular studies of the neuronal nicotinic acetylcholine receptor family. *Mol. Neurobiol.* **1:** 281.

Lo, M.M.S., P.B. Garland, J. Lamprecht, and E.A. Bernard. 1980. Rotational mobility of the membrane-bound acetylcholine receptor of *Torpedo* electric organ measured by phosphorescence depolarisation. *FEBS Lett.* **111:** 407.

McManaman, J.L., J.C. Blosser, and S.H. Appel. 1982. Inhibitors of membrane depolarization regulate acetylcholine receptor synthesis by a calcium-dependent, cyclic nucleotide independent mechanism. *Biochim. Biophys. Acta* **720:** 28.

Matteoli, M., C. Haimann, F. Torri-Tarelli, J.M. Polak, B. Ceccarelli, and P. De Camilli. 1988. Differential effect of α-latrotoxin on exocytosis from small synaptic vesicles and from large dense-core vesicles containing calcitonin gene-related peptide at the frog neuromuscular junction. *Proc. Natl. Acad. Sci.* **85:** 7366.

Merlie, J.P. and J.M. Kornhauser. 1989. Neural regulation of gene expression by an acetylcholine receptor promoter in muscle of transgenic mice. *Neuron* **2:** 1295.

Merlie, J. and J.R. Sanes. 1985. Concentration of acetylcholine receptor mRNA in synaptic regions of adult muscle fibers. *Nature* **317:** 66.

Merlie, J.P., R. Sebbane, S. Gardner, E. Olson, and J. Lindstrom. 1983. The regulation of acetylcholine receptor expression in mammalian muscle. *Cold Spring Harbor Symp. Quant. Biol.* **48:** 135.

Miledi, R. 1960. The acetylcholine sensitivity of frog muscle fibers after complete or partial denervation. *J. Physiol.* **151:** 1.

Meunier, J.C., R. Sealock, R. Olsen, and J.P. Changeux. 1974. Purification and properties of the cholinergic receptor from *Electrophorus electricus* electric tissue. *Eur. J. Biochem.* **45:** 371.

Mishina, M., T. Takai, K. Imoto, M. Noda, T. Takahashi, S. Numa, C. Methfessel, and B. Sakmann. 1986. Molecular distinction between fetal and adult forms of muscle acetylcholine receptor. *Nature* **321:** 406.

Monod, J. and F. Jacob. 1962. General conclusions: Teleonomic mechanisms in cellular metabolism, growth and differentiation. *Cold Spring Harbor Symp. Quant. Biol.* **26:** 389.

Morgan, J.I. and T. Curran. 1986. Role of ion flux in the control of c-*fos* expression. *Nature* **322:** 552.

Moss, S.J., M.G. Darlison, D.M.W. Beeson, and E.A. Barnard. 1989. Developmental expression of the genes encoding the four subunits of the chicken muscle acetylcholine receptor. *J. Biol. Chem.* **264:** 20199.

Moss, S.J., D.M. Beeson, J.F. Jackson, M.G. Darlison, and E.A. Barnard. 1987. Differential expression of nicotinic acetylcholine receptor genes in innervated and denervated chicken muscle. *EMBO J.* **6:** 3917.

Murre, C., P. Schonleber McCaw, H. Vaessin, M. Caudy, L.Y. Jan, Y.N. Jan, C.V. Cabrera, J.N. Buskin, S.D. Hauschka, A.B. Lassar, H. Weintraub, and D. Baltimore. 1989. Interactions between heterologous helix-loop-helix proteins generate complexes that bind specifically to a common DNA sequence. *Cell* **58:** 537.

Narayan, P. and H.C. Towle. 1985. Stabilization of a specific nuclear mRNA precursor by thyroid hormone. *Mol. Cell Biol.* **5:** 2642.

Nef, P., A. Mauron, R. Stalder, C. Alliod, and M. Ballivet. 1984. Structure, linkage and sequence of the two genes encoding the delta and gamma subunits of the nicotinic acetylcholine receptor. *Proc. Natl. Acad. Sci.* **81:** 7975.

Neubig, R.R., E.H. Krodel, N.D. Boyd, and J.B. Cohen. 1979. Acetylcholine and local anesthetic binding to *Torpedo* nicotinic postsynaptic membranes after removal of nonreceptor peptides. *Proc. Natl. Acad. Sci.* **76:** 690.

New, H.V. and A.W. Mudge. 1986. Calcitonin gene-related peptide regulates muscle acetylcholine receptor synthesis. *Nature* **323:** 809.

Nghiêm, H.O., J. Cartaud, C. Dubreuil, C. Kordeli, G. Buttin, and J.P. Changeux. 1983. Production and characterization of a monoclonal antibody directed against the 43,000-dalton ν_1 polypeptide from *Torpedo marmorata* electric organ. *Proc. Natl. Acad. Sci.* **80:** 6403.

Niedel, J.E. and P.J. Blackshear. 1986. Protein kinase C. In *Phosphoinositides and receptor mechanisms* (ed. J.W. Putney, Jr.), vol. 7, p. 47. A.R Liss, New York.

Noguchi, K., E. Senba, Y. Morita, M. Sato, and M. Tohyama. 1990. α-CGRP and β-CGRP mRNAs are differentially regulated in the rat spinal cord and dorsal root ganglion. *Mol. Brain Res.* **7:** 299.

Olson, E.N., L. Glaser, J.P. Merlie, and J. Lindstrom. 1984. Expression of acetylcholine receptor α-subunit mRNA during differentiation of the BC$_3$H1 muscle cell line. *J. Biol. Chem.* **259:** 3330.

Olson, E.N., L. Glaser, J.P. Merlie, R. Sebanne, and J. Lindstrom. 1983. Regulation of surface expression of acetylcholine receptors in response to serum and cell growth in the BC$_3$H1 muscle cell line. *J. Biol. Chem.* **258:** 13946.

Österlund, M., B. Fontaine, A. Devillers-Thiéry, B. Geoffroy, and J.P. Changeux. 1989. Acetylcholine receptor expression in primary cultures of embryonic chick myotubes. I. discoordinate regulation of α-, γ-, and δ-subunit gene expression by calcitonin gene-related peptide and by muscle electrical activity. *Neuroscience* **32:** 279.

Peng, H.B. and S.C. Froehner. 1985. Association of the postsynaptic 43K protein with newly formed acetylcholine receptor clusters in cultured muscle cells. *J. Cell Biol.* **100:** 1698.

Pezzementi, L. and J. Schmidt. 1981. Rapid modulation of acetylcholine receptor synthesis. *FEBS Lett.* **135:** 103.

Piette, J., A. Klarsfeld, and J.P. Changeux. 1989. Interaction of nuclear factors with the upstream region of the α-subunit gene of chicken muscle acetylcholine receptor: Variations with muscle differentiation and denervation. *EMBO J.* **8:** 687.

Piette, J., J.L. Bessereau, M. Huchet, and J.P. Changeux. 1990. Two adjacent MyoD1-binding sites regulate expression of the acetylcholine receptor α-subunit gene. *Nature* **345:** 353.

Popot, J.L. and J.P. Changeux. 1984. The nicotinic receptor of acetylcholine: Structure of an oligomeric integral membrane protein. *Physiol. Rev.* **64:** 1162.

Popper, P. and P.E. Micevych. 1989. Localization of calcitonin gene-related peptide and its receptors in a striated muscle. *Brain Res.* **496:** 180.

Ranvier, L. 1875. *Traité technique d'histologie.* F. Savy, Paris.

Rhodes, S.J. and S.F. Konieczny. 1989. Identification of MRF4; a new member of the muscle regulatory factor gene family. *Genes Dev.* **3:** 2050.

Richter, E.A., P.J.F. Cleland, S. Rattigan, and M.G. Clark. 1987. Contraction-associated translocation of protein kinase C in rat skeletal muscle. *FEBS Lett.* **217:** 232.

Roa, M. and J.P. Changeux. 1991. Characterization and developmental evolution of a high affinity binding site for calcitonin gene related peptide (CGRP) on chick skeletal muscle membrane. *Neuroscience* (in press).

Robert, B., P. Barton, A. Minty, P. Daubas, A. Weydert, F. Bonhomme, J. Catalan, D. Chazottes, J.L. Guénet, and M. Buckingham. 1985. Investigation of genetic linkage between myosin and actin genes using an interspecific mouse back-cross. *Nature* **314:** 181.

Ross, A.F., M. Rapuano, J.H. Schmidt, and J.M. Prives. 1987. Phosphorylation and assembly of nicotinic acetylcholine receptor subunits in cultured chick muscle cells. *J. Biol. Chem.* **262:** 635.

Rousselet, A., J. Cartaud, and P.F. Devaux. 1979. Importance des interactions protéine-protéine dans le maintien de la structure des fragments excitables de l'organe électrique de *Torpedo marmorata*. *C.R. Acad. Sci. D* **289:** 461.

Rousselet, A., J. Cartaud, P.F. Devaux, and J.P. Changeux. 1982. The rotational diffusion of the acetylcholine receptor in *Torpedo marmorata* membrane fragments studied with a spin-labelled alpha-toxin: Importance of the 43,000 protein(s). *EMBO J.* **1:** 439.

Saitoh, T. and J.P. Changeux. 1980. Phosphorylation *in vitro* of membrane fragments from *Torpedo marmorata* electric organ. *Eur. J. Biochem.* **105:** 51.

Salpeter, M. and R.H. Loring. 1985. Nicotinic acetylcholine receptors in vertebrate muscle: Properties, distribution and neural control. *Prog. Neurobiol.* **25:** 297.

Sanes, J.R., L.M. Marshall, and U.J. McMahan. 1978. Reinnervation of muscle fiber basal lamina after removal of myofibers. Differentiation of regenerating axons at original synaptic sites. *J. Cell Biol.* **78:** 176.

Schuetze, S.M. and L.W. Role. 1987. Developmental regulation of nicotinic acetylcholine receptor. *Annu. Rev. Neurosci.* **10:** 403.

Sealock, R. 1982. Visualization at the mouse neuromuscular junction of a submembrane structure in common with *Torpedo* postsynaptic membranes. *J. Neurosci.* **2:** 918.

Shainberg, A. and M. Burstein. 1976. Decrease of acetylcholine receptor synthesis in muscle cultures by electrical stimulation. *Nature* **264:** 368.

Shainberg, A., S.A. Cohen, and P.G. Nelson. 1976. Induction of acetylcholine receptors in muscle cultures. *Pfluegers Arch. Eur. J. Physiol.* **361:** 255.

Shieh, B.H., M. Ballivet, and J. Schmidt. 1987. Quantitation of an alpha subunit splicing intermediate: Evidence for transcriptional activation in the control of acetylcholine receptor expression in denervated chick skeletal muscle. *J. Cell Biol.* **104:** 1337.

―――. 1988. Acetylcholine receptor synthesis rate and levels of receptor subunit messenger RNAs in chick muscle. *Neuroscience* **24:** 175.

Smilowitz, H., E. Smart, C. Bowik, and R.J. Chang. 1988. Regulation of the number of α-bungarotoxin binding sites in cultured chick myotubes by a 1.4 dihydropyridine calcium channel antagonist. *J. Neurosci. Res.* **19:** 321.

Sobel, A., M. Weber, and J.P. Changeux. 1977. Large scale purification of the acetylcholine receptor protein in its membrane-bound and detergent-extracted forms from *Torpedo marmorata* electric organ. *Eur. J. Biochem.* **80:** 215.

Sobel, A., T. Heidmann, J. Hofler, and J.P. Changeux. 1978. Distinct protein components from *Torpedo marmorata* membranes carry the acetylcholine receptor site and the binding site for local anesthetics and histrionicotoxin. *Proc. Natl. Acad. Sci.* **75:** 510.

St. John, P.A., S.C. Froehner, D.A. Goodenough, and J.B. Cohen. 1982. Nicotinic postsynaptic membranes from *Torpedo*: Sidedness, permeability to macromolecules, and topography of major polypeptides. *J. Cell. Biol.* **92:** 333.

Takami, K., K. Hashimoto, S. Uchida, M. Tohyama, and H. Yoshida. 1986. Effect of calcitonin gene-related peptide on the cyclic AMP level of isolated mouse diaphragm. *Jpn. J. Pharmacol.* **42:** 345.

Takami, K., Y. Kawai, S. Shiosaka, Y. Lee, S. Girgis, C.J. Hillyard, I. MacIntyre, P.C. Emson, and M. Tohyama. 1985a. Immunohistochemical evidence for the coexistence of calcitonin gene-related peptide- and choline acetyltransferase-like immunoreactivity in neurons of the rat hypoglossal, facial and ambiguus nuclei. *Brain Res.* **328:** 386.

Takami, K., Y. Kawai, S. Uchida, M. Tokyama, Y. Shiotani, H. Hoshida, P.C. Emson, S.H. Girgis, C.J. Hillyard, and I. MacIntyre. 1985b. Effect of calcitonin gene-related peptide on contraction of striated muscle in the mouse. *Neurosci. Lett.* **60:** 227.

Tamaoki, T., H. Nomoto, I. Takahashi, Y. Kato, M. Morimoto, and F. Tomita. 1986. Staurosporine, a potent inhibitor of phospholipid/Ca^{++} dependent protein kinase. *Biochem. Biophys. Res. Commun.* **135:** 397.

Thayer, M.J., S.J. Tapscott, R.L. Davis, W.E. Wright, A.B. Lassar, and H. Weintraub. 1989. Positive autoregulation of the myogenic determination gene MyoD1. *Cell* **58:** 241.

Tsay, H.J. and J. Schmidt. 1989. Skeletal muscle denervation activates acetylcholine receptor genes. *J. Cell Biol.* **108:** 1523.

Uchida, S., H. Yamamoto, S. Ilio, N. Matsumoto, X.B. Wang, N. Yonehara, Y. Imai, R. Inoki, and H. Yoshida. 1990. Release of calcitonin gene-related peptide-like immunoreactive substance from neuromuscular junction by nerve excitation and its action on striated muscle. *J. Neurochem.* **54:** 1000.

Usdin, T.B. and G.D. Fischbach. 1986. Purification and characterization of a polypeptide from chick brain that promotes the accumulation of acetylcholine receptors in chick myotubes. *J. Cell Biol.* **103:** 493.

Vandlen, R.L., W.C.S. Wu, J.C. Eisenach, and M.A. Raftery. 1979. Studies of the composition of purified *Torpedo californica* acetylcholine receptor and of its subunits. *Biochemistry* **10:** 1845.

Vergara, J., R.Y. Tsien, and M. Delay. 1985. Inositol 1,4,5-triphosphate; a possible chemical link in excitation-contraction coupling in muscle. *Proc. Natl. Acad. Sci.* **82:** 6352.

Villar, M.J., M. Huchet, T. Hökfelt, J.P. Changeux, J. Fahrenkrug, and J.C. Brown. 1988. Existence and coexistence of calcitonin gene-related peptide, vasoactive intestinal polypeptide- and somatostatin-like immunoreactivities in spinal cord motoneurons of developing embryos and post-hatch chicks. *Neurosci. Lett.* **86:** 114.

Villar, M.J., M. Roa, M. Huchet, T. Hökfelt, J.P. Changeux, J. Fahrenkrug, J.C. Brown, M. Epstein, and L. Hersh. 1989. Immunoreactive calcitonin gene-related peptide, vasoactive intestinal polypeptide, and somatostatin in developing chicken spinal cord motoneurons. Distribution and role in regulation of cAMP in cultured muscle cells. *Eur. J. Neurosci.* **1:** 269.

Wang, X.M., H.J. Tsay, and J. Schmidt. 1990. Expression of the acetylcholine receptor δ-subunit gene in differentiating chick muscle cells is activated by an element that contains two 16 bp copies of a segment of the α-subunit enhancer. *EMBO J.* **9:** 783.

Wang, Y., H.P. Xu, X.M. Wang, M. Ballivet, and J. Schmidt. 1988. A cell type-specific enhancer drives expression of the chick muscle acetylcholine receptor α-subunit gene. *Neuron* **1:** 527.

Witzemann, V., G. Richardson, and C. Boustead. 1983. Characterization and distribution of acetylcholine receptors and acetylcholinesterase during electric organ development in *Torpedo marmorata*. *Neuroscience* **8:** 333.

Witzemann, V., B. Barg, Y. Nishikawa, B. Sakmann, and S. Numa. 1987. Differential regulation of muscle acetylcholine receptor gamma and epsilon subunits mRNAs. *FEBS Lett.* **223:** 104.

Wennogle, L.P. and J.P. Changeux. 1980. Transmembrane orientation of proteins present in acetylcholine receptor-rich membranes from *Torpedo marmorata* studied by selective proteolysis. *Eur. J. Biochem.* **106:** 381.

Woodruff, M.L., J. Theriot, and S.J. Burden. 1987. 300-kD subsynaptic protein copurifies with acetylcholine receptor-rich membranes and is concentrated at neuromuscular synapses. *J. Cell Biol.* **104:** 939.

Wright, W., D.A. Sassoon, and V.K. Lin. 1989. Myogenin, a factor regulating myogenesis, has a domain homologous to MyoD. *Cell* **56:** 607.

M_r 42,000 ARIA: A Protein That May Regulate the Accumulation of Acetylcholine Receptors at Developing Chick Neuromuscular Junctions

D.L. FALLS,* D.A. HARRIS, F.A. JOHNSON,* M.M. MORGAN,
G. CORFAS,* AND G.D. FISCHBACH*
Department of Anatomy and Neurobiology, Washington University School of Medicine, St. Louis, Missouri 63110

At the neuromuscular junction (NMJ), as at other chemical synapses, the number and distribution of neurotransmitter receptors are critical factors determining the response to presynaptic stimulation. A cardinal event in the formation of the NMJ is the accumulation of acetylcholine receptors (AChRs) in the muscle membrane opposed to the nerve terminal. At the mature junction, receptors are packed in the postsynaptic membrane at a density in excess of $10,000/\mu m^2$. The localization is striking in that more than 70% of the receptors are restricted to the endplate, a region that comprises less than 0.1% of the muscle-surface membrane. In this paper, we review our work directed at elucidating the structure, function, and biological role of a protein purified from chick brain on the basis of its ability to increase the rate of insertion of AChRs into the surface membrane of cultured chick myotubes. This protein, which we designate an ARIA for its *a*cetylcholine *r*eceptor-*i*nducing *a*ctivity, may act at developing and mature neuromuscular junctions. It may also act at chemical synapses in the brain.

Evidence for a Motor Neuron AChR-inducing Activity

Although AChRs and AChR clusters are present on uninnervated embryonic myotubes and myoblasts, it is clear that ingrowing motor nerves induce new receptor clusters rather than seeking out preexisting ones (Anderson et al. 1977; Frank and Fischbach 1979). Interestingly, at early times after addition of neurons to myotube cultures, receptor clusters are found at >80% of growth cone-muscle contacts (Role et al. 1987), an incidence that cannot be explained by a random distribution of receptor clusters along nerve processes. Furthermore, muscle cells are not promiscuous in regard to AChR cluster formation; to date, only cholinergic neurons have been shown to induce clusters. We have compared cholinergic spinal cord motor neurons and ciliary ganglion neurons with noncholinergic spinal cord interneurons (Role et al. 1985). Motor neurons and ciliary ganglion neurons induced many neurite-associated receptor patches (NARPs) with a mean of

1.2 NARPS per 100 μm of neurite-myotube contact. Interneurons were associated with <0.1 receptor clusters/100 μm of contact, a value that is near the background level of clusters on uninnervated myotubes. We have also found that chick sensory neurons (noncholinergic) dissociated from dorsal root ganglia do not induce receptor clusters, confirming an earlier finding made in *Xenopus* cultures (Cohen and Weldon 1980).

Taken together, these investigations suggest that the accumulation of AChRs at the endplate results from a specific interaction between the motor neuron growth cone and the muscle, and the following questions are raised: (1) By what mechanism is the endplate cluster formed, and (2) what is the nature of the interaction between the nerve and muscle?

Chick NARPs form by the directed insertion of newly synthesized AChRs. At least two processes contribute to the accumulation of AChRs at developing junctions (for review, see Schuetze and Role 1987). First, there is a local increase in the rate of AChR synthesis and insertion. Second, AChRs, which can diffuse in the lipid bilayer, become trapped at developing junctions, presumably by binding to sites within the cytoskeleton and/or extracellular matrix. At *Xenopus* junctions, aggregation of surface receptors appears to play the most significant role at early times (Anderson and Cohen 1977).

At chick junctions, on the other hand, an increased rate of local insertion of newly synthesized receptors plays the predominate role at early times (Role et al. 1985; Dubinsky et al. 1989). Myotube cultures were treated with unlabeled α-bungarotoxin (BgTx) to block existing (old) surface receptors. At several intervals between 8 and 17 hours after adding dissociated ciliary neurons to myotube cultures, new AChRs were labeled with rhodamine-BgTx, and all receptors (new plus old) were labeled with monoclonal antibody 35 (MAb 35), a rat monoclonal antibody (provided by J. Lindstrom, Salk Institute), and a fluorescein-labeled goat anti-rat secondary antibody. Normalized rhodamine/fluorescein intensity ratios measured on digitized images indicated that the great majority of AChRs at developing NARPs were not present on the surface membrane prior to nerve-muscle contact.

These results were extended by examining the pat-

---

*Present address: Department of Neurobiology, Harvard Medical School, Boston, Massachusetts 02115.

tern of newly inserted AChRs into NARPs only 1 hour after blocking the existing surface receptors with unlabeled BgTx. For each of the 73 NARPs examined, the pattern of new receptors could be superimposed on the template of total receptors identified with MAb 35, consistent with the idea that NARPs are composed of locally inserted receptors. None of the NARPs demonstrated a rim of new receptors, indicative of trapping mobile receptors at the perimeter of the NARP. It can be further concluded from the data of Dubinsky et al. (1989) that the rate of addition of new AChRs into the membrane of young NARPs greatly exceeds the basal rate of insertion of AChRs per unit area of membrane (see also Role et al. 1985).

Evidence for a diffusible AChR-inducing factor. Early in vitro experiments implicated diffusible factors in the regulation of chick myotube AChR levels (Cohen and Fischbach 1977). Myotubes located close to spinal cord explants were more sensitive to iontophoretically applied ACh, and they bound more ^{125}I-labeled BgTx than did myotubes located some distance away. We have recently obtained in vivo evidence for diffusible AChR-inducing factors acting prior to NMJ formation (Morgan 1990). After labeling the nerve with dioctadecyl tetramethyl indocarbocyanine (DiI), intact chick limb buds were serially sectioned at 100-μm intervals. On embryonic (E) days 5 and 6, most of the limb muscle AChR clusters were adjacent to the nerve trunk but were not contacted by axons or growth cones. These results suggest both the release of diffusible AChR-inducing factors from the invading cholinergic nerves prior to the period of NMJ formation and responsiveness to such factors at this early developmental stage.

Purification of a 42-kD ARIA

Progress has been made in identifying putative trophic factors that can increase the rate of receptor insertion or that promote receptor aggregation. We have focused on the former in light of the findings described above and have purified an AChR-inducing activity more than 10^5-fold from acid extracts of adult chicken brains by ion exchange, size exclusion, and reverse-phase high-performance liquid chromatography (Jessell et al. 1979; Buc-Caron et al. 1983; Usdin and Fischbach 1986). The purification was based on a sensitive, reliable assay in which the initial rate of appearance of new surface membrane AChRs was measured with ^{125}I-labeled BgTx 4 hours after blocking all exposed (old) receptors with unlabeled BgTx (Devreotes and Fambrough 1975). From a preparation starting with 500 chicken brains, only 0.5 μg of protein was recovered in active fractions eluted from the final column. In these early experiments, no protein could be detected in the final column fractions by silver stain of SDS polyacrylamide gels, but after radioiodinating the most active fraction, a single, broad band centered at about M_r 42,000 was evident (Usdin and Fischbach

1986). When fractions from an earlier stage of the purification were electrophoresed, receptor-inducing activity could be eluted from gel slices representing this same mobility range. The most pure material increased the rate of receptor insertion ≥5-fold with a half-maximal concentration of approximately 15 pM. The M_r 42,000 band migrated more rapidly after digestion with neuraminidase or an endoglycosidase preparation, and the bioactivity was destroyed following exposure to

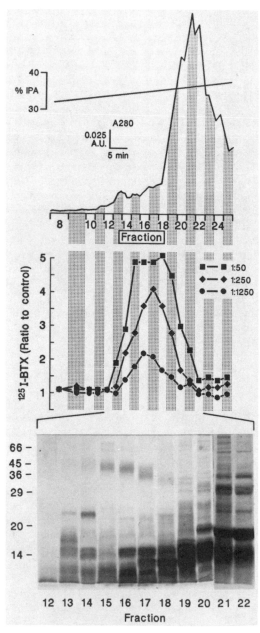

Figure 1. Partial purification of chick brain ARIA through step 5 ("C4/HFBA" column): (*Top*) Chromatogram; (*middle*) bioactivity in the indicated fractions; (*bottom*) silver-stained SDS-polyacrylamide gel of fractions 12–22 (within the bracket). For the fractions with peak bioactivity, the protein concentration tested in the bioassay at the 1:1250 dilution was approximately 60 ng/ml.

trypsin. On the basis of this evidence, we concluded that the bioactivity in the active fractions of the final column was due to a 42-kD sialoglycoprotein.

The purification has now been modified and scaled up. The current protocol is as follows: (1) delipidation of 1000 chicken brains by acetone and ether extraction; (2) extraction of the residual brain "mud" with a cocktail containing trifluoroacetic acid (TFA), formic acid, hydrochloric acid, sodium chloride, and several protease inhibitors followed by adsorption onto Vydac C18 and batch elution with acetonitrile to desalt and further defat; (3) ion-exchange chromatography on CM Sepharose eluted with a linear salt gradient; (4) reverse-phase (RP) chromatography on a semipreparative Vydac C4 column eluted with a gradient of isopropyl alcohol (IPA) in TFA; (5) RP chromatography on the semipreparative Vydac C4 eluted with a gradient of IPA in heptafluorobutyric acid (HFBA); (6) size-exclusion chromatography on a TSK3000SW column; and (7) analytical RP chromatography on a microbore Vydac C18 column eluted with a gradient of acetonitrile in TFA.

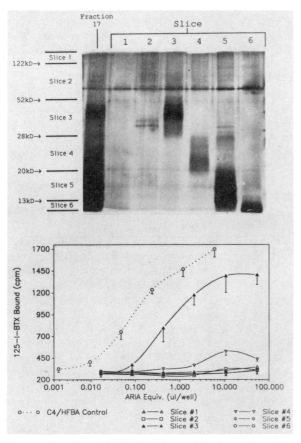

Figure 2. Elution of AChR-inducing activity from slices of an SDS polyacrylamide gel. (*Top*) Slice boundaries are shown to the left of the lane that contains a sample of fraction 17 (see Fig. 1). (Lanes *1–6*) The protein eluted from the corresponding slices. (*Bottom*) AChR-incorporation rate dose-response curves demonstrating that the bioactivity is principally in slice 3, which contains the M_r 33,000–45,000 band. Dotted line is the preelectrophoresis control.

To minimize losses, many of our experiments begin with ARIA purified through step 5 (referred to as C4/HFBA fractions). Receptor-inducing activity elutes from this C4 column as a symmetric, broad peak just before the main protein peak. Figure 1 (top) shows a typical elution in which each fraction was assayed at three doses (Fig. 1, middle). In silver-stained gels of the same fractions (Fig. 1, bottom), a descending staircase of broad bands ranging between M_r 45,000 and M_r 35,000 was evident in the successive active fractions through fraction 18. The same pattern has been observed in C4/HFBA bioactive fractions from more than 20 different extractions. After digesting active fractions with N-glycanase (Genzyme; peptide:N-glycosidase F), an enzyme that cleaves asparagine-linked glycans, all of the bands migrate at the same rate ($\sim M_r$ 33,000), suggesting that the staircase is due to variable glycosylation of the same core protein. Removal of N-linked sugars does not, however, eliminate all heterogeneity within the band: After N-glycanase digestion, analysis by SDS-PAGE (nonequilibrium IEF, first dimension; SDS-PAGE, second dimension) reveals a cluster of spots in the M_r 33,000 two-dimensional range at the basic end of the gel.

To confirm that C4/HFBA receptor-inducing activity migrated in the M_r 35,000–45,0000 range, we separated the components of one fraction (Fig. 1, fraction 17) by SDS-PAGE. Gel slices were homogenized and eluted, and the eluent was chloroform/methanol precipitated to remove SDS (Wessel and Flügge 1984) prior to bioassay. Although the AChR-inducing activity eluted is reduced approximately tenfold compared with the C4/HFBA material (Fig. 2, dotted line), essentially all of the recovered activity appeared in the same gel slice that contained the protein of interest (Fig. 2). The gels were run without reducing agents, since no activity could be recovered following exposure to 50 mM dithiothreitol or 700 mM β-mercaptoethanol.

The apparent molecular weight of the bioactivity shifts along with the M_r 35,000–45,000 protein band following removal of N-linked sugars. In the experiment shown in Figure 3, most of the activity in an undigested sample was present in slice 2 of the gel. Some activity and a faint band were present in slice 4. After digestion with N-glycanase, the heaviest band staining was shifted into slice g14, and the bioactivity in slice g14 was greater than in C4, the parallel control slice. A corollary of this result is that N-linked sugars are not essential for receptor-inducing activity.

ARIA Selectively Increases the Level of AChR α-Subunit mRNA

C4/HFBA bioactive fractions and preparations of similar specific activity have been used to investigate the mechanism by which ARIA increases the AChR-incorporation rate and to begin studies of other biological effects of ARIA.

Earlier experiments had shown that chicken brain ARIA does not increase total protein synthesis (Usdin

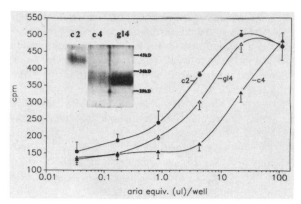

Figure 3. Shift of apparent molecular weight of ARIA after digestion of C4/HFBA material with *N*-glycanase. A C4/HFBA fraction sample digested with *N*-glycanase and a control sample were compared in a gel-elution experiment (see Fig. 2 and text; note, however, that different slice boundaries were used in this experiment and that of Fig. 2). The bioassay results for control slices 2 and 4 (c2, c4) and for *N*-glycanase-treated C4/HFBA slice 4 (gl4) are presented. (*Inset*) A silver stain of the same samples run on an SDS gel.

and Fischbach 1986) or alter the degradation rate of surface receptors. We have recently found that the effect of ARIA is specific even in regard to individual subunits of the AChR (Harris et al. 1988). Nuclease protection assays after solution hybridization with ^{32}P-labeled cRNA probes for the α-, γ-, and δ-subunits (prepared from genomic AChR clones provided by M. Ballivet, University of Geneva) were performed on RNA prepared from myotube cultures. Compared with untreated cultures, samples from ARIA-treated cultures showed a large increase in a 224-nucleotide probe fragment protected by α-mRNA with essentially no change in the fragments protected by the γ- and δ-mRNAs. A 285-nucleotide α-probe fragment, which may represent a partially spliced nuclear precursor of the mature α-mRNA (Shieh et al. 1987), was also increased, suggesting that ARIA acts at the level of gene transcription. The selective effect of ARIA on α-mRNA has also been documented by in situ hybridization (Harris et al. 1989).

In situ hybridization experiments also made evident the fact that the levels of α-mRNA associated with myotube nuclei in ARIA-treated cultures varied dramatically. Large differences in grain density were observed even between nuclei separated by only 50 μm within the same cytoplasm. This heterogeneity among nuclei is probably not due to an uneven distribution of ARIA receptors on the cell surface because the same result was obtained after induction of AChR synthesis by tetrodotoxin (TTX). Thus, some nuclei and hence some regions of each myotube may be more inducible than others. Moreover, untreated myotubes also vary in the amount of α-mRNA associated with nuclei (Bursztajn et al. 1989; Harris et al. 1989). Thus, variability in basal transcription levels and inducibility by ARIA may be related. In this regard, it is noteworthy that the total number of AChRs within different

NARPs ranges over three orders of magnitude (Dubinsky et al. 1988). No consistent trend of NARP intensity or area along the length of individual neurites was evident. Moreover, the same wide range in total receptor number was observed among receptor clusters (hot spots) on uninnervated myotubes. These observations suggest that the variation in NARP size and density may result from regional variation in the ability of multinucleated myotubes to respond rather than from variation of the local concentration of AChR-inducing activity. If so, the heterogeneity in responsiveness might reflect the uneven distribution of regulatory factors within multinucleated myotubes. It will be important to identify such factors to determine whether they are associated with nuclei of a particular myoblast lineage and to define the relationship between sites of nerve-muscle synapse formation and regions of ARIA responsiveness.

Spinal cord explants also increase α-subunit mRNA in cocultured myotubes (Bursztajn et al. 1990). As observed in ARIA-treated cultures, the amount of α-mRNA associated with different myotube nuclei in the cocultures varies dramatically. In the same study, it was shown that ciliary neurons (cholinergic) also induce α-mRNA, but dorsal root ganglion cells (noncholinergic) do not. Importantly, the ciliary neurons increased the level of α-mRNA even when prevented from directly contacting the myotubes by the interposition of a 0.4-μm membrane.

It is likely that the effects of ARIA are mediated by a specific receptor acting through a second messenger pathway. We have not yet attempted to identify receptors, and little can be said about ARIA second messengers. cAMP, Ca^{++}, and protein kinase C have all been implicated as potential regulators of AChR levels (Shainberg et al. 1976; Birnbaum et al. 1980; McManaman et al. 1981; Fontaine et al. 1987; Shieh et al. 1988; Klarsfeld et al. 1989). Of these, we have to date investigated only the relationship of cAMP to the action of ARIA and have found that cAMP is unlikely to play a role (Johnson et al. 1990). cAMP levels in cultures treated with ARIA were compared with cAMP levels in cultures treated with several other factors known to modulate AChR levels. Fibroblast-free myotube cultures were treated with ARIA, calcitonin gene-related peptide (CGRP), or forskolin; cAMP was measured by a radioimmunoassay. Forskolin increased cAMP 17-fold, CGRP increased cAMP 4.5-fold, and ARIA produced no change. In parallel cultures, forskolin increased AChR incorporation 4.3-fold, CGRP increased AChR incorporation 1.1-fold (10%), and ARIA increased AChR incorporation 3.2-fold. Thus, ARIA probably does not act through a cAMP-dependent mechanism.

Other Effects of ARIA on AChR Biosynthesis?

A 42-kD ARIA-like molecule may regulate the type of AChRs synthesized and the overall rate of AChR synthesis. At rat endplates, AChRs undergo an increase in channel conductance and a decrease in mean channel open time during the first 3 weeks after birth (for review, see Schuetze and Role 1987). This change in phenotype appears to be due to expression of the gene for a fifth receptor subunit, the ε-subunit gene (Mishina et al. 1986; Witzemann et al. 1987). The switch in ACh channel conductance and kinetics does not occur if muscles are denervated shortly after birth (Brenner et al. 1983; Brenner and Sakmann 1983; Schuetze and Vicini 1986), so the change in phenotype may be under neurotrophic control. Recent experiments in collaboration with J.-C. Martinou and J. Merlie (Washington University) have shown that addition of chick brain ARIA to primary cultures of mouse myotubes may increase the level of ε-subunit mRNA by sevenfold. Significantly, TTX at doses sufficient to prevent contraction and produce a clear increase in α-mRNA had no effect on ε-mRNA. Likewise, CGRP increased α-mRNA but did not increase ε-mRNA.

Other Proteins Concentrated at the Motor Endplate

The motor neuron induces not just the formation of a junctional receptor cluster, but rather the assembly of an intricately organized synaptic machinery with many molecular components. It is certainly possible that the formation and maintenance of a neuromuscular junction require coordinate regulation of the synthesis and processing of these molecules. Characterization of the effects of ARIA on other synaptic molecules will give insight into both the spectrum of action of ARIA and patterns of regulation at the NMJ.

A number of proteins are known to accumulate at the mature motor endplate. Voltage-gated Na^+ channels are concentrated in the troughs of junctional folds and also in the perijunctional membrane (Beam et al. 1985; Flucher and Daniels 1989). The cytoplasmic surface of the postsynaptic membrane is associated with proteins of 43 kD, 51 kD, 87 kD, and 270 kD (Carr et al. 1989) that are thought to play a role in receptor immobilization, perhaps by anchoring AChRs to the underlying cytoskeleton (for review, see Froehner 1986), and with ankyrin, which is codistributed with Na^+ channels (Flucher and Daniels 1989). The synaptic cleft contains high concentrations of acetylcholinesterase (AChE), agrin, S-laminin, at least two proteoglycans, neural cell adhesion molecule (N-CAM), and several other determinants (for review, see Sanes 1989). Among the molecules in the cleft, agrin is of particular interest in regard to the initial accumulation of AChRs. Agrin is present in spinal cord motor neurons (Magill-Solc and McMahan 1988), but at least one

form of agrin is present in (and synthesized by) embryonic myotubes (Godfrey et al. 1988; Fallon and Gelfman 1989; Lieth et al. 1989). Recent experiments with species-specific anti-agrin antibodies have shown that muscle-derived agrin accumulates at newly formed nerve muscle synapses in vitro (Lieth et al. 1989).

We are now studying the effect of ARIA on the number of voltage-gated Na^+ channels. Using radiolabeled saxitoxin ([^{3}H]STX, provided by W. Catteral), we found that in three of four experiments, ARIA increased the number of STX-binding sites in cultured myotubes almost to the same extent as BgTx-binding sites.

An ARIA Candidate Protein

Amino-terminal sequence determination. Employing material obtained using the scaled-up preparation (see above), the amino-terminal sequence of the broad band centered at M_r 42,000 was determined in several ways. First, a reversed-phase column fraction, comparable to the C4/HFBA fraction described above, was analyzed by SDS-PAGE, electroblotted onto a polyvinylidine difluoride (PVDF) membrane (Matsudaira 1987), and the segment of PVDF that contained the M_r 35,000–45,000 band was placed directly in the sample chamber of an Applied Biosystems 410A gas phase sequencer. Second, pooled active fractions from the C4/HFBA column were further purified by gel filtration through a TSK column (step 6). An active fraction from this column that contained little protein detectable by silver stain other than the broad band of interest was concentrated, applied to a polybrene-coated glass-fiber filter, and sequenced. Third, a preparation was carried through the C18 microbore stage of the purification (step 7). The final A214 trace of this scaled-up preparation showed a complex of three peaks over the range of bioactive fractions rather than the one small peak observed in a previous study (Usdin and Fischbach 1986). The fraction from each peak with the maximal absorbance at 214 nm was sequenced. The sequences at the bottom of the page were obtained with, in every case, only one amino acid evident at each cycle. Thus, it appears that we are dealing with the same sequenceable protein in each preparation. In step 7, receptor-inducing activity was maximal in peak 2, whereas most of the mass was in peak 1. This result suggests that some forms of the protein are not biologically active, a possibility that is discussed further below.

Immunoblots provided additional evidence for the identity of the staircase of bands in successive C4/HFBA fractions. An antiserum raised against a synthe-

M_r 35,000–45,000 band:	K K G K G K P S G G G E G
TSK fraction:	K K G K G K P S G G G ? G A G S H ? Q P S Y P ? Q P G
C18-peak 1:	K K G K G K P S G G
C18-peak 2:	K K G K G K P ? G G
C18-peak 3:	? ? G K ? K

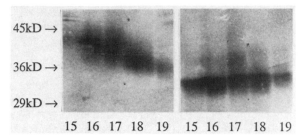

Figure 4. Western blot of sequential C4/HFBA fractions probed with a rabbit antiserum raised against a synthetic peptide corresponding to the amino-terminal 11-amino-acid sequence determined by Edman degradation. (*Left*) Undigested fractions; (*right*) the same fractions digested with *N*-glycanase.

tic peptide corresponding to the first 11 amino acids labeled each component of the staircase (Fig. 4, left), and after *N*-glycanase digestion, the antiserum stained the bands aligned at M_r 33,000 (Fig. 4, right). No staining was detected with preimmune serum or with immune serum that had been preincubated with excess peptide. These results were an important confirmation of our conclusions based on the silver-stained gels (see above).

Molecular cloning of an ARIA candidate protein. The polymerase chain reaction (PCR) was used with degenerate 5′ and 3′ primers (corresponding to amino acids 1–7 and 19–23 of the chemically determined sequence) to amplify from chicken brain poly(A)$^+$ RNA a 34-nucleotide segment that encodes amino acids 8–18. PCR products were separated by polyacrylamide gel electrophoresis, and bands of approximately the expected size were eluted, ligated into pBluescript II (STRATAGENE), and transfected into *Escherichia coli*. Clones that appeared to contain inserts of exactly the right length, determined by high-resolution gel electrophoresis, were sequenced by the dideoxy chain termination method. The amino acid sequence predicted by translating the PCR-amplified segment corresponded to the sequence determined by Edman degradation. It indicated that residue 12 is tryptophan and residue 18 is arginine. A synthetic 34-mer probe with the identical sequence was used to screen an embryonic chick brain cDNA library in λgt10 phage (obtained from D. Fambrough, Johns Hopkins). From 250,000 phage, four positive clones were obtained: three that were 2.2 kb long and one that was 1.9 kb long. Sequence analysis revealed that all three 2.2-kb clones had identical 5′ and 3′ ends; the 1.9-kb clone shared the same 3′ end but was truncated by 300 nucleotides at its 5′ end.

One of the 2.2-kb inserts, which we designate 65-21, was sequenced in its entirety. This clone contains a coding region that predicts a protein of 267 amino acids flanked by 3′ and 5′ untranslated regions of 1216 nucleotides and 171 nucleotides, respectively. The protein includes the entire sequence of the 27 amino acids determined by Edman degradation. Thus, there can be

no doubt that 65-21 corresponds to the protein that we partially sequenced chemically.

The first methionine upstream of the chemically determined sequence is followed by a relatively hydrophobic, 24-amino-acid sequence that is characteristic of signal peptides, and the amino-terminal lysine of the chemically determined sequence (residue 25) follows a predicted signal sequence cleavage site (Folz and Gordon 1987). Several other features of the deduced amino acid sequence are noteworthy (Fig. 5). There is a series of eight imperfect hexapeptide repeats in the amino-terminal half of the molecule in which every third residue is proline and every sixth residue is glycine. An uninterrupted stretch of 20 nonpolar amino acids flanked by charged residues is located near the middle of the sequence, and a shorter region rich in hydrophobic residues is located near the carboxyl terminus. There are four potential asparagine-linked glycosylation sites in the molecule. The sequence also contains two cysteine residues with the potential therefore for disulfide bond formation.

A computer search of the NBRF protein data base revealed that the chick 65-21 protein is related to the mammalian prion protein (PrP), a normal component of the nervous system, which in modified form has been implicated in the pathogenesis of a group of transmissible neurodegenerative diseases (for a recent review, see Prusiner 1989). The sequence predicted by 65-21 and the sequence of a mouse PrP (Westaway et al. 1987) are shown aligned in Figure 6. With one gap in the 65-21 sequence and five in the prion sequence, the two proteins are identical at 33% of the amino acid positions (lines). The degree of similarity rises to 43% when conservative substitutions are taken into account (closed diamonds). With one exception, a stretch of 24 amino acids that includes most of the central hydrophobic region is identical in the chick and mouse proteins. All 24 match the sequence of the PrP from a different mouse strain (Westaway et al. 1987). The close relationship of these proteins is also evident at the level of structural domains. Both contain proline- and glycine-rich repeats in the amino-terminal half of the molecule and both contain central and carboxy-terminal hydrophobic regions. The 65-21 protein and PrP each contain two cysteine residues, and after optimal alignment, one

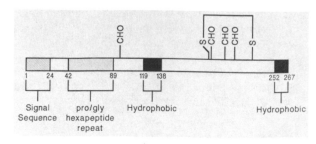

Figure 5. Schematic of 65-21 protein structural features. CHO signifies potential asparagine-linked glycosylation sites. The relative positions of the two cysteines (S) are indicated, and they are represented as forming an intramolecular disulfide bond (which, however, has not been directly demonstrated).

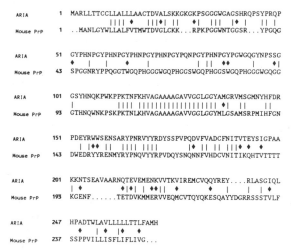

```
ARIA       1  MARLLTTCCLLALLLAACTDVALSKKGKGKPSGGGWGAGSHRQPSYPRQP
                  ||||  ♦    |||♦|  ||   ♦|  |||  |♦ |   ||| |
Mouse PrP  1  ..MANLGYWLLALFVTMWTDVGLCKK...RPKPGGWNTGGSR...YPGQG

ARIA      51  GYPHNPGYPHNPGYPHNPGYPHNPGYPQNPGYPHNPGYPGWGQGYNPSSG
                 ♦   |   |   ♦   |        | ||  ♦♦     ♦     ♦|
Mouse PrP 43  SPGGNRYPPQGGTWGQPHGGGWGQPHGGSWGQPHGGSWGQPHGGGWGQGG

ARIA     101  GSYHNQKPWKPPKTNFKHVAGAAAAGAVVGGLGGYAMGRVMSGMNYHFDR
              |        ||||  ||||||||||||||||||| ♦|  ||    ||
Mouse PrP 93  GTHNQWNKPSKPKTNLKHVAGAAAAGAVVGGLGGYMLGSAMSRPMIHFGN

ARIA     151  PDEYRWWSENSARYPNRVYYRDYSSPVPQDVFVADCFNITVTEYSIGPAA
              |  |♦♦  ||  ||||  |||  |♦ ||  ||  |  |||♦ ♦  ♦
Mouse PrP 143 DWEDRYYRENMYRYPNQVYYRPVDQYSNQNNFVHDCVNITIKQHTVTTTT

ARIA     201  KKNTSEAVAARNQTEVEMENKVVTKVIREMCVQQYREY....RLASGIQL
              | ♦      ♦|♦| | ♦♦|| ♦     ♦      |   | ♦    |
Mouse PrP 193 KGENF......TETDVKMMERVVEQMCVTQYQKESQAYYDGRRSSSTVLF

ARIA     247  HPADTWLAVLLLLLTTLFAMH
              ♦  |  |♦  |♦  ♦
Mouse PrP 237 SSPPVILLISFLIFLIVG...
```

Figure 6. Predicted amino acid sequence of 65-21 aligned with that of a mouse PrP. The PrP sequence is from Westaway et al. (1987). **Note added in proof:** The sequence labeled "ARIA" should instead be labeled "65-21 protein". Based on further evaluation of the nucleic acid sequence data, we have interpreted residue 111 of the 65-21 protein to be alanine, not (as shown in the figure) arginine.

of the cysteines is located in the same position in both proteins (65-21 residue 186) and the other is separated by four residues. One of the two potential *N*-glycosylation sites in PrP occurs at the same position as one of the four 65-21 protein sites, and the second differs in position by only one residue. Finally, we have found that as with PrP, the 65-21 protein may be attached to the surface membrane by a phosphatidylinositol-glycan anchor (see below).

Tissue distribution and developmental time course of 65-21. The predominant mRNA species detected on Northern blots hybridized with radiolabeled 65-21 is 2.9 kb. In chicken spinal cord and brain (the source of ARIA), the amount of this message increased during embryonic development and reached maximal values in adult animals. It is significant that the mRNA is expressed in the spinal cord as early as E6 because it is at this time that motor axons first invade the primitive muscle masses in the limb and functional nerve-muscle

synapses can be demonstrated (Landmesser and Morris 1975). In adult animals, the 2.9-kb mRNA was highly concentrated in the central nervous system, and with the exception of the kidney, little or no signal was detected in nonneuronal tissues. In embryos, the 2.9-kb mRNA was most concentrated in the brain and spinal cord, but significant levels were present in nonneuronal tissues. In situ hybridization of sections from E18 and adult spinal cords using ^{35}S-labeled cRNA probe revealed that 65-21 mRNA is concentrated in the ventral horn (Fig. 7). Label above the level produced by a control sense-strand probe was evident throughout the cord, but clusters of grains over large cells in the ventral gray matter, presumably motor neurons, were striking.

We raised rabbit anti-sera and mouse monoclonal antibodies against synthetic peptides that correspond to sequences within the protein encoded by 65-21. In our initial immunohistological studies, we have found that several of the monoclonal antibodies that recognized C4/HFBA material on ELISA label determinants that are concentrated in motor neurons of E18 spinal cord (Fig. 8), a result in agreement with the in situ findings.

Does 65-21 Encode an ARIA?

The following evidence supports the hypothesis that the 65-21-encoded protein is the 42-kD ARIA: (1) A single, broad band in this molecular weight range is evident in silver-stained gels of nearly all active fractions. (2) ARIA can be eluted from gel slices that contain this band. (3) The band and the bioactivity migrate more rapidly after *N*-glycanase digestion. (4) Only one amino-terminal sequence was detected in gel slices or column fractions that contained bioactivity (and the band). (5) The distribution of 65-21 protein and mRNA is consistent with a possible role in neuromuscular junction formation. Determinants recognized by monoclonal antibodies raised against three different peptides that correspond to predicted sequences within 65-21 are concentrated in anterior horn motor neurons, in ciliary ganglion neurons, and perhaps in other cholinergic neurons, as well. mRNA recognized by 65-21 is concentrated in motor neurons, and it is expressed in the spinal cord at the time AChR-inducing

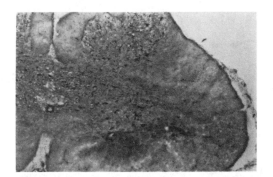
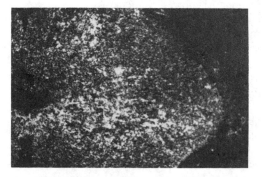

Figure 7. Localization of 65-21 mRNA by in situ hybridization in a 10-μm frozen section of chick E18 spinal cord. (*Left*) Thionin stain (a Nissl stain) visualized with bright-field optics; (*right*) dark-field illumination. The ^{35}S-labeled probe was derived from the 3' noncoding region. Ventral is at the bottom of the figure; lateral is to the right.

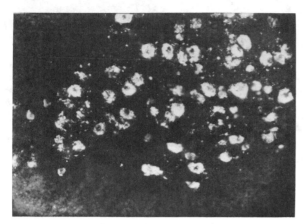

Figure 8. Immunohistochemistry localization of 65-21 protein. A frozen section of E18 spinal cord was incubated with MAb 5.1, a mouse monoclonal raised against a synthetic peptide corresponding to an internal 13-amino-acid segment of the 65-21 protein. Note the concentration of label in large neurons of the anterior horn. The same pattern of staining has been seen with other antibodies raised against synthetic peptides corresponding to different regions of the 65-21 protein. Ventral is at the bottom of the figure; lateral is to the left.

activity is first evident in the limb. (6) The predicted protein includes a signal sequence, which is consistent with the notion that ARIA is a secreted protein.

More definitive proof depends on immunoprecipitation of ARIA or expression of the bioactivity following transfection with 65-21. Unfortunately, we have not yet succeeded on either front. A brief summary of our efforts to date follows.

None of the antipeptide sera or monoclonal antibodies now in hand precipitated the receptor-inducing activity or a significant amount of the M_r 35,000–45,000 protein, and none of the peptides or antibodies blocked the effect of ARIA. Using the pET (plasmid for *Ex*pression by *T*7 RNA polymerase) vector system (Rosenberg et al. 1987), a bacterial fusion protein was constructed that includes the entire coding region of 65-21. A rabbit antiserum raised against the fusion protein (designated 024) did precipitate most of the material recognized on Western blots, but the bioactivity in the supernatant was not decreased compared with the preimmune control. Similarly, we have not consistently been able to recover more bioactivity from the immune pellet than from the prebleed pellet. These results raise a question about the identity of 65-21 protein and ARIA. Either 024 and the antipeptide antibodies recognize an inactive form of ARIA or ARIA is a different protein, perhaps with a blocked amino terminus, whose physical properties are similar enough to the 65-21 protein that ARIA and the 65-21 protein remain associated through the entire purification procedure. We favor the idea that we are dealing with a single protein, the bulk of which is inactive either because of the lack of crucial posttranslational modification or as a result of our rigorous purification protocol. It would certainly not be surprising that anti-

bodies directed against a bacterial fusion protein or short peptide fragments do not recognize the protein in its native, folded conformation (Lerner 1984).

We have used a transient transfection protocol in attempts to express AChR-inducing activity. Metabolic labeling experiments indicated that COS cells transfected with a vector containing the entire 65-21 coding region were not processing the 65-21 protein in the expected manner: Several discrete bands between M_r 25,000 and M_r 35,000 were evident rather than a broad band centered at M_r 42,000. Therefore, we introduced the same expression vector construct into a more "neuronal" cell line: neuroblastoma N2a. In contrast with the COS cells, transfected N2a cells synthesize a broad band of labeled protein in the M_r 35,000–45,000 range. The band was seen both in medium conditioned by 65-21-transfected N2a cells and in SDS extracts of these cells. Since the mammalian PrP can be attached to the cell membrane by a phosphatidylinositol glycolipid anchor (Stahl et al. 1987), we treated a preparation of transfected N2a cells with phosphatidylinositol-specific phospholipase C (PIPLC). A protein that reacts with anti-65-21 antisera was released into the medium following digestion of intact cells with this enzyme. No receptor-inducing activity was recovered in cell extracts, conditioned medium, or in the medium collected after digestion with the PIPLC. However, calculations based on ARIA dose-response curves and Western blots indicate that in these experiments, the transiently transfected N2a cells produced, at the most, 1/100 the amount of protein required to produce an effect in our bioassay (assuming that the specific activity of the recombinant protein is similar to that of the protein purified from brain). Additional expression studies with stably transfected cell lines and with postmitotic neurons are now under way.

Following a conclusive demonstration of the molecular identity of the chicken brain ARIA, it will remain to be demonstrated that this molecule has a physiological role in neuromuscular junction formation. This question will be approached through detailed immunohistochemical and in situ hybridization studies and by attempting to perturb synaptogenesis in vitro and in vivo with blocking antibodies and antisense RNA.

CONCLUSIONS

We have purified (to apparent homogeneity) a protein from chicken brain that increases the rate of AChR synthesis severalfold with a half maximal response of about 15 pM (Jessell et al. 1979; Buc-Caron et al. 1983; Usdin and Fischbach 1986). This protein selectively increases the level of mRNA that encodes the AChR α-subunit (Harris et al. 1988, 1989). An amino-terminal amino acid sequence has been determined by Edman degradation, and the entire amino acid sequence of an ARIA candidate protein has been deduced from a full-length cDNA clone (named 65-21) isolated from an embryonic chick cDNA library. A number of lines of evidence suggest that the cloned protein is the AChR-inducing activity in our extract. However, a puzzle remains to be resolved before concluding that ARIA is identical to the protein encoded by 65-21: To date, we have failed to immunoprecipitate AChR-inducing activity, and we have not expressed bioactivity by transfecting cells with 65-21-containing plasmids.

The predicted amino acid sequence is homologous to the mammalian PrP, a glycoprotein found in normal brain but whose function is unknown. The 65-21-encoded protein may be the chicken homolog of the mammalian PrP or possibly a member of a family of prion-like proteins. A modified form of the prion protein (PrP^{Sc}) is thought to be involved in the pathogenesis of scrapie in sheep and rodents and in several human neurodegenerative diseases (Prusiner 1989). It is attractive to think that an AChR-inducing factor also plays a crucial trophic role in the brain and that neuronal degeneration results from the accumulation of an inactive form of the protein.

ACKNOWLEDGMENTS

We thank Rebecca Cole, Rebecca Dill-Devor, Sepideh (Dawn) Lavasani, and William Walsh for their excellent technical assistance. This work was supported by the National Institute of Neurological Diseases and Strokes (NINDS), the McKnight Foundation, and the McDonnell Center for Cellular and Molecular Neurobiology at Washington University. D.L.F. is the recipient of a Physician Scientist Award from the National Institute of Child Health and Human Development, and D.A.H. is the recipient of a Clinical Investigator Development Award from the NINDS.

REFERENCES

Anderson, M.J. and M.W. Cohen. 1977. Nerve-induced and spontaneous redistribution of acetylcholine receptors on cultured muscle cells. *J. Physiol.* **268**: 757.

Anderson, M.J., M.W. Cohen, and E. Zorychta. 1977. Effects of innervation on the distribution of acetylcholine receptors on cultured muscle cells. *J. Physiol.* **268**: 731.

Beam, K.J., J.H. Caldwell, and D.J. Campbell. 1985. Na channels in skeletal muscle concentrated near the neuromuscular junction. *Nature* **313**: 588.

Birnbaum, M., M.A. Reis, and A. Shainberg. 1980. Role of calcium in the regulation of acetylcholine receptor synthesis in cultured muscle cells. *Pfluegers Arch. Eur. J. Physiol.* **385**: 37.

Brenner, H.R. and B. Sakmann. 1983. Neurotrophic control of channel properties at neuromuscular synapses of rat muscle. *J. Physiol.* **337**: 159.

Brenner, H.R., T. Meier, and B. Widmer. 1983. Early action of nerve determines motor endplate differentiation in rat muscle. *Nature* **305**: 536.

Buc-Caron, M.H., P. Nystrom, and G.D. Fischbach. 1983. Induction of acetylcholine receptor synthesis and aggregation: Partial purification of low molecular weight activity. *Dev. Biol.* **95**: 378.

Bursztajn, S., S.A. Berman, and W. Gilbert. 1989. Differential expression of acetylcholine receptor mRNA in cultured myotube nuclei. *Proc. Natl. Acad. Sci.* **86**: 2928.

———. 1990. Factors released by ciliary neurons and spinal cord explants induce acetylcholine receptor mRNA expression cultured muscle cells. *J. Neurobiol.* **21**: 387.

Carr, C., G.D. Fischbach, and J.B. Cohen. 1989. A novel 87,000-M_r protein associated with acetylcholine receptors in *Torpedo* electric organ and vertebrate skeletal muscle. *J. Cell Biol.* **109**: 1753.

Cohen, M.W. and P.R. Weldon. 1980. Localization of acetylcholine receptors and synaptic ultrastructure at nerve-muscle contacts in culture: Dependence on nerve type. *J. Cell Biol.* **86**: 388.

Cohen, S.A. and G.D. Fischbach. 1977. Clusters of acetylcholine receptors located at identified nerve-muscle synapses *in vitro*. *Dev. Biol.* **59**: 24.

Devreotes, P.N. and D.M. Fambrough. 1975. Acetylcholine receptor turnover in membranes of developing muscle fibers. *J. Cell Biol.* **65**: 335.

Dubinsky, J.M., M. Morgan, and G.D. Fischbach. 1988. Variation among acetylcholine receptor clusters induced by ciliary ganglion neurons *in vitro*. *Dev. Biol.* **130**: 209.

Dubinsky, J.M., D.J. Loftus, G.D. Fischbach, and E.L. Elson. 1989. Formation of acetylcholine receptor clusters in chick myotubes: Migration or new insertion? *J. Cell. Biol.* **109**: 1733.

Fallon, J.R. and C.E. Gelfman. 1989. Agrin-related molecules are concentrated at AchR clusters in normal and aneural developing muscle. *J. Cell Biol.* **108**: 1527.

Flucher, B.E. and M.P. Daniels. 1989. Distribution of Na$^+$ channels and ankyrin in neuromuscular junctions is complementary to that of acetylcholine receptors and the 43kd protein. *Neuron* **3**: 163.

Folz, R.J. and J.I. Gordon. 1987. Computer-assisted predictions of signal peptidase processing sites. *Biochem. Biophys. Res. Commun.* **146**: 870.

Fontaine, B., A. Klarsfeld, and J. Changeux. 1987. Calcitonin gene-related peptide and muscle activity regulate acetylcholine receptor α-subunit mRNA levels by distinct intracellular pathways. *J. Cell Biol.* **105**: 1337.

Frank, E. and G.D. Fischbach. 1979. Early events in neuromuscular junction formation *in vitro*. Induction of acetylcholine receptor clusters in the postsynaptic membrane and morphology of newly formed nerve-muscle synapses. *J. Cell Biol.* **83**: 143.

Froehner, S.C. 1986. The role of the postsynaptic cytoskeleton in AchR organization. *Trends Neurosci.* **9**: 37.

Godfrey, E.W., R.E. Siebenlist, P.A. Wallskog, L.M. Walters, D.L. Bolander, and D.E. Yorde. 1988. Basal lamina components are concentrated in premuscle masses and at early acetylcholine receptor clusters in chick embryo hindlimb muscles. *Dev. Biol.* **130**: 471.

Harris, D.A., D.L. Falls, and G.D. Fischbach. 1989. Differential activation of myotube nuclei following exposure to an acetylcholine receptor-inducing factor. *Nature* **337**: 173.

Harris, D.A., D.L. Falls, R.M. Dill-Devor, and G.D. Fischbach. 1988. Acetylcholine receptor-inducing factor from chicken brain increases the level of mRNA encoding the receptor α-subunit. *Proc. Natl. Acad. Sci.* **85**: 1893.

Jessell, T.M., R.E. Siegel, and G.D. Fischbach. 1979. Induction of acetylcholine receptors on cultured skeletal muscle by a factor extracted from brain and spinal cord. *Proc. Natl. Acad. Sci.* **76**: 5397.

Johnson, F.A., D.L. Falls, and G.D. Fischbach. 1990. Acetylcholine receptor-inducing activity does not increase intracellular cAMP in chick myotubes. *Soc. Neurosci. Abstr.* **16**: 412.

Klarsfeld, A., R. Laufer, B. Fontaine, A. Deuillers-Thiery, C. Dubreuil, and J.P. Changeux. 1989. Regulation of muscle AchR α subunit gene expression by electrical activity: Involvement of protein kinase C and Ca^{2+}. *Neuron* **2**: 1229.

Landmesser, L.T. and D.G. Morris. 1975. The development of functional innervation in the hind limb of the chick embryo. *J. Physiol.* **249**: 301.

Lerner, R.A. 1984. Antibodies of predetermined specificity in biology and medicine. *Adv. Immunol.* **36**: 1.

Lieth, E., A.C. Missias, E. Yang, and J. Fallon. 1989. Agrin-related molecules at the developing neuromuscular junction. In *The assembly of the nervous system* (ed. L.T. Landmesser), p. 213. A.R. Liss, New York.

Magill-Solc, C. and U. J. McMahan. 1988. Motor neurons contain agrin-like molecules. *J. Cell Biol.* **107:** 1825.

Matsudaira, P. 1987. Sequence from picomole quantities of proteins electroblotted onto polyvinylidene diflouride membranes. *J. Biochem.* **262:** 10035.

McManaman, J.L., J.C. Blosser, and S.H. Appel. 1981. The effects of calcium on acetylcholine receptor synthesis. *J. Neurosci.* **1:** 771.

Mishina, M., T. Takai, K. Imoto, M. Noda, T. Takahashi, S. Numa, C. Methfessel, and B. Sakmann. 1986. Molecular distinction between fetal and adult forms of muscle acetylcholine receptor. *Nature* **321:** 406.

Morgan, M.M. 1990. "A study in early myogenesis: Acetylcholine receptor expression by mononucleated muscle cells of the chick." Ph.D. thesis, Washington University, St. Louis, Missouri.

Prusiner, S.B. 1989. Scrapie prions. *Annu. Rev. Microbiol.* **43:** 345.

Role, L.W., D. Roufa, and G.D. Fischbach. 1987. The distribution of acetylcholine receptor clusters and sites of transmitter release along chick ciliary ganglion neurite-myotube contacts in culture. *J. Cell Biol.* **104:** 371.

Role, L.W., V.R. Matossian, R.J. O'Brien, and G.D. Fischbach. 1985. On the mechanism of acetylcholine receptor accumulation at newly formed synapses on chick myotubes. *J. Neurosci.* **5:** 2197.

Rosenberg, A.H., B.N. Lade, D. Chui, S. Lin, J.J. Dunn, and F.W. Studier. 1987. Vectors for selective expression of cloned DNAs by T7 RNA polymerase. *Gene* **56:** 125.

Sanes, J.R. 1989. Extracellular matrix molecules that influence neural development. *Annu. Rev. Neurosci.* **12:** 491.

Schuetze, S.M. and L.W. Role. 1987. Developmental regulation of nicotinic acetylcholine receptors. *Annu. Rev. Neurosci.* **10:** 403.

Schuetze, S.M. and S. Vicini. 1986. Apparent acetylcholine receptor channel conversion at individual rat soleus endplates *in vitro. J. Physiol.* **375:** 153.

Shainberg, A., S.A. Cohen, and P.G. Nelson. 1976. Induction of acetylcholine receptors in muscle cultures. *Pfluegers. Arch. Eur. J. Physiol.* **361:** 255.

Shieh, B.H., M. Ballivet, and J. Schmidt. 1987. Quantitation of an alpha subunit splicing intermediate: Evidence for transcriptional activation in the control of acetylcholine receptor expression in denervated chick skeletal muscle. *J. Cell Biol.* **104:** 1337.

———. 1988. Acetylcholine receptor synthesis rate and levels of receptor subunit messenger RNAs in chick muscle. *Neuroscience* **24:** 175.

Stahl, N., D.R. Borchelt, K. Hsiao, and S.B. Prusiner. 1987. Scrapie prion protein contains a phosphatidylinositol glycolipid. *Cell* **51:** 229.

Usdin, T.B. and G.D. Fischbach. 1986. Purification and characterization of a polypeptide from chick brain that promotes the accumulation of acetylcholine receptors in chick myotubes. *J. Cell Biol.* **103:** 493.

Wessel, D. and I.T. Flügge. 1984. A method for the quantitative recovery of protein in dilute solution in the presence of detergents and lipids. *Anal. Biochem.* **138:** 141.

Westaway, D., P. Goodman, C. Mirenda, M.P. McKinley, G. Carlson, and S. Prusiner. 1987. Distinct prion proteins in short and long scrapie incubation period mice. *Cell* **51:** 651.

Witzemann, V., B. Barg, Y. Nishikawa, B. Sakmann, and S. Numa. 1987. Differential regulation of muscle acetylcholine receptor γ- and ϵ-subunit mRNAs. *FEBS Lett.* **223:** 104.

The Agrin Hypothesis

U.J. McMahan

Department of Neurobiology, Stanford University School of Medicine, Stanford, California 94305-5401

The surface of the muscle fiber at vertebrate neuro-muscular junctions is characterized by aggregates of molecules and organelles that, altogether, comprise the postsynaptic apparatus. Some of these aggregates play a direct role in synaptic transmission and thus are crucial for neuromuscular function. For example, the plasma membrane of the muscle fiber has aggregates of receptors (AChRs) for the neurotransmitter, acetylcholine, whereas the basal lamina of the myofiber has a high concentration of acetylcholinesterase (AChE).

During the last 20 years, considerable effort has been devoted to understanding how the postsynaptic apparatus forms in the embryo, how it is regulated in the adult, and how it reforms during regeneration. One finding from these studies is that the formation and maintenance of the postsynaptic apparatus is dependent on molecules provided by the axon (for review, see Dennis 1981). Studies conducted in my laboratory have led to the hypothesis that agrin, a protein we have purified and begun to characterize, is such a molecule. The agrin hypothesis (Nitkin et al. 1987; Magill-Solc and McMahan 1988; McMahan and Wallace 1989) is as follows: Agrin, or a protein very similar to it, is synthesized in the cell bodies of motor neurons and transported in their axons to muscle. During embryogenesis, as motor axons approach and grow over the surface of developing myofibers, they release agrin. When agrin binds to an agrin receptor on the myotube surface, it causes AChRs, AChE, and other components of the postsynaptic apparatus, including components of the synaptic basal lamina, to aggregate on the myotube surface in the vicinity of the activated receptor. Agrin becomes associated with this nascent synaptic basal lamina and thus is bound at the synaptic site, where it can continue to interact with its receptor on the myofiber. Release of agrin from motor nerve terminals at the adult neuromuscular junction and its incorporation into the synaptic basal lamina help maintain the postsynaptic apparatus by ensuring that newly synthesized components become concentrated at the synaptic site, whereas release of agrin by regenerating axons accounts for their ability to induce postsynaptic apparatus at ectopic sites on denervated myofibers. Agrin that persists in basal lamina after myofibers are damaged is believed to account for the ability of the synaptic basal lamina to induce the formation of AChR and AChE aggregates in regenerating muscle fibers, even in the absence of axon terminals. Here, I review the characteristics of agrin and the results of experiments that led to the hypothesis, and I describe recent experiments that have led to and resulted from the cloning of agrin cDNA.

Agrin and Its Effects on Cultured Myotubes

Agrin was purified from basal-lamina-containing extracts of the electric organ of the marine ray *Torpedo californica* (Rubin and McMahan 1982; Godfrey et al. 1984; Nitkin et al. 1987). We selected the electric organ as a tissue source because it is enriched in cholinergic synapses and it had been useful for identifying and characterizing other synaptic molecules such as AChRs and AChE. Basal lamina extracts were used because our previous studies (Burden et al. 1979; McMahan and Slater 1984; Anglister and McMahan 1985) had demonstrated that synaptic basal lamina at the neuromuscular junction has stably bound to it molecules that cause AChRs and AChE to aggregate on regenerating myofibers.

The basal lamina-containing extracts of the electric organ caused a 3- to 20-fold increase in the number of AChR aggregates (Fig. 1) on cultured chick myotubes (Godfrey et al. 1984). The extracts had little or no effect on myotube size, the total number of AChRs on the myotube surface, or the rate of AChR degradation. The AChR-aggregating effect was dose-dependent and due, at least in part, to lateral migration of AChRs present in the muscle cell plasma membrane at the time the extracts were applied. The aggregation of AChRs at developing neuromuscular junctions also occurs, at least in part, by lateral migration (Anderson and Cohen 1977; Ziskind-Conhaim et al. 1984; Role et al. 1985). The increase in number of receptor aggregates was first seen 2–4 hours after the extracts were added to the cultures, and it was maximal by 24 hours (Godfrey et al. 1984). A library of monoclonal antibodies was made that immunoprecipitated the AChR-aggregating molecules in our electric organ extracts (Reist et al. 1987). Each of five different monoclonal antibodies tested immunoprecipitated polypeptides with molecular masses of 150, 135, 95, and 70 kD (Nitkin et al. 1987). Gel-filtration chromatography of electric organ extracts revealed two peaks of AChR-aggregating activity; one comigrated with the 150-kD polypeptide, the other with the 95-kD polypeptide. The 135- and 70-kD polypeptides did not cause AChR aggregation. On the basis of these molecular characteristics and the pattern of staining seen in sections labeled with the monoclonal antibodies, we concluded that the electric organ AChR-aggregating factor (150 and 95 kD) was distinct

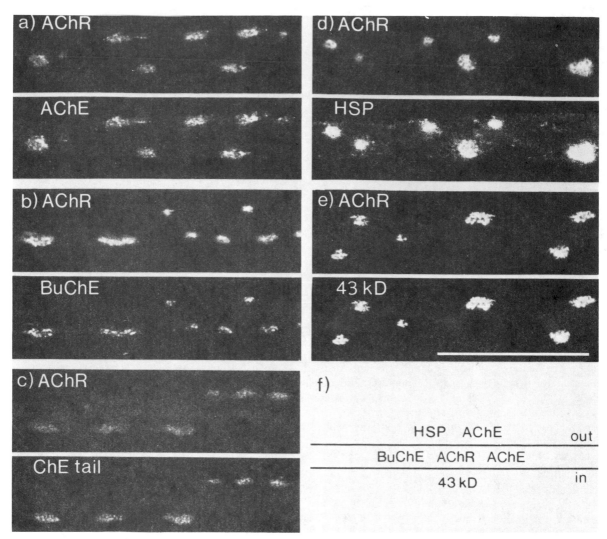

Figure 1. Agrin-induced specializations in cultured chick myotubes contain extracellular matrix, membrane, and cytoplasmic components of the postsynaptic apparatus. (a–e) Fluorescence micrographs of segments of myotubes from agrin-treated cultures labeled with rhodamine-α-bungarotoxin to visualize AChRs and antibodies to AChE catalytic subunit (a), BuChE catalytic subunit (b), collagen-like tail of A_{12} ChE (c), heparan sulfate proteoglycan (HSP) (d), and 43-kD AChR-associated protein (43 kD) (e) and visualized with fluorescein-conjugated second antibody. Each panel shows the same myotube segment under rhodamine optics (*top*) and fluorescein optics (*bottom*). Bar, 50 mm. (f) Schematic representation of an agrin-induced specialization, indicating that it contains at least two extracellular matrix components (heparan sulfate proteoglycan and A_{12} AChE), three membrane components (AChR and globular forms of AChE and BuChE), and one cytoplasmic component (43-kD AChR-associated protein) of the postsynaptic apparatus (McMahan and Wallace 1989).

from previously identified molecules at the neuromuscular junction and we named it "agrin" (Nitkin et al. 1987).

As illustrated in Figure 1, extracts containing agrin also caused the formation of aggregates of AChE, butyrylcholinesterase (BuChE), heparan sulfate proteoglycan (a basal lamina component), and a 43-kD AChR-associated protein (Wallace et al. 1985; Nitkin et al. 1987; McMahan and Wallace 1989; Wallace 1989). All are components of the postsynaptic apparatus at the neuromuscular junction. Each of the components accumulated with a time course similar to that of AChR aggregation, and the aggregates tended to be coextensive. Several lines of evidence indicated

that agrin caused the accumulation of all these components. For example, gel filtration chromatography revealed that there were two forms of each activity, one comigrating with the 150-kD agrin polypeptide and the other with the 95-kD agrin polypeptide. Moreover, five different monoclonal antibodies recognizing at least four different epitopes on agrin immunoprecipitated all the activities.

The formation of AChR aggregates induced by agrin was not prevented by inhibition of protein synthesis (Wallace 1988), consistent with our finding that agrin-induced accumulation of AChRs occurred by lateral migration (Godfrey et al. 1984). The accumulation of components of the extracellular matrix, such as heparan sulfate proteoglycan, would seem less likely to occur by lateral migration, and therefore might require release of newly synthesized proteins. Indeed, formation of aggregates of heparan sulfate proteoglycan was prevented by inhibitors of protein synthesis (Wallace 1989). Thus, different components of the postsynaptic apparatus accumulate in agrin-induced specializations by different mechanisms.

Agrin-induced AChR aggregation was prevented by inhibitors of energy metabolism (Wallace 1988). The dependence on metabolic energy indicates that agrin-induced AChR aggregation is a more complex process than simple cross-linking of surface receptors by a multivalent ligand (such as occurs during patching on lymphocytes), which does not rely on energy metabolism. Moreover, we estimate that for every molecule of agrin we add to the culture medium, 160 AChRs are induced to aggregate (Nitkin et al. 1987). This stoichiometry, together with the finding that agrin-induced specializations contain high concentrations of several other components of the postsynaptic apparatus, suggests that agrin acts catalytically, for example, by binding to a receptor on the surface of myotubes and triggering a cascade of intracellular events that results in the formation of a postsynaptic specialization (Nitkin et al. 1987).

One consequence of the interaction of agrin with myotubes is an increase in phosphorylation of surface AChRs. This was the first and so far the only biochemical change detected in agrin-treated myotubes. Using subunit-specific monoclonal antibodies, B.G. Wallace in this laboratory has observed that agrin causes a slight increase in phosphorylation of the γ and δ AChR subunits and a three- to fourfold increase in phosphorylation of the β subunit (Wallace 1991). More recently, Wallace has learned that agrin-induced phosphorylation of the β subunit begins within 30 minutes of adding agrin, before there is any detectable change in AChR distribution, and reaches a plateau by 4 hours, at which time agrin-induced receptor aggregation is just beginning. Agrin-induced AChR phosphorylation is blocked by low pH and by activation of protein kinase C with TPA, two treatments that block agrin-induced AChR aggregation. Together, these findings indicate that agrin-induced phosphorylation is unlikely to be a consequence of receptor aggregation and raise the possibility that phosphorylation plays a causal role in the formation of AChR aggregates.

Agrin-like Molecules in Synaptic Basal Lamina

We found that extracts from *Torpedo* skeletal muscle also caused the formation of AChR aggregates on cultured chick myotubes (Godfrey et al. 1984). The maximal effect was the same as that for extracts from the electric organ. Moreover, monoclonal antibodies against different epitopes on agrin blocked and immunoprecipitated the AChR-aggregating activity from muscle (Fallon et al. 1985). Thus, muscle contains agrin, but in lower amounts than the electric organ, as

might be expected, since the electric organ has a much higher concentration of synapses.

Of the 14 anti-agrin monoclonal antibodies in our library, 13 stain neuromuscular junctions in *Torpedo*; 4 also stain neuromuscular junctions in frog and/or chicken (Reist et al. 1987). In all cases, the distribution of stain is the same; it fills the synaptic cleft and junctional folds, and lines the surface of the Schwann cells that cap the axon terminals (Fig. 2a). In chicken and *Torpedo*, the monoclonal antibodies stain the basal lamina both in the extrajunctional region of slow muscle fibers and on smooth muscle fibers of blood vessels (Reist et al. 1987). Antibodies to agrin also have been shown to bind to basement membranes in several other tissues (Godfrey et al. 1988). Thus, molecules antigenically related to agrin are not restricted to the neuromuscular junction, but at the junction, agrin-like molecules are highly concentrated in the synaptic cleft, the site where molecules that cause AChR and AChE aggregation on regenerating muscle fibers are known to be.

The molecules recognized by the monoclonal antibodies are stably bound to the basal lamina, as demonstrated by crush-damaging frog muscle so that all cells at the neuromuscular junction—muscle fibers, axon terminals, and their Schwann cells—degenerated while leaving much of the basal lamina intact (Reist et al. 1987). Regeneration was prevented. After 3 weeks, when the cellular debris had been phagocytized, the empty basal lamina sheaths were treated with anti-agrin monoclonal antibodies. As illustrated in Figure 2b, the synaptic regions of the muscle fiber basal lamina and Schwann cell basal lamina are stained (cf. Fig. 2a).

Agrin-like Molecules in the Cell Bodies of Motor Neurons

Figure 3 shows a frozen cross section from the spinal cord of a chick embryo that was incubated with anti-agrin monoclonal antibodies and processed for immunohistochemistry. Motor neurons are clearly stained. Such staining was also observed in the electric lobe of the neonatal *Torpedo* brain, the part of the brain that innervates the electric organ, and in the spinal cords of neonatal *Torpedo* and adult frogs (Magill-Solc and McMahan 1988). A search for staining in the lumbosacral region of the chick spinal cord at early developmental stages (Fig. 3, inset) revealed that motor neurons stained as early as embryonic day 5, the time at which motor neurons in this region begin to form neuromuscular junctions (Landmesser and Morris 1975).

Regardless of the age or species of animal, the stain in motor neurons, as observed by light microscopy, was concentrated in patches in the cytoplasm, suggesting that it was associated with cytoplasmic organelles. Electron microscopy on adult frog spinal cords (Magill-Solc and McMahan 1988) revealed that the stain was concentrated in the Golgi apparatus of the motor neuron, the site where proteins destined for transport to the cell surface are processed.

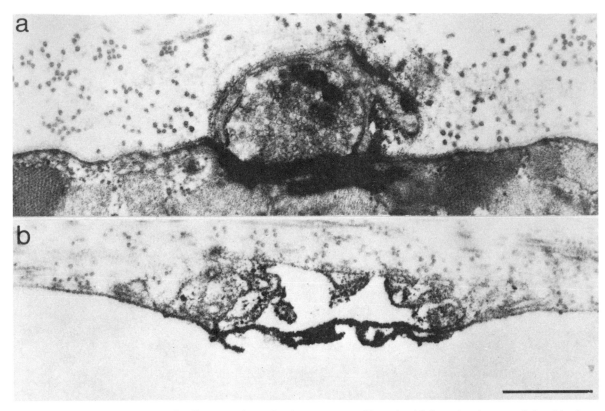

Figure 2. Anti-agrin monoclonal antibodies recognize molecules concentrated in and stably bound to the synaptic basal lamina at neuromuscular junctions. (*a*) Normal neuromuscular junction in cutaneous pectoris muscle of frog. (*b*) Site of a neuromuscular junction 3 weeks after the cutaneous pectoris muscle was damaged by crushing. Myofiber, axon terminal, and Schwann cell degenerated and were phagocytized in response to the trauma, but the basal lamina of the myofiber and Schwann cell persisted. Antibody binding in the damaged muscle is localized to the synaptic portion of the myofiber basal lamina and to the Schwann cell basal lamina, presenting a staining pattern identical to that at the normal neuromuscular junction. Bar, 1 mm.

We observed no neuronal staining with anti-agrin monoclonal antibodies in regions of the brain and spinal cord that did not contain motor neurons. On the other hand, capillaries throughout the central nervous system (CNS) were outlined by the stain, as was the surface of the brain and spinal cord (Fig. 3). Electron microscopy of the frog spinal cord revealed that the stain associated with capillaries was concentrated in the basal lamina that lies between the capillaries and the endfoot processes of astrocytes (Magill-Solc and McMahan 1988). Thus, in the CNS, molecules antigenically similar to agrin are not confined to motor neurons, but motor neurons are distinct among neurons in that they have a high concentration of such molecules in their cell bodies.

Extracts of the electric lobes of adult *Torpedo* brains and the spinal cords of adult *Torpedo* and frogs and day-18 chick embryos caused the aggregation of AChRs on cultured chick myotubes (Magill-Solc and McMahan 1988; see also Godfrey et al. 1988). The extract from the electric lobe also caused AChE aggregation. To determine whether the AChR- and AChE-aggregating activities in the electric lobe extracts were antigenically related to agrin, we assayed the ability of anti-agrin antibodies to immunoprecipitate the activities (Magill-Solc and McMahan 1988). For these

experiments, we used five monoclonal antibodies, each directed against a different epitope on agrin. Each of the monoclonal antibodies immunoprecipitated nearly all the AChR-aggregating activity from the extracts of electric lobe of *Torpedo* brain, as they did agrin from electric organ extracts. Two of these monoclonal antibodies (the only ones tested) also immunoprecipitated electric lobe AChE-aggregating activity, as expected. AChR-aggregating activity in extracts of the spinal cords of *Torpedo*, frogs, and chicks also was immunoprecipitated by anti-agrin antibodies. Thus, the AChR- and AChE-aggregating molecules in extracts of the electric lobe and spinal cord are antigenically similar to agrin.

To learn whether any of the AChR-aggregating activity detected in spinal cord extracts is derived from motor neurons, we separated motor neurons from other cellular components in the spinal cord of day-6 chick embryos (Magill-Solc and McMahan 1988). The separation procedure results in two cellular fractions: one in which more than 95% of the cells are motor neurons and one which is enriched in non-motor neurons (Dohrmann et al. 1986). When extracts of each fraction were made and tested for AChR-aggregating activity, we found that the specific activity of the motor-neuron-containing fraction was sevenfold greater than

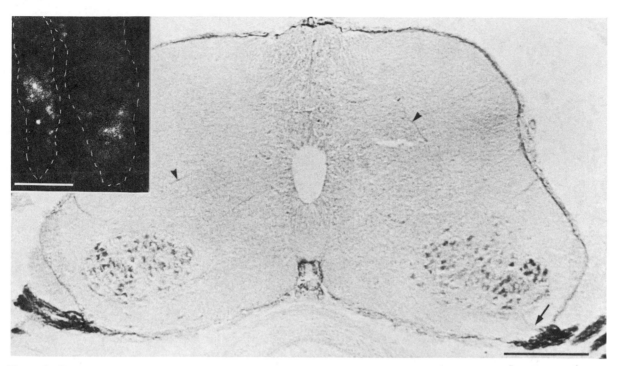

Figure 3. Cross section of the lumbosacral region of a spinal cord from a day-10 chick embryo incubated with an anti-agrin monoclonal antibody. Motor neurons and the pial surface of the spinal cord are intensely stained. Capillaries (arrowheads) are lightly stained. Glial cells and other neurons are not stained. The intensely stained structures outside the spinal cord are ventral roots; much of the stain is probably in the Schwann cell basal lamina, which is known to stain intensely in the adult. The lightly stained region (arrow) of the spinal cord extending from the right motor column to the right ventral root was observed at higher magnification to be composed of narrow cell processes having a nearly uniform diameter, probably motor axons. Bar, 200 mm. (*Inset*) Portions of two motor neurons (outlined by dashed lines) in the lumbosacral region of the spinal cord of a day-6 chick embryo labeled with an anti-agrin monoclonal antibody. Similar but less intense staining was seen in motor neurons of the lumbosacral region at embryonic day 5, the time at which motor neurons in this region begin to form neuromuscular junctions. Bar, 10 μm.

that of the non-motor-neuron-containing fraction. Moreover, most of this activity was immunoprecipitated by anti-agrin antibodies. Thus, motor neurons contain AChR-aggregating molecules antigenically related to agrin, and the agrin-like molecules are present from the time neuromuscular synapses are beginning to form.

Anterograde Transport of Agrin-like Molecules in Motor Axons

The presence of agrin-like molecules in the Golgi apparatus of motor neurons strongly suggests that agrin is synthesized in motor neuron cell bodies and transported anterogradely along axons to their terminals. However, as discussed above, anti-agrin antibodies also stain extrajunctional regions of certain muscle fibers in *Torpedo* and chick muscles and in aneural limbs of chick embryos (Fallon et al. 1985; Reist et al. 1987; Fallon and Gelfman 1989), raising the possibility that the agrin-like molecules detected in motor neurons are produced by myofibers and transported retrogradely along their axons to the cell body. To determine whether agrin-like molecules are transported from motor neuron cell bodies to axon terminals, we ligated

the sciatic nerve in the frog and examined the distribution of agrin-like molecules on both sides of the ligature (Magill-Solc 1990; Magill-Solc and McMahan 1990). Experiments by other workers (Grafstein and Forman 1980) have revealed that material synthesized in neuron cell bodies and transported to their terminals accumulates on the cell body side of such a ligature. In normal frog sciatic nerve, there is no anti-agrin monoclonal antibody staining, except on the axonal surface at nodes of Ranvier (Reist et al. 1987). However, in ligated nerves, a large fraction of the axonal cytoplasm stained on the cell body side of the ligature (Fig. 4). Such staining was not observed if the ventral roots supplying the sciatic nerve were severed 3 days prior to ligation, indicating that the stained material in nerves with intact ventral roots had accumulated in motor axons as expected. In extracts of normal nerves, we detected no AChR-aggregating activity; however, in ligated nerves, much higher levels of activity could be detected on the cell body side of the ligature than on the terminal side. Moreover, the activity was immunoprecipitated with anti-agrin monoclonal antibodies and was absent in ligated nerves in which the motor axons had been severed 3 days prior to ligation. These findings, coupled with our in situ hybridization studies

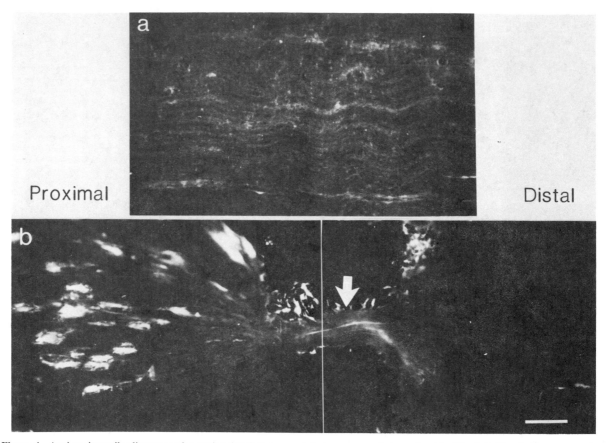

Figure 4. Anti-agrin antibodies recognize molecules that accumulate in axons on the proximal (cell body) side of a ligature on the sciatic nerve of the frog. (*a*) Longitudinal section through a segment of normal nerve stained with anti-agrin monoclonal antibodies. (*b*) Anti-agrin monoclonal-antibody-stained longitudinal section through a segment of nerve ligated for 2 days. Bar, 100 μm.

using the cDNA that encodes agrin and agrin-like molecules (see below), are fully consistent with the hypothesis that agrin is synthesized in motor neuron cell bodies and transported along their axons to muscle.

Anti-agrin Serum Inhibits Neuron-induced AChR Aggregation on Cultured Myotubes

If chick motor neurons are cocultured with myotubes, they induce the formation of AChR patches on the surface of the myotubes at and near regions of neuromuscular contact. Reist (1990) found that when cocultures were grown in the presence of IgG purified from anti-agrin serum, the formation of such aggregates was 80–90% inhibited (Fig. 5). The inhibition was dose-dependent, and the IgG had no other obvious effects on muscle fibers or neurons; e.g., it did not inhibit the low-level spontaneous formation of AChR aggregates commonly encountered in untreated muscle cultures (Godfrey et al. 1984). Thus, agrin is directly involved in the formation of the postsynaptic apparatus at developing neuromuscular synapses.

cDNA Encoding Agrin

The function and regulation of expression of agrin-like proteins at the neuromuscular junction can best be studied with reagents that can only be obtained using molecular genetic techniques. Accordingly, a cDNA library constructed in λgt11 from poly(A)$^+$ RNA isolated from the electric lobe of *Dyscopyge ommata*, an electric ray closely related to *Torpedo*, was screened with our serum raised against agrin. One of four clones initially isolated was determined by epitope selection of the antiserum to encode a fusion protein containing antigenic determinants shared with all four *Torpedo* agrin (150, 95 kD) and agrin-like (135, 70 kD) proteins. This cDNA clone, called OL4, has an insert of 4.5 kb and has been characterized by sequence analysis (M.A. Smith et al., in prep.). The cDNA encodes a protein with an amino acid sequence that is very similar to the amino-terminal sequence of the 95-kD form of agrin and 70-kD form of inactive agrin-like protein in *Torpedo* electric organ extracts. Eleven of fourteen amino acids are identical; one exchange is due to the conservative mutation from valine to leucine. This homology is many orders of magnitude beyond random expectation, and the minor differences in the sequence are expected to be due to the fact that different species of marine rays were used for the cloning and protein determination. Interestingly, this sequence begins at a lysine residue, and the DNA sequence predicts an arginine just upstream. The sequence of two basic residues such as arginine-lysine is often the site of endo-

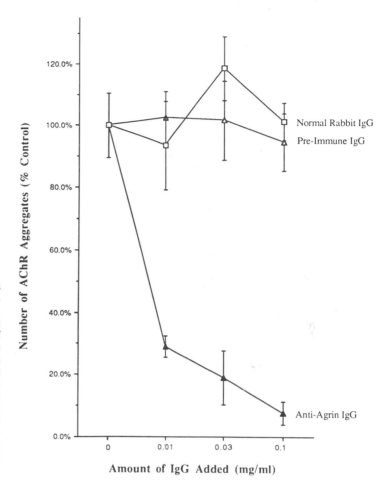

Figure 5. IgG from anti-agrin serum inhibits motor-neuron-induced formation of AChR aggregates in chick motor neuron/myotube cocultures. Dissociated motor neurons were cultured with myotubes for 3 days in the presence or absence of IgG from normal rabbits or IgG from rabbits immunized against electric organ polypeptides immunoprecipitated by monoclonal antibodies against agrin. Myotube AChR aggregates labeled by rhodamine-α-bungarotoxin were counted in the vicinity of neurite/myotube contacts. The mean number of AChR aggregates in IgG-treated cultures was divided by the mean number of aggregates in cultures grown without IgG and expressed as percentage of control. Values represent the mean of 6 dishes (2 platings) ± S.E.M.

proteolytic cleavages that release biologically active peptides from larger precursors.

Searches of both the GenBank (Release 61) and the National Biomedical Research Foundation (Release 19) sequence data bases indicate that OL4 encodes a unique protein. However, several domains of the deduced amino acid sequence show similarity to other previously characterized proteins. For example, there are four distinct classes of epidermal growth factor (EGF)-like repeats; EGF repeats have been observed in other extracellular matrix molecules, and certain of the repeats in the predicted protein are homologous to those in laminin (see, e.g., Montell and Goodman 1988). There are two tripeptide domains, RGD and LRE, that are also common to other extracellular matrix molecules (see, e.g., Hunter et al. 1989). Unexpectedly, there are domains that have significant similarity to members of the pancreatic secretory trypsin inhibitor family. Northern blots reveal two transcripts of approximately 9.5 kb and 7 kb; they are expressed in both neuronal (brain, spinal cord) and nonneuronal tissues (skeletal muscle, liver, heart) of adult *D. ommata*, but the level of expression of the 7-kb transcript is positively correlated with regions of the CNS that have high concentrations of motor neurons.

Using the electric ray OL4 clone as a probe, homologous cDNA clones were isolated from a chick brain library (K. Tsim et al., in prep.) and rat spinal cord library (R. Rupp et al., in prep.). Both have been sequenced and show strong homology ($>60\%$) with the OL4 clone. Northern blot analysis indicates that corresponding message in both species is 8–9 kb and is concentrated in brain and spinal cord of embryos. The rat cDNA is judged to be full length on the basis of size, initiation site, signal sequence, and continuous open reading frame. On the basis of Northern blot analysis, the chick cDNA is nearly full length. We have developed an expression system for chick agrin cDNA. The 5' end of a 4.7-kb cDNA was coupled to an initiation site and signal sequence and transfected into COS-7 cells (K. Tsim et al., in prep.). The transfected cells secreted a protein that induced AChR aggregation in a manner indistinguishable from that of authentic *Torpedo* agrin (Fig. 6). Moreover, the active protein was immunoprecipitated by anti-agrin antibodies. This expression of a functionally active protein recognized by anti-agrin monoclonal antibodies demonstrates that chick cDNA encodes agrin. Whether or not the *Torpedo* and rat cDNAs encode agrin or an inactive agrin-related protein remains to be determined.

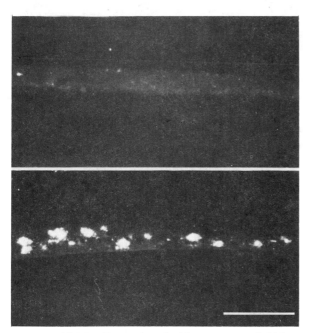

Figure 6. COS-7 cells transfected with a construct of chicken agrin cDNA secrete a protein with AChR-aggregating activity. SR-α-based pJFE14 (Elliot et al. 1990) was modified by cloning a leader sequence derived from hemagglutinin of the avian influenza virus FPV into the polylinker site. Chick agrin cDNA was subcloned in frame with this leader sequence using the *Eco*RI site in the polylinker. Orientation and the correct reading frame were confirmed by sequencing the 5′ end of the constructs. COS-7 cells were transiently transfected using a modified version of a DEAE-dextran procedure. After 3 days in culture, the conditioned medium was collected, cleared of cell debris by centrifugation, and assayed for AChR-aggregating activity on cultured chick myotubes (Nitkin et al. 1987). (*Top*) Conditioned medium from COS-7 cells transfected with the modified expression vector pJFE14. (*Bottom*) Conditioned medium from COS-7 cells transfected with chick agrin cDNA in modified pJFE14. Bar, 50 μm.

Transcripts Homologous to Agrin cDNA Are Concentrated in Motor Neurons

Our studies with anti-agrin antibodies provide strong evidence that motor neurons synthesize agrin. Accordingly, one might expect that probes for agrin mRNA would hybridize with motor neuron mRNA in tissue sections. Indeed, in situ hybridizations done on frozen sections of spinal cord of adult *D. ommata*, embryonic rat (Magill-Solc 1990; Magill and McMahan 1990; M.A. Smith et al., in prep.), and both embryonic and 1-month-old chicks (K. Tsim et al., in prep.) result in heavy antisense labeling of motor neurons (Fig. 7). Motor neurons are also labeled in motor nuclei of the brain stem and, in *D. ommata*, in the electric lobe of the medulla, the region that innervates the electric organ (Fig. 7). We also observed in *D. ommata* and in chick embryos labeling of cells other than motor neurons. For example, in *D. ommata*, there were heavily labeled cells in the habenula, a small nucleus of the thalamus, and in the Purkinje layer of the cerebellar cortex. In chick embryos, the ganglion cell layer of the

retina was heavily labeled. Lower, but above-background, labeling was nearly uniformly distributed throughout all sections of the CNS, in agreement with Northern blot analysis, indicating that whereas mRNA recognized by agrin mRNA antisense is highly concentrated in motor neurons, it is broadly distributed in the CNS. Finally, we have noted that for both motor neurons and retinal ganglion cells in chick, the concentration of agrin-like transcripts is developmentally regulated; i.e., labeling of these cells by in situ hybridization is far greater during certain stages of development than at other stages. For example, labeling was first detected in motor neurons in the lumbosacral region of the spinal cord between embryonic days 5 and 6, the time at which these motor neurons begin to make neuromuscular junctions. Maximal labeling was observed between embryonic days 10 and 13. By embryonic day 19, the labeling was greatly decreased, and by postnatal day 30, it was reduced even further but was still above background.

AChRs Accumulate at Sites of Agrin-Myofiber Interaction

The agrin hypothesis predicts that agrin induces AChRs and other components of the postsynaptic apparatus to aggregate at the site where agrin interacts with its receptor on the myofiber. We tested this part of the hypothesis by using molecular genetic techniques in the following way (S. Kroger et al., in prep.): Cell-free basal lamina sheets were prepared from the retinas of day-10 chick embryos (Halfter et al. 1987). The sheets were placed flat onto the bottom of polylysine-coated petri dishes and extracted with 0.2 M bicarbonate buffer (pH 9.0) overnight at 4°C. COS cells transfected with chick agrin cDNA constructs were seeded 24 hours after transfection onto the basal lamina sheets at low density. The COS cells were removed from the sheets after 24 hours by extraction with 2% Triton X-100 detergent. Patches of agrin deposited by the COS cells remained adherent to the basal lamina during the extraction procedure. Myoblasts were then plated onto the agrin-conditioned basal lamina sheets. After 5 days, when the myoblasts had fused to form myotubes, the preparations were stained with anti-agrin monoclonal antibodies to mark the agrin patches in the basal lamina and with rhodamine-α-bungarotoxin to mark the AChR aggregates of the myofibers. We compared such cultures with control cultures preplated with COS cells that had been transfected with a chick agrin cDNA construct that generated a protein which was inactive but was nevertheless deposited in the basal lamina and stained with anti-agrin monoclonal antibodies. It was clear that the active basal-lamina-bound agrin induced the formation of AChR aggregates in the myotubes. Moreover, more than 80% of the induced aggregates were coextensive with the agrin patches (Fig. 8), indicating that AChRs had preferentially accumulated at sites where the agrin interacted with the myotubes.

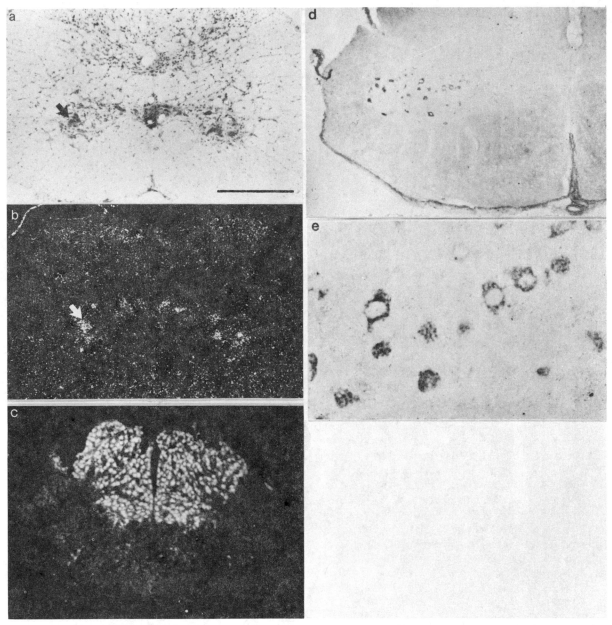

Figure 7. Localization of agrin mRNA in motor neurons by in situ hybridization. (*a*) Bright-field micrograph of a cross section from adult *D. ommata* spinal cord stained with cresyl violet to reveal neurons. As in other vertebrates, motor neurons (arrow) are the largest neurons in the spinal cord and are situated in the ventral horn of the gray matter. (*b*) Dark-field autoradiograph of adjacent section from *D. ommata* spinal cord after hybridizing with ^{35}S-labeled agrin antisense mRNA. Aggregates of grains (arrow) having the size, frequency, and distribution of motor neurons are situated over the ventral horn. (*c*) Cross section from medulla of adult *D. ommata*. Dark-field autoradiograph after hybridizing with ^{35}S-labeled antisense mRNA. Grains are concentrated over the electromotor neurons of the electric lobe. (*d*) Cross section through the ventral quadrant of a 1-month-old chick spinal cord. Bright-field micrograph after hybridizing with digoxigenin-linked agrin antisense mRNA, treating with an alkaline phosphatase-linked anti-digoxigenin antibody, and staining for alkaline phosphatase. Cells in ventral horn are heavily stained. (*e*) Higher-power view of section in *c* showing that the labeled cells have the characteristics of motor neurons. Bar: (*a* and *b*) 400 μm; (*c*) 1.1 mm; (*d*) 100 μm; (*e*) 500 μm.

DISCUSSION

Findings that are consistent with the major parts of the agrin hypothesis can be summarized in the following way.

1. *Agrin is synthesized in the cell bodies of motor neurons:* Anti-agrin monoclonal antibodies stain Gol-

gi apparatus in the cell bodies of motor neurons (Magill-Solc and McMahan 1988). Extracts of motor-neuron-enriched fractions of spinal cord are enriched in molecules that induce AChR aggregation in cultured myotubes. The active proteins are immunoprecipitated by anti-agrin monoclonal antibodies (Magill-Solc and McMahan 1988). Agrin an-

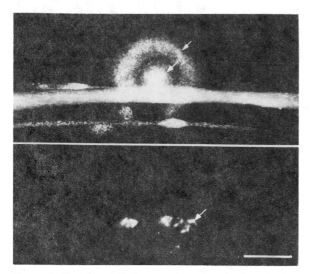

Figure 8. Myotube AChRs aggregate at agrin deposits in a basal lamina substrate. (*Top*) Agrin-like protein deposited by a transfected COS cell into isolated chick retina basal lamina is shown at arrows. The protein was stained with anti-agrin antibody and viewed with fluorescein optics. The COS cell was removed by detergent extraction, and myotubes formed from myoblasts were seeded onto the basal lamina after the extraction. (*Bottom*) Same field as shown above but viewed with rhodamine optics after labeling AChRs with rhodamine-conjugated α-bungarotoxin. AChR aggregates (arrow) are at the point where a muscle fiber lies adjacent to an agrin patch. Bar, 50 μm.

tisense recognizes mRNA in cell bodies of motor neurons (Magill-Solc and McMahan 1990).

2. *Agrin is transported in motor axons to muscle:* Anti-agrin monoclonal antibodies stain in motor axons molecules that accumulate on the CNS side of a ligature placed on the nerve in which the axons run (Magill-Solc and McMahan 1990). Extracts of ligated nerves reveal that, on the CNS side of the ligation, motor axons are enriched in AChR-aggregating molecules that are immunoprecipitated by anti-agrin monoclonal antibodies (Magill-Solc and McMahan 1990).

3. *Agrin binds to synaptic basal lamina:* Agrin is extracted from basal lamina fractions of the electric organ (Godfrey et al. 1984; Nitkin et al. 1987). Muscle extracts similar to those of the electric organ contain molecules having AChR-aggregating activity that can be immunoprecipitated by anti-agrin antibodies (Godfrey et al. 1984; Fallon et al. 1985). Anti-agrin monoclonal antibodies stain synaptic basal lamina in the electric organ and muscle; antigenic molecules remain bound to basal lamina for weeks after muscle fibers and axons degenerate (Reist et al. 1987). Molecules with AChR- and AChE-aggregating activity remain bound to synaptic basal lamina for weeks after degeneration of muscle fibers and axon terminals (McMahan and Slater 1984).

4. *Agrin mediates nerve-induced aggregation of molecules that comprise the postsynaptic apparatus:* Agrin induces cultured myotubes to form patches on

their surface that have a high concentration of extracellular matrix (heparin sulfate proteoglycan, AChE), plasma membrane (AChR, AChE, and BuChE), and cytoplasmic (43-kD protein) components of the postsynaptic apparatus (McMahan and Wallace 1989; Wallace 1989). Anti-agrin IgG inhibits motor-neuron-induced aggregation of AChRs on cultured myotubes (Reist 1990).

5. *Agrin directs the formation of the postsynaptic apparatus by interaction with a muscle fiber receptor:* Agrin-induced AChR aggregation is prevented by inhibitors of energy metabolism (Wallace 1988). A few molecules of agrin cause the aggregation of a far greater number of AChRs and other postsynaptic proteins (Nitkin et al. 1987). Agrin-induced AChR aggregation does not require protein synthesis, but agrin-induced heparan sulfate proteoglycan aggregation does (Wallace 1989). Agrin-induced AChR aggregation is inhibited by activation of protein kinase C with TPA (Wallace 1988). Agrin causes phosphorylation of AChR (Wallace 1991), which apparently occurs just prior to AChR aggregation.

6. *Agrin-induced aggregation of AChRs occurs at the site where agrin binds to its receptor:* Myotube AChRs aggregate at deposits of agrin-like protein in a basal lamina substrate (S. Kroger at al., in prep.).

A brief glance at the above list raises several questions that provide opportunities to test the hypothesis. For example: Is agrin released by motor axons? If so, is it the motor-neuron-released agrin that directs the formation of the postsynaptic apparatus? What role, if any, do the agrin-related molecules produced by skeletal myotubes play in forming the postsynaptic apparatus? One problem in answering such questions directly is that so far, no marker is known to be specific for agrin. All the anti-agrin monoclonal antibodies and antisera that we have prepared recognize not only agrin, but also inactive agrin-related polypeptides in extracts of the electric organ. One explanation might be that there is only one molecule in situ recognized by anti-agrin antibodies and that the inactive agrin-related polypeptides in our extracts are proteolytic fragments of agrin digested during tissue preparation. On the other hand, agrin could be a member of a family of molecules of which only it, agrin, is active in directing the formation of the postsynaptic apparatus. Indeed, we have isolated from the chick brain library a cDNA that is highly homologous to the chick agrin cDNA (M. Ruegg et al., in prep.). When transfected into COS cells, it codes for a secreted protein that is immunoprecipitated by anti-agrin antibodies, but unlike protein encoded by agrin cDNA, it does not induce the formation of AChR aggregates on cultured myotubes (M. Ruegg et al., in prep.). Another homolog, also encoding for inactive protein but antigenically similar to agrin, has been isolated from a chick muscle library (M. Ruegg et al., in prep.). These findings are consistent with the possibility that agrin is a member of a family of molecules with differing functions. By using molecular genetic techniques to identify the active site(s) in agrin, it may be possible to make markers that specifically recognize agrin, which should enable more direct studies on it than heretofore possible.

The agrin hypothesis does not eliminate the need for factors other than agrin in regulating the formation and maintenance of the postsynaptic apparatus in skeletal muscles. For example, electromechanical activity is known to regulate the extent to which AChE accumulates at synaptic sites (Dennis 1981). In addition, molecules such as ARIA (Usdin and Fischbach 1986) or CGRP (Fontaine at al. 1986; New and Mudge 1986) may be released by axon terminals to control the rate of synthesis of AChRs, and components of the cytoskeleton of the myofiber may be crucial for immobilizing and/or stabilizing AChR aggregates. The agrin hypothesis, as it now stands, simply predicts that agrin released by the axon interacts with a receptor on the muscle fiber to trigger a cascade of second-messenger-mediated events, leading to the aggregation of AChRs and other postsynaptic components at the site of the agrin/agrin receptor interaction. Thus, the agrin/agrin receptor interaction specifies *where* nerve-induced postsynaptic apparatus forms and, provided the second-messenger-mediated cascade is functional, *when* it begins to form. Nonphysiological activation of the agrin receptor or the cascade may explain how nonphysiological materials, such as latex beads (Peng and Cheng 1982), and nonphysiological conditions, such as denervation (Ko et al. 1977; McMahan and Slater 1984), cause the aggregation of AChRs and other postsynaptic components on muscle fibers in the absence of agrin.

Because this is a volume about the brain, it is relevant to raise the question of whether agrin might play a role in the formation and regulation of postsynaptic apparatus at neuron-to-neuron synapses in the CNS. Receptor aggregates have been described at cholinergic, GABA-ergic, glycine-ergic, and adrenergic neuron-to-neuron synapses (Marshall 1981; Jacob et al. 1984; Triller et al. 1985; Aoki et al. 1987; Richards et al. 1987). Moreover, most neuron-to-neuron synapses have an aggregate of proteins lining the cytoplasmic surface of the postsynaptic membrane known as the postsynaptic density. Such postsynaptic specializations make it likely that there are molecules at neuron-to-neuron synapses that function similarly to agrin at the neuromuscular junction. Indeed, we have extracted AChR-aggregating molecules that can be immunoprecipitated by anti-agrin monoclonal antibodies from regions of the brain where motor neurons are in such low abundance as to seem unlikely to be able to account for the activity (Magill-Solc and McMahan 1988). Such molecules could be derived from nonmotor neurons and their synapses and/or basal lamina associated with brain capillaries, which is stained by anti-agrin antibodies (Magill-Solc and McMahan 1987). To date, we have not observed staining of CNS synapses by our anti-agrin antibodies. Accordingly, agrin may be present at CNS synapses but in such low concentrations that we cannot detect it, or agrin may be present at CNS synapses but not tightly bound to synaptic cleft material so that it diffuses away during tissue preparation. Our in situ hybridization studies indicate that agrin or agrin-like molecules are produced by neurons other than motor neurons, including retinal ganglion cells. Our finding that the agrin-like mRNA in retinal ganglion cells and motor neurons is developmentally regulated raises the further possibility that close examination of different regions of the nervous system during different stages of development may reveal other groups of neurons that express agrin or agrin-like molecules. The problem of determining whether there is agrin at CNS synapses is directly related to the larger problems of understanding how postsynaptic apparatus having one type of receptor aggregate forms alongside postsynaptic apparatus having another receptor type on the same neuron, and of determining the sequence of steps and mechanisms involved in CNS synapse remodeling.

REFERENCES

Anderson, M.J. and M.W. Cohen. 1977. Nerve-induced and spontaneous redistribution of acetylcholine receptors on cultured muscle cells. *J. Physiol.* **268:** 757.

Anglister, L. and U.J. McMahan. 1985. Basal lamina directs acetylcholin-esterase accumulation at synaptic sites in regenerating muscle. *J. Cell Biol.* **101:** 735.

Aoki, C., T.H. Joh, and V.M. Pickel. 1987. Ultrastructural localization of β-adrenergic receptor-like immunoreactivity in the cortex and neostriatum of rat brain. *Brain Res.* **437:** 264.

Burden, S.J., P.B. Sargent, and U.J. McMahan. 1979. Acetylcholine receptors in regenerating muscle accumulate at original synaptic sites in the absence of the nerve. *J. Cell Biol.* **82:** 412.

Dennis, M.J. 1981. Development of the neuromuscular junction. *Annu. Rev. Neurosci.* **4:** 43.

Dohrmann, U., D. Edgar, M. Sendtner, and H. Thoenen. 1986. Muscle-derived factors that support survival and promote fiber outgrowth from embryonic chick spinal motor neurons in culture. *Dev. Biol.* **118:** 209.

Elliot, J.F., G.R. Albrecht, A. Gilladoga, S.M. Handunnetti, J. Neequaye, G. Lallinger, J.N. Minjas, and R.J. Howard. 1990. Genes for *Plasmodium falciparum* surface antigens cloned by expression in COS cells. *Proc. Natl. Acad. Sci.* **87:** 6363.

Fallon, J.R. and C.E. Gelfman. 1989. Agrin-related molecules are concentrated at acetylcholine receptor clusters in normal and aneural developing muscle. *J. Cell Biol.* **108:** 1527.

Fallon, J.R, R.M. Nitkin, N.E. Reist, B.G. Wallace, and U.J. McMahan. 1985. Acetylcholine receptor-aggregating factor is similar to molecules concentrated at neuromuscular junctions. *Nature* **315:** 571.

Fontaine, B., A. Klarsfeld, T. Hokefelt, and J.-P. Changeaux. 1986. Calcitonin gene-related peptide, a peptide present in spinal cord motoneurons, increases the number of acetylcholine receptors in primary cultures of chick embryo myotubes. *Neurosci. Lett.* **71:** 59.

Godfrey, E.W., M.E. Deitz, A.L. Morstad, P.A. Wallskog, and D.E. Yorde. 1988. Acetylcholine receptor-aggregating proteins are associated with the extracellular matrix of many tissues in *Torpedo*. *J. Cell Biol.* **106:** 1263.

Godfrey, E.W., R.M. Nitkin, B.G. Wallace, L.L. Rubin, and U.J. McMahan. 1984. Components of *Torpedo* electric organ and muscle that cause aggregation of acetylcholine receptors on cultured muscle cells. *J. Cell Biol.* **99:** 615.

Grafstein, B. and D.S. For man. 1980. Intracellular transport in neurons. *Physiol. Rev.* **60:** 1167.

Halfter, W., W. Reckhaus, and S. Kroger. 1987. Nondirected axonal growth on basal lamina from avian embryonic neurol retina. *J. Neurosci.* **7:** 3712.

Hunter, D.D., B.E. Porter, J.W. Bulock, S.P. Adams, J.P. Merlie, and J.R. Sanes. 1989. Primary sequence of a motor neurons-selective adhesive site in the synaptic basal lamina protein S-laminin. *Cell* **59:** 905.

Jacob, M.H., D.K. Berg, and J.M. Lindstrom. 1984. Shared antigenic determinant between the *Electrophorus* acetylcholine receptor and a synaptic component on chicken ciliary ganglion neurons. *Proc. Natl. Acad. Sci.* **81:** 3223.

Ko, P.K., M.J. Anderson, and M.W. Cohen. 1977. Denervated skeletal muscle fibers develop discrete patches of high acetylcholine receptor density. *Science* **196:** 540.

Landmesser, L. and D.G. Morris. 1975. The development of functional innervation in the hindlimb of the chick embryo. *J. Physiol.* **249:** 301.

Magill-Solc, C. 1990. "Molecules in motor neurons that direct the aggregation of acetylcholine receptors on skeletal muscle fibers." Ph.D. thesis, Neurosciences Program, Stanford University, California.

Magill-Solc, C. and U.J. McMahan. 1988. Motor neurons contain agrin-like molecules. *J. Cell Biol.* **107:** 1825.

———. 1990. Synthesis and transport of agrin-like molecules in motor neurons. *J. Exp. Res.* **153:** 1.

Marshall, L. M. 1981. Synaptic localization of α-bungarotoxin binding which blocks nicotinic transmission at frog sympathetic neurons. *Proc. Natl. Acad. Sci.* **78:** 1948.

McMahan, U.J. and C.R. Slater. 1984. The influence of basal lamina on the accumulation of acetylcholine receptors at synaptic sites in regenerating muscle. *J. Cell Biol.* **98:** 1452.

McMahan, U.J. and B.G. Wallace. 1989. Molecules in basal lamina that direct the formation of synaptic specializations at neuromuscular junctions. *Dev. Neurosci.* **11:** 227.

Montell, D.J. and C.S. Goodman 1988. *Drosophila* substrate adhesion molecule: Sequence of laminin B1 chain reveals domains of homology with mouse. *Cell* **53:** 463.

New, H.V. and A.W. Mudge. 1986. Calcitonin gene-related peptide regulates muscle acetylcholine receptor synthesis. *Nature* **323:** 809.

Nitkin, R.M., M.A. Smith, C. Magill, J.R. Fallon, Y.-M.M. Yao, B.G. Wallace, and U.J. McMahan. 1987. Identification of agrin, a synaptic organizing protein from *Torpedo* electric organ. *J. Cell Biol.* **105:** 2471.

Peng, H.B. and P.-C. Cheng. 1982. Formation of postsynaptic specializations induced by latex beads in cultured muscle cells. *J. Neurosci.* **2:** 1760.

Reist, N.W. 1990. "Molecules that direct the neuron-induced formation of postsynaptic specializations at the neuromuscular junction." Ph.D. thesis, Neurosciences Program, Stanford University, California.

Reist, N.E., C. Magill, and U.J. McMahan. 1987. Agrin-like molecules at synaptic sites in normal, denervated and damaged skeletal muscles. *J. Cell Biol.* **105:** 2457.

Richards, J.G., P. Schoch, P. Haring, B. Takacs, and H. Mohler. 1987. Resolving GABA$_a$/benzodiazapine receptors. Cellular and subcellular localization in the CNS with monoclonal antibodies. *J. Neurosci.* **7:** 1886.

Role, L.W., R.R. Matossian, R.J. O'Brien, and G.D. Fischbach. 1985. On the mechanism of acetylcholine receptor accumulation at newly formed synapses of chick myotubes. *J. Neurosci.* **5:** 2197.

Rubin, L.L. and U.J. McMahan. 1982. Regeneration of the neuromuscular junction: Steps toward defining the molecular basis of the interaction between nerve and muscle. In *Disorders of the motor unit* (ed. D.L. Schotland), p. 187. Wiley, New York.

Triller, A., F. Cluzeaud, F. Pfeiffer, H. Betz, and H. Korn. 1985. Distribution of glycine receptors at central synapses: An immunoelectron microscopy study. *J. Cell Biol.* **101:** 683.

Usdin, T.B. and G.D. Fischbach. 1986. Purification and characterization of a polypeptide from chick brain that promotes the accumulation of acetylcholine receptors in chick myotubes. *J. Cell Biol.* **103:** 493.

Wallace, B.G. 1988. Regulation of agrin-induced acetylcholine receptor aggregation by Ca^{++} and phorbol ester. *J. Cell Biol.* **107:** 267.

———. 1989. Agrin-induced specializations contain cytoplasmic, membrane, and extracellular matrix-associated components of the postsynaptic apparatus. *J. Neurosci.* **9:** 1294.

———. 1991. The mechanism of agrin-induced acetylcholine receptor aggregation. *Philos. Trans. R. Soc. Lond. B Biol. Sci.* (in press).

Wallace, B.G., R.M. Nitkin, N.E. Reist, J.R. Fallon, N.N. Moayeri, and U.J. McMahan. 1985. Aggregates of acetylcholinesterase induced by acetylcholine receptor-aggregating factor. *Nature* **315:** 574.

Ziskind-Conhaim, L., I. Geffen, and Z.W. Hall. 1984. Redistribution of acetylcholine receptors on developing rat myotubes. *J. Neurosci.* **4:** 2346.

S-Laminin

J.R. Sanes,* D.D. Hunter,*‡ T.L. Green,* and J.P. Merlie †
*Departments of Anatomy and Neurobiology and of †Pharmacology, Washington University Medical Center,
St. Louis, Missouri 63110

A variety of processes contribute to generating patterns of connectivity in the nervous system. These include the production of appropriate numbers and types of cells at particular times and places, the expression of intrinsic programs by neurons, the guided outgrowth of axons to appropriate targets, and the selection of appropriate postsynaptic partners by individual neurites. With the aim of discovering some of the molecules that determine where and when axons make synapses, we have focused on the vertebrate skeletal neuromuscular junction. As the most accessible of vertebrate synapses, the neuromuscular junction has been the subject of numerous histological, physiological, and molecular studies, so a wealth of information is available about its structure, function, and development (Salpeter 1987; Fernandez and Donoso 1988). It is the only synapse at which several pre- and postsynaptic molecules have been identified, localized, and cloned (J.R. Sanes and J.P. Merlie, in prep.). Furthermore, motor axons can successfully reinnervate adult muscle following nerve injury, facilitating studies of synaptogenesis in a convenient postembryonic environment (Sanes and Covault 1985).

Most important for the studies reported here, reinnervation of muscle is topographically selective: Regenerating axons preferentially reinnervate original synaptic sites (Fig. 1a–c) (Tello 1907; Bennett and Pettigrew 1976). For example, in some muscles, more than 95% of the regenerated synapses form on the approximately 0.1% of the muscle fiber surface that was originally synaptic (Letinsky et al. 1976; Sanes et al. 1978). Other experiments have shown that "foreign" motor axons can form synapses at new or "ectopic" sites if they are implanted far from original synaptic sites but that this happens only if the muscle is already denervated (Elsberg 1917; Frank et al. 1975). Together, these results suggest that muscle provides at least three types of information to the regenerating axon. First, because ectopic synapses form only on denervated muscle, there must be some difference between innervated and denervated muscles that axons recognize. Second, because the original synaptic sites are so small that axons would not often find them by chance alone, there is probably some mechanism to bias axonal growth toward these sites. Third, because

the reinnervation of original sites is precise to a submicron level, some signal must be localized at these sites.

These three cues could, in principle, be carried by separate molecules or by variations in the distribution of a single molecule. Our current view, summarized in Figure 2, is that many more than three molecular species are involved. We believe that these molecules are arranged in at least four different groups, such that muscles are increasingly attractive to regenerating axons with decreasing distance from original sites (Covault et al. 1987; Sanes et al. 1990b). First, there is evidence that denervated muscle secretes soluble growth or trophic factors that can attract axons from a distance. These factors have not yet been identified, but recent studies implicate the insulin-like growth factors in this process (Ishii 1989; Caroni and Grandes 1990 and references therein). Second, two cell adhesion molecules (CAMs), neural CAM (N-CAM) and N-cadherin, which are concentrated at synaptic sites in innervated muscle, appear all along the muscle fiber surface after denervation (Covault and Sanes 1985; Rieger et al. 1985; Covault et al. 1986; Hahn and Covault 1989; L. Scott et al., unpubl.). Given the evidence from several laboratories that these molecules are involved in nerve-muscle interactions in vitro (see, e.g., Bixby et al. 1987), it seems possible that they mediate the enhanced susceptibility of denervated muscle to reinnervation in vivo (also see Booth et al. 1990). Third, a set of adhesive macromolecules, most notably tenascin, accumulates outside of muscle fibers following denervation (Sanes et al. 1986). These extracellular or interstitial deposits are not found throughout the muscle, however, but are concentrated in perisynaptic areas and appear to be products of a unique class of fibroblasts that are located near synapses and are activated when the nerve is injured (Gatchalian et al. 1989; Weis et al. 1990). These perisynaptic accumulations may act, along with elements of the nerve trunk (Scherer and Easter 1984; Kuffler 1986), to guide regenerating axons back to original synaptic sites. Finally, there is a group of molecules that are concentrated precisely at synaptic sites in innervated muscle and remain localized at these sites following denervation (for review, see Sanes 1989; Sanes et al. 1990a). We suspect that the molecules responsible for the recognition of synaptic sites by regenerating axons are members of this group. The remainder of this paper concentrates on one such molecule, s-laminin.

‡Present address: Neuroscience Laboratories, Tufts University School of Medicine, Boston, Massachusetts 02111.

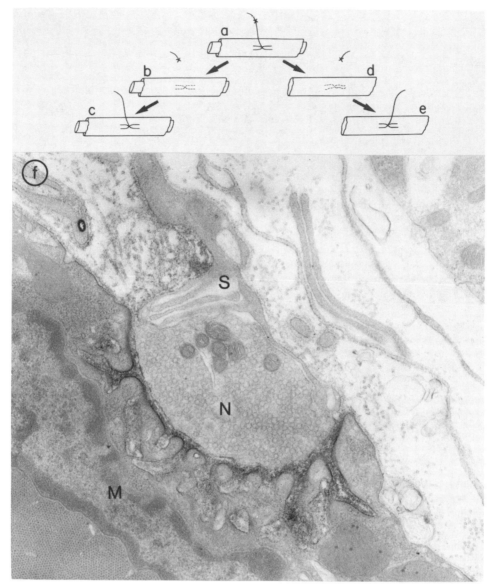

Figure 1. (*a–e*) Regenerating motor axons preferentially reinnervate original synaptic sites on denervated muscle fibers (*a–c*) and on BL sheaths from which muscle fibers have been removed (*d, e*). (*f*) S-laminin is concentrated in synaptic BL. Electron micrograph of a neuromuscular junction from a muscle stained with MAb C1 plus horseradish-peroxidase-second antibody. Reaction product is concentrated in synaptic BL between nerve terminal (N) and muscle fiber (M); extrasynaptic and Schwann cell (S) BLs are not detectably stained.

Identification of S-Laminin

Evidence on the subcellular localization of synapse-associated factors that regenerating motor axons recognize was provided by the experiment diagrammed in Figure 1, a, d, and e. Each muscle fiber is ensheathed by a layer of basal lamina (BL) that extends through the synaptic cleft at the neuromuscular junction. Muscles were damaged and denervated in vivo in a way that caused the muscle fibers to degenerate but permitted their BLs to survive. Light and electron microscopy were then used to identify original synaptic sites and to follow axonal regeneration. Axons that grew into the region of damage contacted synaptic sites on the BL

"ghosts" as selectively as they would have in the presence of intact muscle fibers (Sanes et al. 1978). Furthermore, in areas where they contacted synaptic BL, axons differentiated into nerve terminals, as judged by morphological, immunocytochemical, and physiological criteria (Glicksman and Sanes 1983). Thus, at least some of the site-specific factors that influence regenerating axons are tightly associated with synaptic BL.

Isolation of synaptic BL in pure form proved infeasible, and convenient bioassays of synaptic selectivity were not available. We therefore adopted an immunohistochemical approach to seek molecular correlates of the functional specialization demonstrable during rein-

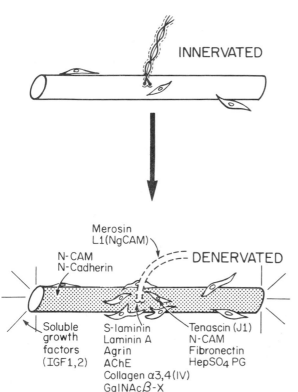

Figure 2. Denervated muscles express a variety of molecules with which regenerating motor axons may interact. Increasing numbers of molecular species are present with decreasing distance from original synaptic sites. (Adapted from Covault et al. 1987; Sanes et al. 1990b.)

nervation. The protein we now call s-laminin was initially defined by antisera to an alkali digest of lens capsule, which is a particularly thick and easily isolated BL. These sera, subsequently named junction-specific-1 (JS-1), stained synaptic BL more intensely than extrasynaptic BL in adult rat muscle (Sanes and Hall 1979). Because the antisera were inadequate for biochemical studies (they were not monospecific), we used the same immunogen to generate three monoclonal antibodies (MAbs), C4, D5, and D7, that also stained synaptic BL selectively; a fourth, similar MAb, C1, was obtained using muscle BL as the immunogen (Fig. 1f) (Sanes and Chiu 1983; Hunter et al. 1987). Staining by each MAb was blocked by preincubation of sections with JS-1, the MAbs all stained the same subset of nonmuscle BLs, and they all recognized the same polypeptide (see below). However, the antibodies differed in species cross-reactivity and in their ability to recognize fixed or denatured antigen, indicating that they recognized distinct epitopes. The selective staining of synaptic sites by this group of antibodies therefore appeared to reflect the restricted distribution of the JS-1 antigen, rather than selective exposure of one particular determinant on a uniformly distributed component.

One of the nonmuscle BLs that all JS-1 antibodies stained was glomerular BL in kidney. Because glomeruli are more abundant in kidney than synaptic sites are

in muscle, we used glomerular extracts to identify the antigen. MAbs C4, D5, and D7 recognized a 190-kD protein on immunoblots of glomerular extracts; C1 did not react with immunoblots but did precipitate a 190-kD, C4-reactive antigen. The solubility properties of the antigen and its sensitivity to a variety of hydrolases indicated that it was a noncollagenous glycoprotein tightly associated with the matrix by a combination of hydrophobic and disulfide bonds. These properties suggested that the JS-1 antigen was an integral component of BL.

Partially purified antigen was used to raise a new group of MAbs, and the complete set was used to screen a λgt11 cDNA library from rat kidney. cDNAs encoding D5-reactive fusion proteins recognized a single mRNA of about 5.7 kb on Northern blot analysis. These were used to isolate longer clones, and the process was repeated until the entire mRNA had been cloned. Reactivity of fusion proteins with several MAbs and reactivity of kidney-derived antigen with antisera to fusion protein confirmed that the cDNAs encoded the JS-1 antigen. Subsequently, cDNAs encoding JS-1 were isolated from muscle-derived libraries and found to be identical in sequence to the kidney-derived cDNAs. These results, along with results of Northern blot and RNase analyses, suggest that the predominant (and possible sole) form of JS-1 in muscle is identical in primary structure to that in kidney.

The most striking feature of the JS-1 sequence was its homology with the subunits of laminin. Because of this homology and the restriction of JS-1 to a subset of BLs including synaptic BL, we renamed it s-laminin (Hunter et al. 1989a). Laminin purified from tumor cells is a cruciform trimer of A, B1, and B2 subunits (Timpl 1989) (Fig. 3, top). All of the subunits are related to each other, and accordingly, s-laminin is related to all of them. However, in both primary sequence and predicted secondary structure, s-laminin's closest relative is the B1 subunit (Fig. 3, bottom). We have since found that a few MAbs to s-laminin (e.g., C4) cross-react weakly with laminin B1 and that some polyclonal antisera to laminin cross-react weakly with s-laminin. Most antibodies we have tested, however, show no detectable cross-reactivity among subunits.

The homology of s-laminin with laminin has been informative in three ways. First, the discovery that the laminins form a multigene family extending beyond the A, B1, and B2 genes alerts us to the possibility that other laminin-like genes exist. Second, previous work on the structure and assembly of laminin subunits suggests testable hypotheses about the structure of native s-laminin. Finally, and perhaps most important, the large body of work showing that laminin is a potent promoter of neurite outgrowth (Sanes 1989) provides ways to assess the functions of s-laminin.

Function of S-Laminin

For initial functional studies of s-laminin, we employed a short-term assay of cell attachment. We used

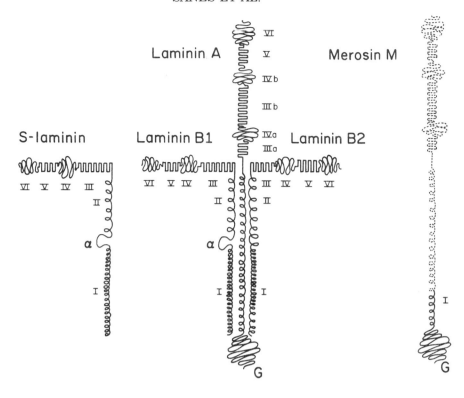

Figure 3. S-laminin is homologous to the B1 subunit of laminin. (*Top*) Domain structures of laminin subunits and their diagrammatic representations are adapted from Sasaki et al. (1988 and references therein). Homology of merosin M with laminin A is documented by Ehrig et al. (1990); dashed line indicates region that has not been sequenced. (*Bottom*) Percentage of identity between s-laminin and laminin subunit amino acid sequences. Values of >35% are boxed. Values in parentheses include conservative substitutions. (The bottom portion of Fig. 3 is modified from Hunter et al. 1989a.)

	VI	V	IV	III	II	α	I	TOTAL
MOUSE B1	72	65	42	60	28	52	38	52 (68)
HUMAN B1	71	65	40	60	28	49	39	51 (68)
DROSOPHILA B1	58	56	28	49	27	61	23	41 (56)
MOUSE B2	22	40	13	41	13	–	17	25 (46)
MOUSE A	20	36	14	38	16	–	15	24 (41)
HUMAN M							24	24 (38)

neurons from embryonic chick ciliary ganglia for these experiments because ciliary neurons innervate striated muscle in vivo and form conventional cholinergic neuromuscular junctions. In addition, we had previously shown that ciliary neurons recognize original synaptic sites on fragments of adult skeletal muscle in vitro (Covault et al. 1987). Thus, ciliary neurons are somatic motoneurons, but they are much easier to isolate than spinal motoneurons. Dissociated ciliary neurons were incubated for 1–2 hours on dishes that had been coated with s-laminin or with laminin. The plates were then washed, and the attached cells were counted. In this assay, neurons adhered as well to s-laminin purified from kidney as to laminin. Subsequently, we found that neurons adhered to a recombinant protein comprising the carboxy-terminal 80 kD (40%) of s-laminin. This adhesion was specific in that it was blocked by antibod-

ies to s-laminin and was not mimicked by other proteins such as bovine serum albumin (Hunter et al. 1989b). These results indicate that at least one adhesive site for motoneurons is present in the carboxy-terminal 40% of s-laminin.

Our interest in this adhesive site increased when we compared the behavior of ciliary neurons with that of other cell types. Under conditions where several types of neurons (e.g., tectal, sensory, and ciliary neurons), neuron-like cells (e.g., PC12, B35, and B104 cells), and nonneuronal cells (e.g., fibroblasts, myoblasts, and glomerular epithelial cells) adhered well to laminin, only ciliary motoneurons attached significantly to the s-laminin fusion protein. This cell-type specificity fits well with the functional selectivity expected for synaptic BL: Nerves that innervate and reinnervate muscles often contain as many sensory and sympathetic axons as motor axons; yet, as far as is known, only motor axons recognize muscle fibers. The adhesive site present in the carboxy-terminal portion of s-laminin could, in principle, mediate this selectivity. We therefore defined this site in detail (Fig. 4). First, we found that a smaller recombinant fragment comprising the carboxy-terminal 20 kD or 10% of s-laminin was as adhesive and cell-type-specific as the longer fusion protein. We then synthesized nine peptides to span this approximately 200-amino-acid stretch and asked which if any could inhibit adhesion to the immobilized fragment. A single 21-amino-acid-long peptide spanning residues 1666–1686 in the full sequence was inhibitory, placing an adhesive site within this region. This assay was repeated with smaller and smaller peptides until we found a tripeptide, leucine-arginine-glutamate (LRE), that inhibited adhesion of ciliary neurons to the recombinant fragment. The potency of LRE in molar terms is approximately equal to that of the 21-amino-acid-long peptide, indicating that LRE defines a crucial determinant of a motoneuron-selective adhesive site (Hunter et al. 1989b).

An implication of these results is that motoneurons bear a receptor specific for LRE. With the long-term goal of isolating such a receptor, we screened a number of cell lines for their ability to recognize the s-laminin-derived fusion protein and/or LRE-protein conjugates. So far, only one cell line has been found to be capable of LRE-dependent adhesion. This line, NSC-34, is derived from a fusion of rat spinal cord cells to a neuroblastoma line. It resembles spinal motoneurons by several neurochemical and functional criteria (Cashman et al. 1987); the ability of NSC-34 cells to recognize s-laminin is additional evidence that they are derived from a spinal motoneuron.

Adhesion of many neuronal and nonneuronal cells to many extracellular matrix molecules is now known to be mediated by cell-surface receptors encoded by a multigene family, the integrins. In many cases, integrins recognize short peptide sequences within their substrates, for example, RGD in fibronectin (Ruoslahti

and Pierschbacher 1987). For these reasons, it seemed likely that the LRE receptor would be an integrin. In all cases studied so far, the activity of integrins is strictly dependent on divalent cations, particularly magnesium. We therefore assayed the cation dependence of adhesion to s-laminin as a simple diagnostic test for the involvement of integrins. As expected, adhesion of NSC-34 cells to laminin was entirely dependent on extracellular magnesium ions but was unaffected by calcium ions. Interestingly, however, adhesion of NSC-34 cells to the s-laminin fragment was robust in the presence of chelating agents, was unaffected by extracellular magnesium, and was inhibited by the presence of extracellular calcium (Fig. 5A,B) (D.D. Hunter et al., in prep.). To our knowledge, no receptors for extracellular matrix molecules have been described that display this pattern of divalent ion dependence. Although identification of the LRE receptor awaits its purification, our results are not consistent with it being a member of the integrin family. In addition, the effect of calcium suggests a novel mechanism for regulation of LRE-dependent adhesion in situ: Adhesion might be strengthened if extracellular calcium concentrations fell as may happen, for example, consequent to calcium influx during synaptic transmission (Attwell and Iles 1979).

Although LRE-containing peptides may eventually be useful in the isolation of the LRE receptor, a more pressing question is, What purpose does the LRE-dependent adhesive interaction serve? As a first step in addressing this issue, we extended the short-term adhesion assay to longer incubation times to ask how ciliary neurons and NSC-34 cells behaved on substrata coated with laminin, s-laminin, or LRE-protein conjugates. In one variant of this experiment, we found that NSC-34 cells soon extended neurites on laminin but not on LRE-protein conjugates, although similar numbers of cells adhered to both substrata. It was not merely that the LRE-conjugate fails to support process outgrowth, however; rather, the conjugate inhibited process outgrowth on laminin (Fig. 5C,D). One implication of this result is that s-laminin might arrest neurite outgrowth promoted by laminin. Experiments in which ciliary neurons growing on laminin failed to cross an overlaid stripe of s-laminin are consistent with this idea (Weis et al. 1989). These results suggest the working hypothesis that, whereas laminin promotes the outgrowth of regenerating axons back to and along the muscle fiber surface, s-laminin is one of the components of synaptic BL that causes axons to stop growing at original synaptic sites (and possibly to initiate their differentiation into nerve terminals at these sites).

Structure of S-Laminin

More informative tests of the function of s-laminin will require assaying the molecule in its native, full-length, glycosylated form. To this end, we ligated several cDNAs to generate an expression vector that contains the entire s-laminin coding region. Muscle cells

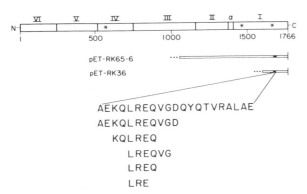

Figure 4. Mapping an adhesive site for ciliary neurons on s-laminin. Fusion proteins (pET-36 and pET-65-6) and synthetic peptides to which ciliary neurons bind are shown relative to the deduced amino acid sequence and domain structure of s-laminin. Positions of three LREs in s-laminin are indicated by asterisks. (Adapted from Hunter et al. 1989b.)

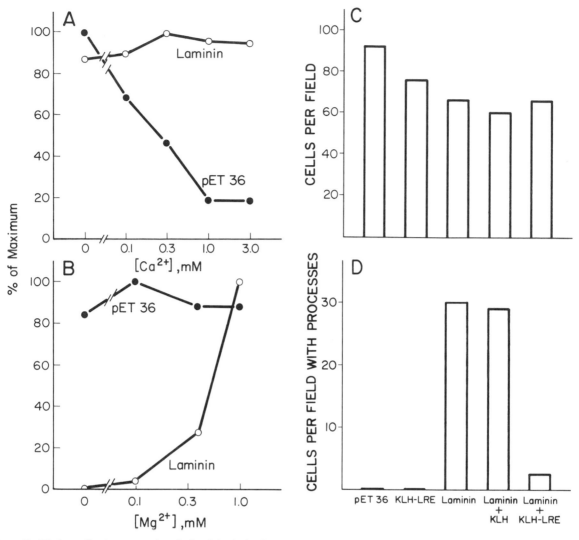

Figure 5. Distinct adhesive properties of s-laminin-derived peptides and laminin. (*A,B*) Adhesion of NSC-34 (motoneuron-like) cells to laminin requires magnesium ions but is calcium-independent. In contrast, adhesion to the LRE-containing pET-36 fusion protein (see Fig. 4) is unaffected by extracellular magnesium ions but inhibited by calcium ions. These results suggest that LRE-dependent adhesion is not mediated by any hitherto described integrin, all of which are magnesium-dependent. (*C,D*) Laminin, pET-36, and an LRE-protein conjugate (keyhole limpet hemocyanin-CKQLREQ; KLH-LRE) all support adhesion of NSC-34 cells to a similar extent. However, KLH-LRE inhibits the neurite outgrowth promoted by laminin.

transfected with this plasmid produce a protein that is identical in size to native s-laminin and is recognized by antibodies to s-laminin on immunoblots (Fig. 6a). Purification of this recombinant s-laminin for tests in vitro is in progress.

In parallel, we used the expression vector to generate several lines of transgenic mice in which rat s-laminin is expressed under the control of a myosin-light-chain promoter, which we previously showed to promote skeletal-muscle-specific expression (Rosenthal et al. 1989). We then studied the transgenic animals using antibodies that recognize rat but not mouse s-laminin. In one such line, we were surprised to find that immunoreactive s-laminin was concentrated in the basal lamina of intramuscular blood vessels but was not detectable in extramuscular blood vessels or in the basal lamina of muscle fibers themselves (Fig. 6d–f). One

interpretation of this result is that other proteins are required for s-laminin to be delivered to and/or incorporated in BL. Perhaps extrasynaptic regions of the muscle fiber, which are normally devoid of s-laminin, lack such proteins, whereas vascular and synaptic BL, which are normally rich in s-laminin, contain such proteins. S-laminin made and secreted by muscle fibers might remain soluble until bound to appropriate components of vascular membranes or BL.

One specific possibility along these lines is suggested by the trimeric structure of laminin (Fig. 3, bottom): Perhaps s-laminin occurs in a complex with other laminin-like subunits, some of which are absent from extrasynaptic BL. As a first test of this idea, we used a panel of monoclonal antibodies specific for individual laminin subunits to stain a variety of muscle and nonmuscle BLs. In addition, we examined the distribution

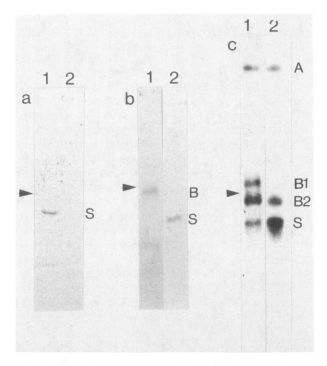

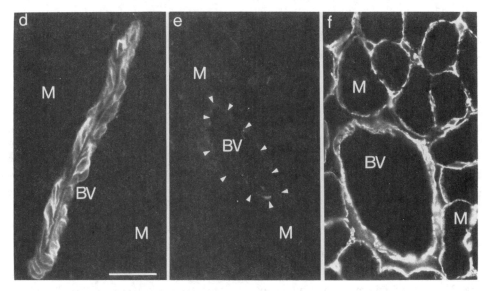

Figure 6. (*a*) Muscle cells transfected with full-length rat s-laminin cDNA express s-laminin. Extracts of normal and transfected mouse C2 cells were immunoblotted with a MAb (D5) that recognized rat but not mouse s-laminin. (Lane *1*) Transfected cells; (lane *2*) untransfected cells. (*b,c*) S-laminin occurs in a complex with other laminin subunits. (*b*) Immunoblotting demonstrates specificity of antibodies to s-laminin (lane *1*) and laminin (lane *2*). (*c*) Immunoprecipitation of metabolically labeled material from a rat muscle cell line reveals the presence of specific oligomers. Anti-B2 coprecipitates B1, s-laminin, and an A-like chain (lane *1*), whereas anti-s-laminin coprecipitates laminin B2 and an A-like chain but not B1 (lane *1*). Arrows indicate position of 200-kD marker (myosin). (*d–f*) Transgenic mice carrying the rat s-laminin cDNA controlled by a myosin-light-chain promoter accumulate s-laminin in the BL of intramuscular arterial vessels. (*d*) Transgenic muscle stained with an antibody to rat s-laminin that does not cross-react with mouse s-laminin. (*e*) Control muscle stained with anti-rat s-laminin. (*f*) Transgenic muscle stained with anti-mouse laminin. A blood vessel (BV) and two muscle fibers (M) are marked in each part, and the vessel is outlined in *e*. Bar: (*d*) 100 μm.

of the protein merosin M, which was recently shown to be a homolog of the laminin A subunit (Ehrig et al. 1990). This immunohistochemical study revealed an unexpected heterogeneity of BLs in several tissues. At least five of the seven BLs studied have distinct patterns of laminin isoforms, and all five laminin-like subunits

have distinct distributions (Fig. 7). Specifically, the synaptic and extrasynaptic portions of the muscle fiber's sheath are more different from each other than we previously thought. Thus, not only s-laminin, but also the laminin A subunit is concentrated in synaptic basal lamina. In contrast, laminin B1 is abundant in ex-

SANES ET AL.

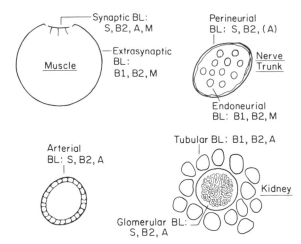

Figure 7. Laminin subunits and homologs are differentially distributed in various BLs. Sketches summarize distribution of laminin subunits and homologs in several BLs. (Adapted from Sanes et al. 1990a.)

trasynaptic basal lamina but is not detectable synaptically. The B2 and M subunits are present throughout the muscle fiber BL. In parallel, we have found that the component chains of collagen IV, $\alpha1-\alpha4$, are also differentially distributed among BLs (Sanes et al. 1990a). Together, these results suggest a revision of the prevailing view that all BLs, including synaptic and extrasynaptic BL in muscle (Sanes 1982), contain an identical set of major structural components. Instead, we now conclude that each BL contains some laminin-like and some collagen IV-like molecules but that these vary from one BL to another. It may be that the laminins and collagen IV play similar structural roles in all BLs but that the unique properties of each BL are determined by its isotype.

Our results are consistent with the idea that laminin molecules generally occur as trimers of a B1-like, an A-like, and a B2-like subunit. In these trimers, B1 and s-laminin can substitute for each other, as can merosin M for laminin A; other laminin-like subunits may remain to be discovered. To obtain direct evidence for this scheme, we immunoprecipitated native and recombinant s-laminin from cultured cells using subunit-specific antibodies. Initial results, shown in Figure 6 (b and c), are consistent with our hypothesis. Antibodies to laminin B2 coprecipitate laminin B1 and s-laminin, as well as a laminin A-like subunit. In contrast, a monoclonal antibody to s-laminin coprecipitates B2 and an A-like subunit but not B1 (Green et al. 1990). Thus, muscle cells appear to assemble a B1, B2, A trimer and an s-laminin, B2, A trimer. Analysis of placental laminins also supports the idea that subunits can combine to form several distinct heterotrimers (Engvall et al. 1990). Further experiments are required to catalog the full range of laminin isotypes that are permissible, to determine the identity of the A-like subunit in muscle, and to ask whether other subunits exist.

A Common Motif in Synaptic BL Proteins

Why might laminin-like subunits be differentially combined in a common trimeric structure? Individual subunits have now been found to bear several potential active sites that can be recognized by cellular receptors. These include a potential integrin-binding site (RGD) in laminin A, neurite-outgrowth promoting sites in A and B2, at least two discrete sites in B1 that bind nonneural cells, and the LRE site described above. The variations among BLs described here imply that the BLs in peripheral nerve and muscle contain different combinations of these sites. Thus, the variable arrangements of laminin isoforms of the BLs that regenerating axons encounter may serve to display different combinations of active sites to axons at different points along their path, influencing axonal growth and differentiation in complex ways.

Specifically, the differential distribution of laminins between synaptic and extrasynaptic BL appears to concentrate LREs at synaptic sites. There are, in fact, several occurrences of LRE in the laminin family. S-laminin itself bears three LREs, laminin A bears one, and laminin B2 bears two. In contrast, there is no LRE in laminin B1 or in the portion of merosin M that has been sequenced so far. Synaptic BL substitutes LRE-rich s-laminin for LRE-free laminin B1 and adds LRE-containing laminin A to merosin M. Laminin B2 contains two LREs and is present both synaptically and extrasynaptically; however, recent studies with synthetic peptides suggest that negatively charged residues flanking these LREs render them inactive in adhesion assays (R. Morris-Valero and J.R. Sanes, unpubl.). Thus, the laminin of the synaptic cleft is particularly rich in the motoneuron-adhesive sequence LRE.

The speculation that LRE-dependent adhesion is important for synapse formation or maintenance receives further support from the sequences of other components of the muscle fiber surface that have recently been cloned. Six proteins have now been shown to be concentrated in synaptic BL: s-laminin, laminin A, agrin, acetylcholinesterase, and collagens $\alpha3$ (IV) and $\alpha4$ (IV) (see Fig. 2). (McMahan and Wallace 1989; Sanes 1989; Sanes et al. 1990a). Of these, the first four have been sequenced and all bear LREs. S-laminin bears three, laminin A (mouse) bears one, agrin (rat) bears two, and acetylcholinesterase (*Torpedo* and human) bears one (Hunter et al. 1989b; R. Scheller, pers. comm.). In contrast, sequenced proteins that are concentrated at synaptic sites in innervated muscle but appear extrasynaptically following denervation lack LRE; these include N-CAM, N-cadherin, and the subunits of the acetylcholine receptor (see Hunter et al. 1989b). Although LRE would appear occasionally in random sequences ($\sim$ 1 occurrence per 500 kD; Hunter et al. 1989a), the observed frequency (7 occurrences in $\sim$ 800 kD of synaptic BL sequence) is unlikely to have occurred by chance alone. We therefore suggest that the concentration of several LRE-containing proteins at synaptic sites in muscle fibers may contribute importantly to the attractiveness of those sites for regenerating motor axons.

S-Laminin in Embryonic Muscle

Before considering roles that s-laminin might play in embryonic muscle, it is important to know when and where it appears, which cells make it, and how its accumulation is regulated. To answer the first of these questions, we stained sections of embryonic rat intercostal muscle with MAbs to s-laminin (then called JS-1), as well as to laminin, collagen IV, collagen VI, fibronectin, and a heparan sulfate proteoglycan (Chiu and Sanes 1984). S-laminin-like immunoreactivity was detectable predominantly at synaptic sites; little or none accumulated in nonsynaptic areas. Furthermore, s-laminin appeared only *after* acetylcholine receptors (stained with rhodamine-α-bungarotoxin) clustered in the postsynaptic membrane, and a rudimentary BL (stained with anti-laminin and anti-proteoglycan) formed in the synaptic cleft. The late appearance of s-laminin has been confirmed with the newer MAbs described above, indicating that it does not reflect a peculiarity of the single MAb (C1) used in the first study. Interestingly, a MAb (C21) believed to recognize laminin B1 (Sanes et al. 1990a) stains both synaptic and extrasynaptic BL at early stages but ceases to stain synaptic sites as they become s-laminin-positive (Chiu and Sanes 1984). Thus, the laminins at embryonic synaptic sites become distinguishable from those in extrasynaptic areas only after synapses form.

These results are not consistent with the simplest view of s-laminin's role—that its accumulation prefigures sites of synaptic contact. However, despite some controversy, there is no convincing evidence that embryonic muscles have predetermined sites of innervation (for discussion, see Sanes and Chiu 1983). Instead, it is likely that synapses initially form at random, and that subsequent elongation of myotubes from both ends leads to the adult arrangement in which synapses are concentrated in a central band (Bennett and Pettigrew 1976). Once synapses form, nerve and muscle collaborate to deposit a specialized matrix at points of contact. Similarly, when ectopic synapses form in adult muscle (see above), s-laminin is detectable only after functional transmission is established and acetylcholine receptors aggregate in the postsynaptic membrane (Weinberg et al. 1981).

How might the motor axon determine the sites at which s-laminin accumulates? The two possibilities are that the motoneuron synthesizes s-laminin (as has been proposed for agrin; McMahan and Wallace 1989) or that it organizes postsynaptic differentiation (as is the case for acetylcholine receptors; Schuetze and Role 1987). These possibilities are not mutually exclusive, and we have no evidence for or against the first of them. However, muscle cells cultured without neurons can synthesize s-laminin (Fig. 6c) and incorporate it

into a BL (Sanes and Lawrence 1983). Furthermore, whereas laminin is present throughout the BL that cultured myotubes assemble, s-laminin is concentrated at the acetylcholine-receptor-rich "hot spots" that form even when no neurons are present in the cultures (Silberstein et al. 1982; Sanes and Lawrence 1983). These hot spots are also enriched in other "synaptic" features, such as acetylcholinesterase, cytoskeletal elements, and junctional folds, indicating that myotubes are capable of assembling an elaborate postsynaptic apparatus on their own (Sanes et al. 1984). However, treatment of such cultures with neural extracts or with agents that modulate electrical activity, i.e., treatments that mimic likely effects of innervation, not only affect the formation of s-laminin- and acetylcholine-receptor-rich hot spots, but also differentially affect the deposition of synaptic and extrasynaptic BL components (Sanes and Lawrence 1983; Sanes et al. 1984). The particular patterns of regulation observed suggest a model wherein myotubes make BL but axons use a combination of activity-dependent and -independent means to confine the deposition of s-laminin to synaptic sites (Sanes et al. 1984).

If s-laminin accumulates under neural control and only after synapses form, what purpose could it serve? One possibility is that s-laminin (and/or other components of synaptic BL) could promote the maturation of synapses once they have formed. In fact, newly formed nerve terminals are morphologically unspecialized; most active zones form, and vesicles accumulate after the time at which s-laminin appears. In that components of synaptic BL are known to organize presynaptic differentiation during reinnervation (Glicksman and Sanes 1983), it is reasonable to imagine that similar molecules could play similar roles in the embryo. A second possibility is that s-laminin-rich areas induced at initially formed synapses become preferred sites of attachment for later arriving axons. Each developing myotube transiently receives inputs from several motor axons, all of which converge at a single synaptic site. Subsequently, all inputs but one are eliminated by a competitive process that is distance-dependent. By confining all of a myotube's inputs to a limited area, synaptic BL could sharpen the competitive interactions that lead to the adult pattern of innervation. Although speculative, these possibilities (discussed more fully in Chiu and Sanes 1984) are consistent with the known facts of neuromuscular development and with models that have been proposed to explain synaptic dynamics (Van Essen et al. 1990 and references therein). Thus, they may serve as good starting points for experimental tests of s-laminin's role now that appropriate reagents are in hand.

S-Laminin in the CNS

We hope that some of the molecules characterized in studies of neuromuscular synaptogenesis will eventually prove to be involved in the development of the less experimentally accessible central nervous system (CNS). For the CAMs shown in Figure 2, this premise is amply supported: Many of these molecules were first isolated from brain tissue, and their roles in CNS development are being actively investigated in many laboratories (for review, see Rutishauser and Jessell 1988). On the other hand, the brain's BLs are confined to meningeal surfaces and blood vessels, and the CNS was long thought to be otherwise devoid of extracellular matrix. However, as antibodies have become available that recognize matrix-associated molecules in the periphery, it has become apparent that many of these molecules, including laminin, are also present in the developing CNS (for review, see Sanes 1989). We therefore asked whether s-laminin is also expressed in the CNS. Our studies to date have revealed three intriguing sites of expression (D.D. Hunter et al., in prep.).

First, s-laminin is transiently present in the embryonic cerebral cortex. It appears in punctate deposits, as has been seen for laminin in subcortical regions (Letourneau et al. 1988; Liesi and Silver 1988; Gordon-Weeks et al. 1989), and is concentrated in the cortical subplate, as has been reported for fibronectin (Stewart and Pearlman 1987; Chun and Shatz 1988). In general, the distribution of s-laminin parallels that of laminin in cortex. (We used a polyclonal serum to detect laminin and do not yet know which subunits are present.) However, detectable s-laminin-like immunoreactivity appears later and disappears earlier than does laminin and, at any given stage, only a subset of the laminin-positive areas are s-laminin-positive. Because the subplate is an area in which neuroblasts migrate, axons grow, and transient synapses form (for review, see Shatz et al. 1988), it is tempting to speculate that s-laminin plays a role in guiding one or more of these processes.

Second, s-laminin is concentrated on the ventromedial surface of the developing spinal cord. Whereas a laminin-positive layer encircles the entire cord, anti-s-laminin selectively stains the small strip of subpial material that caps the floor plate (Fig. 8). Neuroanatomical studies have indicated that the axons of intraspinal commissural neurons are attracted to and influenced by elements associated with the floor plate (see, e.g., Ramon y Cajal 1909; Dodd and Jessell 1988; Chuang and Lagenaur 1990). It is possible that these axons, which are likely to contact the s-laminin-rich surface as they grow (Ramon y Cajal, 1909), are influenced by the s-laminin that they encounter there.

Third, whereas most capillaries in the periphery are s-laminin-negative (Sanes et al. 1990a), the BLs of capillaries in the brain and spinal cord are s-laminin-positive. However, detectable s-laminin appears in these capillaries late in development. In the embryo, elements of the vessel walls, presumably BLs, are laminin-positive but s-laminin-negative (Fig. 8b,c); only postnatally does s-laminin appear at these sites. In light of evidence that the blood-brain barrier matures late in development (Risau et al. 1986), it is possible

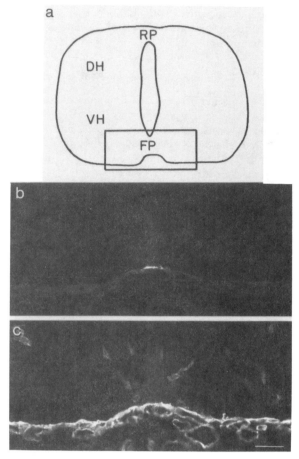

Figure 8. S-laminin is concentrated at the pial surface of the floor plate in embryonic (day 15) rat spinal cord. A cryostat section was doubly stained with mouse anti-s-laminin and fluorescein-anti-mouse immunoglobulin G (IgG) (*b*) plus rabbit anti-laminin and rhodamine-anti-rabbit IgG (*c*). *a* shows orientation of micrographs. (DH) Dorsal horn; (VH) ventral horn; (FP) floor plate; (RP) roof plate. Bar, 100 μm.

that s-laminin plays a role in organizing or maintaining some elements of this barrier.

In summary, in the CNS as in the periphery, s-laminin occurs in a distinct subset of laminin-containing structures. The spatial and temporal patterns of s-laminin expression in the CNS suggest several roles that it may play, but the questions of what these roles are and of whether laminin isoforms in general are important for central neural development remain to be answered.

ACKNOWLEDGMENTS

We thank Steve Adams, Joe Bulock, Jeanette Cunningham, Dorothy Dill, Eva Engvall, Rafael Llinas, Robin-Morris Valero, Jacqueline Mudd, Brenda Porter, Vandana Shah, and Joachim Weis for important contributions to this work. We are grateful to National Institutes of Health, the Muscular Distrophy Association, and the Monsanto-Washington University Alliance for support.

REFERENCES

Attwell, D. and J.F. Iles. 1979. Synaptic transmission: Ion concentration changes in the synaptic cleft. *Proc. R. Soc. Lond. B Biol. Soc.* **206:** 115.

Bennett, M.R. and A.G. Pettigrew. 1976. The formation of neuromuscular synapses. *Cold Spring Harbor Symp. Quant. Biol.* **40:** 409.

Bixby, J.L., R.S. Pratt, J. Lilien, and L.F. Reichardt. 1987. Neurite outgrowth on muscle cell surfaces involves extracellular matrix receptors as well as calcium-dependent and independent cell adhesion molecules. *Proc. Natl. Acad. Sci.* **84:** 2555.

Booth, C.M., S.K. Kemplay, and M.C. Brown. 1990. Antibody to neural cell adhesion molecule impairs motor nerve terminal sporting in a mouse muscle locally paralyzed with botulinum toxin. *Neuroscience* **35:** 85.

Caroni, P. and P. Grandes. 1990. Nerve sprouting in innervated adult skeletal muscle induced by exposure to elevated levels of insulin-like growth factors. *J. Cell Biol.* **110:** 1307.

Cashman, N.R., S. Balet, and J. Antel. 1987. Clonal cell lines from neuroblastoma-spinal cord cell hybridization. *Soc. Neurosci. Abstr.* **13:** 1511.

Chiu, A.Y. and J.R. Sanes. 1984. Differentiation of basal lamina in synaptic and extrasynaptic portions of embryonic rat muscle. *Dev. Biol.* **103:** 456.

Chuang, W. and C.F. Lagenaur. 1990. Central nervous system antigen P84 can serve as a substrate for neurite outgrowth. *Dev. Biol.* **137:** 219.

Chun, J.J.M. and C.J. Shatz. 1988. A fibronectin-like molecule is present in the developing cat cerebral cortex and is correlated with subplate neurons. *J. Cell. Biol.* **106:** 857.

Covault, J. and J.R. Sanes. 1985. Neural cell adhesion molecule (N-CAM) accumulates in denervated and paralyzed skeletal muscles. *Proc. Natl. Acad. Sci.* **82:** 4544.

Covault, J., J.M. Cunningham, and J.R. Sanes. 1987. Neurite outgrowth on cryostat sections of innervated and denervated skeletal muscle. *J. Cell Biol.* **105:** 2479.

Covault, J., J.P. Merlie, C. Goridis, and J.R. Sanes. 1986. Molecular forms of N-CAM and its RNA in developing and denervated skeletal muscle. *J. Cell Biol.* **102:** 731.

Dodd, J. and T.M. Jessell. 1988. Axon guidance and the patterning of neuronal projections in vertebrates. *Science* **242:** 692.

Ehrig, K., I. Leivo, W.S. Argraves, E. Ruoslahti, and E. Engvall. 1990. Merosin, a tissue-like specific basement membrane protein, is a laminin-like protein. *Proc. Natl. Acad. Sci.* **87:** 3264.

Elsberg, C.A. 1917. Experiments on motor nerve regeneration and the direct neurotization of paralyzed muscles by their own and by foreign nerves. *Science* **45:** 318.

Engvall, E., D. Earwicker, T. Haaparanta, E. Ruoslahti, and J. R. Sanes. 1990. Distribution and isolation of four laminin variants; tissue restricted distribution of heterotrimers assembled from five different subunits. *Cell Regul.* (in press).

Fernandez, H.L. and J.A. Donoso. 1988. *Nerve-muscle cell trophic communication.* CRC Press, Boca Raton, Florida.

Frank, E., J.K.S. Jansen, T. Lomo, and R.H. Westgaard. 1975. The interaction between foreign and original motor nerves innervating the soleus muscle of rats. *J. Physiol.* **247:** 725.

Gatchalian, C.L., M. Schachner, and J.R. Sanes. 1989. Fibroblasts that proliferate near denervated synaptic site in skeletal muscle synthesize the adhesive molecules tenascin/J1, NCAM, fibronectin, and a heparan sulfate proteoglycan. *J. Cell Biol.* **108:** 1973.

Glicksman, M. and J.R. Sanes. 1983. Development of motor nerve terminals formed in the absence of muscle fibers. *J. Neurocytol.* **12:** 661.

Gordon-Weeks, P.R., N. Giffin, S.E. Weekes, and C. Barben.

1989. Transient expression of laminin immunoreactivity in the developing rat hippocampus. *J. Neurocytol.* **18:** 451.

Green, T.L., D.D. Hunter, W. Chan, J.P. Merlie, and J.R. Sanes. 1990. Expression of the synaptic cleft protein s-laminin in cell lines. *Soc. Neurosci. Abstr.* **16:** 1011.

Hahn, C.G. and J. Covault. 1989. Activity-dependent regulation of muscle N-cadherin. *Soc. Neurosci. Abstr.* **15:** 1365.

Hunter, D.D., J.R. Sanes, and A.Y. Chiu. 1987. An antigen concentrated in the basal lamina of the neuromuscular junction. *Soc. Neurosci. Abstr.* **13:** 375.

Hunter, D.D., V. Shah, J.P. Merlie, and J.R. Sanes. 1989a. Laminin-like adhesive protein concentrated in the synaptic cleft of the neuromuscular junction. *Nature* **338:** 229.

Hunter, D.D., B.E. Porter, J.W. Bulock, S.P. Adams, J.P. Merlie, and J.R. Sanes. 1989b. Primary sequence of a motor neuron-selective adhesive site in the synaptic basal lamina protein s-laminin. *Cell* **59:** 905.

Ishii, D.N. 1989. Relationship of insulin-like growth factor II gene expression in muscle to synaptogenesis. *Proc. Natl. Acad. Sci.* **86:** 2898.

Kuffler, D.P. 1986. Isolated satellite cells of a peripheral nerve direct the growth of regenerating frog axons. *J. Comp. Neurol.* **249:** 57.

Letinsky, M.K., D.G. Fischbach, and U.J. McMahan. 1976. Precision of reinnervation of original postsynaptic sites in muscle after a nerve crush. *J. Neurocytol.* **5:** 691.

Letourneau, P.C., A.M. Madsen, S.L. Palm, and L.T. Furch. 1988. Immunoreactivity for laminin in the developing ventral longitudinal pathway of the brain. *Dev. Biol.* **125:** 135.

Liesi, P. and J. Silver. 1988. Is astrocyte laminin involved in axon guidance in the mammalian CNS? *Dev. Biol.* **130:** 774.

McMahan, U.J. and B.G. Wallace. 1989. Molecules in basal lamina that direct the formation of synaptic specializations at neuromuscular junctions. *Dev. Neurosci.* **11:** 227.

Ramon y Cajal, S. 1909. *Histologie du systeme nerveux de l'homme et des vertebres.* Malone, Paris. (Reprinted 1972 by Institute Ramon y Cajal, Madrid.)

Rieger, F., M. Grumet, and G.M. Edelman. 1985. N-CAM at the vertebrate neuromuscular junction. *J. Cell Biol.* **101:** 285.

Risau, W., R. Hallman, and U. Albrecht. 1986. Differentiation-dependent expression of proteins in brain endothelium during development of the blood-brain barrier. *Dev. Biol.* **117:** 537.

Rosenthal, N., J.M. Kornhauser, M. Donoghue, K.M. Rosen, and J.P. Merlie. 1989. Myosin light chain enhancer activates muscle-specific, developmentally regulated gene expression in transgenic mice. *Proc. Natl. Acad. Sci.* **86:** 7780.

Ruoslahti, E. and M.D. Pierschbacher. 1987. New perspectives in cell adhesion: RGD and integrins. *Science* **238:** 491.

Rutishauser, U. and T.M. Jessell. 1988. Cell adhesion molecules in vertebrate neural development. *Physiol. Rev.* **68:** 819.

Salpeter, M.M., ed. 1987. *The vertebrate neuromuscular junction.* A.R. Liss, New York.

Sanes, J.R. 1982. Laminin, fibronectin and collagen in synaptic and extrasynaptic portions of muscle fiber basement membrane. *J. Cell Biol.* **93:** 442.

———. 1989. Extracellular matrix molecules that influence neural development. *Annu. Rev. Neurosci.* **12:** 521.

Sanes, J.R. and A.Y. Chiu. 1983. The basal lamina of the neuromuscular junction. *Cold Spring Harbor Symp. Quant. Biol.* **48:** 667.

Sanes, J.R. and J. Covault. 1985. Axon guidance during reinnervation of skeletal muscle. *Trends Neurosci.* **8:** 523.

Sanes, J.R. and Z.W. Hall. 1979. Antibodies that bind specifically to synaptic sites on muscle fiber basal lamina. *J. Cell Biol.* **83:** 357.

Sanes, J.R. and J.C. Lawrence. 1983. Activity-dependent accumulation of basal lamina by cultured rat myotubes. *Dev. Biol.* **97**: 123.

Sanes, J.R., L.M. Marshall, and U.J. McMahan. 1978. Reinnervation of muscle fiber basal lamina after removal of myofibers. Differentiation of regenerating axons at original synaptic sites. *J. Cell Biol.* **78**: 176.

Sanes, J.R., M. Schachner, and J. Covault. 1986. Expression of several adhesive macromolecules (N-CAM, L1, J1, NILE, uvomorulin, laminin, fibronectin, and a heparan sulfate proteoglycan) in embryonic, adult and denervated adult skeletal muscles. *J. Cell Biol.* **102**: 420.

Sanes, J.R., E. Engvall, R. Butkowski, and D.D. Hunter. 1990a. Molecular heterogeneity of basal laminae: Isoforms of laminin and collagen IV at the neuromuscular junction and elsewhere. *J. Cell Biol.* **11**: 1685.

Sanes, J.R., D.H. Feldman, J.M. Cheney, and J.C. Lawrence. 1984. Brain extract induces synaptic characteristics in the basal lamina of cultured myotubes. *J. Neurosci.* **4**: 464.

Sanes, J.R., J. Covault, C.L. Gatchalian, D.D. Hunter, M.B. Laskowski, and J.P. Merlie. 1990b. Regulation of synaptogenesis in adult skeletal muscle. In *Morphoregulatory molecules* (ed. J.P. Thiery et al.), p. 401. Wiley, New York.

Sasaki, M., H.K. Kleinman, H. Huber, R. Deutzmann, and Y. Yamada. 1988. Laminin, a multidomain protein. The A chain has a unique globular domain and homology with the basement membrane proteoglycan and the laminin B chains. *J. Biol. Chem.* **263**: 16536.

Scherer, S.S. and S.S. Easter, Jr. 1984. Degenerative and regenerative changes in the trochlear nerve of goldfish. *J. Neurocytol.* **13**: 519.

Schuetze, S.M. and L.W. Role. 1987. Developmental regulation of nicotinic acetylcholine receptors. *Annu. Rev. Neurosci.* **10**: 403.

Shatz, C.J., J.J. Chun, and M.B. Luskin. 1988. The role of the subplate in the development of the mammalian telencephalon. In *Cerebral cortex* (ed. A. Peters and E.G. Jones), vol. 7, p. 35. Plenum Press, New York.

Silberstein, L., N.C. Inestrosa, and Z.W. Hall. 1982. Aneural muscle cell cultures make synaptic basal lamina components. *Nature* **295**: 143.

Stewart, G.R. and A.L. Pearlman. 1987. Fibronectin-like immunoreactivity in the developing cerebral cortex. *J. Neurosci.* **7**: 3325.

Tello, F. 1907. Degeneration et regeneration des plaques motrices après la section des nerfs. *Trav. Lab. Recherche Biol.* **5**: 117.

Timpl, R. 1989. Structure and biological activity of basement membrane proteins. *Eur. J. Biochem.* **180**: 487.

Van Essen, D.C., H. Gordon, J.M. Soha, and S.E. Fraser. 1990. Synaptic dynamics at the neuromuscular junction: Mechanisms and models. *J. Neurobiol.* **21**: 223.

Weinberg, C.B., J.R. Sanes, and Z.W. Hall. 1981. Formation of neuromuscular junctions in adult rats: Accumulation of acetylcholine receptors, aceylcholinesterase, and components of synaptic basal lamina. *Dev. Biol.* **84**: 255.

Weis, J., S. Fine, and J.R. Sanes. 1990. Development of perisynaptic cells in skeletal muscles of transgenic mice. *Soc. Neurosci. Abstr.* **16**: 802.

Weis, J., D.D. Hunter, J.P. Merlie, and J.R. Sanes. 1989. S-laminin inhibits neurite extension promoted by laminin. *Soc. Neurosci. Abstr.* **15**: 164.

NMDA Receptor as a Mediator of Activity-dependent Synaptogenesis in the Developing Brain

M. CONSTANTINE-PATON

Department of Biology, Yale University, New Haven, Connecticut 06511

The synapses that exist in the adult vertebrate brain are the survivors of a rigorous, competitive sorting process that occurs during a discrete period of development and that uses activity patterns in convergent pathways. Numerous experiments have manipulated activity to demonstrate that the refined topographic projections and the segregated stimulus response properties of the mature central nervous system (CNS) are sculpted during development by a process that appears to stabilize converging synapses that cooperate in driving common target cells. That the local circuitry within each brain region may be organized by similar "Hebbian" rules has recently been suggested by a number of computational models of neural self-organization. Thus, activity, long relegated to the role of functional validator of other developmental interactions, is slowly emerging as a prominent structuring parameter in the complex process of neural circuit differentiation.

Retinotectal Projection as a Model System for Studies of Developmental Restructuring of CNS Synapses

In investigating the role of activity during synaptogenesis, my laboratory uses the projection from the retina to the optic tectal lobes of the developing frog. The retinal ganglion cells are the major input to the optic tectum, and their terminals are readily accessible from embryonic stages. The tectum itself shows many properties, such as topographic and columnar organization, complex reciprocal connections, and locally arborizing axon collaterals, that are usually associated with much more complex cortically organized regions of the CNS. In addition, the retinotectal system of cold-blooded vertebrates uses the same excitatory amino acid (EAA) transmitters/receptor systems (Milson and Mitchell 1977; Langdon and Freeman 1986, 1987; Debski et al. 1987; Fox and Fraser 1987; Schmidt 1990) and shows functional synaptic plasticity similar to that seen in the neocortex and hippocampus of mammals (Udin and Fawcett 1988; Constantine-Paton et al. 1990).

The single most important property of the retinotectal system for our studies, however, is that the dynamics of normal synaptogenesis are better understood in the tectum than in any other structure of the vertebrate brain. Electron microscopy studies of the developing retinotectal neuropil have demonstrated that synapses between the retina and tectum are present from the earliest developmental stages, that they are located on growth-cone-bearing processes, and that they are concentrated on the most distal branches of retinal ganglion cell terminal arbors. Single retinal ganglion cell terminals growing within the tectum of developing *Xenopus* have also been examined over time using vital dye marking, laser confocal microscopy, and image intensification. The studies have documented a previously inferred process of continual sprouting and retraction of the synapse-bearing distal branches in these synaptic arbors (O'Rourke and Fraser 1990). The significance of this dynamic state is that, in the developing tectum, the organization of the retinotectal terminal field is a function of the relative lifetimes of synapses at particular locales. Ganglion cell synaptic lifetimes are long if converging synapses arise from neurons that are retinal neighbors and short if nonneighboring cells coinnervate a common target. This differential distribution of synaptic lifetimes maintains the coherence, or retinotopy, of the retinotectal projection in the face of disparately expanding retinal and tectal neuron populations.

It now seems clear that the differential distribution of synapse lifetime is a developmental translation of the Hebbian rule: High temporal correlations in activity patterns of ganglion cells are associated with their close spatial proximity within the retina (Arnett 1978; Arnett and Spraker 1981; Mastronarde 1983a,b) and result in increased synaptic lifetimes when their synapses converge on a common target. Stabilization of synapses from retinal neighbors becomes disrupted in all experimental manipulations that mask (Stryker and Strictland 1984; Schmidt and Eisele 1985; Cook and Rankin 1986) or eliminate these correlations in activity (Meyer 1982, 1983; Schmidt and Edwards 1983; Boss and Schmidt 1984; Stryker and Harris 1986). The dynamic properties of the retinotectal map require that the activity-dependent processes that stabilize synapses from retinal neighbors must be continually active throughout the long period of retinotectal growth. Thus, any manipulation that selectively disrupts these activity-dependent processes should produce a progressive disordering of nearest-neighbor relations among ganglion cell synapses and a progressive degradation of topography.

We have used a slow release plastic to treat continuously the developing frog (*Rana pipiens*) with low concentrations ($\sim 10^{-6}$ to 10^{-7} M) of agonists specific to the *N*-methyl-D-aspartate (NMDA) subtype of glutamate receptor. The continuous presence of these drugs has a disruptive effect on both the overall topography of the retinotectal projection and the relative ordering of single retinal terminals without damaging ganglion cells or tectal neurons and without slowing the growth of the projection as a whole (Cline and Constantine-Paton 1989). It therefore appears that NMDA receptor function is critical to the stabilization of synapses from coinnervating retinal neighbors. Here, we briefly review the salient features of our work. We also present a specific but generalizable model that links the dynamic properties of process extension and withdrawal within synaptic arbors to synaptic convergence, synapse stabilization, and the establishment of topographic order within the developing CNS.

EAA Transmission between the Retina and the Tectum

Several different laboratories have now demonstrated that the general glutamate or aspartate receptor blocker, kynurenic acid, will reversibly eliminate the postsynaptic component of the field potential generated in the retinotectal neuropil as a result of electrical stimulation of the optic nerve (Langdon and Freeman 1986; Debski et al. 1987). Quantitative autoradiographic receptor-binding studies, in both the goldfish and the frog, indicate the presence of the NMDA and at least one non-NMDA, quisqualate-sensitive receptor subtype (McDonald et al. 1989). The presence of an NMDA receptor in developing tectal neurons has recently been verified in whole-cell voltage clamp recordings from tadpole brain slices that allow diencephalic stimulation of the optic tract and bath application of EAA agonists and antagonists (Hickmott and Constantine-Paton 1990). The current/voltage curves taken from the late phase of the excitatory postsynaptic current (EPSC) of many of these cells show the negative slope conductance (Fig. 1b) characteristic of the mammalian NMDA receptor and the amphibian NMDA receptor studied previously in dissociated spinal cord cultures (Mayer and Westbrook 1987). This late phase of the EPSC is eliminated reversibly by low concentrations of the NMDA receptor antagonist D,L-2-amino-5-phosphonovaleric acid (APV) (Fig. 1a). An important point in these traces is that APV does not markedly decrement the amplitude of this postsynaptic current. In fact, in the particular cell shown, agonist application was actually associated with an increased excitability and a "spike-like" fast inward current. Failure of low levels of APV to decrease retinotectal synaptic transmission has also been observed in extracellular analyses of the effects of this antagonist on the postsynaptic components of the optic-nerve-evoked field potential in the tectum (Debski and Constantine-Paton 1988; Schmidt 1990) and in analyses of APV effects

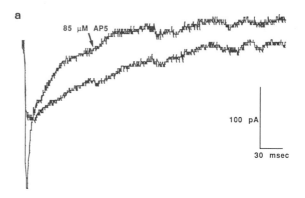

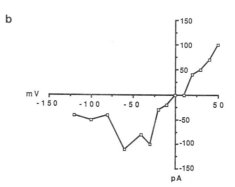

Figure 1. Examples of data on NMDA-receptor-mediated responses obtained from whole-cell voltage clamp of tectal neurons in the slice preparation. (*a*) Effect of APV (AP5) in a spiking cell. What we are calling spikes are large, very rapid inward currents that frequently appear at the peak of the EPSC at holding potentials more negative than −40 mV and are probably due to activation of the standard voltage-gated Na current. This cell had a resting potential of −58 mV. Recordings were made at a holding potential of −40 mV. In response to optic tract stimulation, the EPSC showed a short latency and a sustained component. Bath application of 85 μM APV in normal Mg^{++} saline (3 mM) for 20 min (reversible with 30 min of wash) caused a block of the late, sustained component of the EPSC; however, in this cell, APV actually caused a spike at the peak of the EPSC. Each record is the digital average of five individual traces in response to maximal electrical stimulation in the optic tract. (*b*) An example of an I/V plot of the long-latency (150 msec) NMDA-dependent current in normal Mg^{++} saline (3.0 mM). The plot shows a distinct region of negative slope conductance, corresponding to voltage-dependent block of the NMDA channel by Mg^{++}, as has been seen in other systems. Reducing Mg^{++} from 3 mM to 0.5 mM abolishes this region, yielding a fairly linear plot (data not shown). The curve also has a reversal potential of around 0 mV, as would be expected for the NMDA current.

on retinotectal synaptic transmission as assayed from the ipsilateral retinotectal projection relayed through the nucleus isthmus (Scherer and Udin 1989; S.B. Udin and M. Constantine-Paton in prep.). This situation in the frog tectum contrasts with that in the postnatal cat, where a significant proportion of the visual drive to cortical neurons is blocked by APV, which makes it difficult to dissociate the effects of blocking postsynaptic cell activation from the effects of selectively interfering with NMDA receptor activation (Kleinschmidt et al. 1987; Miller et al. 1989; Bear et al. 1990).

Induced Tectal Ocular Dominance Columns as an Assay for Selective Synapse Stabilization

The doubly innervated tectum of three-eyed frogs is a preparation that has been uniquely important to our studies of NMDA receptor involvement in synaptogenesis because it provides a macrocellular assay for a functional synapse stabilization mechanism. Tecta innervated from the earliest developmental stages by two retinas are produced by adding a supernumerary eye primordium to the forebrain region of neural tube stage embryos. As the animals grow, retinal terminals from retinotopically equivalent regions of a host and the supernumerary eye must compete for synaptic space within the developing tectal neuropil. In this situation, the result of the selective stabilization of synapses from retinal neighbors is an active segregation of the synaptic fields of the two retinas into interdigitating "striped" ocular dominance zones (Constantine-Paton and Law 1978; Law and Constantine-Paton 1981), and any manipulation that selectively disrupts the stabilization mechanism should be manifest as a gradual desegregation of the stripes. We have used the stripe desegregation assay to show that the continuous presence of APV (Fig. 2), as well as the continuous presence of NMDA plus the active NMDA channel blocker MK801, will disrupt synapse stabilization. Both of these treatments will also produce a significant decrement in the resolution of the retinotopic map in normal tecta as assayed by a marked increase in the retinal area occupied by retinal ganglion cell bodies backfilled from a single locus in the tectal lobe. The biologically inactive L-isomer of APV or the independent application of NMDA or MK801 (Fig. 3) fails to disrupt both retinotopy and the eye-specific terminal segregation characteristic of doubly innervated tectal lobes (Cline and Constantine-Paton 1989, 1990b; Cline et al. 1987).

Double innervation produces more subtle modifications of normal activity patterns and cellular interactions that may also be important to our understanding of the mechanism through which the NMDA receptor mediates selective synapse stabilization. Quantitative light microscopic analyses on three-eyed frogs with one singly innervated and one striped tectum have shown, that, in the absence of any obvious rerouting of retinal ganglion cell (RGC) axons to other brain regions, the RGCs surviving in the supernumerary or host retinas are not significantly different. Thus, tecta innervated by two retinas actually receive input from nearly twice the number of RGCs compared with the normal tectum of the same animal. However, the volume of the doubly innervated tectal lobes increases, on average, by only 33%, indicating a relatively pronounced compression of each of the doubly innervating retinal projections (Constantine-Paton and Ferrari-Eastman 1987). Furthermore, the compression of these projections occurs in the absence of any decrease in the tangential extent of individual RGC terminal arbors (Fig. 4), which implies an increased overlap of retinal terminals and a

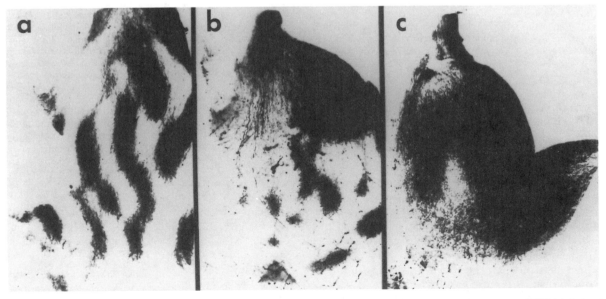

Figure 2. Effect of chronic treatment of striped tectal lobes with the competitive blocker of the NMDA receptor APV. (*a*) Striped tecta treated for 4 weeks with a slab of the slow-release plastic Elvax-P40 show no disruption of the striped segregation pattern between the terminal zones of the doubly innervating retinas. (*b*) Two and one-half weeks of treatment with Elvax-P40 infiltrated with 10^{-4} M APV causes a disruption of the segregation pattern, although signs of retina-specific clumping are still evident. (*c*) Four weeks of treatment with Elvax-P40 infiltrated with 10^{-4} M APV causes a complete desegregation of the terminal zones of the two retinas. In all cases, the retinal projection of the supernumerary eye was labeled by placing a pledglet of horseradish peroxidase (HRP) on the cut supernumary optic nerve at least 24 hours prior to sacrificing the animal and reacting the unsectioned brain to visualize the HRP product. The tectal lobes are subsequently split at their rostral and caudal pole and flattened between two coverslips in order to visualize the termination pattern in one plane. (Reprinted, with permission, from Cline et al. 1987.)

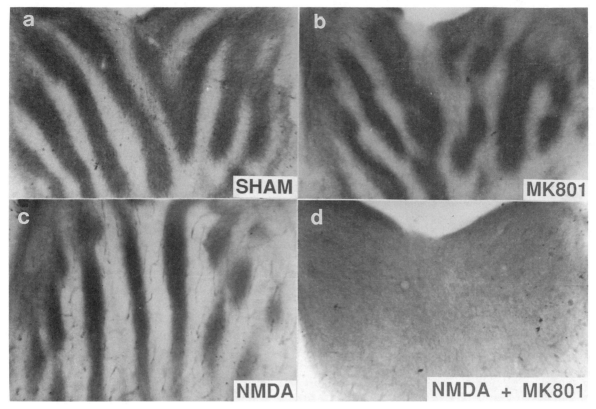

Figure 3. Effect of chronic treatment of striped tectal lobes with MK801, the noncompetitive, open-channel blocker of the NMDA receptor, and with NMDA itself. (*a*) Striped tectum treated with uninfiltrated Elvax-P40. (*b*) Striped tecta treated with Elvax-P40 infiltrated with 10^{-4} M MK801 (a gift from Miles Laboratories) show no sign of desegregation. (*c*) Striped tecta treated with Elvax-P40 infiltrated with 10^{-4} M NMDA show increased segregation, evidenced as a sharpening of stripe boundaries. (*d*) Striped tecta treated with Elvax P-40 infiltrated with both 10^{-4} M MK801 and NMDA show desegregation similar to that seen with APV. The effectiveness of simultaneous treatment with the agonist and noncompetitive antagonist suggests that, in the normal operating tectum, the NMDA channel is not open for periods of time sufficient to obtain effective open-channel blocking. Simultaneous treatment with the agonist would increase the amount of time tectal NMDA channels are in the open configuration and makes them more vulnerable to MK801 blockade. All treatments are for 4 weeks. Processing as in Fig. 2. (Data from Cline et al. 1987; Cline and Constantine-Paton 1990b.)

larger retinal area represented by converging synapses even within the stripes of each eye. An important implication of this situation for activity-dependent synapse stabilization arises because the degree of activity correlation among RGCs is directly related to their retinal proximity. Thus, both correlated activity per unit volume of neuropil and the amount of NMDA receptor activation should be considerably decreased in striped tecta as compared with normal tecta. Stripe boundaries are regions of poor activity correlation because nonneighboring terminals from the two different retinas must interact. Furthermore, even within each stripe, synapses from more distant and less synchronized retinal locales are situated closer together than in the normal animal.

Several morphological differences between doubly and singly innervated tectal lobes may actually result from these decreases in correlated activity. For example, the ratio of synapse number in the retinotectal neuropil to innervating ganglion cells is markedly reduced in striped as compared with normal tecta (Constantine-Paton and Norden 1986; J.J. Norden and M.

Constantine-Paton, in prep.). This could reflect decreased numbers of stabilized synapses per ganglion cell as a result of less effective driving of NMDA receptors. In addition, we have found that the number of branches within individual RGC arbors is significantly increased in striped as compared with normal tecta (Fig. 4). This initially unexpected association of increased branch initiation with a situation in which decreased NMDA receptor activation is expected has contributed to our current working hypothesis linking specific structural changes in RGC terminals to activation of this receptor system (Cline and Constantine-Paton 1990b).

Effects of Chronic NMDA Treatment

Studies with antagonists of the NMDA receptor have also included a series of animals in which tecta were treated chronically with low concentrations of NMDA itself. On the basis of cell counts in both the retina and the tectum, experiments with a wide range of NMDA doses and analyses of the morphology of single RGC

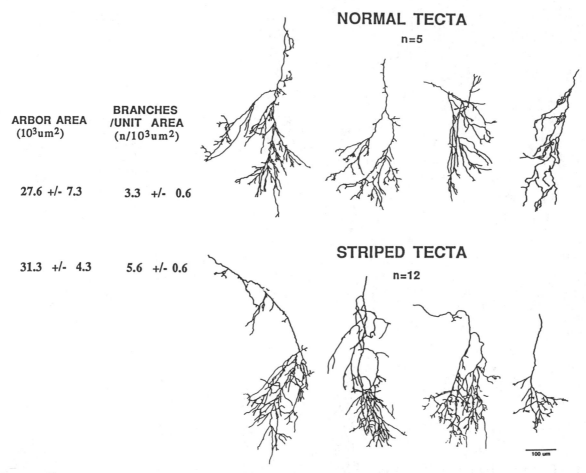

NORMAL TECTA
n=5

ARBOR AREA (10^3um^2)	BRANCHES /UNIT AREA (n/10^3um^2)
27.6 +/- 7.3	3.3 +/- 0.6
31.3 +/- 4.3	5.6 +/- 0.6

STRIPED TECTA
n=12

100 um

Figure 4. Comparison of RGC terminal arbor morphology observed in flattened tecta after HRP-labeling individual terminals in normal tadpole lobes and in doubly innervated striped lobes. The range of terminal arbor sizes observed in the middle laminae of the retinotectal synaptic zone are illustrated on the right-hand side of the figure for both the doubly innervated and normal lobes. The morphometric data for both types of lobes are shown on the left-hand side of the figure. Although the tangential areas covered by the terminals in both types of tecta are the same, the number of terminal branches in doubly innervated lobes is significantly increased over normal. (Data from Cline and Constantine-Paton 1989, 1990b.)

terminals, we are fairly confident that toxic effects of NMDA are absent from our material. Nevertheless, in all striped tecta treated chronically with the agonist, segregation of the two retinal terminal zones is consistently and significantly increased (Fig. 3c). Moreover, on the level of single RGC terminals, the tangential extent of the arbors remained constant, but the number of fine terminal branches was markedly reduced, resulting in a significant decrease in arborization density (Cline and Constantine-Paton 1990b). These observations were initially perplexing. Comparable analyses on normal tecta showed no significant effect on either arbor area or density with chronic NMDA or APV treatments (Cline and Constantine-Paton 1989). Furthermore, chronic APV treatment of doubly innervated tecta sufficient to produce complete desegregation of the striped innervation zone showed some decreases in the branch density of individual RGC terminal arbors, but these decreases were far less pronounced than those produced by treatment with NMDA for comparable periods of time (Fig. 5) (Cline and Constantine-Paton 1990b).

The piece of information that has most helped us to clarify this puzzling set of data and generate some testable predictions as to how NMDA receptor function is associated with RGC synaptic terminal morphology came from physiological, rather than anatomical, assays of the effects of NMDA treatment. These studies used the field potential evoked by electrical stimulation of the optic nerve in a tadpole tectal preparation where the vasculature is cannulated through the heart. This allowed ion substitution studies, which dissected presynaptic versus postsynaptic components of the response (Debski and Constantine-Paton 1990) and delivered reproducible amounts of low concentrations of drugs. With this preparation, we generated dose-response curves of the tectal neuron population response to NMDA and APV. In normal tadpole tecta, concentrations of APV specific for the NMDA receptor subtype (< 100 μM) fail to decrement and actually produce a slight increase in the postsynaptic components of tectal field potential. Low, fully reversible concentrations of NMDA (2–20 μM) increase spontaneous activity but actually decrease the same post-

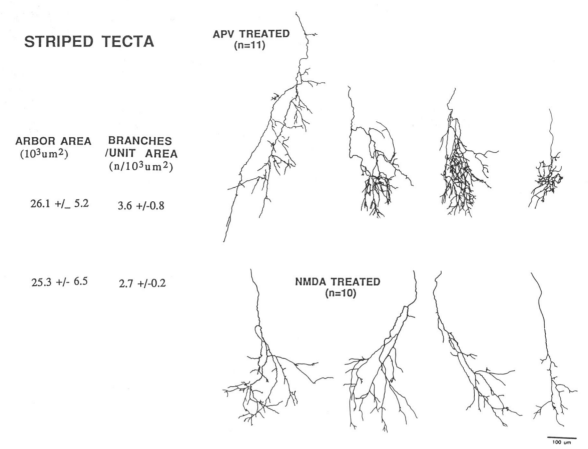

STRIPED TECTA

APV TREATED
(n=11)

ARBOR AREA (10^3 um^2)	BRANCHES /UNIT AREA (n/10^3um^2)
26.1 +/_ 5.2	3.6 +/-0.8
25.3 +/- 6.5	2.7 +/-0.2

NMDA TREATED
(n=10)

100 um

Figure 5. Comparison of RGC terminal morphology after HRP-labeling individual terminals in doubly innervated tectal lobes treated either with 10^{-4} M APV in Elvax or 10^{-4} M NMDA in Elvax. Neither treatment significantly effects the tangential extent of the arbors. However, compared with terminals in untreated doubly innervated tecta (see Fig. 4), NMDA has a much more pronounced effect in reducing branch number than does APV. Format and processing as in Fig. 4. (Data from Cline and Constantine-Paton 1990b.)

synaptic components (Debski and Constantine-Paton 1988; E.A. Debski et al., in prep.). The reasons for this dose-dependent decrement are complex. Postexcitatory depression of cells driven strongly by the increased spontaneous activity probably plays a role. However, excitation of NMDA receptor bearing inhibitory interneurons would also be consistent with the extremely low effective doses and with the increased response amplitude observed with APV. Regardless of the precise circuitry that may produce these tectal population responses, their important attribute is that they are extremely stable, and thus dose responses are reproducible throughout the course of an experiment and from animal to animal. Thus, using the NMDA dose-response curves of normal tecta as references, we explored the sensitivity of the postsynaptic components of the evoked response in tecta treated chronically with either APV or NMDA. Chronic APV treatment produced a small increase in the NMDA sensitivity of one of these components and no change in another. When summed together, the effect of chronic APV treatment on the NMDA dose-response curve is barely discernible (see Fig. 6b). However, chronic treatment with NMDA produced a pronounced and highly significant

upward shift in both postsynaptic components of this response, indicating a marked decrease in the physiological effectiveness of tectal NMDA receptors as a result of chronic exposure to low doses of the drug (Fig. 6a) (Debski et al. 1989). This decrease is significantly different in two respects from the simple desensitization in response to an agonist seen for many other receptor systems. First, the decreased effectiveness is stable over time. It remains unchanged throughout the course of the recording sessions regardless of the many saline washes and control responses to which the neurons are exposed during this period. Second, the decrease does not appear to arise from a decrease in the number of NMDA receptors expressed in the retinotectal neuropil. Quantitative autoradiographic receptor-binding studies on the chronically treated neuropil have failed to reveal any significant differences between normal and either APV- or NMDA-treated tectal lobes (E.A. Debski et al., in prep.).

Instead, we have suggested that these changes may reflect a normal, highly adaptive feedback response of the developing nervous system to increased driving of NMDA receptors. Too much NMDA receptor activation could produce the well-characterized Ca^{++}-

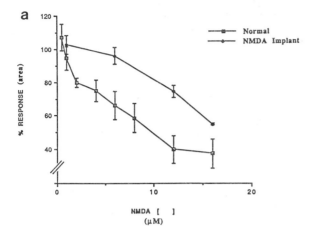

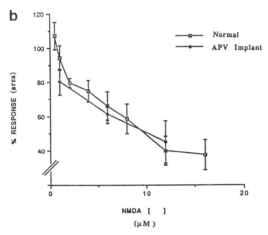

Figure 6. Effect of acute application of NMDA on the post-synaptic components recorded in the tectum following optic nerve stimulation of normal animals and animals whose tecta have been chronically treated with either NMDA or APV. The area under the curve of the postsynaptic components for each drug concentration examined was measured before (control), while the drug was pumped through the cannulated tadpole brain preparation (experimental), and then 15 or 30 min after the preparation had been returned to normal saline solution (wash). Percentage of response is calculated as the area under the curve during drug treatment, divided by the average of the control and wash responses × 100. Control, experimental, and wash responses are each the average of ten evoked potentials. (*a*) In normal animals (□), low concentrations of NMDA produce a pronounced decrease in the postsynaptic components of the optic-nerve-evoked response. Acute application of NMDA also decreases the postsynaptic components of tecta chronically treated for 4–6 weeks with 10^{-4} M NMDA in Elvax (◆). However, in these chronically treated tectal lobes, a significantly higher concentration of NMDA must be applied to produce the same decrease in the postsynaptic components. (*b*) The response of tecta treated chronically with 10^{-4} M APV in Elvax is not different from that of normal animals. Each point represents an average of at least three different measurements from at least three different preparations. (Data from E.A. Debski et al., in prep.)

mediated neurotoxicity of this agonist (Choi and Rothman 1990). However, if the proposed functional link between NMDA receptor activation and synapse stabilization is correct, then too little receptor activation would not allow young synapses invading a zone of

relatively poorly correlated activity to become stabilized. The shifting and sorting of synaptic contacts necessary to optimize convergence and produce functionally effective inputs could not occur.

In short, we think that by chronically treating tecta with NMDA, we have triggered a down-regulation of NMDA receptor effectiveness that may be the normal response of the developing nervous system to increased refinement of projections and increased convergence of synapses whose activity is highly correlated in time. Increased segregation of ocular dominance columns and the marked changes in RGC terminal morphology following chronic NMDA treatment of striped tectal lobes are fully consistent with a down-regulation of NMDA receptor effectiveness that somehow buffers all the effects of Ca^{++} influx through the channel. The three specific postulates of our model linking modulation of RGC terminal arbor growth and synapse stabilization to NMDA receptor activation are given below, followed by a relatively detailed explanation of our data in terms of these postulates.

A Model for NMDA Receptor Function in Synapse Stabilization

The central tenet of the NMDA receptor hypothesis for synapse stabilization is that the onset of a barrage of correlated activity will depolarize the membrane through non-NMDA receptors, removing the Mg^{++} block on the channel. This allows the release of glutamate by subsequent action potentials to permit Ca^{++} influx through the NMDA channel. It is this Ca^{++} influx that initiates a series of events that ultimately feedback on the effective inputs and stabilize them selectively (Cline et al. 1987; Kleinschmidt et al. 1987). This is essentially the same role that Wigstrom and Gustafsson (1985) proposed for NMDA receptors in initiating hippocampal long-term potentiation. Three extensions of this hypothesis pertain to developing visual projections. (1) Local circuitry in the retina gives rise to the activity correlations among retinal neighbors. These correlations will fall off with increasing retinal separation and are used by retinal synapses in the tectum to drive NMDA receptors (Arnett 1978; Arnett and Spraker 1981; Mastronarde 1983a,b). (2) NMDA receptor activation increases the lifetimes of the synapses producing the activation and, indirectly, of the synaptic arbor branches containing those synapses. Thus, the factor determining the lifetime of each new terminal branch within the synaptic arbor of a visual afferent should be the amount of NMDA receptor activation it can participate in within a newly invaded region of neuropil. The positions of newly generated synaptic arbor branches may be random, but their lifetimes will be determined by the number of coactive converging synaptic neighbors they encounter in each region. Stable positions are very likely to be the ones shared by ganglion cells who are retinal neighbors. (3) Low levels of NMDA receptor activation are causally related to a high probability that new branches will be initiated from adjacent, "ineffective" regions of synaptic terminal arbors. This postulate need not imply a direct effect of NMDA receptor activation. Nevertheless, in a situation where neurites are known to be continuously sprouting, a means of both up- and down-regulating motility based on correlated activity would increase the efficiency of the activity-dependent tuning process. In the retinotectal system, this would greatly facilitate the movement of arbors away from regions of poorly correlated activity.

The operation of these NMDA-receptor-mediated effects in sculpting RGC terminal arbor position and thereby establishing and maintaining the coherence of the retinotopic map during normal retinotectal development is diagramed in Figure 7. These postulates are also consistent with the structural differences between normal and striped tecta. Postulate 1 relates the lower NMDA receptor activation expected in striped as compared with normal tecta to the lower correlated activity per unit volume of neuropil expected in those

lobes. Postulate 2 may be reflected in the smaller number of synapses per ganglion cell in doubly versus singly innervated tecta (Constantine-Paton and Norden 1986; J.J. Norden and M. Constantine-Paton, in prep.). Postulate 3 would account for the increased number of terminal branches revealed by our light microscope analyses of RGC arbors in doubly innervated versus singly innervated tecta (Cline and Constantine-Paton 1990b).

The effects of chronic drug treatment on retinal termination pattern and terminal morphology are also consistent with these postulates. APV treatment disrupts retinotopy and eye-specific segregation because it blocks the selective stabilization of RGC synapses and terminal branches that are coactive with converging synapses from retinal neighbors (Postulates 1 and 2). At the individual RGC level in normal tecta, this does not significantly alter arbor area or branch number because the lifetimes of short terminal branches are decreased (Postulate 2) at the same time that many

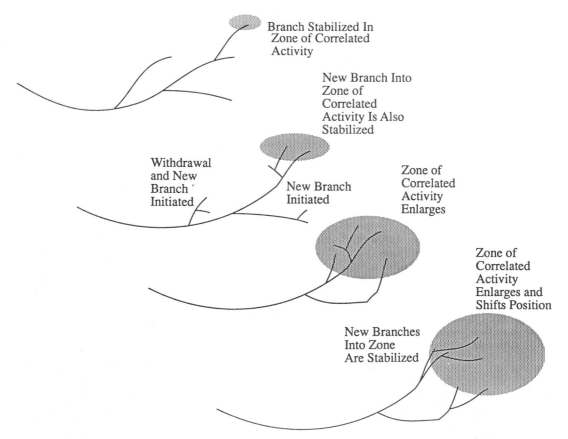

Figure 7. RGC axon terminals shift their position within the tectum on the basis of where their branches colocalize with branches from retinal neighbors that carry correlated activity. The relationship between synapse and RGC process stabilization in regions of correlated activity (stippled ellipses) and sprouting or withdrawal of branches in regions of poorly correlated activity is shown schematically for one terminal at several increasingly later times within a normal tectal lobe. The size of the region of correlated activity here is assumed to become larger over time as the trial and error sorting process proceeds to make the topographic map more coherent. The zone of correlated activity is shown to shift over time to illustrate the caudalward shift of the retinotectal projection as a result of poorly correlated new ganglion cell terminals arriving in rostral tectum (to the right in the diagram). Notice that the three rules postulated for the effects of NMDA receptor activation on RGC branch behavior (e.g., stabilization in regions of correlated activity, sprouting, or withdrawal in regions of poorly correlated activity; see text for details) will determine not only the structure of the terminal, but also where its dense arborizations are positioned relative to other retinal inputs carrying activity patterns that are either well or poorly correlated in time with the pictured terminal.

new branches are initiated to replace them (Postulate 3). In striped tecta where correlations in activity and NMDA receptor activation are lower to begin with (Postulate 3), we suggest that the effect of APV on decreasing lifetime of terminal branches outweighs its effects in increasing new branch initiation. The older regions, constituting the proximal branches of the arbor, will always have more highly correlated neighbors because, compared with the new distal branches, they have had more time to collect these neighbors by trial and error. Thus, RGC arbors in APV-treated striped tecta, as compared with untreated striped tecta, show a small but significant decrease in terminal branches. This is because many of the distal arbor branches are lost, whereas residual, unblocked NMDA receptors and the higher correlations in activity in more proximal arbor regions prevent new branch initiation at a rate sufficient to replace them (Cline and Constantine-Paton 1990b).

The situation is more complicated in tecta treated chronically with NMDA. The continuous presence of low levels of NMDA should mean that even brief synaptic events, as long as they are sufficient to remove the Mg^{++} block on the NMDA channel (Mayer et al. 1984), will be able to activate the channel. However, in these same tecta, the "effectiveness" of the NMDA receptors is reduced (E.A. Debski et al., in prep.). We suggest that this decreased, physiologically measured effectiveness also decreases the ability of NMDA receptors to exert their effects on branch survival and branch initiation. In chronically treated normal tecta, these two opposite effects cancel out, resulting in no change in either topography or the tangential extent and branch number of individual RGC arbors. In striped tecta, however, decreases in NMDA receptor effectiveness, superimposed on an already decreased level of correlated activity, should place all regions of RGC arbors with normally low probabilities of encountering correlated activity in jeopardy of being pruned. Thus, stripe borders are sharpened by RGC branch withdrawal, and on the individual arbor level, the youngest (most distal) terminal arbor branches should be eliminated. The continuous presence of NMDA would make little difference to the survival of these branches because the degree of correlated activity in the newly invaded neuropil regions would be insufficient to remove the Mg^{++} block of the channel. However, the continuous presence of the agonist should make a difference in the more proximal regions of the arbor where the terminal has existed for a period sufficient to "collect" well-correlated neighbors. In this region, the effect of every instance of correlated convergent release of an excitatory transmitter should be prolonged, thereby stabilizing these regions of the arbor (Postulate 2) and decreasing the probability (Postulate 3) that new branches will be initiated to replace the ones that are withdrawn. The result is the extremely sparse RGC arbors we observe in striped tecta chronically treated with NMDA.

Clearly, this three-part model is largely generated post hoc from the data briefly presented above. It should also be clear that it is largely incomplete. For example, we cannot specify whether all the important NMDA receptors are located postsynaptically or whether any other transmitter systems play a significant role in the stabilization or branch initiation process. We have also avoided any mention of the possible responses of postsynaptic dendrites, although we know from studies of dendritic morphology relative to stripe boundaries that many dendritic branches fail to cross stripe boundaries (Katz and Constantine-Paton 1988). Nevertheless, these ideas have generated several specific predictions about lifetimes of retinotectal contacts and retinal axon responsiveness to active NMDA receptors that we are now prepared to test in tissue culture. They have also generated predictions about changes in NMDA receptor effectiveness under chronic treatment and in striped tecta that it should be possible to test at the single-cell level using whole-cell voltage clamping in the tectal slice. Furthermore, at least one of the assumptions made in our interpretation of the original data, that the majority of synapses that survive in striped tecta treated chronically with NMDA should be especially stable, seems to be borne out in very recent electron microscopy analyses of chronically treated neuropil. As hoped, we found no evidence of NMDA toxicity in this tissue, but we also noted a significant increase (46%) over normal tecta (27%) in the number of synaptic profiles showing multiple presynaptic terminals converging on a single postsynaptic site (Yen and Constantine-Paton 1990). Increased clustering of converging synapses is the likely morphological correlate of synapses that are very well stabilized. As a result of having longer lifetimes, these synapses should be able to collect larger numbers of well-correlated neighbors. The synapses in NMDA-treated striped tecta also show a marked increase in the size of the synaptic densities when compared with those of untreated tecta (Fig. 8). These observations raise the possibility that the amount of synaptic convergence and the size of the synaptic densities are morphological indicators of synapse stability.

CONCLUSION

An assumption implicit in our concentration of effort on the primary visual projection of the frog is that the understanding of synapse stabilization and NMDA receptor function derived from this relatively simple visual projection will generalize to the less accessible central projections of other vertebrates. Our work and that of other CNS developmental neurobiologists have increasingly demonstrated similarities rather than differences between warm- and cold-blooded vertebrate visual development and plasticity. Thus, early retinal projections in chicks (Nakamura and O'Leary 1989) and rats (Simon and O'Leary 1990) now appear to undergo a period of rigorous synaptic plasticity that is similar in principle if not in overall geometry to the well-established shift of projections in fish (Steurmer and Easter

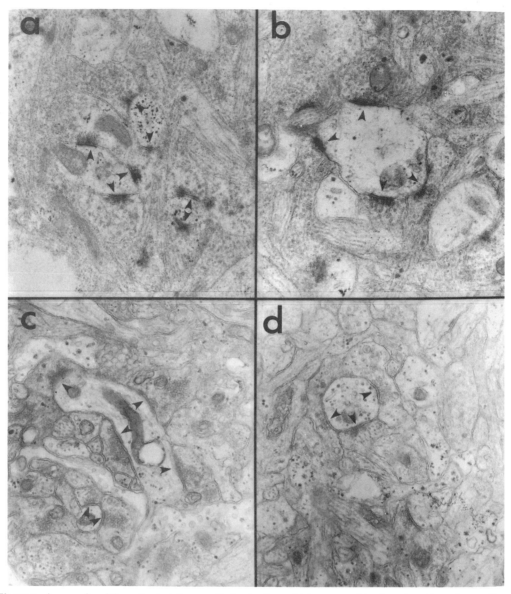

Figure 8. Electron micrographs of the retinotectal neuropil of striped tectal lobes treated for 4 weeks with 10^{-4} M NMDA in Elvax (*a*, *b*) and untreated striped tectal lobes (*c*, *d*). The treatment with low doses of NMDA ($\sim 10^{-7}$ M per day) has no obvious degenerative effect on the neuropil. However, the postsynaptic thickenings in the tecta treated with NMDA are much more pronounced than those in the comparably stained untreated tectal neuropil. In addition, stereological counting of synapses in over 4500 μm^2 of the untreated tectal lobe and a similar area in the NMDA-treated tectal lobe revealed no difference in overall synapse density. Nevertheless, more synapses (46%) in the NMDA-treated tectal neuropil were in arrays where two or more presynaptic terminals converged on a single postsynaptic profile when compared with the untreated tectal lobe (27%).

1984) and frogs (Gaze et al. 1979; Reh and Constantine-Paton 1984). Binocular convergence appears to have a critical period in *Xenopus* (Keating and Feldman 1975) quite similar to the analogous critical periods in cats and monkeys. Eye-specific segregation is similar in both form and mechanism across the vertebrate phyla, and most recently, the NMDA receptor has been implicated in the activity-dependent synaptic competition that establishes retinotopy, afferent segregation, and afferent convergence in fish, frogs, ferrets, and cats (Constantine-Paton et al. 1990).

In goldfish, high NMDA sensitivity is found during

the final stages of optic nerve regeneration, when activity patterns in the retina are critical to refinement of the retinotopic map. During this period, a form of enhanced synaptic efficacy can be induced by frequent stimulation of the optic nerve. Both the enhanced synaptic efficacy and the retinotopic refinement can be blocked with APV at concentrations that do not appear to block retinotectal transmission (Schmidt 1990). In *Xenopus laevis*, APV treatment of a developing tectal lobe blocks the indirect cholinergic retinal projection from converging on the locus of the tectum carrying similar activity patterns from the same region of visual space through the direct retinal projection of the contralateral eye (Scherer and Udin 1989). In developing ferrets, chronic treatment with APV will block the normal segregation of on-center and off-center visual responses to different sublaminae that normally occur in the lateral genticulate nucleus (Hahm et al. 1990). Thus, the results in all three of these other vertebrate systems are highly consistent with our own observations and ideas.

In attempting to generalize the effects of NMDA receptor function to nontectal systems, it is important to recognize that our understanding of the cytoplasmic cascades tied to the active NMDA receptor in the tectum is in its infancy (Cline and Constantine-Paton 1990a). The immediate events triggered by active NMDA receptors in the visual system become particularly important when attempting to extend the tectal data to NMDA-related visual plasticity in the neocortex. The fact that APV can block interocular segregation, a structural reflection of binocular competition in the tectum, without blocking retinotectal synaptic transmission, is strong evidence that the active NMDA receptor can function developmentally as a selective detector of correlated activity. Nevertheless, a significant controversy still surrounds NMDA receptor function in mediating binocular competition and stimulus selectivity within the developing cortex. APV treatment of the developing cortex blocks the monocular takeover of cortical neurons by the nondeprived eye in the monocular deprivation paradigm. The treatment also blocks the development of stimulus selectivity and the responsiveness of many cortical neurons to any retinal input (Kleinschmidt et al. 1987; Bear et al. 1990). Thus, it has been argued (Miller et al. 1989) that the NMDA receptor may be merely functioning as another excitatory receptor in this cortex and that APV is exerting its effects by blocking activation, not by blocking the specific detection and reinforcement of inputs that are coactive with their postsynaptic target. Dominant roles for the NMDA receptor as an excitatory transmitter in the mammalian cortex and as a selective detector of correlated activity in that same structure are not mutually exclusive, but until the cytoplasmic changes associated with NMDA receptor activation and synapse stabilization are known, there will be no way of rigorously testing this possibility.

One potentially important observation is in danger of being overlooked as a result of this controversy: Namely, the amount of retinal excitation transmitted to neurons in afferent cortical layers via the NMDA channel appears to decrease progressively in the postnatal kitten, whereas NMDA sensitivity of neurons in other cortical layers remains high throughout life (Tsumoto et al. 1987; Fox et al. 1989). Moreover, the decrease in NMDA sensitivity of layer IV parallels the structural segregation of left and right eye ocular dominance columns in this layer. Dark rearing, which delays ocular dominance segregation, also delays the decrease in NMDA sensitivity (Fox et al. 1990). The observations are completely consistent with our suggestions arising

from striped tectal lobes chronically treated with NMDA. Perhaps, both in afferent cortical layers and in the retinotectal terminal field, NMDA receptor function must be tied to Ca^{++} fluxes sufficient to alter cytoskeletal elements and produce large-scale restructuring of connections. In such regions, it would be adaptive to have large amounts of NMDA receptor activation cause a protective down-regulation of NMDA receptor effectiveness. This would simultaneously cause a decreased ability of visual afferents to attain stabilized synapses and maintain processes in zones of relatively poorly correlated activity. Thus, afferent processes are pruned, the ability to shift and sort synaptic position is lost, and the only remaining synapses exist in the well-segregated eye-specific zones, where correlated activity is high. If this idea is correct, there are several interesting correlates. First, the unknown biochemical processes that decrease the effectiveness of NMDA receptors in afferent zones with increased use will also be extremely important in the regulation of structural synaptic plasticity. Second, cytoplasmic events linked to the active NMDA receptor in afferent zones may be quite different from the events linked to NMDA receptor function in local circuits that must show changes in synaptic effectiveness throughout life. In short, an understanding of the cytoplasmic cascades specifically associated with the numerous different instances of NMDA receptor function and plasticity is badly needed. The significance of these data would extend far beyond an understanding of developmental synapse stabilization. They might tell us, for example, how to reintroduce developmental synaptic plasticity to the damaged adult brain. They might also tie the developmental functions of the NMDA receptor into a comprehensive understanding of the receptor's role in cognitive functions such as learning and memory.

ACKNOWLEDGMENT

Work in M. Constantine-Paton's laboratory was supported by National Institutes of Health grant RO1-EY06039.

REFERENCES

Arnett, D.W. 1978. Statistical dependence between neighboring retinal ganglion cells in goldfish. *Exp. Brain Res.* **32:** 49.

Arnett, D.W. and T.E. Spraker 1981. Cross-correlation analysis of the maintained discharge of rabbit retinal ganglion cells. *J. Physiol.* **317:** 29.

Bear, M., A., Kleinschmidt, Q. Gu, and W. Singer. 1990. Disruption of experience-dependent modifications in striate cortex by infusion of an NMDA receptor antagonist. *J. Neurosci.* **10:** 909.

Boss, V.C. and J.T. Schmidt. 1984. Activity and the formation of ocular dominance patches in dually innervated tectum of goldfish. *J. Neurosci.* **4:** 2891.

Choi, D.W. and S.M. Rothman. 1990. The role of glutamate neurotoxicity in hypocicischemic neuronal death. *Annu. Rev. Neurosci.* **13:** 171.

Cline, H.T. and M. Constantine-Paton. 1989. NMDA receptor antagonists disrupt the retinotectal topographic map. *Neuron* **3:** 413.

———. 1990a. The differential influence of protein kinase inhibitors on retinal arbor morphology and eye-specific stripes in the frog retinotectal system. *Neuron* (in press).

———. 1990b. NMDA receptor agonist and antagonists alter RGC terminal morphology in the frog retinotectal projection. *J. Neurosci.* **10:** 1197.

Cline, H.T., E. Debski, and M. Constantine-Paton. 1987. NMDA receptor antagonist desegregates eye specific strips. *Proc. Natl. Acad. Sci.* **84:** 4342.

Constantine-Paton, M. and P. Ferrari-Eastman. 1987. Pre- and postsynaptic correlates of interocular competition and segregation in the frog. *J. Comp. Neurol.* **225:** 178.

Constantine-Paton, M. and M.I. Law. 1978. Eye-specific termination bands in tecta of three-eyed frogs. *Science* **202:** 639.

Constantine-Paton, M. and J.J. Norden. 1986. Synapse regulation in the developing visual system. In *Development of order in the visual system* (ed. S.R. Hilfer and J.B. Sheffield), p. 1. Springer-Verlag, New York.

Constantine-Paton, M., H.T. Cline, and E.A. Debski. 1990. Patterned activity, synaptic convergence and the NMDA receptor in developing visual pathways. *Annu. Rev. Neurosci.* **13:** 129.

Cook, J.E. and E.C.C. Rankin. 1986. Impaired refinement of the regenerated retinotectal projection of the goldfish in stroboscopic light: A quantitative WGA-HRP study. *Exp. Brain Res.* **63:** 421.

Debski, E.A. and M. Constantine-Paton. 1988. The effects of glutamate receptor agonists and antagonists on the evoked tectal potential in *Rana pipiens*. *Soc. Neurosci. Abstr.* **15:** 495.

———. 1990b. Evoked pre- and post-synaptic activity in the optic tectum of the cannulated tadpole. *J. Comp. Physiol.* (in press).

Debski, E.A., H.T. Cline, and M. Constantine-Paton. 1987. Kynurenic acid blocks retinal-tectal transmission in *Rana pipiens*. *Soc. Neurosci. Abstr.* **14:** 674.

———. 1989. Chronic application of NMDA or AP5 affects the NMDA sensitivity of the evoked tectal response in *Rana pipiens*. *Soc. Neurosci. Abstr.* **14:** 495.

Fox, B.E.S. and S.E. Fraser. 1987. Excitatory amino acids in the retinotectal system of *Xenopus laevis*. *Soc. Neurosci. Abstr.* **13:** 766.

Fox, K., N. Daw, and D. Ezepita. 1990. Dark-rearing kittens delays the developmental decrease in cortical NMDA receptor efficacy. *Soc. Neurosci. Abstr.* **16:** 798.

Fox, K., H. Sato, and N. Daw. 1989. The location and function of NMDA receptors in cat and kitten visual cortex. *J. Neurosci.* **9:** 2443.

Gaze, R.M., M.J. Keating, A. Ostberg, and S.H. Chung. 1979. The relationship between retinal and tectal growth in larval *Xenopus*. Implication for the development of the retinotectal projection. *J. Embryol. Exp. Morphol.* **53:** 103.

Hahm, J.-O., R.B. Langdon, and M. Sur. 1990. NMDA antagonists prevent segregation of retinal afferents in on- and off-sublaminae in ferret lateral geniculate nucleus. *Invest. Opthalmol.* (suppl.) **31:** 395.

Hickmott, P.W. and M. Constantine-Paton. 1990. Physiology and morphology of neurons in *Rana pipiens* tectal slices. *Soc. Neurosci. Abstr.* **16:** 985.

Katz, L.C. and M. Constantine-Paton. 1988. Relationships between segregated afferents and postsynaptic neurons in the optic tectum of three-eyed frogs. *J. Neurosci.* **8:** 3160.

Keating, M.J. and J. Feldman. 1975. Visual deprivation and intertectal neuronal connections in *Xenopus laevis*. *Proc. R. Soc. Lond. B Biol. Sci.* **191:** 467.

Kleinschmidt, A., M.F. Bear, and W. Singer. 1987. Blockade of NMDA receptors disrupts experience-dependent plasticity of kitten striate cortex. *Nature* **238:** 355.

Langdon, R.B. and J.A. Freeman. 1986. Antagonists of glutaminergic neurotransmission block retinotectal transmission in goldfish. *Brain Res.* **398:** 169.

———. 1987. Pharmacology of retinotectal transmission in the goldfish: Effects of nicotinic ligands strychnine and kynurenic acid. *J. Neurosci.* **7:** 760.

Law, M.I. and M. Constantine-Paton. 1981. Anatomy and physiology of experimentally produced striped tecta. *J. Neurosci.* **1:** 741.

Mastronarde, D.N. 1983a. Correlated firing of cat retinal ganglion cells. I. Spontaneously active inputs to X- and Y-cells. *J. Neurophysiol.* **49:** 303.

———. 1983b. Correlated firing of cat retinal ganglion cells. II. Responses of X- and Y-cells to single quantal events. *J. Neurophysiol.* **49:** 325.

Mayer, M.L. and G.L. Westbrook. 1987. The physiology of excitatory amino acids in the vertebrate central nervous system. *Prog. Neurobiol.* **28:** 197.

Mayer, M.L., G.L. Westbrook, and P.B. Gutherie. 1984. Voltage-dependent block by Mg^{++} of NMDA responses in spinal cord neurons. *Nature* **309:** 261.

McDonald, J.W., H.T. Cline, M. Constantine-Paton, W.E. Maragos, M.V. Johnston, and A.B. Young. 1989. Quantitative autoradiographic localization of NMDA, quisqualate and PCP receptors in the frog tectum. *Brain Res.* **482:** 155.

Meyer, R.L. 1982. Tetrodotoxin blocks the formation of ocular dominance columns in goldfish. *Science* **218:** 589.

———. 1983. Tetrodotoxin inhibits the formation of refined retinotopography in goldfish. *Dev. Brain Res.* **6:** 293.

Miller, K.D., B. Chapman, and M.P. Stryker. 1989. Visual responses in adult cat visual cortex depend on N-methyl-D-aspartate receptors. *Proc. Natl. Acad. Sci.* **86:** 5183.

Milson, J.A. and J.F. Mitchell. 1977. Action of amino acids on evoked responses in the frog optic tectum. *Br. J. Pharmacol.* **59:** 484.

Nakamura, H. and D.D.M. O'Leary. 1989. Inaccuracies in initial growth and arborization of chick retinotectal axons followed by course corrections and axon remodeling to develop topographic order. *J. Neurosci.* **9:** 3776.

O'Rourke, N.A. and S.E. Fraser. 1990. Dynamic changes in optic fiber terminal arbors lead to retinotopic map formation: An in vivo confocal microscopic study. *Neuron* **5:** 159.

Reh, T.A. and M. Constantine-Paton. 1984. Retinal ganglion cell terminals change their projection sites during larval development of *Rana pipiens*. *J. Neurosci.* **4:** 442.

Scherer, W.J. and S.B. Udin. 1989. N-methyl-D-aspartate antagonists prevent interaction of binocular maps in *Xenopus* tectum. *J. Neurosci.* **9:** 3837.

Schmidt, J.T. 1990. Long-term potentiation and activity dependent retinotopic sharpening in the regenerating retinotectal projection of goldfish: Common sensitive perios and sensitivity to NMDA blockers. *J. Neurosci.* **10:** 233.

Schmidt, J.T. and D.L. Edwards. 1983. Activity sharpens the map during the regeneration of the retinotectal projection in goldfish. *Brain Res.* **269:** 29.

Schmidt, J.T. and L.E. Eisele. 1985. Stroboscopic illumination and dark rearing block the sharpening of the regenerated retinotectal map in goldfish. *Neuroscience* **14:** 535.

Simon, D.K. and D.D.M. O'Leary. 1990. Limited topographic specificity in the targeting and branching of mammalian retinal axons. *Dev. Biol.* **137:** 125.

Steurmer, C.A.O. and S.S. Easter. 1984. Rules of order in the retinotectal fascicles of goldfish. *J. Neurosci.* **4:** 1045.

Stryker, M.P. and W.A. Harris. 1986. Binocular impulse blockade prevents formation of ocular dominance columns in cat visual cortex. *J. Neurosci.* **6:** 2117.

Stryker, M.P. and S.L. Strictland. 1984. Physiological segregation of ocular dominance columns depends on the pattern of afferent electrical activity. *Invest. Opthalmol.* (suppl.) **25:** 278.

Tsumoto, T., K. Hagihara, H. Sato, and Y. Hata. 1987. NMDA receptors in the visual cortex of young kittens are more effective than those of adult cats. *Nature* **327:** 513.

Udin, S.B. and J.W. Fawcett. 1988. Formation of topographic maps. *Annu. Rev. Neurosci.* **11:** 289.

Wigstrom, H. and B. Gustafsson. 1985. On long-lasting potentiation in the hippocampus: A proposed mechanism for its dependence on coincident pre- and post-synaptic activity. *Acta Physiol. Scand.* **123:** 519.

Yen, L.-H. and M. Constantine-Paton. 1990. EM analysis of NMDA-treated tecta in three-eyed *Rana pipiens*. *Soc. Neurosci. Abstr.* **16:** 1288.

Construction of Modular Circuits in the Mammalian Brain

D. PURVES AND A.-S. LaMANTIA

Department of Neurobiology, Duke University Medical Center, Durham, North Carolina 27710

Neurobiologists have long appreciated that many regions of the mammalian brain are organized into repeating units or modules (Golgi 1874; Lorente de Nó 1949; Hubel et al. 1977; Mountcastle 1978; Szentagothai 1978; Goldman-Rakic 1984; Hubel 1988). The first example of this principle was recognized more than a century ago when C. Golgi (1874) described glomeruli in the olfactory bulb. More recently, various classes of columns and patches have been discovered in the cerebral cortex, the most thoroughly studied of which are orientation columns, ocular dominance columns, and blobs in the primary visual cortex of primates (Hubel 1988). The development of these units, however, is not fully understood. For instance, a simple question that remains unanswered is whether the number of modular circuits increases, decreases, or remains stable during postnatal life. This question bears on issues as diverse as the explanation of critical periods, the response of the nervous system to injury, and the long-term storage of information.

An obvious fact pertinent to the development of modules is that the mammalian brain grows substantially during postnatal life. The brain of the rhesus monkey, for example, doubles in weight between birth and adulthood (Purves and LaMantia 1990), and the weight of the human brain increases about fourfold between birth and the 20th year of life (Copoletta and Wolbach 1932; Pakkenberg and Voigt 1964; Dekaban and Sadowsky 1978). Even the brain of a mouse increases in weight by a factor of about 4 between birth and maturity (Pomeroy et al. 1990). There are at least three ways in which the development of modules could be related to brain growth: (1) The postnatal growth of the brain could reflect the commensurate growth of a fixed complement of modular circuits; (2) the number of these functional units could decrease in concert with other regressive events in neural development (for review, see Purves and Lichtman 1980, 1985; Cowan et al. 1984); and (3) brain growth could reflect the addition of new functional units and their constituent elements.

Here, we report the use of a variety of methods, including in vivo microscopic imaging of the brain, to distinguish between these three possibilities. Our approach has been to monitor the generation of modular circuits in two very different parts of the central nervous system: the rodent olfactory bulb and the monkey visual cortex. The evidence we have obtained favors the last of these three alternatives, namely, that novel circuits continue to be constructed during postnatal life. Finally, we suggest that activity-dependent trophic interactions may provide a basis for the formation of diverse modular circuits.

METHODS

To determine whether there is a net change in the number of modules and their constituent elements in the olfactory system, we first carried out an analysis of glomeruli in the olfactory bulb of developing and adult mice. Glomeruli are spherical regions of superficial neuropil comprising an intense efflorescence of the apical dendrites of mitral cells and their dense innervation by olfactory afferent (and other) axon terminals. We examined the development of this region of the telencephalon by measuring the numbers of glomeruli and their constituent cellular elements with light and electron microscopy. These techniques are described in detail elsewhere (Pomeroy et al. 1990).

In parallel with these in vitro studies, we assessed the postnatal development of modular circuits in the olfactory system of living mice using vital staining and confocal microscopy. Our purpose in this component of the study was to determine whether particular modules persist or whether some of these units are lost during development. Newborn animals were anesthetized and placed on the stage of a scanning confocal microscope adapted for in vivo imaging (LaMantia and Purves 1989). To visualize olfactory glomeruli in situ, one of the bulbs was exposed through a window made in the overlying bone. The diffusion barrier presented by the meninges was transiently breached by brief treatment with hypertonic saline solution, and the glomeruli were stained by topical application of a dilute solution of the styryl dye RH414 to the intact dura (for details, see LaMantia and Purves 1989). The animals were then allowed to recover. After an interval of up to several weeks, a second image of the bulb was made by perfusing mice with aldehyde fixatives and staining the glomeruli with Sudan Black. In this way, we obtained a more permanent record of the glomerular pattern at a particular time after the acquisition of an initial in vivo image. The two images could then be compared quantitatively to determine the degree of change in the number and pattern of modular units.

To assess the development of modules in the cerebral cortex, we examined another class of iterated circuits called blobs. Blobs are cytochrome-oxidase-positive patches that form an orderly array in the primary visual cortex of primates. To visualize these units in histological sections, neonatal or adult rhesus monkeys were sedated with ketamine, deeply anesthetized with barbiturate, and perfused with cold phosphate-buffered saline, followed by a solution of 2.5% paraformaldehyde and 0.5% glutaraldehyde in phosphate buffer. The residual fixative was then rinsed from the tissues by further perfusion with phosphate-buffered saline. The brains were rapidly removed from the skull, weighed, photographed, and divided in the mid-sagittal plane. The blobs were visualized in the left hemisphere using cytochrome oxidase histochemistry (Wong-Riley 1979), and their density was determined. The right hemisphere was sectioned serially to measure the surface area of the striate cortex. These procedures are fully described elsewhere (Purves and LaMantia 1990).

RESULTS

Analysis of Module Development in the Olfactory Bulb

The olfactory bulbs have several features that recommend them for an analysis of the development of brain circuitry. First, they are clearly bounded and compact. Second, the bulbs comprise only four basic cell types and one major source of extrinsic innervation. Third,

and most important, the major processing circuits of the olfactory bulbs, the glomeruli, are quite distinct. Accordingly, one can follow quantitatively the development of these itcrated modules both in histological preparations and in the living animal (Fig. 1).

The questions that we wished to address initially were the following: (1) Does the postnatal growth of this part of the mammalian central nervous system involve the addition of neural circuits and their constituent elements? (2) Is there any evidence that modules like glomeruli are eliminated during development? Our analysis of the numbers of complex circuits, neuronal branches, and synapses as a function of postnatal age in the olfactory bulbs showed that this region of the central nervous system is gradually constructed for at least the first 2–3 months of the mouse's postnatal life (Fig. 2). Thus, between birth and the time mice reach their full adult dimensions at about 12 weeks of age, each bulb increases in size by a factor of 8, the number of glomeruli increases by a factor of 4–5, the length of mitral cell dendritic branches increases by a factor of 11, and the number of glomerular and extraglomerular synapses increases by factors of 90 and 170, respectively (Pomeroy et al. 1990). Each of these parameters increases steadily from birth through sexual maturity and beyond, in concert with the enlargement of the olfactory mucosa and the growth of the brain and the entire animal. On the basis of these histological and ultrastructural measures, the developmental strategy for establishing the neural circuitry of this part of the mouse brain appears to be one of ongoing construction.

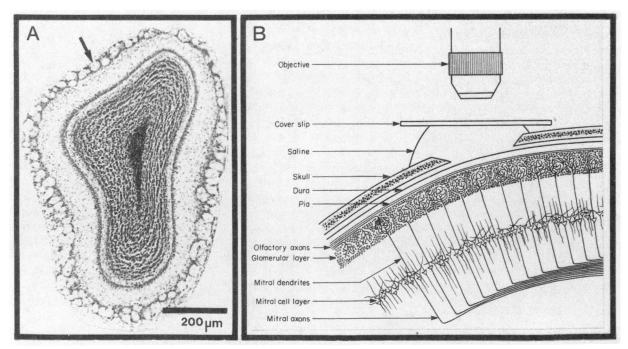

Figure 1. Olfactory glomeruli in the adult mouse. (*A*) Frontal section (50 μm) through the right olfactory bulb of a young adult mouse after aldehyde fixation and staining with cresyl violet (dorsal surface is up, lateral to the left). The outer layer of the mammalian bulb comprises spherical units of neuropil (glomeruli), the borders of which are defined by a continuous rind of closely packed periglomerular cells. There are about 1800 such modules in each olfactory bulb of an adult mouse (see Fig. 2). (*B*) Diagram of the method of visualizing glomeruli in the living mouse.

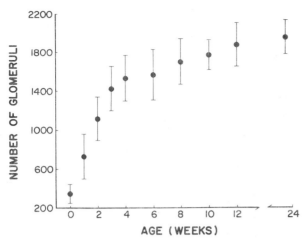

Figure 2. Number of olfactory glomeruli in the developing bulbs of CF1 male mice from birth to 24 weeks of age. Each point represents the mean of counts in ten bulbs from at least five different animals; error bars show the standard deviation. The addition of these modules continues throughout the full period of maturation (male mice are sexually competent at 6–7 weeks of age). (Reprinted, with permission, from Pomeroy et al. 1990.)

These observations in the fixed brain imply that the development of modules involves their progressive addition without elimination of units already formed. This inference, however, can only be validated by observing the same brain repeatedly in a living animal: In vivo imaging enables a direct assessment of whether the initial modules persist and which units (if any) are lost as an animal matures. We therefore examined the pattern of identified glomeruli in the olfactory bulb of individual mice on two separate occasions during postnatal development (LaMantia and Purves 1989).

To monitor the formation of glomeruli, we adapted vital staining and imaging techniques first used in the peripheral nervous system (for review, see Purves and Voyvodic 1987). Visualizing the living brain over time, however, presents special problems. First, glomeruli are located well beneath the brain surface. Second, the meninges must remain intact to preserve the integrity of the brain during the interval between observations. These membranes limit the access of vital dyes to the brain and present a substantial impediment to microscopical imaging. Such difficulties are minimized in the mouse olfactory bulb, where the glomeruli are near the surface of the brain and where the overlying membranes are relatively thin. Histological, ultrastructural, and electrophysiological evaluation of the integrity of bulbs stained and imaged in this way showed no adverse effects of the procedure.

Our results with vital fluorescence staining and confocal microscopy demonstrate that the formation of iterated modules in the brain can indeed be observed directly during postnatal development (Fig. 3). Comparison of images obtained in the same animal after an interval of 1 hour or less revealed identical patterns of glomeruli. After intervals of 1–3 weeks, however, newly formed modules were apparent among the glomeruli initially observed. Moreover, none of the original glomeruli (over 600 in a series of animals) were ever lost, at least over an interval spanning the first several weeks of a mouse's life. We have therefore

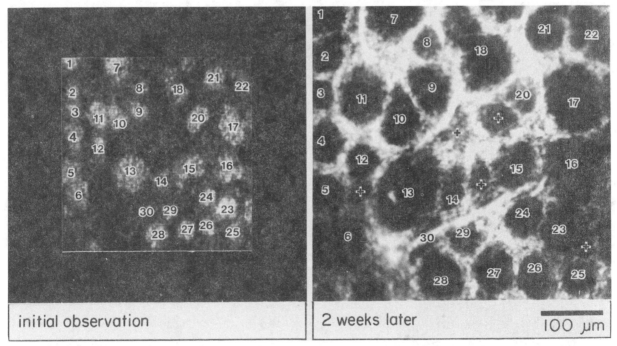

Figure 3. Representative images of the pattern of olfactory glomeruli observed in a living newborn mouse (*left*) and again in the same animal after an interval of 2 weeks (*right*). The glomeruli in the neonate have been vitally stained with the styryl dye RH414 (see Fig. 1B); the final pattern is observed by staining with Sudan Black. Numbers show corresponding glomeruli; pluses indicate glomeruli added during the interval between observations. (Reprinted, with permission, from LaMantia and Purves 1989.)

concluded that modular circuits in this part of the mouse brain are established gradually during postnatal development by the addition of new functional units, without deletions from the original population. Examination of glomerular patterns in adult mice suggests that there is no further change in the basic arrangement of glomeruli once the final number of modules has been established (LaMantia et al. 1989).

On the basis of this evidence in the olfactory system, we have proposed that a similar addition of modular circuits may occur in other regions of the growing mammalian brain (Pomeroy et al. 1990). However, some peculiar features of the olfactory bulb—particularly the postnatal addition of receptor neurons and interneurons (Hinds 1967; Graziadei and Monti-Graziadei 1979a,b, 1980)—limit the ability to generalize from the results summarized here. Accordingly, we have begun to examine the postnatal elaboration of neural circuitry in the primate cerebral cortex where several other classes of modules have been described previously (for reviews, see Goldman-Rakic 1984; Hendrikson 1985; Hubel 1988) and where neurogenesis is complete early in development (Rakic 1985).

Analysis of Module Development in the Visual Cortex

To study the development of modules in the cerebral cortex of the rhesus monkey, we chose another class of histologically visible neural circuit, the blobs in the primary visual cortex (Fig. 4) (Horton and Hubel 1981; Carroll and Wong-Riley 1984; Horton 1984; Livingstone and Hubel 1984). Blobs were first noticed by M. Wong-Riley in area 17 of the monkey cortex after cytochrome oxidase staining (see Livingstone and Hubel 1984). The morphology and distribution of blobs was subsequently studied in detail in various primates (Horton 1984; Hendrickson 1985), and the physiological role of these modules was explored (Livingstone and Hubel 1984, 1987). Blobs are evident in the visual cortex of prosimians, old and new world monkeys, and

humans; they are not, however, found in a variety of other mammals (Horton 1984; Horton and Hedley-Whyte 1984; Condo and Casagrande 1990). Although the function of blobs is not entirely clear, many of the neurons within them respond to color but not to specific stimulus orientations (Livingstone and Hubel 1984, 1987; but see Condo and Casagrande 1990). Blobs also project specifically to a subset of cytochrome-oxidase-positive stripes in area 18. Thus, these units are physiologically and anatomically distinct.

Blobs are particularly well suited for our studies because, like glomeruli, they can be visualized and counted using procedures that do not rely on the injection and transport of tracers or the uncertainties of immunohistochemistry. In newborn monkeys, the density of blobs is about $5/mm^2$ (Fig. 4 and Table 1). The area occupied by each primary visual cortex is about $800\ mm^2$ (see also Van Essen et al. 1984). Accordingly, there are about 4000 blobs in each hemisphere of a newborn monkey. In the adult rhesus monkey, the density of blobs is also about $5/mm^2$ (Fig. 4 and Table 1). The extent of area 17, however, is substantially more than at birth, being about $1200\ mm^2$ on average (Fig. 5). Thus, each hemisphere of the adult monkey contains about 6000 blobs. These results indicate that blobs are added to the cortex during postnatal maturation, although to a less marked degree than are glomeruli in the olfactory bulb (cf. Fig. 2).

DISCUSSION

A comparison of the two very different types of modules we have studied—glomeruli in the olfactory system and blobs in the visual cortex—raises the possibility that the numbers (and patterns) of such iterated circuits are generated by a common developmental mechanism. In both these systems, novel circuits continue to be constructed over a period that extends into postnatal life. Thus, the postnatal increase in the size of mammalian brains, which is usually attributed to glial proliferation, angiogenesis, myelination, and other fac-

Table 1. Brain Growth and Module Number in the Monkey Visual Cortex

	Age	Brain weight (g)	Area of striate cortex (mm^2)	Opercular blob density ($/mm^2$)	Overall number of blobs/hemisphere
Neonatal animals					
	3 days	50	670	4.6	3082
	4 days	50	825	6.0	4950
	5 days	64	910	5.0	4550
					Mean = 4194 ± 568 ±S.E.M.)
Adult animals					
	7 years	106	1210	4.2	5082
	8 years	105	1148	5.8	6658
	12 years	101	1246	4.9	6105
					Mean = 5948 ± 462 ± S.E.M)[a]

[a]Despite the small sample size, the difference between the means of neonatal and adult animals is significant ($p = 0.0373$).

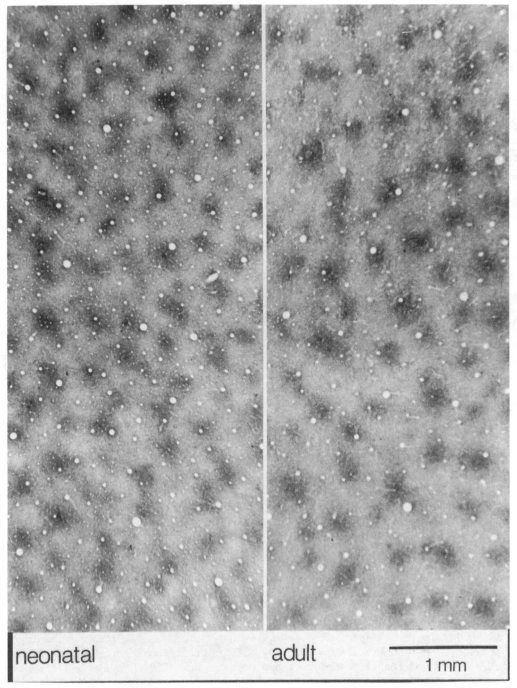

Figure 4. Density of cytochrome-oxidase-positive blobs in the opercular region of the striate cortex of an infant rhesus monkey (*left*) and an adult monkey (*right*). The density of blobs is about the same at both ages (see also Table 1).

tors that are independent of neural circuitry, may also reflect the ongoing addition of modular and other processing units to the maturing brain (see also Constantine-Paton and Law 1978). A contrasting interpretation of brain development is that the full complement of neural circuits, or even a surfeit of such circuits, is present in early life. In this view, neural development involves selection from this initial repertoire: Useful circuits are stabilized to form the mature patterns of connections, and less useful ones are removed (Young 1979; Changeux 1985; Edelman 1987). The present results, whether considered in the olfactory or the visual system, argue against this interpretation.

Our evidence that modules are added progressively during the period of animal maturation and brain growth may be pertinent to rationalizing several neurobiological phenomena that are still poorly understood. One such phenomenon is the widespread occurrence of

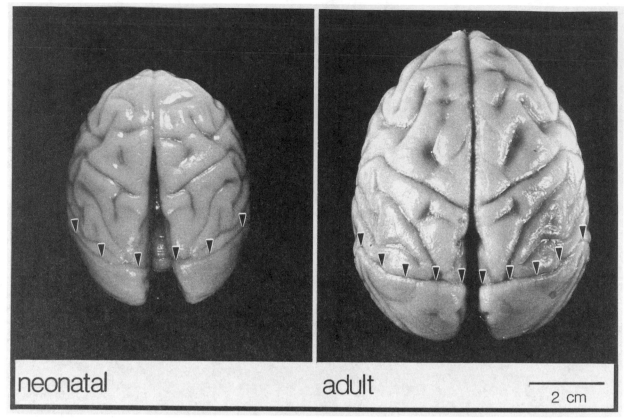

Figure 5. Dorsal view of a rhesus monkey brain at birth (*left*) and at maturity (*right*). The exposed portion of the striate cortex lies posterior to the lunate sulcus (arrowheads). The size of the portion of the visual cortex that can be seen in this view is evidently larger in the adult (as is the overall size of the brain). Measurements of serial sections of area 17 in infant and adult monkeys confirm this impression (see Table 1). (Reprinted, with permission, from Purves and LaMantia 1990.)

critical periods, epochs in early life when the brain is particularly susceptible to the effects of experience. If the postnatal construction of circuits is indeed prevalent in the developing brain, the occurrence of critical periods may reflect the normal duration of this process. Similarly, the more efficient recovery from neural injury in early life (Kennard 1942) may be explained by the normally greater capacity for postnatal circuit construction in early life compared with that in adulthood. Finally, it is apparent from both ethological and psychological studies that the juvenile brain is especially capable of storing new information (for review, see Marler and Terrace 1984). The ongoing construction of neural circuits during maturation may provide a neurobiological substrate for this ability as well.

If ongoing circuit construction is an integral part of brain maturation, what general mechanism might drive this process and determine its gradual waning during the later stages of postnatal development (see Fig. 2, for example)? One possibility is the modulation of neuritic growth. From a structural perspective, iterated units in the olfactory and visual systems apparently represent periodic fluctuations in the organization of neuropil. Thus, each glomerulus is a dense tangle of specific classes of axon terminals and dendrites; the surrounding rind of nerve and glial cells appears to have been excluded from the tangle by the proliferating

neuritic arborizations and their synaptic connections (Pomeroy et al. 1990). The cytological differences that define blobs in the striate cortex are much less distinct (and less well understood). Nevertheless, blobs may also represent the preferential growth of specific axonal and dendritic elements. Modules may therefore represent foci of neuritic growth.

Another common feature of blobs and glomeruli concerns the relative intensity of their electrical activity. Both these classes of modular circuits are labeled by activity-dependent markers such as 2-deoxyglucose (2-DG) in the absence of any specific stimulus paradigm (Stewart et al. 1979; Humphrey and Hendrikson 1983). This metabolic difference implies that the circuit elements within modules are constitutively more active than the surrounding neuropil (Sokoloff 1984). For blobs, 2-DG labeling is enhanced by the presentation of colored stimuli (Livingstone and Hubel 1984, 1987); for glomeruli, specific odors stimulate increased 2-DG labeling of particular units (Stewart et al. 1979; Coopersmith and Leon 1984). The enhanced metabolic labeling of such modules, in both quiescent and stimulated animals, raises the possibility that differential neural activity is in part responsible for the accelerated growth of modular neuropil during development.

These common characteristics of glomeruli and blobs suggest that module formation may be stimulated by the activity-driven trophic interplay of axons and their synaptic targets. Trophic interactions are, by definition, neuronal dependencies in which the growth and stability of pre- and postsynaptic neurites are governed by specific molecules provided by the synaptic partners (for review, see Purves 1988). In the peripheral nervous system, the trophic agent nerve growth factor is known to affect the elaboration of both axonal and dendritic arborizations of responsive neurons via local interaction (Purves et al. 1988). Many of these effects are influenced by activity (for review, see Purves 1988). Although the molecular biology of trophic dependencies is less well understood in the central nervous system, several nerve growth factors have now been identified in the brain, where they appear to exercise effects similar to those observed in the peripheral nervous system (Leibrock et al. 1989; Maisonpierre et al. 1990). Trophic interactions therefore provide a plausible basis for the periodic differences in brain neuropil that characterize at least some classes of modules. Finally, since trophic dependencies typically become less intense as development proceeds, the diminished construction of novel circuits in maturity might be explained by the diminished vigor of trophic interactions.

If the formation and maintenance of iterated units do depend on trophic interactions, the prevalence of iterated circuits in the brain may be better interpreted as the result of developmental rules rather than functional imperatives. In the case of blobs, for example, the arrangement of modules may reflect differential patterns of activity and their trophic consequences, rather than, as most people believe, a functional need to segregate color and form channels. This alternative interpretation could explain the following observations: (1) that blobs are present in some orders (primates) and not in others (carnivores), (2) that other classes of modules (e.g., ocular dominance columns) are present in some monkeys but not in others (Hendrikson 1985), (3) that modular circuits are prominent in some brain regions but not in others, (4) that novel modular circuits can be created experimentally by altering developmental circumstances (implanting an extra eye in tadpole, for example) (Constantine-Paton and Law 1978), and (5) that modules such as blobs are present in the absence of retinal input (Kuljis and Rakic 1990).

SUMMARY

Comparison of seemingly different modular units in the mammalian brain raises the possibility of a common mechanism for their formation: the growth of neuropil mediated by trophic interactions. The ongoing postnatal construction of modular circuits according to trophic interplay may in turn account for the remarkable plasticity of the juvenile brain. By the same token, the normal waning of circuit construction during postnatal development may explain the end of critical periods, the diminished ability to recover from injury in older animals, and the decline with increasing age in the ability of mammals to learn complex skills.

REFERENCES

Carroll, E.W. and M.T.T. Wong-Riley. 1984. Quantitative light and electron microscopic analysis of cytochrome oxidase-rich zones in the striate cortex of the squirrel monkey. *J. Comp. Neurol.* **222:** 1.

Changeux, J.-P. 1985. *Neuronal man: The Biology of mind* (transl. by L. Garey). Pantheon, New York.

Condo, G.. and V.A. Casagrande. 1990. Organization of cytochrome oxidase staining in the visual cortex of nocturnal primates *(Galago crassicaudatus* and *Galago senegalensis)*. I. Adult patterns. *J. Comp. Neurol.* **293:** 632.

Constantine-Paton, M. and M.I. Law. 1978. Eye-specific termination bands in tecta of three eyed frogs. *Science* **202:** 639.

Coopersmith, R. and M. Leon. 1984. Enhanced neural response to familiar olfactory cues. *Science* **225:** 849.

Copoletta, J.M. and S.B. Wolbach. 1932. Body length and organ weight of infants and children. *Am. J. Pathol.* **9:** 55.

Cowan, W.M., J.W. Fawcett, D.D.M. O'Leary, and B.B. Stanfield. 1984. Regressive events in neurogenesis. *Science* **225:** 1258.

Dekaban, A.S. and D. Sadowsky. 1978. Changes in brain weights during the span of human life: Relation of brain weights to body heights and body weights. *Ann. Neurol.* **4:** 345.

Edelman, G.M. 1987. *Neural Darwinism: The Theory of Neuronal Group Selection.* Basic Books, New York.

Goldman-Rakic, P. 1984. Modular organization of pre-frontal cortex. *Trends Neurosci.* **7:** 419.

Golgi, C. 1874. Sulla fina struttura dei bulbi olfattorii. *Riv. Sper. Freniatr. Med. Leg. Alienazioni Ment.* **1:** 405.

Graziadei, P.P.C. and G.A. Monti-Graziadei. 1979a. Neurogenesis and neuron regeneration in the olfactory system of mammals. I. Morphological aspects of differentiation and structural organization of the olfactory sensory neurons. *J. Neurocytol.* **8:** 1.

———. 1979b. Neurogenesis and neuron regeneration in the olfactory system of mammals. II. Degeneration and reconstitution of the olfactory sensory neurons after axotomy. *J. Neurocytol.* **8:** 197.

———. 1980. Neurogenesis and neuron regeneration in the olfactory system of mammals. III. Deafferentation and reinnervation of the olfactory bulb following section of the *fila olfactoria* in rat. *J. Neurocytol.* **9:** 145.

Hendrickson, A.E. 1985. Dots, stripes and columns in monkey visual cortex. *Trends Neurosci.* **7:** 406.

Hinds, J.W. 1967. Autoradiographic study of histogenesis in the mouse olfactory bulb. I. Time of origin of neurons and neuroglia. *J. Comp. Neurol.* **134:** 287.

Horton, J.C. 1984. Cytochrome oxidase patches: A new cytoarchitectonic feature of monkey visual cortex. *Philos. Trans. R. Soc. Lond. B Biol. Sci.* **304:** 199.

Horton, J.C. and E.T. Hedley-Whyte 1984. Mapping of cytochrome oxidase patches and ocular dominance columns in human visual cortex. *Philos. Trans. R. Soc. Lond. B Biol. Sci.* **304:** 255.

Horton, J.C. and D.H. Hubel. 1981. Regular patchy distribution of cytochrome oxidase staining in primary visual cortex of macaque monkey. *Nature* **292:** 762.

Hubel, D.H. 1988. *Eye, brain, and vision.* Scientific American Library, New York.

Hubel, D.H., T.N. Wiesel, and S. LeVay. 1977. Plasticity of ocular dominance columns in the monkey striate cortex. *Philos. Trans. R. Soc. Lond. B Biol. Sci.* **278:** 377.

Humphrey, A.L. and A.E. Hendrickson. 1983. Background and stimulus induced patterns of high metabolic activity in the visual cortex (area 17) of the squirrel and macaque monkey. *J. Neurosci.* **3:** 345.

Kennard, M.A. 1942. Cortical reorganization of motor function. Studies on series of monkeys of various ages from infancy to maturity. *Arch. Neurol. Psychiatry* **48:** 227.

Kuljis, R.0. and P. Rakic. 1990. Hypercolumns in primate visual cortex can develop in the absence of cues from photoreceptors. *Proc. Natl. Acad. Sci.* **87:** 5303.

LaMantia, A.-S. and D. Purves. 1989. Development of glomerular pattern visualized in the olfactory bulbs of living mice. *Nature* **341:** 646.

LaMantia, A.-S., S.L. Pomeroy, and D. Purves. 1989. Direct observation of the olfactory bulb over time in developing and adult mice. *Soc. Neurosci. Abstr.* **15:** 809.

Leibrock, I., F. Lottspeich, A. Hohn, M. Hofer, B. Hengerer, P. Masiakowski, H. Thoenen, and Y.-A Barde. 1989. Molecular cloning and expression of brain-derived neurotrophic factor. *Nature* **341:** 149.

Livingstone, M.S. and D.S. Hubel. 1984. Anatomy and physiology of a color system in the primate visual cortex. *J. Neurosci.* **4:** 309.

———. 1987. Connections between layer 4B of area 17 and the thick cytochrome oxidase stripes of area 18 in the squirrel monkey. *J. Neurosci.* **7:** 3371.

Lorente de Nó, R. 1949. The structure of cerebral cortex. In *Physiology of the nervous system*, 3rd edition (ed. J. Fulton), p. 288. Oxford University Press, New York.

Maisonpierre, P.C., L. Belluscio, S. Squinto, N.Y. Ip, M.E. Furth, R.M. Lindsay, and G.D. Yancopoulos. 1990. Neurotrophin-3: A neurotrophic factor related to NGF and BDNF. *Science* **24:** 1446.

Marler, P. and H.S. Terrace. 1984. *The biology of learning* (Dahlem Workshop Reports). *Life Sci. Res. Rep.* **29.**

Mountcastle, V.B. 1978. An organizing principle for cerebral function: The unit module and the distributed system. In *The mindful brain: Cortical organization and the group-selective theory of higher brain function* (ed. G.M. Edelman and V.B. Mountcastle), p. 7. MIT Press, Cambridge, Massachusetts.

Pakkenberg, H. and J. Voigt. 1964. Brain weight of the Danes. *Acta Anat.* **56:** 297.

Pomeroy, S.L., A.-S. LaMantia, and D. Purves. 1990. Post-natal construction of neural circuitry in mouse olfactory bulb. *J. Neurosci.* **10:** 1952.

Purves, D. 1988. *Body and brain: A trophic theory of neural connections.* Harvard University Press, Cambridge, Massachusetts.

Purves, D. and A.-S. LaMantia. 1990. Numbers of blobs in the primary visual cortex of neonatal and adult monkeys. *Proc. Natl. Acad. Sci.* **87:** 5764.

Purves, D. and J.W. Lichtman. 1980. Elimination of synaptic connections in the developing nervous system. *Science* **210:** 153.

———. 1985. *Principles of neural development.* Sinauer Associates, Sunderland, Massachusetts.

Purves, D. and J.T. Voyvodic. 1987. Imaging mammalian nerve cells and their connections over time in living animals. *Trends Neurosci.* **10:** 398.

Purves, D., W.D. Snider, and J.T. Voyvodic. 1988. Trophic regulation of nerve cell morphology and innervation in the autonomic nervous system. *Nature* **336:** 123.

Rakic, P. 1985. Limits of neurogenesis in primates. *Science* **227:** 154.

Sokoloff, L. 1984. *Metabolic probes of central nervous system activity in experimental animals and man.* (Magnes Lecture Ser., vol. 1). Sinauer Associates, Sunderland, Massachusetts.

Stewart, W.B., J.S. Kauer, and G.M. Shepherd. 1979. Functional organization of rat olfactory bulb, analyzed by the 2-deoxyglucose method. *J. Comp. Neurol.* **185:** 715.

Szentagothai, J. 1978. The neuron network of the cerebral cortex: A functional interpretation. *Proc. R. Soc. Lond. B Biol. Sci.* **201:** 219.

Van Essen, D.C., W.T. Newsome, and J.H.R. Maunsell. 1984. The visual field representation in the striate cortex of the macaque monkey: Asymmetrics, anisotropics and individual variability. *Vision Res.* **24:** 426.

Wong-Riley, M. 1979. Changes in the visual system of monocularly sutured or enucleated cats demonstrable with cytochrome oxidase histochemistry. *Brain Res.* **171:** 11.

Young, J.Z. 1979. Learning as a process of selection and amplification. *J. R. Soc. Med.* **72:** 801.

Target Selection by Cortical Axons: Alternative Mechanisms to Establish Axonal Connections in the Developing Brain

D.D.M. O'Leary,* A.R. Bicknese, J.A. De Carlos, C.D. Heffner,
S.E. Koester, L.J. Kutka, and T. Terashima
*Departments of Anatomy and Neurobiology and of Neurology and Neurological Surgery,
Washington University School of Medicine, St. Louis, Missouri 63110*

A fundamental issue in developmental neurobiology is the mechanism by which specific connections are established between neuronal populations and their targets. Much of what is known about this subject has come from the study of simple neural systems, both vertebrate and invertebrate, both in vivo and in vitro (Purves and Lichtman 1985). These studies have led to a number of generalizations regarding the behavior of developing axons. First, the growth cone is essential for neurite elongation, directional pathfinding, and target recognition (Kater and Guthrie, this volume). Second, the branching of the primary axon of neurons that form divergent collateral projections is achieved by the bifurcation of the axonal growth cone at specific points in its pathway (Shaw and Bray 1971; Bray 1973; Wessells and Nuttall 1978; Raper et al. 1983). Finally, these behaviors of the growth cone are made in response to local molecular cues encoded within, or that develop within, the axonal pathway (Hamburger 1988). It has only recently been realized that major populations of developing axons do not behave in this stereotyped manner. We describe here our studies of the development of axonal projections from layer 5 of the rat neocortex to subcortical targets to illustrate alternative mechanisms that axons use to establish their connections.

Layer 5 is an important output layer of the neocortex, being the only source of cortical projections to targets in the midbrain, hindbrain, and spinal cord. We have been particularly interested in determining how layer-5 neurons select their targets, form collateral projections to widely divergent targets, and establish the differences in patterns of layer-5 projections between areas of the adult neocortex. In pursuit of these questions, we have identified three stages in the development of layer-5 projections (Fig. 1). First, layer-5 axons extend out of the cortex toward the spinal cord, bypassing their subcortical targets. Second, the subcortical targets are exclusively contacted by axon collaterals that develop by a "delayed interstitial branching" off the flank of a spinally directed primary axon. Layer-5 neurons in diverse cortical areas initially develop a common set of branches. Third, specific branches and segments of the primary axon are selectively eliminated to yield the mature projections functionally appropriate for the area of cortex in which the layer-5 neuron resides. Thus, in this system, unlike in others studied to date, the primary growth cone is not responsible for target selection or for axon branching. The limited role of the growth cone of primary layer-5 axons is to select the appropriate pathway to exit cortex and then to

---

* Present address: Molecular Neurobiology Laboratory, The Salk Institute, La Jolla, California 92037.

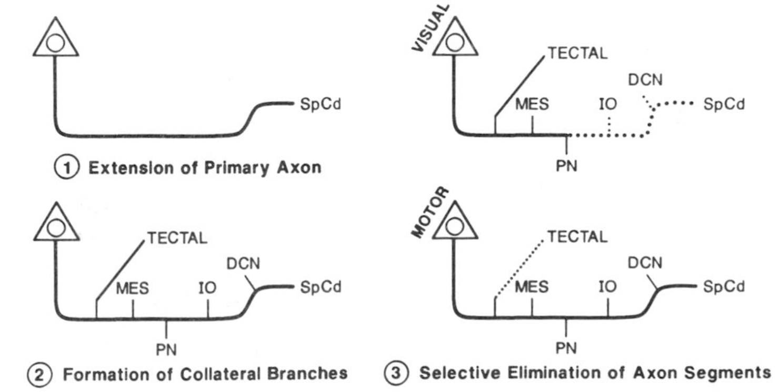

Figure 1. Development of subcortical projections of layer-5 neurons has three phases. (*1*) Primary layer-5 axons extend out of cortex toward the spinal cord, bypassing their subcortical targets. (*2*) Subcortical targets are later contacted exclusively by axon collaterals that develop by a delayed interstitial branching of the spinally directed primary axon. Layer-5 neurons in motor and visual cortex develop a common set of branches. (*3*) Specific branches and segments of the primary axon are selectively eliminated (dotted lines) to yield the mature projections functionally appropriate for the area of cortex in which the layer-5 neuron resides. Collateral branch abbreviations: (TECTAL) Includes several targets, with the superior colliculus being the major and most distal one; (MES), i.e., mesencephalic, includes several midbrain nuclei, the red nucleus being a major one; (PN) basilar pons, a major structure in the pons; (IO) inferior olive, a nucleus in the medulla; (DCN) dorsal column nuclei, nuclei in caudal medulla; (SpCd) spinal cord, most distal target of the primary cortical layer-5 axons.

continue an undeviated growth spinally along a single, prominent tract. In vitro studies, supported by additional evidence from in vivo experiments, indicate that one of the subcortical targets, the basilar pons, promotes its own innervation by releasing a diffusible signal that induces the interstitial formation of collateral branches from the primary layer-5 axons and directs their ingrowth.

Development of Area-specific Patterns of Layer-5 Projections

Different regions of the adult neocortex have unique patterns of layer-5 projections to subcortical targets. For example, layer-5 neurons in the primary motor and visual areas project to distinct, but overlapping, sets of subcortical targets; this important feature of cortical organization is schematized in Figure 2. In the adult, a proportion of layer-5 neurons have branching axons that innervate more than one subcortical target (Jones 1984). To determine how these area-specific patterns of layer-5 projections develop, we focused our attention on the corticospinal projection and five major corticofugal projections to the midbrain and hindbrain. In rostral-to-caudal order, these brain-stem projections are tectal (includes several targets, with the superior colliculus as the most distal one), mesencephalic (includes several midbrain nuclei, such as the red nucleus), pontine (specifically, the basilar pons), inferior olive, and dorsal column nuclei. Using the anterograde axon tracer DiI (Honig and Hume 1986), we first established that during development, layer-5 projections to brain-stem targets are formed exclusively by collateral branches of spinally directed axons (O'Leary and Terashima 1988, 1989). We next addressed whether the area-distinct patterns of layer-5 subcortical projections in the adult reflect developmentally distinct patterns of axon branching or, alternatively, whether they are selected from an initially common pattern of axon branching. This determination is of interest because it defines whether layer-5 axons from different cortical areas respond differentially to cues that may govern their branching, and thus branch only at area-specific locations, or whether they initially behave in a similar way. We find that as a population, layer-5 neurons in motor and visual cortex initially develop comparable sets of collateral branches (Fig. 2). Although a layer-5 neuron may initially develop more collateral branches than it will permanently retain, branches only form at specific and stereotypic positions along the axon tract (O'Leary and Terashima 1988, 1989). This observation indicates that specific cues initiate branching and that such cues operate only at selective positions along the axon tract. These cues are recognized by layer-5 neurons in motor and visual cortex independent of whether the collateral projection subsequently formed is functionally appropriate for the cortical area in which the neuron is located.

Area-specific, layer-5 projections are achieved later in postnatal development through the selective retention of different subsets of the initial complement of branched projections. For example, layer-5 neurons in motor cortex will lose their tectal branch, whereas those in visual cortex will lose the "spinal" segment of their primary axon caudal to the pontine branch point, even if it forms branches to the inferior olive and dorsal column nuclei (see Stanfield et al. 1982; O'Leary and Stanfield 1985; Stanfield and O'Leary 1985a; O'Leary and Terashima 1988, 1989). The remodeling of the initial common projection pattern is not a fixed property of layer-5 neurons but is dependent on their location in the developing cortex (Stanfield and O'Leary 1985b; O'Leary and Stanfield 1989). Late fetal motor and visual cortex transplanted heterotopically into the cortex of newborn rats permanently retain subcortical projections characteristic of their new location: Motor cortical neurons placed in the visual area will initially extend a spinal axon but lose it and keep a tectal projection; visual cortical neurons placed in the motor region will retain a spinal projection. Thus, layer-5 subcortically projecting neurons in motor and visual areas of cortex appear to belong to the same general class of cortical projection neuron.

Do layer-5 subcortically projecting neurons found in all areas of developing neocortex have a similar axon growth and branching program? Evidence from retrograde labeling studies, interpreted in the context of our findings using DiI to label anterogradely developing layer-5 axons, suggest that they do. Fast Blue injected into the spinomedullary junction of adult rats labels

Projection Patterns of Mature
Layer 5 Subcortically Projecting Neurons

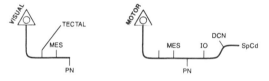

Distinct Projection Patterns are
Selected from a Common, Early Pattern

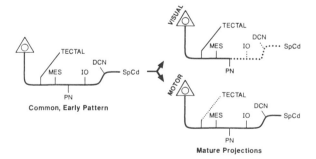

Figure 2. (*Top*) Schematic illustration of basic subcortical projection patterns of layer-5 neurons in motor and visual cortex in adult rats. (*Bottom*) Layer-5 neurons in motor and visual cortex initially develop similar patterns of branched projections. Dotted lines indicate collateral branches and segments of the primary axon that are later selectively lost to generate area-specific projections characteristic of motor and visual cortex.

corticospinal neurons confined to layer 5 of sensorimotor regions of the cortex (Fig. 3A). However, similar injections done during the first postnatal week label a continuous band of layer-5 neurons extending across the entire neocortex (Fig. 3B) (Stanfield et al. 1982; Terashima and O'Leary 1988). Therefore, layer-5 neurons in *all* areas of the developing neocortex extend a spinal axon. Thus, the foundation exists, in the form of the extension of the "primary," spinally directed axon, for layer-5 neurons in all neocortical areas to form a common, early set of axon branches. Additional retrograde labeling studies indicate that layer-5 neurons in all neocortical areas do indeed form several of the major collateral projections (Bicknese and O'Leary 1990). The retrograde dye Fast Blue was injected into the superior colliculus (tectal branch), the

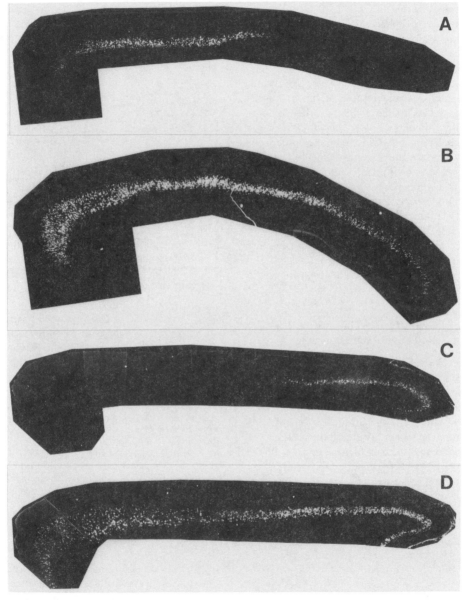

Figure 3. Distributions of corticospinal and corticotectal neurons in adult and developing rats. (*A–D*) Fluorescence montages of sagittal sections spanning the entire rostral to caudal length of the cortex. Rostral is to the left and dorsal is to the right. *A* and *C* are at the same magnification. *B* and *D* are increased in magnification to match the length of the young cortex with the adult. (*A*) Corticospinal neurons labeled with Fast Blue injected into the spinomedullary junction in an adult rat. Labeled cells are restricted to layer 5 of sensorimotor areas of cortex. (*B*) Corticospinal neurons labeled in a developing rat with a similar Fast Blue injection as in *A*, but made on P5. Labeled cells are restricted to layer 5 but are distributed throughout the neocortex. Thus, layer 5 neurons in all areas of the neocortex initially extend a spinally directed primary axon. (*C*) Corticotectal neurons labeled with Fast Blue injected into the superior colliculus in an adult rat. Labeled cells are restricted to layer 5 and are primarily found in visual cortical areas. (*D*) Corticotectal neurons labeled in a developing rat with a similar injection as in *C*, but made on P2. The labeled cells are again restricted to layer 5 but are distributed throughout the cortex. Therefore, layer-5 neurons in all areas of cortex initially develop the tectal branch from the primary spinally directed axon. See text for further discussion.

region of the red nucleus (mesencephalic branch), or the dorsal column nuclei of neonatal and adult rats. Although in adult animals, the distribution of layer-5 neurons labeled from each site is limited to specific cortical regions, in neonatal rats, they are present throughout the neocortex. Examples of representative cases in which Fast Blue was injected into the superior colliculus are shown in Figure 3, C and D. These findings, taken together with those obtained with DiI, demonstrate that as a population, developing layer-5 neurons in all areas of cortex extend a spinally directed axon, and from this primary axon send branches to major targets in the midbrain and hindbrain. Direct support for this conclusion comes from double retrograde labeling experiments using Fast Blue and Diamidino Yellow (Bicknese and O'Leary 1990). Individual layer-5 neurons in all regions of the developing cortex can be double-labeled, with one dye injected into the superior colliculus or dorsal column nuclei and the other into the spinal cord. Double-labeled neurons are also observed when the superior colliculus and the dorsal column nuclei are injected with different dyes. Thus, individual layer-5 neurons can also form branches off the spinally directed primary axon to more than one target. These findings suggest that subcortically projecting layer-5 neurons throughout the developing neocortex have similar potentials in axon targeting and belong to the same neuronal class, although they may ultimately have distinct projection patterns in the adult.

The Primary Growth Cone Plays No Role in Target Selection or Axon Branching

As a rule, cortical neurons innervate multiple targets through collateral projections. Although collateral projections are common throughout the adult nervous system, little is known about the developmental mechanisms involved in collateral formation. Previous studies have pointed to growth cone bifurcation as the predominant mechanism of axon branching (see Introduction). However, using DiI as an anterograde axon tracer in developing rats, we find that the collateral projections of layer-5 neurons form by a novel mechanism, the "delayed interstitial budding" of collateral branches from primary cortical axons days after they extend past the branch point (O'Leary and Terashima 1988, 1989). For example, as summarized in Figure 4, the corticopontine projection develops from preexisting corticospinal axons by an interstitial budding of collateral branches, rather than through a direct ingrowth of the primary axons or of branches formed by the bifurcation of their growth cones (O'Leary and Terashima 1988). Initially, layer-5 axons grow caudally past the pons toward the spinal cord, apparently not recognizing their basilar pontine target. Days later, collateral branches begin to bud from the axons at specific locations in the axon tract overlying the basilar pons. The collaterals then grow directly into their pontine target. Interestingly, the actively growing pontine

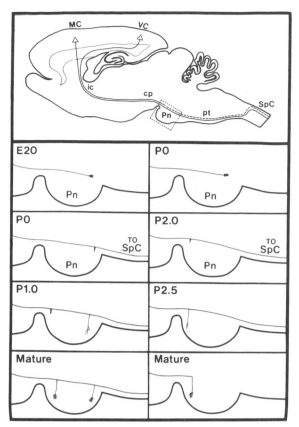

Figure 4. The corticopontine projection develops by a delayed interstitial budding of collateral branches from corticospinal axons. (*Top panel*) Sagittal view of trajectory of corticospinal axons arising from layer-5 neurons in developing motor (MC) and visual cortex (VC) of rats. Corticospinal axons leave cortex via the internal capsule (ic) and grow through the cerebral peduncle (cp) and pyramidal tract enroute to the spinal cord (SpC). Corticospinal axons from the VC are later eliminated (dashed line) beyond the collateral branch that innervates the basilar pons (Pn). The area enclosed by the dashed box, which includes the basilar pons and the part of the corticospinal axon tract overlying it, is enlarged below to show the development of the corticopontine projection from MC (*left*) and VC (*right*). Corticospinal axons reach the pons on E20 (MC) or P2 (VC) but grow caudally past it. Days later, branches bud from the corticospinal axons at positions in the axon tract directly overlying the basilar pons. Collateral budding differs in time and location depending on the cortical origin of the corticospinal axon. The post-pontine segment of the corticospinal axon forms a permanent (MC) or transient projection (VC) to the spinal cord. Dorsal is to the top and caudal is to the right.

collaterals lack a morphologically definable growth cone, although the distal end of the branch is a motile tip. At the time of collateral budding, the growth cones of the still elongating primary axons are more than 4 mm caudal to the pons. This major cortical projection develops in the same fashion regardless of whether the primary, spinally directed layer-5 axon is permanent (as for motor cortex) or transient (as for visual cortex). In the latter case, the pontine projection is the most caudal connection of mature visual layer-5 neurons.

These observations imply that the growth cone of the primary layer-5 axon fails to recognize the basilar pons as a target appropriate for cortical innervation. Our further observations using similar methods indicate that the growth cone of the primary axon ignores every subcortical target of layer-5 neurons (O'Leary and Terashima 1989). Layer-5 axons extend out of cortex via the internal capsule and continue to grow caudally through the cerebral peduncle, pyramidal tract, and into the spinal cord, bypassing their targets in the midbrain and hindbrain. As summarized in Figure 5, branches begin to bud well after the primary axons have grown past the future branch points. During the entire phase of interstitial axon branching, the primary axons continue to extend caudally. We have been unable to relate the timing of collateral branching to a specific behavior of the primary growth cones, e.g., a stopping or dramatic slowing of axon extension or reaching a particular point in the subcortical pathway. We have not seen any indication that the growth cones of primary layer-5 axons recognize their future branch points, nor do filopodial remnants mark them. Our impression, which is based on the examination of static images of DiI-labeled axons at various developmental stages, is that branches bud de novo from smooth segments of cortical axons.

Our observations establish that the growth cone of the primary layer-5 axon plays no role in target selection, a conclusion that is confirmed by our analysis of growth cone morphology. Previous studies carried out

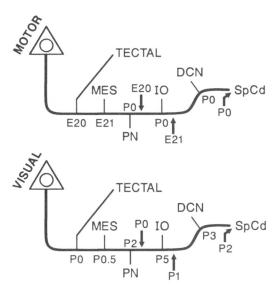

Figure 5. Subcortical targets of layer-5 neurons are contacted exclusively by collateral branches that develop from primary, spinally directed axons by a mechanism of delayed interstitial axon branching. The thick line represents the primary axon. Each collateral branch begins to bud well after the primary cortical axon has grown caudally past the branch point. Ages on either side of the thick line indicate the time at which that particular collateral branch begins to bud interstitially from the primary axon. The ages associated with the bold arrows mark the point of extension of the primary axon at the age indicated. For example, in motor cortex cases, at E20, when the tectal branch begins to bud from the primary axon, the distal end of the primary axon has already grown past the basilar pons.

both in vertebrates (Tosney and Landmesser 1985; Bovolenta and Mason 1987) and in invertebrates (Taghert et al. 1982; Bentley and Caudy 1983) have found that growth cone morphology changes dramatically as developing axons extend along their pathway. These studies report that the growth cone increases in complexity when it reaches a "decision point" in the pathway, whether the decision is to select and extend down one of several potential paths (Taghert et al. 1982; Tosney and Landmesser 1985) or to leave the pathway and invade an appropriate target nucleus that lies along the axon tract (Bovolenta and Mason 1987). The increased complexity features a broadening and shortening of the growth cone and the extension of more prominent lamellapodia and numerous filopodia. It has been proposed that these changes in growth cone morphology are in response to specific, local cues selectively present within the axon tract at decision points.

Using the method of DiI labeling in aldehyde-fixed tissue (Godement et al. 1987), we have studied changes in the morphology of cortical growth cones as they extend out of cortex and grow past the first of the prominent branch points, the site of the future tectal branch (J.A. De Carlos and D.D.M. O'Leary, unpubl.). The growth cones of primary cortical axons have expansive lamellapodia and numerous filopodia extended in many directions as they approach the interface of the cortical intermediate zone with the internal capsule, the pathway through which axons exit the cortex (Fig. 6A,E,F). As we describe below, this is a decision point for cortical axons, and their morphologies resemble those described for growth cones at decision points in other vertebrate systems. However, the growth cones quickly become elongated and more simple in appearance as they leave this decision region (Fig. 6G) and retain this appearance as they extend caudally through the cerebral peduncle and past the region of the axon tract at which the tectal branch will later develop (Fig. 6C,D,H). Although this region of the axon tract will be a decision point for cortical axons, even at this level of resolution, we cannot detect a response of the primary growth cones. Assuming that the growth cones are receptive to the cues that mark the branch points, it is not clear why they fail to respond. The possibilities are that they prefer the axonal pathway or pass by the branch point too rapidly to be adequately influenced or perhaps the cues have not yet developed at the time the growth cones arrive. On the other hand, it is possible that the growth cones are not receptive to the cues that mark branch points, although the length of axon millimeters behind them clearly is both receptive and responsive.

In Vitro Demonstration That a Target-derived Diffusible, Chemotropic Activity Initiates and Directs Cortical Axon Branches

Studies of axon branching and target recognition have focused almost exclusively on the behavior of the growth cone of the primary axon (Landmesser 1984;

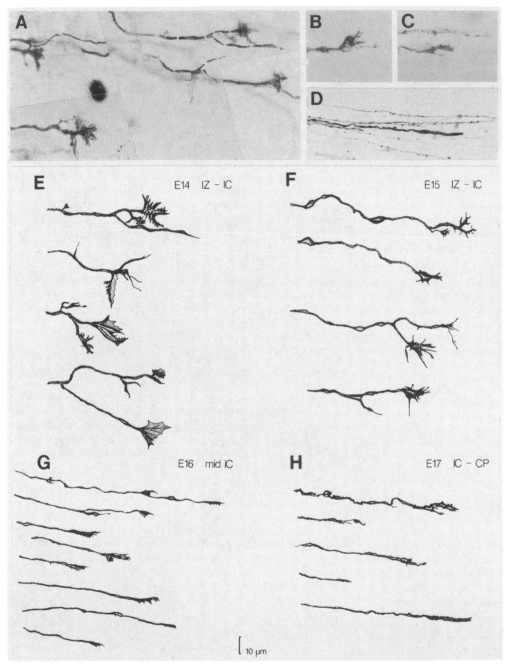

Figure 6. Morphologies of growth cones of primary cortical axons in subcortical pathways. Fetal rats were aldehyde-fixed from E13 to birth. Growth cones were then labeled by anterograde DiI filling and photoconverted in the presence of DAB (see Sandell and Masland 1988). (*A*) E14 growth cones in the intermediate zone (IZ) near the interface with the nascent internal capsule (IC). This region is a presumed decision point in the axon path. They have extensive lamellapodia and filopodia extended in many directions. These are the growth cones of the first axons to leave the cortex and belong to preplate (i.e., subplate) neurons (De Carlos and O'Leary 1990). (*B*) A later-arriving E15 growth cone that has extended a short distance into the nascent IC. (*C,D*) E17 growth cones in the caudal part of IC and rostral part of the CP, within the region of the axon path that the tectal branch will first form on E20. Their morphologies are simple. (*E-H*) Camera lucida drawings of representative growth cones in different regions of the subcortical pathway. (*E*) At E14. Growth cones in the cortical decision region, the interface between the IZ and the nascent IC. They have complex morphologies. (*F*) At E15. Growth cones in the same decision region as in *E*. Their morphologies are similar to those at E14. (*G*) At E16. Growth cones in the mid and caudal part of the IC. They are elongated and simple. (*H*) At E17. Growth cones in caudal IC and rostral CP, the region where the tectal branch will later form. They have mainly elongated morphologies. Filopodia tend to be extended in the direction of growth. (CP) Cerebral peduncle; (IC) internal capsule; (IZ) intermediate zone.

458

Dodd and Jessell 1988). However, target selection by layer-5 axons and the requisite branching are *not* responsibilities of the growth cone of the primary axon. This feature poses unique problems to be resolved in the course of defining the process of target recognition in this system. Our studies thus far have focused on defining the mechanism that directs the formation of the collateral branch that innervates the basilar pons. This immediate goal has two objectives: (1) to determine the cues that provide the directional guidance of pontine collateral branches to their target, the basilar pons, and (2) to identify the cues that mark branch points and initiate interstitial branching. The former objective addresses a problem common to the targeting of all axons, whereas the latter objective is particularly important since collateral budding is the first visible sign that the primary cortical axon recognizes a target appropriate for cortical innervation.

What is the nature of the cues that govern the budding and directed growth of pontine collaterals? One possibility is that pontine collaterals are produced at predetermined points along the primary cortical axons according to a program intrinsic to layer-5 cortical neurons. Such an intrinsic program appears to govern the geometry of axonal bifurcation in certain neurons of the leech (Acklin and Nicholls 1990). Alternatively, the process could be controlled by local cues, i.e., "signals encoded in the structure in which the growth cone is in direct contact" (Hamburger 1988), which develop selectively in the region of the axon tract overlying the basilar pons. A further possibility is that a molecular signal is released by the basilar pons and diffuses into the overlying axon tract to interact, either directly or indirectly, with cortical axons to induce their interstitial branching and direct collateral extension. Chemotropic guidance of axons was first proposed late in the last century by Ramon y Cajal (1894), but, due to a lack of supporting evidence, has been largely ignored until recently.

An effective method to distinguish between these possibilities is to coculture at a distance within three-dimensional collagen matrices cortical explants with target explants of basilar pons and a control tissue. Since the explants are firmly embedded within the collagen matrix and do not contact one another, any possible action of local cues is effectively excluded. Therefore, the consistent observation that cortical axon outgrowth is directed across the intervening matrix preferentially toward a target explant would necessitate that the target is releasing a diffusible, chemotropic activity to which the cortical axons respond. This procedure has been used to demonstrate that a diffusible signal emanating from the maxillary process attracts axons of trigeminal ganglion neurons (Lumsden and Davies 1983, 1986) and that a different signal released by the spinal floor plate provides directional cues for commissural axons (Tessier-Lavigne et al. 1988).

In our initial study (Heffner et al. 1990), full thickness, rectangular explants of cortex, extending from the pia to the ventricle, were taken from motor and visual cortical areas and either cultured alone or cocultured with target explants of basilar pons and a control tissue for 24–48 hours. Control tissues used were mammillary bodies, other parts of the hypothalamus, olfactory bulb (none of which receive neocortical innervation), and pieces of neocortex. All explants were taken from P0 or P1 rats, the developmental stage at which pontine collateral branches are budding from corticospinal axons in vivo. The target explants were placed on the opposite sides of the cortical explant at a distance of 150–300 μm. Although the pia to ventricular orientation was maintained, the sidedness was entirely random.

When cortex is cultured by itself in the collagen gel, axon outgrowth is predominantly from the ventricular surface, with some growth extending from the sides of the explant; most axons grow in an inferior direction (Fig. 7A). However, when cortex is cocultured with basilar pons and a control tissue, axon outgrowth is consistently enhanced from the side of the cortical explant facing the basilar pons; this growth is strongly directed toward pontine explant but not toward the control explant (Fig. 7B) (motor and visual cortex respond similarly). Qualitative assessment from phase-contrast observations of 201 cocultures shows that axon growth extends predominantly from the side of the cortical explant facing the basilar pons in 86% of the cases and from the side facing the control explant in about 2% of the cases. The remaining 12% of the cocultures had near-equal growth from the two sides of the cortical explant. These findings indicate that the basilar pons releases a diffusible activity that influences the directional growth of cortical axons in a target-specific manner. Quantitative measurements of axon behavior in 122 cocultures support this conclusion. First, 2564 cortical axons were scored as having a trajectory that, if continued, would intercept either the pontine or control tissue explant; 79% of these axons are directed toward the basilar pons. Second, 593 cortical axons, with an initial trajectory that would miss the two target explants, were scored as turning greater than 30° toward one or the other target explant; 96% of these axons turn toward the pontine explant. These numbers underestimate the influence of the pontine explant on the directionality of cortical axon growth, since we scored only axons whose growth cones were obvious; thus, the many axons that had already contacted the pontine explant were excluded from this analysis—very few axons contact the control tissue explant.

To visualize axon behavior within the cortical explant and to identify the parent cells of cortical axons that extend into the collagen matrix, as well as those that contact the target explants, cultures were fixed with aldehyde, and the fluorescent axon tracer DiI was injected into the collagen matrix in the path of the axons extending from the ventricular surface of cortical explants cultured alone ($n = 67$); in cocultures, DiI was injected into the pontine ($n = 97$) or control tissue explant ($n = 53$). DiI is especially useful in this context, since when applied in fixed tissue to the axon or an

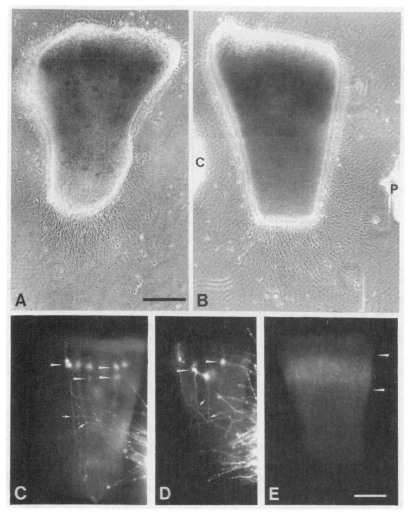

Figure 7. Directed cortical axon growth in three-dimensional collagen matrices after 24 hr in culture. (*A,B*) Phase-contrast images. (*A*) Motor cortex cultured alone. Most axon growth is directed inferiorly from the ventricular surface of the explant (pial surface is to the top). (*B*) Motor cortex cocultured with control tissue (C) to the left and basilar pons (P) to the right. Cortical axon growth extends predominantly from the side facing the pons and is directed laterally toward the basilar pons. Cortical axons growing on the control side maintain their inferior direction of growth. Bar: (*A,B*) 200 μm. (*C,D*) Fluorescence images of axon branching in cortical explants. In each, motor cortex is cocultured with control tissue to the left and basilar pons to the right as in *B*. Only the cortical explant is in the field of view. After aldehyde fixation, DiI was injected into the pontine explant. In the examples illustrated, the pontine explants were only partially filled with DiI to facilitate observations. Because of explant thickness, only some labeling is in focus at any focal plane; segments of labeled axons are not visible when well out of the focal plane. Retrogradely labeled cell bodies in the cortical explants (some marked with arrowheads) are in the layer-5 region (compare with *E*). Many retrogradely labeled cortical neurons contact the pontine explant by collateral branches; some branch points visible in the cortical explant are marked with arrows. (*E*) An explant of motor cortex taken 24 hr after rhodamine isothiocyanate was injected into the spinomedullary junction of a newborn rat to label retrogradely the band of corticospinal/corticopontine neurons in layer 5 (marked with arrowheads). Bar: (*C–E*) 200 μm.

axonal branch, it will label by diffusion the entire neuronal membrane, including the axon and all of its branches (Godement et al. 1987). DiI labeling from the pontine explant shows that cortical axons contact it in one of two ways and indicates that much of the pontine-directed growth of cortical axons across the intervening collagen matrix orients within the cortical explant. Some ventricularly directed cortical axons turn within the cortical explant and emerge from the side facing the pontine explant. Many cortical axons, however, maintain their ventricularly directed growth but extend col-

lateral branches that grow laterally to emerge from the pontine-facing side of the cortical explant (Fig. 7C,D).

Further observations suggest that the tropic effect of the basilar pons is specific for the axons of layer-5 neurons, the neurons that form the corticopontine projection in vivo. DiI injected into the path of axons extending from the ventricular surface of cortical explants cultured alone labels cell bodies distributed widely over the pial to ventricular extent of the explant. However, most of the cell bodies retrogradely labeled from the pontine explant are found within a narrow band that runs across the width of the cortical explant (Fig. 7C,D). Therefore, cells throughout the cortical explant send axons into the collagen matrix, but only the axons of a select group of cortical neurons respond to the pontine-derived signal. To compare the distribution of this group to that of identified layer-5 corticospinal-pontine neurons in similar explants, we injected the retrograde tracer RITC into the path of their axons at the spinomedullary junction in P0 rats; 24 hours later, full thickness, rectangular explants of motor and visual cortex were embedded into three-dimensional collagen matrices (Fig. 7E). The distribution of most cortical neurons retrogradely labeled in vitro from the pontine explant is coincident with that of the layer-5 corticospinal-pontine neurons prelabeled in vivo (in Fig. 7, compare C and D to E). DiI injected into the control tissue explants only occasionally labels cortical axons and rarely labels branches, and the few labeled cortical cells are widely scattered. Thus, in vitro, a chemotropic signal derived from the basilar pons can operate over a distance and specifically affect the directional growth of layer-5 cortical axons, either directly or by conditioning the substrate.

Although these collagen matrix coculture experiments demonstrate that layer-5 cortical axons extend collateral branches preferentially toward the basilar pons in response to a diffusible signal emanating from it, they provide only suggestive evidence that the pontine-derived signal can induce the formation of the collateral branches. It is possible, for example, that branches form spontaneously or in response to other undefined influences and then are attracted by the chemotropic activity released by the basilar pons. To determine whether the pontine-derived activity can initiate branch formation, we carried out an additional set of in vitro experiments using a modification of the three-dimensional collagen gel method (Heffner and O'Leary 1990). For these experiments, full-thickness pieces of P0 or P1 cortical explants were cultured alone within the collagen matrix and allowed to extend axons. As described above, the majority of axon growth is directed inferiorly from the ventricular surface of the isolated cortical explants; 24 hours later, a target explant of basilar pons or of a control tissue (same as used previously) was embedded in the collagen gel lateral to the axons already extending from the ventricular sur-

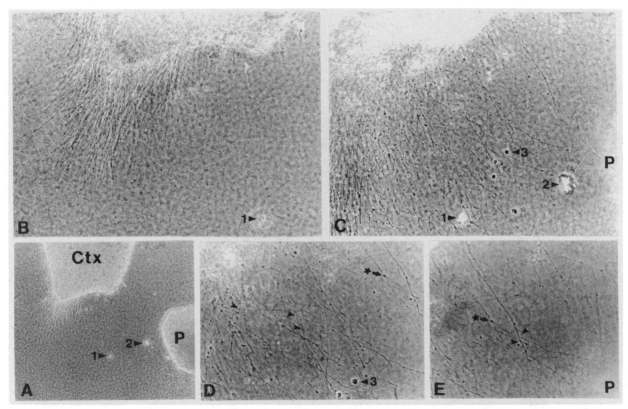

Figure 8. Phase-contrast images of directed cortical axon growth and branch formation in delayed cocultures of cortex and basilar pons in three-dimensional collagen matrices. (*A*) Low-power photo taken immediately after the explant of basilar pons (P) was embedded into the matrix. The motor cortex explant (Ctx) was embedded in the matrix and cultured for 24 hr prior to this. At the time the pons was added, axons were extending off the ventricular surface in an inferior direction. (*B*) Higher-power photo of the cortical axon growth at the time the pontine explant was added. (*C*) Same culture and magnification as those in *B*, but 24 hr after adding the pontine explant. Cortical axons not present at the time the pontine explant was added are directed laterally toward it. (*D,E*) Higher-power views of regions of *C*. Many of the axons directed laterally toward the pontine explant are collateral branches. Some branch points are marked by arrowheads. The branch point indicated by the asterisk is marked in *D* and *E*. Blemishes in the collagen are marked in *A–D* for reference points.

face of the cortical explant (Fig. 8A,B). After a further 24 hours of growth, the cultures were fixed with aldehyde. Examination using phase-contrast optics reveals that a contingent of cortical axons not present at the time the pontine explant was added is directed laterally through the collagen gel toward the pontine explant (Fig. 8C). The growth of these axons tends to be orthogonal to that of the axons that had already extended from the ventricular surface of the cortical explant at the time the pontine explant was added. Many of these later arising, laterally growing cortical axons are branches that form in the collagen matrix (Fig. 8D,E). Such directed, de novo growth of cortical axons is not observed in similar delayed cocultures of cortex and control tissue explants, nor in cases in which cortex is cultured alone for 48 hours.

In a representative series of cultures, DiI labeling was used to quantify the presence of branches (both within the collagen gel and within the cortical explant), the directional growth of the branches, and the laminar location of their cells of origin. DiI was injected into the delayed target explant, pontine and control, or in cases in which no target explant was later added, directly into the collagen gel in the path of the outgrowing cortical axons. Our data are presented in Table 1. In cultures of cortex alone ($n = 67$), DiI labeling did not reveal branch formation within the collagen gel. Occasional branches do form in the cortical explant and extend equally to the left or right (directional coefficient $= 0.04$). The retrogradely labeled parent cells are distributed throughout much of the cortical explant, with 32% found in layer 5. Since phase-contrast observations show that very few axons contact the control target, small injections of DiI made into the control explant in delayed cocultures ($n = 29$; delayed control set A in Table 1) retrogradely fill few axons.

Therefore, in other delayed cocultures ($n = 36$; delayed control set B in Table 1), larger DiI injections were made into the control tissue explant and the neighboring collagen gel to involve more axons extending from the cortical explant. The resultant labeling qualitatively and quantitatively resembles that described for cultures of cortex alone. A small number of randomly directed branches are labeled in the cortical explant (directional coefficient $= 0.04$), and branches are rarely seen in the collagen gel. Again, the labeled cells of origin are distributed widely within the cortical explant, with only 22% found in the layer-5 region. Thus, DiI labeling confirms that the later addition of a target explant of control tissue has little effect on the directional growth or branching of the cortical axons.

Although the delayed addition of a control target explant does not appear to affect the growth and branching of cortical axons, their behavior is greatly influenced by the addition of the basilar pons as a target explant (Table 1). Small DiI injections made into the pontine explant in delayed cocultures ($n = 58$) reveal that within the cortical explant, the number of branches formed per labeled cell is increased five- to eightfold over that seen in cultures of cortex alone or in cocultures with a control target added; the great majority of these branches are also directed toward the pontine explant (directional coefficient $= 0.78$). This result again suggests that the pontine-derived activity stimulates cortical axon branching. However, a further observation provides more definitive evidence. The same small DiI injections show that a substantial proportion of cortical axons branch in the collagen gel, and all of these branches are directed toward the pontine explant (directional coefficient $= 1.00$). Of the cortical neurons retrogradely labeled from the pontine explant in these delayed cocultures, 86% are found in the layer-5 re-

Table 1. Quantitative Analysis of DiI Labeling in Delayed Cocultures

Culture situation	No. of cases	Labeled cells in cortex		Branches in cortex			Branches in matrix	
		total	% layer 5	no.	per cell	direc coeff	no.	per cell
Cortex alone	67	638	32%	52	0.08	0.04	0	0.00
Cortex + Delayed Control (set A)	29	7	0%	0	0.00	—	0	0.00
Cortex + Delayed Control (set B)	36	465	22%	25	0.05	0.04	3	0.01
Cortex + Delayed Pons	58	345	86%	145	0.42	0.78	86	0.25

Explants of P0–P1 motor cortex were cultured for 48 hr in three-dimensional collagen matrices, either alone or in the presence of a P0–P1 target explant of basilar pons or a control tissue for the final 24 hr (see Fig. 8). Cultures were fixed with aldehyde, and DiI was injected either into the target explant (delayed pontine or delayed control set A), into the control explant and neighboring collagen matrix (delayed control set B), or into the path of axons extending from the ventricular surface of the cortical explant in cultures of cortex grown alone. Number of retrogradely labeled cortical cells were counted, and the percentage in layer 5 was determined. Branches extended from DiI-filled axons, within either the cortical explant or matrix, were also counted. Branches per cell equal number of branches formed by labeled axons divided by number of retrogradely labeled cortical cells. (Direc Coeff) Directional coefficient: In delayed cocultures, a Direc Coeff of 1 indicates that all branches extend to the side on which the target explant is placed. A Direc Coeff of 0 indicates that branches extend equally to the side toward or away from the target explant. Calculation of Direc Coeff: (number of branches extending toward side of target explant minus number extending toward opposite side) divided by total number of branches. In cases of cortex grown alone, branch extension to the left or right was substituted for toward or away from the target explant (the highest value was used for toward the target).

gion, supporting our earlier determination that layer-5 axons preferentially respond to the pontine-derived activity. From these findings, we conclude that the basilar pons induces at a distance the interstitial branching of layer-5 cortical axons through the release of a diffusible activity.

The diffusible signal released by the basilar pons influences cortical axons in two ways. First, it promotes the directional growth of cortical axons and their branches; this response defines a tropic activity. Second, it initiates the budding of collateral branches interstitially along the length of cortical axons. This response is a novel action for a chemotropic signal and may be an entirely distinct phenomenon from that of directed axon outgrowth. However, if the initiation of an axon branch is the first step in a cascade of events that results in the directional growth of collateral branches toward the source of a diffusible tropic signal, then branch induction could be classified as a chemotropic response. Nevertheless, the dual action of the pontine-derived signal raises the possibility that it is composed of multiple molecules that carry out distinct functions.

In Vivo Evidence for Target Control of the Interstitial Formation and Directional Growth of Collateral Branches

The corticopontine projection forms from corticospinal axons by a delayed interstitial budding of collateral branches within the axon tract directly overlying the basilar pons (O'Leary and Terashima 1988). Our observations made on cocultures of cortex and basilar pons grown in three-dimensional collagen gels (Heffner et al. 1990; Heffner and O'Leary 1990) closely resemble those made in vivo and suggest that the formation of the corticopontine projection may be controlled by the basilar pons through the release of a diffusible chemotropic signal. To evaluate whether such a chemotropic mechanism may operate in situ during normal brain development, we have carried out two sets of in vivo experiments (Missias et al. 1990).

The first set of experiments tests two hypotheses. First, if local cues govern the branching of layer-5 axons within the axon tract overlying the basilar pons, layer-5 neurons should still branch at this location even in the absence of the basilar pons itself. Second, if the basilar pons controls the branching of layer-5 axons, branches should form even at aberrant locations along layer-5 axons if they overlie ectopically positioned aggregations of basilar pontine neurons. These anatomical anomalies were achieved by X-irradiating pregnant rats during the period of genesis and migration of basilar pontine neurons; X-irradiation has been shown to kill proliferating cells and induce migrational defects (D'Amato and Hicks 1980; Jensen and Killackey 1984). Although there is some overlap in the production of layer-5 and basilar pontine neurons, this experiment can be effectively carried out since virtually all layer-5 neurons are born on E14 and E15 (Bruckner et al. 1976), prior to the peak production of basilar pon-

tine neurons. Basilar pontine neurons are generated in the lateral recess of the fourth ventricle on the dorsal aspect of the medulla from E15 to E18, with more than 90% born on E16 and later (Altman and Bayer 1978). The postmitotic neurons leave the proliferative zone, migrate ventrally around the circumference of the medulla and rostrally along its ventral surface, and aggregate beneath the pons proper.

X-irradiation on a single gestational day, either E16 or E17, results in a small reduction in the size of the basilar pons. In animals irradiated on both E16 and E17, the basilar pons is substantially reduced in size, often to about 10% of its normal volume. In a number of rats irradiated on E16 and E17, multiple, discrete aggregations of cells are found on the ventral surface of the hindbrain underlying the cerebral peduncle or pyramidal tract (the pathway of layer-5 cortical axons along the ventral surface of the pons and medulla). In some cases, multiple aggregations are found at the appropriate location for the basilar pons, beneath the cerebral peduncle of the pons proper, but in other cases, they are also located more caudally at ectopic positions beneath the medullary pyramidal tract. The hindbrain from such a case, and from an age-matched control, is shown in Figure 9, A and B. In this P3 animal, the rostralmost aggregation is located beneath the pontine cerebral peduncle (marked C in Fig. 9B) but is greatly reduced in size and occupies a position that corresponds to the caudal part of the basilar pons in a normal P3 rat. Two other aggregations are found caudally at ectopic positions underlying the medullary pyramidal tract (marked D and E in Fig. 9B).

Although in the absence of basilar pons-specific markers it is difficult to be certain of the identity of the neurons that compose the ectopic aggregations, several lines of evidence lead to the conclusion that they are indeed basilar pontine neurons. First, basilar pontine neurons are the only neurons generated in the hindbrain during or after the time of X-irradiation (Altman and Bayer 1978). They would then be the only hindbrain neurons affected by the radiation. Second, the ectopic aggregations are found along the normal migratory path of basilar pontine neurons. This migratory path is unique to basilar pontine neurons, and the basilar pons is the only neuronal structure present on the ventral surface of the pons and medulla beneath the cerebral peduncle and pyramidal tract. Third, the morphology, size, and Nissl-staining characteristics of the cells in the ectopic aggregations are comparable to those of the neurons that form the normal basilar pons, as well as the small aggregations of neurons found at the location appropriate for the basilar pons in irradiated animals.

In the irradiated cases, the location of branch formation by layer-5 corticospinal-pontine axons is tightly coupled with the positioning of the aggregations of pontine neurons. In the P3 case illustrated in Figure 9B, DiI was injected into the visual cortex to label anterogradely layer-5 axons and their branches; P3 is early in the development of visual corticopontine collat-

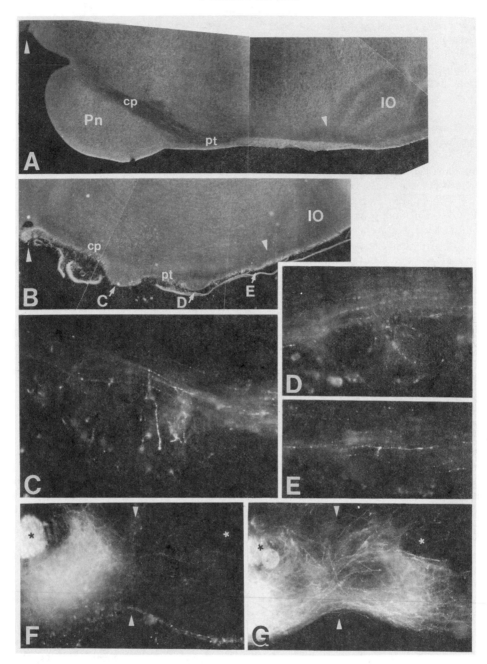

Figure 9. In vivo evidence for the chemotropic influence of basilar pons on cortical axons. (*A*) Sagittal section through the hindbrain of a normal, P3 rat. The basilar pons lies beneath the cerebral peduncle (cp). The primary layer-5 axons extend caudally through the cerebral peduncle, continue down the pyramidal tract (pt) of the medulla, and into the spinal cord. (*B*) Sagittal section of the hindbrain from a P3 X-irradiated on E16 and E17; same magnification as *A*. Arrowheads mark corresponding points on *A* and *B*. (IO) Inferior olive. Caudal is to the right and dorsal is to the top. Arrows indicate the three aggregations of pontine neurons. The aggregation marked *C* underlies the region of the cerebral peduncle that caudal basilar pons does in a normal rat. Aggregations marked *D* and *E* are found in ectopic locations. (*C,D,E*) Fluorescence images of the three aggregations. Layer-5 axons, labeled with the fluorescent axon tracer DiI, injected into the visual cortex, form branches over each aggregation. (*F,G*) Fluorescence images of coronal sections from P6 rats; the corticopontine projection is labeled with DiI injected into the left motor cortex. (*F*) Few labeled axons cross from the left to right basilar pons in a normal, P6 rat. (*G*) Large numbers cross when the cortical input to the right basilar pons is prevented from forming. Arrowheads mark the midline between the left and right basilar pons. Dorsal is to the top. Asterisks mark the cerebral peduncles.

erals (see Fig. 4). The branching of visual layer-5 axons occurs within the axon tract directly over both the reduced basilar pons and the two ectopic aggregations of basilar pontine neurons (Fig. 9C,D,E). The branches extend ventrally across the axon tract and into the underlying aggregations. Thus, visual cortical axons

develop ventrally directed branches at aberrant points along their length, apparently in response to the aggregations of pontine neurons. No ventrally directed branches are found in the region of the axon tract that would normally overlie rostral basilar pons, the location at which visual cortical axons normally branch, nor at positions between the three aggregations of pontine neurons. An occasional branch extends dorsally into the overlying pontine or medullary tegmentum (which appears affected by the irradiation), a sparse projection present in normal rats.

These observations indicate that the location of cortical axon branching is not intrinsic to the axon and strongly suggest that local cues do not govern the formation of the pontine collateral branch. Some caution is warranted here since we cannot rule out the possibility that the locations of aggregations of pontine neurons and cortical axon branching are determined by the same or colocalized set of local cues, the spatial expression of which is altered by the X-irradiation. However, the most straightforward interpretation of these findings is that the basilar pons controls the formation of the collateral branches that innervate it.

In the second set of in vivo experiments, we took advantage of two anatomical features of the basilar pons: It is a bilaterally symmetrical, midline structure, and virtually its entire cortical input arises from the ipsilateral cortex. We reasoned that if the basilar pons attracts its cortical innervation through the release of a diffusible, chemotropic signal, then a basilar pons deprived of its normal cortical input should attract contralateral layer-5 axons across the midline. In a series of P2, P4, and P6 control rats, anterograde DiI labeling of layer-5 axons from motor and visual cortex was used to determine the laterality of cortical input to the basilar pons during normal development. In all cases, few or no labeled axons are found to cross the midline and enter the opposite basilar pons. The normal case with the largest number of labeled crossing axons (from a P6 rat) is shown in Figure 9F. In experimental animals, cortical axons were unilaterally removed prior to their extension of collateral branches into the basilar pons on the right side of the brain. For this, the right cortical hemisphere and the white matter overlying the internal capsule were lesioned in a series of newborn rat pups to destroy all layer-5 axons exiting that side of the cortex. The laterality of the corticopontine projection from the intact (left) hemisphere was determined at P6. DiI injected into the left motor or visual cortex labels an abnormally large number of layer-5 axons that cross the midline and enter the opposite (right) basilar pons. All axons cross at the level of the basilar pons; no labeled axons are observed to arrive at the right basilar pons by extending down the right cerebral peduncle. A representative case is shown in Figure 9G. The sparse labeling seen in the contralateral pons following unilateral cortical DiI injections in control rats rules out that the dense contralateral labeling seen in the experimental cases is due to a failure of retraction of a normally transient projection. The magnitude of the axonal response and the finding that these axons cross at the level of the basilar pons and not rostral to it suggest that the aberrantly crossing axons are responding to a chemoattractant diffusing across the midline from the denervated basilar pons. An alternative explanation is that some form of axonal competition between the left and right corticopontine collaterals occurring at the

midline normally prevents them from crossing to the opposite basilar pons. This explanation is less attractive since the corticopontine projection tends to be displaced from the midline in normal animals, whereas medial lemniscal axons from the dorsal column nuclei terminate densely in the most medial part of the basilar pons. This midline lemniscal input is intact in the experimental animals.

Taken together, the in vitro and in vivo evidence presented here indicates that in the developing brain, the basilar pons becomes innervated by controlling at a distance the budding and directed ingrowth of cortical axon collaterals through the release of a diffusible molecule. Whether collateral branches extended to other subcortical targets of layer-5 neurons are formed in response to diffusible, chemotropic signals remains to be determined.

Role of the Growth Cones of the Primary Axons of Layer-5 Neurons

Since the growth cones of primary layer-5 axons play no role in target selection, what role do they have in the development of layer-5 projections? The answer to this question may be found in the cortex, itself. Layer 5 contains a heterogeneous population of neurons, including two major classes of projection neurons: those that project subcortically and those that send an axon through the corpus callosum to the contralateral cortex. In adult rats, callosal and subcortically projecting neurons are separate populations (Catsman-Berrevoets et al. 1980). We have confirmed this adult segregation and examined its development using double labeling with retrograde fluorescent dyes (Koester and O'Leary 1989). In the same animals, Fast Blue was injected into the pyramidal decussation to label retrogradely layer-5 subcortically projecting neurons through their primary, spinally directed axon, and Diamidino Yellow was injected into the contralateral cortex to label retrogradely callosal neurons. In the noninjected cortex of adults, all neurons are single-labeled, confirming that callosal and subcortically projecting neurons are two distinct projection classes (Fig. 10A).

We then addressed the means by which these two projection populations become segregated during development. One possibility is that layer-5 neurons initially establish both connections and then lose one or the other. Large numbers of neurons in both neuronal populations, callosal and subcortically projecting, have been demonstrated to lose their long axon selectively during postnatal development (Innocenti 1981; O'Leary et al. 1981; Ivy and Killackey 1982; Stanfield et al. 1982). To test whether long transient collaterals to both targets are initially extended with one or the other subsequently eliminated, we applied the double retrograde labeling paradigm to neonatal rats prior to the described elimination of transient callosal and subcortical axons. Figure 10, C and D, shows the radial distribution of the labeled neurons. Fast-Blue-labeled subcortically projecting cells are located exclusively in layer 5, and Diamidino-Yellow-labeled callosal neurons

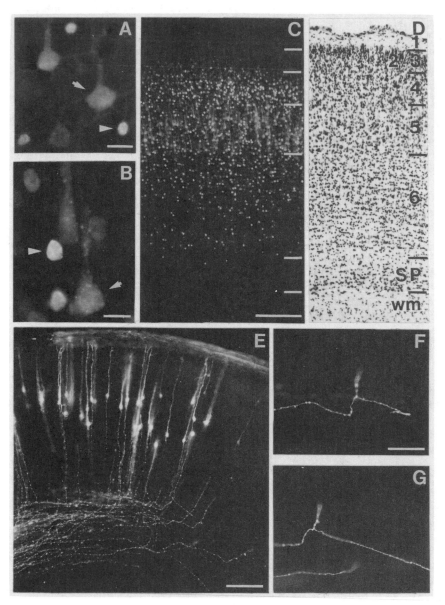

Figure 10. Connectional distinctions between callosal and subcortically projecting layer-5 neurons. (*A–D*) Fast Blue was injected into the spinomedullary junction to label the primary, spinally directed axon of subcortically projecting layer-5 neurons; Diamidino Yellow was injected into contralateral cortex to label callosally projecting neurons. (*A*) Retrogradely labeled layer-5 neurons in an adult rat. (*B*) Layer-5 neurons labeled in a P5 rat. In *A* and *B*, arrowheads mark Diamidino-Yellow-labeled nuclei and arrows mark Fast-Blue-labeled cell bodies. (*C*) A low-power view of the laminar distribution of callosal neurons and layer-5 subcortically projecting neurons in a P5 rat. (*D*) The same section as in *C* after Nissl staining. Cortical layers are marked on *C* and *D*. Fast-Blue-labeled (subcortically projecting) neurons are restricted to layer 5; Diamidino Yellow (callosal) neurons are present throughout the layers 4, 5, and 6. At this age, although unlike at later ages, few callosal cells are labeled in the still differentiating layers 2/3. (*E*) A coronal section from an E19 rat. Neurons that sent an axon through the corpus callosum were retrogradely filled with DiI injected into the contralateral cortex after the brain was aldehyde-fixed. On the basis of their position and developmental state, these neurons are layer 5/6 neurons. The corpus callosum is to the left (medially). Dorsal is to the top. (*F, G*) Branching axons of neurons filled with DiI in E19 (*F*) and E21 (*G*) aldehyde-fixed brains. The process to the left is the main axon that extends through the corpus callosum. The process extending to the right is a laterally directed branch. In *G*, the branch extends laterally to end in an another cortical region on the same side. Bars: (*A*) 20 μm; (*B*) 10 μm; (*C, D, E*) 200 μm; (*F, G*) 50 μm.

are distributed throughout layers 2–6. Cells single-labeled with one or the other dye are intermingled within layer 5 (Fig. 10B). However, neurons are not double-labeled. Thus, individual neurons do not extend long axons both callosally and subcortically.

Short axon collaterals that do not reach the dye-injection sites, however, would go undetected in these

experiments. Therefore, we have used the fluorescent axon tracer DiI to fill projection neurons in aldehyde-fixed brains of late-stage fetuses and early postnatal rats. Large injections of DiI were made into one cortical hemisphere. The noninjected hemisphere of cortex was later examined for the presence of retrogradely filled callosal neurons with axon branches extending into the internal capsule, the pathway through which axons exit cortex to subcortical targets. Figure 10E shows a representative E19 case, an age shortly after cortical axons cross the corpus callosum, and a few days after layer-5 axons first exit the cortex. Many of the cells labeled at this age are likely to be layer-5 neurons, since more superficial cells have yet to extend axons to the contralateral cortex. Axons arising from these labeled cells grow ventrally into the intermediate zone, turn sharply, and extend toward and through the corpus callosum. Some callosal axons extend branches laterally to other parts of the ipsilateral cortex (Fig. 10F,G), but none ever enter the internal capsule. Thus, even at early stages of axon extension in this system, the callosal projection is segregated from the subcortical one.

The connectional distinctions seen between callosal and layer-5 subcortically projecting neurons in the adult are apparent at early stages of axon elongation. These early connectional distinctions establish that callosal and subcortically projecting populations of cortical neurons comprise two distinct classes of projection neurons. Although both callosal and subcortically projecting neurons extend axon collaterals to more targets than they will retain, the sets of distant targets to which they initially project are separate and are appropriate targets for that specific class of cortical neuron. Since both classes are found in layer 5, they are likely generated at the same stage of development and are presumably exposed to the same sets of cues for axon pathfinding. Therefore, the growth cones of callosally and subcortically projecting neurons must respond differentially to cues associated with their common growth substrate. These differential responses are the basis of a neuron's "decision" to send an axon across the corpus callosum or out of cortex through the internal capsule. Indeed, as described earlier (Fig. 6), cortical growth cones have transiently complicated morphologies within this decision region of their pathway, an indication in other systems that a growth cone is making a targeting decision (Tosney and Landmesser 1985; Bovolenta and Mason 1987). The decision of layer-5 axons to exit the cortex is likely mediated by local guidance cues associated with their pathway or possibly by an earlier growing population of axons extended by cortical subplate neurons (McConnell et al. 1989; De Carlos and O'Leary 1990). We conclude that the major role of the growth cone of a subcortically projecting, layer-5 neuron is to direct its primary axon into the internal capsule and then to continue an undeviated growth spinally along a single, prominent tract.

SUMMARY

We have described our studies of the development of projections from layer 5 of the rat neocortex to subcortical targets in the midbrain and hindbrain. The major points are briefly summarized here.

1. Layer-5 neurons extend a primary axon out of cortex and along a spinally directed trajectory, bypassing all of their targets in the midbrain and hindbrain. These targets are later contacted exclusively by collaterals formed by a delayed interstitial branching of the primary axon, not by growth cone bifurcation.

2. Collateral branches only form at stereotypic positions, not randomly along the length of the axon. Thus, specific cues identify branch points, and the length of the primary axon well behind its growth cone responds to these cues.

3. Layer-5 neurons in diverse areas of cortex initially develop the same basic set of collateral branches, although they will permanently retain different subsets of the initial common set. Therefore, branch cues are recognized by layer-5 neurons independent of whether the collateral projection formed is functionally appropriate for the cortical region in which the neuron resides.

4. In vitro and in vivo evidence indicates that one of the major branches, which forms the corticopontine projection, is induced and directed into its target, the basilar pons, by a diffusible, target-derived, tropic signal. Thus, a chemotropic cue promotes recognition of the basilar pontine target by the primary layer-5 axons.

5. In this system, then, target selection is not the responsibility of the growth cone of the primary axon. On the basis of morphological changes and growth trajectory of the growth cones of primary layer-5 axons, we conclude that their major role is to direct the axons out of cortex and maintain an undeviated growth down a single, common path.

ACKNOWLEDGMENTS

We thank Brad Schlaggar for his helpful comments on the manuscript. The work summarized here was supported by National Institutes of Health grant EY-07025 from the National Eye Institute, the McKnight Endowment Fund for Neuroscience, and the Alfred P. Sloan Foundation. J.A.D. was supported by a Spanish predoctoral fellowship from the Ministero de Educacion y Ciencia, and S.E.K. was supported by a National Science Foundation predoctoral fellowship.

REFERENCES

Acklin, S.E. and J.G. Nicholls. 1990. Intrinsic and extrinsic factors influencing properties and growth patterns of identified leech neurons in culture. *J. Neurosci.* **10:** 1082.

Altman, J. and S.A. Bayer. 1978. Prenatal development of the cerebellar system in the rat-cytogenesis and histogenesis of the inferior olive, pontine gray, and the precerebellar reticular nuclei. *J. Comp. Neurol.* **179:** 49.

Bentley, D. and M. Caudy. 1983. Navigational substrates for peripheral pioneer growth cones: Limb-axis polarity cues, limb-segment boundaries, and guidepost neurons. *Cold Spring Harbor Symp. Quant. Biol.* **48:** 573.

Bicknese, A.R. and D.D.M. O'Leary. 1990. Axon targeting potentials of layer-5 projection neurons across the developing cortex. *Soc. Neurosci. Abstr.* **16:** 311.

Bovolenta, P. and C. Mason. 1987. Growth cone morphology varies with position in the developing mouse visual pathway from retina to first targets. *J. Neurosci.* **7:** 1447.

Bray, D. 1973. Branching patterns of individual sympathetic neurons in culture. *J. Cell Biol.* **56:** 702.

Bruckner, G., V. Mares, and D. Bieshold. 1976. Neurogenesis in the visual system of the rat. An autoradiographic investigation. *J. Comp. Neurol.* **166:** 245.

Catsman-Berrevoets, C.E., R.N. Lemon, C.A. Verburgh, M. Bentivoglio, and H.G.J.M. Kuypers. 1980. Absence of callosal collaterals derived from rat corticospinal neurons. *Exp. Brain Res.* **39:** 433.

D'Amato, C.J. and S.P. Hicks. 1980. Development of the motor system: Effects of radiation on developing corticospinal neurons and locomotor function. *Exp. Neurol.* **70:** 1.

Dodd, J. and T.M. Jessell. 1988. Axon guidance and the patterning of neuronal projections in vertebrates. *Science* **242:** 692.

De Carlos, J.A. and D.D.M. O'Leary. 1990. Subplate neurons "pioneer" the output pathway of rat cortex but not pathways to brainstem or spinal targets. *Soc. Neurosci. Abstr.* **16:** 311.

Godement, P., J. Vanselow, S. Thanos, and F. Bonhoeffer. 1987. A study in developing nervous systems with a new method of staining neurones and their processes in fixed tissue. *Development* **101:** 697.

Hamburger, V. 1988. Ontogeny of neuroembryology. *J. Neurosci.* **8:** 3535.

Heffner, C.D. and D.D.M. O'Leary. 1990. Chemotropic induction of axon collateral branch formation by target tissue in vitro. *Soc. Neurosci. Abstr.* **16:** 151.

Heffner, C.D., A.G.S. Lumsden, and D.D.M. O'Leary. 1990. Target control of collateral extension and directional axon growth in the mammalian brain. *Science* **247:** 217.

Honig, M.G. and R.I. Hume. 1986. Fluorescent carbocyanine dyes allow living neurons of identified origin to be studied in long-term cultures. *J. Cell Biol.* **103:** 171.

Innocenti, G.M. 1981. Growth and reshaping of axons in the establishment of visual callosal connections. *Science* **212:** 824.

Ivy, G.O. and H.P. Killackey. 1982. Ontogenetic changes in the projections of neocortical neurons. *J. Neurosci.* **2:** 735.

Jensen, K.F. and H.P. Killackey. 1984. Subcortical projections from ectopic neocortical neurons. *Proc. Natl. Acad. Sci.* **81:** 964.

Jones, E.G. 1984. Laminar distributions of cortical efferent cells. In *Cerebral cortex,* vol. 1: *Cellular components of the cerebral cortex* (ed. A. Peters and E.G. Jones), p. 521. Plenum Press, New York.

Koester, S.E. and D.D.M. O'Leary 1989. Selective axon growth not axon loss produces connectional distinctions between callosal and subcortically projecting layer 5 cortical neurons. *Soc. Neurosci. Abtsr.* **15:** 960.

Landmesser, L.T. 1984. The development of specific motor pathways in the chick embryo. *Trends Neurosci.* **7:** 336.

Lumsden, A.G.S. and A.M. Davies. 1983. Earliest sensory nerve fibers are guided to peripheral targets by attractants other than nerve growth factor. *Nature* **306:** 786.

———. 1986. Chemotropic effect of specific target epithelium in developing mammalian nervous system. *Nature* **323:** 538.

McConnell, S.K., A. Gosh, and C.J. Shatz. 1989. Subplate neurons pioneer the first axon pathway from the cerebral cortex. *Science* **245:** 978.

Missias, A., L.J. Kutka, B.S. Reinoso, and D.D.M. O'Leary. 1990. In vivo evidence for target control of collateral formation and directional axon growth in mammalian brain. *Soc. Neurosci. Abstr.* **16:** 311.

O'Leary, D.D.M. and B.B. Stanfield. 1985. Occipital cortical neurons with transient pyramidal tract axons extend and maintain collaterals to subcortical but not intracortical targets. *Brain Res.* **336:** 326.

———. 1989. Selective elimination of axons extended by developing cortical neurons is dependent on regional locale. Experiments utilizing fetal cortical transplants. *J Neurosci.* **9:** 2230.

O'Leary, D.D.M. and T. Terashima. 1988. Cortical axons branch to multiple subcortical targets by interstitial axon budding: Implications for target recognition and "waiting periods." *Neuron* **1:** 901.

———. 1989. Growth and branching of cortical axons: Implications for target selection by developing axons. *Soc. Neurosci. Abtsr.* **15:** 875.

O'Leary, D.D.M., B.B. Stanfield, and W.M. Cowan. 1981. Evidence that early postnatal restriction of the cells of origin of the callosal projection is due to the elimination of axonal collaterals rather than to the death of neurons. *Dev. Brain Res.* **1:** 607.

Purves, D. and J.W. Lichtman. 1985. *Principles of neural development.* A. Sinauer, Sunderland, Massachusetts.

Ramon y Cajal, S. 1894. *Les nouvelles idees sur la structure du systeme nerveux chez l'homme et chez vertebres.* Reinwald, Paris.

Raper, J.A., M. Bastiani, and C.S. Goodman. 1983. Pathfinding by neuronal growth cones in grasshopper embryos. I. Divergent choices made by the growth cones of sibling neurons. *J. Neurosci.* **3:** 20.

Sandell, J.H. and R.H. Masland. 1988. Photoconversion of some fluorescent markers to a diaminobenzidine product. *J. Histochem. Cytochem.* **36:** 555.

Shaw, G. and D. Bray. 1971. Movement and extension of isolated growth cones. *Exp. Cell Res.* **104:** 55.

Stanfield, B.B. and D.D.M. O'Leary. 1985a. The transient corticospinal projection from the occipital cortex during the postnatal development of the rat. *J. Comp. Neurol.* **238:** 236.

———. 1985b. Fetal occipital cortical neurons transplanted to the rostral cortex can extend and maintain a pyramidal tract axon. *Nature* **313:** 135.

Stanfield, B.B., D.D.M. O'Leary, and C. Fricks. 1982. Selective collateral elimination in early postnatal development restricts cortical distribution of rat pyramidal tract neurones. *Nature* **298:** 371.

Taghert, P.H., M.J. Bastiani, R.K. Ho, and G.S. Goodman. 1982. Guidance of pioneer growth cones: Filopodial contacts and coupling revealed with an antibody to lucifer yellow. *Dev. Biol.* **94:** 391.

Terashima, T. and D.D.M. O'Leary 1988. Quantitative analysis of the cortical distribution of pyramidal tract neurons in young and adult rats. *Anat. Rec.* **220:** 96A.

Tessier-Lavigne, M., M. Plackzek, A.G.S. Lumsden, J. Dodd, and T.M. Jessell. 1988. Chemotropic guidance of developing axons in the mammalian central nervous system. *Nature* **336:** 775.

Tosney, K.W. and L.T. Landmesser 1985. Growth cone morphology and trajectory in the lumbosacral region of the chick embryo. *J. Neurosci.* **5:** 2345.

Wessells, N.K. and R.P. Nuttall. 1978. Normal branching, induced branching, and steering of cultured parasympathetic motor neurons. *Exp. Cell Res.* **115:** 111.

Pioneer Neurons and Target Selection in Cerebral Cortical Development

C.J. Shatz, A. Ghosh, S.K. McConnell, K.L. Allendoerfer, E. Friauf, and A. Antonini

Department of Neurobiology, Stanford University School of Medicine, Stanford, California 94305-5401

The construction of any nervous system from that of the simplest invertebrate to that of the most complex mammal requires the solution of several major problems. Neurons must be generated in appropriate numbers and locations, axons must select correct pathways to their targets, and, once there, the appropriate patterns of connections must be formed. In invertebrates, many observations suggest that axonal pathways are laid down very early, when distances are small, as the axons of pioneer neurons navigate terrain traversed subsequently by appropriate subsets of later-generated axons (Goodman et al. 1984). The early formation of many axonal pathways also occurs in mammalian nervous system development. For example, in the adult visual system, retinal ganglion cells project to the lateral geniculate nucleus (LGN), which in turn projects to the neurons of layer 4 of the primary visual cortex. During development, ganglion cells and LGN neurons are generated at about the same time, and both sets of neurons immediately grow axonal projections toward their targets (Rakic 1977; Shatz 1983; Walsh et al. 1983; Hickey and Hitchcock 1984; Shatz and Luskin 1986), suggesting that, here too, connections are formed as early as possible in order to minimize the considerable problems of pathfinding and target selection posed by the progressive growth of the brain.

In the development of the mammalian cerebral cortex, an additional logistical complexity is added to the set of problems mentioned above. To produce the millions of neurons required for the adult cortex requires a very prolonged period of neurogenesis, lasting from weeks to months, depending on the species (rodents to primates). Neurons, once postmitotic, must also migrate over increasingly longer distances to reach their final locations within the cortical plate (for reviews, see Rakic 1975; McConnell 1988). Thus, unlike the retinal ganglion cells and LGN neurons, many cortical neurons are generated very late in development, often well after their targets have been formed and their axonal inputs have arrived. In this paper, we consider the logistical problem posed by the prolonged period of neurogenesis in the cortex, and we present evidence that the problem is solved in part by the construction of a transient neural scaffold early in development.

RESULTS AND DISCUSSION

Geniculocortical Axons Wait in the Subplate Prior to Invading the Cortical Plate

The temporal mismatch between cortical neurogenesis and incoming axonal projections is exemplified in the development of the geniculocortical projection system: Axons from the LGN arrive within the developing cerebral wall well before their ultimate target neurons in cortical layer 4 have completed migration and assumed their final position within the cortical plate just above the previously generated neurons of layers 5 and 6 (Lund and Mustari 1977; Rakic 1977; Shatz and Luskin 1986). In the cat's visual system, for example, anterograde tracing experiments using tritiated amino acids injected in vivo (Shatz and Luskin 1986) or the lipophilic tracer DiI injected in aldehyde-fixed brains (A. Ghosh and C.J. Shatz, in prep.) have shown that the growth cones of LGN axons have entered the internal capsule by embryonic day 30 (E30; gestation is 65 days in the cat). Axons grow through the intermediate zone (future white matter) of the cerebral cortical wall, and the first ones arrive just below the forming visual cortex at about E36. Then, rather than grow directly into the cortical plate, the majority of LGN axons accumulate within the intermediate zone immediately below the cortical plate; this zone is called the *subplate*. During the ensuing 2–3 weeks, vast numbers of LGN axons remain confined within the subplate until about E50, when a few can also be detected within layer 6 of the cortex. The accumulation of LGN axons within the subplate at E50 is shown in Figure 1. By about E55, massive numbers of LGN axons have invaded the cortical plate and some have arrived at last within layer 4. By birth, most axons have left the subplate and have extended significant branches within layer 4 (Shatz and Luskin 1986; for review, see Shatz et al. 1988; A. Ghosh and C.J. Shatz, unpubl.). Similar axonal "waiting periods" of different durations have been described in the development of the rodent (about 1 week: Lund and Mustari 1977) and primate (about 6 weeks: Rakic 1977) geniculocortical projection. In fact, such periods may be a common feature of cortical development, since they are also present in the de-

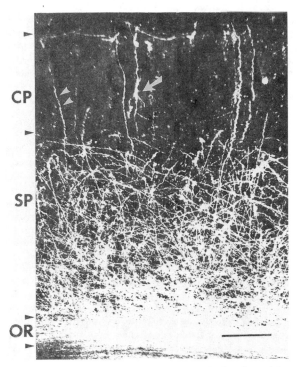

Figure 1. Pattern of labeling within the cerebral wall resulting from an injection of DiI into the LGN of an aldehyde-fixed cat brain at E50. Many geniculocortical axons are labeled as they run within the optic radiations (OR) and then fan out to enter the subplate (SP). At this age, very few axons leave the subplate to enter the cortical plate (CP) and those that do so either traverse the CP entirely without branching (double arrowheads) to enter the marginal zone or have just entered the base of layer 6. The somata and dendrites of an occasional retrogradely labeled pyramidal cell can also be seen (arrow). Bar, 200 μm.

velopment of the axonal projection from somatosensory (Wise et al. 1977) and auditory (A. Ghosh and C.J. Shatz, unpubl.) thalamus and in the development of interhemispheric connections via the corpus callosum (Wise and Jones 1978; Innocenti 1981).

At present, it is not known why ingrowing axonal systems accumulate within the subplate and wait before invading the cortical plate. However, tritiated thymidine birth-dating studies have shown that at E36 in the cat, when the first LGN axons have just arrived, the cortex itself consists only of future layer 6 (Luskin and Shatz 1985a). The first neurons belonging to cortical layer 4 are not generated within the ventricular zone of the lateral ventricle until about E37 and do not complete their migrations to the cortical plate until about E52 (Shatz and Luskin 1986; for review, see Shatz et al. 1988). Thus, it may be that axons wait within the subplate until their target neurons have completed migrating and assumed their final position within the appropriate cortical layer.

The existence of significant axonal waiting periods raises the important question of how axons can "wait," or for that matter even survive, in the absence of their adult neuronal targets. To understand the mechanisms responsible for this exceptional behavior, it is essential to learn more about the cellular environment of the

zone in which the axons wait: the subplate. Here, we present evidence that the subplate contains a set of the earliest-generated neurons of the cerebral cortex. Subplate neurons pioneer the first axon pathways between cortex and subcortical targets, they mature to participate in complex neural circuits well before the neurons of the adult cortical layers, and they are required for the normal development of connections between LGN axons and layer 4 cortical neurons. Then, most are eliminated by programmed cell death. These observations suggest that subplate neurons play an essential but transient role in cerebral cortical development.

The First Postmitotic Neurons of the Cerebral Cortex Are the Subplate and Marginal Zone Neurons

The cerebral cortex, like other parts of the mammalian central nervous system (CNS), arises as postmitotic neurons migrate away from a germinal zone at the ventricular surface: the ventricular zone. Tritiated thymidine birth-dating studies have shown that neurons comprising the cortical layers are generated sequentially, with those constituting the deepest cortical layer (layer 6) generated first and those occupying the most superficial cellular layers (layers 2 and 3) generated last (for review, see McConnell 1988). In the cat, cortical neurogenesis extends from E30 to E57. However, [³H]thymidine given at any time during the week prior to E30 labels a very small population of cells located either in the white matter below the cortex or in layer 1 just under the pial surface, but no labeled cells are present within the adult cortical layers (Luskin and Shatz 1985a). Thus, the neurons of the adult cortical layers are not the first neurons to leave the mitotic cycle and migrate away from the ventricular zone.

To learn more about these early-generated cells, [³H]thymidine was given at times between E24 and E28, which labels these cells exclusively without involving the neurons of cortical layer 6; the migration and position of these cells were examined autoradiographically at subsequent fetal or neonatal ages (Luskin and Shatz 1985b). The results of these experiments are summarized in Figure 2. By E30, many early-generated cells have already migrated away from the ventricular zone to assume initial positions immediately beneath the pial surface within the marginal and intermediate zones. By E40, the early-generated population has been split into two regions—the marginal zone and the subplate—due to the subsequent genesis and migration of the neurons that will belong to the deeper cellular layers (layers 5 and 6) of the adult cortex. By birth, the cortical plate has thickened further as neurogenesis ceases and migration to the superficial cortical layers nears completion; many [³H]thymidine-labeled subplate and marginal zone cells persist at this age. In contrast, by about 2 months postnatal, very few early-generated cells remain, based on the presence of [³H]thymidine labeling. As discussed below, we believe that many of the early-generated cells are eliminated by cell death.

These observations indicate that the pattern of gene-

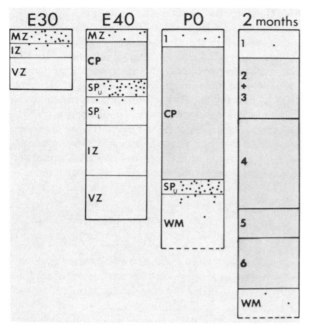

Figure 2. Summary diagram of the developmental history of the earliest generated cells (●) of the cat's visual cortex. These cells undergo their last round of DNA synthesis and cell division between E24 and E30, and by E30, some have already completed their migration away from the ventricular zone (VZ) to assemble in a loose "preplate" within the marginal and intermediate zones (MZ, IZ). By E40, as the later-generated cells of the adult cortical plate (CP) insert themselves, this early-generated population is split apart into one group that resides in the MZ and another that resides below the CP in the subplate (SP$_u$ = upper part of the subplate; SP$_l$ = lower part). By birth (P0), the cortical plate has thickened further, and the early-generated cells are still present in large numbers within the SP and MZ. However, by 2 months postnatal, many have disappeared, the intermediate zone has matured into the white matter (WM), and the cortical plate has matured into the six-layered cortex. (Reprinted, with permission, from Luskin and Shatz 1985b.)

sis of the cerebral cortex does not follow a strict inside-first, outside-last gradient. Rather, the adult cortical layers are initially sandwiched between an earlier-generated cell population that disappears, as judged from [³H]thymidine labeling. Furthermore, since [³H]thymidine given before E24 does not result in heavily labeled cells anywhere in the telencephalon, the cells produced between E24 and E30 are the first post-mitotic cells of the neocortex (Luskin and Shatz 1985a,b). In view of their early birth dates and their appropriate location within the waiting zone, the subplate cells could interact with early-arriving geniculocortical axons, perhaps acting as temporary targets, until the final targets, the neurons of cortical layer 4, are generated and complete their migrations. The possibility that there are interactions between subplate cells and afferent axons will be considered more fully below.

Most, if not all, of the early-generated population residing in the subplate and marginal zones are neurons. Because neurons belonging to the adult cortical layers 2–6 are generated only after E30 in the cat, it is possible to identify the early-generated population un-

ambiguously using [³H]thymidine injections given any time between E24 and E28. Cells were therefore tagged on their birth dates with [³H]thymidine and later immunostained with neuron-specific antibodies such as those against neurotransmitters, neuropeptides, or cytoskeletal constituents, such as microtubule-associated protein 2 (MAP2), which is located only in the somata and dendrites of neurons. Many subplate and marginal zone cells marked with [³H]thymidine could also be labeled with antibodies against neuropeptide Y (NPY), choleocystokinin, somatostatin, glutamic acid decarboxylase (GAD), or GABA; virtually all [³H]thymidine-labeled subplate and marginal zone cells could be double-labeled with MAP2 (Chun et al. 1987; Chun and Shatz 1989a).

At present, we cannot say with certainty whether a similar pattern of neurogenesis is present in the neocortex of all mammals, although we consider it most likely. The uncertainty arises because strictly analogous birth-dating experiments have not been performed in other mammals. For instance, in primates, Kostovic and Rakic (1980) examined adult animals and found that early injections of [³H]thymidine labels cells both in layer 6 and in the white matter. We would predict that still earlier injections would have labeled exclusively cells in the white matter and layer 1, particularly if older fetal or neonatal animals were examined (rather than adults). In rodents, the extremely rapid pace of cortical neurogenesis (days, versus weeks in cats and monkeys) makes it difficult in principle to obtain the time resolution necessary to detect an early-generated population that is spatially distinct from the cortical plate, since a single pulse of [³H]thymidine always labels cells located within more than one cortical layer (see, e.g., Miller 1988). Nevertheless, it should be possible to determine the earliest time at which [³H]thymidine labels the cells of the fetal neocortex, and then by examining some of these labeled animals at subsequent times during fetal life through adulthood, to determine whether a substantial proportion of the population disappears. Unfortunately, despite recent studies of neurogenesis in rodent neocortex (see, e.g., Bayer and Altman 1990), this exact sequence of necessary experiments has not been performed. However, a recent study by Al-Ghoul and Miller (1989) suggests that of the rat neocortical cells generated at E12, few remain by about 3 weeks postnatal. Thus, cells generated at this time could be subplate neurons in view of their early birth date, location at the base of the cortical plate, and disappearance in postnatal life. The issues of whether these cells are in fact the first generated, and whether most disappear by adulthood as in the cat, or rather remain as constituents of layer 6b in rodents, are still unresolved.

Subplate Neurons Undergo Programmed Cell Death

As shown in Figure 2, many of the early-generated cells disappear by about 2 months postnatal in the cat, as judged from the loss of the [³H]thymidine tag. This observation raises the possibility that subplate neurons are eliminated by cell death during the neonatal period. Several lines of evidence strongly support this possibility. Valverde and Facal-Valverde (1988) have observed at the electron microscopic level degenerating neurons in the subplate of the temporal lobe of the neonatal cat; these neurons resemble morphologically many of the subplate neurons that we have studied using immuno-histochemical staining techniques (see, e.g., Chun and Shatz 1989a,b). Kostovic and Rakic (1980) have made similar observations in the monkey neocortex. Moreover, the density of subplate neurons immunostained for neuropeptides or for MAP2 decreases dramatically during the immediate postnatal period (Chun and Shatz 1989b). For example, the density of MAP2-immunoreactive neurons remaining in the white matter of the lateral gyrus (immediately below cat visual cortex) at 25 weeks postnatal is only about 15% of that present at birth, and due to the techniques used, we believe this to be a conservative estimate (see Chun and Shatz 1989b). In contrast, the area of the white matter increases by about twofold at most. Thus, it is not possible to account for the fall in subplate neuron number entirely on the basis of dilution by growth. Nor is it likely that subplate neurons down-regulate the expression of MAP2 (as is possible for the neuro-peptides), since MAP2 is a stable cytoskeletal marker. The most reasonable interpretation of these observations is that a large proportion of the subplate neurons, perhaps as much as 80–90% in visual cortex, are eliminated by cell death during the immediate postnatal period. Combined [³H]thymidine labeling and im-munohistochemistry have shown that the remaining MAP2 and neuropeptide-immunoreactive neurons persist within the white matter to adulthood (Chun and Shatz 1989b), to become the interstitial neurons of Cajal (Ramon y Cajal 1911; Kostovic and Rakic 1980).

The cellular mechanisms responsible for the death of subplate neurons are not known. The time of onset of cell death, however, is correlated with the period during which thalamocortical axons leave the subplate and grow into cortical layer 4, as shown in the time lines of Figure 3 (see also Shatz et al. 1988), raising the possibility that interactions between waiting axons and sub-plate neurons may be critical in regulating the survival of subplate neurons. However, it is equally possible that subplate neurons begin to die first, thereby permit-ting the "waiting" axons to leave the subplate and enter the cortical plate. At present, these alternatives cannot be distinguished; nor is it currently known whether, by analogy with insect nervous system development (Fahr-bach and Truman 1987), global hormonal changes, perhaps such as those associated with birth, might trig-ger the death of subplate neurons entirely indepen-dent of interactions with waiting afferent axonal systems.

Recently, we (Allendoerfer et al. 1990) discovered that subplate neurons express immunoreactivity for the nerve growth factor (NGF) receptor, raising the addi-tional possibility that dependence on NGF or a related molecule (Maisonpierre et al. 1990; Rodriguez-Tebar et al. 1990) may regulate the survival and subsequent death of these cells. Throughout development, virtually all immunostaining for the NGF receptor in the cat and ferret neocortex is associated with subplate neurons. Immunostaining can be detected as early as E30 in the cat, just after the first subplate neurons become post-mitotic and postmigratory. As shown in Figure 3, levels of immunostaining remain high until about E50, when

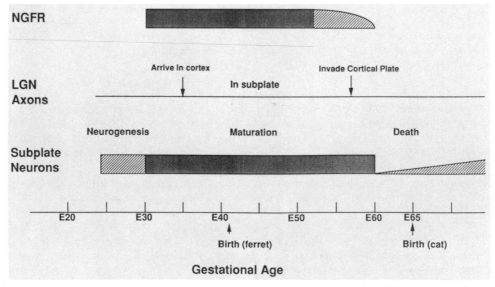

Figure 3. Time lines for three separate developmental events in cat visual cortex. (*Top*) Time course of appearance and disappearance of subplate neuron immunostaining for the nerve growth factor receptor (NGFR). Hatching indicates a decline in staining intensity. (*Middle*) Time course of development of the geniculocortical projection (LGN axons). (*Bottom*) Life history of subplate neurons is summarized. They are generated between E24 and E30 (hatching), mature anatomically and functionally between E30 and E60, and then begin to die in increasing numbers (hatched ramp) thereafter.

staining intensity begins to decline; by E60, immuno-staining is undetectable despite the continued presence of many subplate neurons. Loss of the NGF receptor is closely followed by death of subplate neurons beginning about 1 week thereafter, suggesting that receptor loss could be the first step in a cascade of events that eventually leads to programmed cell death.

Subplate Neurons Express Neurotransmitter Phenotypes and Function in Synaptic Microcircuits during Fetal Life

During the month-long period between E30, after most subplate neurons have migrated away from the ventricular zone to take up their locations below the forming cortical plate, and birth, when they begin to die, subplate neurons differentiate and participate in complex neural circuits. As mentioned above, these neurons, along with their cogenerated counterparts in the marginal zone, express immunoreactivity for GAD, GABA, and several neuropeptides (Chun et al. 1987; Wahle and Meyer 1987; Chun and Shatz 1989a; for review, see Shatz et al. 1988). Many subplate neurons

can be immunostained for somatostatin or NPY during fetal life well before neurons of the cortical plate become immunoreactive. Moreover, there appears to be a relationship between radial position and neuropeptide phenotype: Those subplate neurons located at the base of the cortical plate tend to be immunoreactive for somatostatin, whereas the majority of NPY-immunoreactive subplate neurons tend to reside in deeper portions of the subplate (Chun and Shatz 1989a).

Results from many separate anatomical experiments indicate that the processes of subplate neurons during fetal and neonatal life make extensive local ramifications, both within the subplate and directly above within the cortical plate (see Figs. 4 and 6) (Marin-Padilla 1972; Wahle and Meyer 1987; Chun and Shatz 1989a; Friauf et al. 1990; for review, see Shatz et al. 1988). By means of retrograde tracing, we also discovered that subplate neurons can extend axons to distant targets, including the opposite hemisphere (Chun et al. 1987), and the thalamus and superior colliculus (McConnell et al. 1989). Some of these morphological features of subplate neurons in the cat are shown at E50 in Figure 4. Thus, subplate neurons resemble the neurons of the

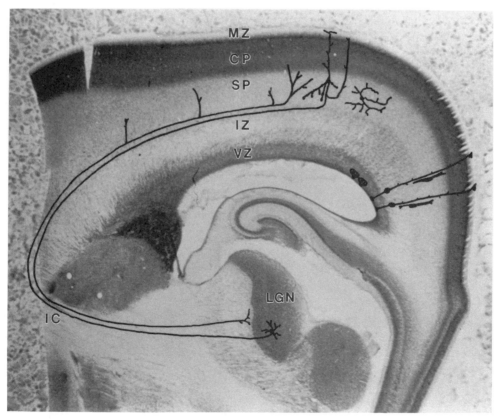

Figure 4. A cartoon-photograph showing the cellular constituents of the developing wall of the cerebral hemisphere and the relationship between subplate (SP) neurons and geniculocortical axons at about 2 weeks before birth in the cat (E50). One LGN neuron is shown sending its axon to the subplate below visual cortex. A generic subplate neuron sends a long projecting axon back to the LGN and also a recurrent collateral into the cortical plate (CP). Both sets of axons travel within the intermediate zone (IZ) of the cerebral wall and traverse the internal capsule (IC) to reach the thalamus. A local circuit subplate neuron is also shown. Other constituents of the intermediate zone include radial glial cells and migrating neurons (right). Based on Marin-Padilla (1971), Rakic (1975), Shatz and Luskin (1986), McConnell et al. (1989), Friauf et al. (1990), and Antonini and Shatz (1990). (MZ) Marginal zone; (VZ) ventricular zone. See text for further details.

adult cortical layers in that they can be either local circuit or projection neurons.

Together, these observations raised the question of whether, as in the adult cerebral cortex, there is a relationship between the neurotransmitter phenotype and the axonal projection pattern of subplate neurons. In the adult, interneurons are immunoreactive for GABA and frequently colocalize a neuropeptide such as somatostatin, NPY, or CCK (Hendry et al. 1984; Somogyi et al. 1984), whereas at least some projection neurons are likely to use excitatory amino acids (Baughman and Gilbert 1981; Dori et al. 1989). To investigate whether subplate neurons exhibit similar subtypes, we (Antonini and Shatz 1990) injected retrograde tracers into the subplate, cortical plate, or distant targets such as the thalamus or opposite hemisphere and then immunostained sections for various neuropeptides (NPY, somatostatin). Results indicated that at least some of the local circuit subplate neurons are peptide-immunoreactive, whereas subplate neurons with long projections are not. Rather, subplate neurons with thalamic or interhemispheric projections could be retrogradely labeled with [³H]aspartate, indicating that, like the neurons of the cortical plate later on, they too may use an excitatory amino acid as a transmitter

(Baughman and Gilbert 1981; Streit 1980). These observations suggest that the subplate exhibits basic features of cortical organization later echoed in the layers of the adult cerebral cortex.

As described above, several different sets of observations indicate that subplate neurons achieve a high degree of morphological maturity during the developmental period preceding the onset of programmed cell death. (And those subplate neurons that survive the period of cell death retain at least some of their characteristic transmitter phenotypes into adulthood; see Chun and Shatz 1989b.) In addition, subplate neurons receive synaptic contacts (Chun et al. 1987), an observation that illuminates previous ultrastructural studies showing that the first synapses to form in the telencephalon are found early in fetal life within the subplate (and marginal zone), well before synapses can be detected within the cortical plate (Molliver et al. 1973; Cragg 1975; Kostovic and Rakic 1980; Chun and Shatz 1988a). Thus, the subplate is a synaptic neuropil during development, with subplate neurons acting as postsynaptic partners to presynaptic inputs, whose origins are currently unknown. There are, however, several likely candidates, including the axonal processes of other subplate neurons and afferent axonal systems

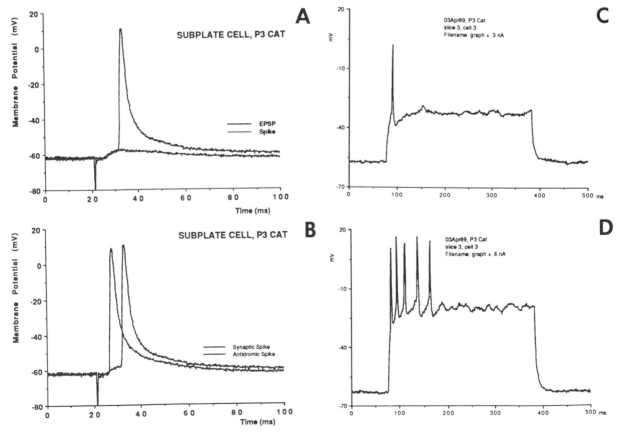

Figure 5. Intracellular microelectrode recordings in vitro from a subplate neuron identified by filling it with biocytin at postnatal day 3 (P3) in the cat. (*A, B*) Electrical stimulation of the optic radiations evoke orthodromic and antidromic (at higher threshold: *B*) action potentials or synaptic potentials (at low threshold: *A*). (*C, D*) Action potentials evoked by different levels of intracellular current injection. This particular neuron fired a single action potential at low levels of depolarization (*C*) and several spikes that adapted at higher levels (*D*). (Modified from Friauf et al. 1990.)

such as the thalamocortical axons that are waiting in the subplate. Definitive identification of the presynaptic elements requires that they be labeled selectively and studied at the electron microscopic level. In the case of the thalamic axons, this poses a significant problem since the thalamus and subplate are reciprocally connected during development, as shown in Figure 4. Consequently, the injection of any tracer that labels the waiting axons anterogradely will also label the axons and recurrent collaterals of subplate neurons by means of retrograde transport, making a conclusive identification of a labeled presynaptic terminal difficult.

The above observations suggest that the anatomical substrates for functional synaptic interactions are present within the subplate early in fetal life. To investigate whether subplate neurons are capable of firing action potentials and whether they receive functional synaptic inputs, we made intracellular microelectrode recordings from subplate neurons in slices of fetal and neonatal cat visual cortex maintained in vitro (Friauf et al. 1990). Stimulating electrodes were placed in the intermediate zone in the approximate location where thalamocortical axons arising from the LGN are known to travel (the optic radiations; see Fig. 1). Biocytin was injected into each neuron in order to verify its identity as a subplate neuron on the basis of its location beneath the cortical plate. As early as E50, subplate neurons received excitatory postsynaptic potentials and fired action potentials to electrical stimulation of the optic

radiations, indicating that some of the synapses seen in the electron microscope are indeed capable of functional transmission. Recordings from a subplate neuron studied at postnatal day 3 are shown in Figure 5. This neuron is typical of those recorded in that it receives synaptic input (Fig. 5A), fires orthodromic and antidromic action potentials (Fig. 5B), and has a characteristic spiking pattern to intracellularly applied current (Fig. 5C,D).

Biocytin injections into recorded subplate neurons revealed that they are a morphologically heterogeneous population with respect to their dendritic branching patterns (Friauf et al. 1990). About half were inverted pyramids, the classic subplate neuron morphology (Chun et al. 1987; Chun and Shatz 1989a; McConnell et al. 1989), and others were fusiform in appearance. The axonal arborization patterns of subplate neurons were remarkable in that they not only branched within the subplate, but many entered the cortical plate and terminated within the marginal zone and cortical layer 4, particularly at older fetal and neonatal ages. An example of such a cell at postnatal day 1 is shown in Figure 6. The presence of axonal processes within both subplate and cortical plate suggests that subplate neurons could establish a neural scaffold or framework in which cellular elements of the adult cerebral cortex develop.

In sum, the results of these anatomical and physiological experiments indicate that subplate neurons can function in transient microcircuits during development.

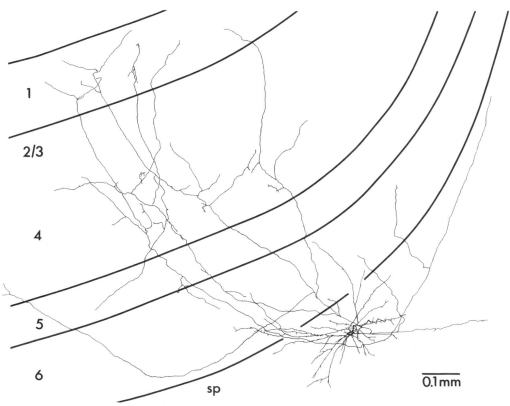

Figure 6. Reconstruction of a biocytin-injected subplate neuron at P1 beneath the cat's visual cortex. The dendrites of this cell are almost exclusively confined to the subplate, whereas the axon branches not only within the subplate, but also extensively within the cortical plate. Note the collaterals given off within layers 1 and 4. (Modified from Friauf et al. 1990.)

They receive synaptic inputs, some of which may be supplied by the waiting thalamocortical axons. Some axonal projections of subplate neurons are made to the cortical plate above, raising the possibility that they might send direct inputs to developing cortical neurons, especially to those of layer 4. Thus, subplate neurons may function as a crucial but transient synaptic link between developing thalamic axons and their ultimate target cells in the cortex. In view of the observations that fetal retinal ganglion cells are spontaneously active (Galli and Maffei 1988), and that retinogeniculate transmission is operational in utero (Shatz and Kirkwood 1984), we consider it quite likely that visual subplate neurons are also spontaneously active. If so, then the proper functioning of this circuit during fetal development, driven by spontaneously evoked action potential activity, could be required for the normal formation of connections between thalamus and cortex well before the familiar activity-dependent sorting of geniculocortical axons to form the system of ocular dominance columns takes place postnatally (Stryker and Harris 1986).

Subplate Neurons Pioneer the First Axon Pathways from the Cerebral Cortex

The fact that subplate neurons belong to the first postmitotic population of the neocortex and that they have long-distance axonal projections to the thalamus, superior colliculus, and opposite hemisphere made us wonder whether the axons of subplate neurons might form the initial pathways to some or all of these targets very early in development, when distances are short and the problems of pathfinding and target selection are at a minimum. To investigate this possibility, we took advantage of the unique birth dates of subplate neurons and performed anterograde and retrograde labeling experiments at times before the neurons of the adult cortical layers were present. Following their migration away from the ventricular zone, the first postmitotic neurons take up positions just below the pial surface, where they form a loose layer of cells known as the "preplate" or the primordial plexiform layer (Marin-Padilla 1971). At E30 in the cat, this layer is made up exclusively of cells that will later reside either in the subplate or in the marginal zone, since the cells that belong to the adult cortical layers are just being generated at the ventricular surface at this time (see Fig. 2) (Luskin and Shatz 1985a,b). Therefore, we first injected the lipophilic tracer DiI directly into the wall of the cerebral hemisphere in aldehyde-fixed brains at E30 in order to label anterogradely the axons of any neurons projecting out of the cortex (McConnell et al. 1989). After injections into the lateral wall of the cerebral hemisphere, DiI-labeled axons could be traced within the intermediate zone as they traveled toward and traversed the internal capsule to enter the thalamus. In contrast, at E26, no axons could be traced into the thalamus (nor could any thalamic neurons be retrogradely labeled). Thus, the axons labeled at E30

must indeed traverse this pathway first, suggesting that they are pioneers in the sense originally defined from studies in insect nervous systems (Bate 1976; Bentley and Keshishian 1982; Ho and Goodman 1982).

To learn which cortical neurons supply the pioneering axons, DiI was placed in the thalamus or internal capsule at E30 in order to label retrogradely any neurons that may have sent axons from cortex to thalamus (McConnell et al. 1989). As shown in Figure 7, neurons situated in the preplate within the lateral wall of the cerebral hemisphere were retrogradely labeled, indicating that the early-generated population indeed sends axons to the thalamus even before neurons of the adult cortical layers are generated. Because, at later times, only subplate (and not marginal zone) neurons can be retrogradely labeled by similar thalamic injections, we believe that this early projection is formed primarily if not exclusively by the axons of the subplate neurons. The results of the anterograde and retrograde labeling experiments taken together indicate that the axons of subplate neurons pioneer pathways between thalamus and cortex. In view of the fact that subplate neurons in older animals can be retrogradely labeled by injections into the superior colliculus or opposite hemisphere, it could be that these and other long-distance cortical projection pathways are also pioneered by the axons of subplate neurons.

By forming these first subcortical axons, subplate neurons may help to solve a major logistical problem of cerebral cortical development: How to form appropri-

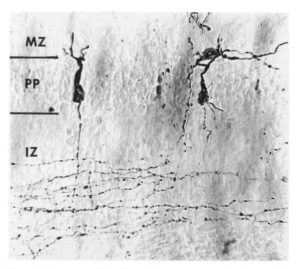

Figure 7. Pattern of labeling within the cerebral wall resulting from an injection of DiI into the internal capsule in an aldehyde-fixed cat brain at E30. Three neurons located just below the marginal zone (MZ) within the preplate (PP) are retrogradely labeled. At this age, the only neurons present are the early-generated population, consisting of subplate and marginal zone cells. Their axons leave the PP and join the axons of other retrogradely labeled subplate neurons as they run within the intermediate zone (IZ) toward the internal capsule. The DiI fluorescence was converted by incubating with diaminobenzidine to a permanent reaction product visible in transmitted light (for method, see McConnell et al. 1989).

ate connections with very distant targets. Later-generated neurons in cortical layers 5 and 6, which form the bulk of the adult descending projection to subcortical targets, could conceivably be guided by the early subplate axon pathway to their targets; an analogous mechanism is used in the formation of pathways in the grasshopper or zebrafish embryo (Goodman et al. 1984; Kuwada 1986). Ablation studies in zebrafish and grasshopper indicate that pioneer neurons are in fact required for the normal development of later-forming pathways (Goodman et al. 1984; Kuwada 1986; Klose and Bentley 1989), and in the future, it will be essential to see whether ablating subplate neurons during the early period in which their axons are pioneering subcortical pathways can disrupt the subsequent development of cortico-subcortical projections in an analogous fashion.

Subplate Neurons Are Required for the Formation of Thalamocortical Connections

Throughout fetal life, subplate neurons and thalamocortical axons are closely interrelated spatially. Their axons travel along the same or similar pathways between thalamus and cortex, and just as LGN axons accumulate in the subplate, so too do subplate axons accumulate just outside the LGN (McConnell and Shatz 1988 and in prep.). Although, as mentioned above, there is no direct evidence to show that LGN axons make synaptic contacts with subplate neurons, it is likely that the two sets of cells interact with each other throughout an extended period of fetal life. We therefore wondered whether subplate neurons might be required for the development of connections between thalamus and cortex.

To investigate this possibility, we (Ghosh et al. 1989, 1990) deleted subplate neurons at E43, a time when LGN axons have just begun to accumulate within the subplate underlying visual cortex. We then examined the consequences for the subsequent development of the geniculocortical projection by labeling LGN axons with DiI at a variety of times following the lesion. Subplate neurons could be selectively eliminated at E43 by injection of the excitotoxin kainic acid (Chun and Shatz 1988b). However, [^{3}H]thymidine autoradiography showed that neurons belonging to the adult cortical layers, in particular layer 4, are not affected by the injection, presumably because they are too immature to express glutamate receptors (Coyle et al. 1981). In addition, immunohistochemistry for glial fibrillary acidic protein or vimentin showed that the radial glia, and the subsequent development of astrocytes, proceeded normally.

It was remarkable to find that deleting subplate neurons from a restricted region underlying visual cortex prevented LGN axons from invading that region, despite the presence of layer 4 neurons. Rather, LGN axons remained within a tight fascicle and traveled within the white matter for long distances (millimeters), well past visual cortex until they could not be traced

further. To date, we have examined the consequences of subplate neuron deletion at E43 on the geniculocortical projection at E50, E60, E63, and postnatal day 5. In each case, those LGN axons that were diverted from their normal visual cortical target area by the subplate lesion had not invaded cortex anywhere else. An example is shown in Figure 8, in which LGN axons were labeled with DiI at postnatal day 5, subsequent to a kainic acid injection made into the subplate at E43. At this age in normal animals (Fig. 8A), a DiI injection into the LGN results in massive labeling within the cortical plate: Anterogradely labeled thalamocortical axons traverse the deeper cortical layers to branch within cortical layer 4, and the somata and dendrites of layer 6 pyramidal cells are retrogradely labeled. In contrast, in the region where subplate neurons have been deleted (verified by MAP2 immunostaining), DiI-labeled LGN axons fail to invade the cortical plate, and few if any pyramidal neurons are retrogradely labeled (Fig. 8B). These observations provide direct support for the suggestion that interactions between subplate neurons and waiting LGN axons are necessary for the normal development of thalamocortical connections. Moreover, the absence of retrogradely labeled pyramidal neurons supports the suggestion made in the preceding section that subplate neurons, or the pathway formed by their axons, may also be required for the development and maintenance of the recurrent projection from the layer 6 pyramidal cells to the LGN. Finally, the results of this experiment suggest that the cortical plate alone does not contain sufficient information to permit growing thalamocortical axons from different thalamic nuclei to recognize and select their appropriate cortical target area—the participation of subplate neurons is apparently required.

The nature of the interactions within the subplate that might mediate the normal process of cortical target selection and ingrowth by thalamic axons is currently unknown. One possibility, mentioned above, is that activity-dependent synaptic interactions within the subplate, between ingrowing axons and subplate neurons, may be involved. Another is that subplate neurons, by releasing their (putative) transmitters and neuropeptides, may control the growth states of axons and perhaps even cortical neurons in a manner similar to that observed for dissociated cells in vitro (for review, see Lipton and Kater 1989). Subplate neurons could also be necessary for maintaining an extracellular milieu that promotes appropriate interactions. Previous studies have shown that the subplate is densely immunoreactive for fibronectin, which disappears as subplate neurons are eliminated during programmed cell death (Stewart and Pearlman 1987; Chun and Shatz 1988b). When subplate neurons are deleted prematurely by kainic acid injections, fibronectin immunostaining also disappears, indicating that the presence of subplate neurons is required for its expression (probably by the radial glial cells; see Pearlman et al. 1988). Thus, subplate neurons and other cell types may create extracellular substrates that support the interactions necessary

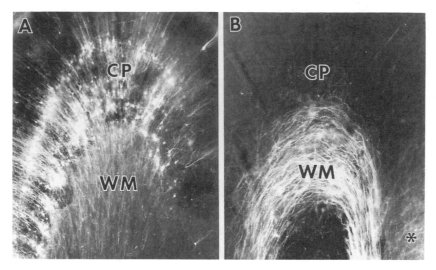

Figure 8. Consequences of deleting subplate neurons below visual cortex on E43 for the subsequent neonatal organization of the geniculocortical projection. To visualize the projection, DiI was placed into the LGN in aldehyde-fixed brains. (*A*) The pattern of DiI labeling in normal cat visual cortex (apex of the lateral gyrus) at postnatal day 2. Layers 4–6 of cortical plate (CP) are filled with fluorescent processes belonging to anterogradely labeled LGN axons and the dendrites and somata of retrogradely labeled cortical neurons making subcortical projections to the LGN and superior colliculus. (*B*) Pattern of DiI labeling in visual cortex at postnatal day 5 resulting from an injection of kainic acid into the visual subplate at E43. Anterogradely labeled geniculocortical axons remain bundled within the white matter (WM) and fail to enter the cortical plate immediately above the lesion. (At the lower right [asterisk], however, LGN axons can enter a region of visual cortex where subplate neurons remain, as verified by MAP2 immunostaining of the adjacent section.) Retrogradely labeled neurons are missing from the cortical plate.

for normal axonal development. At present, it is not possible to distinguish between these alternatives, and in fact, it might be most reasonable to imagine that all may contribute to the process of axonal target selection and ingrowth during cortical development.

CONCLUSION

The construction of the cerebral cortex and elaboration of its inputs, outputs, and intrinsic connections is a major undertaking in the development of the mammalian CNS. Here, we have presented evidence that cerebral cortical development proceeds along a plan similar to that used in the construction of a city skyscraper: An initial scaffold is established in which building construction proceeds. Upon completion, the scaffold is dismantled, leaving little or no trace behind. For the cerebral cortex, the subplate neurons and their processes may provide a comparable neural scaffold. Their axons pioneer pathways to subcortical targets, thereby establishing routes that could be followed by later-forming axonal projections. Within the subplate, their processes may act as temporary targets for ingrowing thalamocortical axons and other afferent axonal systems. The axonal arborizations of subplate neurons traverse the cortical plate, reaching the marginal zone and also branching within layer 4 at later ages, thereby establishing a projection to the final targets of the ingrowing thalamocortical axons. Thus, throughout development, subplate neurons maintain a dynamic and intimate relationship with the sets of neurons that ultimately will be connected directly to each other in the adult. Although the precise cellular interactions

subserving this relationship are currently unknown, its importance to normal cortical development is underscored by the experimental observation that deletion of subplate neurons during the period of axonal waiting prevents thalamocortical axons from selecting and invading their appropriate cortical target area.

Many previous morphological studies of mammalian cerebral cortical development have led to the conclusion that the subplate and marginal zone neurons together represent a phylogenetically older form of cortical organization (Marin-Padilla 1971), which, during ensuing development, is subsequently replaced by the phylogenetically younger neocortex. Whether and how such a transition might occur both in ontogeny and phylogeny remains a mystery, but perhaps a mutation affecting the control of the cell cycle and number of divisions undergone by individual stem cells in the ventricular zone might be sufficient. If cells continue to divide, thereby inserting large numbers of additional neurons into the scaffold formed by the early-generated population, it is conceivable that epigenetic factors could be entirely responsible for the ensuing remodeling, leading to the appearance of the mature neocortex. Whatever the case, the subplate is not merely a "phylogenetic remnant" during cortical development. Here, we have presented many lines of evidence to suggest that subplate neurons mature to function in a complex microcircuit in the fetal brain. Moreover, subplate neurons are essential for the formation of the adult pattern of connections. Thus, subplate neurons play a crucial role in neocortical development, and future experiments will elucidate the cellular and molecular mechanisms that mediate this role.

ACKNOWLEDGMENTS

The authors acknowledge Drs. Jerold Chun and Marla Luskin, whose earlier contributions have been essential to this work. Research from the authors' laboratory was supported by National Institutes of Health grants EY-02858 to C.J.S., NRSA EY-06028 to S.K.M., a National Science Foundation predoctoral fellowship to K.L.A., and a NATO/DAAD postdoctoral fellowship to E.F.

REFERENCES

Al-Ghoul, W.M. and M.W. Miller. 1989. Transient expression of Alz-50 immunoreactivity in developing rat neocortex: A marker for naturally occurring neuronal death? *Brain Res.* **481**: 361.

Allendoerfer, K.L., D.L. Shelton, E.M. Shooter, and C.J. Shatz. 1990. Nerve growth factor immunoreactivity is transiently associated with the subplate neurons of the mammalian cerebral cortex. *Proc. Natl. Acad. Sci.* **87**: 187.

Antonini, A. and C.J. Shatz. 1990. Relation between putative transmitter phenotypes and connectivity of subplate neurons during cerebral cortical development. *Eur. J. Neurosci.* **2**: (in press).

Bate, C.M. 1976. Pioneer neurons in an insect embryo. *Nature* **260**: 54.

Baughman, R.W. and C.D. Gilbert. 1981. Aspartate and glutamate as possible neurotransmitters in the visual cortex. *J. Neurosci.* **1**: 427.

Bayer, S.A. and J. Altman. 1990. Development of layer I and the subplate in the rat neocortex. *Exp. Neurol.* **107**: 48.

Bentley, D. and H. Keshishian. 1982. Pathfinding by peripheral pioneer neurons in grasshoppers. *Science* **218**: 1082.

Chun, J.J.M. and C.J. Shatz. 1988a. Distribution of synaptic vesicle antigens is correlated with the disappearance of a transient synaptic zone in the developing cerebral cortex. *Neuron* **1**: 297.

———. 1988b. A fibronectin-like molecule is present within the developing cat cerebral cortex and is correlated with subplate neurons. *J. Cell Biol.* **106**: 857.

———. 1989a. The earliest-generated neurons of the cat cerebral cortex: Characterization by MAP2 and neurotransmitter immunohistochemistry during fetal life. *J. Neurosci.* **9**: 1648.

———. 1989b. Interstitial cells of the adult neocortical white matter are the remnant of the early generated subplate neuron population. *J. Comp. Neurol.* **282**: 555.

Chun, J.J.M., M.J. Nakamura, and C.J. Shatz. 1987. Transient cells of the developing mammalian telencephalon are peptide immunoreactive neurons. *Nature* **325**: 617.

Coyle, J.T., S.J. Bird, R.H. Evans, R.L. Gulley, J.V. Nadler, W.J. Nicklas, and J.W. Olney. 1981. Excitatory amino acid neurotoxins: Selectivity, specificity and mechanisms of action. *Neurosci. Res. Program Bull.* **19**: 331.

Cragg, B.G. 1975. The development of synapses in the visual system of the cat. *J. Comp. Neurol.* **160**: 147.

Dori, I., M. Petrou, and J.G. Parnavelas. 1989. Excitatory transmitter amino acid-containing neurons in the rat visual cortex: A light and electron microscopic immunocytochemical study. *J. Comp. Neurol.* **290**: 169.

Fahrbach, S.E. and J.W. Truman. 1987. Mechanisms for programmed cell death in the nervous system of a moth. Selective neuronal death. *Ciba Found. Symp.* **126**: 65.

Friauf, E., S.K. McConnell, and C.J. Shatz. 1990. Functional synaptic circuits in the subplate during fetal and early postnatal development of cat visual cortex. *J. Neurosci.* **10**: 2601.

Galli, L. and L. Maffei. 1988. Spontaneous impulse activity of rat retinal ganglion cells in prenatal life. *Science* **242**: 90.

Ghosh, A., A. Antonini, S.K. McConnell, and C.J. Shatz. 1989. Ablation of subplate neurons alters the development of geniculocortical axons. *Soc. Neurosci. Abstr.* **15**: 960.

———. 1990. Subpate neurons are required for the formation of thalamocortical connections. *Nature* (in press).

Goodman, C.S., M.J. Bastiani, C.Q. Doe, S. duLac, S. Helfand, J.Y. Kuwada, and J.B. Thomas. 1984. Cell recognition during neuronal development. *Science* **225**: 1271.

Hendry, S.H.C., E.G. Jones, J. DeFelipe, D. Schmechel, C. Brandon, and P.C. Emson. 1984. Neuropeptide containing neurons of the cerebral cortex are also GABAergic. *Proc. Natl. Acad. Sci.* **81**: 6526.

Hickey, T.L. and P.F. Hitchcock. 1984. Genesis of neurons in the dorsal lateral nucleus of the cat. *J. Comp. Neurol.* **228**: 186.

Ho, R.K. and C.S. Goodman. 1982. Peripheral pathways are pioneered by an array of central and peripheral neurons in grasshopper embryos. *Nature* **297**: 404.

Innocenti, G. 1981. Growth and reshaping of axons in the establishment of visual callosal connections. *Science* **212**: 824.

Klose, M. and D. Bentley. 1989. Transient pioneer neurons are essential for formation of an embryonic peripheral nerve. *Science* **245**: 982.

Kostovic, I. and P. Rakic. 1980. Cytology and time of origin of interstitial neurons in the white matter in infant and adult human and monkey telencephalon. *J. Neurocytol.* **9**: 219.

Kuwada, J.Y. 1986. Cell recognition by neuronal growth cones in a simple vertebrate embryo. *Science* **233**: 740.

Lipton, S.A. and S.B. Kater. 1989. Neurotransmitter regulation of neuronal outgrowth, plasticity and survival. *Trends Neurosci.* **12**: 265.

Lund, R.D. and M.J. Mustari. 1977. Development of the geniculocortical pathway in rats. *J. Comp. Neurol.* **173**: 289.

Luskin, M.B. and C.J. Shatz. 1985a. Neurogenesis of the cat's primary visual cortex. *J. Comp. Neurol.* **242**: 611.

———. 1985b. Studies of the earliest-generated cells of the cat's visual cortex: Cogeneration of subplate and marginal zones. *J. Neurosci.* **5**: 1062.

Maisonpierre, P.C., L. Belluscio, S. Squinto, N.Y. Ip, M.E. Furth, R.M. Lindsay, and G.D. Yancopoulos. 1990. Neurotrophin-3: A neurotrophic factor related to NGF and BDNF. *Science* **247**: 1446.

Marin-Padilla, M. 1971. Early prenatal ontogenesis of the cerebral cortex (neocortex) of the cat (*Felis domestica*). A Golgi study. I. The primordial neocortical organization. *Z. Anat. Entwicklungsgesch.* **134**: 117.

———. 1972. Prenatal ontogenetic history of the principal neurons of the neocortex of the cat (*Felis domestica*). A Golgi study. II. Developmental differences and their significance. *Z. Anat. Entwicklungsgesch.* **136**: 125.

McConnell, S.K. 1988. Development and decision-making in the mammalian cerebral cortex. *Brain Res. Rev.* **13**: 1.

McConnell, S.K. and C.J. Shatz. 1988. Prenatal development of axonal projections from the cat's visual cortex. *Soc. Neurosci. Abstr.* **14**: 743.

McConnell, S.K., A. Ghosh, and C.J. Shatz. 1989. Subplate neurons pioneer to first axon pathway from the cerebral cortex. *Science* **245**: 978.

Miller, M.W. 1988. Development of projection and local circuit neurons in cerebral cortex. In *Cerebral cortex: Development and maturation of cerebral cortex* (ed. A. Peters and E.G. Jones), vol. 7, p. 133. Plenum Press, New York.

Molliver, M.E., I. Kostovic, and H. Van der Loos. 1973. The development of synapses in the cerebral cortex of the human fetus. *Brain Res.* **50**: 403.

Pearlman, A.L., J. Cohen, and W. Puckett. 1988. Radial glia: A cellular source for fibronectin during early cortical development. *Soc. Neurosci. Abstr.* **11**: 748.

Rakic, P. 1975. Timing of major ontogenetic events in the visual cortex of the rhesus monkey. In *Brain mechanisms in mental retardation* (ed. N.A. Buchwald and M. Brazier), p. 3. Academic Press, New York.

———. 1977. Prenatal development of the visual system in the rhesus monkey. *Philos. Trans. R. Soc. Lond. B* **278**: 245.

Ramon y Cajal, S. 1911. *Histologie du systeme nerveux de l'homme et des vertebres,* vol. 2. Maloine, Paris (reprinted Madrid, 1952).

Rodriguez-Tebar, A., G. Dechant, and Y.-A. Barde. 1990. Binding of brain-derived neurotrophic factor to the nerve growth factor receptor. *Neuron* **4:** 487.

Shatz, C.J. 1983. The prenatal development of the cat's retinogeniculate pathway. *J. Neurosci.* **3:** 482.

Shatz, C.J. and P.A. Kirkwood. 1984. Prenatal development of functional connections in the cat's retinogeniculate pathway. *J. Neurosci.* **4:** 1378.

Shatz, C.J. and M.B. Luskin. 1986. Relationship between the geniculocortical afferents and their cortical target cells during development of the cat's primary visual cortex. *J. Neurosci.* **6:** 3655.

Shatz, C.J., J.J.M. Chun, and M.B. Luskin. 1988. The role of the subplate in the development of the mammalian telencephalon. In *Cerebral cortex: Development and maturation of cerebral cortex* (ed. A. Peters and E.G. Jones), vol. 7, p. 35. Plenum Press, New York.

Somogyi, P., A.J. Hodgson, A.D. Smith, G.M. Nunzi, A. Gorio, and J.-Y. Wu. 1984. Different populations of GABAergic neurons in visual cortex and hippocampus of cat contain somatostatin- or choleocystokinin-immunoreactive material. *J. Neurosci.* **4:** 2590.

Stewart, G.R. and A.L. Pearlman. 1987. Fibronectin-like immunoreactivity in the developing cerebral cortex. *J. Neurosci.* **7:** 3325.

Streit, P. 1980. Selective retrograde tracing indicating the transmitter of neuronal pathways. *J. Comp. Neurol.* **191:** 429.

Stryker, M.P. and W.A. Harris. 1986. Binocular impulse blockade prevents the formation of ocular dominance columns in cat visual cortex. *J. Neurosci.* **6:** 2117.

Valverde, F. and M.V. Facal-Valverde. 1988. Postnatal development of interstitial (subplate) cells in the white matter of the temporal cortex of kittens: A correlated golgi and electron microscopic study. *J. Comp. Neurol.* **269:** 168.

Wahle, P. and G. Meyer. 1987. Morphology and quantitative changes of transient NPY-ir neuronal populations during early postnatal development of the cat visual cortex. *J. Comp. Neurol.* **161:** 165.

Walsh, C., E.H. Polley, T.L. Hickey, and R.W. Guillery. 1983. Generation of cat retinal ganglion cells in relation to central pathways. *Nature* **302:** 611.

Wise, S.P. and E.G. Jones. 1978. Developmental studies of thalamocortical and commissural connections in the rat somatic sensory cortex. *J. Comp. Neurol.* **175:** 187.

Wise, S.P., S.H.C. Hendry, and E.G. Jones. 1977. Prenatal development of sensorimotor cortical projections in cats. *Brain Res.* **138:** 538.

Activity-dependent Regulation of Gene Expression in Adult Monkey Visual Cortex

E.G. Jones,* D.L. Benson,* S.H.C. Hendry,* and P.J. Isackson*†
*Departments of *Anatomy and Neurobiology and †Biological Chemistry, University of California, Irvine, California 92717*

Neural activity exercises a powerful influence over the development of the nervous system. In the visual cortex of monkeys, the onset of spontaneous retinal ganglion cell activity (Mastronade 1989) appears to be temporally correlated with the commencement of segregation of geniculo-cortical afferents into eye dominance domains (Rakic 1976), and anatomical and physiological plasticity of their terminations can be induced by perturbed visual experience during a critical period in the first few months of life (Hubel and Wiesel 1977; Hubel et al. 1977; LeVay et al. 1980). Certain effects may even be seen into the second year (Blakemore et al. 1978). Although originally considered to be a developmentally regulated process, plasticity appears to continue into adult life, for retinal activity continues to exert a strong influence over the visual cortex even in adult monkeys. A brief period of monocular deprivation brought about in adult monkeys by eye removal, or by action potential blockade due to intraocular tetrodotoxin injections, quickly leads, in the deprived-eye columns of the visual cortex, to reductions in cellular and terminal levels of immunocytochemically detectable γ-aminobutyric acid (GABA); its synthesizing enzyme, glutamic acid decarboxylase (GAD); the $GABA_A$ receptor; and certain tachykinins (Hendry and Jones 1986; Hendry et al. 1988, 1990). Over the same time period, immunocytochemically detectable levels of type II calcium calmodulin-dependent protein kinase (CaM II kinase) increase in the deprived-eye columns (Hendry and Kennedy 1986). The GABA/GAD effect is rapidly reversible, and the maintenance of normal levels of these and other molecules depends on the maintenance of action potentials in the optic nerve (Hendry and Jones 1988).

Studies in the peripheral nervous system (see, e.g., LaGamma et al. 1984; Black et al. 1985; LaGamma and Black 1989) suggest that activity-dependent up or down regulation of gene transcription underlies certain parallel changes that occur in gene expression for enzymes involved in catecholamine synthesis and for the precursors of certain neuropeptides. The present study was therefore devoted to determining if the activity-dependent changes in GAD and the second-messenger-related protein, CaM II kinase, could be regulated by changes in gene transcription. This work is being published in full elsewhere (Benson et al. 1990).

METHODS

Preparation of cDNA clones. GAD and CaM II kinase cDNAs derived from monkey mRNA were amplified by the polymerase chain reaction (PCR), using synthetic oligonucleotide primers that corresponded to conserved regions.

Oligonucleotides synthesized for GAD PCR amplification contained 21 bases of sequence identical in cat GAD cDNA (Kobayashi et al. 1987) and human GAD cDNA (D.L. Benson et al., unpubl.). The 5' sense oligonucleotide (5'-GGATCCCCTCACAA-GATGATGGGCGTG-3') contained a BamHI site and 21 bases corresponding to bases 1324–1344 of cat cDNA (Kobayashi et al. 1987), which encompasses the sequence encoding the pyridoxal phosphate-binding region of GAD. The 3' antisense oligonucleotide (5'-GAGGCTTTGTGGAATATACCA-3') contained 21 bases corresponding to bases 1663–1683 of cat GAD cDNA.

Oligonucleotides synthesized for CaM II kinase PCR amplification flanked the region of greatest subunit variability between the α, β, and β' sequences of rat CaM II kinase (Bennett and Kennedy 1987; Lin et al. 1987). The 5' sense oligonucleotide (5'-GGATCCCT-GAAGAAGTTCAATGCCAGG-3') contained a Bam-HI site and 21 bases in sequence corresponding to bases 869–889 of the rat α-subunit cDNA (Lin et al. 1987). This segment is 95% identical in the α, β, and β' subunits and encompasses the kinase domain. The 3' antisense oligonucleotide (5'-GTCGACATGAA-AGTCCAGGCCCTCGAC-3') contained a SalI site and 21 bases of sequence (bases 1165–1185 of the α subunit) from a moderately conserved region (76% identical) downstream from the region of greatest variability. All of the oligonucleotides were modified to contain restriction sites for cloning directly into pBluescribe (pBS; Stratagene) (Scharf et al. 1986). This contains bacteriophage T3 and T7 RNA polymerase-binding sites and the universal and reverse primer sequence.

RNA was extracted from monkey visual cortex (GAD) or frontal cortex (CaM II kinase) according to the method of Chirgwin et al. (1979); 10 μg was primed with oligo(dT) and reverse transcribed with 27 units of AMV reverse transcriptase (Boehringer Mannheim Biochemicals). Half of the resulting single-stranded cDNA was amplified by 35 cycles of PCR (Saiki et al. 1985, 1988). In the first cycle, the template was denatured for 5 minutes at 90°C and then cooled to 55°C; 2.5 units of *Taq* DNA polymerase (from *Thermus aquaticus* YTl; Perkin-Elmer Cetus) was then added, and the temperature was increased to 72°C for 3 minutes of nucleotide extension. The remaining 34 cycles each consisted of 30 seconds denaturing at 90°C, 1 minute of oligonucleotide annealing at 55°C, and 3 minutes of polymerization.

Amplified cDNA was restricted with *Bam*HI and *Eco*RI for GAD and with *Bam*HI and *Sal*I for CaM II kinase. It was purified by electroelution from a polyacrylamide gel, ligated to *Bam*HI/*Eco*RI- or *Bam*HI/*Sal*I-digested pBS, and transformed into 71.18 cells. Plasmids containing inserts were sequenced using the dideoxy chain termination method with modified bacteriophage T7 DNA polymerase and with [α-^{32}P]dATP as label (Sanger et al. 1977; Tabor and Richardson 1987).

Cloning. Six of eight PCR-generated CaM II kinase α cDNA clones (CaM II kinase α) had 95% sequence identity with rat CaM II kinase in the comparable region (Lin et al. 1987). Two of the clones (CaM II kinase α-33) contained a 33-bp insert at the point where rat CaM II kinase α, β, and γ' subunit sequences diverge (Bulleit et al. 1988) (Fig. 1A,B) but were otherwise identical to the six CaM II kinase clones. Three 360-bp monkey GAD cDNA clones generated contained at the 5' end the proposed pyridoxal phosphate-binding region, which is conserved between pig DOPA decarboxylase cDNA (Bossa et al. 1977) and cat GAD cDNA (Kobayashi et al. 1987). There was 97% sequence homology with cat GAD cDNA in this region.

Labeling probes. Antisense GAD riboprobes were prepared as follows: The pBSGAD clone was linearized with *Bam*HI and transcribed with T7 RNA polymerase. This yielded a 365-nucleotide, antisense riboprobe for in situ hybridization studies, which was transcription-labeled with [α-^{35}S]UTP. Sense-strand control riboprobes were transcribed from *Pvu*II-digested pBSGAD using T3 RNA polymerase.

Antisense CaM II kinase riboprobes were transcribed with T3 RNA polymerase from a *Bam*HI-restricted pBSCKII α-33 clone. The plasmid yielded a 373-nucleotide riboprobe that was labeled with [α-^{35}S]UTP. Sense-strand control riboprobes were transcribed from the *Pvu*II-digested plasmid, transcribed with T7 RNA polymerase, and labeled with [α-^{35}S]UTP.

In situ hybridization. Ten adult macaque monkeys (seven *Macaca fuscata*, two *Macaca fascicularis*, and one *Macaca arctoides*) ranging in age from 3 to 20 years were used. Six animals were deprived of vision in one eye for varying periods ranging from 48 hours to 5 days by injecting 15 μg of the sodium channel blocker, tetrodotoxin (TTX), into the vitreous cavity under ketamine anesthesia. Two of the animals that survived for 4 and 5 days were given a second TTX injection on

the fourth day; in one, under ketamine anesthesia, the retinal ganglion cells were destroyed by a single intraocular injection of 0.3 ml of 100 mM cobalt chloride 15 days before sacrifice (see Malpeli and Schiller 1979), and in one animal, under barbiturate anesthesia, one eye was removed 5 days prior to sacrifice. Material from 20 other animals, monocularly deprived for varying periods by the same methods and in which the visual cortex was stained immunocytochemically to show changes in GAD and CaM II kinase protein levels, was available for comparison (Hendry and Jones 1986, 1988; Hendry and Kennedy 1986). Two normal animals served as controls. All animals were given an overdose of Nembutal and perfused through the heart with 4% paraformaldehyde in 0.5 M PO$_4$ buffer at pH 7.4. Brains were postfixed overnight in 4% paraformaldehyde and then immersed in 20% sucrose in 4% paraformaldehyde.

Blocks of the visual cortex were frozen on dry ice, and 25 μm of serial sections were cut on a sliding microtome in the frontal plane or in a plane parallel to the lateral surface of the occipital lobe and collected in cold 0.1 M phosphate buffer. Regular series were labeled with the antisense GAD probe and with the antisense CaM II kinase probe, or they were stained with 0.25% thionin or for cytochrome oxidase (CO) (Wong-Riley 1979).

Free-floating sections were washed twice in 0.1 M glycine in 0.1 M PO$_4$ buffer (pH 7.2) for 6 minutes at room temperature, followed by proteinase K (1 μg/ml in 50 mM EDTA/0.1 M Tris, pH 8) for 30 minutes at 30°C, then in 0.25% acetic anhydride in 2× SSC (saline sodium citrate) at room temperature. Sections were next incubated in hybridization buffer containing 50% deionized formamide, 10% dextran sulfate, 0.7% Ficoll, 0.7% polyvinyl pyrrolidone, 350 mg/ml bovine serum albumin (BSA), 0.15 mg/ml yeast tRNA, 0.33 mg/ml denatured herring sperm DNA, and 20 mM dithiothreitol (DTT) for 1 hour at 60°C. They were then transferred to fresh hybridization buffer containing an additional 20 mM DTT and 1 × 10^4 cpm/μl of the [α-^{35}S] antisense riboprobe for at least 20 hours at 60°C.

Following hybridization, sections were washed in 4× SSC, digested with ribonuclease A, 920 μg/ml of 10 mM Tris-saline, pH 8, 1 mM EDTA) for 30 minutes at 45°C, and washed through descending concentrations of SSC with 5 mM DTT to a final stringency of 0.1× SSC at 60°C for 1 hour. Sections were mounted on gelatin-coated slides, dried, and exposed to Amersham βmax film for 1–4 days. After developing the film, lipids were extracted from the sections by soaking them in chloroform. The slides were then dipped in Kodak NTB2 emulsion (diluted 1:1), exposed for 7–15 days at 4°C, developed in Kodak D19, fixed, and stained with cresyl violet. Film densitometry was carried out using a Microcomputer Imaging Device (Imaging Research). Each autoradiographic image was calibrated to ^{14}C-labeled, brain paste standards exposed on the film. Sense-strand radiolabeled RNA probes were hybridized to sections as controls for the in situ hybridization. In these, the visual cortex showed no labeling above background.

RESULTS

Deprivation Effects Shown by Immunocytochemistry

To date in this laboratory, monocular deprivation in adult monkeys has been found to affect immunocytochemically detectable levels of several transmitters, peptides, or proteins and levels of at least one receptor, as detected by immunocytochemistry or receptor binding. Increased levels of immunoreactivity have been detected for the α subunit of CaM II kinase, and decreased levels have been detected for GABA and its synthesizing enzyme GAD, as well as for tachykinins (Hendry and Jones 1986, 1988; Hendry and Kennedy 1986; Hendry et al. 1987, 1988) and the $GABA_A$ receptor, as localized by immunocytochemistry, using a monoclonal antibody (Vitorica et al. 1988) and by ^3H-labeled flunitrazepam and ^3H-labeled muscimol binding (Hendry et al. 1990).

All of the effects of monocular deprivation are particularly evident in layer IVC of area 17, a layer characterized by the presence of large numbers of terminals of geniculocortical afferents, by high concentrations of GABA and GABA-tachykinin cells and of $GABA_A$ receptor density, and by intense histochemical staining for the mitochondrial enzyme, CO. The CO staining indicates a high level of metabolic activity and provides a useful marker for identifying deprived and nondeprived ocular dominance columns in sections adjacent to those showing localization of molecular or other probes.

Although the most readily detectable effects on the markers indicated above occur in layer IVC, effects can also be shown to extend to other layers as well, especially layers IVA, III, and VI. These will not be considered further here. The effects can be detected after eye removal, after injection of TTX into an eye, and after monocular eyelid suture. They are just as robust in each case but appear within 2 days of eye removal or TTX injection and only after 4–6 weeks of eyelid suture. The effects in layer IVC are characterized by enhanced immunoreactive staining for CaM II kinase α in the deprived-eye dominance columns and by reductions in immunoreactive staining for GAD, GABA, and the $GABA_A$ receptor and for tachykinins in the same columns. $GABA_A$ receptor density, as determined by ligand binding, is reduced by approximately 25% in the deprived columns.

The effects on GABA and GAD immunoreactivity are such that 50% of the GABA cells in layer IVC of a deprived column fail to stain (Figs. 1 and 2). Preliminary evidence suggests that all the GABA-tachykinin cells fail to stain for tachykinin immunoreactivity. These effects are not determined by cell death, for cell counts reveal that the total cell population is un-

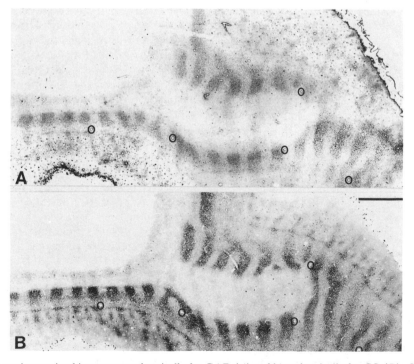

Figure 1. Alternate sections stained immunocytochemically for GAD (*A*) and histochemically for CO (*B*). Circles indicate same blood vessels. Sections were taken from an animal subjected to monocular deprivation and show reductions in immunocytochemically detectable GAD levels in the deprived ocular dominance columns. Bar, 1 mm. (Reprinted, with permission, from Hendry and Jones 1988.)

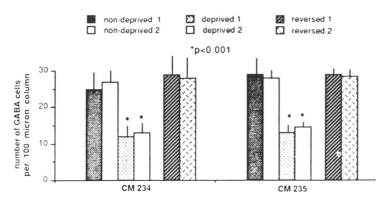

TTX LAYER IVCB DEPRIVATION REVERSAL

Figure 2. Counts of GABA immunoreactive cells per 100-μm-wide column spanning layer IV from deprived and nondeprived ocular dominance columns, as seen in biopsies (left pairs of each set of histograms) taken from the visual cortices of two animals monocularly deprived by TTX injection. Right columns of each set of histograms show return to normal levels as seen in the opposite cortex after cessation of TTX and a renewed period of binocular visual experience. (Reprinted, with permission, from Hendry and Jones 1988.)

changed. Moreover, the effect is reversible. Cessation of TTX injection or re-opening of the eyelids returns the immunocytochemical staining patterns to normal (Fig. 2). The effects are not age-dependent and can be induced as readily in monkeys from 2 years to more than 20 years of age.

Transcript Localization by In Situ Hybridization in Monkey Visual Cortex

CaM II kinase. *Normal*: In area 17 of the normal visual cortex, hybridization of the radioactively labeled CaM II kinase riboprobes is very dense in layers II through VI. In each layer, the density of autoradiographic grains is relatively homogeneous (Fig. 3), and even at very short exposure times, the level of labeling is exceedingly high, making it difficult to localize the silver grains to individual cell somata. Despite this, differences in density enable individual cortical laminae to be discerned and their borders to be delineated. There is an unusually large amount of labeling over the neuropil. Comparison with the underlying Nissl-stained pattern and with adjacent CO-stained sections shows that layers II and IVB contain the greatest amount of CaM II kinase mRNA labeling. Layers III, IVCβ, and VI contain somewhat lesser amounts, although a narrow band in the upper portion of layer VI is more densely labeled. Levels are low in layers IVCα and V, and the lowest levels are found in layers IVA and I and in a narrow strip at the border between layers IVC and V. Within a layer, no periodicities could be detected in the labeling pattern in radial or surface-parallel sections.

In area 18, hybridization of CaM II kinase is dense in layers II and III. Layer IV is homogeneously labeled at a level approximately equal to layer IVCα in area 17. Layer VI is more intensely labeled than in area 17, and its border with layer V is more distinct. The level of neuropil hybridization is, again, particularly high. Hybridization with radioactively labeled sense-strand riboprobes revealed no labeling above background levels in areas 17 or 18.

Deprived: After brief periods of monocular deprivation by TTX injection, retinal destruction, or eye re-

moval, the pattern of CaM II kinase mRNA localization changes dramatically irrespective of survival time and of the age of the animal. The level of CaM II kinase cRNA hybridization becomes greatly enhanced in regular columns that extend through the thickness of layers II through VI in area 17. These alternate with similar columns showing lower levels of labeling (Figs. 1 and 3). In sections cut parallel to the pial surface, the alternating dense and less-dense columns appear as long stripes that are especially visible in layer IVC. Here, they correlate closely with the ocular dominance columns seen in the adjacent CO-stained sections. The long stripes of light and dark CO staining that appear in layer IVC can be superimposed on those found in the adjacent autoradiograph using the cut profiles of blood vessels that enter the cortex along radial trajectories as guides. This comparison shows that the stripes of enhanced in situ hybridization correspond to the lightly stained CO stripes, representing deprived ocular dominance columns, and the stripes showing weaker hybridization correspond to the darker CO stripes, representing nondeprived columns (Wong-Riley 1979; Horton and Hubel 1981). Enhanced CaM II kinase mRNA levels in the deprived-eye columns are apparent 48 hours after monocular deprivation and are still evident after 15 days of monocular deprivation. Beyond that time, although the CO-stained sections show a maximal effect, there is less distinction between deprived and nondeprived columns in the autoradiographs.

In layers II and III, which show homogeneous labeling in normal area 17, continuous stripes of higher autoradiographic grain density, approximately 500 μm wide, alternate with less-dense stripes approximately 300 μm wide in the monocularly deprived animals. Correlation with the adjacent CO-stained sections reveals that the denser stripes of hybridization in layers II and III lie over rows of CO-stained periodicities ("blobs") that lie at the centers of ocular dominance columns in these layers (Horton and Hubel 1981; Horton 1984). The patches of CO staining in the rows of deprived-eye periodicities become shrunken in longer-deprived animals (Horton 1984), and direct correlation of the stripes of labeling with the rows of periodicities reveals that wider, denser stripes of hybridization lie

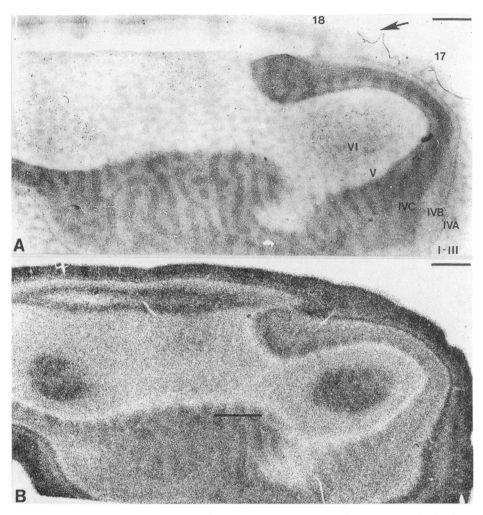

Figure 3. Paired CO-stained (*A*) and autoradiographic (*B*) sections from areas 17 and 18 of a monocularly deprived monkey showing (in *B*) enhanced levels of in situ hybridization that reveal increased levels of CaM II kinase mRNA in the deprived-eye dominance columns. Line in *B* indicates region quantified in Fig. 4. Bar, 1 mm. (Reprinted, with permission, from Benson et al. 1990.)

over the rows of shrunken CO-stained periodicities that represent the deprived eye, whereas the narrower, less-dense stripes of hybridization lie over the intervening rows of nonshrunken periodicities that represent the nondeprived eye (see Benson et al. 1990).

In layers IVB, V, and VI, slightly wider stripes of enhanced hybridization also alternate with narrower stripes of less-dense hybridization. The dense stripes in layer VI are denser than those in the other two layers. In all cases, the stripes are aligned with rows of CO-stained periodicities detectable in these layers (Horton 1984), and the denser stripes of hybridized label coincide with rows of periodicities that lie above (layer IVB) or below (layers V and VI) the dense stripes of label representing deprived-eye dominance columns in layer IVC. Quantification by image density analysis shows that hybridization density over deprived-eye columns is up to four or five times greater than that over normal eye columns (Fig. 4). No inhomogeneities in

the hybridization pattern can be detected in area 18 of normal or monocularly deprived monkeys (Fig. 2).

GAD. *Normal:* In contrast with the CaM II kinase hybridization pattern, autoradiographic grains associated with hybridized antisense GAD riboprobes are distinctly localized over cell somata. Large and small clusters of silver grains are associated with underlying Nissl-stained cell nuclei, and large (21 μm) and small (10 μm) grain clusters correspond to large and small cells, respectively.

In the autoradiographs, laminae of differential grain density correspond to laminae and sublaminae of the normal area 17, as seen in Nissl- and CO-stained sections. Small clusters with few grains are observed throughout layer I. Large and small clusters are found through layers II and III. Layer IVA is a thin, densely labeled band. Layer IVB shows a line of large clusters that form a thin strip in the middle of the layer. Layer IVC is characterized by small clusters indicative of

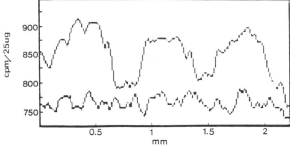

Figure 4. Comparison of CaM II kinase mRNA levels in the region indicated by the line in Fig. 3 (upper trace). This shows enhanced levels (peaks) over the three deprived columns included in the traverse. Valleys, representing normal columns, show levels close to normal. Normal levels are shown by lower trace taken from section of a similar region of area 17 of a normal monkey, hybridized at the same time and exposed on the same sheet of X-ray film. (Reprinted, with permission, from Benson et al. 1990.)

lightly labeled small cells. Differential GAD in situ hybridization reveals sublaminae in layers IVCα and IVCβ. Layer IVC has an upper sublamina that is wider and more densely labeled and a thinner, less densely labeled sublamina. Layer IVCβ has three sublaminae: two relatively densely labeled superficial and deep bands separated by a less dense, intermediate band. Layer V shows a decrease in overall grain density and the reappearance of large clusters of grains. Layer VI is subdivided into three laminae; superficial and deep bands are more heavily labeled than an intermediate, less dense band.

In area 18, GAD mRNA labeling in layers I, II, and III is approximately equal to that in area 17. Hybridization in layer IV is slightly denser than in the overlying layers, but no sublaminae are seen. Layers V and VI resemble those in area 17. Sections of areas 17 and 18 cut parallel to the pial surface reveal no periodicities in the hybridization pattern. Control sections hybridized with sense-strand probes show no labeling above background levels.

Deprived: Monocular deprivation in the same animals as those used for the CaM II kinase studies described above resulted in no detectable change in the pattern of GAD mRNA hybridization in area 17 or area 18 (see Benson et al. 1990). No irregularities that could be associated with deprived- or nondeprived-eye dominance columns, demonstrable in the adjacent CO-stained sections could be seen (Fig. 5). No statistical difference between hybridization in deprived and nondeprived ocular dominance columns was detected in layer IV by quantitative image analysis (level of significance = 0.01). S1 nuclease protection studies, using ^{32}P-labeled GAD cRNA probes, also revealed no change in GAD mRNA levels in monocularly deprived visual cortex (see Benson et al. 1990).

DISCUSSION

This study suggests that increases in CaM II kinase immunoreactivity, which have been demonstrated in

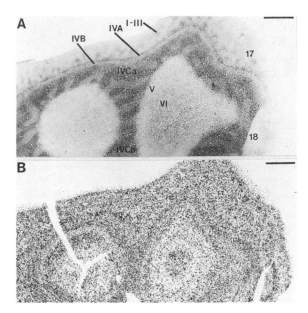

Figure 5. Paired CO-stained (*A*) and anteroradiographic (*B*) sections from a monocularly deprived monkey showing lack of change in GAD mRNA levels, as indicated by in situ hybridization. Bar, 1 mm. (Reprinted, with permission, from Benson 1990.)

nondeprived eye columns of adult monkey visual cortex following periods of monocular deprivation (Hendry and Kennedy 1986), derive from corresponding increases in mRNA levels; this, in turn, implies that the CaM II kinase deprivation effect is mediated at transcriptional levels. In contrast, the large decreases in GAD immunoreactivity that occur in deprived-eye columns of adult monkey visual cortex following monocular deprivation (Hendry and Jones 1986, 1988) are not accompanied by detectable changes in GAD mRNA levels; this implies that the deprivation effect on GAD protein levels is likely to be mediated at a posttranscriptional level.

CaM II kinase is an abundant protein and makes up at least 1% of all forebrain protein in the rat (Erondu and Kennedy 1985). A similar abundance in monkeys is reflected in the dense CaM II kinase hybridization pattern. The high mRNA levels in the neuropil are most likely to be in the large, densely packed apical and basal dendritic systems of cortical pyramidal cells. These are the cells primarily delineated by CaM II kinase immunoreactivity (D.L. Benson et al., unpubl.).

The dendrites of cortical pyramidal cells contain significant amounts of free and attached ribosomes (Peters et al. 1976) so that CaM II kinase mRNA may therefore be translated at these sites as well as in the soma. Because CaM II kinase is associated with postsynaptic densities (Kennedy et al. 1983; Kelly et al. 1984), it may be specifically associated with the large numbers of dendritic spines and their associated asymmetrical synapses. Dendritic ribosomes and dendritic spines have previously been associated in pyramidal cells of the rat hippocampal formation, where both may be involved in dendritic plasticity during reinnervation (Steward 1983).

Activity-dependent Regulation of CaM II Kinase

Immunoreactivity for CaM II kinase α increases in deprived-eye dominance columns of layer IVC as early as 2 days following eye removal or monocular TTX injection and after about 9 weeks of monocular eyelid suture (Hendry and Kennedy 1986; S.H.C. Hendry et al., unpubl.). The present results would imply that this increase in immunocytochemically detectable protein levels would result from an increase in CaM II kinase gene transcription in cells of the deprived-eye columns. The present results also appear to indicate that the increase in immunoreactivity seen under deprived conditions reflects an increase in protein levels and not increased phosphorylation of the enzyme (which immunocytochemistry would also detect) (Erondu and Kennedy 1985). CaM II kinase mRNA in the deprived columns is increased within 48 hours and can still be distinguished as late as 15 days following monocular deprivation but seems to be less apparent at the later time. The more prolonged increase in CaM II kinase protein known to occur following monocular deprivation might therefore be maintained by increased protein stability or other mechanisms.

Neuronal activity has been already shown to be important in regulating gene transcription in the peripheral nervous system. In explanted sympathetic ganglia of rats, increases in presynaptic activity, which result in depolarization of the cells, elicit increases in mRNA for tyrosine hydroxylase (TH) followed by increases in TH protein levels. This is accompanied by decreases in preprotachykinin mRNA and in substance-P levels (Kessler and Black 1982; Black et al. 1985; Roach et al. 1987). Reduction in afferent activity, in contrast, is accompanied by an increase in preprotachykinin mRNA and no change in TH mRNA (Roach et al. 1987). TH and proenkephalin and their mRNAs also appear to be differentially regulated in a similar manner in the adrenal medulla (Kilpatrick et al. 1984; LaGamma et al. 1984; Kanamatsu et al. 1986; LaGamma and Black 1989). In the central nervous system, enhanced neural activity accompanying epileptiform activity increases in proenkephalin and proneuropeptide-Y mRNAs and by changes in levels of a number of immunocytochemically detectable peptides (White et al. 1987; White and Gall 1987; Gall and Isackson 1989). In the visual cortex of monocularly deprived monkeys, the increase in CaM II kinase gene expression revealed by in situ hybridization extends from layer IVC into the parts of deprived-eye dominance columns that occupy layers II through VI (Hendry and Kennedy 1986). The extent of the effect is greater than would be predicted from the immunocytochemical observations, which showed changes only in layer IVC (Hendry and Kennedy 1986). This presumably reflects differences in the sensitivity of the two techniques. In regions corresponding to rows of CO-stained deprived-eye patches

and in parts of the inter-row regions adjacent to them, hybridization of CaM II kinase cRNA is enhanced relative to levels in the alternating rows of nondeprived eye patches. This indicates that CaM II kinase mRNA levels increase in the regions of decreased CO activity that reflect reduced metabolic activity presumably carried along the vertically oriented synaptic circuits that pass out of layer IVC into over- and underlying layers.

Changes in CaM II kinase levels are likely to have effects that are potentially long-lasting. The kinase can phosphorylate many substrates, including synapsin I, MAP2, TH, and tryptophan hydroxylase (Bennett et al. 1983; Yamauchi and Fujisawa 1983; Schulman 1984; Vulleit et al. 1984). It also enhances transmitter release from the presynaptic terminal at the squid giant synapse, probably in association with synapsin I (Llinás et al. 1985), and by increasing vesicle mobility (McGuiness et al. 1989). It is a major postsynaptic density protein (Kennedy et al. 1983; Kelly et al. 1984), although it has not yet been associated with a specific type of synapse. In the hippocampus, it is thought to be essential for the induction of long-term potentiation (Malenka et al. 1989; Malinow et al. 1989). Effects of monocular deprivation mediated by CaM II kinase may therefore affect synapse function in both the short and long terms and may even have structural consequences. Increases in CaM II kinase transcription resulting from visual deprivation in the adult monkey are likely to be indicative of changes in other second-messenger-related intracellular events set in motion by reduced activity in cells of deprived-eye dominance columns. These events probably also play a role in the regulation of levels of the other proteins and peptides found by immunocytochemistry. The regulation of immediate-early genes, whose gene products will be involved in the later regulation of gene transcription for CaM II kinase and other intracellular proteins, is also likely to be a concomitant of visual deprivation. Several immediate-early genes have been shown to be induced in response to increased neuronal activity in other systems as well as to mitogens and growth factors (Greenberg et al. 1985; Morgan and Curran 1986; Kujubu et al. 1987; Milbrandt 1987; White and Gall. 1987; Saffen et al. 1988; Cole et al. 1989; Gall and Isackson 1989).

GAD Distribution

The pattern of GAD and GABA immunoreactivity, which is confined to nonpyramidal neurons of both large and small sizes in all layers of the primate cortex (Hendrickson et al. 1981; Hendry and Jones 1986; Fitzpatrick et al. 1987; Hendry et al. 1987), is reflected in the distribution of large and small grain clusters in the in situ hybridization using GAD riboprobes. The in situ approach revealed distinct sublaminae in layers IVCα, IVCβ, and VI. The two subdivisions of layer IVCα are the same as those shown by Fitzpatrick et al. (1987) in immunocytochemical preparations, but no subdivisions comparable to those detected by in situ hybridization in layers IVCβ or VI have been described by immunocytochemistry.

GAD Expression following Monocular Deprivation

In contrast to the activity-dependent regulation of CaM II kinase α gene transcription, levels of GAD gene transcription appear to be maintained in deprived-eye columns following monocular deprivation. This maintenance of GAD gene expression in the face of monocular deprivation is also seen in adult cat visual cortex (Benson et al. 1989). These results are surprising in view of the fact that following 4 days of monocular deprivation by eye removal or TTX injection and 7–9 weeks of monocular deprivation by eyelid suture, approximately 50% of the GABAergic neurons in the deprived-eye dominance columns of monkey area 17 fail to show immunocytochemically detectable levels of GAD or GABA (Hendry and Jones 1986, 1988; Hendry et al. 1987). The effects are reversible upon recovery from TTX or after reopening of the eyelids and are not due to cell death (Hendry and Jones 1988; E.G. Jones et al., unpubl.); instead, they depend on the presence or absence of impulse activity in the optic nerve.

There are three potential explanations for failure to detect changes in GAD mRNA levels in the present experiments. First, GAD enzyme levels could be regulated by neuronal activity at a posttranslational level. Effects such as deamidation, methylation, or limited proteolysis could render the enzyme less stable or undetectable by immunocytochemistry (for review, see Benyon 1980).

Second, events occurring between DNA transcription and posttranslational processing could be specifically regulated. These could include covalent modifications of mRNA, transcript splicing, and the initiation of mRNA translation. Changes in mRNA maturation are not likely to be the cause of the changes in GAD protein levels, since changes in polyadenylation or 5′ capping would affect mRNA stability and would therefore be detected by in situ hybridization studies as an increase or decrease in hybridization levels. Although GAD gene expression could be regulated by an alternative splicing event, there is no present evidence to indicate that alternative splicing is a method utilized by cells to regulate protein levels. Instead, mature functional GAD mRNA may be prevented from being translated, thus regulating protein levels.

Two GAD genes have recently been discovered, one encoding a 65-kD protein and the other a 68-kD protein (Kaufman et al. 1989; A.J. Tobin, pers. comm.). Immunocytochemical studies indicate that the proteins are colocalized in GABA cells, although with different intracellular distributions (Houser et al. 1989). The GAD probes used in the present study would localize the transcript of the GAD gene that corresponds to the 65-kD protein. Although it is conceivable that the GAD gene corresponding to the 65-kD protein maintains normal transcription levels and that correspond-

ing to the 68-kD protein is differentially regulated in response to monocular deprivation, this is unlikely. One of the polyclonal antisera used in earlier studies to demonstrate a decrease in GAD protein immunoreactivity following monocular deprivation preferentially binds the smaller GAD protein. Therefore, it is unlikely that changes in the remaining 68-kD protein could be solely responsible for the decrease in GAD immunoreactivity. However, two additional GAD mRNAs have been identified in cats and rats. These may represent alternative splicing products or additional GAD genes that could be differentially regulated (Bond et al. 1988; Benson et al. 1989).

CONCLUSIONS

Immunocytochemistry and receptor binding reveal that the levels of a large number of neuroactive molecules in the adult primate visual cortex are regulated in an activity-dependent manner. These seem to be manifestations of a widespread general effect whereby neural activity regulates transmitter, receptor, and second-messenger-related functions throughout the nervous system. The regulatory mechanisms involved may be complex and varied, and the present results suggest that activity-dependent changes may be effected at both transcriptional and posttranscriptional levels. The changes in protein levels associated with changes in neural activity, although remarkably robust, are not necessarily attributable directly to changes in gene transcription. The interplay between the many potential mechanisms is probably the key to understanding how neural activity regulates neuronal gene expression under activity-dependent conditions.

ACKNOWLEDGMENTS

This work was supported by grant number EY-07193 from the National Institutes of Health, U.S. Public Health Service.

REFERENCES

Bennett, M.K. and M.B. Kennedy. 1987. Deduced primary structure of the α subunit of brain type II Ca++ calmodulin-dependent protein kinase determined by molecular cloning. *Proc. Natl. Acad. Sci.* **84:** 1794.

Bennett, M.K., N.E. Erondu, and M.B. Kennedy. 1983. Purification and characterization of a calmodulin-dependent protein kinase that is highly concentrated in brain. *J. Biol. Chem.* **258:** 12735.

Benson, D.L., P.J. Isackson, C. Gall, and E.G. Jones. 1990. Differential effects of monocular deprivation on glutamic acid decarboxylase and type II calcium-calmodulin dependent protein kinase gene expression in adult monkey visual cortex. *J. Neurosci.* (in press).

Benson, D.L., P.J. Isackson, S.H.C. Hendry, and E.G. Jones. 1989. Expression of glutamic acid decarboxylase mRNA in normal and monocularly deprived cat visual cortex. *Mol. Brain Res.* **5:** 279.

Benyon, R.J. 1980. Protein modification and the control of intracellular protein degradation. In *The enzymology of post-translational modification of proteins* (ed. R.F. Freedman and H.C. Hawkins), p. 363. Academic Press, New York.

Black, I.B., D.M. Chikaraishi, and E.J. Lewis. 1985. Trans-synaptic increase in RNA coding for tyrosine hydroxylase in a rat sympathetic ganglion. *Brain Res.* **339:** 151.

Blakemore, C., L.J. Garey, and F. Vital-Durant. 1978. The physiological effects of monocular deprivation and their reversal in the monkey's visual cortex. *J. Physiol.* **283:** 223.

Bond, R.W., K.R. Jansen, and D.J. Gottleib. 1988. Pattern of expression of glutamic acid decarboxylase mRNA in the developing rat brain. *Proc. Natl. Acad. Sci.* **85:** 3231.

Bossa, R., F. Martini, D. Barra, C. Borri Voltattorni, A. Minelli, and C. Turano. 1977. The chymotryptic phos-phopyridoxyl peptide of dopa decarboxylase from pig kidney. *Biochem. Biophys. Res. Commun.* **78:** 177.

Bulleit, R.F., M.K. Bennett, S.S. Malloy, J.B. Hurley, and M.B. Kennedy. 1988. Conserved and variable regions in the subunits of brain type II Ca^{2+}/calmodulin-dependent protein kinase. *Neuron* **1:** 63.

Chirgwin, J.M., A.E. Przblya, R.J. MacDonald, and W.J. Rutter. 1979. Isolation of biologically active ribonucleic acid from sources enriched in ribonuclease. *Biochemistry* **18:** 5294.

Cole, A.J., D.W. Saffen, J.M. Baraban, and P.F. Worley. 1989. Rapid increase of an immediate early gene mes-senger RNA in hippocampal neurons by NMDA receptor activation. *Nature* **340:** 474.

Erondu, N.E. and M.B. Kennedy. 1985. Regional distribution of type II Ca^{2+}/calmodulin dependent protein kinase in rat brain. *J. Neurosci.* **5:** 3270.

Fitzpatrick, D., J.S. Lund, D.E. Schmechel, and A.C. Tow-les. 1987. Distribution of GABAergic neurons and axon terminals in the macaque striate cortex. *J. Comp. Neurol.* **264:** 73.

Gall, C.M. and P.J. Isackson. 1989. Limbic seizures increase neuronal production of messenger RNA for nerve-growth factor. *Science* **245:** 758.

Greenberg, M.E., L.A. Greene, and E.B. Ziff. 1985. Nerve growth factor and epidermal growth factor induce rapid transient changes in proto-oncogene transcription in PC12 cells. *J. Biol. Chem.* **260:** 14101.

Hendrickson, A.E., S.P. Hunt, and J.-Y. Wu. 1981. Immuno-cytochemical localization of glutamic acid decarboxylase in monkey striate cortex. *Nature* **292:** 605.

Hendry, S.H.C. and E.G. Jones. 1986. Reduction in number of immunostained GABAergic neurons in deprived-eye dominance columns of monkey area 17. *Nature* **320:** 750.

———. 1988. Activity dependent regulation of GABA ex-pression in the visual cortex of adult monkeys. *Neuron* **1:** 701

Hendry, S.H.C. and M.B. Kennedy. 1986. Immunoreactivity for a calmodulin-dependent protein kinase is selectively increased in macaque striate cortex after monocular depri-vation. *Proc. Natl. Acad. Sci.* **83:** 1536.

Hendry, S.H.C., E.G. Jones, and N. Burstein. 1988. Activity-dependent regulation of tachykinin-like immunoreactivity in neurons of monkey visual cortex. *J. Neurosci.* **8:** 1225.

Hendry, S.H.C., J. Fuchs, A.L. De Blas, and E.G. Jones. 1990. Organization and plasticity of immunocytochemical-ly localized $GABA_A$ receptors in adult monkey visual cortex. *J. Neurosci.* **10:** 2438.

Hendry, S.H.C., H.D. Schwark, E.G. Jones, and J. Yan. 1987. Numbers and proportions of GABA immunoreac-tive neurons in different areas of monkey cerebral cortex. *J. Neurosci.* **7:** 1503.

Horton, J.C. 1984. Cytochrome oxidase patches: A new cyto-architectonic feature of monkey visual cortex. *Philos. Trans. R. Soc. Lond. B Biol. Sci.* **304:** 199.

Horton, J.C. and D.H. Hubel. 1981. Regular patchy distribu-tion of cytochrome oxidase staining in primary visual cor-tex of macaque monkey. *Nature* **292:** 762.

Houser, C.R., J.E. Miyashiro, D.L. Kaufman, and A.J. Tobin. 1989. Immunocytochemical studies using a new

antiserum against bacterially produced feline glutamate decarboxylase. *Soc. Neurosci. Abstr.* **15:** 488.

Hubel, D.H. and T.N. Wiesel. 1977. Functional architecture of macaque monkey visual cortex. *Proc. R. Soc. Lond. B Biol. Sci.* **198:** 1.

Hubel, D.H., T.N. Wiesel, and S. LeVay. 1977. Plasticity of ocular dominance columns in monkey striate cortex. *Philos. Trans. R. Soc. Lond. B Biol. Sci.* **278:** 377.

Kanamatsu, T., C.D. Unsworth, E.J. Diliberto, Jr., O.H. Viveros, and J.S. Hong. 1986. Reflex splanchnic nerve stimulation increases levels of proenkephalin A mRNA and proenkephalin A related peptides in the rat adrenal medulla. *Proc. Natl. Acad. Sci.* **83:** 9245.

Kaufman, D.L., C.R. Houser, and A.J. Tobin. 1989. Two forms of glutamic acid decarboxylase (GAD), with differ-ent N-terminal sequences, have distinct intraneuronal dis-tributions. *Soc. Neurosci. Abstr.* **15:** 487.

Kelly, P.T., T.L. McGuinness, and P. Greengard. 1984. Evi-dence that the major postsynaptic density protein is a component of a Ca^{2+}/calmodulin dependent protein ki-nase. *Proc. Natl. Acad. Sci.* **81:** 945.

Kennedy, M.B., M.K. Bennett, and N.E. Erondu. 1983. Bio-chemical and immunochemical evidence that the "major postsynaptic density protein" is a subunit of a calmodulin-dependent protein kinase. *Proc. Natl. Acad. Sci.* **80:** 7357.

Kessler, J.A. and I.B. Black. 1982. Regulation of substance P in adult rat sympathetic ganglia. *Brain Res.* **234:** 182.

Kilpatrick, D.L., I.B. Howells, G. Fleminger, and S. Uden-friend. 1984. Denervation of rat adrenal glands markedly increases preproenkaphalin mRNA. *Proc. Natl. Acad. Sci.* **81:** 7221.

Kobayashi, Y., D.L. Kaufman, and A.J. Tobin. 1987. Glutamic acid decarboxylase cDNA: Nucleotide sequence encoding an enzymatically active fusion protein. *J. Neuro-sci.* **7:** 2769.

Kujubu, D.A., R.W. Lim, B.C. Varnum, and H.R. Herschman. 1987. Induction of transiently expressed genes in PC12 pheochromocytoma cells. *Oncogene* **1:** 257.

LaGamma, E.F. and I.B. Black. 1989. Transcriptional control of adrenal catecholamine and opiate transmitter genes. *Mol. Brain Res.* **5:** 17.

LaGamma, E.F., J.E. Adler, and I.B. Black. 1984. Impulse activity differentially regulates [Leu] enkephalin and cat-echolamine characters in the adrenal medulla. *Science* **224:** 1102.

LeVay, S., T.N. Wiesel, and D.H. Hubel. 1980. The develop-ment of ocular dominance columns in normal and visually deprived monkeys. *J. Comp. Neurol.* **191:** 1.

Lin, C.R., M.S. Kapiloff, S. Durgerain, K. Tatemoto, A.F. Russo, P. Hanson, H. Schulman, and M.G. Rosenfeld. 1987. Molecular cloning of a brain-specific calcium-calmodulin-dependent protein kinase. *Proc. Natl. Acad. Sci.* **84:** 5962.

Llinás, R., T.L. McGuinness, C.S. Leonard, M. Sugimori, and P. Greengard. 1985. Intraterminal injection of synap-sin I or calcium/calmodulin-dependent protein kinase II alters neurotransmitter release at the squid giant synapse. *Proc. Natl. Acad. Sci.* **82:** 3035.

Malenka, R.C., J.A. Kauer, D.J. Perkel, M.D. Mauk, P.T. Kelly, R.A. Nicoll, and M.N. Waxham. 1989. An essential role for postsynaptic calmodulin and protein kinase activity in long-term potentiation. *Nature* **340:** 554.

Malinow, R., H. Schulman, and R.W. Tsien. 1989. Inhibition of postsynaptic PKC or CaMKII blocks induction but not expression of LTP. *Science* **245:** 862.

Malpeli, J.G. and P.H. Schiller. 1979. A method of reversible inactivation of small regions of brain tissue. *J. Neurosci. Methods* **1:** 143.

Mastronade, D.N. 1989. Correlated firing of cat retinal gangli-on cells. I. Spontaneously active inputs to X- and Y-cells. *J. Neurophysiol.* **49:** 303.

McGuinness, T.L., S.T. Brady, J.A. Gruner, M. Sugimori, R. Llinás, and P. Greengard. 1989. Phosphorylation-dependent inhibition by synapsin 1 of organelle movement in squid axoplasm. *J. Neurosci.* **9:** 4139.

Milbrandt, J. 1987. A nerve growth factor-induced gene encodes a possible transcriptional regulatory factor. *Science* **238:** 797.

Morgan, J.I. and T. Curran. 1986. Role of ion flux in the control of c-*fos* expression. *Nature* **322:** 552.

Peters, A., S.L. Palay, and H.D. Webster. 1976. *The fine structure of the nervous system: The neurons and supporting cells.* Saunders, Philadelphia.

Rakic, P. 1976. Prenatal genesis of connections subserving ocular dominance in the rhesus monkey. *Nature* **261:** 467.

Roach, A., J.E. Adler, and I.B. Black. 1987. Depolarizing influences regulate preprotachykinin mRNA in sympathetic neurons. *Proc. Natl. Acad. Sci.* **84:** 5078.

Saffen, D.W., A.J. Cole, P.F. Worley, B.A. Christy, K. Ryder, and J.M. Baraban. 1988. Convulsant-induced increase in transcription factor messenger RNAs in rat brain. *Proc. Natl. Acad. Sci.* **85:** 7795.

Saiki, R.K., S. Scharf, F. Faloona, K.B. Mullis, G.T. Horn, H.A. Erlich, and N. Arnheim. 1985. Enzymatic amplification of β-globin genomic sequences and restriction site analysis for diagnosis of sickle-cell anemia. *Science* **230:** 1350.

Saiki, R.K., D.H. Gelfand, S. Stoffel., S.J. Scharf, R. Higuchi, G.T. Horn, K.B Mullis, and H.A. Erlich. 1988. Primer directed enzymatic amplification of DNA with a thermostable DNA polymerase. *Science* **239:** 487.

Sanger, F., S. Nicklen, and A.R. Coulson. 1977. DNA sequencing with chain terminating inhibitors. *Proc. Natl. Acad. Sci.* **74:** 5463.

Scharf, S.J., G.T. Horn, and H.A. Erlich. 1986. Direct cloning and sequence analysis of enzymatically amplified genomic sequences. *Science* **233:** 1076.

Schulman, H. 1984. Phosphorylation of microtubule-associated proteins by a Ca^{2+}/calmodulin-dependent protein kinase. *J. Cell Biol.* **99:** 11.

Steward, O. 1983. Alterations in polyribosomes associated with dendritic spines during reinnervation of the dentate gyrus of the adult rat. *J. Neurosci.* **3:** 177.

Tabor, S. and C.C. Richardson. 1987. DNA sequence analysis with a modified bacteriophage T7 DNA polymerase. *Proc. Natl. Acad. Sci.* **84:** 4767.

Vitorica, J., D. Park, G. Chin, and A.L. De Blas. 1988. Monoclonal antibodies and conventional antisera to the $GABA_A$ receptor/benzodiazepine receptor/Cl^- channel complex. *J. Neurosci.* **8:** 615.

Vulliet, P.R., J.R. Woodgett, and P. Cohen. 1984. Phosphorylation of tyrosine hydroxylase by calmodulin-dependent multiprotein kinase. *J. Biol. Chem.* **259:** 13680.

White, J.D. and C.M. Gall. 1987. Differential regulation of neuropeptide and proto-oncogene mRNA content in the hippocampus following recurrent seizures. *Mol. Brain Res.* **3:** 21.

White, J.D., C.M. Gall, and J.F. McKelvy. 1987. Enkephalin biosynthesis and enkephalin gene expression are increased in hippocampal mossy fibers following a unilateral lesion of the hilus. *J. Neurosci.* **7:** 753.

Wong-Riley, M.T.T. 1979. Changes in the visual system of monocularly sutured or enucleated kittens demonstrable with cytochrome oxidase histochemistry. *Brain Res.* **171:** 11.

Yamauchi, T. and H. Fujisawa. 1983. Purification and characterization of the brain calmodulin-dependent protein kinase (kinase II), which is involved in the activation of tryptophan 5-monooxygenase. *Eur. J. Biochem.* **132:** 15.

Factors Involved in the Establishment of Specific Interconnections between Thalamus and Cerebral Cortex

C. BLAKEMORE AND Z. MOLNÁR

University Laboratory of Physiology, Oxford OX1 3PT, United Kingdom

How, during development, do nerve fibers from one part of the brain find their way to the appropriate target cells? This problem seems particularly acute for the cerebral cortex, which is characterized by the remarkable diversity but exquisite specificity of its afferent inputs and efferent outputs. In humans, this vast sheet of tissue is about 2000 cm^2 in area, is 3–4 mm thick, and contains perhaps 20 billion neurons. Although there is morphological similarity across the entire neocortex (everywhere it has a six-layered structure with the same basic types of differentiated neurons), there are distinctive regional variations in the proportions of different cell types and the relative thickness of layers.

As early as 1909, Brodmann classified the human cortex into dozens of specialized cytoarchitectural areas, purely on the basis of these local differences in histological appearance. The major sensory and motor fields can be identified in all mammalian species, and differences in the overall size of the cerebral hemispheres are at least partly explained by differences in the number of distinct cytoarchitectural zones. It is a testimony to the power of anatomical description that Brodmann's numbering schemes are still widely used by physiologists as well as by modern neuroanatomists who now have methods to examine the afferent and efferent connections of each area.

In general, each cortical field, recognized by its histological specialization, has its own distinctive interconnections with other cortical and subcortical structures, which lead to its individual functional role. There is a special relationship between cortical fields and the thalamus, the great mass of relay nuclei in the diencephalon through which virtually all afferent input to the cortex passes. Most cortical areas are specifically interconnected with their own particular thalamic nuclei: area 17 (the primary visual cortex) with the dorsal lateral geniculate nucleus (LGN), area 4 (the primary motor cortex) with the ventrobasal nucleus, the primary auditory cortex (areas 41 and 42) with the medial geniculate nucleus, and so on. In each field, specific thalamocortical input terminates mainly in layer 4 of the cortex, and neurons of layer 6 of that area send corticofugal projections back to the same thalamic nucleus.

Neurogenesis and the Formation of the Cortical Plate

During embryogenesis, a wave of development sweeps through each sensory system from periphery to cortex. In rhesus monkeys, for which the gestation period is about 165 days, Rakic (1977) has shown with cell birth-date labeling techniques that the first retinal ganglion cells are generated about the 30th day of gestation (E30), whereas those destined to form the LGN start to be born around E36. Cortical neurons are generated from cells of the proliferative neuroepithelium near the surface of the cerebral ventricle, and they migrate up along the processes of radial glial cells toward the surface of the cerebral wall. Neurogenesis of the cells of the primary visual cortex in the monkey takes place between about E43 and E102.

The first postmitotic cells entering the cerebral wall form a layer under the pial surface called the *preplate*, most of whose neurons (in monkeys and cats at least) die before or shortly after birth. Further waves of migrating juvenile neurons penetrate the preplate, dividing it into an upper layer, which becomes the cell-sparse layer 1 of the mature cortex, and the *subplate*, a population of cells lying below the cortical plate proper in what will become the white matter, most of which have been shown, in several species, to die shortly after birth (see Shatz et al. 1988). The layers of the cortex itself are formed in an inside-out sequence, each successive generation of immature neurons migrating through the existing layers to take its place under layer 1. In rodents, despite the much shorter gestation period (21–22 days in the rat), all neurons appear to be generated by birth, but migration of cortical cells is not complete until the end of the first postnatal week.

There is little hint of regional specialization at the earliest stages in the development of the cerebral cortex. Apart from anteroposterior and lateromedial gradients in the timing of overall maturation, all regions of the developing cortex appear similar until some time after the arrival of axons from the thalamus. There is currently great interest in the possibility that committed cortical fields emerge from an undifferentiated, more or less equipotential *protocortex* (see

McConnell 1989; O'Leary 1989). Regional differentiation might be imposed on each field by some local environmental influence. Such a process of induced differentiation could simplify the huge problem of genetic determination of such a complex structure, because the distinctive characteristics of each cortical zone would not have to be prespecified directly at the birth of each neuron in the germinal epithelium. One obvious candidate for such a local inducing agent is the afferent input, particularly the specific thalamic projection that each area receives at around the time that its idiosyncratic histological appearance begins. The regional specialization of the cerebral cortex might result from self-organization, stimulated by only one specified event during embryogenesis—the guidance of thalamic axons from each nucleus of the thalamus to their appropriate location in the cortex. We have been interested in the nature of that guidance.

Prenatal Development of Thalamocortical Interconnection

In all mammalian species so far examined, thalamic axons reach their cortical target zones by the time of birth. In monkeys, LGN fibers fan up toward the cortex in the optic radiation as early as halfway through gestation (Rakic 1977). However, the axons gather in the subplate below the occipital cortical plate and do not penetrate the plate itself until some time later (Shatz et al. 1988). LGN axons are visible throughout the lower layers of the primary visual cortex 3 weeks before birth, and terminals are beginning to concentrate in the lower part of layer 4 (Rakic 1977). Even at this early stage, the thalamic axons are quite precisely directed toward their target area; the accumulation of LGN axons below and in the cortical plate stops abruptly at the boundary between putative area 17 and the immediately adjacent area 18.

In animals with shorter gestation periods, thalamocortical innervation is less mature at birth, but even in rodents, LGN axons accumulate beneath the appropriate region of occipital cortex some days before birth (Lund and Mustari 1977). On the day of birth in the cat (before the photoreceptors begin to function), all the major pathways into and out of the primary visual cortex are present (Price and Blakemore 1985; Henderson and Blakemore 1986), although they vary in their state of maturity and degree of topographic precision. At the earliest stages, corticocortical and interhemispheric connections are characterized by exuberance of axon distribution (see Innocenti 1981; Dehay et al. 1985) and aberrance of arrangement of the cells of origin (Price and Blakemore 1985), but the ascending and descending interconnections with subcortical structures are more precisely and correctly arranged (Henderson and Blakemore 1986).

Figure 1 shows two coronal sections through the posterior part of the right cerebral hemisphere of a kitten, where area 17 occupies the medial bank of the marginal gyrus. On the day of birth, 24 hours earlier, a small amount of a mixture of the anterograde tracer tritiated proline and the retrogradely transported tracer horseradish peroxidase (HRP) had been injected into the lateral part of the LGN, which represents the peripheral part of the visual field in the adult. In the dark-field autoradiograph of Figure 1B, labeled LGN axons are seen streaming up through the white matter, running radially through the deep layers of the cortex, and are already concentrating and forming terminals in layer 4. Two patches of invasion are visible: a prominent one in area 17, deep in the medial bank of the gyrus, and a less dense one in area 18, the second visual area (which also receives geniculate input in cats). In both areas, the innervation lies in a region that will come to represent the peripheral visual field.

The section in Figure 1A was processed for HRP, which appears as a bright reaction product in the cell bodies of corticogeniculate neurons with axons terminating in the injected region of the LGN. They lie in a dense band in layer 6 (just as in the adult animal) of area 17 and a sparser band in area 18, in roughly the same positions as the thalamocortical innervation.

We can conclude that both thalamocortical and corticothalamic projections are basically constructed before birth, linking thalamic nuclei and their corresponding cortical fields. They are both at least roughly topographically organized and are in register, and they terminate in and originate from the correct cortical layers. How, then, are these interconnections guided? To tackle that question, we have been using a combination of techniques: tissue culture and the labeling of projections in the fetal brain.

METHODS

Coculture. We used techniques for culturing similar to those recently described by Romijn et al. (1988). Explants were cut from neocortex, diencephalon, and other areas of the brain of fetal or early postnatal Sprague-Dawley rats. The fetal animals were obtained from time-mated females by caesarian section under pentobarbital anesthesia (100 mg/kg, intraperitoneal); surgery on postnatal animals was performed under hypothermia or, at later ages, pentobarbital anesthesia. Coronal slices of neocortex or hippocampus, or sagittal slices of cerebellum, 350–400-μm thick, cut with a hand-held tissue chopper, were placed on collagen-coated microporous membranes in culture chambers with N2 hormone-supplemented, serum-free medium just covering the explant, at 36°C in 5% CO_2. Such slices survive well for many weeks, preserving their organotypic characteristics and undergoing obvious cellular maturation. They become slightly thinner and spread a little but do not collapse to virtual monolayers as with the roller-tube method (Gähwiler, 1988). Electron microscopy (in collaboration with P.R. Loewenstein, University of Dundee) shows their appearance to be remarkably normal even at the ultrastructural level.

To study the formation of connections, slices of cortex, hippocampus, or cerebellum were cocultured with

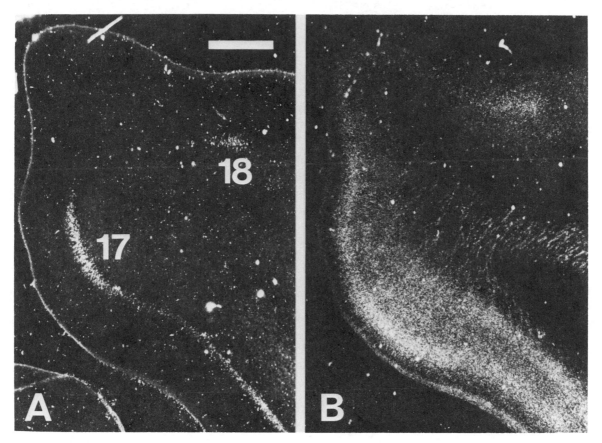

Figure 1. Coronal sections (25 μm for A, 50 μm for B) through the marginal gyrus of the right hemisphere of a kitten in which, 24 hr earlier, on the day of birth, a single injection (0.05–0.1 μl) of a mixture of 25 μCi/μl [^{3}H]proline and 10% HRP conjugated to wheat-germ agglutinin had been made into the lateral half of the LGN (which represents the peripheral visual field in the adult). (A) Dark-field micrograph of a section processed for HRP histochemistry. Cortical neurons with axons projecting to the injection site are filled with reaction product and appear bright. They lie virtually exclusively in layer 6 (as do corticothalamic cells in the adult), deep in the medial part of area 17 and in the lateral part of area 18, both of which represent the peripheral visual field. (B) Dark-field autoradiograph showing labeled LGN fibers in the white matter and streaming radially into the cortical plate in the same two regions of the cortex. Terminal label is beginning to concentrate over layer 4. Bar, 1 mm. From the study of Henderson and Blakemore (1986).

neighboring explants of thalamus rapidly dissected from E15–17 fetuses with a microsurgical knife. The thalamic block, as small as 0.5 mm × 0.5 mm × 0.3 mm, was taken from the dorsolateral aspect of the posterior diencephalon (fetal LGN), from an equivalent position more anterior in the thalamus (corresponding to nuclei that become connected to frontal cortical fields), or from other parts of the developing thalamus. To learn how to recognize the position of the LGN and, hence, other parts of the thalamus reliably from surface landmarks, we started by exposing a number of E16 fetal rats by hysterotomy, and we injected one eye with HRP. These fetuses were delivered by caesarian section 1 day later, and sections of the brains were processed for HRP histochemistry to reveal the terminal fields of optic nerve axons in the LGN. We proved the reliability of our localization of the thalamic tissue removed for culture by cutting, staining, and examining sections of the remaining part of the diencephalon to be sure that we had removed the desired

region. This experience enabled us to become confident of the identification of the major divisions of the thalamus from surface landmarks.

Thalamic explants also survive well for long periods in culture, although they tend to spread laterally somewhat more than cortical slices. Figure 2 summarizes schematically the procedure for the preparation of cocultures. This paper is based on the examination of almost 350 successful cocultures.

One of the explants in each coculture group was labeled with the lipophilic carbocyanine dye, DiI (Honig and Hume 1986), usually by briefly preincubating the explant in a solution of DiI in alcohol and dimethylsulfoxide before rinsing it in Hank's balanced salt solution and placing it into the culture chamber. Any axons that grew out of this explant were intensely labeled with the fluorescent dye for a period of about 5 days (after which the label became concentrated back in the cell body membranes, presumably because of membrane recycling). We examined the labeled axons

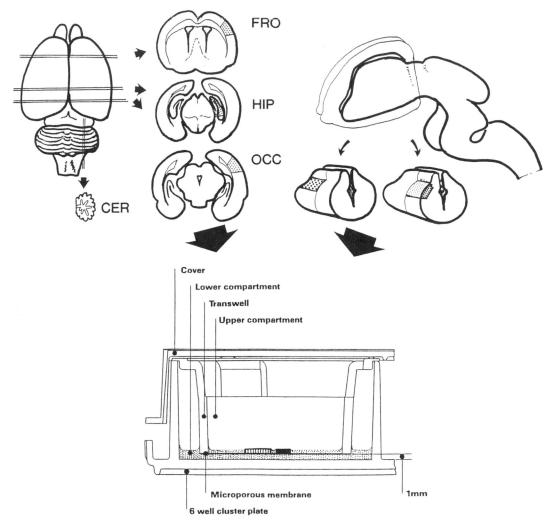

Figure 2. Schematic diagram of the procedure for the collection of tissue for coculture. At the top are drawings of the neonatal rat brain (*left*) and the fetal brain (*right*). Small thalamic blocks were taken from E15–17 rat fetuses, usually from the dorsolateral aspect of the diencephalon, as shown on the top right. The posterior blocks (shown very schematically in light stippling) contained almost exclusively LGN, whereas the more anterior blocks (heavy stippling) definitely excluded LGN and consisted of small fragments of thalamic nuclei that would normally have connected to more frontal areas of cortex. In some cases, more ventral and lateral thalamus was explanted. The thalamic explant was placed on the collagen-coated microporous membrane of a Colstar Transwell-COL culture chamber (lower diagram) close to one or more slices of tissue from fetal (E15–18) or postnatal (P0–11) rats. The upper left illustration of the neonatal rat brain shows the positions from which slices were cut. Slices of frontal (FRO) cortex (putative sensorimotor cortex), hippocampus (HIP), and occipital (OCC) cortex (putative area 17) were excised, as shown by the stippled regions, from coronal sections cut at the anteroposterior levels indicated. In some experiments, sagittally cut slices of cerebellum (CER) were used.

by epifluorescent microscopy after fixing the coculture in 4% paraformaldehyde. To study the distribution of axons at later stages, we fixed unlabeled cocultures, placed one or more small crystals of DiI directly into one of the explants, and stored the coculture for several weeks to allow diffusion of the dye along the fixed axons (Godement et al. 1987).

In many experiments, we were interested in comparing the patterns of innervation in various target tissues. To maximize the chances of revealing even small differences in the attraction of targets, we devised a "choice" paradigm in which each thalamic block was flanked by two different slices, and the ingrowth of axons was compared.

Pathway tracing in the fetal brain. We exploited the capacity of carbocyanine dyes to diffuse along axons in fixed tissue to trace pathways between thalamus and cortex in whole fixed fetal rat brains of different ages, from E13 to birth. Fetuses delivered by caesarian section under pentobarbital anesthesia were perfused with 4% paraformaldehyde in 0.1 M phosphate buffer (pH 7.4). We placed one or more of a variety of dyes (DiI, DiO, DiA, etc.) as small crystals into the surface of the neocortex or, after sagittal transection of the fixed brain, into the developing thalamus. After incubation in fixative for several weeks, 100–200-μm coronal or horizontal sections were cut and viewed under epifluorescent illumination with appropriate filters to reveal the different dyes. Sections were counterstained with bisbenzamide to reveal laminae and the boundaries of nuclei.

RESULTS

Pattern of Geniculocortical Innervation in Culture

Yamamoto et al. (1989), who used techniques similar to ours, recently reported the successful coculture of explants of fetal rat LGN and immediately postnatal visual cortex, with invasion of the cortex by thalamic fibers and innervation of the LGN by the axons of cells in the lower layers of the cortex. Bolz et al. (1990), using the roller-tube method, have also described the formation of corticofugal projections from cells in immediately postnatal visual cortex when cultured with another explant of the same gestational age. The morphology and laminar distribution of the cells of origin of these projections were different (in ways similar to the situation in vivo), depending on whether the neighboring explant was a block of LGN or another slice of cortex.

We decided to investigate whether the tendency of thalamic explants to innervate cortical slices is affected by the relative ages of the donor animals, the state of laminar development of the cortex, and the position within the thalamus and cortex from which the explants are taken. It is important to emphasize that, with culturing in serum-free medium on a collagen-coated substrate, there is little spontaneous neurite extension in the absence of a neighboring target explant. Therefore, any substantial invasion of one structure by axons from another is presumably an indication of a trophic, or at least a permissive, influence of the one on the other. Rapid axon invasion occurs only if the explants are separated by less than about 2 mm (although the neurites can span larger gaps if the cultures are grown on a laminin-coated membrane). The involvement of diffusible trophic factors is further suggested by the manner of axon outgrowth in such cocultures. Axons do not initially sprout in all directions from the innervating explant; they stream out specifically toward the attractive target. If the distance between the two structures is more than about 1 mm, the growing axons tend to fasciculate to form dense fiber bundles bridging the gap.

In an attempt to optimize thalamocortical innervation, we tried to mimic the timing of events in vivo by placing explants of E16 thalamus (which the results of Lund and Mustari [1977] suggested is the stage of initial outgrowth of thalamic axons) next to the ventricular surface of slices of neonatal (P0–3) occipital cortex. Within 1 day, DiI-labeled axons were seen sprouting from the side of the LGN explant close to the cortical slice. The axons ran into the white matter and up through the cortical plate at a rate of up to 1 mm per day: Most ran radially, although some took more oblique or irregular routes. They penetrated the cortical

tissue and did not simply grow over the surface of the slice. The general pattern of innervation appeared remarkably normal, except that the axons did not terminate in the middle of the cortical plate, as the majority of thalamic fibers do in vivo, but grew up to reach the marginal zone after about 3 days in culture. Figure 3, top, is a fluorescence micrograph showing axons from an explant of E16 LGN invading a slice of P3 occipital cortex after just 4 days in culture. Most of the fibers have reached the pial surface, and some are starting to ramify over it. One axon (far right) has turned through 90° and has coursed horizontally more than 1.5 mm through the upper layers: At its tip (far left) is a bright expanded growth cone. Figure 3, bottom, is a high-power view of growth cones at the growing ends of axons below the pial surface.

We left some cocultures for longer periods, up to several weeks, and then fixed them and applied DiI as crystals to the LGN explant to trace the distribution of axons after the 5 days for which they can be followed in prestained material. Even after long periods, many axons still extended to the cortical surface, although some had become restricted to lower layers and had varicosities, which might represent synaptic boutons, along their length and at their tips.

Removal of the occipital cortex in a newborn rat in vivo results in virtually total degeneration of the LGN. However, Cunningham et al. (1987) found that more geniculate cells survive if gel impregnated with culture medium conditioned by explants of embryonic occipital cortex is implanted into the cavity of such a cortical lesion. They interpreted this to mean that the cortex produces a diffusible proteinaceous trophic factor that promotes the survival of axotomized LGN cells.

It seems clear from our results in culture that neonatal visual cortex also produces a factor that stimulates neurite outgrowth from the fetal LGN (conceivably the same substance that rescues axotomized cells). The growth of axons is rapid and is directed toward the cortical plate. As in vivo, invading thalamic axons in such cocultures encounter first the intermediate zone of the white matter, then the subplate layer, and finally, the cortical plate itself. However, innervation is not dependent on that particular sequence of contact. If the LGN explant is placed against the radially cut end of a cortical slice, many axons pass horizontally into the white matter, coursing along under the cortex and then turning up to run radially into the cortical plate, much like normal thalamic axons growing up from the diencephalon. However, in such cultures, a substantial fraction of LGN fibers pass straight into the gray matter of the cortex, running parallel to the layer in which they enter it.

Invasion even occurs if the LGN block is placed next to the pial surface (as long as the pia itself is removed), and the fibers run radially or diagonally down toward the white matter. In this case, all axons invade the cortical plate without prior contact with the intermediate zone or subplate cells.

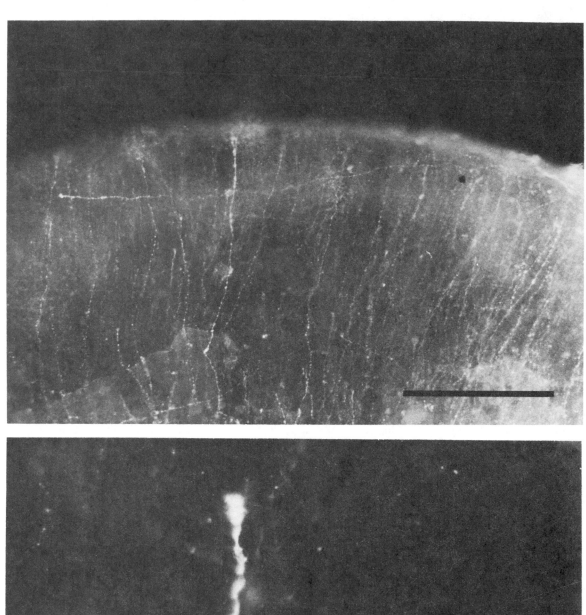

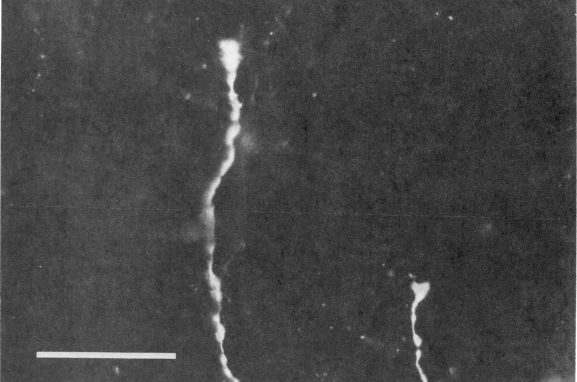

Figure 3. Fluorescence photomicrographs of DiI-labeled axons from an E16 LGN explant growing into a slice of P0 occipital cortex after 4 days in culture. (*Top*) Low-power view of the entire thickness of the cortical plate, showing axons running radially to the top of the cortex, where some have turned laterally to run in the marginal zone or across the pial surface. Bar, 0.5 mm. (*Bottom*) High-power view of individual axons in the cortex with expanded growth cones at their tips. Bar, 50 μm.

496

Emergence of Laminar Specificity

We wondered whether the tendency of LGN axons to grow through the whole thickness of the cortical plate when cultured with immediately postnatal visual cortex might reflect the incomplete development of cortical laminae at birth in the rat. According to the thymidine birth-dating study of Lund and Mustari (1977), migration of immature cortical cells is far from complete at birth. They found cells born on E17, which ultimately contribute substantially to layer 4, scattered through all layers on the day of birth, with a concentration under the marginal zone. Those generated at later fetal ages, which mainly form the supragranular layers, were presumed to be at an even earlier stage in the process of migration at the time of birth. Migration of cells continued during the first postnatal week, concurrent with the invasion of the cortical plate by thalamic fibers, the majority of which terminated in layer 4 by the end of the first week.

Unless migration continues in culture, these results suggest that slices taken shortly after birth should have abnormal lamination. In fact, Bolz et al. (1990) have shown, by means of birth-date labeling with bromodeoxyuridine, that cells born on E16 and E18 have distributions through the cortex that look fairly similar in normal animals more than 12 days old and in slices taken shortly after birth and cultured for 2–3 weeks. However, we thought that innervation by LGN explants might be more normal if they were cocultured with slices of cortex taken toward the end of the first week of life, when migration should be complete. Indeed, the pattern of ingrowth was very different when older cortical slices were used. With E16 LGN and P5 occipital cortex, initial invasion was somewhat slower, and after 4 days in culture, many axons appeared to have branched locally, lost their growth cones, and terminated 300–400 μm below the pial surface, at the depth of layer 4. Just as in vivo, some axons extended to the marginal zone (Fig. 4).

This general pattern of innervation occurred for all later postnatal slices of occipital cortex, up to P11, the oldest explant taken. To be sure that these results with older slices were not accounted for by differences in culturing conditions, we employed the "choice" paradigm (see Methods), culturing an E16 LGN explant flanked by two cortical slices, one P3, the other P6. Both were innervated by the LGN but with different patterns, as found with single cocultures. Thus, it appears that sometime between P3 and P5, the cortex starts to express a specific signal that makes thalamic fibers branch and terminate around layer 4 and that prevents the majority from continuing to advance to the pial surface. When we placed E16 LGN next to the cleaned pial surface of older cortical slices, axons readily grew in through the supragranular layers and again tended to terminate in the middle of the cortical plate. Therefore, this expressed signal is not one that simply discourages axon growth in the upper layers: It seems likely that, at about postnatal day 4, neurons of layer 4,

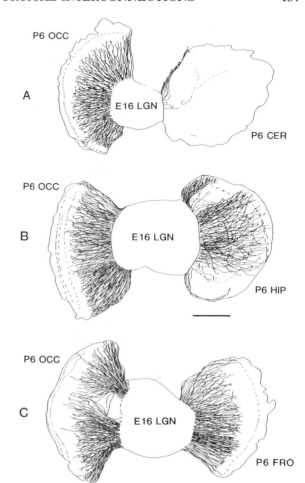

Figure 4. Results of the "choice" paradigm in which each explant of E16 LGN was cultured next to two different slices. Camera lucida drawings show DiI-labeled thalamic axons after 5 days in culture. (*A*) Confronted by P6 occipital cortex (OCC) and cerebellum (CER), geniculate innervation was almost entirely restricted to the slice of neocortex, in which a few axons reached the marginal zone, but most terminated in what appeared to be layer 4, about 400 μm below the surface. Of the few axons that sprouted toward the cerebellar slice, most ran around one border of the slice. (*B*) When cultured with P6 occipital cortex and hippocampus (HIP), the density of innervation from E16 LGN was much more similar, but in the hippocampus the axons did not terminate in a distinct zone and mainly extended toward the surface. (*C*) With P6 occipital and frontal cortex (FRO), geniculate axons invaded both slices densely with very similar patterns. In both cases, a few axons reached the marginal zone, but most terminated around layer 4. Bar, 1 mm.

which have reached their correct position and matured considerably, express a specific "stop signal," which encourages thalamic axons to arborize and terminate.

Target Selectivity of Thalamic Innervation in Culture

So far, we have merely shown that a piece of occipital cortex is a more attractive medium for axon invasion than the collagen-coated membrane that makes up the rest of the LGN explant's environment in the culture chamber. To test whether the trophic influence is specific, we cultured E16 LGN with slices of other tissue. In fact, we used the choice paradigm to compare the innervation of different structures. Figure 4 shows the results of culturing E16 LGN for 5 days with various choices. The most dramatic result is the contrast between the florid invasion of P6 occipital cortex and the virtual avoidance of a slice of P6 cerebellum (Fig. 4A). In more than 20 cocultures involving LGN and cerebellum (from P1–8), we have seen only a tiny number of axons *penetrating* the cerebellum. Axon growth was mainly restricted to a few fasciculated bundles running around the edge of the cerebellar slice or across its surface.

Given the choice between P6 occipital cortex and P6 hippocampus, LGN axons showed little preference (Fig. 4B). Hippocampal slices were innervated almost as densely as neocortical slices, but, interestingly, the axons continued up to the surface of the hippocampus and did not tend to terminate specifically in the middle layers, as in occipital cortex of this age. This implies that the hippocampus, a region of allocortex, exerts a general trophic influence similar to that of neocortex but has no equivalent to the stop signal expressed by cortical layer 4.

Positional Selectivity of Thalamocortical Innervation in Culture

Our starting question concerned the mechanism by which thalamic axons from different nuclei find their way to the appropriate cortical fields. We have shown a trophic influence of occipital cortex on LGN, and we now ask whether different cortical areas selectively attract fibers from their particular thalamic nuclei. We used the choice paradigm to test this by culturing explants of either LGN or some other region of the developing thalamus, each flanked by slices of two different regions of cortex. The result was unequivocal: The pattern of innervation was indistinguishable whatever regions of thalamus and cortex were combined. For example, Figure 4C shows the very similar axonal outgrowth from an E16 LGN explant into P6 occipital cortex and P6 frontal cortex (which the LGN never innervates in vivo). Equally, explants of anterior thalamus and more ventral thalamus sent axons in a similar pattern into occipital, frontal, or any other region of cortex.

One might imagine that regional chemospecificity need be evident only at an earlier age, before thalamic axons fully invade the cortical plate in vivo, in order to guide them to the appropriate area of cortex. However, we saw no hint of positional preference, even when we cultured slices of P0 cortex in combination with fetal thalamus.

Early Corticothalamic Projections in Culture

Recently, McConnell et al. (1989) showed that cells of the cortical subplate, the first postmitotic neurons of the developing cerebrum, send a pioneering projection down toward the thalamus in the cat before the cells of the lower layers of the cortical plate proper have even been born (see Shatz et al., this volume). They suggested that this pioneer pathway may then guide subsequent thalamocortical innervation. This is an attractive notion, and it would remove the need for any positionally specific cortical trophic influence on thalamic axons. However, it remains to be established that this subplate projection is positionally ordered, with each cortical zone sending its subplate axons only to the appropriate region of the thalamus. Even if this were the case, it would simply displace the need for a mechanism of positional guidance from thalamocortical to corticothalamic projections.

We started to look at these problems in the rat by culturing thalamic explants with slices of embryonic cortex, taken as early as E15, when the first neurons of the cortex proper are being born (Miller 1988) and only the preplate cells have completed their migration. We preincubated the cortical slice with DiI to label corticofugal axons. Figure 5 summarizes the results. Innervation of thalamus by embryonic cortex, presumably from subplate cells, did occur but was less profuse than the thalamocortical innervation described above. However, again there was no obvious positional preference. Any region of embryonic cortex innervated equally any region of developing thalamus.

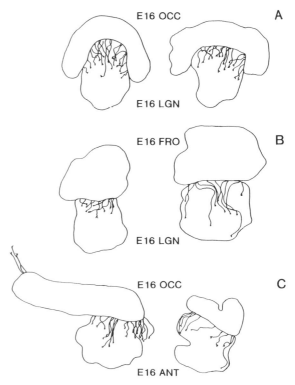

Figure 5. Camera lucida drawings of axon outgrowth from E16 cortical explants cultured for 4 days with thalamic explants of the same age. Two examples of each combination are shown. (*A*) Occipital cortex (OCC) sends axons (presumably from subplate cells) into LGN. (*B*) Frontal cortex (FRO) also innervates LGN. (*C*) Occipital cortex innervates anterior thalamus (ANT).

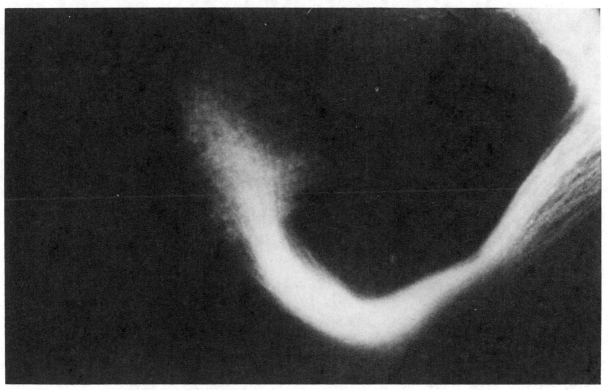

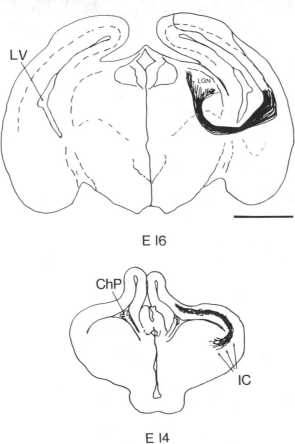

E 16

E 14

Figure 6. DiI diffusion from a crystal placed on the occipital cortex of fixed fetal brains to reveal connection with the thalamus. (*Top*) Fluorescence micrograph of an E16 brain, showing the labeled bundle of fibers running in the intermediate zone (upper right), turning medially, narrowing as it passes through the internal capsule and then sweeping up to surround the LGN. (*Middle*) Camera lucida drawing of an entire coronal section through the brain of the same animal (LV, lateral ventricle). Bar, 1 mm. (*Bottom*) Coronal section of the labeled bundle seen after placement of a crystal on occipital cortex of an E14 brain. Descending axons are just passing through the primitive internal capsule (IC) and have growth cones at their tips (ChP, choroid plexus).

499

If these results apply in vivo, and if fibers from subplate to thalamus do indeed establish guidance paths along which thalamic axons grow to the correct areas of cortex, they must do so by means of some mechanism other than positionally specific trophic attraction.

Ordered Interconnection of Cortex and Thalamus in the Developing Brain

To trace the routes taken by the early projections from cortex to thalamus and vice versa, we placed small crystals of variously colored carbocyanine dyes at different positions in fixed fetal rat brains (E13 to birth) and examined the axons stained by diffusion after several weeks. Early on E14, a crystal of DiI on the occipital cortex densely stained the thin preplate and the radial glia extending down to the ventricular zone, but no axons were visible leaving the cortex. Application of dye just a few hours later revealed a short bundle of axons leaving the preplate, presumably from subplate neurons, and turning 90° in the intermediate zone to direct their growth cones toward the primitive internal capsule, the gateway between telencephalon and diencephalon. By the end of the 14th day, the bundle of corticofugal axons is passing through the primitive internal capsule (Fig. 6, bottom), and 1 day later, it has turned sharply upward and embraced the developing LGN (Fig. 6, top and middle). Placement of dye on other cortical regions revealed similar neatly organized tracts, each heading toward the appropriate area of the thalamus. The timing of outgrowth varies systematically. More lateral regions of cortex send out axons up to a day before those from more medial regions, and they lie more lateral in the intermediate zone, run lower in the internal capsule, and head for more ventral parts of the thalamus.

Figure 6, top, is a fluorescence micrograph of a coronal section at the level of the LGN after placement of a crystal of DiI on the occipital cortex at E16 (Fig. 6, middle, is a camera lucida drawing of a nearby section from the same brain). The stained tract runs down in the intermediate zone (upper right part of Fig. 6, top), turns medially, narrows as it approaches the internal capsule, and then bends up as it emerges in the diencephalon to run to the LGN.

At first, we thought that the pathways from subplate to thalamic nuclei were completely established before the outgrowth of thalamocortical fibers (which would obviously have reinforced the notion that the former guide the entire growth of the latter). However, when we left such sections several weeks longer for dye diffusion, we saw stained cell bodies in the LGN, presumably retrogradely labeled along thalamic axons that had already reached the occipital cortex. This impression was confirmed by experiments in which crystals were placed in various parts of the thalamus. Axons appear to leave the thalamus at the same time that the first fibers are leaving the cortex (early on E14 for the geniculocortical pathway), and the corresponding af-

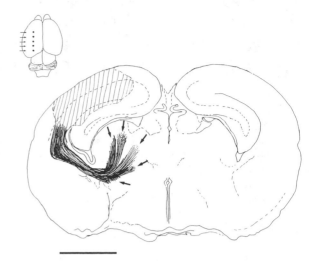

Figure 7. Bundles of axons linking cortex and thalamus were revealed by application of five carbocyanine dyes at points in a parasagittal row along the left hemisphere of a fixed E20 rat brain (inset diagram of surface view). After several weeks for anterograde and retrograde diffusion, 250-μm-thick coronal sections were examined with different filters in the fluorescence microscope to reveal the various dyes. Five distinct bundles were clearly visible passing through the primitive internal capsule without mixing or crossing, and running to different thalamic nuclei: The tip of each bundle is marked with an arrow. This coronal section was at the level of termination of the bundles from the two caudal crystal placements, and retrogradely labeled thalamic cells were visible at the end of each bundle. The tracts labeled from the more anterior crystals ended at more rostral and ventral levels in the thalamus. Bar, 1 mm.

ferent and efferent bundles meet in the intermediate zone close to the internal capsule (at around E14/15 for the occipital cortex). Thus, the descending and ascending axons each pioneer the pathway through their own segment of the brain and, after a "handshake" near the internal capsule, each may guide the growth of the other over the distal part of its trajectory (Molnár and Blakemore 1990). LGN axons have reached the occipital cortex by E16, 2 days earlier than the original estimate of Lund and Mustari (1977).

By E16, the earliest afferent and efferent fibers to and from any cortical point are closely intermingled to form a single bundle, which is expected if they have acted as mutual guides. Placement of dye on any position in the cortex between E16 and birth, which labels both the ascending and descending pathways, always leads to a single stained tract. Figure 7 shows an E20 brain in which five dyes were placed in a parasagittal row. In this thick coronal section, five separate bundles, each recognized by its distinctive color under different fluorescence filters, were seen passing through the internal capsule and diverging in the diencephalon. The more posterior the cortical point, the more dorsal and posterior its target in the thalamus.

DISCUSSION

Rather than each cortical field exerting a specific attraction only for its own thalamic afferents or each thalamic nucleus attracting the subplate axons of its own field, our coculture experiments suggest that there are powerful but positionally nonspecific trophic interactions between the two tissues. In the search for a mechanism of guidance for thalamic innervation of the cortex, the spotlight falls on the closely coordinated expeditions of subplate and thalamic axons at the earliest stages of their growth. Each set of fibers appears to grow as a tight, ordered bundle toward the internal capsule, taking its place next to its neighbors in a position dependent on its site of origin. It is important to emphasize how small the brain is and how simple its anatomical relationships are at this stage of coordinated growth. At E14, the cerebral hemispheres are essentially a flat sheet wrapped around the ball of the diencephalon (Fig. 6, bottom). Fibers from the cortex need only run down through the intermediate zone, maintaining their position in the growing array to set up a strictly topographic distribution, those from dorsal cortex lying more medial, those from lateral cortex more lateral. Likewise, axons from different thalamic nuclei need only grow straight toward the internal capsule, not crossing their neighbors, to establish a similarly ordered pattern. After they have met, the rapid growth of the forebrain begins to impose complex bends and twists on both sets of fibers (Fig. 6, top and middle), but each pioneer bundle may guide its counterpart over the final, increasingly distorted part of its journey.

The key, then, to selective afferent innervation of cortical fields may lie in some quite simple property of the extracellular matrix between thalamus and cortex, determining the direction of growth of both sets of fibers toward the internal capsule. That, combined with a strict sequence of outgrowth and a tendency of fibers not to cross their neighbors, might be enough to establish the two ordered patterns of pioneers, which then guide each other home.

Such a mechanism, based on a simple algorithm specifying the rough direction of growth and maintaining fiber order, might explain the distribution of afferent axons from specific thalamic nuclei to their target areas in the cortex. It might also account for the spontaneous emergence of extra cortical fields, especially for each of the senses, which is such a compelling feature of the evolution of the forebrain. Any mutation that causes the appearance of a new population of thalamic

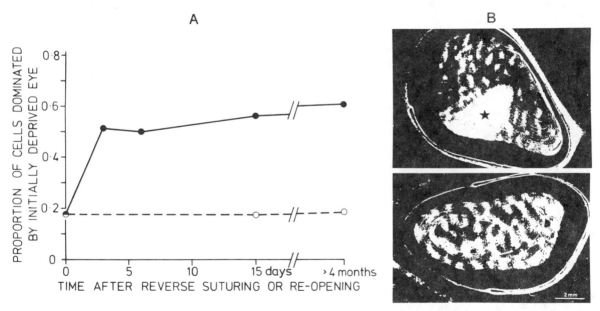

Figure 8. Summary of electrophysiological and anatomical results of Blakemore et al. (1981) and Swindale et al. (1981), showing the capacity of geniculate axons to reinnervate layer 4, on the basis of competitive interaction between the two eyes. Monkeys were deprived of vision by closing the lids of the right eye for 3–4 weeks; then that eye was reopened and, in some cases, the left eye was closed for a period of time (reverse suturing) before single cells were recorded in area 17 and their ocular dominance was determined. (*A*) The graph plots the proportion of cells recorded in layer 4c that were dominated by the initially deprived right eye. In a control animal recorded at the end of the initial deprivation (zero on the abscissa), less than 20% of cells were dominated by the deprived eye, and they occurred in small clusters along each tangential penetration through layer 4c. Simply reopening the right eye, restoring binocular vision, did not improve the situation (open circles and dashed line), but reverse suturing (filled circles, continuous line) caused a rapid increase in the size of the clusters of cells driven by the initially deprived eye. (*B*) The initially deprived right eye of each animal had been injected with 1–1.5 mCi of tritiated proline 11–19 days before perfusion, in order to perform transneuronal autoradiography (see LeVay et al. 1980). Tangential sections of the cortex were coated with emulsion to study the regions of termination of axons from the right-eye layers of the LGN. Above is a darkfield montage of an autoradiograph showing part of the right calcarine cortex of a control animal, which was simply monocularly deprived for 23 days. The patches of right-eye terminals (white areas) are grossly shrunken (except for the large patch marked with a star, which presumably corresponds to the optic disc of the other eye, where there can be no competition between the two eyes). The lower montage is from the calcarine cortex of an animal deprived in the right eye for 26 days and then reverse sutured for only 6 days. This has been sufficient to cause expansion of the terminal fields and the reestablishment of clear ocular dominance "stripes."

cells with input from a sense organ might, through the operation of this kind of relational guidance system, lead the axons of those additional thalamic cells to colonize an area of cortex adjacent to the target field of their immediate thalamic neighbors. That captured region of cortex might in turn become differentiated to process the sensory information that it receives from the thalamus and from other cortical regions (perhaps automatically directed to it by similar simple algorithms of connectivity).

It is difficult to imagine that such a mechanism could establish the remarkably precise topographic representations that exist *within* sensory areas, especially the primary visual cortex. In area 17, there is a "map" of the visual field, globally distorted because of over-representation of the fovea, but locally remarkably precise. For the central field, each millimeter of the cortical surface is equivalent to the width of just a few cones in the fovea, and some cortical cells have receptive fields with central summating regions equivalent in width to only one or two cones (see Blakemore 1990;

Hawken and Parker 1990). There is strong evidence that sensory stimulation after birth can regulate the arborization of afferent axons, synaptogenesis, and the strength of synapses, hence controlling the local precision of afferent input.

Although geniculate axons already lie under the visual cortex at birth and have even started to innervate layer 4 in monkeys and cats (Fig. 1), much consolidation of input continues after birth. In both cats and monkeys, an active reorganization takes place during the first 6–8 weeks after birth (LeVay et al. 1980). In the adult monkey, fibers from right-eye and left-eye layers of the LGN terminate in a pattern of alternating "ocular dominance stripes," each about 0.3 mm across, visible in autoradiographs of tangential sections through layer 4 after injection of one eye with tritiated amino acid. But at birth, fibers from the two eyes are intermingled in layer 4, with only slight variation in relative density. The process of ocular segregation, which can be viewed as local regulation of the topography of thalamic input, is dependent on activity in

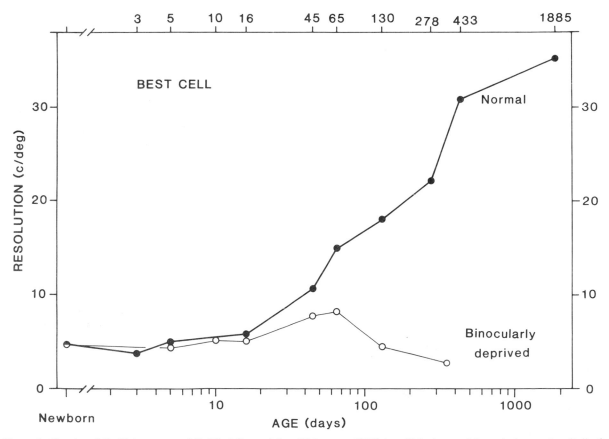

Figure 9. Results of C. Blakemore and F. Vital-Durand (see Blakemore 1990) in which the spatial resolution or "acuity" of individual cells in monkey area 17 was determined by stimulating the receptive field of each cell with drifting, high-contrast gratings and increasing the spatial frequency (the number of cycles of the grating per degree of visual angle) until the cell just stopped responding. Resolution is plotted against the age of the animal (log scale) for normal monkeys (filled circles) and for monkeys that had been binocularly deprived by lid suture since the day of birth (open circles). Results are shown only for the best-resolving cell recorded in the foveal projection area, but these data are representative, since significant numbers of cells in each animal had performance similar to that of the best. Deprivation grossly interferes with the normal substantial postnatal improvement of neuronal acuity, presumably indicating that cortical cells require stimulation with well-focused retinal images in order to maintain synaptic input from a well-localized ensemble of LGN axons.

the two sets of axons: If a monkey or cat is reared with one eye closed, the LGN terminals carrying signals from that eye become restricted to small, shrunken patches (see Fig. 8B), while the other eye's input occupies the remaining space, leading to cortical cells becoming functionally dominated by input from the nondeprived eye (Fig. 8A). The process of competition between the two sets of axons is dynamically regulated on the basis of their *relative* activity. Reversing the competitive advantage at an early age by reopening a deprived eye and closing the other causes rapid expansion of the territory occupied in layer 4 by the originally deprived axons (Fig. 8).

At the level of individual cortical neurons, there appear to be even more subtle local mechanisms for the regulation of effective afferent input, which might depend on synaptic strengthening on the basis of correlated presynaptic and postsynaptic activity. For instance, in the foveal representation area of the visual cortex of an adult monkey, some individual neurons have receptive fields with summating centers little more than a single foveal cone in width. They are thus able to detect a grating pattern moving across the receptive field when the individual bars of the grating are approximately the same size as a single cone (see Hawken and Parker 1990). This property demands remarkable precision in the arrangement of afferent input onto individual cortical cells, and it seems that the maintenance of such precise convergence is regulated through synaptic plasticity early in life (see Blakemore 1990). In monkeys reared with both eyes closed (abolishing fine spatial detail in the retinal image), cortical cells fail to undergo the normal developmental improvement in the "acuity" of their receptive fields (Fig. 9).

In conclusion, the mechanisms that determine thalamic innervation of target cells in the cortex are several. Factors in the extracellular environment may initially direct the axons toward the internal capsule, whence they might grow over their corticofugal counterparts to reach their cortical field. A nonspecific trophic influence of the cortex attracts them in, and a carefully timed stop signal from layer 4 terminates their growth. Local competitive interaction, dependent on the relative activity of different classes of fibers, can adjust their distribution locally. Finally, synaptic modulation, exaggerated during a specific early sensitive period in some areas of cortex but perhaps continuing throughout life in others, refines the input to individual neurons in ways that are presumably crucial for establishing the computational operations that the cortex performs.

ACKNOWLEDGMENTS

Our laboratory, which belongs to the Oxford McDonnell-Pew Centre for Cognitive Neuroscience, is supported by grants from the Medical Research Council and the Wellcome Trust. For his first year in Oxford, Z.M. held a Soros-Hungarian Academy of Sciences Scholarship.

REFERENCES

Blakemore, C., ed. 1990. Maturation of mechanisms for efficient spatial vision. In *Vision: Coding and efficiency*, p. 254. Cambridge University Press, Cambridge, England.

Blakemore, C., F. Vital-Durand, and L.J. Garey. 1981. Recovery from monocular deprivation in the monkey. I. Reversal of physiological effects in the visual cortex. *Proc. R. Soc. Lond. B Biol. Sci.* 213: 399.

Bolz, J., N. Novak, M. Gotz, and T. Bonhoeffer. 1990. Formation of target specific neuronal projections in organotypic slice cultures from rat visual cortex. *Nature* 346: 359.

Brodmann, K. 1909. *Vergleichende Lokalisationslehre der Grosshirnrinde in ihren prinzipien dargestellt auf Grund des Zellenbaues.* J.A. Barth, Leipzig.

Cunningham, T.J., F. Haun, and P.D. Chantler. 1987. Diffusible proteins prolong survival of dorsal lateral geniculate neurons following occipital cortex lesions in newborn rats. *Dev. Brain Res.* 37: 133.

Dehay, C., J. Bullier, and H. Kennedy. 1985. Transient projections from the fronto-parietal and temporal cortex to areas 17, 18 and 19 in the kitten. *Exp. Brain. Res.* 57: 208.

Gähwiler, B.H. 1988. Organotypic cultures of neural tissue. *Trends Neurosci.* 11: 484.

Godement, P., J. Vaneslow, S. Thanos, and F. Bonhoeffer. 1987. A study in developing visual systems with a new method of staining neurones and their processes in fixed tissue. *Development* 101: 697.

Hawken, M.J. and A.J. Parker. 1990. Detection and discrimination mechanisms in the striate cortex of the Old-World monkey. In *Vision: Coding and efficiency* (ed. C. Blakemore), p. 103. Cambridge University Press, Cambridge, England.

Henderson, Z. and C. Blakemore. 1986. Organization of the visual pathways in the newborn kitten. *Neurosci. Res.* 3: 628.

Honig, M.G. and R.I. Hume. 1986. Fluorescent carbocyanine dyes allow living neurons of identified origin to be studied in long-term cultures. *J. Cell Biol.* 103: 171.

Innocenti, G.M. 1981. Growth and reshaping of axons in the establishment of visual callosal connections. *Science* 212: 824.

LeVay, S., T.N. Wiesel, and D.H. Hubel. 1980. The development of ocular dominance columns in normal and visually deprived monkeys. *J. Comp. Neurol.* 191: 1.

Lund, R.D. and M.J. Mustari. 1977. Development of the geniculocortical pathway in rats. *J. Comp. Neurol.* 173: 289.

McConnell, S.K. 1989. The determination of neuronal fate in the cerebral cortex. *Trends Neurosci.* 12: 342.

McConnell, S.K., A. Ghosh, and C.J. Shatz. 1989. Subplate neurons pioneer the first axon pathway from the cerebral cortex. *Science* 245: 978.

Miller, M.W. 1988. Development of projection and local circuit neurons in neocortex. In *Cerebral cortex: Development and maturation of cerebral cortex* (ed. A. Peters and E.G. Jones), vol. 7, p. 133. Plenum Press, New York.

Molnár, Z. and C. Blakemore. 1990. Relationship of corticofugal and corticopetal projections in the prenatal establishment of projections from thalamic nuclei to specific cortical areas of the rat. *J. Physiol.* 430: 104P.

O'Leary, D.D.M. 1989. Do cortical areas emerge from a protocortex? *Trends Neurosci.* 12: 400.

Price, D.J. and C. Blakemore. 1985. The postnatal development of the association projection from visual cortical area 17 to area 18 in the cat. *J. Neurosci.* 5: 2443.

Rakic, P. 1977. Prenatal development of the visual system in rhesus monkey. *Philos. Trans. R. Soc. Lond. B Biol. Sci.* 278: 245.

Romijn, H.J., B.M. De Jong, and J.M. Ruijter. 1988. A procedure for culturing rat neocortex explants in a serum-free nutrient medium. *J. Neurosci. Methods* 23: 75.

Shatz, C.J., J.J.M. Chun, and M.B. Luskin. 1988. The role of the subplate in the development of the mammalian telencephalon. In *Cerebral cortex: Development and maturation of cerebral cortex* (ed. A. Peters and E.G. Jones), vol. 7, p. 35. Plenum Press, New York.

Swindale, N.V., F. Vital-Durand, and C. Blakemore. 1981. Recovery from monocular deprivation in the monkey. III. Reversal of anatomical effects in the visual cortex. *Proc. R. Soc. Lond. B Biol. Sci.* **213**:435.

Yamamoto, N., T. Kurotani, and K. Toyama. 1989. Neural connections between the lateral geniculate nucleus and visual cortex in vitro. *Science* **245:** 192.

Expression of Neural Proteoglycans Correlates with the Acquisition of Mature Neuronal Properties in the Mammalian Brain

S. Hockfield, R.G. Kalb, S. Zaremba, and H. Fryer

Section of Neuroanatomy, Yale University School of Medicine, New Haven, Connecticut 06510

The neurons in the mature mammalian central nervous system (CNS) are an enormously diverse group of cells. The acquisition of mature, differentiated neuronal properties takes place over an extended developmental period, through a number of different mechanisms. Some of the very last events in neuronal development occur late in the postnatal period, when the mature set of synapses between neurons and their targets is selected and the adult anatomical and physiological properties of neurons are acquired. Experiments in many different systems have shown that the mature set of synapses is selected from an initial set by selective stabilization of some synapses and elimination of others (for review, see Purves and Lichtman 1985). The process of synapse selection is governed, at least in part, by neuronal activity. Temporal matching of pre- and postsynaptic activity is thought to be critical in determining whether a synapse will be retained or lost. Environmental stimuli (such as visual or auditory signals) can be extremely effective in evoking the neuronal activity that mediates synapse selection and the acquisition of mature neuronal properties.

The period in development during which the activity of a neuron, evoked by environmental stimuli, can influence mature neuronal phenotype has been called the critical or sensitive period. Critical periods in development are circumscribed, so that an immature, relatively plastic state of a neuron is followed by a mature, relatively nonplastic state. Synapse selection and stabilization are critical components of the transition from the immature and plastic state to the mature and nonplastic state. The mechanisms by which the mature set of synapses is stabilized are little understood. We have been exploring the possibility that the change in neuronal phenotype from an immature, plastic state to a mature, less plastic state might be reflected by changes in the molecular properties of neurons. Identification of proteins that are expressed at the close of the critical period could advance our understanding of the biological processes underlying the loss of synaptic plasticity in development.

One class of molecules that may play a role in stabilizing mature neuronal structure are the elements of the extracellular matrix (ECM). In many tissues, the ECM serves to stabilize intercellular interactions and helps to maintain tissue integrity (for review, see Ruoslahti 1989; Hockfield 1990). Most extracellular matrices

are rich in proteoglycans, glycoproteins that are extensively modified by characteristic long, unbranched chains, called glycosaminoglycans, composed of repeating disaccharide units. We have identified a chondroitin sulfate proteoglycan in the mammalian CNS that shares many features with components of nonneural ECM. Here, we describe our studies showing that this proteoglycan is expressed at the end of the period of synaptic plasticity and that its expression is regulated by patterned neuronal activity during development. We provide evidence that this chondroitin sulfate proteoglycan is one member of a larger family of neural proteoglycans, many of which exhibit exquisite cell-type specificity in the mammalian CNS. Our results suggest that the loss of plasticity during development is accompanied, and possibly subserved, by the elaboration of an ECM. This matrix may also play a role in maintaining the mature, differentiated properties of neurons.

METHODS

The generation and characterization of monoclonal antibody Cat-301 and its antigen have been described previously (McKay and Hockfield 1982; Zaremba et al. 1989). For immunochemistry, antigen was partially purified from urea extracts of cat cortex membranes by DEAE chromatography and Sepharose CL-2B gel filtration (Zaremba et al. 1989). Fractions from the Sepharose column containing the Cat-301 antigen were pooled. A second pool was made of fractions eluting at the column void volume. Aliquots of both pools were analyzed for proteoglycan content by incubation with chondroitinase, followed by electrophoresis and immunoblotting with Cat-301 or antibodies to chondroitin sulfate (see below). Final purification of the Cat-301 antigen was performed on a Cat-301 antibody affinity column (Guimaraes et al. 1990). Other methods for immunohistochemical and immunochemical analyses were performed as reported previously (Hockfield and McKay 1983; Kalb and Hockfield 1988; Zaremba et al. 1989; Guimaraes et al. 1990).

Antibodies to chondroitin sulfate were obtained from ICN and as a generous gift from B. Caterson (Couchman et al. 1984) and were used according to Watanabe (Watanabe et al. 1989). Antibodies 3B3/C1 (anti-6S), 2B6 (anti-4S), and 1B5/C5 (anti-0S) recognize, respectively, 6 sulfated, 4 sulfated, and unsulfated chondroitin and dermatan sulfate proteoglycans. Purified aggrecan from bovine cartilage was a generous gift from J. Hassell and J. Sandy.

RESULTS
Cat-301 Recognizes a Chondroitin Sulfate Proteoglycan

Biochemical analyses demonstrate that Cat-301 recognizes a chondroitin sulfate proteoglycan. The apparent molecular weight of the antigen on reducing SDS-PAGE is approximately 680,000 and is shifted to 580,000 upon digestion with chondroitinase (Zaremba et al. 1989), an enzyme that specifically removes chondroitin sulfate glycosaminoglycans. Furthermore, after Cat-301 antibody affinity chromatography, the purified antigen reacts with monoclonal antibodies to chondroitin sulfate (Fig. 1). Together, these results demonstrate that the Cat-301 antigen is a proteoglycan of the chondroitin sulfate class.

Since proteoglycans have been shown to be important constituents of ECM in many tissues, we were interested in determining whether the Cat-301 proteoglycan might be related to other previously described, nonneural ECM proteoglycans. Cat-301 immunoreactivity is not detected in most nonneural tissues from the cat, including liver, kidney, and muscle. It is, however, found at high concentrations in cartilagenous tissues, including trachea, articular cartilage, and tendon (H. Fryer et al., in prep.). Many of the nonneural tissues that are Cat-301-positive also express the large, aggregating chondroitin sulfate-proteoglycan from cartilage, called aggrecan (Doege et al. 1988, 1990). We have now demonstrated that the Cat-301 antigen from brain is related to aggrecan by at least two

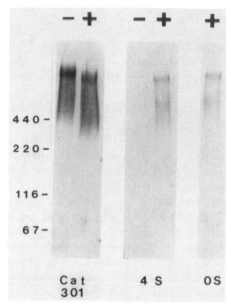

Figure 1. Cat-301 immunoprecipitates a chondroitin sulfate proteoglycan. Antigen was purified by Cat-301 antibody affinity chromatography, incubated overnight in the absence (−) or presence (+) of chondroitinase, and subjected to Western blot analysis with Cat-301 or anti-stub antibodies. Chondroitinase treatment results in a shift in the apparent molecular weight of the Cat-301 reactive band and exposure of the epitope reactive with the anti-4S chondroitin sulfate antibody. The affinity-purified, chondroitinase-treated antigen also reacts with anti-0S and anti-6S antibodies (not shown).

criteria. First, both aggrecan (Sandy and Plaas 1989) and the Cat-301 antigen from brain form aggregates with hyaluronic acid (H. Fryer et al., in prep.). This has been demonstrated in two ways: (1) the Cat-301 antigen from brain has a higher buoyant density on cesium chloride gradients in the presence of exogenous

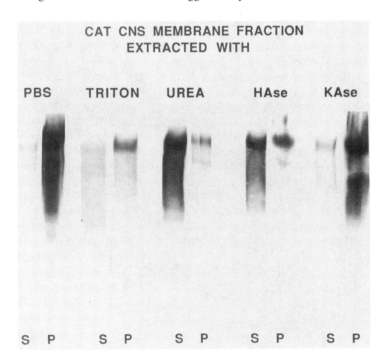

Figure 2. The Cat-301 antigen is bound to an insoluble extracellular matrix and is released by digestion with hyaluronidase. Cat CNS membrane fractions, prepared as described previously (Zaremba et al. 1989), were resuspended and incubated overnight in phosphate-buffered saline (PBS), PBS with 1% Triton X-100 (TRITON), PBS with 8 M urea (UREA), PBS with 250 units/ml leech hyaluronidase (HAse), or PBS with 2.5 units/ml keratanase (KAse). The samples were centrifuged at 30,000g for 30 min, separated into supernatant (S) and particulate (P) fractions, and assayed for Cat-301 immunoreactivity. Immunoreactivity is released from membrane fractions into the supernatant by urea or HAse.

hyaluronic acid than it does in the absence of hyaluronic acid or in the presence of exogenous chondroitin sulfate and (2) the Cat-301 antigen from brain is released from membrane preparations by digestion with hyaluronidase, but not by digestion with keratanase (Fig. 2). Second, purified aggrecan from cat and bovine articular cartilage is immunologically related to the brain Cat-301 proteoglycan.

Cat-301 Recognizes a Surface-associated Proteoglycan Expressed on Subsets of Neurons in the Mammalian CNS

Monoclonal antibody Cat-301 was initially generated to gray matter from the cat CNS (McKay and Hockfield 1982). Cat-301 recognizes a cell-surface antigen (Fig. 3) on subsets of neurons in many areas of the CNS of several mammalian species (Hockfield et al. 1983, 1990; Kalb and Hockfield 1988; DeYoe et al. 1990). In each area, the set of Cat-301-positive neurons is restricted and characteristic for that area. In central visual areas of the cat and primate, Cat-301 recognizes

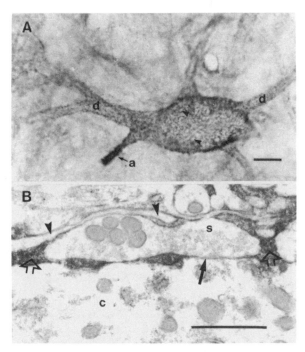

Figure 3. Cat-301 recognizes a surface-associated extrasynaptic antigen. (*A*) Cat-301 immunoreactivity is nonuniformly distributed over the surface of a neuron from the cat spinal cord ventral horn. Small, unstained fenestrae (arrowheads) interrupt the surface staining. These fenestrae represent the sites of synaptic contact seen in *B*. Immunoreactivity covers the cell body and extends out over proximal dendrites (d). The initial segment of the axon (a) is intensely immunoreactive. Bar, 20 μm. (*B*) At the electron microscopic level, immunoreactivity (open arrows) is localized to the extracellular surface of a neuron cell body (c). A synapse, filled with small, clear synaptic vesicles (s) is made onto the cell, and areas of synaptic contact (arrow) are devoid of antibody staining. The astrocytic sheath around the synapse (arrowheads) is outside the region of perisynaptic immunoreactivity. Bar, 1 μm.

anatomically and physiologically defined neuron classes. For example, in the cat and monkey dorsal lateral geniculate nucleus (LGN, the visual thalamus), neurons associated with processing the motion component of a visual stimulus, the Y cells in the cat LGN (Sur et al. 1988; Hockfield and Sur 1990) and the magnocellular neurons in the monkey LGN (Hockfield et al. 1983; Hendry et al. 1984) express high levels of the Cat-301 antigen. Neurons that process the form and color components of a visual stimulus express far lower levels of the antigen. This relatively selective association of Cat-301 immunoreactivity with the "motion," or "magnocellular," pathway is further preserved through several orders of cortical processing. In the primary (area V1 or 17) and secondary (area V2) visual cortex of monkey (DeYoe et al. 1990) and humans (Hockfield et al. 1990), Cat-301-positive neurons are most dense in layers or subdivisions that receive input (either directly or indirectly) from magnocellular LGN. Similarly, in association visual cortex, those areas implicated in processing the motion component of visual stimuli (the middle temporal and medial superior temporal areas) contain far greater densities of Cat-301-positive neurons than those areas implicated in processing the form or color components (such as inferio-temporal cortex and area V4) (DeYoe et al. 1990). These results provide evidence that neurons within a functionally defined pathway can share molecular properties. Similar observations have been made for a glycoprotein named LAMP (limbic-system-associated membrane protein) which identifies neurons in several areas of the mammalian limbic system (Levitt 1984; Zacco et al. 1990).

Cat-301 immunoreactivity is associated with the surface of neurons. Analysis at the electron microscopic level has shown that the antigen is localized along the surface of neurons but is excluded from regions of synaptic contact (Fig. 3). Cat-301 binds to live cells, demonstrating that the Cat-301 epitope is located on the extracellular surface of neurons (Zaremba et al. 1989). Extraction and detergent partitioning criteria further show that the Cat-301 proteoglycan lacks an integral membrane domain (Zaremba et al. 1989). The extracellular localization of the Cat-301 epitope, combined with the absence of a membrane-spanning domain, indicates that the entire antigen must be extracellular. This is consistent with the Cat-301 antigen being a component of the extracellular matrix.

Neuronal Activity Regulates the Expression of the Cat-301 Proteoglycan in Central Visual Areas

Cat-301 expression is first detected relatively late in neuronal development. In every case examined to date, neurons do not express Cat-301 immunoreactivity until well into postnatal life. In the cat LGN, for example, surface-associated Cat-301 immunoreactivity is first seen around postnatal day 30. Adult levels of immunoreactivity are not reached until postnatal day 90 (Sur et al. 1988). The time course of antigen expression parallels the previously described maturation of the electrophysiological properties of Y cells (Daniels et al. 1978; Mangel et al. 1983), the subset of cat neurons associated with the motion pathway described above. Several experiments have demonstrated that Cat-301 selectively recognizes Y cells (Sur et al. 1988; Hockfield and Sur 1990).

The acquisition of mature Y-cell electrophysiological properties requires visual experience during a circumscribed period in postnatal life (for review, see Movshon and Van Sluyters 1981; Sherman and Spear 1982). Cats deprived of normal visual experience during this critical period do not develop normal visual function and lack a normal complement of physiologically mature LGN Y cells. In a large series of experiments, we have shown that manipulations of the visual system that prevent the normal maturation of Y cells also reduce Cat-301 immunoreactivity in the cat LGN (Sur et al. 1988; A.J. Sheetz et al.; P. Kind et al.; both unpubl.). For example, LGN from cats raised with one eye sutured closed show reduced levels of Cat-301 immunoreactivity in the layers that receive input from the closed eye (Fig. 4). Previous experiments have shown that this manipulation also results in a marked reduction in the complement of Y cells in deprived layers (Sherman et al. 1972; Hofmann and Cynader 1977).

The reduction in Cat-301 expression is not tied simply to levels of neuronal activity but expressly to neuronal activity during early postnatal life (Hockfield et al. 1989). A reduction in neuronal activity in adult animals can produce a reduction in the level of a number of neural proteins (Hendry and Kennedy 1986; Hevner and Wong-Riley 1990; Jones et al., this volume), without the profound effects on neuronal anatomy and physiology seen in neonates. However, deprivation of normal visual input in adult animals for extended periods of time has no effect on Cat-301 expression. Significantly, animals initially deprived of normal visual input during the postnatal (critical) period and subsequently exposed to normal visual input do not express the Cat-301 antigen at normal levels. For exam-

ple, in the LGN of animals that received intraocular injections of tetrodotoxin (which blocks Na$^+$ channels and therefore blocks neuronal conduction) for the first 7 weeks of life and then allowed to survive (without tetrodotoxin or its effects) for another 17 weeks, there is an almost complete depletion of Cat-301 from the LGN layers that receive input from the injected eye (A.J. Sheetz et al., unpubl.). Here again, the inability to "rescue" Cat-301 expression parallels the inability to "rescue" normal physiological properties of neurons in central visual areas following visual deprivation during the critical period (Sherman et al. 1972; Dubin et al. 1986).

A reduction in immunoreactivity for a monoclonal antibody could be a consequence of either a reduced level of the antigen itself or a masking or alteration of the epitope recognized by that antibody. As described briefly above, a second monoclonal antibody, Cat-304, recognizes the Cat-301 proteoglycan, but at a different site from that recognized by Cat-301 (Zaremba et al. 1989). We have shown that the decrease in levels of immunoreactivity following visual deprivation is identical for both these antibodies (Guimaraes et al. 1990). This result strongly suggests that the reduction in the Cat-301 proteoglycan following activity deprivation reflects a down-regulation of the proteoglycan itself and not simply a loss of the Cat-301 epitope.

Cat-301 Expression on Spinal Motor Neurons Requires Normal Patterns of Activity during a Circumscribed Period in the Postnatal Period

To determine whether the activity-dependent regulation of Cat-301 expression observed in the visual system reflects a general property of neuronal maturation, we next examined the regulation of antigen expression on another set of neurons, spinal motor neurons. In adult hamsters, all motor neurons with axons in the sciatic nerve express the surface-associated Cat-301 immunoreactivity (Kalb and Hockfield 1988). Sciatic motor neurons are Cat-301-negative at postnatal day 7, and by

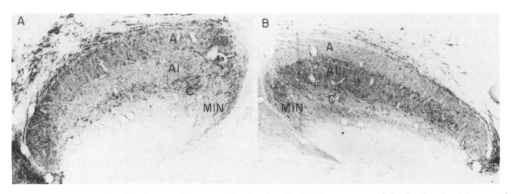

Figure 4. Neonatal monocular deprivation produces a reduction in Cat-301 immunoreactivity in deprived layers of cat LGN. Sections of the LGN from a cat with a left monocular suture from birth show reduced staining in LGN layers receiving input from the deprived (left) eye. In the left LGN (*A*), reduced Cat-301 staining is seen in layer A1, whereas in the right LGN (*B*), reduced staining is seen in layers A and C.

postnatal day 14, all sciatic motor neurons are Cat-301-positive. Manipulations of the neuromuscular unit that disrupt the normal pattern of motor neuron activity between postnatal days 5 and 21 prevent the normal development of the expression of the Cat-301 antigen. Sciatic nerve lesion, dorsal rhizotomy, decortication, and cordotomy performed during the early postnatal period all result in a marked reduction in the percentage of sciatic motor neurons that are Cat-301-positive.

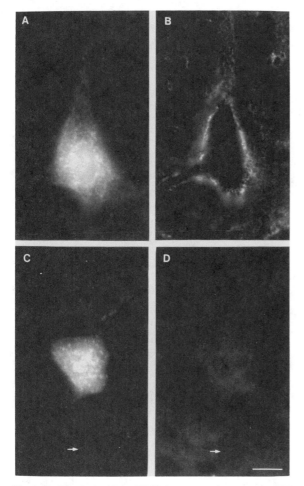

Figure 5. Blockade of the NMDA receptor in neonates inhibits Cat-301 expression on sciatic motor neurons. APV, an NMDA receptor antagonist, inhibits Cat-301 expression in neonatal (C, D) animals but not in adult (A, B) animals. (A) Section of the spinal cord from an APV-treated adult hamster viewed for fast blue staining under UV optics shows a retrogradely labeled sciatic motor neuron. (B) The same field as in A viewed under FITC optics for Cat-301 immunoreactivity shows that this sciatic motor neuron is Cat-301-positive. (C) Section of the spinal cord from an APV-treated neonatal hamster viewed for fast blue staining under UV optics shows a retrogradely labeled sciatic motor neuron. (D) The same field as in C viewed under FITC optics for Cat-301 immunoreactivity shows that this sciatic motor neuron is Cat-301-negative following APV administration. The arrows in C and D identify the same blood vessel as a reference point. APV was continuously administered for 14 days by implanting a slow-release polymer (Elvax) containing 10 mM APV in the subarachnoid space over the lumbar enlargement. Bar, 14 μm.

When performed on adult animals, none of these lesions have any effect on Cat-301 expression (Kalb and Hockfield 1988, 1990b). Cat-301 expression therefore defines a critical period for motor neuron development, during which alterations in activity of the neuromuscular unit influence the acquisition of mature molecular properties of motor neurons.

Experiments designed to dissect further the components of the neuromuscular unit required for Cat-301 expression indicate that large-diameter, but not small-diameter, primary afferent inputs mediate activity-dependent Cat-301 expression (Kalb and Hockfield 1990b). The neurotransmitter of some of the large-diameter afferents is glutamate (Salt and Hill 1983). Recent experiments have shown that blockade of the NMDA subclass of glutamate receptor during the critical period inhibits Cat-301 expression on motor neurons (Fig. 5) (Kalb and Hockfield 1990a). To ensure that the NMDA receptor antagonists do not depress spinal synaptic transmission nonspecifically, we assayed the H-reflex (a monosynaptic reflex that measures motor neuron excitability) and its relation to the M-response (the orthogradely generated compound muscle action potential) (Kimura 1983). No differences were observed between NMDA-antagonist-treated and vehicle-treated animals in the latency, maximal amplitude, or rectified area under the curve for the H-reflex or the M-response (Fig. 6). Neither was there any difference in H-latency/M-latency, H-max/M-max, or H-area/M-area. These results suggest that chronic blockade of the NMDA receptor does not block synaptic transmission between primary afferents and motor neurons.

These experiments provide evidence that NMDA-receptor-mediated events are involved in activity-dependent maturation of motor neurons. The mechanisms of this process may be similar to other systems where the NMDA receptor has been implicated in mediating long-lasting, activity-dependent modifications of neuronal properties, including the segregation of retino-tectal projections in the frog (Cline et al. 1987; Cline and Constantine-Paton 1990), the acquisition of response properties of visual cortical neurons in the developing cat (Bear et al. 1990), and the generation of long-term potentiation in the rodent hippocampus (for review, see Nicoll et al. 1988).

Antigenically Distinct Chondroitin Sulfate Proteoglycans Identify Subsets of Neurons

Our results on the regulation of the Cat-301 proteoglycan suggest that the expression of extracellular proteoglycans reflects late events in neuronal maturation. The Cat-301 proteoglycan is expressed on only a limited subset of neurons, yet late developmental mechanisms must be a general feature of neuronal maturation. This suggests that other neurons might express surface-associated proteoglycans distinct from that recognized by Cat-301. We have used antibodies to other proteoglycans to explore the possibility that dif-

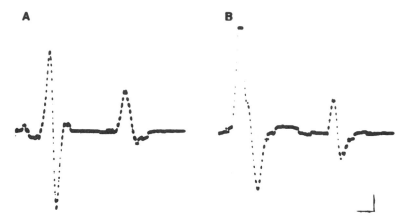

Figure 6. Chronic blockade of the NMDA receptor does not block synaptic activation of motor neurons. Representative recordings of the H-reflex obtained from 19-day old hamsters that had been treated with saline-Elvax (*A*) or APV-Elvax (*B*) from postnatal day 7. The first response is the orthograde compound action potential (M-response) and the late response is the H-reflex. There was no significant difference between saline- and APV-treated animals in a variety of measures (see text for details). Bars: Horizontal, 2 msec; vertical, 100 μV.

ferent neuronal subsets express distinct classes of proteoglycans.

Antibodies to the sugar stub remaining after chondroitinase digestion of proteoglycans detect heterogeneity in the position of sulfate substitution on the hexose rings of chondroitin sulfate glycosaminoglycans (Couchman et al. 1984). We have used these antibodies to examine the cellular distribution of different chondroitin sulfate proteoglycans in the mammalian CNS. Two antibodies directed to different sugar residues reveal distinct subpopulations of immunoreactive neurons. In the cat visual cortex (Figs. 7A–C), for example, Cat-301 recognizes a dense band of neurons in layer 4 and fewer neurons in superficial (2 and 3) and deep (5 and 6) layers. Anti-6S recognizes a large number of neurons in layers 2 through 6, with few antibody-positive neurons in layers 1 and 5. Anti-4S recognizes a much smaller population of neurons, largely restricted to layers 4 and 6. Western blot analyses of cat brain support this suggestion of diversity among proteoglycans by revealing a number of bands that react with antibodies to 4S, 0S, or 6S, but not with Cat-301 (Fig. 7D). Further diversity among CNS proteoglycans is observed using antibodies to keratan sulfate (a different glycosaminoglycan modification of proteoglycans) which also identify neuronal subsets (Zaremba et al. 1990a,b). All of these antibodies recognize surface-associated antigens, demonstrating heterogeneity in the surface proteoglycans expressed by mammalian CNS neurons.

DISCUSSION

Monoclonal antibody Cat-301 recognizes a chondroitin sulfate proteoglycan expressed on the surface of subsets of neurons in the mammalian CNS. The onset of Cat-301 expression correlates with the end of the period of synaptic plasticity in two systems, the cat LGN and the hamster sciatic neuromuscular unit. The Cat-301 proteoglycan is a positive molecular marker for the acquisition of normal mature properties of neurons, as its expression is regulated by neuronal activity during development: When deprived of normal patterns of activity during a critical period in development, LGN Y cells do not go on to develop normal physiological properties, nor do they express the Cat-301 proteoglycan. Similar observations have been made for motor neurons in the hamster spinal cord. These results suggest that the onset of Cat-301 immunoreactivity reflects a general phenomenon in neuronal maturation, i.e., the activity-driven acquisition of normal, mature neuronal phenotype.

The Cat-301 proteoglycan has biochemical properties that indicate that it is a component of extracellular material in the mature mammalian CNS. We have shown that it is not an integral membrane protein and that a substantial fraction of the proteoglycan is incorporated into an insoluble material in the mature CNS. These properties are similar to components of ECM in other tissues. The CNS had been believed to lack a standard ECM, because electron microscopy has failed to show electron-dense material in intercellular spaces (Peters et al. 1976). Antibodies to ECM components reveal that although the mature CNS is largely lacking in some standard ECM components, such as collagen, laminin, and fibronectin (or standard forms of these components), it is a rich source of proteoglycans (Carlson and Wight 1987; Oohira et al. 1988; Margolis and Margolis 1989; Watanabe et al. 1989). Some proteoglycans are generally distributed, such as the chondroitin sulfate proteoglycan PG-1000 (S.S. Carlson, pers. comm.), whereas others such as those described here and by Fujita and Watanabe (Fujita et al. 1989; Watanabe et al. 1989) are restricted in distribution to neuronal subsets. The complement of CNS proteoglycans changes dramatically during development (Hoffman et al. 1988; Herndon and Lander 1990) so that the proteoglycans expressed late in development differ sub-

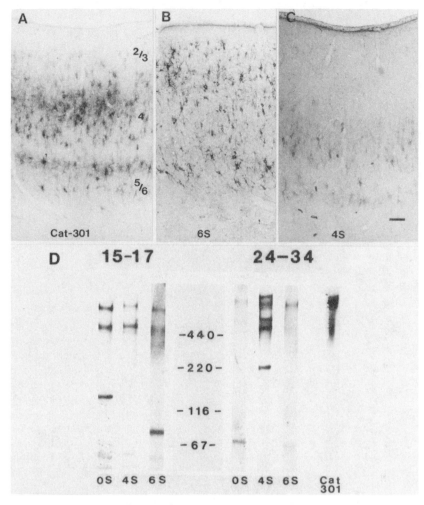

Figure 7. Cat cortex contains a family of chondroitin sulfate proteoglycans. Sections of cat visual cortex were stained with Cat-301 (*A*), anti-6S (*B*), and anti-4S (*C*). Each antibody recognizes a restricted subset of neurons. (*A*) Intense Cat-301 immunoreactivity is seen in layer 4, and a second band of staining is seen in layer 5/6. Layer 2/3 has far less staining. (*B*) Anti-6S stains neurons in all layers of area 17, with more labeling in the superficial layers than is seen with Cat-301. (*C*) Anti-4S stains a limited number of neurons, with far more staining in deeper layers than in superficial layers. Layers 2, 3, and 5 contain very few anti-4S-labeled neurons. Bar, 100 μm. (*D*) Biochemical evidence for heterogeneity among chondroitin sulfate proteoglycans from cat cortex. Enriched proteoglycan fractions were made from a urea extract of cat cortex by DEAE ion-exchange chromatography, followed by gel filtration on Sepharose CL-2B (Zaremba et al. 1989). Fractions eluting in the void volume (15–17) were pooled separately from fractions containing the Cat-301 antigen (24–34), treated with chondroitinase, and examined on Western blots. Both the void volume pool and the Cat-301 antigen pool exhibit a diverse set of antigens reactive with the different antibodies to chondroitin sulfate stubs (anti-0S, -4S, and -6S).

stantially from those expressed early in development. Such changes in molecular composition suggest that CNS proteoglycans play a variety of roles in CNS development and function.

The CNS proteoglycans we have studied are expressed late in development. For the Cat-301 proteoglycan, we have shown that expression first occurs at the end of the period of synaptic plasticity and that the pattern of neuronal activity during the plastic period regulates expression of the proteoglycan. The basic synaptic connections between neurons are established during the plastic period and, under normal conditions, are subject to little modification in the adult animal. Together, our observations suggest the following hypothesis (Fig. 8). Early in development, synaptic con-

nections are initially established and then undergo a period of activity-dependent "refinement" by which some synapses are stabilized and others are eliminated. These synaptic modifications take place in a relatively fluid extracellular environment, characterized by larger extracellular spaces than are present in the mature CNS (Vaughn 1989). Following the period during which synaptic modifications occur, a more mature, relatively nonplastic period commences that lasts the life of an animal. The stabilization of synaptic structure is accompanied by the elaboration of an ECM, composed, in part, of proteoglycans, some of which are associated with specific classes of neuron. This mature matrix is relatively insoluble and could serve to stabilize synaptic structure through interactions with cell-surface mole-

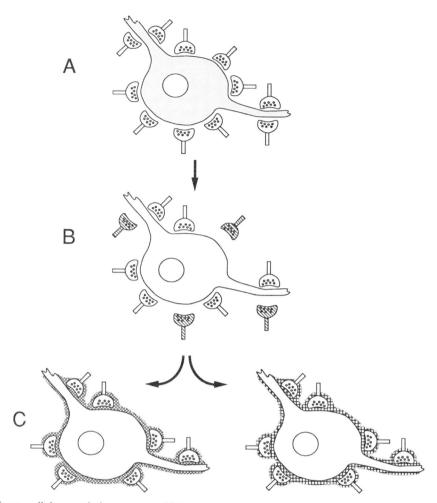

Figure 8. Role of extracellular matrix in synapse stabilization. (*A*) Early in development, synapses are made on a neuron, only some of which will be retained into adulthood. (*B*) Over the course of development, some synapses are retained (clear synapses) and some are lost (crosshatched synapses). The selection of which synapses are retained and which are lost is determined, in part, by the correlation in activation of a synapse and the postsynaptic cell. The final number of synapses on a neuron may not actually decrease, as new synapses can be made during the period of synapse selection. (*C*) Following the selection of the appropriate set of synapses, an extracellular matrix is elaborated that serves to stabilize the mature structure. The extracellular matrix is heterogeneous, so that different types of neurons express matrices of different compositions. (See text for details.)

cules (adhesive mechanisms) or by acting as inhibitors of further neurite growth (inhibitory or repulsive mechanisms). The pattern of activity of a neuron during the critical period determines which set of synapses is selected, which in turn determines some features of mature neuronal phenotype. Our results suggest that (1) Cat-301 is one member of a larger family of neural ECM proteoglycans, (2) neurons that are Cat-301-negative express alternate members of this family, and (3) neuronal differentiation is reflected by the expression of specific cell-surface proteoglycans.

Proteoglycans are large molecules with many different functional domains and have been described as a "multipurpose glue" (Ruoslahti 1989). They can bind a number of other kinds of molecules, including other components of ECM and cell-surface proteins (Hoffman et al. 1988; Clement et al. 1989; Perides et al. 1989; Sandy and Plaas 1989; Sun et al. 1989) and differentiation and growth factors (Andres et al. 1989; Cheifetz and Massagué 1989; Bernfield and Sanderson

1990). Proteoglycans can influence cellular differentiation and proliferation (Andres et al. 1989; Bernfield and Sanderson 1990). The large size and high charge of these molecules can act to regulate diffusion or concentration of other molecules through and in the extracellular space (Lindahl and Hook 1978). These characteristics of proteoglycans enable them to organize the extracellular environment. The restricted distribution of CNS proteoglycans demonstrated here suggests that the immediate extracellular environment of an individual neuron can be exquisitely regulated. Regulation of the immediate extracellular environment may play a role in maintaining mature differentiated neuronal properties.

ACKNOWLEDGMENTS

We thank Gail Kelly for expert technical assistance. This work was supported by National Institutes of Health grants EY-06511 (S.H.), EY-05855 (S.Z.), NS-

01247 (R.G.K.), and by National Science Foundation grant BNS-8812163 (S.H.).

REFERENCES

Andres, J.L., K. Stanley, S. Cheifetz, and J. Massagué. 1989. Membrane-anchored and soluble forms of betaglycan, a polymorphic proteoglycan that binds transforming growth factor-β. *J. Cell Biol.* **109:** 3137.

Bear, M.F., A. Kleinschmidt, Q. Gu, and W. Singer. 1990. Disruption of experience-dependent synaptic modifications in striate cortex by infusion of an NMDA receptor antagonist. *J. Neurosci.* **10:** 909.

Bernfield, M. and R.D. Sanderson. 1990. Syndecan, a developmentally regulated cell surface proteoglycan that binds extracellular matrix and growth factors. *Philos. Trans. R. Soc. Lond. B Sci.* **327:** 171.

Carlson, S.S. and T.N. Wight. 1987. Nerve terminal anchorage protein one (TAP-1) is a chondroitin sulfate proteoglycan: Biochemical and electron microscopic characterization. *J. Cell Biol.* **105:** 3075.

Cheifetz, S. and J. Massagué. 1989. Transforming growth factor-β (TGF-β) receptor proteoglycan. Cell surface expression and ligand binding in the absence of glycosaminoglycan chains. *J. Biol. Chem.* **264:** 12025.

Clement, B., B. Segui-Real, J.R. Hassell, G.R. Martin, and Y. Yamada. 1989. Identification of a cell surface-binding protein for the core protein of the basement membrane proteoglycan. *J. Biol. Chem.* **264:** 12467.

Cline, H.T. and M. Constantine-Paton. 1990. NMDA receptor agonist and antagonists alter retinal ganglion cell arbor structure in the developing frog retinotectal projection. *J. Neurosci.* **10:** 1197.

Cline, H.T., E.A. Debski, and M. Constantine-Paton. 1987. N-methyl-D-aspartate receptor antagonist desegregates eye-specific columns. *Proc. Natl. Acad. Sci.* **84:** 4342.

Couchman, J.R., B. Caterson, J.E. Christner, and J.R. Baker. 1984. Mapping by monoclonal antibody detection of glycosaminoglycans in connective tissues. *Nature* **307:** 650.

Daniels, J.D., J.D. Pettigrew, and J.L. Norman. 1978. Development of single-neuron responses in kitten's lateral geniculate nucleus. *J. Neurophysiol.* **41:** 1373.

DeYoe, E.A., S. Hockfield, H. Garren, and D. Van Essen. 1990. Antibody labeling of functional subdivisions in visual cortex: Cat-301 immunoreactivity in striate and extrastriate cortex of the macaque monkey. *Vis. Neurosci.* **5:** 67.

Doege, K., M. Sasaki, and Y. Yamada. 1990. Rat and human cartilage proteoglycan (aggrecan) gene structure. *Biochem. Soc. Trans.* **18:** 200.

Doege, K., M. Sasaki, E. Horigan, J.R. Hassell, and Y. Yamada. 1988. Complete primary structure of the rat cartilage proteoglycan core protein deduced from cDNA clones. *J. Biol. Chem.* **262:** 17757.

Dubin, M.W., L.A. Stark, and S.M. Archer. 1986. A role for action-potential activity in the development of neuronal connections in the kitten retinogeniculate pathway. *J. Neurosci.* **6:** 1021.

Fujita, S.C., Y. Tada, F. Murakami, M. Hayashi, and M. Matsumura. 1989. Glycosaminoglycan-related epitopes surrounding different subsets of mammalian central neurons. *Neurosci. Res.* **7:** 117.

Guimaraes, A., S. Zaremba, and S. Hockfield. 1990. Molecular and morphological changes in cat lateral geniculate nucleus and visual cortex induced by visual deprivation are revealed by monoclonal antibodies Cat-301 and Cat-304. *J. Neurosci.* **10:** 3014.

Hendry, S.H.C. and M.B. Kennedy. 1986. Immunoreactivity for calmodulin-dependent protein kinase is selectively increased in macaque striate cortex after monocular deprivation. *Proc. Natl. Acad. Sci.* **83:** 1536.

Hendry, S.H.C., S. Hockfield, E.G. Jones, and R.D.G. McKay. 1984. A monoclonal antibody that identifies subsets of neurons in the central visual system of the monkey and cat. *Nature* **307:** 267.

Herndon, M.E. and A.D. Lander. 1990. A diverse set of developmentally regulated proteoglycans is expressed in the rat central nervous system. *Neuron* **4:** 949.

Hevner, R.F. and M.T.T. Wong-Riley. 1990. Regulation of cytochrome oxidase protein levels by functional activity in the macaque monkey visual system. *J. Neurosci.* **10:** 1331.

Hockfield, S. 1990. Proteoglycans in neural development. *Semin. Dev. Biol.* **1:** 55.

Hockfield, S. and R.D.G. McKay. 1983. A surface antigen expressed by a subset of neurons in the vertebrate central nervous system. *Proc. Natl. Acad. Sci.* **80:** 5758.

Hockfield, S. and M. Sur. 1990. Monoclonal antibody Cat-301 identifies Y-cells in the dorsal lateral geniculate nucleus of the cat. *J. Comp. Neurol.* **300:** 320.

Hockfield, S., R.G. Kalb, and A. Guimaraes. 1989. Experience-dependent expression of neuronal cell surface molecules. In *Neuroimmune networks: Physiology and diseases* (ed. E.J. Goetz and N.H. Spector), p. 57. A.R. Liss, New York.

Hockfield, S., R.B.H. Tootell, and S. Zaremba. 1990. Molecular differences among neurons reveal an organization of human visual cortex. *Proc. Natl. Acad. Sci.* **87:** 3027.

Hockfield, S., R. McKay, S.H.C. Hendry, and E.G. Jones. 1983. A surface antigen that identifies ocular dominance columns in cortical area 17 and laminar features of the lateral geniculate nucleus. *Cold Spring Harbor Symp. Quant. Biol.* **48:** 877.

Hoffman, S., K.L. Crossin, and G.M. Edelman. 1988. Molecular forms, binding functions and developmental expression patterns of cytotactin and cytotactin-binding proteoglycan, an interactive pair of extracellular matrix molecules. *J. Cell. Biol.* **106:** 519.

Hofmann, K.P. and M. Cynader. 1977. Functional aspects of plasticity in the visual system of adult cats after early monocular deprivation. *Philos. Trans. R. Soc. Lond. B. Biol. Sci.* **278:** 411.

Kalb, R.G. and S. Hockfield. 1988. Molecular evidence for early activity-dependent development of hamster motor neurons. *J. Neurosci.* **8:** 2350.

———. 1990a. Induction of a neuronal proteoglycan by the NMDA receptor in the developing spinal cord. *Science* **250:** 294.

———. 1990b. Large diameter primary afferent input is required for expression of the Cat-301 proteoglycan on the surface of motor neurons. *Neuroscience* **34:** 391.

Kimura, J. 1983. The H-reflex and other late responses. In *Electrodiagnosis in diseases of nerve and muscle: Principles and practice*, p. 379. F.A. Davis, Philadelphia.

Levitt, P. 1984. A monoclonal antibody to limbic system neurons. *Science* **223:** 299.

Lindahl, U. and M. Hook. 1978. Glycosaminoglycans and their binding to biological macromolecules. *Annu. Rev. Biochem.* **47:** 385.

Mangel, S.C., J.R. Wilson, and S.M. Sherman. 1983. Development of neuronal response properties in the cat dorsal lateral geniculate nucleus during monocular deprivation. *J. Neurophysiol.* **50:** 240.

Margolis, R.U. and R.K. Margolis. 1989. Nervous tissue proteoglycans. *Dev. Neurosci.* **11:** 276.

McKay, R.D.G. and S. Hockfield. 1982. Monoclonal antibodies distinguish antigenically discrete neuronal types in the vertebrate central nervous system. *Proc. Natl. Acad. Sci.* **79:** 6747.

Movshon, J.A. and R.C. Van Sluyters. 1981. Visual neural development. *Annu. Rev. Psychol.* **32:** 477.

Nicoll, R.A., J.A. Kauer, and R.C. Malenka. 1988. The current excitement in long-term potentiation. *Neuron* **1:** 97.

Oohira, A., F. Matsui, M. Matsuda, Y. Takida, and Y.

Kuboki. 1988. Occurrence of three distinct molecular species of chondroitin sulfate proteoglycan in the developing rat brain. *J. Biol. Chem.* **263:** 10240.

Perides, G., W.S. Lane, D. Andrews, D. Dahl, and A. Bignami. 1989. Isolation and partial characterization of a glial hyaluronate-binding protein. *J. Biol. Chem.* **264:** 5981.

Peters, A., S.L. Palay, and H.D. Webster. 1976. *The fine structure of the nervous system: The neurons and supporting cells.* W.B. Saunders, Philadelphia.

Purves, D. and J.W. Lichtman. 1985. *Principles of neural development.* Sinauer Associates, Sunderland, Massachusetts.

Ruoslahti, E. 1989. Proteoglycans in cell regulation. *J. Biol. Chem.* **264:** 13369.

Salt, T.E. and R.G. Hill. 1983. Neurotransmitter candidates of primary afferent somatosensory fibers. *Neuroscience* **10:** 1083.

Sandy, J.D. and A.H.K. Plaas. 1989. Studies on the hyaluronate binding properties of newly synthesized proteoglycans purified from articular chrondrocyte cultures. *Arch. Biochem. Biophys.* **271:** 300.

Sherman, S.M. and P.D. Spear. 1982. Organization of visual pathways in normal and visually deprived cats. *Physiol. Rev.* **62:** 738.

Sherman, S.M., K.P. Hofmann, and J. Stone. 1972. Loss of a specific cell type from dorsal lateral geniculate nucleus in visually deprived cats. *J. Neurophysiol.* **35:** 352.

Sun, X. D.F. Mosher, and A. Rapraeger. 1989. Heparan sulfate-mediated binding of epithelial cell surface proteoglycan to thrombospondin. *J. Biol. Chem.* **264:** 2885.

Sur, M., D. Frost, and S. Hockfield. 1988. Expression of a cell surface antigen on Y-cells in the cat lateral geniculate nucleus is regulated by visual experience. *J. Neurosci.* **8:** 874.

Vaughn, J.E. 1989. Fine structure of synaptogenesis in the vertebrate central nervous system. *Synapse* **3:** 255.

Watanabe, E., S.C. Fujita, F. Murakami, M. Hayashi, and M. Matsumura. 1989. A monoclonal antibody identifies a novel epitope surrounding a subpopulation of the mammalian central neurons. *Neuroscience* **29:** 645.

Zacco, A., V. Cooper, P.D. Chantler, S. Fisher-Hyland, H.L. Horton, and P. Levitt. 1990. Isolation, biochemical characterization and ultrastructural analysis of the limbic system associated membrane protein (LAMP), a protein expressed by neurons comprising functional neural circuits. *J. Neurosci.* **10:** 73.

Zaremba, S., A. Guimaraes, R.G. Kalb, and S. Hockfield. 1989. Characterization of an activity-dependent, neuronal surface proteoglycan identified with monoclonal antibody Cat-301. *Neuron* **2:** 1207.

Zaremba, S., G. Kelly, R.G. Kalb, and S. Hockfield. 1990a. Keratan sulfate proteoglycans associated with neuronal surfaces in CNS. *Soc. Neurosci. Abstr.* **16:** 496.

Zaremba, S., J.R. Naegele, C.J. Barnstable, and S. Hockfield. 1990b. Neuronal subsets express multiple high-molecular weight cell-surface glycoconjugates defined by monoclonal antibodies Cat-301 and VC1.1. *J. Neurosci.* **10:** 2985.

Experimental and Theoretical Studies of the Organization of Afferents to Single Orientation Columns in Visual Cortex

M.P. STRYKER, B. CHAPMAN, K.D. MILLER, AND K.R. ZAHS

Department of Physiology and Neuroscience Graduate Program, University of California,
San Francisco, California 94143-0444

In the visual cortex, as in other neocortical areas in mammals, neuronal response properties are arranged in columns. Cortical columns were described in the earliest experiments of Hubel and Wiesel (1962), who demonstrated that all of the neurons within each radial column in the primary visual cortex respond selectively to elongated edges of a particular angle or orientation. Since then, a number of visual response properties, in addition to selectivity for stimulus orientation, have been found to be shared by the neurons within single cortical columns. Each column is specific for *topography*, in that all neurons have their receptive fields in a particular portion of the visual field; for *ocular dominance*, in that all neurons in a particular column will tend to respond more strongly to one eye than to the other eye; and (in many species) for *on- or off-center-type*, in that the neurons within a column will tend to respond better to bright stimuli than to dark stimuli, or vice versa. Neighboring columns differ from one another in a systematic fashion, generally in a manner that makes changes in response properties as gradual and progressive as possible as one proceeds from column to column in the tangential direction. Thus, the columns of the visual cortex are precisely organized both radially and tangentially with respect to three (or, in many species, all four) of the response properties noted above.

To understand how this organization arises in development, we must know something about the anatomical connections responsible for these columns. The structural basis for the organization of topography and ocular-dominance columns has been reasonably well understood for more than a decade (Hubel et al. 1977). Direct anatomical and physiological experiments have revealed that topography and ocular-dominance columns are not merely products of intracortical circuitry. Instead, the major afferent input to the visual cortex from the lateral geniculate nucleus is precisely ordered with respect to topography and ocular dominance. For the ocular dominance columns, at least, the progressive reorganization of this afferent pathway in development appears to be the mechanism by which the orderly arrangement of cortical columns is established. Relatively simple mechanisms of activity-dependent synapse rearrangement can account for the principal features of afferent organization with respect to topography and ocular-dominance columns, and the plasticity exhibited by the developing visual cortex is consistent with the existence of such mechanisms (for review, see Miller and Stryker 1990).

Approaches to the Microcircuitry of Cortical Orientation Selectivity

The structural basis of the orientation columns has remained elusive and difficult to establish with confidence. The original model of Hubel and Wiesel (1962) proposed that neurons with simple-type receptive fields were endowed with orientation selectivity by virtue of the alignment in the visual field of the receptive fields of the lateral geniculate nucleus neurons from which the simple cell received its input. Figure 1 shows the circularly symmetric receptive field of an *on*-center geniculate neuron at the top left, with locations in the center giving *on* responses marked with closed plus signs and locations in the surround giving *off* responses marked with open minus signs. At the right are shown the overlapping receptive fields of four such geniculocortical afferents that are aligned at an angle of about 40° from the vertical. The hypothesis regarding the afferent convergence that produces simple-cell receptive fields is illustrated by the dotted axons of these four geniculate cells, terminating on a single stellate neuron in the visual cortex. The dashed rectangle indicates the size and position of an optimal bright-bar stimulus for the hypothesized cell. In this case, the arrangement of afferents could constitute a structural basis for the orientation columns, just as they do for the other sorts of cortical columns. Later models (Creutzfeldt et al. 1974; Sillito 1975) proposed that orientation selectivity was produced largely or completely by intracortical circuitry. In this latter case, the arrangement of afferents might have nothing to do with orientation columns, making them fundamentally different from the other types of cortical columns.

The Hubel and Wiesel (1962) model was supported by several lines of evidence. First, Hubel and Wiesel noted that the major geniculate input terminated most heavily in layer IV and, to a much lesser extent, in layer VI. These were precisely the layers in which cells with simple-type receptive fields were found. The structure of the simple-cell receptive field was readily explicable

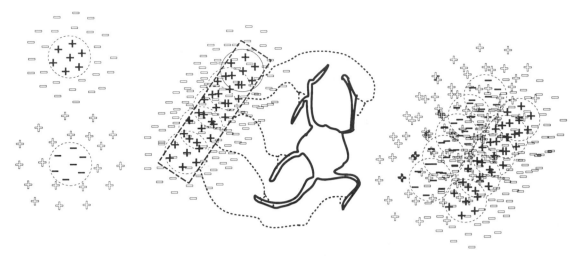

Figure 1. Original model for neuronal circuitry underlying cortical orientation selectivity redrawn with changes from Hubel and Wiesel (1962). (*Left*) Receptive fields of two lateral geniculate nucleus neurons, an *on*-center cell above and an *off*-center cell below. Responses of the cells' center mechanism are indicated with closed pluses or minuses; responses of the cells' surround mechanism are indicated with open pluses or minuses. Pluses indicate responses to light onset or to sustained local brightness; minuses indicate responses to light offset or to sustained local darkness. (*Center*) Proposed convergence of five geniculocortical afferents (the receptive fields are identical to those illustrated at left and are aligned in the visual field) onto a cortical simple cell to endow that cell with selective responses to bars or edges of light oriented at approximately 40° clockwise from the vertical. The optimum size for a light bar projected onto the simple-cell's receptive field is indicated by the dashed rectangle; the hypothesis is that this rectangle also activates the geniculocortical afferents in the manner illustrated, falling simultaneously on all their centers. Axons (dashed lines) of the geniculocortical afferents are hypothesized to make synaptic connections onto the cortical stellate cell shown in the right half of the center panel. Note the parallel arrangements of areas responsive to light onset or light offset in the cortical receptive field. (*Right*) A second kind of simple cell hypothesized to receive inputs from *on*- and *off*-center geniculocortical afferents that occupy parallel rows in the visual field.

by the hypothesis that it received convergent input from a collection of geniculocortical afferents whose receptive fields were aligned. The spatially separate *on* and *off* areas of simple-cell receptive fields would then correspond to the *on* and *off* areas of the receptive fields of their geniculate inputs. Responses to the separate *on* and *off* areas appeared to summate more or less linearly, so that the optimal *on* stimulus was one that filled all of the *on* regions simultaneously with minimal intrusion into the *off* regions, and vice versa for *off* stimuli. All of these findings were consistent with the Hubel and Wiesel model.

The orientation-selective cells that predominated in the other layers of the cortex had receptive fields that were termed complex because they could not easily be explained by convergent input from geniculate afferents. Although complex cells were orientation-selective, they commonly responded poorly to flashed lights, and they generally lacked separate *on* and *off* areas whose alignment could account for the preferred orientation. Even when complex cells responded to flashed lights, the optimal stimulus size could not be predicted from (and was usually much smaller than) the areas responsive to small, flashed lights. The properties of complex cells were, however, readily explained by the hypothesis that they received convergent inputs from a collection of simple cells in the same orientation column. This hypothesis accorded with the sparse or absent geniculocortical afferent inputs to the layers of cortex in which complex cells predominate. The struc-

ture of receptive fields, together with the anatomy of afferent pathways, was then seen to be consistent with a hierarchical arrangement in which geniculocortical afferents converge in their major zone of termination on simple cells that themselves provide convergent excitatory input to complex cells up and down the cortical column.

The emphasis in the Hubel and Wiesel (1962) hypothesis was on the pattern of convergence of excitatory inputs consistent with known anatomy that could explain the visual response properties of cortical neurons. An alternative hypothesis for explaining orientation selectivity emphasized the role of inhibitory inputs. The cross-orientation inhibition model assumed that excitatory thalamocortical inputs to cortical cells were not aligned in the visual field with the precision needed to make cortical cells orientation-selective. Instead, the cortical cells were hypothesized not to be selective or to be only weakly selective on the basis of their thalamocortical inputs, and intracortical inhibitory connections between neurons with orthogonal orientation preferences was hypothesized to account for cortical cell orientation specificity (Blakemore and Tobin 1972; Creutzfeldt et al. 1974). The orderly arrangement of cortical columns, with neighboring columns having similar preferred orientations and more distant columns generally having gradually increasing differences in preferred orientation, appeared to be consistent with a simple model in which local corticocortical excitation and more remote corticocortical inhibition would cooperate to create or refine orientation selectivity. Such a model is illustrated in Figure 2, which shows a hypothetical surface view of a 1.6-mm square of visual cortex. The bold lines and stippled figures indicate neuronal responses as a polar function of stimulus orientation in each of nine different cortical columns, four of which are selective for the same orientation as the central one and four of which are selective for the orthogonal orientation. The synaptic connections hypothesized in this model are illustrated as well; when the corticocortical inputs illustrated are active, orientation selectivity is made more precise. Orientation selectivity is minimal or absent without inhibitory inputs from columns representing orthogonal orientations (for details, see Fig. 2).

Experimental tests of the cross-orientation inhibition model have provided mixed results. The principal experimental finding in support of the cross-orientation inhibition model is the effect of reducing or eliminating local γ-aminobutyric acid (GABA)-mediated inhibition. Treatment of visual cortex with bicuculline or other pharmacological agents designed to remove intracortical inhibition reduced or eliminated orientation selectivity in the majority of cortical cells (Tsumoto et al. 1979; Sillito et al. 1980; other studies revealed much smaller effects, Pettigrew and Daniels 1973; Albus and Baumfalk 1989; Eysel et al. 1989). In addition, the excitatory regions that were revealed by blocking or reducing corticocortical inhibition did not appear to be elongated parallel to the axis of preferred orientation. Both the reduction of orientation selectivity and the apparently circular excitatory receptive fields were surprising, if one accepts the Hubel and Wiesel (1962) model.

It has not been possible directly to confirm or deny the Hubel and Wiesel and cross-orientation inhibition hypotheses. Each of these hypotheses deals with mi-

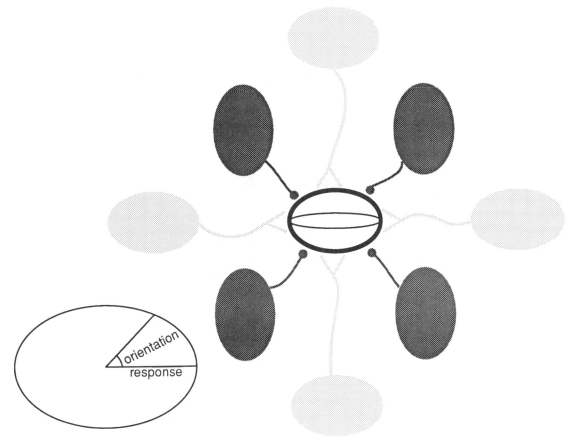

Figure 2. Model for the establishment or refinement of orientation selectivity by an intracortical network. Each oval indicated the weak selectivity for stimulus orientation that would be present in a central region of the cortex and eight neighboring regions if they did not have orientation- selective excitatory and inhibitory corticocortical synaptic connections. The perimeters of the ovals indicate in polar coordinates the response expected from each region as a function of stimulus orientation. The four regions with identical orientation preferences (light stippling, horizontal elongation) are hypothesized to make mutually excitatory connections. The four regions with orthogonal orientation preference (dark stippling, vertical elongation) are hypothesized to make inhibitory connections with neurons in the central region. The very eccentric thin oval in the central region indicates the precise orientation selectivity expected under the assumptions of this model when the corticocortical connections are active and effective. The initial selectivity may be hypothesized to result from asymmetric convergence of *on*- and *off*-center thalamocortical inputs (Heggelund 1986), or it may be hypothesized to be vanishingly small (and perhaps a consequence of the ellipsoidal nature of afferent receptive fields, as proposed by Vidyasagar and Urbas [1982], and Shou and Leventhal [1989]), so that the network bootstraps itself over the course of a few seconds through stages of increasing selectivity.

crocircuitry, i.e., the details of the sources of synaptic inputs to an individual cortical cell. We simply lack methods for studying the receptive fields of the population of neurons that provide input to one particular neuron. Anatomical techniques lack the resolution to label such a population selectively. In any case, labeling such a population of neurons would be only half the job; one would still have to map the receptive fields of this population.

Two major physiological approaches have been applied to this problem. The first is to identify the neurons that provide input to a particular neuron recorded extracellularly by analyzing the cross-correlations in their discharge patterns. Such cross-correlations can provide strong evidence for monosynaptic excitation or inhibition between two cells or for common inputs to the two cells. The cross-correlation analysis of Tanaka (1983) of geniculate and cortical neuronal responses revealed little evidence for elongated collections of geniculocortical inputs to single simple cells but did show *on-* and *off-*center geniculate inputs to distinct *on-* and *off-*regions of simple-cell receptive fields. In nearly all cases, however, only a small number of inputs to a given cell could be found. The largest of these inputs accounted for, on average, only 11% of the simple-type cortical cell's discharge, suggesting that each cortical cell received at least nine such inputs or, perhaps, very many more if the additional inputs were much smaller. Only if a comparable number of inputs could be found would one expect to be able to determine whether the receptive fields of the collection of inputs were aligned in the visual field, as hypothesized by the Hubel and Wiesel (1962) model. Cross-correlation studies of corticocortical connections revealed the strongest connections, both excitatory and inhibitory, between neurons in the same cortical column (Toyama et al. 1981), with the frequency and strength of connections decreasing as cortical neurons were more widely separated. Cross-orientation inhibition was not prominent; instead, Hata et al. (1988) found the strongest and most frequent inhibitory connections between neurons with preferred orientations that differed by less than 45°. This study found almost no inhibition between orthogonal orientations. From the cross-correlation studies alone, it is not clear whether the predominance of same- and near-orientation inhibition reflects principally that the closest recording sites tend to be both most strongly interconnected (and therefore the investigator is most likely to find individual units that are sufficiently powerfully connected to detect inhibitory inputs with cross-correlation) and most likely to have similar orientations or whether the net inhibition is actually much less at orthogonal orientations than at similar or neighboring orientations.

Cross-correlation studies did reveal, however, the effects of what appeared to be long-distance excitatory connections (T'so et al. 1986). These effects appeared largely to result from common inputs to cortical columns of the same orientation separated by as much as several millimeters. These effects were proposed to result from the periodic patchy interconnections that connect columns of similar orientation (Gilbert and Wiesel 1989). Taken together, cross-correlation experiments have shown excitatory corticocortical connections that do respect orientation columns, consistent with a corticocortical model for the refinement of orientation selectivity, but they have not supported either the Hubel and Wiesel (1962) model of geniculocortical afferent convergence onto simple cells or a model in which corticocortical inhibition from the orthogonal orientation produces orientation specificity.

A second physiological approach to the microcircuitry of orientation selectivity has been to record synaptic potentials intracellularly in an effort to study the receptive fields of the units producing the synaptic potentials. By injecting current into a cell, it is possible to isolate either excitatory postsynaptic potentials ([EPSPs] by hyperpolarizing) or inhibitory postsynaptic potentials ([IPSPs] by depolarizing). Ferster (1986) demonstrated the selectivity of these techniques for revealing one or the other sort of synaptic potential by testing the responses to electrical stimulation of the optic tract or radiations—typically, a monosynaptic excitation followed by disynaptic inhibition. Ferster then examined the orientation tuning of the EPSPs and IPSPs isolated in this fashion. Not surprisingly, the EPSPs were selective for stimulus orientation in a manner very similar to the cortical cell when it was allowed to spike. More surprisingly, IPSPs showed very similar orientation tuning. This result is very different from that predicted by the cross-orientation inhibition model, which suggests that IPSPs would be elicited preferentially by stimuli oriented orthogonal to the preferred orientation of the cell. Although it is uncertain whether all PSPs are adequately isolated by these techniques (Martin 1988), Ferster's findings are consistent with the idea that the overwhelming majority of input, even to cortical simple cells, comes from within the same or closely similar orientation columns, and in that respect, they are in accord with the conclusions from the cross-correlation studies noted above. Since the cellular origin of the PSPs observed in these studies could not be identified, however, these results can only support but do not demonstrate that the geniculocortical input is arranged as hypothesized in the Hubel and Wiesel (1962) model. A quantitative model of geniculocortical excitatory convergence is consistent with the PSP recordings and the other properties of cortical simple cells (Ferster 1987).

Experimental Studies of Afferents to Single Orientation Columns

We have now investigated the arrangement of the geniculocortical afferents that provide the thalamic input to orientation columns by recording from afferent terminal arbors in the major input layer, layer IV, of the visual cortex of the ferret (Chapman et al. 1989, 1991). The organization of the cortex in this species is similar to that of the more widely studied carnivore, the cat (Law et al. 1988). In intact cortex, one can rarely record isolated electrical signals of more than one or two geniculocortical afferents in a single vertical penetration through cortical layer IV. As originally pointed out by Helen Sherk (University of Washington), the factor that prevents isolation of the electrical activity produced by the many afferent terminal arbors through which a microelectrode must pass on its way through the cortex is not the small size of their extracellularly recorded action potentials in comparison with the intrinsic electrical noise of the microelectrode, since the microelectrode noise can be as little as 5 μV, whereas afferent spikes are 10–100 μV. Instead, it is the ongoing discharge of cortical cells that produces spikes of some hundreds of microvolts that prevents recognition of most of the signals from afferents. We applied drugs to silence the cortical cell discharge and thereby made it routine to record and plot 10–40 afferent receptive fields on a single vertical penetration through the visual cortex.

The design of our experiment is illustrated in Figure 3. The procedure was to align a microelectrode so that it passed down a single orientation column in the primary visual cortex of the ferret. Recordings were made at a series of cortical depths to guarantee this alignment by observing that preferred orientation was the same (or nearly so) throughout all the layers of the cortex. Plots of neuronal response as a function of stimulus orientation, like those shown at the right side of the figure, allowed us accurately to determine the preferred orientation of the cortical cells. In the earlier experiments, the electrode was withdrawn from the cortex, and cortical cells were then silenced by killing them, using superfusion of the excitotoxin kainic acid (Zahs and Stryker 1988). In the later experiments, the electrode was withdrawn to a position in layer III just above the major input to layer IV; the cortical cells were then silenced more quickly and with less damage by superfusing them with muscimol, a potent analog of the inhibitory neurotransmitter, GABA, that acts on the postsynaptic GABA$_A$ receptors to inhibit all cortical neurons. Once the cortical cells were silent, the microelectrode was advanced again slowly into and through layer IV, where the action potentials of many

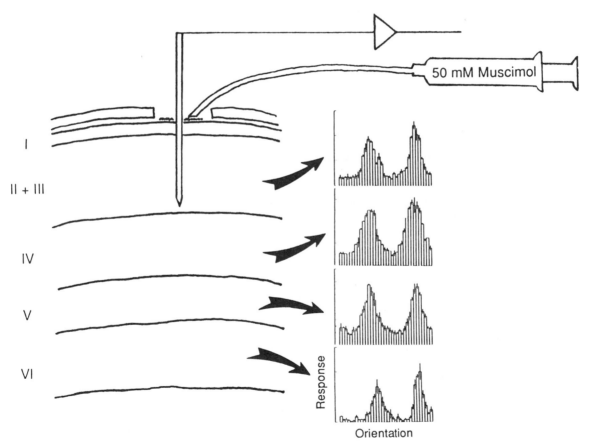

Figure 3. Experimental setup for study of Chapman et al. (1991) illustrating cortical cell orientation-tuning histograms. A radial microelectrode penetration through the depth of cortical area 17 is shown. Orientation-tuning histograms for four single-unit recordings from cells located at the end of the arrow's tails are shown on the right. Each histogram shows the mean response in spikes per second to three presentations of 36 randomly interleaved orientations of moving light bars swept across the cell's receptive field. Orientation conventions are the same as those described in Fig. 2. After these recordings were made, the electrode was withdrawn to approximately the depth shown, just above layer IV. Muscimol (50 mM) was then superfused onto gelfoam surrounding the electrode for several hours to silence cortical cell activity prior to advancing the electrode again down through layer IV to record the responses of geniculocortical afferents.

afferent single units were individually discriminable. These units had visual response properties identical to those of the parent cell bodies recorded in the lateral geniculate nucleus (LGN), and their responses to electrical stimulation of the LGN confirmed that they were the terminals of geniculate cells. In most experiments, the use of a blind procedure ensured that the plotting of the afferent receptive fields was not influenced by knowledge of the prior results from the cortical cells.

Figure 4 shows the results of this experiment for three cases. In the cases illustrated, the afferent receptive fields, shown as ellipses, occupied an elongated region of the visual field, and the axes of elongation matched the preferred orientations of the cortical cells. Both of these findings were generally true. We can examine the degree of elongation of geniculocortical afferent input to a typical orientation column by plotting the entire collection of geniculocortical afferent receptive field centers from the 18 such experiments that we performed, after rotating the sample from each penetration by an angle that puts the preferred orientation of the cortical cells at the horizontal. This universe of geniculocortical input, shown in Figure 5, gives our best estimate of the coverage of the visual field by the inputs to a single orientation column (plotted as if it were a column selective for the horizontal orientation). The number of geniculate inputs illustrated is of the same order as Martin's (1988) estimate of the true number of geniculocortical afferents that terminate around a single thin column in the cat's visual cortex. In any one experiment, of course, we saw only about 5–10% of the number illustrated, and our analysis depends on the assumption that the sample obtained in this experiment is a random sample from the larger universe of afferent inputs.

A quantitative Monte-Carlo analysis of the individual penetrations showed that the afferent receptive fields were significantly elongated with better than 90% confi-

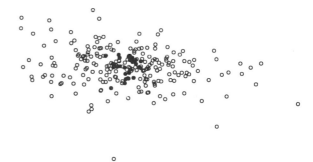

Figure 5. A universe of afferent receptive field positions was constructed from the 18 afferent receptive field arrays obtained in Chapman et al. (1991). Afferent receptive field locations were normalized for magnification factor by calculating the mean radius of the receptive fields encountered in each penetration and then multiplying the distance of each receptive field center from the center of the array by the average mean radius for all penetrations divided by the mean radius for that particular penetration. All the arrays were placed in register so that their geometric centers were superimposed, and they were individually rotated by an amount that rotated the preferred orientation of their associated cortical cell to the horizontal orientation. Afferent receptive field centers (not the whole fields) are shown. (○) Receptive field centers from 16 penetrations in which afferents were significantly aligned; (●) unaligned afferent arrays that were not significantly aligned (encountered in two penetrations). This universe represents our best estimate of the extent of afferent input to a single orientation column. Note the similarity to the central simple cell shown in Fig. 1.

dence in 16 of the 18 experiments and with at least 99.99% confidence in 13 of the 16 cases. The agreement between cortical orientation selectivity and the principal axis of elongation of the collection of afferent receptive fields is illustrated for these 16 cases in Figure 6. Although there are three cases of mismatches by as much 25°, overall, the matches are good, as indicated by the proximity of the data points to the line of the

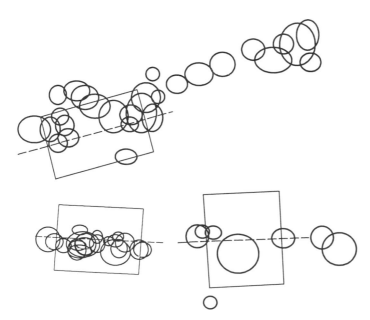

Figure 4. Receptive fields of cortical cells and geniculocortical afferents recorded in three microelectrode penetrations using the techniques illustrated in Fig. 3. *On*-center afferents are shown as solid ovals. For each penetration, the receptive field of a cortical cell recorded at the top of layer IV is shown (rectangle), with its preferred orientation, determined from its orientation-tuning histogram (dashed line). Note the alignment of the collection of afferent receptive fields in each case with the preferred orientation of the cortical neuron.

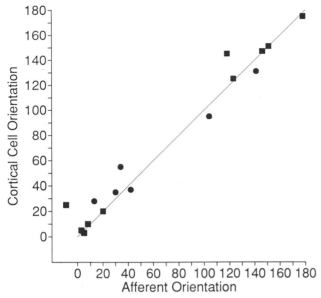

Figure 6. Correspondence between the cortical cell orientation preference and the angle of the principal axis of afferent receptive field arrays. Orientations are plotted following the normal mathematical conventions for angles: Zero degrees represents horizontal, with other orientations measured counterclockwise from the horizontal orientation. (■) Data collected under the blind protocol; (●) data collected when the experimenter plotting afferent receptive fields knew the orientation preference of the cortical cells at that site. The diagonal line ($x = y$) indicates the predicted result if cortical and afferent best orientations matched perfectly. (Data from Chapman et al. 1991.)

prediction of perfect agreement between the orientation of the collection of afferent receptive fields and that of the cortical cells.

The findings of this experiment are exactly as would be predicted by the Hubel and Weisel (1962) model. These findings would appear to be surprising, at least at first sight, if orientation selectivity were produced purely by intracortical mechanisms. This experiment thus provides strong evidence that, at least in adult animals, orientation columns are similar to the other cortical columns in that their arrangements correspond to, and may be determined by, the arrangement of their geniculocortical afferent inputs. As discussed below, however, such an arrangement of input might also be expected if orientation selectivity were produced early in development by some intracortical mechanism, after which afferent terminals were allowed to refine or stabilize in a manner that depends on the correlation between cortical and afferent activity. This possibility is consistent with the early emergence of periodic patchy corticocortical connections reminiscent of those that in adults connect columns of like orientation selectivity (Luhmann et al. 1986; Gilbert and Wiesel 1989; Callaway and Katz 1990). Thus, the finding of orientation specificity in the array of geniculocortical afferent input to a single orientation column in adult animals does not answer the chicken and egg question of who organizes whom—do the afferents come first and organize the

cortical columns, or vice versa? For that, we need to turn to studies of development.

Mechanisms of Geniculocortical Afferent Organization in Development

The earliest features of central nervous system organization, including the generation of appropriate numbers of target neurons, their migration to appropriate positions, the outgrowth of axons, their navigation along appropriate pathways, their recognition of the target structure, and their formation of at least coarsely topographic maps, all appear to be governed by molecular mechanisms of specificity, and all take place normally in the absence of neuronal activity (for review, see Harris and Holt 1990). Thalamocortical organization does not appear to violate these general rules, insofar as they are understood. A special feature of thalamocortical organization is the subplate zone of the cortex, which contains many neurons that normally die at later stages of development. At least a coarse topographic specificity appears to be present when the afferent arbors finally grow into the cortical plate from the subplate zone, within which they may have become organized during a waiting period of as long as several weeks (Shatz and Luskin 1986). Neurons in the subplate make and receive synaptic connections very early and have been hypothesized to play a pioneer role in the development of corticofugal and corticopetal pathways (McConnell et al. 1989; Ghosh et al. 1990).

In several respects, however, the geniculocortical afferents appear to exhibit little specificity in their initial growth into the cortical plate, and a number of results suggest that afferents organize under the influence of patterns of neural activity. These phenomena have been studied most intensively in the case of the ocular-dominance columns. In particular, the initial growth of eye-specific inputs into the visual cortex does not take place in the form of ocular-dominance patches. Instead, geniculocortical afferents serving the two eyes initially make connections to the cortex in a completely overlapping pattern (Hubel et al. 1977; Rakic 1977; LeVay et al. 1978, 1980). Ocular-dominance patches then develop by the progressive segregation of these initially overlapping inputs (LeVay and Stryker 1979).

The development of the ocular-dominance columns proceeds abnormally if the normal patterns of neural activity are disrupted. These abnormalities were first evident physiologically. Most neurons in the cat's visual cortex ordinarily respond to stimulation through either eye (Hubel and Wiesel 1962). Such binocular responses in the visual cortex are unaffected by even years of monocular visual deprivation in adult animals, but as little as a few days or weeks of monocular visual experience during a sensitive period in early life leaves most cortical neurons unresponsive to the eye whose vision had been occluded (Wiesel and Hubel 1963a; Hubel and Wiesel 1970). In young monocularly deprived animals, the two eyes were entirely normal, and neurons driven by the deprived eye in the lateral geniculate nucleus, which is the major source of input to the visual cortex, appeared to be nearly normal (Wiesel and Hubel 1963b). Thus, neonatal monocular visual deprivation produces a rapid and powerful change in the visual cortex, where inputs from the two eyes first have the opportunity to interact on single neurons, rather than at some more peripheral stage of the visual system. These changes are produced most powerfully during a sensitive period in early life at and slightly after the time that major rearrangements of geniculocortical afferent arbors would be taking place in normal development. Studies of binocular visual deprivation and discordant binocular inputs suggest that the plasticity is a result of a competitive interaction between the geniculocortical afferents serving the two eyes that depends on patterns of neural activity (for review, see Stryker 1990). The plasticity produced by various visual deprivation procedures may thus represent the outcome of normal developmental mechanisms in the presence of abnormal patterns of activity.

Consistent with this notion is the fact that ocular-dominance columns do not form at all when neural activity is blocked (Stryker and Harris 1986). Instead of segregating, geniculocortical afferents appear to remain in their infantile state of complete overlap. These experiments suggest that the normal developmental rearrangement of geniculocortical synaptic connections to form ocular-dominance columns requires neural activity. Since ocular-dominance columns form, to a considerable extent, in utero in the monkey (Rakic 1977; DesRosiers et al. 1978; LeVay et al. 1980) and in cats raised with bilateral lid suture or in total darkness, it appears that the maintained activity of retinal ganglion cells in darkness is sufficient for segregation and that visually driven activity is not required. Even in darkness, however, there is information in the pattern of maintained activity of retinal ganglion and geniculate cells. Neighboring ganglion cells of the same center type tend to fire together over time periods of a millisecond to a few tens of milliseconds in adult cats (Mastronarde 1983), and activity is also correlated over longer time scales (Levick and Williams 1964; Rodieck and Smith 1966). Even before the retinal circuitry has developed in utero, ganglion cells have rhythmic activity, and the activities of neighboring neurons may be correlated (Maffei and Galli-Resta 1990). Such correlated activity within one eye and its absence between the two eyes could be the source of the information used by the developing visual system to distinguish the afferents serving one eye from those serving the other.

Stent (1973) and Changeux and Danchin (1976) proposed mechanisms to account for the effects of visual deprivation during early life. These mechanisms were formally similar to the rule described by Hebb (1949) which postulates that synapses are strengthened to the extent that the activities of pre- and postsynaptic neurons are correlated and that synapses are weakened otherwise. A Hebb rule for the adjustment of

geniculocortical synaptic strengths would be expected to allow the geniculocortical afferents serving each eye to remain together in normal development, since their correlated activities would allow them to cooperate in activating the cortical cells to which they provided input. The absence of correlation between activity in the two eyes would not allow cooperative activation of cortical cells and would therefore cause the two eyes' afferents to segregate from one another. Such a rule could also explain the effects of early monocular and binocular visual deprivation, discordant binocular inputs, and the effects of binocular activity blockade.

A number of experiments were designed to test crucial assumptions of the Hebb synapse mechanism. A difference between the neural activity in the two eyes, but not necessarily vision, was found to be necessary for ocular-dominance plasticity (Chapman et al. 1986), consistent with a Hebb synapse explanation of development, in which the statistics of neural activity are sufficient to account for ocular-dominance plasticity. By introducing controlled patterns of activity into the two optic nerves using electrical stimulation, Stryker (1986) showed that ocular-dominance columns did not form when activity in the two eyes was simultaneous, but that an equal amount of activity delivered alternately to the two eyes did allow ocular-dominance segregation. These experiments were consistent with the Hebb synapse prediction that development and plasticity were controlled by the timing of neural activity. Reiter et al. (1986) then showed that blocking both pre- and postsynaptic activity in the cortex completely prevented plasticity, thereby confirming the cortex as the crucial locus of the changes in development. To investigate whether presynaptic geniculocortical afferent activity, postsynaptic cortical activity, or both (as postulated by a Hebb synapse mechanism) are important in ocular-dominance plasticity, Reiter and Stryker (1988) selectively blocked postsynaptic activity during a period of monocular deprivation by pharmacologically inhibiting the cortical cells. In the region of cortex in which postsynaptic action potentials were blocked not only was the normal synaptic plasticity prevented, but inputs from the less-active, occluded eye came to dominate over those from the more active, nondeprived eye, exactly as predicted by a Hebb synapse model, since the activity of the less-active, occluded eye is better correlated with that of the inhibited postsynaptic cortical cells than is the activity of the more-active open eye. The role of the postsynaptic cells appears therefore to be crucial because identical patterns of afferent activity produced opposite types of plasticity, depending on whether the postsynaptic cortical cells were able to respond to their inputs.

Mathematical Model of Ocular-dominance Columns

By explaining, at a qualitative level, how a simple neural mechanism could produce precise patterns of connections in development, the Hebb rule was tremendously appealing. Quantitatively, however, it was not clear whether such an explanation would work with realistic elements. It was also not clear what degree or extent of correlated activity in the retina or LGN would be necessary, what pattern of initial connections was possible, and what the role of intracortical interconnections would be in the process. Finally, a genuine model of development should allow one to predict the widths of the ocular-dominance columns from the input parameters.

Miller et al. (1989) constructed and analyzed a mathematical model of the development of ocular-dominance columns capable of addressing such quantitative questions. The model incorporates a minimal set of features consistent with the experiments above: (1) two sets of afferents, corresponding to the two eyes or to the layers of the LGN that serve the two eyes, that initially make widespread overlapping connections, some of which become ineffective or are removed in development; (2) correlated activity among afferents serving one eye, and the absence of correlation between the two eyes; and (3) postsynaptic activity in the cortex that is communicated via intracortical synaptic connections. These features are described by model parameters A (for the geniculocortical afferent terminal *arbor*), C (for *correlations* in the patterns of discharge activity), and I (corticortical *interaction*). The strength S of each synaptic connection between the afferents and the cortical cells was hypothesized to change by a Hebb rule, and the model was carried forward in time from its initial state of coarsely topographic but otherwise random and near-uniform connections.

This model was analyzed mathematically, and the evolution of its neural connections was simulated in the computer. The model robustly reproduces many of the biological phenomena described above. Ocular-dominance columns indistinguishable in form from real ones were reproduced with a characteristic spacing in the presence of activity, and the model reproduced the known effects of monocular deprivation on column size and spacing. Receptive fields were refined during development, and afferent arbors broke up into patches resembling those observed anatomically. All of these similarities between the model and biological development indicate that a simple rule for synaptic plasticity in a system with initial connectivity such as that of the developing visual cortex can, at least in principle, account for the rich structure of ocular-dominance patches observed biologically. Mathematical analysis revealed that the spacing of the ocular-dominance columns was determined by the corticortical interaction I function, if that function selected a spacing small enough to contain the initial afferent arbor A. If the corticortical interaction function I selected for a spacing that was too large, the spacing would be constrained by the maximum that could be sustained by the arbor function A. A sufficient spread of the correlation function C was important for allowing monocular cortical neurons to develop at all, but beyond that, its role was purely permissive, and it played no role in setting the spacing of ocular-dominance patches.

Each of the three parameters A, C, and I of the model can be, and has been to a limited extent, measured by straightforward anatomical and physiological experiments. The ocular-dominance column spacings observed experimentally fall well within the range of the spacing predicted by the model from our best experimental estimates of these three model parameters (for discussion, see Miller 1990a; Miller and Stryker 1990).

One surprising finding from the mathematical analysis was that the same mathematics could be used to model development under any of a wide range of biological mechanisms of synaptic plasticity. In fact, all of the biologically plausible mechanisms of synaptic plasticity that, to our knowledge, had been proposed to underlie ocular dominance plasticity could be described in the same mathematical framework that we had used to analyze the Hebb synapse model. Therefore all of the mechanisms could with appropriate values of the parameters equally well mimic biological development. As one extreme example, the model was applied to a hypothetical mechanism in which the afferent terminals interact with one another through diffusible tropic or trophic substances and the postsynaptic cells play no role in synaptic plasticity (Miller et al. 1989b). The difference between the model's treatment of the various hypotheses is the biological interpretation of the model parameters. For example, in the original model, the corticortical interaction function I represented the net synaptic interaction among cortical cells as a function of their separation. In the mathematically identical presynaptic trophic substance model, the I function represented the release, diffusion, degradation, and uptake of the hypothetical trophic factor or factors. In either case, the mathematical model tells us what the spatial extent of the net interactions between synapses on different cells had to be to produce ocular-dominance columns of the experimentally observed spacing. However, it does not tell us the biological mechanism by which such interactions are effected. The *quantitative* description obtained from the mathematical model allows one to measure experimentally the value of the model parameters under different assumptions about biological mechanisms of plasticity and to rule out most proposed mechanisms on the basis that they would not predict ocular-dominance patches of the observed spacing. If a proposed mechanism of synaptic plasticity does not operate in development, it is unlikely that the measured values of the model parameters would agree with the ones required by the model except by chance, and if they do not agree, the mechanism simply cannot be the correct one.

Model of the Development of Orientation Columns

Our studies of the ocular-dominance columns indicate that a quite general mechanism of synaptic plasticity in conjunction with the known architecture of the developing cortex and initially rather diffuse patterns of neural connections that are only statistically regular can give rise to eye-specific patterns of geniculocortical afferent connections such as those observed biologically. What sort of explanation could then be offered for the other aspects of afferent and cortical organization, such as the refinement of topographic maps, the formation in some species of *on/off* patches, and the organization of orientation columns? Perhaps surprisingly, it now appears that all of these phenomena could be produced by the same mechanisms of plasticity, responding to changing patterns of neural activity and connections as development proceeds. von der Malsburg (1979), Fraser (1980), and other investigators have modeled map refinement and binocular segregation in the retinotectal system using similar principles, and the experiments from the Constantine-Paton and Udin laboratories, among others (for review, see Constantine-Paton et al. 1990), provide strong support for the operation of similar principles in that system.

Miller (1989, 1990b, and in prep.) has recently proposed a model for the development of orientation columns in which the pattern of activity in *on*-center and *off*-center geniculocortical afferents, together with corticocortical interactions and arbor functions such as those in the ocular-dominance column model, can give rise to an arrangement of orientation columns and a partial segregation of *on* and *off* afferents such as that observed experimentally. This model is illustrated in Figure 7. The model is nearly identical formally to the ocular-dominance column model described above with one major exception, the correlation structure of *on*-center and *off*-center geniculocortical afferent activity. The hypothesis is that the activities of afferents of the same center type are highly correlated when their receptive fields are very near, but as the separation of receptive field centers increases, they become anticorrelated with one another. This is illustrated for two *on*-center afferents in the middle panel of Figure 8. When the receptive fields of the afferents are close to one another, the two centers overlap, and they will be driven in near synchrony by the same visual stimulus or spontaneous retinal input. When the receptive fields of the two afferents are separated by a greater distance, note that the *off*-surround of each afferent lies on top of the *on*-center of the other. In this situation, the afferent activities will then be anticorrelated, since any visual stimulus or localized spontaneous retinal activity that excited one of the afferents would inhibit the other. At greater distances still, the afferents would be uncorrelated. Note further what happens with two afferents of opposite center type, illustrated in the lower panel of Figure 8. When the receptive field centers of *on* and *off* afferents overlie one another, their activities will, of course, be anticorrelated. However, when the two receptive fields of opposite center type are separated by one center-diameter, the *on*-center of the one afferent lies on the *on*-surround of the other, and the *off*-surround of the one afferent is superimposed on the

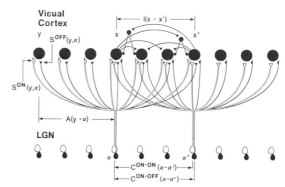

Figure 7. Elements of the model of Miller (1989, 1990, and in prep.) for the development of cortical orientation selectivity. (*1*) Afferents from the lateral geniculate nucleus (LGN) project to the visual cortex. *On*-center and *off*-center afferents (open and closed ellipses, respectively) make equivalent initial projections to the cortex. Synaptic interconnections among cortical cells (●) may be either excitatory (more local, direct connections) or inhibitory (more distant connections via inhibitory interneurons). (*2*) The afferents project to all cortical cells in a compact region, making a terminal arborization; the strength of the connection between a cortical point y and a geniculate point α is given by the arbor function A $(y-\alpha)$, which is zero outside the arbor radius. (*3*) The degree of correlation in firing among incoming afferents from retinotopic positions α and α' is represented by the correlation functions $C^{ON-OFF}(\alpha-\alpha')$ and $C^{ON-ON}(\alpha-\alpha')$ ($C^{OFF-OFF}$ is present but is not illustrated), where $C^{ON-OFF}(\alpha-\alpha')$ gives the correlation between an *on*-center afferent from α and an *off*-center afferent from α', etc. (*4*) Each synapse has a physiological strength that varies with time during development. This is illustrated by the functions $S^{ON}(y, \alpha)$ and $S^{OFF}(y, \alpha)$. (*5*) Finally, there is some influence of activity at a cortical point x' on the strength of synapses at a cortical point x. This spread of influence, as a function of distance, is summarized in the corticocortical interaction function I $(x-x')$ that may be both excitatory and inhibitory at different distances. See text for discussion.

off-center of the other. The activities of the two opposite-type afferents will therefore be correlated with one another at this receptive-field separation, since a visual stimulus or spontaneous event in the retina would drive the two in synchrony.

The result of this peculiar correlation structure can be understood as favoring the development of traditional simple-cell receptive fields, such as that illustrated in Figure 1, with parallel rows of *on*-center and *off*-center afferents providing inputs to single cells. Computer simulations of the model with this correlation structure, starting from an initial state of diffuse, coarsely topographic connections without elongated patterns of afferent input or any organization of cortical orientation, produce patterns of tangential organization of orientation columns that resemble the ones observed in deoxyglucose or optical images of the orientation columns in monkeys and cats (Hubel and Wiesel 1963a; Hubel et al. 1978; Schoppman and Stryker 1981; Singer 1981; Blasdel and Salama 1986; Grinvald et al. 1986; Lowel et al. 1988; Redies et al. 1990). The model exhibits elongated collections of *on*- and *off*-center inputs to single orientation columns such

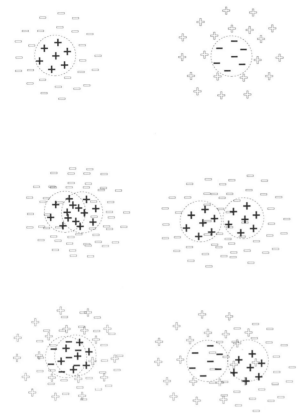

Figure 8. *On-* and *off*-center geniculocortical afferent receptive fields drawn individually (*top left* and *top right*) and with varying extents of superimposition (*below*). Conventions for symbols are the same as those in Fig. 1. (*Middle*) Two *on*-center receptive fields close together and at a separation of one receptive field center diameter. Note that cells will be activated simultaneously by light falling on their common center on the left-hand side of the figure but that they will rarely be activated together when their receptive fields are separated by the distance indicated on the right-hand side. (*Bottom*) One *off*-center and one *on*-center afferent at small separations to left and a separation of one receptive-field diameter at right. Note that these two cells will be driven in synchrony by visual stimuli when their receptive fields are disposed as indicated on the right-hand side of the bottom panel. This figure illustrates the synergistic action of opposite center types at appropriate receptive field separations. Note the similarity of the arrangement shown at the bottom right-hand side of this figure to the right-hand side simple cell illustrated in Fig. 1.

as those observed in Figure 4. The model also exhibits a patchy organization of regions dominated by *on-* and *off*-center inputs such as that described by Zahs and Stryker (1988) in ferret visual cortex.

In the orientation model, the periodicity of the pattern that develops depends on both the corticocortical interaction function I and the afferent correlation function C. In the ocular-dominance model, we noted above that the afferent correlation function C was merely permissive; as long as it was sufficiently broad, it played no role in setting the size of the ocular-dominance patches. This difference between the two outcomes is consistent with the different spacings ob-

served experimentally for orientation and ocular-dominance columns in the same cortex (Hubel et al. 1978; Blasdel and Salama 1986; Grinvald et al. 1986; Lowel et al. 1988).

This model has as yet little direct experimental support, but it is straightforward to test. Predictions of such a model are that orientation columns should not develop if activity of the cortex or of the afferents is blocked or if the correlation structure of the *on-* and *off*-center afferents is dramatically altered, for example, by chronic electrical stimulation that excites both kinds of afferents in synchrony. If these predictions are not borne out, the model must be wrong. As described above, the organization of the orientation columns in the visual cortex of the cat appears to be laid down by the time of the earliest microelectrode recordings made soon after birth and before ocular-dominance columns begin to form (Hubel and Wiesel 1963b). For this reason, we have begun to study the development of orientation columns in the ferret, which is born sufficiently early that one can record from its visual cortex and manipulate activity before orientation-selective responses are present. Orientation selectivity is clearly evident before the time of natural eye opening, and Chapman's preliminary findings suggest that neural activity is essential for the normal development of orientation selectivity. This activity takes place at a time in the animal's life when it would ordinarily live in a subterranean nest in total darkness, similar with respect to visual stimulation to the environment of animals still in utero (Sherk and Stryker 1976). Thus, the nonvisual maintained or "spontaneous" neural activity in the developing visual system may play a role for the cortex such as that suggested for prenatal activity in the formation of layers in the lateral geniculate nucleus (Shatz and Stryker 1988).

CONCLUSIONS

We have seen that the geniculocortical afferent inputs to single-orientation columns mirror and may underlie the specificity of the cortical responses, just as the afferent inputs to the ocular-dominance columns do. Models of the development of specificity in afferent connections and cortical responses are consistent with a unifying notion that the same mechanisms of synaptic plasticity give rise to all four aspects of cortical organization discussed above: refined topography, ocular-dominance columns, *on/off* patches, and orientation columns. Although we will not have conclusive evidence for this hypothesis until we understand the cellular and molecular mechanisms of plasticity in more detail than we do at present, we may nevertheless design experiments that would be difficult to reconcile with other mechanisms. For example, if we could create columns with dramatically abnormal spacing by selectively perturbing corticocortical synaptic interactions, we would have compelling evidence that the columns did emerge by a self-organizing process such as the one we have modeled.

Directly interfering, at a molecular level, with proposed mechanisms of plasticity is another approach of potentially great value. However, it is an approach that is also fraught with difficulty because some of the molecular machinery responsible for plasticity may contribute significantly to neuronal activity as well, and alterations of activity may affect plasticity by any of a variety of mechanisms. Recent investigations on blocking the N-methyl-D-asparate receptor (which currently appears to be the most promising molecular candidate for the correlation detector required by a Hebb synapse) have illustrated these difficulties (compare the interpretations of Kleinschmidt et al. 1987 with those of Miller et al. 1989a). Eventually, we should have the molecular tools to interfere with plasticity at a stage beyond that of blocking transmembrane currents. By altering plasticity without affecting neural activity, such tools will allow us to determine whether the same mechanisms of plasticity give rise to the various forms of afferent and cortical organization.

The combination of experimental studies of the development of cortical and afferent organization in vivo with theoretical studies of the classes of mechanisms that could account for such development has proved powerful. With the addition to these of molecular and cellular approaches in vitro, the future promises a genuine understanding of how the richness of cortical organization responsible for our perception and behavior arises.

ACKNOWLEDGMENTS

The studies reviewed here were carried out with the support of the National Eye Institute, the System Development Foundation, and the Human Frontiers Science Program.

REFERENCES

Albus, K. and U. Baumfalk. 1989. Bicuculline induced changes in excitability and orientation selectivity of striate cortical neurones. Soc. Neurosci. Abstr. 15: 324.

Blakemore, C. and E.A. Tobin. 1972. Lateral inhibition between orientation detectors in the cats visual cortex. Exp. Brain Res. 15: 439.

Blasdel, G.G. and G. Salama. 1986. Voltage-sensitive dyes reveal a modular organization in monkey striate cortex. Nature 321: 579.

Callaway, E.M. and L.C. Katz. 1990. Emergence and refinement of clustered horizontal connections in cat striate cortex. J. Neurosci. 10: 1134.

Changeux, J.P. and A. Danchin. 1976. Selective stabilization of developing synapses as a mechanism for the specification of neuronal networks. Nature 264: 705.

Chapman, B., K.R. Zahs, and M.P. Stryker. 1989. Receptive fields of geniculocortical afferents tend to be aligned along preferred orientation of cortical cells. Soc. Neurosci. Abstr. 15: 1055.

————. 1991. Relation of cortical cell orientation selectivity to alignment of receptive fields of geniculocortical afferents that arborize within a single orientation column in ferret visual cortex. J. Neurosci. 11: (in press).

Chapman, B., M.D. Jacobson, H.O. Reiter, and M.P. Stryker. 1986. Ocular dominance shift in kitten visual cor-

tex caused by imbalance in retinal electrical activity. Nature 324: 154.

Constantine-Paton, M., H.T. Cline, and E. Debski. 1990. Patterned activity, synaptic convergence, and the NMDA receptor in developing visual pathways. Annu. Rev. Neurosci. 13: 129.

Creutzfeldt, O.D., U. Kuhnt, and L.A. Benevento. 1974. An intracellular analysis of visual cortical neurones response to moving stimuli: Response in cooperative neural network. Exp. Brain Res. 21: 251.

DesRosiers, M.H., O. Sakurada, T. Jehle, M. Shinohara, C. Kennedy, and L. Sokoloff. 1978. Demonstration of functional plasticity in the immature striate cortex of the monkey by means of ^{14}C-deoxyglucose method. Science 200: 447.

Eysel, U.T., J.M. Crook, and H.F. Machemer. 1989. Orientation tuning in cat striate cortex involves intracortical suppression of cross-orientation excitation. Soc. Neurosci. Abstr. 15: 324.

Ferster, D. 1986. Orientation selectivity of synaptic potentials in neurons of cat primary visual cortex. J. Neurosci. 6: 1284.

————. 1987. Origin of orientation-selective EPSPs in simple cells of cat visual cortex. J. Neurosci. 7: 1780.

Fraser, S.E. 1980. Differential adhesion approach to the patterning of nerve connections. Dev. Biol. 79: 453.

Gilbert, C.D. and T.N. Wiesel. 1989. Columnar specificity of intrinsic horizontal and corticocortical connections in cat visual cortex. J. Neurosci. 9: 2432.

Ghosh, A., A. Antonini, S.K. McConnell, and C.J. Shatz. 1990. Requirement for subplate neurons in the formation of thalamocortical connections. Nature 347: 179.

Grinvald, A., E. Lieke, R.D. Frostig, C.D. Gilbert, and T.N. Wiesel. 1986. Functional architecture of cortex revealed by optical imaging of intrinsic signals. Nature 324: 361.

Harris, W.A. and C.E. Holt. 1990. Early events in the embryogenesis of the vertebrate visual system: Cellular determination and pathfinding. Annu. Rev. Neurosci. 13: 155.

Hata, Y., T. Tsumoto, H. Sato, K. Hagihara, and H. Tamura. 1988. Inhibition contributes to orientation selectivity in visual cortex of cat. Nature 335: 815.

Hebb, D.O. 1949. The organization of behaviour. Wiley, New York.

Heggelund, P. 1986. Quantitative studies of the discharge fields of single cells in cat striate cortex. J. Physiol. 373: 277.

Hubel, D.H. and T.N. Wiesel. 1962. Receptive fields, binocular interaction and functional architecture in the cat's visual cortex. J. Physiol. 160: 106.

————. 1963a. Shape and arrangement of columns in cat's striate cortex. J. Physiol. 165: 559.

————. 1963b. Receptive fields of cells in striate cortex of very young, visually inexperienced kittens. J. Neurophysiol. 26: 994.

————. 1970. The period of susceptibility to the physiological effects of unilateral eye closure in kittens. J. Physiol. 206: 419.

Hubel, D.H., T.N. Wiesel, and S. LeVay. 1977. Plasticity of ocular dominance columns in monkey striate cortex. Philos. Trans. R. Soc. Lond. B 278: 377.

Hubel, D.H., T.N. Wiesel, and M.P. Stryker. 1978. Anatomical demonstration of orientation columns in macaque monkey. J. Comp. Neurol. 177: 361.

Kleinschmidt, A., M.F. Bear, and W. Singer. 1987. Blockade of "NMDA" receptors disrupts experience-dependent plasticity of kitten striate cortex. Science 238: 355.

Law, M.I., K.R. Zahs, and M.P. Stryker. 1988. Organization of primary visual cortex (area 17) in the ferret. J. Comp. Neurol. 278: 157.

LeVay, S. and M.P. Stryker. 1979. The development of ocular dominance columns in the cat. In Aspects of Developmental Neurobiology Society for Neuroscience Symposia (ed.

J.A. Ferrendelli), vol. 4, p. 83. Society for Neuroscience, Bethesda, Maryland.

LeVay, S., M.P. Stryker, and C.J. Shatz. 1978. Ocular dominance columns and their development in layer IV of the cat's visual cortex: A quantitative study. *J. Comp. Neurol.* **179:** 223.

LeVay, S., T.N. Wiesel, and D.H. Hubel. 1980. The development of ocular dominance columns in normal and visually deprived monkeys. *J. Comp. Neurol.* **191:** 1.

Levick, W.R. and W.O. Williams. 1964. Maintained activity of lateral geniculate neurones in darkness. *J. Physiol.* **170:** 582.

Lowel, S., H.J. Bischof, B. Leutenecker, and W. Singer. 1988. Topographic relations between ocular dominance and orientation columns in the cat striate cortex. *Exp. Brain Res.* **71:** 33.

Luhmann, H.J., L. Martinez Millan, and W. Singer. 1986. Development of horizontal intrinsic connections in cat striate cortex. *Exp. Brain Res.* **63:** 443.

Maffei, L. and L. Galli-Resta. 1990. Correlation in the discharges of neighboring rat retinal ganglion cells during prenatal life. *Proc. Natl. Acad. Sci.* **87:** 2861.

Martin, K.A.C. 1988. The Wellcome prize lecture: From single cells to simple circuits in the cerebral cortex. *Quart. J. Exp. Physiol.* **73:** 637.

Mastronarde, D.N. 1983. Correlated firing of retinal ganglion cells I. Spontaneously active inputs to X and Y cells. *J. Neurophysiol.* **49:** 303.

McConnell, S.K., A. Ghosh, and C.J. Shatz. 1989. Subplate neurons pioneer the first axon pathway from the cerebral cortex. *Science* **245:** 978.

Miller, K.D. 1989. Orientation-selective cells can emerge from a hebbian mechanism through interactions between ON and OFF center inputs. *Soc. Neurosci. Abstr.* **15:** 794.

———. 1990a. Correlation-based models of neural development. In *Neuroscience and connectionist models* (ed. M.A. Gluck and D.E. Rumelhart), p. 267. Lawrence Erlbaum, Hillsdale, New Jersey.

———. 1990b. Cortical organization of orientation selectivity emerges from interactions between on- and off-center inputs. *Soc. Neurosci. Abstr.* **16:** 798.

Miller, K.D. and M.P. Stryker. 1990. Development of ocular dominance columns: Mechanisms and models. In *Connectionist modeling and brain function: The developing interface* (ed. S.J. Hanson and C.R. Olson), p. 255. MIT Press, Cambridge, Massachusetts.

Miller, K.D., B. Chapman, and M.P. Stryker. 1989a. Visual responses in adult cat visual cortex depend on N-methyl-D-asparate receptors. *Proc. Natl. Acad. Sci.* **856:** 5183.

Miller, K.D., J.B. Keller, and M.P. Stryker. 1989b. Ocular dominance column development: Analysis and simulation. *Science* **245:** 605.

Pettigrew, J.D. and J.D. Daniels. 1973. GABA antagonism in visual cortex: Different effects on simple, complex, and hypercomplex neurons. *Science* **182:** 81.

Rakic, P. 1977. Prenatal development of the visual system in the rhesus monkey. *Philos. Trans. Roy. Soc. Lond. B* **278:** 245.

Redies, C., M. Diksic, and H. Riml. 1990. Functional organization in the ferret visual cortex: A double-label 2-deoxyglucose study. *J. Neurosci.* **10:** 2791.

Reiter, H.O. and M.P. Stryker. 1988. Neural plasticity without postsynaptic action potentials: Less-active inputs become dominant when kitten visual cortical cells are pharmacologically inhibited. *Proc. Natl. Acad. Sci.* **85:** 3623.

Reiter, H.O., D.M. Waitzman, and M.P. Stryker. 1986. Cortical activity blockade prevents ocular dominance plasticity in the kitten visual cortex. *Exp. Brain Res.* **65:** 182.

Rodieck, R.W. and P.S. Smith. 1966. Slow dark discharge rhythms of cat retinal ganglion cells. *J. Neurophysiol.* **29:** 942.

Schoppmann, A. and M.P. Stryker. 1981. Physiological evidence that the 2-deoxyglucose method reveals orientation columns in cat visual cortex. *Nature* **293:** 574.

Shatz, C.J. and M.B. Luskin. 1986. The relationship between the geniculocortical afferents and their cortical target cells during development of the cat's primary visual cortex. *J. Neurosci.* **6:** 3655.

Shatz, C.J. and M.P. Stryker. 1988. Prenatal tetrodotoxin infusion blocks segregation of retinogeniculate afferents. *Science* **242:** 87.

Sherk, H. and M.P. Stryker. 1976. Quantitative study of cortical orientation selectivity in visually inexperienced kitten. *J. Neurophysiol.* **39:** 63.

Shou, T. and A.G. Leventhal. 1989. Organized arrangement of orientation-sensitive relay cells in the cat's dorsal lateral geniculate nucleus. *J. Neurosci.* **9:** 4287.

Sillito, A.M. 1975. The contribution of inhibitory mechanisms to the receptive field properties of neurones in the striate cortex of the cat. *J. Physiol.* **250:** 305.

Sillito, A.M., J.A. Kemp, J.A. Milson, and N. Berardi. 1980. A re-evaluation of the mechanisms underlying simple cell orientation selectivity. *Brain Res.* **194:** 517.

Singer, W. 1981. Topographic organization of orientation columns in the cat visual cortex. *Exp. Brain Res.* **44:** 431.

Stent, G.S. 1973. A physiological mechanism of Hebb's postulate of learning. *Proc. Natl. Acad. Sci.* **84:** 3936.

Stryker, M.P. 1986. The role of neural activity in rearranging connections in the central visual system. In *The biology of change in otolaryngology* (ed. R.W. Ruben et al.), p. 211. Elsevier, Amsterdam.

———. 1990. Activity-dependent reorganization of afferents in the developing mammalian visual system. In *Development of the visual system* (ed. D.M.K. Lam and C.J. Shatz), p. 267. MIT Press, Cambridge, Massachusetts.

Stryker, M.P. and W.A. Harris. 1986. Binocular impulse blockade prevents formation of ocular dominance columns in the cat's visual cortex. *J. Neurosci.* **6:** 2117.

Tanaka, K. 1983. Cross-correlation analysis of geniculostriate neuronal relationships in cats. *J. Neurophysiol.* **49:** 1303.

Toyama, K., M. Kimura, and K. Tanaka. 1981. Cross-correlation analysis of interneural activity in cat visual cortex. *J. Neurophys.* **46:** 191.

T'so, D.Y., C.D. Gilbert, and T.N. Wiesel. 1986. Relationships between horizontal interactions and functional architecture as revealed by cross-correlation analysis. *J. Neurosci.* **6:** 1160.

Tsumoto, T., W. Eckart, and O.D. Creutzfeldt. 1979. Modification of orientation sensitivity of cat visual cortex neurones by removal of GABA mediated inhibition. *Exp. Brain Res.* **34:** 351.

von der Malsburg, C. 1979. Development of ocularity domains and growth behavior of axon terminals. *Biol. Cybernet.* **32:** 49.

Wiesel, T.N. and D.H. Hubel. 1963a. Single-cell responses in striate cortex of kittens deprived of vision in one eye. *J. Neurophysiol.* **26:** 978.

———. 1963b. Effects of visual deprivation on morphology and physiology of cells in the cat's lateral geniculate body. *J. Neurophysiol.* **26:** 978.

Vidyasagar, T.R. and J.V. Urbas. 1982. Orientation sensitivity of cat LGN neurones with and without inputs from visual cortical areas 17 and 18. *Exp. Brain Res.* **46:** 157.

Zahs, K.R. and M.P. Stryker. 1988. Segregation of ON and OFF afferents to ferret visual cortex. *J. Neurophysiol.* **59:** 1410.

Chemosensory Cell Function in the Behavior and Development of *Caenorhabditis elegans*

C.I. Bargmann,* J.H. Thomas,*† and H.R. Horvitz*
Howard Hughes Medical Institute, Department of Biology, Massachusetts Institute of Technology, Cambridge, Massachusetts 02139; †Department of Genetics, University of Washington, Seattle, Washington 98195

Chemosensation enables organisms to detect food, predators, potential mates, and other indicators of environmental quality. Organisms ranging in complexity from bacteria to mammals identify chemicals as attractants or repellents and modify their behaviors accordingly (Adler 1975). In bacteria, the identity and regulation of chemosensory receptors has been elegantly elucidated (Koshland 1988; Simon et al. 1989). More recently, chemosensory cAMP receptors in the slime mold *Dictyostelium discoideum* (Klein et al. 1988) and pheromone receptors in yeast (Burkholder and Hartwell 1985; Hagen et al. 1986) have been identified. Less is known about the molecules and mechanisms of chemosensation in metazoan organisms.

Multicellular animals sense chemicals using specialized cells in the nervous system. In vertebrates, different categories of chemosensory cells are known to recognize different molecules. Some small, water-soluble compounds are sensed by neurons in the taste bud papillae, a variety of volatile odorants are sensed by olfactory neurons, mammalian pheromones are sensed by the vomeronasal neurons, and irritant chemicals are sensed by nocioceptive neurons in the oral cavity (Finger and Silver 1987). How many types of cells are included in each of these categories, how chemosensory neurons identify stimuli using receptor molecules, and how this information is processed and integrated by the sensory neurons and the central nervous system are not fully understood.

At some level, any neuron that responds to a chemical neurotransmitter could be considered a chemosensory neuron. However, neurons that sense environmental chemical stimuli face special problems. Many different chemicals can be presented by the environment, so a variety of molecules should be recognized by an effective chemosensory system. In addition, concentrations of sensed environmental molecules are unlikely to be as uniform as concentrations of molecules released by a neighboring cell during neurotransmission. Indeed, the absolute level of a molecule in the environment might be less important than whether its concentration is changing and the direction of the change.

We are studying chemosensation in the small soil nematode *Caenorhabditis elegans*. The adult hermaphrodite has only 302 neurons in its nervous system, and the anatomies and morphological connections of all of these neurons were described previously (Albertson and Thomson 1976; White et al. 1976, 1986). Combining this anatomical information with genetic analysis and laser microsurgery should allow the characterization of each of the neurons involved in a particular behavioral response (see, e.g., Chalfie et al. 1985; Avery and Horvitz 1989). *C. elegans* is sensitive to numerous environmental chemical stimuli: An animal can chemotax to an attractive compound, avoid a noxious compound, and modify its movement, egg-laying, feeding, defecation, and development based on the availability of food (Ward 1973; Dusenbery 1974; Cassada and Russell 1975; Culotti and Russell 1978; Horvitz et al. 1982; Avery and Horvitz 1990; Thomas 1990). Table 1 lists some responses that are regulated by chemical signals in the environment and some chemicals to which *C. elegans* responds. We have focused our studies on the identification and characterization of the sensory neurons required for several of these responses.

C. elegans Can Chemotax to Many Compounds

C. elegans can chemotax to bacteria, its food source, and to a variety of small water-soluble molecules, including cAMP, biotin, several amino acids, Na^+ and Cl^- ions, and basic pH (Ward 1973; Dusenbery 1974; C.I. Bargmann and H.R. Horvitz, in prep.). This behavior can be observed by placing an animal within a petri plate containing agar with a gradient of an attractive molecule. Wild-type animals will orient their movement along the surface of the agar and migrate to the peak of the gradient (Fig. 1).

In addition, we have found that *C. elegans* will chemotax to many volatile odorants, including organic alcohols, ketones, esters, ethers, and aromatic molecules (C.I. Bargmann and H.R. Horvitz, in prep.). This behavior is similar to chemotaxis to the water-soluble molecules described above. However, whereas water-soluble molecules must be allowed to diffuse within the agar over many hours, a volatile attractant can be presented by suspending it over the agar surface immediately before the assay. Our analysis of chemosensory cells and mutants indicates that the response to volatile odorants is distinct from that to water-soluble small molecules (see below). Both volatile and water-soluble attractants are probably produced by the soil bacteria that *C. elegans* consumes.

The observed behaviors appear to be genuine chemotaxis (oriented movement) and not the trapping

Table 1. Regulation of Behavior by External Stimuli

Behavior	With bacteria	Without bacteria	References
Pharyngeal pumping (feeding)	rapid	slow	1, 2
Egg laying	rapid	slow	1
Movement	inactive	active	1
Defecation cycle	rapid	slow	3

Compounds to which *C. elegans* will chemotax	References
Cl^-, SO_4^-, NO_3^-, Br^-, I^-	4, 5
Na^+, K^+, Li^+, Ca^{++}, Mg^{++}	4, 5
cAMP, cGMP	4
Biotin	6
Lysine, histidine, cysteine, serotonin	4, 6
Basic pH	4, 5
Pyridine	7
Benzaldehyde, 2-butanone, isoamyl alcohol	8

Substances that *C. elegans* will avoid	
Acid pH	5
High osmotic strength	9
Extract of garlic	10
Extract of dead *C. elegans* ("avoidance factor")	11
Copper ions	12
Sodium dodecyl sulfate	12
D-Tryptophan	13

References: (1) Horvitz et al. 1982; (2) Avery and Horvitz 1990; (3) Thomas 1990; (4) Ward 1973; (5) Dusenbery 1974; (6) C.I. Bargmann and H.R. Horvitz, in prep. (7) Dusenbery 1976; (8) C.I. Bargmann and H.R. Horvitz in prep.; (9) Culotti and Russell 1978; (10) J. Culotti, pers. comm.; (11) J.H. Thomas and H.R. Horvitz in prep. (12) J. Thomas, unpubl.; (13) Dusenbery 1975.

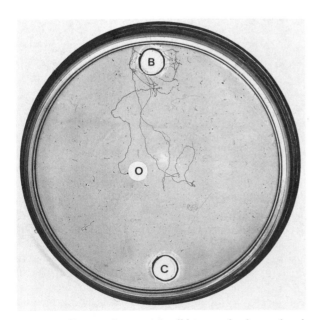

Figure 1. Chemotaxis assay. A wild-type animal was placed on agar on a petri plate at the origin marked O in the presence of the attractant biotin (B, at top). A control area equidistant from the origin is marked C (bottom). After 1 hr, the animal was removed, and the plate was photographed. The tracks made by the movement of the nematode on the agar are visible. This animal moved directly to the biotin and then wandered away from and back to the attractant several times during the assay.

or accumulation of animals at the highest concentration of an attractant (Ward 1973). One critical component of chemotaxis is alignment of the head so that movement is perpendicular to the gradient of attractant. When animals with a kinked neck ("bent head" mutants) are placed in a gradient in which wild-type animals would approach the attractant in a direct line, the bent head mutants approach the attractant in a spiral pattern (Ward 1973). This observation indicates that *C. elegans* chemotaxes by placing its head in a particular relationship to the sensed gradient of attractant, rather than by maximizing the speed at which it approaches the attractant.

The comparison of concentrations of attractants by different chemosensory neurons is unlikely to be a component of chemotaxis in *C. elegans*. Chemotaxis proceeds normally in the absence of functional tail chemosensory neurons (Ward 1973; C.I. Bargmann and H.R. Horvitz, in prep.), so attractant concentrations at the head and tail need not be compared for the orientation of movement. All chemosensory neurons in *C. elegans* belong to left-right symmetrical pairs of cells, but the two sides of the head are probably not compared to each other: The animal moves on a solid surface lying on its side, so the left and right sensory openings lie one on top of the other and presumably encounter similar concentrations of attractants. Movement on a solid substrate is propagated through dorsal-

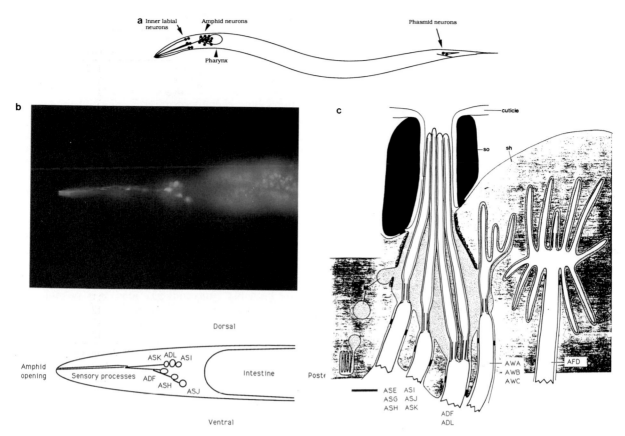

Figure 2. Sensory neuron structure in *C. elegans*. (*a*) Positions and morphologies of sensory neurons in *C. elegans*. A nematode is diagramed lying on its side, so that the sensory neurons on the left are visible; a similar set of neurons are found on the right side of the animal. Within the major ganglia of the head lie the cell bodies of the inner labial neurons (IL1 and IL2) and the amphid neurons (AWA, AWB, AWC, AFD, ASE, ADF, ASG, ASH, ASI, ASJ, ASK, and ADL). The sensory processes of the amphid neurons run anteriorly to the tip of the nose, where some are exposed through the two amphid channel openings (one amphid each on the left and right). The sensory processes of the inner labial neurons also run anteriorly to the tip of the nose, where the IL2 endings are exposed through the six radially arranged inner labial openings. The lumbar ganglia contain the cell bodies of the phasmid neurons (PHA and PHB). The sensory processes of the phasmid neurons run posteriorly toward the tail, where they are exposed through the two phasmid openings (one phasmid each on the left and right). For more details about sensory structures, see below and Ward et al. 1975 and Ware et al. 1975. (*b*) FITC-filling of amphid sensory neurons. A live adult animal that was soaked in the dye FITC is shown visualized by epifluorescence. Anterior is at left and posterior is at right; this picture shows about the anterior one third of the animal. Six cells (ASK, ADL, ASI, ADF, ASH, and ASJ) on this side of the head have taken up the fluorescent dye (Hedgecock et al. 1985). Their sensory endings run to the anterior tip of the animal, where they are exposed. Their cell bodies can be seen in this plane of focus. The autofluorescent granules of the intestine are also visible. The six cells on the other side of the head and the two pairs of cells in the tail that also take up FITC are not visible in this photograph. (*c*) Schematic diagram of the amphid sensillum, adapted from Perkins et al. 1986. This cross-section illustrates some of the ciliated sensory endings of the chemosensory neurons at the opening where they are exposed to the environment. A cuticle surrounding the animal is pierced by the socket cell (so), a toroid-shaped cell that forms the amphid channel opening. Adjacent to and under the socket cell is the sheath cell (sh), a support cell that encases the sensory endings and secretes matrix material (M) into the amphid channel. The sensory endings of the neurons ASE, ADF, ASG, ASH, ASI, ASJ, ASK, and ADL protrude through the sheath and socket cell to be presented to the environment. ASE, ASG, ASH, ASI, ASJ, and ASK have single exposed cilia (two of these neurons are diagramed), whereas the ADF and ADL endings branch to form two cilia at their transition zones (narrow region) (one of these neurons is diagramed). The sensory endings of the neurons AWA, AWB, and AWC are enveloped by the sheath cell, in a space continuous with the opening of the amphid channel (the AWA neuron is diagramed). The sensory endings of the AFD neuron also protrude into the sheath cell. The phasmid and inner labial sensilla are similar to the amphid sensilla in general organization. The IL2, PHA, and PHB endings are exposed to the environment, whereas the IL1 endings are slightly displaced from the opening of the inner labial sensilla. Bar, 1.0 μm.

ventral head bends. It is possible that comparisons are made between dorsal and ventral positions of the head, although there is no obvious dorsal-ventral asymmetry in the chemosensory structures. Alternatively, differences in attractant concentrations may be sensed directly over time.

Analysis of Chemosensory Cell Function

Eleven classes of cells in *C. elegans* have been proposed to be chemosensory, based on the observation that they have endings exposed to the environment through specialized structures in the cuticle (Fig. 2)

(Ward et al. 1975; Ware et al. 1975). Ten of these classes (ASE, ADF, ASG, ASH, ASI, ASJ, ASK, ADL, PHA, PHB) each consist of a pair of bilaterally symmetric neurons, whereas the eleventh class (IL2) consists of six neurons, for a total of 26 exposed cells. In addition, there are three bilaterally symmetric pairs of neurons (AWA, AWB, AWC) and six IL1 neurons with endings that are continuous with openings in the cuticle, although the endings are not exposed directly. Also contained within the same sensilla as many of these neurons are the bilaterally symmetric pair of AFD neurons, which have endings near openings in the cuticle. All of these cells are diagramed in Figure 2.

The role of each of these cell types in a given response can be examined by killing individual cells or groups of cells using a laser microbeam. When the nucleus of a neuron is killed in young animals, the cell usually ceases to function by the time the animal reaches adulthood 3 days later (Chalfie and Sulston 1981; Chalfie et al., 1985; Avery and Horvitz 1987, 1989). It is possible to target individual cells for laser ablation without disrupting the function of adjacent cells (Avery and Horvitz 1989).

Several Kinds of Neurons with Overlapping Functions Direct Chemotaxis to Small Molecules

When a single class of chemosensory cells, the ASE neurons, is killed, chemotaxis to cAMP, biotin, Na^+ ions, and Cl^- ions is compromised (C.I. Bargmann and H.R. Horvitz, in prep.). No other individual chemosensory cell type is essential for these responses. These results suggest that the ASE neurons can sense several chemically distinct attractants.

Although killing the ASE cells reduces chemotaxis to cAMP, biotin, Na^+, and Cl^- ions substantially, a residual chemotaxis response to all of these compounds remains after the ASE cells are killed. This response is abolished if the ADF, ASG, and ASI cells are killed in addition to the ASE cells (C.I. Bargmann and H.R. Horvitz, in prep.). Since killing the ADF, ASG, and ASI cells without killing the ASE cells does not result in a chemotaxis defect, it appears that these four cell types are redundant in their abilities to sense this group of attractants.

The cells that are required for chemotaxis to lysine overlap with, but are distinct from, the cells that are required for chemotaxis to cAMP, biotin, Na^+, and Cl^- ions. To abolish chemotaxis to lysine, the ASE, ASG, ASI, and ASK cells must be killed. The simplest interpretation of these results is that three cell types (ASE, ASG, and ASI) sense lysine as well as cAMP and the other attractants, one cell type (ADF) senses cAMP, biotin, and Na^+, and Cl^- ions without sensing lysine, and one cell type (ASK) senses lysine but not cAMP and the other attractants.

The specificity of the effects of killing particular cell types strongly supports the idea that their chemosen-

sory function is assayed in these experiments. An alternative explanation might be that the death of a cell leads to a nonspecific defect in chemotaxis; for example, a particular cell type might be required for any coordinated movement. Such general effects are unlikely to explain the defects in chemotaxis observed after killing chemosensory cells. Since chemotaxis to lysine can occur after the ASE, ADF, ASG, and ASI cells have been killed, the mechanism for directed movement must still be operational in these animals, but it cannot be recruited for movement toward cAMP, biotin, Na^+, or Cl^- ions. This observation is consistent with specific sensory roles of those four cell types in the responses to cAMP, biotin, Na^+, and Cl^- ions.

C. elegans can discriminate among attractants recognized by a single cell type. For example, an animal will chemotax to Na^+ ions in the presence of a concentration of Cl^- ions sufficient to saturate the response to Cl^- ions (Ward 1973). Since the ASE neurons recognize both Na^+ ions and Cl^- ions, it is possible that discrimination among attractants takes place within a single cell type, such as the ASE neurons. Alternatively, there could be specialized neurons that discriminate among attractants but are not themselves required for chemotaxis.

All of the exposed chemosensory cells, including the five described above that sense various identified attractants, can be killed without diminishing the response to volatile odorants (C.I. Bargmann and H.R. Horvitz, in prep.). In contrast, when the AWC neurons are killed, chemotaxis to the volatile odorants benzaldehyde and 2-butanone becomes inefficient, whereas chemotaxis to Cl^- ions is unaffected. This result implicates the AWC cells as neurons that sense volatile odorants. The AWC cells have flattened, extended cilia that are not directly exposed to the environment but rather are encased in a pocket that is continuous with an opening in the cuticle (Fig. 2c) (Ward et al. 1975; Ware et al. 1975). Volatile odorants may be transported through that opening to the endings of the AWC cells, or the odorants may diffuse directly through the cuticle to reach the AWC cell cilia.

ASH Neurons Participate in Avoidance of Several Noxious Stimuli

When *C. elegans* is presented with noxious chemical stimuli, it displays a stereotypical behavior to avoid the repellent (Culotti and Russell 1978). The animal moves backward briefly and then changes its orientation and proceeds to move forward in a new direction. The response takes a few seconds and is repeated each time the animal encounters a repellent. Avoidance behavior can be assayed by placing an animal in a small ring of the repellent. The animal will remain trapped for minutes to hours if avoidance responses prevent it from crossing the ring (Fig. 3).

C. elegans will avoid acid pH, copper ions, sodium dodecyl sulfate, and unidentified repellents present in garlic and extracts of dead *C. elegans* (Ward 1973; Dusenbery 1975; J.H. Thomas and H.R. Horvitz, in prep.; J. Culotti, pers. comm.; J. Thomas, unpubl.). In a different type of avoidance assay, *C. elegans* appears to avoid D-tryptophan (Dusenbery 1975). In addition, the animal avoids high concentrations of salts, sugars, and other molecules (Culotti and Russell 1978). This latter response is probably due to a general avoidance of high osmotic strength.

Individual sensory cell types have been killed to examine their roles in several avoidance responses (J.H. Thomas and H.R. Horvitz, in prep.). Killing the ASH neurons leads to reduced avoidance of high osmotic strength and of extract of dead nematodes. Killing the ASH and ADL neurons together leads to a defect in garlic avoidance. These results show that a single cell type, the ASH cell, is involved in the avoidance of several noxious stimuli.

Although the ASH cells have an important function in avoidance, killing these neurons does not completely eliminate the responses to high osmotic strength, garlic, and probably the response to dead nematodes (J.H. Thomas and H.R. Horvitz, in prep.). Other cells (including ADL, in the case of garlic avoidance) probably function in these residual avoidance responses. These minor cells are most likely chemosensory neurons because their function is disrupted by killing the support cells that ensheath the chemosensory cilia in the head (J.H. Thomas and H.R. Horvitz, in prep.). Thus, the avoidance of at least some noxious chemicals is mediated through specific chemosensory cells and not

through general toxic effects of the avoided compounds.

Chemosensory Cells Control a Developmental Decision by *C. elegans*

The development of *C. elegans* and other nematodes can proceed along either of two alternative life cycles (Cassada and Russell 1975; Golden and Riddle 1984). When raised at low population densities, animals grow to adulthood through four larval stages (L1–L4) in about 3 days. Under conditions of crowding and starvation, animals differentiate and arrest in an alternative third larval stage called a dauer larva. The dauer larva is specialized to survive in and escape from harsh conditions and can persist for several months without feeding. It cannot reproduce. When sufficient food becomes available, a dauer larva resumes development and becomes a fertile adult. Thus, there are two developmental decisions based on environmental conditions: whether to become a dauer larva, and, if a dauer larva is formed, whether and when to recover from the dauer stage.

A subset of the chemosensory cells is involved in deciding whether to become a dauer larva (C.I. Bargmann and H.R. Horvitz, in prep.). When the ADF, ASG, and ASI cells are killed together in young animals, the animals form dauer larvae regardless of crowding or availability of food. These dauer larvae recover within a day to grow to adulthood when food is available. If either the ADF or the ASI cells are intact, animals grow to adulthood without passing through a dauer stage. Thus, ADF and ASI appear to function redundantly to prevent dauer formation in the presence of adequate food. When only ADF and ASI are killed, dauer larvae sometimes form. The percentage of animals that form dauer larvae is increased if the ASG cells are also killed, so the ASG cells probably have a (minor) role in the decision to form dauer larvae.

The ASJ cells are crucial for recovery from the dauer stage. If the ASJ neurons are killed in dauer larvae, most animals do not recover when food is presented (C.I. Bargmann and H.R. Horvitz, in prep.). In contrast, the ADF, ASG, and ASI neurons can be killed without inhibiting recovery from the dauer stage.

When the ADF, ASG, ASI, and ASJ cells are killed together in young larvae, animals arrest as dauer larvae and do not recover. Presumably, this irreversible arrest results from the combination of inappropriate dauer formation caused by the deaths of the ADF, ASG, and ASI cells and inability to recover caused by the deaths of the ASJ cells. Thus, the activity of some chemosensory cells is required for *C. elegans* to develop to adulthood.

How do the chemosensory cells function in dauer formation? Positive and negative environmental signals are evaluated in the decision to form a dauer larva. A pheromone that is released by all stages of *C. elegans* and presumably is indicative of population density pro-

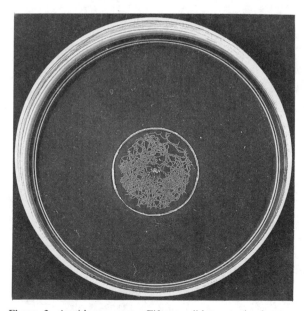

Figure 3. Avoidance assay. Fifteen wild-type animals were placed in the center of a petri plate containing agar within a ring of 60% glycerol, visualized with xylene cyanol. After 15 min, the animals were killed by exposure to chloroform, and the plate was photographed. Of the animals, 0/15 crossed the glycerol ring, although they moved actively throughout the duration of the assay. Their tracks are visible within the osmotic ring.

motes dauer formation, whereas food (bacteria) prevents dauer formation. The food and pheromone levels together determine the developmental outcome (Golden and Riddle 1984). The chemosensory neurons might detect either or both of these stimuli and transmit information to the other cell types in the animal that are altered during dauer formation. One plausible model, suggested by the results of the laser ablation experiments, is that chemosensory cells are stimulated by food and inhibited by the pheromone. If food exceeds pheromone, the chemosensory cells actively prevent dauer formation, whereas, if pheromone exceeds food, these cells are inhibited and dauer formation proceeds by default.

Changes that occur in the dauer larva affect many cell types, including cells of the nervous system, epidermis, pharynx, and intestine (Cassada and Russell 1975; Riddle 1988). Dauer formation is a striking example of neuronal regulation of the development of both neuronal and nonneuronal tissues. It is known that the activity of neurons can influence the differentiation and survival of their synaptic targets, including both neurons and muscle (Buller et al. 1960; Cowan et al. 1984), and of neuron-associated sensory structures (Zalewski 1969). It is possible that general regulation of development by the nervous system is widespread in other organisms. Indeed, the differentiation of specialized shrimp claws depends on their innervation (Mellon and Stephens 1978), and the regeneration of limbs in amphibians usually requires innervation of the regenerating tissue (Brockes 1984).

Mutations That Lead to General Defects in Chemosensory Cell Function

When wild-type animals are incubated in the dye fluorescein isothiocyanate (FITC), eight chemosensory cell types take up the dye and stain brightly (Fig. 2b) (Hedgecock et al. 1985; Perkins et al. 1986). Screening for animals that are defective in FITC-filling has allowed the isolation of mutations that affect the chemosensory neurons (Perkins et al. 1986). Screens for animals defective in chemotaxis (Dusenbery et al. 1975; Lewis and Hodgkin 1977) or avoidance (Culotti and Russell 1978; J. Thomas, unpubl.) have also yielded mutants with defective chemosensory cells. Many of the mutants identified by FITC-filling defects or behavioral defects are pleiotropically abnormal in FITC-filling, chemotaxis, avoidance, and dauer formation (Lewis and Hodgkin 1977; Culotti and Russell 1978; Perkins et al. 1986). The examination of serial electron micrographs of such mutants has revealed that they have defects in the ciliated sensory endings of the chemosensory cells or in the structural cells that form the opening through which those endings are exposed to the environment.

At least 11 genes, and probably more, can mutate to produce structural abnormalities in the ciliated endings of many chemosensory neurons (Perkins et al. 1986).

The cilia of the chemosensory neurons and other putative sensory neurons are the only cilia found in *C. elegans* hermaphrodites (White et al. 1986). Therefore, mutations in any gene that is required specifically to construct cilia would cause a defect in these particular cell types. Mutants with shortened or abnormal cilia might be defective in such genes (Lewis and Hodgkin 1977; Albert et al. 1981; Perkins et al. 1986).

As discussed above, the analysis of chemotaxis and avoidance responses at the cellular level indicates that multiple cell types must be inactivated to eliminate any particular response (C.I. Bargmann and H.R. Horvitz; J.H. Thomas and H.R. Horvitz; both in prep.). This observation might explain why most of the mutants isolated in behavioral screens have pleiotropic defects in many chemosensory neurons.

Chemosensory Cells and the Genetics of Dauer Formation

Most of the mutations described above that cause structural defects in the ciliated sensory neurons also cause a dauer-defective phenotype, in which animals fail to form dauer larvae in response to crowding and starvation (Albert et al. 1981; Perkins et al. 1986). Indeed, several genes that can mutate to result in structural abnormalities of the chemosensory cells were first identified in screens for mutants that fail to form dauer larvae (Riddle et al. 1981). The failure of dauer formation in chemosensory mutants suggests that when environmental signals cannot be sensed by the animals, they grow to adulthood rather than forming dauer larvae.

In contrast (see above), killing certain chemosensory neurons with the laser results in the opposite phenotype: Animals form dauer larvae inappropriately under favorable conditions (C.I. Bargmann and H.R. Horvitz, in prep.). If these same chemosensory cells are killed in mutants with defects in the chemosensory endings of those cells, dauer larvae form (C.I. Bargmann and H.R. Horvitz, in prep.). Thus, the chemosensory cells prevent dauer formation even in mutants in which the sensory endings of these cells are defective. These results suggest that these chemosensory cells are active in the absence of environmental stimulation.

Screens for mutants defective in dauer formation have also identified many genes that can mutate to cause a dauer-defective phenotype without obvious abnormalities in the chemosensory cells (Riddle et al. 1981). The dauer-defective phenotype of most of those mutants is independent of chemosensory cell function: Unlike wild-type animals, these mutants fail to form dauer larvae when the chemosensory cells are killed (C.I. Bargmann and H.R. Horvitz, in prep.). The mutations identified in these screens could alter the target cells for chemosensory cell activity so that they are unaffected by chemosensory cell signals, or they could allow different cells to provide the activity of chemosensory cells required for development to adulthood.

The laser ablation experiments described above demonstrate functional redundancy among cells in various chemosensory processes. This cellular redundancy could result in genetic redundancy in those responses. If two different mutations each inactivate one of two redundant cells involved in a particular response, that response would be normal in animals bearing either individual mutation. However, an animal bearing both mutations would display a synthetic defect in that response.

Such genetic redundancy has been observed in studies of genes that affect dauer formation. Animals bearing mutations in either *unc-31* (unc, *unc*oordinated) or *aex-3* (aex, *a*nterior body contraction and *ex*pulsion defective) are apparently normal in their development, but animals mutant in both *unc-31* and *aex-3* are dauer-constitutive: They form dauer larvae inappropriately under favorable conditions (Thomas 1990; L. Avery, pers. comm.). A synthetic dauer-constitutive phenotype is also expressed by animals doubly mutant in the genes *unc-31* and *unc-3* (C.I. Bargmann, unpubl.). Each of the genes *unc-31* and *aex-3* or *unc-3* might be required in one of two sets of cells that function in parallel, as do the chemosensory cells. Alternatively, these genes could encode redundant products that act within the same cell types.

Mutations That Affect Subsets of Chemosensory Functions

To analyze the genetic requirements for chemosensation in greater detail, it is helpful to distinguish mutants with specific defects in chemosensory neurons from mutants that have general problems with coordination or viability. Mutations that affect some but not all responses are likely to alter particular components in chemosensory behaviors. Therefore, we are seeking mutants with defects in a subset of chemotaxis and avoidance behaviors.

A screen for mutants defective in the osmotic avoidance response has yielded mutants that do not have structural defects in the chemosensory cells as visualized by FITC-filling (J. Thomas, in prep.). One mutant, *osm-10(n1602)* (osm, *osm*otic avoidance-defective) appears to be specifically defective in the osmotic avoidance response, as *osm-10* animals are normal for all other avoidance and chemotaxis responses that have been assayed. Since the ASH cells are used both in osmotic avoidance and in other avoidance responses, *osm-10* is unlikely to eliminate completely the function of a particular chemosensory cell type. Rather, it seems likely that *osm-10* encodes a molecule, possibly within the ASH cells, required for the response to high osmotic strength but not for the response to other repellents. Detailed analysis of this and other mutants could lead to the identification of molecules that are involved in chemoreception of noxious stimuli.

Mutants with specific chemotaxis defects have also been isolated (C.I. Bargmann, unpubl.). For example,

the mutation *che(n1851sd)* (che, *che*motaxis-defective) causes a strong defect in chemotaxis to cAMP and Cl⁻ ions, without eliminating chemotaxis to any other attractant studied. Since cAMP and Na^+ are sensed by the same group of cells (ASE, ADF, ASG, and ASI) and the Na^+ response is normal, whereas the cAMP response is eliminated, the *che(n1851sd)* mutation might disrupt the ability of the ASE, ADF, ASG, and ASI cells to sense or respond to a subset of their normal stimuli.

The isolation of mutants defective in their abilities to sense volatile odorants has identified mutations that cause defects in the response to volatile odorants without affecting chemotaxis to cAMP, Na^+, or Cl⁻ ions (C.I. Bargmann and H.R. Horvitz, in prep.). The molecular receptors for volatile odorants have not been identified in any animal, nor is the mechanism of signal transduction in olfactory neurons well understood (Reed 1990). Molecular characterization of mutants defective in responses to volatile odorants might lead to an understanding of odorant reception in *C. elegans*.

CONCLUSIONS

Different *C. elegans* chemosensory neurons function in different chemical responses. So far, we have identified functions for nine different classes of chemosensory neurons (Table 2). The ASE, ASG, and ASI cells are important in chemotaxis to several small molecules; the ADF and ASK cells participate in chemotaxis to subsets of those small molecules; AWC is involved in chemotaxis to volatile odorants; ASH and ADL mediate avoidance of several repellents; ADF, ASG, and ASI regulate dauer larva formation; and ASJ regulates dauer larva recovery. Although this description of neuronal function is no doubt incomplete, it is possible to make some generalizations about the nature of chemosensory processing in *C. elegans* based on the existing data.

First, different cell types are critical in different kinds of sensations and responses. The cells that are most important in avoidance, the ASH and ADL cells, do not overlap with the cells that are important in chemotaxis. In addition, among the cells that recognize attractive compounds, different classes of cells recognize water-soluble compounds and volatile odorants. In vertebrates, irritants, volatiles (odorants), and water-soluble molecules (tasted compounds) are also recognized by different chemosensory neuron types (Finger and Silver 1987). It is possible that the properties of these categories of chemical stimuli demand different cell types for recognition.

Second, single cell types can recognize distinct chemicals. The ASH cells mediate avoidance of several repellents, and the ASE cells direct chemotaxis to at least five distinct attractants, including attractants that can be discriminated by the animal (Ward 1973; C.I. Bargmann and H.R. Horvitz, in prep.). This versatility of single neurons may allow the animal to sense and

Table 2. Functions of Chemosensory Cells of *C. elegans*

Neuron	Chemotaxis to cAMP, biotin, Cl⁻, Na⁺	Chemotaxis to lysine	Chemotaxis to volatile odorants	Dauer formation	Dauer recovery	Chemical avoidance
ASE	+	+				
ADF	+			+		
ASG	+	+		+		
ASI	+	+		+		
ASK		+				
ASJ					+	
ASH						+
ADL						+
AWC			+			

All cells listed above have sensory endings contained within the amphid sensilla (see Fig. 2), which also contain the endings of the neurons AWA, AWB, and AFD. The ASE, ADF, ASG, ASH, ASI, ASJ, ASK, and ADL neuron endings are exposed through the opening of the amphid channel. The AWC neuron endings are enveloped in the processes of the amphid sheath cell but continuous with the opening of the amphid channel. References: Chemotaxis to cAMP, biotin, Cl⁻, Na⁺, and lysine; C.I. Bargmann and H.R. Horvitz, in prep.; chemotaxis to volatile odorants: C.I. Bargmann and H.R. Horvitz, in prep.; dauer formation and recovery: C.I. Bargmann and H.R. Horvitz, in prep.; chemical avoidance: J.H. Thomas and H.R. Horvitz, in prep.

respond to diverse environments with a small nervous system. In fact, multifunctional chemosensory cells are probably present even in organisms with large numbers of chemosensory neurons. Physiological data from the olfactory and gustatory neurons in both vertebrates and invertebrates indicate that single cells typically respond to several distinguishable odorants or tastes (West and Bernard 1978; Sicard and Holley 1984; Scott and Chang 1984; Siddiqi 1987).

The recognition of different attractants by single cells indicates that some integration of information about the environment occurs within single neurons. Each sensory cell may encode a characteristic part of the combinations of attractants and repellents that may be present at different times.

Third, single cell types regulate distinct responses. The most striking example is provided by the ADF, ASG, and ASI cells. These neurons function both in the behavioral regulation of chemotaxis and in the developmental regulation of dauer formation. Dauer formation ultimately affects the development of many neuronal and nonneuronal cell types, whereas chemotaxis specifically affects movement. Nevertheless, these two different processes use several of the same chemosensory cell types. Since some responses to chemical stimuli have not yet been localized to chemosensory cells (including minor components of avoidance, dauer recovery, and chemotaxis to volatiles), there may be additional cases of multiple responses controlled by single chemosensory neurons. Preliminary results suggest that the ASH neurons might regulate egg-laying as well as avoidance responses (C.I. Bargmann, unpubl.).

Our experiments demonstrate considerable redundancy or overlap in the functions of chemosensory neurons. Even in the small nervous system of *C. elegans*, several classes of cells must be killed to eliminate most chemosensory responses. Similarly, multiple classes of *C. elegans* sensory neurons that mediate a response to touch are functionally redundant (Chalfie and Sulston 1981; Chalfie et al. 1985). In both of these

systems, several sensory cell types act as parallel processors of external stimuli.

The accuracy of sensory processing could be greatly increased by allowing several cells to identify a particular stimulus. The levels of chemical or tactile stimulation probably vary over time and space so that relatively subtle differences indicate that a food source or predator is nearby. Therefore, small differences in stimulus strength must be accurately sensed. If several cells sense a stimulus, the sensitivity for that response could be increased. For example, if a single cell detects a small difference in stimulus strength 50% of the time, and any of four cells can detect and respond to that stimulus, then at least one of the cells will respond over 90% of the time. Thus, the effective threshold for the response of the organism to the stimulus could be lower than that for any one cell. This sort of mechanism might well be operating in chemotaxis, since killing either the left or the right ASE neuron leads to a reduction in the fidelity of the response that is less pronounced than the effect of killing both ASE neurons (C.I. Bargmann and H.R. Horvitz, in prep.). This observation suggests that the activities of the two ASE neurons are additive in some way.

In addition, the presence of several cells of related function might increase the fidelity of a response by increasing the signal-to-noise ratio for chemosensation. If the simultaneous activation of two cells stimulated a response synergistically, the background level of response due to random fluctuations in the activities of those cells would be substantially reduced.

A close examination of sensory processing suggests more complex relationships between cell functions than simple redundancy. In the sensation of repellent and attractive compounds and in the sensation of touch, there are clearly cells that contribute to the responses to different extents. The most important cells (ASE for attractants and ASH for repellents) might have a lower threshold for the stimulus than the others, or it might be better able to deliver that information to the motor system. Some data support the idea that redundant cells may have different stimulus thresholds; thus, the ASE cells are more important for chemotaxis to low concentrations than to high concentrations of NaCl (C.I. Bargmann and H.R. Horvitz, in prep.), and the PVD cells direct avoidance of heavy touch but not of light touch (Way and Chalfie 1989).

Further behavioral analyses of the chemosensory nervous system should elucidate the contribution of each cell to particular behaviors. In addition, the genetic and molecular analyses of mutants defective in sensory behaviors should allow the identification of molecules important in different steps of sensory neuron function. Mutations that lead to defective sensory cilia might disrupt the function of microtubules or microtubule-associated proteins required for the formation of a cilium; mutations that lead to defects in responses to a subset of the stimuli recognized by a single cell type might disrupt the chemosensory receptor molecules or signal-transduction apparatus within the sensory cell. Mutations that cause defects in all the functions of a single cell type might disrupt the development or signaling properties of that cell.

Different chemosensory responses of *C. elegans* can be modulated by experience. Repeated or continuous exposure of an animal to a chemical attractant leads to a loss of the response to that attractant (Ward 1973 and C.I. Bargmann and H.R. Horvitz, in prep.), and starvation under crowded conditions leads to changes in the responses to several attractants (C.I. Bargmann, unpubl.). These behavioral changes might correspond to sensory adaptation and nonassociative learning. The cellular and genetic requirements for modulation of these simple behaviors should be accessible to further study.

ACKNOWLEDGMENTS

We are grateful to Michael Basson, Laird Bloom, Scott Clark, Gian Garriga, Michel Labouesse, and Steve McIntire for comments on this manuscript. This work was supported by U.S. Public Health Service research grant GM-24663. C.I.B. was supported by the Helen Hay Whitney foundation. J.H.T. was supported by the American Cancer Society (Massachusetts division) and is a Searle Scholar. H.R.H. is an investigator of the Howard Hughes Medical Institute.

REFERENCES

Adler, J. 1975. Chemotaxis in bacteria. *Annu. Rev. Biochem.* **44:** 341.

Albert, P.S., S.J. Brown, and D.L. Riddle. 1981. Sensory control of dauer larva formation in *Caenorhabditis elegans* dauer larva. *J. Comp. Neurol.* **198:** 435.

Albertson, D.G., and J.N. Thomson. 1976. The pharynx of *Caenorhabditis elegans. Philos. Trans. R. Soc. Lond. B* **275:** 299.

Avery, L., and H.R. Horvitz. 1987. A cell that dies during wild-type *C. elegans* development can function as a neuron in a *ced-3* mutant. *Cell* **51:** 1071.

————. 1989. Effects of killing identified pharyngeal neurons on feeding behavior in *Caenorhabditis elegans. Neuron* **3:** 473.

————. 1990. Effects of starvation and neuroactive drugs on feeding in *Caenorhabditis elegans. J. Exp. Zool.* **253:** 263.

Brockes, J.P. 1984. Mitogenic growth factors and nerve dependence of limb regeneration. *Science* **225:** 1280.

Buller, A.J., J.C. Eccles, and R.M. Eccles. 1960. Interactions between motoneurones and muscles in respect of the characteristic speeds of their responses. *J. Physiol.* **150:** 417.

Burkholder, A.C., and L.H. Hartwell. 1985. The yeast alpha-factor receptor: Structural properties deduced from the sequence of the STE2 gene. *Nucleic Acids Res.* **13:** 8463.

Cassada, R.C. and R.L. Russell. 1975. The dauer larva, a post-embryonic developmental variant of the nematode *Caenorhabditis elegans. Dev. Biol.* **46:** 326.

Chalfie, M. and J. Sulston. 1981. Developmental genetics of the mechanosensory neurons of *Caenorhabditis elegans. Dev. Biol.* **82:** 358.

Chalfie, M., J.E. Sulston, J.G. White, E. Southgate, J.N. Thomson, and S. Brenner. 1985. The neural circuit for touch sensitivity in *Caenorhabditis elegans. J. Neurosci.* **5:** 956.

Cowan, W.M., J.W. Fawcett, D.D.M. O'Leary, and B.B. Stanfield. 1984. Regressive events in neurogenesis. *Science* **225:** 1258.

Culotti, J.G. and R.L. Russell. 1978. Osmotic avoidance defective mutants of the nematode *Caenorhabditis elegans. Genetics* **90:** 243.

Dusenbery, D.B. 1974. Analysis of chemotaxis in the nematode *Caenorhabditis elegans* by countercurrent separation. *J. Exp. Zool.* **188:** 41.

————. 1975. The avoidance of D-tryptophan by the nematode *Caenorhabditis elegans. J. Exp. Zool.* **193:** 413.

————. 1976. Attraction of the nematode *Caenorhabditis elegans* to pyridine. *Comp. Biochem. Physiol.* **53C:** 1.

Dusenbery, D.B., R.E. Sheridan, and R.L. Russell. 1975. Chemotaxis-defective mutants of the nematode *Caenorhabditis elegans. Genetics* **80:** 297.

Finger, T.E. and W.L. Silver. 1987. Chemical sensitivity and sensibility: Overview and introduction. In *Neurobiology of taste and smell* (ed. T.E. Finger and W.L. Silver), p. 3. Wiley, New York.

Golden, J.W., and D.L. Riddle. 1984. The *Caenorhabditis elegans* dauer larva: Developmental effects of pheromone, food, and temperature. *Dev. Biol.* **102:** 368.

Hagen, H.C., G. McCaffrey, and G.F. Sprague, Jr. 1986. Evidence the yeast STE3 gene encodes a receptor for peptide pheromone a-factor: Gene sequence and implications for the presumed receptor. *Proc. Natl. Acad. Sci.* **85:** 1418.

Hedgecock, E.M., J.G. Culotti, J.N. Thomson, and L.A. Perkins. 1985. Axonal guidance mutants of *Caenorhabditis elegans* identified by filling sensory neurons with fluorescent dyes. *Dev. Biol.* **111:** 158.

Horvitz, H.R., M. Chalfie, C. Trent, J. Sulston, and P.D. Evans. 1982. Serotonin and octopamine in the nematode *Caenorhabditis elegans. Science* **216:** 1012.

Klein, P.S., T.J. Sun, C.L. Saxe, A.R. Kimmel, R.L. Johnson, and P.N. Devreotes. 1988. A chemoattractant receptor controls development in *Dictyostelium discoideum. Science* **241:** 1467.

Koshland, D.E. 1988. Chemotaxis as a model second messenger system. *Biochemistry* **27:** 5829.

Lewis, J.A. and J.A. Hodgkin. 1977. Specific neuroanatomical changes in chemosensory mutants of the nematode *Caenorhabditis elegans. J. Comp. Neurol.* **172:** 489.

Mellon, D.F. and P.J. Stephens. 1978. Limb morphology and function are transformed by contralateral nerve section in snapping shrimps. *Nature* **272:** 246.

Perkins, L.A., E.M. Hedgecock, J.N. Thomson, and J.G. Culotti. 1986. Mutant sensory cilia in the nematode *Caenorhabditis elegans. Dev. Biol.* **117:** 456.

Reed, R.R. 1990. How does the nose know? *Cell* **60**: 1.

Riddle, D.L. 1988. The dauer larva. In *The nematode* Caenorhabditis elegans (ed. W.B. Wood), p.393. Cold Spring Harbor Laboratory, Cold Spring Harbor, New York.

Riddle, D.L., M.M. Swanson, and P.S. Albert. 1981. Interacting genes in nematode dauer larva formation. *Nature* **290**: 668.

Scott, T.R., and F.-C.T. Chang. 1984. The state of gustatory neural coding. *Chem. Senses* **8**: 297.

Sicard, G. and A. Holley. 1984. Receptor cell responses to odorants: Similarities and differences among odorants. *Brain Res.* **292**: 283.

Siddiqi, O. 1987. Neurogenetics of olfaction in *Drosophila melanogaster*. *Trends Genet.* **3**: 137.

Simon, M.I., K.A. Borkovich, R.B. Bourret, and J.F. Hess. 1989. Protein phosphorylation in the bacterial chemotaxis system. *Biochimie* **71**: 1013.

Thomas, J.H. 1990. Genetic analysis of defecation in *Caenorhabditis elegans*. *Genetics* **124**: 855.

Ward, S. 1973. Chemotaxis by the nematode *Caenorhabditis elegans*: Identification of attractants and analysis of the response by use of mutants. *Proc. Natl. Acad. Sci.* **70**: 817.

Ward, S., N. Thomson, J.G. White, and S. Brenner. 1975. Electron microscopical reconstruction of the anterior sensory anatomy of the nematode *Caenorhabditis elegans*. *J. Comp. Neurol.* **160**: 313.

Ware, R.W., D. Clark, K. Crossland, and R.L. Russell. 1975. The nerve ring of the nematode *Caenorhabditis elegans*: Sensory input and motor output. *J. Comp. Neurol.* **162**: 71.

Way, J.C. and M. Chalfie. 1989. The *mec-3* gene of *Caenorhabditis elegans* requires its own product for maintained expression and is expressed in three neuronal cell types. *Genes Dev.* **3**: 1823.

West, C.H.K. and R.A. Bernard. 1978. Intracellular characteristics and responses of taste bud and lingual cells of the mudpuppy. *J. Gen. Physiol.* **72**: 305.

White, J.G., E. Southgate, J.N. Thomson, and S. Brenner. 1976. The structure of the ventral nerve cord of *Caenorhabditis elegans*. *Philos. Trans. R. Soc. Lond. B* **275**: 327.

———. 1986. The structure of the nervous system of the nematode *Caenorhabditis elegans*. *Philos. Trans. R. Soc. Lond. B* **314**: 1.

Zalewski, A.A. 1969. Combined effects of testosterone and motor, sensory, or gustatory nerve reinnervation on the regeneration of taste buds. *Exp. Neurol.* **24**: 285.

Bacterial Microprocessing

H.C. Berg

*Department of Cellular and Developmental Biology, Harvard University, Cambridge, Massachusetts 02138;
The Rowland Institute for Science, Cambridge, Massachusetts 02142*

To someone trying to understand the brain, the bacterium *Escherichia coli* must be an awesome beast. Its talents are legion, but its size is miniscule. *E. coli* is a cylindrical organism less than 1 μm in diameter by 2 μm long—20 would fit end-to-end in a single rod cell of the human retina or some 3000 in that of a frog. Yet, it is adept at counting molecules of specific sugars, amino acids, or dipeptides; at integration of similar or dissimilar sensory inputs over space and time; at comparing counts taken over the recent and the not so recent past; at triggering an all-or-nothing response; at swimming in a viscous medium; and as we shall see, even at pattern formation.

At the 53rd Symposium, I presented an overview of sensory transduction in bacterial chemotaxis (Berg 1988), describing the kinds of measurements that *E. coli* makes on its surroundings and noting how this strategy matches the physical constraints imposed by small size in an aqueous environment (i.e., by life at low Reynolds number; see Purcell 1977). I will restate that case briefly, comment on progress made in the field during the past 2 years, and mention some of the work going on in my own laboratory.

Behavioral Strategy

E. coli is propelled by about six helical filaments, each driven at its base by a reversible rotary motor. When the motors turn counterclockwise (CCW), the filaments form a bundle that pushes the cell steadily forward (for cells grown on a rich medium, ~ 35 μm/sec), and the cell is said to "run." When the motors turn clockwise (CW), the bundle flies apart, the filaments move the cell this way and that with little net displacement, and the cell is said to "tumble." Runs are relatively long (mean ~ 1 sec), and tumbles are relatively short (mean ~ 0.1 sec). Both are distributed exponentially with the shorter intervals the more probable. In the wild type, the motors spin alternately CCW and CW. Thus, the track of a cell appears as a three-dimensional random walk with relatively straight segments of mean length about 35 μm, interrupted by nearly random changes in direction (Berg and Brown 1972; Lowe et al. 1987). However, the runs are not perfectly straight because the cell suffers from rotational Brownian movement and is destined to wander off course by as much as 90° in 10 seconds. Nor are the changes in direction precisely random; the distribution of angles between successive runs peaks slightly in the forward direction.

E. coli measures concentrations of chemicals for which it has receptors as a function of time and then decides whether life is getting better or worse; it samples its environment as it moves along and makes temporal comparisons (Brown and Berg 1974). If the concentration of an attractant increases or if the concentration of a repellent decreases, the cell extends its runs; otherwise, it does nothing. Thus, it drifts in a favorable direction by biasing the random walk. The bias is positive: The runs get longer not shorter.

In principle, *E. coli* could make spatial comparisons, given enough time. However, to do so, it would have to move very slowly. A cell that moves rapidly through a medium containing molecules that it absorbs encounters more of these molecules in front than behind (Berg and Purcell 1977). Therefore, if such a cell compares concentrations measured in front with those behind, it always finds new directions favorable. In any event, measurements of concentration take time; the precision of the measurement increases with the square-root of the total count, i.e., with the product of the concentration and the integration time. With a cell the size of *E. coli*, the integration time is limited by Brownian motion, as noted earlier. Thus, a chemical cannot be sensed at an arbitrarily low concentration. This is why the dissociation constants for the most sensitive chemoreceptors in *E. coli* are in the micromolar range, rather than in the nano- or picomolar range.

By following the direction of rotation of a flagellar motor in a tethered cell (a cell fixed to a glass slide by a single flagellar filament; Silverman and Simon 1974) and stimulating the cell iontophoretically with short pulses or small steps, one can show that a wild-type cell compares the concentration measured over the past second with that measured over the previous 3 seconds and responds to the difference (Block et al. 1982; Segall et al. 1986; Berg 1988). As the concentration of an attractant increases or as the concentration of a repellent decreases, the probability of CCW rotation goes up. Otherwise, it reverts to the value observed in the absence of a stimulus. An exception occurs if the concentration of an attractant decreases (or if that of a repellent increases) rapidly enough for the difference to exceed a substantial threshold. In that event, the probability of CCW rotation falls below the baseline (Block et al. 1982). It is easy to exceed this threshold in the laboratory by mixing chemicals (see, e.g., Macnab and Koshland 1972) but not in the wild, where abrupt spatial inhomogeneities are smoothed out by diffusion.

Biochemical Machinery

Figure 1 is a biochemist's section through *E. coli* (for general reviews, see Macnab 1987a,b; Stewart and Dahlquist 1987). Responses to chemicals are mediated by three convergent pathways, one thought to involve changes in protonmotive force, servicing electron acceptors such as O_2, nitrate, and fumarate (Fig. 1, bottom; cf. Shioi et al. 1987) and also proline (Clancy et al. 1981), a second thought to involve changes in the levels of phosphorylation of proteins linked to sugar phosphotransferases (Fig. 1, left; cf. Lengeler and Vogler 1989), and a third involving proteins that span the cytoplasmic membrane, known as transducers or methyl-accepting chemotaxis proteins (MCPs) (Fig. 1, top). The latter system has been studied most intensively. The transducers interact either directly with chemicals that diffuse through the outer membrane, such as serine or aspartate, or indirectly via binding proteins found in the periplasmic space (the region between the outer and inner membranes). These pro-

teins mediate responses to dipeptides and to the sugars maltose, ribose, and galactose. The transducers also are involved in chemotaxis toward salts (Qi and Adler 1989) or away from a variety of repellents (see the general reviews), as well as in temperature sensing (cf. Lee et al. 1988). A recent breakthrough has been the discovery that the transducers are linked to the flagellar motors via a phosphorylation cascade (Fig. 1, right). This cascade ends with a small cytoplasmic protein called CheY, which when phosphorylated interacts with the switch at the base of the flagellar motor, increasing the probability that the motor spins CW. The kinase, CheA, and its substrates, CheY and CheB, have been shown to be members of a large family of two-component bacterial regulatory systems, most of which control gene expression (for recent reviews, see Bourret et al. 1989; Stock et al. 1989, 1990). Another cytoplasmic component, CheZ, is a phosphatase that hydrolyzes CheY-P. The coupling between the transducers and CheA is not well understood; however, it is known to involve CheW (Borkovich et al. 1989; Conley et al.

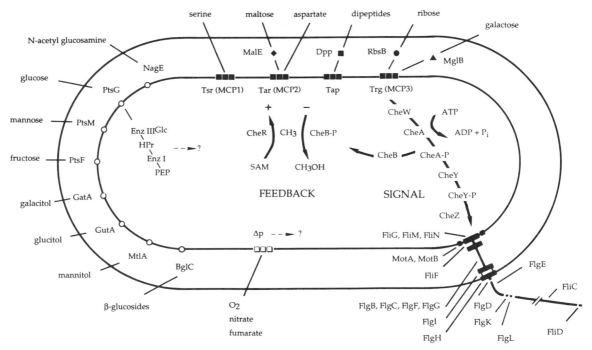

Figure 1. Machinery for chemotaxis in *E. coli* that has been identified thus far (compare Berg 1988, Fig. 6). More is now known about the signaling pathway (*right*) and some of the components of the flagellar motor (*lower right*). Also, the nomenclature for the flagellar genes has been unified (Iino et al. 1988). The chemoreceptors are binding proteins found in the periplasmic space, such as MalE (which binds maltose), proteins that span the cytoplasmic membrane, such as Tsr (which binds serine), or the enzymes II of the sugar phosphotransferase system, such as MtlA (which binds mannitol). Information about receptor occupancy is passed across the cytoplasmic membrane and eventually to the base of the flagellar motors, where it changes the probabilities that the motors turn CW or CCW. This signaling occurs through a cascade of events involving the cytoplasmic proteins CheW, CheA (which autophosphorylates to yield CheA-P), CheY (which is phosphorylated by CheA-P to yield CheY-P), and CheZ. A negative feedback loop counteracts the effects of this signal, enabling the cells to adapt. In the system studied most extensively, which involves the transducers Tsr, Tar, Tap, and Trg (also called MCPs), this feedback is effected by multiple methylation of cytoplasmic domains. When more attractant is bound, methyl groups (CH_3) are transferred from *S*-adenosyl methionine (SAM) to glutamyl residues via a methyl transferase (CheR). When less attractant is bound, these methyl groups are removed by a methylesterase (CheB-P, following activation of CheB by CheA-P), liberating methanol (CH_3OH). In the Pts and O_2 systems, the signal and feedback pathways are not known, although signaling in the latter system is thought to involve changes in protonmotive force (Δp). Fli and Flg components are required for flagellar assembly; only those thought to be part of the final structure are shown. FliG, FliM, and FliN comprise the switch that enables a motor to change direction. MotA and MotB are required for force generation.

1989; Liu and Parkinson 1989; Sanders et al. 1989). Everyone would be delighted if CheW turned out to be a G protein, but the evidence for this is scant. CheW might have a binding site for purine nucleotides (Stock et al. 1987), but the transducers have two, rather than seven, transmembrane α-helices (Krikos et al. 1983; Russo and Koshland 1983), and they function as dimers (Milligan and Koshland 1988).

The phosphorylation cascade explains why signaling in filamentous cells has a short space constant ($\sim 2 \mu m$ in cells that are wild type for chemotaxis, $\sim 6 \mu m$ in cheZ mutants; Segall et al. 1985). By using a signal that can diffuse a few micrometers before being inactivated, the cell can both couple inputs from receptors of the same kind (and thus improve the total count; see above) and integrate inputs from receptors of different kinds. Clearly, it is more important for E. coli to be able to respond quickly (to have a signal that decays rapidly, i.e., on a 0.1-sec time scale) than to signal over a long range (to have a signal with a long decay length). However, we still do not understand how the cell is able to integrate inputs over periods as long as 1 second or why the signaling pathway has such high gain (see Berg 1988).

To make temporal comparisons, the cell requires more machinery, namely, a feedback loop involving methylation and demethylation (Fig. 1, middle). Cells carrying null mutations in both cheR, the gene that specifies the methyltransferase, and cheB, the gene that specifies the methylesterase, still respond to and integrate inputs, but they do not make short-term temporal comparisons (Segall et al. 1986). A wild-type cell adapts to a small step stimulus within about 4 seconds; some cheRcheB cells do not adapt at all, and others partially adapt but comparatively slowly.

The question of whether cheRcheB mutants are chemotactic has been controversial. Stock et al. (1985) isolated second-site revertants of cheR cells on soft agar by selecting cells that swarmed more rapidly. These proved to be cheRcheB cells. However, a more rapid swarm rate does not necessarily mean that cells are chemotactic, because cheR cells only run, whereas cheRcheB cells run and tumble. Cells that can tumble swarm more rapidly because tumbles enable them to back away from obstructions in the agar (Wolfe and Berg 1989). Stock et al. (1985) also reported small responses of cheRcheB cells to relatively shallow gradients of aspartate, but not serine, in the capillary assay (see also Weis et al. 1990). However, such responses were not seen in shallow gradients in the layered-gradient assay (Weis and Koshland 1988). We have developed a new assay in which the flux of bacteria through a microchannel plate (a fused array of capillary tubes) separating two identical stirred chambers is determined from light scattered out of a beam of a laser diode (Berg and Turner 1990). Gradients are imposed by adding an attractant or a repellent to one of the chambers. Weak chemotactic responses are assessed from ratios of fluxes observed in paired experiments in which the sign of the gradient is reversed. In this assay,

cheRcheB cells do not respond to steep gradients of either aspartate or serine. The question remains whether cells without CheR or CheB are defective for reasons that have nothing to do with methylation or demethylation. This alternative has been ruled out by Hazelbauer et al. (1989), who used site-directed mutagenesis to remove the methylation sites in the transducer Trg. Cells loaded with these defective Trg molecules failed to follow gradients of galactose, unless they also carried transducers for other attractants with functional methyl-accepting sites. So, the evidence at hand strongly favors the view that methylation and demethylation are required for bacterial chemotaxis.

It should be noted that adaptation in E. coli plays a more limited role than it does in the retinal rod. Cells do not respond to a given attractant over a wide range of concentrations. The response is proportional to the time-rate of change of receptor occupancy, with the concentration of receptors and the values of their dissociation constants fixed (Brown and Berg 1974; Block et al. 1983). If the concentration of the ligand is too small to affect receptor occupancy or if the receptors are saturated, then the cells fail to respond. At intermediate concentrations, the signal generated by the transducers is computed somehow from the difference between the present concentration, indicated by receptor occupancy, and the past concentration, indicated by the level of receptor methylation (i.e., by a comparison of parameters that change rapidly or slowly, cf. Delbrück and Reichardt 1956). Presumably, the difference in the size of the response observed when a cell swims up a gradient of an attractant, as opposed to that observed when it swims down, has to do with the fact that methylation is relatively slow and demethylation is relatively rapid (for review, see Springer et al. 1979); repellent stimuli are subject to a substantial threshold (Block et al. 1983).

Alternative Strategies

The question of whether an organism can accumulate in a region that it finds more favorable by swimming at a constant speed and modulating its tumbling frequency on the basis of measurements of the local concentration of an attractant has been a matter of debate for many years. Fraenkel and Gunn (1940) defined this strategy as "klinokinesis" (without adaptation) and asserted that it would not work. Patlak (1953), on the basis of an elaborate mathematical analysis, claimed otherwise. Confusion has reigned ever since. We have reconsidered this matter and find that different assumptions about the microscopic behavior of organisms demand distinct diffusion equations (Schnitzer et al. 1990). As long as the swimming speed is constant, one always obtains Fick's equation for the flux, $J = -D(\partial C/\partial x)$, where J is the net number of cells per unit area and unit time moving in the $+x$ direction at position x, D is the diffusion coefficient at position x, and C is the number of cells per unit volume at position x. At equilibrium, $J = 0$ and C is constant: There is no accumulation.

However, if the swimming speed varies, cells will accumulate in regions in which the speed is low: The equilibrium distribution is inversely proportional to speed. Fraenkel and Gunn (1940) defined the latter strategy as "orthokinesis" and asserted correctly that it would work. The appropriate diffusion equation for this case depends on whether one varies speed by changing the microscopic step length or step time. Thus, Fraenkel and Gunn were right, and Patlak was wrong. If the speed is constant, there is no flypaper effect, as it has been called in the literature on bacteria (Stock and Stock 1987).

The situation is more complicated if cells suppress tumbles in response to concentrations sensed over the past. If such cells do not make temporal comparisons, we find by Montecarlo simulation that they swim down rather than up a gradient of an attractant. They remember where they have been, but they do not have a standard for comparison. If the cells do make temporal comparisons, then they swim up the gradient as expected. Strictly speaking, this strategy, which is used by *E. coli*, should be called "chemoklinokinesis with adaptation." However, Pfeffer (1884) used the term "chemotaxis" at a time when he believed that bacteria could steer directly toward the source of an attractant (for review, see Berg 1975), and this term has remained in use.

Flagellar Motors

A detailed treatment of these remarkable machines is outside the scope of the present survey. However, for some of our ideas about how they might work, see Meister et al. (1989). For general reviews, see Macnab (1987a, 1988) or Macnab and DeRosier (1988). In *E. coli* and other common bacteria, the motors are driven by a proton flux. In alkalophilic or marine organisms, sodium ions are used instead (cf. Imae and Atsumi 1989). If the external viscous drag is high, as in a tethered cell, the motor turns slowly at a few Hz but exerts high torque ($\sim 3 \times 10^{-11}$ dyne cm). In this regime, the motor works at high efficiency as a reversible engine close to thermodynamic equilibrium. If the protonmotive force is fixed, the torque is insensitive to changes in temperature or of hydrogen isotope. If the external viscous drag is low, as in a mutant lacking a flagellar filament or, surprisingly, when the filament works in a bundle, the motor turns rapidly at a few hundred Hz and exerts low torque. In this regime, it works at low efficiency far from thermodynamic equilibrium; the torque increases with temperature and decreases when the cells are shifted from H_2O to D_2O. Most of the evidence to date suggests that the motor is tightly coupled, i.e., that a fixed number of protons carries it through one revolution. Under normal operating conditions, protons always flow from the outside to the inside of the cell, regardless of whether the motor spins CW or CCW. The motor runs in either direction at about the same speed; however, it some-

times pauses when it switches from CCW to CW (Eisenbach et al. 1990).

Our interest has focused on the proteins MotA and MotB (Fig. 1, lower right). These proteins are not required for the assembly of the flagellum, but they can activate preexisting basal structures, incrementing the torque in a series of eight equally spaced steps (Blair and Berg 1988). This implies that the motor contains eight independent, force-generating elements composed, at least in part, of MotA and MotB. Studies of a series of *motA* mutants suggest that MotA is a proton channel (Blair and Berg 1990). David Blair has sequenced 53 dominant mutants (mutants that block or severely impair motility when expressed in wild-type cells), and he has found that they correspond to 30 different alleles. All except two of these encode amino-acid substitutions that cluster in or near four hydrophobic and presumably membrane-spanning α-helical segments that make up only one third of the length of the polypeptide chain (Fig. 2). We think that MotA functions as a monomer, since the torque generated in cells in which wild-type and mutant proteins are mixed is proportional to the fraction of protein that is wild type. If so, there are not enough polar amino acids available to build transmembrane hydrogen-bonded chains, so we probably are dealing with an aqueous channel (D.F. Blair and H.C. Berg, in prep.).

David Blair also has isolated a number of *motB* mutants. Most of these amino acid substitutions fall in

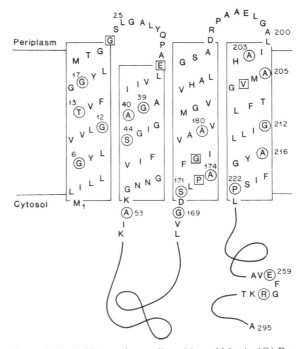

Figure 2. Probable membrane disposition of MotA. (◯) Residues altered in nonfunctional dominant alleles. (▢) Residues altered in severely impaired dominant alleles. The structure is based on the sequence data and hydropathy profile of Dean et al. (1984), and it corresponds to the more conventional of the two alternative structures that they proposed. The fraction of the protein that is in the cytosol is relatively large (note the residue numbers).

the MotB periplasmic domain (see Chun and Parkinson 1988). It is possible that MotB is an elastic element that links MotA to the cell wall, but this might be wishful thinking because such an element is an essential feature in our model for the rotary motor (Meister et al. 1989).

In the interest of completeness, note that both voltage- and stretch-sensitive channels have been found in patch-clamp studies of *E. coli* spheroplasts (reviewed by Saimi et al. 1988). However, their physiological functions are not known. In cases in which the distinction has been made, they are found in the outer membrane, rather than in the inner membrane (Delcour et al. 1989). As far as we know, channels are not involved in the sensory systems outlined in Figure 1. Electrogenic mechanisms for coupling the transducers to the flagella have been ruled out by the experiments with filamentous cells described earlier (Segall et al. 1985) and also by valinomycin-induced voltage clamp (Margolin and Eisenbach 1984). For an entré to recent work on development of the flageller organelle, see Kutsukake et al. (1990) and Jones and Macnab (1990).

Pattern Formation

When swimming in large numbers, *E. coli* can generate complex and intriguing patterns. The best known of these are the traveling bands that arise when chemotactic strains are inoculated near the center of a petri plate in soft agar containing metabolizable attractants. As the cells take up these attractants, grow, and divide, they generate spatial gradients, which they subsequently chase, swarming outward in concentric bands (cf. Adler 1966; Nossal 1972; Wolfe and Berg 1989). The bands are sufficiently dense to be seen by scattered light. Something rather different is shown in Figure 3. This quasi-periodic array of groups of cells was generated in 2 days at 25°C from an inoculum of cells of strain HCB317 (a *tsr* deletion mutant; Wolfe et al. 1987) taken from a single-colony isolate. The cells were placed near the center of a petri plate containing a layer of agar (0.3%, Difco) about 2-mm thick, prepared in M9 minimal salts medium (Miller 1972) containing 4.5 mM sodium succinate (Sigma). The spots, which are stationary, developed behind the circular front, which moved outward at a constant speed. Initially, the spots were relatively bright and contained cells that were vigorously motile. Later on, they faded somewhat as the cells stopped swimming. Since the diffusion coefficient of a nonmotile cell is quite small, the pattern behind the front is stable. Although gradients of succinate can be sensed by serine-blind mutants (Mesibov and Adler 1972), the bacteria do not appear to be chasing succinate. Similar patterns can be obtained with α-ketoglutarate, which is not an attractant. Also, the patterns fail to develop at concentrations of succinate (< 2.5 mM) that are still well above the chemotactic threshold. However, chemotaxis is involved, since formation of the pattern is blocked by addition of a nonmetabolizable analog of aspartate, α-methyl-D,L-aspartate. These studies were initiated by Elena Bud-

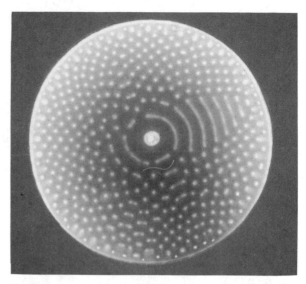

Figure 3. A pattern of small compact colonies generated by migration of a serine-blind mutant of *E. coli* on a soft-agar plate containing a defined medium with a single carbon source. The pattern was generated by active accumulation of cells in the wake of the circular front, not by seeding and subsequent growth (see text). The outer ring is 6.2 cm in diameter. This is a copy of a Polaroid photograph; the outer regions of the plate have been covered by a mask.

rene, who first saw such patterns while working at Moscow State University. She has brought the problem to Harvard. It would be interesting if we are dealing with a bacterial pheromone, but it seems unlikely that the chemoattractant will prove to be species specific.

SUMMARY

E. coli is a remarkable creature that has honed its sensory talents in the face of daunting physical constraints. Although not a model for the brain (Berg 1981), it demands our admiration and respect (Berg 1988). It is teaching us about behavioral strategies, sensory receptors, signal transduction, adaptation, chemomechanical energy conversion, rotary engines, development, and even pattern formation.

ACKNOWLEDGMENTS

This work was supported by the Rowland Institute for Science and by grants from the National Science Foundation (DCB-8903690) and the National Institute of Allergy and Infectious Diseases (AI-16478).

REFERENCES

Adler, J. 1966. Chemotaxis in bacteria. *Science* **153:** 701.
Berg, H.C. 1975. Chemotaxis in bacteria. *Annu. Rev. Biophys. Bioeng.* **4:** 119.
———. 1981. Of bugs and brains. *Nature* **292:** 870.
———. 1988. A physicist looks at bacterial chemotaxis. *Cold Spring Harbor Symp. Quant. Biol.* **53:** 1.
Berg, H.C. and D.A. Brown. 1972. Chemotaxis in *Escherichia coli* analysed by three-dimensional tracking. *Nature* **239:** 500.

Berg, H.C. and E.M. Purcell. 1977. Physics of chemoreception. *Biophys. J.* **20**: 193.

Berg, H.C. and L. Turner. 1990. Chemotaxis of bacteria in glass capillary arrays. *Biophys. J.* (in press).

Blair, D.F. and H.C. Berg. 1988. Restoration of torque in defective flagellar motors. *Science* **242**: 1678.

———. 1990. The MotA protein of *E. coli* is a proton-conducting component of the flagellar motor. *Cell* **60**: 439.

Block, S.M., J.E. Segall, and H.C. Berg. 1982. Impulse responses in bacterial chemotaxis. *Cell* **31**: 215.

———. 1983. Adaptation kinetics in bacterial chemotaxis. *J. Bacteriol.* **154**: 312.

Borkovich, K.A., N. Kaplan, J.F. Hess, and M.I. Simon. 1989. Transmembrane signal transduction in bacterial chemotaxis involves ligand-dependent activation of phosphate group transfer. *Proc. Natl. Acad. Sci.* **86**: 1208.

Bourret, R.B., J.F. Hess, K.A. Borkovich, A.A. Pakula, and M.I. Simon. 1989. Protein phosphorylation in chemotaxis and two-component regulatory systems of bacteria. *J. Biol. Chem.* **264**: 7085.

Brown, D.A. and H.C. Berg. 1974. Temporal stimulation of chemotaxis in *Escherichia coli. Proc. Natl. Acad. Sci.* **71**: 1388.

Chun, S.Y. and J.S. Parkinson. 1988. Bacterial motility: Membrane topology of the *Escherichia coli* MotB protein. *Science* **239**: 276.

Clancy, M., K.A. Madill, and J.M. Wood. 1981. Genetic and biochemical requirements for chemotaxis to L-proline in *Escherichia coli. J. Bacteriol.* **146**: 902.

Conley, M.P., A.J. Wolfe, D.F. Blair, and H.C. Berg. 1989. Both CheA and CheW are required for reconstitution of chemotactic signaling in *Escherichia coli. J. Bacteriol.* **171**: 5190.

Dean, G.E., R.M. Macnab, J. Stader, P. Matsumura, and C. Burks. 1984. Gene sequence and predicted amino acid sequence of the *motA* protein, a membrane-associated protein required for flagellar rotation in *Escherichia coli. J. Bacteriol.* **159**: 991.

Delbrück, M. and W. Reichardt. 1956. System analysis for the light growth reactions of *Phycomyces.* In *Cellular mechanisms in differentiation and growth* (ed. D. Rudnick), p. 3. Princeton University Press, New Jersey.

Delcour, A.N., B. Martinac, J. Adler, and C. Kung. 1989. Modified reconstitution method used in patch-clamp studies of *Escherichia coli* ion channels. *Biophys. J.* **56**: 631.

Eisenbach, M., A. Wolf, M. Welch, S.R. Caplan, I.R. Lapidus, R.M. Macnab, H. Aloni, and O. Asher. 1990. Pausing, switching and speed fluctuation of the bacterial flagellar motor and their relation to motility and chemotaxis. *J. Mol. Biol.* **211**: 551.

Fraenkel, G.S., and D.L. Gunn. 1940. *The orientation of animals: Kineses, taxes and compass reactions.* Clarendon Press, Oxford. (Reprinted with additional notes in 1961 by Dover Publications, New York.)

Hazelbauer, G.L., C. Park, and D.M. Nowlin. 1989. Adaptational "crosstalk" and the crucial role of methylation in chemotactic migration by *Escherichia coli. Proc. Natl. Acad. Sci.* **86**: 1448.

Iino, T., Y. Komeda, K. Kutsukake, R.M. Macnab, P. Matsumura, J.S. Parkinson, M.I. Simon, and S. Yamaguchi. 1988. New unified nomenclature for the flagellar genes of *Escherichia coli* and *Salmonella typhimurium. Microbiol Rev.* **52**: 533.

Imae, Y. and T. Atsumi. 1989. Na^+-driven bacterial flagellar motors. *J. Bioenerg. Biomem.* **21**: 705.

Jones, C.J. and R.M. Macnab. 1990. Flagellar assembly in *Salmonella typhimurium:* Analysis with temperature-sensitive mutants. *J. Bacteriol.* **172**: 1327.

Krikos, A., N. Mutoh, A. Boyd, and M.I. Simon. 1983. Sensory transducers of *E. coli* are composed of discrete structural and functional domains. *Cell* **33**: 615.

Kutsukake, K., Y. Ohya, and T. Iino. 1990. Transcriptional

analysis of the flagellar regulon of *Salmonella typhimurium. J. Bacteriol.* **172**: 741.

Lee, L., T. Mizuno, and Y. Imae. 1988. Thermosensing properties of *Escherichia coli tsr* mutants defective in serine chemoreception. *J. Bacteriol.* **170**: 4769.

Lengeler, J.W. and A.P. Vogler. 1989. Molecular mechanisms of bacterial chemotaxis towards PTS-carbohydrates. *FEMS Microbiol. Rev.* **63**: 81.

Liu, J. and J.S. Parkinson. 1989. Role of CheW protein in coupling membrane receptors to the intracellular signaling system of bacterial chemotaxis. *Proc. Natl. Acad. Sci.* **86**: 8703.

Lowe, G., M. Meister, and H.C. Berg. 1987. Rapid rotation of flagellar bundles in swimming bacteria. *Nature* **325**: 637.

Macnab, R.M. 1987a. Flagella. In *Escherichia coli and Salmonella typhimurium: Cellular and molecular biology* (ed. F.C. Neidhardt), vol. 1, p. 70. American Society for Microbiology, Washington, D.C.

———. 1987b. Motility and chemotaxis. In *Escherichia coli and Salmonella typhimurium: Cellular and molecular biology* (ed. F.C. Neidhardt), vol. 1, p. 732. American Society for Microbiology, Washington, D.C.

———. 1988. The end of the line in bacterial sensing: The flagellar motor. *Cold Spring Harbor Symp. Quant. Biol.* **53**: 67.

Macnab, R.M. and D.J. DeRosier. 1988. Bacterial flagellar structure and function. *Can. J. Microbiol.* **34**: 442.

Macnab, R.M. and D.E. Koshland, Jr. 1972. The gradient-sensing mechanism in bacterial chemotaxis. *Proc. Natl. Acad. Sci.* **69**: 2509.

Margolin, Y. and M. Eisenbach. 1984. Voltage clamp effects on bacterial chemotaxis. *J. Bacteriol.* **159**: 605.

Meister, M., S.R. Caplan, and H.C. Berg. 1989. Dynamics of a tightly coupled mechanism for flagellar rotation. *Biophys. J.* **55**: 905.

Mesibov, R. and J. Adler. 1972. Chemotaxis toward amino acids in *Escherichia coli. J. Bacteriol.* **112**: 315.

Miller, J.H. 1972. *Experiments in molecular genetics*, p. 431. Cold Spring Harbor Laboratory, Cold Spring Harbor.

Milligan, D.L. and D.E. Koshland, Jr. 1988. Site directed cross-linking: Establishing the dimeric structure of the aspartate receptor of bacterial chemotaxis. *J. Biol. Chem.* **263**: 6268.

Nossal, R. 1972. Growth and movement of rings of chemotactic bacteria. *Exp. Cell. Res.* **75**: 138.

Patlak, C.S. 1953. Random walk with persistence and external bias. *Bull. Math. Biophys.* **15**: 311.

Pfeffer, W. 1884. Locomotorische Richtungsbewegungen durch chemische Reize. *Unters. Bot. Inst. Tübingen* **1**: 363.

Purcell, E.M. 1977. Life at low Reynolds number. *Am. J. Phys.* **45**: 3.

Qi, Y. and J. Adler. 1989. Salt taxis in *Escherichia coli* bacteria and its lack in mutants. *Proc. Natl. Acad. Sci.* **86**: 8358.

Russo, A.F. and D.E. Koshland, Jr. 1983. Separation of signal transduction and adaptation functions of the aspartate receptor in bacterial sensing. *Science* **220**: 1016.

Saimi, Y., B. Martinac, M.C. Gustin, M.R. Culbertson, J. Adler, and C. Kung. 1988. Ion channels in *Paramecium*, yeast and *Escherichia coli. Trends Biochem. Sci.* **13**: 304.

Sanders, D.A., B. Mendez, and D.E. Koshland, Jr. 1989. Role of the CheW protein in bacterial chemotaxis: Overexpression is equivalent to absence. *J. Bacteriol.* **171**: 6271.

Schnitzer, M.J., S.M. Block, H.C. Berg, and E.M. Purcell. 1990. Strategies for chemotaxis. *Symp. Soc. Gen. Microbiol.* (in press).

Segall, J.E., S.M. Block, and H.C. Berg. 1986. Temporal comparisons in bacterial chemotaxis. *Proc. Natl. Acad. Sci.* **83**: 8987.

Segall, J.E., A. Ishihara, and H.C. Berg. 1985. Chemotactic signaling in filamentous cells of *Escherichia coli. J. Bacteriol.* **161**: 51.

Shioi, J., C.V. Dang, and B.L. Taylor. 1987. Oxygen as attractant and repellent in bacterial chemotaxis. *J. Bacteriol.* **169:** 3118.

Silverman, M. and M. Simon. 1974. Flagellar rotation and the mechanism of bacterial motility. *Nature* **249:** 73.

Springer, M.S., M.F. Goy, and J. Adler. 1979. Protein methylation in behavioural control mechanisms and in signal transduction. *Nature* **280:** 279.

Stewart, R.C. and F.W. Dahlquist. 1987. Molecular components of bacterial chemotaxis. *Chem. Rev.* **87:** 997.

Stock, A., J. Mottonen, T. Chen, and J. Stock. 1987. Identification of a possible nucleotide binding site in CheW, a protein required for sensory transduction in bacterial chemotaxis. *J. Biol. Chem.* **262:** 535.

Stock, J. and A. Stock. 1987. What is the role of receptor methylation in bacterial chemotaxis. *Trends Biochem. Sci.* **12:** 371.

Stock, J.B., A.J. Ninfa, and A.M. Stock. 1989. Protein phosphorylation and regulation of adaptive responses in bacteria. *Microbiol. Rev.* **53:** 450.

Stock, J.B., A.M. Stock, and J.M. Mottonen. 1990. Signal transduction in bacteria. *Nature* **344:** 395.

Stock, J., A. Borczuk, F. Chiou, and J.E.B. Burchenal. 1985. Compensatory mutations in receptor function: A reevaluation of the role of methylation in bacterial chemotaxis. *Proc. Natl. Acad. Sci.* **82:** 8364.

Weis, R.M., S. Chasalow, and D.E. Koshland, Jr. 1990. The role of methylation in chemotaxis: An explanation of outstanding anomalies. *J. Biol. Chem.* **265:** 6817.

Weis, R.M. and D.E. Koshland, Jr. 1988. Reversible receptor methylation is essential for normal chemotaxis of *Escherichia coli* in gradients of aspartic acid. *Proc. Natl. Acad. Sci.* **85:** 83.

Wolfe, A.J. and H.C. Berg. 1989. Migration of bacteria in semisolid agar. *Proc. Natl. Acad. Sci.* **86:** 6973.

Wolfe, A.J., M.P. Conley, T.J. Kramer, and H.C. Berg. 1987. Reconstitution of signaling in bacterial chemotaxis. *J. Bacteriol.* **169:** 1878.

Ultrastructural Correlates of Mechanoelectrical Transduction in Hair Cells of the Bullfrog's Internal Ear

R.A. Jacobs and A.J. Hudspeth

*Department of Cell Biology and Neuroscience, University of Texas Southwestern
Medical Center, Dallas, Texas 75235-9039*

Hair cells are the receptors of the internal ear and the lateral-line organ. These cells are accordingly key elements in the sensitivities of vertebrates to sound, angular acceleration, linear acceleration, seismic vibration, and water motion. In every known organ of the acousticolateralis sensory system, hair cells act as strain gauges that produce electrical responses when subjected to mechanical forces derived from the relevant stimuli.

Mechanoelectrical transduction occurs in a specialized receptor organelle, the hair bundle, whose stereotyped structure is discussed in detail below. Deflection of the hair bundle by a mechanical stimulus opens force-sensitive transduction channels (for reviews, see Hudspeth 1983a, 1985, 1989; Howard et al. 1988; Roberts et al. 1988). The ensuing flow of ionic current into the hair cell produces a receptor potential, which in turn regulates the release of synaptic transmitter and hence the activity of one or more eighth-nerve fibers.

The biophysical basis of mechanoelectrical transduction has been most extensively investigated in the sacculus of the bullfrog (Hudspeth and Corey 1977). Hair cells from this organ are advantageous for electrophysiological studies because they can readily be dissected and maintained in vitro, they are large and robust enough to endure a variety of recording procedures, and they are sufficiently typical in structure and operation to serve as models for hair cells in general. The present study, a morphological investigation of the bullfrog's saccular macula, extends the valuable earlier descriptions of this organ (Hillman 1969, 1976; Hillman and Lewis 1971; Lewis and Li 1973, 1975) and relates the structures of hair cells and adjoining cells to the processes of mechanoelectrical transduction and synaptic signaling.

EXPERIMENTAL PROCEDURES

Preparation of hair cells. Saccular epithelia, dissected from the ears of adult bullfrogs (*Rana catesbeiana* Shaw) of both sexes, were maintained in a standard saline solution containing 110 mM Na^+, 2 mM K^+, 4 mM Ca^{++}, 118 mM Cl^-, 5 mM HEPES, and 3 mM D-glucose (Kroese et al. 1989). After the pH was adjusted to 7.25, the solution's osmotic strength was 220 mmoles/kg. Except as noted below, all procedures were conducted at room temperature (22–25°C). To facilitate removal of otolithic membranes from saccular maculae, some samples were treated for 30–60 minutes with 50 mg/liter subtilopeptidase BPN′ (Sigma Chemical Co., St. Louis, Missouri); the otolithic membrane could then be dissected free without trauma to hair bundles.

For light-microscopic observation of hair bundles, living cells were enzymatically dissociated with papain (Lewis and Hudspeth 1983; Hudspeth and Lewis 1988a) and allowed to settle onto the coverglass bottom of a 500-μl experimental chamber. These cells were observed with a mechanically stabilized, inverted microscope (IM35, Carl Zeiss, Oberkochen, Federal Republic of Germany) equipped with differential-interference-contrast optics, a 63 × oil-immersion objective lens (numerical aperture 1.4), and a 40 × water-immersion objective lens (numerical aperture 0.75) used as a condenser.

Fixation. Whole saccular maculae, prepared as described above, were stretched flat in a small chamber, and their otolithic membranes were dissected with or without prior enzymatic digestion. The tissue was fixed for 60–120 minutes at 4°C in a solution containing 200 mM glutaraldehyde and 5 mM $CaCl_2$. This primary fixative was either buffered at pH 7.4 with 80 mM sodium cacodylate or buffered at pH 7.2 with 45 mM HEPES. After a short rinse in Ca^{++}-containing buffer, the tissue was postfixed for 30 seconds to 60 minutes at 0°C with 40 mM OsO_4 in Ca^{++}-containing buffer, rinsed again in the buffer solution, and dehydrated in a graded series of ethanol concentrations. The samples were stained en bloc for 60 minutes at 4°C with 10 mM uranyl acetate in 95% ethanol, further dehydrated in absolute ethanol and propylene oxide, and embedded in epoxy plastic (EMbed 812, Electron Microscopy Sciences, Fort Washington, Pennsylvania).

Transmission electron microscopy. Sections were cut on a diamond knife at a thickness of 50–100 nm (Ultracut E ultramicrotome, Reichert-Jung, Vienna, Austria) and collected on uncoated 300-mesh grids. After staining with saturated aqueous uranyl acetate and 0.2% lead citrate, the sections were examined by electron microscopy (JEM-100C, JEOL Ltd., Tokyo, Japan or Philips EM 300, Philips' Gloeilampenfabrieken, Eindhoven, The Netherlands) at an accelerating voltage of 80 kV.

Freeze-fracture electron microscopy. Whole saccular maculae with intact otolithic membranes were subjected to glutaraldehyde fixation for 60 minutes as described above. After a brief rinse in Ca^{++}-containing buffer solution, the specimens were cryoprotected for 120 minutes at 4°C with 23% glycerol in Ca^{++}-containing buffer solution. The sacculi were then mounted in double-replica holders and frozen by abrupt immersion in melting chlorodifluoromethane (Freon-22, DuPont, Wilmington, Delaware).

At a temperature of −100°C and a pressure less than 130 μPa, each frozen specimen was fractured in a freeze-fracture unit (BAF 300 or BAF 400T, Balzers AG, Liechtenstein). An electron-beam evaporation gun was then used to shadow the fractured surface with a platinum-carbon layer about 5 nm thick, as determined by a thin-film gauge. After the replicas were strengthened by carbon shadowing, they were removed from the vacuum, warmed to room temperature, and cleansed of residual tissue in 30% household bleach. The replicas were then rinsed in distilled water, mounted on Formvar-coated grids, and examined at an accelerating voltage of 80 kV by electron microscopy (JEM-100C or Philips EM 300).

Scanning electron microscopy. Saccular epithelia were subjected to glutaraldehyde primary fixation and OsO_4 postfixation according to the protocol described above. After dehydration in ethanol, specimens were critical-point dried from liquid CO_2, sputter-coated with gold-palladium, and examined by scanning electron microscopy (Autoscan, ETEC Corp., Hayward, California, or JSM 840, JEOL Ltd.) at an accelerating voltage of 20–35 kV.

Figure 3, A and B, was obtained from rapidly frozen sacculi of the closely related leopard frog (*Rana pipiens* Schreber). Each macula was placed in approximately 10 μl of saline solution on a thin copper specimen holder and then frozen in a propane-jet apparatus (QFD-101, Balzers AG). The apparatus was modified to produce a single, vertical jet of liquid propane (Plattner and Bachmann 1982). After freeze-substitution in 1% OsO_4 in acetone for 92 hours at −55°C, the tissue was warmed in successive 1-hour steps to −20°C, −4°C, 4°C, and room temperature. After three rinses in acetone and four in ethanol, each specimen was critical-point dried and prepared for microscopic observation as described above.

RESULTS AND DISCUSSION

The Saccular Macula

The bullfrog's sacculus is a detector of seismic vibration at frequencies below 100 Hz (Koyama et al. 1982). The organ, an oblate ellipsoid about 3 mm in greatest length, is essentially an epithelial pouch surrounded by a layer of connective tissue. The central cavity of the sacculus is filled with otoconia, which are dense, microcrystalline, calcareous masses a few micrometers in length. Embedded in a gelatinous matrix, the otoconia constitute an inertial mass that shifts position during accelerations, thereby initiating the sacculus's response.

The wall of the sacculus is thickened on its medial surface, the site of the organ's sensory region, the macula. A discoidal structure about 1 mm across, the macula contains some 3000 hair cells disposed among approximately twice as many supporting cells (Fig. 1A). The saccular nerve, a branch of the eighth cranial nerve, inserts in the macular region; the macula is also extensively vascularized.

The Hair Bundle

From the apical surface of each hair cell extends its mechanoreceptive organelle, the hair bundle (Fig. 2A). In a large hair cell, this bundle comprises about 60 processes, whose lengths increase monotonically from one edge of the bundle to the opposite edge. This gradient in height confers on the bundle not only a plane of mirror symmetry, but also a vectorial sensitivity to stimulation. Pushing the bundle in the positive direction, toward its taller processes, leads to a depolarizing receptor potential and increased firing in the afferent nerve fibers, whereas deflection in the negative direction, toward the bundle's short edge, hyperpolarizes the hair cell and inhibits neuronal activity (Shotwell et al. 1981). So that stimuli in any conceivable direction can be detected, every possible hair-bundle orientation is represented within the plane of the saccular macula (Fig. 1B).

The processes of a hair bundle occur in a hexagonal array, which can be demonstrated both by thin sections across the bundle (Fig. 2B) and by freeze-fracture views of the bundle's insertion at the cellular apex (Fig. 2C). At the center of the bundle's tall edge stands the solitary kinocilium, which is distinctive because its shaft contains an axoneme, or 9 + 2 array of microtubules (Figs. 2B and 4G,H). The kinocilium's distal end forms a bulbous swelling (Figs. 2A, 4G,H, and 6A) that is the site at which mechanical stimuli impinge on the hair

Figure 1. The saccular macula of the bullfrog. (*A*) A scanning electron micrograph of the macular region reveals ∼3000 hair bundles protruding from the epithelial surface. Although the otolithic membrane has been dissected away, a few loose crystalline otoconia overlie the macula. (*B*) A map of hair-bundle polarities in the preparation shown in *A* reveals that all orientations occur in the saccular macula. Each arrow indicates the direction of maximal mechanical sensitivity of the marked hair bundle. Note that the bundles reverse in orientation at the striola, the irregular arc that divides the macula into a neural (lower) portion and an abneural (upper) portion. Magnification: (*A*) 210 × .

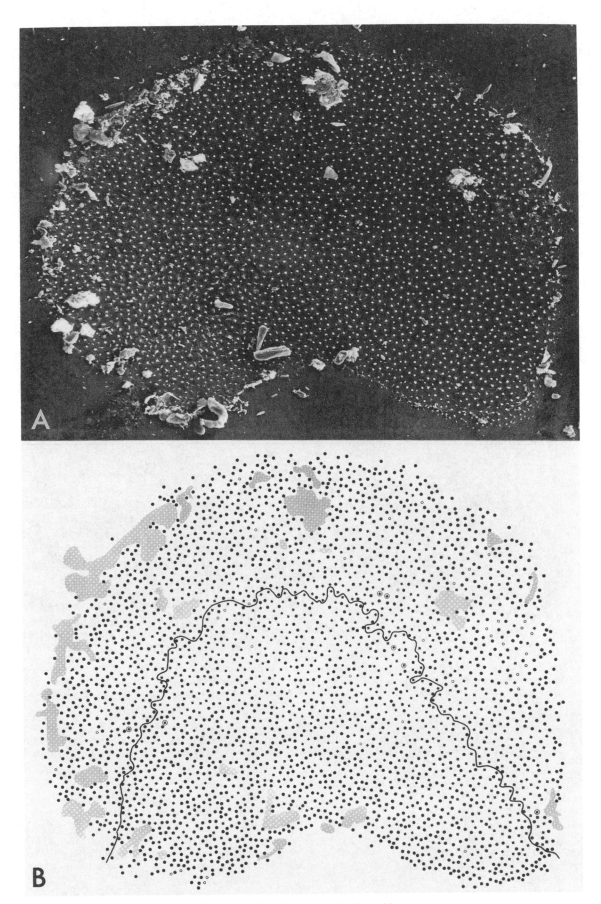

Figure 1. (*See facing page for legend.*)

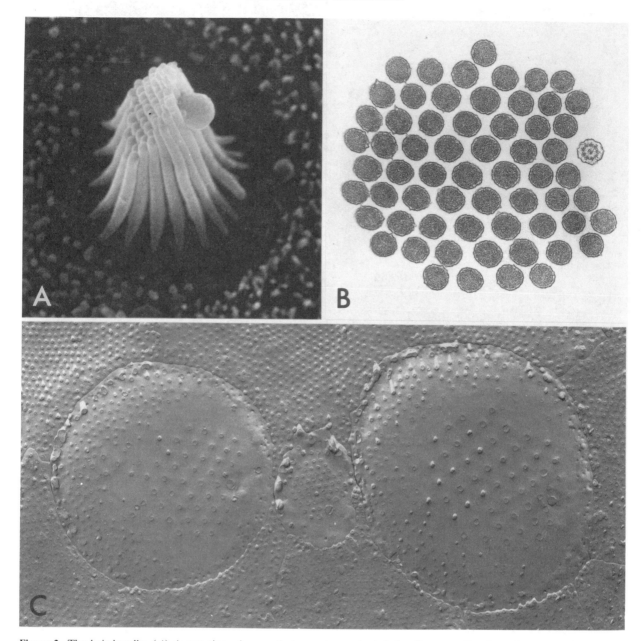

Figure 2. The hair bundle. (*A*) A scanning micrograph demonstrates the hair bundle protruding from the apical surface of a saccular hair cell. The lengths of the ~ 60 stereocilia increase systematically from the left to the right edge of the bundle. The single kinocilium, which occurs at the bundle's tall edge, terminates in a bulbous swelling. (*B*) A thin section across a hair bundle reveals the hexagonal packing of the constituent processes. The kinocilium is distinguished by its cytoskeleton of axonemal microtubules; the stereocilia contain rods of cross-linked microfilaments. (*C*) A freeze-fracture view of the apical surfaces of three hair cells illustrates the hexagonal packing of the stereociliary and kinociliary insertions. The supporting cells around the hair cells are covered with microvilli, which are more closely packed than the processes in the hair bundles. This micrograph shows the rare juxtaposition of hair cells without an intervening supporting cell. Magnifications: (*A*) 13,500 × ; (*B*) 23,000 × ; (*C*) 8,500 × .

bundle. The remaining processes of the bundle are stereocilia, each of which consists of a cross-linked fascicle of actin microfilaments enveloped by a tube of plasmalemma (Figs. 2B and 4). The stereociliary plasmalemma contains numerous, large, randomly distributed intramembrane particles. In addition, treatment with the antibiotic filipin suggests that this membrane is relatively rich in cholesterol (Fig. 6A) (Forge et al. 1988). Each stereocilium is about 450 nm in diameter along most of its length, but it tapers to a diameter of about 100 nm in approximately 1 μm above its insertion into the cellular apex (Figs. 4A,C,D and 6A). Concomitant with this tapering, the microfilaments of the stereociliary core decrease in number from about 600 in the shaft of the stereocilium to only about 30 in the rootlet that penetrates into the cuticular plate (Fig. 4C), a filamentous network in the hair cell's apical cytoplasm.

The Otolithic Membrane

The otolithic membrane is an extracellular sheet, roughly coextensive with the macular surface (Fig. 3A) that couples hair bundles to the mass of calcareous otoconia filling the sacculus. The membrane consists of a feltwork of filaments, which is punctuated by cylindrical holes into which the hair bundles extend (Fig. 3B). When an animal is subjected to acceleration, such as that due to gravity or to a vibrating substrate, the mass of dense otoconia shifts with respect to the animal's body in the direction opposite the acceleration. This motion displaces the otolithic membrane, which in turn deflects the attached hair bundles.

Transmission electron micrographs reveal a tenuous substance filling the 6-μm gap between the apical surfaces of the supporting cells and the lower surface of the compact otolithic membrane (Fig. 3C). At high magnification, it is apparent that this material consists of numerous fine filaments. Favorably oriented sections suggest that these filaments are regularly attached to the surface membranes of the supporting cells between the microvilli (Fig. 3D). The extraordinary regularity in the position of the filaments is best appreciated from tangential sections across the microvilli at the apices of the supporting cells (Fig. 3E). It is evident that two strands occur midway between each pair of microvilli. Because of the hexagonal packing of these organelles, each microvillus is therefore surrounded by 12 filaments. The array is essentially perfect except where the regular packing of the microvilli themselves is interrupted by a cellular boundary, a dislocation in the microvillar array, or the presence of a degenerate cilium near each cell's center.

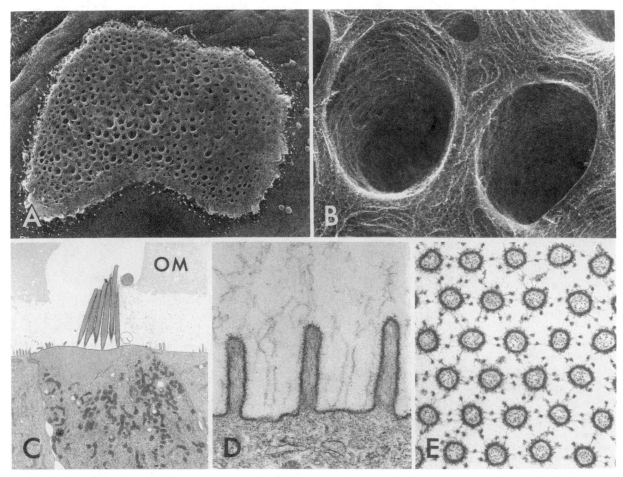

Figure 3. The otolithic membrane. (*A*) The intact otolithic membrane covers all the hair cells of the sacculus, save the few at the macular periphery that had been newly formed by mitosis. This and the adjacent scanning micrograph are from the sacculi of leopard frogs. (*B*) The otolithic membrane is interrupted by a cylindrical cavity above each hair bundle. The filamentous nature of the compact otolithic membrane is evident in this specimen, which was prepared by the propane-jet freezing technique. (*C*) This low-power transmission electron micrograph illustrates the otolithic membrane's contact with the kinociliary bulb of the hair bundle. Fine strands, extending from the apices of supporting cells, connect the compact portion of the otolithic membrane (OM) to the macular surface. (*D*) A high-magnification view of the apical surface of a supporting cell shows the filaments that extend to the compact otolithic membrane. Note that two filaments insert into the plasmalemma between each pair of microvilli. (*E*) A tangential section across the apical surface of a supporting cell displays the regularity with which paired filaments lie in the hexagonal array of microvilli. Magnifications: (*A*) 170 × ; (*B*) 3,500 × ; (*C*) 3,300 × ; (*D*) 50,000 × ; (*E*) 65,000 × .

These observations raise the possibility that the sites of filamentous attachment are molecular grommets, sites through which successively synthesized monomers are fed to join the filaments that ascend to and perhaps form the otolithic membrane. Freeze-fracture preparations do not show unusual intramembrane structures at the sites of the filaments' attachments. Although this could indicate that there is no transmembrane component associated with the strands, it remains possible that the attachment sites are among the anonymous throng of intramembrane particles on the P fracture faces of supporting cells (Figs. 2C and 6F).

Connections of the Hair Bundle

The processes of the hair bundle participate in filamentous linkages of five distinct types (Fig. 4A). Stimulus forces propagate from the otolithic membrane to hair bundles through uniform, 50-nm-long strands that connect the kinociliary bulb to the otolithic membrane (Fig. 4G,H). Over a distance of about 1 μm along its shaft, the single kinocilium is in turn ligated to the five tallest stereocilia (Fig. 4G,H) (Hillman 1969; Hillman and Lewis 1971). This connection, which occurs as a series of dense filamentous linkages at intervals of about 40 nm, presumably transmits force from the kinocilium to the stereocilia.

Stereocilia are interconnected in three ways. About 1 μm above their insertions into the apical cellular surface, each is attached by fibrils to the six stereocilia that surround it (Fig. 4B,C) (Csukas et al. 1987). These connections, as well as the dense glycocalyx that protrudes from the stereociliary membranes, are largely destroyed by the protease digestion ordinarily employed to prepare hair cells for physiological recording (Fig. 4D) (Hudspeth and Corey 1977; Kroese et al. 1989). Although they may be important in holding the stereocilia upright and preventing torque of the bundle, the basal stereociliary connections accordingly do not seem necessary for mechanoelectrical transduction.

Along the distal surfaces of the stereocilia, where they come into close approximation with one another, occur lateral interstereociliary contacts of a second type. These are highly variable, amorphous, osmiophilic mats that fill the space between the stereocilia over about 250-nm regions of apposition (Fig. 4E). It is

uncertain whether contacts of this sort represent local specializations of the stereociliary surfaces or simply the interdigitation of the glycocalyces of the processes involved. The apical, lateral contacts may prove important, however, in the propagation of stimulus forces across the hair bundle (Howard et al. 1988).

The final type of contact, and the most interesting, occurs at the hair bundle's top: The tip of each stereocilium is attached to the flank of the longest adjacent stereocilium by a single, fine filament (Fig. 4F) (Pickles et al. 1984). The link's insertions are marked by densities beneath the plasma membranes; the large, irregular particles seen in freeze-fracture preparations of stereociliary tips (Fig. 6C) may represent the sites of insertion (Forge et al. 1988). In sectioned specimens, such tip links are characteristically about 5 nm in diameter and about 150 nm long. Because they occur at the site where transduction current enters a hair cell (Hudspeth 1982) and because their orientation accords with the axis along which a bundle is sensitive (Shotwell et al. 1981), these tip links are thought to be involved in mechanoelectrical transduction. More specifically, each tip link may be an elastic gating spring (Corey and Hudspeth 1983a). Stretched by the shear between stereocilia when the bundle is pushed in the excitatory direction, this link may pull open the molecular gates of transduction channels attached to one or both of its ends (for reviews, see Howard et al. 1988; Roberts et al. 1988; Hudspeth 1989). Channel gating by such a direct means is consistent with the short response latency of hair cells, which is in the microsecond range (Corey and Hudspeth 1979a, 1983a). This model for transduction also accords with the observation that each hair cell possesses approximately as many tip links as it has transduction channels (Holton and Hudspeth 1986; Howard and Hudspeth 1988).

Motion within the Hair Bundle

If a tip link is a gating spring, it is of interest to know what strain it experiences during the hair-bundle motions encountered during normal stimulation. The intricate, three-dimensional stacking of processes within a hair bundle complicates modeling of the bundle's behavior. Nevertheless, the essential features of movement can be understood by considering only the

---

Figure 4. Connections of the hair bundle. (A) This vertical section through a saccular hair bundle illustrates the sites of the five types of connections in a bundle, each of which is labeled according to the panel below in which it is illustrated at higher magnification. (B) Basal connections, which link stereocilia along all three hexagonal axes of the bundle, are prominent in a tangential section near the base of a tannic-acid-treated hair bundle. (C) The basal connections join stereocilia ~1 μm above their basal insertions in the upper portions of the stereociliary tapers. (D) Exposure of a macula to subtilopeptidase BPN', a routine preparative treatment for physiological recordings, removes the basal connections and much of the glycocalyx. (E) Amorphous material ($\rightarrow$) joins the lateral aspects of stereocilia near their distal ends. (F) Each stereocilium possesses a single tip link ($\rightarrow$) that extends to the side of the longest adjacent stereocilium. Both insertions of each link are characterized by distortions of the membrane and local cytoplasmic densities. (G) The bulbous tip of the kinocilium is attached to the compact otolithic membrane (OM) by uniform fibers ($\rightarrow$). Note that the axonemal microtubules apparently extend into the kinociliary bulb as dissociated protofilaments. A tip link connects the stereocilia at the extreme left. (H) A transverse section across the kinociliary bulb illustrates both the fibrils that link the kinocilium to the otolithic membrane and the dense junctions ($\rightarrow$) between the kinocilium and the five longest stereocilia. Magnifications: (A) 12,500 ×; (B) 100,000 ×; (C) 70,000 ×; (D) 47,000 ×; (E) 90,000 ×; (F) 90,000 ×; (G) 76,000 ×; (H) 47,000 ×.

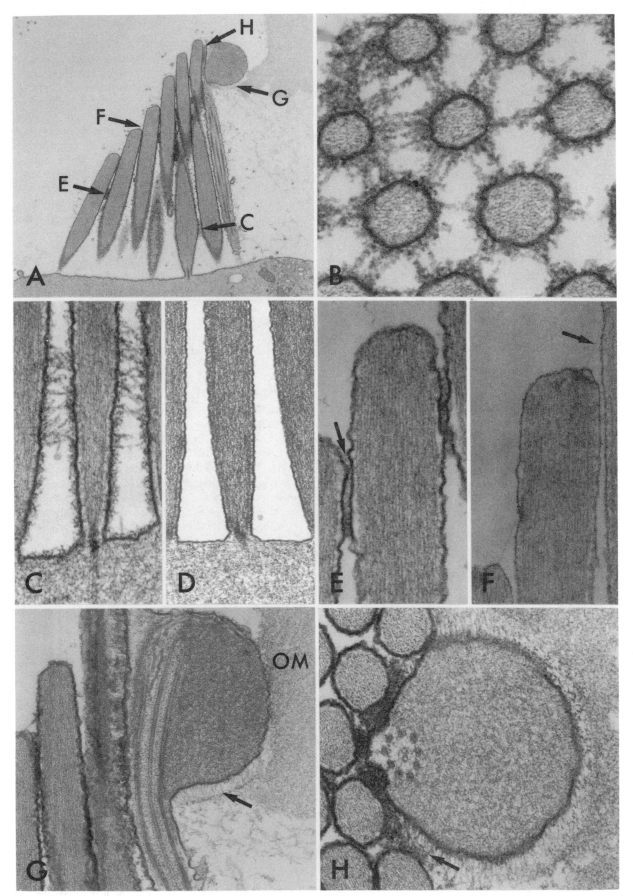

Figure 4. (*See facing page for legend.*)

stereocilia that lie within the bundle's plane of mirror symmetry and by considering each stereocilium to be a rigid, right circular cylinder that pivots about a punctate attachment at its base (Fig. 5A).

The movement of the stereocilia can be calculated by imposing a displacement at the tip of the longest stereocilium, the position where force is actually transferred from the kinocilium, and by calculating the ensuing motions of successively shorter stereocilia. Suppose that a stimulus probe, attached at a height H to the kinociliary bulb, moves horizontally a distance X in the hair bundle's mirror plane. If the stereocilium immediately behind the kinocilium initially rests at an angle ϕ_r with respect to the plane of the apical epithelial surface, that stereocilium's angle after stimulation ϕ_1 is

$$\phi_1 = \tan^{-1}\left[\frac{H}{H/\tan(\phi_r) + X}\right]$$

If the angle between one stereocilium (the nth) and the plane of the apical epithelial surface is ϕ_n, the angle assumed by the adjacent, shorter stereocilium ϕ_{n+1} is

$$\phi_{n+1} = \phi_n - \frac{\pi}{2} + \tan^{-1}\left(\frac{r}{l_{n+1}}\right)$$
$$+ \cos^{-1}\left\{\frac{s_{n+1} \cdot \sin\phi_n + d_{n+1} \cdot \cos\phi_n - r}{[(l_{n+1})^2 + r^2]^{1/2}}\right\}$$

in which r is the radius of each stereocilium, l_{n+1} is the length of the shorter stereocilium, s_{n+1} is the space between the two stereocilia in the plane of the apical epithelial surface, and d_{n+1} is the depression of the shorter stereocilium's base with respect to that of the

longer because of the roughly circular curvature of the hair cell's apex (Figs. 3C, 4A, and 6A) (Hudspeth 1983a).

When measurements of hair-bundle dimensions (Table 1) are employed in the computer model, simulation of bundle motion produces images (Fig. 5A) that closely resemble those obtained upon deflection of a living bundle (Hudspeth 1983b). If it is then supposed that tip links are elastic structures that are elongated or shortened as the bundle moves, the model may be used to estimate their lengths as a function of bundle displacement. The results demonstrate that, over the physiological range of stimulation, each link's extension is essentially proportional to the bundle's motion (Fig. 5B). Moreover, despite the differing heights of the stereocilia, all of the links throughout a bundle undergo very nearly the same elongation when a bundle is displaced. This result buttresses an important assumption of the current model for mechanoelectrical transduction (Corey and Hudspeth 1983a; Holton and Hudspeth 1986; Howard and Hudspeth 1988; Howard et al. 1988), that the gating springs on every stereocilium receive the same stimulus when a bundle is moved.

Although the detailed formulae above are necessary to describe the full range of hair-bundle motions, physiological stimuli move the stereocilia only 1–6° from their resting positions (Roberts et al. 1988; Rüsch and Thurm 1989). Over this narrow range of deflections, small-angle approximations may reasonably be applied to trigonometric relations. The shear between the tips of any two adjacent stereocilia can therefore be approximated as $x = (s/h) \cdot X = \gamma \cdot X$, in which s is the interstereociliary spacing, h is the height of the stereocilia at

A

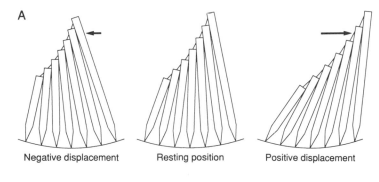

Negative displacement   Resting position   Positive displacement

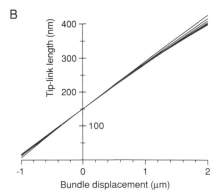

Figure 5. Computer simulation of hair-bundle motion. (*A*) Each diagram depicts the positions of seven stereocilia along a bundle's plane of mirror symmetry. (*Middle*) The bundle in its resting position. (*Left and right*) Bundle positions following horizontally directed stimuli (→), of −1 μm and +2 μm, applied to the bundle at the height of the kinociliary bulb, 6.7 μm above the apical epithelial plane, respectively. The bundles' dimensions are based on the data of Table 1 and on the assumption that stereocilia are 450 nm in diameter. For graphical clarity in these panels, the tip links have been lengthened and their lower insertions have been displaced to the centers of the stereociliary tips. (*B*) The simulation program was used to calculate the lengths of tip links between successive stereocilia; the resting tip-link length was set at 150 nm. Over the very large stimulus range of 3 μm, the changes in tip-link lengths are approximately proportional to the bundle's deflection. Within the physiological operating range of approximately ±100 nm, each link is extended about 14% of the distance that the bundle is displaced.

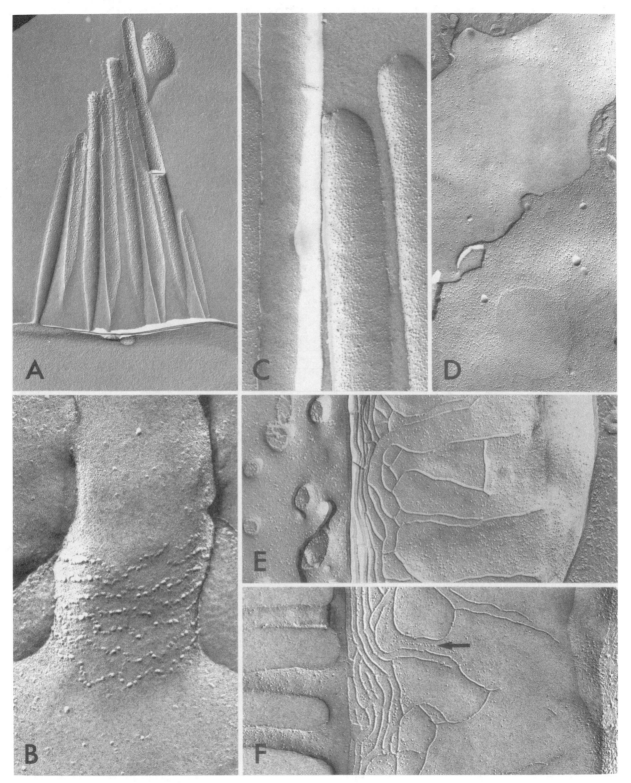

Figure 6. Freeze-fracture preparations of hair and supporting cells. (*A*) A low-power view of a hair bundle treated with filipin, a drug that marks cholesterol-rich membranes, demonstrates characteristic membrane lesions on the plasmalemma of the kinociliary bulb. Although the membrane covering the upper portions of the stereocilia is cholesterol-rich, the basal, tapered regions display few filipin lesions. (*B*) The insertion of the kinocilium is marked by a ciliary necklace, a set of circumferential rings of intramembrane particles, similar to that found on motile cilia. (*C*) The *P* faces of the distal shanks of stereocilia are studded with intramembrane particles. The stereociliary tips are irregular in contour and have a few large intramembrane particles. (*D*) The lateral aspects of supporting cells are interconnected by massive gap junctions, here seen on both the *E* and the *P* faces of apposed cells. (*E*) The *P* face of the tight junction between a hair cell and a supporting cell consists of ~6 complete intramembrane strands. (*F*) At the apical contact between two supporting cells, small aggregates of intramembrane particles (→), perhaps the connections of gap junctions, occur among the strands of the tight junction. Magnifications: (*A*) 10,000×; (*B*) 135,000×; (*C*) 70,000×; (*D*) 30,000×; (*E*) 65,000×; (*F*) 65,000×.

Table 1. Dimensions of Hair Bundles in the Bullfrog's Sacculus

Number of stereocilia in bundle	Mean inter-stereociliary spacing (μm)	Longest stereocilium (μm)	Shortest stereocilium (μm)	Angle of longest stereocilium (in degrees)	Angle of shortest stereocilium (in degrees)	Height of kinociliary bulb (μm)
65	0.94	7.4	4.0	101	65	7.2
58	1.00	6.9	3.5	101	73	7.0
50	0.97	7.6	4.2	105	63	6.2
81	0.86	7.8	3.7	99	69	6.8
57	0.96	7.8	4.6	101	65	8.0
67	0.90	8.1	3.5	99	68	6.4
61	0.98	8.3	2.6	105	71	7.5
52	0.80	8.6	4.0	93	63	6.8
52	0.89	7.6	3.0	106	85	7.1
69	0.95	8.8	2.3	101	69	6.6
53	0.91	8.6	2.8	102	66	7.1
51	1.09	9.3	3.0	99	69	6.8
69	0.97	8.1	2.6	100	75	6.8
68	1.00	8.6	3.7	96	72	6.8
62	—	9.8	5.5	—	—	6.2
57	—	8.8	3.1	—	—	6.5
57	—	9.1	2.6	—	—	5.5
55	—	8.6	4.3	—	—	5.5
60	—	8.8	3.7	—	—	6.4
57	—	9.1	3.0	—	—	5.8
60 ± 2	0.94 ± 0.02	8.4 ± 0.2	3.5 ± 0.2	101 ± 1	70 ± 2	6.7 ± 0.1

Counts of stereocilia were made from freeze-fracture and transverse-section micrographs of hair bundles (e.g., Fig. 2B,C). All other measurements were made from differential-interference-contrast photomicrographs of enzymatically isolated living hair cells and were calibrated against a 10-μm stage micrometer (Carl Zeiss, Oberkochen, Federal Republic of Germany). Each entry for interciliary spacing is the mean measured along a row of 4–5 stereocilia in a bundle's plane of bilateral symmetry. The final values are reported as means ± standard errors of means (S.E.M). The data in each column were taken from different cells, except that the same cells supplied paired measurements for the fifth and sixth columns. On the basis of light-microscopic observations and of computer modeling of the stacking of stereocilia in hair bundles (Fig. 5A), the diameter of individual, unfixed stereocilia is ~450 nm. A large hair cell of the bullfrog's sacculus, typical of those used in physiological recordings, has a single kinocilium and ~60 stereocilia in its hair bundle. The stereocilia occur in ranks whose heights differ by approximately equal increments of ~325 nm; in descending order of height, the ranks typically contain 2, 4, 3, 4, 5, 4, 5, 4, 5, 4, 5, 4, 3, 4, 3, and 1 stereocilia, so the mean stereociliary length is ~6.0 μm.

the point of shear, and X is the displacement applied at the hair bundle's tip. The geometrical gain factor for the bundle, $\gamma = s/h$, relates approximate tip-length extension to hair-bundle deflection; for hair cells of the bullfrog's sacculus, $\gamma = (0.94\ \mu\text{m})\ /\ (6.7\ \mu\text{m}) = 0.14$ (Table 1) (Howard et al. 1988).

The tip links of an undisturbed hair cell in the bullfrog's sacculus are about 150 nm in length (Fig. 4F). The range of bundle deflections over which a cell responds to transient stimuli, about ±100 nm, therefore corresponds to changes in tip-link length of ±14 nm or a strain (change in length divided by original length) of only 0.09 (Howard et al. 1988). Even when the transduction apparatus is saturated by continuous ±500-nm stimuli, the tip links' strain is 0.5 at most. Because strains of this magnitude can be accommodated by biological fibers such as elastin and collagen (Burton 1954), it is plausible that tip links can bear stimuli of physiological magnitudes. Large, maintained deflections of a hair bundle induce adaptation of the transduction process (Eatock et al. 1987), which may protect hair cells against overstimulation. Measurements of hair bundles' mechanical properties suggest that adaptation involves a reduction in gating-spring strain (Howard and Hudspeth 1987a; Assad et al. 1989; Hacohen et al. 1989), possibly by relocation of the tip

links' insertions (Howard and Hudspeth 1987b; Hudspeth 1989).

Supporting Cells

Each hair cell of the saccular epithelium is suspended among six supporting cells, which are attached around the hair cell's apical perimeter by a junctional complex. A hair cell accordingly does not rest on the basal lamina but occupies a cylindrical pouch formed by the supporting cells. The geometrical relation between hair and supporting cells is highly regular. Hair cells form a hexagonal array with a center-to-center spacing of about 12 μm; the boundaries between the intervening supporting cells run along the three axes of the hair cells' hexagonal lattice. A similar array occurs in many other acousticolateralis organs in which the epithelial tiling pattern can be discerned. Even the cellular packing of the mammalian organ of Corti (Gulley and Reese 1976) is in part a plastically distorted variant of this theme.

The packing pattern of hair and supporting cells has two interesting consequences. First, hair cells ordinarily do not contact one another. On rare occasions when two hair cells do abut, one of the pair is inevitably stunted as if suppressed by its neighbor (Fig. 2C).

Second, whereas adjacent supporting cells form extensive junctions with one another, the normal lattice rarely contains points at which three (or more) supporting cells meet. Because such trigonal contacts must inevitably arise when a hair cell dies and is extruded from the epithelium, it is conceivable that they somehow initiate the mitogenic signal that leads to intercalary hair cell replacement in mitotically competent organs, such as the avian basilar papilla (Corwin and Cotanche 1988). Viewed in another way, an additional hair cell is called for whenever a supporting cell makes two adjacent junctions with other supporting cells, rather than contacting alternately a hair and a supporting cell. In organs apparently incapable of mitosis after ontogeny, such as the organ of Corti, trigonal junctions persist as recognizable scars (Bredberg 1968).

Intercellular Junctions

Around their apical perimeters, the epithelial cells of the saccular macula are attached to one another by junctional complexes that consist of tight junctions (*zonulae occludentes*) and intermediate junctions (*zonulae adherentes*). The basolateral membrane surfaces of both hair and supporting cells are focally joined by desmosomes (*maculae adherentes*). Adjacent supporting cells additionally make extensive gap junctions with one another (Fig. 6D) (Jahnke 1975; Gulley and Reese 1976; Hama 1980). Gap junctions occur on hair cells only rarely and at the periphery of the macula, where they link supporting cells to hair cells that have recently differentiated from mitotic precursors (Lewis and Li 1973; Ginzberg and Gilula 1979).

In every acousticolateralis organ that has been investigated, the fluids bathing the apical and the basolateral surfaces of cells are different. The apical surface of a hair cell is characteristically exposed to a K^+-rich, Na^+- and Ca^{++}-poor fluid (which is termed endolymph in the internal ear), whereas the basolateral surface faces a solution similar in composition to other extracellular fluids (which is termed perilymph in the internal ear). Tight junctions separate the dissimilar solutions bathing the two epithelial surfaces (Jahnke 1975; Gulley and Reese 1976). In the bullfrog's sacculus, these junctions comprise about six anastomotic intramembrane strands, which resemble those in other physiologically tight epithelia (Claude and Goodenough 1973). The junctions between hair and supporting cells, however, differ from those interconnecting supporting cells. Whereas the former possess only the linear intramembrane strands characteristic of tight junctions (Fig. 6E), the junctions between supporting cells are embellished with small, linear clusters of coarse intramembrane particles (Fig. 6F). Because of their similarity in size and packing density to the connexons of the extensive gap junctions between supporting cells (Fig. 6D), these particles appear to represent small gap junctions intercalated among the tight junctional strands (Revel et al. 1973).

The tight junctions of the saccular macula are doubtlessly important in maintaining the high-K^+ environment in which hair bundles are situated. Because the transduction channels of hair cells can pass cations of a wide range of sizes (Corey and Hudspeth 1979b; Ohmori 1985), it remains uncertain why an elevated K^+ concentration is important. The poor ionic discrimination of transduction channels allows them to be plugged by ototoxic drugs such as the aminoglycoside antibiotics (Kroese et al. 1989). Tight junctions may protect the internal ear by slowing the access of harmful substances to the endolymph (Tran Ba Huy et al. 1981). The resistance of tight junctions in the sacculus is also important in the generation of the microphonic potential, an electrical response that arises when the summed transduction currents of numerous stimulated hair cells flow across the junctions (Corey and Hudspeth 1983b).

The Afferent Synapse

Hair cells excite afferent nerve fibers by the quantal release of chemical synaptic transmitters (Ishii et al. 1971). On its basolateral surface, each saccular hair cell forms multiple afferent synapses (Fig. 7A) with striking presynaptic specializations. A synaptic contact has a 400-nm-diameter presynaptic dense body, which is surrounded by a halo of lucent, spherical, 40-nm-diameter synaptic vesicles (Fig. 7B) (Gleisner et al. 1973; Hama and Saito 1977). The plasma membrane adjacent to this dense body is endowed with a presynaptic density that usually forms three, parallel, 250-nm-long strips. Large intramembrane particles, which occur in the same pattern (Fig. 7D) (Gulley and Reese 1977; Hama 1980), are presumably coextensive with the strips of presynaptic density (Fig. 7C). The postsynaptic membrane opposite an active zone possesses coarse intramembrane particles (Fig. 7E) that could represent receptors for the synaptic transmitter, probably glutamate (Cochran et al. 1987).

At the hair cell's afferent synapse, an influx of Ca^{++} through voltage-activated channels triggers transmitter release by exocytosis of the contents of synaptic vesicles (Fig. 7B,D). The Ca^{++} channels of hair cells in the bullfrog serve a second function as well. Each of these cells is tuned to a specific frequency of stimulation by an electrical resonance in its membrane, which results from the interplay of inward current through voltage-activated Ca^{++} channels and outward current through Ca^{++}-activated K^+ channels (Lewis and Hudspeth 1983; Hudspeth and Lewis 1988a,b). For resonance to occur at frequencies near 100 Hz, Ca^{++} can diffuse only a very short distance from the Ca^{++} channels through which it enters a cell to the K^+ channels that it activates. Consistent with this requirement, the Ca^{++} and K^+ channels of hair cells are not randomly disposed on the membrane surface but occur together in clusters (Roberts and Hudspeth 1987a,b) that may correspond to the grouped intramembrane particles at

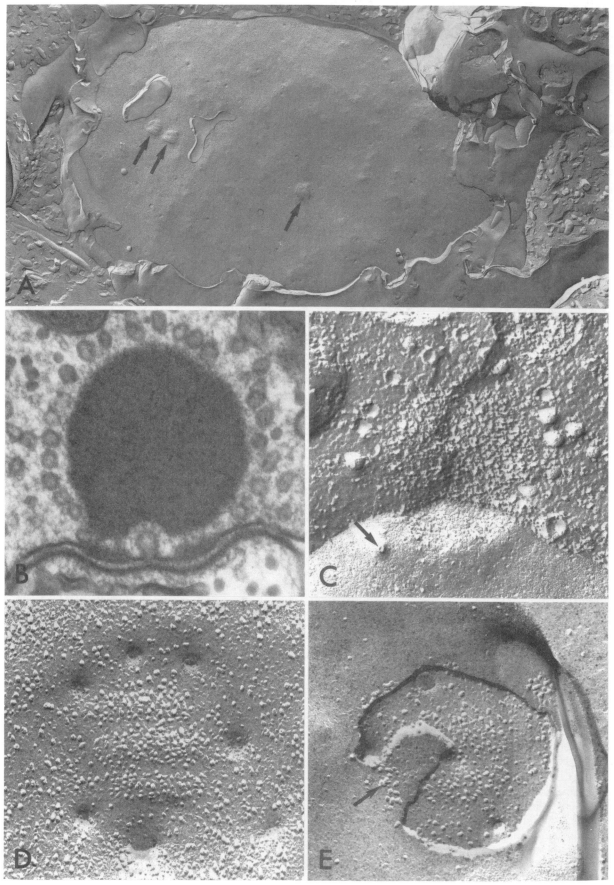

Figure 7. (*See facing page for legend.*)

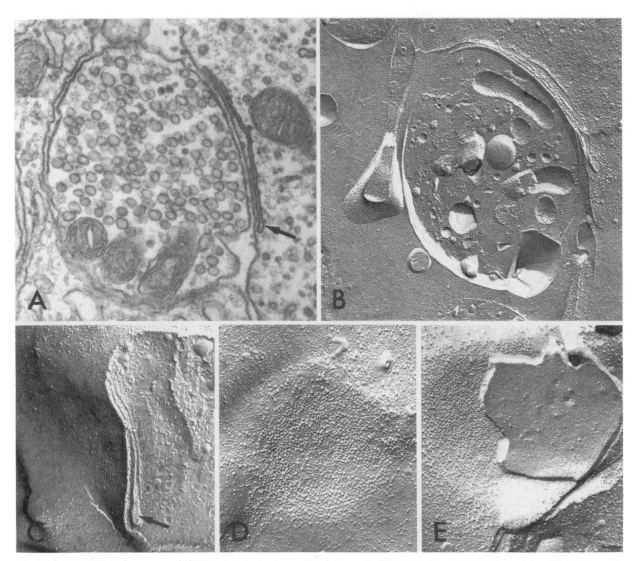

Figure 8. The efferent synapse. (*A*) The terminal of an efferent axon is filled with lucent synaptic vesicles. The pre- and postsynaptic densities are not prominent, but the synapse is distinguished by a single membranous cisterna (→) in the hair cell's cytoplasm. (*B*) A freeze-fracture view of an efferent synapse demonstrates the pre- and postsynaptic features encountered in a similar orientation in *A*. (*C*) This high-power, freeze-fracture preparation reveals a cluster of postsynaptic particles in the hair cell's plasmalemma, to the right of which lie the membrane surfaces of the cisterna (→). (*D*) The *P* fracture face of the postsynaptic membrane is marked by a dense aggregation of intramembrane particles that presumably include the receptors for acetylcholine. (*E*) This fracture plane intersected not only the *P* face of the hair cell's plasmalemma, but also the presynaptic *E* face of the efferent terminal. The transmitter-release site is marked by a pitted fracture face with a few large particles. Magnifications: (*A*) 60,000 ×; (*B*) 38,000 ×; (*C*) 64,000 ×; (*D*) 70,000 ×; (*E*) 55,000 ×.

Figure 7. The afferent synapse. (*A*) In this freeze-fracture view of the basal surface of a hair cell, clusters of intramembrane particles (→) mark the sites of three afferent synaptic contacts. (*B*) A high-power view of a thin section through an afferent synapse shows an osmiophilic, presynaptic dense body surrounded by synaptic vesicles. Between two obliquely sectioned strips of presynaptic density, a vesicle has fused with the plasmalemma. The afferent nerve terminal displays a postsynaptic density; fine strands also interpenetrate the intercellular space of the synaptic gap. (*C*) This freeze-fracture view reveals the granular interior of a dense body, which is surrounded by synaptic vesicles. The pitted *E* fracture face of the presynaptic membrane reveals the cross-fractured neck of a fusing vesicle (arrow). (*D*) The *P* fracture face of a hair cell's presynaptic membrane, marked by three strips of large intramembrane particles, is surrounded by numerous sites of vesicle fusion. (*E*) The fracture plane of this specimen intersected the *E* face of the postsynaptic membrane, which contains irregular clumps of large particles (→). The deeper plane of fracture, which reveals the particles clustered on the *P* face of a hair cell, identifies this site as an afferent synapse. Magnifications: (*A*) 11,000 ×; (*B*) 125,000 ×; (*C*) 125,000 ×; (*D*) 125,000 ×; (*E*) 125,000 ×.

synaptic sites (Pumplin et al. 1981; Roberts et al. 1990a). The concerted opening of Ca^{++} channels can produce a high local Ca^{++} concentration at synaptic active zones (Simon and Llinás 1985; Smith and Augustine 1988); at the afferent synapse of the frog's hair cell, the Ca^{++} concentration may transiently exceed 1 mM (Roberts et al. 1990a, b).

The Efferent Synapse

Most hair cells receive efferent synaptic inputs from neurons in the brainstem or cerebellum; the synaptic transmitter at such synapses is acetylcholine, which may be coreleased with calcitonin-gene-related peptide or other substances (Adams et al. 1987). Although activation of the efferent innervation generally desensitizes hair cells and reduces their frequency selectivity (Art et al. 1982; Brown et al. 1983), the efferent system has a stimulatory effect in some instances (Goldberg and Fernández 1980).

Efferent nerve endings on saccular hair cells are characteristically filled with lucent, spherical vesicles about 50 nm in diameter (Fig. 8A,B) (Gulley and Reese 1977). Although both the pre- and postsynaptic densities are modest, the postsynaptic region of the hair cell is marked by a single intracellular cisterna, whose spatial extent roughly matches that of the efferent terminal (Fig. 8A,B,C). The *P* face of the postsynaptic membrane contains a circular plaque of large, closely spaced intramembrane particles that may correspond to receptors for the chemical transmitter (Fig. 8C,D,E) (Gulley and Reese 1977). The external fracture face of the presynaptic membrane is lightly pitted and occasionally displays apparent exocytotic fusions of synaptic vesicles (Fig. 8E).

ACKNOWLEDGMENTS

We thank Mr. D. Raizen and Drs. J.L. Allen, P.G. Gillespie, and L.F.A. Jaramillo for comments on the manuscript. Dr. J.H.R. Maunsell helped the authors with geometrical calculations on hair-bundle motion, Mr. P. Koen provided outstanding maintenance of several of the electron microscopes, and Mr. M. Jacobson contributed to the freeze-fracture investigation of bundle structure. The research on which the present results are based was supported by National Institutes of Health grants DC-00241 (previously NS-13154 and NS-20429) and DC-00317 (the erstwhile NS-22389), by the System Development Foundation, and by the Perot Family Foundation.

REFERENCES

Adams, J.C., E.A. Mroz, and W.F. Sewell. 1987. A possible neurotransmitter role for CGRP in a hair-cell sensory organ. *Brain Res.* **419:** 347.
Art, J.J., A.C. Crawford, R. Fettiplace, and P.A. Fuchs. 1982. Efferent regulation of hair cells in the turtle cochlea. *Proc. R. Soc. Lond. B Biol. Sci.* **216:** 377.
Assad, J.A., N. Hacohen, and D.P. Corey. 1989. Voltage dependence of adaptation and active bundle movement in bullfrog saccular hair cells. *Proc. Natl. Acad. Sci.* **86:** 2918.
Bredberg, G. 1968. Cellular pattern and nerve supply of the human organ of Corti. *Acta Otolaryngol.* (suppl.) **236:** 1.
Brown, M.C., A.L. Nuttall, and R.I. Masta. 1983. Intracellular recordings from cochlear inner hair cells: Effects of stimulation of the crossed olivocochlear efferents. *Science* **222:** 69.
Burton, A.C. 1954. Relation of structure to function of the tissues of the wall of blood vessels. *Physiol. Rev.* **34:** 619.
Claude, P. and D.A. Goodenough. 1973. Fracture faces of zonulae occludentes from "tight" and "leaky" epithelia. *J. Cell Biol.* **58:** 390.
Cochran, S.L., P. Kasik, and W. Precht. 1987. Pharmacological aspects of excitatory synaptic transmission to second-order vestibular neurons in the frog. *Synapse* **1:** 102.
Corey, D.P. and A.J. Hudspeth. 1979a. Response latency of vertebrate hair cells. *Biophys. J.* **26:** 499.
———. 1979b. Ionic basis of the receptor potential in a vertebrate hair cell. *Nature* **281:** 675.
———. 1983a. Kinetics of the receptor current in bullfrog saccular hair cells. *J. Neurosci.* **3:** 962.
———. 1983b. Analysis of the microphonic potential of the bullfrog's sacculus. *J. Neurosci.* **3:** 942.
Corwin, J.T. and D.A. Cotanche. 1988. Regeneration of sensory hair cells after acoustic trauma. *Science* **240:** 1772.
Csukas, S.R., T.H. Rosenquist, and M.J. Mulroy. 1987. Connections between stereocilia in auditory hair cells of the alligator lizard. *Hearing Res.* **30:** 147.
Eatock, R.A., D.P. Corey, and A.J. Hudspeth. 1987. Adaptation of mechanoelectrical transduction in hair cells of the bullfrog's sacculus. *J. Neurosci.* **7:** 2821.
Forge, A., S. Davies, and G. Zajic. 1988. Characteristics of the membrane of the stereocilia and cell apex in cochlear hair cells. *J. Neurocytol.* **17:** 325.
Ginzberg, R.D. and N.B. Gilula. 1979. Modulation of cell junctions during differentiation of the chicken otocyst sensory epithelium. *Dev. Biol.* **68:** 110.
Gleisner, L., Å. Flock, and J. Wersäll. 1973. The ultrastructure of the afferent synapse on hair cells in the frog labyrinth. *Acta Otolaryngol.* **76:** 199.
Goldberg, J.M. and C. Fernández. 1980. Efferent vestibular system in the squirrel monkey: Anatomical location and influence on afferent activity. *J. Neurophysiol.* **43:** 986.
Gulley, R.L. and T.S. Reese. 1976. Intercellular junctions in the reticular lamina of the organ of Corti. *J. Neurocytol.* **5:** 479.
Gulley, R.L. and T.S. Reese. 1977. Freeze-fracture studies on the synapses in the organ of Corti. *J. Comp. Neurol.* **171:** 517.
Hacohen, N., J.A. Assad, W.J. Smith, and D.P. Corey. 1989. Regulation of tension on hair-cell transduction channels: Displacement and calcium dependence. *J. Neurosci.* **9:** 3988.
Hama, K. 1980. Fine structure of the afferent synapse and gap junctions on the sensory hair cell in the saccular macula of goldfish: A freeze-fracture study. *J. Neurocytol.* **9:** 845.
Hama, K. and K. Saito. 1977. Fine structure of the afferent synapse of the hair cells in the saccular macula of the goldfish, with special reference to the anastomosing tubules. *J. Neurocytol.* **6:** 361.
Hillman, D.E. 1969. New ultrastructural findings regarding a vestibular ciliary apparatus and its possible functional significance. *Brain Res.* **13:** 407.
———. 1976. Vestibular and lateral line system. 14. Morphology of peripheral and central vestibular systems. In *Frog neurobiology* (ed. R. Llinás and W. Precht), p. 452. Springer-Verlag, Berlin.
Hillman, D.E. and E.R. Lewis. 1971. Morphological basis for a mechanical linkage in otolithic receptor transduction in the frog. *Science* **174:** 416.
Holton, T. and A.J. Hudspeth. 1986. The transduction chan-

nel of hair cells from the bull-frog characterized by noise analysis. *J. Physiol.* **375**: 195.

Howard, J. and A.J. Hudspeth. 1987a. Mechanical relaxation of the hair bundle mediates adaptation in mechanoelectrical transduction by the bullfrog's saccular hair cell. *Proc. Natl. Acad. Sci.* **84**: 3064.

———. 1987b. Adaptation of mechanoelectrical transduction in hair cells. In *Sensory transduction* (ed. A.J. Hudspeth et al.), p. 138. Fondation pour l'Etude du Système Nerveux Central et Périphérique, Geneva.

———. 1988. Compliance of the hair bundle associated with gating of mechanoelectrical transduction channels in the bullfrog's saccular hair cell. *Neuron* **1**: 189.

Howard, J., W.M. Roberts, and A.J. Hudspeth. 1988. Mechanoelectrical transduction by hair cells. *Annu. Rev. Biophys. Biophys. Chem.* **17**: 99.

Hudspeth, A.J. 1982. Extracellular current flow and the site of transduction by vertebrate hair cells. *J. Neurosci.* **2**: 1.

———. 1983a. Mechanoelectrical transduction by hair cells in the acousticolateralis sensory system. *Annu. Rev. Neurosci.* **6**: 187.

———. 1983b. The hair cells of the inner ear. *Sci. Am.* **248**: 54.

———. 1985. The cellular basis of hearing: The biophysics of hair cells. *Science* **230**: 745.

———. 1989. How the ear's works work. *Nature* **341**: 397.

Hudspeth, A.J. and D.P. Corey. 1977. Sensitivity, polarity, and conductance change in the response of vertebrate hair cells to controlled mechanical stimuli. *Proc. Natl. Acad. Sci.* **74**: 2407.

Hudspeth, A.J. and R.S. Lewis. 1988a. Kinetic analysis of voltage- and ion-dependent conductances in saccular hair cells of the bull-frog, *Rana catesbeiana. J. Physiol.* **400**: 237.

———. 1988b. A model for electrical resonance and frequency tuning in saccular hair cells of the bull-frog, *Rana catesbeiana. J. Physiol.* **400**: 275.

Ishii, Y., S. Matsuura, and T. Furukawa. 1971. Quantal nature of transmission at the synapse between hair cells and eighth nerve fibers. *Jpn. J. Physiol.* **21**: 79.

Jahnke, K. 1975. The fine structure of freeze-fractured intercellular junctions in the guinea pig inner ear. *Acta Otolaryngol.* (suppl.) **336**: 1.

Koyama, H., E.R. Lewis, E.L. Leverenz, and R.A. Baird. 1982. Acute seismic sensitivity in the bullfrog ear. *Brain Res.* **250**: 168.

Kroese, A.B.A., A. Das, and A.J. Hudspeth. 1989. Blockage of the transduction channels of hair cells in the bullfrog's sacculus by aminoglycoside antibiotics. *Hearing Res.* **37**: 203.

Lewis, E.R. and C.W. Li. 1973. Evidence concerning the morphogenesis of saccular receptors in the bullfrog (*Rana catesbeiana*). *J. Morphol.* **139**: 351.

———. 1975. Hair cell types and distributions in the otolithic and auditory organs of the bullfrog. *Brain Res.* **83**: 35.

Lewis, R.S. and A.J. Hudspeth. 1983. Voltage- and ion-dependent conductances in solitary vertebrate hair cells. *Nature* **304**: 538.

Ohmori, H. 1985. Mechano-electrical transduction currents in isolated vestibular hair cells of the chick. *J. Physiol.* **359**: 189.

Pickles, J.O., S.D. Comis, and M.P. Osborne. 1984. Cross-links between stereocilia in the guinea pig organ of Corti, and their possible relation to sensory transduction. *Hearing Res.* **15**: 103.

Plattner, H. and L. Bachmann. 1982. Cryofixation: A tool in biological ultrastructural research. *Int. Rev. Cytol.* **79**: 237.

Pumplin, D.W., T.S. Reese, and R. Llinás. 1981. Are the presynaptic membrane particles the calcium channels? *Proc. Natl. Acad. Sci.* **78**: 7210.

Revel, J.-P., P. Yip, and L.L. Chang. 1973. Cell junctions in the early chick embryo—a freeze etch study. *Dev. Biol.* **35**: 302.

Roberts, W.M. and A.J. Hudspeth. 1987a. Spatial distribution of ion channels in hair cells of the bullfrog's sacculus. *Biophys. J.* **51**: 203a.

———. 1987b. Co-localization of Ca^{2+} channels with Ca^{2+}-activated K^+ channels in hair cells of the bullfrog's sacculus. *Soc. Neurosci. Abstr.* **13**: 177.

Roberts, W.M., J. Howard, and A.J. Hudspeth. 1988. Mechanoelectrical transduction, frequency tuning, and synaptic transmission by hair cells. *Annu. Rev. Cell Biol.* **4**: 63.

Roberts, W.M., R.A. Jacobs, and A.J. Hudspeth. 1990a. Co-localization of ion channels involved in frequency selectivity and synaptic transmission at presynaptic active zones of hair cells. *J. Neurosci.* **10**: 3664.

———. 1990b. Presynaptic calcium concentration exceeds one millimolar in frog saccular hair cells. *Biophys. J.* **57**: 303a.

Rüsch, A. and U. Thurm. 1989. Cupula displacement, hair bundle deflection, and physiological responses in the transparent semicircular canal of young eel. *Pflügers Arch.* **413**: 533.

Shotwell, S.L., R. Jacobs, and A.J. Hudspeth. 1981. Directional sensitivity of individual vertebrate hair cells to controlled deflection of their hair bundles. *Annu. N.Y. Acad. Sci.* **374**: 1.

Simon, S.M. and R.R. Llinás. 1985. Compartmentalization of the submembrane calcium activity during calcium influx and its significance in transmitter release. *Biophys. J.* **48**: 485.

Smith, S.J. and G.J. Augustine. 1988. Calcium ions, active zones and synaptic transmitter release. *Trends Neurosci.* **11**: 458.

Tran Ba Huy, P., C. Manuel, A. Meulemans, O. Sterkers, and C. Amiel. 1981. Pharmacokinetics of gentamicin in perilymph and endolymph of the rat as determined by radioimmunoassay. *J. Infect. Dis.* **143**: 476.

Model of Phototransduction in Retinal Rods

V. TORRE,* S. FORTI,† A. MENINI,‡ AND M. CAMPANI*

*Dipartimento di Fisica, Universita' di Genova, 16146 Genova, Italy; †Istituto per la Ricerca Scientifica
e Tecnologica, Trento, Italy; ‡Istituto di Cibernetica e Biofisica, Consiglio Nazionale delle
Ricerche, 16146 Genova, Italy

Phototransduction is the process by which the absorption of a photon by a molecule of rhodopsin in a photoreceptor is transformed into an electrical signal. This electrical signal is caused by the modulation of a current, usually called photocurrent, flowing across the light-sensitive channels in the plasma membrane of outer segments. Na^+ carries the large fraction of this current, but Ca^{++} also contributes by about one fourth of the photocurrent. Phototransduction occurs through changes in the concentration of a substance, usually referred to as the internal messenger, recently identified as guanosine 3',5'-cyclic monophosphate (cGMP) (Caretta and Cavaggioni 1983; Fesenko et al. 1985; Yau and Nakatani 1985; Haynes et al. 1986; Zimmermann and Baylor 1986). It is now known that Ca^{++} is not a positive transmitter (Matthews et al. 1985; Lamb et al. 1986), as originally proposed (Hagins 1972), but plays a crucial role in light adaptation (Torre et al. 1986; Matthews et al. 1988; Nakatani and Yau 1988c). It is also well established that cGMP controls the current induced in excised patches from outer segments of photoreceptors in a cooperative way (Fesenko et al. 1985; Haynes et al. 1986; Zimmermann and Baylor 1986).

The purpose of this paper is to extend the comparison between a model of phototransduction presented in detail previously (Forti et al. 1989) and a variety of experimental results already published or obtained in our laboratory. The original model was developed to explain phototransduction in rods of the newt (*Triturus cristatus*), but it also seems to be adequate to reproduce phototransduction in rods of many amphibians and reptiles. In the experiments reported, the light-sensitive current, or photocurrent, was usually measured with a suction electrode (Baylor et al. 1979a,b; Lamb et al. 1986).

THEORETICAL SECTION

We now briefly review the different mechanisms involved in phototransduction and in light adaptation. A detailed explanation for the derivation of the proposed model has been published previously (Forti et al. 1989), and here we recall the main pathways controlling intracellular Ca^{++} and cGMP metabolism. We assume that the main site of action of intracellular Ca^{++} is the guanylate cyclase (Lolley and Racz 1982; Pepe et al. 1986; Koch and Stryer 1988; Rispoli et al. 1988). A list of the symbols and their meanings, as used

in this text, appears before the Acknowledgments in this paper.

Changes of Intracellular Ca^{++}

Intracellular Ca^{++} is buffered (McNaughton et al. 1986), and its changes $\dot{c}$ are controlled by the influx through light-sensitive channels (Yau and Nakatani 1984a; Hodgkin et al. 1985; Nakatani and Yau 1988a; Menini et al. 1988), by its extrusion by the Na^+/Ca^{++} exchange (Yau and Nakatani 1984b; Hodgkin et al. 1987; Lagnado et al. 1988), and finally by binding and unbinding to internal buffers. The equations describing these mechanisms are

$$\dot{c} = \frac{J_{Ca}}{2Fv} - \gamma_{Ca}c - k_1(e_T - c_b)c + k_2c_b \quad (1)$$

$$\dot{c}_b = k_1(e_T - c_b)c - k_2c_b \quad (2)$$

where J_{Ca} is the total Ca^{++} current, F the Faraday constant, v the free volume of the rod, e_T the total buffer concentration, c_b the Ca^{++} concentration bound to the buffer, γ_{Ca} the rate of Ca^{++} extrusion mediated by the Na^+/Ca^{++} exchange, and k_1 and k_2 the "on" and "off" rate for the binding of Ca^{++} to the internal buffer. The majority of the influx of Ca^{++} occurs through the light-sensitive channels, and it is about one fourth of the total light-sensitive current (Menini et al. 1988).

Equations 1 and 2 describe the Ca^{++} extrusion through the Na^+/Ca^{++} exchange by a simple first-order mechanism, neglecting the Ca^{++} entry through the exchange itself, which will be relevant when $[Ca^{++}]_i$ is very low. As pointed out by Blaustein and Hodgkin (1969), at equilibrium and when $[Ca^{++}]_i$ is entirely controlled by the activity of the exchanger, the intracellular level of free Ca^{++} c_0 is set by

$$c_0 = [Ca^{++}]_i = [Ca^{++}]_0 \frac{[Na^+]_i^3}{[Na^+]_0^3} e^{V_mF/RT} \quad (3)$$

taking $[Na^+]_i = 12$ mM (Torre 1982) and $V_m = -60$ mV, a value of c_0 equal to about 100 nM is obtained.

Consequently, Equation 1 can be more appropriately rewritten as

$$\dot{c} = \frac{J_{Ca}}{2Fv} - \gamma_{Ca}(c - c_0) - k_1(e_T - c_b)c + k_2c_b \quad (4)$$

Changes of Intracellular cGMP

In the dark, cGMP is continuously produced by the enzyme guanylate cyclase at a rate A and is hydrolyzed by the enzyme phosphodiesterase (PDE) at a rate $\bar{V}$. The rate of cGMP hydrolysis is increased by light proportionally to the activated phosphodiesterase PDE^* (Liebman and Pugh 1982). Therefore, we can describe changes of free cGMP g as

$$\dot{g} = A - g(\bar{V} + \sigma PDE^*) \qquad (5)$$

where σ is a proportionality constant, assumed for simplicity to be $1\ \sec^{-1}\ \mu M^{-1}$. The resting level of cGMP was assumed to be $2\ \mu M$ (Stryer 1986; Nakatani and Yau 1988b). The activity of the cyclase is controlled by intracellular Ca^{++} in a cooperative way (Lolley and Racz 1982; Pepe et al. 1986; Koch and Stryer 1988; Rispoli et al. 1988), and the simplest way to describe this effect is to assume that

$$A = \frac{A_{max}}{1 + \left(\dfrac{c}{K_c}\right)^m} \qquad (6)$$

where A_{max} is the maximal activity of the cyclase, K_c is the intracellular Ca^{++} concentration producing half inhibition of the cyclase activity, and m is the number of Ca^{++} molecules necessary to inhibit a cyclase molecule. According to Koch and Stryer (1988), m is close to 4, and K_c is about $0.1\ \mu M$. Since the resting level of free intracellular Ca^{++} in darkness is about 300 nM (Ratto et al. 1988), the modulating action of Ca^{++} on the cyclase is expected to be high in darkness but, in the presence of steady bright lights, when intracellular free Ca^{++} has substantially dropped, the activity of the cyclase is affected to a lesser extent by intracellular Ca^{++}.

Reconstruction of the Kinetics of Photoresponses

Let us now attempt to provide a kinetic scheme able to reproduce several aspects of phototransduction. Our aim is not to obtain a perfect fitting of the experimental recordings, but to explain the major features of the kinetics of phototransduction using a parsimonious model that considers the known biochemistry of the cGMP cascade and of changes of intracellular Ca^{++}.

The light-sensitive channel is activated by cGMP, and experiments with excised patches (Haynes et al. 1986; Zimmerman and Baylor 1986) have shown that the cGMP-activated current J depends on the concentration g of cGMP as

$$\frac{J}{J_{max}} = \frac{g^3}{K^3 + g^3} \qquad (7)$$

where J_{max} is the maximal cGMP-dependent current that can be recorded in an excised patch, and K is the cGMP concentration half-activating the maximal current J_{max}. Equation 7 suggests that at least three molecules of cGMP must bind to the channel before opening it.

A characteristic feature of photoresponses is the slow time course of the electrical response to the absorption of a photon, usually explained as being caused by a series of slow stages involved in phototransduction. In an analysis of the kinetics of light responses in Limulus photoreceptors, Fuortes and Hodgkin (1964) identified the slow stages as activations but also as inactivations of the internal transmitter. Therefore, a slow stage in phototransduction (Baylor et al. 1974; Cervetto et al. 1977; Baylor et al. 1979a; Lamb 1986) of vertebrate rods could be a slow activation in the cGMP cascade but might also be a slow inactivation. In Figure 1, we have reported the known biochemical events involved in the control of free intracellular cGMP.

The pathway for the activation of PDE^* is known in great detail, but the values of rate constants of different biochemical steps in the intact cell have yet to be established precisely. Light activates rhodopsin very quickly. Activated rhodopsin is inactivated by the encounter with the two proteins, rhodopsin kinase and the 48-kD protein (Applebury and Chabre 1986; Stryer 1986). It is assumed that the inactivation of photo-excited rhodopsin Rh is reversible, thus giving origin to the late response. The inactivation of Rh is a slow process and is likely to be one of the slow stages in phototransduction.

It is well known that one activated rhodopsin is able to activate about 500 transducins per second (Bennett et al. 1982; Vuong and Stryer 1984), and one transducin activates one PDE within 100 msec (Liebman and Evanzuk 1982), therefore indicating that the activation of PDE by transducins is another slow stage in phototransduction. The only known pathway for PDE^* inactivation is through inactivation of transducin, which again could be another slow stage in phototransduction

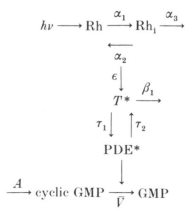

Figure 1. Scheme of biochemical events involved in the control of intracellular cGMP. $h\nu$ is a photon. Rh and Rh_i are the activated and inactivated rhodopsin, respectively. T^* and PDE^* are the active transducin and phosphodiesterase, respectively.

(Applebury and Chabre 1986; Stryer 1986). From Figure 1, we obtain the following set of equations:

$$\dot{Rh} = J_{h\nu}(t) - \alpha_1 Rh + \alpha_2 Rh_i \quad (8.1)$$

$$\dot{Rh}_i = \alpha_1 Rh - (\alpha_2 + \alpha_3)Rh_i \quad (8.2)$$

$$\dot{T}^* = \epsilon Rh(T_{Tot} - T^*) - \beta_1 T^* + \tau_2 PDE^* \quad (8.3)$$

$$\dot{PDE}^* = \tau_1 T^*(PDE_{Tot} - PDE^*) - \tau_2 PDE^* \quad (8.4)$$

where Rh and Rh_i are the photoexcited and inactive rhodopsin concentration, T_{Tot} and T^* are the total and activated transducin concentration, PDE_{Tot} and PDE^* are the total and the active phosphodiesterase concentration, and $J_{h\nu}(t)$ is the flux of rhodopsin photoisomerizations. In Equations 8, we have assumed that the concentrations of excitable rhodopsin are unlimited and that the maximal amount of excitable transducin T_{Tot} and phosphodiesterase PDE_{Tot} are 1000 μM and 100 μM, respectively (for a justification of these assumptions, see Stryer 1986). The values of the rate constants α_1, α_2, α_3, β_1, τ_1, and τ_2 were chosen to be equal to 20 sec^{-1}, 0.0005 sec^{-1}, 0.05 sec^{-1}, 10.6 sec^{-1}, 0.1 sec^{-1} μM^{-1}, and 10 sec^{-1}, respectively. The values for α_2 and α_3 were selected to produce the time course and amplitude of the late response (see Forti et al. 1989). The values for α_1, β_1, τ_1, and τ_2 were primarily selected to account for the kinetics of dim flash responses.

To reconstruct fully the kinetics of phototransduction, the four differential Equations 8 describing the activation of phosphodiesterase and the following Equations 9–12 were solved

$$\dot{c} = bJ - \gamma_{Ca}(c - c_0) - k_1(e_T - c_b)c + k_2 c_b \quad (9)$$

$$\dot{c}_b = k_1(e_T - c_b)c - k_2 c_b \quad (10)$$

$$\dot{g} = \frac{A_{max}}{1 + \left(\dfrac{c}{K_c}\right)^4} - g(\bar{V} + \sigma PDE^*) \quad (11)$$

$$J = J_{max} \frac{g^3}{g^3 + K^3} \quad (12)$$

The value of different parameters and the reason for their choice are given in Table 1.

The differential equations were numerically integrated with the following initial conditions: $g(0) = 2\,\mu$M, $c(0) = 300$ nM, $c_b(0) = 500/(1 + 4/0.3)\,\mu$M = 34.9 μM, $Rh(0) = 0$, $Rh_i(0) = 0$, $T^*(0) = 0$, and $PDE^*(0) = 0$.

EXPERIMENTAL SECTION

In this section, we compare the model with a variety of experimental results obtained in recent years in amphibian rods. It will be shown that the model reproduces many features of phototransduction and light adaptation. Moreover, the model is consistent with experiments in which the extracellular or intracellular medium of the rod is changed. In the model, the

Table 1. Value and Reason of Choice of Parameters Used in the Model

Parameter	Value	Reason of choice
α_1	20 sec^{-1}	to fit the time course of photoresponses to dim flash of light
α_2	0.0005 sec^{-1}	see Forti et al. (1989)
α_3	0.05 sec^{-1}	see Forti et al. (1989)
ϵ	0.5 sec^{-1} μM^{-1}	from Bennett et al. (1982)
T_{Tot}	1000 μM	from Stryer (1986)
β_1	10.6 sec^{-1}	to fit the time course of fast reactivation of the photocurrent at the cessation of a step of light
τ_1	0.1 sec^{-1} μM^{-1}	to fit the time course of photoresponse to dim flash of light
τ_2	10 sec^{-1}	
PDE_{Tot}	100 μM	from Stryer (1986)
σ	1 sec^{-1} μM^{-1}	unitary proportionality constant
γ_{Ca}	50 sec^{-1}	see Forti et al. (1989)
c_0	100 nM	from Equation 3
b	0.625 μM sec^{-1} pA^{-1}	see Forti et al. (1989)
k_1	0.2 sec^{-1} μM^{-1}	to reproduce the kinetics of the reactivation of the photocurrent with steps of light and to have an affinity buffer with K_D close to 10 μM (Hodgkin et al. 1987)
k_2	0.8 sec^{-1}	
e_T	500 μM	
$\bar{V}$	0.4 sec^{-1}	from Hodgkin and Nunn (1988)
A_{max}	65.6 μM sec^{-1}	to have 2 μM for the resting level of free cGMP
K_c	100 nM	from Koch and Stryer (1988)
K^3	1000 μM^3	from Zimmerman and Baylor (1986)
J_{max}	5040 pA	see Forti et al. (1989)

light intensity is expressed in $Rh_t^* sec^{-1}$ corresponding to about 2000–4000 photoisomerization sec^{-1} $(Rh_s^* sec^{-1})$.

Responses to Flashes and Steps of Light

Figure 2 illustrates the results of experiments from rods of the newt. Families of photoresponses to brief flashes of light in darkness and in the presence of a steady light equivalent to the 1300 $Rh^* sec^{-1}$ are shown. The circulating photocurrent was 30 pA in darkness and was reduced to 15 pA by the steady light. In darkness, the time to peak of the dim flash response was 950 msec and decreased to 650 msec by increasing the light intensity by 100 times. When flashes are superimposed on backgrounds of steady light, the time to peak of dim flash responses shortens to 330 msec, and the acceleration of the time to peak with brighter flashes is not observed with very bright steady lights.

Photoresponses to steps of light of 60 seconds of increasing intensity are shown in Figure 2, E and G. Photoresponses to intermediate and bright light intensities reach a peak within 1 or 2 seconds, and at later times, present a partial reactivation of the photocurrent. This delayed reactivation of the photocurrent is the major mechanism underlying light adaptation. When the step of light is switched off, the photocurrent reactivates with a complex time course. In the presence of brighter lights, the photocurrent remains fully suppressed for a few seconds before commencing to reactivate. After a partial fast recovery of the photocurrent, a long-lasting component of the photoresponse is observed, as shown in Figure 2E.

Photoresponses to steps of light of 60 seconds of increasing intensity, in the presence of a steady light equivalent to 1050 $Rh^+ sec^{-1}$, are shown in Figure 2G. The effect of the steady light on the kinetics of photoresponses is mostly pronounced at the cessation of the steps of light where an overshoot can be observed and the kinetics of the late response is slightly accelerated. The time course of the reactivation of the photocurrent, observed with steps of light initially blocking a large fraction of the circulating current, is not accelerated. Similarly, the time course of reactivation of the photocurrent at the termination of nonsaturating steps of light is hardly affected.

A family of traces obtained by solving the set of differential Equations 8–12 in which the flux of photoisomerization $J_{hv}(t)$ had a duration of 10 msec is illustrated in Figure 2B. The theoretical curves have a time course similar to the experimental traces shown in Figure 2A. The time-to-peak of theoretical traces, which is about 1080 msec for dim lights, shortens to 690 msec for bright lights, which is similar to the experimental behavior. The time to peak shortens because as intracellular Ca^{++} drops, the cyclase is stimulated, thus more efficiently counteracting the light-induced phosphodiesterase activation. The amplitude of photocurrent recorded with a suction pipette is usually 60% of the photocurrent recorded with a patch pipette; therefore,

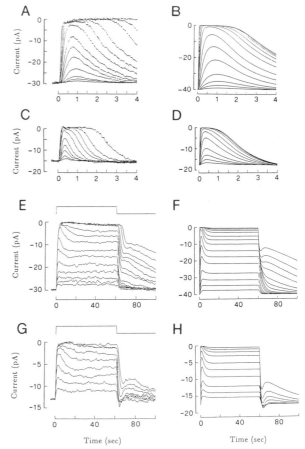

Figure 2. Families of responses to brief flashes in darkness (A) and superimposed on a steady light equivalent to 1300 $Rh^* sec^{-1}$ (C). Flash intensities in A were 3, 6, 12, 25, 58, 115, 230, 600, 1150, 2350, 6100, 12,500, and 24,000 Rh^*, and in C they were 58, 115, 230, 600, 1150, 2350, 6100, 12,500, 24,000, and 50,000 Rh^*. In B and D, theoretical curves obtained from Equations 8–12 are plotted. Theoretical photocurrents obtained with pulses of $J_{hv}(t)$ of duration 10 msec were equal to (B) 0.2, 0.5, 1, 2, 5, 10, 20, 50, 100, 200, 500, 1000, 2000 and $Rh_t^* sec^{-1}$ or equal to (D) 2, 5, 10, 20, 50, 100, 200, 500, 1000, and 2000 $Rh_t^* sec^{-1}$, superimposed on a steady light equivalent to 0.1 $Rh_t^* sec^{-1}$. In E and G, photoresponses to steps of light of 60 sec of duration are reproduced. In E, the intensities of steady lights were equivalent to 5, 11, 20, 45, 100, 210, 480, 1050, 2200, 4500, 11,500, 22,000, 45,000, 110,000, and 220,000 $Rh^* sec^{-1}$. In G, photoresponses to steps of light of 60 sec in the presence of a steady light were equivalent to 1050 $Rh_s^* sec^{-1}$. The intensities of steps of light were 480, 1050, 2200, 4500, 11,500, 22,000, 45,000, 110,000, and 220,000 $Rh^* sec^{-1}$. In F and H, theoretical curves obtained from Equations 8–12 with steps of $J_{hv}(t)$ of 60 sec duration are plotted. In F, the theoretical photocurrents obtained with $J_{hv}(t)$ are equal to 0.002, 0.005, 0.01, 0.02, 0.05, 0.1, 0.2, 0.5, 1, 2, 5, 10, 20, and 50 $Rh_t^* sec^{-1}$. In H, the theoretical photocurrents obtained with steps of $J_{hv}(t)$ of 60 sec of duration superimposed on a steady light were equivalent to 0.1 $Rh_t^* sec^{-1}$. The intensities of $J_{hv}(t)$ were 0.05, 0.1, 0.2, 0.5, 1, 2, 5, 10, 20, and 50 $Rh_t^* sec^{-1}$.

in the model, the various parameters were set so that the amplitude of the theoretical photocurrent is about 30% larger than the photocurrent recorded with a suction pipette.

The theoretical families of photocurrents, obtained by simulating a pulse superimposed on a steady flux of photoisomerizations are shown in Figure 2D. In agreement with the experimental traces, the time-to-peak of the dim flash response shortens to 450 msec and does not accelerate with brighter flashes (compare with the experimental traces of Figure 2A,C). The experimental traces obtained in response to bright flashes of light have a longer plateau than the theoretical traces.

A family of theoretical traces, simulating a flux of photoisomerizations of 60 seconds, is shown in Figure 2F. In agreement with the experimental traces (see Fig. 2E), the photocurrent, after a partial or complete suppression, reactivates with a delay. This reactivation is produced by the second slow fall of intracellular Ca^{++}, caused by the Ca^{++} uptake by the internal buffer. At the termination of the light, the theoretical curves show almost the same behavior as the experimental traces, where the photocurrent reactivates with a fast and a late or slow component. The fast reactivation of the photocurrent is due to the substantial depletion of intracellular Ca^{++}, which activates the cyclase (Hodgkin and Nunn 1988). This enzyme remains activated even during the 2 or 3 seconds of the fast reactivation because the influx of Ca^{++} through light-sensitive channels is absorbed by the intracellular Ca^{++} buffer. The slow component is probably caused by the reversible inactivation of photoactivated rhodopsin.

A defect of the model evident in the traces shown in Figure 2F is the almost instantaneous reactivation of the photocurrent at the cessation of the step of light. A more complex scheme for the inactivation cascade is likely to remove this defect.

Figure 2H reproduces theoretical traces simulating a step of light of 60 seconds but in the presence of a steady light. The theoretical traces reproduce the time course of the experimental recordings shown in Figure 2G quite well. The presence of a steady light in the model does not accelerate the time course of the reactivation of the photocurrent, in agreement with the experimental observation. As with the experimental traces of Figure 2G, a similar rebound of the photocurrent is observed at the cessation of the step of light.

Amplitude of Photoresponse and Light Intensity

The relation between normalized photoresponse $\Delta J / J_s$ and light intensity I, which is an essential feature of phototransduction and light adaptation, is usually explained by several theoretical curves (Baylor et al. 1974; Lamb et al. 1981; Forti et al. 1989). The Michaelis-Menten equation

$$\frac{\Delta J}{J_s} = \frac{I}{I + I_0} \qquad (13)$$

has been used in many circumstances, but the exponential equation

$$\frac{\Delta J}{J_s} = 1 - e^{-I} \qquad (14)$$

seems to reproduce the experimental data better

(Lamb et al. 1981). The equation

$$\frac{\Delta J}{J_s} = 1 - \left(\frac{I_0}{I + I_0} \right)^n \qquad (15)$$

where n is an integer, has been proposed recently (Forti et al. 1989) because it can be derived by a simple scheme taking into account the cooperativity among cGMP molecules in opening light-sensitive channels.

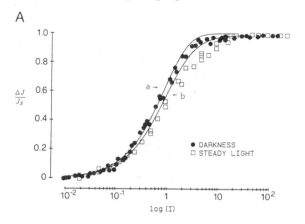

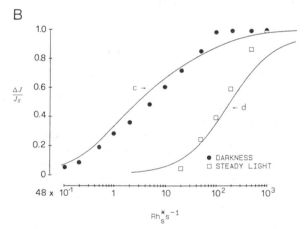

Figure 3. Relation between $\Delta J / J_s$ and light intensity I. $\Delta J = J_s - J$, where J_s is the steady circulating photocurrent, and J is the circulating current at the time of the measurement. (*A*) The experimental points of Forti et al. (1989) illustrated in Fig. 2B obtained with flashes of light in darkness (●). The experimental points of Forti et al. (1989) illustrated in Figure 2C obtained with flashes of light in the presence of a steady light equivalent to 110,000 $Rh_s^* sec^{-1}$ (○). The continuous line indicated by a was obtained by the model considering the relation $\Delta J / J_s$ at 0.4 sec following the onset of the flash of light. The continuous line indicated by b was obtained by the model in the presence of a steady light equivalent to 1 $Rh_t^* sec^{-1}$ and measuring the relation $\Delta J / J_s$ at 0.2 sec following the onset of the flash of light. Theoretical curves were shifted to have the rising phase matching the experimental points. (*B*) The relation between $\Delta J / J_s$ and light intensity 16 sec after the onset of a step of light. The experimental points of Forti et al. (1989) in Fig. 7 obtained in darkness (●) and in the presence of a steady light (□) are equivalent to 51,000 $Rh_s^* sec^{-1}$. The continuous line indicated by c was obtained by the model with steps of light from 0.002 $Rh_t^* sec^{-1}$ to 100 $Rh_t^* sec^{-1}$. The continuous line indicated by d was obtained by the model in the presence of a steady light of 2 $Rh_t^* sec^{-1}$ and with steps of light from 0.5 $Rh_t^* sec^{-1}$ to 300 $Rh_t^* sec^{-1}$.

Figure 3A reproduces the experimental points obtained by Forti et al. (1989) (data from Fig. 2B,C) in darkness and in the presence of a bright light equivalent to 110,000 $Rh_s sec^{-1}$. The experimental relation between $\Delta J/J_s$ and I in darkness is well reproduced by the exponential Equation 14 (not shown in the figure) and by the model. The same experimental relation in the presence of a bright steady light is less steep and is poorly fitted by the exponential Equation 14 (not shown). The relation obtained by the model does not exactly fit the experimental points, but it is consistent with the less steep behavior observed experimentally.

Figure 3B reproduces the relation between $\Delta J/J_s$ and light intensity measured 16 seconds after the onset of a step of light in darkness and in the presence of a steady light equivalent to 51,000 $Rh_s^* sec^{-1}$. Data are from Figure 7 of Forti et al. (1989). In darkness, the relation obtained with steps of light is less steep than the relation obtained with flashes of light because light adaptation had the time to develop fully. As a consequence of light adaptation, the operating range of the rod is expanded by about 1 log unit. The same relation obtained by the model, under similar conditions, is consistent with this broadening of the operating range. In the presence of a bright steady light, the operating range of light is similarly reduced in the rod and in the model.

Light Adaptation

When a steady light impinges on a photoreceptor, several processes are initiated leading to light adaptation. Light adaptation consists in a broadening of the operating range (see previous section), in a desensitization, and in a speeding up of phototransduction. These last two features are usually characterized by the decreased flash sensitivity S_F relative to the sensitivity in darkness $_D S_F$ and the acceleration of the time course of photoresponses in the linear range (Baylor and Hodgkin 1974). The decrease of sensitivity is usually described as the Weber-Fechner law, which has the analytical form

$$\frac{S_F}{_D S_F} = \frac{1}{1 + \dfrac{I}{\bar{I}}} \tag{16}$$

where $\bar{I}$ is the light intensity halving the flash sensitivity. Figure 4A compares the relative change of the flash sensitivity $S_F/_D S_F$ with steady lights, as obtained by the model and experimental results obtained from six rods of the newt. Each symbol corresponds to data from a rod. The experimental points are very well fitted by Equation 16 with the value 40 $Rh_s^* sec^{-1}$ for I (not shown in the figure) and by the model. The light intensity in the model halving the flash sensitivity is about 0.011 $Rh_t^* sec^{-1}$. Figure 4B shows that the acceleration of the time-to-peak of photoresponse in the linear range obtained from six different rods is very similar to the behavior shown by the model. In the presence of very bright steady lights, however, the time-to-peak in

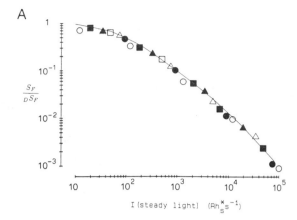

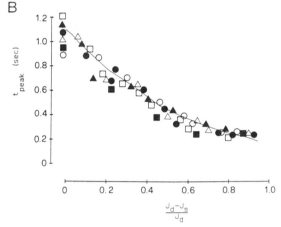

Figure 4. (*A*) Relation between $S_F/_D S_F$ and steady light intensity I, where $_D S_F$ is the flash sensitivity in darkness, and S_F is the flash sensitivity in the presence of a steady light. Each symbol corresponds to experimental points from a rod of the newt. The continuous line was obtained by the model with a steady light halving the flash sensitivity equal to about 0.011 $Rh_t^* sec^{-1}$. (*B*) The relation between the time-to-peak in the linear range t_{peak} and normalized suppressed current ($J_D - J_S/J_D$, where J_D is the circulating current in darkness, and J_S is the circulating current in the presence of a steady light. Each symbol corresponds to experimental points from a rod of the newt. The continuous line was obtained by the model.

rods of the newt is shortened to about 300 msec, whereas in the model, the time-to-peak is reduced to 230 msec. The results shown in Figure 4 indicate that the model reproduces the essence of light adaptation remarkably well.

Antagonism between Steady Light and PDE Inhibitor

The kinetics of photoresponses is accelerated by steady lights but is slowed down when the activity of PDE is reduced by the addition to the bathing medium of inhibitors of the enzyme PDE, such as the compound 3-isobutyl-1-methylxanthine (IBMX) (Capovilla et al. 1983; Cervetto and McNaughton 1986). Figure 5, A, B, and C, reproduces experimental recordings from rods of the toad (*Bufo marinus*) obtained by Cervetto and McNaughton (1986). The addition of 20 μM IBMX to

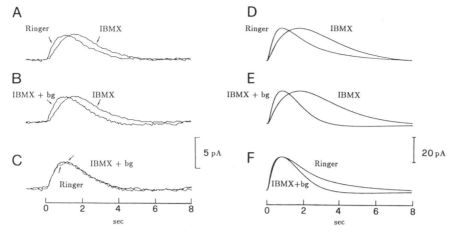

Figure 5. Interaction between background light and 20 μM IBMX. Dim flash responses scaled to the same height for comparison of time course. (*A*) Responses in Ringer solution and in IBMX, both in darkness. (*B*) Responses in IBMX, in darkness and in the presence of a bright background (bg). (*C*) Responses in Ringer solution, in darkness, and in IBMX with a bright background light. (Reprinted, with permission, from Cervetto and McNaughton 1986.) (*D, E, F*) Theoretical curves obtained with Equations 8–10, 12, and 17 with a value of 20 μM for [*IBMX*].

the bathing medium caused an increase in the light-sensitive current and a prolongation of the time course of the responses that were neutralized by background lights. In Figure 5, the dim flash responses have all been scaled to the same height to facilitate comparison of the time course. Figure 5 shows responses in darkness, the effect of a bright background light in IBMX, and that this light was sufficient to neutralize exactly the effects of IBMX on the time course.

The inhibitory effect of IBMX on the PDE activity can be accounted for in the model by replacing Equation 11 with Equation 17

$$\dot{g} = \frac{A_{max}}{1 + \left(\dfrac{c}{K_c}\right)^4} - g\,\frac{\bar{V} + \sigma PDE^*}{1 + \dfrac{[IBMX]}{K_I}} \qquad (17)$$

where [*IBMX*] is the IBMX concentration in the bathing medium and K_I is the concentration of IBMX halving the PDE activity. The value of K_I has been taken to be 3 μM as stated in Capovilla et al. (1983). Figure 5, D, E, and F, illustrates traces obtained by the model when Equation 11 has been substituted with Equation 17 with the value of [*IBMX*] equal to 20 μM. It is evident that the model reproduces the effect of IBMX and steady light on the time-to-peak of photoresponses rather well.

Effect of Inhibiting the Na$^+$/Ca^{++} Exchange

Figure 6, A, B, and C, illustrates the results of experiments obtained by Hodgkin et al. (1985) from rods of the toad (*Bufo marinus*) when extracellular Na$^+$ was replaced with Li$^+$. The photocurrent initially increased because Li$^+$ is more permeable than Na$^+$ through the light-sensitive channels, but the initial current was not maintained and declined to a small value with a time constant of about 1.4 seconds (Fig. 6A).

The time constant of the decline of current was prolonged to 5.4 seconds by the addition of 10 μM IBMX (Fig. 6B), and it was shortened to 0.6 second in a dim background light (Fig. 6C). These results were explained qualitatively by Hodgkin et al. (1985), assuming that (1) a rise in internal Ca^{++} leads to a reduction in the light-sensitive current, (2) internal Ca^{++} is maintained at a low level by a Na$^+$/Ca^{++} exchange mechanism, and (3) Li$^+$ cannot substitute Na$^+$ in the exchange with Ca^{++}.

It is now shown that the proposed model of phototransduction can quantitatively reproduce the results of Hodgkin et al. (1985) very well. The inability of Li$^+$ to substitute Na$^+$ in the Na$^+$/Ca^{++} exchange was taken into account in the model by setting γ_{Ca}, the rate constant of Ca^{++} extrusion through the Na$^+$/Ca^{++} exchange, equal to 0 in Equation 9 for the time when Na$^+$ is removed from the bathing medium, and the effect of IBMX was described using Equation 17 instead of Equation 11. Figure 6, D, E, and F, reproduces the obtained curves. It is evident that the basic features of the experiments illustrated in Figure 6, A, B, and C, are well reproduced by the model. The theoretical time constant of the decline of the photocurrent, when Na$^+$ is removed, is 1.7 seconds, in the presence of IBMX, it is prolonged to 2.8 seconds, and a steady light accelerates it to 0.6 second. The transient increase of the photocurrent observed when Na$^+$ is replaced with Li$^+$ is not reproduced by the model because Na$^+$ and Li$^+$ were assumed, for simplicity, to be equally permeable through the light-sensitive channel.

Effect of Increasing Ca^{++} Buffering Capacity

When a photoreceptor is loaded with the Ca^{++} chelator 1,2-bis (0-aminophenoxy) ethane-*N, N, N', N'*-tetraacetic acid (BAPTA) (Tsien 1980), the time course of photoresponses is affected significantly

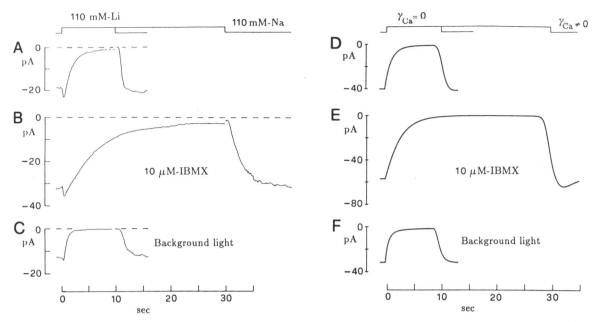

Figure 6. Effect of 10 μM IBMX and dim light on the rate of decrease of light-sensitive current after removing external Na$^+$. (*A*) Response to 10-sec application of 110 μM Li$^+$ solution in darkness in the absence of IBMX. (*B*) A 30 sec application of Li$^+$ in the presence of 10 μM IBMX throughout. (*C*) Repeat of *A* in dim light (5.4 photoisomerizations sec^{-1}). Timing of solution changes shown at the top. (Reprinted, with permission, from Hodgkin et al. 1985) (*D, E, F*) Theoretical curves obtained with Equations 8–10, 12, and 17 with a value of 10 μM for [*IBMX*]. $\gamma_{Ca} = 0$ for simulating the substitution of external Na$^+$ with Li$^+$ that is unable to replace Na$^+$ in the Na$^+$/Ca^{++} exchange. In *F*, the theoretical steady light was 0.01 Rh$^*_\ast$sec^{-1}.

(Lamb et al. 1986; Torre et al. 1986). Figure 7, A, B, and C, illustrates the results of the experiments obtained by Torre et al. (1986) from rods of the salamander (*Ambystoma tigrinum*). Figure 7A shows a typical family of photocurrent responses to flashes of increasing intensity and exhibits a characteristic acceleration of time-to-peak with increasing flash intensity. Figure 7B shows the same experiment after entrapment of BAPTA (10 mM in patch pipette): The responses to dim flashes were prolonged, the normal acceleration of responses with brighter flashes disappeared, the responses to intense flashes remained saturated longer, and a pronounced overshoot occurred at all intensities. In Figure 7C, the individual responses for three flash intensities from the control and trapped BAPTA families plotted as normalized responses have been superimposed.

A further test of the proposed model is to see whether the introduction into the model of a high-affinity Ca^{++} buffer with the on and off rates h_1 and h_2 equal to 100 sec^{-1} μM^{-1} and 10 sec^{-1} as with BAPTA (Tsien 1980) reproduces the changes of the kinetics of photoresponses experimentally observed by infusing BAPTA into the rod. The theoretical model is accordingly changed by substituting Equation 9 with the two Equations 18 and 19

$$\dot{c} = \frac{J_{Ca}}{zFV} - \gamma_{Ca}(c - c_0) - k_1(c_T - c_b)c$$
$$+ k_2 c_b - h_1(h_T - h_b)c + h_2 h_b \quad (18)$$

$$\dot{h}_b = h_1(h_T - h_b)c - h_2 h_b \quad (19)$$

where h_T is the total concentration of the high-affinity buffer and h_b is the Ca^{++} concentration bound to the high-affinity buffer. Families of theoretical photoresponses obtained under control conditions or by simulating the infusion of 1000 μM BAPTA are shown in D and E of Figure 7, respectively. Figure 7F compares traces generated by the model without the high-affinity buffer and traces obtained with a model including 1000 μM BAPTA. The theoretical curves reproduce quite accurately the experimental recordings shown in Figure 7, A, B, and C. The increase of sensitivity, the rebound at the termination of the photoresponse, the lengthening of the photoresponse, the lack of the acceleration of the time to peak with flashes of increasing intensity are all features shared by the experimental traces and the theoretical curves.

CONCLUSIONS

In this paper, a quantitative reconstruction of the kinetics of phototransduction has been attempted, obtaining a satisfactory agreement between theoretical and experimental curves. A noticeable feature of the proposed model is the relatively small modulation of internal messengers, while preserving the ability of the photoreceptor to transduce light intensity over a 4-log-unit range. The level of free cGMP during a steady light does not fall below the level set by the maximal activity of PDE and cyclase, and from Equation 9, intracellular Ca^{++} cannot fall below 100 nM (i.e., the value of c_0). From Equation 11, at the steady state, the lower level of cGMP is

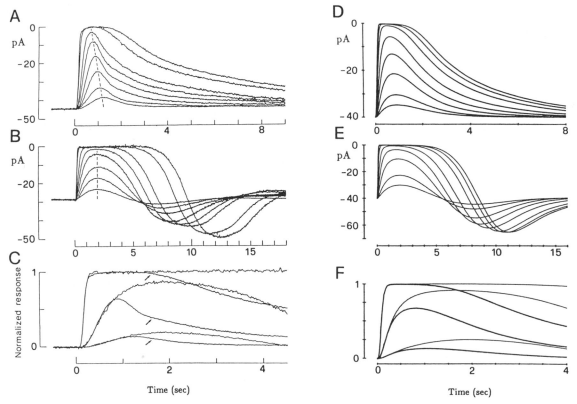

Figure 7. Effect of trapped BAPTA on the flash responses of a rod. (*A*) Control conditions. Responses recorded for brief flashes of light delivered at time zero. Flash intensities increased in steps of approximately a factor of 2 from ~ 10 to 1900 isomerizations. (*B*) After trapping BAPTA. Responses from the same cell with the same series of flashes. (*C*) Normalized response (i.e., response divided by circulating dark current) for three flash intensities. Broken lines in *A* and *B* show the trends in time-to-peak. (Reprinted, with permission, from Torre et al. 1986.) (*D*) Theoretical curves in control conditions obtained with Equations 8–12 and pulses of $J_{hv}(t)$ of duration of 10 msec equal to 1, 2, 5, 10, 20, 50, 100, 200 Rh$^*_t$sec^{-1}. (*E*) Theoretical curves obtained with Equations 8, 11, 12, 18, and 19 simulating the infusion of 1000 μM BAPTA and the same pulses as in *D*. (*F*) Superimposed traces obtained with (lighter traces) and without infusion of BAPTA (heavy traces) and pulses of $J_{hv}(t)$ equal to 2, 20, and 200 Rh$^*_t$sec^{-1}.

$$\frac{A_{max}}{\left(1 + \left(\frac{c_0}{k_c}\right)^4\right)(\bar{V} + \sigma PDE_{Tot})} \quad (20)$$

which from the values of Table 1 is 0.33 μM, and so consequently at the steady state, the level of free cGMP decreases by a factor of only 6. This ability to modulate the response over a rather wide range of light intensity with small changes in the concentration of internal transmitters is due to the cooperative action of cGMP on the channel and of Ca^{++} on the cyclase activity. These observations may suggest that any transduction mechanism is unlikely to require large changes of internal second messengers, such as a rise or a fall of free Ca^{++} by several log units, and so, consequently, the obvious design to increase the operating range of the transduction process would be to use highly cooperative mechanisms.

The model is able to account for many features of the kinetics of phototransduction but not all the details, as discussed in the Experimental Section. The main defect of the model, evident in Figure 2, consists of a faster reactivation of the photocurrent after a bright light. This defect also manifests itself in Figures 5 and 6,

where an overshoot of the theoretical photocurrent is observed in the presence of IBMX. This defect after all is not surprising, as the biochemical events involved in the reactivation of the photocurrent are the least understood.

List of Symbols

I	light intensity (in arbitrary units)
I_0	light intensity producing a photoresponse of half amplitude (in arbitrary units)
J	photocurrent or cGMP gated current in excised patches (pA)
J_S	steady circulating photocurrent (pA)
g	concentration of cGMP (μM)
K	half activation of the cGMP-gated current in excised patches (μM)
J_{max}	maximal cGMP-gated current in excised patches (pA)
t	time
hv	photons
F	Faraday constant
v	rod volume (l)

J_{Ca}	Ca^{++} influx (μM sec^{-1})
γ_{Ca}	rate constant of Ca^{++} extrusion in the absence of Ca^{++} buffers mediated by the Na^+/Ca^{++} exchanger (sec^{-1})
e_T	low-affinity Ca^{++} buffer concentration (μM)
c	intracellular free Ca^{++} concentration (μM)
c_b	intracellular Ca^{++} concentration bound to the low affinity buffer (μM)
k_1, k_2	on and off rate constants for the binding of Ca^{++} to the buffer (μM^{-1} sec^{-1} and sec^{-1}, respectively)
$K_D =$	K_2/K_1 μM
c_0	intracellular Ca^{++} concentration at the steady state (μM)
V_m	membrane potential (mV)
A	guanylate cyclase activity (μM sec^{-1})
$\bar{V}$	cGMP hydrolysis in dark (sec^{-1})
V	cGMP hydrolysis (sec^{-1})
PDE^*	activated phosphodiesterase (μM)
σ	proportionality constant (μM^{-1} sec^{-1})
PDE_{Tot}	total phosphodiesterase (μM)
b	proportionality constant between Ca^{++} influx and photocurrent (μM sec^{-1} pA^{-1})
A_{max}	maximal activity of guanylate cyclase (μM sec^{-1})
K_c	intracellular Ca^{++} concentration halving the cyclase activity
α_1	rate constant of Rh* inactivation (sec^{-1})
α_2	rate constant of the reaction Rh$_i$ $\rightarrow$ Rh* (sec^{-1})
α_3	rate constant of the decay of inactive rhodopsin (sec^{-1})
Rh	active rhodopsin (μM)
Rh$_i$	inactive rhodopsin (μM)
Rh*	effective photoisomerizations
ϵ	rate constant of T^* activation (μM^{-1} sec^{-1})
β_1	rate constant of T^* inactivation (sec^{-1})
τ_1	rate constant of PDE activation (sec^{-1} μM^{-1})
τ_2	rate constant of PDE inactivation (sec^{-1})
T^*	active transducin (μM)
T_{Tot}	total transducin (μM)
$J_{h\nu}(t)$	theoretical flux of photoisomerization (Rh$_t^*$ sec^{-1})
h_1, h_2	on and off rate constants for the binding of Ca^{++} to the high-affinity buffer (μM^{-1} sec^{-1} and sec^{-1}, respectively)
h_b	intracellular Ca^{++} concentration bound to the high-affinity buffer (μM)
h_T	high-affinity Ca^{++} buffer concentration (μM)
K_I	IBMX concentration halving the phosphodiesterase activity (μM)

ACKNOWLEDGMENTS

We thank Ms. Cristina Rosati for doing the artwork and for providing editorial assistance and Ms. Marta Zanini for help in typing the manuscript. Clive Prestt checked the English.

REFERENCES

Applebury, M.L. and M. Chabre. 1986. Interaction of photo-activated rhodopsin with photoreceptors proteins: The cyclic GMP cascade. In *The molecular mechanism of photoreception* (ed. H. Stieve), p. 51. Springer-Verlag, Berlin.

Baylor, D.A. and A.L. Hodgkin. 1974. Changes in time scale and sensitivity in turtle photoreceptors. *J. Physiol.* **242:** 729.

Baylor, D.A., A.L. Hodgkin, and T.D. Lamb. 1974. The electrical response of turtle cones to flashes and steps of light. *J. Physiol.* **242:** 685.

Baylor, D.A., T.D. Lamb, and K.W. Yau. 1979a. The membrane current of single rod outer segments. *J. Physiol.* **288:** 589.

————. 1979b. Responses of retinal rods to single photons. *J. Physiol.* **288:** 613.

Bennett, N., M. Michel-Villaz, and H. Kuhn. 1982. Light induced interaction between rhodopsin and the GTP-binding protein: Metarhodopsin II is the major photoproduct involved. *Eur. J. Biochem.* **127:** 97.

Blaustein, M.P. and A.L. Hodgkin. 1969. The effect of cyanide on the efflux of calcium from squid axons. *J. Physiol.* **200:** 497.

Capovilla, M., L. Cervetto, and V. Torre. 1983. The effects of phosphodiesterase inhibitors on the electrical activity of toad rods. *J. Physiol.* **343:** 277.

Caretta, A. and A. Cavaggioni. 1983. Fast ionic flux activated by cyclic GMP in the membrane of cattle rod outer segments. *Eur. J. Biochem.* **132:** 1.

Cervetto, L. and P.A. McNaughton. 1986. The effects of phosphodiesterase inhibitors and lanthanum ions on the light-sensitive current of toad retinal rods. *J. Physiol.* **370:** 9.

Cervetto, L., E. Pasino, and V. Torre. 1977. Electrical responses of rods in the retina of *Bufo marinus*. *J. Physiol.* **267:** 17.

Fesenko, E.E., S.S. Kolesnikov, and A.L. Lyubarsky. 1985. Induction by cyclic GMP of cationic conductance in plasma membrane of retinal rod outer segment. *Nature* **313:** 310.

Forti, S., A. Menini, G. Rispoli, and V. Torre. 1989. Kinetics of phototransduction in retinal rods of the newt *Triturus cristatus*. *J. Physiol.* **419:** 265.

Fuortes, M.G.F. and A.L. Hodgkin. 1964. Changes in time scale and sensitivity in the ommatidia of Limulus. *J. Physiol.* **172:** 239.

Hagins, W.A. 1972. The visual process: Excitatory mechanisms in the primary receptor cells. *Annu. Rev. Biophys. Bioeng.* **1:** 131.

Haynes, L.W., A.R. Kay, and K.W. Yau. 1986. Single cyclic GMP-activated channel activity in excised patches of rod outer segment membrane. *Nature* **321:** 66.

Hodgkin, A.L. and B.J. Nunn. 1988. Control of light-sensitive current in salamander rods. *J. Physiol.* **403:** 439.

Hodgkin, A.L. P.A. McNaughton, and B.J. Nunn. 1985. The ionic selectivity and calcium dependence of the light-sensitive pathway in toad rods. *J. Physiol.* **358:** 447.

————. 1987. Measurement of sodium calcium exchange in salamander rods. *J. Physiol.* **391:** 347.

Koch, K.W. and L. Stryer. 1988. Highly cooperative feedback control of retinal rod guanylate cyclase by calcium ions. *Nature* **334:** 64.

Lagnado, L., L. Cervetto, and P.A. McNaughton. 1988. Ion transport by the Na-Ca exchange in isolated rod outer segments. *Proc. Natl. Acad. Sci.* **85:** 4548.

Lamb, T.D. 1986. Photoreceptor adaptation—Vertebrates. In *The molecular mechanism of photoreception* (ed. H. Stieve), p. 267. Springer-Verlag, Berlin.

Lamb, T.D., H.R. Matthews, and V. Torre. 1986. Incorporation of calcium buffers into salamander retinal rods: A rejection of the calcium hypothesis of phototransduction. *J. Physiol.* **372:** 315.

Lamb, T.D., P.A. McNaughton, and K.W. Yau. 1981. Spatial spread of activation and background desensitization in toad rod outer segments. *J. Physiol.* **319:** 463.

Liebman, P.A. and A.T. Evanzuk. 1982. Real time array of rod disk membrane cyclic GMP phosphodiesterase and its controller enzymes. *Methods Enzymol.* **81:** 532.

Liebman, P.A. and E.N. Pugh. 1982. Gain, speed, and sensitivity of GTP binding vs. PDE activation in visual excitation. *Vision Res.* **22:** 1475.

Lolley, R.H. and E. Racz. 1982. Calcium modulation of cyclic GMP synthesis in rat visual cells. *Vision Res.* **22:** 1481.

Matthews, H.R., V. Torre, and T.D. Lamb. 1985. Effects on photoresponse of calcium buffers and cyclic GMP incorporated into the cytoplasm of retinal rods. *Nature* **313:** 582.

Matthews, H.R., R.I. Murphy, G.I. Fain, and T.D. Lamb. 1988. Photoreceptor light adaptation is mediated in isolated rods of the tiger salamander. *Nature* **334:** 67.

McNaughton, P.A., L. Cervetto, and B.J. Nunn. 1986. Measurement of the intracellular free calcium concentration in salamander rods. *Nature* **322:** 261.

Menini, A., G. Rispoli, and V. Torre. 1988. The ionic selectivity of the light-sensitive current in isolated rods of the tiger salamander. *J. Physiol.* **402:** 279.

Nakatani, K. and K.W. Yau. 1988a. Calcium and magnesium fluxes across the plasma membrane of the toad rod outer segment. *J. Physiol.* **395:** 695.

———. 1988b. Guanosine 3′, 5′-cyclic monophosphate-activated conductance studied in a truncated rod outer segment of the toad. *J. Physiol.* **395:** 731.

———. 1988c. Calcium and light adaptation in retinal rods and cones. *Nature* **334:** 69.

Pepe, I.M., I. Panfoli, and C. Cugnoli. 1986. Guanylate cyclase in rod outer segments of the toad retina. *Fed. Eur. Biochem. Soc. Lett.* **203:** 73.

Ratto, G.M., R. Payne, W.G. Owen, and R.Y. Tsien. 1988. The concentration of cytosolic free Ca^{2+} in vertebrate rod outer segments measured with Fura 2. *J. Neurosci.* **8:** 3240.

Rispoli, G., W.A. Sather, and P.B. Detwiler. 1988. Effect of triphosphate nucleotides in the response of detached rod outer segments to low external calcium. *Biophys. J.* **53:** 388a.

Stryer, L. 1986. Cyclic GMP cascade of vision. *Annu. Rev. Neurosci.* **9:** 87.

Torre, V. 1982. The contribution of the electrogenic Na-K pump to the electrical activity of toad rods. *J. Physiol.* **333:** 315.

Torre, V., H.R. Matthews, and T.D. Lamb. 1986. Role of calcium in regulating the cyclic GMP cascade of phototransduction in retinal rods. *Proc. Natl. Acad. Sci.* **83:** 7109.

Tsien, R.Y. 1980. New calcium indicating and buffers with high selectivity against magnesium and proton: Design, synthesis and properties of prototype structures. *Biochemistry* **19:** 2396.

Vuong, T.M. and L. Stryer. 1984. Millisecond activation of transducin in the cyclic nucleotide cascade of vision. *Nature* **311:** 659.

Yau, K.W. and K. Nakatani. 1984a. Cation selectivity of light-sensitive conductance in retinal rods. *Nature* **309:** 352.

———. 1984b. Electrogenic Na-Ca exchange in retinal rod outer segment. *Nature* **311:** 661.

———. 1985. Light-suppressible, cyclic GMP-sensitive conductance in the plasma membrane of a truncated rod outer segment. *Nature* **317:** 252.

Zimmerman, A.L. and D.A. Baylor. 1986. Cyclic-GMP sensitive conductance of retinal rods consists of aqueous pores. *Nature* **321:** 70.

Similar Algorithms in Different Sensory Systems and Animals

M. KONISHI

Division of Biology, California Institute of Technology, Pasadena, California 91125

Animals must both recognize and localize the sensory signals essential for their survival and reproduction. Certain cues contained in a signal define its identity and location. Such cues include, for example, the temporal pattern of song for species recognition in crickets and binaural disparities for sound localization in owls. One can predict potential cues and the methods of using them from consideration of the physical attributes of the signal for the task. The discovery of the real cue that is used by the animal, however, requires study of the animal's response to different potential cues.

Once the real cue is identified, the next question is how is it encoded in the language of the nervous system? One can develop an algorithm for the solution of the coding problem. There are, however, many possible ways of solving the same problem. There is, however, no theoretical means of identifying the real algorithm. Analysis of neuronal responses to stimuli and study of the connections between neurons may inform us about the coding scheme because the connections and signals between neurons underlie the coding mechanisms, but what neurons tell depends on what question the investigator asks. As Barlow (1972) pointed out, "...neurophysiology and sensation are best linked by looking at the flow of information rather than simpler measures of neuronal activity."

A neurophysiological investigation of how information is transformed from lower- to higher-order stations may be difficult because information processing is highly nonlinear. Going in the opposite direction, the "top-down" approach is easier in some systems because one starts with the knowledge of what is encoded at the top or at a relatively higher station. The criterion for encoding is the stimulus selectivity of single neurons. The flow of information is therefore inferred from the stimulus selectivities recorded in interconnected stations. For example, the neurons of the external nucleus of the inferior colliculus in the barn owl respond selectively to a combination of interaural time and intensity differences. The neuronal selectivities for these binaural cues have been traced from this nucleus back to the first sites where the selectivities emerge and the pathways for the flow of information be established (Konishi et al. 1988).

The approach that looks for the flow of information has been used only in a few complex neural systems including the visual system of the macaque monkey (for review, see Van Essen 1985; Hubel and Livingstone 1987; Maunsell and Newsome 1987; De Yoe and Van Essen 1988; Livingstone and Hubel 1987, 1988), the auditory system of the barn owl (hereafter referred to as the owl) (for review, see Konishi et al. 1988), and the electrosensory system of the weakly electric fish, *Eigenmannia* (hereafter referred to as the electric fish) (for review, see Heiligenberg 1986). Also, the top-down approach from the auditory cortex to lower-order nuclei in the mustached bat is rapidly achieving the same level of understanding that has been reached in the owl and electric fish (Suga 1984, 1988; N. Suga et al., this volume). The coding processes and the behavioral significance of neurophysiological and anatomical findings are, however, better understood in the owl and electric fish than in any other vertebrate system. Comparisons of these systems show that different sensory systems and different animals use similar procedures in the processing of biological signals, although their neural implementations may vary. Similar comparisons have been made previously (Ulinski 1984; Carr 1986). This paper discusses some of these procedures for sensory processing and their implications for the theory of neural coding.

Separation of Neural Codes for Different Stimulus Variables

Sensory systems separate neural codes for different stimulus variables and configurations. Although a single neuron can carry more than one pulse code as in the auditory nerve of the owl, the processing of different stimulus variables eventually requires the separation of relevant codes. Initial separation of codes occurs in sense organs, ganglia, or in the first station of the brain (Ulinski 1984). The owl's auditory system detects interaural time and intensity differences for sound localization (Fig. 1) (Moiseff and Konishi 1981; Moiseff 1989). The owl's auditory nerve carries the codes for the amplitude, phase, and frequency of sound. Amplitude and phase are encoded by the rate and timing of nerve impulses, respectively. The codes for frequencies are separated in the auditory nerve, since different primary auditory fibers respond to different frequencies. On the other hand, the amplitude and phase codes are not separated in the auditory nerve. Separation of these codes occurs in the cochlear nuclei, the first station in the brain. The owl's cochlear nucleus consists of two

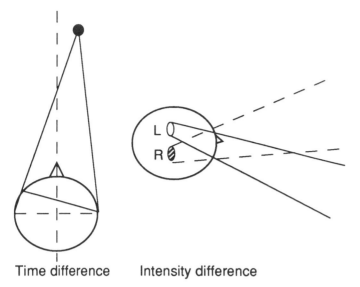

Time difference   Intensity difference

Figure 1. Binaural disparity cues for sound localization. A difference in the length of sound path between the two ears produces an interaural time difference, which varies as a function of the incidence angle of sound relative to the midsagittal plane of the head. The owl uses this function for localization in azimuth. A difference in the amplitude of sound between the two ears results both from the shadowing effects of the head and from differences in the directionality of the two ears. In the barn owl, the left ear is located higher than the right ear relative to eye level, and the two ears are sensitive in different directions. This asymmetry enables the owl to use interaural intensity differences for localization in the vertical plane. Each two-dimensional locus in space is thus uniquely defined by a combination of interaural time and intensity differences.

spatially separate populations of neurons. Both populations receive both the amplitude and phase codes, but one, nucleus angularis, preserves only the amplitude code, and the other, nucleus magnocellularis, largely preserves the phase code (Sullivan and Konishi 1984; Takahashi et al. 1984). The projections from these nuclei to the midbrain station, the inferior colliculus, are separate (Takahashi and Konishi 1989a,b). There are therefore two parallel pathways in the brainstem of the owl.

The electric fish uses sinusoidal electrical signals to orient and navigate in murky water. Fish avoid jamming one another by raising or lowering the frequency of their signals, always changing in the direction that maximizes the frequency difference between the two. A fish detects changes in the amplitude and phase of the beat waveform, resulting from the adding of its own signal and the signal of the neighbor, to determine whether it should lower or raise its frequency to avoid jamming (Fig. 2) (Heiligenberg 1986). Two different classes of electroreceptors encode amplitude and phase. Although these receptors are intermixed over the entire body surface, the neurons that receive input from the receptors are separated in different layers of the electrosensory lateral line lobe, the first station of the brain electrosensory pathway. These layers give rise to separate pathways for amplitude and phase, as in the owl.

Similarly, visual neurons sensitive to different stimulus variables are separated in different layers of the retina, the optic tectum, the lateral geniculate body, and the visual cortex (Maturana et al. 1960; Lettvin et al. 1961; for review, see Rodieck 1979). In the macaque monkey's visual system, magnocellular and parvocellular optic ganglion cells have different morphological and physiological properties (Bowling and Michael 1980; Michael 1988). Magnocellular neurons are fast responding and are sensitive to contrast, but they are color blind and poor in spatial resolution, whereas parvocellular neurons are characterized by color selectivity, high spatial resolution, slow response, and low contrast sensitivity. Magnocellular neurons project to the bottom two layers, and parvocellular neurons project to the top four layers of the lateral geniculate body (Kaplan and Shapley 1982; Perry et al. 1984; Michael 1988).

Specialized Neural Circuits for Salient Cues

The brain contains special circuits to detect salient cues that are not directly encoded in single primary sensory neurons. Examples of these cues include binaural and binocular disparities, orientation, velocity, and echo delays. Although the existence of special circuits for the detection of salient cues would seem obvious, a single neural network that detects more than one such cue cannot be excluded. For example, the oscillator circuits of invertebrates can produce more than one pattern of output by chemical modulation of the synapses and membrane ion channels of selected neurons (Getting 1989; Marder 1989). Whether this sort of modulation regulates the property of sensory detector circuits remains to be investigated.

The existence of special circuits has been proposed in various models of sensory systems, such as circuits for the detection of the direction of stimulus movement in the compound eye of the fly and the rabbit retina, for binocular disparity in the mammalian visual cortex, and for binaural time differences (Jeffress 1948; Reichardt 1961; Barlow et al. 1964; Julesz 1971). The search for the real circuits of this sort has been generally unsuccessful. The circuit for the detection of interaural time differences in the owl's brainstem is a notable exception. Like Jeffress's model, this circuit consists of delay lines and coincidence detectors (Figs. 3 and 4) (Sullivan and Konishi 1986; Carr and Konishi 1988). In the electric fish, circuits for the comparison of the phase angle and amplitude of electrical signals between different body areas have been identified (Maler 1979; Carr et al. 1986a,b; Shumway and Maler 1989).

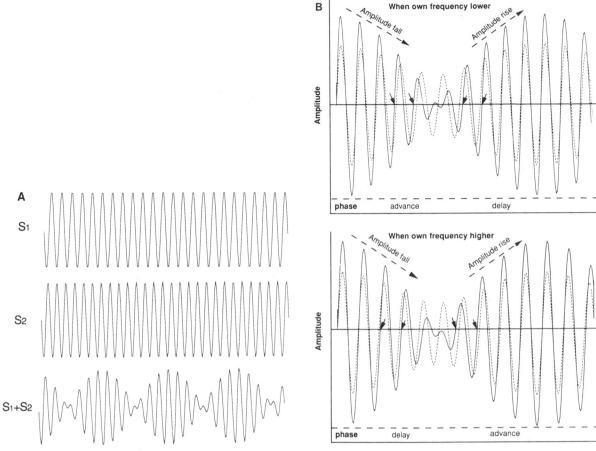

Figure 2. Determination of the sign of frequency differences by electric fish, *Eigenmannia*. (*A*) Electrical signals. *Eigenmannia* generates sinusoidal electrical signals for navigation and orientation. When an individual (S_1) encounters another individual (S_2), they avoid jamming each other by changing the frequency of their signals. The fish uses the beat waveform ($S_1 + S_2$) to determine whether its own frequency is higher or lower. (*B*) The fish uses differences in the phase and amplitude of the beat waveform between different body loci to determine the sign of frequency differences. In this figure, the solid-line and dotted-line waveforms show different degrees of contamination of S_1 by S_2. The solid-line waveform is more contaminated and registered at one body locus, and the dotted-line waveform at another locus. The small arrowheads indicate the phase relationships between the two waveforms. The left-slanted arrowheads indicate that the phase of the solid-line waveform is advanced relative to that of the dotted-line waveform. When these phase relationships and the rise and fall of amplitude are combined, the sign of frequency differences can be uniquely determined. Thus, the sequence, a fall in amplitude with a phase advance followed by a rise in amplitude with a phase delay, indicates that the fish's own frequency is lower than that of the other fish.

Transmission of Information by Coded Lines

Eventual transformation of codes to "coded lines" is a universal operation in all sensory systems. In this scheme, relevant sensory information is transferred from one neuron to the next, not because the recipient neuron sorts out signals encoded in impulses, but simply because the two neurons are connected. The time comparison circuits of owls and electric fish mentioned above receive information about phase from phase-locked spikes. The output of each phase-disparity circuit of the electric fish carries the code for a "phase difference," but this code no longer uses the timing of impulses (cf. Fig. 3). Although the output fibers of the owl's nucleus laminaris carry phase-locked spikes, the phase information so conveyed is not used by the recipient stations. The neurons of these stations lack the morphological specializations necessary for the pre-

servation of phase information such as calycine synapses, yet different neurons respond selectively to different ranges of interaural phase disparities. All higher-order neurons that receive input directly or indirectly from the nucleus laminaris are selective for interaural time difference.

New coded lines emerge at all levels. Sound frequency is not encoded in the number of impulses but by coded lines, which ultimately derive their frequency selectivities from the electromechanical properties of the basilar membrane-hair cell complex. Neuronal selectivities for movement, stimulus orientation, and binocular disparity emerge for the first time in the primary visual cortex in the macaque monkey, and color, movement, and orientation-selective neurons are segregated in different layers or areas. These selectivities are line-coded and conveyed by parallel channels to higher-order stations in the extrastriate visual

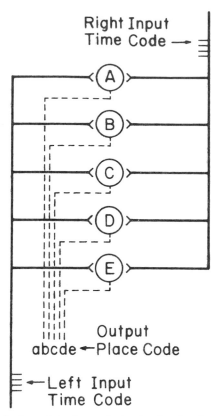

Right Input Time Code →

Output abcde ← Place Code

← Left Input Time Code

Figure 3. A model of neural circuits for the detection of interaural time differences. It uses the principles of coincidence detection and delay lines. Binaural neurons, A, B, C, D, and E, fire maximally only when impulses from the two sides arrive simultaneously. Except for C, the paths for impulse transmission to each neuron are different between the two sides. These asymmetries cause interaural differences in the arrival time of impulses. A neuron fires maximally when an imposed interaural time difference compensates for the asymmetry in impulse transmission time. This array of neurons thus encodes systematically different azimuthal locations of sound.

cortex (Hubel and Livingstone 1987; Maunsell and Newsome 1987; De Yoe and Van Essen 1988; Livingstone and Hubel 1988).

The above comparison of the starting points of coded lines shows that code transformation to coded lines occurs as soon as relevant stimulus properties are detected. Just as neural codes for primary stimulus variables are separated, so are those for line-coded cues. Thus, the establishment of coded lines leads to the separation of neural codes for different cues. Line-coding obviates the need to reproduce at different levels of neural systems the same detection mechanisms every time the relevant information is needed.

Convergence of Parallel Pathways

Parallel pathways for the separate processing of different cues may reunite in higher-order stations. Such convergence serves several different purposes. In the owl's auditory system, interaural time differences are detected in each frequency band by the special circuit

mentioned above. Interaural time differences are measured as phase differences in different frequency channels. These channels are separate in all stations below the external nucleus of the inferior colliculus. In these lower stations, neurons respond to more than one interaural time difference because the time differences separated by integer multiples of the stimulus period give rise to the same phase difference. This phenomenon is termed phase ambiguity. The convergence of different frequency channels on single neurons in the external nucleus of the inferior colliculus eliminates phase ambiguous responses in these neurons, thus enabling them to encode the true interaural time difference (Takahashi and Konishi 1986).

Similarly, the electric fish must gather phase and amplitude information from a large area of its body surface to determine the sign of frequency differences. If a fish is experimentally prevented from receiving electrical signals from a large area of its body surface, it cannot discriminate between the signs of frequency differences. Under these conditions, neurons of the prepacemaker nucleus that are sensitive to differences in frequency fail to detect the sign of frequency differences. These uncertainties are partly due to the fact that phase disparities between different body areas vary with the relative orientation of the two fish. The neurons of the prepacemaker nucleus can determine the sign of frequency differences independently of fish orientation because they normally receive inputs from a large part of the body surface (Kawasaki et al. 1988b; Keller 1988; Keller and Heiligenberg 1989). Similarly, the convergence of parallel channels in the visual system appears to underlie the position-independent responses of neurons to stimulus properties, such as orientation (Hubel and Wiesel 1962), and complex stimulus configurations, such as hands and faces (Gross et al. 1972; Perret et al. 1982; Kendrick and Baldwin 1987).

Another role of convergence is the creation of new coordinate systems and stimulus dimensions in sensory perception. The convergence of the intensity and time-processing pathways in the owl gives rise to neurons that respond neither to interaural time nor to intensity differences alone but to a combination of the two. These neurons encode auditory space because the combinations of time and intensity differences define the coordinates of auditory space in the owl. In the monkey visual system, the magnocellular and parvocellular pathways appear to converge in several different areas of the cortex (Van Essen 1985). These points of convergence may be responsible for such phenomena as the detection of structure from motion and shape from shading (De Yoe and Van Essen 1988).

Hierarchy, Single Neurons, and Networks

Sensory systems process stimuli in hierarchically organized neural networks. When a system contains parallel pathways, each pathway may be hierarchically organized. In a hierarchical system, neurons at higher

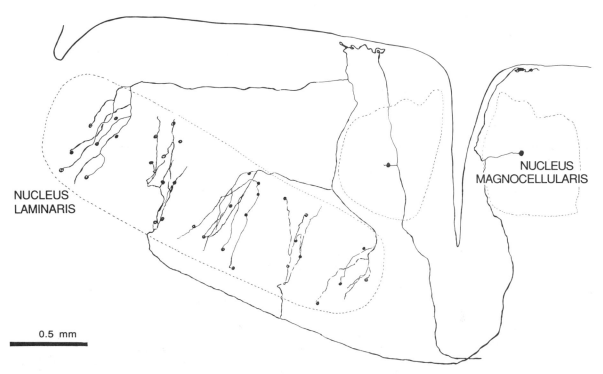

Figure 4. Neural circuits for the detection of interaural time differences. Nucleus magnocellularis is one of the first brain stations in the owl's auditory system. Nucleus laminaris receives inputs from both the ipsilateral and contralateral magnocellular nuclei. The figure shows axon collaterals from single ipsilateral and contralateral neurons projecting into nucleus laminaris, which contain binaural neurons. For the sake of clarity, the ipsilateral and contralateral axons are shown separately, although they interdigitate in reality. These interdigitating axons serve as delay lines, and the laminaris neurons serve as coincidence detectors. Interaural phase differences are computed separately for each frequency band.

stations are selective for more complex combinations and configurations of stimulus variables than those at lower stations. The neuron at the top of the hierarchy represents the results of the sum total of the computations that take place in processing the signal. Sherrington (1941) called such a neuron a "pontifical cell," although he rejected the idea of mind represented by one such cell. The argument against the usefulness of the concept of a pontifical neuron was best expressed by Marr (1982) when he wrote, ". . . Suppose, for example, that one actually found the apocryphal grandmother cell (a cell that fires only when one's grandmother comes into view). Would that really tell us anything much at all? It would tell us that it existed—Gross's hand-detectors tell us almost that—but not why or even how such a thing may be constructed from the outputs of previously discovered cells. Do the single-unit recordings—the simple and complex cells—tell us much about how to detect edges or why one would want to, except in a rather general way through arguments based on economy and redundancy? If we really knew the answers, for example, we should be able to program them on a computer. But finding a hand-detector certainly did not allow us to program one."

One of the problems in the study of these "object-specific" neurons is to identify the salient cues that the neurons and animal detect for the recognition of the object. Once the cues are defined, the origin and trans-

mission of neuronal selectivities for them can be studied. For further discussion of object-specific neurons, there are two points that need clarification. One is the expression, single neurons; a single cell may be selective for a complex stimulus, but it does not perform all the computations necessary for the recognition of the stimulus. A single neuron in a network is nothing but a nodal point, although the point may be a site of complex integrative processes. Tapping of such a point can reveal the results of some of the computations carried out by the network. When a network is hierarchically organized, the neuron at the top of the hierarchy will represent the results of all computations by the network. The second point concerns the idea that there ought to be only one cell at the top of the hierarchy. Because there is no theoretical reason to reject such an idea, one must rely on the results of observational and experimental studies.

In both the owl and electric fish, we know the algorithms for the genesis of the stimulus selectivity of neurons at the top of the hierarchically organized networks. In other words, we know the connections and processes underlying the stimulus selectivity of these object-specific neurons. Figure 5 summarizes the algorithm for sound localization by the owl and that for jamming avoidance response by the electric fish. In this figure, the hierarchy of processing can be compared with that of networks. Thus, in these systems, the neurons at the top of the hierarchy do represent the

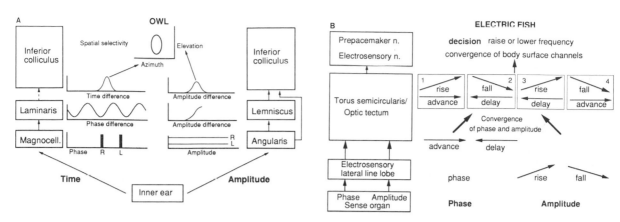

Figure 5. Hierarchical organization. In both the owl's auditory system (*A*) and the electric fish's electrosensory system (*B*), biologically relevant signals are processed in hierarchically organized neural networks. Primary stimulus variables, such as the phase and amplitude of sinusoidal signals, are encoded in the sense organ. The neural codes for these stimulus variables are routed to different parallel pathways in the first brain station. The stimulus configuration for the detection of relevant signals are detected by special neural circuits in higher-order stations. The parallel pathways that process different cues for the detection of the same signal converge in higher-order stations, where neuronal selectivity for a combination of the different cues emerges. In general, neuronal stimulus selectivity becomes narrower and less ambiguous as one ascends the hierarchy. The stimulus selectivity of the neurons at the top of the hierarchy is the result of all the computations that are carried out by the networks. The stimulus selectivity of these neurons is very much like that of the whole animal. In *A*, the ordinate of all graphs shows the number of impulses. The bar histogram shows the sensitivity of neurons to stimulus phase. Phase information is conveyed to both cochlear nuclei, but only the nucleus magnocellularis retains the phase code. The two magnocellular nuclei send the right (R) and left (L) phase values in each frequency band to nucleus laminaris, which detects and encodes phase differences. The sinusoidal curve next to nucleus laminaris shows neuronal responses to interaural time differences that give rise to the same phase difference. The cochlear nucleus angularis abandons the phase code but retains the amplitude code; the line graph shows how a right and left intensity difference is encoded in the discharge rate of angularis neurons. This information is sent to one of the lemniscal nuclei and the inferior colliculus. Partial selectivity to interaural intensity differences emerges in the lemniscal nucleus (Manley et al. 1988). Convergence of the time and intensity pathways in the inferior colliculus creates neurons selective for a combination of intensity and time disparities. These neurons have spatial receptive fields in which the azimuthal and elevational position and dimension are determined, respectively, by the neurons' selectivity to interaural time and intensity differences. In *B*, the arrows pointing to the right and left indicate neurons sensitive to phase advance and delay, respectively. These neurons occur in lamina 6 of the torus semicircularis. Numbers 1, 2, 3, and 4 indicate four different neuron types (in deeper layers of the torus semicircularis) that are selective for four different combinations of phase and amplitude combinations mentioned in Fig. 2B. The prepacemaker nucleus contains neurons that discriminate the sign of frequency differences.

final results of the computations that occur in all of the lower-order networks (Konishi et al. 1988; Rose et al. 1988). In both the owl and the electric fish, experimental disruptions of any of these computational processes have profound effects on the selectivity of the neurons at the top of the hierarchy (Takahashi et al. 1984; Heiligenberg 1986).

The hierarchies shown in Figure 5 appear simple without feedback loops, although such connections are known in the electric fish (Bastian 1986; Carr and Maler 1986; Bastian and Bratton 1990; Bratton and Bastian 1990). Hierarchical organizations are, however, evident in even more complex systems such as the macaque visual system in which reciprocal connections occur between almost all successive levels above the lateral geniculate nucleus. The anatomical hierarchy in this case is recognized by the feedforward and feedback connections that can be recognized in the laminar organization of the cortex (Maunsell and Van Essen 1983). The hierarchy of processing in the monkey visual system can be inferred from the distribution of different stimulus selectivities in interconnected stations. For example, the lateral geniculate nucleus is anatomically one level below the primary visual cortex. The same rank order applies to these stations in terms

of processing because neuronal selectivity for orientation and the direction of movement is not present in the lateral geniculate but emerges for the first time in the primary visual cortex. Similarly, neuronal selectivity for stimulus velocity emerges in the middle temporal (MT) area which is anatomically at least two levels away from the primary visual cortex (Hubel and Livingstone 1987; Maunsell and Newsome 1987; De Yoe and Van Essen, 1988; Livingstone and Hubel 1988), although the contributions of inputs other than the striate cortex and V2 to the stimulus selectivities of MT neurons make a simple serial hierarchy unlikely (Rodman et al. 1989).

Brain Maps and Coding

The owl's space-specific neurons are arranged according to the location of their spatial receptive fields, i.e., they form a map of auditory space (Knudsen and Konishi 1978a). A similar kind of map is found in the mustached bat; this species presumably measures the distance of a target by detecting the time delay between the emitted signal and the echo from the object. In the auditory cortex of this species, echo delays are mapped, i.e., neurons tuned to different echo delays are systematically arranged (Suga and O'Neill 1979).

Neither the map of auditory space nor the map of echo delays is due to a topographical projection of the inner ear, which maps frequency instead of space or time. The maps of auditory space and echo-delays are "centrally synthesized" in contrast with maps that copy the topographical arrangement of sensory cells, such as the tonotopic, retinotopic, and somatotopic maps (Konishi 1986; Knudsen et al. 1987). In a centrally synthesized map, the mapped variable is computed by a special network in a lower-order station or within the station containing the map, and different values of the variable are systematically represented by an orderly array of neurons.

Neuronal maps present an interesting problem for the study of the coding mechanisms. All maps contain place-codes, meaning that spike number, intervals, and other parametric or stochastic attributes do not uniquely distinguish one member neuron from another. Take, for example, two space-specific neurons at some distance apart in the map; they are tuned to different combinations of interaural time and intensity differences, yet they may fire the same number of spikes with the same temporal pattern. The map sites where firing occurs is thus the only code for the location of the sound source. A neuronal map is, however, not just a two-dimensional matrix of independent variables, but an array with connections between the member neurons. Neurophysiological evidence suggests that the neighboring space-specific neurons of the owl interact to produce a receptive field organization consisting of an excitatory center and an inhibitory surround (Knudsen and Konishi 1978b). Such an interaction may be mediated by the presumed "horizontal connections" between space-specific neurons.

Although brain maps would seem most attractive for the study of distributed coding mechanisms, there is no reason to believe that such mechanisms involve the whole map. What is the minimum map area over which integration must take place for relevant sensations to occur? In addressing this question, one can learn much from behavioral studies. For example, the preattentive discrimination of visual textures uses local features rather than the statistical attributes of the textures encompassing the whole visual field (Julesz 1981).

Object-specific Neurons and Perception

The space-specific neurons of the owl and the prepacemaker neurons of the electric fish are selective for the same salient cues that cause the whole animal to experience the percept of the relevant signal or object. The behavioral role of object-specific neurons either can be inferred from comparison between behavioral and neuronal findings or can be studied directly by ablation or stimulation of the neurons. The stimulus requirements and response properties of these neurons may match qualitatively or even quantitatively with the behavioral responses of the animal. This match has been particularly well established in the electric fish. As mentioned above, just as the fish can behaviorally determine the sign of frequency differences independently of the orientation of the electrical field, so can the neurons of the prepacemaker nucleus. This ability contrasts with the inability of neurons in lower-order stations to distinguish unambiguously one sign from the other. The electric fish is extremely sensitive to differences in the phase angles of the electrical signals between different loci on the body surface. Evidence shows that the fish can behaviorally detect a time difference as small as 1 μsec. The prepacemaker neurons are equally sensitive to such small time differences under the same experimental conditions (Rose and Heiligenberg 1985; Kawasaki et al. 1988a).

In the owl, space-specific neurons respond only to sound coming from a restricted area in space because they are tuned to the combination of interaural time and intensity differences that results when the sound source is located in the restricted area. Similarly, a combination of interaural time and intensity differences causes the owl to turn its head in the direction predicted from the binaural disparities. The owl hears two signals, one in each ear, yet it "perceives" a single phantom source, when the two signals are identical except for disparities in time and intensity between the ears. The same phenomenon in man is known as binaural fusion. The connections and signals of the network that the space-specific neurons represent underlie the perception of location, and the activity of these neurons presumably creates the percepts of spatial loci.

Although comparisons of behavior and neuronal responses provide indirect evidence for the perceptual role of object-specific neurons, direct evidence is difficult to obtain. Lesions and stimulation are usually regarded as the ultimate means of testing the behavioral function of neurons. For example, the middle temporal area of the macaque monkey contains many neurons selective for stimulus velocity. A partial lesion of this area temporarily abolishes the learned response of the eye to pursue a moving stimulus and raises the threshold of detecting coherent movement in a random dot display. The recovery from the effects of lesions remains unexplained (Newsome et al. 1985; Newsome and Pare 1988).

Object-specific Neurons in Sensorimotor Transformation

The formation of a percept may cause effector or motor responses, as in the raising or lowering of signal frequency in the electric fish and in the sound-induced head-turning response of the owl. The owl's auditory system transforms binaural disparities into head-centered spatial coordinates. These space-specific neurons project to the optic tectum where they form a joint auditory-visual map of space (Knudsen 1982). In addition, the optic lobe appears to contain maps of head movement vector and speed (Du Lac and Knudsen 1990). How the bimodal map projects to the motor map is not known.

The prepacemaker nucleus of the electric fish is particularly interesting for the discussion of central sensorimotor links (Heiligenberg 1990; Keller et al. 1990). The nucleus contains two classes of neurons: one concerned with the jamming avoidance response and the other with aggression and courtship behavior. The fish modulates its electrical signal to produce "chirps" during courtship. Intracellular stimulation of a single neuron elicits chirps in the fish. Although these neurons fire during spontaneous chirps, an individual neuron may or may not fire. There are about 100–200 such cells in each side of the body, and different subsets of cells might control different chirp patterns. These examples from the owl and electric fish illustrate how object-specific neurons can convey the output of a hierarchically organized sensory system to a specific motor system, which itself is hierarchically organized. In other systems, higher-order interneurons link hierarchically organized sensory and motor systems. Electrical stimulation of a single interneuron in the ventral nerve cord of a crayfish elicits a particular posture or movement (Wiersma and Ikeda 1964). According to recent studies of command neurons in the behaving animal, a group of command fibers contribute to the control of several different motor output patterns, but the amount and nature of the contributions by different fibers vary in different patterns (Hensler 1988; Larimer 1988). Similar principles appear to be used in the cortical control of the arms, hands, and fingers in the macaque monkey (Lemon 1988).

CONCLUDING REMARKS

Contrary to the growing skepticism that the method of single-unit recording is inadequate for the study of complex networks, the proper use of single-unit neurophysiology is in the analysis of network property and function. The two main examples used here show that the single-unit method is a powerful tool for the study of complex networks when certain conditions are met. These prerequisites include knowledge of the salient cues used by the animal, the possibility of manipulating and using the same cues in both behavioral and neurophysiological experiments, and information about the connections between different stations of the neural system in question. The owl and electric fish systems satisfy all of the conditions. The stimulus selectivity of single neurons provides direct access to the coding mechanisms of these systems. Comparisons of the two systems show similar steps and procedures in the genesis of the neural codes for biologically relevant signals. These similarities are not just due to the common evolutionary source from which the auditory and electrosensory systems descended. More complex systems such as the visual system of the macaque monkey appear to use the same basic steps and procedures. These similarities therefore suggest the existence of rules in neural coding that transcend different neural systems,

although the neural implementation of the rules may differ between systems.

Finally, one of the challenges for future research is how to explain dynamic changes in perception such as shifts in attention. In the electric fish, the electrosensory lateral line lobe, the first station in the brain, is controlled by feedback from one of the higher centers, both directly and indirectly via the cerebellum. Preliminary evidence suggests that the indirect feedback pathway may control the gain of all pyramidal neurons, and the direct one may control the gain of local populations of somatotopically arranged pyramidal neurons (Bastian 1986; Bastian and Bratton 1990; Bratton and Bastian 1990). As Heiligenberg (1990) pointed out, local control may help to concentrate attention to the input from a particular part of the body surface. In the case of the owl, it refuses to localize a signal if its head-turning response is repeatedly unrewarded. Similarly, the owl learns to discriminate between rewarding and unrewarding targets presented either simultaneously or separately (Quine and Konishi 1974; Kenuk and Konishi 1975). The site and mechanisms of such decision making and their relationships to the hierarchical system described above remain to be established.

ACKNOWLEDGMENTS

I thank Allison Doupe and Caroly Shumway for reading the manuscript.

REFERENCES

Barlow, H.B. 1972. Single units and sensation: A neuron doctrine for perceptual psychology? *Perception* **1:** 371.
Barlow, H.B., R.M. Hill, and W.R. Levick. 1964. Retinal ganglion cells responding selectively to direction and speed of image motion in the rabbit. *J. Physiol.* **173:** 377.
Bastian, J. 1986. Gain control in the electrosensory system: A role for the descending projections to the electrosensory lateral line lobe. *J. Comp. Physiol. A* **158:** 505.
Bastian, J. and B. Bratton. 1990. Descending control of electroreception. I. Properties of nucleus praeeminentialis neurons projecting indirectly to the electrosensory lateral line lobe. *J. Neurosci.* **10:** 1226.
Bowling, D.B. and C.R. Michael. 1980. Projections of single physiologically characterized optic tract fibres in the cat. *Nature* **286:** 899.
Bratton, B. and J. Bastian. 1990. Descending control of electroreception. II. Properties of nucleus praeeminentialis neurons projecting directly to the electrosensory lateral line lobe. *J. Neurosci.* **10:** 1241.
Carr, C.E. 1986. Time coding in electric fish and barn owls. *Brain Behav. Evol.* **28:** 122.
Carr, C.E. and M. Konishi. 1988. Axonal delay lines for time measurement in the owl's brainstem. *Proc. Natl. Acad. Sci.* **85:** 8311.
Carr, C.E. and L. Maler. 1986. Electroreception in gymnotiform fish. Central anatomy and physiology. In *Electroreception* (ed. T.H. Bullock and W. Heiligenberg), p. 319. Wiley, New York.
Carr, C.E., W. Heiligenberg, and G.J. Rose. 1986a. A time-comparison circuit in the electric fish midbrain. 1. Behavior and physiology. *J. Neurosci.* **6:** 107.
Carr, C.E., L. Maler, and B. Taylor. 1986b. A time-comparison circuit in the electric fish midbrain. II. Functional morphology. *J. Neurosci.* **6:** 1372.

De Yoe, E.A. and D.C. Van Essen. 1988. Concurrent processing streams in monkey visual cortex. *Trends Neurosci.* **11:** 219.

Du Lac, S. and E.I. Knudsen. 1990. Neural maps of head movement vector and speed in the optic tectum of the barn owl. *J. Neurophysiol.* **63:** 131.

Getting, P.A. 1989. Emerging principles governing the operation of neural networks. *Annu. Rev. Neurosci.* **12:** 185.

Gross, C.G., C.E. Rocha-Miranda, and D.B. Bender. 1972. Visual properties of neurons in inferotemporal cortex of the macaque. *J. Neurophysiol.* **35:** 96.

Heiligenberg, W. 1986. Jamming avoidance responses. In *Electroreception* (ed. T.H. Bullock and W. Heiligenberg). p. 613. Wiley, New York.

———. 1990. The neural basis of behavior. A neuroethological view. *Annu. Rev. Neurosci.* **11:** (in press).

Hensler, K. 1988. Intersegmental interneurons involved in the control of head movements in crickets. *J. Comp. Physiol.* **162:** 111.

Hubel, D.H. and M.S. Livingstone. 1987. Segregation of form, color and stereopsis in primate area 18. *J. Neurosci.* **7:** 3378.

Hubel, H.D. and T.N. Wiesel. 1962. Receptive fields, binocular interaction and functional architecture in the cat's visual cortex. *J. Physiol.* **160:** 106.

Jeffress, L.A. 1948. A place theory of sound localization. *J. Comp. Physiol. Psychol.* **41:** 35.

Julesz, B. 1971. *Foundations of cyclopean perception.* University of Chicago Press, Illinois.

———. 1981. Textons, the elements of texture perception, and their interactions. *Nature* **290:** 91.

Kaplan, E. and R.M. Shapley. 1982. X and Y cells in the lateral geniculate nucleus of macaque monkeys. *J. Physiol.* **330:** 125.

Kawasaki, M., G.J. Rose, and W. Heiligenberg. 1988a. Temporal hyperacuity in single neurons of electric fish. *Nature* **336:** 173.

Kawasaki, M., L. Maler, G.J. Rose, and W. Heiligenberg. 1988b. Anatomical and functional organization of the prepacemaker nucleus in gymnotiform electric fish: The accommodation of two behaviors in one nucleus. *J. Comp. Neurol.* **276:** 113.

Keller, C.H. 1988. Stimulus discrimination in the diencephalon of Eigenmannia: The emergence and sharpening of a sensory filter. *J. Comp. Physiol.* **162:** 747.

Keller, C.H. and W. Heiligenberg. 1989. From distributed sensory processing to discrete motor representations in the diencephalone of the electric fish, *Eigenmannia. J. Comp. Physiol. A* **164:** 565.

Keller, C.H., L. Maler, and W. Heiligenberg. 1990. Structural and functional organization of a diencephalic sensory-motor interface in the gymnotiform fish, *Eigenmannia. J. Comp. Neurol.* **293:** 347.

Kendrick, K.M. and B.A. Baldwin. 1987. Cells in temporal cortex of conscious sheep can respond preferentially to the sight of faces. *Science* **236:** 448.

Kenuk, S.A. and M. Konishi. 1975. Discrimination of noise spectra by memory in the barn owl. *J. Comp. Physiol.* **97:** 55.

Konishi, M. 1986. Centrally synthesized maps of sensory space. *Trends Neurosci.* **9:** 163.

Konishi, M., T.T. Takahashi, H. Wagner, W.E. Sullivan, and C.E. Carr. 1988. Neurophysiological and anatomical substrates of sound localization in the owl. In *Auditory function* (ed. G.M. Edelman et al.), p. 721. Wiley, New York.

Knudsen, E.I. 1982. Auditory and visual maps of space in the optic tectum of the owl. *J. Neurosci.* **2:** 1177.

Knudsen, E.I. and M. Konishi. 1978a. A neural map of auditory space in the owl. *Science* **200:** 795.

———. 1978b. Center-surround organization of auditory receptive fields. *Science* **202:** 778.

Knudsen, E.I., S. du Lac, and S.D. Esterly. 1987. Computational maps in the brain. *Annu. Rev. Neurosci.* **10:** 41.

Larimer, J.L.. 1988. The command hypothesis: A new view using an old example. *Trends Neurosci.* **11:** 506.

Lemon, R. 1988. The output map of the primate motor cortex. *Trends Neurosci.* **11:** 501.

Lettvin, J.L., H.R. Maturana, W.H. Pitt, and W.S. McCulloch. 1961. Two remarks on the visual system of the frog. In *Sensory communication* (ed. W.A. Rosenblith). M.I.T. Press, Cambridge, Massachusetts.

Livingstone, M.S. and D.H. Hubel 1987. Psychophysical evidence for separate channels for the perception of form, color, movement, and depth. *J. Neurosci.* **7:** 3416.

———. 1988. Segregation of form, color, movement, and depth: Anatomy, physiology, and perception. *Science* **240:** 740.

Maler, L. 1979. The posterior lateral line lobe of certain gymnotoid fish: Quantitative light microscopy. *J. Comp. Neurol.* **183:** 323.

Manley, G.A., C. Koeppl, and M. Konishi. 1988. A neural map of interaural intensity difference in the brainstem of the barn owl. *J. Neurosci.* **8:** 2665.

Marder, E. 1989. Chemical modulation of an oscillatory neural circuits. In *Neuronal and cellular oscillators* (ed. J.W. Jacklet), p. 317. Marcel Dekker, New York.

Marr, D. 1982. *Vision.* Freeman, San Francisco.

Maturana, H.R., J.L. Lettvin, W.H. Pitt, and W.S. McCulloch. 1960. Physiology and anatomy of vision in the frog. *J. Gen. Physiol.* (suppl.) **43:** 129.

Maunsell, J.H.R. and W.T. Newsome. 1987. Visual processing in monkey extrastriate cortex. *Annu. Rev. Neurosci.* **10:** 363.

Maunsell, J.H.R. and C.D. Van Essen. 1983. The connections of the middle temporal visual area (MT) and their relationship to a cortical hierarchy in the macaque monkey. *J. Neurosci.* **3:** 2526.

Michael, C.R. 1988. Retinal afferent arborization patterns, dendritic field orientations, and the segregation of function in the lateral geniculate nucleus of the monkey. *Proc. Natl. Acad. Sci.* **85:** 4914.

Moiseff, A. 1989. Bi-coordinate sound localization by the barn owl. *J. Comp. Physiol.* **164:** 637.

Moiseff, A. and M. Konishi. 1981. Neuronal and behavioral sensitivity to binaural time difference in the owl. *J. Neurosci.* **1:** 40.

Newsome, W.T. and E.B. Pare. 1988. A selective impairment of motion perception following lesions of the middle temporal visual area (MT). *J. Neurosci.* **8:** 2201.

Newsome, W.T., R.H. Wurtz, M.R. Dursteler, and A. Mikami. 1985. Deficits in visual motion processing following ibotenic acid lesions of the middle temporal visual area of the macaque monkey. *J. Neurosci.* **5:** 825.

Perret, D.I., E.T. Rolls, and W. Caan. 1982. Visual neurons responsive to faces in the monkey temporal cortex. *Exp. Brain Res.* **42:** 319.

Perry, V.H., R. Oehler, and A. Cowey. 1984. Retinal ganglion cells that project to the dorsal lateral geniculate nucleus in the macaque monkey. *Neuroscience* **12:** 1101.

Quine, D.B. and M. Konishi. 1974. Absolute frequency discrimination in the barn owl. *J. Comp. Physiol.* **93:** 347.

Reichardt, W. 1961. Autocorrelation: A principle for the evaluation of sensory information by the central nervous system. In *Sensory communication* (ed. W.A. Rosenblith), p. 303. Wiley, New York.

Rodieck, R.W. 1979. Visual pathways. *Annu. Rev. Neurosci.* **2:** 193.

Rodman, H.R., C.G. Gross, and T.D. Albright. 1989. Afferent basis of visual response properties in area MT of the macaque. I. Effects of striate removal. *J. Neurosci.* **9:** 2033.

Rose, G. and W. Heiligenberg. 1985. Temporal hyperacuity in the electric sense of fish. *Nature* **318:** 178.

Rose, G.J., M. Kawasaki, and W. Heiligenberg. 1988. "Recognition units" at the top of a neuronal hierarchy? Prepacemaker neurons in *Eigenmannia* code the sign of frequency differences unambiguously. *J. Comp. Neurol.* **162:** 759.

Sherrington, C.S. 1941. *Man on his nature.* Cambridge University Press, Cambridge, England.

Shumway, C.A. and L. Maler. 1989. GABAnergic inhibition shapes temporal and spatial response properties of pyramidal cells in the electrolateral line lobe of gymnotoid fish. *J. Comp. Physiol.* **164:** 391.

Suga, N. 1984. The extent to which biosonar information is represented in the bat auditory cortex. In *Dynamic aspects of neocortical function* (ed. G.M. Edelman et al.), p. 315. Wiley, New York.

———. 1988. Auditory neuroethology and speech processing: Complex-sound processing by combination-sensitive neurons. In *Auditory function* (ed. G.M. Edelman et al.), p. 679. Wiley, New York.

Suga, N. and W.E. O'Neill. 1979. Neural axis representing target range in the auditory cortex of the mustache bat. *Science* **206:** 351.

Sullivan, W.E. and M. Konishi. 1984. Segregation of stimulus phase and intensity in the cochlear nuclei of the barn owl. *J. Neurosci.* **4:** 1787.

———. 1986. Neural map of interaural phase difference in the owl's brainstem. *Proc. Natl. Acad. Sci.* **83:** 8400.

Takahashi, T.T. and M. Konishi. 1986. Selectivity for interaural time difference in the owl's midbrain. *J. Neurosci.* **6:** 3413.

———. 1988a. Projections of the cochlear nuclei and nucleus laminaris to the inferior colliculus of the barn owl. *J. Comp. Neurol.* **274:** 190.

———. 1988b. Projections of nucleus angularis and nucleus laminaris to the lateral lemniscal nuclear complex of the barn owl. *J. Comp. Neurol.* **274:** 212.

Takahashi, T., A. Moiseff, and M. Konishi. 1984. Time and intensity cues are processed independently in the auditory system of the owl. *J. Neurosci.* **4:** 1781.

Ulinski, P.S. 1984. Design features in vertebrate sensory systems. *Am. Zool.* **24:** 717.

Van Essen, D.C. 1985. Functional organization of primate visual cortex. In *Cerebral cortex* (ed. A. Peters and E.G. Jones), vol. 3, p. 259. Plenum Press, New York.

Wiersma, C.A.G. and K. Ikeda. 1964. Interneurons commanding movements in the crayfish *Procambarus clarki* (Girard). *Comp. Biochem. Physiol.* **12:** 509.

Specialized Subsystems for Processing Biologically Important Complex Sounds: Cross-correlation Analysis for Ranging in the Bat's Brain

N. Suga, J.F. Olsen,* and J.A. Butman

Department of Biology, Washington University, St. Louis, Missouri 63130

Sensory signals are processed by cross-correlating incoming signals with stored information (arrays of filters) in the brain. For the processing of biosonar information, the central auditory system of the mustached bat contains specialized subsystems. One of the most interesting subsystems performs cross-correlation analysis for the processing of distance information conveyed by echo delays (time intervals). This analysis involves (1) delay lines that shift the neural response to an emitted biosonar pulse in the time domain, (2) a multiplication of the neural response to the echo and the delayed neural response to the emitted pulse by frequency-modulated (FM-FM) neurons acting as coincidence detectors, and (3) the creation of a computational map for the systematic representation of echo delays, i.e., target distances. In this paper, we describe the properties of the biosonar pulse of the mustached bat and the neural mechanisms for the processing of distance information thus far explored. Since the auditory system creates subsystems specialized for process-

ing biologically important complex sounds in a species-specific way, we also describe the difference in the neural mechanisms for ranging between different species of bats and speculate on a subsystem specialized for the processing of speech sounds in humans.

METHODS

Mustached bats (*Pteronotus parnellii parnellii* and *P. p. rubiginosus*) were used in our research in auditory neuroethology, since their biosonar signals are complex and highly stereotyped and since the biosonar information conveyed by individual signal elements is known. Single-unit responses to various types of acoustic stimuli were recorded with tungsten-wire electrodes inserted into the central auditory system of unanesthetized bats. The most frequently used acoustic stimuli were a synthesized pulse (P), echo (E), elements of P and E, and combinations of these sounds (see Fig. 1A). The terms P and E are somewhat arbitrary. P was usually delivered earlier than E and/or was usually lower than E in frequency and/or larger than E in amplitude (see, e.g., Suga et al. 1983). The FM-FM

---

*Present address: Department of Neurobiology, Stanford University Medical School, California 94305-5401.

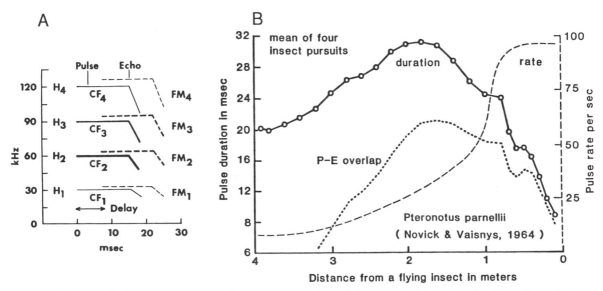

Figure 1. (*A*) Schematized sound spectrogram of a biosonar pulse (—) of the mustached bat and a Doppler-shifted echo (- - -). The pulse consists of four harmonics (H_1–H_4) and eight components (CF_1–CF_4 and FM_1–FM_4). (Adapted from Suga et al. 1983.) (*B*) The duration (—) and emission rate (- - -) of biosonar pulses vary when the bat flies to a flying insect. During this target-directed flight, pulses and echoes overlap as shown by the dotted line. (Adapted from Novick and Vaisnys 1964.)

combination-sensitive neurons described here showed a best response to the P-E pair in which E is delayed from P and is higher in frequency (corresponding to a Doppler shift) and smaller in amplitude than P. In fact, FM-FM neurons show the same response to a pair of self-vocalized pulse and its echo as that to a pair of synthesized pulse and echo (Kawasaki et al. 1988). Therefore, the terms P and E are justifiable by the neural responses.

RESULTS AND DISCUSSION

Biosonar Pulse and Ranging

The mustached bat flies close to vegetation and hunts flying insects with biosonar. Its biosonar pulse is complex, consisting of four harmonics (H_1–H_4), each of which is composed of a long constant-frequency (CF) component and a short frequency-modulated (FM) component. Therefore, there are eight components (CF_1–CF_4 and FM_1–FM_4) in each emitted pulse (Fig. 1A). In the pulse, the first harmonic is the weakest component, containing less than 1% of the total energy, but it can effectively stimulate the bat's own ears by bone conduction. It is expected that the echo's first harmonic is inefficient in stimulating the bat's ears. Accordingly, the bat hears all four harmonics in the pulse but hears only the higher three harmonics in the echo.

The long CF component is suited for velocity measurement because its energy is concentrated at a particular frequency. The short FM component is suited for distance measurement (ranging) because its energy is distributed over a wide band of frequencies. The primary cue for distance measurement is the delay of an echo from an emitted pulse (1.0-msec delay = 17.3-cm distance at 25°C).

The precision of distance measurement for prey-catching, landing, and object-avoidance is probably constrained in several ways: (1) The size of targets for bats is larger than 2 mm. The wing spans of mosquitoes and moths predominantly range from 10 to 40 mm; (2) the bat flies at speeds of 4–9 meters/sec, and the insects also fly at speeds from several centimeters to a few meters per second; (3) on calm days, there is a vertical temperature gradient across the air near the ground. When the bat dives chasing an insect near the ground, for example, the conduction velocity of biosonar pulses and echoes changes 0.6 meter/sec for every degree temperature change. Thus, under natural conditions, the mustached bat can probably resolve differences in distance of several millimeters at best. In fact, the just-noticeable distance difference is about 16 mm for *Pteronotus suapurensis*, a species of the mustached bat family (Simmons 1973).

There is another behavioral observation that relates to distance measurement (Fig. 1B). When the mustached bat approaches a flying insect, it initially lengthens the duration of its biosonar pulse (by increasing the duration of the CF component), presumably to obtain more information conveyed by the CF_2 about wing beat. The bat then systematically reduces its pulse duration (by reducing the CF duration). The rate of pulse emission increases during this target-directed flight. These changes in pulse duration and emission rate begin when the bat is 3–4 meters from the target (Novick and Vaisnys 1964). This indicates that ranging and other biosonar measurements are particularly important at distances less than 3 meters.

If the auditory cortex of the mustached bat has an area specialized for the systematic representation of distance information, how large would it be to represent distances up to 3 meters with a 16-mm resolution? To obtain an idea of the cortical representation of distance information, we assume that the distance neurally represented changes by 32 mm from one column (20 μm wide) to an adjacent column along the distance axis in a specialized cortical area and that the 16-mm resolution is based on the difference between the optimum excitation of a single column and the suboptimum equal excitation of two adjacent columns. Then, the length of the distance axis in this cortical area would be 1.9 mm long to represent distances up to 3.0 meters. Does such a 1.9-mm-long cortical area exist? The auditory cortex of the mustached bat contains the 1.8–2.0-mm-long FM-FM area where a distance axis is formed. In the following, we describe how this distance axis is computed in the central auditory system, after briefly reviewing the basic response properties of FM-FM neurons.

Odotopic Representation in the Auditory Cortex

For echolocation, the bat emits a biosonar pulse (P) and listens to an echo (E). Peripheral neurons respond to P alone and also respond to E alone. The time interval between the two grouped discharges is directly related to the E delay. That is, the target-distance information is coded by the time interval between the grouped discharges. There is no peripheral neuron that is specialized for examining this time interval. In the auditory cortex, however, there are large groups of neurons that respond to neither P alone nor E alone but respond strongly to a P-E pair with a particular E delay. This type of neuron is clustered in the FM-FM (Suga et al. 1978, 1983; O'Neill and Suga 1979, 1982; Suga and O'Neill 1979), dorsal fringe (DF) (Suga and Horikawa 1986) and ventral fringe (VF) areas (Edamatsu et al. 1989) of the auditory cortex.

For example, an FM-FM neuron shows a very weak response with a long latency (15 msec) to P delivered alone, and it shows a very faint response with a short latency (6 msec) to a Doppler-shifted E delivered alone. When P and E are combined with a 9-msec E delay, the weak responses to the individual sounds are superimposed, and the neuron shows a very strong facilitative response. There are 16 signal elements in the P-E pair. By eliminating some of the signal elements from the P-E pair, specific components (e.g., PFM_1 and EFM_2) are found to be essential to excite this neuron. Accordingly, we call this type of neuron an FM$_1$-FM$_2$ combination-sensitive neuron or simply an FM$_1$-FM$_2$ neuron.

By determining the specific components of the P-E pair required to excite a neuron, three major types of combination-sensitive neurons were found in the FM-FM area: FM$_1$-FM$_2$, FM$_1$-FM$_3$, and FM$_1$-FM$_4$. FM$_1$-FM$_2$ neurons are clustered in a ventral band. FM$_1$-FM$_3$ and FM$_1$-FM$_4$ neurons are clustered in dorsal and central bands, respectively. Thus, the FM-FM area consists of three subdivisions. At the boundaries of the bands, there are multi-combination-sensitive neurons such as FM$_1$-FM$_{2,4}$, FM$_1$-FM$_{3,4}$, and, occasionally, FM$_1$-FM$_{2,3,4}$ neurons (Misawa and Suga 1990). Therefore, the FM-FM area has a very interesting functional organization to process complex acoustic signals.

The speed and direction of the frequency sweep in FM signals are important parameters for the excitation of most FM-FM neurons (Suga et al. 1983; Edamatsu and Suga 1989). For example, when PFM$_1$ and EFM$_2$

are delivered as a pair of natural downward sweeps, an FM$_1$-FM$_2$ neuron shows a strong response to each paired stimulus. However, if PFM$_1$ or EFM$_2$ is reversed in sweep direction, the neuron shows no response.

More importantly, FM-FM neurons are tuned to particular echo delays. An FM-FM neuron, for example, shows a weak or no response to P (PFM$_1$) or E (EFM$_n$; $n = 2$, 3, or 4) delivered alone. It shows a strong facilitative response to the P-E (PFM$_1$-EFM$_n$) pair with a particular E (EFM$_n$) delay (e.g., 5 msec) but does not respond to a P-E pair with an E delay either shorter than 4 msec or longer than 7 msec. Its response starts to appear at a 4-msec E delay, is strongest for a 5-msec E delay, and diminishes for E delays longer than 5 msec. The "best delay" to excite this neuron is 5 msec. Each FM-FM neuron is tuned to a particular E delay. In Figure 2, curve a, for example, is a delay-tuning curve of a neuron tuned to a 0.7-msec E delay, and curve e indicates a neuron tuned to a 4.2-msec E

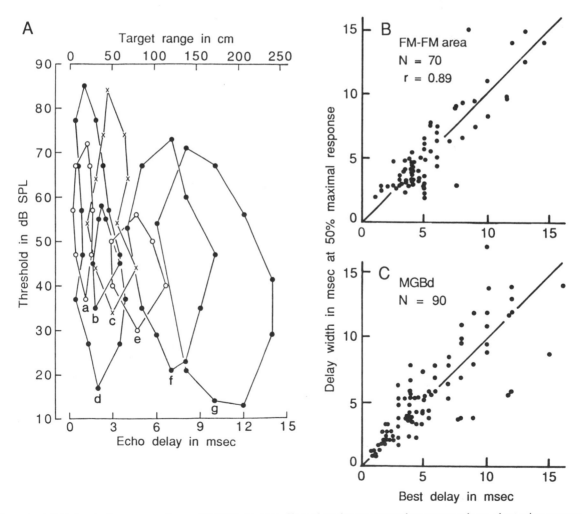

Figure 2. (A) Delay-tuning curves of seven FM-FM neurons. Since they do not respond to strong echoes, the tuning curves are closed at the top. (Adapted from O'Neill and Suga 1982.) (B) The relation between best delays and delay widths of cortical FM-FM neurons (Suga and Horikawa 1986). (C) The relation between best delays and delay widths of thalamic FM-FM neurons. (Adapted from Olsen 1986.)

delay. There is a broad spectrum of delay-tuning curves that span the extent of behaviorally important delays. The widths of delay-tuning curves (delay width) are linearly related to their best delays: the longer the best delay, the wider the delay width (Fig. 2A,B).

Delay-tuning curves are usually spindle shaped or oval (Fig. 2A) because echo amplitude as well as E delay is an important parameter for determining the response of these neurons. For instance, curve e indicates that this particular neuron is tuned to a 4.2-msec E delay and a 43 dB sound pressure level echo. That is, the neuron is tuned to a target of a particular cross-sectional area located at a particular distance.

How is the FM-FM area functionally organized? The FM-FM area is about 900 μm thick, and 40–50 neurons are arranged more or less orthogonally to the surface. When a recording electrode is inserted orthogonally into the FM-FM area, all the neurons recorded in one penetration are tuned to a particular E delay, e.g., 3.5 msec. When an electrode is inserted into a slightly different location, all the neurons recorded are tuned to

a different E delay, e.g., 5.1 msec (Fig. 3B). Therefore, there is a columnar organization in terms of E delay.

How are these columns characterized by particular E delays distributed along the cortical surface? When a recording electrode is inserted rostrocaudally across the FM-FM area, the best delay of a neuron increases (Fig. 3C). Therefore, there is a delay axis. This delay axis is found in each of the three subdivisions of the FM-FM area. It extends from 0.4 msec to about 18 msec. Thus, there is a range axis representing 7–310 cm (odotopic representation). The slope of the range axis up to 150 cm is 20 mm/column, and beyond 150 cm the slope is about 30 mm/column. These neurophysiological data show a beautiful correlation with the behavioral data.

Corticocortical projections indicate that range information flows from the FM-FM area to the DF area and then to the VF area. In both the DF and VF areas, the three main types of FM-FM neurons form separate bands. All of these neurons are tuned to particular echo delays. There is no noticeable difference in response

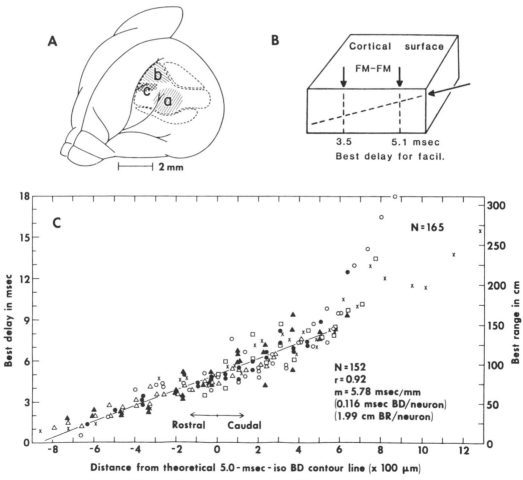

Figure 3. Columnar organization (*B*) and odotopic representation (*C*) in the FM-FM area of the auditory cortex. (*A*) A dorso-lateral view of the left cerebrum. The dotted lines indicate cortical auditory areas. a, b, and c represent the DSCF, FM-FM, and CF/CF areas, respectively. (*B*) Neurons arranged orthogonally to the cortical surface are tuned to an identical echo delay (target distance), e.g., 3.5 msec. (*C*) The best delay (best range) of FM-FM neurons systematically increases along the rostrocaudal axis of the FM-FM area. (Adapted from Suga and O'Neill 1979.)

properties between neurons in these three areas. The DF area is smaller than the FM-FM area, and the VF area is smaller than the DF area. The delay axis extends to 18 msec in the FM-FM area (Suga and O'Neill 1979), 9 msec in the DF area (Suga and Horikawa 1986), and 5 msec in the VF area (Edamatsu et al. 1989). Therefore, range information up to 87 cm is represented three times in the auditory cortex. These multiple odotopic representations may be related to the importance of processing range information at the terminal phase of target-directed flight.

The broader the frequency bandwidth of the signal, the better the signal is for sound localization in elevation and azimuth. Therefore, FM signals are suited not only for ranging, but also for target localization. However, FM-FM neurons are broadly tuned in direction, and their best delays are affected little with changes in the direction of an echo source. They are thus not suited for directional target localization but to target ranging (Suga et al. 1990). Directional information must be processed separately from and in parallel with range information.

Transformation of Temporal Code into Place Code for Ranging

Before the explanation of the basic mechanisms for the transformation of the temporal code of distance information into the place code, two essential points about FM-FM neurons should be clarified. FM-FM neurons are "delay-dependent multipliers," so that the array of FM-FM neurons acts as a cross-correlator for processing distance information. FM-FM neurons extract distance information by comparing EFM_n with PFM_1. FM_1 is the weakest component in the emitted pulse and virtually nonexistent in the echo, so that it is used as the timing reference to measure distances, allowing the bat to distinguish P from E by acoustic parameters alone. Since FM-FM neurons act as delay-dependent multipliers, we have been exploring where and how delay lines are created and where and how multiplication is performed.

Auditory information is conveyed to the auditory cortex through the brainstem auditory nuclei (cochlear nucleus, superior olivary complex, and nucleus of the lateral lemniscus), the inferior colliculus in the midbrain, and the medial geniculate body (MGB) in the thalamus. There are no FM-FM neurons in either the inferior colliculus (O'Neill 1985) or the brachium of the inferior colliculus (Kuwabara and Suga 1988). On the other hand, there are FM-FM neurons in the dorsal (d) division of the MGB (Olsen 1986; Olsen and Suga, 1990). Compared with cortical FM-FM neurons, thalamic FM-FM neurons respond better to individual signal elements in P-E pairs and show less facilitation to P-E pairs. The widths of their delay-tuning curves are

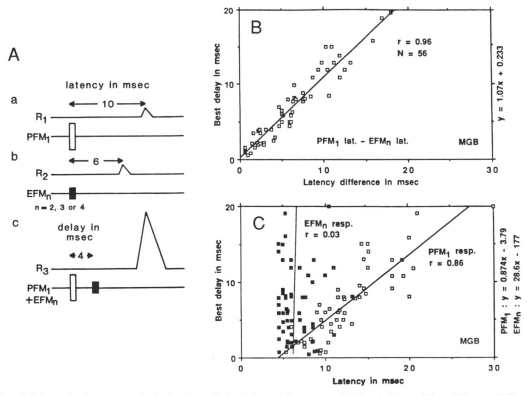

Figure 4. (*A*) Schematized responses (Rs) of a single thalamic FM-FM neuron to PFM_1 (a), EFM_n (b), or $PFM_1 + EFM_n$ (c). (P) Pulse; (E) echo; (*n*) 2, 3, or 4 (Suga 1990a). (*B*) Relation between best delay and latency difference (response latency for PFM_1-response latency for EFM_n). (*C*) Relation between best delay and response latency for either PFM_1 or EFM_n. (Adapted from Olsen 1986.)

very similar to those of cortical delay-tuning curves (Fig. 2). The basic response properties of cortical FM-FM neurons including amplitude selectivity are present in thalamic FM-FM neurons. It is thus clear that signals from FM_1-responding neurons and signals from FM_n-responding neurons in the inferior colliculus converge on the same neurons in the MGBd to create FM-FM neurons and that these thalamic FM-FM neurons project to the FM-FM area of the auditory cortex. These electrophysiological data are verified by the anatomical data (Olsen 1986; Olsen and Suga, 1990).

In the MGB, most FM-FM neurons respond to FM_1 alone and also to FM_n alone. When FM_1 is delivered alone, an FM-FM neuron shows a weak response with a long latency, e.g., 10 msec. When FM_n is delivered alone, the same neuron shows a weak response but with a short latency, e.g., 6 msec (Fig. 4A). Thus, there is a 4-msec latency difference in this example. When FM_1 and FM_n are combined with a 4-msec FM_n (E) delay, the weak responses evoked by the individual sounds coincide and the best facilitative response is evoked. The best delay for the facilitative response is the same as the latency difference.

For thalamic FM-FM neurons, the best delay is linearly related to the latency difference with a slope close to 1.0 (Fig. 4B). Interestingly, the response latency for FM_1 is long and linearly related to the best delay of a neuron, whereas the response latency for FM_n is short and nearly the same regardless of best delay (Fig. 4C). These data indicate that almost all delay lines necessary for cross-correlation analysis are created by neurons tuned to FM_1. However, this correlation is weaker than that between latency difference and best delay, indicating that a small mismatch between a best delay and an FM_1 response latency is adjusted by neurons tuned to FM_n.

As described above, FM-FM neurons are created in the MGB. So, the next question asks, where are delay lines created, in the thalamus or in a subthalamic nucleus? Auditory information is conveyed to the inferior colliculus from the cochlea through the lateral lemniscus and from there to the MGB through the brachium of the inferior colliculus. At the brachium (the output of the inferior colliculus), almost all neurons are tuned to particular single frequencies (i.e., not combination sensitive). Neurons responding to FM_1 show long laten-

cies and a broad distribution of latencies (3.5–15 msec), but neurons responding to FM_n show short latencies and a tight distribution (3.5–6.5 msec). Therefore, the delay lines are created at least to some extent by subthalamic nuclei. Which nucleus does create the delay lines? At the dorsal end of the lateral lemniscus (the input to the inferior colliculus), response latencies are short and nearly the same regardless of whether neurons are tuned to FM_1 or FM_n (3.0–6.2 msec). Therefore, delay lines are created in the inferior colliculus (Kuwabara and Suga 1988).

The inferior colliculus is a huge nucleus and has a latency axis from 4 to 12 msec within its main nucleus. In other words, there are delay lines of up to 8 msec within the inferior colliculus (Hattori and Suga 1989). There are three problems. Delay lines of up to 8 msec exist for neurons responding to FM_n and those responding to FM_1. The distributions of response latencies of collicular neurons do not match those at the brachium of the inferior colliculus. The delay axis of the FM-FM area extends to 18 msec (Suga and O'Neill 1979). The exceptionally long best delay observed is 23 msec for both the auditory cortex (Suga and Horikawa 1986) and the MGB (Olsen 1986). The delay lines in the main nucleus of the inferior colliculus alone are not enough to account for the full range of best delays. In rats, the response latencies of neurons in the dorsal cortex of the inferior colliculus are generally longer than those of neurons in the main nucleus (Horikawa and Murata 1988). In the mustached bat, the response latencies of neurons in the dorsal cortex and their projection to the MGBd remains to be studied.

The data obtained from the MGB (Olsen 1986) and the auditory cortex (Edamatsu and Suga 1989) indicate that the response of FM-FM neurons to a particular E delay is contrasted by lateral inhibition operating in the E-delay domain. In Figure 5, for example, an FM_1-FM_4 neuron shows a very poor response to PFM_1 with a 12-msec latency and a clear response to EFM_4 with a 6-msec latency. When PFM_1 and EFM_4 are paired, there is no response at all for 0- and 1-msec EFM_4 delays. This indicates that the long-latency response to PFM_1 is preceded by inhibition. (This is a reason why the complete pulse containing both FM_1 and FM_n does not excite FM-FM neurons.) It also indicates that the short-latency response to EFM_4 is followed by inhibi-

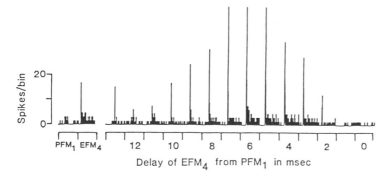

Figure 5. Inhibition and facilitation of the response of a thalamic FM_1-FM_4 neuron to EFM_4 as a function of echo delay. The series of peri-stimulus-time-cumulative (PSTC) histograms represent responses to PFM_1 alone, EFM_4 alone, and PFM_1-EFM_4 pairs with different EFM_4 delays from 13 to 0 msec. The neuron's response to EFM_4 is facilitated at echo delays between 3 and 8 msec (best delay = 6 msec) but is inhibited at shorter and longer echo delays. Each histogram is 50 msec long. (Adapted from Olsen 1986.)

tion. The best delay of this neuron is 6 msec. At 11- and 12-msec EFM_4 delays, the response is smaller than that to EFM_4 alone, indicating that the excitatory response to PFM_1 is also followed by inhibition. In other words, the response of the FM-FM neuron is inhibited to E delays that are too short or too long for the neuron. Delay-tuning curves for facilitative response are often sandwiched between inhibitory delay-tuning curves.

In relation to long delay lines, the inhibition occurring prior to the long-latency PFM_1 response is important. In thalamic FM-FM neurons, best delays longer than 4 msec are usually associated with inhibition (Olsen 1986; J.F. Olsen and N. Suga, in prep.). We thus hypothesized that delay lines shorter than 4 msec are created by axonal and synaptic delays, but those longer than 4 msec are created by synaptic inhibition. The width of a delay-tuning curve is linearly related to best delay: the longer the best delay, the wider is the width of a delay tuning curve (Fig. 2C). This relationship cannot be easily explained by the addition of synaptic jitter through multiple excitatory interneurons but by the assumption that the duration of rebound depolarization is dependent on the duration of the inhibition (the delay line).

A logical reconstruction of the data obtained from subcortical auditory nuclei indicates the computational neural network for ranging shown in Figure 6 (Suga 1990a). For simplicity, circuits for lateral inhibition in the E-delay domain, frequency-sweep selectivity, and amplitude tuning are omitted from the network. In Figure 6, the array of circles at the center represents the array of thalamic FM-FM neurons. In the auditory periphery, there is an array of neurons tuned to different portions of FM_1 (hereafter, the FM_1 channel). The circle at the bottom left of Figure 6 (PFM_1) represents

a peripheral neuron tuned to a particular portion of FM_1. In the FM_1 channel, a peripheral neuron sends signals to a higher-order neuron (neuron "C") through a circuit associated with forward self-inhibition, so that neuron C responds phasically to an FM_1 stimulus when the stimulus sweeps across the frequency-tuning curve of the neuron. The phasic response of neuron C may be produced by fast adaptation rather than inhibition. (Multiple discharges of action potentials, before multiplication takes place, would introduce a large ambiguity in coding distance information.) Neuron C sends signals to the array of FM-FM neurons through neurons "D" and "E" that create delay lines. Shorter delays are created by different lengths and/or diameters of axons and excitatory interneurons, whereas longer delays are created by inhibition with different durations. In this figure, longer delays are located further right along the array of FM-FM neurons.

In the auditory periphery, another array of neurons is tuned to different portions of FM_n (hereafter, the FM_n channel). The circle at the upper left of Figure 6 (EFM_n) represents a peripheral neuron tuned to a particular portion of FM_n. As in the FM_1 channel, a phasic response is created to maintain accurate timing information. Neuron "A" sends signals to the array of FM-FM neurons through neuron "B." These signals arrive simultaneously across the array of FM-FM neurons. This results in a difference in arrival time (latency) between the two inputs of each FM-FM neuron. The latency difference systematically increases from the left to the right along the array of FM-FM neurons, and it is the same as the best delay for the excitation of the FM-FM neuron. The proximity of an echo delay to a neuron's best delay is coded by impulse discharges.

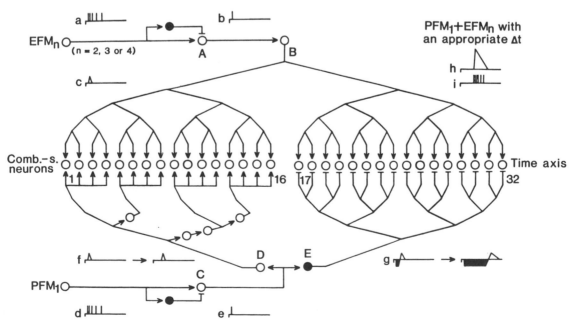

Figure 6. A neural model for processing target-range information by cross-correlation analysis. Essential functional elements in the model are forward self-inhibition (or rapid adaptation), delay lines, and multipliers (Suga 1990a).

For the characterization of delay and multiplication at synapses, we first hypothesized the following synaptic events. PFM_1 and EFM_n each evoke depolarization and hyperpolarization in the system creating FM-FM neurons, as shown in Figure 7A. (This does not mean to suggest that all synaptic events take place in a single thalamic FM-FM neuron. Some of the synaptic events may occur in neurons in subthalamic nuclei to be incorporated into the response of the FM-FM neuron.) The response of FM-FM neurons to P, which contains FM_1 and FM_n, is the result of the superposition of the responses to FM_1 and FM_n, so that it may consist of a faint short-latency, fast depolarization, and/or a faint long-latency depolarization separated by hyperpolarization. The response to E alone is the same or nearly the same as that to FM_n alone because EFM_1 is so weak that it does not excite the FM_1 channel. (Remember that PFM_1 is less than 1% of the total energy of the emitted pulse.) When PFM_1 is followed by EFM_n and the PFM_1-evoked long-latency depolarization is superimposed with the EFM_n-evoked short-latency depolarization, a depolarization consisting of a fast and a slow component is evoked that is respectively mediated by non-N-methyl-D-aspartate (NMDA) and NMDA receptors. The IPSPs are mediated by γ-aminobutyric acid ($GABA_A$) receptors. The PFM_1-evoked IPSP evokes a delayed rebound depolarization. It acts as a delay line. The EFM_n-evoked IPSP shortens the dura-

tion of the facilitative response, so that the responses to P-E pairs at high repetition rates (~ 100 pairs/sec) do not fuse. Both the IPSPs evoked by FM_1 and FM_n contribute to create narrow delay tuning. All these speculations must be tested by iontophoretic applications of various drugs to FM-FM neurons and neurons in the subthalamic nuclei through multibarrel electrodes.

A focal application of bicuculline (a $GABA_A$ antagonist) to thalamic FM-FM neurons should shorten best delays longer than 4 msec, would lengthen the duration of facilitation, and would broaden delay tuning of the neurons, if all the speculated synaptic events are correct and take place in the MGBd. A bicuculline application dramatically increases the duration of facilitation in most thalamic FM-FM neurons tested but has little effect on delay-tuning width. In the FM-FM area of the auditory cortex, a bicuculline application increases the duration of facilitation and widens the delay tuning of most neurons. Therefore, inhibition plays a role in sharpening facilitative delay-tuning in the auditory cortex (Butman and Suga 1989). However, delay width is not different between the cortex and thalamus (Fig. 2). Delay-dependent facilitation is stronger in the cortex than in the thalamus. These data suggest that several thalamic FM-FM neurons converge on single cortical FM-FM neurons to enhance delay-dependent facilitation and that the expected broadening of delay

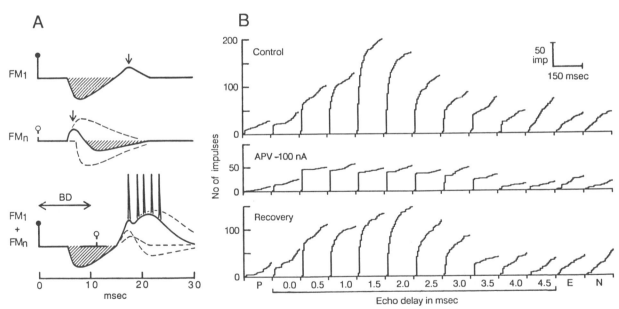

Figure 7. (A) Hypothesis of the synaptic mechanisms for creating a long delay line (long best delay), narrow delay tuning, and facilitation (multiplication). PFM_1 evokes an IPSP followed by a rebound depolarization. EFM_n evokes a fast excitatory postsynaptic potential (EPSP) followed by an inhibitory postsynaptic potential (IPSP). These result from the interaction between the EPSP and IPSP indicated by the dashed lines. The strong facilitative response is evoked when the rebound depolarization evoked by PFM_1 is superimposed with the depolarization evoked by EFM_n. The facilitative response consists of a fast and a slow component. (BD) Best delay. (B) APV (NMDA antagonist) abolishes the slow component of the delay-dependent facilitative responses of a thalamic FM-FM neuron to P-E pairs. Three series of PSTC histograms were obtained 3 min prior to (control), immediately after (APV), and 10 min after (recovery) an iontophoretic application of 100 nA APV. (E) Echo stimulus alone. (N) No stimulus. (P) Pulse stimulus alone. The horizontal bar at the bottom indicates the P-E paired stimuli with different echo delays ranging from 0.0 to 4.5 msec. Each PSTC histogram is 150 msec long. The neuron shows the best response to a 1.5–2.0-msec echo delay.

tuning due to this convergence, however, does not take place because of lateral inhibition.

The facilitative response (multiplication of response) of FM-FM neurons in the MGBd consists of two components: fast and slow. APV (D-L-2-amino-5-phosphonovaleric acid) (NMDA antagonist) abolishes the slow component and makes the facilitative response phasic but does not change the width of a delay-tuning curve. The functional role of the slow component of facilitation is probably to "amplify" the fast component with a burst of discharges and to make the response to a best delay more prominent (Fig. 7B) (Butman and Suga 1990).

Neural Mechanisms of Ranging Differ between Species

The abilities of several species of bats to discriminate target ranges have been accounted for by assuming that these species perform cross-correlation analysis of the FM components of P and E. The neural mechanisms of this cross-correlation analysis differ between species, reflecting the properties of biosonar signals they use. The mustached bat emits CF-FM pulses consisting of eight components (CF_1–CF_4 and FM_1–FM_4), whereas the little brown bat, *Myotis lucifigus*, emits FM pulses with only one harmonic (FM_1) in which frequency sweeps downward about one octave. In the auditory cortex of both species, there are arrays of delay-tuned neurons. As described above, FM-FM neurons in the mustached bat use delay lines created by neurons responding to PFM_1 and extract range information from the combination of PFM_1 and EFM_n ($n = 2$, 3, or 4). The response latency to PFM_1 is always longer than the response latency to EFM_n regardless of PFM_1 amplitude. In contrast, the response latency of FM-FM neurons of the little brown bat is long to a strong stimulus (PFM_1) but short to a weak stimulus (EFM_1). This latency difference is called a "paradoxical" latency shift. These neurons use the paradoxical latency shift (delay line) created by a strong PFM_1 and extract distance information from the combination of the strong PFM_1 and weak EFM_1 (Sullivan 1982a,b; Berkowitz and Suga 1989).

Details of the responses of FM-FM neurons of the little brown bat indicate that neural inhibition is associated with paradoxical latency shift. That is, the strong FM_1 evokes inhibition at short latency and then rebounds excitation (a long-latency excitatory response). In contrast, the weak FM_1 is below the threshold for inhibition but evokes a short latency excitation. When the strong FM_1 (P) and the weak FM_1 (E) are paired so that the long-latency excitation is superimposed on the short-latency excitation, the neuron shows a facilitative response. In the mustached bat, inhibition is associated with a long latency response to FM_1, as already described. Thus, inhibition is a most likely mechanism for creating the delay lines required for the processing of range information in both species.

The big brown bat, *Eptesicus fuscus*, emits short FM pulses with 2–3 harmonics. Higher harmonics appear in later portions of the pulse. In this species, FM-FM neurons are found in the midbrain (Feng et al. 1978). The response properties of these neurons are different from those of FM-FM neurons in the auditory cortex of the mustached bat and of the little brown bat (Dear and Suga 1989).

Parallel-hierarchical Processing of Auditory Information

It has been known that the auditory system consists of anatomically distinct subsystems (see, e.g., Morest 1964). Each nucleus in the ascending auditory system contains several subdivisions or subnuclei. The MGB consists of three major subdivisions: ventral (v), dorsal (d), and medial (m). The MGBv and MGBd are further subdivided. The MGBv projects to the primary auditory cortex (AI), whereas the MGBd and MGBm project to non-AI. In addition to the major projections, complex overlapping projections also exist (see, e.g., Winer 1988). Therefore, there are at least two subsystems. The MGBv and AI may be called the ventral system, whereas the MGBd and non-AI may be called the dorsal system.

The physiological data obtained from bats, cats, monkeys, and rats are still limited, but these data indicate a functional distinction between the ventral and dorsal systems. Neurons in the ventral system show narrow frequency tuning and consistent, strong responses to single tone bursts. The ventral system shows systematic tonotopic representation. The MGBv contains a low density of NMDA receptors. On the other hand, neurons in the dorsal system show broad frequency tuning and inconsistent or weak responses to single tone bursts (see, e.g., Andersen et al. 1980). The dorsal system shows a vague tonotopic representation. The MGBd contains a high density of NMDA receptors (Monaghan and Cotman 1985). NMDA receptors are probably important for plasticity, learning (see, e.g., Collingridge et al. 1983; Kleinschmidt et al. 1987), and creating combination-sensitive neurons. The dorsal system shows much higher plasticity than the ventral system (Diamond and Weinberger 1986; J.-M. Edeline and N.M. Weinberger, in prep.). It has been speculated that neurons in the dorsal system would respond well to particular complex sounds. According to Buchwald et al. (1988), the dorsal division of the cat's MGB is specialized for processing the cat's cries. In the mustached bat, the MGBd is specialized for processing complex biosonar signals (Olsen 1986; Olsen and Suga 1990).

In the mustached bat, the auditory cortex consists of several functional subdivisions: the combination-sensitive areas and the tonotopically organized AI, which belong to the dorsal and ventral systems, respectively (Fig. 8) (Suga 1984, 1988). The arrays of combination-sensitive neurons examine different combinations of information-bearing elements in biologically important

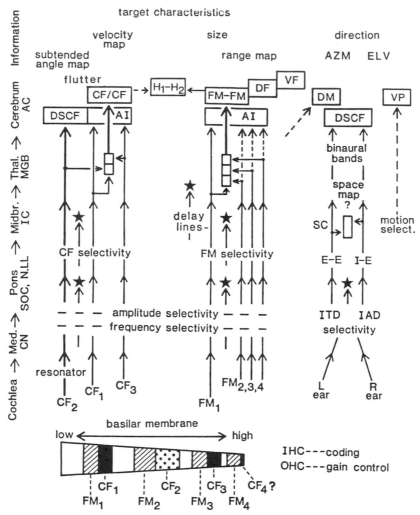

Figure 8. Specialized subsystems perform the parallel-hierarchical processing of different types of biosonar information carried by complex biosonar signals. The CF_1–CF_4 and FM_1–FM_4 of the biosonar pulse and echo are analyzed at different locations along the basilar membrane in the cochlea (*bottom*). The signal elements coded by auditory nerve fibers are sent up to the auditory cortex (AC) through several auditory nuclei (*left-hand side*). During the ascent of the signals, frequency selectivity is increased in some neurons and amplitude, CF and FM selectivities are added to some neurons (arrows with a star). Each star indicates that the addition of selectivity also takes place in the auditory nuclei and cortex. In certain regions of the MGB, two channels processing different signal elements (e.g., CF_1 and CF_2 or FM_1 and FM_2) converge to produce "combination-sensitive" neurons: CF/CF and FM-FM neurons. These combination-sensitive neurons respectively project to the CF/CF and FM-FM areas of the auditory cortex, where target velocity or range information is systematically represented. FM-FM neurons act as delay-dependent multipliers. The delay lines used by them are probably created in the inferior colliculus and in the medial geniculate body. Because of corticocortical connections, the DF, VF, and ventro-anterior areas also consist of combination-sensitive neurons (*center top*). Auditory signals are also projected to the tonotopically organized primary auditory cortex (AI). The AI contains the DSCF area, which has the frequency versus amplitude coordinates to represent velocity and subtended angle of a target. The DSCF area consists of two subdivisions mainly containing I-E or E-E binaural neurons. Signal processing in the auditory system is parallel-hierarchical. (Adapted from Suga 1988.)

complex sounds and extract certain types of auditory information. In this paper, we described the processing of range information by the arrays of FM-FM neurons. In addition, CF/CF combination-sensitive neurons are tuned to combinations of the pulse CF_1 and the echo CF_2 or CF_3 and are specialized for processing velocity information (Suga et al. 1979, 1983; Suga and Tsuzuki 1985). Most of the response properties of FM-FM and CF/CF neurons reflect neural interactions taking place in the MGBd, which utilizes the response properties

created in subthalamic nuclei. For example, amplitude tuning of thalamic FM-FM neurons are mostly created in the inferior colliculus (Kuwabara and Suga 1988). In the mustached bat, the AI is large and contains a specialized area, the Doppler-shifted CF (DSCF) area, where the frequency and amplitude of the CF_2 component of biosonar signals are overrepresented along frequency versus amplitude coordinates (Suga 1977; Suga and Manabe 1982). The DSCF area receives the projection from the MGBv, which shows systematic tonotopic representation (Olsen 1986). The sharp "level-tolerant" frequency tuning and amplitude selectivity of DSCF neurons are created by subcortical nuclei (Suga and Jen 1977; O'Neill 1985; Olsen 1986).

Recent data obtained from the mustached bat indicate that the "electrophysiologically explored" functional cortical areas belonging either to the ventral or dorsal system have different behavioral significances. A bilateral lesion of the DSCF area lengthens the reaction time for Doppler-shift compensation and reduces the amount of this compensation (Gaioni et al. 1988). A bilateral application of muscimol (GABA agonist) to the DSCF area reversibly abolishes fine frequency discrimination (0.05%) near the CF_2 frequency but has no effect on small echo-delay discrimination (Riquimaroux et al. 1989). On the other hand, a bilateral application of muscimol to the FM-FM area reversibly abolishes small echo-delay discrimination (1.0 msec) but has no effect on frequency discrimination (Riquimaroux et al. 1990).

How do these data obtained from the mustached bat and others contribute to the understanding of the central processing of "speech sounds" in the human brain? Speech processing has been understood to be a unique neocortical function. Wernicke's model, based on clinical neurology and adapted by Geschwind (1979), explains fascinating aspects of the processing of spoken and written languages and the programming of speech production. Recent data obtained from positron-emission tomography (PET) studies of human brains indicate that information flow for speech processing within the cerebrum is more complex than that illustrated in Wernicke's model (Petersen et al. 1988). However, the PET studies do not yet give us any information on thalamocortical projections for speech processing.

How do the different subdivisions of the MGB project to different portions of the auditory cortex for speech processing? The anatomical and physiological data obtained from different species of mammals suggest that the information flow from the AI to Wernicke's area is not essential for speech processing. That is, the information flow from the AI to Wernicke's area in Wernicke's model is misleading or even wrong. We believe that speech processing takes place in a specialized subsystem already separated from nonspeech processing at the MGB (Suga 1990b).

The planum temporale contains Wernicke's area, and Heschel's gyrus contains the AI. Since speech processing is usually a function of the left hemisphere, the left planum temporale is much larger than the right. If information flow from the AI to Wernicke's area is essential for speech processing, one would expect that the larger the left planum temporale, the larger the left Heschel's gyrus. However, the opposite is true. When the left planum temporale is much larger than the right, the left Heschel's gyrus is much smaller than the right (Galaburda 1984), suggesting that information flow from the AI to Wernicke's area is not essential for speech processing.

It is difficult to believe that comprehension of complex speech takes place in Wernicke's area with auditory information sent from the tonotopically organized AI (Romani et al. 1982; Pantev et al. 1988) to Wernicke's area. The speech processing system is most likely to be separated from the nonspeech processing system at the MGB. Speech sounds are probably processed to a great extent in the MGBd, which is expected to contain many combination-sensitive neurons. If so, the larger the left planum temporale compared to the right, the larger the left MGBd and/or MGBm are than the right. This anatomical relationship remains to be examined.

The psychoacoustical data obtained by Liberman and Mattingly (1989) strongly suggest that speech sounds are processed independently from nonspeech sounds. Our data obtained from the mustached bat favor this hypothesis. The speech of humans is a specialized species-specific function. Biosonar of bats is also a specialized species-specific function. To understand the specialized function in the human (speech), the studies on specialized functions in animals (e.g., biosonar) may yield important clues. The data obtained from the mustached bat indicate that the specialization is not simply due to a larger population of neurons, but also to the specialized operation of neural circuits and the creation of specialized functional subsystems. The evidence that the central auditory systems of humans and animals share basic principles for processing auditory information will increase with the progress in auditory physiology. We would like to point out that an amplitopic representation in the AI first found in the mustached bat (Suga 1977; Suga and Manabe 1982) has been found in humans (Pantev et al. 1989). (Tunturi [1952] reported threshold representation to the ipsilateral input in the dog's AI. This is quite different from amplitopic representation [Suga 1978].)

If the human central auditory system consists of the above subsystems, psychoacoustical data obtained from humans with stimuli unrelated to speech sounds (e.g., pure tones and clicks) are probably related to the characterization of the ventral system and not the dorsal system. The visual system consists of two subsystems: the magnocellular system for processing motion and depth and the parvocellular system for processing color and form (Livingston and Hubel 1988). We have to test the theory of the dorsal versus ventral systems by incorporating different types of experiments in anatomy, physiology, and psychophysics.

ACKNOWLEDGMENTS

The work described in this paper has been supported by U.S. Public Health Service research grant ROI-NS17333, Office of Naval Research grant N00014-90-J-1068, and Air Force Office for Scientific Research grant 87-0250. J.A.B. has also been supported by National Research Service Award medical scientist-training grant GMO-7200.

REFERENCES

Andersen, R.A., P.L. Knight, and M.M. Merzenich. 1980. The thalamocortical and corticothalamic connections of AI, AII and the anterior auditory field (AAF) in the cat: Evidence for two largely segregated systems of connections. *J. Comp. Neurol.* **194:** 663.

Berkowitz, A. and N. Suga. 1989. Neural mechanisms of ranging are different in two species of bats. *Hear. Res.* **41:** 255.

Buchwald, J., L. Dickerson, J. Harrison, and C. Hinman. 1988. Medial geniculate body unit responses to cat cries. In *Auditory pathway* (ed. J. Syka et al.), p. 319. Plenum Press, New York.

Butman, J.A. and N. Suga. 1989. Bicuculline modifies the delay tuning of FM-FM neurons in the mustached bat. *Soc. Neurosci. Abstr.* **15:** P1293.

———. 1990. NMDA receptors are essential for delay-dependent facilitation in FM-FM neurons in the mustached bat. *Soc. Neurosci. Abstr.* (in press).

Collingridge, G.L., S.J. Kehl, and H. McLennan. 1983. Excitatory amino acids in synaptic transmission in the Schaffer collateral-commissural pathway of the rat hippocampus. *J. Physiol.* **334:** 33.

Dear, S.P. and N. Suga. 1989. Representation of target range in the dorsolateral midbrain tegmentum of the big brown bat. *Soc. Neurosci. Abstr.* **15:** P1293.

Diamond, D.M. and N.M. Weinberger. 1986. Classical conditioning rapidly induced changes in frequency receptive fields of single neurons in secondary and ventral ectosylvian auditory cortical fields. *Brain Res.* **372:** 357.

Edamatsu, H. and N. Suga. 1989. Delay tuning and inhibition of FM-FM combination-sensitive neurons in the ventral fringe area of the mustached bat's auditory cortex. *Assoc. Res. Otolaryngol.* (Abstr.) P38.

Edamatsu, H., M. Kawasaki, and N. Suga. 1989. Distribution of combination-sensitive neurons in the ventral fringe area of the auditory cortex of the mustached bat. *J. Neurophysiol.* **61:** 202.

Feng, A.S., J.A. Simmons, and S.A. Kick. 1978. Echo detection and target-ranging neurons in the auditory system of the bat *Eptesicus fuscus*. *Science* **202:** 645.

Gaioni, S.J., N. Suga, and H. Riquimaroux. 1988. Effects of bilateral ablation of the auditory cortex and/or cingulate cortex on the biosonar behavior of the mustached bat. *Soc. Neurosci. Abstr.* **14:** P1100.

Galaburda, A.M. 1984. Anatomical asymmetries. In *Cerebral dominance* (ed. N. Geschwind and A.M. Galaburda), p. 11. Harvard University Press, Cambridge.

Geschwind, N. 1979. Specialization of the human brain. *Sci. Am.* **241:** 180.

Hattori, T. and N. Suga. 1989. Latency map in the inferior colliculus of the mustached bat. *Assoc. Res. Otolaryngol.* P94 (Abstr.).

Horikawa, J. and K. Murata. 1988. Spatial distribution of response latencies in the rat inferior colliculus. *Proc. Jpn. Acad.* **64B:** 181.

Kawasaki, M., D. Margoliash, and N. Suga. 1988. Delay-tuned combination-sensitive neurons in the auditory cortex of the vocalizing mustached bat. *J. Neurophysiol.* **59:** 623.

Kleinschmidt, A., M.F. Bear, and W. Singer. 1987. Blockade of "NMDA" receptors disrupts experience-dependent plasticity of kitten striate cortex. *Science* **238:** 355.

Kuwabara, N. and N. Suga. 1988. Mechanisms for production of "range-tuned" neurons in the mustached bat: Delay lines and amplitude selectivity are created by the midbrain auditory nuclei. *Assoc. Res. Otolaryngol.* P200 (Abstr.).

Liberman, A.M. and I.G. Mattingly. 1989. A specialization for speech perception. *Science* **243:** 489.

Livingston, M. and D. Hubel. 1988. Segregation of form, color, movement and depth: Anatomy, physiology and perception. *Science* **240:** 740.

Misawa, H. and N. Suga. 1990. Multi-combination-sensitive neurons in the FM-FM area of the auditory cortex of the mustached bat. *Assoc. Res. Otolaryngol.* P274 (Abstr.).

Monaghan, D.T. and C.W. Cotman. 1985. Distribution of *N*-methyl-D-aspartate-sensitive L-[^{3}H]glutamate-binding sites in rat brain. *J. Neurosci.* **5:** 2909.

Morest, D.K. 1964. The neuronal architecture of the medial geniculate body of a cat. *J. Anat.* **99:** 143.

Novick, A. and J.R. Vaisnys. 1964. Echolocation of flying insects by the bat, *Chilonycteris parnellii*. *Biol. Bull.* **127:** 478.

Olsen, J.F. 1986. "Functional organization of the medial geniculate body of the mustached bat." Ph.D. thesis, Washington University, Seattle.

Olsen, J.F. and N. Suga. 1990. Combination-sensitive neurons in the medial geniculate body of the mustached bat: Encoding of target range information. *J. Neurophysiol.* (in press).

O'Neill, W.E. 1985. Responses to pure tones and linear FM components of the CF-FM biosonar signal by single units in the inferior colliculus of the mustached bat. *J. Comp. Physiol.* **157:** 797.

O'Neill, W.E. and N. Suga. 1979. Target range-sensitive neurons in the auditory cortex of the mustache bat. *Science* **203:** 69.

———. 1982. Encoding of target-range information and its representation in the auditory cortex of the mustached bat. *J. Neurosci.* **47:** 225.

Pantev, C., M. Hoke, K. Lehnertz, and B. Lütkenhöner. 1989. Neuromagnetic evidence of an amplitopic organization of the human auditory cortex. *Electroencephalogr. Clin. Neurophysiol.* **72:** 225.

Pantev, C., M. Hoke, K. Lehnertz, B. Lütkenhöner, G. Anogianakis, and W. Wittkowski. 1988. Tonotopic organization of the human auditory cortex revealed by transient auditory evoked magnetic fields. *Electroencephalogr. Clin. Neurophysiol.* **69:** 160.

Petersen, S.E., P.T. Fox, M.I. Posner, M. Mintun, and M.E. Raichle. 1988. Positron emission tomographic studies of the cortical anatomy of single-word processing. *Nature* **331:** 585.

Riquimaroux, H., S.J. Gaioni, and N. Suga. 1989. Muscimol application to the bat's auditory cortex disrupts fine frequency discrimination of biosonar signals. *Soc. Neurosci. Abstr.* **15:** P1292.

———. 1990. Muscimol disrupts temporal discrimination by the FM-FM area of the mustached bat's auditory cortex. *Soc. Neurosci. Abstr.* (in press).

Romani, G.L., S.L. Williamson, and L. Kaufman. 1982. Tonotopic organization of the human auditory cortex. *Science* **216:** 1339.

Simmons, J.A. 1973. The resolution of target range by echolocating bats. *J. Acoust. Soc. Am.* **54:** 157.

Suga, N. 1977. Amplitude-spectrum representation in the Doppler-shifted-CF processing area of the auditory cortex of the mustache bat. *Science* **196:** 64.

———. 1978. Specialization of the auditory system for reception and processing of species-specific sounds. *Fed. Proc.* **37:** 2342.

———. 1984. The extent to which biosonar information is represented in the bat auditory cortex. In *Dynamic aspects of neocortical function* (ed. G.M. Edelman et al.), p. 315. John Wiley, New York.

———. 1988. Auditory neuroethology and speech processing: Complex sound processing by combination-sensitive neurons. In *Functions of the auditory system* (ed. G.M. Edelman et al.), p. 679. John Wiley, New York.

———. 1990a. Cortical computational maps for auditory imaging. *Neural Networks* **3:** 3.

———. 1990b. Subsystems for processing different types of auditory information: Speculation on speech-sound processing. *Assoc. Res. Otolaryngol.* P111 (Abstr.).

Suga, N. and J. Horikawa. 1986. Multiple time axes for representation of echo delays in the auditory cortex of the mustached bat. *J. Neurophysiol.* **55:** 776.

Suga, N. and P.H.-S. Jen. 1977. Further studies on the peripheral auditory system of "CF-FM" bats specialized for fine frequency analysis of Doppler-shifted echoes. *J. Exp. Biol.* **69:** 207.

Suga, N. and T. Manabe. 1982. Neural basis of amplitude-spectrum representation in the auditory cortex of the mustached bat. *J. Neurophysiol.* **47:** 225.

Suga, N. and W.E. O'Neill. 1979. Neural axis representing target range in the auditory cortex of the mustached bat. *Science* **206:** 351.

Suga, N. and K. Tsuzuki. 1985. Inhibition and level-tolerant frequency tuning in the auditory cortex of the mustached bat. *J. Neurophysiol.* **53:** 1109.

Suga, N., M. Kawasaki, and R.F. Burkard. 1990. Delay-tuned neurons in the auditory cortex of the mustached bat are not suited for processing directional information. *J. Neurophysiol.* **64:** 225.

Suga, N., W.E. O'Neill, and T. Manabe. 1978. Cortical neurons sensitive to combinations of information-bearing elements of biosonar signals in the mustached bat. *Science* **200:** 778.

————. 1979. Harmonic-sensitive neurons in the auditory cortex of the mustached bat. *Science* **203:** 270.

Suga, N., W.E. O'Neill, K. Kujirai, and T. Manabe. 1983. Specificity of combination-sensitive neurons for processing of complex biosonar signals in the auditory cortex of the mustached bat. *J. Neurophysiol.* **49:** 1573.

Sullivan, W.E. III. 1982a. Neural representation of target distance in auditory cortex of the echolocating bat *Myotis lucifigus. J. Neurophysiol.* **48:** 1011.

————. 1982b. Possible neural mechanisms of target distance coding in auditory system of the echolocating bat *Myotis Lucifigus. J. Neurophysiol.* **48:** 1033.

Tanturi, A.R. 1952. A difference in the representation of auditory signals for the left and right ears in the iso-frequency contours of the right middle ectosylvian auditory cortex of the dog. *Am. J. Physiol.* **168:** 712.

Winer, J.A. 1988. Anatomy of the medial geniculate body. In *Neurobiology of hearing*, II: *The central auditory system* (ed. R.A. Altschuler et al.), p. 100. Raven Press, New York.

Associative Memory Function in Piriform (Olfactory) Cortex: Computational Modeling and Neuropharmacology

M.E. Hasselmo, M.A. Wilson, B.P. Anderson, and J.M. Bower
Division of Biology, California Institute of Technology, Pasadena, California 91125

A wide range of mammalian behaviors require the recognition of odors. Although the recognition of some olfactory cues may be innate, in many instances animals are capable of learning new odors specific to an individual or object (Halpin 1980; Leon 1987). Rats, for example, display one trial learning in olfactory discrimination tasks (Slotnick and Katz 1974), translating a learning set between different olfactory stimuli with a flexibility usually only seen in the visual behavior of primates. Of course, rats show a preference for using olfactory cues (Nigrosh et al. 1975), but even visually oriented primates are capable of learning subtle discriminations between olfactory stimuli (Takagi 1979; Rabin and Cain 1989).

In our research, we are interested in understanding how the olfactory system of mammals provides the capacity to learn and subsequently recognize complex odor stimuli. The functional requirements of odor identification, coupled with the anatomy and physiology of the olfactory system, have led us to believe that this process may be based on a biological implementation of what is referred to as an autoassociation memory (Haberly 1985; Haberly and Bower 1989; Bower 1990a,b). Abstract models of this type of memory use autocorrelation learning rules to generate stable outputs to complex input patterns (Palm 1980; Kohonen 1984). Such a capacity is important to the olfactory system of mammals, which can identify behaviorally relevant odors consisting of diverse blends of molecules that are sometimes significant only in their relative concentrations (Epple et al. 1989). Abstract autoassociative memories are also capable of generating a previously learned output pattern in response to the associated input pattern even if that pattern is degraded or appears in a different context (Kohonen et al. 1976; Palm 1980; Kohonen 1984). Similarly, mammals show the capacity to recognize odors at very low concentrations or in the context of very different background odors (McCartney 1951).

Beyond these similar functional capabilities of autoassociative memories and the olfactory system, the anatomy and physiology of olfactory networks themselves also suggest an autoassociative basis for olfactory recognition (Haberly and Bower 1989). In particular, several characteristics of the primary olfactory cerebral cortex, or piriform cortex, suggest that this region could be the site of an autoassociative memory (Haber-

ly 1985; Haberly and Bower 1989; Bower 1990a). First, lesions of piriform cortex, which is the largest region of cerebral cortex devoted solely to olfactory processing (Haberly 1985), or its afferent input significantly impair the capacity to learn or retain olfactory discrimination tasks (Slotnick and Berman 1980; Staubli et al. 1987). Second, as shown in Figure 1, the piriform cortex occupies a central position between the sensory periphery and multimodal cortical structures such as the entorhinal cortex and hippocampus (Price 1987), which are

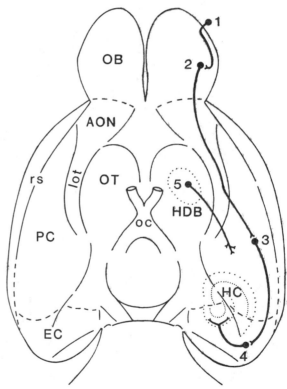

Figure 1. A representation of the ventral surface of the rat brain showing, on the left, the main structures of the olfactory system and, on the right, the main components in the olfactory circuit: (*1*) Receptor cell in olfactory epithelium; (*2*) olfactory bulb mitral cells; (*3*) olfactory cortex pyramidal cell; (*4*) entorhinal cortex pyramidal cell; (*5*) cholinergic neuron in horizontal limb of the diagonal band of Broca. (OB) Olfactory bulb; (AON) anterior olfactory nucleus; (OT) olfactory tubercle; (lot) lateral olfactory tract; (rs) rhinal sulcus; (PC) piriform cortex; (EC) entorhinal cortex; (HDB) horizontal limb of the diagonal band of Broca; (HC) hippocampus.

believed to be fundamental to general memory function (Squire 1986). Third, the afferent input to the piriform cortex from olfactory bulb neurons contains a highly distributed representation of olfactory sensory information because single bulbar neurons respond to a wide variety of odors (Mathews 1972; Tanabe et al. 1975). Such a distributed representation is quite appropriate for subsequent processing by an autoassociation memory (Palm 1980; Kohonen 1984). Finally, the feature of the piriform cortex that is most suggestive of an autoassociative function is its pattern of excitatory neuronal connections. Both the afferent projection from the olfactory bulb and the intrinsic connections within the cortex itself are extensive and diffuse in their distribution (Haberly and Price 1978; Luskin and Price 1983a). As shown in Figure 2, this distributed connectivity is highly reminiscent of more abstract autoassociation memory models (Palm 1980; Kohonen 1984).

In this paper, we describe the interaction of computational modeling and experimental data in our efforts to model the function of olfactory cortex as an autoassociative memory. First, we present results from a structurally realistic computer simulation of the piriform cortex based on previous anatomical and physiological research. We then consider two cases involving the interaction of modeling with results from in vitro brain-slice experiments on the olfactory cortex. In the first case, these experimental techniques were used to confirm the model-based prediction that different piriform cortex synapses would have different synaptic modification properties. In the second case, we present experiments showing synapse-specific cholinergic sup-

pression of excitatory transmission and report preliminary results in which a simplified model of the piriform cortex was used to understand the possible functional significance of this selective cholinergic modulation. Thus, this paper not only describes our recent research results, but also documents several examples of the value of interactions between modeling and physiological techniques in unraveling the functional organization of complex brain circuits.

METHODS

Realistic computer simulation of the piriform cortex. The realistic simulation of the piriform cortex consists of compartmental numerical simulations in which three populations of individual neurons are modeled along with their synaptic interconnections. The properties of the neurons and their connections are taken from real physiological data, and the connectivity pattern is derived from anatomical data. In particular, the models duplicate the extensive and broadly distributed bulbar projections to the cortex, as well as the similarly extensive and diffuse intrinsic excitatory connections within the network itself (Haberly and Price 1978; Luskin and Price 1983a). Typically, the models consist of several thousands of each type of neuron and generate as output physiologically measurable results (e.g., neuronal spike trains, EEGs, and evoked potentials). Figure 3 illustrates the general layout of the model. For details of the mathematical structure of this model, see Wilson and Bower (1989).

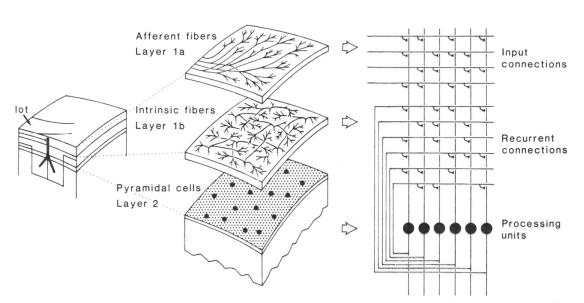

Figure 2. Comparison of the piriform cortex anatomical structure with an autoassociation matrix memory. In layer 1a, afferent input from the LOT forms synapses on the distal dendrites of the piriform cortex pyramidal cells in a diffuse, nontopographic manner. This input may be analogous to the distributed input connections of an autoassociation memory. In layer 1b, intrinsic fibers arising from piriform cortex pyramidal cells in layers 2 and 3 synapse on proximal portions of other pyramidal cell dendrites in a diffuse, nontopographic manner. These synaptic connections may be analogous to the recurrent connections of an autoassociation memory.

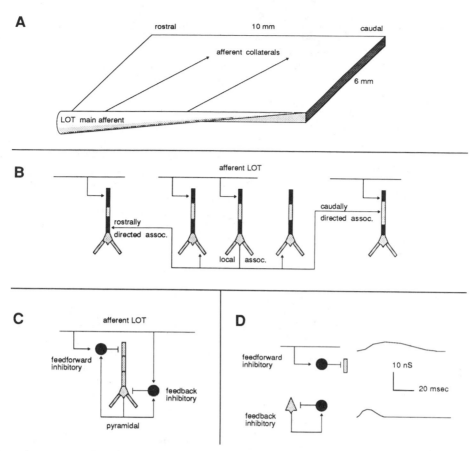

Figure 3. Schematic representation of structurally realistic computational model of the piriform cortex. (*A*) Spatial pattern of afferent input from the LOT. (*B*) Basic circuitry of intrinsic connections arising from piriform cortex pyramidal cells, forming synapses in layers 1b and 3. (*C*) Pattern of interconnection between pyramidal cells and two classes of inhibitory interneurons modeled. (*D*) Temporal properties of inhibitory synaptic conductances induced by the two classes of inhibitory interneurons. (Reprinted, with permission, from Bower 1990a.)

Simplified computational model of piriform cortex. In addition to the structurally complex model of the piriform cortex just described, we also make use of a simplified cortical model to explore more readily the dependence of model results on parameter values. Typically, as in the current example, such a simplified model is used initially to explore a new physiological finding before incorporating the results into the more complex model. In the current case, the simplified model consisted of a set of units with activity levels described by a computational approximation of the following equation

$$a_j(t+1) = \sum_{i=1}^{n} (f[B_{i,j}] - H_{i,j})g(a_i[t]) + A_j$$

Where the activity level a represents the membrane potential of a neuron at a time t. A patterned input A added to this activity represents the effect of afferent synaptic input from the olfactory bulb. A thresholded sigmoid frequency response function $g(a)$ determines the output of all units. The output directly excites other pyramidal cells in the network in proportion to an intrinsic connectivity matrix B, where $f(\ )$ is a saturat-

ing function. It also activates interneurons mediating local feedback inhibition on other pyramidal cells, represented by the inhibitory connectivity matrix H. During the learning phase, a Hebb-type learning rule was instituted at the intrinsic fiber connections with the following formulation

$$\Delta B_{ij} = C^* g(a_i)^*(a_j - x)$$

Where the increment ΔB represents the change in synaptic strength, the constant C determines the sensitivity of the synapse to synaptic modification, and the postsynaptic activity a_j must surpass a threshold x for learning to take place.

In vitro electrophysiology of piriform cortex slices. As described in the introduction, we have used an in vitro brain-slice preparation of the piriform cortex to test model results and to generate new information about the structure of this cortex for use in modeling. Slices were cut perpendicular to the laminar organization of the cortex and maintained following standard procedures (see Hasselmo and Bower 1990 and in prep.). The clear laminar segregation of afferent and intrinsic association fibers in the piriform cortex (Price 1973;

Luskin and Price 1983b) allows differential stimulation of the two fiber systems. Stimulating electrodes placed in layer 1a selectively activate afferent fibers from the lateral olfactory tract (LOT) that terminate on distal portions of pyramidal cell dendrites, whereas electrodes placed in layer 1b activate intrinsic fibers terminating on proximal portions of these same dendrites (Bower and Haberly 1986; Hasselmo and Bower 1990 and in prep.). Extracellular field potential responses to stimulation of layers 1a or 1b were obtained with 3 M NaCl electrodes of about 5-MOhm impedance placed in the layer being stimulated. Individually recorded traces were averaged over a set of 10–30 stimulus trials. Height of synaptic potentials was compared before and after presentation of stimulus trains or before and after perfusion with pharmacological agents at different concentrations.

RESULTS

Olfactory Cortex as Autoassociation Memory

To explore how well the detailed structure of olfactory cortex might support autoassociation memory function, we have spent the last several years building structurally realistic models based on the existing experimental data concerning anatomical and physiological features of the olfactory cortex (Wilson and Bower 1988, 1989, 1990; Bower 1990a). Initially, these models were used to attempt to replicate the periodic or oscillatory behavior induced in the cortex in response to both direct electrical stimulation of its afferents and natural activation of its inputs (Wilson and Bower 1990). Along with suggesting new mechanisms for the generation of this periodic activity, this initial modeling effort also increased confidence that the simulations capture essential structural and physiological features of this cortex. Subsequently, we have investigated the possible functional significance of cortical structure for olfactory object recognition (Wilson and Bower 1988). The following sections briefly summarize several recent results in this regard.

To study the autoassociation memory capacity of the network, the model was provided with input intended to represent loosely the activity of single neurons in the olfactory bulb. Synaptic connections between bulbar neurons and neurons in the olfactory cortex were assigned completely randomly, as were the initial weights of each connection. These connections are depicted diagrammatically in Figure 3. To explore learning in the network, a Hebb-type correlation learning rule was also introduced to govern activity-dependent changes in the synaptic strengths of modeled connections (Wilson and Bower 1988). At the time when these simulations were performed, no information was yet available on the existence or form of synaptic modification in piriform cortex, but evidence for Hebb-type synaptic modification did exist in the closely related hippocampus (Wigstrom et al. 1986), and Hebbian learning rules provide the autocorrelation capacity of many abstract

autoassociative models (Kohonen and Oja 1976; Kohonen et al. 1976; Palm 1980; Kohonen 1984).

Although the learning of natural olfactory stimuli undoubtedly requires quite complex network properties, in our initial investigations of our cortical model, we concentrated on two relatively simple aspects of associative learning. First, we studied the capacity of the model to converge on consistent patterns of neuronal activity in response to particular input patterns. Presumably, if the olfactory cortex is responsible for odor recognition, it should be able to generate consistent neuronal output in the presence of consistent neuronal input. Second, we studied the capacity of the model to generate a stable pattern of neuronal activity in the presence of an incomplete version of the input stimulus. Because the mix of molecules being emitted by any object can vary with, for example, its age or environmental circumstances, it is presumed that olfactory recognition must, to some extent, be insensitive to these variations.

Convergence to stable output. As shown in Figures 4 and 6, the model was capable of learning to generate a stable output when presented with a consistent input pattern. First, in the absence of synaptic modification, repeated presentation of the identical pattern of input activity resulted in a continually varying pattern of cortical activity. However, when synaptic modification was allowed under the same stimulus conditions, the network converged to a stable pattern of neuronal response after several stimulus presentations. For the small network of 100 units modeled in Figure 4, this convergence was relatively rapid, requiring only a small number of presentations. For a larger network of 2500 units, convergence takes longer, as shown in Figure 6. Figure 5A demonstrates that the network could also learn to generate different patterns of activity in response to different patterns of input. The capacity of the structurally complex model of the network has not been rigorously explored, but the simplified model of the piriform cortex described above shows the capacity to store successfully a large number of input patterns.

Pattern completion. The second and perhaps more interesting question addressed with the model was to what extent a stable output, once learned, was resilient to changes in the input pattern. This was tested by reducing the number of active bulbar inputs by half and comparing the response under these conditions to the response of the network to the original full pattern of stimulation. General results are shown in Figure 5B. In the examples, it can be seen that, before learning, reducing the number of active input neurons by 50% resulted in a pattern of activity in the cortex that was only 56% similar to the cortical response to a full stimulus. After learning, however, the same 50% reduction in active bulbar neurons produced a pattern of activity 80% similar to that evoked by the original input. The larger network shows this capacity for completion as well, as discussed below. Accordingly, the model demonstrates that once learned, specific cortical

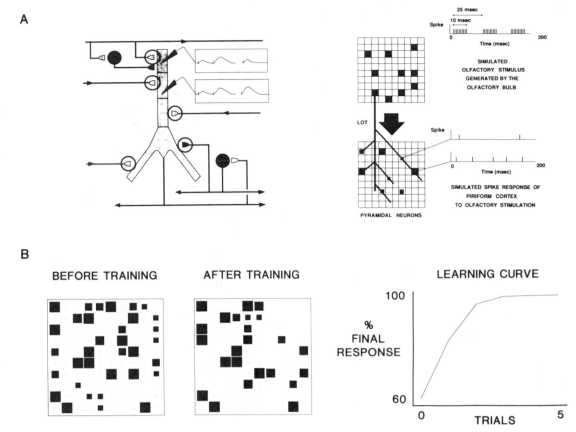

Figure 4. Simulations of the piriform cortex autoassociation memory properties. (*A*) On the left, circled synapses show where the effect of Hebbian modification rules were compared in early simulations. On the right is a diagram of random projection patterns from active bulbar neurons to cortical cells. In the cortex, the size of each black square represents the number of action potentials generated in that cell. (*B*) On the left, the response of the cortex to activity in a random set of ten bulbar neurons before and after learning produced a stable pattern of activity. On the right, activity converges toward the final pattern of activity, expressed as the percentage of similarity with the final response. (Reprinted, with permission, from Bower 1990a.)

patterns can be regenerated when only a partial version of the original stimulus is presented. Again, natural variability in the molecules given off by an object presumably makes this capacity important in the recognition of olfactory stimuli.

Locus of Synaptic Modification

In the first interaction of modeling and experimental work, we considered the locus of synaptic modification rules in the network. With any model as complex as this model of olfactory cortex, the question of parameter sensitivity becomes an important issue (Wilson and Bower 1989). It must be pointed out, however, that many of the structural and physiological parameters used in the current model are constrained by the results of actual anatomical and physiological experiments (Wilson and Bower 1990). Taking advantage of these constraints is one of the motivations for making models structurally realistic (Bower 1990a). However, as mentioned above, one important feature of the model that was not initially constrained by actual data was the type and location of activity-dependent synaptic learning within the network. At the time these simulations were

conducted, it was not yet known which, if any, of the different synapses in the piriform cortex were capable of long-term activity-dependent changes in synaptic strength (Bower and Haberly 1986). Accordingly, the model was used to compare the consequences of learning properties in different synaptic populations.

Modeling. To determine whether learning in the model was dependent on the particular locus of synaptic modification, we compared network performance with a Hebb-type learning rule in either the afferent or intrinsic fiber system synapses (Wilson and Bower 1988). These two fiber systems constitute the major sources of excitatory input in this network (Haberly 1985). The results of these experiments clearly showed that the associative memory capacity of the piriform cortex model was dependent on the presence of Hebb-type learning in the intrinsic fiber synapses (Fig. 6). When synaptic modification was limited to synapses associated with the afferent fiber system, the network did not converge to a stable output pattern in response to a consistent input. The capacity for completion of incomplete input patterns also depended on which set of synapses showed modification. When only afferent

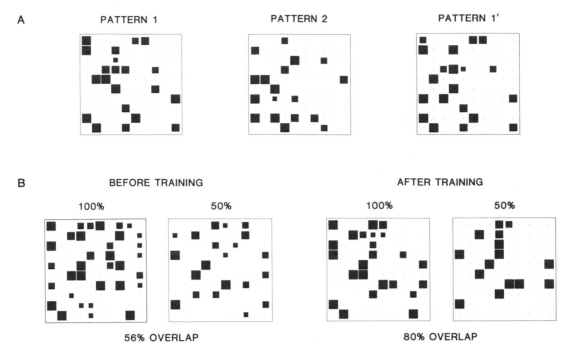

Figure 5. Properties of autoassociative learning of input patterns. (*A*) Cortical response to successive training sessions using two different patterns of afferent input. The diagram at the far right demonstrates that the simulation maintains a relatively stable pattern of response to pattern 1 even after training with pattern 2. (*B*) Cortical response to input patterns at full strength (100%) and with five of the original ten bulbar neurons active (50%). Before training, the response to the degraded stimulus shows only 56% similarity to the nondegraded stimulus. After training, the response to the degraded stimulus shows 80% overlap with the nondegraded response. (Reprinted, with permission, from Bower 1990a.)

fibers were modifiable during learning, the system showed considerably less completion than when intrinsic fiber synapses were modifiable. Doubling the gain of afferent fiber modification actually reduced the level of completion, whereas doubling the gain of the intrinsic fiber learning rule provided almost 100% completion of the input pattern. Accordingly, the clear prediction from these results was that synapses of the intrinsic association fiber system should represent the principal site of synaptic learning in the olfactory cortex.

Electrophysiology. As just described, our model of associative learning in the olfactory cortex makes two predictions that are experimentally testable. First, the model suggests that synapses associated with the afferent projection fibers should be relatively unmodifiable. Second, the model predicts that synapses associated with the intrinsic association fiber system should be capable of much more substantial modification. In the case of the afferent projections, the balance of the data already indicates that these synapses show neither short-term nor substantial long-term potentiation (Racine and Milgram 1983; Racine et al. 1983; Stripling et al. 1988; Kanter and Haberly 1989). However, it has only been recently that careful comparisons between afferent and intrinsic synaptic properties have been made. Motivated by our modeling results, we have conducted a series of experiments that demonstrate that synaptic potentials evoked by intrinsic fiber stimulation show clear and consistent short-term potentia-

tion at frequencies that elicit no change or depression of synaptic potentials evoked by afferent fiber stimulation (Hasselmo and Bower 1990). Furthermore, an in vitro experiment using extracellular recording techniques, performed subsequent to the simulations described above but naive with respect to the modeling results, shows a significantly greater level of long-term potentiation in intrinsic than in afferent fiber synaptic potentials (Kanter and Haberly 1989). These experimental results are clearly in good agreement with the model's prediction that synaptic modification should appear primarily in the intrinsic fiber synapses.

Cholinergic Modulation of Piriform Cortex Function

Having demonstrated that a model structured like the piriform cortex was capable of autoassociative memory function, we were interested in extending the realism of the model by incorporating other network features potentially relevant to this function. In particular, we were interested in exploring any influences on piriform cortex synapses of neuromodulatory agents with known behavioral effects on memory acquisition or retention. Given the previous modeling work, in these studies, we were particularly interested in identifying any differential effects of these agents on afferent and intrinsic fiber systems.

In our first experiments of this type, we have focused on the role of cholinergic innervation of the piriform

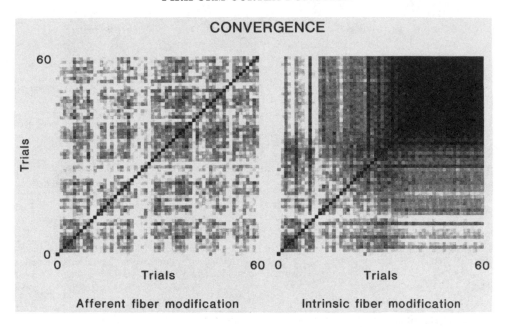

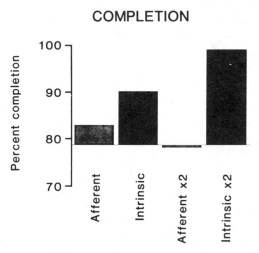

Figure 6. Comparison of effects of synaptic modification at afferent and intrinsic fiber synapses. Top two figures show a correlation matrix for each case. Each square represents the similarity of activity at one trial step of the simulation (x axis) with the activity at a previous or subsequent trial step of the simulation (y axis). Darker squares reflect a greater similarity of activity patterns. Correlation of a trial with itself results in the line of black squares running at a diagonal. On the left, activity patterns show little similarity during the course of afferent fiber modification. On the right, activity converges toward a final stable pattern of activity. On the bottom, the percentage of completion is compared for different loci of synaptic modification.

cortex. Both the piriform cortex and olfactory bulb appear to receive extensive cholinergic innervation from a region of the basal forebrain, the horizontal limb of the diagonal band of Broca (Wenk et al. 1977; Macrides et al. 1981). Cholinergic antagonists have been shown to impair learning of new information in humans (Kopelman 1986). In addition, the memory and cognitive impairments associated with Alzheimer's disease have been proposed to be related to a loss of cholinergic innervation of cortical regions (Coyle et al. 1983). These impairments include a decreased capacity to identify olfactory stimuli (Warner et al. 1986; Doty et al. 1987; Koss et al. 1988).

Electrophysiology. Previously, cholinergic agonists had been shown to suppress synaptic transmission in the piriform cortex (Williams et al. 1985; Williams and Constanti 1988), but this work was performed in slices cut tangential to the cortical surface, preventing a comparison of afferent and intrinsic synapses. Accordingly, we undertook experiments to test specifically whether cholinergic agents might differentially affect afferent and intrinsic fiber synaptic transmission. As shown in Figure 7, we found marked differences in the suppression of transmission between these two synaptic systems. The acetylcholine agonist carbachol strongly suppressed synaptic potentials elicited by intrinsic fiber

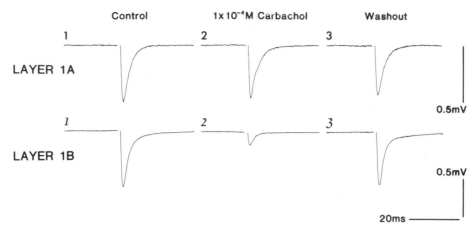

Figure 7. Selective suppression of intrinsic fiber synaptic transmission by the acetylcholine analog carbachol. Extracellular synaptic potentials evoked by stimulation of layer 1a afferent fibers show little decrease in response to perfusion of 100 μM carbachol, whereas extracellular synaptic potentials evoked by stimulation of layer 1b intrinsic fibers show strong suppression in response to 100 μM carbachol.

stimulation, decreasing the height of potentials by over 40% at a concentration of 5 μM and by almost 70% at 100 μM (M.E. Hasselmo and J.M. Bower, in prep.). In contrast, carbachol reduced the height of afferent fiber synaptic potentials by less than 12%, even at a concentration of 500 μM. This differential effect on afferent and intrinsic fiber synaptic potentials appeared whether they were recorded extracellularly from the layer being stimulated or intracellularly from the same piriform cortex pyramidal cell. Thus, cholinergic modulation of synaptic function is directed at precisely those cortical synapses that our previous modeling work suggested are critical for memory function in this network.

Modeling. As a first step in studying the functional significance of the selective suppression of intrinsic fiber synaptic transmission, we have used a simplified version of the piriform cortex model to examine the effect of this suppression on the model's autoassociation memory capacity. In general, the capacity of an associative memory is defined as the number of distinct memories that can be recalled without contamination by other memories. Because memory storage in an autoassociative network is highly distributed, each memory shares some overlapping set of units or neurons with other memories. As the number of memories stored in a particular network increases, the amount of overlap goes up, raising the possibility that a particular input pattern will generate an output composed of a combination of multiple memories. Thus, a chief limitation on the storage capacity of an association memory network of the type considered here is the overlap of patterns stored in the network.

In abstract models of associative memory, the problem of overlap is usually dealt with by constructing input patterns with as little overlap as possible (Palm 1980) or by preprocessing the input with a separate network using anti-Hebbian learning rules (Kohonen and Oja 1976). However, these techniques may be unrealistic for the olfactory system. As noted above,

olfactory bulb neurons projecting to the piriform cortex often respond to a wide variety of odor stimuli. So, the input to the cortex naturally has a high degree of overlap. In addition, in the natural world, it is sometimes necessary to distinguish odors that are molecularly very similar (Halpin 1980; Epple et al. 1989). Accordingly, it seems reasonable to assume that the olfactory cortex employs some active, internal mechanism for reducing the overlap between the response patterns to different olfactory stimuli.

In a class of abstract network models usually considered separately from autoassociative memories, internal connectivity patterns have been used to decrease the overlap between input patterns. Networks of this kind, sometimes referred to as competitive neural networks (Rumelhart and Zipser 1986; Grossberg 1987), use lateral inhibition between active units to increase the sparseness of the activity induced by any particular input pattern. This effectively decreases the likelihood of overlap with other activity patterns. Strong inhibitory feedback connections that could perform this function have been shown to exist within piriform cortex (Tseng and Haberly 1988). However, in our previous simulations of autoassociative behavior, the effect of these inhibitory influences was dominated by the excitatory influences of the extensive intrinsic fiber system. In these simulations, the primary identified action of the inhibitory neurons was to regulate cortical oscillatory activity (Wilson and Bower 1990). Our discovery of a selective cholinergic suppression of intrinsic excitatory synapses raises the possibility that cholinergic agonists could affect the balance of excitation and inhibition in the cortex and thus serve to increase the sparseness of neural activity and increase memory storage capacity.

The effect of cholinergic suppression on the capacity and efficiency of associative storage in our simplified model of piriform cortex was assessed by a number of different criteria. First, we determined the number of memories successfully stored by the network under different degrees of intrinsic fiber synaptic suppression. A successfully stored memory was defined as an input pattern for which the network reduced the level of noise (i.e., the network reached an activity pattern closer to the learned activity pattern than the test input pattern was to the learned input pattern). A further criterion for a successfully stored memory was that it did not completely overlap with other stored memories. In this case, stored memories had to differ by at least one active unit. For successfully stored memories, we also examined the mean amount of noise reduction and the mean percentage of completion of incomplete patterns.

To model the effects of cholinergic modulation, the gain of the intrinsic connectivity matrix B was homogeneously reduced to a percentage of its previous strength. In some simulations, the change in gain was varied at different stages of learning. In the preliminary simulations described here, for each input pattern, the cholinergic modulation shut off intrinsic connections ($B_{i,j} = 0$) for the first five input cycles (i.e., the first five times stimuli were presented to the network). For the subsequent stimulus cycles, intrinsic connections were returned to their full strength and allowed to change in strength using the usual Hebbian learning rule. The results showed that this modulation increased the number of successfully stored "memories" by 40%. Modulation of intrinsic connection strengths also increased the amount of completion and noise reduction in successfully stored memories. Thus, simulations completed to date are consistent with the proposal that cholinergic suppression of intrinsic fiber connectivity strength could serve to increase the capacity and efficiency of associative memory storage.

Recently, we have attempted to replicate the results of the simplified model using the more extensive compartmental model of the piriform cortex. The results show that cholinergic modulation of intrinsic fiber connections in this model results in a more rapid convergence to a stable representation of the input pattern. In addition, a test of learning with different levels of intrinsic fiber strength showed that the level of completion of patterns during the recall phase varied depending on the strength of intrinsic fibers during learning. Interestingly, if the strength of intrinsic connections was too low during learning, completion was not as strong, but completion was even poorer when the strength of intrinsic connections was too high during learning. It would therefore seem that some intermediate range of values for intrinsic fiber strength may be optimal for memory function. If this is true, we would predict that the extent of cholinergic modulation may be varied during memory storage and recall in the real piriform cortex.

DISCUSSION

In this paper, we have outlined several examples of the fruitful interaction between computational modeling and experimental techniques. Results of our work

suggest that piriform cortex may function as an autoassociation memory, with the capacity to form stable representations of olfactory stimuli and to respond to noisy or incomplete forms of these stimuli. To date, the model has been used primarily to explore functional implications of cortical properties, but the model provides a framework for considering results from many different types of experimentation. For example, lesions of the olfactory cortex impair discrimination of complex odors more than simple odors (Staubli et al. 1987). This resembles a property of autoassociative memory models called graceful degradation; damage to the system results in a gradual reduction of memory capacity affecting complex patterns more strongly. At the other end of the experimental spectrum, psychophysical studies reveal complex perceptual interactions in odor mixtures (Laing 1989) that may depend on the familiarity of the olfactory stimuli (Rabin and Cain 1989). These effects could result from the autocorrelation of sensory input that we propose occurs in the piriform cortex. The model can also be used to suggest future experiments. Cells recorded in the olfactory cortex already show the distributed representation of olfactory stimuli expected for an autoassociative memory (Tanabe et al. 1975), but the model suggests that a cell responding to one of two odors could be induced to respond to the other by associative pairing of the two. Thus, the model can be used to tie together multiple levels of inquiry into the process of olfactory discrimination.

The modeling work can also serve to identify network features that may be more generally relevant to other regions of the cortex. For example, we have discussed differences in activity-dependent modification of intrinsic but not afferent fiber synaptic strength, which could be important for other cortical circuits involved in memory. Studies show a clear difference in the role of postsynaptic activity in long-term potentiation of mossy fiber versus association fiber synapses of region CA3 of the hippocampus (Zalutsky and Nicoll 1990), but the functional implications of this difference have not been considered. Our modeling of the cholinergic modulation of the piriform cortex function may also apply to the function of other brain regions. Given the broad cholinergic projections to all regions of the neocortex and the hippocampus (McKinney et al. 1983), it seems worth considering whether the effects on memory capacity and efficiency we have discovered in our models might not be more generally applicable. The final sections of this paper considers how our model relates to other evidence on the involvement of cholinergic modulation in memory formation.

Relation to Other Cholinergic Pharmacological Effects

We have described effects of cholinergic agonists on synaptic transmission mediated by putative presynaptic receptors. However, in these experiments, we have also noted postsynaptic effects of cholinergic agents.

Specifically, acetylcholine and its agonists increase the excitability of the piriform cortex pyramidal cells. Previous descriptions of this result attribute the effect to the shutting down of specific membrane potassium conductances but do not speculate on the functional significance of these changes (Constanti and Galvan 1983; ffrench-Mullen et al. 1983; Constanti and Sim 1985).

When considered in relation to the role we propose for the cholinergic system in enhancing memory formation, it is possible to provide a new interpretation for the functional significance of increases in cell excitability mediated by cholinergic agents. This postsynaptic change could complement the presynaptic effects already discussed in three different ways. First, the partial suppression of intrinsic fiber activity, coupled with greater cellular excitability, would be expected to allow afferent fibers to drive pyramidal cells more effectively. This could serve to assure that the structure of the original input from the olfactory bulb would be more clearly maintained during cortical activity without the intermixing of information expected from the extensive association fiber system. Second, increased excitability in those pyramidal cells receiving significant afferent input could increase the drive on nearby inhibitory interneurons which, in turn, might result in further suppression of marginally active pyramidal cells. This would tip the balance of intrinsic excitation and inhibition further toward inhibition and thereby further enhance the sparseness of the pattern of activity discussed above. Finally, shutting down the membrane potassium currents would result in a more sustained depolarization of active neurons, increasing the likelihood of Hebbian synaptic modification.

Relation to Other Cortical Structures

Beyond the piriform cortex, cholinergic agents have similar effects in the hippocampus, shutting down membrane potassium currents (Benardo and Prince 1982; Halliwell and Adams 1982; Cole and Nicoll 1984; Madison et al. 1987) and suppressing synaptic transmission by putative presynaptic mechanisms (Yamamoto and Kawai 1967; Hounsgaard 1978; Valentino and Dingledine 1981; Sheridan and Sutor 1990). Thus, the network effects suggested for the piriform cortex may apply to the hippocampus as well. However, although differences in modulation of the afferent input to the dentate gyrus have been noted (Kahle and Cotman 1989), no experiments have directly compared cholinergic effects on afferent and intrinsic fiber synaptic transmission in this region or interpreted these results in terms of specific memory function. Interestingly, in the hippocampus, cholinergic agonists have also been shown to initiate θ-type oscillations (Konopacki et al. 1987), which some evidence suggests may be the optimal temporal frequency for inducing long-term potentiation (Larson et al. 1986). In our simulations of the piriform cortex, a slight depolarization of pyramidal cells, such as that induced by cholinergic agonists, increases the oscillatory activity of the network (M.A.

Wilson and J.M. Bower, unpubl.). Thus, cholinergic modulation may also set the temporal characteristics of neuronal activity in this region to those optimal for associative storage. Cholinergic effects have also been investigated in the cingulate cortex. Here, postsynaptic effects on potassium conductances have been noted, in addition to a further proposed specific activation of inhibitory interneurons (McCormick and Prince 1986). Obviously, any cholinergic-induced increase in inhibitory suppression of pyramidal cells will further increase the ratio of inhibitory versus excitatory intrinsic activity, which our modeling suggests increases the capacity and efficiency of memory encoding.

General Behavioral Significance of Cholinergic Modulation

On the basis of the results presented in this paper, we propose that cholinergic modulation may mediate between two different functional states of the network. Our results suggest that cholinergic input enhances the process of storing new information, and accordingly, we propose that this system should be active during periods when new olfactory patterns are being learned. Thus, novel stimuli or stimuli associated with reinforcement would be expected to activate cholinergic projection neurons. On the other hand, our models show that during recall, strong intrinsic connections are useful for completing degraded input patterns or decreasing the effects of background noise. Accordingly, cholinergic activity would be expected to be low during these periods.

As mentioned above, the cholinergic projection to the piriform cortex originates in the horizontal limb of the diagonal band. Although we are unaware of any electrophysiology yet performed on the neurons of the horizontal limb, results of recordings from other related regions of the basal forebrain have demonstrated changes in neuronal activity dependent on the reinforcement value of a stimulus (Richardson and DeLong 1988; Wilson and Rolls 1990a) or its novelty (Wilson and Rolls 1990b). As noted above, this is the activity pattern we would expect for a system modulating storage of new information. Also, anatomical data show that cells of this region project diffusely into the piriform cortex (Luskin and Price 1982). This diffuse projection is in keeping with the putative role of the system in modulating synaptic efficacy across the entire network.

Our proposal also fits well with the results of studies on the role of cholinergic modulation in various tasks requiring memory. The muscarinic cholinergic antagonist scopolamine impairs memory acquisition in a range of behavioral tests in rodents (Spencer and Lal 1983). Of particular interest, injection of scopolamine prior to the presentation of odors appears to decrease the normal habituation to an odor over the first three presentations and prevents the increase in response to subsequent presentation of a novel odor (Hunter and Murray 1989). In human testing, scopolamine has been shown to impair performance in a wide range of memory tasks (Kopelman 1986). In tests of human olfactory perception, scopolamine has been shown to increase the threshold for detection of geraniol but did not affect the identification of 40 familiar odors in the University of Pennsylvania Smell Identification Test (UPSIT) (Serby et al. 1989). Note that this involved a test of previously learned odors, not the acquisition of new olfactory information. The lack of effect of scopolamine on olfactory identification in normal people is somewhat surprising in light of the fact that Alzheimer's disease, which involves a loss of cholinergic innervation throughout the cortex (Coyle et al. 1983), decreases the capacity for identification of odors on the UPSIT test (Warner et al. 1986; Doty et al. 1987; Koss et al. 1988). The difference in effect may be due to damage to noncholinergic structures of the olfactory system in Alzheimer's disease (Esiri and Wilcock 1984; Reyes et al. 1987). However, another interpretation is that the impairment in Alzheimer's disease is due to a long-term buildup of interference between olfactory memories, and that cholinergic-related deficits would be more difficult to detect in the short run. Interestingly, Alzheimer's patients perform worse on later parts of the olfactory identification task, suggesting that they may suffer from increased interference between memories during the course of olfactory testing (Warner et al. 1986). The theoretical framework presented in this paper provides a means of describing these and other behavioral effects in terms of detailed network physiology and may ultimately provide new insights on the role of cholinergic innervation in regulating the cortical processing of sensory information.

ACKNOWLEDGMENTS

This work was supported by Office of Naval Research contract N00014-88-K-0513 and National Institutes of Health postdoctoral training grant NS-07251.

REFERENCES

Benardo, L.S. and D.A. Prince. 1982. Ionic mechanisms of cholinergic excitation in mammalian hippocampal pyramidal cells. *Brain Res.* **249:** 333.

Bower, J.M. 1990a. Reverse engineering the nervous system: An anatomical, physiological, and computer based approach. In *An introduction to neural and electronic networks* (ed. S. Zornetzer et al.), p. 3. Academic Press, New York.

———. 1990b. Associative memory in a biological network: Structural simulations of the olfactory cerebral cortex. In *Neural networks*, vol. II. (ed. S. Miltunovic and M. Antognetti). Prentice Hall, New York. (In press.)

Bower, J.M. and L.B. Haberly. 1986. Facilitating and nonfacilitating synapses on pyramidal cells: A correlation between physiology and morphology. *Proc. Natl. Acad. Sci.* **83:** 1115.

Cole, A.E. and R.A. Nicoll. 1984. Characterization of a slow cholinergic postsynaptic potential recorded in vitro from rat hippocampal pyramidal cells. *J. Physiol.* **352:** 173.

Constanti, A. and M. Galvan. 1983. M-current in voltage-clamped olfactory cortex neurones. *Neurosci. Lett.* **39:** 65.

Constanti, A. and J.A. Sim. 1985. A slow, muscarine-sensitive Ca-dependent K current in guinea-pig olfactory cortex neurones in vitro. *J. Physiol.* **365:** 47P.

Coyle, J.T., D.L. Price, and M.R. DeLong. 1983. Alzheimer's disease: A disorder of cortical cholinergic innervation. *Science* **219:** 1184.

Doty, R.L., P.F. Reyes, and T. Gregor. 1987. Presence of both odor and detection deficits in Alzheimer's disease. *Brain Res. Bull.* **18:** 597.

Epple, G., A. Belcher, K.L. Greenfield, I. Kuderling, K. Nordstrom, and A.B. Smith. 1989. Scent mixtures used as social signals in two primate species: *Saguinus fuscicollis* and *Saguinus o. oedipus*. In *Perception of complex smells and tastes* (ed. D.G. Laing et al.), p. 173. Academic Press, New York.

Esiri, M.M. and P.K. Wilcock. 1984. The olfactory bulb in Alzheimer's disease. *J. Neurol. Neurosurg. Psychiatry* **47:** 56.

ffrench-Mullen, J.M.H., N. Hori, H. Nakanishi, N.T. Slater, and D.O. Carpenter. 1983. Asymmetric distribution of acetylcholine receptors and M channels on prepyriform neurons. *Cell. Mol. Neurobiol.* **3:** 163.

Grossberg, S. 1987. Competitive learning: From interactive activation to adaptive resonance. *Cognit. Sci.* **11:** 23.

Haberly, L.B. 1985. Neuronal circuitry in olfactory cortex: Anatomy and functional implications. *Chem. Senses* **10:** 219.

Haberly, L.B. and J.M. Bower. 1989. Olfactory cortex: Model circuit for study of associative memory? *Trends Neurosci.* **12:** 258.

Haberly, L.B. and J.L. Price. 1978. Association and commissural fiber systems of the olfactory cortex of the rat. I. Systems originating in the piriform cortex and adjacent areas. *J. Comp. Neurol.* **178:** 711.

Halliwell, J.V. and P.R. Adams. 1982. Voltage-clamp analysis of muscarinic excitation in hippocampal neurons. *Brain Res.* **250:** 71.

Halpin, Z.T. 1980. Individual odors and individual recognition: Review and commentary. *Biol. Behav.* **5:** 233.

Hasselmo M.E. and J.M. Bower. 1990. Afferent and association fiber differences in short-term potentiation in piriform (olfactory) cortex of the rat. *J. Neurophysiol.* **64:** 179.

Hounsgaard, J. 1978. Presynaptic inhibitory action of acetylcholine in area CA1 of the hippocampus. *Exp. Neurol.* **62:** 787.

Hunter, A.J. and T.K. Murray. 1989. Cholinergic mechanisms in a simple test of olfactory learning in the rat. *Psychopharmacology* **99:** 270.

Kahle J.S. and C.W. Cotman. 1989. Carbachol depresses the synaptic responses in the medial but not the lateral perforant path. *Brain Res.* **482:** 159.

Kanter, E.D. and L.B. Haberly. 1989. APV dependent induction of long term potentiation in piriform (olfactory) cortex slices. *Soc. Neurosci. Abstr.* **15:** 929.

Kohonen T. 1984. *Self-organization and associative memory.* Springer-Verlag, Berlin.

Kohonen T. and E. Oja. 1976. Fast adaptive transformation of orthogonalizing filters and associative memory in recurrent networks of neuron-like elements. *Biol. Cybern.* **21:** 85.

Kohonen T., E. Reuhkala, K. Makisaran, and L. Vainio. 1976. Associative recall of images. *Biol. Cybern.* **22:** 159.

Konopacki, J., M.B. MacIver, B.H. Bland, and S.H. Roth. 1987. Carbachol-induced EEG "theta" activity in hippocampal brain slices. *Brain Res.* **405:** 196.

Kopelman, M.D. 1986. The cholinergic neurotransmitter system in human memory and dementia: A review. *Q. J. Exp. Psychol.* **38:** 535.

Koss, E., J.M. Weiffenbach, J.V. Haxby, and R.P. Friedland. 1988. Olfactory detection and identification performance are dissociated in early Alzheimer's disease. *Neurology* **38:** 1228.

Laing, D.G. 1989. The role of physicochemical and neural factors in the perception of odor mixtures. In *Perception of complex smells and tastes* (ed. D.G. Laing et al.), p. 173. Academic Press, New York.

Larson, J., D. Wong, and G. Lynch. 1986. Patterned stimulation at the theta frequency is optimal for induction of hippocampal long-term potentiation. *Brain Res.* **368:** 347.

Leon, M. 1987. Plasticity of olfactory output circuits related to early olfactory learning. *Trends Neurosci.* **10:** 434.

Luskin, M.B. and J.L. Price. 1982. The distribution of axon collaterals from the olfactory bulb and the nucleus of the horizontal limb of the diagonal band to the olfactory cortex, demonstrated by double retrograde labeling techniques. *J. Comp. Neurol.* **209:** 249.

———. 1983a. The topographic organization of associational fibers of the olfactory system in the rat, including centrifugal fibers to the olfactory bulb. *J. Comp. Neurol.* **216:** 264.

———. 1983b. The laminar distribution of intracortical fibers originating in the olfactory cortex of the rat. *J. Comp. Neurol.* **216:** 292.

Macrides, F., B.J. Davis, W.M. Youngs, N.S. Nadi, and F.L. Margolis. 1981. Cholinergic and catecholaminergic afferents to the olfactory bulb in the hamster: A neuroanatomical, biochemical and histochemical investigation. *J. Comp. Neurol.* **203:** 495.

Madison, D.V., B. Lancaster, and R.A. Nicoll. 1987. Voltage clamp analysis of cholinergic action in the hippocampus. *J. Neurosci.* **7:** 733.

Mathews, D.F. 1972. Response patterns of single units in the olfactory bulb of the rat to odor. *Brain Res.* **47:** 389.

McCartney, W. 1951. Olfaction in animals. *Int. Perfumer* **4:** 3.

McCormick, D.A. and D.A. Prince. 1986. Mechanisms of action of acetylcholine in the guinea pig cerebral cortex in vitro. *J. Physiol* **375:** 169.

McKinney, M., J.T. Coyle, and J.C. Hedreen. 1983. Topographic analysis of the innervation of the rat neocortex and hippocampus by the basal forebrain cholinergic system. *J. Comp. Neurol.* **217:** 103.

Nigrosh, B.J., B.M. Slotnick, and J.A. Nevin. 1975. Olfactory discrimination, reversal learning, and stimulus control in rats. *J. Comp. Physiol. Psychol.* **89:** 285.

Palm, G. 1980. On associative memory. *Biol. Cybern.* **36:** 19.

Price, J.L. 1973. An autoradiographic study of complementary laminar patterns of termination of afferent fibers to the olfactory cortex. *J. Comp. Neurol.* **150:** 87.

———. 1987. The central olfactory and accessory olfactory systems. In *The neurobiology of taste and smell* (ed. T.E. Finger and W.L. Silver), p. 205. Wiley, New York.

Rabin, M.D. and W.S. Cain. 1989. Attention and learning in the perception of odor mixtures. In *Perception of complex smells and tastes* (ed. D.G. Laing et al.), p. 173. Academic Press, New York.

Racine, R.J. and M.W. Milgram. 1983. Short-term potentiation phenomena in the rat limbic forebrain. *Brain Res.* **260:** 201.

Racine, R.J., M.W. Milgram, and S. Hafner. 1983. Long-term potentiation phenomena in the rat limbic forebrain. *Brain Res.* **260:** 217.

Reyes, P.F., G.T. Golden, P.L. Fagel, R.G. Fariello, L. Katz, and E. Carner. 1987. The prepiriform cortex in dementia of the Alzheimer type. *Arch. Neurol.* **44:** 644.

Richardson, R.T. and M.R. DeLong. 1988. A reappraisal of the functions of the nucleus basalis of Meynert. *Trends Neurosci.* **11:** 264.

Rumelhart D.E. and D. Zipser. 1986. Feature discovery by competitive learning. *Cognit. Sci.* **9:** 75.

Serby, M., C. Flicker, B. Rypma, S. Weber, J.P. Rotrosen, and S.H. Ferris. 1989. Scopolamine and olfactory function. *Biol. Psychiatry* **28:** 79.

Sheridan, R.D. and B. Sutor. 1990. Presynaptic M1 muscarinic cholinoceptors mediate inhibition of excitatory synaptic transmission in the hippocampus in vitro. *Neurosci. Lett.* **108:** 273.

Slotnick, B.M. and H.M. Katz. 1974. Olfactory learning-set formation in rats. *Science* **185:** 796.

Slotnick, B.M. and E.J. Berman. 1980. Transection of the lateral olfactory tract does not produce anosmia. *Brain Res. Bull.* **5:** 141.

Spencer, D.G. and H. Lal. 1983. Effects of anticholinergic drugs on learning and memory. *Drug Dev. Res.* **3:** 489.

Squire, L.R. 1986. Memory: Brain systems and behavior. *Trends Neurosci.* **11:** 170.

Staubli, U., F. Schottler, and D. Nejat-Bina. 1987. Role of dorsomedial thalamic nucleus and piriform cortex in processing olfactory information. *Behav. Brain Res.* **25:** 117.

Stripling, J.S., D.K. Patneau, and C.A. Gramlich. 1988. Selective long-term potentiation in the pyriform cortex. *Brain Res.* **441:** 281.

Takagi, S.F. 1979. Dual systems for sensory olfactory processing in higher primates. *Trends Neurosci.* **2:** 313.

Tanabe, T., M. Iino, and S.F. Takagi. 1975. Discrimination of odors in olfactory bulb, pyriform-amygdaloid areas and orbito-frontal cortex of the monkey. *J. Neurophysiol.* **38:** 1284.

Tseng, G.-F. and L.B. Haberly. 1988. Characterization of synaptically mediated fast and slow inhibitory processes in piriform cortex in an in vitro slice preparation. *J. Neurophysiol.* **59:** 1352.

Valentino, R.J. and R. Dingledine. 1981. Presynaptic inhibitory effect of acetylcholine in the hippocampus. *J. Neurosci.* **1:** 784.

Warner, M.D., C.A. Peabody, J.J. Flattery, and J. Tinklenberg. 1986. Olfactory deficits and Alzheimer's disease. *Biol. Psychiatry* **21:** 116.

Wenk, H., U. Meyer, and V. Bigl. 1977. Centrifugal cholinergic connections in the olfactory system of rats. *Neuroscience* **2:** 797.

Wigstrom H., B. Gustafsson, Y.-Y. Huang, and W.C. Abraham. 1986. Hippocampal long-term potentiation is induced by pairing single afferent volleys with intracellularly injected depolarizing current pulses. *Acta Physiol. Scand.* **126:** 317.

Williams, S.H. and A. Constanti. 1988. Quantitative effects of some muscarinic agonists on evoked surface-negative field potentials recorded from the guinea-pig olfactory cortex slice. *Br. J. Pharmacol.* **93:** 846.

Williams, S.H., A. Constanti, and D.A. Brown. 1985. Muscarinic depression of evoked surface-negative field potentials recorded from guinea-pig olfactory cortex in vitro. *Neurosci. Lett.* **56:** 301.

Wilson, F.A.W. and E.T. Rolls. 1990a. Neuronal responses related to reinforcement in the primate basal forebrain. *Brain Res.* **509:** 213.

———. 1990b. Learning and memory is reflected in the responses of reinforcement-related neurons in the primate basal forebrain. *J. Neurosci.* **10:** 1254.

Wilson M.A. and J.M. Bower. 1988. A computer simulation of olfactory cortex with functional implications for storage and retrieval of olfactory information. In *Neural information processing systems.* (ed. D. Anderson), p. 114. AIP Press, New York.

———. 1989. The simulation of large-scale neuronal networks. In *Methods in neuronal modeling: From synapses to networks.* (ed. C. Koch and I. Segev), p. 291. MIT Press, Cambridge.

———. 1990. Cortical oscillations and temporal interactions in a computer simulation of piriform cortex. *J. Neurophysiol.* (in press).

Yamamoto, C. and N. Kawai. 1967. Presynaptic action of acetylcholine in thin sections from the guinea-pig denate gyrus in vitro. *Exp. Neurol.* **19:** 176.

Zalutsky, R.A. and R.A. Nicoll. 1990. Comparison of two forms of long-term potentiation in single hippocampal neurons. *Science* **248:** 1619.

Neural Image Transformation in the Somatosensory System of the Monkey: Comparison of Neurophysiological Observations with Responses in a Neural Network Model

I.N. Bankman, S.S. Hsiao, and K.O. Johnson

Phillip Bard Laboratories of Neurophysiology, Department of Neuroscience and Department of Biomedical Engineering, The Johns Hopkins University School of Medicine, Baltimore, Maryland 21205

Although the mechanisms of perception are not understood, it seems that there must be a continuous process of matching between incoming neural images and images stored in memory and that this is done in a time frame that amounts to a small number of neuronal input/output cycles. In both the visual and somatosensory systems, the topographic organization of receptors laid out across the retina and the skin dictates that the first neural representation of externally imposed geometric form and the corresponding stimulus are isomorphic. However, pattern matching based on isomorphic images is prohibitively time consuming; identification requires matching between the unknown image and every possible template at every possible location, size, and orientation. The images being matched by the higher mechanisms underlying perception must be in some other form. A primary task of the sensory systems must be to transform neural images from their initial isomorphic form to the form that underlies perception, recognition, and association. The somatosensory system, like other sensory systems, is a large neural network that effects this overall transformation through a series of operations at successive synaptic relay zones. Understanding this transformational process will ultimately require explicit models that can be tested against experimental data. We present one such model in this paper.

The study reported here is part of a larger study of the neural mechanisms underlying tactile pattern recognition. The experimental design is the one pioneered by Mountcastle (Talbot et al. 1968) in which a form of sensory behavior is first studied using psychophysical methods and then followed by neurophysiological studies using exactly the same stimulus conditions. Studies using this experimental design have traditionally been described as neural coding studies. This design addresses the question: What is it in the complex array of neural activity evoked by a stimulus that conveys the information on which behavior is based? The characterization of these studies as "neural coding studies" emphasizes the fact that the brain is an information processor and that information processing in the brain needs to be studied directly. The question that we

address in our study is: How is spatial form coded in the distributed patterns of neural activity evoked by patterns like embossed letters of the alphabet?

Psychophysical studies of tactile letter recognition in humans have characterized tactile letter recognition over a wide range of stimulus conditions (Johnson and Phillips 1981; Loomis 1981, 1982; Phillips et al. 1983), including conditions that are identical to those that we use in our neurophysiological studies (Vega-Bermudez et al. 1989). The psychophysical studies show that tactile pattern recognition is largely independent of the tactual mode (active, passive, scanned, or stationary) and that the threshold for letter recognition, the height producing 50% correct identifications, is 5 mm. This threshold, 5 mm, is close to the limit imposed by the peripheral innervation density of cutaneous SA (slowly adapting) and RA (rapidly adapting) afferents (Johnson and Phillips 1981; Phillips et al. 1983), which implies that the neural representations of letters must be passed through to recognition with little, if any, loss of information. Throughout the neurophysiological experiments reported in this paper, letters 8 mm in height were used. At 8 mm, human performance is nearly perfect; therefore, a clear, highly structured representation must exist at all levels of the pathway to recognition.

The neurophysiological studies have shown that the primary representation of scanned tactile form is an isomorphic neural image of the stimulus in the SA and RA afferent populations (Johnson and Lamb 1981; Phillips et al. 1988). That observation was not unexpected; the topography of the receptor sheet and the small receptive fields of SA and RA afferent fibers predict that conclusion. The unexpected outcome of these studies is that fine form recognition appears to rely on the SA population response (evidence is reviewed in Johnson et al. 1990). The primary data were obtained from the monkey, but comparisons of primary afferent fiber responses to scanned Braille and Braille-like dot patterns in man and monkey show that the responses are nearly identical in the two species (Johnson and Lamb 1981; Phillips et al. 1990).

Neurophysiological studies in cortical areas 3b and 1

of the alert monkey are consistent with the psycho-physical and peripheral neurophysiological studies. The majority of neurons in areas 3b and 1 and particularly those classified as SA respond to scanned letters with highly structured spatiotemporal responses. The primary difference between the cortical and peripheral data is the complexity and heterogeneity of cortical responses.

A neural network model was designed to match the major anatomical, physiological, and psychophysical properties of the somatosensory system. The anatomical structure of the system shows that the overall transformation between the periphery and the neural imagery that enters memory and recognition is effected as a series of partial transformations at successive synaptic relay zones. The term transformation means simply that the neural images leaving each synaptic relay zone, e.g., the ventrobasal complex of the thalamus, are different from those entering the zone. The columnar organization of the cortex and the modular organization of the earlier stages of processing specify modular construction (Mountcastle 1976; Dykes et al. 1982; Jones and Friedman 1982). Receptive field studies require that somatotopy be retained at all levels of processing, that connections be constrained to somatotopically adjacent regions, and that receptive fields become progressively larger and more complex at higher levels of processing (Robinson and Burton 1980; Mountcastle 1984; Pons et al. 1987). The psychophysical data require that each level preserve all the spatial information from the preceding level (Johnson and Phillips 1981; Phillips et al. 1983). These properties do not specify a unique network. The structure of the network presented here is based on the rule that each unit computes either the sum or difference of discharge rates from homologous units in adjacent modules of the preceding level. Although it was not intended to duplicate a known mathematical transform, the transform that is effected by these rules is a two-dimensional Walsh-Hadamard transform (Rao 1985).

In this paper, we show that the discharge patterns produced by intermediate units in the network are similar to discharge patterns that we have observed in a substantial number of cortical neurons. That is, we show that the cortical neurophysiological responses that we observe are like those that occur within a network that is effecting a transformation from isomorphism to some completely distributed representation in which every unit's response is different. The network responses that match neurophysiological responses closely are based on receptive fields with oriented bands of excitation and inhibition, like simple cells in visual cortex, which raises the possibility that form processing mechanisms in touch and vision are similar.

The network simulation does not explain the fundamental mechanisms of tactile pattern recognition. However, it does provide an answer to the question: How will we discover the transformational process that leads to the representations used in memory and recognition? A practical approach is to construct and try

networks that effect transformations of various kinds and to compare the responses of units in those networks with observed neurophysiological responses. Each network is a concrete hypothesis whose successes and failures can be evaluated and used to guide future attempts.

METHODS

The experimental data were obtained from 70 primary afferent fibers in anesthetized monkeys and 174 cortical neurons in Brodmann's areas 3b and 1 in alert monkeys performing a behavioral task unrelated to the tactile stimuli. The methods are described in Johnson and Phillips (1988) and Phillips et al. (1988). All of the neurons had receptive fields on the glabrous skin of a finger pad. Peripheral and cortical neurons with cutaneous receptive fields were classified as SA when they responded to steady, punctate skin indentation with a sustained change in impulse rate and as RA when the response was transient (Talbot et al. 1968). This classification does not imply strict submodality segregation in the ascending pathways. Cortical neurons classified as RAs could have been driven partially or exclusively by peripheral SA afferents, and the cortical SAs could have been driven partially by peripheral RA afferents. However, cortical neurons classed as SA must receive some peripheral SA input to account for their sustained response to sustained indentation.

The tactile stimuli consisted of embossed, sans serif, uppercase letters 8.0-mm high with a relief height of 500 μm, which were attached to the surface of a drum (Johnson and Phillips 1988). During the experiment, the drum was lowered onto the skin region containing the receptive field, rotated at a constant velocity, and translated axially 200 μm after each revolution. The drum surface velocity was 50 mm/sec for all of the data shown in this paper unless specified otherwise. The neural responses are displayed on a raster plot, called a spatial event plot (SEP), in which the action potentials are plotted as ticks at the appropriate stimulus surface coordinates (see Fig. 1).

SEPs reconstructed from single neuron responses can be interpreted in two ways. The conservative interpretation, which is always applicable and involves no assumptions, is that the SEP represents the single neuron's responses to complex moving stimuli. That is, the SEP is viewed simply as a raster plot of the evoked response where space rather than time is the independent variable. A sharp, well-defined isomorphic image implies high temporal and spatial resolution and (for cortical neurons) spatially limited input convergence. An additional interpretation, which is warranted under some conditions, is that the single neuron SEP approximates a spatiotemporal neural image of the stimulus as it would appear distributed across a population of similar neurons. This second interpretation applies when (1) the single neuron is one of a population of neurons with similar response properties but different receptive loci, (2) the receptive loci are distributed more or less

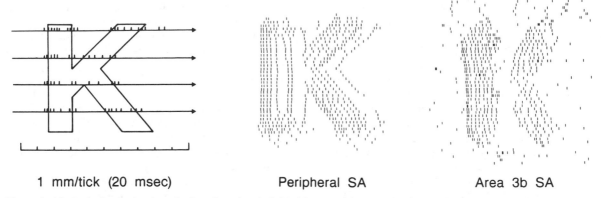

| 1 mm/tick (20 msec) | Peripheral SA | Area 3b SA |

Figure 1. Method of assigning impulse locations (vertical ticks) in a spatial event plot. The embossed letter K (6.0-mm high, 500 μm relief) was repeatedly scanned ($\sim$50 times at 50 mm/sec) across the receptive field of a peripheral SA and an area 3b SA neuron innervating a finger pad. The stimulus moved from right to left across the receptive field (left vertical bar of the K entered the receptive field first on each scan). The stimulus was shifted vertically by 200 μm after each scan.

uniformly across the skin surface, and (3) they are distributed with sufficient density to convey an informative image. The validity of these assumptions is known at the level of the peripheral nerve. The receptive fields of SA and RA afferents are arrayed densely beneath the skin surface (Johansson and Vallbo 1979; Darian-Smith and Kenins 1980), and their responses are quite homogeneous within their respective classes. These facts justify the neural image interpretation for the peripheral SA and RA SEPs.

Neural network model. The model is a three-dimensional, feed-forward, neural network with cascaded stages of inhibitory and excitatory synapses. A two-dimensional version of the neural network model is shown in Figure 2, where the flow of information is from left to right and processing units are connected by synapses whose strengths are +1 and −1. The firing rate of a unit is computed simply as the sum of firing rates of each of the input units weighted by the corresponding synaptic strengths. At each level, there are identical repeating modules, which are two units wide at level 2, four units wide at level 3, and so on. In the two-dimensional network illustrated in Figure 2, half the units within each module compute sums, and half compute differences of rates from homologous units in adjacent modules at the preceding level. The complex receptive fields that emerge can be seen by tracing the connections of internal units back to level 1; for example, by tracing the connections of unit 4c (level 4, row c) back to the primary layer (level 1), it can be seen that its receptive field is + + − − + + − − when expressed in terms of the inputs from units 1a to 1h.

The three-dimensional network used in this study is analogous to the two-dimensional network shown in Figure 2. In the three-dimensional version, each unit receives inputs from four homologous units, one from each of four modules at the preceding level. The connectivity pattern of units in the three-dimensional network can be generated by using the connectivity pattern of the two-dimensional network. Considering the

two basic connection patterns in the two-dimensional network as two distinct vectors, i.e., (1 1) and (1 −1), the four possible outer product matrices determine the four basic connection patterns in the three-dimensional network. These are illustrated in Figure 5. The result is a pattern of connectivity in which one fourth of the units in a module sum inputs from homologous units in preceding modules, whereas three fourths compute differences. The primary layer (level 1) consists of receptor units spaced at 0.8 mm to match the primary afferent innervation density in monkeys (Darian-Smith and Kenins 1980).

The input to the network consisted of spike trains that had been recorded from monkey peripheral SA

Level

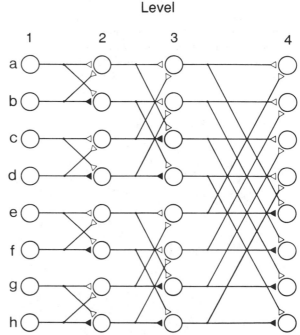

Figure 2. Two-dimensional version of the three-dimensional network used in this study. ($\triangle$) Excitatory (+1) synaptic junctions. ($\blacktriangle$) Inhibitory (−1) junctions.

afferent fibers. The spike trains were fed into the primary units to simulate the neural population discharge that occurs when stimulus letters are scanned at 50 mm/sec. The result was a neural image moving at 50 mm/sec across the receptor units of the network. As in the neurophysiological experiments, the image was swept repeatedly with 200-μm shifts between sweeps.

Impulse trains were replaced at the first synaptic junction by a continuous activation function based on instantaneous, inverse interspike intervals. From there onward, these activation functions were added and subtracted according to the synaptic weights in the network. The activation values transmitted from one level to the next were allowed to take negative as well as positive values (see Discussion). The predicted discharge pattern for each network node was computed using a Poisson impulse generator with an absolute refractory period of 1.0 msec, which matches the stochastic properties of the cortical neuronal firing patterns (K.O. Johnson, unpubl.). The only adjustments were done at this final step. The rate was scaled, and a background rate added to compare the model discharge patterns with individual cortical neurons having different background rates and response intensities. None of the synaptic weights were adjusted.

RESULTS

Discharge patterns from typical peripheral SA and RA afferent fibers are displayed in Figure 3. Some of the features of cortical neuronal responses to scanned letters are accounted for by primary transduction mechanisms. SA afferent fibers resolve spatial detail more acutely than do the RA afferents. Both SA and RA afferents are more sensitive to leading and trailing features than to internal features. Horizontal segments (segments aligned with the scanning direction) evoke relatively few impulses in both SA and RA afferents. Because the SA SEPs from different neurons are similar to one another, as are the RA SEPs, it can be inferred that the population response is a sampled version of the images shown in Figure 3 and that the primary representation of form in the somatosensory system is a pair of neural images that look like the SA and RA SEPs illustrated in Figure 3. The SA discharge pattern illustrated in Figure 3 was used in the simulations reported here.

Discharge patterns from four cortical area 3b SA neurons are shown in Figure 4. They are typical of the entire sample of 64 3b SA neurons in several ways. First, they display the high level of spatiotemporal structure that is characteristic of neurons in this sample. Second, and more importantly, they display some of the variety of cortical neuronal responses that were observed. In some cases, the underlying pattern of excitation and inhibition can be inferred by inspection. For example, the response illustrated at the top of Figure 4 is composed of a double image of the stimulus letters, one shifted down and to the right of the other. That is particularly evident in the response to the letter J but also in the responses to C and G. To account for this kind of response in terms of the peripheral responses illustrated in Figure 3, the receptive field of this neuron must have a band of inhibition between the two diagonally offset zones of excitation. In other cases, such as the response displayed in the third row of Figure 4, it is evident that the response is the result of complex processing whose form is not easily inferred from the SEP. A large fraction of the area 3b SA neurons that we have studied showed responses that are as diverse and complex as those shown in Figure 4.

Three-dimensional versions of the two-dimensional network illustrated in Figure 2 and its complement (excitation replaced with inhibition and vice versa) were simulated using the SA afferent discharge illustrated in Figure 3 as input. These networks, which consisted of 2 × 2 modules at level 2, 4 × 4 modules at level 3, and so forth (see Methods), produced discharge patterns that were compared with observed cortical neuronal discharge patterns. The neuronal responses

Peripheral SA

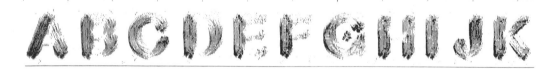

Peripheral RA

Figure 3. Spatial event plots reconstructed from one SA and one RA peripheral afferent fiber. Velocity: 50 mm/sec; letter height: 8.0 mm; contact force: 60g.

Area 3b SA's

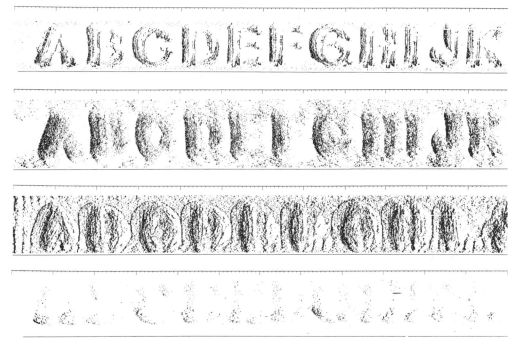

Figure 4. Spatial event plots derived from four slowly adapting cortical neurons in area 3b of awake monkey. Letter height: 8.0 mm; scanning velocity: 50 mm/sec with the exception of panel 3 for which the letter height and scanning velocity were 6.0 mm and 20 mm/sec, respectively. Contact force: 60g. (Adapted from Phillips et al. 1988.)

displayed in the remainder of this section were selected as follows. Every area 3b and 1 neuronal response (174 neurons) was examined and classified as having response properties like one of the model responses or not. Of the neuronal responses, 37% (64/174) were judged to resemble one of the model responses, 40% were classed as not matching one of the responses, whereas the remainder were judged to be too weakly structured for classification. Among area 3b SA neurons, only 8% (5/64) fell in this weakly structured category; the remainder were evenly split between

those that matched one of the model responses and those that did not. In each of the comparisons illustrated in this paper (Figs. 5, 6, and 7), the neuronal response is the best match for the model network response.

The discharge patterns produced by the four different patterns of synaptic weighting at level 2 of the network are illustrated in Figure 5. The unit illustrated in Figure 5a receives excitatory inputs from four adjacent units in level 1. The spatial averaging effected by this unit produces a simulated output that is a blurred

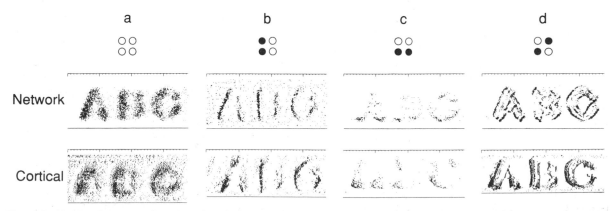

Figure 5. Simulated responses from level 2 of the network (*top*) and responses of cortical neurons (*bottom*) with similar discharge patterns. The 2 × 2 pattern of open and closed circles above each pair of spatial event plots represents the kernel for one unit at level 2, i.e., the pattern of inhibition and excitation from four primary units in the preceding layer. (○) Excitatory input from a single primary afferent unit. (●) Inhibition. The four kernels represent the four patterns of excitation and inhibition that occur at level 2.

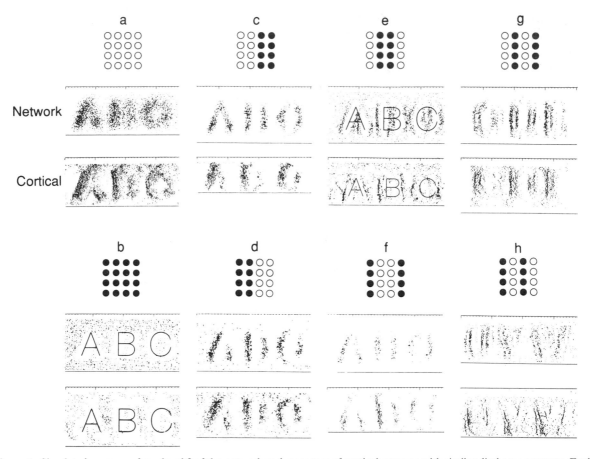

Figure 6. Simulated responses from level 3 of the network and responses of cortical neurons with similar discharge patterns. Each 4 × 4 kernel represents the cumulative pattern of excitation (○) and inhibition (●) traced back to single primary units.

replica of the peripheral input. Beneath it is the response of a cortical area 3b SA neuron to the scanned letters A, B, and C. In all of the results reported here, the peripheral neural discharge pattern passed from right to left across the input layer as though the finger were scanned from left to right across the letters.

Figure 5b illustrates the discharge of another type of unit at level 2 together with a corresponding cortical neuron whose discharge is similar. The orientation of the open (excitatory) and closed (inhibitory) circles indicates that the leading edge of the letters passed first into the vertical pair of excitatory inputs and then into the trailing inhibitory pair. The narrow leading response to each letter is accounted for by the trailing inhibition, which shuts off the broad discharge zone in the input pattern (see Fig. 3). Notice that the vertical orientation of the excitatory pair causes a small vertical spatial smearing, which closes the gap in the letter C.

Figure 5, c and d, illustrates the two remaining unit types at level 2 of the network. The excitatory inputs at the top of the receptive field shown in Figure 5c cause it to respond to the bottoms of the letters and then, at points further up the letters, only at locations where the excitatory elements are activated but not the inhibitory elements as in the center of the C. The matching cortical neuron (3b SA) responds more at the lower left and upper right, suggesting that the neuron's receptive field

was oriented differently than the receptive field of the network unit illustrated in Figure 5c. The network unit response illustrated in Figure 5d is composed of two positive images displaced diagonally by 1.1 mm with an inhibitory band between them. The cortical neuronal response selected as being most similar was discussed earlier (Fig. 4, top row). Of cortical neurons, 6% (11/174) yielded responses that were judged to be most similar to discharge patterns produced by level 2 units.

At level 3 of the network, the modules are 4 × 4, and the network and its complement each contain 16 unit types. Eight of those unit types and neuronal responses that were judged to be good matches are displayed in Figure 6. As in Figure 5, the weighting pattern (kernel) above each pair of plots identifies the unit from which the simulated results were obtained. As in Figure 5, the vertical bands of excitation elongate the vertical features of the letters. The neuronal response illustrated in Figure 6c appears to be an exception but it is not; the neuron whose response best matched the network response was studied with letters that were 6.0 mm high, rather than 8.0 mm high, and that accounts for their smaller size. The responses to letters CDE and UVW were chosen for comparison in Figure 6, g and h, because they show the finely structured on-off-on responses more clearly than do the responses to ABC (in both the network and neuronal responses).

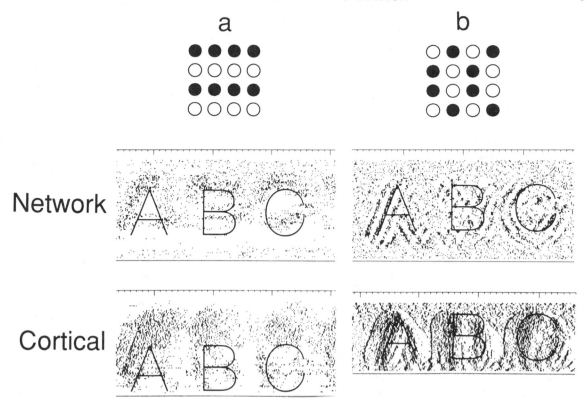

Figure 7. Simulated responses from a level 3 unit with a horizontally banded kernel (*a*) and one with a complex kernel (*b*). Beneath are two cortical neuronal responses.

There were many matches for units with vertically banded kernels (i.e., bands at right angles to the scanning direction, which was proximal to distal along the long axis of the finger) but relatively few good matches for units with kernels of other types. Network units with horizontally banded kernels produce discharge patterns with horizontal bands of firing. A few cortical neurons exhibited such bands; one is illustrated in Figure 7a. The neuronal and network responses match in terms of the activity above the letters (because of the excitatory row across the bottom of the receptive field), the lack of activity below the letters (because of the inhibitory row across the top), the activity to the left of the A (because of the preponderance of excitation when the field is approached from the lower right), and the internal horizontal bands of activity.

Figure 7b illustrates a typical response of the type that occurs in network units with more complex kernels, which constitute 9/16 of all units at level 3. The spatial event plots derived from the simulated responses for these kernels are dominated by high spatial frequencies and, as in many of the cortical responses, the relationship to the stimulus waveform is only evident when the stimulus pattern is overlaid. None of the cortical neuronal responses were well matched to any of these simulated responses. The cortical neuronal response at the bottom of Figure 7b was not classed as matching a network response, but it is included here to show the closest match to the responses of the more complex network kernels. The

neuronal SEP has a quasi-isomorphic appearance with an overlay of bidirectional banding like that in the simulated response. The neuronal response may be like that which would be expected if the weighting pattern were Gabor-like (Jones and Palmer 1987; Daugman 1988), i.e., the product of a Gaussian with the kernel illustrated at the top of Figure 7b.

DISCUSSION

Network Design

The network illustrated in Figure 2 evolved in two steps. First, a network implementation of the fast Fourier transform (FFT) algorithm (Oppenheim and Schafer 1975) was considered because of similarities between its architecture and the architecture of the somatosensory system. The FFT achieves an enormous reduction in the number of computations through a series of small stepwise transformations with modest computational requirements between steps. Algorithms like the FFT exist for most well-known mathematical transformations, and each has a network equivalent based on repeating modular units and sparse connectivity between levels. The enormous saving in number of computations in the stepwise, fast algorithms relative to direct, single-step algorithms is paralleled by enormous savings in the connectivity of the analogous stepwise networks relative to single-step networks. It is interesting to speculate that a process of efficient, stepwise transformation may be operating in the somatosensory system and that it makes feasible the transformations that occur there.

The reduction in connectivity required to effect a complete, distributed transform can be seen by comparing the cross-sectional areas of networks that effect transformations in single and multiple steps. At any level of a network, the cross-sectional area required by all of the connections between one level and the next is at least ndA, where n is the number of units in the first layer, d is the divergence number (the average number of units in layer i + 1 contacted by each unit in layer i), and A is the cross-sectional area of a single connection. We assume that the number of output units is at least as great as the number of input units (which is required for completeness). If the transformation is effected in one step, the divergence number must be at least n and the cross-sectional area must be at least n^2A. In the FFT and the network simulated in this paper, the divergence number, d, is 4 and the total cross-sectional area is $4nA$. From these considerations, it can be seen that the reduction in cross-sectional area achieved by stepwise transformation is $n:d$. In the somatosensory system, the number of primary afferents in each dorsal column is approximately $n = 10^6$. The divergence number is not known, but it is small relative to 10^6. If it were 4, as in the network simulated here, the reduction ratio would be 250,000:1, i.e., a single-step transformation would require a cross-sectional area 250,000 times larger than the area of one dorsal column. The real divergence number is likely to be larger than 4, but even if it were 1000, the stepwise architecture would achieve a 1000:1 reduction in cross-sectional area. These calculations suggest that some form of efficient calculation is essential and that this is the purpose of stepwise processing in the brain.

The FFT algorithm was not simulated because it seemed arbitrary, and the standard forms of the algorithm involve widespread convergence at the first stage of processing. The network presented in this paper evolved from the FFT and takes into consideration the anatomical, physiological, and psychophysical constraints stated above. In this network and all efficient stepwise networks, the structure of the first few steps reveals the entire structure. If the transformations effected by the somatosensory system are accomplished by a form of repeated, modular connection, as in the efficient transformation algorithms, then discovery of the final representational form might be possible by a process of inference. This is our primary reason for considering these networks as models for sensory processing.

One of the criteria used in the construction of the network, completeness, requires some comment. The fact that spatial acuity for complex patterns is near the limits imposed by the primary afferent spacing at the fingertip (Johnson and Phillips 1981; Phillips et al. 1983) suggests that no sensory data are lost in the somatosensory pathways innervating the fingers. If the final neural image is not a complete representation of the primary neural image, there is a loss of dimensionality relative to the primary representation, i.e., dimensions whose variations are not transmitted through the system (called a null space in operator theory [Shilov 1961]). There is no evidence of a stimulus dimension above the limits of acuity that cannot be differentiated in a psychophysical task. Thus, we assume that completeness is a property of the transformational process operating on the neural images that subserve tactile letter recognition.

The spacing between primary nodes, 0.8 mm, was selected to match the current best estimate of the innervation density of primary SA afferents in the monkey (Darian-Smith and Kenins 1980). Other spacings (0.6, 1.0, and 1.2 mm) were tried but were found to degrade the matches.

The synaptic weights were chosen as the simplest possible weights that produce a complete, distributed transformation. In the two-dimensional form illustrated in Figure 2, the weighting patterns compute spatial sums and differences (gradients) from homologous units at the preceding level. In the full three-dimensional network, the application of sums and differences in two directions produces four 2×2 patterns of weighting, which are illustrated in Figure 5. The 2×2 weighting pattern illustrated in Figure 5a produces a spatial average of the homologous computational result in each of four adjacent modules at the preceding level. The weighting patterns in Figure 5, b and c, compute spatial gradients of homologous computational results. The pattern in Figure 5d computes the oriented spatial curvature. The result of repeated application of these rules of connectivity is exhibited in Figures 6 and 7.

Explanatory Power of the Model

The network accounts for the responses of a substantial fraction of area 3b and 1 neurons in terms of banded inhibitory and excitatory receptive fields like those of simple cells in visual cortex (Hubel and Wiesel 1968; Mullikin et al. 1984). The question that we cannot answer with certainty is the one of uniqueness: Can those same responses be accounted for by some other form of receptive field? A hypothesis that has to be examined further is that spatial form processing and the final representation of letters of the alphabet are the same in the visual and somatosensory systems. It might be surprising if the two systems were not similar. There are anatomical (Jones and Powell 1969; Friedman et al. 1986; Pons et al. 1987), psychophysical (Craig 1979; Loomis 1982; Phillips et al. 1983), and evolutionary (Gregory 1967) reasons to believe that they might be similar.

A major difference between the results of our study and previous neurophysiological investigations is the prevalence of cortical neurons in the finger region of area 3b that exhibit complex inhibitory and excitatory interactions. In our study, the majority of responses to scanned letters exhibit spatiotemporal structure that could only be the result of an interaction between excitation and inhibition. Inhibitory interneurons are a major part of the anatomical structure at all levels of the system (Hendry et al. 1987; Westman 1990). The effects of these inhibitory neurons were uncovered only when we examined the responses to scanned letters. In our own manual probing of receptive fields with punctate probes, we found evidence of inhibition in only a small number of neurons. Among those displayed in this paper, neither inhibition nor directional selectivity was uncovered by manual probing except for the neuron displayed in Figure 6b.

The network illustrated in Figure 2 provides an explanation for these contradictory results. The receptive fields of primary afferents are 2–4 mm in diameter, i.e., 3–5 mean primary afferent spacings (Talbot et al. 1968). A small punctate probe would activate a dozen primary afferents. Activation of the network in an analogous manner would produce little, if any, evidence of inhibition because inhibition is balanced by excitation through the network. In the network shown in Figure 2, only units 3c, 3g, and 4e would exhibit an inhibitory effect when 3–5 primary units are activated. Even those units would yield evidence of inhibition only if they possessed a background discharge rate. The evidence of structured inhibition shows up in scanning because a dynamic, structured pattern of neural activity moves across the distal circuitry that drives a single neuron. Inhibition and excitation show up in the spatial event plots because of the systematic way that primary afferent fibers are activated by the stimulus. Neurons in areas 3b and 1 routinely respond much more vigorously to stroking than to punctate indentation (as do peripheral afferents). When using a punctate probe, the inhibition would be manifested as an irregularity in the discharge that would be difficult to detect. Direct demonstration of detailed spatiotemporal patterns of excitation and inhibition in the receptive fields of somatosensory cortical neurons will require a dense array of closely spaced probes capable of generating the appropriate spatial stimulus patterns.

On a larger scale, somatotopy and the growth of receptive field size and complexity were designed into the model so it cannot be credited with explaining them. However, it makes quantitative predictions about the growth of receptive field size and the granularity of somatotopy. Somatotopy is preserved at a fine-grained level within areas 3b and 1 of the macaque (Pons et al. 1987), which means (according to the model) that modules in 3b and 1 are small and that SI cortex resides at an early stage of processing. However, the quantitative properties of somatotopy and receptive field size have not been studied in sufficient detail to draw any conclusions about the correspondence between models like the one presented here and the somatosensory system. Qualitatively, there is no contradiction. Somatotopy disappears slowly in the somatosensory system and in the network considered here. For example, in the layer that is three synapses before the final layer (which exhibits no somatotopy) in the model, the body surface is represented by 64 somatotopically adjacent modules.

Lack of Fit

There are responses produced by the network that we did not observe in the neurophysiological studies and neurophysiological responses that could not be matched by the network. The matches that we found were all assigned to network units with uniform excitation (13/174), uniform inhibition (5/174), vertical bands of excitation and inhibition (42/174), or horizontal bands (4/174). Those groups only account for 14 out of 32 unit types at level 3 of the excitatory network and its complement. Only one cortical neuron, which is illustrated in Figure 7b, yielded a response with some properties resembling the responses produced by the other 18 network units.

The network simulation produced discharge patterns of a kind that would be expected in a network based on linear spatial mechanisms. Such a network can only effect place shifted addition and subtraction of its inputs. Many neurons yielded responses that were more structured than any response produced by the network (two are illustrated in Figs. 5d and 6h) and were of a kind that we think could only be accounted for by nonlinear mechanisms.

The network, as shown, violates basic physiological constraints. It should be regarded as symbolizing a slightly more complex but equivalent network that is constructed as follows. First, to satisfy Dale's law, every inhibitory synapse needs to be replaced by an excitatory synapse and an inhibitory interneuron. A more significant modification is required to account for the fact that neurons cannot transmit negative activation levels through negative impulse rates. The network axons illustrated in Figure 2 transmit negative as well as positive effects from one level to the next. Thus, the effect transmitted from one level to the next cannot be interpreted directly as impulse frequency. In a network composed of more realistic elements, which only transmit positive impulse frequencies, each node needs to be replaced with two parallel units. The first of these would be connected as in Figure 2 but only transmit the synaptic drive when it is positive. The second unit would be inserted with complementary synaptic inputs and outputs. These units would form a complementary pair with one firing only when the original unit was transmitting a positive effect and the other firing only when the original unit was transmitting a negative effect.

A final item relates to position and size invariance. Subjects in psychophysical experiments recognize letters immediately regardless of location and size (for sizes above threshold). The network illustrated in Figure 2 cannot account for those important psychophysical facts. Because it produces a transformed but complete representation of the input image, changes in size and location are registered as changes in the output image. No part of the output image is size or position invariant. However, a small, physiologically realizable modification of the network does yield position invariance (Reitbock and Brody 1969). That is one of the variations that will be simulated in future studies.

CONCLUSION

The study presented here had two objectives. One was to compare cortical neuronal responses to scanned letters against those produced by a network effecting a complete, distributed transformation. The results are consistent with the hypothesis that the somatosensory system effects a major transformation of the neural representation of form in a stepwise manner and that the heterogeneity of response types observed in areas 3b and 1 is exactly that which would be expected within such a transformational process. The second objective was to undertake a form of modeling that seems to us to be critical if the sensory systems are to be understood as systems. Each sensory system is a stepwise network producing one or more transformations of the primary neural images. The prospect of understanding these networks up to some intermediate level of processing holds promise for understanding the form of representation that underlies pattern recognition.

ACKNOWLEDGMENT

This research was supported by National Institutes of Health grant NS-18787.

REFERENCES

Craig, J.C. 1979. A confusion matrix for tactually presented letters. *Percept. Psychophys.* **26:** 409.
Darian-Smith, I. and P. Kenins. 1980. Innervation density of mechanoreceptive fibers supplying glabrous skin of the monkey's index finger. *J. Physiol.* **309:** 147.
Daugman, J.G. 1988. Complete discrete 2-D Gabor transforms by neural networks for image analysis and compression. *IEEE Trans. Acoust. Speech Sig. Process.* **36:** 1169.
Dykes, R.W., D.D. Rasmusson, D. Stretavan, and N.B. Rehman. 1982. Submodality segregation and receptive field sequences in the cuneate, gracile, and the external cuneate nuclei of the cat. *J. Neurophysiol.* **47:** 389.
Friedman, D.P., E.A. Murray, J.B. O'Neill, and M. Mishkin. 1986. Cortical connections of the somatosensory fields of the lateral sulcus of macaques: Evidence for a corticolimbic pathway for touch. *J. Comp. Neurol.* **252:** 323.
Gregory, R.L. 1967. Origin of eyes and brains. *Nature* **213:** 369.
Hendry, S.H.C., H.D. Schwark, E.G. Jones, and Y. Jan. 1987. Numbers and proportions of GABA-immunoreactive neurons in different areas of monkey cerebral cortex. *J. Neurosci.* **7:** 1503.
Hubel, D.H. and T.N. Wiesel. 1968. Receptive fields and functional architecture of monkey striate cortex. *J. Physiol.* **195:** 215.
Johansson, R.S. and A. Vallbo. 1979. Tactile sensitivity in the human hand: Relative and absolute densities of four types of mechanoreceptive units in glabrous skin. *J. Physiol.* **286:** 283.
Johnson, K.O. and G.D. Lamb. 1981. Neural mechanisms of spatial tactile discrimination: Neural patterns evoked by Braille-like dot patterns in the monkey. *J. Physiol.* **310:** 117.

Johnson, K.O. and J.R. Phillips. 1981. Tactile spatial resolution: I. Two-point discrimination, gap detection, grating resolution, and letter recognition. *J. Neurophysiol.* **46:** 1177.
———. 1988. A rotating drum stimulator for scanning embossed patterns and textures across the skin. J. Neurosci. Methods **22:** 221.
Johnson, K.O., J.R. Phillips, S.S. Hsiao, and I.N. Bankman. 1990. Tactile pattern recognition. In *Information processing in the somatosensory system* (ed. O. Franzen and J. Westman). Macmillan, London. (In press.)
Jones, E.G. and D.P. Friedman. 1982. Projection pattern of functional components of thalamic ventrobasal complex upon monkey somatic sensory cortex. *J. Neurophysiol.* **48:** 521.
Jones, E.G. and T.P.S. Powell. 1969. Connexions of the somatic sensory cortex of the rhesus monkey. I. Ipsilateral cortical connexions. *Brain* **92:** 477.
Jones, J.P. and L.A. Palmer. 1987. An evaluation of the two-dimensional Gabor filter model of simple receptive fields in cat striate cortex. *J. Neurophysiol.* **58:** 1233.
Loomis, J.M. 1981. On the tangibility of letters and Braille. *Percept. Psychophys.* **29:** 37.
———. 1982. Analysis of tactile and visual confusion matrices. *Percept. Psychophys.* **31:** 41.
Mountcastle, V.B. 1976. An organizing principle for cerebral function: The unit module and the distributed system. In *The mindful brain* (ed. G.M. Edelman and V.B. Mountcastle), p. 7. MIT Press, Cambridge.
———. 1984. Central nervous mechanisms in mechanoreceptive sensibility. In *Handbook of physiology—The nervous system III* (ed. I. Darian-Smith), p. 789. American Physiological Society, Bethesda, Maryland.
Mullikin, W.H., J.P. Jones, and L.A. Palmer. 1984. Periodic simple cells in cat area 17. *J. Neurophysiol.* **52:** 372.
Oppenheim, A.V. and R.W. Schafer. 1975. *Digital signal processing.* Prentice-Hall, Engelwood Cliffs.
Phillips, J.R., K.O. Johnson, and H. Browne. 1983. A comparison of visual and two modes of tactual letter recognition. *Percept. Psychophys.* **34:** 243.
Phillips, J.R., R.S. Johansson, and K.O. Johnson. 1990. Representation of Braille characters in human nerve fibers. *Exp. Brain Res.* (in press).
Phillips, J.R., K.O. Johnson, and S.S. Hsiao. 1988. Spatial pattern representation and transformation in monkey somatosensory cortex. *Proc. Natl. Acad. Sci.* **85:** 1317.
Pons, T.P., J.T. Wall, P.E. Garraghty, C.G. Cusick, and J.H. Kaas. 1987. Consistent features of the representation of the hand in area 3b of macaque monkeys. *Somatosens. Res.* **4:** 309.
Rao, K.R. 1985. *Discrete transforms and their applications.* Van Nostrand Reinhold, New York.
Reitbock, H. and T.P. Brody. 1969. A transformation with invariance under cyclic permutation for applications in pattern recognition. *Control* **15:** 130.
Robinson, C.J. and H. Burton. 1980. Organization of somatosensory receptive fields in cortical areas 7b, retroinsula, postauditory and granular insula of *M. fascicularis*. *J. Comp. Neurol.* **192:** 69.
Shilov, G.E. 1961. *An introduction to the theory of linear spaces.* Prentice-Hall, Engelwood Cliffs.
Talbot, W.H., I. Darian-Smith, H.H. Kornhuber, and V.B. Mountcastle. 1968. The sense of flutter-vibration: Comparison of the human capacity with response patterns of mechanoreceptive afferents from the monkey hand. *J. Neurophysiol.* **31:** 301.
Vega-Bermudez, F., K.O. Johnson, K.H. Fasman, and S.S. Hsiao. 1989. Active vs passive touch in a letter recognition task: Human performance and velocity effects. *Soc. Neurosci. Abstr.* **15:** 313.
Westman, J. 1990. GABAergic neurons and terminals in the dorsal column nuclei and lateral cervical nucleus. In *Information processing in the somatosensory system* (ed. O. Franzen and J. Westman). Macmillan, London. (In press.)

Protein-Chromophore Interactions in Rhodopsin Studied by Site-directed Mutagenesis

J. NATHANS

Howard Hughes Medical Institute, Department of Molecular Biology and Genetics and Department of Neuroscience, Johns Hopkins University School of Medicine, Baltimore, Maryland 21205

Visual pigments are the light-absorbing proteins in the retina that initiate phototransduction. Each consists of an integral membrane protein, opsin, covalently joined via a protonated Schiff's base to a chromophore, 11-*cis* retinal (or in some instances, a closely related retinal). Visual pigments are members of a large family of cell-surface receptors, including many hormone receptors, that convey and amplify stimulus information by activating G proteins. Upon photoexcitation, the visual pigment chromophore, 11-*cis* retinal, is isomerized in situ from *cis* to *trans* (Fig. 1A). This isomerization and the accompanying activation of the visual pigment are analogous to the replacement of an an-

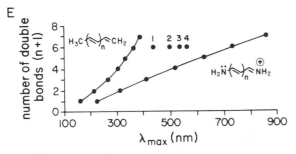

Figure 1. Retinal, polyene, and cyanine structures and absorbance maxima. (*A*) Photoisomerization of a protonated retinylidene Schiff's base from 11-*cis* to all-*trans*. (*B*) Major (*upper*) and minor (*lower*) resonance structures of a protonated retinylidene Schiff's base. (*C*) Major (*upper*) and minor (*lower*) resonance structures of a polyene. (*D*) Equivalent resonance structures of a cyanine. (*E*) Absorbance maxima as a function of number of double bonds for polyenes (*left*), cyanines (*right*), and human visual pigments (*center*: 1, blue pigment; 2, rhodopsin; 3, green pigment; 4, red pigment [Dartnall et al. 1983; Schnapf et al. 1987]).

tagonist by an agonist in the binding pocket of one of the related hormone receptors.

The absorbance spectra of a large number of visual pigments have been determined, and these spectra have in common a broad bell shape, closely resembling the shape of a protonated Schiff's base of retinal free in solution. The pigment spectra differ from one another and from that of the free chromophore in their positions along the wavelength axis: Points of maximal absorbance have been found throughout the visible range, from far red to near ultraviolet (Liebman 1971). Presumably, amino acid sequence differences among the visual pigments determine their distinctive absorbance spectra.

Recently, the amino acid sequences of a number of visual pigments have been determined, including bovine (Hargrave et al. 1983; Nathans and Hogness 1983; Ovchinnikov et al. 1983), chicken (Takao et al. 1988), human (Nathans and Hogness 1984), mouse (Baehr et al. 1988), octopus (Ovchinnikov et al. 1988), and *Drosophila* (O'Tousa et al. 1985; Zuker et al. 1985, 1987; Cowman et al. 1986; Fryxell and Meyerwitz 1987; Montell et al. 1987) rhodopsins; and the three human cone pigments (Nathans et al. 1986). These sequences define a family of homologous proteins and provide a data base to guide future experiments. It is reasonable to suppose that highly conserved properties such as efficient isomerization and G-protein activation will be reflected in the conservation of single amino acids or protein domains. Conversely, those properties that differ between pigments, for example, the absorbance spectrum, will be reflected in protein sequence differences.

All visual pigment sequences reveal seven predominantly hydrophobic stretches of amino acids. These are presumed to form a bundle of seven membrane-spanning α-helical segments, an arrangement consistent with protein modification experiments using water-soluble probes (for a recent review, see Nathans 1987). 11-*cis* retinal is covalently attached to lysine 296 (in the bovine rhodopsin numbering system) in the center of the seventh hydrophobic stretch (Bownds 1967; Wang et al. 1980). Rhodopsin's polarized absorbance in oriented rod outer segments indicates that 11-*cis* retinal lies parallel to the plane of the bilayer (Chabre et al. 1982). Fluorescence energy transfer experiments indicate that the chromophore is close to the center of the bilayer (Thomas and Stryer 1982), consistent with its site of covalent attachment. These and other experiments suggest that the seven membrane-spanning segments form a ring around a central retinal-binding pocket. This model predicts that amino acids in several or all of these segments may come into close proximity to the chromophore. Most likely, amino acids that protrude beyond the membrane do not contact the chromophore.

How does binding to a visual pigment modify the absorbance spectrum of 11-*cis* retinal? To answer this question, we first need to consider the photochemical properties of retinal. Like all conjugated compounds, retinal exists as a mixture of resonance states (Fig. 1B). Resonance distributes π electrons more evenly along the carbon chain: Double bonds acquire a partially single bond character, and single bonds acquire a partially double bond character. Molecular orbital calculations and a large body of experimental data indicate that an increase in π electron delocalization results in a lower energy difference between ground and photoexcited states, i.e., a red shift in absorbance (Suzuki 1967; Mathies and Stryer 1976). This effect is apparent in comparing the absorbance maxima of polyenes and cyanines. As shown in Figure 1C, polyenes exist predominantly in one resonance state; alternate resonance states produce an unfavorable charge separation. As a consequence, polyenes exhibit pronounced alternations in bond length and have a large energy difference between ground and photoexcited states, i.e., they absorb at short wavelengths. In contrast, cyanines exist as an equal mixture of two energetically equivalent resonance states (Fig. 1D). Cyanines show no bond length alternation and have absorbance maxima at significantly longer wavelengths than polyenes (Fig. 1E).

The difference in absorbance maxima between free 11-*cis* retinal and the visual pigments derives in part from Schiff's base formation. When measured in methanol, free retinal has an absorbance maximum of 380 nm, whereas the chloride salt of a protonated *N*-butylamine Schiff's base of retinal absorbs maximally at 440 nm (Pitt et al. 1955). (The latter compound is the standard against which the visual pigments and other retinal derivatives are compared.) In protonated Schiff's bases of retinal, resonance structures such as the one shown in Figure 1B are energetically favorable because they partially delocalize the positive charge throughout the π electron system. As seen in Figure 1, a protonated Schiff's base of retinal is in essence a hybrid between a cyanine and a polyene; the degree of electron delocalization and bond alternation is intermediate between those of polyenes and cyanines. As a consequence, the absorbance maxima of all visual pigments fall within the intervals defined by the polyene and cyanine absorbance maxima. This is shown in Figure 1E for the absorbance maxima of the four human visual pigments.

During the past 30 years, a number of plausible models have been advanced to account for the spectral tuning of retinal (Hubbard and Sperling 1973; Kakitani et al. 1985). Most models propose that a negatively charged amino acid serves as the Schiff's base counterion. Alternatively, the protonated Schiff's base in the visual pigment could be paired to a counterion from solution, for instance chloride, or could be stabilized by a surrounding shell of polar residues. Changes in the distance or charge density of the putative counterion have been hypothesized to play a role in generating the differences in absorbance maxima that distinguish the visual pigments from one another, from their photoexcited intermediates, and from the reference protonated Schiff's base (Blatz et al. 1972; Baasov and Sheves 1986; Fukada et al. 1990). With respect to interactions along the polyene chain, one model proposes that in bovine rhodopsin a negatively charged amino acid selectively stabilizes the photoexcited state by contacting the polyene chain near carbon 13 (Honig et al. 1976, 1979; Kakitani et al. 1985). This point charge model is consistent with the red shifts seen in comparing a series of dehydroretinal analogs of bovine rhodopsin to the corresponding *N*-butylamine salts (Koutalos et al. 1989). Interactions along the polyene chain that do not involve charged residues have also been considered. Twisting of the chromophore about double or single bonds would produce, respectively, a red shift or a blue shift (Blatz and Liebman 1973); polarizable groups near the chromophore would stabilize the photoexcited state by compensatory electronic movements and therefore produce a red shift; polar groups would produce either a red shift or a blue shift, depending on their orientation with respect to the dipole moment of the chromophore (Irving et al. 1969, 1970; Hays et al. 1980).

To test these models, I have studied the properties of rhodopsin derivatives in which various residues have been altered by site-directed mutagenesis (Nathans 1990a,b). In these experiments, I have chosen to study bovine rather than human rhodopsin because it is the better characterized of the two visual pigments. I would anticipate similar results with human rhodopsin, given that the two are 94% identical at the amino acid level, have identical charged residues, and have absorbance maxima within several nanometers of one another (Crescitelli and Dartnall 1953; Wald and Brown 1958).

MATERIALS AND METHODS

Plasmids and cells. The rhodopsin expression plasmid pCIS-cRho contains a bovine rhodopsin-coding region (Nathans and Hogness 1983) under the control of a human cytomegalovirus immediate-early enhancer and promoter, an SV40 poly(A) addition site, and an SV40 origin of DNA replication (Nathans et al. 1989; Gorman et al. 1990). In a typical experiment, 100 μg of a pCIS-cRho mutant plasmid and 10 μg of pRSV-TAg (an SV40 T-antigen expression plasmid) were coprecipitated onto 20 10-cm diameter plates of 293S cells (a suspension-adapted variant of a human embryonic kidney cell line; ATCC CRL 1573) by the calcium phosphate method (Gorman 1985).

In vitro mutagenesis. Mutagenic oligonucleotides were used to prime DNA synthesis on a single-stranded pCIS-cRho template as described previously (Carter 1987). Covalently closed double-stranded circular products were gel purified and transfected into an *Escherichia coli* mutant deficient in the mismatch repair gene *mutL* (Glickman and Radman 1980). After overnight growth in liquid culture, plasmid DNA was harvested from the pool of *mutL* transformants; the rhodopsin-coding region was excised, gel purified, ligated to the parental pCIS plasmid, and introduced into wild-type *E. coli*. Single colonies harboring mutant plasmids were identified by colony hybridization using the mutagenic oligonucleotides as probes. For each mutant, the entire rhodopsin-coding region was sequenced on one strand by the dideoxy method, both to confirm the predicted nucleotide changes and to rule out spurious ones.

*Membrane preparation and joining to 11-*cis* retinal.* Solutions for membrane preparation were chilled on ice, and all centrifugation steps were performed at 4°C. Sixty hours after transfection, the cells were collected by vigorously washing the plates with phosphate-buffered saline (PBS) containing 5 mM EDTA. The cells were centrifuged at 1000g for 10 minutes, washed once with 20 ml of PBS, and resuspended in 10 ml of 0.1 M sodium phosphate (pH 6.5), 1 mM EDTA, 250 mM sucrose, and 0.2 mM PMSF. The cell suspension was homogenized for 30 seconds in a Polytron homogenizer (Brinkmann) at a setting of 5.5, diluted to 25 ml with the same buffer, and then layered on top of a 10-ml 1.15 M sucrose cushion containing 0.1 M sodium phosphate (pH 6.5) and 1 mM EDTA. The homogenate was centrifuged in a swinging-bucket rotor (SW28) at 105,000g for 30 minutes. Membranes were collected from the interface between the homogenization buffer and the sucrose cushion, diluted with 8 volumes of 0.1 M sodium phosphate (pH 6.5) and 1 mM EDTA, and centrifuged in a swinging-bucket rotor (SW28) at 105,000g for 30 minutes. The resulting membrane pellet was solubilized in 0.3 ml of 0.1 M sodium phosphate (pH 6.5), 1 mM EDTA, and 5% digitonin (Kodak) at 23°C.

All manipulations involving 11-*cis* retinal were performed under dim red light. 11-*cis* retinal (stored dry in the dark under argon at −80°C) was first dissolved in ethanol to a concentration of 4×10^{-3} M and then diluted with 20 volumes of 0.1 M sodium phosphate (pH 6.5), 1 mM EDTA, and 5% digitonin; 0.1 ml of the aqueous 11-*cis* retinal solution was added to the solubilized preparation and incubated at 23°C for 2 hours in the dark. The reaction was terminated by the addition of 0.05 ml of 0.6 M hydroxylamine (adjusted to pH 6.0 with sodium hydroxide), and the sample was incubated for an additional 30 minutes at 23°C (Hubbard et al. 1971).

For measuring the reaction rate with hydroxylamine and for monitoring the effect of halide addition, the protocol was modified as follows. Reconstitution with 11-*cis* retinal was performed in the presence of 1 mM DTT at 23°C overnight with membranes collected from the sucrose step gradient. To remove excess 11-*cis* retinal, the membranes were diluted with 8 volumes of 0.1 M sodium phosphate (pH 6.0) containing 4% bovine serum albumin and centrifuged in a swinging bucket rotor (SW28) at 105,000g for 30 minutes. The resulting membrane pellet was solubilized in 0.3 ml of 0.1 M sodium phosphate (pH 6.0) and 5% digitonin at 23°C.

Absorbance spectra. Before measuring the absorbance spectrum, samples were centrifuged at 11,000 rpm in an Eppendorf microfuge for 5 minutes. Spectra were obtained on the supernatant before and after 10 minutes of photobleaching with a 15-W incandescent bulb placed behind a glass shield and a 495-nm short-wave cutoff filter approximately 10 cm from the cuvette. Spectra were recorded in a water-jacketed cuvette holder at 20°C with a Kontron Instruments Uvikon spectrophotometer. Kontron Instruments software was used to calculate the difference spectra and determine the absorbance maxima shown in Figures 4 and 12. Earlier work has shown that for absorbance maxima averaging 0.075 ODU, this method has a mean variation in duplicate experiments of 2.4 nm (Nathans 1990a). For the halide addition experiments shown in Table 1 and Figures 7, 8, and 9, approximately twofold greater accuracy in estimating absorbance maxima was obtained by transferring the photobleaching difference spectra to a MacIntosh computer and calculating for each spectrum the best-fitting fifth-order polynomial.

Table 1. Visual Pigment Absorbance Maxima Determined from Difference Spectra

Halide added	Wild type[a] +halide, ±hv (n = 3)	E113Q[a] +halide, ±hv (n = 5)	E113Q[b] ±halide, −hv (n = 3)
Chloride	498.0 ± 1.0	495.0 ± 2.0	487.5 ± 1.5
Bromide	499.0 ± 1.0	498.5 ± 1.5	490.0 ± 2.0
Iodide	498.5 ± 2.0	504.5 ± 2.5	497.0 ± 2.5

Absorbance maxima (in nm) are presented as the mean ± s.d.; the number of independent experiments are shown in parentheses.

[a]Derived from photobleaching difference spectra in the presence of 0.1 M of the indicated halide (Fig. 8).

[b]Derived from difference spectra obtained by subtracting the absorbance before halide addition from the one obtained after halide addition (Fig. 7).

Protein blots. Membrane samples containing expressed opsin were diluted with three volumes of SDS sample buffer, electrophoresed on an SDS/12% polyacrylamide gel, and electroblotted onto nitrocellulose (Burnette 1981). Opsin was detected by using a mouse monoclonal antibody directed against residues 3–14 of bovine rhodopsin (B6-30; gift from Dr. Paul Hargrave) and an alkaline-phosphatase-conjugated goat anti-mouse second antibody.

RESULTS

Expression of Bovine Rhodopsin in Tissue-culture Cells

To produce rhodopsin by expression of cloned cDNA, I have used the mammalian tissue-culture system developed by Dr. Cornelia Gorman (Gorman et al. 1990). Bovine rhodopsin-coding sequences were introduced into a human embryonic kidney cell line under the control of a cytomegalovirus immediate-early enhancer and promoter. Stable cell lines obtained by cotransfection of the expression plasmid and a plasmid conferring G418 resistance (Southern and Berg 1982) produce 100–200 μg of bovine opsin per liter of saturated growth medium ($\sim 10^9$ cells). Transient cotransfection of the expression plasmid and a plasmid directing expression of SV40 large T-antigen produces a comparable level of protein, typically 1–3 μg per 10-cm dish (10^7 cells). This level corresponds to 3×10^6 molecules per cell. Expressed opsin is membrane associated and heterogeneously glycosylated (Fig. 2). In one stable cell line examined by immunoelectron microscopy, opsin was seen to accumulate in the plasma membrane (Nathans et al. 1989).

In a typical experiment, total cell membranes are purified from 20 10-cm plates of transiently transfected cells. The membranes are solubilized in digitonin and incubated in the dark with 11-*cis* retinal. Several hours later, hydroxylamine is added to convert excess free retinal into retinal oxime (Hubbard et al. 1971). Retinal that has bound to opsin to form rhodopsin is resistant to attack by hydroxylamine. Absorbance spectra are recorded before and after the sample is exposed to light of greater than 495 nm (Fig. 2). Irradiation isomerizes the 11-*cis* retinal in rhodopsin to all-*trans* retinal, which then dissociates and is converted to retinal oxime. The difference between the absorbance spectra obtained before and after light exposure reveals a positive absorbance peak in the visible region (rhodopsin) and a negative peak in the ultraviolet region (retinal oxime). Endogenous cellular constituents give only trace absorbance in the visible region, none of which appears to be photolabile. When expressed in this tissue-culture system, wild-type rhodopsin produces a photobleaching difference spectrum identical to that produced by bovine rhodopsin isolated from cattle retinas.

Aspartate and Glutamate Mutants

Because current models of transmembrane topography and of the retinal-binding pocket are still preliminary, a study was undertaken to systematically test the role of each of the 22 negatively charged amino acids in determining the absorbance spectrum of bovine rhodopsin. Each glutamate was replaced by glutamine and each aspartate by asparagine. A triple substitution mutant was constructed at positions 330, 331, and 332; at all other positions, single substitution mutants were constructed. Figure 3 shows the locations of these residues in a transmembrane model of rhodopsin. The model is based on hydropathy, known sites of proteolytic cleavage, and the experiments presented below regarding the role of glutamate 113. Similar models have been proposed by Hargrave et al. (1983), Ovchinnikov et al. (1982), and Nathans and Hogness (1983). Mutants are referred to by the single letter amino acid designation of the wild-type residue followed by the position number in the polypeptide chain followed by the single letter amino acid designation of the introduced residue; e.g., E201Q refers to the substitution of glutamate 201 by glutamine.

In an initial series of reconstitution experiments, total cell membranes were prepared in sodium phosphate and EDTA; solubilized in sodium phosphate,

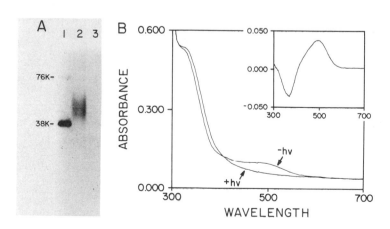

Figure 2. Protein blot and absorbance spectra of wild-type bovine rhodopsin expressed in human embryonic kidney cells. *(A)* Nitrocellulose blot of a SDS/12% polyacrylamide gel visualized with a mouse monoclonal anti-bovine rhodopsin primary antibody and an alkaline-phosphatase-conjugated goat anti-mouse secondary antibody. *(1)* Bovine rod outer segments containing 200 ng rhodopsin; *(2)* total cell membranes from 2×10^6 embryonic kidney cells stably transformed with the rhodopsin expression plasmid; *(3)* total cell membranes from 2×10^6 embryonic kidney cells. *(B)* Absorbance spectra of expressed wild-type bovine rhodopsin after joining in vitro to 11-*cis* retinal, both before (*−hv*) and after (*+hv*) light exposure; *(inset)* photobleaching difference spectrum derived by subtracting the two spectra shown in the main panel.

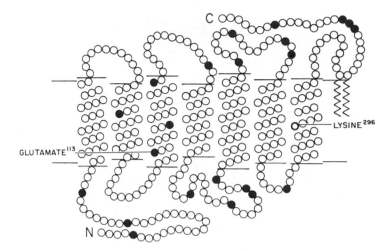

Figure 3. Transmembrane model of bovine rhodopsin. Each aspartate and glutamate is indicated by a filled circle. Lysine 296 is the residue to which retinal is covalently bound; glutamate 113 is the protonated retinylidene Schiff's base counterion. (*Bottom*) Extracellular; (*top*) intracellular.

GLUTAMATE¹¹³

LYSINE²⁹⁶

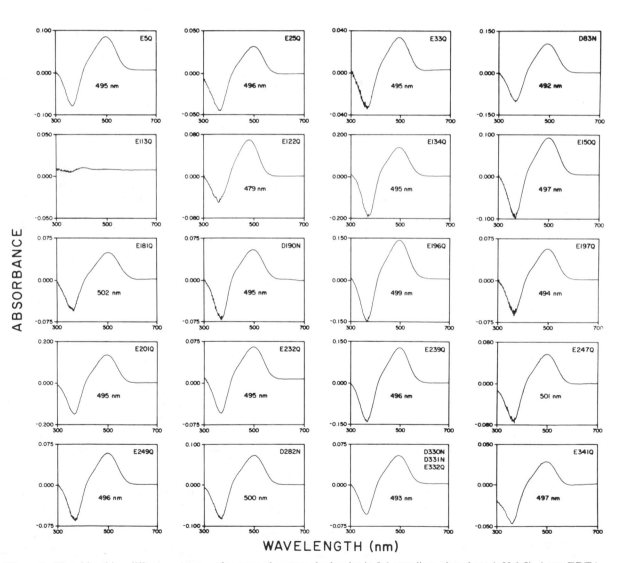

Figure 4. Photobleaching difference spectra of expressed mutant rhodopsins in 0.1 M sodium phosphate (pH 6.5), 1 mM EDTA, 5% digitonin, and 50 mM hydroxylamine. The absorbance maximum is indicated below each spectrum.

EDTA, and digitonin; and incubated in the dark with 11-*cis* retinal. To convert excess retinal to retinal oxime, hydroxylamine was then added to 50 mM, and the samples were incubated for an additional 30 minutes at room temperature. Absorbance spectra were recorded before and after photobleaching, and the difference spectra were calculated (Fig. 4). Of the 20 mutants, 19 have photobleaching difference spectra closely resembling that of wild-type rhodopsin: 18 mutants have absorbance maxima within 8 nm of the wild type; E122Q is blue-shifted 17 nm. Under these conditions, E113Q differs markedly from the wild type: It does not show an absorbance peak in the visible region, and it exhibits no change in absorbance after exposure to light. To further characterize the anomalous behavior of E113Q, photobleaching difference spectra were obtained as described above except in the absence of hydroxylamine (Fig. 5). Under these conditions, E113Q also produces no absorbance change upon exposure to light. Figure 6 shows that the E113Q apoprotein accumulates to a comparable level and is glycosylated to the same extent as E25Q.

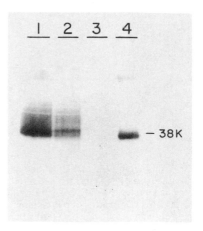

Figure 6. Protein blot of expressed rhodopsin mutants. Each lane of an SDS/12% polyacrylamide gel was loaded with the equivalent of 4% of the sample used for spectrophotometry and visualized with a monoclonal mouse anti-bovine rhodopsin primary antibody and alkaline phosphatase-conjugated goat anti-mouse secondary antibody. (*1*) E25Q; (*2*) E113Q; (*3*) mock transfected control; (*4*) bovine rod outer segments containing 300 ng rhodopsin.

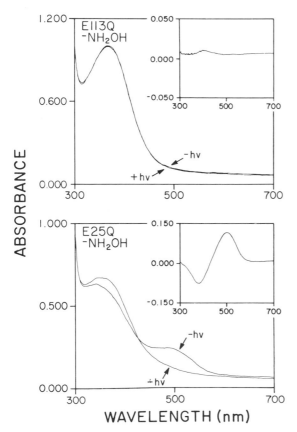

Figure 5. Absorbance spectra before and after photobleaching in the absence of hydroxylamine (*main panel*) and photobleaching difference spectra (*inset*) of rhodopsin mutants E113Q and E25Q. The sample contains 0.1 M sodium phosphate (pH 6.5), 1 mM EDTA, and 5% digitonin.

E113Q: Effect of Halides and Hydroxylamine

The experiments described above suggest a model in which glutamate 113 provides a negative charge that is essential for normal visual pigment formation. This model assumes that the anions present in solution, phosphate and EDTA, are unable to substitute for the missing negative charge. To examine the possibility that a smaller anion could substitute for the charge normally present at position 113, chloride (sodium chloride, 0.1 M final concentration) was added to a sample of E113Q that had been incubated with 11-*cis* retinal. An increase in absorbance in the visible region, maximal at 487 nm, and a concomitant decrease in the ultraviolet, maximal at 380 nm, were observed (Fig. 7). The chloride-dependent absorbance change was complete before a spectrum could be recorded, a delay of approximately 15 seconds. The chloride-dependent peak in the visible region resembles that of bovine rhodopsin in its absorbance maximum (487 nm vs. 498 nm) and photolability (Fig. 8). Photobleaching generates a product that is identical in its absorbance spectrum to free all-*trans* retinal. The magnitude of the chloride-dependent absorbance change is greater at pH 6.0 than at pH 7.0. The experiments described below were therefore performed at pH 6.0.

Chloride addition converts E113Q from a form that absorbs maximally at 380 nm to one that absorbs maximally at 487 nm. The 380-nm absorbance peak matches that of an unprotonated Schiff's base of retinal, as seen in metarhodopsin II and in Schiff's bases of retinal in solution, all of which absorb at wavelengths less than 400 nm. The 487-nm absorbance peak is presumed to derive from a protonated Schiff's base, as seen in wild-type rhodopsin and in protonated Schiff's bases of retinal in solution, which absorb at wavelengths greater than 400 nm. The simplest interpretation of this experi-

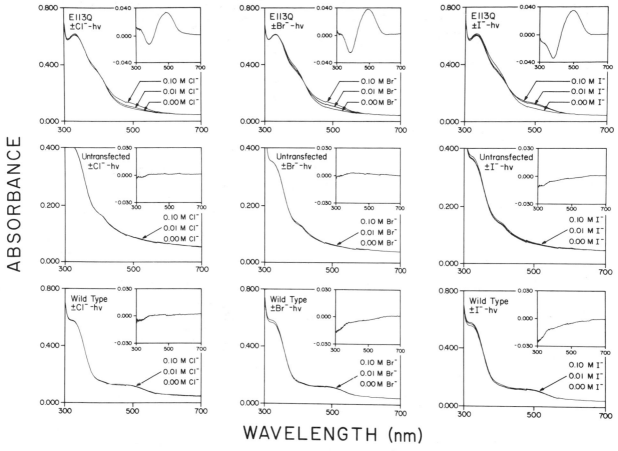

Figure 7. Absorbance spectra before and after addition of sodium chloride, bromide, or iodide to final concentrations of 10 mM and 100 mM (main panels). The insets show difference spectra in which the 0 mM halide absorbance spectrum has been subtracted from the 100 mM halide absorbance spectrum. The samples contained 0.1 M sodium phosphate (pH 6.0) and 5% digitonin. (*Top panels*) E113Q; (*middle panels*) untransfected cell membranes; (*bottom panels*) wild-type rhodopsin expressed in 293S cells.

ment is that glutamate 113 normally serves as the Schiff's base counterion. Mutation of glutamate 113 to glutamine favors deprotonation of the Schiff's base. Addition of chloride to E113Q leads to protonation of the Schiff's base because chloride serves as a surrogate counterion. Presumably, phosphate and EDTA, the two other solution anions present in the sample, are too bulky to enter the retinal-binding site.

To test this interpretation, the absorbance spectra and the photobleaching difference spectra of E113Q

were measured following addition of either chloride, bromide, or iodide to 0.1 M (Figs. 7, 8, and 9). This experiment was inspired by the observation of Blatz et al. (1972) that the absorbance maxima of *N*-butylamine-protonated Schiff's bases of retinal move to progressively longer wavelengths when paired with halide counterions of increasing atomic radius. For example, in benzene, the chloride salt absorbs maximally at 437 nm, the bromide salt at 448 nm, and the iodide salt at 457 nm. In tetrahydrofuran, the absorbance

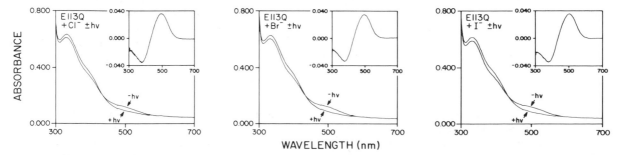

Figure 8. Absorbance spectra before and after photobleaching (*main panels*) and photobleaching difference spectra (*insets*) of rhodopsin mutant E113Q in the presence of 100 mM sodium chloride, bromide, or iodide. The samples were prepared as in Fig. 7.

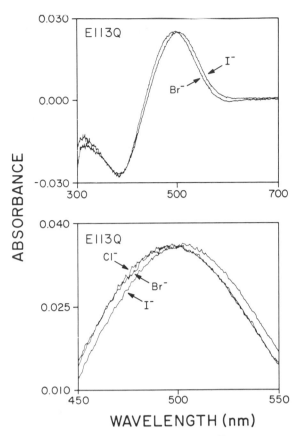

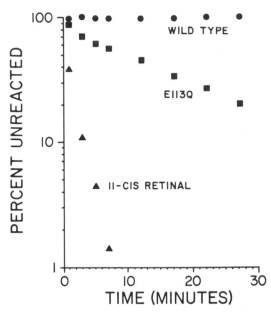

Figure 10. Time course of hydroxylamine reactivity with wild-type rhodopsin, rhodopsin mutant E113Q, and free 11-*cis* retinal at 20°C. All samples contained equal amounts of 293S membranes, 0.1 M sodium phosphate (pH 6.0), 5% digitonin, and 0.1 M sodium chloride. The reaction was initiated by addition of hydroxylamine to a final concentration of 50 mM.

Figure 9. Superposition of photobleaching difference spectra of rhodopsin mutant E113Q in 100 mM sodium iodide or bromide (*upper panel*), and 100 mM sodium iodide, bromide, or chloride (*lower panel*, enlarged). The samples were prepared as in Figs. 7 and 8.

maxima are 430 nm, 432 nm, and 441 nm, respectively. The red shifts in absorbance reflect an increase in π electron delocalization.

When added to E113Q, each halide induces a rapid conversion of the 380-nm species to one absorbing maximally near 495 nm. Table 1 lists the absorbance maxima derived from difference spectra following halide addition in the absence of light (Fig. 7; 3 independent experiments) and following photobleaching in the presence of 0.1 M halide (Figs. 8 and 9; 5 independent experiments). There is a reproducible 7–8-nm difference between the absorbance maxima measured from the two types of difference spectra. The cause of this discrepancy is not known. In discussing these pigments, the photobleaching absorbance maxima will be considered the true maxima. Control samples prepared identically from untransfected cells or from cells expressing wild-type rhodopsin showed no significant absorbance change upon halide addition. Table 1 lists the absorbance maxima derived from photobleaching difference spectra of wild-type rhodopsin in the presence of chloride, bromide, and iodide. These values are identical within experimental error.

The hypothesis that halides act as counterions in E113Q predicts that the Schiff's base in E113Q should

be accessible to other small molecules in the aqueous environment. To test this prediction, the time course of reaction between hydroxylamine and the chromophore in E113Q was determined (Fig. 10). At 20°C in 0.1 M chloride, the half life of E113Q in 50 mM hydroxylamine is 12 minutes, as measured by the disappearance of the absorbance peak at 487 nm. Under identical conditions, free 11-*cis* retinal and wild-type rhodopsin have half lives of 1 minute and > 10 hours, respectively.

Charged Amino Acids That Differ between Visual Pigments

The starting point for these experiments is the spectral absorbance and amino acid sequence data for the four human visual pigments. Human rhodopsin, which mediates vision in dim light, peaks at 493–497 nm (Crescitelli and Dartnall 1953; Wald and Brown 1958); the three human cone pigments, which mediate color vision, peak at approximately 420–440 nm, 530 nm, and 560 nm (referred to as blue, green, and red pigments, respectively [Dartnall et al. 1983; Schnapf et al. 1987]). Comparison of the red and green pigment amino acid sequences shows 96% identity, whereas all other pairwise comparisons show approximately 40% identity (Nathans et al. 1986).

To examine the possibility that differences in charged amino acids play a role in spectral tuning, the locations of charged residues in the four human pigments were compared (Fig. 11). If we include histidine as a potentially charged residue, there are four positions of interest in the putative transmembrane segments at which

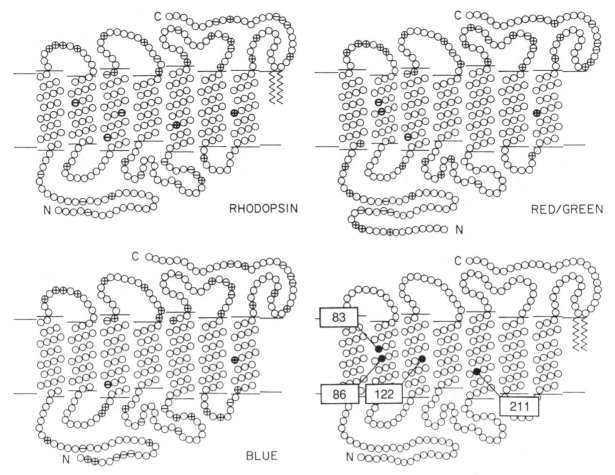

Figure 11. Charged amino acids in human visual pigments. Arginine, histidine, and lysine are indicated by (+); glutamate and aspartate by (−). Variable residues in the putative transmembrane segments are numbered using the bovine rhodopsin numbering system.

charged residues appear. Excluded from this group are the conserved lysine 296, to which 11-*cis* retinal binds, and glutamate 113, which is presumed to function in each pigment as the Schiff's base counterion as shown above for bovine rhodopsin. In the putative transmembrane regions, the blue pigment has none of the four charges, the red and green pigments have two charged residues, and rhodopsin has three charged residues, one of which (aspartate 83) is shared with the red and green pigments. Table 2 lists the amino acids at these four positions for each of the pigments. (Number-

ing of amino acids follows the bovine rhodopsin sequence.)

Nine site-directed mutants were constructed to produce the cone pigment charge distributions at the four variable positions. All of the single amino acid substitutions were constructed: D83G, M86E, E122I, and H211C. In addition, single substitution mutants were constructed that minimize structural perturbations not related to charge: D83N, E122Q, and E211F. Two double mutants were constructed by sequential mutagenesis to produce the charge distributions corre-

Table 2. Nonconserved Charged Amino Acids in the Putative Transmembrane Segments of Bovine and Human Rhodopsin and the Four Human Cone Pigments

Amino acid position	Human/bovine rhodopsin	Human blue	Human red/green
83	Asp	Gly	Asp
86	Met	Leu	Glu
122	Glu	Leu	Ile
211	His	Cys	Cys

The bovine rhodopsin numbering system is used.

sponding to the blue pigment (E122I D83G) and the red and green pigments (E122I M86E).

Upon incubation with 11-*cis* retinal, all of the mutant opsins produce photolabile pigments with absorbance spectra similar in shape to that of rhodopsin (Fig. 12; see Fig. 4 for D86N and E122Q spectra). All of the pigments are stable in the presence of 50 mM hydroxylamine for 30 minutes at room temperature.

The absorbance maximum of each mutant pigment will be taken as the average of the two experimental determinations, one of which is shown in Figs. 4 and 8. The maxima show a mean variation in two trials of 2.4 nm, the greatest spread being 5 nm. Relative to wild-type rhodopsin (absorbance maximum, 498 nm), substitution of aspartate 83 with glycine or asparagine leads to shifts of +1.5 nm and −8.5 nm, respectively; substitution of glutamate 122 with isoleucine or glutamine leads to shifts of −2 and −17 nm, respectively; substitution of aspartate 83 with glycine together with substitution of glutamate 122 with isoleucine leads to a shift of −1.5 nm; and substitution of histidine 211 with phenylalanine or cysteine leads to shifts of −4.5 nm and −5 nm, respectively. These amino acid alterations mimic the charge distribution seen in the human blue cone pigment, the absorbance maximum of which is shifted −68 ± 10 nm with respect to rhodopsin.

Substitution of methionine 86 with glutamate leads to a shift of −5.5 nm and substitution of methionine 86 with glutamate together with substitution of glutamate 122 with isoleucine leads to a shift of −7 nm. These

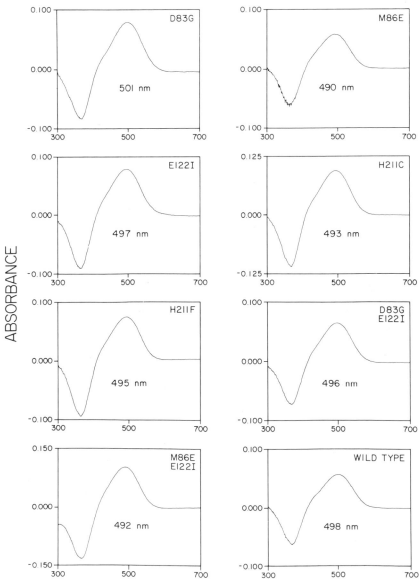

Figure 12. Photobleaching difference spectra of expressed mutant rhodopsins in 0.1 M sodium phosphate (pH 6.5), 1 mM EDTA, 5% digitonin, and 50 mM hydroxylamine. The absorbance maximum is indicated below each spectrum.

amino acid alterations, together with E122Q, E122I, H211F, and H211C described above, mimic the charge distribution seen in the human green and red pigments, the absorbance maxima of which are shifted +32 nm and +62 nm, respectively, relative to rhodopsin.

DISCUSSION

Charged amino acids have been hypothesized to play two distinct roles in spectral tuning. One negatively charged residue is presumed to be near the protonated Schiff's base nitrogen and to serve as its counterion (Honig et al. 1976). A second negatively charged residue is postulated to lie near the polyene chain to stabilize excited state resonance structures (the point charge model; Kropf and Hubbard 1958; Honig et al. 1976, 1979; Kakitani et al. 1985). In bovine rhodopsin, the second negatively charged residue is hypothesized to be near carbon 13 of 11-*cis* retinal, based on the spectral shifts observed when dehydroretinal analogs are used to reconstitute the pigment (Koutalos et al. 1989). Analogous experiments with chicken iodopsin (absorbance maximum, 562 nm) have led to the hypothesis that a negatively charged residue in that pigment is near the β-ionone ring (Chen et al. 1989). Substitution of the putative point charge by a neutral residue should lead to a blue shift in the absorbance spectrum, reflecting a decrease in π electron delocalization. Substitution of the putative Schiff's base counterion by a neutral residue should lead either to a red shift, reflecting an increase in π electron delocalization, and/or a deprotonation of the Schiff's base. Unprotonated retinylidene Schiff's bases absorb at approximately 380 nm.

Identification of the Retinylidene Schiff's Base Counterion

To test the role of negatively charged residues in spectral tuning, each aspartate and glutamate was mutated to asparagine and glutamine, respectively. (In designing these experiments, only aspartate and glutamate were considered as negatively charged residues; the possibility exists, however, that one or more tyrosinates may be present in bovine rhodopsin or other visual pigments.) Of these, E113Q is the only mutant that differs markedly from the wild type. Upon reconstitution with 11-*cis* retinal and in the absence of small solution anions, E113Q forms a pigment absorbing at 380 nm. This pigment is presumed to contain an unprotonated retinylidene Schiff's base. In the presence of halides, the absorbance of E113Q shifts to approximately 495 nm, reflecting the protonation of the Schiff's base. In these experiments, the UV-absorbing form of E113Q has not been observed directly; its existence is inferred by the shift from UV to visible absorbance upon halide addition.

It appears that in E113Q the normal Schiff's base counterion is absent, and that a halide from solution can serve as a surrogate Schiff's base counterion. This

interpretation is supported by the observation of a progressive red shift upon addition of halides with progressively larger atomic radii (chloride vs. bromide vs. iodide). The direction and magnitude of the red shifts resemble those seen by Blatz et al. (1972) with protonated Schiff's bases of retinal in solution, in particular in tetrahydrofuran. Halides have no effect on the absorbance spectrum of wild-type rhodopsin. These characteristics of E113Q, together with the nearly wild-type behavior of all of the other glutamate and aspartate mutants, identify glutamate 113 as the retinylidene Schiff's base counterion in bovine rhodopsin. Alternative mechanisms for stabilizing the protonated Schiff's base in wild-type rhodopsin—i.e., pairing to a counterion from solution or interacting with favorably disposed dipoles—are unlikely to be relevant. Zhukovsky and Oprian (1989) and Sakmar et al. (1989) have arrived at the same conclusion on the basis of a related series of experiments. Glutamate is present at the homologous location in all of the other vertebrate pigments sequenced to date: chicken (Takao et al. 1988), mouse (Baehr et al. 1988), and human (Nathans and Hogness 1984) rhodopsins; and the three human cone pigments (Nathans et al. 1986). It is interesting that aspartate 113 in the β-adrenergic receptor, which is located at a position similar to that of glutamate 113 in bovine rhodopsin, is proposed to ion-pair with the primary amine in adrenergic ligands (Strader et al. 1987, 1988).

The identification of glutamate 113 as the Schiff's base counterion provides a constraint on the spatial proximity of two positions (113 and 296) that are widely separated on the linear sequence. A second constraint of this type has been defined by Karnik et al. (1988) between cysteine 110 and cysteine 187, which form a disulfide bond. These constraints provide two useful starting points for tertiary structure prediction.

Mechanisms of Spectral Tuning

The halide salts of E113Q can be compared to the corresponding halide salts of a protonated retinylidene Schiff's base in solution without the confounding effect of a change in counterion. This comparison suggests that the red shift induced in 11-*cis* retinal upon forming the halide salts of E113Q is not caused by a decrease in counterion charge density or an increase in counterion distance relative to that of the reference protonated Schiff's base in methanol. Given the nearly identical red shifts induced in 11-*cis* retinal upon joining to wild-type rhodopsin or to E113Q in the presence of halides, it appears that the tuning mechanisms operating in E113Q can account for the full extent of the wild-type red shift. This observation is consistent with dehydroretinal experiments that implicate an electrostatic perturbation along the polyene chain in spectral tuning (Koutalos et al. 1989).

With respect to the charged amino acids that differ between pigments, alterations at each of the four candidate positions in the putative transmembrane segments produce absorbance shifts far smaller than those seen between pigments. Mutant E122Q produced the largest spectral shift, -17 nm. However, a more drastic substitution at that same position, E122I, produced only a -2-nm shift, implying that glutamate 122 is not intimately involved in spectral tuning. These results rule out a significant role for these residues in spectral tuning.

The present set of mutants eliminate all aspartate and glutamate residues as candidates for a point charge lying along the polyene chain. Instead, they are consistent with a more general interpretation of the dehydroretinal data, namely, that spectral tuning could be due to either charged, polar, or polarizable residues in the neighborhood of the chromophore. Future experiments will be aimed at testing the latter two possibilities.

ACKNOWLEDGMENTS

I thank Ms. Carol Davenport for assistance in DNA sequencing; Dr. Cornelia Gorman, Dr. Arthur Levinson, and Mr. Robert Kline (Genentech) for advice on tissue-culture expression systems and for making available the CIS vector and 293s cell line used in this work; Dr. Lubert Stryer (Stanford University) and the Hoffmann-La Roche Company for gifts of 11-*cis* retinal; Dr. Paul Hargrave (University of Florida) for the gift of monoclonal anti-bovine rhodopsin antibody; Dr. Clark Riley, Ms. Anatoli Amarantidis, and Ms. Cynthia Wendling for synthesis of oligonucleotides; Ms. Jimo Borjigin, Dr. Isabel Chiu, Ms. Shannath Merbs, Dr. Ching-Hwa Sung, Ms. Yanshu Wang, Dr. Charles Weitz, and Dr. Donald Zack for helpful discussions; and Ms. Teri Chase for assistance in preparing the manuscript. This work was supported by the National Eye Institute of the National Institutes of Health and by the Howard Hughes Medical Institute.

REFERENCES

Baasov, T. and M. Sheves. 1986. Alteration of pKa of the bacteriorhodopsin protonated Schiff base. A study with model compounds. *Biochemistry* **25:** 5249.

Baehr, W., J.D. Falk, K. Bugra, J.T. Triantafyllos, and J.F. McGinnis. 1988. Isolation and analysis of the mouse opsin gene. *FEBS Lett.* **238:** 253.

Blatz, P.E. and P.A. Liebman. 1973. Wavelength regulation in visual pigments. *Exp. Eye Res.* **17:** 573.

Blatz, P.E., J. Mohler, and H. Navangul. 1972. Anion-induced wavelength regulation of absorption maxima of Schiff bases of retinal. *Biochemistry* **11:** 848.

Bowmaker, J.K. and H.J.A. Dartnall. 1980. Visual pigments of rods and cones in a human retina. *J. Physiol.* **298:** 501.

Bownds, D. 1967. Site of attachment of retinal in rhodopsin. *Nature* **216:** 1178.

Burnette, W.N. 1981. "Western" blotting: Electrophoretic transfer of proteins from SDS-polyacrylamide gels to unmodified nitrocellulose and radiographic detection with antibody and radioiodinated protein A. *Anal. Biochem.* **112:** 195.

Carter, P. 1987. Improved oligonucleotide-directed mutagenesis using M13 vectors. *Methods Enzymol.* **154:** 382.

Chabre, M., J. Breton, M. Michel-Villaz, and H. Saibil. 1982. Linear dichroism studies in the visible, UV, and IR on oriented rod suspensions. *Methods Enzymol.* **81:** 605.

Chen, J.G., T. Nakamura, T.G. Ebrey, H. Ok, K. Konno, F. Derguini, K. Nakanishi, and B. Honig. 1989. Wavelength regulation in iodopsin, a cone pigment. *Biophys. J.* **55:** 725.

Cowman, A.C., C.S. Zuker, and G.M. Rubin. 1986. An opsin gene expressed in only one photoreceptor cell type of the *Drosophila* eye. *Cell* **44:** 705.

Crescitelli, F. and H.J.A. Dartnall. 1953. Human visual purple. *Nature* **172:** 195.

Dartnall, H.J.A., J.K. Bowmaker, and J.D. Mollon. 1983. Human visual pigments: Microspectrophotometric results from the eyes of seven persons. *Proc. R. Soc. Lond. B* **220:** 115.

Fryxell, K.J. and E.M. Meyerowitz. 1987. An opsin gene that is expressed only in the R7 photoreceptor cell of *Drosophila. EMBO J.* **6:** 443.

Fukada, Y., T. Okano, Y. Shichida, T. Yoshizawa, A. Trehan, D. Mead, M. Denny, A.E. Asato, and R.S.H. Liu. 1990. Comparative study on the chromophore binding sites of rod and red-sensitive cone visual pigments by use of synthetic retinal isomers and analogues. *Biochemistry* **29:** 3133.

Glickman, B.W. and M. Radman. 1980. *Escherichia coli* mutator mutants deficient in methylation-instructed DNA mismatch repair. *Proc. Natl. Acad. Sci.* **77:** 1063.

Gorman, C. 1985. High efficiency gene transfer into mammalian cells. In *DNA cloning* (ed. D.M. Glover), vol. II, p 143. IRL Press, Oxford.

Gorman, C., D.R. Gies, and G. McCray. 1990. Transient production of proteins using an adenovirus transformed cell line. *DNA Protein Eng. Techniq.* **2:** 3.

Hargrave, P.A., J.H. McDowell, D.R. Curtis, J.K. Wang, E. Juszczak, S.L. Fong, J.K. Mohanna Rao, and P. Argos. 1983. The structure of bovine rhodopsin. *Biophys. Struct. Mech.* **9:** 235.

Hays, T.R., S.H. Lin, and H. Eyring. 1980. Wavelength regulation in rhodopsin: Effects of dipoles and amino acid side chains. *Proc. Natl. Acad. Sci.* **77:** 6314.

Honig, B., A. Greenberg, V. Dinur, and T. Ebrey. 1976. Visual pigment spectra: Implications of the protonation of the retinal Schiff base. *Biochemistry* **15:** 4593.

Honig, B., U. Dinur, K. Nakanishi, V. Balough-Nair, M.A. Gawinowicz, M. Arnaboldi, and M.G. Motto. 1979. An external point charge model for wavelength regulation in visual pigments. *J. Am. Chem. Soc.* **101:** 7084.

Hubbard, R. and L. Sperling. 1973. The colors of the visual pigment chromophores. *Exp. Eye Res.* **17:** 581.

Hubbard, R., P.K. Brown, and D. Bownds. 1971. Methodology of vitamin A and visual pigments. *Methods Enzymol.* **18:** 615.

Irving, C.S., G.W. Byers, and P.A. Leermakers. 1969. Effect of solvent polarizability on the absorption spectrum of all-*trans* retinylpyrrolidiniminium perchlorate. *J. Am. Chem. Soc.* **91:** 2141.

———. 1970. Spectroscopic model for the visual pigments. Influence of microenvironmental polarizability. *Biochemistry* **9:** 858.

Kakitani, H., T. Kakitani, H. Rodman, and B. Honig. 1985. On the mechanism of wavelength regulation in visual pigments. *Photochem. Photobiol.* **41:** 471.

Karnik, S.S., T.P. Sakmar, H.-B. Chen, and H.G. Khorana. 1988. Cysteine residues 110 and 187 are essential for the formation of correct structure in bovine rhodopsin. *Proc. Natl. Acad. Sci.* **85:** 8459.

Koutalos, Y., T.G. Ebrey, M. Tsuda, K. Odashima, T. Lien, M.H. Park, N. Shimizu, F. Derguini, K. Nakanishi, H.R. Gilson, and B. Honig. 1989. Regeneration of bovine and octopus opsins in situ with natural and artificial retinals. *Biochemistry* **28:** 2732.

Kropf, A. and R. Hubbard. 1958. The mechanism of bleaching rhodopsin. *Ann. N.Y. Acad. Sci.* **74:** 266.

Liebman, P.A. 1971. Microspectrophotometry of photoreceptors. *Handb. Sensory. Physiol.* **7:** 482.

Mathies, R. and L. Stryer 1976. Retinal has a highly dipolar vertically excited singlet state: Implications for vision. *Proc. Natl. Acad. Sci.* **73:** 2169.

Montell, C., K. Jones, C. Zuker, and G.M. Rubin. 1987. A second opsin gene expressed in the ultraviolet sensitive R7 photoreceptor cells of *Drosophila melanogaster. J. Neurosci.* **7:** 1558.

Nathans, J. 1987. Molecular biology of visual pigments. *Annu. Rev. Neurosci.* **10:** 163.

———. 1990a. Determinants of visual pigment absorbance: Role of charged amino acids in the putative transmembrane segments. *Biochemistry* **29:** 937.

———. 1990b. Determinants of visual pigment absorbance: Identification of the retinylidene Schiff's base counterion in bovine rhodopsin. *Biochemistry* (in press).

Nathans, J. and D.S. Hogness. 1983. Isolation, sequence analysis, and intron-exon arrangement of the gene encoding bovine rhodopsin. *Cell* **34:** 807.

———. 1984. Isolation and nucleotide sequence of the gene encoding human rhodopsin. *Proc. Natl. Acad. Sci.* **81:** 4851.

Nathans, J., D. Thomas, and D.S. Hogness. 1986. Molecular genetics of human color vision: The genes encoding blue, green, and red pigments. *Science* **232:** 193.

Nathans, J., C.J. Weitz, N. Agarwal, I. Nir, and D.S. Papermaster. 1989. Production of bovine rhodopsin by mammalian cell lines expressing cloned cDNA: Spectrophotometry and subcellular localization. *Vision Res.* **29:** 907.

O'Tousa, J.E., W. Baehr, R.L. Martin, J. Hirsh, W.L. Pak, and M.W. Applebury. 1985. The *Drosophila* ninaE gene encodes an opsin. *Cell* **40:** 839.

Ovchinnikov, Y.A., N.G. Abdulaev, A.S. Zolotarev, I.D. Artamov, I.A. Bespalov, A.E. Dergachev, and M. Tsuda. 1988. Octopus rhodopsin: Amino acid sequence deduced from cDNA. *FEBS Lett.* **232:** 69.

Ovchinnikov, Y.A., N.G. Abdulaev, M.Y. Feigina, I.D. Artamonov, A.S. Bogachuk, A.S. Zolotarev, E.R. Eganyan, and P.V. Kostetskii. 1983. Visual rhodopsin III: Complete amino acid sequence and topography in the membrane. *Bioorg. Khim.* **9:** 1331.

Pitt, G.A.J., F.D. Collins, R.A. Morton, and P. Stok. 1955. Studies on rhodopsin. *Biochem. J.* **59:** 122.

Sakmar, T.P., R.R. Franke, and H.G. Khorana. 1989. Glutamic acid-113 serves as the retinylidene Schiff base counterion in bovine rhodopsin. *Proc. Natl. Acad. Sci.* **86:** 8309.

Schnapf, J.L., T.W. Kraft, and D.A. Baylor. 1987. Spectral sensitivity of human cone photoreceptors. *Nature* **325:** 439.

Southern, P.J. and P. Berg. 1982. Transformation of mammalian cells to antibiotic resistance with a bacterial gene under control of the SV40 early region promoter. *J. Mol. Appl. Genet.* **1:** 327.

Strader, C.D., I.S. Sigal, M.R. Candelore, E. Rands, W.S. Hill, and R.A.F. Dixon. 1988. Conserved aspartic acid residues 79 and 113 of the beta-adrenergic receptor have different roles in receptor function. *J. Biol. Chem.* **263:** 10267.

Strader, C.D., I.S. Sigal, R.B. Register, M.R. Candelore, E. Rands, and R.A.F. Dixon. 1987. Identification of residues required for ligand binding to the beta-adrenergic receptor. *Proc. Natl. Acad. Sci.* **84:** 4384.

Suzuki, H. 1967. *Electronic absorption spectra and geometry of organic molecules.* Academic Press, New York.

Takao, M., A. Yasui, and F. Tokunaga. 1988. Isolation and sequence determination of the chicken rhodopsin gene. *Vision Res.* **28:** 471.

Thomas, D.D. and L. Stryer. 1982. The transverse location of the retinal chromophore of rhodopsin in rod outer segment disc membranes. *J. Mol. Biol.* **154:** 145.

Wald, G. and P.K. Brown 1958. Human rhodopsin. *Science* **127:** 222.

Wang, J.K., J.H. McDowell, and P.A. Hargrave. 1980. Site of attachment of 11-*cis* retinal in bovine rhodopsin. *Biochemistry* **19:** 5111.

Zuker, C.S., A.F., Cowman, and G.M. Rubin. 1985. Isolation and structure of a rhodopsin gene from *D. melanogaster. Cell* **40:** 851.

Zuker, C.S., C. Montell, K.R. Jones, T. Laverty, and G.M. Rubin. 1987. A rhodopsin gene expressed in photoreceptor cell R7 of the *Drosophila* eye: Homologies with other signal transducing molecules. *J. Neurosci.* **7:** 1550.

Zhukovsky, E.A. and D.D. Oprian. 1989. Effect of carboxylic acid side chains on the absorption maximum of visual pigments. *Science* **246:** 928.

Cone Excitations and Color Vision

T.W. KRAFT,* C.L. MAKINO,† R.A. MATHIES,‡ J. LUGTENBURG,§
J.L. SCHNAPF,* AND D.A. BAYLOR†

*Departments of Ophthalmology and Physiology, University of California, San Francisco, California 94143;
†Department of Neurobiology, Stanford Medical School, Stanford, California 94305; ‡Department of
Chemistry, University of California, Berkeley, California 94702; §Department of Chemistry,
State University of Leiden, Leiden, The Netherlands

The brain computes the colors in visual images by comparing the excitations of three types of retinal cones, each sensitive in a different region of the spectrum. Nearly two centuries after trichromacy was enunciated by Thomas Young (1802), Nathans et al. (1986) established its molecular basis by cloning the genes for the three cone pigments. Despite this achievement, it has been difficult to define the wavelength dependence of the cone excitations and to delineate the molecular mechanism of wavelength selectivity. Microspectrophotometry (for review, see Bowmaker 1984, 1990) has been used to measure the spectral absorption of single cones, but the small quantity of pigment in one cell restricts the measurements to wavelengths where the absorption is strong. Suitable expression systems for the cone pigments are not yet available.

We have used physiological methods to study the light-evoked cone excitations of the primate retina. In particular, we have asked:

1. How sensitive is each cone pigment to light of different wavelengths?
2. Does one cone contain only one pigment?
3. How do physiological and psychophysical estimates of cone spectral sensitivity compare?
4. What mechanisms determine the band of wavelengths to which a particular pigment responds?

Spectral Sensitivities of Macaque and Human Cones

We measured the spectral sensitivities of single cones by recording their electrical responses to monochromatic light. A cone's membrane current was measured by drawing the outer segment into a fire-polished pipette (see Fig. 1). The sensitivity to photons of a given wavelength was determined from the reciprocal of the flash strength required to evoke a response of criterion amplitude (see Fig. 2). The sensitivity determined in this way is proportional to the wavelength-dependent probability that the pigment in the cone will absorb a photon (Baylor et al. 1987). Figure 2 demonstrates that a cone encoded the number of photons absorbed but not their wavelength. Thus, after suitable adjustment of the flash strength, light at 500 nm and 659 nm evoked identical responses. All the cones studied behaved in this way, signaling only the number of photons absorbed.

Figure 3 summarizes the results of spectral sensitivity measurements on 41 cones of the monkey *Macaca fascicularis*. The three curves have maxima near 430 nm, 530 nm, and 560 nm. For simplicity, we term these types blue, green, and red, respectively. The ratio of the excitations of the three cones is the elementary color signal analyzed by the brain. At any wavelength, this ratio is proportional to the separation of the curves on the log ordinate scale.

Two features of the results in Figure 3 are noteworthy. First, at 600 nm, the blue curve lies five log units below the red and green curves. We interpret this to indicate that the pigment in the blue cone is very pure, less than 1 molecule in 10^5 being of red or green type. One cell, therefore, seems to express one and only one pigment gene, an appropriate strategy to make the best use of the pigments in wavelength discriminations. Second, the individual spectra within a class were remarkably similar. Although group averages are plotted in Figure 3, analysis indicated that the positions on the abscissa of individual spectra within a group varied by less than 1.5 nm (S.D.). Thus, across cells and animals (9 macaques were used), pigment molecules of a given type appeared to absorb identically.

The spectra of red and green cones from a surgical specimen of human retina (Schnapf et al. 1987) were indistinguishable from the corresponding macaque spectra. This confirms the suggestion from color-matching experiments (DeValois et al. 1974) that macaque and human cones are similar. The spectral sensitivity of human blue cones has not yet been determined.

Cone Spectra and Psychophysics

The monkey cone spectra satisfactorily predicted the results of several kinds of psychophysical experiments on human color vision. In the classic color-matching experiments of Stiles and Burch (1959), a subject viewed a divided field (diagram at top of Fig. 4). A monochromatic test light of selected wavelength was presented in the left side of the field. The subject adjusted the intensities of monochromatic lights at long, middle, and short wavelength in the right half of the field until the entire field appeared uniform. Within each cone class, the excitation was then the same throughout the field. The smooth curves at the bottom

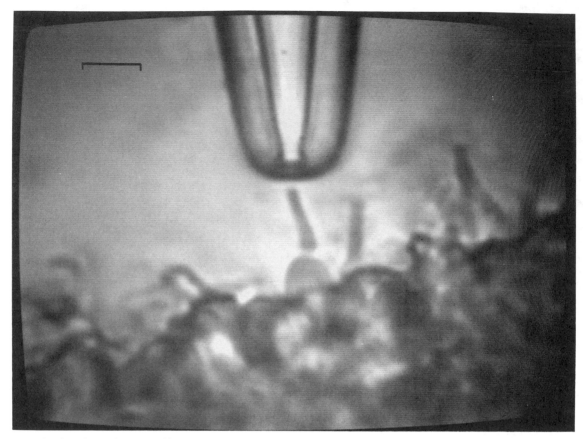

Figure 1. Suction electrode approaching a red cone of the macaque retina, as photographed from the video monitor during an experiment. The cone's response to light was recorded by drawing the outer segment into the electrode and measuring the light-induced reduction in inward membrane current. Bar, 10 μm.

of Figure 4 plot the measured matching intensities as a function of the wavelength of the test light. The symbols show our prediction (Baylor et al. 1987), based on the measured sensitivities of the monkey cones. To make the prediction, the intensities of the three matching lights were obtained from three simultaneous equations expressing the equality of each cone response to the stimuli on the right and left.

Figure 5 shows an attempt to fit the photopic luminosity function, a psychophysically measured quantity that expresses the relative ability of photons to excite cone vision. The continuous curve is the psychophysical function, whereas the symbols were calculated as a weighted sum of the corrected spectral sensitivities of human red and green cones (Schnapf et al. 1988). The fit is satisfactory with the red contribution weighted 1.9 times as heavily as the green. What this weighting means remains to be determined. One possibility is that red cones are roughly twice as numerous as green cones in the cone mosaic.

Brindley (1955) discovered that the apparent hue of a monochromatic light reddens with increasing wavelength to 700 nm but progressively yellows beyond 700 nm; certain wavelength pairs straddling 700 nm appeared identical. The shapes of the red and green cone spectra provide a physiological basis for Brindley's findings. Figure 6 shows the red cone sensitivity relative to the green cone sensitivity as a function of wavelength. The curve has a maximum at about 700 nm. The curve declines at wavelengths beyond 700 nm, because here the red spectrum declines slightly more rapidly than the green spectrum. At long wavelength, where the brain can only measure the excitations of the red and green cones, there are pairs of wavelengths on either side of 700 nm that excite the red and green cones in the same ratio and thus appear identical.

Molecular Basis of Spectral Sensitivities

The molecular mechanisms that regulate light absorption by the three cone pigments are not well understood. In all three pigments, light is absorbed by the same 11-*cis* retinal chromophore. The proteins redshift the chromophore's absorption to the appropriate regions of the spectrum. In the blue pigment, the redshift seems to depend largely on the presence of a protonated Schiff base linkage between retinal and protein (Loppnow et al. 1989). What produces the additional redshift in the red and green pigments, and what causes the 30-nm separation between their spectra? The notion that negative charges in the cone proteins may redshift retinal's absorption (Chen et al. 1989) has not

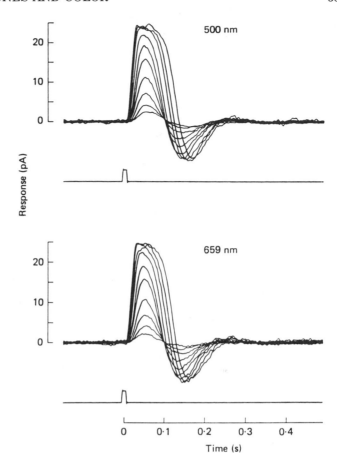

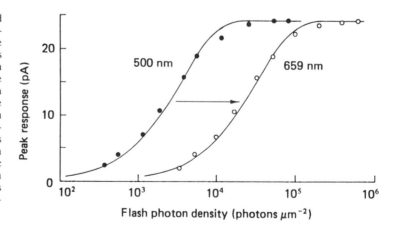

Figure 2. Determination of a macaque red cone's relative quantum sensitivity at two wavelengths from its electrical response to light. The upper panels show the cell's averaged responses to monochromatic flashes of increasing strength at 500 nm and 659 nm. The change in membrane current from the level in darkness is plotted as a function of time, with a flash monitor trace below the responses. The graph at the bottom gives the dependence of peak response amplitude on flash strength. The smooth curves fitted to the points have the same shape. From their horizontal displacement on the logarithmic abscissa (arrow), the cone's sensitivity at 659 nm was determined to be 9 times lower than its sensitivity at 500 nm. (Reprinted, with permission, from Baylor et al. 1987.)

been confirmed by site-directed mutagenesis in rhodopsin (Nathans 1990). Additional evidence against different tuning charges as a basis for the different absorptions of red and green pigments is provided by the primary structure of the opsins, in which the charged residues thought to lie near the chromophore are identical (Nathans et al. 1986).

Alternatively, the different spectral absorptions of the green and red pigments might arise from protein-induced differences in twist at the 6–7 carbon bond of retinal. In free solution, retinal adopts a twisted 6-*s*-*cis*

configuration, in which the angle between the ring and side chain is 40–120° out of plane (Honig et al. 1971). In bacteriorhodopsin, the protein twists the chromophore into the planar *s*-*trans* configuration at the 6–7 carbon bond (Harbison et al. 1985; van der Steen et al. 1986). Planarity improves the effective conjugation in the double bond system and redshifts the absorption by 30 nm. Does a similar mechanism produce the additional redshift of the red cone pigment? We tested this possibility (Makino et al. 1990) by replacing the retinal chromophore in red and green cones with a

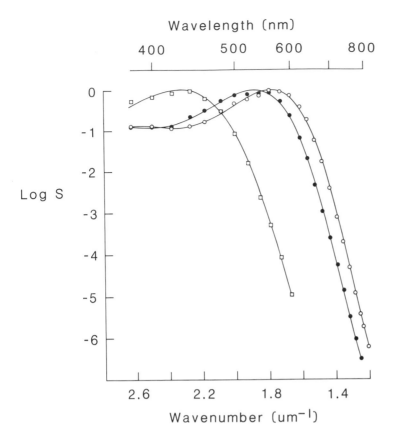

Figure 3. Spectral sensitivities of macaque cones. Relative sensitivity to a quantum plotted on a log scale as a function of wave number (or wavelength). The curves have maxima near 430 nm (blue cones), 530 nm (green), and 560 nm (red). Points are averages from measurements on 5 blue, 20 green, and 16 red cones from retinas of 9 macaques. Continuous curves drawn by eye.

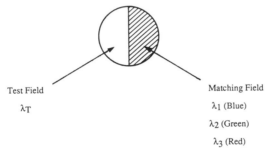

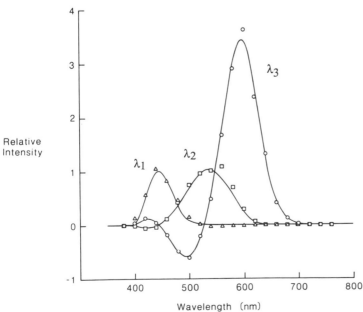

Figure 4. Color-matching functions measured psychophysically by Stiles and Burch (1959, continuous curves) compared with those calculated from the measured spectral sensitivities of monkey cones (points). The stimuli for the psychophysical experiment are diagrammed above. A monochromatic test light of wavelength λ_T was presented at unit intensity in the left half of the field. The subject adjusted the intensities of matching lights λ_1 (444 nm), λ_2 (526 nm), and λ_3 (645 nm) in the right half of the field until the entire field appeared uniform. The graph below gives the quantum intensities of the matching lights as a function of the wavelength of the test light. In the calculation, the monkey cone spectral sensitivities were modified to allow for absorption of light by the human lens and macular pigment and for self-screening in the cone pigment. (Reprinted, with permission, from Baylor et al. 1987.)

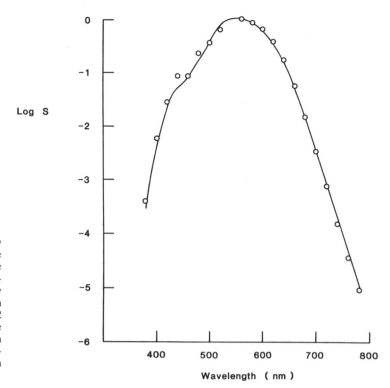

Figure 5. Photopic luminosity function fitted by a weighted sum of the spectral sensitivities of the red and green cones. The continuous curve is the photopic luminosity function of Vos (1978), expressed on a quantum basis. The symbols show the sum of the measured human red and green cone sensitivities, with the red weighted 1.92 times as heavily as the green. As in Fig. 4, the cone sensitivities were corrected for absorption by the lens and macular pigment and for self-screening. (Reprinted, with permission, from Schnapf et al. 1988.)

retinal analog that could not rotate about the 6–7 carbon bond (see structure in Fig. 7). This compound was the synthetic, planar-locked 6-s-cis, 9-cis retinal (van der Steen et al. 1989). It has not yet been possible to synthesize the corresponding 11-cis retinal analog; we assume that the 9-cis analog might behave similarly to locked 11-cis retinal.

The locked analog was introduced into red and green monkey cones in the following way. The inner segment

of an isolated cone was drawn into a suction electrode, which recorded the cell's photocurrent. After the cone's spectral type was determined, its pigment was bleached by applying an intense white light for a few minutes. The retinal chromophore photoisomerized to the all-*trans* configuration and dissociated from the protein. At this stage, the cell was unresponsive to light. The retinal analog, in phospholipid vesicles, was then perfused over the outer segment, which protruded

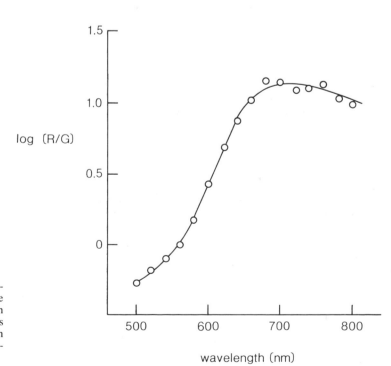

Figure 6. Sensitivity of macaque red cones relative to that of green cones plotted on a log scale as a function of wavelength. The points are from the sensitivities plotted in Fig. 3. The continuous curve was drawn by eye. Wavelengths at which the ordinate is the same have the same appearance.

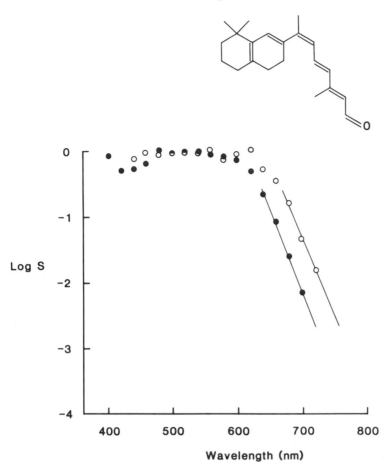

Ring-locked 6-s-cis 9-cis retinal

Figure 7. Spectral sensitivities of macaque red (○) and green (●) cones containing the planar-locked 6-*s-cis*, 9-*cis* retinal analog (structure shown above). Points are averages from experiments on two red and three green cones. Separation between linear regression lines at long wavelength is 31 nm.

from the suction electrode. Formation of a new pigment was signaled by the appearance of responses to light flashes and was confirmed by a new spectral sensitivity curve.

Figure 7 (bottom) shows that the spectral sensitivities of monkey red and green cones containing the locked analog were still separated by 30 nm. This result is not consistent with the idea that different twists at the 6–7 carbon bond of retinal produce the different absorptions in the red and green pigments. We hope to confirm this interpretation and test other tuning mechanisms by using other retinal analogs.

CONCLUSIONS

Physiological measurements have provided a quantitative description of how the wavelength of the light is encoded by the excitations of three types of retinal cones. The cone excitations had a highly reproducible wavelength dependence in our sample, apparently because one cone expresses only one pigment and because the spectral absorptions of the pigments are stereotyped across different cones and different individuals. The spectral sensitivities of the cones provide a physiological basis for several psychophysical results on human color vision, including the results of color-matching experiments, the form of the photopic luminosity function, and the paradoxical hue shift. The molecular mechanism of tuning in cone pigments remains to be determined. Experiments with a locked retinal analog argue against the notion that the difference between the red and green pigment absorptions results from different protein-induced twists at the 6–7 carbon bond of retinal.

ACKNOWLEDGMENTS

This work was supported by research grants EY-05750 and EY-02051 and National Research Service awards EY-05956 and EY-06195 from the National Eye Institute, U.S.Public Health Service. We thank Robert Schneeveis for excellent technical assistance.

REFERENCES

Baylor, D.A., B.J. Nunn, and J.L. Schnapf. 1987. Spectral sensitivity of cones of the monkey *Macaca fascicularis*. *J. Physiol.* **390:** 145.
Bowmaker, J.K. 1984. Microspectrophotometry of vertebrate photoreceptors: A brief review. *Vision Res.* **24:** 1641.
———. 1990. Visual pigments: Colour vision, opsin structure and evolution. *Semin. Neurosci.* **2:** 25.

Brindley, G.S. 1955. The colour of light of very long wavelength. *J. Physiol.* **130:** 35.

Chen, J.G., T. Nakamura, T.G. Ebrey, H. Ok, K. Konno, F. Derguini, K. Nakanishi, and B. Honig. 1989. Wavelength regulation in iodopsin, a cone pigment. *Biophys. J.* **55:** 725.

DeValois, R.L., H.C. Morgan, M.C. Polson, W.R. Mead, and E.M. Hull. 1974. Psychophysical studies of monkey vision. I. Macaque luminosity and color vision tests. *Vision Res.* **14:** 53.

Harbison, G.S., S.O. Smith, J.A. Pardoen, J.M.L. Courtin, J. Lugtenburg, J. Herzfeld, R.A. Mathies, and R.G. Griffin. 1985. Solid-state ^{13}C NMR detection of a perturbed 6-s-trans chromophore in bacteriorhodopsin. *Biochemistry* **24:** 6955.

Honig, B., B. Hudson, B.D. Sykes, and M. Karplus. 1971. Ring orientation in β-ionone and retinals. *Proc. Natl. Acad. Sci.* **68:** 1289.

Loppnow, G.R., B.A. Barry, and R.A. Mathies. 1989. Why are blue visual pigments blue? A resonance Raman microprobe study. *Proc. Natl. Acad. Sci.* **86:** 1515.

Makino, C.L., T.W. Kraft, R.A. Mathies, J. Lugtenburg, M.E. Miley, R. van der Steen, and D.A. Baylor. 1990. Effects of modified chromophores on the spectral sensitivity of salamander, squirrel and macaque cones. *J. Physiol.* **424:** 545.

Nathans, J. 1990. Determinants of visual pigment absorbance: Role of charged amino acids in the putative transmembrane segments. *Biochemistry* **29:** 937.

Nathans, J., D. Thomas, and D.S. Hogness. 1986. Molecular genetics of human color vision: The genes encoding blue, green, and red pigments. *Science* **232:** 193.

Schnapf, J.L., T.W. Kraft, and D.A. Baylor. 1987. Spectral sensitivity of human cone photoreceptors. *Nature* **325:** 439.

Schnapf, J.L., T.W. Kraft, B.J. Nunn, and D.A. Baylor. 1988. Spectral sensitivity of primate photoreceptors. *Vis. Neurosci.* **1:** 255.

Stiles, W.S. and J.M. Burch. 1959. N. P. L. colour-matching investigation: Final report (1958). *Optica Acta* **6:** 1.

van der Steen, R., P. L. Biesheuvel, R.A. Mathies, and J. Lugtenburg. 1986. Retinal analogues with locked 6-7 conformations show that bacteriorhodopsin requires the 6-s-trans conformation of the chromophore. *J. Am. Chem. Soc.* **108:** 6410.

van der Steen, R., P.L. Biesheuvel, C. Erkelens, R.A. Mathies, and J. Lugtenburg. 1989. 8, 16- and 8, 18-methanobacteriorhodopsin. Synthesis and spectroscopy of 8, 16- and 8, 18-methanoretinal and their interaction with bacterioopsin. *Recl. Trav. Chim. Pays-Bas. Belg.* **108:** 83.

Vos, J.J. 1978. Colorimetric and photometric properties of a 2° fundamental observer. *Color Res. Appl.* **3:** 125.

Young, T. 1802. On the theory of light and colours. *Philos. Trans. R. Soc. Lond. B* **92:** 12.

Color Puzzles

D. HUBEL AND M. LIVINGSTONE

Department of Neurobiology, Harvard Medical School, Boston, Massachusetts 02115

The first systematic studies of the visual cortex of mammals with well-developed color vision presented an intriguing, and as yet unsolved puzzle. Most retinal ganglion cells and most cells in the lateral geniculate body are color coded; most cells in the primary visual cortex (V1) are not (Wiesel and Hubel 1966; Hubel and Wiesel 1968). In the lateral geniculate body, most cells are overtly color opponent. They are activated by light over one range of wavelengths, suppressed by other wavelengths, and less responsive to white. Presumably, all or very nearly all the signals coming from the lateral geniculate to our occipital lobes must pass through the primary visual cortex. Why, then, are color-coded cells so scarce there?

For physiologists interested in color, the lateral geniculate body had already presented two major related puzzles. The commonest cell type in the parvocellular layers of the geniculate is known as type 1. Its receptive field has a small center, excitatory (on) or inhibitory (off), and an antagonistic (off or on) surround. The center and surround are color opponent, and this color opponency is of two subtypes, depending on the cones that supply the center and surround. The red (long wavelength) cones are in opposition to the green (middle wavelength) cones, or the blue (short wavelength) cones are opposed to the red and green cones combined. (For cells in which blue is opposed to red + green, i.e., yellow, the center almost always is fed by blue cones and is almost always "on.") Because these cells show both spatial and chromatic opponency, they can obviously carry both luminance and wavelength information (Fig. 1). It is surprising, in view of the somewhat subsidiary role of color in primate vision, that 80% of cortical inputs should be color coded.

The second geniculate puzzle concerned the relationship of the organization of type 1 receptive fields to what was known about the psychophysics of color perception. The opponency of red versus green and blue versus yellow corresponds well with Hering's psychophysics (1874), but the receptive-field organization seems exactly wrong for mediating color contrast and color constancy—the fact that colors of objects, in contradistinction to the wavelength composition of the light they reflect, can be largely independent of the wavelength composition of the incident light. To mediate red-green spatial effects, we would expect a cell with a red excitatory center to have a green *excitatory* surround, not a green *inhibitory* surround.

It is far easier to imagine a role in color perception for the less common geniculate type 2 cell, in which the opponent cone inputs have the same spatial distributions. They, too, come in red versus green and yellow versus blue subtypes, and in any given region of the visual field, the combined activity of these two types of color opponency determines unambiguously a point in a chromaticity plane. Since these cells lack center-surround opponency, they cannot carry the lateral interactions needed for color constancy. The receptive fields of type 2 cells are larger than the field centers of type 1 cells.

A third, also less common, type of parvocellular cell, the type 3, lacks color coding altogether. Like type 1 cells, these have center-surround fields, but the red and green cone inputs (perhaps also blue) to the receptive-field center are not opponent but of the same sign, either both excitatory or both inhibitory. Moreover, the spatially antagonistic surround also receives input from both red and green cones. These cells are often termed "broadband."

Cells in the magnocellular layers share some properties with parvocellular cells, but in many respects, they are quite different. They are similar in that their receptive fields are radially symmetric and have a center-surround organization. They differ in four major ways: in their temporal characteristics, color selectivity, contrast sensitivity, and spatial resolution.

1. Magno cells respond faster and more transiently than parvo cells (Wiesel and Hubel 1966; Gouras 1968, 1969; deMonasterio and Gouras 1975; Dreher et al. 1976; Schiller and Malpeli 1978; Hicks et al. 1983). Responses of most magno cells to a long-duration stimulus are brief. A minority show a sustained response component, but even these give a brisk burst of impulses at the onset of the stimulus. This sensitivity to the temporal aspects of a visual stimulus suggests that the magno system may play a special role in detecting movement. Many cells at higher levels in this pathway are indeed selective for direction of movement (Dubner and Zeki 1971; Maunsell and Van Essen 1983).

2. Most parvocellular cells are color opponent, whereas magnocellular cells are not, at least for the more conspicuous, transient part of the response; they have broadband receptive-field centers, like the parvocellular type 3 cells (DeValois et al. 1966; Wiesel and Hubel 1966; Gouras 1968, 1969; deMonasterio and Gouras 1975; DeValois et al. 1977; Schiller and Malpeli 1978; Derrington et al. 1984). In the macaque monkey, many magnocellular cells, both

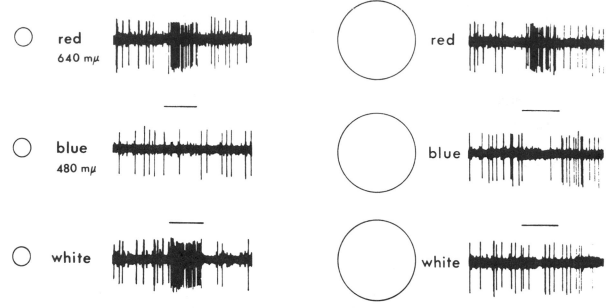

Figure 1. Response properties of a typical parvocellular type 1 cell, demonstrating both its color opponency and spatial opponency. This cell receives excitatory input from red cones over a small central region and inhibitory input from green cones over a larger surrounding area. It shows color opponency in that it is excited by red spots (either small or large) and inhibited by large blue or green spots; it shows spatial opponency in that it is excited by small white spots and not by large ones. (Reprinted, with permission, from Wiesel and Hubel 1966.)

on-center and off-center, show a characteristic sustained suppression of their resting activity in response to a diffuse red light, but not to diffuse white light. To this extent, many magno cells do show color opponency, but what the consequences are in perceptual terms we have no idea.

3. For magno cells, the response as a function of contrast rises much more steeply than for parvo cells, and it saturates at lower contrasts (Shapley et al. 1981; Kaplan and Shapley 1982, 1986; Derrington and Lennie 1984).

4. The final difference between magno and parvo cells is their field-center sizes. At any given eccentricity, magnocellular centers are about twice as large as the centers of the parvo type 1 or type 3 cells (Derrington and Lennie 1984).

Since most parvocellular cells are color opponent and most magno cells are not (except in the sense mentioned above), cells in these two subdivisions respond quite differently to changes in the wavelength of a spot, or to moving color-contrast borders. A type 1 cell will respond when a spot covering the field center is replaced by a spot of a different wavelength, unless the two colors have equal effects on the single type of cone that feeds into the center. The relative intensities at which the effects are equal are, of course, directly predicable from the spectral sensitivity of the center cone type and will be very different for the three types of cones (Fig. 2) (Hubel and Livingstone 1990). Mag-

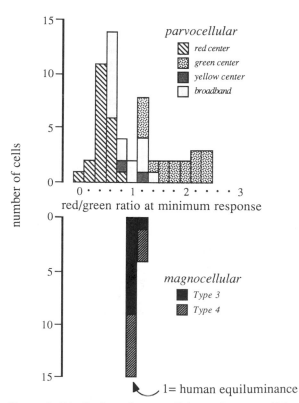

Figure 2. Distribution of parvocellular and magnocellular neurons according to the red/green brightness ratio giving a minimum response. (Reprinted, with permission, from Hubel and Livingstone 1990.)

nocellular receptive-field centers, on the other hand, receive an input of the same sign, either excitatory or inhibitory, from both red and green cones; one would therefore expect these cells to be insensitive to the alternation of two colors whose relative brightnesses are such that the sum of the effects on the two cones is the same. If, from cell to cell, the relative influences of the red and green cones feeding into the center are close to the same, then the positions of the minima that occur as relative brightnesses are varied should all be similar. This is indeed the case, as shown in Figure 2. Krüger (1979) and later the two of us (Hubel and Livingstone 1990) found that magnocellular geniculate cells show a response minimum to a moving color-contrast border at a particular relative brightness—a brightness ratio that is close to a human observer's equiluminant point. (Logothetis et al. [1990] have shown, and we have confirmed, that many magno cells, although showing a minimum at some setting of relative intensities, do not null completely at equiluminance, but respond briefly and weakly at both the red-to-green and the green-to-red transition. Evidently, the effects of removing one color are not precisely matched by introducing the other. Thus, some color sensitivity does persist, although the cells are insensitive to sign of the color contrast.) The fact that magnocellular cells respond so poorly at equiluminance was one of several lines of reasoning that prompted our hypothesis that the aspects of visual perception that deteriorate at equiluminance do so because they are carried predominantly by the magno system (Livingstone and Hubel 1987).

In the primary visual cortex, the pathways stemming from the two major geniculate subdivisions, magnocellular and parvocellular, seem to keep their separate identities. Several anatomical possibilities for cross talk do exist (Lund and Boothe 1975), and indeed it would be hard to imagine a complete independence, given the fact that at least two columnar systems, for ocular dominance and orientation, extend through the entire cortical thickness. So far, however, we have no other convincing physiological indications for extensive interactions.

In the cortex, cells in layers derived from the magnocellular system again show a marked decline or loss of responsiveness at the red-green intensity ratio that corresponds to human equiluminance. In the parvocellular system, things are more complicated, as one might expect from the wide variety of parvo geniculate cells. Here, we confine our discussion to layers 2 and 3. These represent the part of the (mainly) parvocellular path in V1 that projects to other cortical areas and are thus presumably involved more directly in perception than the subcortically projecting infragranular layers (5 and 6).

Leaving aside for the moment the blob system in layers 2 and 3, there are still some exceptions to our opening statement that cells in V1 lack color coding. A few upper-layer cells, although showing about as much orientation selectivity as their neighbors, give far stronger responses to colored bars than to white bars. Such cells make up about 10% of the upper-layer population and may be located at the edges of blobs (Livingstone and Hubel 1984; Hubel and Livingstone 1990). Curiously, of the cells that prefer colored bars, those that prefer red bars are by far the commonest. Over many years, we have seen one or two that preferred blue, and none that preferred green. Many cells respond well to a black bar on a light background, and hardly at all to a light bar on a dark background. The great majority, however, show no color preference and respond about as well to light bars as to dark.

In 1979, Gouras and Krüger made the remarkable observation that many cortical cells that show no overt color preference do carry color information of a more subtle kind. When they used a red bar on a green background to test cells that responded well to both dark and light bars, about half of the cells responded well at all red-to-green intensity ratios. This meant that the color information coming into the cortex from the geniculate had not been entirely lost. We have recently replicated their result (Fig. 3) not only with bars, but also with red-green sine-wave gratings at low spatial frequencies, at which chromatic-aberration effects are negligible. It therefore seems clear that interblob cells in layers 2 and 3 can detect borders on the basis of either luminance or color. Although subtle, this is probably the most prevalent form of color coding in the striate cortex.

In the early 1980s, we discovered a completely distinct color system in the upper layers of V1 (Livingstone and Hubel 1984). About half the cells in the cytochrome-oxidase blobs were overtly color coded, and all the blob cells showed poor orientation selectivity or none. Some of the color-coded cells were similar to type 2 geniculate cells, with color opponency but no receptive-field surround. Most, however, had more complex receptive fields, with a receptive-field center like that of a type 2 cell, but also a surround that suppressed the response at all wavelengths (Fig. 4). A typical cell of this type might give on responses to a small red spot, suppression of firing and off responses to a small green spot, and little or no response to a white spot of any size, or to a large spot at any wavelength. Such cells were reminiscent of the "double opponent" cells that had been seen by Nigel Daw (1968) in goldfish retina.

Several questions remain unresolved concerning the physiology of these blob cells:

1. The use of the term "double opponent" has been criticized (T'so and Gilbert 1988). One objection to its use has been that annular stimuli, confined to the field surround, often produce no response. Yet the absence or weakness of an explicit surround response is a common feature in all types of center-surround cells in both cat and monkey, and also in simple cortical cells. It was first emphasized by Barlow (1953), who pointed out that even in cells that showed no response to annuli, the surround re-

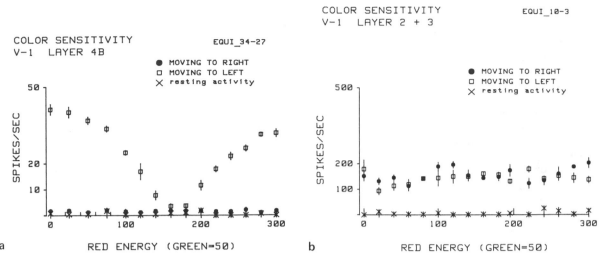

Figure 3. Responses of cortical cells to a red bar moving across a green background as the red brightness is varied. Red = 150 corresponds to human equiluminance as determined by flicker photometry. (*a*) Typical layer 4B cell. Cells in layer 4B, which receive predominantly magnocellular input, show deep minima at equiluminance. (*b*) Response of a typical layer 2/3 cell to the same stimulus. This cell does not show a response decrement at any particular red/green ratio. About half the cells in layers 2 and 3 respond well at all red/green ratios. (Reprinted, with permission, from Hubel and Livingstone 1990.)

sponses could be brought out by tonic illumination of the field center. Explicit responses from the field surround seem to be easier to elicit in the goldfish, but even there they may be weak (N.W. Daw, pers. comm.).

2. The surrounds of these receptive fields present a more perplexing difficulty, noted by T'so and Gilbert (1988). The simple description of the cell's behavior just given—color opponency plus failure to respond to large spots—led us to think of the receptive field of, say, an R⁺ G⁻ center cell as having an R⁻ G⁺ surround. If such a summary diagram is taken literally, then we would expect the cell to give an especially powerful response to a red center-size spot surrounded by green. In most cells, however, the response to a center-size red spot is strongly suppressed by a green annulus. Clearly, no simple summation of responses can adequately characterize such a cell. T'so and Gilbert (1988) call these cells "modified type 2" and describe them as having a broadband inhibitory surround. This seems to us inappropriate, since "inhibitory" does not adequately describe a surround that suppresses both on and off responses. Moreover, we found that in some cells, a red surround is more powerful than a green in inhibiting the response to red stimuli in the receptive-field center, and a green surround is more powerful than a red in inhibiting the green center response. Such cells may therefore be suited to building up the kinds of responses needed for the perception of color contrast and color constancy.

3. About half the cells in the blobs lack any obvious color coding; qualitatively, they are similar to the broadband type 3 cells in the geniculate, except that they tend to have larger field centers. It is not clear whether these cells get their input from broadband

geniculate cells and, if so, whether magnocellular or parvocellular.

4. A full understanding of the blob cells and their relation to color vision depends on knowing their inputs. In the squirrel monkey, Fitzpatrick et al. (1983) have provided evidence that the interlaminar plexuses of the geniculate project selectively to the blobs. For the macaque monkey, we have hints of the same thing. The type 2 cells we have recorded from have tended to be near the interlaminar plexuses (Livingstone and Hubel 1982, 1984, and unpubl.), and these cells are the most logical candidate for building up double-opponent cells. This system may have its origin in the small-cell population of retinal ganglion cells (W-cells) (Casagrande et al. 1990).

Although our present knowledge of the anatomy and physiology of the pathway subserving color is too fragmentary to justify any firm pronouncements, it may be useful to propose a hypothesis that has the merit of being testable. If it evokes as lively a response as our recent ideas on the role of the magnocellular system in movement and depth perception, we will feel fully vindicated!

Our notion is that color vision, in the sense of recognizing and distinguishing colors, as opposed to recognizing shapes or borders through the use of wavelength differences, may depend on the relatively rare type 2 cell (center only, with color opponency) and not on the far commoner type 1 cells (center-surround, with color opponency). We propose that inputs from type 1 cells are pooled in the interblob regions of the upper layers of V1; this pooling of color-opponent inputs results in the loss of sensitivity to the sign of color contrast while retaining responsiveness to color borders at all relative

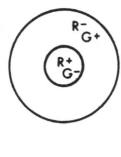

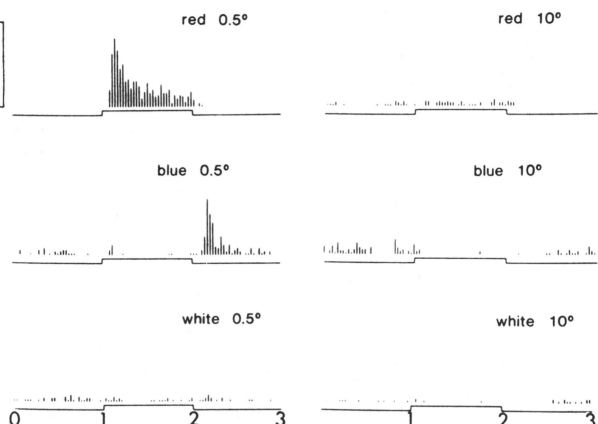

Figure 4. Responses of a double-opponent cell in a cytochrome-oxidase blob of V1. Although annuli alone give no responses, the surround inhibition is apparent as a reduction in the response to larger spots for both red and blue light. Since the surround antagonizes both the on-center and the off-center responses, it cannot be simply a broadband inhibition. (Reprinted, with permission, from Livingstone and Hubel 1984.)

intensities. Upper-layer interblob cells can thus use color contrast as well as luminance contrast for perception. To camouflage itself, a plant or animal must blend in with its background, and this is obviously harder to do for both luminance and wavelength than for luminance alone. We suggest that it is the type 2 cells and the double-opponent cells in the blobs that are responsible for the perception of color as such.

The following observations would seem to support this idea:

1. The low resolution of our color vision, as psychophysically determined, matches the large field size of type 2 cells. The much tinier centers of type 1 cells are a better match for our spatial resolution.

2. It may seem perverse to imagine that the obvious color coding of the type 1 geniculate cells is thrown away, or at least not used for our color sense as usually construed, but rather for the seemingly more humble task of defeating camouflage in the high-spatial-resolution form system. The color opponency of type 1 cells may, however, simply be a by-product of their high spatial discrimination. In the fovea, at least, it seems clear on anatomical grounds that each receptive field center receives input from only a single cone (Polyak 1941; Boycott and Dowling 1969). That single cone must be of one kind or other—specifically either a red cone or a green cone, given the absence of blue cones in the fovea (König 1894; Wald 1967). This cone purity of the

field center is by itself enough to make the cell a carrier of color information. It is less clear why the receptive field surround should be selective for the opponent color rather than broadband. Yet the evidence that type 1 cells have color-opponent surrounds seems clear (Fig. 1). With long-wavelength stimuli, a red on center cell gives on responses of equal magnitude to small and large spots, whereas with short wavelengths it gives a much weaker response to a large spot than to a small. Moreover, spectral sensitivity curves of the surround (Wiesel and Hubel 1966) seem to indicate that they are not broadband. This wavelength selectivity of the surround poses another puzzle. Horizontal cells in the monkey are thought on anatomical and physiological grounds to receive inputs of the same sign from all cone types (Boycott et al. 1987; Dacheux and Raviola 1990); they should therefore be broadband. If both the anatomy and physiology are correct, we may be forced to ask whether the field surrounds of type 1 cells in primates are dependent on amacrine cells rather than on horizontal cells.

3. Using a technique developed by R. Savoy and M. Burns (pers. comm.), we can change the three phosphors of a color monitor in such a way that when a red spot replaces a gray spot, the activity in only the red cones is changed; similarly, a spot can be made to turn from gray to green and change activity only in the green cones, or gray to violet and affect only the blue cones. A protanope is quite blind to a large spot as red as a tomato, and similarly for a deuteranope and an unripe tomato. If we attempt to drive our cortical cells with such stimuli, we find that whereas type 2 cells typically respond vigorously, type 1 cells respond grudgingly or not at all. The contrasts that can be obtained with such stimuli are limited by the maximum brightnesses obtainable with the TV phosphors, and by the fact that the lowest one can go in intensity is to turn the phosphor off. Type 1 cells, whose contrast sensitivities are low, are apparently too insensitive to respond. The fact that a stimulus we have no trouble seeing as colored fails to drive type 1 cells seems to be further evidence that we can see colors without them.

On anatomical and physiological grounds, the blobs project to the thin dark stripes of visual area 2, which in turn project to area V4 (Livingstone and Hubel 1984; DeYoe and Van Essen 1985; Shipp and Zeki 1985). Area V4 may be homologous to the region in the human inferior occipital lobe whose destruction leads to achromatopsia (Pearlman et al. 1979; Damasio et al. 1980). In this rather rare condition, color perception, in the sense of recognition or discrimination of colors, may be completely destroyed with little or no impairment of form vision. Such patients should still be able to use their type-1-to-interblob color information to detect color-contrast borders at all relative brightness, while unable to tell the colors that make up the border. We hope to test this prediction.

We do not know the mechanisms responsible for color contrast or color constancy, or even whether the necessary circuits are present in V1. Evidence from Zeki's work indicates that V4 is involved (Zeki 1980, 1983). Wherever the circuits are, they are presumably fed by cells in the striate cortex, and one should at least expect those cells to have properties not incompatible with color constancy. As already mentioned, type 2 cells are compatible.

We have tried to describe how, despite the enormous amount of information we have about the organization, function, and development of the retina, the geniculate, and the visual cortical areas, color perception still is largely a puzzle. It is hardly any consolation that form perception is even more of a mystery.

REFERENCES

Barlow, H.B. 1953. Summation and inhibition in the frog's retina. *J. Physiol.* **119:** 69.

Boycott, B.B. and J.E. Dowling. 1969. Organization of the primate retina: Light microscopy. *Philos. Trans. R. Soc. Lond. B Biol. Sci.* **255:** 109.

Boycott, B.B., J.M. Hopkins, and G.H. Sperling. 1987. Cone connections of the horizontal cells of the rhesus monkey's retina. *Proc. R. Soc. Lond. B Biol. Sci.* **229:** 345.

Casagrande, V.A., P.D. Beck, G.J. Condo, and E.A. Lachica. 1990. Intrinsic connections of CO blobs in striate cortex of primates. *Invest. Ophthalmol. Visual Sci.* **31:** 1945.

Dacheux, R.R. and E. Raviola. 1990. Physiology of H1 horizontal cells in the primate retina. *Proc. R. Soc. Lond. B Biol Sci.* **239:** 213.

Damasio, A., T. Yamada, H. Damasio, J. Corbett, and J. McKee. 1980. Central achromatopsia: Behavioral, anatomic, and physiologic aspects. *Neurology* **30:** 1064.

Daw, N.W. 1968. Colour-coded ganglion cells in the goldfish retina: Extension of their receptive fields by means of new stimuli. *J. Physiol.* **197:** 567.

deMonasterio, F.M. and P. Gouras. 1975. Functional properties of ganglion cells of the rhesus monkey retina. *J. Physiol.* **251:** 167.

Derrington, A.M. and P. Lennie. 1984. Spatial and temporal contrast sensitivities of neurones in lateral geniculate nucleus of macaque. *J. Physiol.* **357:** 219.

Derrington, A.M., J. Krauskopf, and P. Lennie. 1984. Chromatic mechanisms in lateral geniculate nucleus of macaque. *J. Physiol.* **357:** 241.

DeValois, R.L., I. Abramov, and G.H. Jacobs. 1966. Analysis of response patterns of LGN cells. *J. Opt. Soc. Am.* **56:** 966.

DeValois, R.L., D.M. Snodderly, E.W. Yund, and N.K. Hepler. 1977. Responses of macaque lateral geniculate cells to luminance and color figures. *Sens. Processes* **1:** 244.

DeYoe, E.A. and D.C. Van Essen. 1985. Segregation of efferent connections and receptive field properties in visual area V2 of the macaque. *Nature* **317:** 58.

Dreher, B., Y. Fukada, and R.W. Rodieck. 1976. Identification, classification, and anatomical segregation of cells with X-like and Y-like properties in the lateral geniculate nucleus of old-world primates. *J. Physiol.* **258:** 433.

Dubner, R. and S.M. Zeki. 1971. Response properties and receptive fields of cells in an anatomically defined region of the superior temporal sulcus. *Brain Res.* **35:** 528.

Fitzpatrick, D., K. Itoh, and I.T. Diamond. 1983. The laminar organization of the lateral geniculate body and the striate cortex in the squirrel monkey (*Saimiri sciureus*). *J. Neurosci.* **3:** 673.

Gouras, P. 1968. Identification of cone mechanisms in monkey ganglion cells. *J. Physiol.* **199:** 533.

———. 1969. Antidromic responses of orthodromically identified ganglion cells in monkey retina. *J. Physiol.* **204:** 407.

Gouras, P. and J. Krüger. 1979. Responses of cells in foveal visual cortex of the monkey to pure color contrast. *J. Neurophysiol.* **42:** 850.

Hering, E. 1874. Sizungsberichte der Wiener Akademie. *Math. Naturwiss. Klin.* **69:** S131.

Hicks, T.P., B.B. Lee, and T.R. Vidyasagar. 1983. The responses of cells in macaque lateral geniculate nucleus to sinusoidal gratings. *J. Physiol.* **337:** 183.

Hubel, D.H. and M.S. Livingstone. 1990. Color and contrast sensitivity in the lateral geniculate body and primary visual cortex of the macaque monkey. *J. Neurosci.* **10:** 2223.

Hubel, D.H. and T.N. Wiesel. 1968. Receptive fields and functional architecture of monkey striate cortex. *J. Physiol.* **95:** 215.

Kaplan, E. and R.M. Shapley. 1982. X and Y cells in the lateral geniculate nucleus of the macaque monkey. *J. Physiol.* **330:** 125.

———. 1986. The primate retina contains two types of ganglion cells, with high and low contrast sensitivity. *Proc. Natl. Acad. Sci.* **83:** 2755.

König, A. 1894. *Uber den menschlichen Sehpurpur und seine Bedeutung für das sehen*, vol. 30, p. 577. S.B. Akad. Wissenshaft, Berlin.

Krüger, J. 1979. Responses to wavelength contrast in the afferent visual systems of the cat and the rhesus monkey. *Vision Res.* **19:** 1351.

Livingstone, M.S. and D.H. Hubel. 1982. Thalamic inputs to cytochrome oxidase-rich regions in monkey visual cortex. *Proc. Natl. Acad. Sci.* **79:** 6098.

———. 1984. Anatomy and physiology of a color system in the primate visual cortex. *J. Neurosci.* **4:** 309.

———. 1987. Psychophysical evidence for separate channels for the perception of form, color, movement, and depth. *J. Neurosci.* **7:** 3416.

Logothetis, N.K., P.H. Schiller, E.R. Charles, and A.C. Hurlbert. 1990. Perceptual deficits and the activity of the color-opponent and broad-band pathways at isoluminance. *Science* **247:** 214.

Lund, J.S. and R.G. Boothe. 1975. Interlaminar connections and pyramidal neuron organization in the visual cortex, area 17, of the macaque monkey. *J. Comp. Neurol.* **159:** 305.

Maunsell, J.H.R. and D.C. Van Essen. 1983. Functional properties of neurons in middle temporal visual area of the macaque monkey. I. Selectivity for stimulus direction, speed, and orientation. *J. Neurophysiol.* **49:** 1127.

Pearlman, A.L., J. Birch, and J.C. Meadows. 1979. Cerebral colorblindness: An acquired defect in hue discrimination. *Annu. Neurol.* **5:** 253.

Polyak, S.L. 1941. *The retina.* University of Chicago Press, Illinois.

Schiller, P.H. and J.G. Malpeli. 1978. Functional specificity of lateral geniculate nucleus laminae of the rhesus monkey. *J. Neurophysiol.* **41:** 788.

Shapley, R.M., E. Kaplan, and R. Soodak. 1981. Spatial summation and contrast sensitivity of X and Y cells in the lateral geniculate nucleus of the macaque. *Nature* **292:** 543.

Shipp, S. and S. Zeki. 1985. Segregation of pathways leading from area V2 to areas V4 and V5 of macaque monkey visual cortex. *Nature* **315:** 322.

T'so, D.Y. and C.D. Gilbert. 1988. The organization of chromatic and spatial interactions in the primate striate cortex. *J. Neurosci.* **8:** 1712.

Wald, B. 1967. Blue-blindness in the normal fovea. *J. Opt. Soc. Am.* **57:** 1289.

Wiesel, T.N. and D.H. Hubel. 1966. Spatial and chromatic interactions in the lateral geniculate body of the rhesus monkey. *J. Neurophysiol.* **29:** 1115.

Zeki, S.M. 1980. The representation of colours in the cerebral cortex. *Nature* **284:** 412.

———. 1983. The distribution of wavelength and orientation selectivity in different areas of monkey visual cortex. *Proc. R. Soc. Lond. B Biol. Sci.* **207:** 239.

Parallelism and Functional Specialization in Human Visual Cortex

S. ZEKI

University College London, London, United Kingdom

The last Cold Spring Harbor Symposium to address problems of sensory representation in the cerebral cortex was entitled *The Synapse* and was held in 1975. It was an exciting meeting for me, for many of the ideas that I was to exploit in the ensuing years had just begun to germinate then. At the time (Zeki 1976), I summarized these ideas as follows:

1. *Parallelism*, a notion rooted in the observation that every "point" of the primary visual cortex (area V1), which receives the predominant input from the retina through the lateral geniculate nucleus, has parallel and independent outputs to different visual areas of the prestriate visual cortex. This suggested that different signals are received by different visual areas.

2. *Functional specialization*, which is a direct consequence, at least logically, of the parallel outputs. This was established by direct recording from the areas to which V1 projects (Zeki 1974b, 1978a). Collectively, this evidence showed that the hierarchical strategy of increasing elaboration, whereby each area analyzes all the aspects of the visual image but at a higher level of complexity than the antecedent area (Hubel and Wiesel 1965), cannot be the sole strategy that the visual cortex employs to construct the visual image.

3. A more general *functional segregation* in the visual system, which, again logically, was a natural consequence of observing the functional specialization in the visual areas of the prestriate cortex and the parallel inputs to them. This led me to the prediction that, in addition to the functions that had then been ascribed to V1 by Hubel and Wiesel, it must have another function, namely that of segregating the incoming signals and parceling them out to the different, functionally specialized, visual areas of the prestriate cortex for further processing (Zeki 1976). In fact, parallelism has since been found to be a ubiquitous feature of cortical connectivity, and functional segregation in the visual system has turned out to be a feature that can be traced right back to the retina itself. Fifteen years on, in a Cold Spring Harbor Symposium on *The Brain*, it thus seems interesting to consider briefly whether these ideas apply to the most complex of all brains, that of man, and whether they can be used to account for some apparently bizarre visual syndromes.

FUNCTIONAL SPECIALIZATION IN HUMAN VISUAL CORTEX

Specialization for Color and for Motion

Color and motion were the two visual submodalities that allowed me to establish the principle of functional specialization in primate visual cortex (Zeki 1974a,b, 1976, 1978a). The separation of form was added later (Zeki 1978b). This was perhaps not entirely fortuitous. Color and motion are probably computationally more separate from each other than either is from form vision. In the macaque monkey, the functional specialization was demonstrated by using a combination of anatomical and physiological techniques—the anatomical definition of the relevant area and the physiological characterization of cells within it. The cells of one area, V5, are overwhelmingly directionally selective and none is concerned with the color of the stimulus (Zeki 1974a; Gattass and Gross 1981). In contrast, the overwhelming majority of cells in V4 are wavelength selective, to a greater or lesser degree. The more prominent the wavelength selectivity, the less is the orientation specificity and vice versa. Few cells are directionally selective (see Zeki 1976, 1978a, 1983; Desimone and Schein 1987). Thus, two visual areas that are anatomically distinct turn out to be also functionally distinct, a demonstration that led directly to the concept of functional specialization. That functional specialization may also be a feature of human visual cortex was suggested by early clinical evidence, which purported to show that color vision can be specifically compromised following discrete cortical lesions. This evidence was rapidly discounted and dismissed, mainly for conceptual reasons (see Zeki 1990a). It lay dormant for over 80 years, until functional specialization was discovered in the monkey brain.

There are at least three ways of demonstrating functional specialization in the human brain. One method relies on pathological material, the chance destruction of a specific visual center through a vascular accident or a gunshot wound. Such lesions are only very rarely restricted to a single cortical field, making interpretation awkward. Indeed, this was one of the difficulties that made the early clinical evidence for achromatopsia (cerebral color blindness) so easy to dismiss. Another method relies on the psychophysical technique of equiluminance, pioneered by Lu and Fender (1972) and recently used on an almost industrial scale. The technique relies on abolishing the luminance difference between objects and forcing human subjects to discriminate them by color alone. Under these conditions, the detection of motion becomes difficult and even impossible (see Ramachandran and Gregory 1978; Cavanagh et al. 1984). The method tells us nothing about whether the cortical mechanisms dealing with the different attributes of vision are located in separate cortical areas, nor does it distinguish between the operation and the output. The third technique relies on measuring changes in regional cerebral blood flow when human subjects undertake particular tasks, through the technique of positron emission tomography (PET). On the principle that, if there are several ways of solving a problem, of which some are easier than others, one should always choose the easiest method, my collaborators and I opted for the last method.

In a collaboration with Richard Frackowiak and his team at the Hammersmith Hospital, London, we asked subjects to view multicolored Land Mondrian displays, and compared the activity in their brains with that obtained when the same subjects viewed the same displays, but this time consisting of equiluminous grays and whites. Subtraction and comparison of the scans obtained under these two conditions revealed that the area which was maximally active when subjects had been viewing the color displays was located in the region of the lingual and fusiform gyri, just outside the striate cortex (Fig. 1). The increase in blood flow was more prominent in the left hemisphere, regardless of handedness. This is the very cortical region that had been implicated in color vision in the forgotten clinical evidence. We refer to this area as human V4. In a similar study, we asked subjects to view a pattern of random black and white squares, each subtending about 1°, when it was stationary and when it was moving in different directions at 6° per second. Subtraction and comparison of the scans obtained under these two conditions showed that the region of maximal activity when the subjects had been viewing the moving stimulus occurred in a different area, situated more laterally at the junction of Brodmann's areas 19 and 37 and which we refer to as human V5 (Lueck et al. 1989; Cunningham et al. 1990; S. Zeki et al., in prep.) (Fig. 1). The two areas, V4 and V5, are so clearly separated from each other that there can be little doubt of their functional specialization. It is likely that more specialized visual areas will be demonstrated in the future, but this direct demonstration establishes directly the general principle of functional specialization in human visual cortex.

It is important to note that in both conditions a large region, corresponding to area V1 and the immediately adjoining prestriate cortex (probably V2), was also active (Fig. 1). This shows that V1 feeds both of the specialized visual areas in man, as it does in monkey, and that parallelism is therefore also a feature of human visual cortex. This latter view is reinforced by a more detailed study of the covariation between the active regions in the above studies (S. Zeki et al., in prep.). In the covariation studies, our approach was to choose a pixel situated within regions of high changes in V4 or V5 and ask which other pixels in the scans covaried systematically with the chosen pixel. In the color study, we found that V4 covaried systematically and positively with V1/V2, showing that it is anatomically connected with it. Similarly, in the motion study, V5 covaried positively and systematically with V1/V2, suggesting that it, too, is connected to it, and therefore, that V1/V2 have parallel outputs, at least to these two areas. It is probable that further studies will reveal other outputs from human V1, since in the macaque monkey, V1 also projects to V3 and V3A (Cragg 1969; Zeki 1969, 1980a) and possibly to other areas as well.

Parallelism in Human Visual Cortex

The parallel outputs from human striate cortex are implicit not only in the covariation studies referred to above, but also in the architecture and connections of areas V1 and V2. The cytochrome oxidase architecture of human area V1 is similar to that of the macaque monkey (Horton 1984; Horton and Hedley-Whyte 1984; Livingstone and Hubel 1984), and what little is known of the cytochrome oxidase architecture of human V2 also suggests that it is similar to that of the macaque monkey (Tootell et al. 1983; Burkhalter and Bernardo 1989; Hockfield et al. 1990). Combined anatomical and physiological studies of these two areas in the macaque monkey show that cells concerned with different attributes of the visual scene, such as form, color, and motion, are segregated in both areas and that the connections between them are organized along the "like with like" principle. In V1, cells preferring low spatial frequencies and selective for wavelengths are concentrated in the blobs, which are especially prominent in layers 2 and 3, whereas cells more selective for orientation but largely indifferent to the wavelength of the stimulus are concentrated in the interblob zones (Livingstone and Hubel 1984). The input to both sets of cells is derived principally from the parvocellular or P layers of the lateral geniculate nucleus. The input to layer 4B is derived principally from the magnocellular or M layers of the lateral geniculate nucleus. Here the cells that project to V5 (presumably the orientation and directionally selective ones) are grouped together and separated from cells that project elsewhere (Shipp and Zeki 1989a).

The functional segregation is also prominent in the adjoining area V2 (Cragg 1969; Zeki 1969), which has been shown to have a distinctive, and different, cytochrome oxidase architecture (Tootell et al. 1983). This consists of a set of darkly staining thick and thin stripes, separated from each other by the more lightly staining interstripes. Wavelength selective cells and those with a preference for low spatial frequencies are concentrated in the thin stripes, directionally selective cells in the thick stripes, and orientation selective cells in both

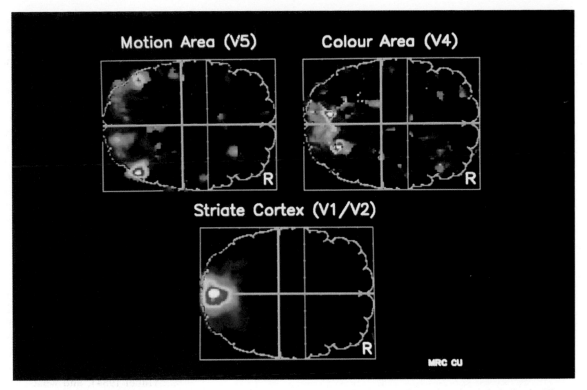

Figure 1. Statistical parametric maps of activity in the cerebral cortex, seen in horizontal slices taken through the brain. The maps were generated by comparing the mean cerebral activity across the different conditions (motion vs. stationary random dot pattern, *upper left*; color vs. gray, *upper right*; and vision vs. nonvision, *below*), using the *t*-statistic following an analysis of covariance (for details of the technique, see Friston et al. 1990). The horizontal slices of the brain are taken at the level of a line connecting the anterior commissure to the posterior commissure. Three subjects were used in each study. The vision vs. nonvision map was generated by comparing the mean cerebral activity when subjects had their eye closed and when they viewed the visual stimuli. The images have been arbitrarily scaled such that white is equal to the change of greatest significance. These images demonstrate the unique profile of changed significance attributable to the three separate activations. Note the difference in position between the loci of maximal changes in the color and the motion studies. The striate cortex, which is difficult to separate from area V2 in these scans, is active in both conditions. For further details, see text.

thick stripes and interstripes. The great majority of cells in the latter two stripes are not selective for the wavelength of the stimulus (Shipp and Zeki 1985; Hubel and Livingstone 1987; but for a less clear-cut result, see DeYoe and Van Essen 1985). The connections of V1 with V2, summarized in Figure 2, reveal not only their parallel nature but also the "like with like" principle. The connections of both areas with the specialized visual areas of the prestriate cortex, also summarized in Figure 2, once again reveal the parallel nature of the outputs from these two areas. In short, the directionally selective cells of layer 4B of V1 project to V5 and to the thick stripes of V2, which in turn project to V5; the orientation selective cells of layer 4B project to V3 and the thick stripes of V2, which also project to V3, whereas the blobs and interblobs project to the thin stripes and interstripes of V2, respectively, both of which project to V4, which also receives a direct input from foveal V1, probably from the blobs (Zeki 1978c; Livingstone and Hubel 1984; Shipp and Zeki 1989a,b; Zeki and Shipp 1989).

Area V3 and the M Form System

The arguments given above make it reasonable to suppose that the organization of human visual cortex is similar to that of the monkey, and that parallelism is also a prominent feature of that organization. Taken in conjunction with the direct demonstration of the specialized motion and color centers in the human brain, they allow us to enquire into the neurological basis of two conditions, achromatopsia and akinetopsia, and to try to account for some of the more bizarre symptoms related to the perceptions of color and of motion. Before doing so, it is important to discuss the role of area V3 (see Fig. 2). It seems likely, given the similarities described above, that human visual cortex will probably be found to contain an area similar in its organization and connections to area V3 of the macaque monkey. Although defined and characterized many years ago (Cragg 1969; Zeki 1969, 1978b), this area has made little impression on neurophysiologists and neuroanatomists. Most of its cells are orientation

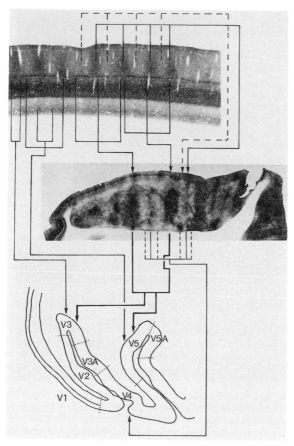

Figure 2. Separate pathways leading from V1 through V2 to the specialized areas V3, V4, and V5 of the prestriate visual cortex, and their relation to metabolic activity revealed by staining sections through V1 and V2 for the metabolic enzyme cytochrome oxidase. Sections through V1 and V2, taken at angles that most clearly reveal their cytochrome oxidase architecture, are shown at the top and center, respectively. Below is a drawing of a horizontal section through the posterior part of the right cerebral hemisphere, to show the position of the prestriate visual areas and of V1. The M pathway includes the output from layers 4B and upper layer 6, directly to V5 and V3 and indirectly to the same areas through the thick stripes of V2 (heavy lines). The dark blobs and lighter interblobs of the upper layers of V1 are part of the P pathway. The blobs project through the thin dark stripes of V2 to area V4 (thin lines), and the interblobs project through the paler interstripes of V2 to V4 (dashed lines). A smaller direct projection from the upper layers of V1 to V4 is not shown. (Reprinted, with permission, from Zeki and Shipp 1988.)

selective and indifferent to the color of the stimulus (Zeki 1978c; Felleman and Van Essen 1987). Although it is therefore presumably involved with form vision in some way, it is fed from the M layers, through layer 4B of V1, and not from the P layers through layers 2 and 3 of V1. It is intimately related to area V3A, which is also characterized by high concentrations of orientation-selective cells that are indifferent to the color of the stimulus (Zeki 1978b). Area V3A also forms part of this form system. In addition, it is an area that com-

bines the "what" and the "where" pathways in one, since many cells in it will only respond if the monkey gazes in a particular direction (Galletti and Battaglini 1989). Knowledge of these facts may turn out to be important in interpreting the characteristics of cerebral achromatopsia and other visual syndromes of cortical origin.

CEREBRAL ACHROMATOPSIA

Cerebral achromatopsia refers to a condition in which the capacity to see colors is lost following cerebral lesions. It is to be distinguished from color agnosia, when colors are seen but not recognized, and from color anomia, the inability to name colors. As well, it is distinct from color confusion syndromes, or dyschromatopsia, although some authors have used the latter term to refer to achromatopsia. It has an interesting history. First described with supporting postmortem studies by Verrey (1888), it was dismissed repeatedly until it "vanished" (Damasio 1985) from the clinical literature, only to reappear after the description of functional specialization in the monkey brain, including one for color (Zeki 1973, 1974b). The reason for this dismissal constitutes an interesting insight into the history of neurology and neurologists and is reviewed at length elsewhere (Zeki 1990a). Verrey believed his "color center" to be located in the lingual and fusiform gyri (Fig. 3), which he mistakenly believed to form part of the primary visual cortex, at a time when that cortex had not yet been definitively equated with the striate cortex. Whether human V4, as demonstrated by PET studies, is located in the lingual or fusiform gyri, or both, is not certain, because both gyri are active under conditions of color stimulation. Separating the two is therefore difficult with the relatively low spatial resolution of PET scans. However, lesions of the fusiform gyrus alone do lead to achromatopsia (Lenz 1921). Moreover, the striate cortex in the lower lip of the calcarine sulcus emerges onto the lingual gyrus, where one would assume V2, which should be active during all types of visual stimulation and which should be located next to V1, to be situated. We are inclined to the view that human V4 is located in the fusiform gyrus, although we cannot be certain of this with the presently available evidence (S. Zeki et al., in prep.). Whether it is located in one or both gyri, the presence of an area in human brain homologous to monkey V4 renders the syndrome of cerebral achromatopsia more comprehensible. Lesions affecting human V4 alone (e.g., the cases of Kolmel 1988) would lead to an absolute achromatopsia, without affecting the other submodalities of vision. In the macaque monkey, it is the contralateral hemifield that is represented in each V4 (Zeki 1977) which accounts for the syndrome of hemiachromatopsia when the lesion is unilateral in humans (e.g., the case of Verrey [1888] and those of Kolmel [1988]).

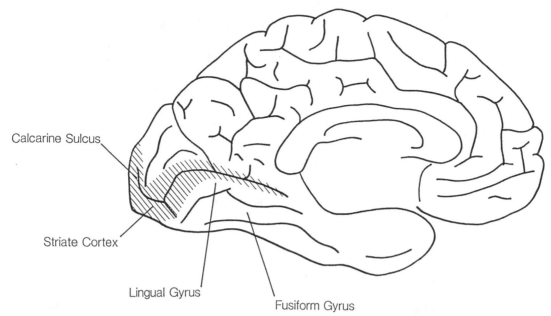

Figure 3. Drawing of the medial side of the left hemisphere of a human brain to show the relationship of the calcarine sulcus and the striate cortex to the lingual and fusiform gyri. The hatched area indicates the limits of the striate cortex.

Form Vision in Achromatopsia

Here intervenes an awkward problem of interpretation if one wishes to push the homology between human and monkey brains further. Monkey V4 receives an input from the thin stripes of V2, where wavelength selective cells and those with a preference for low spatial frequencies are concentrated. It also receives an input from the interstripes of V2, where cells are orientation, but not wavelength, selective. Indeed, there are two patterns of connections between V2 and V4 (Fig. 4). In type 1, which is the more common pattern, the output to V4 is from the thin stripes, whereas in type 2 it is from the interstripes (Zeki and Shipp 1989). Form, or at any rate boundaries, constitute an important ingredient for the construction of color, and a form input to V4 is therefore not surprising. The fact that most cells of V4, whether orientation selective or not, are also wavelength selective to varying degrees (Zeki 1976, 1983; Desimone and Schein 1987) implies that the latter characteristic is conferred on them within V4, either by convergent connections from V2 or by some system of intracortical connections. At any rate, this pattern of connectivity can be interpreted to mean that V4, in addition to being involved with color, is also involved with form vision, especially form in association with color. If form vision were to be a function of V4, then one would expect (assuming the homology with monkey brain) that, following lesions in human V4, form vision will be com-

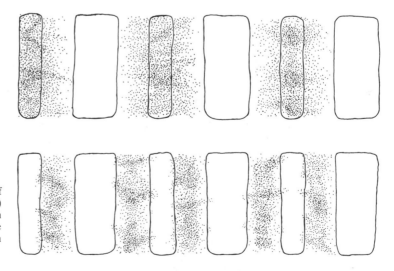

Figure 4. Schematic diagram of the two types of connectivity between V2 and V4. In type 1 (*top*) the V4 efferent cells are centered on the thin stripes, whereas in type 2 (*bottom*) they are centered on the interstripes. (Reprinted, with permission, from Zeki and Shipp 1989.)

promised along with color vision. Yet there are several cases on record which show that form vision can remain intact in cerebral achromatopsia. The recent cases of Kolmel (1988) and Sacks et al. (1988) are good examples.

Two Form Systems

It would be difficult to account for this condition by supposing that vascular lesions selectively spare the subcompartments of V4 in which orientation selective cells are concentrated. It is much easier to suppose that, following lesions to human V4, subjects use the other form system, derived from the M system and based on V3 with its broadband cells, to detect and construct forms. There are several features one might expect if this is the case, although the suggestion being new (Zeki 1990a), the experiments have not been really tried out in any detail. The first feature is that achromatopsic subjects should be able to detect and grade correctly the different lightnesses in a multicolored scene, as when Land color Mondrians are viewed in light of one wave band only. They should also be able to register the change of lightnesses and grade them correctly when the color display is illuminated by light of another wave band. In fact, the achromatopsic patient that I have tested with Oliver Sacks and his colleagues (Sacks et al. 1988) was able to undertake these tasks with ease. This patient, like almost all other achromatopsic patients, described the world in shades of gray. To him there was no difference between a multicolored Mondrian viewed in full illumination and the same Mondrian viewed in middle wave light alone, suggesting that he was using an achromatic channel with maximal sensitivity to middle wave light. However, when the Mondrians were viewed in long or short wave light, they were reported to be very different in terms of their shades of gray from their colored counterpart. When we constructed a black-white-gray Mondrian that was identical in shape and configuration to the multicolored Mondrian, the different grays made to approximate as closely as possible the different lightnesses of the multicolored Mondrian when viewed in middle wave light alone, the patient reported the colored Mondrian and its gray counterpart, both now viewed in full illumination, to be identical. If the M form system is the one mediating form perception in such patients, then one would expect his perception of dynamic form (structure from motion) to be unimpaired. One should also expect that prolonged fixation would fatigue him. Both these predictions were true of our patient. I am aware of the fact that this is a single case study, and the predictions must be tested on other patients. However, the proposal that achromatopsic patients use an alternative form system is perhaps the simplest way to account for why their perception of forms can remain unimpaired. The presence of two form systems may also help to account for why a specific loss of form vision is rarely, if ever, encountered. An alternative explanation is that the functional specialization demonstrated in the macaque monkey brain (Zeki 1974b, 1978a) is carried further in the human brain, with the human homolog of V4 not receiving input from the interstripes of V4, but from the thin stripes alone. Given the pronounced similarities between the early visual areas in the two brains, referred to above, this would seem to be unlikely, although it must be considered as another possibility until discounted.

Transient Achromatopsia

The parallel pathways through the visual cortex are based on cortical sites that differ in their metabolic activity. In V1, for example, the color pathway uses the metabolically rich blobs, whereas the form pathway uses the interblobs and layer 4B, both lower in metabolic activity. Such an organization may be used to account for a syndrome such as transient achromatopsia, described by Lapresle et al. (1977). The achromatopsia in this condition was correlated with falling attacks and was very likely to have been caused by transient arterial insufficiency through the system, the posterior cerebral artery, that irrigates both the cerebellum and the occipital lobe. One may postulate that in such conditions, the metabolically more active cortical sites, the blobs, may be more vulnerable than the interblobs. It is also possible that prolonged arterial insufficiency may damage the vulnerable blobs more permanently, thus depriving the thin stripes of V2 and area V4 of their input. Indeed, brain scans of the patient of Sacks et al. (1988) did not reveal any lesion, and the possibility suggested above must be considered. There are arguments against such an interpretation. One might expect, for example, that the metabolically active layer 4C, which receives the geniculate afferents, should also be affected, leading to a more general and pronounced visual defect. Unfortunately, we have little information on the relative richness of the blood supply to the different layers, and the suggestion must therefore remain conjectural.

Chromatopsia

I use the term chromatopsia to refer to the obverse of achromatopsia, that is to say a condition in which a patient is visually impaired in all submodalities except color vision, which is either unaffected or relatively spared. The condition has been described several times in the clinical literature, the first unequivocal case being that of Wechsler (1933). It has made no impression whatsoever on clinicians, and it is difficult to find a reference to it. The syndrome is associated with severe carbon monoxide poisoning. The consequence is that patients use color to identify objects and in the process commonly misidentify them. One might be tempted to suppose that in such conditions, the blobs and the thin stripes are selectively spared. Their richer blood supply might cushion them from the effects of hypoxia, but no one knows whether this is so. Moreover, such an explanation contradicts the one given above for transient achromatopsia, which supposes that the blobs are more vulnerable to a reduction in blood supply. However, it is not at present possible to resolve this contradiction, unless it can be shown that carboxemia and reduced blood flow have different effects. However, it is at least possible to think about such disorders in terms of the parallel pathways of the human cerebral cortex.

CEREBRAL AKINETOPSIA

Just as color vision can be specifically compromised following specific cortical lesions, so can the perception of motion, leading to the condition of "motion blindness," which I refer to as akinetopsia, to bring it more into terminological line with achromatopsia (Zeki 1991). The best case on record is that of Zihl et al. (1983), whose study represents some kind of landmark in neurological history. It is one of the very few, possibly the only, paper based on a single case study to be accepted by neurologists. This is in contrast to the syndrome of achromatopsia, whose existence was first disputed on the grounds that it was based on only a few cases, and accepted as a syndrome only after the demonstration of functional specialization in the macaque monkey. With akinetopsia, the sequence was reversed, convincing clinical evidence in its favor coming only after the demonstration of functional specialization in the macaque monkey brain, including a specialization for visual motion. The bilateral lesions in the patient of Zihl et al. included the territory where human V5 is found to be located from the PET studies (Cunningham et al. 1990; S. Zeki et al., in prep.). These lesions were a good deal more extensive, although they spared the calcarine or striate cortex. It seems likely, therefore, that territory beyond V5 was involved. Given the specificity of the visual disturbance, it is very likely that the damaged cortex outside V5 is also motion related. In the monkey, V5 is surrounded by other motion-related areas, which are fed through V5 (Zeki 1980b; Maunsell and Van Essen 1983; Desimone and Ungerleider 1986; Tanaka et al. 1986; Komatsu and Wurtz 1988). The role of these areas in processing motion-related information is different from that of V5. Their human counterparts have yet to be delineated. They are likely to be defined in the future, with further refinement of the noninvasive techniques for localization of cortical activity.

Kinetopsia

Just as achromatopsia has its obverse, so does akinetopsia. This consists of a syndrome in which patients are able to see movements in their otherwise scotomatous fields. Riddoch (1917) was the first to describe the condition, which led him to the conclusion that "Movement may be recognized as a special visual perception." He tried to account for the phenomenon by reference to the striate cortex alone, even though it

is likely that the gunshot wounds in some of his patients went beyond area 17. Perhaps for this reason, Holmes (1918) and Teuber (1960), who were in any case hostile to the notion of a functional specialization in the visual cortex, dismissed the claim, which also appears to have vanished from the literature, although like the syndrome of achromatopsia it is now resurfacing. Just as Holmes (1918) had written that "...an isolated loss or dissociation of colour vision is not produced by cerebral lesions," so he asserted that "...the condition described by Riddoch should not be spoken of as a dissociation of the elements of visual sensation." Again, just as Teuber et al. (1960) had written that "There is thus no evidence for a genuine dissociation...of color and form vision," so Teuber (1960) wrote that "Actual measurements...demonstrate that motion perception is impaired *pari passu* with defects in the forming of contours," leading him later to the conclusion that "There was no evidence that one could dissociate detection of moving and stationary targets" (Koerner and Teuber 1973).

In fact, Holmes and Teuber may have been quite right in believing that kinetopsia cannot be accounted for in terms of sparing of motion mechanisms within the striate cortex, even though they were both hostile to the notion of a functional specialization in the visual cortex. To account for Riddoch's results in the context of the striate cortex alone, one would have to suppose that the gunshot wounds were superficial and did not involve layer 4B of V1, in itself a difficult supposition, given the deep nature of the wounds in Riddoch's patients. Moreover, one would also have to suppose that the wounds spared the directionally selective cells of layer 4B, and selectively incapacitated the orientation selective cells, the ones that project to V3. It is hard to imagine how this could be achieved with such indiscriminate lesions. It is perhaps more likely that Riddoch was revealing a subcortical mechanism involved in motion, or possibly a phenomenon analogous to residual vision or blindsight (Pöppel et al. 1973; Perenin and Jeannerod 1978; Weiskrantz 1986).

Although there are still many problems to be solved, it is surprising and gratifying to learn of the progress made in the 15 years separating *The Brain* from *The Synapse*. I never imagined in 1975 that the parallel pathways and the specialized areas that I described at that time would have been worked out in sufficient detail to enable us to account in neuroanatomical and neurophysiological terms for so many syndromes that, even a few years ago, were ascribed to hysterical states. The advances made impel me, perhaps recklessly, to look forward to the next Cold Spring Harbor Symposium, which will surely be entitled *The Mind*. A critical problem then will almost certainly be how the brain succeeds in bringing all the signals in these separate parallel pathways and areas together to give us our unitary experience of vision. More than that, it will consider how signals in parts of the brain representing different functions are assembled together to give rise to consciousness. Discussions of problems such as the neurological nature of hallucinations and dreams will no longer be disreputable. In preparation for that millennial future, it is interesting to address the problem of integration in the visual cortex.

A THEORY OF MULTISTAGE INTEGRATION IN THE VISUAL CORTEX

One might have supposed, naively, that all the specialized visual areas would report to a single master area, which would be the site of integration. Such a supposition, which would logically be a direct consequence of an exclusively hierarchical strategy, has two problems attached to it. The first is that there is no master area to which all the visual areas report; the second is that, even if there were and even if the visual image was finally synthesized there, that would still leave us with the problem of who/what views and interprets that image. These difficulties are not resolved by the modern variant of the exclusive hierarchical doctrine, the two pathway hypothesis of Mishkin et al. (1983).

We suppose that perception of the visual image is due to the simultaneous activity of several of the specialized areas, which therefore must be connected with each other. The problem of the master area, to which all areas must report, is neatly circumvented by the observation that the specialized visual areas can communicate with each other at several different levels. These can be divided into three separate levels: backward, forward, and intermediate (see Zeki and Shipp 1988; Zeki 1990b).

Integration within the M System

The input to specialized areas such as V3, V4, and V5 is highly segregated. V3 and V5 receive their input from separate cells in layer 4B of V1, which is itself principally fed by the M system. They also receive input from the thick stripes of V2, which are in turn fed by layer 4B of V1. However, the return projection from V5 to layer 4B of V1 is not quite so segregated (Shipp and Zeki 1989a). Instead, it involves large parts of the layer which do not themselves project to area V5 (Fig. 5A). In short, through this return projection, area V5 is able to influence not only cells in layer 4B that project to it, but also cells in the same layer that project to area V3. It is thus able to unite two subdivisions of the M system, one concerned principally with motion and the other principally with form. One can readily imagine the importance of such a system in generating one construct from another, for example, form from motion. We expect that in such a system, not only V5 and V3 will be active, but that activity in V1 will be double that obtained when one is stimulating with form alone or with motion alone, since both areas will interact partly through layer 4B of V1. It is a supposition that we are actively testing.

Combination of P and M Inputs

Although there are anatomical opportunities for the P and the M systems to connect within V1 (for review, see Zeki and Shipp 1988), a major combination of P and M inputs seems to be deferred until area V2 (Shipp and Zeki 1989b). The outputs from the stripes of V2 are segregated (see above), but the return inputs to them from V4 and V5 are more widespread and encompass the territory of all stripes, not just the ones projecting to them (Fig. 5B). V5 receives input from the thick stripes of V2, but the return input from V5 to V2, although densest in the territory of the thick stripes, also invades the thin stripes and the interstripes (Shipp and Zeki 1989b). The same pattern prevails for the return projection from V4 (Zeki and Shipp 1989). This thus provides an opportunity for the P and the M systems to converse directly.

The specialized areas have other interconnections. They have direct connections with each other, each of the specialized areas being reciprocally connected with the others (Zeki and Shipp 1988). On the whole, these connections, although consistently present, are relatively weak. They may come under the category of a speculative type of connection, which I have called the operational connection (Zeki 1990c). More importantly, all the specialized areas communicate, either directly or indirectly, with parietal and temporal areas. Most of the projection from area V5 is to the parietal cortex, but there is also a consistent projection to the temporal cortex (Zeki 1990c). Most of the projection from V4 is to the temporal cortex, but there is also a consistent projection to parietal cortex (Zeki 1977). Area V3 projects both to V4 and V5, as well as to V3A (Zeki 1971), which in turn project to parietal and temporal areas, which are interconnected (Seltzer and Pandya 1984). Thus, temporal and parietal areas are able to draw on different specialized areas to undertake their own specialized tasks.

This vast system of interconnections between the specialized parallel pathways establishes a framework within which we can think of how signals are brought together to lead to a coherent percept, one in which all the attributes of the visual scene are seen in precise spatiotemporal registration. It is obvious that activity in any one of these areas can be readily communicated to several other areas through the interconnecting links. One can go a step further and suggest that simultaneous firing of the relevant cells in the different areas *constitutes the percept*.

The backward connections from the specialized visual areas, each of which contains a relatively eroded retinal topography, to areas such as V1 and V2, which have a detailed retinal topography, may constitute a means of maintaining the local sign, that is, of signaling the precise location of an object whose attributes have been determined in the specialized areas. But this reentrant input may also constitute a system for reentering centrally generated constructs into the visual cortex, as

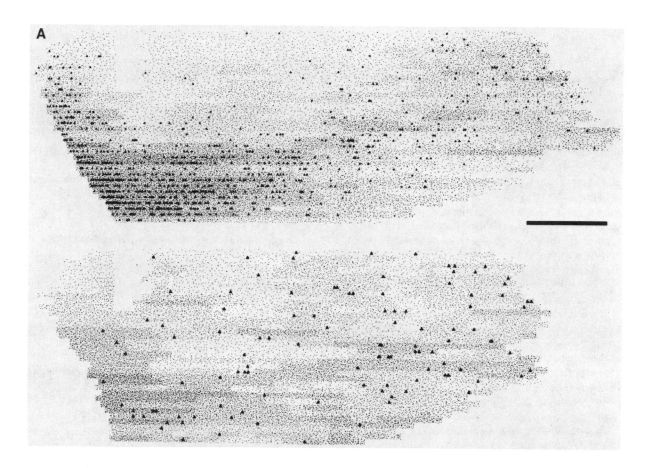

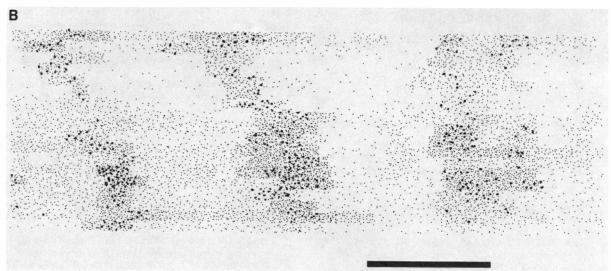

Figure 5. (*A*) Computer-aided, two-dimensional reconstruction of the distribution of cells and fibers in layers 4 B (*above*) and upper layer 6 (*below*) of V1, following an injection of wheat germ agglutinin horseradish peroxidase into area V5. The triangles represent the labeled cells projecting to V5, and the stippling represents the distribution of the return projection from V5 to these layers of V1. (Reprinted, with permission, from Shipp and Zeki 1989a.) (*B*) Computer-aided, two-dimensional reconstruction of the distribution of labeled cells and fibers in area V2, following an injection of wheat germ agglutinin horseradish peroxidase into area V5. Conventions are the same as those in *A*. Bars: (*A*) 5 mm; (*B*) 2 mm. (Reprinted, with permission, from Shipp and Zeki 1989b.)

if they were coming from outside. This occurs in dreams and hallucinations and, to a lesser extent, in visual imagery. The study of such phenomena is likely to become important and provide a rich hunting ground for understanding the physiology of the visual cortex.

Finally, one might want to consider why integration is a multistage process. There are several successive steps within each specialized pathway; for example, the color pathways leading from V2 to V4 (see above). The responses of cells at each level may contribute to perception explicitly, and that contribution must consequently become available to other explicit contributions derived from other sources. The simplest way of achieving this is to allow integration to occur at that stage, rather than a later stage, when the output of the cells may have been further transformed by other influences. Moreover, the signal present at an earlier level may be sufficient, when combined with one at a later stage, to generate a percept without the need to resort to higher areas. Structure from motion provides a good example, in which the output from V3 and V5 can be directed backward to V1, in the reentrant pathway.

Naturally, the theory of multistage integration is still based almost exclusively on anatomical connections and now awaits detailed physiological studies. It is a measure of how much we have achieved over the past 15 years that we are able to invoke specific and well-defined visual pathways to account for specific percepts. The theory may require amplification or modification; it may turn out to be wrong; but it should generate a lot of new experiments and results in preparation for *The Mind*.

ACKNOWLEDGMENT

The author's work reported above was supported by the Wellcome Trust, London.

REFERENCES

Burkhalter, A. and K.L. Bernardo. 1989. Organization of cortico-cortical connections in human visual cortex. *Proc. Natl. Acad. Sci.* **86:** 1071.

Cavanagh, P., C.W. Tyler, and O.E. Favreau. 1984. Perceived velocity of moving chromatic gratings. *J. Opt. Soc. Am.* **1:** 893.

Cragg, B.G. 1969. The topography of the afferent projections in the circumstriate visual cortex (C.V.C.) of the monkey studied by the Nauta method. *Vision Res.* **9:** 733.

Cunningham, V.J., M.P. Deiber, R.S.J. Frackowiak, K.J. Friston, C. Kennard, A.A. Lammertsma, C.J. Lueck, J. Romaya, and S. Zeki. 1990. The motion area (area V5) of human visual cortex. *J. Physiol.* **423:** 101.

Damasio, A.R. 1985. Disorders of complex visual processing: Agnosias, achromatopsia, Balint's syndrome, and related difficulties of orientation and construction. In *Principles of behavioral neurology* (ed. M.M. Mesulam), p. 259. F.H. Davis, Philadelphia.

Desimone, R. and S.J. Schein. 1987. Visual properties of neurons in area V4 of the macaque: Sensitivity to stimulus form. *J. Neurophysiol.* **57:** 835.

Desimone, R. and L.G. Ungerleider. 1986. Multiple visual areas in the caudal superior temporal sulcus of the macaque. *J. Comp. Neurol.* **248:** 164.

DeYoe, E.A. and D.C. Van Essen. 1985. Segregation of efferent connections and receptive field properties in visual area V2 of the macaque. *Nature* **317:** 58.

Felleman, D.J. and D.C. Van Essen. 1987. Receptive field properties of neurons in area V3 of macaque monkey extrastriate cortex. *J. Neurophysiol.* **57:** 889.

Friston, K.J., C.D. Frith, P.F. Liddle, R.J. Dolan, A.A. Lammertsma, and R.S.J. Frackowiak. 1990. The relationship between global and local changes in PET scans. *J. Cereb. Blood Flow Metab.* **10:** 458.

Galletti, C. and P.P. Battaglini. 1989. Gaze dependent visual neurons in area V3A of monkey prestriate cortex. *J. Neurosci.* **9:** 1112.

Gattass, R. and C.G. Gross. 1981. Visual topography of striate projection zone (MT) in posterior superior temporal sulcus of the macaque. *J. Neurophysiol.* **46:** 621.

Hockfield, S., R.B.H. Tootell, and S. Zaremba. 1990. Molecular differences among neurons reveal an organization of human visual cortex. *Proc. Natl. Acad. Sci.* **87:** 3027.

Holmes, G. 1918. Disturbances of vision by cerebral lesions. *Br. J. Ophthalmol.* **2:** 253.

Hubel, D.H. and M.S. Livingstone. 1987. Segregation of form, color and stereopsis in primate area 18. *J. Neurosci.* **7:** 3378.

Hubel, D.H. and T.N. Wiesel. 1965. Receptive fields and functional architecture in two non striate visual areas (18 and 19) of the cat. *J. Neurophysiol.* **28:** 229.

Horton, J.C. 1984. Cytochrome oxidase patches: A new cytoarchitectonic feature of monkey visual cortex. *Philos. Trans. R. Soc. Lond. B Biol. Sci.* **304:** 199.

Horton, J.C. and E.T. Hedley-Whyte. 1984. Mapping of cytochrome oxidase patches and ocular dominance columns in human visual cortex. *Philos. Trans. R. Soc. Lond. B Biol. Sci.* **304:** 255.

Koerner, F. and H.-L. Teuber. 1973. Visual field defects after missile injuries to the geniculo-striate pathway in man. *Exp. Brain Res.* **18:** 88.

Kolmel, H.W. 1988. Pure homonymous hemiachromatopsia. *Eur. Arch. Psychiatry Neurol. Sci.* **237:** 237.

Komatsu, H. and R.H. Wurtz. 1988. Relation of cortical areas MT and MST to pursuit eye movements. I. Localization and visual properties of neurons. *J. Neurophysiol.* **60:** 580.

Lapresle, J., R. Metreau, and A. Annabi. 1977. Transient achromatopsia in vertebrobasilar insufficiency. *J. Neurol.* **215:** 155.

Lenz, G. 1921. Zwei Sektionsfälle doppelseitiger zentraler Farbenhemianopsie. *Z. Gesamte Neurol. Psychiatr.* **71:** 135.

Livingstone, M.S. and D.H. Hubel. 1984. Anatomy and physiology of a color system in primate visual cortex. *J. Neurosci.* **4:** 309.

Lu, C. and D.H. Fender. 1972. The interaction of color and luminance in stereoscopic vision. *Invest. Ophthalmol.* **11:** 482.

Lueck, C.J., S. Zeki, K.J. Friston, M.-P. Deiber, P. Cope, V.J. Cunningham, A.A. Lammertsma, C. Kennard, and R.S.J. Frackowiak. 1989. The colour centre in the cerebral cortex of man. *Nature* **340:** 386.

Maunsell, J.H.R. and D.C. Van Essen. 1983. The connections of the middle temporal visual area (MT) and their relationship to a cortical hierarchy in the macaque monkey. *J. Neurosci.* **3:** 2563.

Mishkin, M., L.G. Ungerleider, and K.A. Macko. 1983. Object vision and spatial vision: Two cortical pathways. *Trends Neurosci.* **6:** 414.

Perenin, M.T. and M. Jeannerod. 1978. Visual function within the hemianopic field following early cerebral hemidecortication in man. I. Spatial localization. *Neuropsychologia* **16:** 1.

Pöppel, E., R. Held, and D. Frost. 1973. Residual visual

function after brain wounds involving the central visual pathways in man. *Nature* **243**: 295.

Ramachandran, V.S. and R.L. Gregory. 1978. Does colour provide an input to human motion perception? *Nature* **275**: 55.

Riddoch, G. 1917. Dissociation of visual perception due to occipital injuries, with especial reference to appreciation of movement. *Brain* **40**: 15.

Sacks, O., R.L. Wasserman, S. Zeki, and R.M. Seigel. 1988. Sudden color blindness of cerebral origin. *Soc. Neurosci. Abstr.* **14**: 1251.

Seltzer, B. and D.N. Pandya. 1984. Further observations on parieto-temporal connections in the rhesus monkey. *Exp. Brain Res.* **55**: 301.

Shipp, S. and S. Zeki. 1985. Segregation of pathways leading from area V2 to areas V4 and V5 of macaque monkey visual cortex. *Nature* **315**: 322.

———. 1989a. The organization of connections between areas V5 and V1 in macaque monkey visual cortex. *Eur. J. Neurosci.* **1**: 309.

———. 1989b. The organization of connections between areas V5 and V2 in macaque monkey visual cortex. *Eur. J. Neurosci.* **1**: 333.

Tanaka, K., K. Hirosaka, H.A. Saito, M. Yukie, Y. Fukada, and E. Iwai. 1986. Analysis of local and wide-field movements in the superior temporal visual areas of the macaque monkey. *J. Neurosci.* **6**: 134.

Teuber, H.-L. 1960. Perception. *Handb. Physiol.* **3 (1)**: 1595.

Teuber, H.-L., W.S. Battersby, and M.B. Bender. 1960. *Visual field defects after penetrating missile wounds of the brain.* Harvard University Press, Cambridge, Massachusetts.

Tootell, R.B.H., M.S. Silverman, R.L. De Valois, and G.H. Jacobs. 1983. Functional organization of the second cortical visual area in primates. *Science* **220**: 737.

Verrey. 1888. Hémiachromatopsie droite absolue. *Arch. d'Ophthal.* **8**: 289.

Wechsler, I.S. 1933. Partial cortical blindness with preservation of color vision. *Arch. Ophthal.* **9**: 957.

Weiskrantz, L. 1986. *Blindsight.* Oxford University Press, London.

Zeki, S. 1969. Representation of central visual fields in prestriate cortex of monkey. *Brain Res.* **14**: 271.

———. 1971. Cortical projections from two prestriate areas in the monkey. *Brain Res.* **34**: 19.

———. 1973. Colour coding in rhesus monkey prestriate cortex. *Brain Res.* **53**: 422.

———. 1974a. Functional organization of a visual area in the posterior bank of the superior temporal sulcus of the rhesus monkey. *J. Physiol.* **236**: 549.

———. 1974b. The mosaic organization of the visual cortex in the monkey. In *Essays on the nervous system* (ed. R. Bellairs and E.G. Gray), p. 327. Clarendon Press, Oxford, England.

———. 1976. The functional organization of projections from striate to prestriate visual cortex in the rhesus monkey. *Cold Spring Harbor Symp. Quant. Biol.* **40**: 591.

———. 1977. Colour coding in the superior temporal sulcus of rhesus monkey visual cortex. *Proc. Roy. Soc. Lond. B Biol. Sci.* **197**: 195.

———. 1978a. Functional specialisation in the visual cortex of the rhesus monkey. *Nature* **274**: 423.

———. 1978b. The cortical projections of foveal striate cortex in the rhesus monkey. *J. Physiol.* **277**: 227.

———. 1978c. The third visual complex of rhesus monkey prestriate cortex. *J. Physiol.* **277**: 245.

———.1980a. A direct projection from area V1 to area V3A of rhesus monkey visual cortex. *Proc. R. Soc. Lond. B Biol. Sci.* **207**: 499.

———. 1980b. The responses of cells in the anterior bank of the superior temporal sulcus in macaque monkeys. *J. Physiol.* **308**: 85P.

———. 1983. The distribution of wavelength and orientation selective cells in different areas of monkey visual cortex. *Proc. Roy. Soc. Lond. B Biol. Sci.* **217**: 449.

———. 1990a. A century of cerebral achromatopsia. *Brain* (in press).

———. 1990b. A theory of multistage integration in the visual cortex. In *Principles of design and operation of the brain* (ed. J.C. Eccles and O. Creutzfeldt). Pontifical Academy, Citta del Vaticano, Italy.

———. 1990c. The motion pathways of the cerebral cortex. In *Vision: Coding and efficiency* (ed. C. Blakemore). University Press, Cambridge, England.

———. 1991. Cerebral akinetopsia (visual motion blindness). *Brain* (in press).

Zeki, S. and S. Shipp. 1988. The functional logic of cortical connections. *Nature* **335**: 311.

———. 1989. Modular connections between areas V2 and V4 of macaque monkey visual cortex. *Eur. J. Neurosci.* **1**: 494.

Zihl, J., D. Von Cramon, and N. Mai. 1983. Selective disturbance of movement vision after bilateral brain damage. *Brain* **106**: 313.

Lateral Interactions in Visual Cortex

C.D. GILBERT, J.A. HIRSCH, AND T.N. WIESEL

The Rockefeller University, New York, New York 10021-6399

A common pattern of connections seen in cortex is a plexus of long-range projections, intrinsic to the cortical areas in which the projecting cells reside. These connections were initially discovered with the use of intracellular injection techniques. The evidence from earlier Golgi studies led to the idea that cortical connections were primarily vertical, running across the cortical layers and with relatively little lateral spread. This view coincided with studies showing columnar functional architecture of cortex. The subsequent finding of the long-range horizontal connections seemed to violate the principles of retinotopic order of visual cortex, since they allow cells to integrate information over a much larger part of visual field than one would expect from their receptive field maps. These connections also make one question how columnar properties could be maintained, considering that they cross columnar boundaries. In this paper, we present evidence that the horizontal connections bear a specific relationship to the columnar functional architecture, that they may mediate the sensitivity of cells' responses to the context in which a visual stimulus is presented, and that the functional properties of cortical cells are dynamic over the short and long term.

To put the characterization of the horizontal connections in the proper context, it is worth reviewing a few points concerning receptive field properties and the functional architecture of cortex. Using simple stimuli, such as a short oriented line segment, receptive fields appear to be quite small. In the superficial layers of monkey striate cortex, a typical receptive field at 4° eccentricity is around 1/4° in diameter. Most cortical cells show selectivity for the orientation of a line stimulus (Hubel and Wiesel 1959). Cells range from those having sharply tuned orientation selectivity to those with no orientation preference, with the sharpest tuning curves having a half bandwidth of 20°. With respect to cortical functional architecture, the first thing one notices is that the visual cortex is retinotopically organized: If one records from cells in electrode penetrations running perpendicular to the cortical surface, the receptive fields of the cells have, with a little scatter, the same visual field location. If one moves an electrode in directions parallel to the cortical surface, there is a gradual movement in receptive field position such that after about 1.5 mm, the receptive fields, taking into account receptive field size and scatter, no longer overlap with those at the beginning of the penetration. The cortex is also organized into columns of cells showing the same orientation specificity, and one

sees a regular clockwise or counterclockwise shift in orientation preference as one moves in 50-μm steps parallel to the cortical surface. Cells are also organized into ocular dominance columns (Hubel and Wiesel 1962, 1963, 1968, 1977). One full cycle of orientation columns, known as a hypercolumn, covers around 750 μm. There is a fixed relationship in striate cortex between cortical distance traveled in hypercolumns and distance traveled in the visual space represented by the hypercolumns: Whether one looks near the foveal representation, where receptive field size and scatter are small, or in the periphery, where they are much larger, the receptive fields of cells separated by a distance of two hypercolumns are nonoverlapping (Hubel and Wiesel 1974). It is because of these principles of cortical topography and columnar functional architecture that the discovery of long-range horizontal connections seemed so surprising.

Anatomy of Horizontal Connections

The longest-range connections in visual cortex are mediated by pyramidal cells. Figure 1 shows the axon of a pyramidal cell in the superficial layers of monkey striate cortex. In this transverse view, the cell, located in layer 3, extended its axon within layers 2 and 3 in directions parallel to the cortical surface. The axon's collaterals were distributed in a series of discrete clusters. The axon extended along the anteroposterior cortical axis, with the long axis running parallel to the ocular dominance columns. The relationship of the axon to the orientation columns is not known.

The first suggestion of the presence of fibers traveling for long distances laterally within the cortex came from degeneration studies (Fisken et al. 1975). Intracellular horseradish peroxidase (HRP) injections, such as that shown in Figure 1, showed that these long-range connections originated in the same cortical area, that the cells of origin were pyramidal, and that the collaterals had a clustered distribution (Gilbert and Wiesel 1979, 1983; Landry et al. 1980; Martin and Whitteridge 1984). Extracellular pathway tracing techniques, using HRP or fluorescent labels, subsequently showed that the horizontal connections were also highly convergent and that the input to a small injection site in the cortex originated from clusters of cells covering a large area (Rockland and Lund 1982, 1983; Gilbert and Wiesel 1989). We will discuss this in greater detail in comparing the distribution of the horizontal connections to the columnar functional architecture.

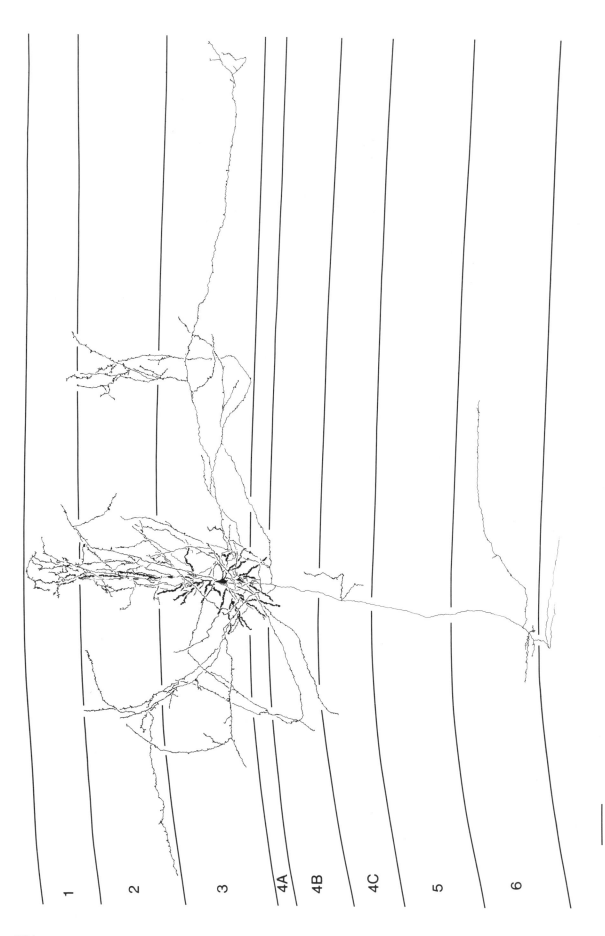

Figure 1. (*See facing page for legend.*)

Using anatomical criteria, we attempted to establish whether the long-range connections were likely to be excitatory or inhibitory. Since pyramidal cells are thought to be excitatory (they tend to show high-affinity uptake for glutamate and glutamate analogs, and form the excitatory type I synapses), the critical question is whether they contact other excitatory (pyramidal) cells or inhibitory interneurons (smooth stellate cells). We made serial electron microscopy reconstructions in the monkey of cells that were postsynaptic to the axon collaterals of superficial layer pyramidal cells at varying distances from the pyramidal somata (McGuire et al. 1991). The ratio of pyramidal to smooth stellate cells that were postsynaptic to the labeled axon terminals was 80% to 20%. This is roughly equivalent to the overall proportion of these two cell types in the cortex, indicating that there was no preference for a given cell type as a target for the horizontal connections. Moreover, the proportion of axospinous contacts is similar to the overall proportion of axospinous type I terminals in the cortex. Other studies have found that the horizontal connections in the cat visual cortex showed a slightly larger preference for contacts with pyramidal cells (Kisvarday et al. 1986; Gabbott et al. 1987). Although the majority of the targets were excitatory, this does not necessarily imply that the net effect of the horizontal connections is excitatory. The effect of the input to smooth stellate cells may be amplified by the position of the synapses relative to the soma, and the number and distribution of the synapses formed by the smooth stellate cells on *their* target neurons. In fact, we found in the tissue slice experiments (see below) that the synaptic potentials produced by the horizontal connections were a mixture of inhibitory and excitatory potentials.

Another feature of the horizontal connections revealed by our ultrastructural study was the sparsity of connections between individual cells. The axons of the pyramidal cells that we studied hop from cell to cell, usually making only a single contact with a given postsynaptic cell. The horizontal connections would therefore operate by "mass action," with hundreds of cells in one cortical column contacting hundreds of cells in another. Another intriguing aspect of the postsynaptic targets was that they tended to be vertical dendrites, such as the apical dendrites of pyramidal cells.

The clustering of axon collaterals seen in the intracellular injections suggested a possible relationship to the functional architecture of cortex. The nature of this relationship may hold a clue to the functional consequences of the horizontal connections. We will show below two lines of evidence from the cat showing the relationship of the clusters of axon collaterals to the orientation columns. A useful tool for visualizing the

horizontal connections used in some of these studies is that of retrograde transport following extracellular dye injection. This technique demonstrates that the horizontal connections, in addition to being highly divergent and clustered in nature, are highly convergent, bringing input from clusters of cells to a particular site.

The region of labeled cells in a tangential cortical section made 2 weeks after a small (150 μm in diameter) injection of rhodamine-filled latex microspheres ("beads") in striate cortex extended for 8 mm in the longest dimension. When one compares this dimension to cortical maps made at this eccentricity (Tusa et al. 1978), the labeled area can be shown to represent approximately 10° of visual angle. This area over which the cells at the injection site collect input is quite large in comparison to the receptive field diameter of these cells, which in the cat is on the order of 1–2°.

After such an injection, the labeled cells are distributed in a number of clusters, having a periodicity of roughly 1 mm. The clustering pattern was compared to that of the orientation columns by labeling the columns with 2-deoxyglucose autoradiography (Fig. 2). Using this approach, we could visualize the orientation columns in the same section as the one from which the distribution of labeled cells is obtained. The bead label injection was made in an orientation column of determined specificity. In the example shown, the injection was made in a vertical orientation column, and the vertical orientation columns were labeled by the 2-deoxyglucose technique. When the pattern of cell clusters is superimposed with the autoradiograph, one can see that there is a close registration in the patterns, with the clusters lying over the darker label, and the areas of lightest label in the autoradiograph being devoid of labeled cells. This then presents a picture of connectivity between columns of similar orientation specificity.

A similar pattern of convergent connections is seen in the connections between different cortical areas. Retrograde labeling of cells in area 17 after an injection of HRP or beads in area 18 produces a large area of clusters of labeled cells (Gilbert and Kelly 1975; Bullier et al. 1984; Ferrer et al. 1988; Gilbert and Wiesel 1989). This is a general feature of corticocortical connections seen in other visual areas, in cortical areas serving other sensory modalities, and in frontal cortex (Goldman and Nauta 1977; Imig and Brugge 1978; Jones et al. 1978; Wong-Riley 1979; Montero 1980; Imig and Reale 1981; Tigges et al. 1981; Goldman-Rakic and Schwartz 1982). Using the combined retrograde labeling/2-deoxyglucose technique, we find a similar rule governing corticocortical connections as in the case of intra-areal connections, with 'connections between columns of similar orientation specificity (Fig. 2, D–F). The picture that emerges from these experi-

---

Figure 1. Layer 3 pyramidal cell in monkey primary visual cortex. The dendrite, studded with spines, is represented by the thicker lines, with the apical dendrite extending toward the pial surface. The axon, covered with boutons, is shown by the thinner lines, and extends for several millimeters parallel to the cortical surface. Note the clustered distribution of the axon collaterals. Bar, 100 μm. (Adapted from McGuire et al. 1991.)

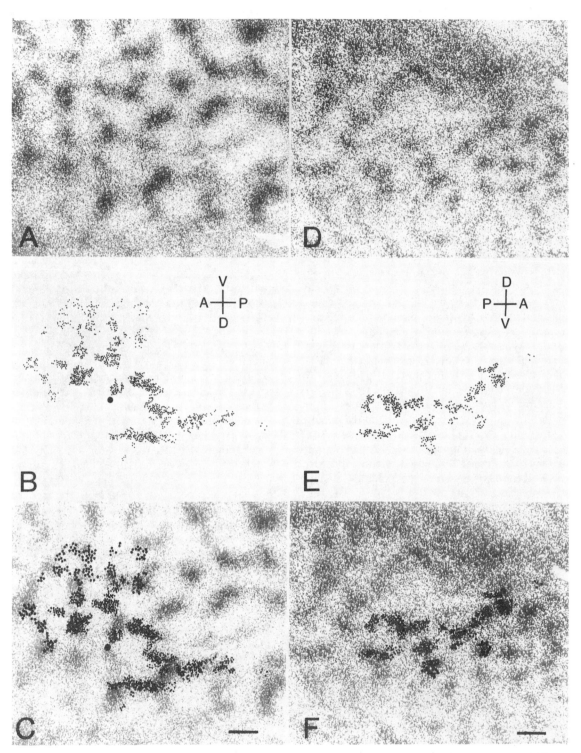

Figure 2. Comparison of distributions of horizontal connections and orientation columns (*A, B, C*) and corticocortical connections and orientation columns (*D, E, F*) in cat primary visual cortex. Connections are labeled by retrograde transport following small (150 μm in diameter) rhodamine-filled latex bead injections in area 17 and area 18. [^{14}C]2-deoxyglucose autoradiography indicates distribution of vertical orientation columns (*A, C; D, F*). Area 17 injection, made in a vertical orientation column, resulted in labeling of clusters of cells occupying a large area within area 17, $\sim$ 8 mm in diameter (*B*). The labeled cell clusters lie over vertical orientation columns, indicating a pattern of projection between columns of similar orientation specificity. A similar rule is seen for corticocortical connections. The injection in area 18 was made in a vertical orientation column and the labeled clusters in area 17 lie over the vertical orientation columns labeled by deoxyglucose autoradiography. Bar, 1 mm. (Adapted from Gilbert and Wiesel 1989.)

ments is a cascade of widespread lateral connections covering increasingly larger parts of the visual field: long-range horizontal connections in one area followed by converging and divergent corticocortical connections (which are, by the way, reciprocal), another stage of long-range horizontal connections in the second area, and so on.

Physiological Measurements of Horizontal Connections

The horizontal connections were studied by two physiological techniques: cross-correlation analysis and intracellular recording in cortical slices. The cross-correlation technique is a statistical technique that enables one to measure the synaptic interactions between cells (Perkel et al. 1967a,b). To some degree, it allows one to distinguish monosynaptic interactions from common input excitation (Michalski et al. 1983), although the anatomy of the system described here would lead one to expect a mixture of these interactions.

In our application of the cross-correlation technique, we did not attempt to differentiate systematically between the kinds of neural interactions observed (monosynaptic vs. common input), but rather to determine the relationships in receptive field properties for a population of cells showing correlated firing versus those firing independently of one another. In these experiments, we recorded from one site with one electrode throughout the experiment, and correlated the firing of a cell at that site with cells encountered by a second electrode along a tangential penetration (Ts'o et al. 1986). As one moves along the electrode track, one sees alternations between peaked and flat correlograms (peaked correlograms indicate interactions between the recorded cells). This waxing and waning in the peaks of the correlograms is reminiscent of the clustering in the pattern of horizontal connections. The two have similar range and periodicity. Peaked correlograms are observed between cells having matching receptive field properties: most notably, similar orientation preference (Ts'o et al. 1986; Ts'o and Gilbert 1988). An additional feature of the interactions between the cells that is revealed by the correlograms is that they are excitatory in nature (as seen in the upward direction of the peaks in the correlograms). A rather curious finding, not unexpected in view of the extent of the horizontal connections, is that correlated firing was observed between cells with nonoverlapping receptive fields. This finding once again emphasizes the implication that the horizontal connections allow cells to integrate input over a larger part of the visual field than their receptive field maps would indicate.

The cross-correlation experiments also provide a measure of the strength of connection between the cell pairs, known as the contribution or effectiveness of the input. The contribution of the horizontal connections in the cat was generally a few percent. Weaker contributions were seen when the electrodes and the receptive fields were farther apart. The small size of the functional connection between the cells is concordant with the sparseness of the connections seen anatomically. Although the strength of horizontal connections between any two sites may be weak (an order of magnitude weaker than interlaminar connections, for example: Toyama et al. 1981a,b), when one takes into account all of the horizontal inputs converging on a cell, the overall effect can be quite substantial.

The synaptic potentials produced by activating the horizontal connections were observed also by recording intracellularly in a tissue slice preparation. In this technique, coronal slices of cat visual cortex, 400 μm thick, were maintained in vitro, enabling us to surgically isolate the horizontal connections and selectively activate different inputs to superficial layer cortical cells. One of the main points learned with this approach is that the influence of the horizontal connections changes according to the concomitant synaptic input that a cell receives from other sources, and that the synaptic potentials elicited by activating the horizontal connections change according to the degree of recruitment of horizontal inputs. These points are illustrated in Figure 3. The intracellular recording electrode in the examples shown was located in the superficial layers, and a cut was made at the boundary between layer 2 + 3 and layer 4 in order to look specifically at horizontal and not interlaminar inputs. In the top panel of part a of the figure, we show the synaptic response to stimulating at a horizontal displacement of 1.2 mm from the impaled cell. In this instance, the response was predominantly excitatory. When the cell was depolarized approximately 15 mV from its resting potential of −72 mV to mimic the effects of converging excitatory inputs, the excitatory postsynaptic potential (EPSP) increased fourfold in area. This enhancement is likely due to voltage-dependent Na^+ channels within the cell membrane (Staftstrom et al. 1985). When a second cell in the same preparation (bottom panel of part a) was injected with the Na^+ channel blocker QX-314 (Connors and Prince 1982), the EPSP assumed a conventional relationship with membrane voltage, decreasing with depolarization. In recordings made in a third cell (part b), we showed specifically that, below threshold for firing, NMDA receptors do not markedly contribute to the depolarization-induced enhancement of the EPSP: That is, the magnitude of the response was not reduced by application of the NMDA antagonist APV (Watkins and Evans 1981). This gives further indication that the enhancement of the EPSP by depolarization is mediated by intrinsic membrane conductances.

One can modify not only the magnitude of the horizontal synaptic potentials, but also the relative balance between excitation and inhibition, by varying the number of horizontal fibers recruited. In part c, at low stimulus strengths the synaptic potential was almost exclusively excitatory. As stimulus voltage was raised, inhibition came to dominate the response. Thus, the effect of activating the horizontal input is not fixed, but can change according to the degree of recruitment and to the state of activation of the postsynaptic cell.

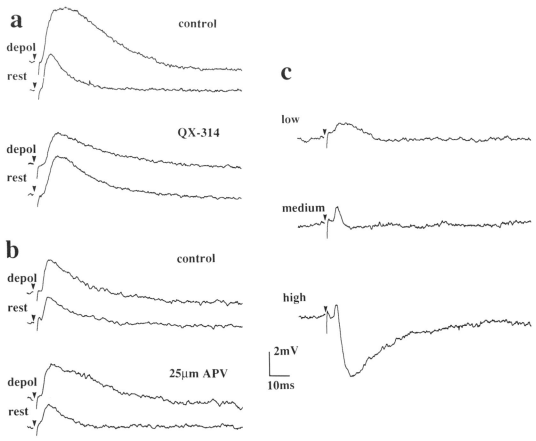

Figure 3. Modification of the synaptic potentials seen in superficial layer pyramidal cells when stimulating horizontal connections in the same layer. A cut was made at the boundary between layers 2 + 3 and 4 in order to isolate the horizontal inputs to the recorded cell. The stimulating electrode was placed 1.2 mm away from the intracellular electrode, remaining in the same layer. Synaptic potentials in *a*, a control cell, and in another cell in the same preparation injected with QX-314; *b*, a cell in control medium and the same cell superfused with 25 μm APV; *c*, the effect of recruiting horizontal inputs by increasing stimulus strength on a single cell. Larger EPSPs are seen in depolarized cells than at rest, and the voltage dependency is blocked by QX-314 (a voltage-dependent Na$^+$-channel blocker) but not by APV (an NMDA-receptor blocker), indicating that the enhancement of the EPSP by depolarization is mediated by intrinsic membrane conductances. The EPSP is partly overlapped by an inhibitory postsynaptic potential (IPSP), and thus has a different shape than those shown in *a*. Part *c* shows that the balance between excitation and inhibition is affected by the stimulus strength. Resting potentials of the cell in *a* (upper), −72 mV; *a* (lower), −74 mV; *b*, −73 mV; *c*, −83 mV. Each trace is the average of three responses to a 100-μsec shock, marked by the arrows. (Adapted from J.A. Hirsch and C.D. Gilbert, in prep.)

Short-term Functional Consequences: Contextual Influences

Although the relationship between the clustering pattern of the horizontal connections and the columnar functional architecture accounts for how these connections are consistent with, and would not disrupt, the cortical columns, we are still left with the problem of the discrepancy between receptive field size and the visuotopic area over which cells receive input. This may be explained by the idea that the definition of receptive field is stimulus dependent. To observe the functional consequences of activating the horizontal connections, one needs to use the appropriate stimulus. From the extent of the horizontal connections in retinotopic terms, it is likely that stimuli placed outside the receptive field, although not capable of activating the cell, may modulate the response of the cell to stimuli placed within the receptive field. The way in which visual attributes in one retinal location are modified by the context in which a feature is presented has long been known from psychophysical studies. A number of studies show that perception of position, depth, and orientation can be altered by the presence of neighboring points or contours (Westheimer et al. 1976; Westheimer and McKee 1977; Butler and Westheimer 1978; Westheimer 1986). Perhaps most relevant to our current consideration is the tilt illusion, where our percept of line orientation is influenced by the presence of nearby lines of differing orientation (Gibson and Radner 1937; Westheimer 1990; for review, see Howard 1986). The fact that the horizontal connections show specificity for orientation, and that they relate disparate visual field positions, raises the possibility that the neuronal substrate for the tilt illusion may be found at as early a stage as the striate cortex.

In a study designed to test this hypothesis, we determined the effect of placing a set of oriented lines outside the receptive field on the excitability and orientation tuning of the cell to a line placed within the receptive field (Gilbert and Wiesel 1990). We refer to the line inside the receptive field as the "center" bar and those outside the receptive field as the "surround" bars. As has been reported in earlier studies, these lines tended to inhibit the response of the cell, although on occasions we have also observed facilitation. It has long been known that, surrounding the excitatory part of the receptive field, there are inhibitory surrounds, either along the orientation axis (producing end-inhibition, Hubel and Wiesel 1965), or along the movement axis (side-band inhibition, Bishop et al. 1973). Although previous studies differ in the relationship between the orientation of the center and that of the inhibitory surrounds (Hubel and Wiesel 1965; Bishop et al. 1973; Maffei and Fiorentini 1976; Fries et al. 1977; Nelson and Frost 1978,1985; Orban et al. 1979; Albus and Fries 1980; Ferster 1981; Morrone et al. 1982), we find that this relationship varies from cell to cell, ranging from iso-orientation inhibition to cross-orientation inhibition. It should be noted, however, that what may appear to be cross-orientation inhibition may instead be an iso-orientation facilitation or disinhibition sitting on top of an inhibition that is not orientation tuned (perhaps originating at earlier stages in the visual pathway).

A rather intriguing phenomenon occurred when we measured orientation tuning to the center bar in the presence of surround bars of various orientations, and is shown in Figure 4. The cell shown in the figure had an optimal orientation of 10°, and its tuning curve is indicated by the bold outline. For many surround orientations, the tuning curve was either suppressed or facilitated to varying degrees, as expected from the orientation tuning of the surround, and is shown in the thinner outlines. When the surround was oriented 30° clockwise from the optimal orientation of the center (to 0°), the peak in the orientation tuning curve shifted 10° from its original position, in a direction away from the orientation of the surround. Moreover, the tuning curve increased in bandwidth. The shift was reversible, returning to the original peak value in the presence of other surrounds or with no surround, and shifting again in the presence of a 0° surround. This was repeated several times.

Another example of a cell showing shifts in orientation tuning is shown in Figure 5. Here, the optimal orientation shifted 15° from the original peak, away from the orientation of the surround. In distinction to the cell in the previous example, this cell showed hysteresis in the orientation shift. After the surround was removed, the cell did not return to its original orientation but had a greatly increased bandwidth. The orientation specificity showed no sign of changing from this tuning for half an hour, and finally was returned to its original state by stimulating the surround with lines of varying orientation.

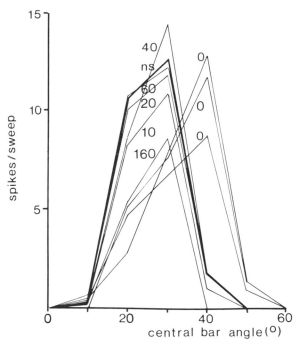

Figure 4. Altering a cell's orientation preference by lines surrounding its receptive field. The surround lines consisted of two groups of 4 in a diamond-shaped configuration, lying adjacent to the receptive field perpendicular to the orientation axis. Each tuning curve is made by changing the orientation of a bar lying within the receptive field center in the presence of surround bars of a fixed orientation. Without surround lines, the cell's tuning curve peaked at 30° (bold line). Surround lines of various orientations inhibited or facilitated the cell's response, and surround lines at 0° orientation shifted the peak response of the cell to 40°. (Reprinted, with permission, from Gilbert and Wiesel 1990.)

Most of the cells in our sample ($n = 36$) showed some change in response to stimulating the surround, either inhibition or facilitation, shifting orientation preference away from or toward the surround, and change in the bandwidth of orientation tuning. We attempted to relate the changes in orientation tuning at the single-cell level to the perceived changes in orientation seen psychophysically by using a model based on an ensemble of oriented cells, each representing a "filter" with a given peak orientation and tuning bandwidth (Fig. 6). The model assumes that estimation of orientation is influenced by the relative activity of all the filters that are activated by the stimulus. The activity of each filter is represented as a vector pointing in the direction of the optimal orientation for the filter and whose length is proportional to the strength of firing. The estimate of orientation is the vector sum. If all the filters in the ensemble have tuning curves of the same bandwidth and height, and if they are spaced at constant shifts in orientation, the estimate of orientation is an accurate reflection of the stimulus orientation. If, however, members of the ensemble are perturbed by changes in the height, optimal orientation, or bandwidth, there will be a disparity between the stimulus orientation and estimate of orientation. In the model, the changes in properties of individual filters that are consistent with

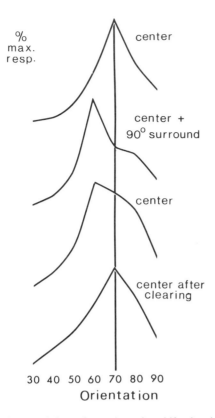

Figure 5. Surround-dependent orientation shifts showing hysteresis. The cell's response initially peaked at 70°. Surround lines of 90° orientation shifted the peak to the left. Removing the surround lines did not return the cell to its original state, but instead, the tuning curve broadened. After stimulating the cell's surround with lines of varying orientation, the tuning curve returned to its original position and width. (Reprinted, with permission, from Gilbert and Wiesel 1990.)

the psychophysical orientation tilt are iso-orientation inhibition (Fig. 7b), attractive shifts in preferred orientation of some of the filters toward the orientation of the surround (Fig. 7c), and increase in orientation tuning bandwidth of filters that peak at orientations away from that of the surround (Fig. 7d, sharpening of the orientation tuning for filters with the same orientation as the surround has a similar effect).

We have observed all of these effects and cannot say at present which of them are the most common or most likely to be related to the perceptual changes. In fact, some of the effects observed, such as "repulsive" shifts in optimal orientation, away from the orientation of the surround, would work in a direction opposite to that expected for the perceptual changes. The relationship between the observed changes and the fact that the long-range horizontal clustered connections run between columns of similar orientation specificity remains unknown. It raises the possibility that the horizontal connections may play a role in gating other inputs to the cell. For example, if the cell receives input from other cells having a range in orientation specificities, the ones that are expressed may be dependent on the state of activation of the horizontal connections. Whatever the precise mechanisms involved, our results suggest that the filter characteristics of cortical cells are not fixed, but are dependent on context, and that the response of a cell to a complex visual environment cannot be predicted from its response to simple visual stimuli. The result is that rather than having cells with fixed filter characteristics, responsive to a restricted part of the visual field, we have a population of cells having dynamic response properties, sensitive to the context in which local features are presented.

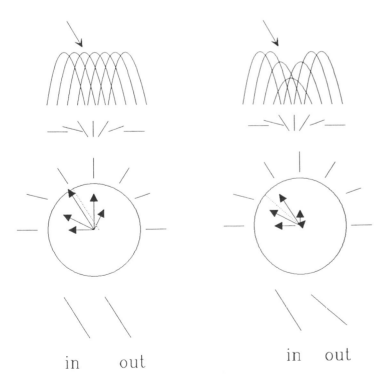

Figure 6. Model for estimation of line orientation based on an ensemble of orientation-selective cells (or orientation "filters"). Each cell responds over a range of orientations but peaks at a particular orientation. The tuning used for the implementation of the model in Fig. 7 is a Gaussian. When the cells are activated by a line of a given orientation (the line sitting on top of the tuning curves), the cells are activated to different levels of excitation, depending on the peak position and breadth of their tuning curves. Each cell constitutes a labeled line, and its firing is represented as a vector pointing in the direction of the orientation of the line and with a length proportional to its firing rate (middle). The estimation of orientation is then taken as the vector sum (dotted line). When the filters are spaced at constant intervals, and have the same height and width (left), the estimation of orientation is equivalent to the stimulus orientation (bottom left). When some of the filters are perturbed (in the example shown on the right, a few are inhibited), the vectors change in length (middle right), and consequently the estimation of orientation is shifted away from the stimulus orientation (bottom right). (Reprinted, with permission, from Gilbert and Wiesel 1990.)

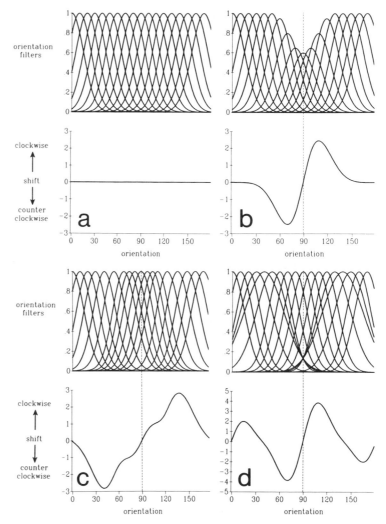

Figure 7. The use of the model shown in Fig. 6 to relate changes in orientation tuning of cells within the ensemble of oriented cells, caused by surround stimulation, to orientation tilt illusions. The top curves represent the 18 filters tuned to different orientations. In the model one can change their height, position, and bandwidth. The bottom curves represent the resultant shifts in perceived orientation for lines of different orientation, with the upward direction representing clockwise shifts, and the downward direction representing counterclockwise shifts. The vertical dotted lines represent the orientation of the surround. (*a*) Filters of uniform height and width and distributed at constant intervals of 10°. At all orientations the estimated orientation is the same as the stimulus orientation. The following perturbations in the ensemble can produce the "repulsive" orientation shift, or tilt illusion, observed psychophysically: (*b*) Inhibition of filters at the same orientation as the surround; (*c*) attractive shift in peak orientations toward the surround orientation; (*d*) broadening of filters at orientations different from that of the surround. (Sharpening of filters at orientations close to that of the surround produces a similar effect.) (Adapted from Gilbert and Wiesel 1990.)

Long-term Modifications in the Horizontal Inputs

Beyond the acute changes in the tuning properties of cells that are mediated by changes in context, we have observed sustained changes in cortical maps produced by permanently modifying the cortical input. These effects may be related to long-term potentiation observed in cortical slices.

The tissue slice results described above demonstrate the state dependency of the horizontal input in the short term. We have also found that under the appropriate circumstances, one can produce a sustained change in the synaptic effectiveness of horizontal input activation, in analogy to that seen in the hippocampus following tetanization of the perforant pathway (Bliss and Lomo 1973). In the experiment shown in Figure 8, both the interlaminar and horizontal inputs are left intact, and one can see the effect of conditioning either input. The protocol for conditioning was to repetitively pair synaptic activation with a pulse of current sufficient to make the cell fire several action potentials (Bindman et al. 1988). For this cell, conditioning of the horizontal input produces a 30% enhancement of the peak post-

synaptic response from the horizontal input and no change in the synaptic response from the interlaminar input. Pairing with interlaminar stimulation produced no increase in the homotypic synaptic response (if anything a slight reduction), and there was no effect on the heterotypic, horizontal input. For other cells, we were able to facilitate the interlaminar response by this protocol. For some cells, both the interlaminar and horizontal input could be enhanced by conditioning the homotypic input.

The experiment we chose to explore long-term changes in visual functional properties was modeled on work in the somatosensory system. There, removal of a finger leads to a shift in that finger's cortical representation to adjacent fingers (Merzenich et al. 1984, 1988). There are several stages in the somatosensory pathway where the remapping may take place, including spinal cord, thalamus, and cortex. Even in the spinal cord, there are widespread connections formed by sensory fibers, and spinal cord sensory maps have been shown to change following peripheral nerve injury (Wall and Werman 1976; Devor and Wall 1978). In our preliminary experiments, we first wished to ascertain the exis-

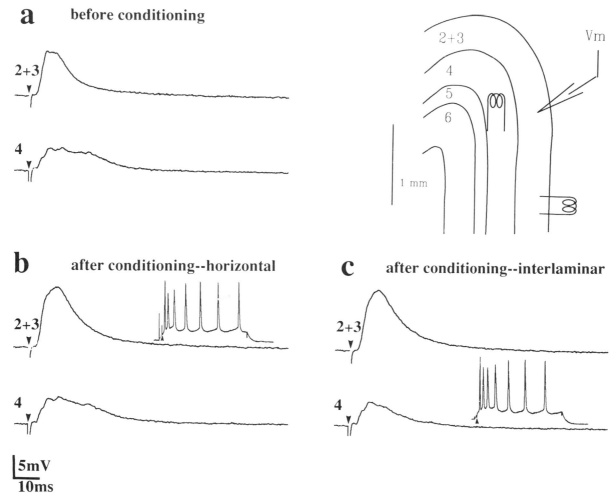

a   **before conditioning**

2+3

4

2+3

4

5

6

1 mm

Vm

b   **after conditioning--horizontal**

2+3

4

c   **after conditioning--interlaminar**

2+3

4

5mV
10ms

Figure 8. Long-term changes in synaptic potentials produced by stimulating horizontal and interlaminar inputs to a superficial layer pyramidal cell. The conditioning stimulus is a pairing of synaptic activation with a pulse of current sufficient to make the cell fire several action potentials. (*a*) Synaptic potentials seen after stimulating horizontal (2 + 3) and interlaminar (4) connections before conditioning; (*b*) postsynaptic responses seen after conditioning the horizontal connections—a 30% increase in the peak of the horizontally evoked PSP is seen, and the interlaminar PSP is unchanged; (*c*) postsynaptic responses seen in the same cell after conditioning the interlaminar connections—the horizontal PSP remains at its enhanced level, and the interlaminar PSP is, if anything, reduced in size. The resting potential of the cell is −77 mV and each trace is the average of 5 trials. The insets show samples of the pairs used for conditioning (Hirsch and Gilbert 1990).

tence and character of topographical reorganization in the visual cortex following retinal lesions. Similar experiments have been done in the cat, either by monocular lesions involving destruction of retinal ganglion cells (Eysel et al. 1981), or monocular lesion with contralateral eye removal (Kass et al. 1990).

The permanent alteration in sensory input was produced by focal laser lesions in the retinae of the two eyes at homologous retinal positions. The lesions, approximately 3–5° in diameter, were made parafoveally, such that their cortical representation would lie on the opercular surface. As expected, immediately after producing the lesion, a large area of the opercular surface could not be visually activated. Over time, however, visual responses returned to a degree, but with some interesting changes, as shown in Figures 9 and 10. The progression in the return of activity is shown in Figure 9a. At the beginning of recording, there was a large

area of cortex unresponsive to visual input. The penetrations done on day 1 are shown in the figure as square symbols, with the filled symbols over visually responsive cortex and the open symbols over cortex where we could not elicit visual responses. The dotted line demarcates the approximate border between the responsive and unresponsive regions. When next recorded at 3 weeks post-lesion, visual responses were found at numerous sites over previously unresponsive cortex (filled triangles). When last tested, at 8 weeks, we found a shift in the boundary between responsive and unresponsive cortex of approximately 3 mm.

The receptive field sizes and locations of the recording sites are shown in Figure 9b. In the figure we mapped the edges of the lesion by back projection with a fundus camera, and the lesion is represented as a dotted line. Initially, we saw a steady shift in receptive field position as we moved across the cortical surface,

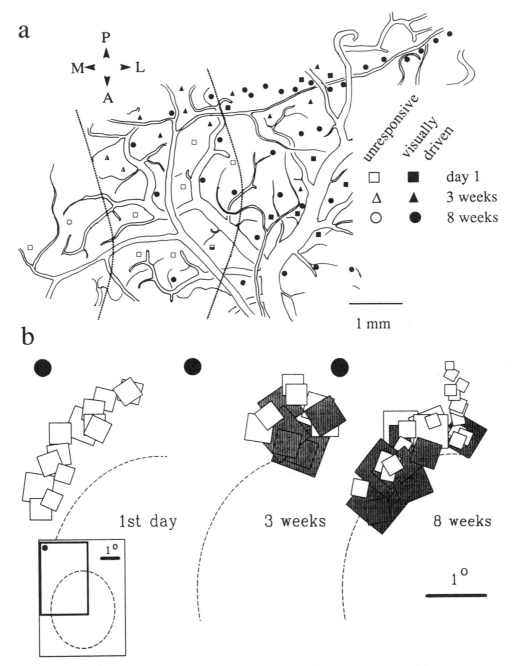

Figure 9. Striate cortical reorganization following focal binocular laser-induced retinal lesions. (*a*) Surface map of the cortical vasculature, with symbols marking the sites of electrode penetrations made on the day of the lesion (squares); after the lesion was made, at 3 weeks postlesion (triangles); and 8 weeks postlesion (circles). Filled symbols represent visually driven activity observed at a penetration at the site indicated, open symbols indicate lack of visual responses. The dotted line to the right indicates the boundary between active and unresponsive cortex immediately following the lesion; the dotted line on the left indicates an approximate 3-mm shift in the active/inactive boundary observed 8 weeks postlesion. (*b*) Receptive fields of cells at the recording sites shown in *a*. The visuotopic boundary of the lesion is indicated by a dotted line and the center of the fovea by a black spot (the inset at lower left indicates the extent of the lesion and the relative position of the fovea). The receptive fields in the part of cortex that initially retained visually driven activity immediately following the lesion are indicated by the open boxes. The fields of cells in cortex that recovered visually driven activity at 3 and 8 weeks postlesion are indicated by the shaded squares.

until we came across the boundary of the cortical "scotoma." At 3 weeks, and to a greater degree at 8 weeks, we found the fields to slow in their visual field progression as the electrode entered the original region of scotoma. Cells as far as 3 mm from the edge of the scotoma (receptive fields found within the original scotoma are cross-hatched) had receptive fields overlapping with those of cells on the originally responsive side of the scotoma. They were orientation specific, but were larger in diameter. There is also a suggestion of shifts in receptive field position in the part of cortex that was originally responsive (Fig. 9b, open boxes),

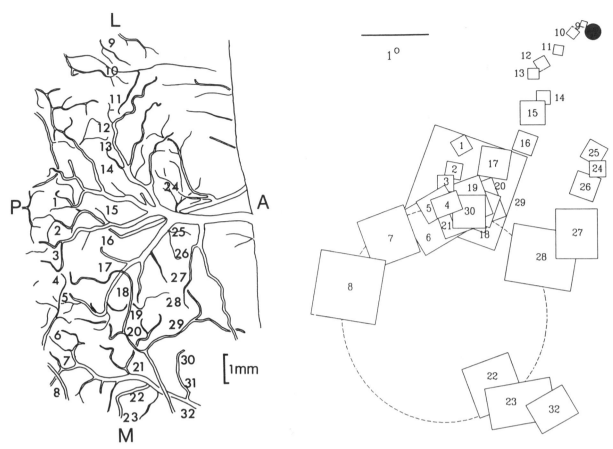

Figure 10. Progression in receptive field position with regular shifts in cortical recording sites in striate cortex, 8 weeks following binocular retinal lesion. (*Left*) Surface map of the cortical vasculature, with the sites of the electrode penetrations indicated by numbers. The boundary of the lesion is indicated by a dotted line. The receptive fields tend to slow in their progression as they approach the visuotopic representation of the lesion boundary (cf. 9–21), and then hop over to the other side of the lesion (cf. 22–23). In other sequences the fields tend to bend around the side of the lesion (cf. 1–8). At this stage, nearly all cortex received visual input, with no silent gaps.

although this finding requires further experiments for confirmation.

Another example of a cortex 8 weeks after retinal laser lesion is shown in Figure 10. The electrode penetrations were made at regular intervals, spaced approximately 400 μm across. The succession of receptive field positions at the recording sites is shown in the right half of the figure, with the lesion represented as a dashed ellipse and the center of the fovea represented as a black spot. As one moves in cortical position from lateral to medial in penetrations 9–23, one moves in field position from the fovea toward the lesion. There is a regular shift in receptive field position, with the distance between fields increasing as one gets farther from the fovea. When the fields approach the area of lesion, however, the progression in field position slows and ultimately stops. The fields, still oriented, increase greatly in receptive field diameter. At one point in the succession of penetrations, the field positions jump across the lesion and resume on the opposite site. An adjacent series of penetrations (1–8), farther from the representation of the vertical meridian (the V1/V2 border), shows the field positions to bend around the

contralateral edge of the lesion. In the third sequence of penetrations (24–32), there is a similar sequence of slowing and jumping in field position as with the first. On occasion, we have found cells with bipartite receptive fields, with one subfield on either side of the lesion.

From these results, one can conclude that the laser lesion has produced in the cortex an expanded representation of the part of the retina surrounding the lesion. Possible perceptual consequences of such reorganization are suggested in the observations of Craik (1966), who made a self-induced retinal lesion by staring at the sun through one eye. This produced, after a period of 6 months, distortions in the thickness of lines passing through the lesion. Interestingly, lines viewed through the lesioned eye were thicker over the course of the line passing through the lesion, and when viewed through the normal eye, lines passing through the homologous location appeared thinner. Although the reasons for the interocular effects are not known, one can imagine that the distortions may be a result of changes in cortical magnification factor that would be a consequence of the reorganization we observed following binocular retinal lesions. We would like to suggest that the retinal input to the deafferented areas of cortex arises from the long-range horizontal connections. The horizontal input to the cortical scotoma, originally modulatory in nature, has become potentiated to the degree that it can now drive the postsynaptic cells. The fact that all the fields we mapped in the experiments shown in Figures 9 and 10 were oriented (even though we made many penetrations through layer 4, which has cells with nonoriented receptive fields) suggests that the reorganization occurs outside the layer receiving geniculate input, and therefore that input to the scotoma arises from horizontal connections within the cortex, rather than by reorganization at earlier stages or by convergence of afferent input to the cortex. In further support of this idea is the finding from the tissue slice studies that the strength of horizontal inputs can be increased by conditioning.

SUMMARY

The findings presented in these studies have brought out different ideas concerning the mechanisms of processing in primary visual cortex than were held at the outset. Rather than thinking of receptive fields as being restricted in their extent, with the process of integration of the components of an image occurring at a much later stage along the visual pathway, we have shown that the integrative process is a progressive one, beginning in the primary visual cortex (or perhaps even earlier) and building up in a cascading series of converging and diverging connections. Rather than thinking of the filter characteristics of a cell as being fixed, it is apparent that they are dynamic and can be modified by the context in which features are presented. Finally, rather than a cortex with a functional architecture that is fixed after a critical period ending in infancy, we find that perturbing the system can lead to long-term topographical reorganization.

Other examples of contextual interactions have been demonstrated in the submodalities of motion, where a cell's directional selectivity is modulated by the presence of movement in the surround (Allman et al. 1985; Tanaka et al. 1986; Gulyas et al. 1987; Orban et al. 1987). In the domain of color, the phenomenon of color constancy, reported for cells in visual area V4 (Zeki 1983), also requires lateral interactions in visual space, comparing the wavelength distribution of light coming from surfaces in different parts of the visual field. The influences presented in these studies, as in our own work in the domain of orientation, are modulatory. The long-term changes in cortical topography following removal of somatosensory input (Merzenich et al. 1984, 1988) or by retinal lesions suggest that with the appropriate manipulations the lateral interactions can be enhanced to the point of activating the postsynaptic cells. Although retinal lesions clearly represent an abnormal disruption of sensory input, they may nevertheless be representative of long-term reorganizations of neural networks occurring under normal circumstances, such as those required for memory.

ACKNOWLEDGMENTS

We thank Peter Pierce for photography, Kaare Christian for computer programming, and Melodie Winauer for histology. The work was supported by National Institutes of Health grants EY-07968, EY-05253, and NS-22789; National Science Foundation grant BNS-8918951; and an award from the Rita Allen Foundation.

REFERENCES

Albus, K. and W. Fries. 1980. Inhibitory sidebands of complex receptive fields in the cat's striate cortex. *Vision Res.* **20:** 369.

Allman, J.M., F. Miezin, and E. McGuinnes. 1985. Direction and velocity specific surround in three cortical visual areas of the owl monkey. *Perception* **14:** 105.

Badcock, D.R. and G. Westheimer. 1985. Spatial location and hyperacuity: The centre-surround localization function has two substrates. *Vision Res.* **25:** 1259.

Bindman, L.J., K.P.S.J. Murphy, and S. Pockett. 1988. Postsynaptic control of the induction of long-term changes in the efficacy of transmission at neocortical synapses in slices of the rat brain. *J. Neurophysiol.* **60:** 1053.

Bishop, P.O., J.S. Coombs, and G.H. Henry. 1973. Receptive fields of simple cells in the cat striate cortex. *J. Physiol.* **231:** 31.

Bliss, T.V.P. and T. Lomo. 1973. Long-lasting potentiation of synaptic transmission in the dentate area of the anesthetized rabbit following stimulation of the perforant path. *J. Physiol.* **232:** 332.

Bullier, J., H. Kennedy, and W. Salinger. 1984. Branching and laminar origin of projections between visual cortical areas in the cat. *J. Comp. Neurol.* **228:** 329.

Butler, T. and G. Westheimer. 1978. Interference with stereoscopic acuity: Spatial, temporal, disparity tuning. *Vision Res.* **18:** 387.

Connors, B.W. and D.A. Prince. 1982. Effects of local anaesthetic QX-314 on the membrane properties of hippocampal pyramidal neurons. *J. Pharmacol. Exp. Ther.* **220:** 476.

Craik, K.J.W. 1966. Localized aniseikonia following eclipse blindness. In *The nature of psychology* (ed. S.L. Sherwood), p. 102. Cambridge University Press, United Kingdom.

Devor, M. and P.D. Wall. 1978. Reorganisation of spinal cord sensory map after peripheral nerve injury. *Nature* **276:** 75.

Eysel, U.T., F. Gonzalez-Aguilar, and U. Mayer. 1981. Time-dependent decrease in the extent of visual deafferentation in the lateral geniculate nucleus of adult cats with small retinal lesions. *Exp. Brain Res.* **41:** 256.

Ferrer, J.M.R., D.J. Price, and C. Blakemore. 1988. The organization of corticocortical projections from area 17 to area 18 of the cat's visual cortex. *Proc. R. Soc. Lond. B* **233:** 77.

Ferster, D. 1981. A comparison of binocular depth mechanisms in areas 17 and 18 of the cat visual cortex. *J. Physiol.* **311:** 623.

Fries, W., K. Albus, and O.D. Creutzfeldt. 1977. Effects of interacting visual patterns on single cell responses in cat's striate cortex. *Vision Res.* **17:** 1001.

Fisken, R.A., L.J. Garey, and T.P.S. Powell. 1975. The intrinsic, association and commissural connections of area 17 of the visual cortex. *Philos. Trans. R. Soc. Lond. Ser. B* **272:** 487.

Gabbott, P.L.A., K.A.C. Martin, and D. Whitteridge. 1987. Connections between pyramidal neurons in layer 5 of cat visual cortex (area 17). *J. Comp. Neurol.* **259:** 364.

Gibson, J.J. and M. Radner. 1937. Adaptation, after-effect and contrast in the perception of tilted lines. *J. Exp. Psychol.* **20:** 453.

Gilbert, C.D. and J.P. Kelly. 1975. The projections of cells in different layers of the cat's visual cortex. *J. Comp. Neurol.* **163:** 81.

Gilbert, C.D. and T.N. Wiesel. 1979. Morphology and intracortical projections of functionally identified neurons in cat visual cortex. *Nature* **280:** 120.

——. 1983. Clustered intrinsic connections in cat visual cortex. *J. Neurosci.* **3:** 1116.

——. 1989. Columnar specificity of intrinsic connections in cat visual cortex. *J. Neurosci.* **9:** 2432.

——. 1990. The influence of contextual stimuli on the orientation selectivity of cells in primary visual cortex of the cat. *Vision Res.* (in press).

Goldman, P.S. and W.J.H. Nauta. 1977. Columnar distribution of cortico-cortical fibers in the frontal association, limbic and motor cortex of the developing rhesus monkey. *Brain Res.* **122:** 393.

Goldman-Rakic, P.S. and M.L. Schwartz. 1982. Interdigitation of contralateral and ipsilateral columnar projections to frontal association cortex in primates. *Science* **216:** 755.

Gulyas, B., G.A. Orban, J. Duysens, and N. Maes. 1987. The suppressive influence of moving texture background on responses of cat striate neurons to moving bars. *J. Physiol.* **57:** 1767.

Hirsch, J.A. and C.D. Gilbert. 1990. Interactions and stimulus-dependent changes of synaptic potentials evoked by activating interlaminar and horizontal pathways in the cat's striate cortex. *Soc. Neurosci. Abstr.* **16:** (in press).

Howard, I.P. 1986. The perception of posture, self-motion and the visual vertical. In *Handbook of perception and human performance* (ed. K.R. Boff), vol. 1, p. 18-1. John Wiley, New York.

Hubel, D.H. and T.N. Wiesel. 1959. Receptive fields of single neurones in the cat's striate cortex. *J. Physiol.* **148:** 574.

——. 1962. Receptive fields, binocular interaction and functional architecture in the cat's visual cortex. *J. Physiol.* **160:** 106.

——. 1963. Shape and arrangement of columns in cat's striate cortex. *J. Physiol.* **165:** 559.

——. 1965. Receptive fields and functional architecture in two nonstriate visual areas (18 and 19) of the cat. *J. Neurophysiol.* **38:** 229.

——. 1968. Receptive fields and functional architecture in monkey striate cortex. *J. Physiol.* **195:** 215.

——. 1974. Uniformity of monkey striate cortex: A parallel relationship between field size, scatter and magnification factor. *J. Comp. Neurol.* **158:** 295.

——. 1977. Functional architecture of macaque monkey visual cortex. *Proc. R. Soc. Lond. B.* **198:** 1.

Imig, T.J. and J.F. Brugge. 1978. Sources and terminations of callosal axons related to binaural and frequency maps in primary auditory cortex of the cat. *J. Comp. Neurol.* **182:** 637.

Imig, T.J. and R.A. Reale. 1981. Ipsilateral corticocortical projections related to binaural columns in cat primary auditory cortex. *J. Comp. Neurol.* **203:** 1.

Jones, E.G., J.D. Coulter, and S.H.C. Hendry. 1978. Intracortical connectivity of architectonic fields in the somatic sensory, motor and parietal cortex of monkeys. *J. Comp. Neurol.* **181:** 291.

Kaas, J.H., L.A. Krubitzer, Y.M. Chino, A.L. Langston, E.H. Polley, and N. Blair. 1990. Reorganization of retinotopic cortical maps in adult mammals after lesions of the retina. *Science* **248:** 229.

Kisvarday, Z.F., K.A.C. Martin, T.F. Freund, Z. Magloczky, D. Whitteridge, and P. Somogyi. 1986. Synaptic targets of HRP-filled layer III pyramidal cells in the cat striate cortex. *Exp. Brain Res.* **64:** 541.

Landry, P., A. Labelle, and M. Deschenes. 1980. Intracortical distribution of axonal collaterals of pyramidal tract cells in the cat motor cortex. *Brain Res.* **191:** 327.

Maffei, L. and A. Fiorentini. 1976. The unresponsive regions of visual cortical receptive fields. *Vision Res.* **16:** 1131.

Martin, K.A.C. and D. Whitteridge. 1984. Form, function and intracortical projections of spiny neurones in the striate visual cortex of the cat. *J. Physiol.* **353:** 463.

McGuire, B.A., C.D. Gilbert, P.K. Rivlin, and T.N. Wiesel. 1991. Targets of horizontal connections in macaque primary visual cortex. *J. Comp. Neurol.* (in press).

Michalski, A., G.L. Gerstein, J. Czarkowska, and R. Tarnecki. 1983. Interactions between cat striate cortex neurons. *Exp. Brain Res.* **51:** 97.

Merzenich, M.M., G. Recanzone, W.M. Jenkins, T.T. Allard, and R.J. Nudo. 1988. Cortical representational plasticity. In *Neurobiology of neocortex* (ed. P. Rakic and W. Singer), p. 41. Wiley, Chichester, England.

Merzenich, M.M., R.J. Nelson, M.P. Stryker, M.S. Cynader, A. Schoppmann, and J.M. Zook. 1984. Somatosensory cortical map changes following digital amputation in adult monkeys. *J. Comp. Neurol.* **224:** 591.

Montero, V.M. 1980. Patterns of connections from the striate cortex to cortical visual areas in superior temporal sulcus of macaque and middle temporal gyrus of owl monkey. *J. Comp. Neurol.* **189:** 45.

Morrone, M.C., D.C. Burr, and L. Maffei. 1982. Functional implications of cross-orientation inhibition of cortical visual cells. I. Neurophysiological evidence. *Proc. R. Soc. Lond. B* **216:** 335.

Nelson, J.I. and B. Frost. 1978. Orientation selective inhibition from beyond the classic visual receptive field. *Brain Res.* **139:** 359.

——. 1985. Intracortical facilitation among co-oriented, co-axially aligned simple cells in cat striate cortex. *Exp. Brain Res.* **61:** 54.

Orban, G.A., B. Gulyas, and R. Vogels. 1987. Influence of a moving textured background on direction selectivity of cat striate neurons. *J. Neurophysiol.* **57:** 1792.

Orban, G.A., H. Kato, and P.O. Bishop. 1979. Dimensions are properties of end-zone inhibitory areas in receptive fields of hypercomplex cells in cat striate cortex. *J. Neurophysiol.* **42:** 833.

Perkel, D.H., G.L. Gerstein, and G.P. Moore. 1967a. Neuronal spike trains and stochastic point processes. I. The single spike train. *Biophys. J.* **7:** 391.

——. 1967b. Neuronal spike trains and stochastic point processes. II. Simultaneous spike trains. *Biophys. J.* **7:** 419.

Rockland, K.S. and J.S. Lund. 1982. Widespread periodic intrinsic connections in the tree shrew visual cortex. *Brain Res.* **169:** 19.

——. 1983. Intrinsic laminar lattice connections in primate visual cortex. *J. Comp. Neurol.* **216:** 303.

Staftstrom, C.E., P.C. Schwindt, M.C. Chubb, and W.E. Crill. 1985. Properties of persistent sodium conductance and calcium conductance of layer V neurons from cat sensorimotor cortex. *J. Neurophysiol.* **53:** 153.

Tanaka, K., K. Hikosaka, H. Saito, M. Yukie, Y. Fukada, and E. Iwai. 1986. Analysis of local and wide-field movements in the superior temporal visual areas of the macaque monkey. *J. Neurosci.* **6:** 134.

Tigges, J., M. Tigges, S. Anschel, H.A. Cross, W.D. Letbetter, and R.L. McBride. 1981. Areal and laminar distribution of neurons interconnecting the central visual cortical areas 17, 18, 19 and MT in Squirrel monkey (Saimiri). *J. Comp. Neurol.* **202:** 539.

Toyama, K., M. Kimura, and K. Tanaka. 1981a. Cross-correlation analysis of interneuronal connectivity in cat visual cortex. *J. Neurophysiol.* **46:** 191.

——. 1981b. Organization of cat visual cortex as investigated by cross-correlation techniques. *J. Neurophysiol.* **46:** 202.

Ts'o, D. and C. Gilbert. 1988. The organization of chromatic and spatial interactions in the primate striate cortex. *J. Neurosci.* **8:** 1712.

Ts'o, D., C. Gilbert, and T.N. Wiesel. 1986. Relationships between horizontal connections and functional architecture in cat striate cortex as revealed by cross-correlation analysis. *J. Neurosci.* **6:** 1160.

Tusa, R.J., L.A. Palmer, and A.C. Rosenquist. 1978. The retinotopic organization of area 17 (striate cortex) in the cat. *J. Comp. Neurol.* **177:** 213.

Wall, P.D. and R. Werman. 1976. The physiology and anatomy of long ranging afferent fibres within the spinal cord. *J. Physiol.* **255:** 321.

Watkins, J.C. and R.H. Evans. 1981. Excitatory amino acid transmitters. *Annu. Rev. Pharmacol. Toxicol.* **21:** 165.

Westheimer, G. 1986. Spatial interaction in the domain of disparity signals in human stereoscopic vision. *J. Physiol.* **370:** 619.

———. 1990. Simultaneous orientation contrast for lines in the human fovea. *Vision Res.* (in press).

Westheimer, G. and S.P. McKee. 1977. Spatial configurations for visual hyperacuity. *Vision Res.* **17:** 941.

Westheimer, G., K. Shimamura, and S. McKee. 1976. Interference with line orientation sensitivity. *J. Opt. Soc. Am.* **66:** 332.

Wong-Riley, M. 1979. Columnar cortico-cortical interconnections within the visual system of the squirrel and macaque monkeys. *Brain Res.* **162:** 201.

Zeki, S.M. 1983. Colour coding in the cerebral cortex: The reaction of cells in monkey visual cortex to wavelengths and colours. *Neuroscience* **9:** 741.

Modular and Hierarchical Organization of Extrastriate Visual Cortex in the Macaque Monkey

D.C. Van Essen,* D.J. Felleman,† E.A. DeYoe,‡ J. Olavarria,*§ and J. Knierim*

*Biology Division, California Institute of Technology, Pasadena, California 91125;
†Department of Neurobiology and Anatomy, University of Texas, Houston, Texas 77030;
‡Department of Anatomy and Cellular Biology, Medical College of Wisconsin, Milwaukee, Wisconsin 53226;
§Department of Psychology, University of Washington, Seattle, Washington 98195

In the 1970s, a quiet revolution began in our understanding of how information processing occurs in regions beyond the primary visual cortex. Work from several laboratories indicated that there were more visual areas than just the three proposed by classic neuroanatomists. The number of extrastriate areas identified around that time was about a half dozen in various species (Zeki 1976; Allman 1977; Van Essen 1979; Tusa et al. 1981). It also became apparent during this period that the connectivity among visual areas was more complex than the simple serial processing sequence that many investigators expected to encounter.

In the ensuing decade, there has been an explosion of information about the organization and function of extrastriate visual cortex. Although several of the basic principles articulated in the previous decade remain largely correct, it is now apparent that the visual cortex is far more complex and intricate in its organization than had been appreciated. In this paper, we discuss recent evidence concerning three important principles: hierarchical organization, modularity within areas, and concurrent processing streams.

METHODS

Anatomical and physiological experiments were carried out on macaque monkeys (*Macaca fascicularis*), using procedures that are described in several previous reports (Maunsell and Van Essen 1983a,b; Van Essen et al. 1986; Felleman and Van Essen 1987; DeYoe et al. 1990). Surgical procedures were carried out under Nembutal or Pentothal anesthesia. Anatomical injections of the tracers bisbenzimide, nuclear yellow, diamidino yellow, horseradish peroxidase, and [³H]-proline were made through a modified Hamilton syringe. Electrophysiological recordings were made from animals anesthetized with nitrous oxide (75%) and paralyzed with a continuous intravenous infusion of Flaxedil. The adequacy of anesthesia was assessed by continuous monitoring of the EKG and routine testing for an absence of an EKG response to noxious stimuli. Visual stimuli were generated by an optical projection system, and receptive fields were plotted manually on a tangent screen. At the end of the experiment, the animal was given an overdose of Nembutal and perfused with formaldehyde and/or glutaraldehyde fixa-

tive in concentrations that were appropriate for the particular histological procedures to be used in a given experiment. In some experiments, large regions of cortex were unfolded and flattened according to the procedure of Olavarria and Van Sluyters (1985) and then sectioned tangential to the cortical surface. In other experiments, the brain was blocked and cut in the horizontal, sagittal, or oblique plane. In most experiments, one series of sections was mounted without coverslipping for scoring of fluorescence labeling, and intervening sections were processed for various histological procedures, including cytochrome oxidase (CO) histochemistry and Cat-301 immunocytochemistry.

Anatomical data were recorded and analyzed using a computerized neuroanatomy system. Histological sections were examined under a Leitz microscope having a motorized stage that was coupled to an IBM PC-XT by an electronic interface (Stahl Instruments). The locations and identifying characteristics of labeled neurons, section outlines, and various fiducial marks were entered using customized software. An immediate hard copy of the data was obtained with a pen plotter that printed the locations of cells onto an enlarged photograph of the original section. Data represented in this fashion were transferred manually to two-dimensional cortical maps (Van Essen and Zeki 1978; Van Essen and Maunsell 1980). The data contained in the PC-XT could also be transported to an IRIS graphics workstation for subsequent analysis of two-dimensional and three-dimensional relationships using customized software. This was particularly useful for data contained in sections of V2 that had been flattened and sectioned tangentially.

RESULTS

Modularity of Areas V2 and V4

We begin with a discussion of the modular organization of V2 and V4, with particular emphasis on the geometry, topology, and connectivity of different compartments. To place these results in perspective, it is useful to review a few key points about area V1 (striate cortex), whose modularity is intimately related to that found at higher levels.

The realization that an individual cortical area can be internally heterogeneous in its architecture and its connections, despite a uniform appearance in conventional cell and myelin stains, first came from studies of V1 in the macaque. Hubel and Wiesel (1972) found that the afferent inputs from the lateral geniculate nucleus (LGN) are arranged in an alternating set of "ocular dominance stripes" within layer 4. Each ocular dominance stripe is about 0.5 mm wide (1 mm/pair), but in any local region, there can be a two- to threefold fluctuation in stripe width, and the stripes in the far peripheral representation are only about half the width of those representing central fields (LeVay et al. 1985). Along the V1/V2 border, the total number of ocular dominance pairs has been estimated at 118 (LeVay et al. 1985).

Another critical finding was that the enzyme CO (Carroll and Wong-Riley 1984) is distributed nonuniformly in the tangential domain, revealing a pattern of CO-enriched "blobs" surrounded by pale-staining "interblobs" (Livingstone and Hubel 1984). The blobs are spaced about 0.4 mm apart on average, and they are situated along the middle of each ocular dominance stripe. The anatomical modularity suggested by these observations is correlated with a highly specific pattern of intrinsic and extrinsic connections for each compartment and with a distinctive constellation of receptive field characteristics. Both the blobs and the interblobs are dominated by inputs from the parvocellular (P cell) populations of retinal ganglion cells and LGN cells that are relayed through layer 4Cb, and they represent components of what we have elsewhere termed the P-B (parvo-blob) and P-I (parvo-interblob) streams, respectively (DeYoe and Van Essen 1988). Complementing these is a third processing stream, the M stream, which includes layers 4Ca and 4B of V1 and is dominated by inputs from the magnocellular (M cell) populations of retinal ganglion cells and LGN cells.

Striate cortex is a highly specialized region of neocortex, especially in primates, and a decade ago it was not at all obvious whether analogous types of modularity were likely to be encountered in extrastriate areas. Interestingly, CO histochemistry proved as useful for V2 as it had for V1, in that it revealed a relatively coarse and stripe-like arrangement of compartments, consisting of CO-rich thick stripes and thin stripes separated by CO-sparse interstripes (Tootell et al. 1983; Livingstone and Hubel 1984). Just as information about the numbers, dimensions, and geometric relationships of blobs and ocular dominance stripes is instructive in understanding the organization of V1, it is of interest to know the overall layout of stripes in V2. The analysis is more difficult, however, because V2 occupies a more convoluted region of cortex and also because the stripes are technically harder to visualize.

Geometry of V2 stripes. We visualized the pattern of stripes over large regions of V2 by using a physical unfolding technique (Olavarria and Van Sluyters 1985) to flatten the cortex prior to sectioning and histochemi-cal staining. In addition to carrying out CO histochemistry, we also examined immunoreactivity for the monoclonal antibody Cat-301, which preferentially labels the thick stripes in V2 (Hendry et al. 1988; DeYoe et al. 1990). Results for the CO pattern in one hemisphere are shown in Figure 1 for tangentially cut sections of dorsal V2 (top) and ventral V2 (bottom). Stripes are visible over nearly the full extent of V2, and there is a pronounced dorsoventral asymmetry in the stripe pattern that has not previously been reported.

In dorsal V2, the CO stripes run fairly directly from the border with V1 on the left to the border with V3 on the right. Most of the stripes extend nearly the full width of dorsal V2, which is fairly constant at about 10 mm in this hemisphere. Altogether, there are 29 CO-dense stripes in this region, which includes nearly the full extent of dorsal V2. The alternation between thick and thin CO stripes is apparent in most regions, but as others have noted (Shipp and Zeki 1989), alternate stripes are sometimes quite similar in width. By examining Cat-301 immunoreactivity in neighboring sections (not shown), we determined that every alternate stripe was rich in Cat-301-positive cells and that there were 14 "thick" stripes in all based on this criterion. Despite the fact that the intrinsic identity of the stripes is better correlated to immunoreactivity and connectivity (see below) than to physical dimensions, we will persist in using the terms "thick stripe" and "thin stripe" as convenient descriptive handles.

In ventral V2, the CO stripes emanate from the V1/V2 border approximately at right angles, just as in dorsal V2. However, they do not simply run directly across to the anterior border of V2 with area VP. Rather, the CO stripes that start in the foveal region bend around those from more peripheral regions, outflanking them and eventually running roughly parallel with the adjoining area VP before they terminate. Thus, in the midportion of ventral V2, some of the stripes are oriented approximately at right angles to others. The total width of ventral V2 in this hemisphere is 13–14 mm, which is somewhat wider than dorsal V2, but the disparity in stripe length is even greater. Several of the stripes are slightly more than 20 mm in length, whereas others are only 5–6 mm long. A total of 14 Cat-301 immunoreactive thick stripes were identified in ventral V2 of this hemisphere. The total number of CO-dense stripes was more difficult to determine, owing to uncertainties in the peripheral representation (bottom of figure). In the opposite hemisphere, the staining was clearer in the periphery, and there were 27 CO-dense stripes in all of ventral V2, 14 of which were Cat-301 immunoreactive thick stripes.

We examined the pattern of CO stripes in a total of five hemispheres for dorsal V2 and eight hemispheres for ventral V2 (Olavarria et al. 1989 and in prep.). In all instances, the stripes in dorsal V2 ran fairly directly from the border with V1 to the border with V3. In ventral V2, there was somewhat greater variability. Wrapping of the central (lateral) CO stripes around the more peripheral (medial) ones was pronounced in four

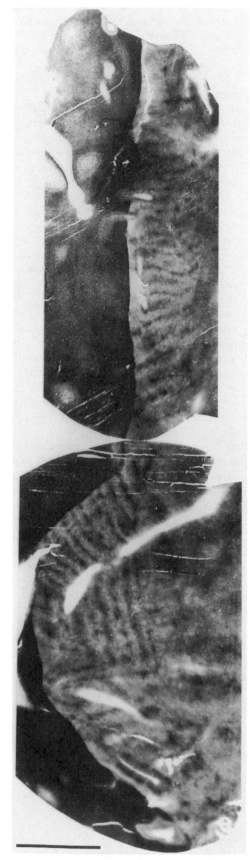

Figure 1. The overall pattern of cytochrome oxidase (CO) stripes in dorsal and ventral V2 (case 90A-L). The photograph is a montage from two sections taken from separate blocks containing all of dorsal and ventral V2, along with large portions of surrounding cortex. Area V1 is the darkly staining region situated posteriorly (to the left). The representation of the periphery is in the uppermost and lowermost regions of unfolded V2, representing inferior and superior visual quadrants, respectively. The foveal representation (in lateral V2) is in the middle of the montage, where the photographs of the two sections are adjoined; no actual tissue is missing in this region. Several pale streaks are visible in regions of folding where the cortex is relatively thin. This is most noticeable ventrally, along the fundus of the inferior occipital sulcus (diagonal streak near the middle). For optimal unfolding and subsequent histochemistry, the brain was perfused with 1% paraformaldehyde and 0.1% glutaraldehyde in 0.1 M phosphate buffer for a period of 7–8 min, followed by 10% sucrose in the same buffer. Bar, 1 cm.

681

hemispheres (counting that in Fig. 1) and present to a lower degree in three of the remaining four hemispheres. In the cases that had less stripe bending, the stripes in ventral V2 ran oblique to the V1/V2 border and were therefore still longer than those in dorsal V2.

Altogether, we estimate that V2 contains about 56 CO-dense stripes and 28 complete sets of stripes (one thick, one thin, and two interstripes), counting both dorsal and ventral V2 subdivisions. Fewer sets were seen in other hemispheres, but this was mainly because the staining in the region of the periphery was less satisfactory owing to the greater complexity of cortical folding. The total length of V2 was approximately 110 mm, indicating an average of 4 mm per set of stripes, which is in agreement with other reports (Shipp and Zeki 1989; Tootell and Hamilton 1989; DeYoe et al. 1990). Unlike the situation in V1, where the ocular dominance stripes and blob spacing decrease in the periphery (Livingstone and Hubel 1984; LeVay et al. 1985), we did not discern any systematic change in stripe periodicity in peripheral V2. A modest effect might have gone undetected, however, because of the greater difficulty in visualizing stripes in this region. There are some fluctuations in stripe periodicity from one region to another, just as is seen for ocular dominance stripes in V1.

The marked dorsoventral asymmetry in V2 stripe geometry adds to a growing list of differences between regions of cortex associated with lower versus upper visual fields (Burkhalter et al. 1986; Van Essen et al. 1986; Previc 1990). The functional significance, if any, of the asymmetry of stripes in V2 is unclear, but it conceivably is linked to the relationships among visual topography, areal boundaries, and the nature of the mapping from V1 to V2 (cf. Carman 1990a,b).

A basic feature of topographic organization in V2 is that lines of constant eccentricity (isoeccentricity contours) run approximately orthogonal to its two boundaries, i.e., from the vertical meridian representation along the V1/V2 boundary to the horizontal meridian representation along the boundary with V3 and VP (Gattass et al. 1981; Van Essen et al. 1986). Thus, in dorsal V2, the isoeccentricity contours run approximately parallel to the CO stripes illustrated in Figure 1 (top). In ventral V2, however, the CO stripes do not simply run parallel to isoeccentricity lines. Rather, any given stripe represents one particular eccentricity near the V1/V2 boundary and spirals out to represent a considerably higher eccentricity as it approaches the boundary with VP. For comparison, the ocular dominance stripes in V1 also have a systematic, but not entirely simple relationship with visual topography. In peripheral portions of the visual field, the ocular dominance stripes run approximately (but not perfectly) parallel to isoeccentricity contours, but in the representation of the central 5°–10°, the relationship is much less orderly (Hubel and Freeman 1977; LeVay et al. 1985). Thus, the main asymmetry in V1 is between central and peripheral representations, whereas that in V2 is between upper and lower field representations.

The geometry of V2 stripes is also of interest from a developmental standpoint. It has previously been suggested that the tendency of ocular dominance stripes to run in a consistent direction requires the presence of some form of external, anisotropic ordering influence that modulates the growth and retraction of geniculocortical arbors (von der Malsburg 1979; Swindale 1980; Fraser 1984). For example, the fact that CO stripes tend to run directly across the short axis of V2 in squirrel monkeys (Livingstone and Hubel 1984), owl monkeys (Tootell et al. 1985), and in the dorsal portion of V2 in the macaque (present results) suggests possible explanations based on an anisotropy in the steepness of the chemospecificity gradients involved in establishing an orderly topographic map (von der Malsburg 1979; Fraser 1984; LeVay et al. 1985). However, our finding that CO stripes are oblique to (and sometimes approximately parallel to) the border of ventral V2 with VP in the macaque clearly indicates that a different explanation is needed for the anisotropy in this region. Interestingly, in cats, there seems no need to invoke any anisotropy at all, in that there is little tendency for ocular dominance stripes to run in a systematic direction (Anderson et al. 1988), even though the overall shape of (unfolded) V1 is as elongated as it is in the macaque.

Connectivity of stripes. It is known from previous work in the macaque that thick stripes project heavily to MT and that both thin stripes and interstripes project to V4 (DeYoe and Van Essen 1985; Shipp and Zeki 1985). Obviously, it is of interest to know whether the projections from thin stripes and interstripes terminate in separate or in overlapping regions within V4.

Our findings (DeYoe et al. 1988) and those of Zeki and Shipp (1989) indicate a high degree of segregation, suggesting that V4 may have a form of modularity akin to that for V1 and V2. Zeki and Shipp inferred this from single tracer injections, which in some cases labeled predominantly interstripes and in other cases labeled predominantly thin stripes. Our approach has been to use multiple tracers in the same hemisphere. This has the advantage of providing a more direct and precise measure of the degree to which projections overlap, and it also gives useful information about the spacing between sites having differential inputs.

Figure 2A illustrates an experiment in which the fluorescent tracers nuclear yellow (NY) and bisbenzimide (BB) were placed at two sites approximately 5 mm apart in V4 on the prelunate gyrus. Receptive fields for the two injection sites were overlapping and at a representation of 3°–4° eccentricity. Both injections led to extensive retrograde labeling that formed a stripe-like pattern in a region of dorsal V2 that was appropriate for the receptive field locations in V4. Over this entire region, there was remarkably little spatial overlap of regions labeled with the two tracers.

The relationship of the fluorescent-labeled stripes to the CO pattern in the same hemisphere can be seen by comparison with the lower panel of Figure 2A, which shows the outline of stripes of high CO activity seen in appropriately reacted nearby sections. Clearly, there is a strong correlation between the two patterns. There are eight elongated regions of heavy blue (BB) labeling, and each of these is closely aligned with an interstripe. The yellow (NY) labeling also occurs mainly as elongated regions, and the five major ones are aligned with alternating CO-dense stripes. In this hemisphere, it was not possible to distinguish between thick and thin stripes simply on the basis of their width. However, we were able to determine stripe identity by examining the pattern of Cat-301 labeling, as described in the preceding section. Strongly Cat-301-positive cells are indicated by green dots in the lower panel of Figure 2A. It is evident that they are concentrated in the CO stripes that lack retrograde label. As noted above, these Cat-301-positive stripes correspond to the thick stripes known to project to MT, which in turn implies that it is the thin stripes which contain the NY-labeled cells projecting to V4.

The stripe pattern in this hemisphere conforms for the most part to the expected four-step sequence of thick-stripe/interstripe/thin-stripe/interstripe. However, there are a few interesting irregularities that merit specific mention. In the large NY-labeled thin stripe in the center of the upper panel, there is a narrow finger of BB-labeled cells cutting completely across the presumed thin stripe. We saw no corresponding gap in the CO pattern. Just to the right of this irregularity, and just below the downward (open) arrow, there is a notable absence of BB-labeled cells in the region where an interstripe would be expected. Interestingly, the CO pattern did seem to show a partial fusion between neighboring thin and thick stripes in this region. More ventrally (at the bottom of the upper panel), there is nearly complete continuity of retrograde labeling over three complete stripe cycles. This indicates that the thick stripes do not extend as far ventrally as the other stripes in this region, a conclusion that is supported by the Cat-301 and CO patterns. Finally, the CO stripe indicated by the upward (solid) arrow on the far right (laterally, near the foveal representation in V2) is heterogeneous and is separable into two patches that apparently have different identities. The upper portion is Cat-301-positive and lacks retrogradely labeled cells. Its lower portion has few Cat-301-positive cells and contains a small but dense clump of NY-labeled cells. The CO pattern in this region was more like two discrete patches rather than a single stripe, as though a thick and a thin stripe abutted one another without completely fusing. Altogether, we conclude that there are a variety of irregular but interesting features of compartmental organization in V2. These can most convincingly be analyzed by using a combination of labels to reveal connectivity, histochemistry, and molecular specificity in the same hemisphere.

The availability of double retrograde labeling in a single hemisphere also allowed us to address the issue of whether modules are completely discrete entities or whether they represent a waxing and waning of prop-

erties that vary continuously when measured parallel to the surface of V2. When one examines the density of CO reaction product (cf. Fig. 1), it often appears more like a smoothly varying sinusoid than a square wave with sharp borders. In this respect, our strategy of drawing lines to indicate the apparent borders of the CO stripes (Fig. 2A) is somewhat arbitrary and quite possibly an oversimplification. If the stripe compartments in V2 have sharply defined borders, one would expect there to be almost perfect segregation of clusters projecting to different parts of V4, even if these borders run an irregular course in places. If, on the other hand, the borders are inherently fuzzy, one would expect to find extensive and consistent intermixing in the transition region of cells projecting to different V4 subregions. This intermixing might be manifested by a high incidence of double-labeled cells, indicating that single cells project to both subregions, or by a "salt-and-pepper" intermixing of cells labeled by one color or the other.

Examination of the patterns shown in Figure 2A at higher magnification indicates that there are definitely some double-labeled cells and that there are some regions where a noticeable degree of intermixing occurs. However, our overall impression is that the degree of intermingling and of double-labeling is rather modest. In many regions, the transition from cells labeled almost exclusively with one color to cells labeled almost exclusively with the other color occurs over distances of only 100–200 μm, which is relatively small in comparison to the values of 500–1000 μm for the width of individual thin stripes and interstripes. Although the issue deserves a more extensive quantitative analysis, our results suggest that V2 stripes have fairly sharply defined borders, rather than having a broad transition region that is intermediate in its connectivity characteristics. However, this does not imply that each stripe is homogeneous in all of its internal characteristics. We have noted already that stripes often show mottling or other nonuniformities in well-stained CO sections (Fig. 1). Patchy nonuniformities within individual stripes have also been reported in a 2-deoxyglucose study of V2 (Tootell and Hamilton 1989).

We analyzed results from a total of ten V4 injections in six hemispheres. In six of the ten injections, labeled cells in V2 were found in multiple stripe-like clusters predominantly confined to a single CO subregion. The labeling was associated mainly with thin stripes in three of these cases and with interstripes in the other three. Conjoint labeling of both thin stripes and interstripes was observed in the remaining four cases, which we attribute to the injection site encroaching on more than one V4 compartment (see below).

The pattern of V2 labeling resulting from each tracer injection could not be predicted from the location of the injection site on the prelunate gyrus. For example, we found that an injection placed close to the lunate sulcus could label thin stripes or interstripes or both. Similarly, more anteriorly placed injections could also label either V2 subregion. This suggests that the projections from thin stripes and interstripes terminate in a number of discrete, segregated regions in V4. Some regions evidently receive input predominantly from the thin stripes, whereas others receive input from the interstripes of V2. We strongly suspect that this pattern represents modular organization within V4, rather than the presence of a pair of visual areas whose border runs across the prelunate gyrus (cf. Maguire and Baizer 1984). Unless this border ran an especially tortuous course, it would be unlikely for similarly placed pairs of injections in V4 to produce complementary labeling patterns in V2 in different experiments (i.e., thin stripes labeled from the posterior injection in one case and from the anterior injection in another).

Our results provide no evidence concerning the topology of the compartments within V4, i.e., whether the pattern involves stripes, checkerboard arrays, patches within a matrix (e.g., blobs within a "sea" of interblobs), or some less regular configuration. However, we can place approximate lower and upper bounds on the average width of the subregions. The estimate for the lower bound is based on the fact that most of the V4 injections (6 of 10) led to labeling predominantly within a single type of V2 stripe. Our injection sites were generally 1–2 mm in diameter, and they presumably were placed randomly with regard to compartmental boundaries. If the compartments were only 1–2 mm wide, most injections would have crossed a compartmental border and would have led to labeling of both types of V2 stripe. Given that this did not occur, we infer that the V4 compartments are at least 2 mm wide. Our estimate of the upper bound is based on the fact that compartmental boundaries were either crossed or hit in all three cases involving multiple tracer injections (two hemispheres with a dual tracer injection and one with a triple tracer). This outcome would be unlikely if the compartments were markedly larger than

the spacing of 3–6 mm between injection sites and if the injections were randomly placed with regard to boundaries, but we acknowledge that this latter assumption is not necessarily valid.

These observations suggest that the compartments in V4 may be on the order of 2–4 mm wide. This is somewhat coarser than the 0.5–2 mm per stripe characteristic of V2, which in turn is coarser than the 0.3–0.6 mm per stripe in V1. The relationship between stripes in V2 and their target areas V4 and MT is illustrated in the schematic diagram shown in Figure 3, in which the relative sizes of the different compartments are roughly preserved. Interestingly, the apparent increase in the size of compartments in V4 is not matched by an increase in total surface area, as V4 is only about half the size of V1 and V2 (Felleman and Van Essen 1991; see below). On the other hand, the progressive increase in compartment size is matched by increases in the sizes of classic receptive fields going from V1 to V2 and V4.

Given the evidence that V4 contains distinct compartments associated with the P-B and P-I streams by virtue of their differential inputs from V2 stripes, we were naturally interested in whether a comparable degree of segregation exists for the connections that V4 is known to have with higher cortical areas in the temporal and parietal lobes. One could envision that connections of different V4 compartments are (1) strongly intermixed at higher levels; (2) distributed so that one compartment is linked mainly to parietal cortex and the other to inferotemporal cortex (IT); or (3) differentially distributed with specific subregions in inferotemporal and/or parietal cortex. Our results from the same case illustrated in Figure 2A support the last of these possibilities. Retrograde labeling from both tracer injections was minimal in parietal cortex, but very strong in IT. The pattern in posterior IT showed considerable

---

Figure 2. Retrograde labeling patterns in extrastriate visual cortex following dual injections of fluorescent tracers in V4. (*A*) Distribution of retrogradely labeled cells in area V2 following paired tracer injections in dorsal V4 (case 85E-L). The upper panel shows a computer reconstruction of six superimposed sections of flattened V2 from the posterior bank of the lunate sulcus. Dorsal (toward the vertical meridian representation) is upward, and lateral (toward the foveal representation) is to the right. The precise positions of cells labeled with nuclear yellow (yellow dots), bisbenzimide (blue dots), or both (white dots) were recorded in each section using a microscope equipped with a digitally controlled stage (see Methods). Tracers (200 nl each) were injected at two sites in V4 separated by 5 mm in the anterior-posterior direction along the surface of the prelunate gyrus, just dorsal to the tip of the inferior occipital sulcus. The lower panel shows a computer reconstruction of three superimposed sections from the same region of V2 as in the upper panel. Data from two of these sections show stripes and patches of high cytochrome oxidase activity (orange outlines). The third section was processed to reveal Cat-301 immunoreactivity. Intensely reactive cells are indicated by the white dots. Despite the irregularity in width of the CO stripes, the Cat-301 labeling reveals which ones are "thick" stripes (see text). The thick stripes correspond to regions in the upper panel lacking cells projecting to V4. Vertical lines connect corresponding points in adjacent CO stripes, which represent thin stripes having a high density of yellow-labeled cells. (Modified from DeYoe et al. 1990.) Bar, 2 mm. (*B*) Organization of inferotemporal cortex and other extrastriate regions as revealed by paired tracer injections into dorsal and ventral V4 (case 85I-L). Results are displayed on a two-dimensional map of extrastriate cortex in the occipital, temporal, and parietal lobes. Red dots indicate locations of retrogradely labeled cells from an injection of dorsal V4, in the location indicated by the large red spot and the associated injection halo. Blue dots indicate locations of cells labeled from an injection of ventral V4, indicated by the large blue spot and surrounding halo. The ventral injection was made at an eccentricity of 4° near the superior vertical meridian. The dorsal injection was in the lower field representation and relatively close to the fovea. Because of uncertainties in the projection of the fovea, we are unsure of the exact receptive field position, but it would appear to be centered at an eccentricity of 2°–4° based on the labeling in V2 relative to the known topography of V2 (Gattass et al. 1981). (*C*) Computer reconstruction of an individual section from the same case as *B*, to show both the laminar distribution and the degree of spatial intermixing of cells associated with the V4d and V4v injections. Anterior is to the right, and medial is upward. Bar, 2 mm. The contour representing this section intersects the boundaries of the cortical map in panel *B* at the locations indicated by the arrows on the lower right.

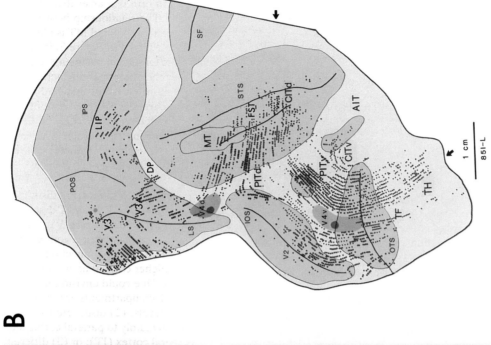

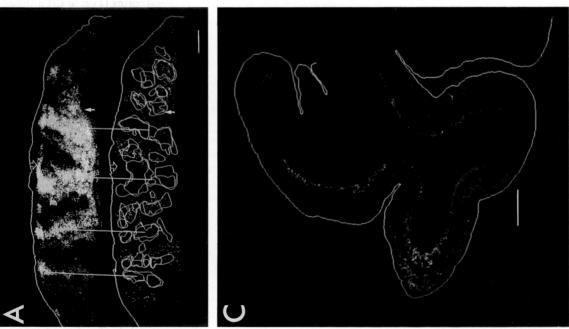

Figure 2. (*See facing page for legend.*)

685

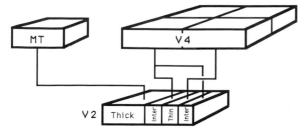

Figure 3. Schematic illustration of the hypothesized compartmental organization of V4 and its relation to the thin stripes and interstripes of V2. Thick stripes project strongly to MT, which also receives a more modest and inconsistent projection from thin stripes (not shown). Thin stripes and interstripes project to separate portions of V4, which are suggested here to be several times wider than the individual V2 stripes. The V4 compartments are drawn in a checkerboard configuration, but we know of no evidence bearing on their actual configuration.

segregation into patches labeled predominantly with one tracer or the other, although the degree of intermixing was certainly greater than that already illustrated for V2. More anteriorly in IT, the retrograde labeling was much more strongly intermixed. These results suggest that the P-B and P-I streams remain distinct over four stages of cortical processing, including areas V1, V2, V4, and posterior IT.

Cells in the P-B and P-I streams differ in their receptive field properties, particularly with regard to selectivity for wavelength, orientation, and spatial frequency (DeYoe and Van Essen 1985; Hubel and Livingstone 1987; Tootell et al. 1988). Presumably, this reflects functionally important differences in the types of information needed by temporal lobe mechanisms involved in visual memory and pattern recognition. However, it is likely that the contributions of different processing streams to perception are intricately intertwined and perhaps somewhat different at successive hierarchical levels (cf. below and DeYoe and Van Essen 1988; Felleman and Van Essen 1991).

One specific indication of this potential complexity was revealed when we injected a "cocktail" of retrograde and anterograde tracers at a single site in V4. The anterogradely labeled terminals in V2 were in register with retrogradely labeled cell bodies in the thin stripes. However, the anterograde label also extended beyond the thin stripes into the adjoining interstripes. This indicates that the feedback connections from V4 to V2 may be more widely distributed than the cell bodies producing the forward projections from V2 to V4. A similar asymmetry has been reported by Shipp and Zeki (1989) and also by Krubitzer and Kaas (1989) for the connections between V2 and MT in the squirrel monkey. Functionally, the wider distribution of feedback connections provides a mechanism for significant interaction of activity from different pathways and could significantly complicate the assignment of function to one stream versus the others.

Organization of IT

The involvement of IT in high-level aspects of pattern recognition was first suggested by lesion studies (cf. Ungerleider and Mishkin 1982) and has received further support from the finding of substantial numbers of cells that show selectivity for faces and other complex patterns (Desimone et al. 1984; Bayliss et al. 1987; Perrett et al. 1987). Previous studies have shown that IT is inhomogeneous in its architecture (Seltzer and Pandya 1978), in its connectivity (Seltzer and Pandya 1978, 1989; Fenstemaker 1986; Iwai and Yukie 1987), in the distribution of receptive field properties (Bayliss et al. 1987; Saito et al. 1987), and in the effects of cooling (Horel et al. 1987). These studies have led to a variety of schemes for the partitioning of IT along the anteroposterior axis, the dorsoventral axis, or combinations thereof. Thus, although there is a general recognition that IT consists of a complex of different areas, a consensus for how it should be partitioned has yet to emerge.

Relationship to area VOT. First, we consider where the posterior border of the IT complex lies in relation to other visual areas. Heretofore, it has been unclear whether IT directly adjoins area V4 (Gattass et al. 1988) or whether there are additional areas interposed (Felleman et al. 1986). We addressed this problem using electrophysiological mapping of visual topography in conjunction with the analysis of interhemispheric connections. Figure 4 shows results from one such experiment that provides evidence for a distinct visual area, which we call VOT (the ventral occipito-temporal area), situated between ventral V4 and IT (Felleman et al. 1986). Stippling on the cortical map in Figure 4 (top) indicates regions receiving interhemispheric connections, as determined by staining for degeneration following transection of the corpus callosum. As has been shown previously for this region, there is a characteristic callosal-free zone almost completely surrounded by a ring of callosal inputs (Van Essen et al. 1982). Within this region, we found two separate representations of the superior visual quadrant. This dual representation is evident in each of the two illustrated sequences of recording sites (Fig. 4, top) and corresponding receptive fields (Fig. 4, bottom). Recording sites A and B (row 1) and G and H (row 2) were situated posteriorly in the callosal-free zone, within what has previously been shown to be ventral V4 (Newsome et al. 1986; Gattass et al. 1988). Their receptive fields were in parafoveal (row 1) or more peripheral (row 2) portions of the superior quadrant. Sites C, D, and I, situated more anteriorly, had receptive fields close to the horizontal meridian. We consider them to be on the V4/VOT border, reflecting an arrangement similar to that which occurs for the V2/V3 and the V2/VP borders (Gattass et al. 1981; Newsome et al. 1986). Sites E and F (row 1) and J and K (row 2) were situated still further anteriorly, and they demonstrate a progression back toward the superior vertical meridian within area VOT. These recording sites are

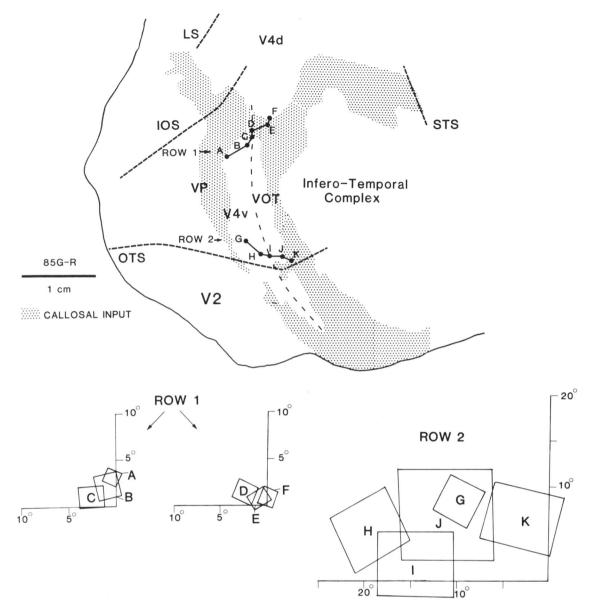

Figure 4. Topographic organization of the ventral occipitotemporal area (VOT) and surrounding cortex. The upper portion shows a two-dimensional map of ventral extrastriate cortex, including the inferior occipital sulcus (IOS), occipitotemporal sulcus (OTS), and superior temporal sulcus (STS). Stippling indicates the regions receiving callosal inputs as revealed by the pattern of degeneration following callosal transection. This allows the approximate locations of areas V2, VP, and V4d, and the inferotemporal complex to be inferred. Multiunit electrophysiological recordings were made in and near the large callosal-free zone and the surrounding callosal-recipient ring in the center of the map. Two rows of recording sites (sequences A–F and G–K) are indicated on the map, and the corresponding receptive fields are shown in the lower part of the figure. In both sequences, there is an orderly progression from upper fields near the vertical meridian, to fields on or near the horizontal meridian, and back toward the vertical meridian. Similar results, albeit with some receptive field scatter from one site to the next, were obtained for a total of 25 recording sites in the vicinity of row 2 and 22 sites in the vicinity of row 1. This indicates that there is a dual representation of the upper quadrant in V4v (situated posteriorly) and VOT (situated anteriorly).

on the portion of the callosal-recipient ring that represents the juncture with IT (see below).

We have not recorded extensively from IT, but instead have used the patterns of connectivity with V4 as a means of deciphering the organization of this region. Previous studies (Desimone et al. 1980; Fenstemaker 1986) have shown that V4 is the major source of visual inputs to IT. To study the connectivity patterns between V4 and IT in greater detail, we made paired

tracer injections into different locations in V4. Figure 2 (B and C) and Figure 5 show results from an experiment in which separate retrograde tracer injections were made into dorsal and ventral V4 at sites that were electrophysiologically confirmed on the basis of receptive field size and topography. The pattern of labeling is plotted on a two-dimensional map of extrastriate cortex in the occipital, temporal, and parietal lobes, with blue dots indicating bisbenzimide-labeled cells from the ven-

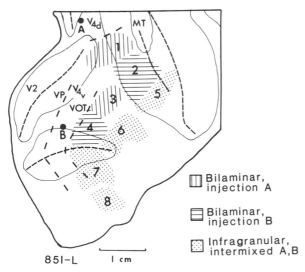

Figure 5. Distribution of labeled cells according to spatial and laminar patterns into eight foci in the temporal lobe following paired injections in V4d (site A) and V4v (site B; Case 85I-L, based on data in Fig. 2B,C). Vertical hatching indicates bilaminar labeling originating from the V4d injection; horizontal hatching indicates bilaminar labeling originating from the V4v injection; and stippling indicates predominantly infragranular labeling originating in a strongly intermixed pattern from both injections.

tral injection and red dots representing nuclear-yellow-labeled cells from the dorsal injection (Fig. 2B).

As expected for tracers placed within V4, both of the injections led to massive retrograde labeling in V2 and in IT, and there was no labeling in V1 (not shown). In addition, there was substantial labeling in a number of other areas. In dorsal extrastriate cortex, the major additional inputs are from areas V3, V3A, LIP, and MT, and probably also DP. In ventral extrastriate cortex, the additional inputs are from areas VP, VOT, FST, TF, and TH. However, our main focus here is on the complex pattern of connections with IT. Four different regions can be identified in IT in this hemisphere on the basis of the laminar organization of connections and on the degree of segregation of inputs from the two injections.

The nature of these distinctions is illustrated in Figure 2C, which shows the distribution of cells labeled with NY (red) and BB (blue) in a single section through the temporal lobe (superior temporal sulcus and occipitotemporal sulcus). Altogether, there are six major patches discernible in this section. Three of the patches contain retrogradely labeled cells essentially all of the same type (all NY or all BB), and in these patches, the cells are distributed in a bilaminar pattern that includes substantial labeling in both superficial and deep layers. In the other three patches (one anteriorly within the superior temporal sulcus and two medial to the occipitotemporal sulcus), the labeling is heavily (albeit not completely) intermixed, and it is largely confined to infragranular layers.

The spatial distribution of these characteristics is indicated more systematically in Figure 5, which con-

tains an expanded view of the ventral portion of the map in Figure 2B. The locations of the injection sites in V4d (site A) and V4v (site B) are shown by solid circles. In this experiment, the corpus callosum had been transected, and we used the pattern of degeneration of interhemispheric connections (see above) as a guide to the locations of several areal boundaries (VP/V4v, VOT/IT, and V4d/IT), as indicated by the coarse dashed lines. Only the labeling in the temporal lobe is shown, and it is divided into eight major foci that are grouped according to the characteristics described in the preceding paragraph. The vertical hatching indicates regions containing almost exclusively cells labeled by the dorsal injection; in these regions, the labeled cells were distributed in a bilaminar pattern. The horizontal hatching indicates regions of bilaminar label associated with the ventral injection. Stippling delineates the combination of predominantly infragranular labeling and of extensive overlap between the two labels.

Foci 1–4 include segregated patches of bilaminar label situated in posterior portions of IT, in the vicinity of what has been called TEO by other investigators (Fenstemaker 1986; Iwai and Yukie 1987). There are two obvious possibilities that might account for the striking degree of segregation in this region. First, patchy inferotemporal labeling might arise if the tracer injections had been into different compartments of V4, as we indeed found for one case described in an earlier section. However, this explanation is unlikely to apply to the present case, because the injections were relatively large and led to labeling in V2 that was quite widespread and very unlikely to have been confined to a single compartment (cf. Fig. 2B). Instead, we favor the alternative interpretation, namely, that the segregation reflects a crude but significant degree of topographic organization in the connections between V4 and posterior IT. This fits with the fact that receptive fields in posterior IT are smaller than in more anterior portions (Desimone and Gross 1979) and with the anatomical observations of Fenstemaker (1986).

The fact that there are two pairs of topographically organized foci suggests that they form two distinct areas, which we have termed PITd and PITv (dorsal and ventral subdivisions of the posterior inferotemporal area). The more anterior pair of foci (5 and 6) differ from PITd and PITv in their lack of anatomically discernible topographic organization and in the laminar organization of their projection back to V4. There is evidence that these two regions differ in their connectivity (Shiwa 1987; Yukie et al. 1988) and in the behavioral effects of inactivation (Horel et al. 1987). We therefore provisionally regard them as different areas, CITd and CITv (dorsal and ventral subdivisions of the central inferotemporal area). In front of the CIT complex is an anterior inferotemporal region that receives only weak projections from V4 (none in this particular case). Like the more posterior regions, there is evidence that it also can be subdivided into dorsal and ventral subregions (AITd and AITv) on the basis of differential connections (Fenstemaker 1986; Shiwa 1987; see also Felleman and Van Essen 1991). Finally, cytoarchitectonic areas TF and TH, situated on the parahippocampal gyrus medial to the occipitotemporal sulcus, are strongly connected to V4 in a manner lacking topographic organization (foci 7 and 8). Thus, there is evidence for six different visual areas within classic IT, plus an additional pair of areas situated more medially.

Overview of Areas and Hierarchical Organization

Visual areas. Having illustrated a variety of specific experiments that add to our understanding of particular visual areas and connections, we now turn to a broader overview that summarizes the layout of different areas and the hierarchical nature of information flow among

them. Based on reports from a number of laboratories, a total of 32 cortical areas in the macaque have been identified and implicated in visual processing on the basis of their visual responsiveness and/or their inputs from other visual areas. Most of these areas are largely or exclusively visual in function, but seven of them (listed in the legend to Fig. 6) are what we consider to be visual association areas because they are also linked to other sensory modalities or to visuomotor functions. The size and location of each area are indicated on the cortical map illustrated in Figure 6. This map shows all of cerebral cortex in the right hemisphere, including transitional, paleocortical, and archicortical regions (635 mm^2 altogether), as well as 9940 mm^2 of neocortex. Visual cortex occupies an estimated 5385 mm^2, or 54% of neocortex. Nearly half of visual cortex is occupied by areas V1 and V2, and the remaining areas

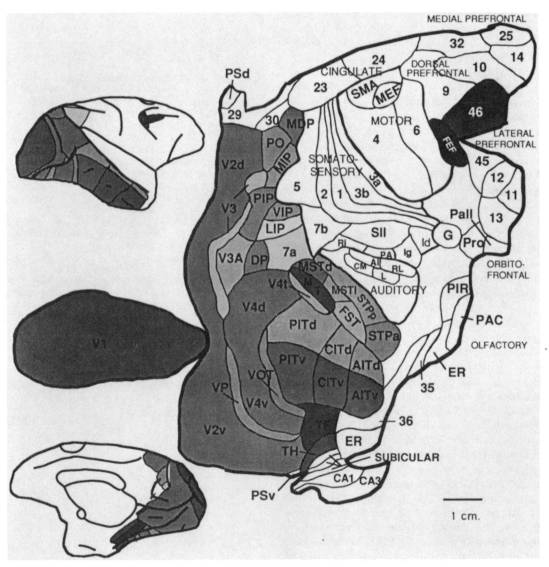

Figure 6. Summary map to show the location and size of visual and other cortical areas on a two-dimensional map of the entire cerebral cortex in the macaque. (Modified from D.J. Felleman and D.C. Van Essen, in prep.) Visual association areas include 7a, STPp, STPa, TF, TH, FEF, and 46.

range in size from 3% to 45% of the size of these larger areas. The map also shows regions devoted to somatosensory, motor, and auditory processing, which, respectively, occupy 11%, 8%, and 3% of neocortex. Additional information on the layout of cortical areas, plus the references on which their identification and characterization are based, is given elsewhere (Felleman and Van Essen 1991).

Less than half of the identified visual areas are topographically organized, in the sense of containing an orderly mapping of the visual field that can be discerned with conventional physiological and anatomical techniques. Area V1 has an extremely precise map of the visual field, but as one moves to areas more anterior (to the right) on the map, topography generally becomes coarser and more irregular. In addition, some areas contain only representations of the upper visual field (VP and VOT) or lower visual field (V3 and V4t). The topographically organized areas occupy all of the occipital lobe and a small portion of inferotemporal and posterior parietal cortex, in a configuration that bears strong similarities to the representation in topographically organized visual areas of the owl monkey (Sereno and Allman 1990). Our best estimate of the way in which the visual field is mapped in these areas is indicated in Figure 7, which summarizes results from many different mapping studies in the macaque monkey (see figure legend). Different symbols are used to show the approximate locations of the representation of the vertical meridian (V), horizontal meridian (H), foveal representation (F), far periphery (P), lower quadrant (−), upper quadrant (+), and the 10° isoeccentricity line (fine stipple), plus the 2° and 40° isoeccentricity lines for area V1 (coarse stipple). For areas having only a very crude topography, plus and minus signs are positioned to indicate where the upper and lower quadrants are represented. Areas lacking any discernible topography are indicated by closely apposed plus and minus symbols. The names of the individual visual areas have been omitted for lack of space, but their identity can be determined by making comparisons with Figure 6.

One interesting point that emerges from inspection of this map is that the 10° isoeccentricity line can be traced as a single swath passing through nearly all of the topographically organized visual areas. Starting ventrally, it passes through areas VOT, V4v, VP, and V2v, jumps across the artificial discontinuity to V1, across another discontinuity to V2d, then to V3, V3A, V4d, V4t, and finally MT. Along this swath, there are a total of ten reversals in the visual field progression, six occurring along a vertical meridian representation and four along the horizontal meridian. The finite thickness of the isoeccentricity representation reflects several factors, including the known variability in topographic organization from one individual to the next, the known irregularities in representation within a single individual, and the uncertainties in transposing experimental data onto a summary map. The four topographically organized areas not included on this

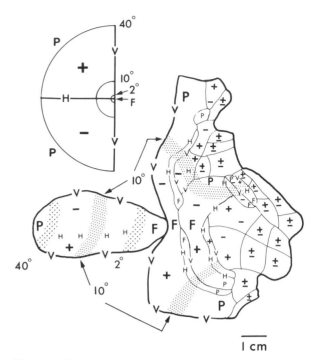

Figure 7. Topographic organization of visual cortex in the macaque. The map outlines all of the visual areas in the occipital, temporal, and parietal lobes, and they can be individually identified by comparison with the preceding figure. Major features of visual topography are indicated for each area as indicated in the drawing of the visual hemifield (upper left) and explained in the text. The primary references on which this summary is based are: V1 (Van Essen et al. 1984); V2 (Gattass et al. 1981; Van Essen et al. 1986); V3, VP, and V4 (Maguire and Baizer 1984; Newsome et al. 1986; Van Essen et al. 1986; Gattass et al. 1988); VOT (Felleman et al. 1985, this paper); V3A and PIP (Van Essen and Zeki 1978; Felleman et al. 1987; Colby et al. 1988); V4t and MT (Van Essen et al. 1981; Desimone and Ungerleider 1986; Maunsell and Van Essen 1987; Gattass et al. 1988); inferotemporal areas (Desimone and Gross 1979; Felleman et al. 1986; Fenstemaker 1986; and this paper); MSTd, MSTl, and FST (Desimone and Ungerleider 1986; Komatsu and Wurtz 1988); PO, MDP, and MIP (Colby et al. 1988); and VIP, LIP, and 7a (Andersen et al. 1985, 1990).

swath are PITd, PITv, PIP, and PO. In none of these is the topography well enough studied to draw isoeccentricity lines with any confidence. Indeed, even in the better-studied areas, the irregularities and uncertainties are relatively large, and the positioning of other isoeccentricity contours (e.g., 2° and 40°) can only be done with confidence for area V1, as illustrated, and for MT (not shown). This issue is of importance for understanding whether there are large differences among areas in the relative amounts of cortex devoted to different eccentricities. It appears from Figure 7 that the emphasis on central versus peripheral vision may be smaller in V2 than in V1, but greater in V4 than in V1. However, even this interpretation should be made with caution until more quantitative data are available for these and other extrastriate areas.

Hierarchical processing. The number of identified connections between specific visual cortical areas has literally exploded in recent years. A decade ago, a summary of connections among visual areas in the macaque included only 13 identified pathways (Van Essen 1979). Now, thanks to the advent of highly sensitive pathway-tracing techniques, and to the increase in the number of identified visual areas, more than 300 pathways have been reported between specific areas in the visual cortex (Felleman and Van Essen 1991). On the basis of data from well-studied areas, it appears that each cortical area typically receives direct inputs from about ten other areas and sends its outputs to about ten areas. This principle is not restricted to the visual system. For example, in the somatosensory and motor cortex, which has not been nearly as intensively studied, 62 pathways have already been identified that interlink the 13 known areas. With such a plethora of connections throughout cerebral cortex, it is important to search for general characteristics that may reflect fundamental aspects of information flow. Three such characteristics appear to be particularly important.

1. Connectivity within the visual cortex is highly reciprocal in nature. This was first appreciated by Tigges et al. (1973, 1981) and by Rockland and Pandya (1979). In nearly all cases that have been examined systematically, a projection from one area to another is matched by a projection in the reverse direction.
2. The laminar organization of these reciprocal connections is usually asymmetric. For the great majority of linkages, the projections terminate preferentially in layer 4 in one direction, and they preferentially avoid layer 4 in the opposite direction. This asymmetry has been suggested to reflect ascending and descending directions of information flow (Rockland and Pandya 1979; Friedman 1983; Maunsell and Van Essen 1983b). In addition, some pathways show a columnar termination pattern (uniform density in most layers, including layer 4), which has been proposed to represent information flow in a lateral direction.
3. By applying this notion of ascending, descending, and lateral relationships across all pairs of interconnected areas, it is possible to generate schemes for an overall hierarchy of cortical areas in the visual system (Maunsell and Van Essen 1983b; Van Essen 1985; Andersen et al. 1990; Boussaud et al. 1990; Felleman and Van Essen 1991) and in the somatosensory-motor system (Friedman et al. 1986; Neal et al. 1987). Moreover, since there are linkages between these two systems, it is possible to combine them into a broader cortical hierarchy that encompasses different modalities.

Figure 8 shows a hierarchical scheme that includes all corticocortical pathways identified as of mid-1990 in the visual and somatosensory-motor systems in the macaque. It includes ten levels of processing in the visual cortex and nine in the somatosensory-motor cortex. In addition, there are two subcortical stages in the visual system (the retina and the lateral geniculate

nucleus) and three stages (dorsal root ganglia, dorsal column nuclei, and ventrobasal nucleus) for the somatosensory system (not shown). Finally, there are several stages at the top of the hierarchy that represent connections of sensory systems to higher centers associated with the limbic system, namely, areas 35 and 36, entorhinal cortex, and the hippocampal complex.

It is important to emphasize that this anatomical picture is not without some complications and apparent internal inconsistencies. In particular, there are a couple of dozen pathways among the hundreds of identified ones (i.e., less than 10%) that do not fit within this scheme for one reason or another (see Felleman and Van Essen 1991). These occur somewhat more frequently at higher levels of the hierarchy, but it is not simply a consequence of a sudden breakdown at a particular level. Many of these apparent exceptions may reflect technical factors, owing to uncertainties in determining areal boundaries or inaccuracies in reporting laminar patterns. On the other hand, it may well be that unequivocal exceptions will persist when the pathways in question are reexamined. This might lead to altered criteria for distinguishing hierarchical relationships or to the conclusion that hierarchical relationships reflect stochastic biases rather than unbreakable rules governing the formation of corticocortical connections. In any event, this scheme represents a hypothesis about function and information processing that is based strictly on anatomical data. It is also a progress report rather than a final statement of connectivity, as further anatomical studies will certainly lead to many additions to the connectivity pattern and probably also to various refinements and revisions.

Altogether, our interpretation is that well over a dozen stages of processing take place between the acquisition of raw visual and somatosensory information and its utilization by the highest levels of cognitive centers in the primate cerebrum. The number of stages appears to be substantially fewer (four or five) in the olfactory system (cf. Haberly 1985; Swanson et al. 1987; Felleman and Van Essen 1991). In other species, such as the rat, there is evidence for hierarchical organization of visual cortex, but with many fewer levels than in the macaque (Coogan and Burkhalter 1990 and pers. comm.). The factors that determine the appropriate number of processing stages in a given sensory system are not known. One specific possibility is that the number of levels is related to the phenomenon of directed attention, whereby high-level areas involved in pattern recognition (e.g., those in the temporal lobe) are able at any given moment to process information from a restricted portion of the sensory periphery and to shift this "window of attention" rapidly in spatial location and scale. An attractive scheme for mediating this attentional process involves a multistage process of convergence from lower to higher levels in which the routing of information is under dynamic, top-down control (Anderson and Van Essen 1987). In this scheme, the number of hierarchical levels depends on the size of the attentional window relative to the total

692

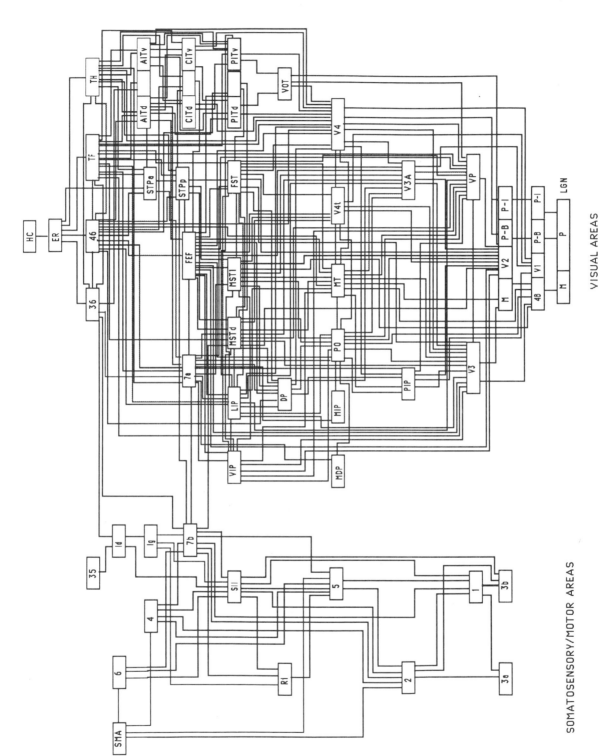

Figure 8. (*See facing page for legend.*)

VISUAL AREAS

SOMATOSENSORY/MOTOR AREAS

extent of the sensory sheet in a manner that fits reasonably well with some of the key organizational features of the primate visual system (Van Essen and Anderson 1990).

The higher centers shown in Figure 8 do not by any means represent the sole outputs of the visual cortex. There are extensive connections with other cortical areas in frontal and cingulate cortex, and also massive connections that every cortical area has with various subcortical centers, including those involved in motor control. They are omitted from the present scheme in part because much less is known about their detailed connections and also because it is not at all clear whether they are organized in a comparable hierarchical fashion. An argument can be made, however, that the pulvinar occupies a relatively low hierarchical level, just above V1, and that the amygdala represents a high level, just below TF and TH (Felleman and Van Essen 1991).

It is unclear whether similar anatomical principles of hierarchical organization apply throughout cerebral cortex. In the auditory cortex, Galaburda and Pandya (1983) have described a dozen architectonic subdivisions and a pattern of connectivity that suggests ascending, descending, and lateral directions when examined one pathway at a time. However, many of the reciprocal relationships they describe are inconsistent with an orderly hierarchy. Similarly, in cingulate cortex, patterns of connectivity have been reported that are difficult to reconcile with an orderly hierarchy involving these areas (Selemon and Goldman-Rakic 1988). Whereas it is entirely possible that large portions of neocortex simply lack any anatomically discernible hierarchical organization, it is important to address the issue using tracer injections that are unequivocally restricted to individual, identified cortical areas.

CONCLUDING REMARKS

In this paper, we have emphasized an anatomical approach to the study of visual cortex, and we have argued that it suggests important principles of cortical organization and information processing. To put the analysis in a broader perspective, we conclude with some brief comments that point to significant issues in the next decade of research on the visual cortex. Specifically, we discuss three topics that in some respects are very different, but perhaps not as disparate as appears at first glance.

Parallel Processing Streams

Within the hierarchical framework illustrated in Figure 8, parallel processing is evident at every level. At the lowest stages of the visual pathway, it is manifested by the P-B, P-I, and M streams discussed in an earlier section. At higher levels, there is an important distinction between inferotemporal areas, which appear to be especially involved in pattern recognition, and posterior parietal areas, which are involved in spatial relationships and the control of visual attention and eye movements (cf. Ungerleider and Mishkin 1982; Maunsell and Newsome 1987; Desimone and Ungerleider 1989). The pathways that interlink these low-level and high-level streams are numerous and complex. To some extent, it appears that the M stream contributes heavily to areas in the parietal lobe, whereas the P-B and P-I streams contribute heavily to inferotemporal cortex. However, there are numerous examples of cross-talk between streams, and these may have important implications for our understanding of visual function (cf. DeYoe and Van Essen 1988; Felleman and Van Essen 1991).

In this connection, an issue that is often raised is whether specific visual functions can be uniquely assigned to individual cortical areas, to compartments within areas, or to particular processing streams that extend across multiple areas. Is MT, for example, a "motion area," or is the P-B stream exclusively and uniquely involved in contributing to the perception of color? These are attractive notions, and physiological and lesion studies are often cited in support of such suggestions. On the other hand, most investigators would probably concur that the issue is not entirely that simple. Motion analysis is not a unitary process, because we use information about image velocity for a variety of perceptual and visuomotor tasks, including motion parallax and structure-from-motion as well as determination of target trajectories. More generally, each low-level sensory cue (e.g., velocity, orientation, spectral composition, and binocular disparity) can contribute to many different aspects of visual perception. Conversely, different types of perception (e.g., distance, form, and surface texture) can derive from several low-level cues operating in isolation or in conjunction (cf. DeYoe and Van Essen 1988; Schiller et al. 1990). Hence, although lesion studies in humans and in laboratory animals provide valuable constraints on the functions to which different areas and compartments contribute, it is important when attempting to interpret these findings to appreciate the number, diversity, and computational complexity of the tasks carried out so effortlessly by the visual system.

Role of Neural Modeling

The cerebral cortex in general and the visual system in particular are too complex to understand from an

---

Figure 8. A unified hierarchy of visual, somatosensory-motor, and higher cortical areas in the macaque. This scheme is based on 305 pathways interlinking visual cortical areas, 62 pathways interlinking somatosensory-motor areas, and additional pathways linking the two systems to one another and to higher cortical centers. The criteria for establishing hierarchical relationships, along with specific connectivity data, appropriate references, and consideration of hierarchical irregularities, are given in D.J. Felleman and D.C. Van Essen (in prep.).

exclusively intuitive analysis. Accordingly, there is a pressing need for specific models which are motivated by biological issues and which capture as much of the underlying structural and physiological data as possible, yet which can account for specific tasks or aspects of system performance (cf. Koch and Segev 1989; Bower 1990). It is also critical that such models be robust and efficient at handling the types of noisy data presented by natural images and other real-world sensory inputs. The visual system is impressively efficient at extracting useful information, discarding irrelevant information, and being minimally disrupted by spurious data contained in the barrage of images that it must continuously process. This efficiency did not arise instantaneously during evolution, and to incorporate it into neural models will require careful attention to basic principles of good engineering (cf. Mead 1989; Van Essen and Anderson 1990).

Need for Data Bases

It might seem curious to conclude with a topic that in a sense is a largely technical matter. However, neuroscientists are rapidly being overwhelmed by a deluge of data that can no longer be efficiently handled exclusively through conventional means. As one specific example, our summaries of the layout of cortical areas and their interconnectivity contained in Figures 6 and 8 will presumably be useful to other investigators, but the utility is restricted by presentation in a static format that cannot readily be updated and is not closely linked to the other types of data contained in the studies from which these summaries were drawn. It would be immensely more useful to have a computerized, graphically oriented data base that could provide flexible, efficient access to information along many dimensions. Using such a data base, one can envision hypothetical scenarios in which, for example, an investigator (1) points to a specific cortical area shown on the computer screen; (2) requests information about its connectivity; (3) views a graphic portrayal of the relevant connections along with a listing of the references on which they are based; and then (4) chooses a particular reference whose text and illustration can be accessed for detailed scrutiny. In a different sequence, the investigator might choose to search for information about the physiology, pharmacology, or development of a particular cortical area or subcortical nucleus and to make comparisons with what is known about this structure in different species, including humans. Attainment of this overall goal, which would have clear utility from clinical and educational standpoints as well as from that of basic research, will be a formidable undertaking. However, most of the critical hardware technology needed to make it feasible have already been developed and are even starting to become within reach economically. These opportunities in information management, if acted on energetically, may contribute importantly in the coming decade to progress in basic neuroscience research and in the way this information may be communicated to the outside world.

ACKNOWLEDGMENTS

This work was supported by grants from the National Institutes of Health (EY-02091) and the Office of Naval Research (N-00014-89-1192). We thank J. Gallant for valuable discussions, K. Tazumi for preparing illustrations, S. Kallenbach for typing, and D. Bilitch for programming the computerized anatomy software.

REFERENCES

Allman, J. 1977. Evolution of the visual system in the early primates. *Prog. Psychobiol. Physiol. Psychol.* **7:** 1.

Andersen, R.A., C. Asanuma, and W.M. Cowan. 1985. Callosal and prefrontal associational projecting cell populations in area 7A of the macaque monkey: A study using retrogradely transported fluorescent dyes. *J. Comp. Neurol.* **232:** 443.

Andersen, R.A., C. Asanuma, G. Essick, and R.M. Siegel. 1990. Cortico-cortical connections of anatomically and physiologically defined subdivisions within the inferior parietal lobule. *J. Comp. Neurol.* **296:** 65.

Anderson, C.H. and D.C. Van Essen. 1987. Shifter circuits: A computational strategy for dynamic aspects of visual processing. *Proc. Natl. Acad. Sci.* **84:** 6297.

Anderson, P.A., J. Olavarria, and R.C. Van Sluyters. 1988. The overall pattern of ocular dominance bands in cat visual cortex. *J. Neurosci.* **8:** 2183.

Baylis, G.C., E.T. Rolls, and C.M. Leonard. 1987. Functional subdivisions of the temporal lobe neocortex. *J. Neurosci.* **7:** 330.

Boussaud, D. L.G. Ungerleider, and R. Desimone. 1990. Pathways for motion analysis: Cortical connections of the medial superior temporal and fundus of the superior temporal visual areas in the macaque. *J. Comp. Neurol.* **296:** 462.

Bower, J.M. 1990. Reverse engineering the nervous system: An anatomical, physiological, and computer based approach. In *An introduction to neural and electronic networks* (ed. S. Zornetzer et al.), p. 3. Academic Press, New York.

Burkhalter, A., D.J. Felleman, W.T. Newsome, and D.C. Van Essen. 1986. Anatomical and physiological asymmetries related to visual areas V3 and VP in macaque extrastriate cortex. *Vision Res.* **26:** 63.

Carman, G.J. 1990a. Mappings of the cerebral cortex. Ph.D. thesis, California Institute of Technology, Pasadena.

———. 1990b. Conformal mapping of the visual pathway. *Soc. Neurosci. Abstr.* **16:** (in press).

Carroll, E. and M. Wong-Riley. 1984. Quantitative light and electron microscopic analysis of cytochrome oxidase-rich zones in the striate cortex of squirrel monkeys. *J. Comp. Neurol.* **222:** 1.

Colby, C.L., R. Gattass, C.R. Olson, and C.G. Gross. 1988. Topographic organization of cortical afferents to extrastriate visual area PO in the macaque: A dual tracer study. *J. Comp. Neurol.* **269:** 392.

Coogan, T.A. and A. Burkhalter. 1990. Conserved patterns of corticocortical connections define areal hierarchy in rat visual cortex. *Exp. Brain Res.* **80:** 49.

Desimone, R. and C.G. Gross. 1979. Visual areas in the temporal cortex of the macaque. *Brain Res.* **178:** 363.

Desimone, R. and L.B. Ungerleider. 1986. Multiple visual areas in the caudal superior temporal sulcus of the macaque. *J. Comp. Neurol.* **248:** 164.

———. 1989. Neural mechanisms of visual processing in monkeys. In *Handbook of neuropsychology* (ed. F. Boller and J. Grafman), vol. 2, p. 267. Elsevier, New York.

Desimone, R., J. Fleming, and C.G. Gross. 1980. Prestriate afferents to inferior temporal cortex: An HRP study. *Brain Res.* **184:** 41.

Desimone, R., T.D. Albright, C.G. Gross, and C. Bruce. 1984. Stimulus-selective properties of inferior temporal neurons in the macaque. *J. Neurosci.* **4**: 2051.

DeYoe, E.A. and D.C. Van Essen. 1985. Segregation of efferent connections and receptive field properties in visual area V2 of the macaque. *Nature* **317**: 58.

———. 1988. Concurrent processing streams in monkey visual cortex. *Trends Neurosci.* **11**: 219.

DeYoe, E.A., S. Hockfield, H. Garren, and D.C. Van Essen. 1990. Antibody labeling of functional subdivisions in visual cortex: CAT-301 immunoreactivity in striate and extrastriate cortex of the macaque monkey. *Vis. Neurosci.* (in press).

DeYoe, E.A., D.J. Felleman, J.J. Knierim, J. Olavarria, and D.C. Van Essen. 1988. Heterogeneous subregions of macaque visual area V4 receive selective projections from V2 thin-stripe and interstripe subregions. *Invest. Ophthalmol. Visual Sci.* (suppl.) **29**: 115.

Felleman, D.J. and D.C. Van Essen. 1987. Receptive field properties of neurons in area V3 of macaque monkey extrastriate cortex. *J. Neurophysiol.* **57**: 889.

———. 1991. Distributed hierarchical processing in primate cerebral cortex. *Cereb. Cortex* (in press).

Felleman, D.J., A. Burkhalter, and D.C. Van Essen. 1987. Visual area PIP: An extrastriate cortical area in the posterior intra-parietal sulcus of macaque monkeys. *Soc. Neurosci. Abstr.* **13**: 626.

Felleman, D.J., E.A. DeYoe, and D.C. Van Essen. 1985. Two topographically organized visual areas in ventral extrastriate cortex of the macaque monkey. *Soc. Neurosci. Abstr.* **11**: 1246.

Felleman, D., J.J. Knierim, and D.C. Van Essen. 1986. Multiple topographic and non-topographic subdivisions of the temporal lobe revealed by the connections of area V4 in macaques. *Soc. Neurosci. Abstr.* **12**: 1182.

Fenstemaker, S.B. 1986. The organization and connections of visual cortical area TEO in the macaque. Ph.D. thesis, Princeton University, New Jersey.

Fraser, S.E. 1984. Cell interactions involved in neuronal patterning: An experimental and theoretical approach. In *Molecular bases of neural development* (ed. G. Edelman et al.), p. 481. John Wiley, New York.

Friedman, D.P. 1983. Laminar patterns of termination of corticocortical afferents in the somatosensory system. *Brain Res.* **273**: 147.

Friedman, D.P., E.A. Murray, J.B. O'Neill, and M. Mishkin. 1986. Cortical connections of the somatosensory fields of the lateral sulcus of macaques: Evidence for a corticolimbic pathway for touch. *J. Comp. Neurol.* **252**: 323.

Galaburda, A.M. and D.N. Pandya. 1983. The intrinsic architectonic and connectional organization of the superior temporal region in the rhesus monkey. *J. Comp. Neurol.* **221**: 169.

Gattass, R., C.G. Gross, and J.H. Sandell. 1981. Visual topography of V2 in the macaque. *J. Comp. Neurol.* **201**: 519.

Gattass, R., A.P.B. Sousa, and C.G. Gross. 1988. Visuotopic organization and extent of V3 and V4 of the macaque. *J. Neurosci.* **8**: 1831.

Haberly, L.B. 1985. Neuronal circuitry in olfactory cortex: Anatomy and functional implications. *Chem. Senses* **10**: 219.

Hendry, S.C.H., E.G. Jones, S. Hockfield, and R.D.G. McKay. 1988. Neuronal populations stained with the monoclonal antibody Cat-301 in the mammalian cerebral cortex and thalamus. *J. Neurosci.* **8**: 518.

Horel, J.A., D.E. Pytko-Joiner, M.L. Voytko, and K. Salsbury. 1987. The performance of visual tasks while segments of the inferotemporal cortex are suppressed by cold. *Behav. Brain Res.* **23**: 29.

Hubel, D.H. and D.C. Freeman. 1977. Projection into the visual field of ocular dominance columns in macaque monkey. *Brain Res.* **122**: 336.

Hubel, D.H. and M.S. Livingstone. 1987. Segregation of form, color, and stereopsis in primate area 18. *J. Neurosci.* **7**: 3378.

Hubel, D.H. and T.N. Wiesel. 1972. Laminar and columnar distribution of geniculo-cortical fibers in the macaque monkey. *J. Comp. Neurol.* **146**: 421.

Iwai, E. and M. Yukie. 1987. Amygdalofugal and amygdalopetal connections with modality-specific visual cortical areas in macaques (*Macaca fuscata*, *M. mulatta*, and *M. fascicularis*). *J. Comp. Neurol.* **261**: 362.

Koch, C. and I. Segev. 1989. *Methods in neuronal modeling: From synapses to networks.* MIT Press, Cambridge.

Komatsu, H. and R.H. Wurtz. 1988. Relation of cortical areas MT and MST to pursuit eye movements. I. Localization and visual properties of neurons. *J. Neurophysiol.* **60**: 580.

Krubitzer, L.A. and J.H. Kaas. 1989. Cortical integration of parallel pathways in the visual system of primates. *Brain Res.* **478**: 161.

LeVay, S., M. Connolly, J. Houde, and D.C. Van Essen. 1985. The complete pattern of ocular dominance stripes in macaque striate cortex and their representation in the visual field. *J. Neurosci.* **5**: 486.

Livingstone, M.S. and D.H. Hubel. 1984. Anatomy and physiology of a color system in the primate visual cortex. *J. Neurosci.* **4**: 309.

Maguire, W.M. and J.S. Baizer. 1984. Visuotopic organization of the prelunate gyrus in rhesus monkey. *J. Neurosci.* **4**: 1690.

Maunsell, J.H.R. and W.T. Newsome. 1987. Visual processing in monkey extrastriate cortex. *Annu. Rev. Neurosci.* **10**: 363.

Maunsell, J.H.R. and D.C. Van Essen. 1983a. Functional properties of neurons in middle temporal visual area (MT) of macaque monkey. I. Selectivity for stimulus direction, velocity and orientation. *J. Neurophysiol.* **49**: 1127.

———. 1983b. The connections of the middle temporal visual area (MT) and their relationship to a cortical hierarchy in the macaque monkey. *J. Neurosci.* **3**: 2563.

———. 1987. Topographic organization of the middle temporal visual area in the macaque monkey: Representational biases and the relationship to callosal connections and myeloarchitectonic boundaries. *J. Comp. Neurol.* **266**: 535.

Mead, C. 1989. *Analog VLSI and neural systems.* Addison-Wesley, Reading, Massachusetts.

Neal, J.W., R.C.A. Pearson, and T.P.S. Powell. 1987. The cortico-cortical connections of area 7b, PF, in the parietal lobe of the monkey. *Brain Res.* **419**: 341.

Newsome, W.T., J.H.R. Maunsell, and D.C. Van Essen. 1986. The ventral posterior visual area of the macaque: Visual topography and areal boundries. *J. Comp. Neurol.* **252**: 139.

Olavarria, J. and R.C. Van Sluyters. 1985. Unfolding and flattening the cortex of gyrencephalic brains. *J. Neurosci. Methods* **15**: 191.

Olavarria, J., E.A. DeYoe, and D.C. Van Essen. 1989. Patterns of cytochrome oxidase staining in the unfolded and flattened V2 of the macaque monkey. *Invest. Ophthalmol. Visual Sci.* (suppl.) **30**: 299.

Perrett, D.I., A.J. Mistlin, and A.J. Chitty. 1987. Visual neurones responsive to faces. *Trends Neurosci.* **10**: 358.

Previc, F.H. 1990. Functional specialization in the upper and lower visual fields in man: Origins and implications. *Behav. Brain Sci.* (in press).

Rockland, K.S. and D.N. Pandya. 1979. Laminar origins and terminations of cortical connections of the occipital lobe in the rhesus monkey. *Brain Res.* **179**: 3.

Saito, N., K. Tanaka, M. Fukumoto, and Y. Fukada. 1987. The inferior temporal cortex of the macaque monkey: II. The level of complexity in the integration of pattern information. *Soc. Neurosci. Abstr.* **13**: 177.

Schiller, P.H., N.K. Logothetis, and E.R. Charles. 1990. Functions of the color opponent and broad-band channels of the visual system. *Nature* **343**: 68.

Selemon, L.D. and P.S. Goldman-Rakic. 1988. Common cortical and subcortical targets of the dorsolateral prefrontal and posterior parietal cortices in the rhesus monkey: Evidence for a distributed neural network subserving spatially guided behavior. *J. Neurosci.* **8:** 4049.

Seltzer, B. and D.N. Pandya. 1978. Afferent cortical connections and architectonics of the superior temporal sulcus and surrounding cortex in the rhesus monkey. *Brain Res.* **149:** 1.

―――. 1989. Intrinsic connections and architectonics of the superior temporal sulcus in the rhesus monkey. *J. Comp. Neurol.* **290:** 451.

Sereno, M.I. and J.M. Allman. 1990. Cortical visual areas in mammals. In *Neural basis of visual function* (ed. A. Levinthal). MacMillan, London. (In press.)

Shipp, S. and S. Zeki. 1985. Segregation of pathways leading from V2 to areas V4 and V5 of macaque monkey visual cortex. *Nature* **315:** 322.

―――. 1989. The organization of connections between areas V2 and V5 of macaque monkey visual cortex. *Eur. J. Neurosci.* **1:** 333.

Shiwa, T. 1987. Corticocortical projections to the monkey temporal lobe with particular reference to the visual processing pathways. *Arch. Ital. Biol.* **125:** 139.

Swanson, L.W., C. Kohler, and A. Bjorklund. 1987. The limbic region. I: The septohippocampal system. In *Handbook of chemical neuroanatomy* (ed. A. Bjorklund et al.), vol. 5, p. 125. Elsevier, New York.

Swindale, N.V. 1980. A model for the formation of ocular dominance stripes. *Proc. R. Soc. Lond. B* **208:** 243.

Tigges, J., W.B. Spatz, and M. Tigges. 1973. Reciprocal point-to-point connections between parastriate and striate cortex in the squirrel monkey (*Saimiri*). *J. Comp. Neurol.* **148:** 481.

Tigges, J., M. Tigges, S. Anschel, N. Cross, W.D. Letbetter, and R.L. McBride. 1981. Areal and laminar distribution of neurons interconnecting the central visual cortical areas 17, 18, 19, and MT in squirrel monkey (*Saimiri*). *J. Comp. Neurol.* **202:** 539.

Tootell, R.B.H. and S.L. Hamilton. 1989. Functional anatomy of the second visual area (V2) in the macaque. *J. Neurosci.* **9:** 2620.

Tootell, R.B.H., S.L. Hamilton, and M.S. Silverman. 1985. Topography of cytochrome oxidase activity in owl monkey cortex. *J. Neurosci.* **5:** 2786.

Tootell, R.B.H., M.S. Silverman, E. Switkes, and R.L. DeValois. 1983. Functional organization of the second cortical visual area of primates. *Science* **220:** 737.

Tootell, R.B.H., M.S. Silverman, S.L. Hamilton, E. Switkes, and R.L. DeValois. 1988. Functional anatomy of macaque striate cortex. V. Spatial frequency. *J. Neurosci.* **8:** 1610.

Tusa, R.J., L.A. Palmer, and A.C. Rosenquist. 1981. Multi-

ple cortical visual areas. In *Cortical sensory organization* (ed. C.N. Woolsey), vol. 2., p. 1. Humana Press, Clifton, New Jersey.

Ungerleider, L.G. and M. Mishkin. 1982. Two cortical visual systems. In *Analysis of visual behavior* (ed. D.G. Ingle et al.), p. 549. MIT Press, Cambridge.

Van Essen, D. 1979. Visual areas of the mammalian cerebral cortex. *Annu. Rev. Neurosci.* **2:** 227.

―――. 1985. Functional organization of primate visual cortex. In *Cerebral cortex* (ed. A. Peters and E.J. Jones), vol. 3, p. 259. Plenum Press, New York.

Van Essen, D.C. and C.H. Anderson. 1990. Information processing strategies and pathways in the primate retina and visual cortex. In *Introduction to neural and electronic networks* (ed. S.F. Zornetzer et al.), p. 43. Academic Press, Orlando, Florida.

Van Essen, D.C. and J.H.R. Maunsell. 1980. Two-dimensional maps of the cerebral cortex. *J. Comp. Neurol.* **191:** 255.

Van Essen, D.C. and S.M. Zeki. 1978. The topographic organization of rhesus monkey prestriate cortex. *J. Physiol.* **277:** 193.

Van Essen, D.C., J.H.R. Maunsell, and J.L. Bixby. 1981. The middle temporal visual area in the macaque: Myeloarchitecture, connections, functional properties and topographic organization. *J. Comp. Neurol.* **199:** 293.

Van Essen, D.C., W.T. Newsome, and J.L. Bixby. 1982. The pattern of interhemispheric connections and its relationship to extrastriate visual areas in the macaque monkey. *J. Neurosci.* **2:** 265.

Van Essen, D.C., W.T. Newsome, and J.H.R. Maunsell. 1984. The visual field representation in striate cortex of the macaque monkey: Asymmetries, anisotropies and individual variability. *Vision Res.* **24:** 429.

Van Essen, D.C., W.T. Newsome, J.H.R. Maunsell, and J.L. Bixby. 1986. The projections from striate cortex (V1) to areas V2 and V3 in the macaque monkey: Asymmetries, areal boundaries, and patchy connections. *J. Comp. Neurol.* **224:** 451.

von der Malsburg, C. 1979. Development of ocularity domains and growth behavior of axon terminals. *Biol. Cybernet.* **32:** 49.

Yukie, M., T. Niida, H. Suyama, and E. Iwai. 1988. Interaction of visual cortical areas with the hippocampus in monkeys. *Neuroscience* **14:** 297.

Zeki, S.M. 1976. The functional organization of projections from striate to prestriate visual cortex in the rhesus monkey. *Cold Spring Harbor Symp. Quant. Biol.* **40:** 591.

Zeki, S. and S. Shipp. 1989. Modular connections between areas V2 and V4 of macaque monkey visual cortex. *Eur. J. Neurosci.* **1:** 494.

Neuronal Mechanisms of Motion Perception

W.T. Newsome, K.H. Britten, C.D. Salzman, and J.A. Movshon*

Department of Neurobiology, Stanford University School of Medicine, Stanford, California 94305;
Center for Neural Science and Department of Psychology, New York University, New York, New York 10003

An enduring problem for sensory neurophysiology is to understand how neural circuits in the cerebral cortex mediate our perception of the visual world. In part, the problem endures because it is difficult; the circuits in visual cortex are formidable both in their number and in their complexity. Of equal importance, however, is that investigation of the visual system has yielded a stream of fascinating insights into the nature of cortical information processing. Perhaps foremost among these insights is that individual cortical neurons, in contrast to retinal photoreceptors, respond selectively to perceptually salient features of the visual scene. For example, neurons in striate cortex (or V1) respond selectively to the orientation of local contours, to the direction of motion of a visual stimulus, or to visual contours that fall on disparate locations in the two retinae (for review, see Hubel 1988).

Selective neurons of this nature are often thought to be related to specific aspects of visual perception. For example, orientation-selective neurons could provide the basic information from which we perceive shape and form, direction-selective neurons might play a prominent role in seeing motion, and disparity-selective neurons could mediate the sensation of stereoscopic depth. Although straightforward links between neuronal physiology and visual perception are intuitively appealing, the evidence for such links is generally indirect (see, e.g., Teller 1984).

The goal of our research is to explore—in as direct a manner as possible—the relationship between the physiological properties of direction-selective cortical neurons and the perception of visual motion. All of the physiological experiments were conducted in the middle temporal area (MT, or V5) of rhesus monkeys, a higher-order visual area that lies near the junction of the occipital, parietal, and temporal lobes as illustrated in Figure 1. We chose MT for these experiments because it contains a conveniently organized population of direction-selective neurons. More than 90% of the neurons in MT are direction-selective (Zeki 1974; Maunsell and Van Essen 1983), and they reside in a series of "direction columns" that systematically represents direction of motion at each point in the visual field (Albright et al. 1984). MT is thus a logical site to investigate the role of direction-selective neurons in motion perception.

Our general strategy is to conduct physiological experiments in rhesus monkeys that are trained to discriminate the direction of motion in a random-dot motion display. In such experiments, we can simultaneously monitor physiological events and perceptual performance. The psychophysical task is designed so that good performance depends on signals of the kind carried by direction-selective cortical neurons. We asked three basic questions during the course of the investigation: (1) Is performance on the direction discrimination task impaired following chemical lesions of MT? (2) Are cortical neurons sufficiently sensitive to the motion signal in the random-dot display to account for psychophysical performance? (3) Can we influence perceptual judgments of motion by manipulating the discharge of directionally selective neurons with electrical microstimulation? The answer to each of these questions is "yes" (Newsome and Paré 1988; Newsome et al. 1989a,b; Salzman et al. 1990); we therefore conclude that under the conditions of our experiments, perceptual judgments of motion direction rely heavily on information carried by direction-selective neurons in MT.

Figure 1. Organization of extrastriate visual areas in the macaque monkey. The middle temporal visual area (MT) is located in the depths of the superior temporal sulcus, which has been opened in this drawing so that normally hidden areas are visible. Thin solid lines indicate borders of visual areas that are known with a reasonable degree of certainty. Dashed lines represent borders that are less well documented. (AIT) Anterior inferotemporal area; (DP) dorsal prelunate area; (MT) middle temporal area; (MST) medial superior temporal area; (PIT) posterior inferotemporal area; (STP) superior temporal polysensory area; (VA) ventral anterior area; (VP) ventral posterior area. (Reprinted, with permission, from Maunsell and Newsome 1987.)

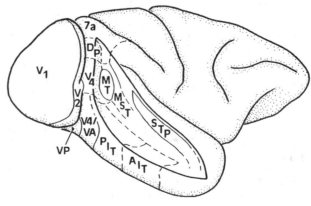

METHODS

We trained five rhesus monkeys (*Macaca mulatta*, three males and two females) on the psychophysical task described below. Prior to training, we surgically implanted each monkey with a search coil for measuring eye movements (Robinson 1963; Judge et al. 1980) and a stainless steel device for immobilizing the head during experiments. After training, a stainless steel recording cylinder was surgically attached to the skull above a craniotomy that permitted microelectrode access to MT. The animals were comfortably seated in a primate chair during daily experimental sessions, and they were returned to their home cages afterward.

Physiological recording. Our general methods for electrophysiological recording in alert monkeys were adapted from those of Wurtz and his colleagues (see, e.g., Mikami et al. 1986). Briefly, the monkey's head was immobilized, and tungsten microelectrodes were advanced into MT using a hydraulic microdrive mounted on the recording cylinder. Action potentials from single MT neurons were isolated, windowed, and displayed on an oscilloscope. The time of occurrence of each action potential, as well as other significant events such as stimulus onset and offset, was stored on a computer disk for subsequent analysis.

Visual stimuli. Each monkey was trained to discriminate the direction of correlated motion in a dynamic random-dot display presented on a CRT screen. The essential feature of this display is that we can vary systematically the signal-to-noise ratio of a unidirectional (or correlated) motion signal within a masking motion noise. The display consists of a stream of randomly positioned dots plotted within a circular aperture. Each dot survives for a brief period of time before being replaced by a partner dot. In one extreme configuration, illustrated in the left-hand panel of Figure 2, each partner dot appeared at a random location on the screen, thus creating random motion noise lacking a correlated motion signal. At the other extreme, illustrated in the right-hand panel of Figure 2, each dot appeared with a fixed displacement in space and time

with respect to its partner so that the motion of each dot was identical across the entire display (100% correlation state). Typically, the monkeys viewed a display that was intermediate between these two extremes. In the display illustrated in the middle panel of Figure 2, for example, 50% of the dots carry the correlated motion signal and 50% of the dots provide a masking motion noise.

Psychophysical procedures. The goal of the psychophysical procedures was to measure the lowest correlation value at which the monkey could successfully discriminate one direction of motion from the direction 180° opposed. The procedures have been described in detail by Newsome and Paré (1988) and are illustrated in Figure 3. On each trial, the monkey was required to maintain its gaze on a central fixation point (FP, Fig. 3A) while attending to the random-dot pattern presented within a display aperture at a peripheral location (large circle). After viewing the display for a brief period, the monkey indicated its judgment of motion direction by making a saccadic eye movement to one of two target LEDs (Pref LED and Null LED) corresponding to the two possible directions of motion. The monkey received a liquid reward for correctly reporting the direction of motion.

Figure 3B illustrates the temporal sequence of events in a single trial. The fixation point appeared at time T1, and the monkey centered its gaze on the fixation point (eye-position trace). After the monkey achieved fixation, the visual display appeared at time T2 and remained visible for 1 or 2 seconds. At time T3, the fixation point and the visual display were extinguished, and the two target LEDs appeared. The monkey indicated its judgment of motion direction by transferring its gaze to the corresponding LED. If the monkey broke fixation prematurely, the trial was aborted and the data were discarded.

In a typical block of trials, the monkey performed the direction discrimination at several correlation levels near psychophysical threshold. The correlation levels were chosen so that the monkey's performance varied from near chance (50% correct) to near perfection.

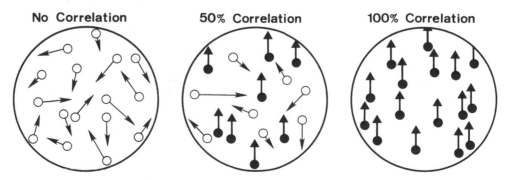

Figure 2. Dynamic random-dot visual display used in the present study. The strength of the motion signal in the display is controlled by specifying the percentage of dots in correlated motion. At 0% correlation (*left* panel), the motion is completely random. At 100% correlation (*right* panel), the motion is completely unidirectional. See text for details. (Reprinted, with permission, from Newsome and Paré 1988.)

A

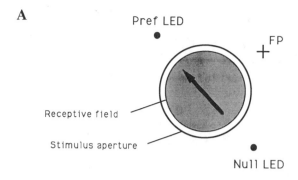

B

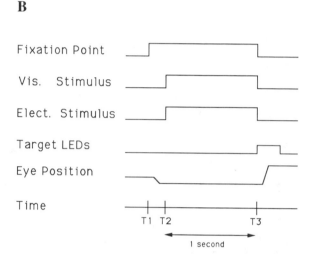

Figure 3. Psychophysical methods employed in the present study. (*A*) Spatial layout of the fixation point (FP), receptive field, stimulus aperture, and target LEDs (Pref LED and Null LED). (*B*) Temporal sequence of events during a single trial. See text for description. (Reprinted, with permission, from Salzman et al. 1990.)

The psychophysical data were compiled into psychometric functions, and sigmoidal curves were fitted to the data. Threshold was considered to be the correlation level at which the monkey made correct decisions on 82% of the trials.

In the single-unit recording experiments, the display aperture was placed directly over the receptive field (shaded circle, Fig. 3A) of the neuron being studied, and the dimensions of the aperture were matched as closely as possible to the dimensions of the receptive field. On each trial, motion was presented in the preferred direction of the neuron (arrow, Fig. 3A) or in the opposite, or null, direction. The speed of the dots in correlated motion was set equal to the preferred speed of the neuron. In this manner, we attempted to create a situation in which the monkey's judgments of motion were likely to depend in part on the responses of the recorded neuron.

In the microstimulation experiments, physiological recordings were obtained from multineuron clusters. The location of the display aperture and the direction and speed of the motion signal were therefore matched

to the properties of the multineuron receptive field. On half of the trials, a train of stimulating pulses (10 μA, 200 Hz, biphasic pulses) began and ended simultaneously with the onset and offset of the random-dot display. Microstimulation effects were assessed by comparing the monkey's performance on stimulated and nonstimulated trials.

In the lesion experiments, it was not necessary to match the visual display in a precise manner to the properties of an individual neuron or group of neurons. Rather, the display aperture was always 10° in diameter and was centered 7° eccentric on the horizontal meridian. Motion was either upward or downward on a given trial, and the direction was randomly chosen from trial to trial. Lesions of MT were made by injecting small volumes (1–4 μl) of the neurotoxin, ibotenic acid (Olney 1983), into MT. The injections were made under physiological control so that the lesion was accurately placed at a point in the visual field map that corresponded to the location in visual space of the stimulus aperture. Histological reconstruction revealed that a single injection of ibotenic acid usually resulted in a lesion restricted to 2–3 mm^2 of cortex.

RESULTS

Figure 4A shows the effect of a unilateral MT lesion on direction-discrimination thresholds in the visual hemifield contralateral to the lesion. Psychophysical threshold is plotted as a function of the speed of the correlated motion signal. The prelesion data, illustrated by the solid curve, represent the mean and standard error of at least ten different threshold measurements at each speed. The postlesion data (dashed line) depict the results of single threshold measurements at three different speeds on the day following the injection of ibotenic acid into MT. MT lesions had a substantial effect on direction-discrimination performance, elevating thresholds by a factor of 3–8 above the mean prelesion level at each speed. Figure 4B shows that the lesion had *no* effect on direction-discrimination thresholds measured at the same time in the hemifield ipsilateral to the lesion. Thus, the threshold elevation illustrated in Figure 4A resulted from the lesion and not from anomalous behavioral variables such as attentional state or degree of water satiation.

This monkey was also trained on an orientation-discrimination task in which he was required to report the orientation of a stationary sine-wave grating that appeared within the same visual display aperture used for the random-dot patterns. We measured contrast thresholds by determining the minimum grating contrast at which the monkey could successfully discriminate orthogonal orientations. Figure 4C shows that the MT lesion had no effect on contrast thresholds measured on the same day as the motion threshold illustrated in Figure 4, A and B. Thus, the MT lesion resulted in striking threshold elevations that appeared to be selective for motion vision and for the hemifield contralateral to the MT lesion. This pattern of results

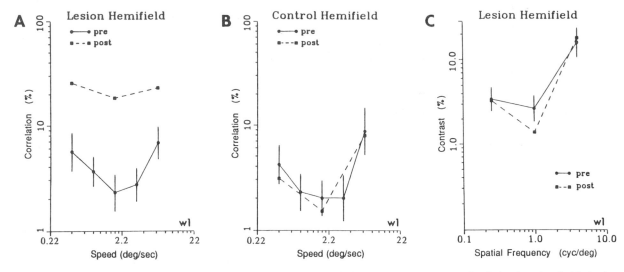

Figure 4. Effects of an MT lesion on psychophysical performance. (*A*) Elevation of direction-discrimination thresholds in the hemifield contralateral to the lesion. The symbols connected by the solid line show the mean of at least ten prelesion thresholds (in percentage of correlated dots) measured for five different stimulus speeds. The error bars indicate standard deviations. The symbols connected by the dashed line show thresholds obtained at three speeds on the first day after an injection of ibotenic acid into MT. (*B*) Lack of effect on direction discrimination thresholds in the ipsilateral hemifield (symbols as in *A*). (*C*) Lack of effect on contrast thresholds in the contralateral hemifield. Thresholds were measured at three different spatial frequencies (symbols as in *A*). (Reprinted, with permission, from Newsome and Paré 1988.)

was observed in a second monkey as well (Newsome and Paré 1988).

The deficit illustrated in Figure 4A was not permanent; with daily practice, the monkey recovered to prelesion performance levels within 1 week of the lesion. That recovery was both quick and complete is partly attributable to the small size of the lesion caused by a single injection of ibotenic acid (2–3 mm² of cortex). In another monkey, we made a complete unilateral MT lesion with multiple injections of ibotenic acid. Direction-discrimination thresholds were permanently elevated in this monkey, although the permanent deficit was smaller than the acute deficit observed during the first week postlesion. Thus, some recovery appears to be mediated by pathways outside MT.

Although the lesion experiments demonstrate that neuronal activity in MT contributes selectively to motion perception, they do not specify the nature of that contribution. A plausible, although extreme, interpretation might hold that MT merely supplies a tonic, nonspecific drive to another visual area, where the critical signals for directional judgments are located. We therefore conducted electrophysiological experiments to determine whether the directional signals in MT could support direction-discrimination performance in our task.

Neuronal Responses during Perceptual Discriminations

We recorded the responses of MT neurons while the monkeys performed a direction-discrimination task that was well matched to the physiological properties of

each neuron (see Methods). A block of trials contained motion stimuli presented in random order in the neuron's preferred or null direction at a range of correlation levels spanning psychophysical threshold. The resulting psychometric function provided a measure of perceptual sensitivity to the motion signal under the conditions of each individual experiment. At the same time, we recorded the response of the MT neuron to the visual stimulus presented on each trial.

Figure 5a illustrates the responses we obtained from one MT neuron during an experiment of this nature. The three histograms show for three correlation levels the number of trials on which the neuron yielded any particular response. In these experiments, the visual stimulus remained on for 2 seconds, and the neuron's response was considered to be the number of action potentials that occurred during the period of stimulus presentation. The hatched bars indicate responses to motion in the neuron's preferred direction, and the solid bars depict responses to motion in the null direction. At the highest correlation level illustrated, 12.8%, the neuron was highly directional: The preferred and null response distributions had little overlap. At the lowest correlation level, 0.8%, the distributions were indistinguishable.

We analyzed these response distributions to obtain a metric of neuronal sensitivity that is directly comparable to the perceptual sensitivity captured by the psychometric function. For this purpose, we employed a simple decision rule to compute the expected performance of an observer who bases his judgments of motion direction on the responses we recorded from the MT neuron under study (Newsome et al. 1989a,b). This expected performance characterizes the sensitivity

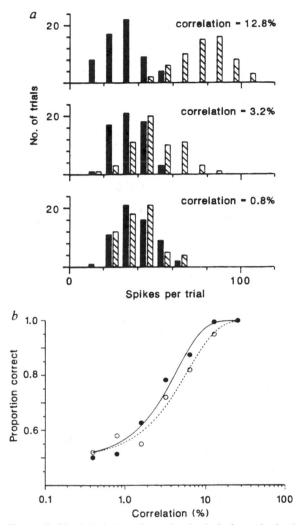

a

b

prefers the opposite direction of motion. Thus, the histograms in Figure 5a represent the responses of both the neuron and the antineuron; the preferred and null directions are simply reversed for the antineuron. If the response of the neuron is larger than that of the antineuron on a particular trial, the decision element chooses motion in the preferred direction of the neuron. If the response of the antineuron is larger, the decision element chooses motion in the preferred direction of the antineuron. At each correlation level, then, the probability of a correct decision is simply the probability that a randomly drawn response from the hatched distribution is larger than a randomly drawn response from the solid distribution. Clearly, this decision rule would yield excellent performance for the data obtained at 12.8% correlation in Figure 5a, while yielding performance near chance (50% correct) at 0.8% correlation.

Using a method derived from signal-detection theory (Green and Swets 1966), we calculated this choice probability at each correlation level for which we obtained data. The resulting neurometric function characterizes the sensitivity of the MT neuron to directional signals in the motion display and is commensurate with the psychometric function that characterizes perceptual sensitivity to the same signals (Tolhurst et al. 1983; Bradley et al. 1987). We obtained both neurometric and psychometric data for a population of 60 neurons in two monkeys. We fitted each data set with a sigmoidal curve according to the method introduced by Quick (1974), and we considered threshold to be the correlation level at which the fitted curve reached 82% correct.

Figure 5b illustrates the neurometric function (closed circles, solid line) computed for the example neuron as well as the psychometric function (open circles, dashed line) obtained on the same set of trials. The two sets of data were statistically indistinguishable ($p > 0.05$). This neuron therefore encoded directional signals with a sensitivity and reliability equal to that with which the monkey discriminated the signals perceptually.

Figure 5. Physiological and psychophysical data obtained simultaneously from an alert rhesus monkey. (*a*) Responses of an MT neuron at three correlation levels near psychophysical threshold. The hatched distributions show responses to motion in the preferred direction; the solid distributions indicate responses to motion in the null direction. Responses were obtained from 60 trials in each direction for each correlation level. As described in the text, we used these response distributions to compute a neurometric function that describes the sensitivity of the neuron to the motion signals in the display. The neurometric function is directly comparable to the psychometric function computed from the monkey's behavioral responses. (*b*) Neurometric (solid symbols, solid curve) and psychometric (open symbols, dashed curve) data obtained on the same set of trials. The psychometric data show the proportion of correct responses obtained from the monkey at each correlation level. Threshold, considered to be the point at which the fitted curve reached 82% correct, was 4.4% correlation for the neuron and 6.1% correlation for the monkey. In other words, the neuron was slightly more sensitive than the monkey. (Reprinted, with permission, from Newsome et al. 1989a.)

of the neuron and may be compared to the actual performance of the monkey on the same block of trials.

We assume that on each trial, a "decision element" compares the responses of two neurons: the one under study and an "antineuron" that differs only in that it

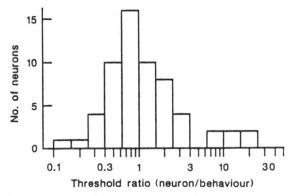

Figure 6. Ratio of neuronal threshold to psychophysical threshold measured during recording experiments from 60 MT neurons. A value of unity indicates perfect correspondence between neurometric and psychometric data. Values near unity were common in our sample. (Reprinted, with permission, from Newsome et al. 1989a.)

Figure 6 illustrates the ratio of neuronal threshold to psychophysical threshold for each of the 60 neurons studied. Neuronal threshold was within a factor of two of psychophysical threshold for 76% of the cells; the neuron illustrated in Figure 5 was therefore typical of the population as a whole.

The physiological data summarized in Figure 6 show that single MT neurons encode directional signals with sufficient sensitivity to account for psychophysical performance. When considered together with the results of the lesion study (above), the data strongly support the notion that perceptual judgments of motion direction are based in large part on the directional signals carried by MT neurons. If this hypothesis is correct, it should be possible to influence judgments of motion direction in a predictable manner by manipulating the responses of MT neurons while a monkey performs the direction-discrimination task. The last experiments were designed to test this possibility.

Influence of Electrical Microstimulation on Perceptual Decisions

In these experiments, we attempted to enhance the representation of a particular direction of motion within the visual cortex by selectively stimulating a population of MT neurons whose preferred directions were similar. Obviously, the major methodological challenge in these experiments was to restrict the microstimulation effects to a physiologically homogeneous group of neurons. The experiment was feasible because MT is organized in a columnar fashion so that neighboring neurons have a common preferred direction. The preferred direction of motion shifts in an orderly manner from column to column so that a complete representation of motion direction exists for each point in the visual field (Albright et al. 1984).

To enhance the representation of a particular direction of motion, we therefore employed microstimulation parameters that activated neurons over distances similar to the dimensions of a typical direction column. We chose parameters (10 μA, 200 Hz, biphasic) that, in a previous study, restricted direct neuronal activation to within approximately 85 μm of the electrode tip (Stoney et al. 1968), and we performed microstimulation experiments at sites in MT where multi-unit recordings maintained a constant preferred direction over at least 150 μm of electrode travel.

Although we attempted to match these dimensions as closely as possible, the exact distribution of stimulated neurons was uncertain. In particular, our physiological exploration of the local geometry of direction columns was restricted to one dimension—the line of electrode travel. We do not know, for example, how the preferred direction may have changed 50 μm to the left or right of the line of electrode travel. In some experiments, then, microstimulation almost certainly affected direction columns other than the target column. In addition, the effects of microstimulation may have spread to other columns, or indeed to other visual areas, by trans-synaptic pathways. However, trans-synaptic spread does not necessarily imply a loss of functional selectivity. Recent experiments in striate cortex (T'so and Gilbert 1988; Gilbert and Wiesel 1989) have shown that individual orientation columns are anatomically connected in a patch-like fashion to other columns with the same preferred orientation. If a similar pattern of local connections exists in MT, it is reasonable to suppose that microstimulation in our experiments activated a *circuit* of neurons related to a particular direction of motion.

Measurements of psychophysical threshold were carried out in our usual manner (see Methods; Fig. 3). The location of the stimulus aperture, the preferred-null axis of motion, and the speed of the correlated dots were matched to the properties of the multi-unit receptive field at the stimulation site. On half of the trials in a block, we applied a train of stimulating pulses that began and ended simultaneously with onset and offset of the random-dot display. The remaining trials provided control measurements of the animal's behavior in the absence of microstimulation. The trials within a block were presented in random order so that the monkey could not anticipate the presence of the stimulating current, the direction of motion, or the correlation level on any given trial.

If MT neurons provide the signals for perceptual judgments of motion direction, we would expect selective microstimulation to bias the animal's decisions toward the preferred direction of the stimulated neurons. Figure 7 shows the results of two experiments in which we observed such an effect. The plots show the proportion of "preferred" decisions (ordinate) as a function of the strength of the motion signal expressed as the percentage of correlated dots (abscissa). A preferred decision is defined as a judgment by the monkey that motion on a particular trial occurred in the preferred direction of the stimulated neurons. Similarly, a "null" decision is a judgment in favor of the null direction. On the abscissa, positive correlations indicate that the stimulus motion was in the preferred direction; negative correlation values signify motion in the null direction. Thus, strong motion signals lie at either end of the abscissa, and weak motion signals fall near the center. The closed symbols illustrate choice performance on stimulated trials and the open symbols depict performance on unstimulated trials. In both experiments, microstimulation caused an increase in the proportion of preferred decisions at each correlation level tested. Summing across correlation levels, microstimulation resulted in a total increase of 43 preferred decisions in Figure 7A and 118 preferred decisions in Figure 7B.

In each experiment illustrated in Figure 7, microstimulation shifted the psychometric function leftward. The magnitude of the leftward shift, expressed in the percentage of correlated dots, provides a measure of the microstimulation effect in units of the visual stimulus. In other words, the leftward shift indicates the visual stimulus that would have yielded a change in choice behavior equivalent to that caused by micro-

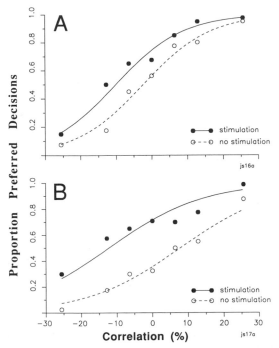

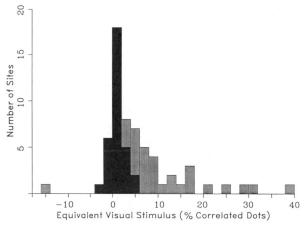

Figure 8. Distribution of microstimulation effects obtained in 62 experiments from three monkeys. In each experiment, the effect of microstimulation was considered to be the shift of the psychometric function in percentage of correlated dots. Positive values on the abscissa indicate leftward shifts (increased preferred decisions); negative values represent rightward shifts (decreased preferred decisions). Experiments that yielded statistically significant shifts (logistic regression, $p < 0.05$) are shown by striped columns. The psychometric function was shifted leftward in 29 of the 30 experiments in which a significant effect was obtained. (Reprinted, with permission, from Salzman et al. 1990.)

Figure 7. Effect of electrical microstimulation in MT on the performance of a rhesus monkey in a direction-discrimination task. The proportion of preferred decisions is plotted against the strength of the motion signal in percentage of correlated dots. Positive correlation values indicate stimulus motion in the preferred direction; negative correlation values represent motion in the null direction. A preferred decision is a judgment by the monkey that stimulus motion on a particular trial was in the preferred direction of the neuron. The open symbols and dashed line represent the monkey's performance on nonstimulated trials; the closed symbols and solid line depict performance on stimulated trials. (*A*) Microstimulation caused a moderate-sized effect in this experiment, shifting the psychometric function leftward by 7.7% correlated dots. (*B*) Microstimulation caused a much larger effect in this experiment; the psychometric function shifted leftward by 20.1% correlated dots. Both effects were statistically significant (logistic regression, $p \leq 0.0001$). (Reprinted, with permission, from Salzman et al. 1990.)

stimulation. We fitted the data in each experiment with sigmoidal curves and used logistic regression analysis (Cox 1970) to estimate the size and statistical significance of the stimulation-induced shift of the psychometric function. In the experiment of Figure 7A, microstimulation caused a leftward shift equivalent to the addition of 7.7% correlated dots to the visual stimulus. The effect was larger in the experiment of Figure 7B, having a stimulus equivalence of 20.1% correlated dots (for both experiments, $p \leq 0.0001$).

We performed such experiments at a total of 62 stimulation sites in three monkeys (Salzman et al. 1990). We observed statistically significant effects ($p < 0.05$) of microstimulation at 18 of 38 sites in one monkey, at 9 of 16 sites in a second monkey, and at 3 of 8 sites in a third. Figure 8 shows the distribution of effects across the entire sample. Positive values correspond to leftward shifts of the psychometric function; negative values indicate rightward shifts. The striped

bars represent experiments in which the effect of microstimulation was statistically significant. In 29 of the 30 experiments with significant effects, the psychometric function was shifted leftward. Thus, microstimulation biased the monkeys' decisions toward the preferred direction of the stimulated neurons in 97% of the experiments in which a significant effect occurred. This result indicates that focal microstimulation selectively enhanced the neural signal related to a particular direction of motion and that the monkey responded to this signal in a meaningful way in the context of the behavioral paradigm.

It is worth noting that a wide range of preferred directions and receptive field locations are represented in the experiments of Figure 8. Within broad limits, we performed the experiment at the first acceptable stimulation site encountered during an experiment without regard to the actual preferred direction or the location of the receptive field. Thus, the metrics of the saccades to the preferred and null target LEDs varied broadly across experiments and were not systematically associated with a particular direction of motion. For this and several other reasons discussed elsewhere (Salzman et al. 1990), it is highly probable that the microstimulation effects resulted from changes in the sensory signals related to motion direction, rather than from changes in motor signals related to the monkey's operant response, a saccadic eye movement.

During this investigation, we were actually surprised that such large perceptual effects could result from a current level that ostensibly activates a region of cortex whose dimensions approximate those of a single column. To interpret the finding properly, it is important to assess the effective spread of the microstimulation current within MT. Two lines of evidence suggest that the effects were well localized. First, we occasionally encountered points in an electrode penetration where the preferred direction of the cluster of neurons shifted abruptly to the opposite direction following a 100-μm advance of the electrode tip. In one penetration, we carried out microstimulation experiments on *both* sides of such a transition point, successfully biasing the monkey's choice behavior in *opposite* directions at stimulation sites separated by only 250 μm. In this experiment, then, direct activation of neurons by the microstimulation current was clearly weighted toward the target column.

Although *direct* excitation appears to be quite local, it may be possible for microstimulation effects to spread *trans*-synaptically within MT, as suggested above. To test this possibility, we required the monkey to perform the psychophysical task in the usual manner, but we applied microstimulation at a topographically noncorresponding site in MT. For example, the stimulating electrode could be placed in the upper quadrant representation in MT while the display aperture was placed in the lower quadrant of the visual hemifield. Under these conditions, the effect of microstimulation was greatly attenuated or eliminated entirely. Microstimulation consistently influenced the monkey's choice behavior only when there was overlap of the display aperture with the receptive field at the microstimulation site. This observation suggests that lateral propagation of directional signals by *trans*-synaptic mechanisms was not widespread within MT, if present at all.

DISCUSSION

The present series of experiments explored the relationship between the responses of direction-selective neurons in extrastriate area MT and the perception of visual motion. We applied several physiological techniques in conjunction with a psychophysical task that required rhesus monkeys to discriminate the direction of motion in a dynamic random-dot display. In an initial set of experiments, lesions of MT caused a selective elevation of thresholds in the direction-discrimination task. The monkeys recovered fully from the effects of partial MT lesions, but a complete unilateral lesion of MT resulted in a permanent impairment. This finding indicates that MT is *necessary* for optimal performance on the direction-discrimination task. In a second set of experiments, a signal-detection analysis of neuronal responses showed that the directional information encoded by MT neurons is *sufficient* to account for psychophysical performance near threshold on the direction-discrimination task. Finally, we found that microstimulation of columns of direction-selective MT neurons can *cause* dramatic changes in a monkey's performance on the direction-discrimination task. When such effects occurred, judgments of motion di-

rection were almost always biased toward the preferred direction of the stimulated neurons.

Although each of these findings suggests further experiments that will permit more precise interpretation, the pattern of results provides compelling evidence that perceptual judgments of motion direction in our psychophysical paradigm are based in part on the activity of direction-selective MT neurons. An important question for future research concerns the neuronal mechanisms that convert such sensory signals into a decision. In our paradigm, the monkey indicates its decision by a saccadic eye movement to one of two locations in space. Clearly, then, neuronal responses in motor centers such as the superior colliculus will reflect the monkey's decision, rather than the strength of the visual stimulus as encoded in the responses of MT neurons. Using anatomy as a guide, it should be possible to determine where this transition occurs in the pathways that link visual cortex to eye movement control centers. Such studies may help localize the decisional mechanisms that integrate sensory and motor functions.

It should be recognized that our results do not require that all, or even most, motion perception is based on the responses of MT neurons. To maximize the chances of establishing a direct link between physiology and perceptual performance, we deliberately selected a visual stimulus that would elicit directional signals in MT neurons in as robust and selective a manner as possible while providing as little information as possible to nondirectional mechanisms. Furthermore, we adjusted the stimulus to be optimal for each neuron or group of neurons that we studied. However, MT is only one locus on an extended cortical pathway that analyzes visual motion information (see Maunsell and Newsome 1987). Whether similar links between neuronal activity and motion vision can be demonstrated at other loci on the pathway is an open and important question.

Finally, it will be of interest to determine whether the general approach employed in the current investigation can be applied to a broader range of questions concerning the physiological basis of visual perception. For example, can we demonstrate that the activity of orientation-selective neurons actually influences perceptual judgments of contour orientation? Can we alter perceptual judgments of relative depth by manipulating the responses of disparity-selective neurons? Clearly, the immediate of goal of such investigations would be to test the intuitive linking assumptions that underlie contemporary research in the physiological basis of vision. A more intriguing possibility, perhaps, is that such investigations will reveal new relationships between physiology and perception that are not apparent at present.

ACKNOWLEDGMENTS

We are grateful to Judy Stein for technical assistance during the course of these experiments. The work was supported by the National Eye Institute (EY-5603 and EY-2017), the Office of Naval Research (N00014-88-K-

0161), and by a McKnight Development Award to W.T.N. C.D.S. is supported by a Medical Student Research Training Fellowship from the Howard Hughes Medical Institute.

REFERENCES

Albright, T.D., R. Desimone, and C.G. Gross. 1984. Columnar organization of directionally selective cells in visual area MT of the macaque. *J. Neurophysiol.* **51:** 16.

Bradley, A., B.C. Skottun, I. Ohzawa, G. Sclar, and R.D. Freeman. 1987. Visual orientation and spatial frequency discrimination: A comparison of single neurons and behavior. *J. Neurophysiol.* **57:** 755.

Cox, D.R. 1970. *Analysis of binary data.* Methuen, London.

Gilbert, C.D. and T.N. Wiesel. 1989. Columnar specificity of intrinsic horizontal and corticocortical connections in cat visual cortex. *J. Neurosci.* **9:** 2432.

Green, D.M. and J.A. Swets. 1966. *Signal detection theory and psychophysics.* Wiley, New York.

Hubel, D.H. 1988. *Eye, brain and vision.* Scientific American, New York.

Judge, S.J., B.J. Richmond, and F.C. Chu. 1980. Implantation of magnetic search coils for measurement of eye position: An improved method. *Vision Res.* **20:**535.

Maunsell, J.H.R. and W.T. Newsome. 1987. Visual processing in primate extrastriate cortex. *Annu. Rev. Neurosci.* **10:** 363.

Maunsell, J.H.R. and D.C. Van Essen. 1983. Functional properties of neurons in the middle temporal visual area (MT) of the macaque monkey. I. Selectivity for stimulus direction, speed and orientation. *J. Neurophysiol.* **49:** 1127.

Mikami, A., W.T. Newsome, and R.H. Wurtz. 1986. Motion selectivity in macaque visual cortex. I. Mechanisms of direction and speed selectivity in extrastriate area MT. *J. Neurophysiol.* **55:** 1308.

Newsome, W.T. and E.B. Paré. 1988. A selective impairment of motion perception following lesions of the middle temporal visual area (MT). *J. Neurosci.* **8:** 2201.

Newsome, W.T., K.H. Britten, and J.A. Movshon. 1989a. Neuronal correlates of a perceptual decision. *Nature* **341:** 52.

Newsome, W.T., K.H. Britten, J.A. Movshon, and M. Shadlen. 1989b. Single neurons and the perception of visual motion. In *Neuronal mechanisms of visual perception* (ed. D. Lam and C.D. Gilbert), p. 171. Portfolio, The Woodlands, Texas.

Olney, J.W. 1983. Excitotoxins: An overview. In *Excitotoxins* (ed. K. Fuxe et al.), p. 82. Macmillan, London.

Quick, R.F. 1974. A vector magnitude model of contrast detection. *Kybernetik* **16:** 65.

Robinson, D.A. 1963. A method of measuring eye movement using a scleral search coil in a magnetic field. *IEEE Trans. Biomed. Eng.* **10:** 137.

Salzman, C.D., K.H. Britten, and W.T. Newsome. 1990. Cortical microstimulation influences perceptual judgments of motion direction. *Nature* **346:** 174.

Stoney, S.D., W.D. Thompson, and H. Asanuma. 1968. Excitation of pyramidal tract cells by intracortical microstimulation: Effective extent of stimulating current. *J. Neurophysiol.* **31:** 659.

Teller, D.Y. 1984. Linking propositions. *Vision Res.* **24:** 1233.

Tolhurst, D.J., J.A. Movshon, and A.F. Dean. 1983. The statistical reliability of signals in single neurons in cat and monkey visual cortex. *Vision Res.* **23:** 775.

T'so, D.Y. and C.D. Gilbert. 1988. The organization of chromatic and spatial interactions in the primate striate cortex. *J. Neurosci.* **8:** 1712.

Zeki, S. 1974. Functional organization of a visual area in the superior temporal sulcus of the rhesus monkey. *J. Physiol.* **236:** 549.

Visual Cortical Signals Supporting Smooth Pursuit Eye Movements

J.A. MOVSHON,* S.G. LISBERGER,† AND R.J. KRAUZLIS†

*Center for Neural Science and Department of Psychology, New York University, New York, New York 10003
†Department of Physiology, W.M. Keck Center for Integrative Neuroscience, and Neuroscience Graduate Program
University of California at San Francisco, California 94143

The visual world is filled with moving objects, and it is therefore no surprise that the visual system contains special mechanisms for the analysis of motion (Hildreth 1983; Nakayama 1985). Visual motion processing has recently been the subject of vigorous neurobiological, psychophysical, and computational analysis. We now have a good understanding of the neuronal mechanisms that represent motion signals in the cerebral cortex (Maunsell and Newsome 1987) and sophisticated models of their function on a number of different levels (Hildreth and Koch 1987). Much interest in visual motion processing mechanisms has come from a desire to link psychophysical studies of motion analysis to their physiological substrate (Newsome et al., this volume). Other investigators have sought to relate computational approaches to motion sensing to biological mechanisms (Adelson and Bergen 1985; Watson and Ahumada 1985). Relatively little attention has been paid to the role that motion signals play in the generation of eye movements. Visual mechanisms that analyze form perform optimally only when the retinal image is stationary or slowly moving (see Graham 1990). One of the main roles of the oculomotor system is to steady the images of moving objects so that they can be properly seen; to perform this stabilization, the oculomotor system must have accurate information about retinal image motion. Signals about motion drive several kinds of eye movements, including the smooth pursuit eye movements that match the velocity of eye movement to the velocity of an attended moving visual target.

There is now good evidence for a cortical pathway specialized for the analysis of visual motion (Maunsell and Newsome 1987). This pathway originates in the M-type (broad-band) cells of the retina and the lateral geniculate nucleus (LGN), passes into the cerebral cortex through V1, and then courses through a complex set of cortical connections to the middle temporal area (MT or V5) and the medial superior temporal area (MST or V5a), which straddle the boundary between the occipital and parietal lobes. The link between the visual motion pathway and pursuit was suggested by the anatomical connections from these areas to the pontine nuclei and accessory optic system, and thence to regions of the cerebellum known to be involved in pursuit eye movements (Brodal 1978, 1979). Focal lesions of MT and MST selectively disrupt pursuit eye move-

ments (Newsome et al. 1985; Dürsteler et al. 1986), producing deficits consistent with the idea that these areas are responsible for providing visual motion signals that support pursuit commands. Although these motion-analyzing neurons are at least six synapses away from the photoreceptors, and the motion information must traverse at least five more synapses to reach extraocular motoneurons, the study of visual motion processing and of the oculomotor system has narrowed the sensorimotor link to the cortico-ponto-cerebellar pathways.

Just as students of motion processing have typically paid little attention to the motor functions associated with motion signals, so those who study pursuit have largely ignored the consequences of visual processing for the kinds of signals available to control pursuit. For example, Robinson et al. (1986) offer a control-theory model of the pursuit system in which the role of the visual system is to produce a replica (delayed 50 msec) of the retinal motion signal. Because their model of visual processing is so simple, Robinson and his colleagues must attribute the dynamic features of pursuit to properties of the motor pathways. Recently, however, it has become clear that many features of pursuit may depend not on motor processing, but on the sensory analysis that precedes it (Lisberger and Westbrook 1985; Lisberger et al. 1987). These insights have come largely from studies that concentrate on analyzing the first "open-loop" phase of pursuit, during which the effects of the pursuit eye movement on retinal target velocity have not yet made themselves felt. Krauzlis and Lisberger (1989) analyzed many of these data and proposed a model with a more elaborate visual "front end." The properties of the visual processing in the model largely account for the dynamics of both open- and closed-loop pursuit, suggesting that much of the detail of the pursuit eye movement response might reflect constraints arising from visual processing, rather than motor output pathways.

The experiments reported in this paper seek to uncover the degree to which signals in the motion sensing pathway can *by themselves* explain the behavior of the pursuit system. Our approach was to study neurons at a high level in the cortical motion pathway, in area MT, with target motion profiles that reveal interesting features of the pursuit system. Our results show that neurons in MT carry signals having many features in common with pursuit, and they suggest that visual, rather than motor, processes may be the determinants of many features of smooth pursuit eye movements.

METHODS

Unit recording. We used conventional methods to record the activity of single isolated units in area MT of anesthetized, paralyzed macaque monkeys (*M. fascicularis*). Tungsten-in-glass microelectrodes (Merrill and Ainsworth 1972) were introduced hydraulically into MT through a craniotomy and durotomy placed over the overlying parietal cortex; unit activity was conventionally amplified and displayed; standard pulses triggered by each action potential were sent to a PDP11 computer for analysis and storage.

The monkeys were anesthetized with an opioid (sufentanil citrate, 4–12 μg/kg/hr) and paralyzed with a curariform muscle relaxant (vecuronium bromide, 0.1 mg/kg/hr), given together with isotonic lactated dextrose in Ringer's solution in intravenous infusion at 10.4 ml/hr. EEG, EKG, end-expiratory P_{CO2}, and body temperature were continuously monitored and maintained in a suitable state to verify that the animal remained properly anesthetized and in good physiological condition.

The corneas were protected with +2D clear contact lenses; supplementary lenses chosen by direct ophthalmoscopy and by optimizing the visual responses of visual units were used to make the retinae conjugate with a CRT display between 30 and 57 cm distant. Visual stimuli were generated on this display by the same PDP11 computer that monitored unit activity and controlled the sequence of stimulus presentations. In the experiments described here, the stimuli were always texture fields consisting of 300–500 randomly positioned bright dots on a dark background; the mean luminance of the display was 10 cd/m^2, and the frame rate was 250 Hz. Suitable motion targets were generated by moving all the dots in a selected region. For most cells, the entire field of dots (subtense: 10–18°) moved; for the minority of cells for which peripheral suppression was noticeable, the motion was confined to the excitatory receptive field, and the dots in the periphery remained stationary. We used extended texture stimuli rather than the single spots typically used in oculomotor work so that we would not need to be concerned in the design of experiments with the location and the timing of the movement of the target; it seems unlikely that this difference would have an important effect on our results. We first established the neuron's direction tuning for our targets; in all the experiments described here, the targets moved in the preferred direction.

The stimuli in a particular experimental series were presented by the computer in a randomly interleaved sequence to attenuate the effects of response variability; average response histograms were calculated and viewed on-line, and the data were stored on disk for later off-line analysis.

We studied 45 neurons from five monkeys in sufficient detail to include in the analysis. All receptive fields were centered within 5° of the fovea. The position of each electrode track was marked with a small electrolytic lesion made by passing current through the electrode tip (2 μA, 2 sec, tip negative). At the end of each experiment, the monkey was killed with an overdose of thiopental sodium and perfused with 4% buffered paraformaldehyde. The region of cortex containing the electrode tracks was blocked, sectioned, and stained for Nissl substance and for myelin. All recording sites were verified to lie within the myeloarchitectural boundaries of MT (Van Essen et al. 1981).

Eye movement recording. Oculomotor data were obtained from a trained rhesus monkey (*Macaca mulatta*), using methods described elsewhere (Lisberger and Westbrook 1985). During experiments, the monkey, with its head restrained, sat in a primate chair facing a tangent screen 114 cm distant, onto which visual targets were projected. The monkey was rewarded for keeping his eye position within 2° of a visual target whose motion was unpredictable from trial to trial; the target was a white spot 0.1–0.3° in diameter viewed against a dark background, and its intensity was set to be several hundred times the threshold of visibility for a human observer. Before the test portion of the trial began, a stationary red 0.1° fixation target of comparable intensity was presented for an unpredictable period of 600–900 msec.

Eye position was recorded using a magnetic search coil technique. Eye position signals were suitably low-pass-filtered, sampled at 1-msec intervals, and stored (along with other relevant timing information) by a PDP11 computer, which also controlled the stimulus display and the behavioral contingencies.

RESULTS

It has long been known that the principal visual signal that drives pursuit is an encoded representation of target direction and speed. Recent analyses have suggested that in addition to signals purely related to speed, the pursuit system also makes use of information about target acceleration and also that its behavior depends on the time course of target presentation. To learn whether these kinds of information were usefully represented in the activity of MT neurons, we examined their responses to targets moving with controlled timings, speeds, and accelerations and compared the results with eye-movement data.

Effects of Target Speed

Representation of target speed. The most useful information on the effect of target speed on pursuit comes from studies using variants of the "step-ramp" paradigm introduced by Rashbass (1961). In experiments of this kind, a stationary visual fixation target simultaneously jumps and begins to move at a constant speed. The pursuit response to step-ramp stimuli consists of a rapid acceleration of the eye to a velocity approximating the target velocity; "catch-up" saccades designed to foveate the moving target can be eliminated by suitable choices of step and ramp parameters. Figure 1 shows pursuit data from a monkey working in a modified step-ramp task. The paradigm is indicated on the left (Fig. 1a): The fixation target was turned on to initiate the trial; then, after an unpredictable interval, the tracking target appeared, stood still for 300 msec, and then moved at a constant speed. The onset of target movement coincided with the offset of the fixation target, which cued the monkey to begin tracking. The traces in Figure 1b show averages of the monkey's eye speed for 400 msec following the beginning of the motion, for seven target speeds. Note that the pursuit

response is graded with speed, becoming both more vigorous and more extended in time at higher target speeds.

Figure 1c shows an analysis of these traces to examine the effects of target speed on eye acceleration during the open-loop phase of pursuit. The value of eye acceleration is plotted for each target speed for an early interval (the first 40 msec of pursuit) and a later interval (the next 60 msec) in each averaged record. Both components of eye acceleration grow monotonically with target speed, with the earliest acceleration component (lower curve) saturating around 15°/sec. At much higher target speeds (in excess of 120°/sec, not shown), the later component of the pursuit response falls off (Lisberger and Westbrook 1985).

This sort of monotonically graded response to target

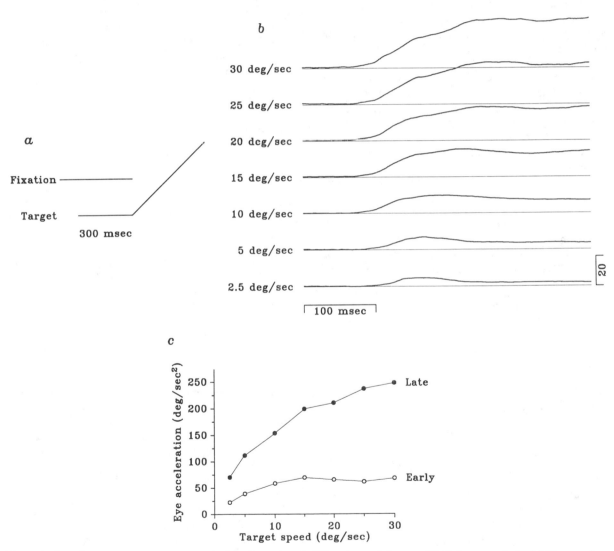

Figure 1. Pursuit eye movement responses to targets moving at different speeds in a modified step-ramp task. (*a*) The monkey viewed a central fixation target before the beginning of each trial. After an unpredictable interval of 600–900 msec, the pursuit target appeared; 300 msec later, the fixation target disappeared and the pursuit target began to move, signaling to the monkey the beginning of the pursuit task. (*b*) Averaged eye-speed traces from trials of the type shown in *a*, for leftward pursuit. Each trace is the average of between 10 and 20 responses. The vertical calibration next to the bottom record is 20°/sec. (*c*) Eye acceleration values derived from the records shown in *b* and similar data for rightward pursuit. The curve marked "early" plots acceleration in the first 40 msec of pursuit; the curve marked "late" plots acceleration in the following 60 msec.

speed has led to the notion that the visual representation of target speed might be similarly graded (see, e.g., Robinson et al. 1986; Krauzlis and Lisberger 1989). Interestingly, the representation of target speed by MT neurons is not graded in this way but is instead based on a multiple-channel strategy in which each neuron is selective for a range of speeds, and neurons having different speed preferences are intermingled (Maunsell and Van Essen 1983). Thus, the visual motion signal driving pursuit responses to different target speeds cannot come from a single neuron or pool of neurons but must derive instead from separate groups of speed-tuned neurons. This transformation of signals from an array of speed-tuned channels to a pursuit command remains unexplored.

Latency dependence on speed. Pursuit responses to targets of different speeds are graded, but responses to low and high speeds are not scaled replicas of one another—there is a systematic effect of target speed on pursuit latency. Inspection of the traces in Figure 1b shows that pursuit begins with a shorter latency for higher target speeds. Figure 2 shows an analysis of this effect, plotting the latency of pursuit against the inverse of target speed; the dependence of latency on speed is approximately linear when represented in this way. The intercept of the plotted regression line is the expected pursuit latency at high target speeds, and the slope may be thought of as the distance through which the target must move before pursuit signals arise. The values for the data shown are 81 msec and 4.1 min of arc, respectively. We were interested to determine whether the onset responses of MT neurons depended on latency in a way that could be related to this aspect of pursuit.

Figure 3 shows data obtained from a single MT neuron. Figure 3a shows averaged response histograms

to a target that remained stationary for 256 msec after it was turned on, and then began to move with the speed indicated under each histogram at the time indicated by the speed trace (bottom) and vertical line. The speed tuning of the cell is evident in the dependence of response magnitude on speed (Fig. 3b). It is also clear that response latency decreased systematically with increasing target speed. This relationship is plotted (again representing speed on an inverse axis) in Figure 3c. The intercept in this case is 49 msec, and the slope is 1.8 min of arc.

Figure 4 compares the derived slope and intercept parameters for 32 MT neurons with the values obtained from the monkey (Fig. 2). The distribution of the value of latency/speed slope for the MT neurons varies fairly widely, but it is centered on the value obtained for the monkey. The shortest asymptotic latencies in the MT cell population are 25–30 msec shorter than the behavioral asymptotic latency, but this difference should be interpreted with caution because of the somewhat different conditions of visual stimulation in the two sets of experiments.

Motion onset delay. Krauzlis and Lisberger (1987, 1989, and unpubl.) have studied an additional factor that influences both the latency and the briskness of pursuit eye movement responses to step-ramp targets: the duration of illumination of the pursuit target before it begins to move. Figure 5 shows the nature and magnitude of this effect. Figure 5a shows a schematic representation of the oculomotor paradigm. At the beginning of a trial, the fixation light was illuminated. The pursuit target then was illuminated; after an unpredictable delay (dashed line), the fixation light was extinguished and the pursuit target began to move at 5°/sec. The monkey was obliged to maintain fixation on the fixation target until it disappeared.

The traces in Figure 5b show averaged eye speed records for the series of delay values indicated beside each histogram. The beginning of each record corresponds to the onset of target motion. The eye-speed records all have the same general form: a rapid rise in eye speed to or slightly beyond the target speed, followed by a more gradual approach to the 5°/sec target speed. Inspection of the records reveals that the onset of the response is delayed and the initial eye acceleration is reduced when the motion onset delay is less than 100 msec or so. This impression is confirmed by Figure 5c, which plots the eye acceleration during the first 40 msec of pursuit as a function of the delay of motion onset from target onset.

Krauzlis and Lisberger (1989) interpreted these data in the context of a mechanism that signals transient acceleration by differentiating an internal representation of target speed, but it is also possible to view this effect in more basic visual terms. When a target flashes on, the transient spreads spatiotemporal energy over the entire range of speeds and directions. If the target starts moving as soon as it appears, one might imagine that accurate information about motion would be

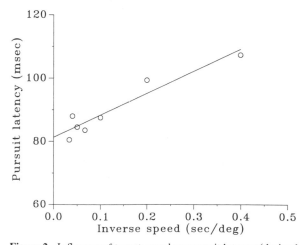

Figure 2. Influence of target speed on pursuit latency (derived from the data shown in Fig. 1b). Latency was determined by identifying the first point in averaged eye-speed records at which speed exceeded the resting value. Speed is plotted on an inverse scale. When represented in this way, the relationship between latency and speed is roughly linear; the solid line is the least-squares regression through the data. The intercept of this function is 81 msec, and its slope is 4.1 min of arc.

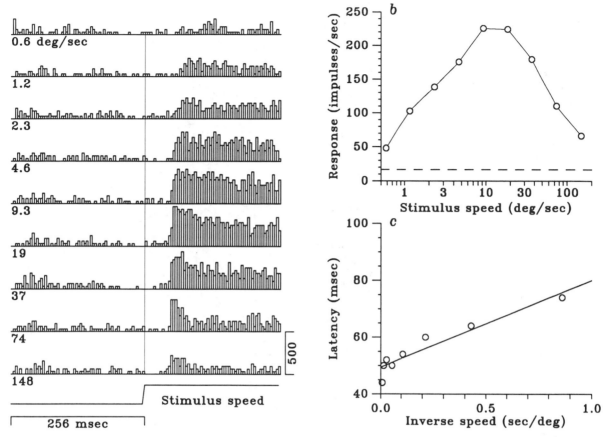

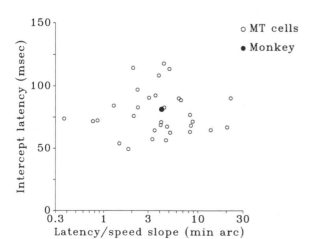

Figure 3. Influence of target speed on the response of a single MT neuron. (*a*) Average response histograms showing the responses to the onset of motion at different speeds (indicated under each histogram). At time 0 (the left end of each histogram), a stationary field of random dots appeared on a previously dark screen. After 256 msec (step in the speed trace at bottom, line through the histograms), the dots began to move at the indicated speed. The vertical calibration beside the bottom histogram is 500 impulses/sec. (*b*) Speed tuning curve for the same neuron, derived from measurements of the neuron's steady-state responses to dot fields drifting at different speeds. The dashed line indicates the maintained discharge measured in the presence of a stationary random dot field. (*c*) Relationship between the latency of neuronal response and stimulus speed, derived from the histograms shown in *a*. As in Fig. 2, speed is plotted on an inverse scale, and the solid line is the least-squares regression line. The intercept in this case is 49 msec, and the slope is 1.8 min arc.

Figure 4. Distributions of the slope and intercept parameters derived from regression fits (Figs. 2 and 3c) for 32 MT neurons (○) compared with the data for the monkey (●).

masked or attenuated by the spatiotemporal "splatter" produced by the flash. If, on the other hand, enough time elapsed between target onset and motion onset for this transient signal to die away, the beginning of target motion could produce an unmasked response. With this explanation in mind, we decided to examine the responses of MT neurons as a function of the delay between target onset and motion onset.

Figure 6 shows the responses of the same MT neuron whose data were shown in Figure 3 to the onset of the motion of a random-dot target that was illuminated for a variable period before it began to move. The extent of the stationary foreperiod is indicated by the leftward extension of each histogram before the time (deflection in the bottom trace) at which target motion began. Clearly, the neuron's response shows an effect of varying motion onset delay that is qualitatively similar to that shown in the eye movement data of Figure 5,

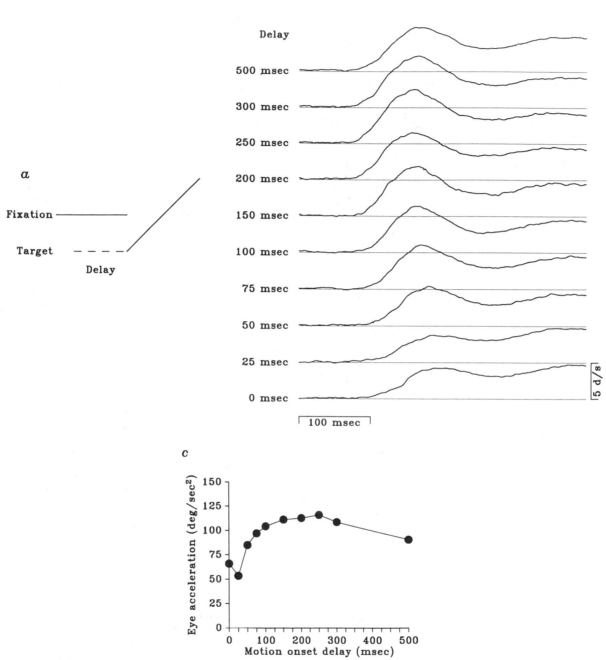

Figure 5. Pursuit eye movement responses to targets whose motion onset was delayed by different amounts. (*a*) Monkey viewed a central fixation target before the beginning of each trial. After an unpredictable interval of 600–900 msec, the pursuit target appeared; a variable delay later, the fixation target disappeared and the pursuit target began to move at 5°/sec. (*b*) Averaged eye-speed traces from trials of the type shown in *a*, for leftward pursuit. Each trace is the average of between 10 and 20 responses. The vertical calibration next to the bottom record is 5°/sec. (*c*) Eye acceleration values during the first 40 msec of pursuit, derived from the data shown in *b*, and from other data for rightward pursuit.

becoming brisker and shorter in latency as the motion onset delay is increased.

To analyze this similarity, we took each histogram, aligned it to the motion onset, and then calculated the difference between the response and the response measured with no onset delay (the bottom record in Fig. 6). We then calculated the peak of this difference

firing rate function as a function of delay. The results of this analysis are shown in Figure 7. Figure 7a shows data from the neuron whose responses are illustrated in Figure 6; Figure 7b shows data from a second neuron that was studied over a wider range of delays. Plainly, both neurons show an effect of motion onset delay that is similar in time course to the effect of such delays on

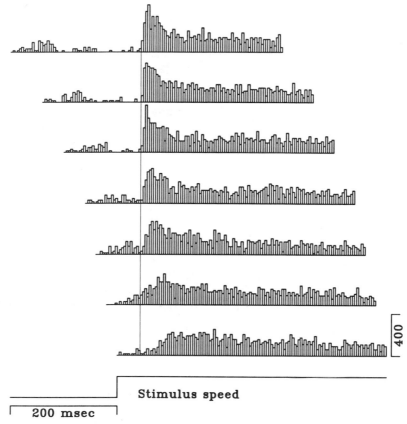

Figure 6. Responses of an MT neuron to target motion beginning with a variable delay after target onset. The target appeared at the beginning of each average response histogram; the histograms have been shifted so that they are aligned on the subsequent onset of target motion (speed trace at bottom). The vertical line marks a time 44 msec after motion onset to facilitate comparison of latency across the histograms. The vertical calibration on the bottom histogram is 400 impulses/sec; the speed for all targets was 37.1°/sec.

eye acceleration (Fig. 5). All the neurons we studied in this way showed similar effects of motion onset delay, although the time course of the effect varied slightly from neuron to neuron.

Effects of Target Acceleration

The data and simulations of Krauzlis and Lisberger (1987, 1989) suggested that the pursuit system might have access to information about both the speed and acceleration of visual targets. We therefore explored the responses of MT neurons to targets whose speed and acceleration varied.

Figure 8 shows the responses of the same MT neuron (data shown in Figs. 3 and 6) to a series of target accelerations and decelerations. The histograms on the left show responses to a 128-msec acceleration pulse that produced a ramp of target speed, from a base speed of 0 (bottom trace). The histograms on the right show responses to a similar deceleration pulse that brought target speed from some value down to 0. The acceleration values are shown under the left-hand histogram of each pair, and the terminal speeds (for acceleration trials) or initial speeds (for deceleration trials) are given under the right-hand histogram. For

low acceleration values, the neuron responded with a simple increase or decrease in firing (for acceleration and deceleration, respectively), suggesting that only speed-related signals were present. When the acceleration values increased, however, the neuron's response developed a distinct pulse coinciding with the period during which speed changed. This response pulse could represent the kind of acceleration-related signal needed to account for the sensitivity of the pursuit system to target acceleration.

Note that the acceleration-related responses do not suggest any particular tuning for acceleration on the part of the neuron. For example, response pulses were evident both for target acceleration and deceleration. Inspection of the data, in combination with the speed tuning of the neuron (Fig. 3b), suggests that these acceleration-related responses could arise as a simple consequence of the neuron's speed tuning. Notice that acceleration-related response pulses occur when the stimulus speed ramps between values that straddle the neuron's optimal speed (roughly 15°/sec; Fig. 3). This response pattern could arise because the stimulus' speed traverse begins at a low (or high) speed ineffective for the neuron, changes to an intermediate value that is more effective, and then ends at a high (or low)

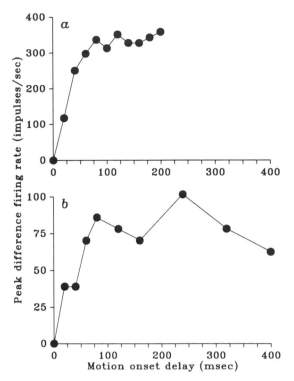

value that is again ineffective. Thus, the "pulse" arises not from a specific sensitivity to acceleration, but from the fact that the stimulus traverses the neuron's speed tuning curve in a way that produces a pulse of excitation. We have attempted to account quantitatively for response waveforms like those shown in Figure 8 by synthesizing predicted responses from the neuron's magnitude and latency of response to different speeds (Fig. 3). In some cases, including the neuron whose data are shown, these predictions are reasonably accurate, but they do not account for the observed asymmetry between responses to acceleration and deceleration. It seems to be necessary to add an additional dynamic stage in order to account properly for the shape of the response, which often includes a markedly greater response to target acceleration than to deceleration.

Another way to determine whether MT neurons are especially sensitive to target acceleration is to try to learn whether their acceleration-related responses are invariant when other stimulus conditions change. Figure 9 shows data (again for the same neuron as in Figs. 3, 6, and 8) from an experiment of this kind, in which we studied the effect of varying the base speed on acceleration-related responses. The left-hand histograms show responses to target accelerations whose durations were adjusted so that speed increased from a base speed of 0°/sec to 18.5°/sec (a value close to optimum: Fig. 3c). The right-hand histograms show responses to an identical acceleration series, but with a base speed of 18.5°/sec and a terminal speed of 37.1°/sec (above optimum). It is clear, first, that base speed

Figure 7. Response enhancement produced by delaying the onset of target motion in two MT neurons. Response histograms like those shown in Fig. 6 were aligned to motion onset and subtracted; the value plotted is the peak of the resulting difference histogram and represents the degree of response enhancement produced by motion onset delay. (a) Responses of the neuron whose data are shown in Fig. 6. (b) Responses of a second neuron studied over a wider range of delays.

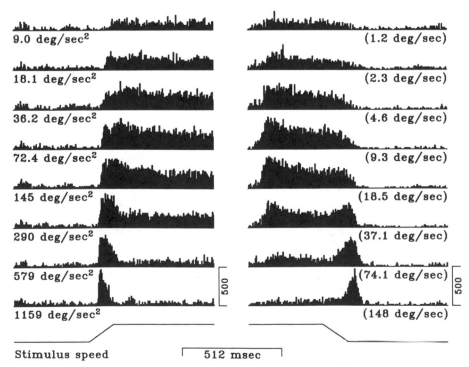

Figure 8. Responses of an MT neuron to target acceleration (left) and deceleration (right). The trace at the bottom of each column gives the time course of stimulus speed throughout the trial; acceleration or deceleration occurred in a 128-msec interval delayed 384 msec from stimulus onset. Stimulus acceleration (or deceleration) is given under the left-hand histogram of each pair; the terminal (or initial) target speed is given under the right-hand histogram of each pair. The initial speed for acceleration trials was 0°/sec, as was the terminal speed for deceleration trials. The calibration next to the bottom histograms is 500 impulses/sec.

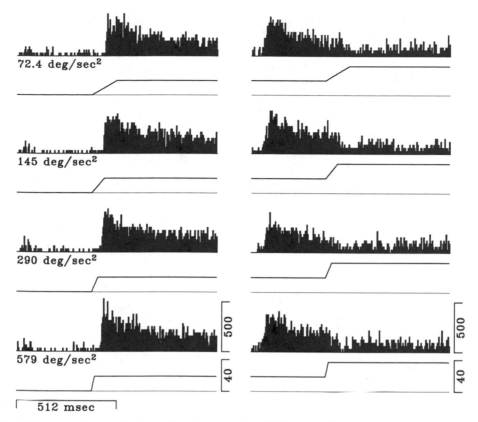

Figure 9. Effect of base speed on acceleration-related responses in an MT neuron. The trace under each histogram shows stimulus speed throughout the trial. For the histograms on the left, the initial speed was 0, and the acceleration duration was adjusted so that the terminal speed was 18.5°/sec. For the histograms on the right, the initial speed was 18.5°/sec and the terminal speed was 37.1°/sec. The acceleration for each pair of histograms is given under the left-hand member of the pair. The calibrations on the lowest histograms and speed traces are 500 impulses/sec and 40°/sec, respectively.

had an important effect on the response. When the target accelerated from 0 to near optimal speed, there was a brisk response including a modest acceleration-related pulse. However, when the target accelerated from near optimal speed to a much higher speed, there was a mild decrease in response. Second, the specific acceleration value had little influence on the response—all the histograms on the left or on the right are rather similar. This pattern of results can again be predicted from the neuron's simple speed tuning (Fig. 3b), by noting that the left-hand histograms show responses to speed modulation between two speeds of very different effectiveness, whereas the right-hand histograms show responses to speed modulation between two speeds of roughly similar effectiveness.

These experiments suggest that MT neurons are not "acceleration-tuned" in the same sense that they are direction- or speed-tuned, because direction and speed tuning depend very little on other stimulus parameters. However, all the neurons we studied showed brisk acceleration-related discharge pulses for suitable choices of base speed and acceleration. These response pulses might well serve the purpose of providing signals like those hypothesized by Krauzlis and Lisberger's (1989) model, in which acceleration signals serve mostly to enhance pursuit commands when retinal velocity changes. They could not serve, however, as the basis for a comprehensive representation of target acceleration in MT.

DISCUSSION

The experiments in this paper were designed to explore the notion that many of the dynamic features of pursuit eye movements are a consequence of fundamentally visual, rather than motor, processes. The results reveal that the response properties of neurons in area MT do indeed have many features in common with the pursuit command signals inferred from studies of the open-loop phase of pursuit in monkeys. In particular, the dependence of MT response latency on target speed is similar to the dependence of pursuit latency on target speed; the effects of introducing delays between the onset of a target and the onset of its motion are similar for MT responses and for pursuit; MT neurons produce acceleration-related responses that may provide the target acceleration signal inferred from analysis of the pursuit system.

A natural question about these results is whether the interesting features of MT responses arise in MT or whether they might be present even earlier in the visual pathway. We have not studied the responses of neurons in V1 to the kinds of stimuli used in these experiments, but it is reasonable to suppose that neurons there might give similar responses. Supporting this is evidence from a series of simulations in which we explored the response of a modified version of the motion energy sensor model of Adelson and Bergen (1985) to motion profiles of the kind used in our experiments. Adelson and Bergen's model is an idealized model of directional mechanisms in primary visual cortex (cf. Emerson et al. 1987). Interestingly, the motion energy simulation seems to capture the dependence of response latency on target speed (Fig. 3) and to generate acceleration-related response pulses under conditions similar to those used to collect the data shown in Figures 8 and 9. The motion energy model does not, however, seem to show any effect of motion onset delay (Fig. 6). Our suggestion that the effect of motion onset delay might arise through interference from transiently elicited signals in sensors having other preferred speeds and directions suggests that interactions among motion sensitive neurons—not included in the Adelson and Bergen model—might be necessary to account for this effect.

A second question concerns the nature of the further processing needed to transform the visual motion signal provided by MT into pursuit commands. Our results suggest that relatively little transformation of the neural signal would be required, other than the transformation from the channel-based representation of speed in MT into the monotonic representation needed to drive eye acceleration (Figs. 1 and 3). A major component of pursuit control, however, is its dependence on conscious decision and motivational processes. For example, the pursuit system must select the components of the visual image that are the target to be tracked and exclude signals related to the movement of other targets or the background. Pursuit also depends strongly on the alertness and attentional state of the animal. Studies of the discharge of cortical neurons during pursuit initiation suggest that few signals of this kind are present in MT neurons. It is possible to imagine that the visual motion signals from MT are combined with or gated by decision-related signals arising elsewhere in the cerebral cortex, to provide suitably formulated signals passing into the ponto-cerebellar pathways, and thence into the cerebellum and brainstem to form motor commands. This scheme would place MT just on the sensory side of the sensory-motor link, and the ponto-cerebellar pathways at the beginning of a set of fundamentally motor pathways. It would appear that by continuing to study visual motion processing in the areas associated with MT, in combination with the decision-related processes arising elsewhere in the pursuit pathways, we can come in time to a full account of the sensory-motor interactions that give rise to this basic class of visuomotor behavior.

ACKNOWLEDGMENTS

This research was supported by National Institutes of Health grants EY-02017 and EY-03878. We are grateful to Suzanne Fenstemaker, Jonathan Levitt, and Nicholas Port for their assistance.

REFERENCES

Adelson, E.H. and J.R. Bergen. 1985. Spatiotemporal energy models for the perception of motion. *J. Opt. Soc. Am. A* **2:** 284.

Brodal, P. 1978. The corticopontine projection in the rhesus monkey: Origin and principles of organization. *Brain* **101:** 251.

———. 1979. The pontocerebellar projection in the rhesus monkey: An experimental study with retrograde axonal transport of horseradish peroxidase. *Neuroscience* **4:** 193.

Dürsteler, M.R., R.H. Wurtz, and W.T. Newsome. 1986. Directional and retinotopic pursuit deficits following lesions of the foveal representation within the superior temporal sulcus of the macaque monkey. *J. Neurophysiol.* **57:** 1262.

Emerson, R.C., J.R. Bergen, and E.H. Adelson. 1987. Movement models and directionally selective neurons in the cat's visual cortex. *Soc. Neurosci. Abstr.* **13:** 1623.

Graham, N.V. 1990. *Visual pattern analyzers.* Oxford University Press, New York.

Hildreth, E.C. 1983. *The measurement of visual motion.* MIT Press, Cambridge, Massachusetts.

Hildreth, E.C. and C. Koch. 1987. The analysis of visual motion: From computational theory to visual mechanisms. *Annu. Rev. Neurosci.* **10:** 477.

Krauzlis, R.J. and S.G. Lisberger. 1987. Smooth pursuit eye movements are not driven simply by target velocity. *Soc. Neurosci. Abstr.* **13:** 170.

———. 1989. A control systems model of smooth pursuit eye movements with realistic emergent properties. *Neural Computat.* **1:** 114.

Lisberger, S.G. and L.E. Westbrook. 1985. Properties of visual inputs that initiate horizontal smooth pursuit eye movements in monkeys. *J. Neurosci.* **5:** 1662.

Lisberger, S.G., E.J. Morris, and L. Tychsen. 1987. Visual motion processing and sensory-motor integration for smooth pursuit eye movements. *Annu. Rev. Neurosci.* **10:** 97.

Maunsell, J.H.R and W.T. Newsome. 1987. Visual processing in monkey extrastriate cortex. *Annu. Rev. Neurosci.* **10:** 363.

Maunsell, J.H.R. and D.C. Van Essen. 1983. Functional properties of neurons in the middle temporal visual area (MT) of the macaque monkey. I. Selectivity for stimulus direction, speed and orientation. *J. Neurophysiol.* **49:** 1127.

Merrill, E.G. and A. Ainsworth. 1972. Glass-coated platinum-plated microelectrodes. *Med. Biol. Eng.* **10:** 662.

Nakayama, K. 1985. Biological motion processing: A review. *Vision Res.* **25:** 625.

Newsome, W.T., R.H. Wurtz, M.R. Dürsteler, and A. Mikami. 1985. Deficits in visual motion processing following ibotenic acid lesions of the middle temporal visual area of the macaque monkey. *J. Neurosci.* **5:** 825.

Rashbass, C. 1961. The relationship between saccadic and smooth tracking eye movements. *J. Physiol.* **159:** 326.

Robinson, D.A., J.L. Gordon, and S.E. Gordon. 1986. A model of the smooth pursuit eye movement system. *Biol. Cybern.* **55:** 43.

Van Essen, D.C., J.H.R. Maunsell, and J.R. Bixby. 1981. The middle temporal visual area in the macaque: Myeloarchitecture, connections, functional properties and topographic organization. *J. Comp. Neurol.* **199:** 293.

Watson, A.B. and A.J. Ahumada. 1985. Model of human visual-motion sensing. *J. Opt. Soc. Am. A* **2:** 322.

Functional Specialization for Visual Motion Processing in Primate Cerebral Cortex

R.H. Wurtz, D.S. Yamasaki, C.J. Duffy, and J.-P. Roy
Laboratory of Sensorimotor Research, National Eye Institute, National Institutes of Health, Bethesda, Maryland 20892

The identification of specific areas of extrastriate cortex of the monkey has been an impetus for the study of higher-order processing in the visual system. The identification of additional areas, analysis of their interconnections, and delineation of the visual properties of cells in these areas have strengthened the view that visual processing is carried out in a series of different areas (for review, see Van Essen 1985; Maunsell and Newsome 1987).

The function of these different areas has generally remained less certain than their identification. As Zeki (1974a,b) originally suggested, these areas may make different contributions to different visual functions, such as color, form, and motion. Furthermore, these functionally distinct areas may be grouped into streams of visual processing as first suggested by Ungerleider and Mishkin (1982). These authors argued that a ventral stream passed through area V4 to the inferotemporal cortex, which served color and form perception, and that a dorsal stream passed through the middle temporal (MT) area to parietal cortex, which was devoted to spatial localization. Both of these proposals depend on some degree of specialization of function within specific extrastriate areas.

Evidence for such specialization of function by area has been slow to emerge. The area in which specialization of visual processing has been most clearly demonstrated is MT. The basis of this specificity is the high frequency of cells that show the necessary characteristic for visual motion processing, direction selectivity—a response to stimulus motion in one direction but not in the opposite direction. The next area, the medial superior temporal (MST) area, also has a high frequency of direction-selective cells and receives a projection from MT. Figure 1 shows the location of both of these areas on a flat map of cerebral cortex and their relation to the primary visual cortex (striate cortex or V1).

In this paper, we concentrate on experiments that we think suggest some conclusions about the specialization of function within extrastriate cortex for visual motion processing. In our experiments, we have studied motion processing required for the guidance of movement: that for eye movements which depend on motion processing, smooth pursuit eye movements; and that required for the guidance of self-movement through the visual environment. We think that our experiments and those of other investigators indicate that MT concentrates and refines motion processing used for any mo-

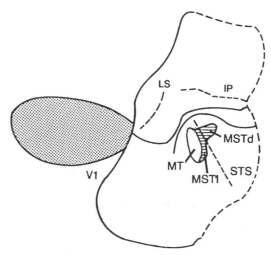

Figure 1. Cortical areas devoted to visual motion processing shown on a flat map of the monkey cerebral cortex. An unfolding process (Van Essen and Maunsell 1980) opens the sulci and displays buried areas. Cortical areas labeled are V1 (the oval area extending to the left, where directionally selective cells are first encountered in cerebral cortex), MT, and MST (areas that have a large proportion of directionally selective cells) (Maunsell and Newsome 1987). Other extrastriate areas also have many directionally selective cells, but for simplicity, these areas are not labeled on the map. A dorsal-medial subregion of MST is indicated as MSTd and a lateral-ventral region as MSTl. Caudal areas are to the left, and rostral areas are to the right. The location of the lunate sulcus (LS), intraparietal sulcus (IP), and superior temporal sulcus (STS) are indicated by dashed lines. Curved solid lines separate the crests of the prelunate gyrus and posterior parietal lobule.

tion-dependent function, be it movement or perception. In contrast, we think our experiments on MST suggest that motion processing there is divided between functionally identifiable subregions that are devoted to specific uses of motion, including the guidance of pursuit eye movements and movement through the environment.

Motion Processing in MT

Besides having a concentration of cells that show direction selectivity, there is also evidence that cells in MT contribute to a higher level of motion analysis than is the case in primary visual cortex (V1). Some MT cells respond to the direction of motion of a complex pattern, rather than to the direction of the component parts, as is the case for all cells studied in striate cortex

(Movshon et al. 1985). Cells in MT respond to those briefly flashed sequential stimuli that lead to a perception of motion (apparent motion), and they maintain the direction selectivity of their response over larger distances between the flashes than do cells in V1 (Mikami et al. 1986a,b; Newsome et al. 1986). That MT is organized for the processing of visual motion is also indicated by evidence of a columnar organization for the axial directions of motion (Albright et al. 1984).

To establish further the extent to which MT contributes to motion processing, several studies have used behaviors of the monkey that are dependent on visual motion processing as a way of probing whether this processing does indeed contribute to those motion-dependent behaviors. One such behavior is a simple eye movement, smooth pursuit, that matches the velocity of the eye to the velocity of a moving target. By training a rhesus monkey (*Macaca mulatta*) to make

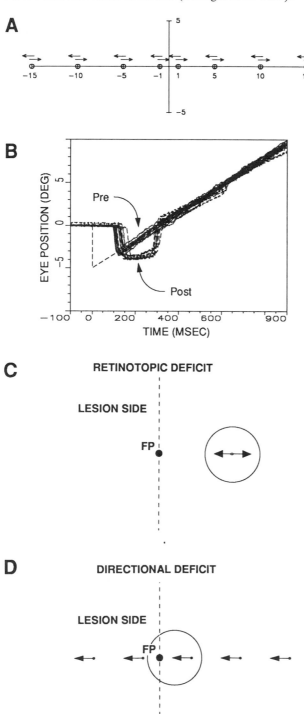

Figure 2. Pursuit deficits following lesions in the superior temporal sulcus (STS). (*A*) Schematic diagram of the tangent screen in front of the monkey showing the central 10° of the vertical meridian and the central 30° of the horizontal meridian, with the fovea centered on the monkey's primary position of gaze. The small circles indicate the sites of the targets in each hemifield, and the arrows indicate that the targets moved either to the right or to the left (16°/sec). The monkey begins a trial by looking at a fixation point at the center of the field and then makes a saccade to the target accompanied by a pursuit movement to match eye speed to target speed. (*B*) Pursuit deficit following a punctate lesion of MT showing ten overlapping prelesion traces (solid lines) and ten postlesion traces (dotted lines) of eye position during pursuit. Prior to the lesion, the monkey made accurate saccades to the moving target, and eye speed matched target speed immediately after the saccade. After the injection, the monkey made long saccades to this target, and eye speed was lower than target speed. Note that once the target was out of the "motion scotoma," the monkey was able to again pursue the target with reasonable accuracy, as indicated by the accurate catchup saccades and higher pursuit speeds. (*C*) The *retinotopic deficit* in pursuit initiation shown on a schematic representation of the visual field. FP indicates the fixation point; the dashed vertical line indicates the vertical meridian of the visual field. When the pursuit target moves within the affected part of the visual field (indicated by the circle contralateral to the side of the lesion), the monkey is unable to match eye speed to target speed or adjust the amplitude of the saccade to reach a moving target. Deficits occur with target motion in any direction (as depicted by the double-headed arrow). The retinotopic deficit follows lesions in extrafoveal MT or MST. (*D*) With a *directional deficit* in the maintenance of pursuit, the monkey's eye speed lags behind the target speed for as long as the target moves toward the side of the brain with the lesion, regardless of where in the visual field the target steps (as indicated by the arrows in both hemifields). A directional deficit in the maintenance of pursuit follows lesions that include MSTl or foveal MT.

such pursuit movements, we were able to show in a series of experiments that the pursuit was impaired by ablation of small regions within MT (Newsome et al. 1985; Dürsteler et al. 1987). Figure 2A shows in schematic outline the behavioral task used in these experiments. The monkey initially looked at a spot of light that appeared at the center of the tangent screen in front of it in order to obtain a reward. We were able to control behavior, accurately record eye position, and record the activity of single cells within the brain using techniques described elsewhere (Komatsu and Wurtz 1988). We used a step-ramp task in which the fixation light went off as another moving spot appeared on the screen at one of the eight locations on the horizontal meridian of the visual field (Fig. 2A). The monkey first made a rapid or saccadic eye movement to bring the fovea close to the target and then a pursuit movement to keep the fovea near the moving target (Fig. 2B). The pursuit movement began as soon as the eye reached the target and, in many cases, even began before the saccade was made to the target. Thus, the monkey used the target motion in one part of the visual field to determine the required velocity of the pursuit eye movement before the eye ever started to move. The practical significance of this early computation is that the motion of the target can be placed in different parts of the visual field and can be used as a probe to determine how well the monkey is able to use the motion information in those parts of the field.

After a punctate chemical lesion in MT (involving an area as small as several millimeters in diameter), a retinotopic area within the contralateral visual field showed a deficit in pursuit initiation. For targets moving in the affected area, the monkey failed to match eye and target speed in the initiation phase of pursuit and to adjust the amplitude of the saccade to compensate for motion of the target, presumably due to a lack of motion information in the affected part of the visual field (Fig. 2B). This deficit affected any direction of target motion from the limited area in the contralateral field related to the cells removed in MT (indicated schematically by the circle in Fig. 2C). This retinotopic deficit was specific for the use of *motion* by the oculomotor system, since when the monkey was required to make a saccade to a *stationary* target, its performance was unimpaired by the lesion (Newsome et al. 1985).

That MT is just as specifically involved in the processing of visual motion information for perception is indicated by the single-cell and ablation experiments of Newsome and his collaborators described elsewhere in this volume. Therefore, single-cell studies indicate that MT concentrates and refines visual motion processing. Selective ablation studies indicate that this motion processing is likely to be used for the control of movement (pursuit) as well as the perception of motion (discrimination). From what we know now, MT can be regarded as a source of motion information for any behavior that requires this information.

Recovery of Function following MT Lesions

A key factor in the question of concentration of motion processing in MT is whether lesions within MT permanently eliminate the functions dependent on motion processing. The deficits in visual motion processing resulting from MT lesions (Newsome et al. 1985; Newsome and Pare 1988) recover rapidly. Recovery of mean performance is nearly complete within a few days, and the deficit is nearly undetectable after 1 week. This rapid recovery is not related to any peculiarity of the chemical lesion, since electrolytic lesions of MT produce the same deficit and rapid recovery of pursuit (D.S. Yamasaki and R.H. Wurtz, in prep.). This finding alone might suggest that MT is not vital for visual motion analysis. But we did find that the larger the area of MT damaged, the slower the recovery. This suggests that the rapid recovery might be related to the small size of the lesions made within MT—certainly the smallest cortical lesions beyond primary sensory areas ever shown to produce a specific behavioral deficit.

To test the notion that the rapid recovery in the monkey's ability to initiate pursuit eye movements is related to the small size of the lesion, we made a much larger lesion in one monkey with the intention of removing all areas devoted to visual motion processing within the superior temporal sulcus (STS): MT on the posterior bank and MST on the abutting anterior bank (D.S. Yamasaki and R.H. Wurtz, in prep.). With multiple injections of the neurotoxin α-amino-3-hydroxy-5-methyl-4-isoxazole propionic acid (AMPA; 15 μg/μl), we succeeded in removing all of MT and all but the very lateral-ventral portion of MST. A small invasion of the intraparietal sulcus spared the ventral intraparietal area (VIP), which also contains directionally selective cells (Colby et al. 1989), and a larger intrusion into the lunate sulcus only partially overlapped the representation of the visual field in which we tested pursuit deficits. The effect of the lesion was dramatic; the recovery was not complete even after more than 7 months. The graphs in Figure 3 show the gradual recovery of eye speed (Fig. 3A) and saccadic error (Fig. 3B). Although there was a gradual improvement of pursuit that approached prelesion levels over the period of months, there was still an oscillation of the performance that hovered about the significance level. This was true for both components of pursuit for as long as we tested, indicating that the monkey never reached full recovery. For a comparison, the dashed lines in Figure 3A,B represent the average recovery profile for smaller AMPA lesions in the STS in two other monkeys. Thus, removal of these motion processing areas, all of MT and most of MST, does more than transiently affect the ability to perform pursuit eye movements; removal produces a continuing deficit. The ability to discriminate the direction of motion also showed a comparably slowed recovery following complete removal of MT alone (Newsome and Pare 1988). These persisting deficits are consistent with the hypothesis that MT (as well as MST) is devoted to visual motion processing.

The effect of large lesions within MT and MST on pursuit eye movements also reveals another factor about the localization of motion processing. Note in the graph in Figure 3A that on the first day after the lesion, the eye speed was greatly reduced, but not to zero. If we assume that the reduced ability of the monkey to perform pursuit just after the lesion reflects the loss of the visual processing used by the normal monkey, the few degrees per second of eye speed remaining immediately after the lesion can then be taken to indicate the contribution that the other undamaged areas normally make to the pursuit system. This residual pursuit, about one-fourth normal pursuit speed, provides some quantitative estimate of the contribution of other cortical areas such as V1, V2, and V3, in which directionally selective cells have been identified (Maunsell and Newsome 1987). The recovery curve would then give an indication of the compensation of other areas to this function over a period of time (Newsome and Wurtz 1988).

Another point to note is that the compensation for the pursuit deficits does not proceed at equal rates for the two deficits: pursuit speed and saccade amplitude. Figure 3 shows that the monkey's ability to match eye

and target speed (Fig. 3A) recovered somewhat faster in the first 100 days after the lesion than did its ability to make an accurate saccade to the moving visual target (Fig. 3B). We have observed this differential rate of recovery in other monkeys as well, and the presence of the two deficits related to visual motion processing allows us to see that the rate of compensation can vary for different uses of the motion information. This in turn raises the possibility that different areas contribute to the recovery of each of these different functions.

Expansion of MT Receptive Fields during Recovery

The shift from rapid recovery with small lesions to a persisting deficit with large lesions emphasizes the contribution of the areas within the STS to the rapid recovery following small lesions. One hypothesis to explain the rapid recovery is that the receptive fields of cells adjacent to the damaged area of MT expand to cover the area of the visual field no longer served by the damaged cells. Since fields of MT neurons are relatively large in the normal monkey (Desimone and Ungerleider 1986; Komatsu and Wurtz 1988), this expansion would not need to be extensive to cover the field affected by small MT lesions. To investigate this possibility, we recorded from cells in regions of MT adjacent to the

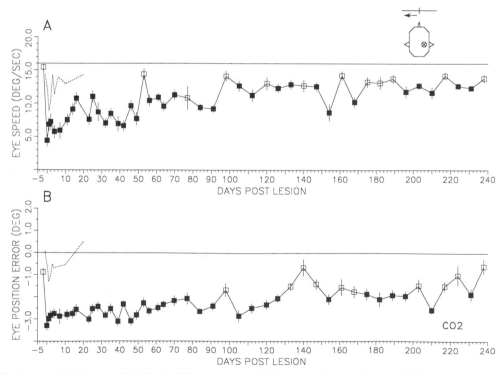

Figure 3. Prolonged deficit in pursuit initiation following a large STS lesion. A large unilateral AMPA lesion produced a pursuit deficit that did not fully recover after more than 7 months (238 days). These graphs plot the eye speed (A) and saccadic eye position error (B) of the monkey's pursuit of one particular step-ramp target (−10° step, leftward motion indicated by the schematic in the upper right corner). Each point is the mean and standard error of ten such trials from each experimental day; (■) a significant difference from prelesion using the Student's t-test ($p < 0.01$). For comparison, the dashed lines in each graph are the averaged recovery profiles for two monkeys that received smaller AMPA lesions in MT and MST. As a reference, the horizontal lines above the data points represent target speed (16°/sec) in A, and zero saccadic error in B. (Adapted from D.S. Yamasaki and R.H. Wurtz, in prep.)

area of a lesion, both before and after we made chemical or electrolytic lesions (D.S. Yamasaki and R.H. Wurtz, in prep.). We implanted guide tubes that directed our recording electrodes to the same sample of cells within MT on successive days and plotted the size of the receptive fields on each of those days. Figure 4A shows the receptive field sizes of a sample set of cells recorded 5 days before an electrolytic lesion and 6 days after the lesion from a guide tube 2 mm from the lesion site. The asterisk shows the location of the average of the receptive field centers recorded at the site of the lesion. The size of a number of the receptive fields clearly increased as indicated by a comparison of the dashed outline of field sizes (prelesion) and the solid outline of field sizes (postlesion). Some fields were larger than any we have seen at that eccentricity within MT in a normal monkey (Komatsu and Wurtz 1988). Although the receptive field sizes expanded, they did not, as we had expected, expand just toward the region of the field with the visual motion deficit, but instead the fields expanded in all directions.

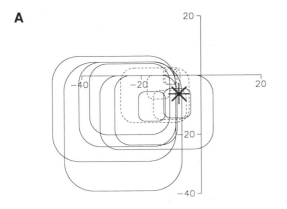

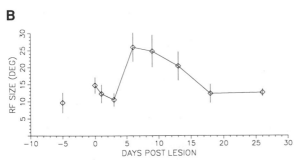

Figure 4. Expansion of receptive fields of MT neurons adjacent to an area of MT damaged by a small electrolytic lesion. (*A*) Dashed lines show receptive fields from a series of cells recorded in MT on prelesion day 5; the solid lines show fields recorded from cells through the same guide tube on postlesion day 6. The large asterisk represents the average of the receptive field centers for the cells recorded at the lesion site before the AMPA injection. Note that the two fields that did not expand were similar in size and location to the prelesion fields, which suggests that we were recording from the same subpopulation of MT cells both prior to and following the lesion. (*B*) Graph of the change of field sizes (the square root of area) from prelesion through each of the postlesion recording days for the same experiment shown in *A*. Each point shows the mean and standard error of the field sizes for the neurons. (Adapted from D.S. Yamasaki and R.H. Wurtz, in prep.)

The amount of the expansion is indicated in Figure 4B, which shows the mean and standard error of the size of the fields (square root of the field area) recorded in one guide tube over a period of more than 3 weeks before and after the electrolytic lesion. The receptive fields showed an initial slight increase, then dramatically increased in size between the third and sixth postlesion days, and then began to contract to their original size. We have observed both the expansion and some indication of a subsequent contraction after either chemical or electrolytic lesions within MT. This expansion was not observed throughout MT but was limited to the receptive fields of cells adjacent to the lesion. Note that the two fields in Figure 4A that did not expand were similar in size and location to the prelesion fields, which suggests that we recorded from the same population of cells before and after the lesion. A similar field expansion was not observed in an experiment by Newsome and Pare (1988). Although the expansion could contribute to the rapid recovery from the lesion, we do not now know whether or not these are simply parallel but unrelated events.

The combination of the slowed recovery following large lesions within MT and MST and the expansion and contraction of the receptive fields of cells in MT does, however, suggest two phases in the recovery process. In the first phase, the receptive fields of the surviving MT neurons adjacent to the lesion expand and compensate for the lesion deficit. This compensation is rapid, occurring within a few days of the lesion. This compensation affects all aspects of motion processing equally (both the pursuit velocity and the amplitude of the saccade to the moving target), which is consistent with the hypothesis that MT provides motion information for any function that requires it. In the second phase, some as yet unidentified areas compensate for the deficit over many months and do so at different rates for different functions. We think that this difference in time course allows us to begin to tease apart two factors: what the ablated area did and what compensation provides. The deficit during the first period probably tells us something about what the damaged brain region did; the change in the deficit in the longer-term recovery period tells us something about the nature of the compensation that occurs within other regions of the brain following damage.

Divisions of MST

MST shares with MT the large proportion of directionally selective cells, and it therefore also is assumed to be concerned with visual motion processing. MST differs from MT in several significant ways. First, the sizes of the receptive fields of many cells in MST are larger than are those in MT (Desimone and Ungerleider 1986; Komatsu and Wurtz 1988). Second, there are at least two areas within MST in which the receptive fields include the fovea, suggesting at least two visual areas within MST. Since cells in these areas include the fovea, it is also not surprising that they discharge during smooth pursuit eye movements when the monkey is attempting to keep a spot of light on the fovea. A third difference between MT and MST is that many of the MST cells that discharge during pursuit eye movements also show evidence of an extraretinal input, one that is not dependent on the visual stimulation considered so far as the only input to these cells. This extraretinal input was revealed by inducing the monkey to continue to perform a pursuit eye movement while removing the visual input to the cell. This was accomplished either by removing the target briefly enough so that the monkey continued the pursuit movement for a few hundred milliseconds in the absence of the target or by stabilizing the image of the target on the retina (Newsome et al. 1988). In both cases, some cells in MST continued to discharge in the absence of the visual stimulus, which we took as evidence of the presence of some other input related to the pursuit eye movement, an extraretinal input. This input might be either proprioceptive or a corollary discharge related to the generation of the pursuit eye movement. Such an input was not seen in MT.

Neurons with the extraretinal input were not equally distributed throughout MST but were concentrated in the same two regions in which the receptive fields of the cells included the fovea. For this reason, we have subsequently regarded MST as comprising two areas. A dorsal medial area that we have referred to as MSTd and a lateral ventral area we have referred to as MSTl. We think the distinctions based on these observations are borne out by the functional differences between these areas considered in the next several sections.

MSTl and Pursuit Maintenance

A number of characteristics of MSTl led to the hypothesis that this area is important for the maintenance phase of pursuit eye movements, i.e., the phase in which the fovea is maintained as close to the moving target as possible. We have reported these observations (Dürsteler et al. 1987; Dürsteler and Wurtz 1988) and provided a summary elsewhere (Wurtz et al. 1990), and will only indicate here the types of observations that have led to this hypothesis. First, MSTl cells have the visual properties that are appropriate to provide input during the maintenance of pursuit: Many cells respond vigorously to small moving spots of light comparable to those used consistently in our experiments on the pursuit system. Second, these cells also have an extraretinal response that occurs during a pursuit eye movement, indicating that they have a movement-related and a visual-related input appropriate for the maintenance of pursuit eye movements.

Third, when we used the same step-ramp task to investigate the contribution of MST to the generation of pursuit as we have used in MT, we found a deficit added onto the retinotopic deficit that we had not seen following lesions of extrafoveal MT. Figure 2D shows this deficit schematically. In this illustration, the target stepped into the right visual field and then moved to the

left. After a lesion was placed in the left MST, there was a clear deficit in the monkey's ability to maintain pursuit of targets moving to the left. The initial pursuit speed was low, and it remained lower than target speed for the duration of the trial. This directional deficit differs from the deficit following an MT lesion in that once the monkey's eye was near the target, it still lagged behind the target; the speed of the eye never matched the speed of the target. This *directional* deficit was present for any step at any point in the visual field as long as the target motion was *toward* the side of the lesion. The directional deficit in the monkey is very similar to the directional deficit first seen in humans in the slow phase of optokinetic nystagmus described by Fox and Holmes (1926). The directional deficit was not seen with all lesions in MST. Lesions that were centered on MSTd had minimal directional deficits (Dürsteler and Wurtz 1988), whereas lesions more closely centered on MSTl had a more profound directional effect.

Fourth, we found that we could modify pursuit when we injected a signal into the system by electrical stimulation. When the monkey was pursuing a target, electrical stimulation produced an acceleration of the pursuit movement toward the side of the brain stimulated (Komatsu and Wurtz 1989). Because of the nature of the neuronal discharge in MSTl to both visual input and eye movement output, because of the nature of the directional deficit that results from ablation of this area, and because of the effects of adding a signal in this area by electrical stimulation, our hypothesis is that MSTl is closely related to the maintenance of pursuit eye movements.

MSTd and Optic Flow

Neurons in MSTd share with MSTl neurons the direction-selective responses to moving stimuli and the extraretinal input associated with pursuit eye movements. However, MSTd neurons also have a salient characteristic that makes them less appropriate for the generation of smooth pursuit: Most MSTd neurons respond better to the motion of a large visual field stimulus than to the motion of small spots of light. In contrast, most MSTl neurons respond better to the motion of small spots of light, although many respond to large-field motion in addition (Komatsu and Wurtz 1988).

Another characteristic of MSTd neurons is their sensitivity to visual stimuli moving in circular or radial patterns (Saito et al. 1986; Tanaka and Saito 1989; Tanaka et al. 1989). The preference of MSTd cells for large-field stimulation combined with their sensitivity to radial stimuli makes these cells appropriate candidates for the visual operations underlying the analysis of optic flow. Such flow stimuli have been recognized as providing critical information for guiding self-movement through the visual environment (Gibson 1950; Koenderink 1986; Warren and Hannon 1990). We studied the responses of MSTd neurons to large-field stimulation covering an area 100° by 100° on a tangent screen in front of the monkey (C.J. Duffy and R.H. Wurtz, in prep.). We used a computer-generated random-dot display projected onto the screen to produce simulations of the patterns of planar, circular, and radial motion that would be seen by an observer moving through the environment.

We found many MSTd neurons that were sensitive to one of these types of motion (planar, circular, or radial) as had been indicated first by the experiments of Saito et al. (1986). Other MSTd neurons responded to more than one type of motion, and several examples of such multiple component neurons are illustrated in Figure 5. The planocircular neuron in the left column responded to both rightward planar motion and to clockwise circular motion. The planoradial neuron in the middle column responded to rightward planar motion and to outward radial motion. Interestingly, we did not find cells that responded to the combination of circular and radial motion. The planocirculoradial neuron in the third column responded to rightward planar motion, counterclockwise circular motion, and outward radial motion. Note that in each of these cases, although the neuron responded to several types of stimulus motion, it still showed direction selectivity within each particular type of motion. For example, the

planocircular neuron responded well to rightward planar motion, but not to leftward planar motion, and to clockwise circular motion, but not to both clockwise and counterclockwise motion. In a sample of over 200 neurons, we found that the cells were divided roughly equally between those that responded primarily to one stimulus component, those that responded to two components, and those that responded to all three components.

These classifications clearly represented the elements of a continuum across neurons, rather than distinct groups. However, we did find differences between neurons that responded to only a single component and those that responded to more than one component. First, single-component neurons showed greater direction selectivity for any planar directional response than did the multicomponent groups. Second, single-component neurons showed stronger direction selectivity within selected components than did double- or triple-component neurons. Third, single-component neurons showed far more inhibitory responses than did the multiple-component neurons. These characteristics led us to suggest that the single-component cells represent a higher level of processing than do the multiple-component cells.

We have also begun to investigate the receptive field

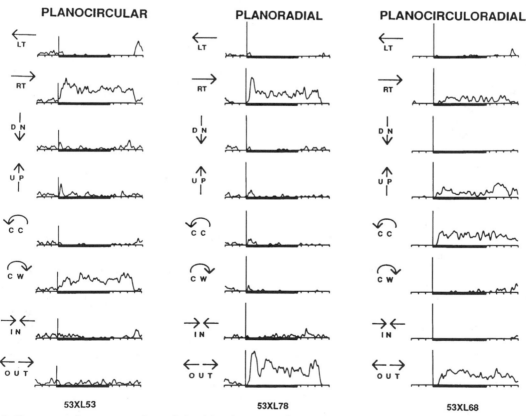

Figure 5. Responses of neurons to planar (left, right, down, or up), circular (counterclockwise, CC, or clockwise, CW), and radial (inward or outward) motion. Each column represents the results for a different cell to each of these stimuli (indicated by the abbreviations to the side of each column). The spike density profiles of each response sums the respo. _ over ten trials (Richmond et al. 1987). The dark line underlying each profile indicates the time that the full-field (100° × 100°) stimulus was on (1.5 sec). The line at the stimulus onset indicates a discharge rate of 100 spikes/sec. (From C.J. Duffy and R.H. Wurtz, in prep.)

organization of MSTd neurons that might account for their sensitivity to circular and radial motion. We have attempted to determine whether the structure of their receptive fields is consistent with either of two hypotheses on the mechanisms of higher-order direction selectivity. One hypothesis, the *direction mosaic hypothesis*, relies on a mosaic of different subfields within the receptive field, each of which has a different planar direction selectivity. For example, for a neuron with outward radial selectivity, the subfield on the right of the visual field would be sensitive to rightward movement and the subfield on the left would be sensitive to leftward movement. This model requires that for the stimulus to be optimally effective, it must cover these multiple subfields and be centered on the receptive field in order for it to maintain its direction selectivity.

Another hypothesis relies on distributed responsiveness throughout the receptive field. This *vector field hypothesis* requires that throughout the receptive field, equal sensitivity be maintained to a specific type of stimulus motion described by vector calculus as the gradient, curl, and divergence of planar, circular, and radial flow fields. Neurons whose receptive fields are organized in this manner would be sensitive to any appropriate flow-field pattern, regardless of the local directions of motion it contained. In addition, circular and radial sensitivity should be stable despite changes in the size and position of the stimulus in the receptive field.

Our initial experiments on this problem have determined the sensitivity of MSTd neurons to higher-order motion within subregions of their receptive fields. Figure 6 shows an example of the results of one such experiment. The response of the cell to large-field (100° × 100°) stimuli is shown schematically in Figure 6A. In this vector summary diagram, the length of the line indicates the amplitude of response in the direction of the stimulus motion, with the horizontal and vertical lines representing planar responses, oblique lines representing radial responses, and the hemicircles representing circular responses. The neuron responded somewhat to rightward and downward planar motions, minimally to circular motion, and best to inward radial motion presented to subregions of the larger field. Figure 6B shows the response of the same stimuli presented to the subfields (33° × 33°). As illustrated, the neuron remained sensitive to radial inward motion throughout the field, although the magnitude of the response changed somewhat within different regions of the field. The responses of this neuron clearly cannot be resolved into separate planar components segregated by direction preference into diffuse regions of the visual field, as would be predicted by the direction mosaic hypothesis. The characteristics of this neuron are more readily described by a vector mosaic model in which the radial inward sensitivity is distributed throughout the entire field as were examples shown by Saito et al. (1986). We think that this neuron represents a higher level of visual integration than the simple planar directional neurons seen in MT and MST.

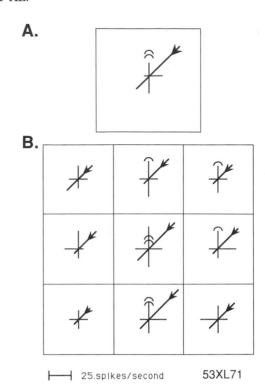

Figure 6. A neuron with a predominantly inward radial response to full-field stimuli that continued to respond to such radial motion to a series of small-field stimuli. (*A*) Representation of the response of an MST cell with leftward, rightward, upward, and downward planar motion indicated by lines in those directions, with clockwise motion indicated by hemicircles, with radial inward motion indicated by the arrow pointing from upper right to lower left toward the center, and with radial outward motion indicated by the line from center to lower left. Size of the response is indicated by the length of the line from the center, with the key for 25 spikes/sec shown at the bottom of the figure. Response is the mean of eight trials in the period from 400 msec after stimulus onset to stimulus offset. (*B*) Response to subfield stimuli covering 33° × 33° areas in nine subregions throughout the larger field. Same schematic representation of response and calibration of that response as in *A*. Although there are shifts in the quantitative response in segments of this field, the radial inward motion persists throughout the entire field. (From C.J. Duffy and R.H. Wurtz, in prep.)

Not all neurons showed this apparent lack of relationship to planar motion. Some neurons showed a clear relationship between planar sensitivity and their circular or radial responses. Particularly with respect to circular sensitivity, there were many cases in which the sensitivity to circular motion could be understood more easily in terms of the direction mosaic model. In general, the neurons that responded to multiple components of motion (planoradial, planocircular, or planocircularoradial) were more likely to show responses to small-field stimuli that are consistent with the direction mosaic hypotheses. In contrast, neurons that responded only to circular or only to radial motion tended to have small-field responses that were more compatible with the vector mosaic hypotheses.

In net, the characteristics of these cells suggest that they have the properties one would expect to find in cells sensitive to optic flow stimulation generated as a person (or a monkey) moves through the visual environment.

MSTd and Disparity

Another major source of information about the depth of objects in the environment is the visual disparity between the images falling on the retinas of the two eyes. Disparity sensitivity is evident in the striate cortex and in several extrastriate visual areas (Poggio 1989). The cells in MT not only have direction selectivity to motion, but also have sensitivity for the depth within the visual field at which this motion occurs (Maunsell and Van Essen 1983). To test the disparity sensitivity of MSTd neurons, we again used the large-field random-dot planar motion stimuli described above. To produce a disparity stimulus, each dot on the screen was represented twice, once by a red dot and once by a green dot, and the monkey wore spectacles with a red filter covering one eye and a green filter covering the other eye. Thus, the red and green dots were seen primarily by one eye or the other. While the monkey continued to look at the white fixation spot on the screen, we could vary the distance between the red and green dots and make the plane of motion of the moving dots appear to be behind the screen (far), on the screen, or in front of the screen (near). We found many MSTd neurons that showed disparity sensitivity, and Figure 7 illustrates one of these neurons (J.-P. Roy and R.H. Wurtz, in prep.). When the stimulus motion appeared to be in front of the screen (near in Fig. 7), the cell responded vigorously to motion in the optimal direction, less well when the motion appeared to be on the screen (screen in Fig. 7), and very little when the stimulus appeared to be behind the screen (far in Fig. 7). This cell was clearly sensitive to near stimuli, and almost all neurons studied were broadly tuned to either near or far stimuli (breadth of the tuning is indicated by the curves shown in Fig. 8). Although there was some variation in the exact shape of the tuning curve, it was

striking that many of the MSTd neurons provided essentially information about whether the planar stimulus motion extended behind the plane of fixation or in front of the plane of fixation, but little information about the exact position of the moving stimulus as in the case for many "tuned" cells in V1 and MT.

So far, the neurons that we have described showed a greater response at a given disparity for motion in the preferred direction of the neuron; motion in the opposite direction produced little if any response regardless of the disparity of the particular stimulus. Other neurons, however, responded to one direction of stimulus motion at one disparity and to the opposite direction of stimulus motion at another disparity (Roy and Wurtz 1990). They were essentially disparity-dependent direction cells. In the example in Figure 8, when motion of the stimulus was to the left (near-left half in Fig. 8), the cell responded when the stimulus appeared to be nearer to the monkey than the screen, whereas with motion of the stimulus to the right, the cell responded optimally when the stimulus was on or behind the screen (far-right side in Fig. 8). Cells with this type of response are able to respond selectively to stimulus motion depending on the position of that motion in depth; stimuli close to the monkey will elicit a response with one direction of motion, while stimuli at another distance from the monkey will elicit a response to motion in the opposite direction. This type of separation between a foreground and a background stimulus should be highly useful for determining the depth of motion in the environment. It is also exactly the type of differentiation required when the subject moves through the environment while fixating on a particular point at a distance, since in this case, objects in front of that point move in one direction on the retina while those behind that point of fixation move in the opposite direction.

In summary, we now know that cells in MSTd provide information about the position of objects in the environment by the use of disparity and by the use of optic flow. In addition, these cells receive an extraretinal signal that we identified during pursuit eye move-

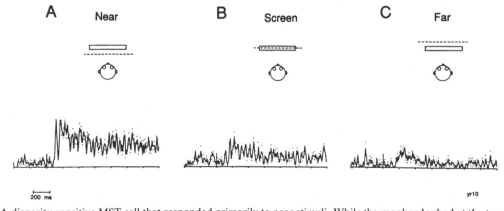

Figure 7. A disparity-sensitive MST cell that responded primarily to near stimuli. While the monkey looked at the tangent screen (rectangles), a random-dot pattern (represented by the dashed lines) moved in the optimum planar direction for this cell and appeared to be in front of the screen (*A*, near), on the screen (*B*, screen), or behind the screen (*C*, far). The spike density displays the response of the cells summed over eight trials. (From J.-P. Roy and R.H. Wurtz, in prep.)

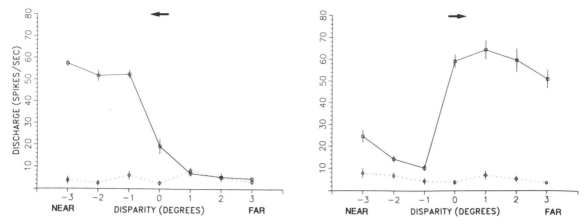

Figure 8. An example of a neuron whose direction preference changed depending on the disparity of the stimulus. For leftward motion, the neuron responded (solid line) above the spontaneous rate (dotted line) when the stimulus appeared to be in front of the screen (near); for rightward motion, it responded when the stimulus appeared to be on or behind the screen (far). Each of the stimuli at seven different disparities was presented five times in a 20° × 20° region within the receptive field of the neuron. Mean and standard errors for the response to each stimulus are for the 600 msec period beginning 400 msec after stimulus onset in order to avoid the initial transient response of the cell. (Adapted from Roy and Wurtz 1990.)

ments. This extraretinal signal might well be related to the type of pursuit that occurs with fixation of gaze on an object in the environment. If this were the case, then the extraretinal signal, the optic flow information, and the disparity information might act together to provide information about the depth of objects as the subject moves in the environment. What we do not know is the extent for which this information is conveyed by an individual neuron as opposed to distributed across many neurons in MSTd.

CONCLUSION: SPECIFICITY OF FUNCTION

The use of movement as an assay for visual motion processing has revealed striking specificity of function in extrastriate areas MT and MST. MT is clearly involved in visual motion processing; the selective responses of these neurons to the direction of visual motion and the effects of the removal of these neurons on behavior indicate a role in both the generation of movement and the perception of motion. Visual processing in MT can best be regarded as pertaining to motion for all occasions. The work on MT to date certainly provides the strongest evidence so far that a specific type of visual processing is concentrated in one extrastriate area. The limitation to this localization is indicated by the small residual motion processing remaining after complete removal of MT, and the gradual recovery after the lesion provides an estimate of the potential contribution of other areas to motion processing.

MST appears to be as devoted to visual motion processing as MT, but we think that the evidence suggests that it is more dedicated to specific functions. In the subregions of MST that have been identified, MSTl and MSTd, experimental evidence suggests that motion processing serves specific behaviors, the maintenance of pursuit eye movements in MSTl, and the guidance

through the visual environment in MSTd. In fact, this close relationship of area to function in MST makes it somewhat easier to evaluate the limits of this specificity. To take MSTl as an example, we cannot say that this area provides all motion information for the maintenance of pursuit; the best hypothesis at this point is that such use of the motion processing is distributed across extrastriate areas but is centered in MSTl. Conversely, we cannot say that MSTl provides motion information only for maintenance of pursuit; we have not tested the relationship of this area enough to other functions that are dependent on motion processing. What we do know is that when we compare the two areas within MST on the same set of motion-related functions, we find striking differences between these areas, and we conclude that these differences reflect remarkable specificity even at our relatively early stage of investigation.

The specificity that we have seen for visual motion processing in MT and MST is far from the classic concept of a generalized association cortex and much closer to the minutely specific localization that has emerged from studies of the primary visual cortex.

REFERENCES

Albright, T.D., R. Desimone, and C.G. Gross. 1984. Columnar organization of directionally selective cells in visual area MT of the macaque. *J. Neurophysiol.* **51:** 16.

Colby, C.L., J.-R. Duhamel, and M.E. Goldberg. 1989. Visual response properties and attentional modulation of neurons in the ventral intraparietal area (VIP) in the alert monkey. *Soc. Neurosci. Abstr.* **15:** 162.

Desimone, R. and L.G. Ungerleider. 1986. Multiple visual areas in the caudal superior temporal sulcus of the macaque. *J. Comp. Neurol.* **248:** 164.

Dürsteler, M.R. and R.H. Wurtz. 1988. Pursuit and optokinetic deficits following chemical lesions of cortical areas MT and MST. *J. Neurophysiol.* **60:** 940.

Dürsteler, M.R., R.H. Wurtz, and W.T. Newsome. 1987. Directional pursuit deficits following lesions of the foveal representation within the superior temporal sulcus of the macaque monkey. *J. Neurophysiol.* **57:** 1262.

Fox, J.C. and G. Holmes. 1926. Optic nystagmus and its value in the localization of cerebral lesions. *Brain* **49**: 333.

Gibson, J.J. 1950. In *The perception of the visual world*. Houghton Mifflin, Boston.

Koenderink, J.J. 1986. Optic flow. *Vision Res.* **26**: 161.

Komatsu, H. and R.H. Wurtz. 1988. Relation of cortical areas MT and MST to pursuit eye movements. I. Localization and visual properties of neurons. *J. Neurophysiol.* **60**: 580.

———. 1989. Modulation of pursuit eye movements by stimulation of cortical areas MT and MST. *J. Neurophysiol.* **62**: 31.

Maunsell, J.H.R. and W.T. Newsome. 1987. Visual processing in monkey extrastriate cortex. *Annu. Rev. Neurosci.* **10**: 363.

Maunsell, J.H.R. and D.C. Van Essen. 1983. Functional properties of neurons in middle temporal visual area of the macaque monkey. II. Binocular interactions and sensitivity to binocular disparity. *J. Neurophysiol.* **49**: 1148.

Mikami, A., W.T. Newsome, and R.H. Wurtz. 1986a. Motion selectivity in macaque visual cortex. I. Mechanisms of direction and speed selectivity in extrastriate area MT. *J. Neurophysiol.* **55**: 1308.

———. 1986b. Motion selectivity in macaque visual cortex. II. Spatio-temporal range of directional interactions in MT and V1. *J. Neurophysiol.* **55**: 1328.

Movshon, J.A., E.H. Adelson, M.S. Gizzi, and W.T. Newsome. 1985. The analysis of moving visual patterns. In *Pattern recognition mechanisms* (ed. C. Chagas et al.). Springer-Verlag, New York.

Newsome, W.T. and E.B. Pare. 1988. A selective impairment of motion perception following lesions of the middle temporal visual area (MT). *J. Neurosci.* **8**: 2201.

Newsome, W.T. and R.H. Wurtz. 1988. Probing visual cortical function with discrete chemical lesions. *Trends Neurosci.* **11**: 394.

Newsome, W.T., A. Mikami, and R.H. Wurtz. 1986. Motion selectivity in macaque visual cortex. III. Psychophysics and physiology of apparent motion. *J. Neurophysiol.* **55**: 1340.

Newsome, W.T., R.H. Wurtz, and H. Komatsu. 1988. Relation of cortical areas MT and MST to pursuit eye movements. II. Differentiation of retinal from extraretinal inputs. *J. Neurophysiol.* **60**: 604.

Newsome, W.T., R.H. Wurtz, M.R. Dürsteler, and A. Mikami. 1985. Deficits in visual motion processing following ibotenic acid lesions of the middle temporal visual area of the macaque monkey. *J. Neurosci.* **5**: 825.

Poggio, G.F. 1989. Neural responses serving stereopsis in the visual cortex of the alert macaque monkey: Position-disparity and image-correlation. In *Sensory processing in the mammalian brain: Neural substrates and experimental strategies* (ed. J.S. Lund), p. 226. Oxford University Press, New York.

Richmond, B.J., L.M. Optican, M. Podell, and H. Spitzer. 1987. Temporal encoding of two-dimensional patterns by single units in primate inferior temporal cortex: I. Response characteristics. *J. Neurophysiol.* **57**: 132.

Roy, J.-P. and R.H. Wurtz. 1990. The role of disparity sensitive cortical neurons in signalling the direction of self-motion. *Nature* (in press).

Saito, H.-A., M. Yukie, K. Tanaka, K. Hikosaka, Y. Fukada, and E. Iwai. 1986. Integration of direction signals of image motion in the superior temporal sulcus of the macaque monkey. *J. Neurosci.* **6**: 145.

Tanaka, K. and H. Saito. 1989. Analysis of motion of the visual field by direction, expansion/contraction, and rotation cells clustered in the dorsal part of the medial superior temporal area of the macaque monkey. *J. Neurophysiol.* **62**: 626.

Tanaka, K., Y. Fukada, and H. Saito. 1989. Underlying mechanisms of the response specificity of expansion/contraction and rotation cells in the dorsal part of the medial superior temporal area of the macaque monkey. *J. Neurophysiol.* **62**: 642.

Ungerleider, L.G. and M. Mishkin. 1982. Two cortical visual systems. In *Analysis of visual behavior* (ed. D.J. Ingle et al.), p. 549. MIT Press, Cambridge, Massachusetts.

Van Essen, D.C. 1985. Functional organization of primate visual cortex. In *Cerebral cortex* (ed. A. Peters and E.G. Jones), vol. 3, p. 259. Plenum, New York.

Van Essen, D.C. and J.H.R. Maunsell. 1980. Two-dimensional maps of the cerebral cortex. *J. Comp. Neurol.* **191**: 255.

Warren, W.H. and D.J. Hannon. 1990. Eye movements and optical flow. *J. Opt. Soc. Am.* **7**: 160.

Wurtz, R.H., H. Komatsu, and D.S.G. Yamasaki. 1990. Cortical visual motion processing for oculomotor control. In *Vision and the brain* (ed. B. Cohen and I. Bodis-Wollner), p. 211. Raven Press, New York.

Zeki, S.M. 1974a. Functional organization of a visual area in the posterior bank of the superior temporal sulcus of the rhesus monkey. *J. Physiol.* **236**: 549.

———. 1974b. Cells responding to changing image size and disparity in the cortex of the rhesus monkey. *J. Physiol.* **242**: 827.

Representation of Visuomotor Space in the Parietal Lobe of the Monkey

M.E. Goldberg, C.L. Colby, and J.-R. Duhamel

Laboratory of Sensorimotor Research, National Eye Institute, Bethesda, Maryland 20892

The concept of representation is basic to our understanding of how the brain works. Since the days of phrenology, specific areas of the brain have been associated with specific perceptual and motor functions. Activity within a representation is the neural equivalent of the represented object: Activity within a visual representation corresponds to the presence of a visual stimulus, and activity within a motor representation predicts the occurrence of the represented movement. All well-understood sensory representations can be described as topological mappings from the receptor surface to the brain area, with some processing constraints superimposed on that representation. Thus, each hemiretina is represented in primary visual cortex (V1), such that a given locus in V1 is activated in response to stimulation of a given retinal locus. Within that locus, individual stimulus features, such as orientation and color, may be represented separately, but the primary organizing principle is retinotopic (Hubel and Wiesel 1977). Similarly, motor representations are organized so that movements are represented contiguously. In the frontal eye field, for example, activity at a given locus of neural tissue corresponds to a particular direction and amplitude of saccade: Saccade amplitude is represented mediolaterally along the arcuate sulcus (Bruce et al. 1985).

Space is a supramodal construct that is not limited to a given kind of sensation, let alone a given receptor surface. We can determine an object's spatial location from many different sensory cues, not only vision, but also somatic sensation, audition, and even olfaction. We calibrate the accuracy of our spatial perception by movement, but the nature of the movement is unimportant: We can look at an object, reach out and touch it, walk over to it, or even throw this book at it. Thus, space is calculated from sensation, calibrated by movement and not linked uniquely to any particular movement or sensation. Almost by definition, if space is represented in the brain explicitly, that representation must differ from simple sensory and motor representations. Analysis of spatial performance may provide insights into the nature of spatial representation. The oculomotor system is particularly well suited to studies of spatial performance, since both monkeys and humans are capable of highly accurate eye movements to visual targets. Previous work from this laboratory has considered how neurons in the frontal eye fields

respond in spatial tasks (Goldberg and Bruce 1990). We have now extended this work to the parietal cortex.

The posterior parietal cortex has long been thought to be important for spatial processing, mainly on the evidence that patients with right parietal lesions neglect contralateral visual space (Critchley 1953). Recordings of single neurons in the posterior parietal cortex also suggest that this region has a function in visuospatial behavior. Parietal neurons discharge in association with visually guided saccades (Mountcastle et al. 1975; Lynch et al. 1977) and respond to visual stimuli (Yin and Mountcastle 1977; Robinson et al. 1978). The visual responsiveness of parietal neurons is enhanced when the monkey makes a saccade to a visual target within its receptive field (Robinson et al. 1978). This enhancement also occurs when the monkey attends to a stimulus in a particular location without making a saccade to it (Bushnell et al. 1981). Unlike enhancement of visual responsiveness in striate cortex, for example, enhancement in parietal cortex is spatially selective. Only when attention is directed to stimuli presented within the receptive field is responsiveness enhanced. Since the enhanced visual response occurs both in the context of moving the eyes to the target and in the case where only the focus of attention is shifted, the output of these cells cannot be read by other neurons as an obligatory command to move the eyes. Rather, this activity must be interpreted as specifying an attentional vector, requiring a shift of attention to a new location regardless of whether or not that shift is accompanied by a change in eye position. These physiological data suggest that posterior parietal cortex is involved in spatially selective attention and complement the clinical impression that it is important in the neural processes underlying general visuospatial attention (Heilman et al. 1987).

The attentional activity in posterior parietal cortex is quite different from the activity in the monkey frontal eye field. In the frontal eye field, neuronal activity is specifically related to saccadic eye movements. Furthermore, frontal eye field neurons discharge only in relation to purposive eye movements: Spontaneous saccades are not associated with any change in discharge rate. Two classes of frontal eye field neurons are of particular interest for understanding spatial processing. Visual neurons show enhanced responses only before saccades and not when the monkey uses the same stimulus in a peripheral attention task (Goldberg and Bushnell 1981). Movement neurons discharge before purposive saccades in the absence of a visual stimulus and have little or no visual responsiveness (Bruce and Goldberg 1985). Movement neurons, but not visual neurons, project to the superior colliculus (Segraves and Goldberg 1987). In contrast to parietal neurons projecting to superior colliculus, which presumably signal an attentional vector, frontal eye field movement neurons signal an intended eye movement. These eye movements are coded in terms of vectors: Stimulation at a given site in the frontal eye field will produce a saccade of a particular amplitude and direction. A given frontal eye field site projects to cells in the superior colliculus from which the same saccade is evoked by electrical stimulation (Bruce et al. 1985; Segraves and Goldberg 1987). Thus, the output of the frontal eye fields is already coded in oculomotor coordinates, i.e., neurons here encode a desired movement.

How does visual input get transformed into oculomotor coordinates? One possibility is that visual input is remapped into an explicit representation of space. The motor coordinates of a desired saccade could then be calculated from this spatial map, which may be coded in head-centered or in inertial coordinates. This formulation requires two coordinate transformations: from visual to spatial coordinates and from spatial to motor coordinates. It also requires an explicit representation of extrapersonal space. A second possibility, and the one that we favor, is that visual input is remapped directly into motor coordinates. This could be accomplished by coding a visual target according to the saccade vector needed to acquire it.

To test these two possibilities, we have used a "double-step" paradigm that allows us to separate the retinal vector of a target from its saccade vector. In this paradigm, introduced by Hallett and Lightstone (1976), the retinal coordinates of a visual target are dissociated from the amplitude and direction of saccade necessary to acquire that target. This dissociation is accomplished by having the subject make two saccades to follow two briefly flashed targets. Because both targets disappear before any eye movement is made, the dimensions of the second saccade cannot be based solely on the retinal location of the second target but must take into account the amplitude and direction of the first saccade. Hallett and Lightstone showed that humans could make accurate saccades in this task: The second saccade is directed to the spatial location of the second target and not to its retinal location. This performance cannot be based on retinal error alone (defined as the difference between the fovea and the retinal position of the target) but must also be based on knowledge of previous saccades or current eye position. This behavior is called "spatially accurate" because saccades are directed to the spatial, rather than to the retinal, location of a target.

Monkeys can also make spatially accurate saccades in a double-step task (Mays and Sparks 1980). The neural mechanisms underlying this ability have been examined in the superior colliculus, the frontal eye fields, and in parietal cortex. Cells in the intermediate layers of the superior colliculus yield movement signals in double-step tasks even though the stimulus acquired by the signaled saccade never appeared in the movement field or the visual receptive field of the neuron (Mays and Sparks 1980). This finding indicates that by the time the oculomotor signal reaches the superior colliculus, it has already been adjusted for the previous saccade. The intermediate layers of the superior colliculus are an output target of both the frontal eye fields and posterior parietal cortex (Lynch et al. 1985; Stanton et al. 1988). The mechanism underlying the transformation from visual to motor coordinates may thus be related to the activity of cells in the frontal eye fields and parietal cortex.

Neurons in the frontal eye fields (Goldberg and Bruce 1990) and in parietal cortex (Gnadt and Andersen 1988) also respond in double-step tasks. In the frontal eye field, visual neurons have response fields that are coded in oculomotor coordinates (Goldberg and Bruce 1990). These visual neurons, which have no independent saccade-related activity, respond selectively to visual stimuli that can be acquired by a particular saccade, regardless of the retinal location of those stimuli. The activity of such cells signals the presence of a visual target not in retinal coordinates, but in motor coordinates. This coordinate transformation could be performed by a vector subtraction of the dimensions of the previous saccade from the retinal location of a target. This mechanism would enable spatially accurate saccades without requiring reference to an explicit coding of target position in space.

In the present experiments, we have recorded from neurons in parietal cortex of the monkey during a number of different visuomotor tasks to approach the question of what aspects of spatial behavior are represented, and what might be the nature of that representation. In this paper, we focus on neurons in a single distinct visual area within parietal cortex, the lateral intraparietal area (LIP), located in the lateral bank of the intraparietal sulcus (Andersen et al. 1985). Neurons in LIP discharge in response to visual stimuli and in association with visually guided and visual-memory-guided saccades (Gnadt and Andersen 1988). The present results suggest that there is an ongoing, dynamic transformation from visual to oculomotor coordinates in which activity in posterior parietal cortex represents the vector for a shift of spatial attention. Like spatial perception itself, this attentional vector does not describe a given movement or sensory datum, but the supramodal construct common to all.

METHODS

Animal preparation. Two rhesus monkeys (*Macaca mulatta*) were trained on a series of visual and oculomotor tasks and surgically prepared under general anesthesia for chronic neurophysiological recording by the implantation of ocular search coils, head-holding devices, and recording chambers, through which electrodes could subsequently be introduced into the cerebral cortex. Behavioral monitoring, eye position and unit sampling, and on-line data analysis were performed by a PDP-11/73 computer (Goldberg 1983). All experimental protocols were approved by the National Eye Institute Animal Care and Use Committee and were certified to be in compliance with the guidelines set forth in the U.S. Public Health Service Guide for the Care and Use of Laboratory Animals.

Physiological methods. Recordings were made with flexible tungsten electrodes introduced through stainless steel guide tubes placed nearly but not quite through the dura, which in turn were stabilized by a nylon grid held rigidly in the recording cylinder (Crist et al. 1988). The grid served as a guide to produce parallel penetrations with a resolution of 0.5 mm. The rigidity of the system and the atraumatic nature of the electrodes allowed us to perform a large number of penetrations at multiple recording sites within intraparietal sulcus. We found that electrode penetrations performed several months apart at the same grid locations yielded neurons with similar response types at similar depths. In one monkey, after having mapped the intraparietal sulcus in both hemispheres, we recorded again at each site and placed a pattern of lesions designed to identify each electrode track and the depth at which specific types of activity were found. By sectioning the brain in the plane of the grid, we were able to reconstruct the location of each of the penetrations. The location of area LIP and a representative section through it are shown in Figure 1.

Behavioral methods. The monkeys were trained on a series of visual, oculomotor, and attentional tasks designed to differentiate sensory and motor correlates of neural activity. All tasks were run in blocks of 16 trials to reinforce the monkey's behavior, except for the learned-saccade task, which was run in blocks long enough to ensure 16 trials each of the randomly intermixed visually triggered and learned saccade trials (Goldberg and Bruce 1990). Cells were studied first on a series of standard tasks, illustrated in Figure 2.

Visual Fixation Task: The monkey gazed at a fixation point and made no eye movement or other discernible response to a second stimulus flashed elsewhere on the tangent screen. The monkey was rewarded either for holding eye position for a certain interval or for releasing a lever to signal a dimming of the fixation point. This task was used to map the receptive field of the cell and to study the visual responsiveness of neurons in a situation where the stimulus had no behavioral significance.

Peripheral Attention Task: The fixation point and receptive field stimulus appeared as in the fixation task, but the monkey had to respond, by releasing a bar, to a dimming of the peripheral stimulus while maintaining central eye position (Wurtz and Mohler 1976). The trial was aborted if the monkey made a saccade to the target. This task was used to study the visual responsiveness of neurons in a situation where the monkey had to attend to a peripheral stimulus but where eye movements to it were expressly forbidden.

Delayed-saccade Task: During the fixation period, the stimulus appeared for 200 msec or less, and the monkey had to continue to look at the fixation point for at least 500 and up to 1500 msec after the stimulus had disappeared. If the monkey made a saccade at the appropriate time (fixation point offset) to the location where the target had been, the target reappeared 200 msec after the saccade, and the monkey was rewarded for holding the new position. This task was used to dissociate activity related to the stimulus from activity related to the movement.

Visually Triggered Saccade Task: The monkey looked at a fixation point until it disappeared, at which time, a peripheral light appeared briefly (less than 50 msec). A 5-msec pause intervened between extinguish-

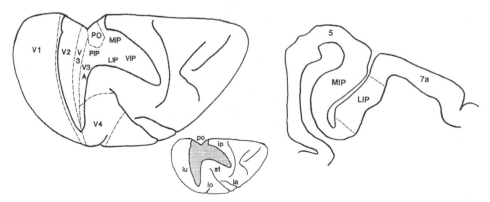

Figure 1. Location of area LIP. The small cartoon at bottom center shows a dorsal view of one hemisphere of macaque cerebral cortex with major sulci labeled. (io) Inferior occipital; (ip) intraparietal; (la) lateral fissure; (lu) lunate; (po) parieto-occipital; (st) superior temporal. The intraparietal, lunate, and parieto-occipital sulci have been opened up to reveal the cortex buried within. In the larger brain at left, the locations of several visual areas are indicated, including the posterior (PIP), the medial (MIP), the ventral (VIP), and the lateral (LIP) intraparietal areas. (Adapted from Colby et al. 1988.) The coronal section on the right shows the location of different divisions within parietal cortex: area 5, MIP, LIP, and area 7a. The dashed lines show the extent of the densely myelinated zone within the lateral bank, which is partially coextensive with area LIP (Andersen et al. 1990).

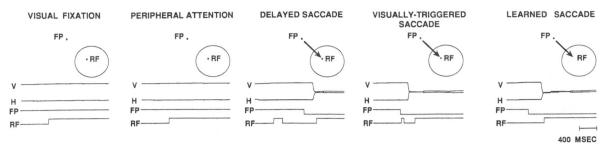

Figure 2. Standard visual and oculomotor tasks. These cartoons illustrate standard tasks used on all LIP neurons. (FP) Fixation point; (RF) receptive field of the cell; (→) requirement that the monkey perform a saccade to the indicated position. Sample eye-movement traces for each task show vertical (V) and horizontal (H) eye displacements over time. Each task begins with the fixation point on. FP and RF time lines indicate onset and offset of visual targets. In the first four tasks, a receptive field stimulus is presented either during or immediately after the fixation period, as indicated by the upward deflection in the RF line. The visual fixation and peripheral attention tasks are identical with regard to initial retinal stimulation, and both require the monkey to maintain central fixation; in the latter task, the monkey must detect the dimming of the peripheral stimulus and respond to that event by releasing a bar. The other three tasks all require the monkey to make a particular saccade. The delayed saccade task requires the monkey to withhold the saccade until the fixation point is extinguished. The visually triggered task requires an immediate saccade to the location where the target is flashed. The target is off during the saccade and reappears after the saccade is completed. In the learned-saccade task, no stimulus ever appears during the trial. The monkey is required to make the same saccade as in the visually triggered tasks. Trials from these two tasks are normally randomly intermingled. In all three of these saccade tasks, the target reappears after the saccade has been performed to help reinforce saccadic accuracy.

ing the fixation point and illuminating the saccade target to ensure that the two lights never appeared simultaneously. The monkey made a saccade to the position of the new target and the target then reappeared. The animal was rewarded for holding the new position or for responding to the dimming of the target. This task was used to study the activity of neurons in association with visually triggered saccades.

Learned-saccade Task: The monkey first made visually triggered saccades to a briefly flashed target. Then, trials in which no target appeared were intermixed with trials having a target. If the monkey made the proper saccade in either case, the target reappeared and the monkey was rewarded as above. This task was used to determine if the neuron had movement-related

activity that was independent of the recent presence of a visual target.

Double-step Task: In this task, which is similar to that devised by Mays and Sparks (1980), the monkey had to make successive eye movements to briefly flashed stimuli outside of the cell's receptive field. This task is illustrated in Figure 3. This paradigm is termed "double step" because the target effectively undergoes two quick step-like displacements. The monkey looked first at the fixation point, for an interval of 700–1200 msec, after which the fixation point disappeared and two stimuli appeared successively, one at A for 100–125 msec and the next at B for 25–50 msec. In the normal double-step task, the combined stimulus duration was sufficiently brief so that both stimuli dis-

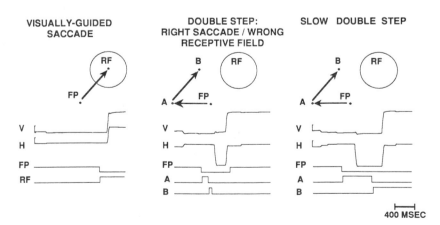

Figure 3. Double-step task. The double-step task is tailored for each cell individually. It is designed to include, as the second saccade, the preferred vector for that cell, as determined in the visually guided saccade task (*left* panel). In the normal double-step task (*center* panel), targets at A and B are flashed on briefly. Both targets are extinguished before the first saccade (from FP to A) begins. Neither target ever appears in the receptive field. In the slow double-step task (*right* panel), the targets are presented in the same sequence but remain on much longer. This allows the monkey to make the saccade from FP to A before target B appears. When B does appear, it is in the receptive field of the cell. This slow version is used to assess activity in relation to the FP to A saccade alone.

appeared before the monkey's eyes began to move. The monkey was required to make two successive saccades, from FP to A and from A to B, and the target reappeared after the second saccade if both saccades were correct. The durations were weighted in favor of the first target because with equal durations, the monkey would usually ignore the first target and make one saccade directly from the fixation point to the second target. Note that the second saccade, A→B, is the same as that in the visually triggered saccade task, FP→RF, but, since both targets are flashed while the eyes are straight ahead, neither of the visual stimuli ever appears in the neuron's receptive field. The second saccade matches the preferred saccade vector of the cell even though the visual target is outside the receptive field. This task dissociates the retinal location of a target from the direction of saccade necessary to acquire that target. A variant of this task, called the "slow double step," requires the monkey to make the same two saccades, but the target at B appears only after the saccade to A has already occurred. This task allows separate examination of responses to targets at A and B.

RESULTS

A total of 282 neurons in LIP were studied in three hemispheres of two rhesus monkeys. Of these, 272 could be driven by a visual stimulus or discharged in association with visually guided saccades. Almost half (125 neurons) had saccade-related activity that was independent of the visual response. For the cells presented here, activity was quantified by counting the number of spikes in a 100-msec epoch starting at the beginning of the burst after a visual stimulus or starting 100 msec before the beginning of the saccade, and then calculating mean discharge frequency, standard deviation, and standard error. For visually guided saccade tasks, anticipatory saccades were discouraged by varying the interval between stimulus onset and the signal to make the saccade. Accordingly, histograms and rasters for these tasks are usually shown twice: once with the rasters aligned on the appearance of the stimulus and again with the rasters aligned on the beginning of the saccade.

Visual, Attentional, and Saccade-related Activity of LIP Neurons

LIP neurons are remarkable for the range of behaviors in which they are active. This range is illustrated in Figure 4. First, this neuron was visually responsive. It gave a brisk response to a visual stimulus (33.33 Hz, s.e.m. 4.75 Hz) in the fixation task, where the monkey looks only at the central fixation point and is free to ignore the stimulus in the receptive field. Second, this visual response was enhanced under two different conditions in which the stimulus had significance for the monkey's behavior. The visual response was larger in both the peripheral attention task (61.88

Hz, s.e.m. 6.66 Hz) and in the delayed-saccade task (45.62 Hz, s.e.m. 2.88). Third, this neuron also discharged immediately before and during the saccade in the delayed-saccade task (30.94 Hz, s.e.m. 2.02). This latter discharge could represent a reactivation of the visual response or true movement-related activity (Boch and Goldberg 1989). To distinguish between these possibilities, we studied the activity of such neurons in the learned-saccade task in which the monkey never sees any target during the fixation period and must make the saccade with no cue except for its memory of the most recent saccade. These learned-saccade trials are intermingled with visually triggered saccade trials. The cell illustrated in Figure 4 discharged before both visually triggered saccades (34.90 Hz, s.e.m. 2.18) and learned saccades (22.50 Hz, s.e.m. 3.10). Although the activity was significantly less in the learned-saccade trials than in the intermixed visually triggered saccade trials ($p < 0.006$, $t = 2.70$, $df = 30$), it was still significantly above the background for this cell ($p < 0.0001$, $t = 7.3$, $df = 30$). Such movement-related activity was seen in 28 of 36 cells studied in both the delayed- and learned-saccade tasks. The converse was quite unusual: Only two cells discharged in a learned-saccade task but not in response to visual stimuli.

Activity of LIP Neurons in Double-step Tasks

Like frontal neurons, some LIP neurons are selective not for the retinal coordinates of the target, but for the oculomotor coordinates that would allow acquisition of the target. This is especially true of neurons with significant activity in the learned-saccade task, but it is also true of some neurons that have either no saccade-related activity or significantly less saccade-related activity than visual activity. Such a neuron is shown in Figure 5. This neuron gave a brisk visual response to stimulus onset in the delayed-saccade task (35.00 Hz, s.e.m. 5.47). The activity level for this cell had returned to baseline at the time of the saccade. Nevertheless, this cell gave a brisk response after the first saccade in the double-step task (26.25 Hz, s.e.m. 5.48). This level of activation is not significantly different from the visual response to a stimulus in the receptive field in the delayed-saccade task. In this double-step experiment, the monkey made successive saccades to stimuli flashed at A and B, neither of which was in the receptive field of the neuron. The neuronal burst occurred before the saccade from A to B, which is the same amplitude and direction as the saccade from FP to RF. This burst could not be attributed to the saccade itself, since the presaccadic activity in the delayed-saccade task (second panel) is at background level. It also cannot be a visual response to the stimulus evoking the first movement nor a postsaccadic response to this first movement, because the neuron does not discharge in association with the first saccade in the slow double-step task (last panel). Note that in the slow double-step task, the cell did give an appropriate response before the second saccade: The second stimulus (B) in this task appears

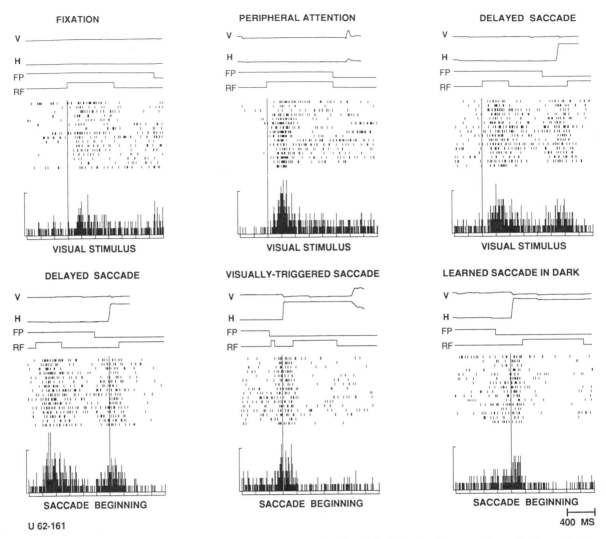

Figure 4. LIP neuron with multiple activities in five standard tasks. In this and the following figures, each panel shows a single eye movement trace from one trial (V and H), the timing of the onset and offset of the fixation point (FP) and receptive field (RF) stimuli, 16 individual rasters, and the associated histogram made from these rasters. The calibration bar at the left of each histogram indicates 100 spikes/sec. The label at the top of each panel indicates the type of trial illustrated, and the label at the bottom indicates the event on which the rasters are aligned. The time of this event is shown by the continuous vertical line extending through both the histogram and the rasters. For the delayed-saccade task, the same rasters are shown twice, first aligned on the onset of the visual stimulus (*top row*) and then aligned on the beginning of the saccade (*bottom row*). This cell has an enhanced visual response in both the peripheral attention and the delayed-saccade tasks (*top row*). It also discharges at the time of the saccade, whether or not a visual stimulus appeared in the course of the trial (*bottom row*).

only after the eye has already moved to A; at this point, stimulus B is in the receptive field of the cell and its onset produces a visual response. Having ruled out the possibility that the double-step response is a visual response to the first stimulus or a motor activation related to either saccade, we conclude that this activity must be a visual response to target B, even though that stimulus never appeared in the neuron's receptive field (as determined in the fixation task). Our explanation for this apparent paradox is that this visual responsiveness depends not on the retinal location of the receptive field, but on the presence of a target that can be acquired by a particular saccade.

Some LIP neurons have both visual and saccade-related activities. For these cells, as for the purely

visual LIP neurons, activity in the double-step task appears to be visual. A neuron with a tonic visual response in the fixation task is illustrated in Figure 6. This neuron also discharged in the delayed-saccade task, giving a brisk burst in response to the stimulus and then maintaining a tonic level of firing that continued until the saccade (top row). In the intermingled visually triggered and learned-saccade trials (middle row), the cell gave a burst in response to the visual stimulus in visually triggered trials, but gave only the sustained response in learned-saccade trials. This cell also had anticipatory activity (bottom row): The cell discharges in anticipation of the onset of the visual stimulus but only in tasks in which the stimulus is significant for the animal's behavior. This anticipatory activity begins

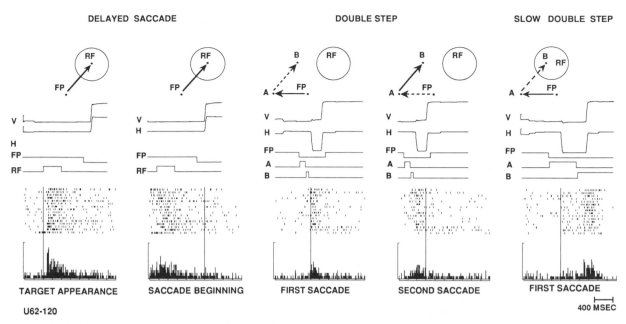

Figure 5. Activity of an LIP neuron in standard and double-step tasks. Solid arrows indicate the current saccade, and dashed arrows indicate either the next or the previous saccade. The first two panels at the left show the response to the visual stimulus when the saccade must be delayed until the fixation point goes off. The visual response to target appearance diminishes at the offset of the stimulus, and there is no activity above baseline at the time of saccade beginning. In the double-step task, the cell discharges after the first saccade and before the second saccade, as though there were a visual stimulus in the receptive field, even though no stimulus ever appeared at that location. In the slow double-step task, there is no activity immediately after the first saccade, indicating that the activity in the normal double-step task is not attributable to postsaccadic firing.

with the start of fixation and continues until the saccade in both the delayed- and learned-saccade tasks. There was no anticipatory activity before stimulus appearance in fixation trials, where the animal is free to ignore the stimulus and does not expect to have to make an eye movement to the stimulus when the fixation point disappears.

The response of this tonic neuron in the double-step task was similar to that for the visual neuron. This cell also discharged during and after the first saccade, and before the second saccade, as shown in Figure 7. The activity in the double-step task (63.08 Hz, s.e.m. 3.04) was significantly higher than the presaccadic activity in the learned-saccade trials (22.62 Hz, s.e.m. 2.88, $p < 0.0001$) but close to the activity in the visually triggered trials of the learned-saccade task (70.00 Hz, s.e.m. 2.415). This activity was not seen when the monkey made single saccades to either one of the stimuli used in the double-step task (slow double step and saccade to second target). As for the previously illustrated cell, we conclude that the activity of this cell in the double-step task represents a visual response to the target at location B, even though this is outside the receptive field of the cell.

We were surprised to find that the stimulus at location B could evoke activity from the neuron even in cases in which the monkey did not perform the double-step saccades correctly. These trials are illustrated in Figure 8. The double-step task is very difficult, and from a long series of double-step trials, we were able to cull a sufficient number of error trials to permit analysis

of neural activity during errors. The monkey tended to make two different kinds of errors: saccades in reversed sequence and saccades direct to the second target, followed by a return to the fixation point. In both of these cases, the cell discharged in response to the second target. In these error trials, the monkey took longer to make the first saccade, and the activity clearly begins before the saccade. Unlike in the correct trials, the activity does not continue until the second saccade, presumably because the B stimulus was no longer the target for an A → B saccade. The activity in these error trials suggests that the stimulus at B can evoke a visual response, as though it were in the receptive field, simply as a result of the paradigm having established a context in which the receptive field would shift.

DISCUSSION

Both humans and monkeys are able to make correct saccades to the spatial location of a target in a double-step task. In this task, the correct saccade cannot be calculated from retinal error alone. This task is therefore useful for gaining insight into how the oculomotor system deals with spatial problems. We have investigated the activity of neurons in LIP during a double-step task. In agreement with previous reports (Gnadt and Andersen 1988), we observe that LIP neurons discharge after the first saccade and before the second saccade. Our main finding is that this activity is a visual response. Parietal neurons give visual responses to

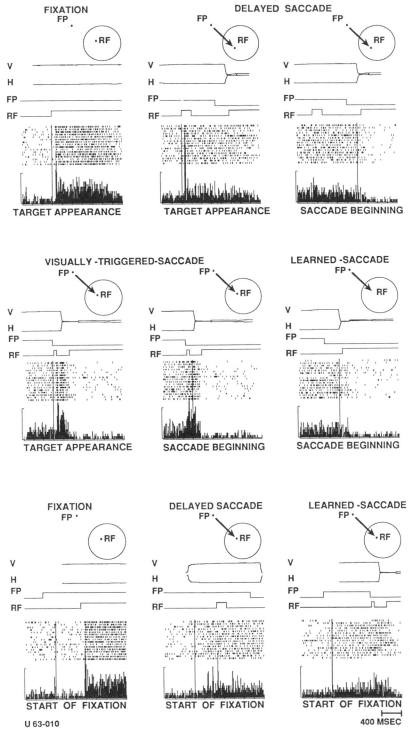

Figure 6. Tonic LIP neuron activity in standard tasks. (*Top row*) Visual response to a target in the receptive field continues from target onset to the end of the trial in the fixation task. In the delayed-saccade task, the activity continues from target onset to initiation of the saccade, even though the target is extinguished well before the saccade. (*Middle row*) Activity in saccade trials continues through the saccade, whether or not there has been a visual stimulus. (*Bottom row*) Activity begins only at target onset when the monkey will not have to perform any saccade (fixation task) but begins to increase at the time of fixation when the monkey anticipates making a saccade, whether or not a visual stimulus occurs (delayed-saccade and learned-saccade tasks).

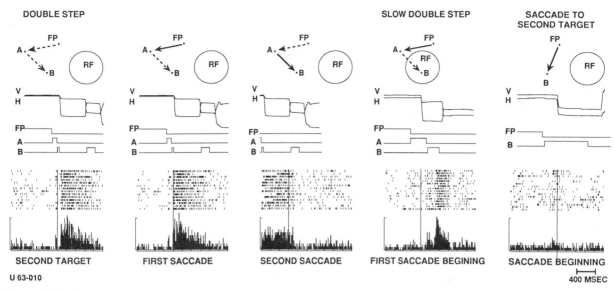

Figure 7. Tonic LIP neuron activity in double-step tasks. The first three panels show the same set of rasters triggered on three different events. The cell fires during the interval between the first saccade and the second saccade. The slow double-step task shows that this is not postsaccadic activation related to the first saccade. The final panel shows that this activity is also not attributable to presaccadic activation related to the second saccade.

targets that dictate a particular saccade when that saccade matches the preferred vector of the cell.

At first glance, it is tempting to interpret this presaccadic activity in motor terms. Two findings from the present study argue against this interpretation. First, some purely visual cells, which have no motor activity in any single-step task, nevertheless discharge between the first and second saccades in a double-step task. Second, some tonic neurons, which normally discharge throughout the period between target and saccade onset in a single-step task, discharge about twice as strongly in the double-step task. We interpret these findings to indicate that the activity observed in the double-step task is visual, and not motor, activity.

If this activity is visual, how can we account for a visual response to a target that never appeared in the cell's receptive field? We suggest that visual activity in parietal cortex is coded not in retinotopic coordinates but in oculomotor coordinates. In any single-step task, the receptive field and the movement field for a given neuron are in register. When these fields are dissociated, as in the double-step task, the cell is driven by targets in the movement field. The signal carried by these cells then says that there exists a target that can be acquired by a particular saccade.

This finding may bear on the question of spatial representation. If the location of a visual stimulus can be represented by a vector, which corresponds to the amplitude and direction of the saccade necessary to acquire it, then it may be unnecessary to invoke an explicit representation of target position in head-centered space. There are at least two different hypotheses as to how the brain produces accurate saccades in the double-step task. The first hypothesis states that the system uses retinal location and eye position to com-

pute an internal representation of target location in head-centered space, from which it then computes the necessary direction of saccade. An alternative possibility is that the brain uses retinal error and the dimensions of a previous eye movement to compute a target vector in saccade coordinates, without computing target position in space explicitly. The transformation of visual input from retinal to motor coordinates is an essential step in the production of spatially accurate eye movements. Visual activity in parietal neurons appears to code target location retinotopically when observed in a simple single-step task. The double-step experiments reveal, however, that these neurons can respond to stimuli presented outside of the retinal receptive field. The first model requires a representation of the position of visual targets in a supraretinal space that is invariant with the movement of the eyes in the orbit (Robinson 1973; Mays and Sparks 1980). Such a representation of target position in space has never been observed, although the information could be calculated from the retinal and orbital position signals that are present (Andersen and Mountcastle 1983; Andersen et al. 1990).

We propose an alternate model which suggests instead that the brain uses the dimensions of the previous saccade and the target position on the retina to compute the required saccade (Goldberg and Colby 1989; Goldberg and Bruce 1990). In this model, there is no unchanging representation of absolute target position. Instead, there is only a representation of the retina and a representation of the previous saccade. Both of these representations have been observed in parietal cortex (Andersen et al. 1990). In the double-step situation, vector subtraction of the first saccade from the retinal location of the second target yields the dimensions of

ERROR TRIALS: SACCADES TO SECOND TARGET AND BACK

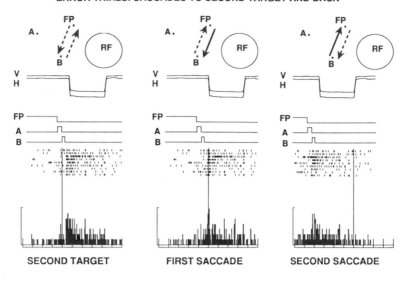

ERROR TRIALS: SACCADES IN REVERSED SEQUENCE

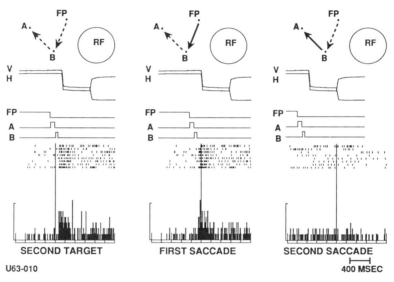

U63-010

400 MSEC

Figure 8. Tonic LIP neuron in error trials from double-step tasks. (*Top row*) Error trials in which the monkey made a saccade directly to the second target and skipped the first target. These three panels show the same set of error trials (culled from a long series of double-step trials) triggered on three different events. The first panel shows neural activity aligned on the onset of the second target (B), before any saccade has occurred. The middle panel shows this same set of trials aligned on the beginning of an incorrect saccade direct to the second target (B). The last panel shows activity aligned on the beginning of the second saccade back to the fixation point. (*Bottom row*) These three panels illustrate activity in relation to a different type of error in which the monkey made saccades to each target but in the reverse sequence. The first saccade in these trials is like the first saccade in the top-row error trials. In both types of error trials, the cell discharge is similar to that observed in correct trials.

the second saccade. The neurons illustrated here derive the bulk of their activity from visual sources: Activity in the double-step task resembles that in visually guided saccade tasks, even though the visual stimulus that evokes the saccade never appears in the visual receptive field of the neuron (as determined in a standard fixation task). This activity cannot arise from post-saccadic processes related to the first saccade of the double step, nor can it arise from premotor processes related to the second saccade, because neither of these events in isolation is associated with sufficient activity.

These parietal neurons thus yield a signal that is visual, in that it is driven by retinal excitation, but that is coded in oculomotor coordinates.

Visual activity in oculomotor coordinates has been demonstrated in the frontal eye field, and the quasivisual cells described in the superior colliculus may also code visual activity in oculomotor coordinates (Mays and Sparks 1980). Cross-modal integration in subcortical and cortical regions may also depend on sensory coding in motor coordinates. Auditory receptive fields in the superior colliculus shift in register with eye position as direction of gaze changes (Jay and Sparks 1984). In the periarcuate region concerned with mouth movements, neurons discharge to stimuli that could be acquired by those mouth movements regardless of the position of the eye in the orbit (Rizzolatti et al. 1981).

In parietal cortex, the actual movement need not take place in order for the transformation to occur. LIP neurons discharge in trials in which the monkey actually made the wrong movements, either by performing the saccades in reversed sequence or by making a saccade to the second target and then returning to the fixation point. These neurons gave the same response as in the correct trials, when the stimulus appeared in a behavioral context suggesting that it would become the target for the proper direction of eye movement. Only when the monkey's error rendered that target no longer appropriate did the cells cease firing. These findings suggest that the computation of oculomotor coordinates is based on the intended, rather than the actual, eye movement and support the idea that parietal neurons specify an attentional vector. This vector is encoded not in absolute spatial terms, but in terms of the movement needed to acquire the target. We propose that the representation of space in posterior parietal cortex is in terms of such attentional vectors.

REFERENCES

Andersen, R.A. and V.B. Mountcastle. 1983. The influence of the angle of gaze upon the excitability of the light-sensitive neurons of the posterior parietal cortex. *J. Neurosci.* **3:** 532.

Andersen, R.A., C. Asanuma, and M. Cowan. 1985. Callosal and prefrontal associational projecting cell in area 7a of the macaque monkey: A study using retrogradely transported fluorescent dyes. *J. Comp. Neurol.* **232:** 443.

Andersen, R.A., R.M. Bracewell, S. Barash, J.W. Gnadt, and L. Fogassi. 1990. Eye position effects on visual, memory, and saccade-related activity in areas LIP and 7a of macaque. *J. Neurosci.* **10:** 1176.

Boch, R.A. and M.E. Goldberg. 1989. Participation of prefrontal neurons in the preparation of visually guided eye movements in the rhesus monkey. *J. Neurophysiol.* **61:** 1064.

Bruce, C.J. and M.E. Goldberg. 1985. Primate frontal eye fields. I. Single neurons discharging before saccades. *J. Neurophysiol.* **53:** 603.

Bruce, C.J., M.E. Goldberg, G.B. Stanton, and M.C. Bushnell. 1985. Primate frontal eye fields. II. Physiological and anatomical correlates of electrically evoked eye movements. *J. Neurophysiol.* **54:** 714.

Bushnell, M.C., M.E. Goldberg, and D.L. Robinson. 1981. Behavioral enhancement of visual responses in monkey cerebral cortex. I. Modulation in posterior parietal cortex related to selective visual attention. *J. Neurophysiol.* **46:** 755.

Colby, C.L., R. Gattass, C.R. Olson, and C.G. Gross. 1988. Topographic organization of cortical afferents to extrastriate visual area PO in the macaque: A dual tracer study. *J. Comp. Neurol.* **238:** 1257.

Crist, C.F., D.S.G. Yamasaki, H. Komatsu, and R.H. Wurtz. 1988. A grid system and a microsyringe for single cell recording. *J. Neurosci. Methods* **26:** 117.

Critchley, M. 1953. *The parietal lobes.* Arnold, London.

Gnadt, J.W. and R.A. Andersen. 1988. Memory related motor planning activity in posterior parietal cortex of macaque. *Exp. Brain Res.* **70:** 216.

Goldberg, M.E. 1983. Studying the neurophysiology of behavior: Methods for recording single neurons in awake behaving monkeys. In *Methods in cellular neurobiology* (ed. J.L. Barker and J.F. McKelvy), vol. 3, p. 225. Wiley, New York.

Goldberg, M.E. and C.J. Bruce. 1990. Primate frontal eye fields. III. Maintenance of a spatially accurate saccade signal. *J. Neurophysiol.* **64:** 489.

Goldberg, M.E. and M.C. Bushnell. 1981. Behavioral enhancement of visual responses in monkey cerebral cortex. II. Modulation in frontal eye fields specifically related to saccades. *J. Neurophysiol.* **46:** 773.

Goldberg, M.E. and C.L. Colby. 1989. The neurophysiology of spatial vision. In *Handbook of neuropsychology* (ed. F. Boller and J. Grafman), vol. 2, p. 301. Elsevier, Amsterdam.

Hallett, P.E. and A.D. Lightstone. 1976. Saccadic eye movements to flashed targets. *Vision Res.* **16:** 107.

Heilman, K.M., R.T. Watson, E. Valenstein, and M.E. Goldberg. 1987. Attention: Behavior and neural mechanisms. In *Handbook of physiology: The nervous system* (ed. F. Plum), sect. 1, vol. 5, p. 461. American Physiological Society, Bethesda, Maryland.

Hubel, D.H. and T.N. Wiesel. 1977. Ferrier lecture: Functional architecture of macaque monkey visual cortex. *Proc. R. Soc. Lond. B Biol. Sci.* **198:** 1.

Jay, M.F. and D.L. Sparks. 1984. Auditory receptive fields in primate superior colliculus shift with changes in eye position. *Nature* **309:** 3450.

Lynch, J.C., A.M. Graybiel, and L.J. Lobeck. 1985. The differential projection of two cytoarchitectonic subregions of the inferior parietal lobule of macaque upon the deep layers of the superior colliculus. *J. Comp. Neurol.* **235:** 241.

Lynch, J.C., V.B. Mountcastle, W.H. Talbot, and T.C.T. Yin. 1977. Parietal lobe mechanisms for directed visual attention. *J. Neurophysiol.* **40:** 362.

Mays, L.E. and D.L. Sparks. 1980. Dissociation of visual and saccade-related responses in superior colliculus neurons. *J. Neurophysiol.* **43:** 207.

Mountcastle, V.B., J.C. Lynch, A. Georgopoulos, H. Sakata, and C. Acuna. 1975. Posterior parietal association cortex of the monkey: Command functions for operations within extrapersonal space. *J. Neurophysiol.* **38:** 871.

Rizzolatti, G., C. Scandolara, M. Matelli, and M. Gentilucci. 1981. Afferent properties of periarcuate neurons in macaque monkeys. II. Visual responses. *Behav. Brain Res.* **2:** 147.

Robinson, D.A. 1973. Models of the saccadic eye movement control system. *Kybernetik* **14:** 71.

Robinson, D.L., M.E. Goldberg, and G.B. Stanton. 1978. Parietal association cortex in the primate: Sensory mechanisms and behavioral modulations. *J. Neurophysiol.* **41:** 910.

Segraves, M.A. and M.E. Goldberg. 1987. Functional properties of corticotectal neurons in the monkey's frontal eye field. *J. Neurophysiol.* **58:** 1387.

Stanton, G.B., C.J. Bruce, and M.E. Goldberg. 1988. Frontal eye field efferents in the macaque monkey. I. Subcortical pathways and topography of striatal and thalamic terminal fields. *J. Comp. Neurol.* **271:** 473.

Wurtz, R.N. and C.W. Mohler. 1976. Organization of monkey superior colliculus: Enhanced visual response of superficial layer cells. *J. Neurophysiol.* **39:** 745.

Yin, T.C.T. and V.B. Mountcastle. 1977. Visual input to the visuomotor mechanisms of the monkey's parietal lobe. *Science* **197:** 1381.

Hierarchical Processing of Motion in the Visual Cortex of Monkey

R.A. ANDERSEN, R.J. SNOWDEN, S. TREUE, AND M. GRAZIANO
Department of Brain and Cognitive Sciences, Massachusetts Institute of Technology,
Cambridge, Massachusetts 02139

Recent work on the visual system of primates has delineated several cortical fields involved in the processing of visual motion. These cortical areas appear to be connected anatomically in stages, which suggests that there is a hierarchy in the machinery for motion perception. In this paper, we outline experiments that we have performed along the most prominent pathway for motion analysis, which begins in area V1 and proceeds through the middle temporal area (MT) to the medial superior temporal area (MST). Our goal has been to demonstrate what sequential processing steps take place at each anatomical stage in this presumably hierarchical system. In the first section, we show how a special class of stimuli, transparent motions, have enabled us to separate distinct and different mechanisms for the processing of directional information in areas V1 and MT. In the second section, we discuss psychophysical experiments that explore the ability to perceive shape from motion. These results indicate that the brain interpolates motion data to form neural representations of moving surfaces, and they have interesting implications for our recording experiments. The last section covers recent work on the possible role of area MST in integrating motion-pattern information. Area MST neurons selective to expanding, contracting, or rotating velocity fields were examined. We found that these cells respond to particular patterns of stimuli irrespective of the location in the receptive field or, to a large extent, the size of the stimulus. These cells may represent a stage in higher-level processing of motion, including the perception of shape from motion.

Motion Transparency

Motion transparency is quite common in natural scenes. It exists whenever two different directions of motion occur at local points in an image. One example of motion transparency is the view one receives looking through a windshield of a moving automobile with rain pouring down the glass. Other less obvious but still common instances of transparency are the motion of a shadow over a textured background, the specular reflections that remain stationary when an object rotates, and the motion discontinuities that occur at the boundaries between a moving object and the background against which it moves. Computer algorithms developed to analyze moving video images have difficulty representing transparent motion because they generally allow only one velocity vector to be present at each pixel in the image. The fact that artificial systems display an inability to analyze motion transparency suggests that the primate visual system has developed a specialized method for its perception.

Motion transparency presents a problem not only to computer algorithms, but also to models of how the nervous system processes motion. The currently prevalent model of motion-direction selectivity employs inhibitory interactions among groups of nerve cells (Barlow and Levick 1965). These inhibitory interactions would suppress motion-selective cells under transparent conditions and render the visual system blind to motion, similar to the artificial systems mentioned above.

To examine how the primate visual system solves this problem, we recorded the activity of motion-selective cells to transparent motion stimuli in areas V1 and MT in behaving monkeys (Erickson et al. 1989; Snowden et al. 1990). Each neuron's preferred direction of movement was assessed by drifting random-dot patterns in different directions through the receptive field. The one eliciting the greatest discharge was termed the preferred direction, and the opposite direction was designated the antipreferred direction (Fig. 1). These two "single-surface" stimuli were then presented in an interleaved block of trials along with a stimulus that was composed of these two stimuli superimposed on one another, producing the transparent condition (Fig. 1). By and large, the direction-selective V1 cells gave a similar response to the preferred direction and to the two-surface stimulus. However, we found that the activity of MT cells stimulated with the two-surface stimulus was always suppressed below the level of that seen to the preferred stimulus alone. We concluded that area V1 direction-selective neurons are only minimally affected under transparent conditions, whereas the activity of MT neurons is suppressed. Thus, there appears to be a hierarchy for directional mechanisms in the motion pathway.

In further experiments, we examined the nature of the inhibitory process in area MT. We "titrated" the effect of excitatory and inhibitory influences by varying the dot density in each of the two directions. It was found that the inhibition appeared to be divisive, reducing the response not by a set number of spikes per second, but rather by a number that increases with the increased firing of the neuron. These interactions may

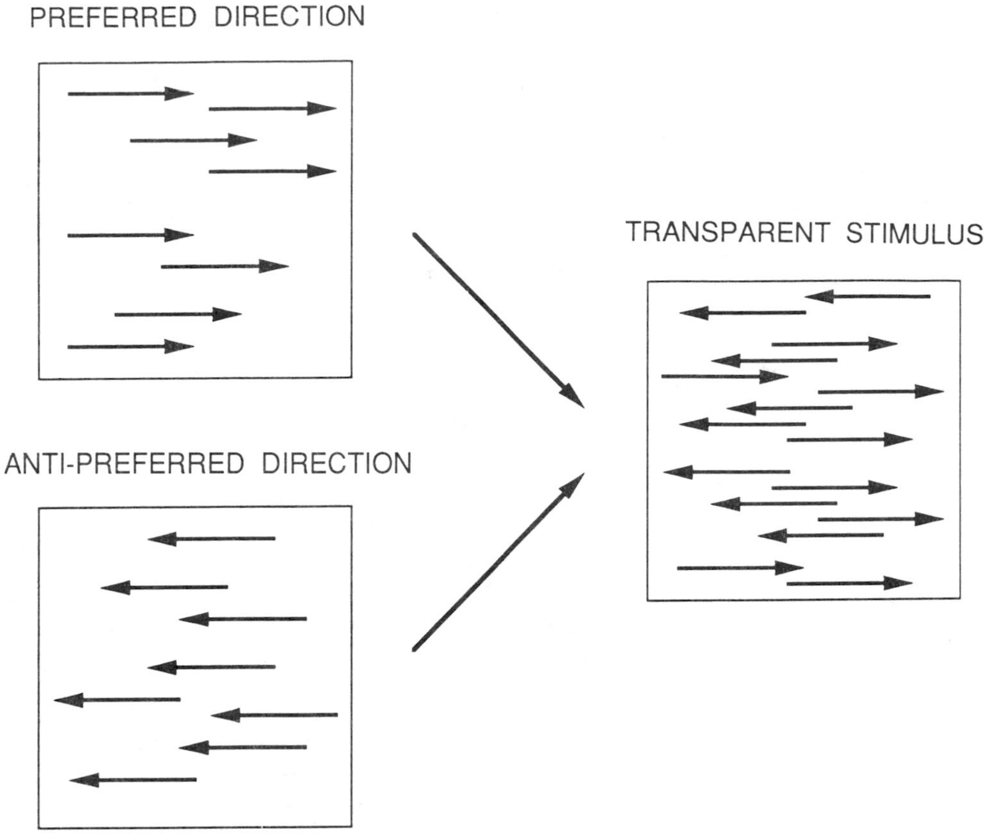

PREFERRED DIRECTION

TRANSPARENT STIMULUS

ANTI-PREFERRED DIRECTION

Figure 1. Example of the transparent motion stimulus used for recording experiments in areas V1 and MT. This stimulus is composed of two sets of dots: one set drifting in the preferred direction of the neuron being recorded from and the other set drifting in the opposite (antipreferred) direction.

be considered a kind of averaging or smoothing of the velocity field.

These results bear upon the issue of how area V1 neurons achieve a directional response. A classic model of how rabbit retinal ganglion cells achieve directional responses postulates that the presence of the anti-preferred stimulus causes a wave of inhibition preceding the arrival of the excitatory signal, vetoing any response (Barlow and Levick 1965). Since this model predicts strong suppressive interactions for our transparent motion condition, the comparative lack of such suppression in primary visual cortex suggests that many primate V1 neurons might achieve directionality by other mechanisms such as facilitation in the preferred direction (Barlow and Levick 1965). Facilitatory mechanisms have occasionally been proposed for directional selectivity in the cat striate cortex, although inhibitory mechanisms are generally believed to predominate there (Goodwin and Henry 1975; Movshon et al. 1978; Sillito 1979; Douglas et al. 1988).

The suppression of the directional response in area MT by nonpreferred directions of motion may result from single MT neurons receiving opposing inputs from different directional cells in the projection from V1 to MT. It is also possible that direction selectivity may be reproduced de novo in MT using inhibitory mechanisms (Rodman and Albright 1989). At present, our

data cannot distinguish between these alternatives. The divisive nature of the inhibition may result from an increase in chloride conductance producing a shunting inhibition (Koch et al. 1986). GABA has been proposed as a likely inhibitory transmitter for producing this type of inhibition for direction-selective neurons in the cat cortex and fly visual system (Sillito 1979; Koch et al. 1986; Egelhaaf et al. 1990).

The two-stage analysis demonstrated in these data has interesting parallels for some models of motion processing in humans and flies (Reichardt 1961; Adelson and Bergen 1985). The first stage of the models for both species measures local motions and the second stage then performs some form of integration, the most common being to average or "smooth" the velocity field. The neurons of area V1 behave like directional filters, extracting their preferred direction of motion from the directions present in the image. Therefore, the transparent motion stimulus appears to activate two separate groups of neurons tuned to opposite directions of movement. This segregation could then form the basis for segmenting the stimulus into two separate moving surfaces. As such, the V1 neurons may correspond to stage 1 of the above models, where local motion measurements are made.

In area MT, the transparent motion stimulus would also activate two subpopulations of neurons tuned for different directions of motion. However, our results show that this activation is considerably less than when each direction is presented alone. If area MT is a major site for the processing of the perception of motion (Siegel and Andersen 1986; Newsome and Paré 1988; Newsome et al. 1989), even under transparent conditions, then the recordings suggest that each direction of motion would be less detectable under transparent conditions, compared to when the direction of motion is presented in isolation. Such a result has been recently reported for transparent motions of orthogonal direction (Snowden 1989). Alternatively, one of several possible parallel motion pathways, such as V1 to V2, V3, or the parieto-occipital area, may be responsible for maintaining the segregation established in V1.

The results point to a two-stage hierarchical process in primate motion perception. The first stage, area V1, takes local velocity measurements and segments the image, and the second, area MT, spatially integrates these measurements. Transparent motion perception may be made possible by allowing separate and multiple independent measures of direction at the initial stage of motion analysis. The reason for the apparent combination of these independent measures with divisive interactions at a later stage in area MT is not clear, but it may perform a smoothing operation that could be important for interpolating surfaces from sparse data (Siegel and Andersen 1988; Husain et al. 1989; Treue et al. 1990), reducing noise, or determining the direction of pattern motion from component motion measurements (Bülthoff et al. 1989; Wang et al. 1989).

Surface Reconstruction for Structure-from-motion Perception

Humans can easily perceive the three-dimensional shape of objects from motion information. For example, the shadow of a wire frame projected onto a flat surface gives little information about the shape of the frame; however, when it is rotated, the three-dimensional shape becomes immediately apparent (Wallach and O'Connell 1953). This ability to recover structure from motion is not a trivial one since, generally, an infinite number of three-dimensional shapes can be given to a two-dimensional image. This structure-from-motion problem can be solved with computer algorithms by introducing certain reasonable constraints, such as the assumption that objects tend to be rigid or continuous. How the brain solves the problem, of course, is another matter. Recent psychophysical work from our laboratory suggests that one aspect of the neural mechanism for computing structure-from-motion is to reconstruct surfaces by interpolating motion cues. We have also extended this idea of surface interpolation to computational algorithms for structure-from-motion analysis.

Psychophysical studies. A task we developed for examining structure-from-motion perception is illustrated in Figure 2. The subjects are to indicate when they see a transition from an unstructured motion field to a motion field that gives the perception of a revolving, hollow cylinder. The time at which the transition occurs is random and unpredicted, and the subjects must release a key as quickly as they can once they perceive the change. To allow for a smooth transition from no structure to structure, the points are on for only a short period of time before being replotted at a new, random location on the screen. When the change in structure occurs, only new points assume the new structure, thus preventing any artifactual cues that would occur if the dots changed speed in midtrajectory. These finite point lifetimes also control for many other potential artifacts such as density and shape cues (see below and Siegel and Andersen 1988, 1990; Andersen and Siegel 1990).

As is illustrated in Figure 3, we found the reaction times in this task to be quite long, usually extending over several point lifetimes (Siegel and Andersen 1988, 1990; Husain et al. 1989; Andersen and Siegel 1990; Treue et al. 1990). This result suggested that the percept of structure from motion builds up over time and that new points were integrated into a representation partially computed from the old points. It is not possible, however, to determine from these data how much of the reaction time is needed as visual input and how much is computation time in the brain or motor reaction time. The surface interpolation hypothesis would predict that more visual input time would improve performance.

To test this idea directly, we presented equal numbers of structured and unstructured stimuli of 40–1700 msec duration in random order and asked subjects to indicate in a two-alternative forced-choice paradigm whether they saw a rotating cylinder or an unstructured noise pattern (Husain et al. 1989; Treue et al. 1990). Figure 4 (closed symbols) shows that performance peaked only after viewing stimuli for more than eight point lifetimes, a result consistent with the surface interpolation idea.

To control for the possibility that the buildup in performance is not due to presentation of new points but to some other process, we performed another experiment (Husain et al. 1989; Treue et al. 1990). After the first point lifetime, the dots were replotted at the beginning of the old trajectory instead of some new, random location. This procedure was repeated in all subsequent point lifetimes, resulting in the repeated presentation of the same motion data that was provided in the first point lifetime. Figure 4 (open symbols) shows that under these conditions, where no new information is supplied, the performance does not build up and remains at chance levels.

Another example supporting the use of surface interpolation comes from experiments in which individual dots in the cylinder were oscillated randomly back and forth along their horizontal trajectory (Treue and Andersen 1990). If the motion system were to follow the individual features of the stimulus, there would be no coherent interpretation of these motions. However,

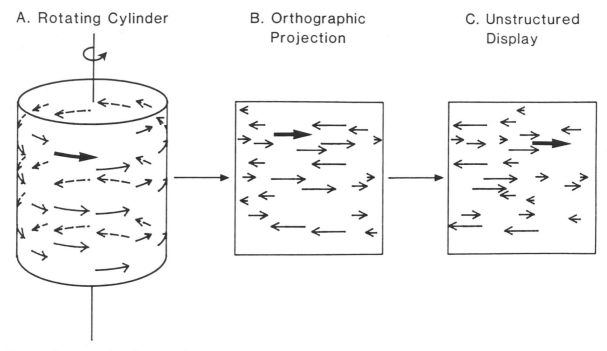

Figure 2. Demonstration of structure-from-motion reaction time task. The velocity of each point is indicated by the length of the arrows. (*A*) The stimuli are generated by first computing the location of points on the surface of the rotating cylinder for each instant in time. (*B*) The points are then parallel (orthographically) projected onto a plane perpendicular to the observer's line of sight. This is the "structured display." (*C*) The unstructured display is computed by taking each point's motion trajectories from the test display and displacing them randomly in a window equal to the width of the display. The fate of an individual motion trajectory for a point crossing the front of the display is shown by the bold arrow. The point density on the surface of the display is kept constant; each point is displayed for a finite amount of time. At the end of this time, the point vanishes and reappears randomly on the screen to follow a new motion trajectory. (Reprinted, with permission, from Siegel and Andersen 1988.)

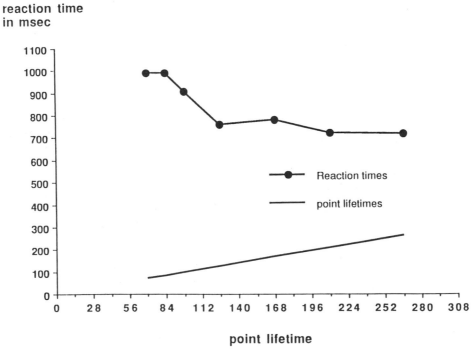

Figure 3. Reaction time as a function of point lifetime. Point lifetime is also plotted to allow easy comparison with reaction time. Note that the reaction time is always many times longer than the point lifetime. (Reprinted, with permission, from Treue et al. 1990.)

744

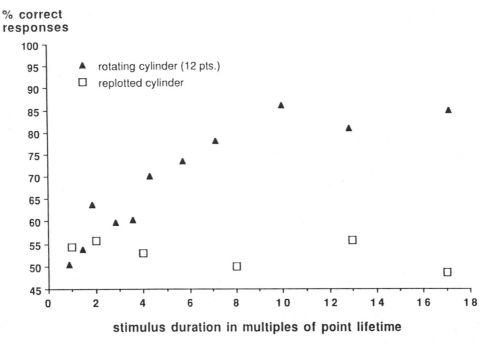

Figure 4. Percentage of correct responses in two alternative forced-choice tasks plotted as a function of stimulus duration. Note the long build up of performance. (□) Percentage of correct responses using 12 points; (▲) percentage of correct responses when points were repeatedly traveling along the same path. (Reprinted, with permission, from Treue et al. 1990.)

subjects simply see a revolving hollow cylinder. This percept can only be easily explained if the structure-from-motion process represents the observed object as two surfaces moving in opposite directions, rather than a collection of individual elements. A given point contributes information to each surface, depending on its direction of motion.

The neural basis for this segmentation of surfaces is suggested by the transparency experiments outlined above. The direction-selective cells in V1 appear to be direction-selective filters that to a large degree ignore motion in the nonpreferred directions. Our stimulus would activate two distinct populations of V1 cells, with each population corresponding to one of the surfaces. As the individual dots oscillated back and forth, they would alternately activate cells in one group and then the other.

Computational studies. Previous computational algorithms developed for analyzing structure-from-motion do not show buildup using short-lived data points. This observation has relevance not only for the biological plausibility of these models, but also for their general performance as image analyzers. In natural situations of object or observer motion, there is often a great deal of occlusion and disocclusion, which is more or less equivalent to the situation of finite point lifetimes. In addition, there is the computationally expensive problem of tracking many individual features over many frames.

We have recently developed a model that combines an extension of Ullman's (1984) incremental rigidity scheme for computing structure-from-motion with a surface interpolation process that reconstructs full three-dimensional surfaces using sparse motion data with finite point lifetimes (Ando et al. 1990). This new algorithm can operate on either displacements or velocities of moving points in an image. Using sequential inputs over time, the algorithm builds up a representation of three-dimensional structure. Each new estimate of the structure is derived by minimizing the overall deviation in structure that is consistent with the present and previous data. As the three-dimensional structure is derived at the locations of the moving points, a smooth surface is filled in between these locations. This constructed surface is saved between views, and individual image points can therefore appear and disappear without affecting the recovery of structure.

This new model has several interesting features from a biological perspective. It initially segregates surfaces based on their two-dimensional image motion before constructing the three-dimensional image. This step is necessary because without it the interpolated surface would average together the back and front surfaces of the cylinder and as a result would average the depth to zero. This "front end" segregation is reminiscent of the segregation in V1 by direction that was found in the motion transparency experiments. This model can also account for the psychophysical data, outlined above, using limited point lifetimes. A similar degradation in performance with fewer points is found in both our model and our psychophysical experiments (Treue et al. 1990), and similar interactions are seen between multiple transparent surfaces in motion and interactions with boundary shape as reported in human experiments by Ramachandran et al. (1988).

Response of Area MST Neurons to Motion Patterns

Several previous studies have reported neurons in area MST that were selective for rotating or expanding or contracting visual stimuli (Sakata et al. 1985, 1986; Saito et al. 1986; Tanaka et al. 1986, 1989; Tanaka and Saito 1989). Examples of these types of stimuli are shown in Figure 5. The stimuli used in these investigations had several potential artifacts. In cases where textured stimuli were used, there was always the potential that the neurons were responding to shape cues in the stimuli and not to their motion. The expansion and contraction stimuli were often generated using dot patterns and zoom lenses, which produce changes in luminance, dot size, and dot density along with the movement. Even natural stimuli produce changes in texture size and density with motion toward or away from the animal. The individual elements of a rotating field have curved trajectories, and for expanding/contracting stimuli, they have accelerations. Moreover, it was not possible to equate the motion speed distributions when testing neurons with these two classes of stimuli. These complications were appreciated by several investigators, and they initiated controls that indicated that it was likely that these neurons were in fact selective to the pattern of motion, rather than the confounding potential artifacts listed above (Tanaka et al. 1989; Tanaka and Saito 1989). However, their presence in the test stimuli have made it difficult to extend these studies due to the linkage of these potential variables with the experimental variables one would like to investigate.

To circumvent this problem, we have recently designed special rotation and expansion stimuli, generated on a high-speed graphics system, which contain only motion-pattern cues (Andersen et al. 1990; Graziano et al. 1990). These stimuli have dots of finite point lifetime, which are randomly, asynchronously replotted so that the static shape cues are constantly, randomly changing. The use of limited point lifetimes also enable an even distribution of points at all times. Each short-lived velocity vector is linear, and thus there are no curvature or acceleration cues. The speed distributions for expansion, contraction, and rotation are equivalent. In short, the only difference between the displays are the local directions of the movement. For expansion, the dots move outward from the center of the display; for rotation, they move tangentially; and for contraction, they move toward the center of the display.

Using these highly controlled stimuli, we confirmed that area MST neurons were often selective for expansion, contraction, clockwise or counterclockwise rotation, or pure translational movement (Graziano et al. 1990). Some cells responded to different combinations of these stimuli, whereas others only responded to one type of movement. Some rotation cells were found to respond to both clockwise and counterclockwise movements.

Using these stimuli, we have been able to examine this motion-pattern selectivity in more detail. If these cells are truly selective for pattern, then they should show position invariance; i.e., the cell should show the same stimulus selectivity regardless of the position the stimulus occupies in the cell's receptive field. Area MST neurons have very large receptive fields, often exceeding 40° in diameter. We tested for position invariance by positioning 10° diameter stimuli at five overlapping locations in the receptive field arranged in a cloverleaf pattern such that the local direction of motion in the areas of overlap was reversed in direction (Andersen et al. 1990). In every case tested, the cells retained the same stimulus selectivity, indicating that they were position-invariant. These cells also showed a degree of size invariance, responding well to 10° and 20° diameter stimuli, although they often tended to respond better to the larger stimuli.

Another parameter we examined was the effect of attention on the response of area MST neurons (Andersen et al. 1990). Attentional modulation was examined using a reaction time task in which the animal was required to release a key in response either to a change in the motion of the stimulus or to a small dimming of the fixation point. The two trial types were randomly interleaved, and the color of the fixation point at the beginning of each trial indicated to the animal which detection was required in a particular trial. Many area MST cells altered their response when the animal attended to the motion cue with a facilitated

Structured Motions

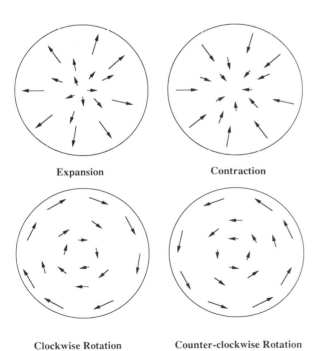

Figure 5. Illustration of expansion, contraction, and rotation stimuli used in recording experiments in area MST by Graziano et al. (1990) and Andersen et al. (1990).

response to the preferred direction of motion, and often a reduced response to the nonpreferred direction of motion. This result suggests that in many cases, the tuning of area MST neurons is sharpened by attention.

CONCLUSIONS

The experiments outlined above provide evidence for hierarchical processing along the cortical visual motion pathway in macaque monkeys. Area V1 direction-selective cells appear to act as directional filters, signaling motion in the preferred direction, with the non-preferred direction having little or no effect. On the other hand, for area MT neurons, the nonpreferred directions powerfully inhibit the response to preferred direction stimuli. We are currently studying the role this inhibitory interaction may play in the spatial integration of motion in area MT.

Our psychophysical experiments suggest that an important step in the analysis of structure-from-motion perception involves surface reconstruction. We are now investigating the role areas MT and MST might play in this surface reconstruction process.

Finally, area MST may play a higher-level role in the processing of motion information with cells selective for particular patterns of motion. The responses of these neurons show pattern position invariance and are also strongly modulated by attention. We are currently asking whether rotation and expansion/contraction are the primary channels used to analyze the structure of the velocity field. An alternative possibility is that there may be a wider range of patterns for which area MST neurons are selective. Thus, in the one case, structure in the velocity field would be decomposed into two basic channels; in the other case, each pattern of motion might activate a large array of different pattern cells by varying amounts.

ACKNOWLEDGMENTS

This work was supported by National Institutes of Health grant EY-07492. Our thanks go to Gail Robertson, Stephen Marchetti, and Richard Keough for technical assistance and to Carol Andersen and Catherine Cooper for editorial assistance.

REFERENCES

Adelson, E.H. and J.R. Bergen. 1985. Spatiotemporal energy models for the perception of motion. *J. Opt. Soc. Am.* **2**: 284.

Andersen, R.A. and R.M. Siegel. 1990. Motion processing in primate cortex. In *Signal and sense: Local and global order in perceptual maps* (ed. G. Edelman et al.). Wiley, New York. (In press.)

Andersen, R.A., M. Graziano, and R.J. Snowden. 1990. Translational invariance and attentional modulation of MST cells. *Soc. Neurosci. Abstr.* (in press).

Ando, H., E.C. Hildreth, S. Treue, and R.A. Andersen. 1990. Recovering 3-D structure from motion with surface reconstruction. *Soc. Neurosci. Abstr.* (in press).

Barlow, H.B. and W.R. Levick. 1965. The mechanism of directionally selective units in the rabbit retina. *J. Physiol.* **178**: 477.

Bülthoff, H., J. Little, and T. Poggio. 1989. A parallel algorithm for real-time computation of optical flow. *Nature* **337**: 549.

Douglas, R.J., K.A.C. Martin, and D. Whitteridge. 1988. Selective responses of visual cortical cells do not depend on shunting inhibition. *Nature* **332**: 642.

Egelhaaf, M., A. Borst, and B. Pilz. 1990. The role of GABA in detecting visual motion. *Brain Res.* **509**: 156.

Erickson, R.G., R.J. Snowden, R.A. Andersen, and S. Treue. 1989. Directional neurons in awake rhesus monkeys: Implications for motion transparency. *Soc. Neurosci. Abstr.* **15**: 323.

Goodwin, A.W. and G.H. Henry. 1975. Direction selectivity of complex cells in a comparison with simple cells. *J. Neurophysiol.* **38**: 1524.

Graziano, M., R.A. Andersen, and R.J. Snowden. 1990. Stimulus selectivity of neurons in macaque MST. *Soc. Neurosci. Abstr.* (in press).

Husain, M., S. Treue, and R.A. Andersen. 1989. Surface interpolation in three-dimensional structure-from-motion perception. *Neural Computat.* **1**: 324.

Koch, C., T. Poggio, and V. Torre. 1986. Computations in the vertebrate retina: Gain enhancement, differentiation and motion discrimination. *Trends Neurosci.* **9**: 204.

Movshon, J.A., I.D. Thompson, and D.J. Tolhurst. 1978. Receptive field organization of complex cells in the cat's striate cortex. *J. Physiol.* **283**: 79.

Newsome, W.T. and E.B. Paré. 1988. A selective impairment of motion perception following lesions of the middle temporal visual area (MT). *J. Neurosci.* **8**: 2201.

Newsome, W.T., K.H. Britten, and I.A. Movshon. 1989. Neuronal correlates of a perceptual decision. *Nature* **341**: 52.

Ramachandran, V.S., S. Cobb, and D. Rogers-Ramachandran. 1988. Perception of 3-D structure from motion: The role of velocity gradients and segmentation boundaries. *Percept. Psychophys.* **44**: 390.

Reichardt, W. 1961. Autocorrelation: A principle of the evaluation of sensory information by the central nervous system. In *Sensory communication* (ed. W.A. Rosenblith), p. 303. Wiley, New York.

Rodman, H.R. and T.D. Albright. 1989. Afferent basis of visual response properties in area MT of the macaque. I. Effects of striate cortex removal. *J. Neurosci.* **9**: 2033.

Saito, H., M. Yukio, K. Tanaka, K. Hikosaka, Y. Fukada, and E. Iwai. 1986. Integration of direction signals of image motion in the superior temporal sulcus of the macaque monkey. *J. Neurosci.* **6**: 145.

Sakata, H., H. Shibutani, Y. Ito, and K. Tsurugai. 1986. Parietal cortical neurons responding to rotary movement of visual stimuli in space. *Exp. Brain Res.* **61**: 658.

Sakata, H., H. Shibutani, K. Kawano, and T. Harrington. 1985. Neural mechanisms of space vision in the parietal association cortex of the monkey. *Vision Res.* **25**: 453.

Siegel, R.M. and R.A. Andersen. 1986. Motion perceptual deficits following ibotenic acid lesions of the middle temporal area in the behaving rhesus monkey. *Soc. Neurosci. Abstr.* **12**: 1183.

———. 1988. Perception of three-dimensional structure from motion in monkey and man. *Nature* **331**: 259.

———. 1990. The perception of structure from visual motion in monkey and man. *J. Cognit. Neurosci.* (in press).

Sillito, A.M. 1979. Pharmological approach to visual cortex. *Trends Neurosci.* **2**: 196.

Snowden, R.J. 1989. Motions in orthogonal directions are mutually suppressive. *J. Opt. Soc. Am.* **6**: 1096.

Snowden, R.J., R.G. Erickson, S. Treue, and R.A. Andersen. 1990. Transparent motion stimuli reveal divisive inhibition in area MT of macaque. *Invest. Opthalmol. Vis. Sci.* (suppl.) **31**: 399.

Tanaka, K. and H. Saito. 1989. Analysis of motion of the

visual field by direction, expansion/contraction, and rotation cells clustered in the dorsal part of the medial superior temporal area of the macaque monkey. *J. Neurophysiol.* **62:** 626.

Tanaka, K., Y. Fukada, and H. Saito. 1989. Underlying mechanisms of the response specificity of the expansion/contraction and rotation cells in the dorsal part of the medial superior temporal area of the macaque monkey. *J. Neurophysiol.* **62:** 642.

Tanaka, K., K. Hikosaka, H. Saito, M. Yukie, Y. Fukada, and E. Iwai. 1986. Analysis of local and wide-field movements in the superior temporal visual areas of the macaque monkey. *J. Neurosci.* **6:** 134.

Treue, S. and R.A. Andersen. 1990. 3-D structure from motion: Rigidity and surface interpolation. *Invest. Opthalmol. Vis. Sci.* (suppl.) **31:** 172.

Treue, S., M. Husain, and R.A. Andersen. 1990. Human perception of structure from motion. *Vision Res.* (in press).

Ullman, S. 1984. Maximizing rigidity: The incremental recovery of 3-D structure from rigid and nonrigid motion. *Perception* **13:** 255.

Wallach, H. and D.N. O'Connell. 1953. The kinetic depth effect. *J. Exp. Psychol.* **45:** 205.

Wang, H.T., B. Mather, and C. Koch. 1989. Computing optical flow in the primate visual system. *Neural Computat.* **1:** 92.

Cortical Neural Mechanisms of Stereopsis Studied with Dynamic Random-dot Stereograms

G.F. POGGIO

The Philip Bard Laboratories of Neurophysiology, Department of Neuroscience and
The Johns Hopkins University School of Medicine, Baltimore, Maryland 21205

In its simplest form, stereopsis provides the capacity for identifying "local" features, a line or a dot, as appearing in front of or behind other similar features from which they differ solely in horizontal disparity (Julesz 1971; Westheimer and McKee 1980). Psychophysical studies with random-dot stereograms, invented by Julesz in 1960, revealed more elaborate disparity processing and proved convincingly that only a difference in the horizontal position of corresponding elements of left and right retinal images is required for the perception of form and movement in stereoscopic depth. Moreover, these studies brought out a major problem of stereoprocessing, the correspondence problem, i.e., how the matching binocular image features are identified. This problem, common in viewing everyday visual scenes, becomes most conspicuous with random-dot stereograms, in which the image of one dot in one eye can be matched with the image of any dot in the other eye. Yet the numerous potential false matches do not disturb the performance of the visual system, and during normal binocular vision, the brain solves the problem of stereoscopic correspondence with ease and precision.

It was the purpose of this study to analyze the responses of single neurons in the visual cortex of the macaque monkey to dynamic random-dot stereopatterns (cyclopean stimuli). Cortical visual neurons "see" the world through two receptive fields, one in each eye, and their activity reflects at all times the interaction of the binocular inputs. The responses of a large proportion of these neurons depend critically on the relative horizontal position of the same image features in the two eyes, an effect called disparity selectivity. Left and right receptive fields of a binocular cortical neuron may be in topographic correspondence in the two eyes, or they may have different relative positions, some pairs with convergent disparities and others with divergent disparities (Barlow et al. 1967; Nikara et al. 1968; Pettigrew et al. 1968; Bishop et al. 1971; Poggio and Fischer 1977; von der Heydt et al. 1978; Fischer and Krueger 1979; Poggio 1980; Ferster 1981; Poggio and Talbot 1981; Poggio and Poggio 1984). In the monkey, disparity-selective neurons have been identified in the striate area (V1) as well as in extrastriate visual areas from V2 to V5 (Hubel and Wiesel 1970; Maunsell and Van Essen 1983; Poggio 1984; Poggio et al. 1985; Burkhalter and Van Essen 1986; Felleman and Van Essen

1987; Hubel and Livingstone 1987). Receptive field disparity is thought to play a basic role in stereopsis, because under conditions of binocular convergent fixation, different cortical neurons are selectively activated by objects at different relative depths (Joshua and Bishop 1970; Bishop and Henry 1971). The mechanisms underlying disparity sensitivity in single neurons are an important biological constraint that greatly limits the number of possible brain operations for deriving depth from flat retinal images. Knowledge of these neural mechanisms is most important for the ultimate goal of understanding how the processing of stereoinformation in the various visual areas is coordinated to produce depth perception.

The observations described below were obtained from an analysis of the impulse activity of single neurons in the striate (V1) and prestriate (V2, V3–V3A) areas of the rhesus monkey under conditions of normal binocular vision and in the absence of anesthetics or other drugs. Macaque monkeys are known to see depth in random-dot stereograms (Bough 1970; Cowey et al. 1975). In the present experiments, however, the monkey was not required to direct its attention to the stimulus presented over the neuron's receptive field, a stimulus that had no relevance for the behavioral visual task the animal was trained to perform. Our initial studies (Poggio 1980; Poggio et al. 1985) revealed neurons in foveal striate and prestriate cortex (V1 and V2) that gave unambiguous responses to dynamic random-dot stereograms. These purely stereoscopic responses were obtained from cells that displayed binocular disparity sensitivity for solid stereo figures (depth neurons), as well as from cells that did not (flat neurons) (Poggio and Fischer 1977; Poggio and Talbot 1981). The results of the present investigation confirm and extend our previous findings, and they suggest that different functional sets of cortical visual neurons subserve different aspects of stereoscopic processing: (1) the zero-disparity, or correspondence, system, which includes neurons narrowly tuned to objects about the distance of fixation, and (2) the near- and the far-disparity systems, composed of neurons tuned to larger disparities (crossed and uncrossed, respectively) and neurons with extended and reciprocal excitatory and inhibitory responses to objects nearer and farther than the fixation distance.

METHODS

Experimental preparation. Six male monkeys, *Macaca mulatta*, with body weights of 3–5 kg were studied. The animals lived in $1.2 \times 1.2 \times 1.2$-meter cages in a room normally housing 12–15 monkeys. All were tuberculin and B-virus-negative. During training or recording sessions, the monkeys sat in primate chairs for 4–6 hours and then returned to their living cages. The animals were deprived of free access to water during the daily sessions; each earned or was given about 30 ml/kg body weight of water each day and allowed access to water 1 day each week. A PDP11/34A minicomputer was used to supervise the animal's behavioral task, to generate and control visual stimulation, and to collect behavioral and neural data. Details of the techniques used in these experiments have been described previously (Poggio et al. 1977, 1988; Poggio and Talbot 1981).

Monkeys were trained to fixate monocularly and binocularly a small target for several seconds and to detect an orientation shift in that target occurring at random times after the beginning of fixation. Correct detections were rewarded with a drop of water. Throughout the recording session, the monkey, its head firmly held, viewed separate display monitors, one with the left eye and the other with the right eye. The position of the eyes was continuously assessed with an infrared optoelectronic system that monitored the position of the corneal light reflex (Poggio and Talbot 1981; Motter and Poggio 1984).

Action potentials from single neurons were recorded from an extracellular position with glass-coated Pt/Ir microelectrodes (Wolbarsht et al. 1960), carried by a Chubbuck microdrive and inserted into the cortex through the intact dura mater via an oil-filled, hydraulically sealed chamber. Recordings were made 6 days per week until thickening of the dura made further successful penetrations difficult (3–4 weeks). The experiment was continued on the right hemisphere after mounting a second recording chamber over the visual cortex. At the end of the experiment, the animal was anesthetized, and the brain was perfused with 4% paraformaldehyde and 0.1% glutaraldehyde (two animals) or simply removed and placed in 10% buffered formalin (four animals). Serial sections of the region of cortex explored in the left and right hemispheres were cut at 20 μm, and stained with 1% thionine. Details of the methods and techniques used for the reconstructions of the microelectrode penetrations were described previously (Poggio et al. 1988).

Visual stimulation. Random-dot patterns were generated by a computer-driven digital subsystem (Julesz et al. 1976) on two high-speed graphic monitors (Hewlett-Packard model 1311A; P4 phosphor), one for each eye. The displays were constructed within a 100×100-dot raster refreshed at 67 frames/sec (interdot separation 0.10°). They included the fixation target and the test stimulus (or figure), both appearing within a larger field or background. The luminance of the display varied linearly with bright-dot density; at 100% density, it was approximately 14 cd/m^2 for the two monkeys on which more extensive observations were made (see Results), and 3–5 cd/m^2 for the other four animals. The bright dot subtended approximately 2.3-minute arc (two monkeys) or 1.2-minute arc (four monkeys).

The *background* field was obtained by intensifying a portion of the dots (typically 20%) randomly selected for each frame of the 100×100 element display (dynamic random-dot background) or by intensifying no dots (dark background). All background fields were square and subtended 10° at the monkey's eye; they were centered over the receptive field of the neuron under observation. The *figure* was a rectangular bar obtained by intensifying all of the dots that fell within its outline (solid bright figure), no dots (solid dark figure), or a randomly selected fraction of them (cyclopean figure). The *fixation target* consisted of two bright bars separated by a narrow dark gap. Target size was typically 0.14° square, with a 0.04° central gap (interdot separation, 0.02°).

Bright bars were used to locate the "minimum-response field" (Barlow et al. 1967) and to define the basic two-dimensional properties of each neuron studied. The size and orientation of the bar were adjusted to evoke optimal binocular responses, and the bar was made to move in opposite directions across the neuron's receptive field (1°/sec to 4°/sec) or was held stationary over it and flashed ON-OFF. The stereoscopic properties of cortical neurons were determined with the three types of stereograms schematically illustrated in Figure 1.

Solid-figure stereograms (SFS) were constructed using as a test stimulus the bright narrow bar of the spatiotemporal configuration previously defined as optimal for the neuron under study. Left and right bars were presented dichoptically at a series of horizontal disparities, uncrossed $(+)$, zero (0), and crossed $(-)$, moving or flashing. They were presented either against a dynamic random-dot background or against a featureless dark field, depending on the amplitude of the response evoked with one or the other (Trotter et al. 1983). The length of the solid bar ranged for different cells between 0.5° and 2.0°, and its width was usually narrow, 0.05° or 0.30°.

Cyclopean stereograms (CYC) of dynamic random dots, constructed as described by Julesz (1960, 1971), were used to test all neurons analyzed in this study. Binocular figures of identical random-dot patterns were displayed within a random-dot background field at a series of disparities including zero. Figure and background had the same dot density, intensity, and interdot separation so that only the presence of a positional difference between the left and the right figures would differentiate these otherwise identical stereopatterns of randomly distributed dots. For any one cell, the size of the cyclopean figure used was often larger than the size of the solid bar figure, because larger cyclopean figures commonly evoked stronger responses and sometimes were needed to elicit any response at all.

SOLID FIGURE (SFS)   CYCLOPEAN (CYC)   UNCORRELATION (UNC)

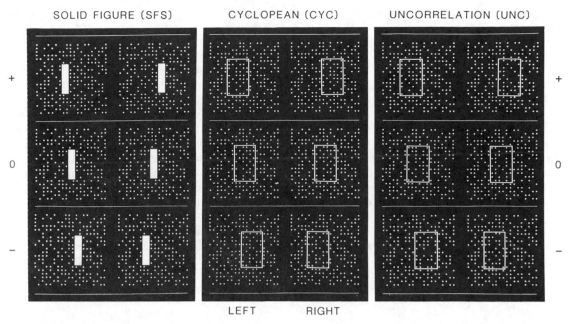

LEFT   RIGHT

Figure 1. Schematic illustration of the three types of displays used for stereoscopic stimulation. For all types, fields of dynamic random dots were generated on two screens (LEFT, RIGHT) seen separately by each eye. A central area formed the test figure, either uniformly bright (SFS) or made up of random dots (CYC, UNC). The figure was presented at a series of disparities, crossed (−), zero (0), and uncrossed (+), against a background of binocularly correlated random dots. The area of the figure in the cyclopean, and the uncorrelation stereograms shown in the illustration, is outlined for emphasis by a *white line*, which, of course, was not present during the experiment.

Uncorrelated stereograms (UNC) of dynamic random dots were utilized in order to separate the effects of positional disparity from those associated with the neuron's sensitivity to binocular image correlation. These stereograms were constructed in the same way as the classic random-dot stereograms described above, with the important differences that the dot patterns within the outline of the two figures were *not* the same—as required by Julesz' cyclopean stereograms— but were randomly different from each other and changing from frame to frame of the display (67/ sec^{-1}).

In this paper, the terms binocular *correlation* and *uncorrelation* refer to the spatial distribution of the dots (texture) over the retinas, the former defining the condition when left and right receptive fields of single cortical neurons are covered by identical image patterns, and the latter defining the condition when the two receptive fields receive different images. The terms binocular *correspondence* and *disparity* identify the topographic relations between the images (or between retinal areas) in the two eyes.

RESULTS

The observations described below are based on the study of 291 neurons isolated in areas V1, V2, and V3–V3A (third visual complex of Zeki [1978]) of the occipital cortex of six male rhesus monkeys. These neurons are a subset of the sample used for our investigation of binocular correlation and disparity selectivity (Poggio et al. 1988). The impulse responses of 125

neurons in areas V1 ($N = 36$), V2 (53), and V3–V3A (36) were analyzed in some detail in two monkeys. In these animals, at least two cortical areas, and often all three, were explored sequentially in the same microelectrode penetration for the purpose of comparing the properties of different areas. In addition, data were available for 166 neurons, nearly all isolated in the striate cortex (V1 = 159; V2 = 7), from a group of four monkeys. In one other monkey, only seven neurons (out of 112 tested in V1) responded to random-dot stereograms, a proportion considerably smaller than that found for any other monkey. Data from this animal were not included in this study; the observation is mentioned here to emphasize the variability in stereoscopic sensitivity that may be observed among rhesus monkeys.

SFS and dynamic random-dot stereopatterns (CYC, UNC) were routinely employed to define the neuron's stereoscopic properties. The neural responses to a series of binocular disparities (crossed and uncrossed) define the disparity selectivity profile of that neuron. It may be assumed that maximal responses obtain when the retinal separation between left and right components of the disparate stimulus corresponds to the binocular separation between the matched subfields in left and right eyes. All types of disparity selectivity profiles obtained with solid contour patterns, and no others, were also found with CYC stereograms. All types were found in all monkeys and in all cortical areas examined; they have been described previously (Poggio and Fischer 1977; Poggio et al. 1988) and are further detailed below.

The number of cells giving differential responses to binocularly disparate stimuli increased from the striate to the prestriate areas (Poggio et al. 1988). Similarly, the proportion of cells responding to CYC patterns rose from 31% in V1 (60/195) to 57% in V2 (34/60) and to 69% in V3–V3A (25/36). This increase was due mainly to neurons with TN/TF (tuned near, tuned far) disparity selectivity, which represented 46% of all depth neurons in V2 and V3–V3A and which were the most frequently sensitive to CYC stimulation (72%). Of the neurons with other disparity sensitivity profiles for solid bars, about 30% responded to random-dot stereograms. The two- and three-dimensional properties of cortical cells appear to be independent of each other, and orientation and directional selectivity occurred with all types of stereoscopic properties. Remarkably, however, the vast majority of neurons (90%) that responded to dynamic CYC stereograms had *complex* receptive field properties (Hubel and Wiesel 1962, 1968), whereas non-CYC neurons were evenly split between simple and complex (Poggio et al. 1985, 1988).

The results of this study confirm and extend previous observations (Poggio 1980, 1984; Poggio et al. 1985, 1988) and give support to the proposition that the early neural processing of stereoscopic information depends on three major functional categories of cortical neurons: the near- and far-disparity systems and the zero-disparity or correspondence system.

Stimulation with Random-dot Stereopatterns

The conditions of binocular stimulation with solid contour figures are self-explanatory and require no comment. CYC and UNC stereograms, on the other hand, have other characteristics that must be taken into consideration for the interpretation of the neural responses.

1. When viewed dichoptically, the two halves of a random-dot stereogram are superimposed. The binocular field of view comprises both a background area, with the same dot pattern in each eye, and an included area, the figure, whose texturally identical left and right members may be in topographic register over the two retinas (zero disparity) or may occupy different retinal positions (crossed or uncrossed disparities) (Fig. 1, middle). The CYC neuron receives and "fuses" the two texturally correlated figures when presented at the appropriate disparities for the binocularly matching subfields within the receptive fields in the two eyes, whereas it receives partially UNC binocular patterns at the other effective disparities. The width of disparity tuning could depend mainly on the size of the subfields (G.F. Poggio and C.E. Connor, in prep.).
2. Binocular correspondence and binocular correlation are operationally interacting aspects of binocular stimulation: Positionally disparate stimuli are uncorrelated for neurons with topographically corre-

sponding receptive fields, and zero-disparity stimuli are uncorrelated for neurons with disparate fields. To observe the effects of the two aspects of the stereoscopic stimulus in some degree of isolation, the responses to CYC stereograms and to UNC stereograms (see Methods) were analyzed. The two types of stereograms differ in that (i) in CYC, the figure has binocularly identical random-dot patterns (correlation), but either it occupies different horizontal positions in the two eyes (disparity) or the figure does not exist at all (zero disparity); (ii) in UNC, the figure has randomly different binocular dot distributions (uncorrelation) irrespective of binocular position. The responses to UNC stereograms are therefore necessarily the same for all disparities, including zero, and comparison of the responses to the two forms of stereoscopic stimulation provides an indication of the differential effects of position and correlation on the neural activity.

Stereoscopic Properties of Cortical Neurons

The near- and far-disparity systems. Neurons of these types give differential responses—excitatory and inhibitory—over adjacent ranges of horizontal disparities. Two main classes have been observed: (1) neurons that give excitatory responses over a relatively narrow disparity range, crossed (tuned near, TN) or uncrossed (tuned far, TF), with peak activation at disparities larger than 0.05° and suppression toward smaller disparities, and (2) neurons with extended asymmetric disparity selectivity, some responding with excitation to crossed disparities and with suppression to uncrossed ones (near neurons, NE), others displaying the reverse profile (far neurons, FA). Typically, the midpoint between excitation and suppression is at, or very close to, zero disparity. The disparity response profiles of these neurons as defined with solid figures versus random-dot patterns were always very similar, but not identical. Maximal responses were obtained at the same disparity, but the range of effective disparities was frequently narrower for CYC than for SFS. Examples are given in Figure 2, in which the response profiles to SFS and CYC stereograms are plotted superimposed for three TN neurons with different tuning widths, one each from the three areas explored.

Figure 3 shows replicas of the binocular responses of two prestriate neurons of the NE system to dynamic CYC stereograms. The cell whose impulse discharges are plotted at the left, an NE cell in V2, gives excitatory responses to stimuli with crossed (−) disparities and inhibitory responses to uncrossed (+) ones. For the cell shown at right, a TN cell in V3, the range of disparities over which differential excitatory and inhibitory responses are obtained is much more limited, with peak excitation at −0.4° and inhibition at +0.2°. As expected, no changes in the ongoing activity of either neuron occur when stereopairs of zero disparity (no cyclopean figure!) are presented over the receptive fields.

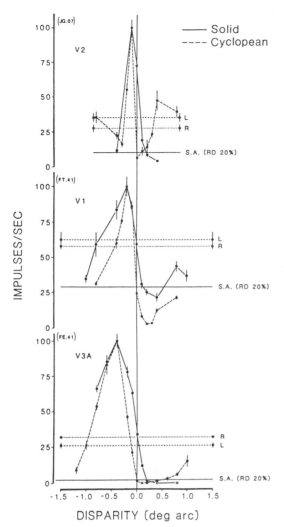

Figure 2. Disparity selectivity profiles for three stereoscopic neurons tuned to crossed disparities (TN neurons), one each from the three cortical areas explored (V1, V2, and V3–V3A). The magnitude and variability of the responses evoked at various positional disparities by *Solid* figure stereograms and *Cyclopean* stereograms are plotted superimposed. All neurons were orientation-selective. The solid figure was a moving bar of optimal configuration (average size 2.0° × 0.3°), and the random-dot figure was square (average size 3.0° × 3.0°) and flashing ON-OFF. The broken horizontal lines (L,R) indicate the level of the responses to monocular stimulation of the left and right eye with the solid bar. The horizontal line near the bottom of each plot marks the level of spontaneous activity (S.A.) of that cell during presentation of a dynamic random-dot background of 20% dot density.

The responses to the different forms of stereoscopic stimulation used in these experiments are illustrated in Figure 4 for two tuned excitatory neurons in area V2. Both neurons respond equally well to SFS and CYC stereopatterns. Neuron KS.07 (left) gives peak excitatory responses at +0.4° (TF) and little or no response to the mirror crossed disparity, −0.4°. Neuron JN.07 (right) displays the reciprocal response behavior (TN): excitation at the crossed disparity and suppression at the uncrossed one. Removal of the binocular correla-

tion between the random-dot figures in the two eyes (UNC) has profound effects on the neural responses. The stereopatterns are now only two binocularly uncorrelated random fields. The responses are predictably the same irrespective of the relative retinal positions of the two uncorrelated figures; they are also smaller in amplitude than the responses evoked by correlated stereopairs of optimal excitatory disparity for the neuron. These effects, although more evident in some neurons than in others, were observed for all TN,TF and NE,FA stereoneurons studied.

The zero-disparity system. Neurons of this stereosystem are sharply tuned to stimuli of zero or near-zero disparity. Some neurons respond with excitation (tuned zero, T0), and others respond with inhibition (tuned inhibitory, TI) to solid-figure stereopairs in retinal correspondence and give the opposite response to disparate stimuli, both farther and nearer. For these neurons, the response profiles that obtain with SFS and CYC figures are predictably different for stereopairs of zero disparity. Figure 5 (CYC) illustrates typical responses of T0 (left) and TI (right) neurons to dynamic random-dot stereograms. No changes in ongoing activity occur with CYC patterns of zero disparity, since left and right members of the stereograms are simply two identical fields of random dots. On the other hand, most evident responses are evoked by disparate CYC figures: The activity of the T0 neurons is suppressed and that of the TI neurons is increased over fairly large and symmetric ranges of crossed and uncrossed disparities.

It is reasonable to presume that neurons of these types have topographically corresponding receptive fields and that they are not sensitive to disparity, but rather signal the textural correlation between the pattern elements over their receptive fields in left and right retinas. Supporting evidence for this is provided by the strong responses that these neurons give when uncorrelation is introduced between binocularly corresponding (zero disparity) dot patterns by making the left and right figures two independent fields of dynamic noise. These responses are shown at the bottom of Figure 5 (UNC).

Neurons insensitive to disparity. Some cortical neurons, more commonly in striate than in prestriate cortex, give similar excitatory responses to SFS stereograms at all disparities, including zero (flat neurons, FL). About one third of these neurons respond also, and in a similar way, to CYC patterns, except, of course, to those of zero disparity (Fig 6, left). The response profile of the FL neuron to CYC is therefore very similar to that of the tuned inhibitory neuron (TI). When the textural correlation between left and right figures is removed (Fig. 6, right), the FL neurons respond equally well at all disparities including zero, their response profile now being the same as that which obtains with SFS. This response behavior suggests that the FL neurons, like the T0 and TI neurons described above, are sensitive to binocular correlation. The lack

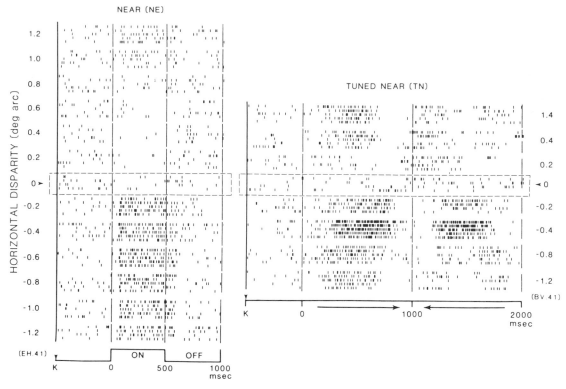

Figure 3. Replicas of sets of impulse sequences evoked at different disparities for two neurons of the NE stereosystem by dynamic random-dot stereograms. In this and following similar illustrations, each upstroke marks the occurrence of an impulse and each horizontal sequence of impulses refers to a single behavioral fixation trial. Initially, the monkey looks at binocularly correlated random-dot background; at *K*, it initiates the trial by pulling the reward key; after a delay of 500 msec (time = 0), the dot pattern within an area in the middle of the display is presented, and either alternates ON-OFF or it moves in opposite directions across the neuron's receptive field. For each stimulus disparity, the activity recorded during several (4–5) successive behavioral trials is represented. (*Left*) NE neuron (EH.41) in area V2; receptive field center (RF) at 5.4° of eccentricity; orientation (OR) = 15° from vertical; bidirectional; test figure size = 4° × 4°. (*Right*) TN neuron (BV.41) in V3; RF at 4.0°; OR = 45°; bidirectional; test figure = 2.9° × 0.6°.

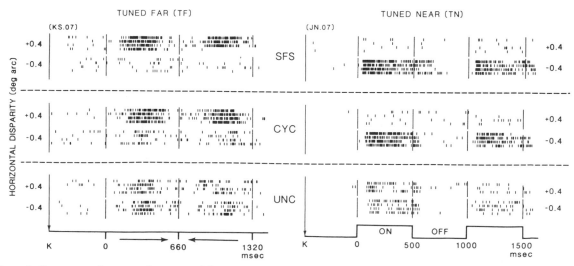

Figure 4. Responses of two tuned neurons of the near- and far-disparity systems to the three different forms of stereograms, SFS, CYC, and UNC. Only the responses to the optimal excitatory disparity and to its reciprocal one are shown. (*Left*) TF neuron (KS.07) in V2; RF at 4.4°; OR = 10°; bidirectional; test figure = 2.1° × 0.4°. (*Right*) TN neuron (JN.07) in V2; RF at 3.4°; OR = 0°; bidirectional; test figure = 2.1° × 0.5°.

DYNAMIC RANDOM-DOT STEREOGRAMS

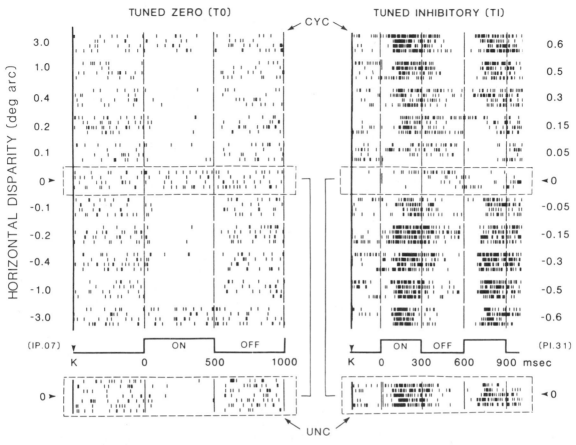

Figure 5. Responses of two neurons of the zero-disparity stereosystem to CYC stereograms at a series of disparities and to UNC stereopairs of zero disparity. The differences in the effects evoked by correlated and uncorrelated patterns at zero disparity are evident, and indeed the responses to the latter (UNC) are for both T0 and TI neurons, identical to those that obtain with texturally correlated (CYC) but positionally disparate stereofigures. (*Left*) T0 neuron (IP.07), in V1; RF at 1.8°; Nonoriented; bidirectional; test figure = 2° × 2°. (*Right*) TI neuron (PI.31) in V1; RF at 2.9°; OR = 65°; direction selective; test figure = 1° × 1°.

of responses to zero-disparity stereofields and their occurrence with disparate patterns also suggest that the receptive fields of these neurons are in retinal correspondence.

DISCUSSION

It was the purpose of this study to investigate the operational mechanisms underlying the stereoscopic properties of binocular neurons in the visual cortex of the alert macaque and, in particular, those mechanisms that subserve the capacity of the visual system to perform fast and precise stereoscopic matchings of the corresponding elements in left and right binocular images of an object in space. The results of psychophysical experiments with random-dot stereograms, in which the object form is seen only under binocular viewing, suggest that the matching problem is resolved at an early stage of visual processing (Julesz 1971). The experimental findings support this notion by showing that a substantial proportion of binocular cortical neurons—typically *complex* neurons—in the striate

(V1) and prestriate (V2, V3–V3A) cortex of the macaque monkey respond most readily and strongly to dynamic random-dot stereograms. Because of their apparent operational capacity of processing binocular matching, these neurons may be termed cyclopean neurons. The cyclopean responses depend chiefly on the relative spatial distribution of the dots over the neuron's receptive fields and ultimately on the contrast correlation between the binocular images. It may be suggested that the anatomic-functional organization that subserves this capacity could result from the spatial arrangements of the neuron's receptive fields in the two eyes, seen as being composed of numerous discrete sites or subfields, with the subfields in one eye functionally linked with subfields of the appropriate positional disparity in the other eye (Poggio and Poggio 1984; Poggio et al. 1988).

Neurons tuned to larger disparities (TN, TF) and neurons giving opposite responses to near and far stimuli (NE, FA) signal the positional disparity of binocular images and may be regarded as processing relative depth information (Disparity systems, near and

DYNAMIC RANDOM-DOT STEREOGRAMS

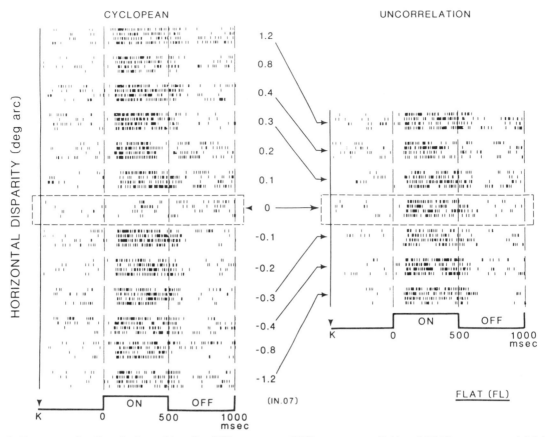

Figure 6. Response of a disparity-insensitive, flat (FL) neuron to CYC stereograms (*left*) and UNC stereograms (*right*). The responses are essentially identical irrespective of correlation or disparity except at the zero disparity when the correlated cyclopean stereopair is not, predictably, associated with any change in the ongoing spontaneous activity of the neuron, whereas the uncorrelated figures evoke a strong excitatory response not different from all other responses in the series. The results indicate that neurons of this type, like the T0 and TI neurons, respond to binocular uncorrelation. Flat neurons (IN.07) in V1; RF at 4.0°; OR = 0°; bidirectional; test figure = 1° × 1°.

far). Neurons tuned at or near-zero disparity (T0, TI), as well as the neurons responding to all disparities (FL), are sensitive to binocular correspondence, and thus signal the reference depth plane about the fixation distance and its immediate surroundings (Correspondence system).

The results of these experiments provide direct physiological support to the hypothesis of Richards (1970, 1971) that the human visual system contains three "pools" of neurons processing stereoscopic information—one for crossed disparities (near), one for uncrossed disparities (far), and one for near-zero disparities—and that at any one time, depth is signaled by the relative activity of the different stereosystems of neurons, especially by the antagonistic action of the near and far systems.

On the basis of their responses to stereoscopic patterns of different configurations, the functional characteristics of the main types of stereoscopic neurons identified in the visual cortex of the macaque may be summarized as follows:

First, tuned neurons of the near- and far-disparity systems (TN, TF), respond to random-dot stereograms

more frequently than any other stereoscopic type (72%). Neurons of these types "see" pairs of stereoimages at disparities other than those at which they are in topographic register with the neuron's receptive fields as uncorrelated stereoimages.

At variance with the other group of tuned neurons, the tuned-zero neurons (T0), the TN and TF neurons respond to uncorrelation with activation and never with suppression. It must be pointed out, however, that the responses of the TN and TF neurons to uncorrelated images are commonly smaller, and never larger, than the responses evoked by correlated images at the disparity of optimal excitatory responses. The depth-response profile of these cells is determined chiefly by positional disparity sensitivity, with image texture correlation playing a less specific role in their stereoselectivity.

Neurons of the near- and far-disparity systems with reciprocal disparity sensitivity to solid bar stereograms (NE, FA) respond less frequently to dynamic random-dot stereograms (30%). Their response profile is qualitatively the same with either form of stimulation, but whereas the excitatory response is always evident (even though usually over a range narrower than that which obtains with solid bars), the inhibitory response may be limited in amplitude and/or extent or it may not be at all evident. The nature and significance of the sensitivity of the NE and FA neurons to random-dot stereograms, and more generally of the organization of their receptive fields, need to be investigated further.

The proposition may be advanced that under conditions of normal binocular vision, neurons of the near- and far-disparity systems signal the relative depth of objects whose identical images project upon the neuron's receptive fields in the two eyes and that in the absence of such objects, they discharge at a level intermediate between the maximal excitatory and inhibitory activity evoked by images at the most effective disparities. The magnitude of the response to uncorrelation is likely to reflect the proportion of binocular element pairs at the optimal disparity for the neuron, a proportion determined by the probabilities involved in combining two independently random patterns presented to the left and right eyes. These populations of TN,TF and NE,FA neurons may operate in the neural processing leading to coarse stereopsis and may also be part of the system controlling binocular vergence. Moreover, the NE and FA neurons could effectively contribute to, or indeed provide the signals for, fine stereopsis by signaling small disparity changes through their finely graded response transition from suppression to facilitation about the horopter (Poggio 1984).

Second, tuned excitatory neurons with disparity tuning peaks within ±3–6 minutes of arc (T0) are activated by correlated stereopatterns of zero or near-zero disparity. Random-dot stereograms of larger disparity, on the other hand, have a strong suppressive effect, which is evoked by the binocular uncorrelation resulting from the mismatch between stereopatterns and receptive field. This is confirmed by the suppression of activity in response to uncorrelated patterns. Tuned inhibitory neurons (TI) give responses opposite to those of the tuned excitatory neurons: suppression by stereopatterns of zero disparity (correlation), and activation by disparate patterns (uncorrelation). These tuned neurons, T0 and TI, may be regarded as contributing in a complementary way to the neural definition of the horopter and of Panum's fusional area. The tuned excitatory neurons are activated and the tuned inhibitory neurons are suppressed by objects about the fixation distance and, reversing their response, respectively, inhibited and excited by nearer or farther objects. The ongoing activity of these two functional sets of neurons, the discharging and the silent ones, may operate in stereopsis by defining the reference distance and may represent the essential neural substrate for binocular single vision, carrying information for fusional sensory mechanisms. Moreover, the activity of these sharply tuned neurons may contribute to the control of disjunctive eye movements and the maintenance of convergent fixation (Poggio and Fischer 1977).

Finally, disparity-insensitive neurons (FL) give strong excitatory responses to disparate random-dot patterns that cover, even partially, their receptive fields. The role, if any, of the FL neurons in stereopsis is unknown.

The observations made in this study show that there are neurons at early stages of cortical processing of binocular information that have cyclopean properties, in that they signal unambiguously positional disparity and texture correlation in dynamic random-dot stereograms. The activity of the cell population engaged by cyclopean stimulation defines the neural representation of the stereogram in the cerebral cortex and provides the conditions leading to the vivid impression of depth and solidity that most human observers experience when viewing binocularly fused random-dot stereograms. It is reasonable to suppose that the same mechanisms operate during binocular vision of the natural world.

ACKNOWLEDGMENTS

This study was supported by grant 5-RO1-EY02966 from the National Institutes of Health, U.S. Public Health Service, and by a grant from the A.P. Sloan Foundation.

REFERENCES

Barlow, H., C. Blakemore, and J.D. Pettigrew. 1967. The neural mechanism of binocular depth discrimination. *J. Physiol.* **193:** 327.
Bishop, P.O. and G.H. Henry. 1971. Spatial vision. *Annu. Rev. Psychol.* **22:** 119.
Bishop, P.O., G.H. Henry, and C.J. Smith. 1971. Binocular interaction fields of single units in the cat striate cortex. *J. Physiol.* **216:** 39.
Bough, E.W. 1970. Stereoscopic vision in the macaque monkey: A behavioral demonstration. *Nature* **225:** 42.
Burkhalter, A. and D.C. Van Essen. 1986. Processing of color, form and disparity information in visual areas VP and V2 of ventral extrastriate cortex in the macaque monkey. *J. Neurosci.* **6:** 2327.
Cowey, A., A.M. Parkinson, and L. Warnick. 1975. Global stereopsis in rhesus monkeys. *Q. J. Exp. Psychol.* **27:** 93.
Felleman, D.J. and D.C. Van Essen. 1987. Receptive field properties of neurons in area V3 of macaque monkey extrastriate cortex. *J. Neurophysiol.* **57:** 889.
Ferster, D. 1981. A comparison of binocular depth mechanisms in area 17 and 18 of the cat visual cortex. *J. Physiol.* **311:** 623.
Fischer, B. and J. Krueger. 1979. Disparity tuning and binocularity of single neurons in the cat visual cortex. *Exp. Brain Res.* **35:** 1.
Hubel, D.H. and M.S. Livingstone. 1987. Segregation of form, color, and stereopsis in primate area 18. *J. Neurosci.* **11:** 3378.
Hubel, D.H. and T.N. Wiesel. 1962. Receptive fields, binocular interaction and functional architecture in the cat's visual cortex. *J. Physiol.* **160:** 106.
———. 1968. Receptive fields and functional architecture of monkey striate cortex. *J. Physiol.* **195:** 215.
———. 1970. Cells sensitive to binocular depth in area 18 of the macaque monkey cortex. *Nature* **225:** 41.
Joshua, D.E. and P.O. Bishop. 1970. Binocular single vision and depth discrimination. Receptive field disparities for central and peripheral vision and binocular interaction on peripheral single units in cat striate cortex. *Exp. Brain Res.* **10:** 389.

Julesz, B. 1960. Binocular depth perception of computer-generated patterns. *Bell Syst. Tech. J.* **39:** 1125.

———. 1971. *Foundations of cyclopean perception.* University of Chicago Press, Illinois.

Julesz, B., B. Breitmeyer, and W. Kropfl. 1976. Binocular-disparity-dependent upper-lower hemifield anisotropy and left-right hemifield isotropy as revealed by dynamic random-dot stereograms. *Perception* **5:** 129.

Maunsell, J.H.R. and D.C. Van Essen. 1983. Functional properties of neurons in middle temporal visual area of the macaque monkey. II. Binocular interaction and sensitivity to binocular disparity. *J. Neurophysiol.* **49:** 1148.

Motter, B.C. and G.F. Poggio. 1984. Binocular fixation in the rhesus monkey: Spatial and temporal characteristics. *Exp. Brain Res.* **54:** 304.

Nikara, T., P.O. Bishop, and J.D. Pettigrew. 1968. Analysis of retinal correspondence by studying receptive fields of binocular single units in cat striate cortex. *Exp. Brain Res.* **6:** 353.

Pettigrew, J.D., T. Nikara, and P.O. Bishop. 1968. Binocular interaction on single units in cat striate cortex: Simultaneous stimulation by single moving slit with receptive fields in correspondence. *Exp. Brain Res.* **6:** 391.

Poggio, G.F. 1980. Neurons sensitive to dynamic random-dot stereograms in areas 17 and 18 of the rhesus monkey cortex. *Soc. Neurosci. Abstr.* **6:** 672.

———. 1984. Processing of stereoscopic information in monkey visual cortex. In *Dynamic aspects of neocortical function* (ed. G.M. Edelman et al.), p. 613. Wiley, New York.

Poggio, G.F. and B. Fischer. 1977. Binocular interaction and depth sensitivity in striate and prestriate cortex of behaving rhesus monkeys. *J. Neurophysiol.* **40:** 1392.

Poggio, G.F. and T. Poggio. 1984. The analysis of stereopsis. *Annu. Rev. Neurosci.* **7:** 379.

Poggio, G.F. and W.H. Talbot. 1981. Neural mechanisms of static and dynamic stereopsis in foveal striate cortex of rhesus monkeys. *J. Physiol.* **315:** 469.

Poggio, G.F., R.W. Doty, and W.H. Talbot. 1977. Foveal striate cortex of behaving monkey: Single-neuron responses to square-wave gratings during fixation of gaze. *J. Neurophysiol.* **40:** 1369.

Poggio, G.F., F. Gonzalez, and F. Krause. 1988. Stereoscopic mechanisms in monkey visual cortex: Binocular correlation and disparity selectivity. *J. Neurosci.* **8:** 4531.

Poggio, G.F., B.C. Motter, S. Squatrito, and Y. Trotter. 1985. Responses of neurons in visual cortex (V1 and V2) of the alert macaque to dynamic random-dot stereograms. *Vision Res.* **25:** 397.

Richards, W.A. 1970. Stereopsis and stereoblindness. *Exp. Brain Res.* **10:** 380.

———. 1971. Anomalous stereoscopic depth perception. *J. Opt. Soc. Am.* **61:** 410.

Trotter, Y., S. Squatrito, B.C. Motter, and G.F. Poggio. 1983. Differential effects of uniform and random-noise backgrounds on the ongoing activity and evoked responses of neurons in foveal A17 and A18 of the macaque. *Soc. Neurosci. Abstr.* **9:** 618.

von der Heydt, R., Cs. Adorjani, P. Haenny, and G. Baumgartner. 1978. Disparity sensitivity and receptive field incongruity of units in cat striate cortex. *Exp. Brain Res.* **31:** 523.

Westheimer, G. and S.P. McKee. 1980. Stereogram design for testing local stereopsis. *Invest. Ophthalmol. Visual Sci.* **19:** 802.

Wolbarsht, M.C., E.F. MacNichol, and H. Wagner. 1960. Glass-insulated platinum micro-electrodes. *Science* **132:** 1309.

Zeki, S.M. 1978. The third visual complex of rhesus monkey prestriate cortex. *J. Physiol.* **277:** 245.

The Grain of Visual Space

G. WESTHEIMER

Division of Neurobiology, Department of Molecular and Cell Biology,
University of California, Berkeley, California 94720

This essay is about an attempt at building a bridge between the hardware of the nervous system, on the one hand, and the behavioral performance of the whole organism, on the other. As practicing scientists, we accept this as a major challenge, and we leave others to agonize over the validity of the enterprise and the possibility of a totally satisfying answer. The bridge has not yet been constructed, but I present here some engineering plans of the approaches from the two sides. The primary proposition, which must be settled at the outset, is the suitability of the terrain for such a task.

In selecting the primate visual system, we have a lot going for us. First, this visual system is nontrivial, the optic nerves accounting for a predominant proportion of all fibers entering the cortex. Second, knowledge of the neuroanatomy and neurophysiology of the primate visual system is quite advanced, in part because of the clear understanding of the nature of the involved stimuli. (Contrast this to the continuing uncertainty surrounding the categorization of olfactory and gustatory stimuli.) Finally, because we are trying to build a bridge and it is important to look at both sides, it is comforting to know that the territory on the behavioral side has been particularly well charted.

Visual space perception was actively investigated well before there was even a rudimentary understanding of the neural pathways from the eye to the brain. This was accomplished via the psychophysical approach, wherein known visual stimuli are presented to the observer and correlated with the perceptual responses they elicit. In modern days, this has become a powerful tool, yielding quantitative data as reliable and repeatable as those in any other area of science. Through introspection and research, aided by the formalism of geometry and other branches of mathematics, and influenced strongly by the physics of the nineteenth century, an effective categorization of the manifold visual stimuli has been achieved. We define the brightness/contrast domain, the color domain with its three components, the time domain, and the space domain, which has three degrees of freedom. All of this was and is done while staying entirely within physics of stimuli, on the one hand, and the subjective response of the observer, on the other.

The advent of structural investigations deepened the comprehension and clarified some issues. Examples to be cited are the identification of the presence and spacing of retinal receptors and the topographic mapping of the retina onto the cortex. But, in principle, a basic understanding of the visual process using physics, anatomy, and psychophysics appears to be a manageable and actually quite successful undertaking.

I want to relate a small part of this story, taking it as far as it is possible with modern techniques of investigation. Only then will I discuss its significance in the context of the larger and more ambitious program of tying together, perhaps even in a causal chain, the knowledge of the functioning of the brain with that of the behavior of the organism confronted with certain kinds of stimuli. The full story of how the visual world is created from the retinal image is, in my view, too complex a problem by far to achieve any reasonable degree of success at this time. But if we segment it properly, we can, with a bit of insight and a lot of luck, make some progress. I have chosen one end of the continuum of visual space for consideration, namely, the smallest detectable increment or change. We come up against a couple of inescapable physical limits here, which need delineation at the outset because we do not want to invoke unknown neural mechanisms where simple physical constraints are really the cause.

The response of the eye's optics to an optical impulse function, i.e., a point source of light, defines the ultimate resolution limit and is known (Fig. 1). The finite size of the elements of the retinal mosaic (Fig. 2) constitutes another constraint and, courtesy of evolutionary convergence, the numerical value of these two factors is almost the same. When it comes to the resolving power of the human visual system, usually called visual acuity, there remains no secret: The limits are set by the eye's optics and the retinal mosaic in the primate

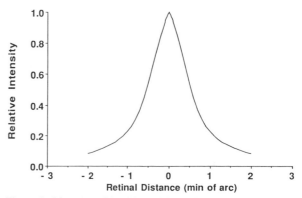

Figure 1. Line-spread function of the optics of the human eye, i.e., light distribution in the retinal image of a very thin line target.

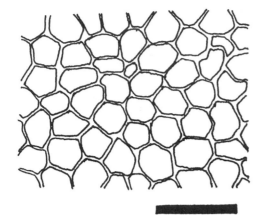

Figure 2. Schematic drawing of the mosaic of retinal cones in the human fovea. Typical values for the width of individual cones is 0.5–0.75 min of arc. (Redrawn from Curcio et al. 1987.)

fovea and little need be demanded by the nervous system beyond preserving the information of the light energy caught by an ensemble of neighboring cones (Fig. 3).

Far from being the end of the story revolving about the smallest limits of spatial discrimination, it is only the beginning. There are, in fact, many visual tasks where an observer can perform spatial judgments much smaller than the above limit, which is on the order of half a minute of arc at best. Although the resolution limit for two stars is on the order of 1 minute of arc, lack of alignment of two abutting lines can be detected when they differ in lateral position by just a few seconds of arc (vernier acuity). There are many

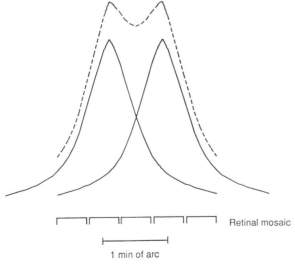

Figure 3. Optical, anatomical, and physiological basis of visual acuity. Two narrow line targets are separated until they can just be resolved. Their line-spread functions (see Fig. 1) then partially overlap and produce a summed light distribution with two humps and a trough. Conditions for resolution are (1) a distinct trough separates the two humps, (2) the two humps and the trough each have the dimension of a receptor width, and (3) the intensity difference between the humps and the trough is detectable physiologically.

capabilities of spatial alignment, distance judgment, shape discriminations, depth judgments, and the like where the threshold may be as little as one-tenth the resolution limit, or perhaps 2–4 seconds of arc. It is this fine grain of visual space, now called hyperacuity, that I think is not only very interesting in itself, but also capable of supporting a bridge between psychophysics and the wet neural sciences.

Conceptually, the simplest experiment in this connection is the following: Present to an observer a vertical line, say 0.5° long, in the fovea and find the minimum step change in line tilt that can be detected. It is about 10 minutes of arc. It is interesting to compare this value with the orientation tuning width of cortical units in the monkey, which is at a minimum 20–30 times larger. For those who would seek immediate correlation between single-unit firing and visual perception, another difficulty needs to be faced. The impulse pattern of a single neuron can be modified in a variety of ways. An oriented unit in the cortex can give more or less of a burst, depending not only on the orientation of the stimulating line, but also on the line's exact position, brightness, length, and probably a host of other factors. Thus, no unique conclusion can be drawn about the orientation of a line stimulus from a single neuron's impulse traffic.

In the psychophysical experiment, one determines the smallest step change in orientation whose direction can be correctly identified, and this even more strongly decouples the situation from the activity of a single neuron. Experiments in progress in R. Vogels' laboratory in Louvain (Vogels and Orban 1990) suggest that, given the excitability and variability of cortical neurons in the alert monkey who is actually performing such tasks, it is likely that the activity of hundreds, perhaps thousands, of neurons must be interrelated to achieve such low thresholds. The situation seems to be similar in the realm of movement control, where the precision of pointing needs encoding in a large population of cells (Georgopoulos, this volume). Finally, to put the matter into perspective, it should be pointed out that similar low thresholds can be obtained with a psychophysical technique, using not just step changes in orientation, but presentations of just single orientations one at a time. A good observer can identify in a sequence of separate presentations which ones are tilted clockwise or counterclockwise with a threshold not too different from those obtained with step stimuli.

When the small value of vernier thresholds was first demonstrated by Wulfing, Hering, the most insightful of sensory physiologists, recognized that neural signals from many elements of the retinal mosaic were required to retrieve the information of spatial offsets as small as those that can be seen by the average observer. For a while it was thought that some averaging process along visual contours might be involved, but in 1953, Ludvigh demonstrated that hyperacuity was not diminished if one shrank the two contours, whose lateral displacement had to be detected, down to a single point each.

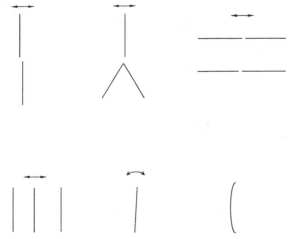

Figure 4. Position differences between feature elements can be detected to a precision almost an order of magnitude smaller than the resolution limit and the size of the elements of the cone mosaic: the hyperacuities. A wide variety of configurations allow these very low thresholds. In each of the patterns shown, just detectable differences are a few seconds of arc. Included are the familiar vernier and similar alignment tasks (*top row*); separation discrimination between pattern elements, e.g., a bisection task (*bottom row left*); orientation discrimination, where a line can be detected as not vertical when its top end has been moved laterally just 6 seconds of arc; and curvature detection, where a line is recognized as being convex left or right when it has a sag of only a few seconds of arc.

After the orientation sensitivity of cortical units was discovered by Hubel and Wiesel, it was thought that the lateral offset of two contours, even two dots, could be tantamount to stimulating a different oriented unit, or different sets of such units, and vernier acuity would thus still remain part of orientation sensitivity. The story is not that simple, however, because there are situations in which the orientation thresholds for line targets are not as good as those for offsets of dot targets, whereas by all indications, lines should stimulate oriented units better than dot targets. Moreover, hyperacuities can be observed for almost any target pattern (Fig. 4). Nor is it necessary to use lateral offsets, since any position changes will do.

Below are listed some of the experimental results that help elucidate the physiological mechanism subserving hyperacuity (Westheimer 1981):

1. Tolerance to motion. A vernier task or a separation discrimination task can be done just as well when the whole pattern moves across the retina at velocities of at least 3°/sec, i.e., differences of target position of a fifth of a receptor diameter can be correctly identified while the whole configuration moves across up to 50 receptors in a 100-msec presentation time (Fig. 5).
2. To detect a vernier offset, it is essential that both pattern elements be presented simultaneously. Asynchronies of 60–80 msec introduce serious loss of performance (Fig. 6).
3. Light signals over a zone of at least 2 minutes of arc are used, and the target elements are assigned a location based on the computation of the centroid of the light distribution making up the target.
4. Thresholds are distance-dependent. When the two targets whose relative positions must be judged are more than a few minutes apart in the fovea (and proportionally larger distances in the retinal periphery), performance suffers.
5. Thresholds deteriorate when competing patterns are too close. A processing zone seems to be needed for good performance, and this processing zone is much larger than the resolution limit.

These and other pieces of evidence imply the following outline of the mechanisms of hyperacuity:

The best spatial thresholds are obtained for the relative localization of two target elements presented to the eye simultaneously. Such thresholds can be as low as 3

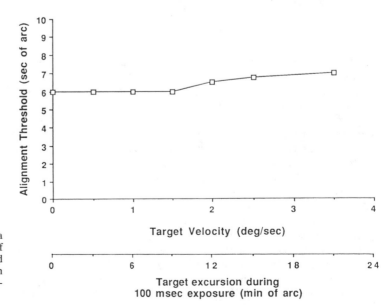

Figure 5. Vernier alignment threshold for a target with retinal image motion of a range of velocities. Target is exposed for 100 msec and sweeps across the retina over the distances on the second axis of abscissae. (Data from Westheimer and McKee 1975.)

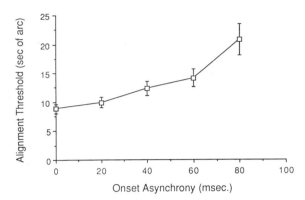

Figure 6. Alignment thresholds for a two-line vernier task when each line is exposed for 200 msec, and the top line has the onset asynchrony with respect to the bottom line shown on the abscissa.

seconds of arc, or one tenth of the spacing of receptors in the fovea. Because there is a wide latitude as to the components of the target pair and there is no need for a fixed position on the retinal mosaic as long as the relative situation of the target elements remain constant, it would be inappropriate to look for a representation of visual space with a grain as fine as hyperacuity thresholds. Rather, one should think of a distinct neural apparatus with the ability to gauge relative position within any target configuration regardless of where it is exactly placed in the fovea, what its detailed light distribution is, and whether it is stationary or in motion. It can be thought of as being of the nature of a differential amplifier, which can detect a small difference signal in the presence of quite a large common signal of the components.

The development of this notion from psychophysical experimentation is a crucial step in the design of appropriate neurophysiological experiments, even if at this stage the latter are as yet only Gedanken experiments. It would seem that the alert primate would be the mandatory preparation, *primate* because the data on which the concepts are based were derived from human experiments (although presumably a similar data bank could be generated for other animals), and *alert* because it seems more than likely that factors such as attention play a significant role here.

Although the emphasis has been on the human spatial visual apparatus, it should be made clear that hyperacuities are not unique to it. There are many instances in which an animal's performance transcends the expectations based on simplistic interpretation of the capabilities of the sensory apparatus. To mention just a few: Wavelength discrimination is less than a nanometer in the face of pigment bandwidth of 100 nm; binaural localization can make use of time differences of just microseconds; and the electric fish can detect incredibly small differences in field strength and frequency. Of the many implications of these findings, two are addressed briefly below.

So far, the predominant strategy in accumulating neurophysiological knowledge of the visual system has been the plotting of receptive fields of single units, and this can be generalized to include such additional attributes as color, motion, and disparity. It should be remembered that this selection of attributes is always preceded by a categorization of stimuli according to criteria external to neurophysiology. The primary ones are, of course, from the mathematical and physical sciences from which we took over concepts of intensity and wavelength of light, the dimensions of space in terms of x, y, and z, or radial distance, elevation and disparity, or the specifications of contours into arc, curvature, or angle.

The original discovery of certain trigger features, such as orientation selectivity of cat cortical cells and directional selectivity of rabbit retinal ganglion cells, was due to serendipity playing on the receptive mind of investigators willing to learn from nature. As the investigations proceed further into the depth of the visual nervous system, serendipity can be relied on less and the categorizations taken over from physics will be less applicable. Their place will be taken by insights from psychophysics and perception, and it is in this context that I wanted to place the results on hyperacuity. The suggested elaboration of visual signals in terms of relative position of features, regardless of feature structure, suggests a whole class of processing mechanisms that were previously unsuspected and that would not ordinarily be found by planning a search of trigger features using criteria taken over from physics. It may, of course, be impossible to demonstrate the presence or operation of such mechanisms when the search is confined to the testing out of single units; progress in this area may have to await newer techniques now being talked and dreamt about (Gilbert et al., this volume). Yet, regardless of the analytical techniques being used, the emphasis has to be on selection of categories, criteria, and attributes to demonstrate the presence of these mechanisms and highlight their operation. It is here that the interaction with psychophysics seems to me to be mandatory. Needed are quantitative findings, not just anecdotal ones, that have their basis in perceptual observations but are given sufficient rigor to allow them to become the basis of detailed neurophysiological investigations.

Finally, it is an interesting exercise to draw some of the consequences of this kind of thinking. Processing mechanisms for visual stimuli in the cortex may involve surprising and rather unsuspected attributes that are only implicit in a physical description of the stimulus, but are brought out overtly by careful psychophysical or perceptual experiments. Let us stay for a moment within the realm of spatial vision. We have seen how likely it is that the fine grain of visual space may not be coded explicitly in terms of an extremely fine mesh of local signs, good everywhere to a few seconds of arc, but rather that hyperacuities arise from a differencing mechanism applied to feature pairs regardless of the details of their configuration or their position. So far, this has been put forward for the discrimination of position and also stereoscopic depth. In other words, we have postulated that within visual space, there is an internal submechanism for position difference detection. I believe that similar conclusions will be inevitable for other attributes within visual space, e.g., parallelism and straightness of lines, continuity of contours, and right-angularity of corners. The problem that bothers me is how any system can handle the concatenation of a massively parallel network of processors within the same domain, all obviously wildly nonlinear, and keep on ending up with a unitary perception of a single visual world. Of course, we allow mild dissonances as in the visual illusions, and we have as yet left out the next stage, viz., that of tying in with the processing of color, motion, and depth, where a similar situation is probably at play. That we perceive a globally unitary external world is therefore a source of continuous wonder and a very fundamental challenge to the neurosciences.

ACKNOWLEDGMENT

Research support from the National Eye Institute under grant R37-EY00220 is gratefully acknowledged.

REFERENCES

Curcio, C.A., K.R. Sloan, O. Packer, A.E. Hendrickson, and R.E. Kalina. 1987. Distribution of cones in human and monkey retina: Individual variability and radial asymmetry. *Science* **236:** 579.

Ludvigh, E. 1953. Direction sense of the eye. *Am. J. Ophthalmol.* **36:** 139.

Vogels, R. and G.A. Orban. 1990. How well do response changes of striate neurons signify differences in orientation? *J. Neurosci.* (in press).

Westheimer, G. 1981. Visual hyperacuity. *Prog. Sens. Physiol.* **1:** 1.

Westheimer, G. and S.P. McKee. 1975. Visual acuity in the presence of retinal-image motion. *J. Opt. Soc. Am.* **65:** 847.

Neural Models of Binocular Depth Perception

S.R. LEHKY,* A. POUGET,† AND T.J. SEJNOWSKI†

*Laboratory of Neuropsychology, National Institute of Mental Health, Bethesda, Maryland 20892;
†Computational Neurobiology Laboratory, The Salk Institute, San Diego, California 92138;
and University of California, San Diego, California 92093

We have known since Wheatstone (1838) that disparities between images presented to the two eyes induce a strong sensation of depth. More recent experiments with random-dot stereograms have shown that disparity is a sufficient cue for stereopsis (Julesz 1960, 1971). Disparity-tuned neurons in visual cortex were first demonstrated in the cat (Barlow et al. 1967; Nikara et al. 1968; Pettigrew et al. 1968) and later in the macaque monkey (Hubel and Wiesel 1970; Poggio and Fischer 1977; Poggio and Poggio 1984). Similar disparity mechanisms probably exist in the human visual cortex.

We have developed a model for the representation of stereo disparity by using a population of neurons that is based on tuning curves similar in shape to those measured physiologically (Lehky and Sejnowski 1990). The model predicts depth discrimination thresholds that agree with human psychophysical data only when the population size representing disparity in a small patch of visual field was in the range of about 20–200 units. This population model of disparity coding at a single spatial location was extended to include lateral interactions, as suggested by psychophysical data on stereo interpolation (Westheimer 1986a).

Disparity is a measure of depth relative to the plane of fixation. Additional sources of information are needed to estimate the distance to the point of fixation, such as that provided by eye vergence, vertical disparity, and accommodation. We have developed a simple model that combines disparity information in a distributed representation and vergence information to compute the absolute depth of objects from the observer (Pouget and Sejnowski 1990). Although these are models of binocular vision, a number of the ideas presented here generalize to the representations of other sensory cues.

Representations of Disparity

In a local representation, disparity is unambiguously represented by the activity of a single neuron. An example of this is shown in Figure 1A, where the value of disparity is indicated by which neuron fires. To cover the entire range of disparities with high resolution, there must be a large number of such narrowly tuned, nonoverlapping units. This form of local representation is called interval encoding and has been used almost universally in models of stereopsis (Marr and Poggio 1976; Mayhew and Frisby 1981). A second form of

local representation is rate encoding (Fig. 1B). Here, a single unit codes all disparity values by its firing rate. As disparity increases, the firing rate of the unit increases monotonically. Examples of models that have used a rate-coded representation of depth are Julesz's dipole model (Julesz 1971) and the model of Marr and Poggio (1979). A third type of encoding, which we use here, is a distributed representation, or population

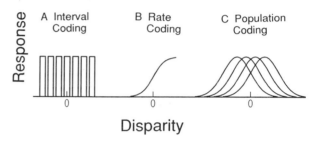

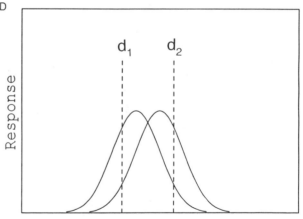

Figure 1. Three methods of encoding disparity and an example of discrimination in a population code. (A) Interval coding: A separate unit is dedicated for each disparity. (B) Rate encoding: Disparity is encoded by the firing rate of a single neuron. (C) Population coding: Disparity is encoded in the pattern of activity in a population having broad, overlapping disparity tuning curves. (D) Population code based on two idealized disparity tuning curves out of a larger population. As stimulus disparity is changed (e.g., from d_1 to d_2), the response of one unit goes up and other goes down, as indicated by the intersection of the dashed lines with the tuning curves. The changes in activities of all units in the population are combined to see if the total change is statistically significant relative to the noise in the units. If so, then the change in disparity is considered perceptually discriminable.

code, in which disparity is encoded by the pattern of activity within a population of neural units, each broadly tuned to disparity and extensively overlapped with each other (Fig. 1C). In a distributed representation, the activity of a single unit is ambiguous.

Neurophysiological Data

Poggio et al. (1985, 1988) have reported that neurons in monkey visual cortex are grouped into three classes on the basis of the their responses to disparity: (1) the "near" neurons, broadly tuned for crossed disparities, (2) the "far" neurons, broadly tuned for uncrossed disparities, and (3) the "tuned" neurons, narrowly tuned for disparities close to zero. The tuned neurons have an average bandwidth of 0.085°, and their peaks are almost entirely restricted to the range ± 0.1°. Near neurons are excited by crossed disparities and inhibited by uncrossed disparities, whereas the opposite holds true for far neurons. In both cases, the response curves have their steepest slope near zero disparity, as they go from excitation to inhibition. The excitatory peaks for far and near neurons are on average at about ± 0.2° (Poggio 1984). This tripartite division is an idealization, and many disparity-tuned neurons are often difficult to fit neatly into any classification scheme. LeVay and Voigt (1988), in their study of disparity tuning in cat visual cortex, emphasize the large number of cells with intermediate properties.

Psychophysical Data

Humans can discriminate small differences of depth near the plane of fixation with an accuracy that is typically around 5 seconds. This is smaller by a factor of about 50 than the width of the narrowest cortical disparity tuning curves and is a factor of 6 smaller than the width of a photoreceptor. Stereoacuity falls off rapidly away from the plane of fixation. The disparity discrimination curve in Figure 2B plots the smallest discriminable change in disparity as a function of stimulus disparity. Disparity increment threshold curves have been measured using a variety of stimuli with similar results, including line patterns (Westheimer 1979), random-dot stereograms (Schumer and Julesz 1984), and difference of Gaussian stimuli (Badcock and Schor 1985).

Another aspect of depth perception is interpolation. In random-dot stereograms, the surface of the square floating in depth appears to be solid, even though the dots may be quite sparse and smooth surfaces are perceived even for complex shapes. This suggests that when a stereogram dot is matched, it influences the perceived depth of neighboring blank locations. Psychophysical experiments have been performed to measure the interactions occurring between two nearby locations (Westheimer 1986a,b; Westheimer and Levy 1987). As shown in Figure 4A, the disparities of two lateral lines (labeled *a*) were set to a series of values by

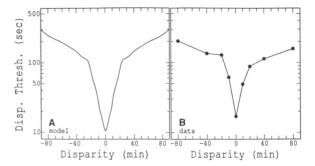

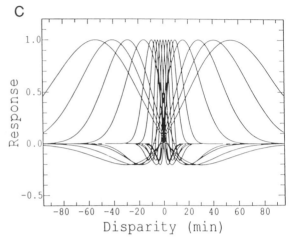

Figure 2. Comparison of a model disparity discrimination curve with a human psychophysical curve. (*A*) The smallest discriminable change in disparity is plotted as a function of a pedestal disparity for a model based on the tuning mechanisms shown in panel *B* and the psychophysical curve measured by Badcock and Schor (1985). (*B*) The smallest population (17 units) judged sufficient to give an adequate representation of the data. Tuning curve width increased with peak location, so that the steepest portions of the near and far curves all fall near zero disparity. Since discriminability depends on tuning curve slope, this organization produced highest discriminability at zero. This population gives a rough indication of the minimum size needed to encode disparity.

the experimenter. The disparities of two nearby inner lines (labeled *b*) were kept at zero. The basic observation was that the presence of depth at *a* warped the perceived depth at *b* to nonzero values. The amount of warping was quantified by having the subject adjust the disparity of the middle line to produce the same apparent depth as the lines at *b*. For small separations, moving the lines at *a* in depth dragged the perceived depth of *b* in the same direction. As the separation increased, this attractive interaction decreased and then reversed so that the two lines appeared to repel each other. This suggests that there are excitatory and inhibitory interactions between pools of neurons representing depth at neighboring locations. In the following section, depth discrimination and depth interpolation are considered in a reference frame relative to fixation. Issues related to depth constancy and absolute depth estimation are discussed in a later section.

MODELING DEPTH DISCRIMINATION

Our model does not attempt to describe how the disparity tuning observed in neurons is synthesized from monocular inputs. Nor do we model the matching process between images to the two eyes, or what aspects of the images may act as tokens during matching. This is the correspondence problem, which we assume the circuitry in the brain has already solved, since neurons have been found that can correctly compute the disparity for lines and random-dot stereograms. We start with model neurons that have the same types of disparity tuning curves found in cortical neurons and ask whether they can account for the psychophysical performance of the visual system.

Threshold for Discrimination

Figure 1D shows a subset of two idealized disparity tuning curves from a much larger population. For disparity d_1, each unit responds at a given level. When the disparity changes to d_2, the response of one unit increases and the response of the other unit decreases. A discriminable change in disparity has occurred if the net change in response summed over all units in the population is significant relative to the noise in the units. Signal detection theory can be used to determine the probability that this change was not produced by chance (Green and Swets 1966). The threshold for discriminability is defined as the value of disparity difference that produces a probability of 0.75 correct discrimination. We applied this method to the idealized tuning curves shown in Figure 2C.

We first attempted, unsuccessfully, to reproduce the human discrimination threshold curve in Figure 2B using just three tuning curves, one from each class. The resulting discrimination curve calculated from signal detection theory had prominent spikes because there was insufficient overlap between mechanisms. More importantly, the best discrimination threshold obtainable with three mechanisms and using the noise observed in neurons was 70 seconds, well below the hyperacuity range. This suggests that there must be more than three units engaged in encoding disparity at a particular location in the visual field.

The next step was to add additional tuning curves to the population. The following rule was found to yield good results: Make the bandwidth of each tuning curve proportional to the disparity of the tuning curve peak. This always placed the steepest portion of the near and far tuning curves near zero disparity, producing fine discrimination at the point of fixation. Thorpe and Pouget (1989) reached a similar conclusion about the importance of the slope of the tuning curve for identifying orientation. The smoothness of the discrimination curve improved as more tuning curves were added; satisfactory results were achieved with a minimum of 17 mechanisms, as shown in Figure 2. It is interesting to note that the fine stereoacuity at zero disparity is produced not by the narrow tuned mechanisms, but by the near and far mechanisms, all of which have their steep portions at zero. Although tuned mechanisms also had steep slopes, they were not concentrated at any one disparity value.

No special significance should be placed on the exact number of mechanisms we used; 17 was just a rough estimate of the minimum size of the population encoding disparity. In addition, no claim is made that the tuning curves presented here are unique. However, more tuning curves can be used. The curve generated by 200 units retained the same shape as that produced by 17 units, but it was shifted down to about 1.0 seconds because of the increased probability summation in the larger population (Lehky and Sejnowski 1990). Any larger population would push stereoacuity to unrealistically low levels. These bounds refer only to the final output that can be assayed by perceptual reports; in particular, this estimate does not include additional binocular units that might be needed for solving the correspondence problem.

Predictions of Interval and Rate Codes

Can models based on interval encoding (Fig. 1A) or rate encoding (Fig. 1B) also account for these data? When some approximation is made to the narrow disparity tuning curves used by Marr and Poggio (1976), as well as many other investigators, the resulting disparity discrimination curve does not resemble the data. The problems are (1) insufficient overlap between mechanisms, leading to a "spiky" appearance of the curve at the fine level, and (2) uniform widths in their tuning, leading to the essential flatness of the curve at a gross level. These are problems independent of the exact shape of the tuning curves. The only way to overcome both of these difficulties is to broaden the tuning curves to overlap more, in effect turning the interval code into a population code. Rate encoding, on the other hand, could account for the psychophysical data very well. The disparity response curve in Figure 1B has a steep slope near zero disparity, leading to fine discriminability, and flattens out for larger disparity values (both positive and negative), where discriminability is poor. With the appropriate flattening function, a V-shaped discrimination curve can be generated. Rate encoding offers the most parsimonious accounting for the psychophysical disparity discrimination data considered in isolation. Unfortunately, there is no evidence for neurons having such monotonic disparity responses, so this form of encoding must be rejected.

MODELING DEPTH INTERPOLATION

In this section, the discrimination model is extended to include interactions between nearby patches of the visual field, which requires the units to influence each other through a network. The opponent spatial organization of depth attraction and repulsion in Westheimer's psychophysical data (Westheimer 1986a;

see introduction) immediately suggests an old idea in neuroscience: short-range excitation and long-range inhibition between neurons (Ratliff 1965). Assume that the entire population of 17 disparity-tuned units used previously (Fig. 2C) is replicated at each spatial location. A unit at one location interacts with units at neighboring locations to form a network. Assume further that a unit interacts only with other units (at different locations) tuned to the same disparity. If units tuned to the same disparity are spatially close, there is mutual excitation; however, if they are farther apart, there is inhibition.

Each encoding population represents disparity for some patch of visual field. For present purposes, the size of these patches may be considered the area subserved by a single cortical column, but this is an empirical question, and in any case, the spatial scale does not affect the formal structure of the model. Similarly, the scale of the lateral interactions is also an empirical question. With these lateral interactions included, the model neurons will adjust their activity levels through a relaxation process. In this manner, the lateral spatial

interactions transform an initial pattern of activity at each position into a new pattern. The responses of a neural population can be shown in an "activity diagram," such as those in Figure 3, which shows the response of each unit by the height of a line relative to spontaneous activity. The line is at a position along the horizontal axis corresponding to the peak of the tuning curve for that unit.

Interpretation of the Population Code

What disparities do the new patterns of activity represent? One possibility is to assign an interpretation based on some weighted average within the population (Georgopoulos et al. 1986). However, this method assigns a unique depth to each point and would run into trouble with transparent surfaces. Another approach, which we adopt, is to consider the pattern of activity in a population as forming a "representational spectrum" irreducible to anything simpler. An interpretation of the pattern is defined by template matching: First, for every possible disparity, a canonical activity pattern is

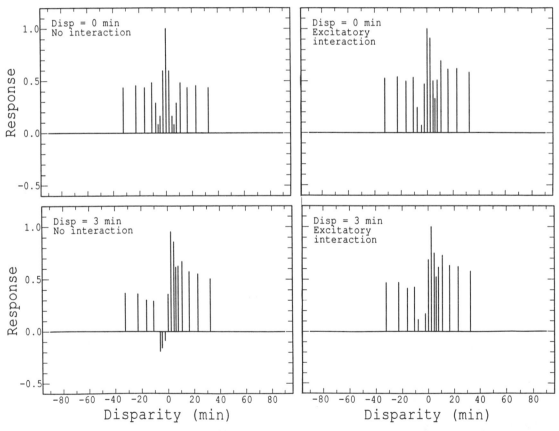

Figure 3. Activity diagrams, showing the patterns of activity when the population of 17 units (Fig. 2C) was presented with different disparities. The height of each line indicates a unit's response. The position of a line along the disparity axis indicates the value of the tuning curve peak for that unit. Each disparity produced a unique pattern of activity, which can be thought of as a representational spectrum. The two left-hand panels show activity patterns when there were no lateral interactions, such as when a single disparity stimulus is presented in isolation. (*Top left*) Response to a disparity of 0.00 min. (*Bottom left*) Response to a disparity of 3.00 min. The two right-hand panels show new activity patterns arising when two disparity stimuli were presented simultaneously at nearby positions, with excitatory interactions between positions. (*Top right*) New pattern in response to 0.00 min, which should be compared to the top left panel. (*Bottom right*) New pattern in response to 3.00 min, which should be compared to bottom left panel.

established, which is simply the pattern produced by a single disparity in the absence of any perturbing lateral influences. Second, the arbitrary activity pattern is matched to the canonical pattern with the minimum root-mean-square (RMS) error between the arbitrary patterns and the canonical patterns.

The mutual excitation between two positions causes an "attractive" effect in the apparent disparities at both positions, as shown in Figure 4B. On the other hand, if the interactions are inhibitory, then there is a "repulsive" effect. The effects described by Westheimer (1986a) are duplicated in the model by using excitatory connections to produce the short-range depth attraction or by using inhibitory connections to produce the longer-range depth repulsion. The model predicts further that if data were collected for larger disparities, the curve would fold over (Fig. 4B).

The model can be easily expanded to three locations. When disparity stimuli are present at only the two lateral locations, the interactions between the populations will indirectly stimulate an intermediate population. This is similar to what happens in a random-dot stereogram, where a solid surface is perceived even though a large fraction of the surface is blank. What pattern of activity was induced in the intermediate position? The answer depended on the disparity gradient (Burt and Julesz 1980): For small disparity differences, the intermediate point was best matched by a disparity that is the average of the two lateral disparities. A very different result occurred when there was a large disparity difference between lateral positions. There was no longer a unique minimum error for the disparity match at the intermediate position; rather, there were two minima. Patterns having two minima can represent two disparities simultaneously at a single position. This nonuniqueness was only seen when there were mutually excitatory interactions between neurons.

There are two circumstances in which multiple disparities could occur simultaneously at a single point. The first is at a depth discontinuity in the surface of an object, and the second is when there are transparent surfaces. What these situations have in common is that nearby points in the visual field may have small spatial separations, yet belong to surfaces at radically different depths. A transition from depth averaging to transparency has been observed psychophysically by Parker and Yang (1989). They measured the depth percept that resulted when random-dot stereograms were constructed by intermixing dots from two depth planes. For small disparity differences, the percept was that of a single surface at the average of the two depths, but for large differences, the percept was that of two simultaneous depths and the appearance of transparency. The disparity difference at the transition from averaging to transparency increased rapidly as a function of the mean disparity of the two sets of dots in both the experiments and the model.

MODELING DEPTH CONSTANCY

An object fixed in the environment does not seem to move around, despite jumps in its retinal location as we continually shift our gaze. This phenomenon, called space constancy, suggests that our internal representation of the world compensates for eye movements. This compensation must also exist for depth as well as location in the visual field, since we also shift the fixation point of our two eyes in depth. Disparity is a relative depth cue as illustrated in Figure 5. When a subject

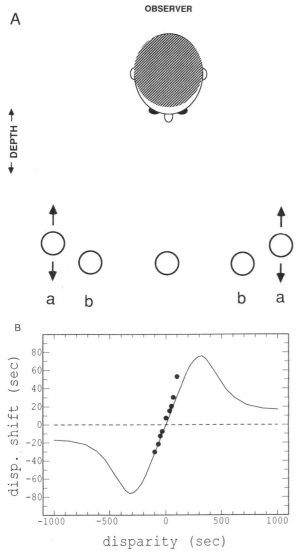

Figure 4. Comparison between human psychophysical measurements of depth interpolation and predictions of a network model. (*A*) Schematic of the setup used by Westheimer (1986a) to measure lateral interactions between nearby stimuli at different depths. The circles represent lines seen by the observer. When the outer lines *a* were moved in depth, the apparent depth of the nearby lines *b* were dragged along with them, although the physical disparities of *b* remained unchanged. For small spatial separations between *a* and *b*, *b* was dragged in the same direction as *a* (attraction), and for larger separations, *b* was repulsed. The central line was used to monitor the apparent depth at *b*. (*B*) Stereo interpolation data (●) from Westheimer (1986a). The apparent shift in disparity at *b* is shown as a function of a real shift in the disparity at *a*. The line shows predictions of the model.

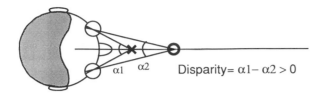

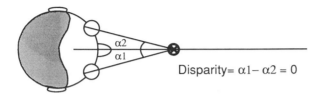

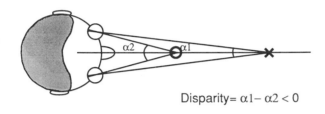

✗ : Fixation Point
O : Object

Figure 5. Schematic drawing of the interaction between disparity and vergence angle. The disparity $(\alpha_2 - \alpha_1)$ of an object depends on the eye vergence α_1. A neuron that is tuned to the depth of an object (O) should respond to (1) far disparities, (2) disparities around zero, and (3) near disparities, depending on the point of fixation of the eyes (✗).

fixates in front of an object, it has a negative disparity, whereas the disparity of the same object is positive when the subject fixates behind it. Although the position of an object along the depth axis is not explicitly represented on the retina, depth can nevertheless be recovered from a variety of other cues, such as eye vergence (Foley and Held 1972; Foley and Richards 1972; Gogel 1961, 1962; von Hofsten 1977), accommodation (Ittelson and Ames 1950), and vertical disparity (Bishop 1989). None of these cues alone can account for depth constancy, which suggests that they normally work in combination, together with monocular cues for depth. However, there are circumstances when each of these cues individually is used to estimate depth, but the extent to which each cue is used under normal circumstances is still debated.

A neural network model for space constancy in the plane of fixation has been proposed by Zipser and Andersen (1988). Physiological data suggest that area 7a in the parietal cortex of the monkey is involved in this transformation (Andersen and Mountcastle 1983).

The goal of our model is to understand the mechanism of space constancy for depth based on the interaction between disparity and vergence cues. Such interactions can be studied by recording from neurons in alert monkeys and determining the disparity tuning curves of neurons for different vergences. In all previous studies, the vergence angle was kept constant. If a neuron were coding depth rather than disparity per se, one should expect a modulation of its disparity tuning with vergence. We make specific predictions for what should be observed.

Network Architecture

A three-layer, feedforward network, completely interconnected between layers (Fig. 6), was trained with the backpropagation algorithm (Rumelhart et al. 1986) to recover absolute depth on the output layer from combinations of 5 eye positions and 21 disparity values. Vergence values were chosen so that the fixation point varied between 20 cm and 50 cm from the subject. Disparity values were limited to the interval $-40°$ to $+4°$. One input unit coded eye vergence with its activity level directly proportional to the vergence angle. This unit was similar to the vergence neurons reported in the parietal cortex (Sakata et al. 1980; Joseph and Giroud 1986) and in the oculomotor nuclei (Mays 1984). The remaining 19 input units encoded disparity with the same representation used in the above model of depth discrimination. There were 25 hidden units in the networks reported here, each of which received inputs from all the input units and projected to all the output units. The 40 output units were trained to compute absolute depth according to a Gaussian curve centered on a position specific to each unit (Fig. 6). Peaks were spread along the whole range of depth tested. Other output representations that were studied gave similar results.

Depth estimation is more accurate at short range. This was taken into account by varying the tuning curve bandwidth with the position of the peak, so that units coding for short distances were more finely tuned than those coding long distances (Fig. 6). We also made the tuning curve bandwidth vary with eye position because stereoacuity is highest near the point of fixation (Westheimer 1979). Thus, an output unit with a peak at 50 cm was trained to produce a narrower Gaussian curve when the fixation point was at 50 cm than when it was elsewhere. This second type of modulation of the output units was effective only for output units in a narrow range around the point of fixation. Although the bandwidths of the output units varied with position and point of fixation, their centers were always fixed.

Properties of the Hidden Units

We studied the hidden units of a mature network that was trained to perform accurately the transformation from relative to absolute depth. The disparity tuning curves were very similar to those of neurons observed

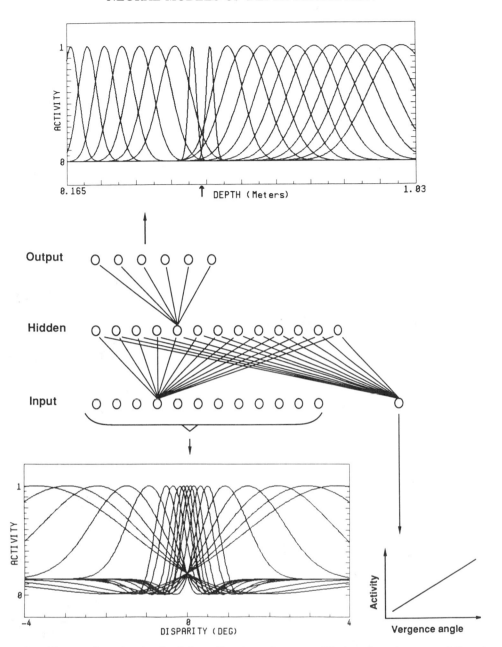

Figure 6. Network architecture for estimating depth from disparity and vergence. The input layer has one unit linearly coding eye vergence (*bottom right*) and a set of units coding disparity using a distributed representation (*bottom left*). The transformation between the input and the output is mediated by a set of hidden units. The output layer is trained to encode distance in a distributed manner (*top*). After training, the tuning curves for each output unit was a gaussian function of depth centered on a value specific to each unit (only every other depth tuning curve is shown here). The bandwidth of the curves increased with depth, except around the fixation point where the curves were narrower. These two types of bandwidth modulation produced depth estimates with relative accuracy similar to that found in humans.

in visual cortex. As shown in Figure 7, they could be roughly classified into three prototypical groups, near, far, and tuned (excitatory and inhibitory), with many intermediate examples (Ferster 1981; LeVay and Voigt 1988; Poggio et al. 1988). Vergence modulated the disparity tuning curves of the hidden units in various ways that fell between two general classes: In the first class, the disparity tuning of the unit remained similar for the five eye positions, but the amplitude of the response was modulated. Figure 7, A and D, shows two

examples of this class, which we call disparity gain-control neurons. These are analogous to translational gain-control neurons in area 7a, whose response is modulated by eye position but not the position of the receptive field (Andersen and Mountcastle 1983). In the second extreme class, the disparity tuning of the unit changed significantly with eye position, even though the shape of the curve remained the same, as illustrated in Figure 7C. For certain eye positions, the tuning curves of these units were completely displaced

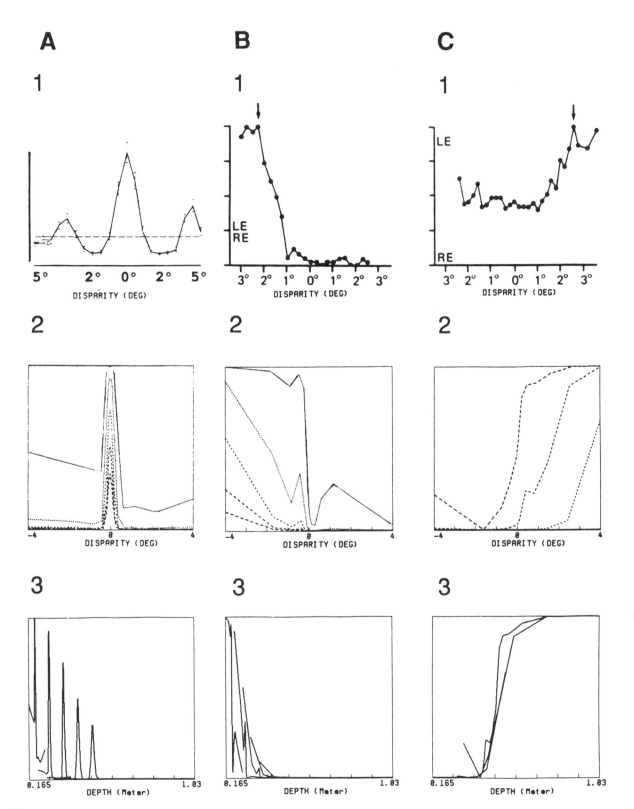

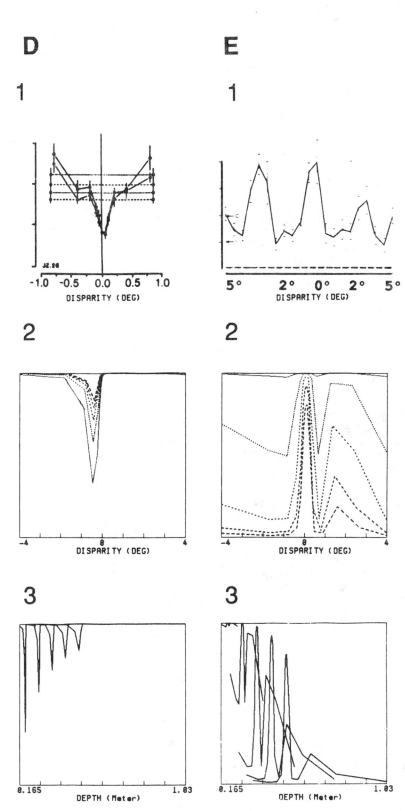

D

1

2

3

E

1

2

3

Figure 7. Comparisons between typical disparity tuning curves for real neurons and for hidden units. (*A*) Excitatory tuned units; (*B*) near units; (*C*) far units; (*D*) inhibitory tuned units; (*E*) intermediate units with multiple peaks. (*Row 1*) Disparity tuning curves for five typical neurons based on recordings from primary visual cortex (*B* and *C*: Ferster 1981 [cat]; *A* and *E*: LeVay and Voigt 1988 [cat]; *D*: Poggio et al. 1988 [monkey]). (*Row 2*) Disparity tuning curves for five equivalent hidden units. Five tuning curves corresponding to the five different eye positions are shown for each unit by dashed and dotted lines. (*A-2, D-2*) Typical disparity gain control units; (*C-2*) example of a unit tuned to depth; (*B-2, E-2*) intermediate type of modulation. Such intermediate units are not perfectly tuned to depth, but the general envelopes of their depth tuning curves do provide useful information for depth estimation. Compare these tuning curves to those of corresponding real neurons in Row *1*. (*Row 3*) Depth tuning curves for the corresponding hidden units. These tuning curves are predictions for what might be found in visual cortex when vergence and disparity tuning are measured in single neurons.

from zero disparity. This has been observed in the cat (see Fig. 7B,C) (Ferster 1981; LeVay and Voigt 1988) and in the monkey (Poggio et al. 1988). Tuned units tend to be in the first class, whereas near and far units tend to belong to the second class. Units exhibiting an intermediate type of modulation are shown in Figure 7, B and E. This second class of hidden units is not unexpected when one considers that the output units completely change their disparity selectivity with eye position (Fig. 5). The surprising result is that so few hidden units change their disparity selectivity with eye position.

The depth tuning curves of the hidden units are shown in Figure 7. The units in the class showing gain control (Fig. 7A) changed their depth sensitivity with vergence, which is an indirect measure of depth. For the units whose disparity selectivity changed completely with vergence (Fig. 7C), the depth tuning is almost perfect. This type of unit is therefore functionally very close to the output units. However, there are usually only 4 or 5 of these hidden units out of 25 hidden units in a single network, and the overall performance of the network does not depend critically on them.

Effect of Higher Depth Acuity around the Fixation Point

The bandwidth of an output unit was designed to vary with the position of the tuning curve relative to the

observer and with its position relative to the fixation point. This mimics the decreasing absolute accuracy of stereopsis with increasing distance and also makes the network more accurate around the fixation point. When a network was not forced to be more accurate around the fixation point, the weights from the sharply tuned unit in the input layer to the hidden units were smaller (Fig. 8). When networks were trained without any modulation of the bandwidth of the output units, the weights were similar to those in networks with bandwidth modulation, but learning was much more difficult and the final error value was higher.

DISCUSSION

The central premise of our modeling was that disparity is encoded by a population of units having broad, overlapping tuning curves. In such a distributed representation, the activity of a single unit gives only a coarse indication of the stimulus parameter. This does not mean that precise information is lost, but only that the information is dispersed over a pattern of activity in the population. The concept of distributed representations arose in nineteenth century psychophysics with the idea that color is encoded by the relative activities in a population of three overlapping color channels. In our model, the parameter is "disparity" rather than "color," and more mechanisms were required to explain the data, but the idea is the same. In a similar

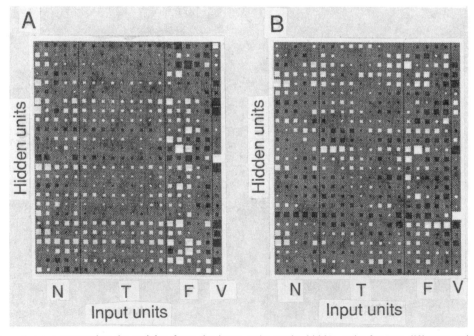

Figure 8. Hinton diagram comparing the weights from the input units to the hidden units for two different training sets. (*A*) Bandwidth of the output units varied only with the position of the center. The weights from the tuned units are small, indicating that these units have little influence on the hidden units. (*B*) Double modulation of the bandwidth of the output units with the position of the center and the position of the fixation point. Tuned input units have more influence on the hidden units as revealed by the higher values of their weights. Each row represents weights from all the input units projecting to a single hidden unit. Each column represents all the weights from a single input unit to all hidden units. The first five columns are from near units (N), the central nine weights are from tuned unit (T), the next five weights are from the far units (F), and the last column corresponds to the vergence unit (V). White weights have positive values and black weights have negative values. The area of the square is directly proportional to the value of the weight.

manner, it is possible to apply the concept to many other parameters. Some consequences of population coding were analyzed by Hinton et al. (1986) in the context of model neurons with only two levels of firing, fully on or fully off. We have extended Hinton's analysis to the case when units have continuous values and noise is the limiting factor rather than width of the tuning curve. We conclude that the population size encoding disparity for a small patch of visual field may be as small as a few tens of units or as large as a few hundred.

Interpreting Population Codes

There are several approaches to the problem of deciding what parameter value a pattern of activity in a population represents. One approach is what we call the "spectrum" method, used in this model of disparity and also in color vision. When assigning a color to the pattern of activity within this small population, the vector of three activities is not reduced to a single number. There is nothing simpler than the pattern itself, which forms a characteristic representational spectrum for each wavelength. In the same manner, our model represents disparity (another one-dimensional parameter) in a high (possibly several hundred)-dimensional space. A second approach is what we call the "averaging" method, used in the population code models of Gelb and Wilson (1983) and Georgopoulos et al. (1986), in which the dimensionality of a representation is reduced during the interpretation process. For example, Georgopoulos et al. (1986) used the averaging method for representing the three-dimensional direction of arm movement. The pattern of activity in a large population was interpreted by collapsing the high-dimensional representational space down to three dimensions by calculating a weighted sum of tuning curve peaks. Their interpretation of population activity is based entirely on this sum and not on any particular spectrum of activity within that population.

Consequences of Using a Population Code for Disparity

In the Marr and Poggio model (1976), which was based on an interval code, false matches were eliminated by using inhibition to shut off all units tuned to the wrong disparities at a given location, a form of winner-take-all circuit. In contrast, the goal in a distributed code is to alter the relative firing rates to produce a new pattern of activity and not to shut off all neurons in a population except one, for a single broadly tuned unit provides little information. The choice of representation also affects the process of interpolation. Grimson (1982) and Terzopoulos (1988) used spline functions to fit through the blank regions between the surface tokens used in the stereomatching process based on an interval code. This procedure also interpolated through real depth discontinuities, shrouding sharp breaks. These models deal with the problem by adding separate

mechanisms that recognize discontinuities and attenuate the interpolation process accordingly (Koch et al. 1986). In our model, interpolation falls out automatically without any shift in parameters or any additional mechanisms.

The discrimination model was concerned in part with the representation of transparent stimuli. It is possible that analogous models can be constructed for other transparency phenomena besides those arising from depth. A specific example involves motion. Adelson and Movshon (1982) have studied the percept of two superimposed gratings drifting in different directions and found conditions under which they "cohered" to form a single drifting plaid or alternatively appeared as two transparent surfaces sliding over each other, depending on how similar the two gratings were in various respects (speed, spatial frequency, contrast, etc.). This might also be understood in terms of a distributed representation for motion formally analogous to the one used for disparity here.

Predictions for Depth Tuning

We have trained a neural network to recover egocentric depth from disparity and vergence information and then determined the response properties of the hidden units to disparity and depth. Similar neural network models have been used to explain the response properties of known neurons in cerebral cortex (Lehky and Sejnowski 1988; Zipser and Andersen 1988). However, this is the first time that such models have been used to make predictions before the physiological results were available. These predictions will soon be tested in experiments by S.J. Thorpe et al. and J. Gnadt (pers. comm.) on alert monkeys. One of the uncertainties of the depth model was the choice of output representation. Fortunately, this choice only affected the relative number of mechanisms of each class found in the hidden layer and not their qualitative properties. We varied the sensitivity of the network to absolute depth and point of fixation by modulating the bandwidths of the output units. The flexibility of this type of distributed coding may be one of the reasons why it is widely used in the cerebral cortex to represent sensory and motor variables.

One point on which our model of stereoacuity and the model of depth estimation differed was the role of the narrowly tuned units. For depth discrimination, the broadly tuned units were primarily responsible for the highest acuity near the plane of fixation. However, in the absolute depth network, the sharply tuned units were important when the output units were modulated to produce fine discrimination around the fixation point. This indicates that different tasks may use different complements from the diverse population of disparity-selective neurons that have been observed in cerebral cortex. There is no reason to assume that the same neurons used to represent relative depth are identical with the neurons used to estimate absolute depth, which is known to be much less accurate. It may be possible to test these predictions by selectively interfering with these tuned disparity neurons in monkeys during the performance of psychophysical tasks.

Psychophysical Consequences

In our network model of depth estimation, we made the assumption that vergence information is accessible to the neural system that judges the depth of objects. One possible consequence of this assumption is that in the absence of other confounding cues, the apparent depth of an object should change as the vergence angle is varied by a prism, even though the actual depth of the object is fixed. Alternatively, the apparent size of an object could change. As the eyes are converged, the object should appear to shrink, since it subtends the same area of the retina, whereas evidence from vergence indicates that it is closer to the observer. Conversely, diverging the eyes should lead to an apparent increase in the size of an object. Ogle (1962) has reported observations that are consistent with these counterintuitive predictions. However, Ogle explained his results differently, and further experiments are needed to choose between various explanations. The vergence effect should also hold for depth seen in random-dot stereograms, since the same argument used for angular size should also hold for disparity. Thus, the apparent height of a single raised dot in a random-dot stereogram should appear to shrink as the eyes are verged and should appear to grow as the eyes are diverged. Experiments using random-dot stereograms of extended objects must control for other depth cues, such as vertical disparities.

In conclusion, we have studied several possible models of binocular organization in the primate visual system. Some models fit only part of the data, such as rate encoding of disparity, which can parsimoniously account for the psychophysical stereoacuity data but is inconsistent with the neurophysiology. Conversely, the psychophysics also constrains interpretation of the neurophysiology. We have further shown that the distributed representation of disparity can both smoothly interpolate between sparse data and incorporate discontinuities and transparency depending on the disparity gradient. Finally, a distributed representation of relative depth can be combined with other cues, such as vergence, to predict the absolute depth of an object. This interaction and mutual constraint between physiological and behavioral data provide a particularly rich environment for the development of neural models.

ACKNOWLEDGMENTS

This research was supported by a grant from the Sloan Foundation to T.J.S. and G.F. Poggio and by grants from the Mathers Foundation and the Drown Foundation to T.J.S. We are grateful to Dr. G.F. Poggio for illuminating discussions about the disparity tuning and response properties of cortical neurons and to S.J. Thorpe for inspiring discussions on the model of depth constancy.

REFERENCES

Adelson, E. and J.A. Movshon. 1982. Phenomenal coherence of moving visual patterns. *Nature* **300:** 523.

Andersen, R. and V. Mountcastle. 1983. The influence of the angle of gaze upon the excitability of the light-sensitive neurons of the posterior parietal cortex. *J. Neurosci.* **3:** 532.

Badcock, D. and C. Schor. 1985. Depth-increment detection function for individual spatial channels. *J. Opt. Soc. Am.* **A2:** 1211.

Barlow, H.B., C. Blakemore, and J.D. Pettigrew. 1967. The neural mechanisms of binocular depth discrimination. *J. Physiol.* **193:** 327.

Bishop, P.O. 1989. Vertical disparity, egocentric distance and stereoscopic depth constancy: A new interpretation. *Proc. R. Soc. Lond. B. Biol. Sci.* **237:** 445.

Burt, P. and B. Julesz. 1980. A disparity gradient limit for binocular fusion. *Science* **208:** 615.

Ferster, D. 1981. A comparison of binocular depth mechanisms in areas 17 and 18 of the cat visual cortex. *J. Physiol.* **311:** 623.

Foley, J.M. and R. Held. 1972. Visually directed pointing as a function of target distance, direction and available cues. *Percept. Psychophys.* **12:** 263.

Foley, J.M. and W. Richards. 1972. Effects of voluntary eye movement and convergence on the binocular appreciation of depth. *Percept. Psychophys.* **11(6):** 423.

Gelb, D. and H. Wilson. 1983. Shifts in perceived size as a function of contrast and temporal modulation. *Vision Res.* **23:** 71.

Georgopoulos, A., A. Schwartz, and R. Kettner. 1986. Neuronal population coding of movement direction. *Science* **233:** 1416.

Gogel, W.C. 1961. Convergence as a cue to absolute distance. *J. Psychol.* **52:** 287.

———. 1962. The effect of convergence on perceived size and distance. *J. Psychol.* **53:** 475.

Green, D. and I. Swets. 1966. *Signal detection theory and psychophysics.* Wiley, New York.

Grimson, W. 1982. A computational theory of visual surface interpolation. *Philos. Trans. R. Soc. Lond. B Biol. Sci.* **298:** 395.

Hinton, G.E., J.L. McClelland, and D.E. Rumelhart. 1986. Distributed representations. In *Parallel distributed processing: Explorations in the microstructure of cognition* (ed. D.E. Rumelhart and J. McClelland), vol. 1, p.77. MIT Press, Cambridge, Massachusetts.

Hubel, D. and T. Wiesel. 1970. Cells sensitive to binocular depth in area 18 of the macaque monkey cortex. *Nature* **225:** 41.

Ittelson, W.H. and A.J. Ames. 1950. Accommodation, convergence and the irrelation to apparent distance. *J. Psychol.* **30:** 43.

Joseph, J.P. and P. Giroud. 1986. Visuomotor properties of neurons of the anterior suprasylvian gyrus in the awake cat. *Exp. Brain Res.* **62:** 355.

Julesz, B. 1960. Binocular depth perception of computer generated patterns. *Bell System Tech. J.* **39:** 1125.

———. 1971. *Foundations of cyclopean vision.* University of Chicago Press, Chicago, Illinois.

Koch, C., J. Marroquin, and A. Yuille. 1986. Analog "neural" networks in early vision. *Proc. Natl. Acad. Sci.* **83:** 4263.

Lehky, S.R. and T.J. Sejnowski. 1988. Network model of shape-from-shading: Neural function arises from both receptive and projective fields. *Nature* **333:** 452.

———. 1990. Neural model of stereoacuity and depth interpolation based on a distributed representation of stereo disparity. *J. Neurosci.* **10:** 2281.

LeVay, S. and T. Voigt. 1988. Ocular dominance and disparity coding in cat visual cortex. *Visual Neurosci.* **1:** 395.

Marr, D. and T. Poggio. 1976. Cooperative computation of stereo disparity. *Science* **194:** 283.

————. 1979. A computational theory of human stereo vision. *Proc. R. Soc. Lond. B Biol. Sci.* **204**: 301.

Mayhew, I. and I. Frisby. 1981. Psychophysical and computational studies towards a theory of human stereopsis. *Artif. Intell.* **16**: 349.

Mays, L.E. 1984. Neural control of vergence eye movements: Convergence and divergence neurons in the midbrain. *J. Neurophys.* **51(5)**: 1091.

Nikara, T., P.O. Bishop, and J.D. Pettigrew. 1968. Analysis of retinal correspondence by studying receptive fields of binocular single units in cat striate cortex. *Exp. Brain. Res.* **6**: 353.

Ogle, K.N. 1962. Perception of distance and size. In *The eye: Visual optics and the optical space sense* (ed. H. Davson), vol. 4, p. 265. Academic Press, New York.

Parker, A.J. and Y. Yang. 1989. Disparity pooling in human stereo vision. *Vision Res.* **29**: 1525.

Pettigrew, J.D., T. Nikara, and P.O. Bishop. 1968. Binocular interaction on single units in cat striate cortex: Simultaneous stimulation by single moving slit with receptive fields in correspondence. *Exp. Brain Res.* **6**: 391.

Poggio, G. 1984. Processing of stereoscopic information in primate visual cortex. In *Dynamic aspects of neocortical function* (ed. G.M. Edelman et al.), p. 613. Wiley, New York.

Poggio, G. and T. Poggio. 1984. The analysis of stereopsis. *Annu. Rev. Neurosci.* **7**: 379.

Poggio, G.F., F. Gonzalez, and F. Krause. 1988. Stereoscopic mechanism in monkey visual cortex: Binocular correlation and disparity selectivity. *J. Neurosci.* **8(12)**: 4531.

Poggio, G., B.C. Motter, S. Squatrito, and Y. Trotter. 1985. Responses of neurons in visual cortex (V1 and V2) of the alert macaque to dynamic random-dot stereograms. *Vision Res.* **25**: 397.

Poggio, T. and B. Fischer. 1977. Binocular interactions and depth sensitivity in striate and prestriate cortex of behaving rhesus monkeys. *J. Neurophysiol.* **40**: 1392.

Pouget, A. and T.J. Sejnowski. 1990. A neural network model for computing depth from stereopsis. *Invest. Ophthalmol. Visual Sci. (suppl.)* **31**: 96.

Ratliff, F. 1965. *Mach bands: Quantitative studies on neural networks in the retina.* Holden-Day, San Francisco.

Rumelhart, D.E., G.E. Hinton, and R.J. Williams. 1986. Learning internal representations by error propagation. In *Parallel distributed processing: Explorations in the microstructure of cognition*, vol. 1, p. 318. MIT Press, Cambridge, Massachusetts.

Sakata, H., H. Shibutani, and K. Kawano. 1980. Spatial properties of visual fixation neurons in posterior parietal cortex of the monkey. *J. Neurophysiol.* **43(6)**: 1654.

Schumer, R. and B. Julesz. 1984. Binocular disparity modulation sensitivity to disparities offset from the plane of fixation. *Vision Res.* **24**: 533.

Terzopoulos, D. 1988. The computation of visible surface representations. *IEEE Trans. Pattern Anal. and Mach. Intell.* **10**: 417.

Thorpe, S.J. and A. Pouget. 1989. Coding of orientation in the visual cortex: Neural network modeling. In *Connectionism in perspective* (ed. R. Pfeifer). Elsevier, Amsterdam.

von Hofsten, C. 1977. Binocular convergence as a determinant of reaching behavior in infancy. *Perception* **6**: 139.

Westheimer, G. 1979. Cooperative neural process involved in stereoscopic acuity. *Exp. Brain Res.* **36**: 585.

————. 1986a. Spatial interaction in the domain of disparity signals in human stereoscopic vision. *J. Physiol.* **370**: 619.

————. 1986b. Panum's phenomenon and the confluence of signals from two eyes in stereoscopy. *Proc. R. Soc. Lond. B Biol. Sci.* **228**: 289.

Westheimer, G. and D. Levi. 1987. Depth attraction and repulsion of disparate foveal stimuli. *Vision Res.* **27**: 1361.

Wheatstone, C. 1838. Contributions to the physiology of vision. 1. On some remarkable and hitherto unobserved phenomena of binocular vision. *Philos. Trans. R. Soc. Lond. B Biol. Sci.* **8**: 39.

Zipser, D. and R. Andersen. 1988. Back propagation learning simulates response properties of a subset of posterior parietal neurons. *Nature* **331**: 679.

Cellular Network Underlying Locomotion as Revealed in a Lower Vertebrate Model: Transmitters, Membrane Properties, Circuitry, and Simulation

S. GRILLNER, P. WALLÉN, AND G. VIANA DI PRISCO

Nobel Institute for Neurophysiology, Karolinska Institutet, S-104 01 Stockholm, Sweden

A great deal of our current understanding of the brain originated from discoveries made at the cellular and molecular levels. However, even with all of the pieces of information at hand, it is very difficult to sort out the relevant mechanisms responsible for the operation of a neural system. Thus, we must use experimental models that are simple enough to understand and yet sufficiently complex to capture essential features of whatever function we want to consider. On the other hand, we need to be able to test the relative contribution of these features and therefore must recur to computer simulations of system models. In this paper, we deal with the motor system used for ambulation. Locomotion is a universal pattern of behavior generated by a family of different neural control systems: (1) generation of the propulsion (rhythmic limb or trunk movements); (2) visuomotor coordination adapting the movements to the environment (e.g., positioning of the limbs in each step cycle); (3) steering movements; (4) equilibrium control during locomotion (e.g., walking with the back upward); and (5) compensation of predicted perturbations before they have occurred, or after the fact.

Propulsive movements are generated by circuits organized in a similar fashion in all vertebrates (cf. Orlovsky and Shik 1976; Grillner 1985). Essentially, spinal pattern generator circuits (central networks with sensory modulation) are controlled by reticulospinal projections, which can be activated from particular brain stem locomotor centers. The mesencephalic locomotor center (see Orlovsky and Shik 1976) can be stimulated in different vertebrates. At low strength, slow locomotion will arise (e.g., walking), and as the stimulation strength is increased, the gait may change to trot and gallop. A very simple type of stimulus can thus elicit propulsion, in which hundreds of different muscles are coordinated to be active, each in their particular phase of the movement. Moreover, as the speed increases, the phase relations may change gradually, or suddenly as in the switch from one type of gait to another.

Stimulation of the locomotor areas in the brain stem can elicit locomotion in all classes of animals, be it tetrapod walking, bird flight, or fish or cyclostome swimming. Figure 1 shows the overall organization of the mammalian control system. Brain stem locomotor centers activate spinal cord central pattern generators, which initiate activity in each group of motoneurons.

The resulting movement will activate sensory receptors, signaling the progress of the movement. These receptors help regulate the duration of the different phases of the movement cycle. Sensory feedback acts on the central pattern generator network (duration of different phases) and the output level (modulation of motoneuron activity), and ascending spinocerebellar projections signal the progress of the actual movement and of the output signals (from the central network) in the form of "efference copy" signals from the pattern generator network to cerebellum.

Cerebellum plays an important part in the final adaptation of the locomotor movements to different types of perturbations, but as indicated in Figure 1, cerebellum is not required for eliciting the basic coordination underlying locomotion. The corticospinal systems appear to be important for the sensory motor coordination involved in the precise positioning of the limbs on uneven surfaces (Georgopoulos and Grillner 1989).

Mesencephalic mammals (without cortex and diencephalon) can coordinate walking movements with some perfection but do not adapt the movements to the external world. Animals with diencephalon, but not cortex intact, behave, on the other hand, in a seemingly normal way. Although their vision is obviously impaired, they can perform goal-directed movements. The interaction between the different output nuclei of the basal ganglia and the mesencephalic locomotor area is now well described. Essentially, GABAergic fibers from ventral and dorsal pallidum and substantia nigrapars reticulata appear to provide a tonic inhibition of the mesencephalic locomotor center and to initiate locomotion by a disinhibition of cells in the mesencephalic area (Garcia-Rill and Skinner 1986; Jordan

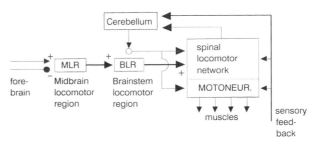

Figure 1. Overall organization of the mammalian control system for locomotion (see text for explanation).

1986). This effect parallels the control of saccadic eye movements from the basal ganglia to the superior colliculus (Waitzman et al. 1988). Whereas propulsive movements can thus be produced by the brain stem–spinal cord, di- and telencephalic structures are important in making the movements behaviorally relevant and goal-directed (Beloozerova and Sirota 1986; Armstrong 1988; Georgopoulos and Grillner 1989; Grillner and Orlovski 1990).

The overall neural control scheme shown in Figure 1 provides important information about the general control strategy used in vertebrate nervous systems. The details of the central pattern generation must obviously differ between species and types of locomotion. But even the timing of the motor output to the muscles of the hindlimbs remains similar among tetrapods of the different classes of vertebrates. During vertebrate evolution, the neuronal circuitry used to control locomotion has gradually been modified in detail and has become more complex and refined to generate the mammalian motor repertoire (Grillner 1985, 1990).

The Lamprey Model

If we are to understand how the networks generating locomotion operate, we need in each case to define (1) which neurons contribute to behavior, (2) the connectivity between relevant neurons, (3) the different types of synaptic mechanisms used, and (4) the membrane properties of relevant neurons. Only with this type of information at hand can one realistically try to understand the basic neural mechanism generating the behavior. Because of the complexity of even the simplest neural circuit, computer simulations have become a necessary tool in the analysis.

With the overall goal to understand complex nervous systems, it is useful to find simpler experimentally amenable models like that of lower vertebrates, which have the same general anatomical organization. The lamprey has a flattened spinal cord, which can be maintained in vitro together with the brain stem over several days. The neural networks underlying a variety of different patterns of behavior can be activated in the isolated nervous system. The in vitro condition permits a detailed analysis of circuitry and synaptic mechanisms. The lamprey nervous system has the ground plan of that of higher vertebrates from the basal ganglia to the spinal cord. The general organization is indeed similar, although the number of cells in each category is much reduced (see Brodin and Grillner 1990; Rovainen 1979, 1982).

Reticulospinal Initiation of Locomotion

In the motor system, the descending control is exerted by reticulospinal neurons, which originate from a posterior, middle, and anterior reticular nucleus and a mesencephalic nucleus. All nuclei contain neurons, which utilize glutamate (excitatory amino acids [EAA]) as a transmitter (see Brodin 1989), and they extend throughout the spinal cord by fibers with a range of different conduction velocities (Rovainen 1982; Kasicki et al. 1988). A large proportion of these cells change their pattern of discharge during locomotion and appear to be involved in the initiation and maintenance of locomotion. These cells have a large fan-like dendritic arbor that covers a large part of the basal plate in a transverse plane (Fig. 2). They can thus easily be activated by all the neuronal traffic up and down the brain stem. Although an increased activity occurs in all reticular nuclei during initiation of locomotion, the posterior nucleus appears to be of particular importance (Kasicki et al. 1988; Ohta and Grillner 1989). The neurons of this nucleus monosynaptically excite motoneurons, as well as the inhibitory and excitatory interneurons, which have been shown to be part of the spinal network generating locomotor activity (Fig. 3).

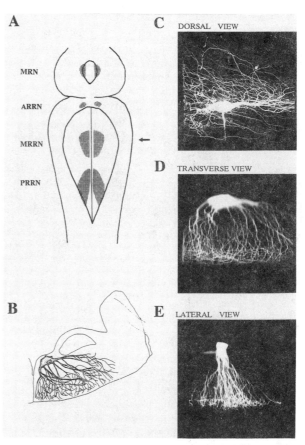

Figure 2. (*A*) The lamprey brain stem contains four different reticular nuclei that control the locomotor networks of the spinal cord. The most rostral nucleus is situated in the mesencephalon (MRN), and three other nuclei are situated in the rhombencephalon: the anterior (ARRN), the middle (MRRN), and the posterior (PRRN). (*B*) A cross-section at the level indicated by the arrow in *A* shows a drawing made by R. Dubuc of a reticulospinal cell. These cells have their cell bodies situated dorsally close to the IV ventricle, and their dendritic trees span ventrally a large portion of the basal plate. (*C–E*) Three-dimensional reconstructions of a reticulospinal neuron made by a confocal laser scanning microscope (objective 20 × /0.75) in three orthogonal viewing directions. The image size is 0.5 mm × 0.5 mm.

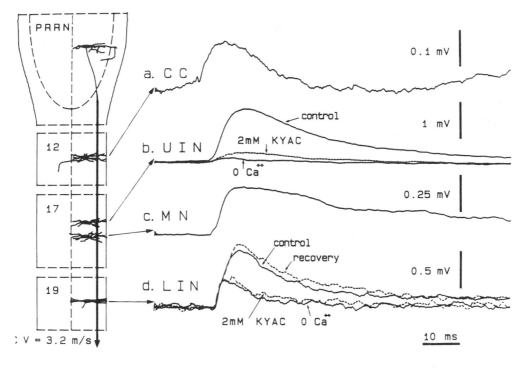

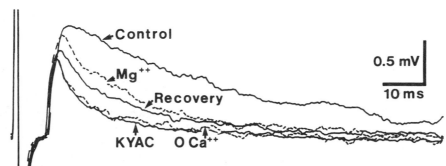

Figure 3. Monosynaptic excitation from a single PRRN neuron to different types of spinal neurons. EPSP is excitatory amino acid (EAA)-mediated, as revealed by blockage with kynurenic acid (KYAC). An electrical component remained in *d* in zero calcium solution. Lower traces demonstrate the presence of an NMDA component, which is blocked by magnesium ions. (Modified from Ohta and Grillner 1989.)

Figure 4 provides a scheme of this circuitry, which is composed of a supraspinal part, a segmental central spinal, and a sensory part. The spinal circuitry feeds information back to the reticular nuclei. In fact, most reticular cells are depolarized in-phase with the rostral ipsilateral ventral root locomotor burst and inhibited with the contralateral burst. This effect is mediated by ascending neurons projecting to the alar plate and then further relayed via small excitatory or inhibitory interneurons projecting to the reticular nucleus (Dubuc and Grillner 1989). This arrangement will tend to make the reticulospinal activity self-sustaining.

In addition to the EAA system discussed here, there are two reticulospinal 5-hydroxytryptamine (5-HT) systems, as well as cholecystokinin (CCK) and peptide YY (PYY) systems, that originate in parts of the anterior and posterior reticular nuclei (Brodin et al. 1986,

1988, 1989). Although we have information about their spinal target neurons (Ohta and Grillner 1989), there is no exact information on their role.

Spinal Locomotor Organization

Although locomotor activity is normally initiated from the brain stem, the motor pattern can be elicited in the isolated spinal cord by stimulation of fiber tracts or by simply increasing the neuronal excitability by adding excitatory amino acids like kainate or *N*-methyl-D-aspartate (NMDA) into the bath (Cohen and Wallén 1980; Grillner et al. 1981b; Brodin et al. 1985). Spinal cord segments in vitro can thus produce the motor output underlying locomotion throughout the normal frequency range (0.25–10 Hz), and this capacity is distributed along the entire spinal cord. It can be di-

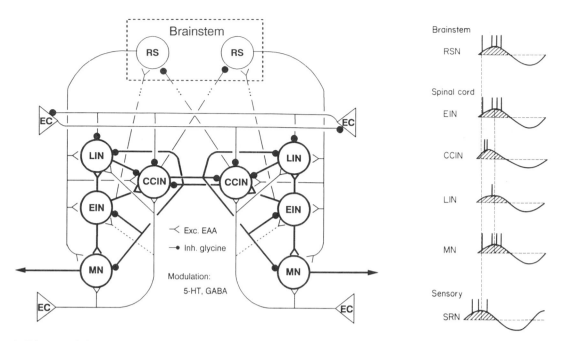

Figure 4. Diagram of the segmental circuitry for locomotion in the lamprey, with its descending and sensory controls (see text for details). The drawing to the right depicts the patterns of discharge in the different types of neurons during a locomotor cycle.

vided into small pieces down to a few segments, each of which can produce rhythmic burst activity and the characteristic intersegmental coordination with a constant phase lag between consecutive segments (Wallén and Williams 1984). Under intact conditions, this results in an undulatory wave traveling down the body, pushing the animal through the water (Grillner 1974; Williams et al. 1989).

Each segment contains about 100 motoneurons, which supply different parts of the myotome. The motoneurons of the left and right sides provide alternating burst activity. As the motoneurons of one side become excited, the motoneurons on the contralateral side become inhibited in a reciprocal fashion. During a swim cycle, each motoneuron thus goes through a phase of excitation, followed by inhibition (Russell and Wallén 1983).

The excitation is derived from excitatory interneurons (EIN), which are phasically active during locomotion (Buchanan and Grillner 1987); they also excite two inhibitory types of interneurons, one of which has an axon that crosses over to the other side (CC interneurons) to inhibit both types of premotor interneurons and motoneurons. The third element in the segmental network is an ipsilateral (LIN) interneuron that inhibits the CC interneurons and thereby contributes to the burst termination (see below and Buchanan and Grillner 1987; Grillner et al. 1988). Figure 4 shows how these different types of neurons discharge in a swim cycle. Thus, locomotion, like other patterns of behavior, is not produced by a simple network of identical elements but by a specific interaction between several heterogeneous groups of neurons, each with morphologically and physiologically distinct properties.

Basic Types of Synaptic Transmission in the Network

Synaptic interactions among the interneurons are due to inhibition via conventional Cl^- IPSPs operated by glycine receptors, whereas excitation is due to glutamate receptors of both kainate/α-amino-3-hydroxy-5-methyl-4-isoxazolepropionate (AMPA) and the NMDA type (Buchanan 1982; Dale and Grillner 1986). Supraspinal and sensory excitatory control is glutamatergic, whereas the sensory inhibitory neurons use glycine receptors (Ohta and Grillner 1989; Viana di Prisco et al. 1990). The basic network interaction uses the conventional neuronal interaction by means of glycine and glutamate receptors. There is additional modulation by 5-HT and GABA (Wallén et al. 1989; Alford et al. 1990; see below), and probably also by the peptidergic systems, the functions of which, however, remain largely unknown (see above).

Operation of the Locomotor Network

Initiation. The segmental network can be turned on by increasing the background excitability to a level at which many neurons in the network would fire action potentials when not actively inhibited. Normally, the reticulospinal EAA systems enhance excitability and thus regulate the level of background excitability and the burst rate produced by the network. Experimentally, the background excitability can also be controlled by adding kainate/AMPA or NMDA to the perfusion fluid. A selective activation of kainate/AMPA receptors after a blockade of NMDA receptors induces locomotor activity in a frequency range of about 1–10

Hz, monotonously increasing with the level of kainate/AMPA receptor activation (see Fig. 5). Activation of NMDA receptors also induces swimming but in the lower frequency range of 0.1–2 Hz (Brodin et al. 1985). As discussed below, this is due to the voltage-dependent properties of the NMDA channels.

Segmental network operation: Qualitative interpretation. Whereas the initiation of activity can be elicited from supraspinal sources, the generation of the motor pattern is due to an interaction among the segmental interneurons. Let us consider the network of Figure 4 and a situation in which the excitability is increased on both the left and right sides such that interneurons would tend to fire action potentials if not actively inhibited. Initially, one of the network sides may become active, and if so, all neurons on that side, whereas the contralateral side then will become inhibited due to a reciprocal inhibition via the CC inter-

neurons. In this way, an asymmetric activity would arise with one active side and one silent side.

Mechanisms for terminating the activity on the active side are thus required. Several factors contribute to the burst termination, such as spike frequency adaptation, plateau properties, and the fact that the lateral interneurons (LIN, see Fig. 4) have a high threshold for activation. When they are discharged, however, they will inhibit the CC interneurons on the same side and thereby disinhibit all neurons on the contralateral side. The crucial factor is thus a disinhibition leading to an excitability increase that causes a discharge of the previously inactive side. The cessation of CC-interneuron activity is thus critical, leading to alternating burst activity.

Simulation of network operation. Qualitative reasoning as above cannot provide more than a very general insight at best. To further evaluate whether the

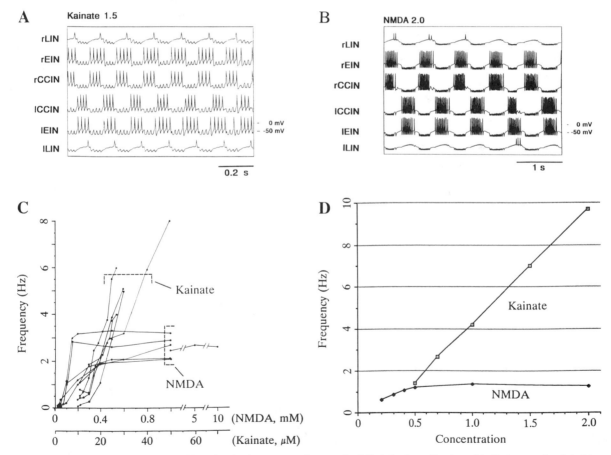

Figure 5. Simulation of EAA-induced bursting in the segmental network. (*A*) A bath application of kainate was simulated by a tonic opening of kainate/AMPA receptor channels (conventional EPSP channels) on the nerve cells of the network in Fig. 4. (*B*) Simulation of NMDA receptor-induced locomotor activity was simulated by a tonic opening of NMDA channels on the network neurons. The NMDA channels had a voltage sensitivity corresponding to a Mg^{++} level of approximately 1.8 mM. The NMDA-induced properties give a powerful contribution to the burst termination, and therefore activity in lateral interneurons (LIN) is not required. (*C*) Experimental data (Brodin et al. 1985) showing the dose-response relationships of fictive locomotion induced by bath application of NMDA and kainate, respectively. (*D*) Relationships between the level of kainate and NMDA receptor activation (arbitrary units) and the response in burst frequency of the simulated segmental network. The dose-response relationships correspond well to those found experimentally (*C*).

network we have defined experimentally can account for the generation of alternating locomotor activity, realistic computer simulations have been performed.

Initial simulations with simplified neurons showed that alternating activity could be generated by a network "hooked up" like the neurons in Figure 4. The neurons of each type were simulated with properties similar to those of the biological cells, but without NMDA receptors and several other features. Such a network could operate in the upper frequency range (above 2 Hz) with the appropriate phasing of the neurons (Grillner et al. 1988).

To make a more realistic simulation, new model neurons have been developed (Ö. Ekeberg et al., in prep.). The passive neurons have a soma and a variable number (three used here) of dendrite compartments. Each compartment may have voltage-dependent Na^+, K^+, and Ca^{++} channels simulated with Hodgkin and Huxley (1952) formalisms. In addition, the intracellular free Ca^{++} levels and Ca^{++}-dependent potassium channels were simulated. For the synaptic interaction, excitations (kainate/AMPA channels) were modeled with a short conductance increase for monovalent cations (Na^+,K^+), and inhibition with a conductance increase for Cl^- ions. A variable conduction delay from the pre- to the postsynaptic cell was generated, and the synapses could be placed at the different compartments. All cells in the network were simulated by giving the model neuron membrane properties that made them closely resemble their biological counterparts in terms of input resistance, shape of action potentials, different phases of after-hyperpolarization, and response to current injection.

In Figure 5, the different model neurons have been combined with synaptic connections similar to those

found experimentally, and the excitability has been increased, again without NMDA receptor activation. The different neurons fire in the same phase relations as during real swimming, and if the background excitability is modified, it will cover a range from about 1.0 to 10 Hz, which is the upper part of the normal range.

When we add NMDA receptors to the network neurons, we then cover a lower burst range from 0.25 to 1.5 Hz, which is the lower part of the normal swim range. Moreover, using NMDA to drive the network, one can see in the graphs of Figure 5 that the burst range reaches a plateau both in the simulation and in the "real" case. The explanation for this plateau most likely lies in the properties of the NMDA channels and their interaction with the remainder of the ion channels in any given cell. Figure 6, A and B, compares conventional kainate/AMPA excitatory postsynaptic potentials (EPSPs) with those of pure NMDA EPSP. The latter is very small at resting membrane potential but is increased on depolarization due to their voltage dependence. These properties in themselves are obviously important for temporal and spatial summation (Ö. Ekeberg et al., in prep.).

The NMDA channels also play another role in that they give rise to plateau or pacemaker-like properties in the individual cells. This is due to an interaction between voltage-dependent NMDA channels that open "explosively" at a threshold value to reach a plateau at a 10–15 mV more depolarized level initially due to the counteraction of voltage-dependent K^+ channels. Since Ca^+ ions will flow in through the open NMDA channels, Ca^{++} will accumulate and open up calcium-dependent K^+ channels, which will gradually pull the membrane potential down to a level at which the

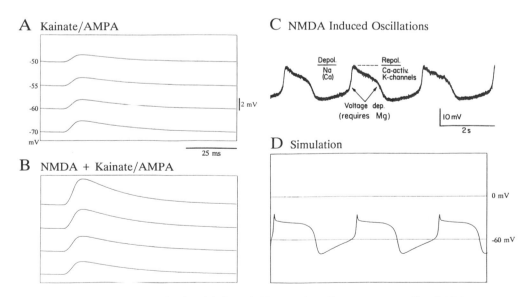

Figure 6. (A,B) Comparison between simulated kainate/AMPA and NMDA receptor-mediated EPSPs. The conventional kainate/AMPA EPSP decreases in size with membrane depolarization (A), whereas the mixed EPSP increases in size (B) due to the voltage dependence of the NMDA channels. (C) Intrinsic, pacemaker-like oscillatory membrane properties induced by NMDA receptor activation. (D) Corresponding simulation of NMDA-induced membrane potential oscillations.

NMDA channels will start to close again (Fig. 6C) (Sigvardt et al. 1985; Grillner and Wallén 1985; Wallén and Grillner 1985, 1987). The model neurons simulate the pacemaker potential and indeed all of their properties (Fig. 6D) (L. Brodin et al., in prep.). The depolarizing plateau can be shortened by hyperpolarizing inputs (inhibitory postsynaptic potentials, IPSPs) and lengthened by depolarizing pulses (EPSPs). The last part of the plateau is labile and readily affected by pulses, whereas the first part is stable and more difficult to influence (Wallén and Grillner 1985). This finding is of obvious relevance as an explanation for the plateau in the graphs of burst rate against background excitation (Fig. 5) observed with NMDA-swimming, and the fact that the burst rate does not exceed 1.5–2.5 Hz in either the NMDA model network or in the biological network.

Intrinsic mechanisms of the network analyzed by simulation. Obviously, the burst termination is of critical importance for the network operation. Let us consider different factors that contribute in this respect. The critical factor for the alternating activity is to terminate the CC-interneuron burst. One obvious factor to consider is spike frequency adaptation. Due to summation of after-hyperpolarization, the first two three-spike intervals will become shorter than the following (see, e.g., Gustafsson 1974), which may be followed by a compensatory pause of sufficient length to disinhibit the contralateral side. This factor can be tested in isolation by decreasing the amplitude of the after-hyperpolarization. With less after-hyperpolarization, everything else being equal, there would be less spike frequency adaption; therefore, if this factor were important, it would lead to longer and more intense bursts and thus a lower frequency. This is indeed what the simulations show and also what is observed experimentally when the after-hyperpolarization is experimentally reduced. The latter can be selectively decreased by administration of 5-HT, and then a slowing of the locomotor burst activity results (Harris-Warrick and Cohen 1985). 5-HT exerts a specific inhibitory effect on the Ca^{++}-dependent K^+ channels, which give rise to the after-hyperpolarization (Wallén et al. 1989).

In addition to the direct effects of intrinsic CC-interneuron spike frequency adaptation, a similar adaptation will also occur in the excitatory interneurons (EINs), leading to a removal of excitation from the CC interneurons. These factors combine to decrease (stop) the CC-interneuron activity.

The connectivity itself provides another mechanism. The lateral interneuron (Fig. 4) has a high threshold, and it fires relatively late during the depolarization (Buchanan and Cohen 1982; Buchanan 1986). When activated, it will inhibit the CC interneuron and directly contribute to the termination of CC-interneuron activity. The large lateral interneurons are present mainly in the rostral part of the spinal cord (Rovainen 1974), but smaller counterparts have also been described (Buchanan and Grillner 1988 and unpubl.).

A third factor is the NMDA plateaus, which act to terminate the bursts during slow regular swimming. The termination of the depolarizing plateau is due to interaction between different channels as discussed above. Although the burst termination is crucial in itself, the contralateral burst initiation must also be considered. The initial critical factor is the disinhibition (from CC interneurons), and then the background excitability that will get the neurons above threshold, which will also open up NMDA channels. The background excitation is further amplified by the intrinsic network excitation from excitatory interneurons. The sensory control will further contribute (see below).

Sensory Fibers Contribute to Network Control

Although the central circuitry can operate in isolation (Figs. 1–5), sensory signals are normally an active part of the control system lamprey, as well as in other vertebrates investigated. Figure 7 shows that even in the notochord–spinal cord preparation, the fictive locomotor activity can be entrained by superimposing movements, simulating in a crude way the laterally directed swimming movements. It is clear that the movements entrain the central activity at frequencies both below and above the rest rate (Grillner et al. 1981a; Grillner and Wallén 1982). This entrainment is due to intraspinal stretch receptor neurons (edge cells) sensing the lateral movements (Grillner et al. 1984). The stretch receptor neurons are of two types (see Fig. 5): those with ipsilateral axons that excite (glutamate) ipsilateral motoneurons and premotoneurons and those with contralateral axons that inhibit (glycine) contralateral neurons (Viana di Prisco et al. 1990). This connectivity can account for the entrainment. Consider a situation when motoneurons on the left side are contracting; then the stretch receptors on the right side will become active. They will then cause an increase of the excitability of the network interneurons on the same side while inhibiting the neurons on the active side. This sensory activity will then clearly contribute to terminate burst activity on the side that is active and to facilitate the ipsilateral burst initiation to short contraction.

Figure 7 shows simulations of the entrainment. Two stretch receptor model neurons are connected to the network (Fig. 7). The middle panel shows rest activity (without "movement"). In the left panel, movement is simulated by injecting sinusoidal current in the two stretch receptor model neurons, which makes them discharge action potentials. The left and right model stretch receptor neurons are 180° out of phase with each other, which leads to a very efficient entrainment at a frequency both above and below the resting burst activity. The established connectivity can thus account for the sensory control. The imposed sinusoidals serve as an oscillator, which is entraining the network oscillation. The phase relations between the two are similar under simulated and biological conditions.

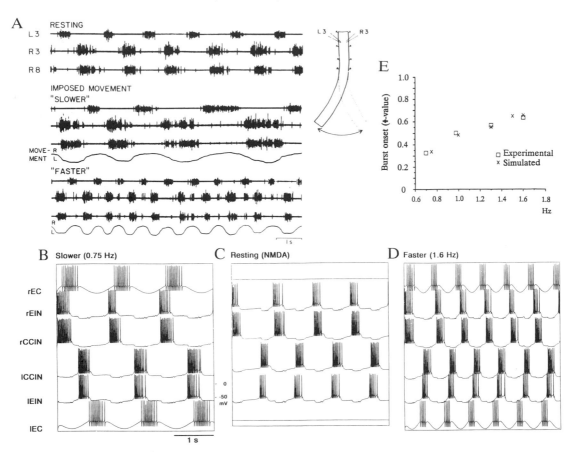

Figure 7. Sensory control of the segmental locomotor network. (*A*) Experimental entrainment of the fictive locomotor rhythm recorded from ventral roots in the in vitro spinal cord preparation (Andersson et al. 1981). Imposed lateral movements, mimicking swimming movements, entrained the rhythm to both slower and faster burst rates. (*B–D*) Simulation of sensory entrainment of the segmental network by edge cells (cf. diagram in Fig. 4). *C* shows the resting rhythm induced by a tonic activation of NMDA receptors on the network neurons. *B* shows the effect of applying a sinusoidal current in the edge cells (EC), which corresponds to application of a lateral bending movement that is slower than the locomotor frequency at rest. A 1:1 entrainment occurs. In *D*, a movement was simulated that had a rate higher than the rest rate, resulting in a 1:1 entrainment to a higher rate. *E* shows plotted values for the phase shift between a fixed point in the movement cycle (applied movement) during 1:1 entrainment of locomotor activity at different movement frequencies. The resting locomotor rate was 1 Hz. The simulated data (crosses) gave a phase curve that was very similar to the experimentally obtained results (squares).

Simulation of the Supraspinal Initiation of Locomotion

The normal initiation of locomotion comes from the reticulospinal neurons, which has been simulated as shown in Figure 8. The descending spinoreticular control is simulated as determined experimentally, whereas the phasic modulation is modeled with alternating excitation and inhibition originating directly from excitatory and CC interneurons, rather than with the additional relay neurons as described above. When the excitability of the reticulospinal neurons was step-increased, the alternating motor pattern was initiated with the appropriate coordination, and thus the connectivity can account as well for the normal initiation.

These findings suggest that the simulations have captured essential features of the normal network and indeed that the connectivity and all properties identified on the segmental level can account for the segmental locomotor behavior. The identified network can

thus provide the backbone of the locomotion, but a number of features have to be added.

Modulation of the Spinal Locomotor Circuitry

Presynaptic modulation via GABAergic mechanisms. In addition to the circuitry discussed above, there is a presynaptic modulation of the synaptic transmission from both excitatory and inhibitory interneurons in the network (Alford et al. 1990; Alford and Grillner 1990). In fact, it appears that segmental GABA interneurons (Brodin et al. 1990a; Christenson et al. 1990b) cause a phasic presynaptic inhibition during each locomotor burst and act via both $GABA_A$ and $GABA_B$ receptors located in the axonal membrane. This modulation is most likely contributing to an efficient intersegmental coordination.

5-HT modulation of the network. Endogenous 5-HT release or bath application of 5-HT gives rise to a

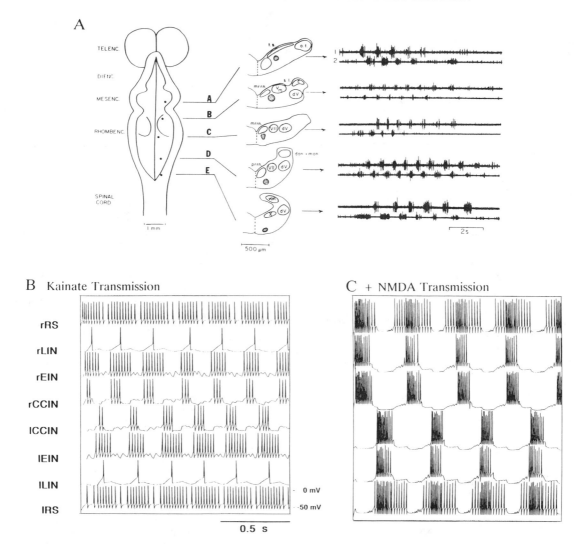

Figure 8. Descending control of the segmental locomotor network. (*A*) Experimental initiation of fictive locomotion by brain stem microstimulation (1-msec pulses at 20 Hz at indicated positions). (Modified from McClellan and Grillner 1984.) (*B,C*) Simulation of the descending control of the network (cf. diagram in Fig. 4). A tonic-depolarizing current was applied to each of the reticulospinal (RS) cells. *B* shows a sequence of rapid locomotor activity in a case where the reticulospinal neurons (as well as all spinal neurons) utilize "conventional" kainate/AMPA receptor-mediated synapses. In *C*, the reticulospinal synapses also involved voltage-sensitive NMDA-mediated components, which resulted in a slow burst pattern. Note the strong phasic modulation of the reticulospinal cells, which results from the ascending excitatory and inhibitory feedback.

depression of the after-hyperpolarization of all cells in the network (Ca^{++}-dependent K channels) (Wallén et al. 1989). This leads to more intense but long-lasting locomotor bursts (Harris-Warrick and Cohen 1985). The 5-HT innervation originates from an intraspinal 5-HT system and also from two descending reticulospinal 5-HT systems (Harris-Warrick et al. 1985; Van Dongen et al. 1985; Brodin et al. 1986). Although the 5-HT innervation is very dense, there appears to be no synaptic specialization formed (Christenson et al. 1990a). The 5-HT systems are fairly well described in terms of target cells and effects, but little is known about their normal pattern of activation or their physiological role.

Intersegmental Coordination

As the lamprey or most fish swim forward (Grillner 1974; Grillner and Kashin 1976; Williams et al. 1989), a mechanical wave is propagated backward on the body, which is due to a constant phase lag between each consecutive segment. The phase lag between adjacent segments is approximately 1% of the cycle duration, whether the latter is 1 second or 0.1 second, which is why it is referred to as a constant phase lag.

The exact mechanisms have not yet been revealed, but it is likely that excitability differences between the leading segments can account for the phase coupling (Grillner 1974; Matsushima and Grillner 1990; Grillner et al. 1991). Simulation of the coupling based on coupled oscillator theory has indicated ways to achieve a phase coupling (Williams et al. 1990).

CONCLUDING REMARKS

In this paper, we have dealt with the neuronal machinery, which can account for propulsion during locomotion in one lower vertebrate. It is shown that the available experimental data are sufficient to account for supraspinal inhibition, sensory modulation, and segmental burst generation. Thus, the available information provides at least the backbone of the full neural machinery. Obviously, more will be learned to form a complete picture. To this burst-generating machinery, we need to integrate the intersegmental coordination and subsequently the control mechanism for body orientation (vestibular; cf. Orlovsky et al. 1990) and steering (tectum).

This simple vertebrate model has thus provided insight into the cellular bases of the basic pattern of behavior in cyclostomes, and new information is also available for the alternating spike pattern of the frog embryo (Roberts et al. 1986; Roberts and Tunstall 1990). One challenge is now to explore which of the different neuronal mechanisms used in these comparatively simple vertebrates have been retained in the transition to locomotion by means of limbs in amphibians and higher vertebrates. In these studies, the new in vitro preparations of mice and neonatal rats will probably become important.

REFERENCES

Alford, S. and S. Grillner. 1990. The involvement of GABA$_B$ receptors and coupled G proteins in spinal GABAergic presynaptic inhibition. *J. Physiol.* (in press).

Alford, S., J. Christenson, and S. Grillner. 1990. Presynaptic GABA$_A$ and GABA$_B$ receptor-mediated phasic modulation in axons of spinal interneurones. *Eur. J. Neurosci.* (in press).

Andersson, O., H. Forssberg, S. Grillner, and P. Wallén. 1981. Peripheral feedback mechanisms acting on the central pattern generators for locomotion in fish and cat. *Can. J. Physiol. Pharmacol.* **59**: 713.

Armstrong, D.M. 1988. The supraspinal control of mammalian locomotion. *J. Physiol.* **405**: 1.

Beloozerova, I.N. and M.G. Sirota. 1986. Activity of neurons of the motor-sensory cortex of the cat during natural locomotion while stepping over obstacles. *Neirofiziologiya* **18**: 546.

Brodin, L. 1989. "Transmitters, receptors and ionic mechanisms in the control of spinal motor circuits. Physiological and morphological studies of the lamprey CNS with special reference to excitatory amino acid transmission." pH.D. thesis, Karolinska Institutet, Stockholm.

Brodin, L. and S. Grillner. 1990. The lamprey CNS in vitro, an experimentally amenable model for synaptic transmission and integrative functions. In *Preparations of vertebrate central nervous systems in vitro* (ed. H. Jahnsen), p. 103. Wiley, New York.

Brodin, L., S. Grillner, and C.M. Rovainen. 1985. N-methyl-D-aspartate (NMDA), kainate and quisqualate receptors and the generation of fictive locomotion in the lamprey spinal cord. *Brain Res.* **325**: 302.

Brodin, L., J.T. Buchanan, T. Hökfelt, S. Grillner, and A.A.J. Verhofstad. 1986. A spinal projection of 5-hydroxytryptamine neurons in the lamprey brainstem. *Neurosci. Lett.* **67**: 53.

Brodin, L., N. Dale, J. Christenson, J. Storm-Mathisen, T. Hökfelt, and S. Grillner. 1990. Three types of GABA-immunoreactive cells in the lamprey spinal cord. *Brain Res.* **508**: 172.

Brodin, L., A. Rawitch, T. Taylor, Y. Ohta, H. Ring, T. Hökfelt, S. Grillner, and L. Terenius. 1989. Multiple forms of pancreatic polypeptide-related compounds in the lamprey CNS: Partial characterization and immunohistochemical localization in the brain stem and spinal cord. *J. Neurosci.* **9**: 3428.

Brodin, L., J.T. Buchanan, T. Hökfelt, S. Grillner, J.F. Rehfeld, P. Frey, A.A.J. Verhofstad, G. Dockray, and J.H. Walsh. 1988. Immunohistochemical studies of cholecystokinin (CCK)-like peptides and their relation to CGRP, 5-HT and Bombesin immunoreactivities in the brainstem and spinal cord of lampreys. *J. Comp. Neurol.* **271**: 1.

Buchanan, J.T. 1982. Identification of interneurons with contralateral caudal axons in the lamprey spinal cord: Synaptic interactions and morphology. *J. Neurophysiol.* **47**: 961.

———. 1986. Premotor interneurons in the lamprey spinal cord: Morphology, synaptic interactions and activities during fictive swimming. In *Neurobiology of vertebrate locomotion* (ed. S. Grillner et al.), p. 321. Macmillan, London.

Buchanan, J.T. and A. Cohen. 1982. Activities of identified interneurons, motoneurons and muscle fibers during fictive swimming in the lamprey and the effects of reticulospinal and dorsal cell stimulation. *J. Neurophysiol.* **47**: 948.

Buchanan, J.T. and S. Grillner. 1987. Newly identified "glutamate interneurons" and their role in locomotion in the lamprey spinal cord. *Science* **236**: 312.

———. 1988. A new class of small inhibitory interneurons in the lamprey spinal cord. *Brain Res.* **438**: 404.

Christenson, J., S. Cullheim, and S. Grillner. 1990a. 5-Hydroxytryptamine immunoreactive varicosities in the lamprey spinal cord have no synaptic specializations—An ultrastructural study. *Brain Res.* **512**: 201.

Christenson, J., F. Bongianni, S. Grillner, and T. Hökfelt. 1990b. GABAergic input to spinal interneurons and primary sensory neurons in the spinal cord as shown by Lucifer Yellow and GABA immunohistochemistry. *Brain Res.* (in press).

Cohen, A.H. and P. Wallén. 1980. The neuron correlate of locomotion in fish. "Fictive swimming" induced in an in vitro preparation of the lamprey spinal cord. *Exp. Brain Res.* **41**: 11.

Dale, N. and S. Grillner. 1986. Dual-component synaptic potentials in the lamprey mediated by excitatory amino acid receptors. *J. Neurosci.* **6**: 2653.

Dubuc, R. and S. Grillner. 1989. The role of spinal cord inputs in modulating the activity of reticulospinal neurons during fictive locomotion in the lamprey. *Brain Res.* **483**: 196.

Garcia-Rill, E. and R.D. Skinner. 1986. The basal ganglia and the mesencephalic locomotor region. In *Neurobiology of vertebrate locomotion* (ed. S. Grillner et al.), p. 77. Macmillan, London.

Georgopoulos, A.P. and S. Grillner. 1989. Visuomotor coordination in reaching and locomotion. *Science* **245**: 1209.

Grillner, S. 1974. On the generation of locomotion in the spinal dogfish. *Exp. Brain Res.* **20**: 459.

———. 1985. Neurobiological bases of rhythmic motor acts in vertebrates. *Science* **228**: 143.

———. 1990. Neurobiology of vertebrate motor behavior—From flexion reflexes and locomotion to manipulative movements. In *Signal and sense: Local and global order in perceptual maps* (ed. S. Hassler), p. 187. Wiley-Liss, New York.

Grillner, S. and S. Kashin. 1976. On the generation and

performance of swimming in fish. In *Neural control of locomotion* (ed. R. Herman et al.), p. 181. Plenum Press, New York.

Grillner, S. and G. Orlovski. 1990. Locomotion, neural networks. In *Encyclopedia of human biology.* Academic Press, New York. (In press.)

Grillner, S. and P. Wallén. 1982. The peripheral control mechanisms acting on the central pattern generators for swimming in the dogfish. *J. Exp. Biol.* **98:** 1.

———. 1985. The ionic mechanisms underlying NMDA receptor induced, TTX-resistant membrane potential oscillations in lamprey neurones active during locomotion. *Neurosci. Lett.* **60:** 289.

Grillner, S., J.T. Buchanan, and A. Lansner. 1988. Simulation of the segmental burst generating network for locomotion in lamprey. *Neurosci. Lett.* **89:** 31.

Grillner, S., A. McClellan, and C. Perret. 1981a. Entrainment of the spinal pattern generators for swimming by mechanosensitive elements in the lamprey spinal cord *in vitro.* *Brain Res.* **217:** 380.

Grillner, S., T.L. Williams, and P.Å. Lagerbäck. 1984. The edge cell, a possible intraspinal mechanoreceptor. *Science* **223:** 500.

Grillner, S., P. Wallén, L. Brodin, and A. Lansner. 1991. Neuronal network generating locomotor behavior in lamprey—Circuitry, transmitters, membrane properties and simulation. *Annu. Rev. Neurosci.* **14:** 169.

Grillner, S., A. McClellan, A. Sigvardt, P. Wallén, and M. Wilén. 1981b. Activation of NMDA receptors elicits "fictive locomotion" in lamprey spinal cord in vitro. *Acta Physiol. Scand.* **113:** 549.

Gustafsson, B. 1974. After hyperpolarization and the control of repetitive firing in spinal neurones of the cat. *Acta Physiol. Scand.* **416.**

Harris-Warrick, R.M. and A.H. Cohen. 1985. Serotonin modulates the central pattern generator for locomotion in the isolated lamprey spinal cord. *J. Exp. Biol.* **116:** 27.

Harris-Warrick, R.M., J.C. McPhee, and J.A. Filler. 1985. Distribution of serotonergic neurons and processes in the lamprey spinal cord. *Neuroscience* **14:** 1127.

Hodgkin, A.L. and A.F. Huxley. 1952. A quantitative description of membrane current and its application to conduction and excitation in nerve. *J. Physiol.* **117:** 500.

Jordan, L. 1986. Initiation of locomotion from the mammalian brainstem. In *Neurobiology of vertebrate locomotion* (ed. S. Grillner et al.), p. 21. Macmillan, London.

Kasicki, S., S. Grillner, Y. Ohta, R. Dubuc, and L. Brodin. 1988. Phasic modulation of reticulospinal neurones during fictive locomotion and other types of motor activity in lamprey. *Brian Res.* **484:** 203.

Matsushima, T. and S. Grillner. 1990 Intersegmental co-ordination of undulatory movements—A "trailing oscillator" hypothesis. *NeuroReport* **1:** 97.

McClellan, A.D. and S. Grillner. 1984. Activation of "fictive swimming" by electric microstimulation of brainstem locomotor regions in an in vitro preparation of the lamprey central nervous system. *Brain Res.* **300:** 357.

Ohta, Y. and S. Grillner. 1989. Monosynaptic excitatory amino acid transmission from the posterior rhombencephalic reticular nucleus to spinal neurons involved in the control of locomotion in lamprey. *J. Neurophysiol.* **62:** 1079.

Orlovsky, G.N. and M.L. Shik. 1976. A neurophysiological analysis of the cat locomotor system. *Int. Rev. Physiol. Neurophysiol.* **10:** 281.

Roberts, A. and M.J. Tunstall. 1990. Mutual re-excitation with post-inhibitory rebound: A simulation study on the mechanisms for locomotor rhythm generation in the spinal cord of *Xenopus* embryos. *Eur. J. Neurosci.* **2:** 11.

Roberts, A., S.R. Soffe, and N. Dale. 1986. Spinal interneurones and swimming in frog embryos. In *Neurobiology of vertebrate locomotion* (ed. S. Grillner et al.), p. 279. Macmillan, London.

Rovainen, C.M. 1972. Synaptic interactions of identified nerve cells in the spinal cord of the sea lamprey. *J. Comp. Neurol.* **154:** 189.

———. 1979. Neurobiology of lampreys. *Physiol. Rev.* **59:** 1007.

———. 1982. Neurophysiology. In *Biology of lampreys* (ed. M.W. Hardisty et al.), p. 1. Academic Press, London.

Russell, D.F. and P. Wallén. 1983. On the control of myotomal motoneurones during "fictive swimming" in the lamprey spinal cord in vitro. *Acta Physiol. Scand.* **117:** 161.

Sigvardt, K.A., S. Grillner, P. Wallén, and P.A.M. Van Dongen. 1985. Activation of NMDA receptors elicits fictive locomotion and bistable membrane properties in the lamprey spinal cord. *Brain Res.* **336:** 390.

Van Dongen, P.A.M., T. Hökfelt, S. Grillner, and A.A.J. Verhofstad, H.W.M. Steinbusch, A.C. Cuello, and A.L. Terenius. 1985. Immunohistochemical demonstration of some putative neurotransmitters in the lamprey spinal cord and spinal ganglia: 5-hydroxytryptamine-, tachykinin-, and neuropeptide Y-immunoreactive neurons and fibers. *J. Comp. Neurol.* **234:** 501.

Viana di Prisco, G., P. Wallén, and S. Grillner. 1990. Synaptic effects of intraspinal stretch receptor neurons mediating movement-related feedback during locomotion. *Brain Res.* (in press).

Waitzman, D.M., T.P. Ma, L.M. Optican, and R.H. Wurtz. 1988. Superior colliculus neurons provide the saccadic motor error signal. *Exp. Brain Res.* **72:** 649.

Wallén, P. and S. Grillner. 1985. The effects of current passage on *N*-methyl-D-aspartate induced, tetrodotoxin-resistant membrane potential oscillations in lamprey neurons active during locomotion. *Neurosci. Lett.* **56:** 87.

———. 1987. *N*-methyl-D-aspartate receptor induced, inherent oscillatory activity in neurons active during fictive locomotion in the lamprey. *J. Neurosci.* **7:** 2745.

Wallén, P. and T.L. Williams. 1984. Fictive locomotion in the lamprey spinal cord in vitro compared with swimming in the intact and spinal animal. *J. Physiol.* **347:** 225.

Wallén, P., J.T. Buchanan, S. Grillner, R.H. Hill, J. Christenson, and T. Hökfelt. 1989. Effects of 5-hydroxytryptamine on the after-hyperpolarization, spike frequency regulation, and oscillatory membrane properties in lamprey spinal cord neurons. *J. Neurophysiol.* **61:** 759.

Williams, T.L., K.A. Sigvardt, N. Kopell, G.B. Ermentrout, and M.P. Remler. 1990. Forcing of coupled non-linear oscillators: Studies of intersegmental coordination in the lamprey locomotor central pattern generator. *J. Neurophysiol.* (in press).

Williams, T.L., S. Grillner, V.V. Smoljaninov, P. Wallén, S. Kashin, and S. Rossignol. 1989. Locomotion in lamprey and trout: The relative timing of activation and movement. *J. Exp. Biol.* **143:** 559.

Understanding Sensorimotor Feedback
through Optimal Control

G.E. LOEB,* W.S. LEVINE,† AND J. HE‡
*Bio-Medical Engineering Unit and Department of Physiology, Queen's University, Kingston, Ontario K7L 3N6,
Canada; †Department of Electrical Engineering, University of Maryland, College Park, Maryland 20734

The general problem of "control" may be divided into two main categories, often designated open-loop and closed-loop (see Fig. 1). We adopt here the convention of using "controller" to designate a device that formulates a set of commands intended to change the state of a system, which commands are executed open-loop, i.e., without modification during the task. (We emphasize that this is a shorthand terminology, not to be confused with the standard usage in control theory denoting both open- and closed-loop components.) We use the term "regulator" to designate a device that attempts to stabilize the state of a system, generating only closed-loop commands, i.e., responses to deviations from the state detected by sensors in the system (Bryson and Ho 1975). Obviously, most complex systems require a mixture of the two types of control.

In sensorimotor neurophysiology, it is common to depict these kinds of controls schematically as if they were separate, even though the anatomical and physiological features of the structures in which they reside suggest a close interrelatedness. For example, the control of locomotion in quadrupeds has been seen as divided between a spinal central pattern generator (CPG), which generates an open-loop program of muscle activation, and various reflexes, also largely spinal, which adjust the activation in response to internal errors and external perturbations. Liddell and Sherrington (1925) first proposed the concept of the motoneuron as the "final common path" whereby the various sources of control signals would be summed to result in the net command to a motor unit. There is now little doubt that the motoneuron, like most central neurons, serves to integrate many disparate sources of input into a single-dimensional output. However, the later notion that these motoneuronal inputs are distinguishable into open-loop and closed-loop types deserves reexamination.

Ironically, Sherrington (1910) himself felt that locomotion was produced primarily through reflex pathways, i.e., from the sequential combination of sensory signals arising from the musculoskeletal mechanics of the limb. The need for an open-loop controller of locomotion was firmly established later by the surprisingly natural temporal patterns of motoneuronal output reported during fictive locomotion in paralyzed, de-

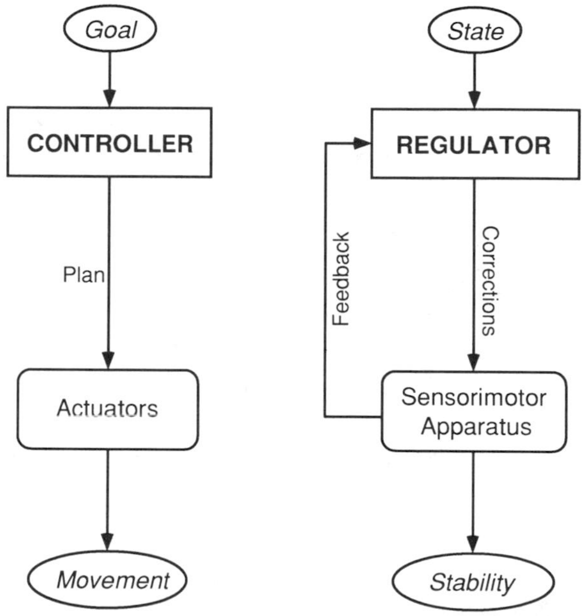

Figure 1. Two basic forms of control: open-loop (*left*) and closed-loop (*right*).

cerebrate cats (Stein 1978; Perret 1983). The identities of the neurons comprising this CPG remain unknown, but they appear to be at least partially coextensive with interneurons receiving primary afferent input. Although the CPG can function without modulated sensory input, such input can modify and reset its output to the motoneurons (Lennard 1985; Conway et al. 1987). Furthermore, the CPG can deeply modulate the gain of most, if not all, of the reflex pathways (see, e.g., Feldman and Orlovsky 1975). Given such relationships, can the theoretically useful concepts of open- and closed-loop control be applied at all to sensorimotor connectivity?

This question assumes even greater significance when applied to control of voluntary behaviors whose basic commands originate in "higher" centers such as motor cortex. As shown in the left panel of Figure 2, the usual schematic assumes that these descending commands (thick arrows) are integrated with the segmental reflexes (dashed arrows) at the final common pathways, the motoneuronal pools controlling each muscle. There are two things wrong with this simple view: (1) The proprioceptive signals from each muscle project largely to

---

‡Present address: Artificial Intelligence Laboratory, Massachusetts Institute of Technology, Cambridge, Massachusetts 02139.

SPINAL INTEGRATION

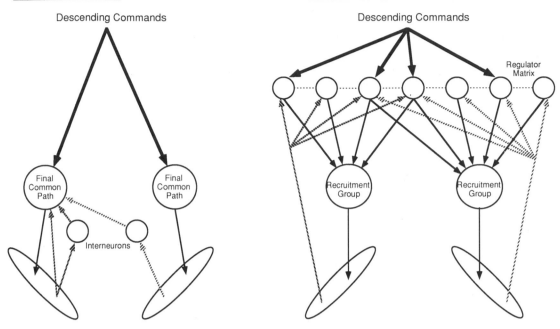

Figure 2. Historical view of spinal cord function (*left*) contrasted with a more contemporary view of the known circuitry (*right*). Dashed lines indicate proprioceptive feedback from muscles (*ovals*).

interneurons in which the signals from many different modalities and loci are combined and then routed to widely separated motor nuclei subserving the entire limb. (2) Most of the descending pathways terminate on these and other interneurons rather than directly onto motoneurons. For example, even in the primate there appears to be no direct corticospinal influence on any motoneurons except those of the digital muscles of the hand (Fetz and Cheney 1980).

The right panel of Figure 2 shows a more realistic schematic, in which both the proprioceptive feedback and the descending commands converge on a matrix of interneurons. We know that among these interneurons, there are at least some distinct subtypes with fairly predictable patterns of input (e.g., Renshaw cells, propriospinal cells, Ib-inhibitory interneurons, reciprocal inhibitory interneurons), but even these permit complex admixtures of widely distributed input signals (for review, see McCrea 1986). We also know of monosynaptic connections that convey signals directly from primary afferents to motoneurons without intercalated interneurons (spindle afferents to homonymous motoneurons), but even this form of connectivity appears to be deeply modulated by presynaptic inhibition from sources as diverse as cutaneous afferents (Jankowska et al. 1981) and the CPG itself (Duenas and Rudomin 1988).

For the above reasons, it seems useful for researchers to consider the possible matrix of connections between sensors and actuators as a blank slate, to be explored

without preconceived notions based on either known reflex pathways or analogies to simple servocontrol of individual torque motors. From the perspective of creating a complex and well-controlled movement despite being limited to such indirect control of motoneurons (Fig. 3), the problem is to find the set of interneurons that, when appropriately enabled and disabled, results in a controller-regulator combination that produces the desired motor output. Note that the behavior of such a hierarchical system is not described completely by the observable trajectory of motion of the limb. Rather, it necessarily includes a complex mechanical impedance to all possible perturbations of position, velocity, and acceleration that might be encountered (as defined by Hogan 1985).

We here describe the use of an engineering technique called "optimal control," which can be combined with models of musculoskeletal systems to generate matrices of such sensorimotor connectivity. For a given system in a given behavioral state, this matrix provides the best set of responses to the set of all possible small perturbations. Best is judged according to performance criteria that assign a weight to factors related to cost (expended effort) and benefit (various measures of stability). By noting the changes in these matrices and their simulated output that are produced by different assumptions about the model components, the external constraints and the performance criteria, one can gain considerable insight into the roles and relative importance of the various components and connections that have been

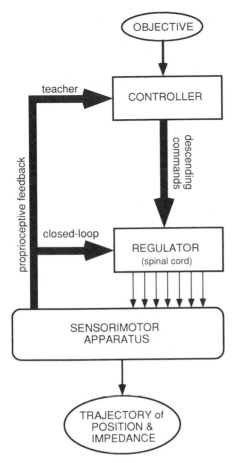

Figure 3. Proposed hierarchical relationship between open-loop controller and closed-loop regulator aspects of motor control.

described by anatomists and physiologists. From this new perspective, we have speculated rather broadly on the computational problems that must be solved by those higher centers that aspire to control such a spinal cord.

METHODS

A description of our model of the musculoskeletal system and techniques for kinesiological data collection and analysis have been published together with a review of other approaches to such modeling (Loeb et al. 1989). Mathematical implementations of models for sensory and motor components and for our application of linear quadratic (LQ) regulator design are described elsewhere (He et al. 1991). A review of technical considerations in the selection of model relationships and our approach to their empirical validation may be found in Loeb et al. (1990). Detailed methods for electrophysiological and neurokinesiological experiments in intact, naturally behaving cats have been published previously (Loeb et al. 1977; Loeb and Gans 1986; Hoffer et al. 1987; Pratt et al. 1990).

Briefly, the application of LQ control requires three types of input:

1. A complete mathematical model of the sensorimotor apparatus, including its mechanical interactions, the response of the actuators (functional groups of motor units) to command and feedback signals, and the sensitivity of sensors for all state variables (or estimators for those state variables built up from available sensors).

2. A target trajectory for the state variables, which we have taken to be their typical values during unperturbed locomotion in intact (albeit chronically instrumented) animals. This includes the trajectories of limb segments and the relative recruitment of individual muscles.

3. Performance criteria, which are the variously weighted ratios of two matrices, a cost matrix R derived from the degree of activation of the muscles, and a benefit matrix Q derived from the deviation of all other state variables from their nominal target trajectory. We have simulated the effects of other, simpler control schemes (e.g., muscle stiffness regulation; Houk 1979) by setting the appropriate terms in the Q matrix to zero.

The LQ method (Stein and Athans 1987) involves two assumptions: (1) that for small enough perturbations, the system is locally linear, and (2) that the appropriate measure of error to be minimized is quadratic, i.e., the sum of the squares of the deviations from the nominal trajectory in all of the state variables. The combination of a linear plant plus quadratic criterion implies linear state feedback control (Athans and Falb 1969); see Discussion.

For the purposes of LQ design, we have simplified the skeletal system into four segments (foot, shank, thigh, and pelvis) linked by three pin joints (ankle, knee, and hip) that permit movement only in the parasagittal plane. There are approximately 45 separately recruitable muscles with significant actions in this plane; these have been collected into 10 groups that have fundamentally different topology with respect to the degrees of freedom of the skeleton (see Fig. 4).

The K matrix contains the predicted gains between all sensors and all actuators at a given phase of the target trajectory and for a given set of performance criteria. In the models described here, each of the three joints had a sensor for joint angle (ϕ) and joint velocity ($\dot{\phi}$) and each of the ten muscle groups had a sensor for combined length and velocity (muscle spindle primary ending, designated Ia), force (Golgi tendon organ, designated Ib), and activation (derived from efference copy via Renshaw cells, designated RC). Thus, the complete K matrix consisted of 36 rows by 10 columns. Individual gains are presented here as signed logarithmic values ranging from ±0.001 (absolute values smaller than this were eliminated) to ±100 (see bar graph in Fig. 4).

The physiological relevance of a particular K matrix was assessed by observing the time course of the response of a simulated hindlimb under the control of this matrix when subjected to various small perturbations in

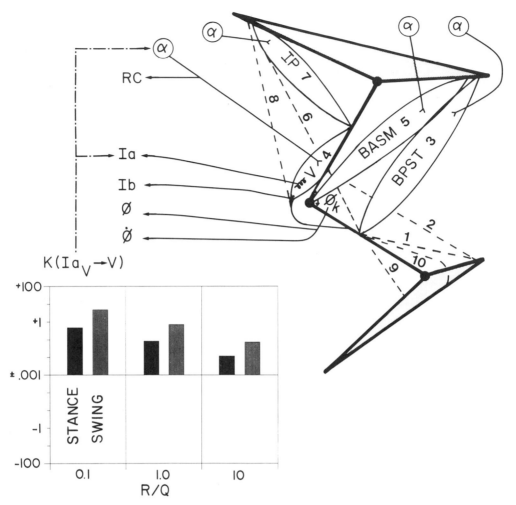

Figure 4. Basic musculoskeletal architecture of the cat hindlimb model, with ten muscle groups: six indicated by dashed lines and four (discussed in Fig. 6) by name ([V] vastus, knee extensor; [IP] iliopsoas, hip flexor; [BASM] biceps anterior and semimembranosus, hip extensor; [BPST] biceps posterior and semitendinosus, knee flexor plus hip extensor). Inset diagram shows typical gains for one element of the feedback matrix K (spindle Ia afferent from vastus muscle to homonymous α motoneurons) for six conditions: three performance criteria (R/Q) ranging from stiff (0.1) to loose (10) and two mechanical states, mid-stance (solid bars) and mid-swing (shaded bars) of walking. Other sources of feedback available include Golgi tendon organs (Ib), Renshaw feedback of motoneuron activity (RC), joint angles (ϕ) and joint velocity ($\dot\phi$).

posture. In particular, we compared the responses of the model system to those measured in intact cats following small horizontal displacements of the foot during quiet standing (Rushmer et al. 1983; Macpherson 1988).

RESULTS

As reported previously (Loeb et al. 1989; He et al. 1991), a relatively natural-appearing response to perturbations during standing could be achieved only by including in the performance criterion the feedback information from all available modalities of sensors and for intermediate R/Q ratios of about 1. Figure 5 depicts the complete K matrix for this condition. Features of note include the generally high positive feedback from homonymous Ia sensors (diagonal line of upward bars in the appropriate region of the matrix) and negative

feedback from homonymous Ib and RC sensors (diagonal lines of downward bars). Heteronymous (off-diagonal) connections are generally weaker, but in toto make up a significant part of the feedback control, particularly for the Ib and RC feedback. All of these are generally consistent with known patterns of reflex connectivity in the lumbosacral spinal cord of the cat (McCrea 1986); it is worth noting that these patterns emerged from a design process that starts out tabula rasa.

One problem with the matrix in Figure 5 is the relatively large gains for the joint angle and angular velocity sensors. There is considerable evidence suggesting that most of the sense of joint position and motion is derived from muscle spindles (Ferrell et al. 1987), probably from both primary and secondary endings. The LQ method requires a sensor or an estimator for all state variables; joint angle and angular velocity

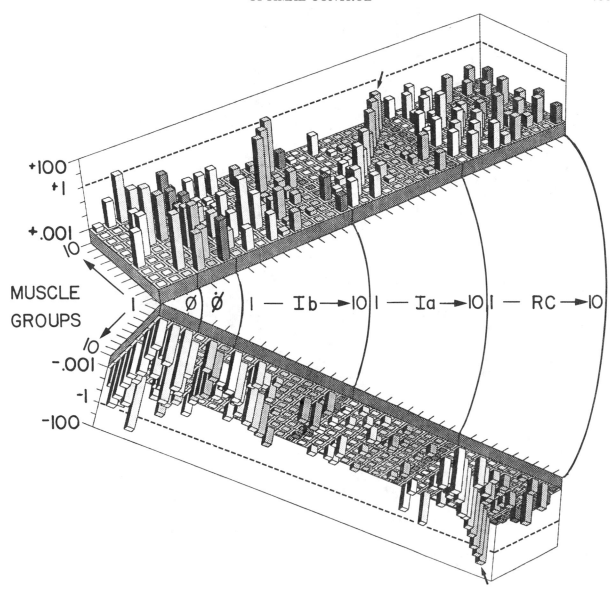

Figure 5. Full K-matrix for mid-stance, R/Q = 1, with positive gains above and negative gains below mirror-line. Afferent sources, identified along horizontal axis, connect at intersections with all muscle groups identified along vertical axis; receptor types and muscle numbers keyed to Fig. 4. Joint afferents ($\phi,\dot{\phi}$) ordered from left to right as hip, knee, and ankle. Small arrows denote tendency for homonymous feedback to be positive from spindle (Ia) afferents and negative from Renshaw cells (RC).

are typically (but not necessarily) used as state variables in equations of motion. In principle, an "optimal estimator" for the joint variables could be determined by appropriately weighting the contribution of all of the muscle spindle afferents (probably requiring a model of the spindle secondary ending as a pure muscle length sensor, which we have not implemented here). However, the prevalence of multiarticular muscles in the cat hindlimb makes this a nontrivial task. An alternative is to rewrite the state equations in coordinates of the actual sensors believed to be present, a task currently under way. Meanwhile, it would be unwise to over-interpret the predicted distribution of the Ia projections (particularly the heteronymous projections) because they probably should include large contributions now buried in the joint sensor projections.

Figure 6 reflects a first attempt to examine the effects of different behavioral tasks and mechanical constraints on regulator design, focusing on just a few selected row-and-column intersections in the full K matrix. The predicted values are shown for mid-stance and mid-swing trajectory and boundary conditions, at three different R/Q values. An R/Q criterion of 1 produces a quite physiological response to perturbations during standing, whereas values of 0.1 and 10 produce behaviors that may be characterized as "too stiff" and "too loose," respectively. Unfortunately, there are no corresponding behavioral data during swing. The swing-phase feedback shows some startling reversals of sign from stance, particularly regarding the relative effects of joint position versus joint velocity and homonymous Ib feedback. Presumably, these reflect

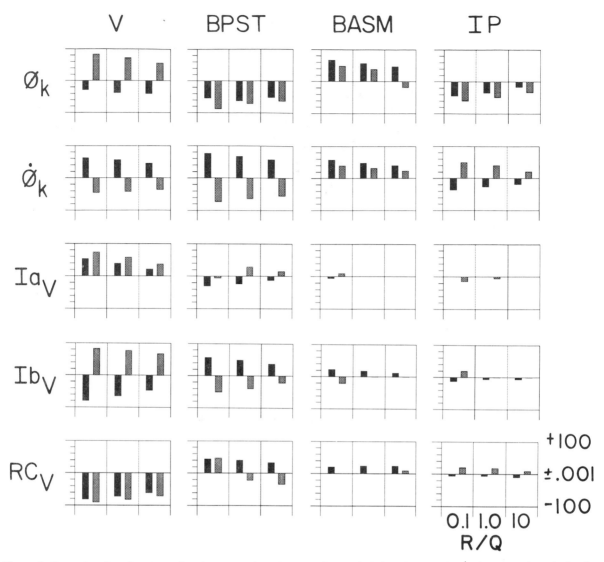

Figure 6. K-matrix values for connections between selected sensors (rows labeled ϕ_k, knee angle; $\dot{\phi}_k$, knee angular velocity; Ia$_V$, vastus spindle primary; Ib$_V$, vastus Golgi tendon organ; RC$_V$, vastus Renshaw cell) and selected muscle groups (columns at top, identified in Fig. 4). Each set of bar graphs indicates gains for different phases (stance, solid bars; swing, shaded bars) and performance criteria R/Q (see inset key in Fig. 4).

the very different mechanical conditions of stance (nearly motionless foot planted on the ground) and swing (rapidly and freely swinging foot).

DISCUSSION

Experimental Testing of Feedback Predictions

We have used comparisons between real and simulated responses to perturbations to gauge the relevance of different performance criteria (He et al. 1991). There are at least three feasible methods to obtain more specific data regarding reflex connectivity and its gating during locomotion:

1. Stimulation of primary afferents while recording electromyographic reflexes in various muscles in walking cats. This method is hampered by the fact

that the thresholds for electrical activation of Ia, Ib, and α motoneurons (projecting to RC) are generally not distinguishable. However, for particular combinations of sensors and actuators, the predicted effects may be robust enough to glean useful information from such mixed inputs.

2. Postsynaptic potential analysis of identified pathways in fictively cycling preparations (see, e.g., Pratt and Jordan 1987). Because of the extremely fine-grain approach and low yield of single-unit recording, it will again be necessary to select for robust predictions. However, information to guide the design of these tedious but critical experiments is one of the main benefits of LQ modeling.

3. Reflex plasticity following changes in musculoskeletal mechanics. Interestingly, the overall locomotor pattern of muscle recruitment appears to be relative-

ly unaffected by surgical changes such as tendon transfers (Sperry 1945; Forssberg and Svartengren 1983), but there is some evidence of changes in reflexes (Yumiya et al. 1979; McMahon and Wall 1989). Again, LQ modeling may be useful in directing the design of relatively long-term experiments that may require chronic instrumentation of young animals.

Limitations of Linear Regulators

The computational methods of linear quadratic regulator design are based on the assumption that even inherently nonlinear systems such as biological limbs can be adequately described by linear approximations when considering their behavior over small enough regions of their state space. From a biological perspective, this translates into four concerns:

1. How large does a perturbation have to be before it requires a response that lies outside the effective range of the regulator? Consider the maintenance of standing posture in bipeds. Small internal or external perturbations give rise to small swaying movements that require a carefully orchestrated distribution of small changes in muscle activation to maintain stability. However, once the center of gravity passes beyond the horizontal extent of the feet, the only viable strategy is the execution of a stepping movement to widen the base of support by relocating one foot (Nashner et al. 1979). A linear regulator would be an excellent choice for controlling sway, but it would have to be supplemented with a triggerable pattern generator to handle the stepping response. Presumably, this generator would reprogram the spinal regulator in the process of executing its response, much as we postulate that the CPG for locomotion prescribes its desired regulator.

2. How frequently during a large movement does the regulator matrix have to be updated? We have generated feedback matrices in which each gain term is not a single value but rather a continuous parameter (actually calculated in small time increments) that changes over the phases of the step cycle. However, it may be that the feedback matrix changes in only a small number of discrete phases during the step cycle. The question of whether locomotion or any other phasic behavior is controlled discretely or continuously is complex and contentious. There is evidence that such behaviors may be driven by oscillators composed of reciprocating "half-centers" (Lundberg 1980), but it is also clear that their elaboration into the detailed recruitment patterns of individual muscles (Abraham and Loeb 1985) and reflex gains (Abraham et al. 1985) introduces a more continuous form of control.

Figure 7 presents one alternative that seems consistent with recent findings about the temporal and spatial distribution of neural activity during fictive locomotion (Jordan 1990) and the effects of sensory

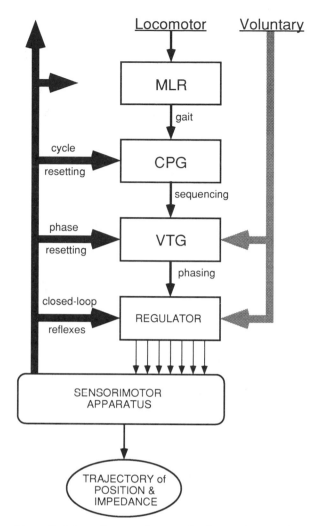

Figure 7. Schematic control system for locomotion, starting with mesencephalic locomotor region (MLR), central pattern generator (CPG), virtual trajectory generator (VTG), and interneuronal regulator matrix controlling the activation of multiple muscle groups (small arrows) in the limb.

perturbations. In the cat hindlimb, locomotion at different speeds can be produced by graded, nonphasic stimulation of the mesencephalic locomotion region (MLR; Severin et al. 1967). MLR neurons project to a group of interneurons beneath the dorsal horn in the lumbar spinal cord that seem likely to be the CPG producing the basic reciprocating drive required for alternating flexion and extension of each limb. However, much of their output does not go directly to the motoneurons in the ventral horn, but rather through interneurons in the intermediate laminae, here designated VTG for virtual trajectory generator. We speculate that these interneurons shape the bistable oscillation of the CPG into the more continuously modulated recruitment of motoneurons and gating of reflexes. Interestingly, different types of somatosensory stimuli introduced during locomotion result in distinctive effects on these putative functions (Lennard 1985). Small or brief proprioceptive inputs give rise to classic short-latency reflexes (e.g., tendon-jerk), whereas large, long-lasting proprioceptive inputs appear to interrupt the CPG, which then restarts its oscillator when the stimulus is removed. Cutaneous stimuli give rise to reflexes that may shorten or lengthen the particular locomotor phase in which they are delivered, but do not reset the basic rhythm.

The relationship between the neurons comprising the VTG and the regulator is not clear. Although they are conceptually distinct processes in control theory and they seem to give rise to different behavioral reflexes (see above), they may actually reflect different emergent properties of the same group of interneurons. This is because the interneurons are connected among themselves as well as receiving inputs from primary afferents and controllers and generating outputs to motoneurons. Such lateral connections probably generate temporal properties such as those responsible for the widespread and consistent patterns of short- and long-latency excitatory reflexes (Forssberg 1979; Abraham et al. 1985).

3. Can the regulator be used to generate point-to-point (e.g. reaching) movements? This question is really a combination of the previous two, viewed from the perspective of a control scheme in which the controller simply provides a target state and then relies on an appropriately programmed regulator. It impacts critically on the potential role of the VTG described above. In principle, the regulator could be directly programmed to achieve stability for the desired final position of the limb, and the movement would be driven solely by the magnitude of the sensory error signal. (This would be akin to equilibrium point control as proposed by Feldman [1966] and Bizzi et al. [1982], but with a distributed regulator to replace the servocontrol of individual muscles.) However, the large initial deviation would be outside the range for which linear regulator design is normally appropriate.

There are three possibilities for generating large movements: (a) The controller could generate a continuous string of nominal positions and associated regulators in small increments (akin to virtual equilibrium point trajectory; Bizzi et al. 1984). However, this would be computationally intensive and vitiates most of the advantages of hierarchical control (see below). (b) Musculotendinous systems have a number of intrinsically stabilizing mechanical properties (Zajac 1990) that may make it feasible for a single regulator to achieve a satisfactory compromise between the dynamics of movement and the statics of posture maintenance. The mathematics for including such compromise criteria in regulator design have yet to be developed; however, intuitively this approach seems likely to lead to at least some unacceptable limitations (e.g., moving quickly but compliantly). (c) The controller could take advantage of the temporal properties of the VTG to introduce phasing into the expression of abruptly shifting regulator designs. This has the attraction of making use of circuitry that seems likely to exist already in the spinal cord and which is under the continuous and local control of resetting reflexes that could handle unforeseen perturbations during the execution of the movement. Furthermore, it seems more consistent with the patterns of activity that have been recorded from motor cortex, which seems more concerned with initiating and terminating movements than with the detailed phasing of muscle recruitment during movements (Fetz et al. 1989; Kalaska et al. 1989).

4. Is linearity a likely or necessary property of neural information processing? There is no question that neural transmission in primary afferents, interneurons, and motoneurons displays a variety of highly nonlinear effects, ranging from the inevitable threshold properties (and associated temporal and spatial summation) to time-dependent effects such as potentiation, depression (Collins et al. 1984), and even bistable switching (Hounsgaard et al. 1988). However, the LQ method does not predict the details of neuronal transmission that must underlie the K matrices. LQ design in this context shares some of the features of linear regression analysis; it can be applied and evaluated in the manner that one would consider a linear curve fit to a noisy data set arising from a complex and poorly understood process. The utility of the analysis depends only on the strength of the correlation, not on any inference of causal relationships. If no reasonable correlation is discovered, then it is up to the researcher's intuition to select a candidate nonlinear regression technique. (Unfortunately, there are no practical methods currently available for nonlinear regulator design, although there is a nonquadratic method called H-infinity that tends to minimize the worst error rather than the mean square error, and hence may be biologically relevant; Francis 1987; Doyle et al. 1989.)

Advantages of Regulator-based Control

Redundancy. Because of the distributed nature of the feedback matrix, no individual sensor or feedback pathway assumes a disproportionate responsibility for responding to any particular perturbation. However, the sudden loss of certain terms could give rise to instability; furthermore, the absence of whole modalities of sensors produces clear and general degradations of performance even when the matrix is recomputed for the optimal control of the reduced system.

Speed. It is axiomatic in servocontrol that delays produce instability and require reductions in permissible gain and, hence, speed of response. It is axiomatic in biological systems that speed often means survival. Thus, one obvious advantage of the controller-regulator hierarchy proposed here is that it permits highly goal-specific reflexes to be programmed into the shortest available neural loops, the spinal-segmental reflexes.

Evidence for such goal-specific spinal reflexes comes from fingertip grasp studied by Cole and Abbs (1987) in humans (ironically, this is virtually the only muscular system in which the neuroanatomy would even permit strictly central control). When the position of the thumb was perturbed, the response was a short-latency (50–60 msec) adjustment of the position of the index finger that was attempting to meet it, even though the muscles controlling the index finger were not perturbed. After allowing for peripheral conduction time, the central delay for this rather clever reflex is 10–15 msec or less, strongly suggesting a spinal pathway. Even faster, goal-specific reflexes have been noted in orofacial muscles perturbed during vocalizations (Gracco and Abbs 1985).

It should be noted that we have not incorporated any neural delay into our models of the regulator for the cat hindlimb. This seems justified in the cat, where most of the total delay for segmental reflexes occurs in the electromechanical activation delay of the muscles (which is included in our component models for muscle dynamics). The inclusion of explicit delay terms in the regulator itself poses a severe computational burden for the regulator design process, which may need to be addressed for other systems.

Growth and functional adaptation. As the musculoskeletal system grows and adapts to different patterns of usage, there will certainly arise the need to adjust the gain of the reflexes. This suggests the need for some local growth rules to adjust the strength of synapses to and from individual interneurons and motoneurons. Although some degree of plasticity has been noted in the spinal cord (Wolpaw and Lee 1989), no general growth rules have been proposed. However, any such changes must interact in an orderly manner with the various sources of descending commands. If higher centers such as motor cortex bypassed these circuits, they would face the double problem of having to make their own detailed adjustments and identifying the changes in the segmental reflex circuits that might affect execution of the descending commands.

Phylogenetic development. It is useful to keep in mind that telencephalons with the capability of programming detailed limb movements are a relatively recent phylogenetic development, whereas spinal cords (and even invertebrate limb ganglia) have been generating and controlling very sophisticated limb movements for a very long time. The higher centers must have evolved incrementally in their needs and capabilities. Thus, it seems likely that their motor planning was based on using as much as possible of the segmental circuitry, even if this led to a proliferation of ad hoc pathways and coordinate frames that would offend a robotic systems designer.

Implications for the Organization of Descending Systems

We might still apply the analogy of a programmable industrial robot to the spinal cord. Its local computer might be expected to contain certain preset motor sequences (e.g., locomotor gaits) that are so frequently needed that it is efficient to encode them into a read-only-memory (e.g., CPG). It would also be capable of producing a virtually unlimited set of motor behaviors, but in this role, it would be largely dependent on programs down-loaded into it by a central controller (where the real "intelligence" would reside). This organization raises two difficult problems for the scientist who must "reverse engineer" such a system (as opposed to designing it from scratch): Namely, how are these programs written and how are they encoded?

If the spinal cord contains essentially all possible regulator and controller designs in its ensemble of interneurons, then the task of the movement designer is to find an acceptable set of interneurons whose net effects result in a controller and regulator combination that is appropriate to the task at hand. If all motor output must be mediated through such a combination (rather than specified directly to the actuators), then there is no way mathematically to invert the desired trajectory to calculate even one of the infinitely many patterns of descending signals that might suffice to perform the task. The method of linear quadratic regulator design that we have used here produces a prediction for the net reflex connectivity between sensors and actuators, but provides no information about how this might be distributed at the single interneuronal level. Furthermore, it is an algebraically intensive approach that is not at all suited to the computational properties of neurons.

Previous approaches to the problem of control system design have interpreted the spinal cord circuitry as a highly constrained and fixed regulator that simplifies the problem of invertability. For example, it has been assumed that the proprioceptive reflexes might "linearize" the complex dynamics of force output by individual muscles (e.g., stiffness regulation; Houk 1979) and that reciprocal neural connections and musculoskeletal mechanics between antagonist muscle pairs forming myotatic units (Lloyd 1946) might provide predictable "equilibrium points" for joint angles (Bizzi et al. 1982). If these regulatory properties are themselves highly dependent on the specifics of each descending program to the spinal interneurons, then such simplifications are not permissible, even if they are sometimes valid descriptors of emergent properties of the system.

This forces us to postulate that descending systems such as cerebral cortex must "learn" to generate each new output program by successive approximation rather than by inversion of the desired trajectory. Of course, this notion is not new (see, e.g., Loeb 1983), but the nature of the spinal cord system that must receive and implement such programs may shed some light on the arrangement and properties of the higher systems that must generate them. In particular, let us consider three preoccupations of cortical neurophysiology: (1) the existence of topical maps; (2) the relationship between the coordinates of these maps and the feature-extracting capabilities of neural networks; and (3) the flow of information that underlies the functional adaptation of these networks. If the cortex uses a singular computational algorithm and the emergent properties of each specific area depend on its particular inputs and outputs (see, e.g., Diamond 1979), then how can such a machine be implemented to accomplish the apparently different tasks of cognition and motor control?

To implement a neural network as the motor controller shown in Figure 3, the input layer would be driven from some premotor region that would specify the objective to be reached, perhaps in coordinates of extrapersonal space, and the output layer would project to the interneurons forming the VTG and regulatory networks of the spinal cord, whose coordinates have no simple physical representation. Sensory feedback would be necessary for at least three functions, all of which are temporally removed from the immediate execution of each motor program: (1) to provide a "teacher" to reinforce network connections when the objective is successfully attained; (2) to signal the suc-

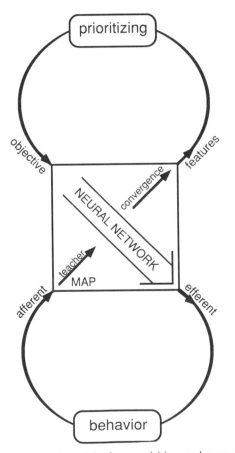

Figure 8. General module for acquisition and perception. Functional schematic of proposed model of a single cerebral cortical area that uses a neural network to translate an input specification of an objective into an efferent search and acquire strategy. Successful completion of the search is signified by afferent information that reinforces the connections defining the search strategy and passes on salient features regarding the acquired objective. It is hypothesized that the coordinate frame of this afferent information defines the topical map of the cortical area.

cessful or unsuccessful completion of a program and thereby to signal readiness for another program; (3) to provide haptic information to characterize objects by the manner in which their loads affect the execution of motor programs. Figure 8 shows such a "motor" network configuration. In contrast, it is usually assumed that the input layer of a cognitive neural network is derived from the representation of the sensory signal, that the output layer goes to other cortical areas, and that any teaching is mediated by "higher" centers. Certainly, there are ample data to suggest that the topicalities of many sensory cortical areas are derived from their sensory input, but such ascending information may not be the only or even the main inputs to a cognitive neural network.

Implications for the General Functions of Cerebral Cortex

The view of sensory cortex as the passive interpreter of sensory data is derived largely from the circumstances of most neurophysiological experiments to date. However, there is growing recognition of the powerful effects of "attention" on the receptive field properties of cortical neurons and on the importance of descending, corticofugal pathways (from sensory as well as motor areas) for shaping the transduction and transmission of information destined for the cerebral cortex (Fetz 1984; Harth et al. 1987; Desimone et al., this volume). This "active" view of perception may be more reconcilable with the operations of motor control. In fact, the scheme shown in Figure 8 can be interpreted as subserving the acquisition of sensory information as well as the attainment of physical goals.

Consider the visual system, in which the representation of the features of a scene must be assembled piecewise by the successive focusing of a high-resolution foveal region on individual regions of interest. The task of decomposing a complex scene is really the development of a series of efficient strategies for the active oculomotor exploration of that scene; the visual feedback from each successive eye movement must inform the interpretation of the last percept and direct the strategy to acquire the next (Ballard 1989). If one were to examine such a process in media res, one would expect to find a neural network that was looking actively for a particular feature that it expected to find and then reporting back whether such an object was found, where it was, and how it deviated from what it was expected to look like. Like motor cortex, sensory (and association) cortex would learn strategies to find and acquire particular objectives; it would report on what it has looked for, not what it is passively looking at. (Note that in many sensory systems, the efferent signals effecting this search may not cause overt movement but rather cause changes in receptor tuning and low-order signal processing, such as in cochlear, retinal, and fusimotor efferents.)

A brain composed of many modules identical to that shown in Figure 8 might be expected to have many desirable emergent properties that are difficult to achieve with the usual configuration of input and output layers in neural networks: (1) It permits (in fact, requires) recursive computation in which the features realized in one cycle would inform the choice of objectives for another cycle. (2) It could thereby generate temporal sequences of motor output such as required for tool-using and other important forms of nondeclarative memory (Squire et al., this volume). (3) It preserves relative location of entities in space and time as intrinsic properties of those entities, which properties are recalled automatically in the process of interpreting a complex situation (e.g., finding sources of food; Allman and Zucker, this volume). (4) It provides a quasi-hierarchical architecture in which information passes freely and in parallel among many areas whose relative position in the chain depends on the nature of the ongoing activity. (5) Its requirement for constant prioritizing of conflicting suggestions about where to direct its receptors leads to the appearance of a single stream of goal-directed, "conscious" behavior.

The establishment of coordinates for the afferent-based map could be driven by an unsupervised neural network, that is, a self-organizing Hebbian network whose representation comes to reflect the inherent frequencies and coherences of patterns that tend to occur in the input data, without regard to any externally imposed goals. The learning task of a higher-order system projecting to such an area would be to discover this coordinate system, much as the motor cortex must discover the organization of the spinal interneurons. The signal specifying the objective to a cortical area would activate those neurons whose aggregate output effects should result in the desired behavior. Points of agreement between the sources of this efferent activity and the resultant afferent activity would then identify the connections to be strengthened, i.e., between those efferent neurons and their cortical inputs specifying the objective. Thus, each module would contain two neural network configurations arranged orthogonally: (1) an unsupervised network to establish the sensory representation and (2) a supervised network employing a knowledge of results that is physiologically plausible (in fact, inevitable) and appropriately configured topically. This arrangement would permit the gradual reassignment of cortical columns to deal with the changing frequency of particular cognitive and motor tasks required over the life of the animal (Merzenich, this volume).

In the specific case of motor cortex, the above analysis tells us more about what not to look for experimentally than about what we might find. It suggests that the topographical coordinates will be neither of the two alternatives that have been the traditional focus of experiments, i.e., neither muscles nor movements. Techniques such as microstimulation (Stoney et al. 1968) and spike-triggered averaging (Fetz and Cheney 1980) have confirmed the broad musculoskeletal topography that is apparent from clinical and experimental lesions, but the divergence of the descending effects of even a single corticospinal neuron belie any attempt to draw such muscle maps more finely. The population vector approach clearly demonstrates the presence of an input signal corresponding to the sort of extrapersonal space coordinates that appear to underlie the topography of some parietal and frontal areas that project to motor cortex (Georgopoulos et al. 1983), but the topographical arrangement of these motor cortical neurons appears not to be strongly related to their contribution to such vectors (A.P. Georgopoulos, pers. comm.). The scheme proposed in Figure 8 suggests that the map should be derived from the afferent information used to reinforce the neural network, but this begs the question of what coordinate scheme has been imposed on this information by its preprocessing in spinal cord, thalamus, and somatosensory cortex. Psychophysical experiments on kinesthesia suggest that we start by considering the orientation of body segments in extrapersonal space (Soechting and Ross 1984), a frame that seems attractive as a compromise between limb-end-point coordinates for the motor-cortical input and the spinal-regulator coordinates of its output. This is at least consistent with the types of information that are conveyed through those regions of the thalamus and sensory cortex that have been demonstrated to produce long-term potentiation in motor cortex (Iriki et al. 1989) and to facilitate learning of motor skills (Sakamoto et al. 1989).

CONCLUSIONS

Optimal controller design has been used to study human and animal jumping (Zajac et al. 1981; Hatze 1981; Pandy et al. 1990) and bipedal walking (Chow and Jacobsen 1971; Yamaguchi 1990), but not in combination with closed-loop regulation. In principle, it should be possible to apply engineering control theory to address questions such as the relative merits of different coordinate schemes for hierarchical systems such as those considered here. However, systems such as outlined in Figure 7 are near or beyond the limits of both current control theory and neurokinesiological methodologies for their exploration. Rather than expecting formal predictions from such modeling, it seems more realistic to use it as a tool to extend and to test our intuition about the workable relationships that might exist between musculoskeletal systems and the neural networks that must control them.

The current resurgence of interest in neural networks stems from several circumstances: (1) They offer a general mechanism that might handle many information-processing problems; (2) they are now sufficiently developed theoretically to anticipate their limitations; and (3) it is feasible to simulate them in computers to observe their interesting and often unpredictable emergent behaviors. We believe that optimal control offers the same three attractions to students of mechanical systems.

Neuroscientists who study sensorimotor control must understand simultaneously the properties of the neural and the mechanical systems. If normal cognition is predominantly an active rather than a passive behavior, then the bidirectional interface between computation and control will turn out to be central to our understanding of much of animal behavior.

ACKNOWLEDGMENTS

This work was supported by grants from the Medical Research Council of Canada (MA-10587), the National Institutes of Health (R0-1 NS-27193), and the Muscular Dystrophy Association of Canada. The authors thank Drs. Apostolos Georgopoulos, John Kalaska, Neville Hogan, Michael Merzenich, and Peter Zarzecki for helpful discussions.

REFERENCES

Abraham, L.D. and G.E. Loeb. 1985. The distal hindlimb musculature of the cat: Patterns of normal use. *Exp. Brain Res.* **58:** 580.

Abraham, L.D., W.B. Marks, and G.E. Loeb. 1985. The distal hindlimb musculature of the cat. II. Cutaneous reflexes during locomotion. *Exp. Brain Res.* **58:** 594.

Athans, M. and P.L. Falb. 1969. *Optimal control.* McGraw Hill, New York.

Ballard, D. 1989. Behavioral constraints on computer vision. *Image Vision Comput.* **7:** 1.

Bizzi, E., W. Chapple, and N. Hogan. 1982. Mechanical properties of muscles: Implication for motor control. *Trends Neurosci.* **5:** 395.

Bizzi, E., N. Accornero, W. Chapple, and N. Hogan. 1984. Posture control and trajectory formation during arm movement. *J. Neurosci.* **4:** 2738.

Bryson, A.E. and Y. Ho. 1975. *Applied optimal control.* Blaisdell Publishing, Waltham, Massachusetts.

Chow, C.K. and D.H. Jacobsen. 1971. Studies of human locomotion via optimal programming. *Math. Biosci.* **10:** 239.

Cole, K.J. and J.H. Abbs. 1987. Kinematic and electromyographic responses to perturbation of a rapid grasp. *J. Neurophysiol.* **57:** 1498.

Collins, W.F., III., M.G. Honig, and L.M. Mendell. 1984. Heterogeneity of group Ia synapses on homonymous a-motoneurons as revealed by high-frequency stimulation of Ia afferent fibers. *J. Neurophysiol.* **52:** 980.

Conway, B.A., H. Hultborn, and O. Kiehn. 1987. Proprioceptive input resets central locomotor rhythm in the spinal cat. *Exp. Brain Res.* **68:** 643.

Diamond, I.T. 1979. The subdivisions of neocortex: A proposal to revise the traditional view of sensory, motor, and association areas. *Prog. Psychobiol. Physiol. Psychol.* **8:** 1.

Doyle, J.C., K. Glover, S.P. Khargonekar, and B.A. Francis. 1989. State space solutions to standard H^2 and $H^\times$ control problems. *IEEE Trans. Automatic Control* **31:** 831.

Duenas, S.H. and P. Rudomin. 1988. Excitability changes of ankle extensor group Ia and Ib fibers during spontaneous fictive locomotion. *Exp. Brain Res.* **70:** 15.

Feldman, A.G. 1966. Functional tuning of the nervous system with control of movement or maintenance of a steady posture. II. Controllable parameters of the muscle. *Biophysics* **11:** 565.

Feldman, A.G. and G.N. Orlovsky. 1975. Activity of interneurons mediating reciprocal Ia inhibition during locomotion. *Brain Res.* **84:** 181.

Ferrell, W.R., S.C. Gandevia, and D.I. McCloskey. 1987. The role of joint receptors in human kinaesthesia when intramuscular receptors cannot contribute. *J. Physiol.* **386:** 63.

Fetz, E.E. 1984. Functional organization of motor and sensory cortex: Symmetries and parallels. In *Dynamic aspects of neocortical function* (ed. G.H. Edelman et al.), p. 453. Wiley, New York.

Fetz, E.E. and P.D. Cheney. 1980. Postspike facilitation of forelimb muscle activity by primate corticomotoneuronal cells. *J. Neurophysiol.* **44:** 751.

Fetz, E.E., P.D. Cheney, K. Mewes, and S. Palmer. 1989. Control of forelimb muscle activity by populations of corticomotoneuronal and rubromotoneuronal cells. *Prog. Brain Res.* **80:** 437.

Forssberg, H. 1979. Stumbling corrective reaction: A phase-dependent compensatory reaction during locomotion. *J. Neurophysiol.* **42:** 936.

Forssberg, H. and G. Svartengren. 1983. Hardwired locomotor network in cat revealed by a retained motor pattern to gastrocnemius after muscle transposition. *Neurosci. Lett.* **41:** 283.

Francis, B.A. 1987. A course in $H^\times$ control theory. Springer-Verlag, Berlin.

Georgopoulos, A.P., R. Caminiti, J.F. Kalaska, and J.T. Massey. 1983. Spatial coding of movement: A hypothesis concerning the coding of movement direction by motor cortical populations. *Exp. Brain Res. (suppl.)* **7:** 327.

Gracco, V.L. and J.H. Abbs. 1985. Dynamic control of the perioral system during speech: Kinematic analyses of autogenic and nonautogenic sensorimotor processes. *J. Neurophysiol.* **54:** 418.

Harth, E., K.P. Unnikrishnan, and A.S. Pandya. 1987. The inversion of sensory processing by feedback pathways: A model of visual cognitive functions. *Science* **237:** 184.

Hatze, H. 1981. A comprehensive model for human motion simulation and its application to the take-off phase of the long jump. *J. Biomech.* **14:** 135.

He, J., W.S. Levine, and G.E. Loeb. 1991. Feedback gains for correcting small perturbations to standing posture. *IEEE Trans. Automatic Control* **518.** (in press.)

Hoffer, J.A., G.E. Loeb, W.B. Marks, M.J. O'Donovan, C.A. Pratt, and N. Sugano. 1987. Cat hindlimb motoneurons during locomotion: I. Destination, axonal conduction velocity and recruitment threshold. *J. Neurophysiol.* **57:** 510.

Hogan, N. 1985. The mechanics of multi-joint posture and movement control. *Biol. Cybern.* **52:** 315.

Houk, J.C. 1979. Regulation of stiffness by skeletomotor reflexes. *Annu. Rev. Physiol.* **41:** 99.

Hounsgaard, J., H. Hultborn, B. Jespersen, and O. Kiehn. 1988. Bistability of a-motoneurones in the decerebrate cat and in the acute spinal cat after intravenous 5-hydroxytryptophan. *J. Physiol.* **405:** 345.

Iriki, A., C. Pavlides, A. Keller, and H. Asanuma. 1989. Long-term potentiation in the motor cortex. *Science* **245:** 1385.

Jankowska, E., D.A. McCrea, P. Rudomin, and E. Sykova. 1981. Observations on neuronal pathways subserving primary afferent depolarization. *J. Neurophysiol.* **46:** 506.

Jordan, L.M. 1990. Brainstem and spinal cord mechanisms for the initiation of locomotion. In *Neurobiological basis of human locomotion* (ed. M. Shimamura et al.). Japan Scientific Societies Press/Springer-Verlag, Tokyo. (In press.)

Kalaska, J.F., D.A.D. Cohen, M.L. Hyde, and M. Prud'homme. 1989. A comparison of movement direction-related versus load direction-related activity in primate motor cortex, using a two-dimensional reaching task. *J. Neurosci.* **9:** 2080.

Lennard, P.R. 1985. Afferent perturbations during "monopodal" swimming movements in the turtle: Phase dependent cutaneous modulation and proprioceptive resetting of the locomotor rhythm. *J. Neurosci.* **5:** 1434.

Liddell, E.G.T. and C.S. Sherrington. 1925. Recruitment and some other factors of reflex inhibition. *Proc. R. Soc. Lond. B.* **97**: 488.

Lloyd, D.P.C. 1946. Integrative pattern of excitation and inhibition in two-neuron reflex arc. *J. Neurophysiol.* **9**: 439.

Loeb, G.E. 1983. Finding common ground between robotics and physiology. *Trends Neurosci.* **6**: 203.

Loeb, G.E. and C. Gans. 1986. *Electromyography for experimentalists.* University of Chicago Press, Chicago.

Loeb, G.E., M.J. Bak, and J. Duysens. 1977. Long-term unit recording from somatosensory neurons in the spinal ganglia of the freely walking cat. *Science* **197**: 1192.

Loeb, G.E., J. He, and W.S. Levine. 1989. Spinal cord circuits: Are they mirrors of musculoskeletal mechanics? *J. Motor Behav.* **21**: 473.

———. 1990. The use of musculoskeletal models to infer principles of sensorimotor control. In *Multiple muscle systems: Biomechanics and movement organization* (ed. J. M. Winters and S.L. Woo), p. 165. First World Congress of Biomechanics. Springer-Verlag, New York.

Lundberg, A. 1980. Half-centres revisited. *Adv. Physiol. Sci.* **1**: 155.

Macpherson, J. 1988. Strategies that simplify the control of quadrupedal stance. I. Forces at the ground. *J. Neurophysiol.* **60**: 204.

McCrea, D.A. 1986. Spinal cord circuitry and motor reflexes. *Exercise Sport Sci. Rev.* **14**: 105.

McMahon, S.B. and P.D. Wall. 1989. Changes in spinal cord reflexes after cross-anastomosis of cutaneous and muscle nerves in the adult rat. *Nature* **342**: 272.

Nashner, L.M., M. Woollacott, and G. Tuma. 1979. Organization of rapid responses to postural and locomotor-like perturbations of standing man. *Exp. Brain Res.* **36**: 463.

Pandy, M.G., F.E. Zajac, E. Sim, and W.S. Levine. 1990. An optimal control model for maximum-height human jumping. *J. Biomech.* (in press).

Perret, C. 1983. Centrally generated pattern of motoneuron activity during locomotion in the cat. In *Neural origin of rhythmic movements: Symposia of the society for experimental biology* (ed. A. Roberts and B. Roberts), p. 405. Cambridge University Press, Cambridge, United Kingdom.

Pratt, C.A. and L.M. Jordan. 1987. Ia inhibitory interneurons and Renshaw cells as contributors to the spinal mechanisms of fictive locomotion. *J. Neurophysiol.* **57**: 56.

Pratt, C.A., C.M. Chanaud, and G.E. Loeb. 1990. Complex muscles of the cat hindlimb. IV. Cutaneous reflex responses in the posterior thigh. *Exp. Brain Res.* (in press).

Rushmer, D.S., C.J. Russell, J.M. Macpherson, J.O. Phillips, and D.C. Dunbar. 1983. Automatic postural responses in the cat: Responses to headward and tailward translation. *Exp. Brain Res.* **50**: 45.

Sakamoto, T., K. Arissian, and H. Asanuma. 1989. Functional role of the sensory cortex in learning motor skills in cats. *Brain Res.* **503**: 258.

Severin, F.V., M.L. Shik, and G.N. Orlovski. 1967. Work of the muscles and single motor neurones during controlled locomotion. *Biofizika* **12**: 660.

Sherrington, C.S. 1910. Flexion-reflex of the limb, crossed extension reflex and reflex stepping and standing. *J. Physiol.* **40**: 28.

Soechting, J.F. and B. Ross. 1984. Psychophysical determination of coordinate representation of human arm orientation. *Neuroscience* **13**: 595.

Sperry, R.W. 1945. The problem of central nervous reorganization after nerve regeneration and muscle transposition. *Q. Rev. Biol.* **20**: 311.

Stein, G. and M. Athans. 1987. The LQG/LTR procedure for multivariable feedback control design. *IEEE Trans. Automatic Control* **32**: 105.

Stein, P.S.G. 1978. Motor systems, with specific reference to the control of locomotion. *Annu. Rev. Neurosci.* **1**: 61.

Stoney, S.D., Jr., W.D. Thompson, and H. Asanuma. 1968. Excitation of pyramidal tract cells by intracortical microstimulation: Effective extent of stimulation current. *J. Neurophysiol.* **31**: 659.

Wolpaw, J.R. and C.L. Lee. 1989. Memory traces in primate spinal cord produced by operant conditioning of H-reflex. *J. Neurophysiol.* **61**: 563.

Yamaguchi, G.T. 1990. Performing whole-body simulations of gait with 3-D, dynamic musculoskeletal models. In *Multiple muscle systems: Biomechanics and movement organization* (ed. J.M. Winters and S.L. Woo), p. 663. Springer-Verlag, New York.

Yumiya, H., K.D. Larsen, and H. Asanuma. 1979. Motor readjustment and input-output relationship of motor cortex following cross-connection of forearm muscles in cats. *Brain Res.* **177**: 566.

Zajac, F.E. 1990. Muscle and tendon: Properties, models, scaling and application to biomechanics and motor control. *CRC Crit. Rev. Biomed. Eng.* **17**: 359.

Zajac, F.E., M.R. Zomlefer, and W.S. Levine. 1981. Hindlimb muscular activity kinetics and kinematics of cats jumping to their maximum achievable heights. *J. Exp. Biol.* **91**: 73.

Population Coding of the Direction, Amplitude, and Velocity of Saccadic Eye Movements by Neurons in the Superior Colliculus

D.L. SPARKS,* C. LEE,† AND W.H. ROHRER‡
*Department of Psychology, University of Pennsylvania, Philadelphia, Pennsylvania 19104-6196;
†Department of Psychology, Seoul National University, Seoul, Korea;
‡Department of Biomedical Engineering, Rutgers University, Busch Campus, Piscataway, New Jersey 08854

Despite the remarkable advances being made by the application of the methods of cell and molecular biology to nervous tissue, molecular approaches to understanding brain function have inherent and severe limitations. Studies restricted to the analysis of the biochemical and biophysical attributes of neurons may produce elegant descriptions of the "hardware" used to perform neural computations, but understanding of the *computations* involved in the analysis and synthesis of sensory signals or the generation of commands for the control of coordinated movements is not likely to come from experiments restricted to the study of neurons in culture, neurons in brain slices, or neurons that are part of homogenized brain tissue. If the operations performed by neurons are to be understood, efforts devoted to describing the neural hardware using molecular techniques must be accompanied by equally intensive attempts devoted to an understanding of the computational algorithms performed by this hardware.

Empirical findings of neurophysiologists (for a recent review, see Knudsen et al. 1987) and conceptual work in artificial intelligence and computer vision (Pitts and McCulloch 1947; Hinton 1981; Feldman and Ballard 1982; Ballard et al. 1983; Baldi and Heiligenberg 1988) indicate that many neural computations are performed by computational maps in the brain. In these maps, neurons may be organized in two- or three-dimensional arrays with systematic variations in the value of a computed parameter (e.g., the angle of orientation of a line segment, the direction or velocity of stimulus movement) across each dimension of the array (Knudsen et al. 1987). Neurons, as elements of the map, may be considered to represent an array of preset processors or filters, each tuned slightly differently, operating in parallel on incoming signals. Consequently, signals are transformed, almost instantaneously, into a place-coded distribution of neural activity where the values of the stimulus parameter are represented as locations of peaks of activity within the map (Knudsen et al. 1987).

Computational maps may also be used for programming movements. Systematic variations in the direction, amplitude, or velocity of a movement can be represented topographically across a neural array. In this paper, we focus on the most thoroughly studied motor map—the map of saccadic eye movements found in the superior colliculus (SC).

Many neurons in the intermediate layers of the SC generate a high-frequency pulse of spike activity that precedes the onset of a saccade by approximately 20 msec (Sparks 1978). These neurons discharge before saccades having a particular range of directions and amplitudes (the movement field of the cell, see Fig. 1A) and, since they are organized according to their movement fields (Wurtz and Goldberg 1972; Robinson 1972; Sparks et al. 1976), form a map of motor (saccadic) space (Fig. 1B). Although, temporally, the high-frequency burst of spike activity generated by many collicular neurons is tightly coupled to saccade onset (Sparks 1978), spatially, the movement fields are usually large and coarsely tuned (Sparks et al. 1976; Sparks and Mays 1980). Because each neuron fires before a broad range of saccades, a large population of neurons is active before each saccade. How are the signals needed to precisely control the direction, amplitude, and velocity of a saccade extracted from the activity of this large population of coarsely tuned cells? One possibility is that the location of the most intense activity within the population is determined at a subsequent stage of neural processing (Knudsen et al. 1987). Another possibility (McIlwain 1976; Sparks et al. 1976; Tweed and Villis 1985; van Gisbergen et al. 1987; van Opstal and van Gisbergen 1989) is that each member of the active population contributes to the movement, and the exact trajectory of a saccade is determined by the average or sum of the population response. Results of recent experiments (Lee et al. 1988), in which small subsets of the active population were reversibly deactivated, support the population-averaging hypothesis.

METHODS

Rhesus monkeys (*Macaca mulatta*) were trained on a saccadic eye movement task in which reinforcement was contingent on looking to a visual target. Animals were prepared for chronic single unit recordings (for details, see Sparks et al. 1976) and an adaptation of the hydraulic microdrive apparatus permitted an insulated, silver-coated glass pipette designed by Malpeli and

A   **B**

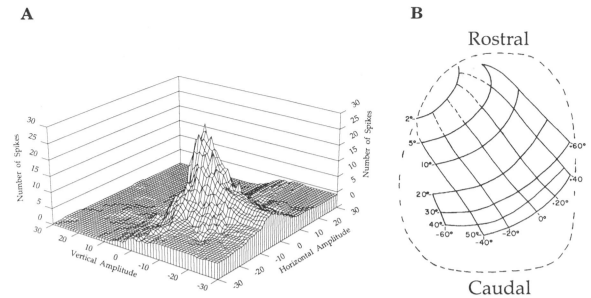

Figure 1. (*A*) Movement field of a saccade-related burst neuron. Three-dimensional representation of the number of spikes in the burst as a function of saccade direction and amplitude. (*B*) Motor map of the SC. Isoamplitude lines (2–50) run from medial to lateral, and isodirection lines (−60 to +60) run from anterior to posterior. From Robinson's microstimulation data (1972).

Schiller (1979) to be lowered into the SC. This probe could be used to record extracellular unit activity, for microstimulation, and for pressure injection of various agents into the SC. Eye position was monitored by the scleral search coil technique (Fuchs and Robinson 1966; Judge et al. 1980). Lidocaine hydrochloride (2%) or bicuculline was delivered by pressure injection; volumes varied from 50 to 200 nl. Bicuculline was prepared as a solution in saline with a concentration of $0.02~\mu g/\mu l$. The location of the pipette tip within the collicular motor map was determined from plots of movement fields and measurements of the direction and amplitude of stimulation-induced saccades. The behavioral effects of the injections were assessed by comparing saccades to a selected set of visual targets before and after the injections.

The general goal of the experiment was to disrupt the spatial and temporal pattern of activity in the motor map and to observe the behavioral consequences of this disruption. The activity can be disrupted by injection of substances which either enhance or depress the activity of cells within a small region of the map. The injection of a local anesthetic (50–100 nl of 2% lidocaine) depresses activity in a local area. An increase in activity can be obtained by small injections of bicuculline, a GABA antagonist. It is known from the work of Hikosaka and Wurtz (1985) that neurons in the substantia nigra pars reticulata (SNpr) exert a tonic inhibitory effect on cells in the intermediate layers of the SC. This inhibition is probably mediated by GABA. Administration of a GABA antagonist such as bicuculline should produce a marked increase in the activity of a subset of the normally active cells by blocking the tonic inhibitory effects normally exerted by the SNpr via the GABAergic pathway. Blocking the tonic inhibitory ef-

fects of the SNpr on the SC by injection of bicuculline should produce an additional peak of activity within the motor map.

Panel 1 of Figure 2 outlines the vector-averaging scheme of Sparks et al. (1976), the hypothesis tested by this experiment. The region of collicular neurons active before a given saccade is assumed to occupy a symmetrical area within the motor map. Only the neurons in the center of the active population discharge maximally before the programmed movement. However, for each subset of active neurons (B) producing a movement tendency with a direction and amplitude other than the programmed movement, there will be a second subset of active neurons (C) producing an opposing tendency such that the resultant of the two movements will have the programmed direction and amplitude. According to this hypothesis, each member of the active population contributes to the ensuing saccade; there is no need to sharpen the population response in order to generate an accurate saccade.

The rationale for the experiment is outlined in panels 2–4 of Figure 2. Suppose a small subset of collicular neurons discharging maximally before straight right saccades 5° in amplitude were inactivated (shown as the darkly shaded area). If the animal were required to make a 5° rightward movement (panel 2), saccade direction and amplitude should be unaffected. The average of the movement tendencies produced by the unaffected neurons in the active population (shown as the larger lightly shaded circle) should result in a saccade having the correct direction and amplitude. However, since the inactivated neurons in the center of the active zone normally discharge earlier than those on the fringe, the latency of the saccade should increase slightly (~30–40 msec). In addition, since recent evidence

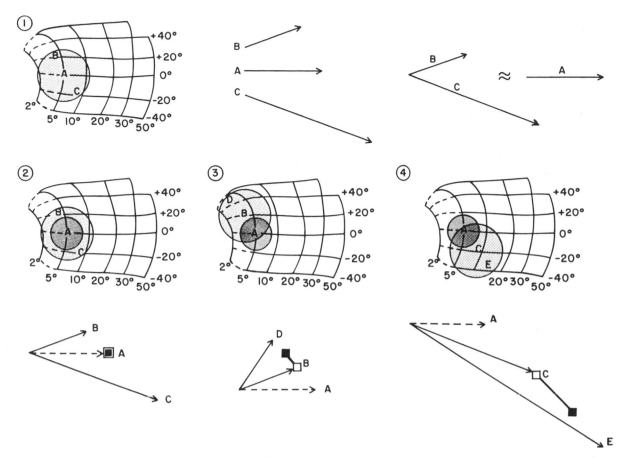

Figure 2. (*1*) Population-averaging scheme of Sparks et al. (1976). (*Left*) Motor map of the left superior colliculus. The stippled area represents the hypothetical extent of cells active before saccades to a target located 5° to the right of the fixation stimulus. The active population is assumed to be symmetrical in shape. (*Middle*) Cells at locations A, B, and C fire most vigorously for the movements shown. (*Right*) Weighted averaging of activity at points B and C yields the same movement as activity at the center of the active population (*A*). (*2–4*) Predicted effect of deactivating a subset of cells in the active population. The site of deactivation (darkly stippled circle) remains the same in each panel, but the location of the active population (lightly stippled area) is different in each panel because saccades to three different targets are required. Beneath each map are the saccade vectors associated with neural activity at each of the locations illustrated. The open square represents the vector of the intended, or programmed, saccade associated with activity in the lightly stippled area. The dashed line represents the vector of the movement tendency produced by neurons at the deactivated site. These neurons will not contribute to the metrics of the saccade, and a saccade to the approximate location of the filled square is predicted. (Reprinted, with permission, from Lee et al. 1988.)

suggests that saccadic velocity may be determined by the level of activity within the active population (Berthoz et al. 1986; Munoz and Guitton 1987; Rohrer et al. 1987), saccadic velocity should be reduced. However, referring to panel 3, with the same region of neurons inactivated, if the animal is now required to make an upward (20° angle) 4° amplitude saccade, the location of the active population shifts, and the inactivated region falls on the periphery of the active zone. Cells in the inactivated region will not balance the activity of cells discharging maximally before saccades having a smaller amplitude and more of an upward component than the programmed saccade. The animal should make a saccade that undershoots the target and has too much of an upward component. Similarly, referring to panel 4, if the animal attempts to make a downward (−20° direction) 9° amplitude saccade, the resulting movement should overshoot the target and have too much of a downward component. Thus, with the same

region of colliculus inactivated, requiring the animal to make different saccades should result in different, but predictable, error patterns.

RESULTS

Injections of 50–200 nl of 2% lidocaine produced measurable modifications of saccadic eye movements lasting from 5 to 20 minutes. The direction and amplitude of movements similar to the "best saccade" (the movement produced by passing small current pulses through the recording/injection probe) were not altered noticeably after the injection (Fig. 3A,B). However, the velocity of movements similar to the best saccade was dramatically reduced (Fig. 3C), and these reductions in velocity were accompanied by increases in duration (Fig. 3D), such that saccadic amplitude remained relatively constant.

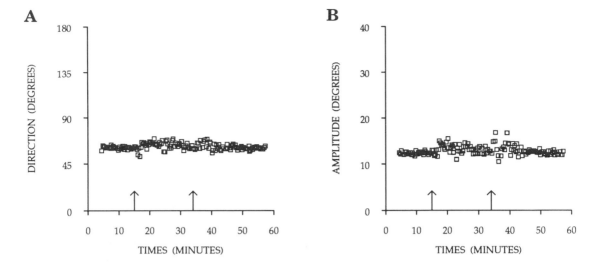

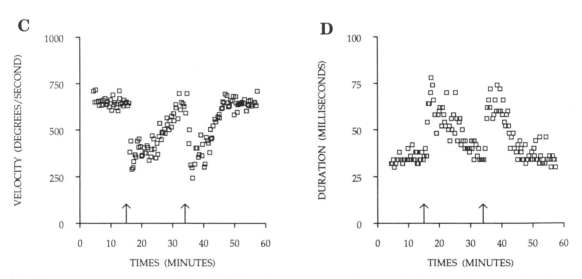

Figure 3. Effects of two injections (each 100 nl of 2% lidocaine) on visually guided saccades similar in direction and amplitude to the best saccade. Each plotted point represents data from a single trial. The time of the injection is indicated by the arrows. For the data plotted, the saccade target was presented at the same location (6° to the right of and 10° above fixation). The reduction in vectorial velocity of ~250°/sec (*C*) was compensated for by an increase in saccadic duration (*D*) so that little effect was observed on saccade direction (*A*) or amplitude (*B*).

As predicted by the population-averaging hypothesis, a systematic pattern of errors in direction and amplitude was observed (Fig. 4A). Saccades to targets requiring more of an upward component than the best saccade had too much of an upward component, and saccades to targets requiring movements with more of a downward component than the best saccade had too much of a downward component. Also as predicted, movements to targets requiring a saccade smaller in amplitude than the best saccade were hypometric; saccades to targets requiring a movement larger than the best saccade were hypermetric. For the injection site represented in Figure 4A, saccades to targets in the

opposite half of the visual field were unaffected, but the range of movements affected varied, depending on the volume of the lidocaine injection.

The pattern of errors observed after injection of bicuculline was also that predicted by a vector-averaging scheme (Fig. 4B). Unlike the lidocaine injections in which the endpoints of postinjection saccades were dispersed away from the endpoint of the stimulation-induced movement, saccades to surrounding targets displayed an "attraction" to this position.

Large changes (~100 msec) in the latency of saccades similar to the best saccade were seen following injections of either lidocaine or bicuculline. Since

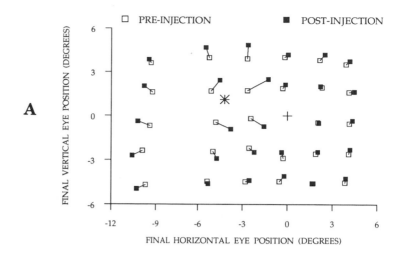

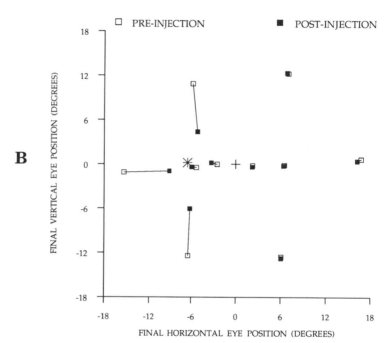

Figure 4. Plots show the positions of the initial fixation (+) and the endpoint (*) of the best saccade. Each symbol represents the average endpoint of 3–5 visually guided saccades. Unfilled symbols represent movements occurring before the injections; filled symbols represent postinjection trials for matching targets. Lines connecting the squares represent the average error introduced by modifying the spatial and temporal pattern of neuronal activity within the SC. (*A*) Effects of a single 200-nl injection of lidocaine. (*B*) Effects of a single 200-nl injection of bicuculline.

neurons in the center of the active population start to fire 20–40 msec before cells on the fringe of the active population, we had expected to see changes on the order of 50 msec. However, the observed latency effects were larger than expected (Fig. 5).

DISCUSSION

Results of these experiments confirm and extend the findings of Hikosaka and Wurtz (1985, 1986) and support the major predictions of the vector-averaging model. Inactivation of collicular neurons produced dramatic reductions in saccadic velocity as well as the predicted pattern of errors in the direction and amplitude of visually guided saccades.

These findings support the hypothesis that saccadic accuracy results from the averaging of the movement

tendencies produced by the entire active population rather than the discharge of a small number of finely tuned cells. Moreover, since the contribution of each neuron to the direction and amplitude of the movement is relatively small, the effects of variability or "noise" in the discharge frequency of a particular neuron are minimized. Thus, the large movement fields (resulting in a large population of neurons being active during a specific movement) may contribute to, rather than detract from, saccadic accuracy.

In general, coarse population coding is efficient, accurate, and relatively insensitive to noise in the discharge of individual units (Hinton 1981; Feldman and Ballard 1982; Ballard et al. 1983). Indeed, the simulations of Baldi and Heiligenberg (1988) produced the apparently paradoxical result that, over a fairly large range, the wider the tuning curve of individual ele-

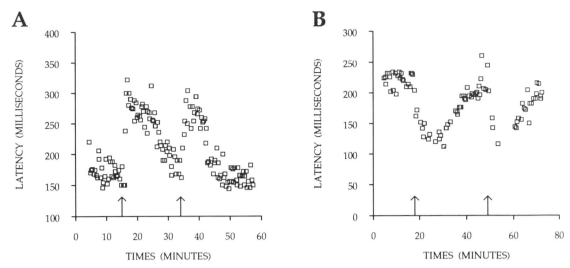

Figure 5. Effects of a single 200-nl injection of lidocaine (*A*) or bicuculline (*B*) on saccadic latency.

ments, i.e., the less precise the single elements, the more robust and precise the overall computation. One disadvantage of coarse coding is difficulty in making two-point discriminations. In this context, it is notable that behavioral experiments (Findlay 1982; Ottes et al. 1984) have shown that when two visual targets are presented close together, the ensuing saccade tends to move the foveal projection to a point between the targets.

Do our findings generalize to other sensory or motor systems? Georgopoulos et al. (1986) have described a distributed population code in the motor cortex for the control of reaching movements of the arm. Ordered arrays of broadly tuned sensory neurons characterize neural maps of several modalities (see Knudsen et al. 1987; Suga et al.; Konishi et al.; Bankman et al.; all this volume).

With respect to the motor map in the SC, much remains to be learned about how signals appropriate for each of the extraocular muscles are extracted from the spatial and temporal pattern of activity observed in the SC (Sparks and Mays 1990). Considerable theoretical and experimental attention is being devoted to this problem, and a more complete understanding of this complex signal transform should be forthcoming.

ACKNOWLEDGMENTS

The research cited from the author's laboratory was supported by National Institutes of Health grant EY-01189 and Alfred P. Sloan Foundation grant 86-10-7.

REFERENCES

Baldi, P. and W. Heiligenberg. 1988. How sensory maps could enhance resolution through ordered arrangements of broadly tuned receivers. *Biol. Cybern.* **59:** 313.
Ballard, D.H., G.E. Hinton, and T.J. Sejnowski. 1983. Parallel visual computation. *Nature* **306:** 21.

Berthoz, A., A. Grantyn, and J. Droulez. 1986. Some collicular efferent neurons code saccadic eye velocity. *Neurosc. Lett.* **72:** 289.
Feldman, J.A. and D.H. Ballard. 1982. Connectionist models and their properties. *Cognit. Sci.* **6:** 205.
Findlay, J.M. 1982. Global visual processing for saccadic eye movements. *Vision Res.* **22:** 1045.
Fuchs, A.F. and D.A. Robinson. 1966. A method for measuring horizontal and vertical eye movement chronically in the monkey. *J. Appl. Physiol.* **21:** 1068.
Georgopoulos, A.P., A.B. Schwartz, and R.E. Kettner. 1986. Neuronal population coding of movement direction. *Science* **233:** 1416.
Hikosaka, O. and R.H. Wurtz. 1985. Modification of saccadic eye movements by GABA-related substances. I. Effect of muscimol and bicuculline in monkey superior colliculus. *J. Neurophysiol.* **53:** 266.
———. 1986. Saccadic eye movements following injection of lidocaine into the superior colliculus. *Exp. Brain Res.* **61:** 531.
Hinton, G.F. 1981. Shape representation in parallel systems. In *Proceedings of the 7th International Joint Conference on Artificial Intelligence*, Vancouver, B.C. p. 1088.
Judge, S.J., B.J. Richmond, and F.C. Chu. 1980. Implantation of magnetic search coils for measurement of eye position: An improved method. *Vision Res.* **20:** 535.
Knudsen, E.I., S. du Lac, and S.D. Esterly. 1987. Computational maps in the brain. *Annu. Rev. Neurosci.* **10:** 41.
Lee, C., W.H. Rohrer, and D.L. Sparks. 1988. Population coding of saccadic eye movements by neurons in the superior colliculus. *Nature* **332:** 357.
Malpeli, J.G. and P.H. Schiller. 1979. A method of reversible inactivation of small regions of brain tissue. *J. Neurosci. Methods* **1:** 143.
McIlwain, J.T. 1976. Large receptive fields and spatial transformations in the visual system. *Int. Rev. Physiol.* **10:** 223.
Munoz, D.P. and D. Guitton. 1987. Tecto-reticulo-spinal neurons have discharges coding the velocity profiles of eye and head orienting movements. *Soc. Neurosci. Abstr.* **13:** 393.
Ottes, F.P., J.A.M. van Gisbergen, and J.J. Eggermont. 1984. Metrics of saccade responses to visual double stimuli: Two different modes. *Vision Res.* **24:** 1169.
Pitts, W. and W.S. McCulloch. 1947. How we know universals: The perception of auditory and visual forms. *Bull. Math. Biophys.* **9:** 127.
Robinson, D.A. 1972. Eye movements evoked by collicular stimulation in the alert monkey. *Vision Res.* **12:** 1795.

Rohrer, W.H., J. White, and D.L. Sparks. 1987. Saccade-related burst cells in the superior colliculus: Relationship of activity with saccadic velocity. *Soc. Neurosc. Abstr.* **13:** 1092.

Sparks, D.L. 1978. Functional properties of neurons in the monkey superior colliculus: Coupling of neuronal activity and saccade onset. *Brain Res.* **158:** 1.

Sparks, D.L. and L.E. Mays. 1980. Movement fields of saccade-related burst neurons in the monkey superior colliculus. *Brain Res.* **190:** 39.

———. 1990. Signal transformations required for the generation of saccadic eye movements. *Annu. Rev. Neurosci.* **13:** 309.

Sparks, D.L., R. Holland, and B.L. Guthrie. 1976. Size and distribution of movement fields in the monkey superior colliculus. *Brain Res.* **113:** 21.

Tweed, D. and T. Vilis. 1985. A two dimensional model for saccade generation. *Biol. Cybern.* **52:** 219.

van Gisbergen, J.A.M., A.J. van Opstal, and A.A.M. Tax. 1987. Collicular ensemble coding of saccades based on vector summation. *Neuroscience* **21:** 541.

van Opstal, A.J. and J.A.M. van Gisbergen. 1989. A non-linear model for collicular spatial interactions underlying the metrical properties of electrically elicited saccades. *Biol. Cybern.* **60:** 171.

Wurtz, R.H. and M.E. Goldberg. 1972. Activity of superior colliculus in behaving monkey. III. Cells discharging before eye movements. *J. Neurophysiol.* **35:** 575.

Properties of Pathways That Mediate Motor Learning in the Vestibulo-ocular Reflex of Monkeys

S.G. Lisberger, D.M. Broussard, and H.M. Bronte-Stewart

Department of Physiology, Neuroscience Graduate Program, and W.M. Keck Center for Integrative Neuroscience, University of California School of Medicine, San Francisco, California 94143

To understand learning in the human brain, we investigate simple behaviors that meet several criteria. These behaviors must have similar properties in humans and experimental animals, must exhibit learning that can be elicited in a simple and reproducible way, and must have neural substrates that are accessible for analysis in awake behaving animals. Eye movement satisfies all of these criteria and has been a model system that, through investigations in behaving monkeys, has yielded much progress in understanding the neural basis for motor activity, including motor learning (Miles and Lisberger 1981; Ito 1982; Fuchs et al. 1985; Lisberger et al. 1987; Robinson 1987).

Learning has been demonstrated in all kinds of eye movements (Miles and Eighmy 1980; Optican and Robinson 1980; Optican et al. 1985; Miles and Kawano 1986; Miles et al. 1987), but the most thorough analysis of the neural basis for learning has focused on one eye movement subsystem called the vestibulo-ocular reflex or VOR (Lisberger 1988). Normally, the VOR generates smooth eye rotation that is equal in amplitude and opposite in direction to any head turn (Keller 1978). As a result, gaze tends to remain stable, and the images from the stationary world are nearly stabilized on the retina. The VOR is active and generates compensatory eye movements in light as well as in darkness. Thus, the primary sensory inputs for the VOR originate in the vestibular apparatus, although the function of the VOR is to help preserve good vision by stabilizing gaze.

Because it is an open-loop system that must perform accurately in the interval before visual feedback, the VOR requires calibration to establish and maintain its normal excellent performance. In the laboratory, we activate the calibration mechanism by fitting monkeys with spectacles that magnify or miniaturize the visual scene (Miles and Fuller 1974). If a monkey views the world through times-two magnifying spectacles, then stability of retinal images from the stationary world requires that the amplitude of eye rotation become twice the amplitude of the head turn. Gradually this occurs. After the monkey has worn the magnifying spectacles for several days, passive head rotation in darkness evokes a VOR that is as large as 1.8 times its original amplitude. Times one-quarter miniaturizing spectacles cause an analogous decrease in the amplitude of the VOR to 0.3 times its original amplitude. The gradual time course of the changes in the VOR and the fact that they are remembered automatically (Miles

and Eighmy 1980) imply that long-term recalibration of the VOR is a form of motor learning and memory.

Figure 1 summarizes our current knowledge about the pathways that underlie the VOR and the basis for motor learning. Inputs to the VOR pathways enter the brain over vestibular primary afferents in the eighth cranial nerve and are transmitted over at least three pathways to motoneurons. The basic VOR pathway is disynaptic and employs VOR interneurons located in the vestibular nucleus (see, e.g., Precht and Baker 1972; Highstein 1973). A second brain stem pathway also receives direct inputs from vestibular afferents (Broussard and Lisberger 1990) but is different in that its interneurons, called flocculus target neurons or FTNs, receive monosynaptic inhibition from the flocculus of the cerebellum (Lisberger and Pavelko 1988). A third VOR pathway transmits vestibular signals through the flocculus. Lesion experiments have shown that the pathway through the flocculus plays only a minor role in the normal VOR but that it is essential for motor learning (Robinson 1976; Ito 1982; Lisberger et al. 1984).

Our previous work (Lisberger 1988) has led to the hypothesis that the site of motor learning is in the vestibular inputs to FTNs across the synapse inside the box in Figure 1. This hypothesis receives support from experiments in which we found that learning was associated with large changes in the responses of FTNs during the VOR induced by passive head turns in the dark (Lisberger and Pavelko 1988). Learning also causes changes in the responses of Purkinje cells in the flocculus during the VOR (Miles et al. 1980; Watanabe 1984), but at latencies that follow the responses of FTNs by an average of 8 msec (Lisberger and Pavelko 1988). The relatively short latency of the responses of FTNs implies that the change in their firing must result from modification within the brain stem vestibular inputs to FTNs and cannot occur merely because of changes in the activity in their inputs from the flocculus. We account for the effect of lesions in the flocculus by suggesting that the visual signals that signal errors in the VOR and guide learning are transmitted through the flocculus (Miles and Lisberger 1981). This suggestion is supported by the finding that signals related to image motion form one of the most important components of the firing of Purkinje cells in the flocculus (Stone and Lisberger 1990).

We are now testing the hypothesis outlined in Figure

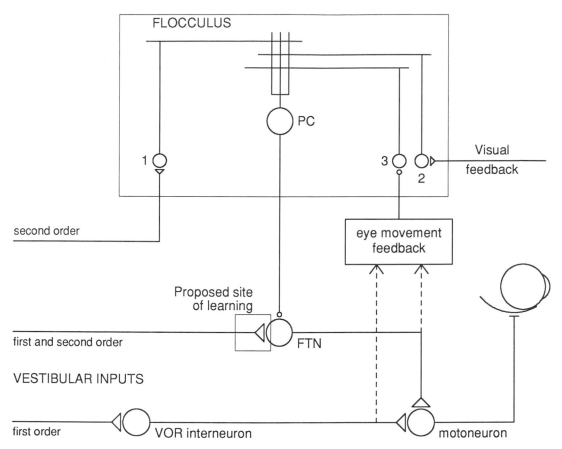

Figure 1. Simplified diagram showing the circuitry of the VOR and the proposed site of motor learning. Vestibular inputs arise on the left side of the diagram and eye movements emerge on the right side. Triangles indicate excitatory synapses, and circles indicate inhibitory circles. Dashed lines indicate pathways that are postulated to exist but whose anatomical basis has not been revealed. (PC) Purkinje cell; (FTN) flocculus target neuron. For simplicity, midline crossings and reciprocal innervation have not been included in the diagram.

1 by using electrical activation of the vestibular apparatus with single shocks. Our goal is to learn more about the synaptic organization of the VOR pathways and to test directly in both the brain stem and cerebellum for synaptic changes that might cause learning. In this paper, we report our initial experiments, in which we have studied the effect of motor learning in the VOR on the eye movements evoked by electrical stimulation of the vestibular apparatus. Our data reveal that only a subset of the VOR pathways are modified in association with learning and that the signals carried by the modified pathways have a different and longer time course than those carried in unmodified pathways.

METHODS

Experiments were conducted on awake rhesus monkeys that had been trained to fixate and track spots of light (for method, see Wurtz 1969). After training had been completed, each monkey was anesthetized with Halothane, and aseptic procedure was used to implant several devices. Bolts were secured to the skull and used to attach a platform that could be used as a mount

for spectacles and to restrain the monkey's head (Miles and Eighmy 1980). A coil of wire was implanted in one eye to allow us to use the magnetic search coil method to monitor horizontal and vertical eye position (Judge et al. 1980).

In a second surgery, the postauricular approach was used to implant a stimulating electrode in the perilymphatic space inside the lumen of the superior semicircular canal (Nelson 1982). A dental burr was used to dissect carefully through the mastoid air cells until the horizontal and superior canals could be visualized. A diamond burr was then used to gently sand the bony labyrinth of the superior canal until it was thin enough to make a tiny hole with a dissecting pin. The electrode was inserted into the hole and secured with Histacryl blue surgical adhesive and dental cement. We implanted the electrodes in the superior canal because they provided excellent electrical activation of afferents from the horizontal canal without compromising the mechanical activation of that canal by natural head turns in the horizontal plane (Bronté-Stewart and Lisberger 1990). Stimulating electrodes were implanted in the superior semicircular canals of three monkeys. In one additional monkey, the stimulating electrode was implanted in the vestibule using a variation of the approach of Goldberg et al. (1984).

During experiments, each monkey sat in a specially designed primate chair. Implanted hardware was used to secure the monkey's head to the ceiling of the chair, and the chair and the coils used to generate a magnetic field were bolted on a servocontrolled turntable that provided passive rotation about the vertical axis. Experiments were run under the control of a laboratory computer that also digitized voltages proportional to horizontal eye position, target position, head velocity, and eye velocity for later analysis. Each channel was digitized at a rate of 500 samples per second. After each experiment, another computer was used to align the responses to multiple presentations of the same stimulus and then to compute the mean and standard error of eye velocity.

Motor learning was induced by fitting monkeys with spectacles that contained either magnifying ($\times 2.2$) or miniaturizing ($\times 0.25$) optics purchased from Designs for Vision in New York. The spectacles were molded to fit each monkey's face and were affixed to the implanted pedestal so that they could be worn continuously in the home cage. Thus, learning was stimulated by the interaction of visual and vestibular stimuli that resulted from the monkeys' active head turns in their home cages. Spectacles were removed for recordings of

the VOR induced by natural and electrical stimuli, but only after the monkey had been transported to the lab and its head had been fixed to the chair.

Experiments consisted of first measuring the VOR evoked by natural vestibular stimuli in darkness and then recording the responses to electrical stimuli at different current intensities. Electrical stimuli consisted of either single shocks or short trains at a frequency of 200 Hz. Natural stimuli consisted of short pulses of head velocity that had a duration of 250 msec and were imposed in darkness (Lisberger and Pavelko 1986). The gain of the VOR was estimated as the mean smooth eye speed during the steady-state of the response divided by the imposed head speed. The experiment was repeated daily, first to ascertain that the responses were consistent for a normal VOR and then to follow changes in the responses during and after the motor learning induced by magnifying or miniaturizing spectacles.

RESULTS

Natural Vestibular Stimulation

Figure 2A illustrates the eye movements evoked by natural vestibular stimulation in darkness before and

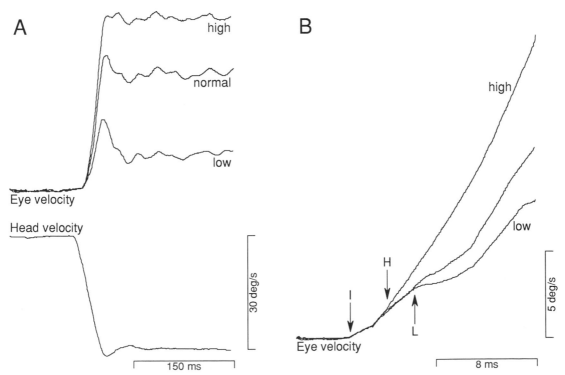

Figure 2. Effect of motor learning in the VOR on the eye movements evoked by a transient, natural vestibular stimulus. Each trace shows the average of 10 traces of eye or head velocity. (*A*) Slow sweep records showing the VOR evoked by rapid changes in head velocity before motor learning (normal) and after learning induced by magnifying (high) or miniaturizing (low) spectacles. (*B*) Fast sweep records showing the events at the initiation of the VOR for the data in *A*. The arrow labeled "I" indicates the initiation of the VOR, and those labeled "H" and "L" point out the times when high-gain and low-gain records of eye velocity diverge from the control record. The gain of the VOR was 0.32, 1.05, and 1.57 for the records labeled low, normal, and high, respectively. Upward deflections are rightward motion.

after motor learning in the VOR. Head velocity was initially zero and then increased rapidly for 50 msec with an average acceleration of 600°/sec² to a steady-state value of 30°/sec to the left. This stimulus, which we call a rapid change in head velocity, evoked a change in eye velocity with a latency that averaged 14 msec (Lisberger 1984). Before learning, the monkey whose data appear in Figure 2A achieved a steady-state eye speed of 31.5°/sec (VOR gain = 1.05). After he had worn the magnifying or miniaturizing spectacles in his cage for several days, there were large changes in the eye movements evoked by the same rapid change in head velocity in darkness. Magnifying spectacles caused the gain of the VOR to increase to 1.57, whereas miniaturizing spectacles caused gain to decrease to 0.32.

The records in Figure 2 reveal two additional effects of motor learning on the eye movements evoked by rapid changes in head velocity. First, the degree of overshoot in eye velocity varied consistently, with a large transient overshoot when the gain of the VOR was low and very little overshoot when the gain of the VOR was high. Second, inspection of the records at higher gain and sweep speed (Fig. 2B) reveals that learning is expressed only after the initial rising phase of the VOR evoked by natural vestibular stimuli. The arrow labeled "I" shows the time of the initiation of the VOR, 14 msec after the onset of head motion. The arrows labeled "H" and "L" show the times when the eye velocity after increases or decreases in VOR gain first deviated from the eye velocity before learning. The first 3.5–6 msec of the response is the same after learning as before, indicating that the VOR pathways that transmit natural stimuli with the shortest latency are not modified during learning. The data in Figure 2 allow us to estimate the total latency of the VOR pathways that are modified by measuring the time when the responses after learning diverge from normal. The total latency of the modified pathways for natural stimuli averaged 19 msec, which is 5 msec longer than the latency of the unmodified pathways (Lisberger 1984).

Electrical Stimulation of the Vestibular Apparatus: Trains

In exploring the effects of electrical stimulation of the labyrinth, we first studied the eye movements evoked by trains of electrical stimuli, to be certain that our electrodes had access to the modified pathways. Figure 3 shows averages of the eye velocities evoked in one monkey. The train of stimuli began at the time indicated by the upward arrow. Before learning, when the gain of the VOR was 0.97, electrical stimulation evoked an initial rapid rise in eye velocity after a latency of 6 msec, followed by a steady plateau at approximately 15°/sec. We show records of eye velocity here, but the response to trains of electrical stimuli was also visible in records of eye position where it appeared as a ramp of eye position before learning.

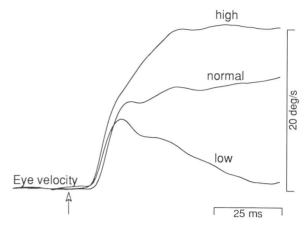

Figure 3. Effect of motor learning on the eye movements evoked by trains of electrical stimuli. The arrow indicates the onset of the train of stimuli. Stimulus parameters were 20 shocks at a frequency of 200 Hz and a current of 300 μA. The gain of the VOR was 0.27, 0.97, and 1.82 for the traces labeled low, normal, and high, respectively. The stimulating electrode was in the left superior semicircular canal. Upward deflections represent rightward eye movement.

Motor learning induced large changes in the steady-state component of the eye velocity evoked by trains of electrical stimuli but caused no change in the latency and only small changes in the initial rising phase of the response. After the gain of the VOR had been reduced to 0.27 with miniaturizing spectacles, eye velocity showed a rapid initial rise but declined back to zero within about 75 msec after the onset of the stimulus (trace labeled "low"). When the gain of the VOR had been increased to 1.82 with magnifying spectacles, eye velocity showed a prolonged rising phase and reached a much higher plateau than it had before learning (trace labeled "high").

Electrical Stimulation of the Vestibular Apparatus: Single Shocks

Because our ultimate goal is to use single electrical shocks to the vestibular apparatus to reveal which synapses are modified during motor learning in the VOR, we have conducted the most thorough analysis of the eye movements evoked by single shocks. Figure 4 compares the responses of one monkey before and after learning. Each trace shows the result of averaging 20 measurements of eye velocity from 20 msec before to 80 msec after the application of single shocks to the labyrinth. Averaging was necessary to obtain reliable estimates of the shape and amplitude of the responses, which were too small to be visible in records of eye position. The left-hand panel shows the profiles of eye velocity evoked before learning by shocks at current intensities ranging from 225 to 425 μA in 50-μA steps. For each stimulus intensity, the profile of eye velocity shows two clear peaks, both of which grow as a function of increases in stimulus current. The right-hand panel shows the eye movements evoked by the same currents

normal   low gain

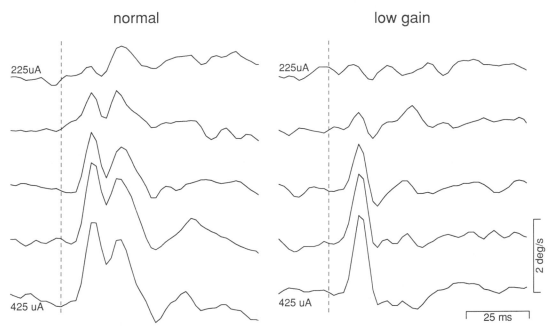

Figure 4. Effect of motor learning on the eye movements evoked by single shocks to the vestibule. Each trace shows eye velocity as a function of time. The traces on the left were obtained when the gain of the VOR was 0.84, and the traces on the right were obtained in the same monkey when the gain of the VOR was 0.38. From top to bottom in each column, the stimulus intensities were 225, 275, 325, 375, and 425 μA. The stimulating electrode was in the left vestibule. Upward deflections represent rightward eye movement.

in the same monkey after motor learning had reduced the gain of the VOR to 0.38. The profile of eye velocity now shows just the early peak, which appears unmodified, and the later peak is gone. This particular implant was atypical both in the small amplitude and the short duration the first peak of eye velocity evoked by single shocks to the labyrinth, because it was placed in the vestibule rather than in the superior semicircular canal. We show the eye movements it evoked because they demonstrate so clearly that there are two components in the VOR evoked by electrical stimulation of the labyrinth and that motor learning affects only the second component.

Figure 5A shows the profile of horizontal eye velocity evoked by the application of single shocks through a typical implant in the superior semicircular canal before motor learning. The twitch has an initial rising phase that moves the eye away from the side of the labyrinth that was stimulated, consistent with the direction of action of the VOR. The rising phase was followed by a deceleration and a small rebound in the other direction. Figure 5B compares the twitches evoked by single shocks at the same current when the gain of the VOR was high, normal, and low. Motor learning had little discernible effect on the rising phase of the response or on the peak eye velocity, but caused marked changes that were evident during the rebound of the twitch. Decreasing the gain of the VOR with miniaturizing

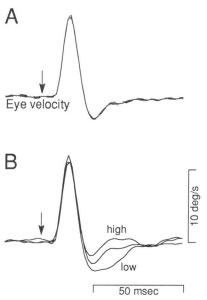

Figure 5. Effect of motor learning on the eye movements evoked by single pulses to the superior semicircular canal. (*A*) Average eye velocity for 20 stimuli before motor learning. Dashed lines indicate one standard error of eye velocity. (*B*) Average eye velocity before motor learning, after adaptation to magnifying spectacles (high), and after adaptation to miniaturizing spectacles (low). Arrows show the time of stimulation. The stimulating electrode was in the left superior semicircular canal. Upward deflections represent rightward eye motion.

spectacles caused the rebound to be larger in amplitude and longer in duration, whereas increasing the gain with magnifying spectacles caused the rebound to become small and short.

We have devised a data analysis procedure to estimate the latency, amplitude, and time course of the component of the response to single shocks that is modified in association with learning. For each stimulus current, we combined the data for responses at different VOR gains but separated the data into groups according to the time after application of the stimulus. We then plotted eye velocity as a function of the gain of the VOR and used linear regression to calculate the slope of the relationship for each millisecond in the averages. The slope of the regression line was taken as an estimate of the effect of the modified pathways on the overall response at that time. A slope of zero indicated that motor learning had no effect at that time; a positive slope indicated that motor learning had some effect; and larger values of the slope indicated greater effects.

Figure 6 shows a family of graphs relating eye velocity to the gain of the VOR for the data shown in Figure 5B. Each graph is labeled according to the time after

application of the stimulus when eye velocity was measured. Thus, the graph in the upper left corner (labeled 0 ms) shows that eye velocity at the time the stimulus was applied was always near zero and was not affected by VOR gain. In the graphs labeled 10 ms and 15 ms, the consistently positive values of eye velocity and of the *y*-intercepts indicate that these times were on the initial, positive part of the eye velocity response. The low values of slope indicate that eye velocity was not affected by motor learning at these early times. For the graphs in the second row, the low values of eye velocity indicate that the peak of the response was over. The positive values of slope indicate that motor learning had a large effect at these later times. The largest effect, indicated by the graph with the steepest slope, occurred 25 msec after the application of the shock. In contrast, eye velocity reached its peak value 12 msec after the application of the stimulus.

To summarize the time course of the component of the response that is due to the modified pathways, we synthesized the family of graphs in Figure 6 into a single trace that plots the slope of the linear regression lines as a function of time. In Figure 7, the two top traces show the results of this analysis for two monkeys, and the

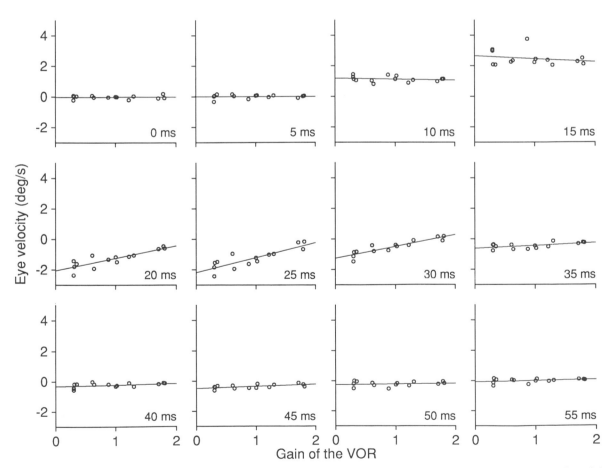

Figure 6. Relationship between eye velocity and the gain of the VOR as a function of time after single pulse stimulation of the labyrinth. Each panel shows eye velocity measured at a given time after the application of the stimulus. Different points represent responses from different days and are plotted as a function of the gain of the VOR. Lines are the result of linear regression analysis. This figure shows the data at 5-msec intervals, but the regression analysis was performed at each msec.

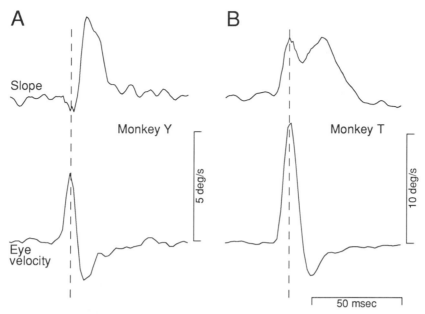

Figure 7. Time course of the modified component of the response to single pulse stimulation of the labyrinth. The upper traces plot the slope of the relationship between eye velocity and the gain of the VOR as a function of time, for every msec from 20 msec before to 80 msec after the application of the stimulus. The lower traces show averages of eye velocity on the same time scale. Vertical dashed lines indicate the time of the peak in eye velocity. The two panels show data from two different monkeys at a stimulus current of 5 times the threshold for evoking an eye movement. Upward deflections represent positive slopes and rightward eye motion.

bottom traces show the twitch of eye velocity on the same time scale. For both monkeys, the modified component of the response had a longer time course than did the eye velocity response. For the monkey whose data appear on the left (Monkey Y), the effect of motor learning appeared only after the peak of the twitch. For the monkey whose data appear on the right (Monkey T), motor learning had an effect on the rising phase and peak of the twitch, but the effect was prolonged well beyond the twitch. These two examples show the extremes in the time course of the modified component of the response in different monkeys. Most of the curves relating slope to time were intermediate. They revealed small changes in the initial part of the response but a time course of changes that was much longer than the time course of the eye velocity response. Even Monkey Y showed some changes in the early part of the response for higher stimulus currents.

To estimate the latency of the modified pathways for electrical stimuli, we measured the time at which the slope of the relationship between VOR gain and eye velocity began to increase. In three of the four monkeys, the latency of the modified pathways was within 1 msec of the latency of the eye velocity response for most stimulus currents. For Monkey Y, the latency was longer for low currents, but equal to the latency of the eye velocity response for high currents.

DISCUSSION

We have used both electrical and natural stimulation of the vestibular apparatus to analyze the pathways that subserve the VOR and to determine the properties of the pathways that are modified when the VOR undergoes motor learning. Natural vestibular stimuli revealed that there are at least two sets of VOR pathways. One set is unmodified and has a total latency for natural vestibular stimuli of 14 msec, whereas the other set is modified and has a total latency of 19 msec. Quantitative analysis of the effects of motor learning on the eye movements evoked by electrical stimuli revealed that the time course of the modified component of the response is quite different from the time course of the overall eye velocity. This confirms the existence of modified and unmodified VOR pathways.

Natural and electrical stimuli activate the VOR pathways in quite different ways and can be used for different purposes. Natural stimuli reveal the normal function of the VOR and the magnitude of the motor learning induced by spectacles. Electrical stimuli are best suited for analysis of the circuitry that mediates the VOR. Yet, the results of both kinds of stimuli must be explained by the same sets of VOR pathways. The purpose of the Discussion will be to describe a simple model of the VOR that is based on the responses to natural vestibular stimuli, and then to evaluate how different parts of the model respond to electrical stimuli.

Figure 8A shows a model that can account for the effect of motor learning on the eye movements evoked by rapid changes in head velocity. Vestibular inputs originate on the left side of the diagram and are transmitted through parallel pathways that have either a fixed gain of 0.3 or an adjustable gain "G." The outputs

A

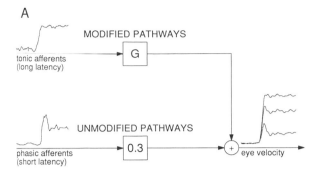

B

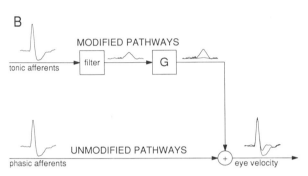

Figure 8. Models showing the activation of the modified and unmodified pathways by natural (*A*) and single pulse electrical (*B*) stimulation of the vestibular apparatus. Signals are conducted along the arrows from left to right. (*A*) Model to account for the VOR evoked by rapid changes in head velocity. The boxes are simple multipliers, and "G" represents the modifications underlying motor learning. The circle with a " + " performs a mathematical addition of its inputs from the modified and unmodified pathways. The traces on the vestibular input pathways at the left of the diagram are the firing rates of tonic and phasic afferents in response to rapid changes in head velocity. The traces at the right show the eye velocity evoked by the same stimulus when the gain of the VOR was low, normal, and high. (*B*) The same model adapted to account for the effect of motor learning on the eye movements evoked by single pulse electrical stimulation of the vestibular apparatus. The box labeled "filter" converts the responses of vestibular primary afferents to single pulses into a more delayed and prolonged signal that is then scaled by the multiplier labeled "G" to alter the gain of the VOR. The traces on the lower right show the eye velocity induced by single shocks after the gain of the VOR was high or low. The traces at the output from "G" show the postulated output from the modified pathways when the gain of the VOR is high or low.

from these two pathways are summed to create a command that is then converted into eye velocity.

The differences in the responses of the modified and unmodified pathways to natural vestibular stimuli can be accounted for by the properties of primary vestibular afferents. Our recordings from afferents during natural vestibular stimuli (Lisberger and Pavelko 1986) revealed that some afferents had latencies as short as 5 msec and exhibited phasic responses in which firing rate during the change in head velocity was much higher than during the subsequent constant head velocity. Other afferents had longer latencies ranging from 9 to 15 msec and had purely tonic responses with no overshoot. Figure 8A shows the firing rate induced by rapid

changes in head velocity in typical phasic and tonic afferents. If the phasic, short-latency afferents project into the unmodified pathways and the tonic long-latency afferents project into the modified pathways, then the earliest part of the VOR will be dominated by the short-latency responses transmitted through the VOR pathways. As we have observed, the first several milliseconds of the VOR evoked by natural stimuli will be unmodified. The differential projections of tonic and phase afferents would also account for the changes we have observed in the overshoot in eye velocity. When the gain of the VOR is reduced by decreasing the value of G to zero, eye velocity will reflect the phasic signals transmitted by the unmodified pathways. When the gain of the VOR is increased by increasing the value of G, the tonic signals emanating from the modified pathways will swamp the phasic signals, and the degree of overshoot should be reduced.

The eye movements evoked by electrical stimulation of the vestibular apparatus reveal further differences between the modified and unmodified pathways. The model in Figure 8B is derived from the analysis of eye movements evoked by natural vestibular stimuli, but is labeled with traces that indicate how single electrical shocks appear to affect the modified and unmodified pathways. Our recordings from the vestibular afferents reveal that both the tonic and the phasic afferents emit a single action potential followed by a pause in activity that is approximately 10 msec in duration (Brontë-Stewart and Lisberger 1990). Therefore, the inputs to both the modified and unmodified pathways are shown as a spike followed by a rebound inhibition. If the vestibular input is transmitted directly through the unmodified pathways, then lowering the gain of the VOR by reducing the value of G to zero will cause single electrical shocks to produce an eye velocity twitch with a substantial rebound, as we have observed.

To produce an effect on eye movements that has a longer time course, the modified pathways must filter the vestibular input. In our data analysis, we estimated the properties of that filter by plotting the slope of the relationship between eye velocity and VOR gain as a function of time. To provide a more graphic estimate of the output from the modified pathways, Figure 8B shows the effect of subtracting the eye velocity twitch at low VOR gain from that obtained at high gain (trace to the right of the box labeled "filter"). Scaling the filtered trace with the box labeled "G" and adding the longer duration output from the modified pathways to the twitch that emanates from the unmodified pathway produces the profile of eye velocity that we measured at high values of VOR gain.

There is an important difference between the effects of motor learning on the eye movements evoked by natural and electrical stimuli. Natural stimuli reveal a difference in the latency of the modified and unmodified pathways. Electrical stimuli revealed differences in the filtering properties of the modified and unmodified pathways, but no consistent differences in latency. We attribute this to differences in the way the two kinds of stimuli activate vestibular afferents. Natural stimuli activate different classes of afferents at different latencies, and the range of latencies across the spectrum of afferents accounts for most of the time delay in the expression of learning (Lisberger and Pavelko 1986). Electrical stimuli activate all afferents with very similar latencies, so that a large time delay in the expression of the learning would not be expected (Bronté-Stewart and Lisberger 1990).

The differences among the effects of motor learning on the eye movements evoked by single current pulses, trains of pulses, and natural vestibular stimuli probably reflect different modes of activation of the same sets of VOR pathways. The magnitude of the changes in VOR gain during motor learning implies that natural vestibular stimuli are transmitted primarily through VOR pathways that are modified. In contrast, learning induces only small and somewhat subtle changes in the eye movements evoked by single electrical pulses. We suspect that electrical stimulation with single pulses activates monosynaptic and disynaptic pathways with the highest efficiency. Thus, the relatively weak contribution of the modified pathways to the eye movements induced by single electrical pulses suggests that the modified VOR pathways are largely polysynaptic. It also suggests that the most direct VOR pathways, including the disynaptic VOR pathway shown in Figure 1, are probably responsible for most of the early twitch in eye velocity and are not modified in association with motor learning. Motor learning had a more pronounced effect on the response to trains of stimuli, presumably reflecting the greater recruitment of indirect pathways and feedback loops.

Our goal is to use electrical stimuli to evaluate the VOR pathways in greater detail and to localize more precisely the site of motor learning in the VOR. The use of discrete stimuli will allow us to establish cause and effect among different neuronal populations by measuring the timing of their responses with high precision. Although firm conclusions will require extensive neural recordings, analysis of the eye movements evoked by electrical stimuli provides some insight into what we might find. For example, the fact that changes in the response to single electrical shocks are apparent at very short latencies suggests that the pathways through the flocculus will have too long a latency to contribute to the early part of the learned response. If we are correct that the site of motor learning is in the vestibular inputs to FTNs in the vestibular nucleus (Lisberger 1988), then it seems likely that the changes are primarily in polysynaptic vestibular inputs to FTNs. However, the presence of monosynaptic vestibular inputs to FTNs (Broussard and Lisberger 1990) could account for the fact that most of our records showed small changes in the peak of the twitch evoked by single shocks.

ACKNOWLEDGMENTS

We are grateful to Dr. Robert Jackler for instruction and guidance in the development of the surgery to implant electrodes in the vestibular apparatus. We thank Terri Pavelko for superb technical assistance. This research was supported by National Institutes of Health grants EY-03878 and K11-EY-00302 and by a Development Award from the McKnight Neuroscience Endowment Fund.

REFERENCES

Bronté-Stewart, H.M. and S.G. Lisberger. 1990. Physiological properties of vestibular afferents participating in the plasticity of the vestibulo-ocular reflex. *Soc. Neurosci. Abstr.* **16:** (in press).

Broussard, D.M. and S.G. Lisberger. 1990. Synaptic inputs to behaviorally characterized neurons in the macaque vestibular nuclei. *Soc. Neurosci. Abstr.* **16:** (in press).

Fuchs, A.F., C.R.S. Kaneko, and C.A. Scudder. 1985. Brainstem control of saccadic eye movements. *Annu. Rev. Neurosci.* **8:** 307.

Goldberg, J.M., C.E. Smith, and C. Fernandez. 1984. Relation between discharge regularity and responses to externally applied galvanic currents in vestibular nerve afferents of the squirrel monkey. *J. Neurophysiol.* **51:** 1236.

Highstein, S.M. 1973. Synaptic linkage in the vestibulo-ocular and cerebello-vestibular pathways to the VIth nucleus in the rabbit. *Exp. Brain Res.* **17:** 301.

Ito, M. 1982. Cerebellar control of the vestibulo-ocular reflex— around the flocculus hypothesis. *Annu. Rev. Neurosci.* **5:** 275.

Judge, S.J., B.J. Richmond, and F.C. Chu. 1980. Implantation of magnetic search coils for measurement of eye position: An improved method. *Vision Res.* **20:** 535.

Keller, E.L. 1978. Gain of the vestibulo-ocular reflex in monkey at high rotational frequencies. *Vision Res.* **18:** 311.

Lisberger, S.G. 1984. The latency of pathways containing the site of motor learning in the monkey vestibulo-ocular reflex. *Science* **225:** 74.

———. 1988. The neural basis for learning of simple motor skills. *Science* **242:** 728.

Lisberger, S.G. and T.A. Pavelko. 1986. Vestibular signals carried by pathways subserving plasticity of the vestibulo-ocular reflex in monkeys. *J. Neurosci.* **6:** 346.

———. 1988. Brain stem neurons in modified pathways for motor learning in the primate vestibulo-ocular reflex. *Science* **242:** 771.

Lisberger, S.G., F.A. Miles, and D.S. Zee. 1984. Signals used to compute errors in the monkey vestibulo-ocular reflex: Possible role of the flocculus. *J. Neurophysiol.* **52:** 1140.

Lisberger, S.G., E.J. Morris, and L. Tychsen. 1987. Visual motion processing and sensory-motor integration for smooth pursuit eye movements. *Annu. Rev. Neurosci.* **10:** 97.

Miles, F.A. and B.E. Eighmy. 1980. Long-term adaptive changes in primate vestibuloocular reflex. I. Behavioral observations. *J. Neurophysiol.* **43:** 1406.

Miles, F.A. and J.H. Fuller. 1974. Adaptive plasticity in the vestibulo-ocular responses of the rhesus monkey. *Brain Res.* **80:** 512.

Miles, F.A. and K. Kawano. 1986. Short-latency ocular following responses of monkey. III. Plasticity. *J. Neurophysiol.* **56:** 1378.

Miles, F.A. and S.G. Lisberger. 1981. Plasticity in the vestibulo-ocular reflex: A new hypothesis. *Annu. Rev. Neurosci.* **4:** 273.

Miles, F.A., D.J. Braltman, and E.M. Dow. 1980. Long-term adaptive changes in primate vestibuloocular reflex. IV. Electrophysiological observation in flocculus of adapted monkeys. *J. Neurophysiol.* **43:** 1477.

Miles, F.A., S.J. Judge, and L.M. Optican. 1987. Optically induced changes in the couplings between vergence and accommodation. *J. Neurosci.* **7:** 2576.

Nelson, R.A. 1982. *Temporal bone surgical dissection manual.* House Ear Institute, Los Angeles, California.

Optican, L.M. and D.A. Robinson. 1980. Cerebellar-dependent adaptive control of primate saccadic system. *J. Neurophysiol.* **44:** 1058.

Optican, L.M., D.S. Zee, and F.C. Chin. 1985. Adaptive response to ocular muscle weakness in human pursuit and saccadic eye movements. *J. Neurophysiol.* **54:** 110.

Precht, W. and R. Baker. 1972. Synaptic organization of the vestibulo-trochlear pathway. *Exp. Brain Res.* **14:** 158.

Robinson, D.A. 1976. Adaptive gain control of the vestibuloocular reflex by the cerebellum. *J. Neurophysiol.* **39:** 954.

————. 1987. The windfalls of technology in the oculomotor system. *Invest. Ophthalmol. Visual Sci.* **28:** 1912.

Stone, L.S. and S.G. Lisberger. 1990. Visual responses of Purkinje cells in the cerebellar flocculus during smooth-pursuit eye movements in monkeys. I. Simple spikes. *J. Neurophysiol.* **63:** 1241.

Watanabe, E. 1984. Neuronal events correlated with long-term adaptation of the horizontal vestibulo-ocular reflex in the primate flocculus. *Brain Res.* **297:** 169.

Wurtz, R.H. 1969. Visual receptive fields of striate cortex neurons in awake monkeys. *J. Neurophysiol.* **32:** 727.

Teaching Neural Networks to Process Temporal Signals for Oculomotor Control

D.B. ARNOLD AND D.A. ROBINSON

Departments of Biomedical Engineering and Ophthalmology, The Johns Hopkins University School of Medicine, Baltimore, Maryland 21205

The vestibulo-ocular reflex moves the eyes in the head whenever the head moves, so that the line of sight does not change in space and images remain relatively stationary on the retina. Visual acuity can thus remain high during movement. Primary vestibular afferents carry the signal of head velocity into the vestibular nuclei. The signal is coded in the modulation of each discharge rate around a steady background rate of about 100 spikes/sec. The motoneurons of the extra-ocular muscles, at the other end, drive the eye with discharge rates, also coded as modulations around a background rate (also about 100 spikes/sec), that are proportional to a combination of desired eye velocity and position: the eye-velocity component overcoming orbital viscosity, the eye-position component counteracting orbital elasticity.

Since the purpose of this reflex is to make eye velocity equal and opposite to head velocity, the sensory head-velocity signal can be reinterpreted as an eye-velocity command and sent directly to the motoneurons to supply the needed component proportional to eye velocity. This is done by second-order vestibular neurons, constituting the central part of the three-neuron arc that forms the skeleton of this reflex. To obtain the needed eye-position command, it is necessary to integrate the eye-velocity signal with respect to time (for review, see Robinson 1989). Schemes involving velocity feedback from muscle spindles can be ruled out, and there is so far no evidence for unique transmitter substances that can make the discharge rate of the post-synaptic cell the time integral of that of the presynaptic axons. Long-term potentiation and depression are multiplicative in action, and, although they involve a form of memory, are not suitable, in the form in which we know them, for building neural networks that integrate in time. A difficulty with schemes involving synapses with clever transmitters is that all the signals in the vestibulo-ocular reflex exist as modulations on a background rate, and it is important that only the modulation be integrated and that the background rate not be integrated. Thus, clever synapses must be clever enough to distinguish between the two.

Lesion studies have located the neural integrator in the bilateral vestibular and prepositus hypoglossi nuclei (Cheron et al. 1986; Cannon and Robinson 1987). Bilateral lesions in this region abolish integrator action. Since the integrator generates the slow phases of vestibular and optokinetic nystagmus, the ramp of smooth pursuit movements, and holds the eye in position after an eccentric saccade, its loss is striking following such lesions. The integrity of the integrator can be measured by the time constant with which it leaks and allows the eye to return to center. Because partial lesions cause partial deterioration of the integrator (decreased time constant), it would appear that the integrator action depends on the collaborative action of many cells; as the connectivity between these cells is gradually lost, so the ability of the network to integrate is gradually lost. This idea is compatible with the idea of positive feedback via systems of reverberating collaterals. If cells excite their neighbors and are excited by them, one has positive feedback, and activity, once started in such a network, would perseverate itself—another way of describing integration.

The most fully developed model of an integrating neural network based on positive feedback was proposed by Cannon et al. (1983). They achieved positive feedback by lateral inhibition. If a cell inhibits its neighbor and is inhibited by that neighbor, the cell excites itself through disinhibition. This arrangement has the natural property of not integrating background rates (they are passed through unmodified) but integrating the push-pull modulation. For best operation, the push and pull signals interdigitate in the network, the signal from the left horizontal canal synapsing on every other cell, that from the right on the remaining cells. This network was robust in that, with 32 neurons, the death of one still allowed reasonable, if not perfect, integration.

Nevertheless, the effect of positive feedback, in engineering terms, is to boost the time constant, τ, of the nerve membrane, taken as 5 msec. The time constant, T, for the whole network can be made as high as 20 sec via the equation T equals $\tau/(1 - W)$, where W is the Fourier transform of the spatial pattern of lateral inhibition. Thus, all the cells and their myriad of synapses go into forming W, and although the loss of a small fraction of them will still permit integration, this global parameter must still be held to a tight tolerance (0.99975). This is not, however, a serious problem. The neural integrator is under the control of motor plasticity. At birth, before vision occurs, the neural integrator in human infants is poor and is still improving its performance (increasing its time constant) at 2 months (Weissman et al. 1989). After lesions that can affect the integrator, there is usually recovery. Thus, some system is monitoring the performance of the integrator, by noting the occurrence of retinal image slip (a signal found in many areas of the brain stem and cerebellum) during head movements and changing synaptic strengths until this source of visual disturbance is acceptably small. In the mature brain, it appears that this function resides in the flocculus, but other experiments suggest that the cerebellum is not required for early development of appropriate brain stem organization. Our theoretical approach does not, at the moment, distinguish between different stages and modalities of motor learning. We note only that integrator function is developed, monitored, and maintained by a neural network that learns through synaptic modification on an hour-to-hour and day-to-day basis. Consequently, we began to develop a model of a neural network that can learn to integrate.

METHODS

Many of the neural networks that have been studied recently (Rumelhart et al. 1986) are designed to learn to recognize spatial input patterns. They do not accept or produce signals that are functions of time. To obtain such signals, one must describe each neuron by a first-order differential equation and then, for n neurons, solve n simultaneous equations. Each neuron responded linearly to the sum of its inputs in proportion to their synaptic weights.

Figure 1 shows the most general basic scheme. All neurons in the pool project to themselves and each other. Each cell receives an input from the left and right semicircular canals and projects to both the left and right motoneurons of a cyclopean eye. Cells may either excite or inhibit their target neurons; Dale's law could be accommodated by inhibitory interneurons if desired. Initially, the synaptic weights are randomized, and all neurons are set to a background discharge rate close to 100 spikes/sec. To train the network, a given synaptic weight is changed by a test amount. The error is the rms difference between the actual output waveform on the motoneuron and the desired waveform (the integral of the input, Fig. 1) integrated over several hundred milliseconds, for both motoneurons. The change in error, for a given weight change divided by the weight change, gives a partial derivative or sensitivity for that synapse. These are measured for every synapse in the network; then a delta rule is applied so that each synaptic weight is changed in proportion to its sensitivity, approximating a steepest-descent method to drive the error to zero.

RESULTS

The learning process almost always converged, and the network learned to integrate. Being linear, it would integrate any function, not just the one on which it was trained. Networks have so far been trained with up to

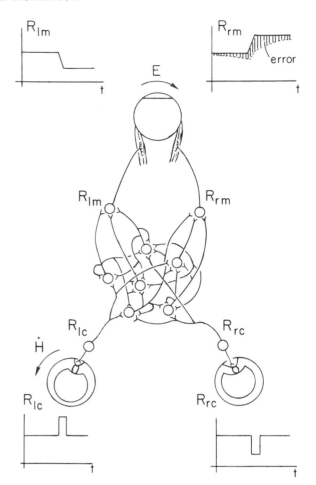

Figure 1. Generic schematic for a neural network to mediate the vestibulo-ocular reflex. R_{lc} and R_{rc} are discharge rates from the left and right semicircular canals that reflect head velocity during a short-duration turn to the left. R_{lm} and R_{rm} are the discharge rates of a left and right motoneuron for a cyclopean eye. ($\dot{H}$) Head velocity; (E) eye position. The schematic suggests that all cells project to all other cells, but the text discusses possible restrictions. The upper right panel helps to visualize the error as the area between the ideal output (solid line) and the actual output (dashed line), although the actual error was the integral of the rms difference.

16 neurons. Loss of one of these neurons causes integrator action to worsen but not disappear. Recovery is much more rapid than initial learning. No solution is unique; rerandomization and relearning produces a different network. The system also learns to recover from unilateral labyrinthectomy.

The system is clearly using positive feedback to achieve integration, but there are so many pathways through the network for a cell to reexcite itself that the final synaptic weights do not show any intuitively obvious pattern. If, as in Figure 1, the motoneuron discharge rates are forced to be the integral of the input, all cells carry the same signal as the output, just at different magnitudes. In some simulations, the motoneuron signal was passed through the oculomotor plant, which can be approximated by a first-order lag, and retinal image slip velocity could then be calculated and used for the error signal. In this arrangement, eye position had to be the integral of the input (head velocity) to eliminate retinal slip. This means that the network not only had to integrate, but also to compensate for the plant dynamics as well by providing the motoneurons with a signal proportional to desired eye velocity (a copy of the input) plus desired eye position (the integral). The network also learned this task, and all the cells in the mature network carried both signals.

It is known that if retinal slip is artificially introduced just at the end of a saccade, one can induce a plastic change in brain stem circuits so that after adaptation (about 10,000 saccades), saccades in the dark are followed by postsaccadic, ocular drifting movements (Kapoula et al. 1989). In this case, the neural network is being asked to produce not just a step in eye movements, but a step followed by a slide. When our model was given this task, it soon learned to produce an impulse response (a saccade) that consisted of a step and a slide so as to continue to drive retinal slip velocity to zero. The main point is that this network is not just learning to integrate, it is learning to produce whatever waveform is necessary, within limits, to eliminate retinal image slip.

To our surprise, although Sherrington's law of reciprocal innervation was imposed on the outputs, these networks did not utilize push-pull behavior in general. Each motoneuron received an input from all n neurons, and all that is necessary is that the sum of these signals, properly weighted, be the desired signal for each motoneuron and, since there are many ways to do this if n is greater than 2, some interneurons end up exciting or inhibiting both motoneurons. Moreover, the interneurons did not always choose to be driven in push-pull by the canals. Some ended up excited or inhibited by both canals. No pathways emerged that could be easily identified as an inhibitory commissural system.

This is contrary to known physiology, which means that the general philosophy, indeed, the main virtue, of neural networks—telling the network what to do but avoiding telling it how to do it—was not working here. Our libertine network persisted in finding unphysiological solutions. The question of push-pullism brings one quickly to the issue of sidedness. A cell being driven in push-pull is excited from the ipsi- (or contra-) side and inhibited from the contra- (or ipsi-) side. Consequently, we divided the cells into left and right and, admitting that much of this wiring was laid down genetically and not by synaptic learning, we forced interneurons to be excited by the ipsilateral canal and inhibited by the contralateral, while exciting contralateral motoneurons and inhibiting ipsilateral motoneurons.

Even with this constraint, the network found solutions in which the position signal was positive for, say, leftward movements, whereas the velocity signal was positive for rightward movements, a phenomenon that has never been reported. If one further constricts the network so that commissural projections are only inhibitory, the incidence of such anomalous cells decreases. All these results are quite preliminary.

DISCUSSION

We had no a priori expectation, just hope, that our method of training the network, which we call the screwdriver approach, would work as consistently as it does. We think that the process resembles postnatal formation of the most basic parts of the oculomotor system, once vision is available, where excitatory and inhibitory synaptic formations are evaluated on a trial and error basis depending on whether retinal image slip increases or decreases. It uses positive feedback through systems of reverberating collaterals of ordinary neurons. Robustness is guaranteed by learning. The model reflects a network of many interconnections, as opposed to exotic synaptic properties, in which larger and larger lesions create a leakier and leakier integrator. Being a learning network, it is not surprising that having once learned how to integrate, it quickly relearns after a lesion, even after a hemilabyrinthectomy.

We are surprised and amused by our need to impose so many constraints on the network to avoid unrealistic neurons. We are amused because in so many neural-network models the units in one, two, or all the layers bear no resemblance to real neurons in the central nervous system. In many applications this is irrelevant; in others, there exists no data base of what real neurons do for comparison. In the vestibulo-ocular reflex, we have a relatively large data base. We know quite well what the input and output neurons do, and we know enough about the interneurons to know what they do not do. Thus, we are in the relatively unique position of, instead of admiring the incredible agility of such networks, rejecting them because they are too fanciful. These networks are amazingly imaginative and will find ingenious ways to get around one's constraints and discover unrealistic solutions.

We are surprised because we have been reduced to hard-wiring much of the network, removing many degrees of freedom. The hard-wired model proposed by Cannon et al. (1983) only raised the question, as most models do, of how many other models would do the same thing. We had hoped to let a freely connected, learning neural network show us other arrangements. Although it did so, most of them were unrealistic, and although our latest version is not hard-wired, it has far more genetic structure than we would have guessed initially. Perhaps we should not be too surprised, considering the venerable age of this reflex, that most of its major tracts are laid down genetically. This is certainly true for the direct, velocity feed-forward pathway from the vestibular nucleus to the motoneurons, but it is more surprising for the neural integrator, where we would have suspected more liberty to get up and do what has to be done. One should, however, bear in mind that our studies here are still very preliminary.

ACKNOWLEDGMENTS

This research was supported by a grant from the Howard Hughes Medical Institute (D.B.A.) and grant

EY-00598 from the National Eye Institute of the National Institutes of Health (D.A.R.). Computer support came from grant EY-01765 and a Whittaker Biomedical Engineering Development Award.

REFERENCES

Cannon, S.C. and D.A. Robinson. 1987. Loss of the neural integrator of the oculomotor system from brain stem lesions in monkey. *J. Neurophysiol.* **57:** 1383.

Cannon, S.C., D.A. Robinson, and S. Shamma. 1983. A proposed neural network for the integrator of the oculomotor system. *Biol. Cybern.* **49:** 127.

Cheron, G., E. Godaux, J.M. Laune, and B. van Derkelen.

1986. Lesions in the cat prepositus: Effects on the vestibulo-ocular reflex and saccades. *J. Physiol.* **372:** 75.

Kapoula, Z., L.M. Optican, and D.A. Robinson. 1989. Visually induced plasticity of postsaccadic ocular drift in normal humans. *J. Neurophysiol.* **61:** 879.

Robinson, D.A. 1989. Integrating with neurons. *Annu. Rev. Neurosci.* **12:** 33.

Rumelhart, D.E., G.E. Hinton, and R.J. Williams. 1986. Learning internal representations by error propagation. In *Parallel distributed processing: Explorations in the microstructure of cognition.* Volume 1: *Foundations* (ed. D.E. Rumelhart and J.L. McClelland), p. 318. MIT Press, Cambridge.

Weissman, B.M., A.O. DiScenna, and R.J. Leigh. 1989. Maturation of the vestibulo-ocular reflex in normal infants during the first 2 months of life. *Neurology* **30:** 534.

Motor-Space Coding in the Central Nervous System

F.A. Mussa-Ivaldi, S.F. Giszter, and E. Bizzi

Department of Brain and Cognitive Sciences, Massachusetts Institute of Technology, Cambridge, Massachusetts 02139

The work presented in this paper is addressed to a motor-control hypothesis known as the "equilibrium-point hypothesis" (Feldman 1974; Bizzi et al. 1984; Hogan 1984). According to this hypothesis, the central nervous system (CNS) takes advantage of the mechanical properties of muscles for solving the complex computational problems related to the control and representation of limb posture and movement.

The equilibrium-point hypothesis is rooted in the observation that muscles are characterized by viscoelastic properties: In other words, when a motor nerve is activated by a train of impulses at a fixed frequency, the force produced by the innervated muscle depends on the length and rate of shortening of the muscle. Under static conditions, the tension developed by the muscle depends on its operating length in a way that is reminiscent of a spring: If we stretch the stimulated muscle, we measure a restoring force that depends on the amount of stretch.

These results were observed in vivo by Rack and Westbury (1969) on the cat's soleus muscle. They described the behavior of the stimulated muscle by presenting a set of "length-tension" curves: For each stimulation frequency, they plotted the tension developed by the muscle at different lengths. These authors took particular care in developing a method of stimulation that was analogous to the natural activation of the motor nerve. Thus, one can conclude from their results that the mechanical effect of the neural input to a muscle is that of selecting a length-tension curve. More recent experiments (Mussa-Ivaldi et al. 1985) have demonstrated that these spring-like muscle properties are directly mirrored in the elastic behavior of the multijoint arm.

Muscles are arranged about the joints in an agonist-antagonist configuration. Hence, a limb's posture is maintained when the torques exerted by opposing muscle groups are equal and opposite. The elastic behavior of the muscles implies that when perturbed by an external force, the limb is displaced by an amount that varies with both the external force and the stiffness of the muscles. When the external force is removed, the limb should return to its original position. Experimental studies of arm movements in monkeys have shown that forearm posture can be seen as an equilibrium point between opposing elastic forces (Bizzi et al. 1976).

The observation that posture is obtained from the interaction between the length-tension properties of opposing muscles led to the equilibrium-point hypoth-

esis. According to this hypothesis (first proposed by Feldman 1974), limb movements result from a shift of the equilibrium point. The studies on the movements of a single joint conducted by Bizzi et al. (1976, 1984), Kelso (1977), and Kelso and Holt (1980) provided the experimental evidence that supports the equilibrium point hypothesis. In particular, Bizzi et al. (1984) demonstrated that the CNS achieves the transition from one arm posture to another by adjusting the relative intensity of neural signals directed to each of the opposing muscles. This result supports the view that a single-joint arm trajectory is generated by neural signals that specify a series of equilibrium positions for the limb.

The equilibrium-point hypothesis has implication both on the control and on the computation of movements. With respect to control, the elastic properties of the muscles provide instantaneous correcting forces when a limb is moved away from the intended trajectory by some external perturbation. With respect to computation, the same elastic properties offer the brain an opportunity to avoid complex dynamical problems.

In particular, we are referring to the problem of deriving the joint torques necessary for producing a desired motion of a limb. This problem requires the solution of an "inverse-dynamics" equation that contains inertial, viscous, and gravitational parameters. According to the equilibrium-point hypothesis, this problem need not be solved explicitly: Once the brain has achieved the ability to represent and control equilibrium postures, it can simply master movements as temporal sequences of such postures. In this context, a representation of inertial, viscous, and gravitational parameters is no longer necessary.

Both the computational value and the control value of the equilibrium-point hypothesis are emphasized when considering multijoint movements. Just to mention one of the peculiar multijoint complexities, the dynamics equations of a multijoint arm are affected by the presence of nonlinear interaction torques between the joints. If the arm has to be driven by an inverse-dynamics computation, these interaction torques could not be neglected without sacrificing the performance (Hollerbach and Flash 1982).

Simulation studies by Flash (1987) have succeeded in reproducing the kinematic features of measured multijoint movements. The simulation implemented the equilibrium-point hypothesis: Hand trajectories were reproduced by moving the equilibrium point on a straight line. At all times, the gap between the equilibrium point and the position of the hand generated an elastic force driving the limb inertia. This very simple computational scheme was sufficient to reproduce fine details of observed trajectories.

Up to this time, however, the experimental evidence for the equilibrium-point hypothesis rested entirely on data derived from psychophysical and behavioral experiments. The goal of the experiment described here was to disclose the neurophysiological underpinnings for the equilibrium-point hypothesis. To this end, we have developed a new experimental paradigm that utilizes spinal frogs.

The spinal frog is a simplified preparation that retains significant multijoint motor abilities (Fukson et al. 1980; Giszter et al. 1989). It is well known, for example, that the spinal frog is capable of generating a coordinated sequence of multijoint hindlimb movements directed to the removal of a noxious stimulus from the skin. This "wiping reflex" requires complex information processing. Thus, the spinal cord must contain circuitry that coordinates the motion of multiple limb segments.

One possible approach to the motor behavior of a spinalized frog consists in postulating that a noxious stimulus on the skin triggers an inverse-dynamics computation within the spinal cord. This computation must ultimately result in the generation of a coordinated pattern of joint torques in the hindlimb. In contrast, according to the equilibrium-point hypothesis, the motion of the hindlimb is generated by the development of neural patterns that specify a sequence of equilibrium points within the limb's workspace (Schotland et al. 1989).

We have addressed these different hypotheses (in a general context rather than examining wiping behavior) by microstimulating the gray matter of spinalized frogs. According to the view that favors inverse dynamics, the activation of a region in the spinal gray is expected to generate a pattern of joint torques. These torques need not define an equilibrium point within the workspace. In fact, for such an equilibrium to occur, it would be necessary that the torques induced in all the joints change from flexion to extension within the range of motion of the limb.

Alternatively, there is a strictly necessary condition for the equilibrium-point hypothesis to be plausible: One must be able to induce a stable equilibrium of the leg within its range of action by activating the spinal gray. Furthermore, the equilibrium-point hypothesis would also imply that a smooth temporal development of neural patterns corresponds to a gradual movement of the equilibrium point.

Our results support the equilibrium-point hypothesis. The stimulation of the premotor layers in the gray matter consistently generated an equilibrium point. Furthermore, this neurally defined equilibrium followed a smooth trajectory during the development of the induced neuromuscular activities. Taken together, these results provide the first neurophysiological evidence for the equilibrium-point hypothesis.

MATERIALS AND METHODS

Surgical Procedures

We have performed microstimulation experiments on 20 spinalized bullfrogs. All surgeries were performed under standard tricaine anesthesia. The spinal cord was transected at the level of the calamus scriptorius. The tectal and other anterior areas were destroyed. Then, the lumbar spinal cord was exposed by removing the spinal arches of the fourth, fifth, and sixth vertebrae. In the same surgical session, we also implanted electromyographic (EMG) electrodes with bipolar leads in 11 leg muscles. The implanted muscles were as follows: gluteus (GL), vastus externus (VE), vastus internus (VI), rectus anticus (RA), rectus internus (RI), biceps (BI), semimembranosus (SM), gastrocnemius (GA), tibialis anticus (TA), sartorius (SA), and adductor magnus (AD). Here, we have used Ecker's nomenclature; the abbreviation for each muscle is in parentheses.

Stimulation Technique

We elicited motor responses by microstimulating the premotor layers in the gray matter of the spinal cord. We used metal stimulating electrodes with impedances ranging from 1 to 10 MΩ. The electrode was placed at depths ranging from 800 to 1400 μm from the dorsal aspect of the spinal cord. We marked electrode locations using electrolytic lesions (10 μA, 15 sec), then visualized these lesions postmortem by examining 30-μm frozen sections stained with cresyl violet. Each stimulus consisted of a train of current impulses. Typically, the train lasted 300 msec. The biphasic impulses had a duration of 1 msec and a frequency of 40 Hz. The current impulses were delivered by a constant-current, linear response stimulus isolator (manufactured by Bak Electronics Inc.). The peak current amplitude ranged between 1 and 6 μA. We chose the current amplitude so as to elicit measurable mechanical responses while remaining close to the threshold of EMG activations.

Data Recording

For each spinal stimulation, we collected the EMG signals from the implanted muscles and the mechanical force at the ankle. An IBM-compatible PC-386 (manufactured by Dell Co.) was used to trigger the stimulation and the data acquisition. The stimulation train was set to begin after 200 msec from the onset of data collection. Both the EMG and the force recording lasted 1.0 second. However, sampling frequencies were different for EMG and force. The raw EMG signals were sampled at a rate of 1000 samples per second. They were subsequently rectified and filtered off-line with a time constant of 20 msec. All the off-line data processing was carried out on a DEC Vax station II.

To measure the mechanical responses, we attached the right ankle of the frog to a six-axis force transducer (Lord LTS-21OF), as shown in Figure 1. The force

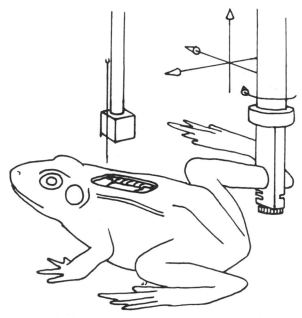

Figure 1. Experimental setup. The stimulating electrode is inserted in the lumbar spinal cord. The right ankle of the spinalized frog is attached to a force transducer. The transducer measures the force and the torque about three orthogonal axes.

transducer was mounted on a two-axis Cartesian manipulator. We determined the location of the frog's ankle (with a resolution of 1 mm) by independently setting the x and y coordinates of this manipulator. The x-y plane corresponded approximately to the horizontal plane. The z-axis was directed upward orthogonally to the x-y plane. The output of the force transducer was a set of three force and three torque components with respect to the x, y, and z axes. The resolution was 0.01 pound (~ 5 gm) for the force components and 0.01 inch-pound for the torque components. The sampling rate for the force signal was 70 Hz. This rate was constrained by the digital communication rate between the sensor controller and the PC. Although we sampled and stored all six force/torque channels, our subsequent analysis was limited to the x and y components of the force vector.

Force Field Analysis

Measurement procedure. The major goal of our experiments was to determine the field of static forces associated with the stimulation of a spinal cord site. To this end, we measured the mechanical response at different ankle locations to the same spinal stimulation. Typically, we recorded the force vectors in a set from 9 to 16 locations forming a regular grid (3×3 or 4×4) over the ankle's workspace. (Here, the term "workspace" is used to indicate the range of movement of the ankle in the horizontal [x-y] plane.) At each grid location, we recorded the force vector elicited by the stimulation of the same spinal-cord locus.

After the mechanical responses had been measured

in all grid locations, the last stimulation was delivered with the ankle placed in the first tested grid location. We then compared the outcome of the last stimulation with the first stimulation. We wish to stress that these two stimulations were delivered at the same spinal site with the ankle at the same grid location. Any visible difference between either the EMG records or the force records in these two stimulations was attributed to some unwanted change in the electrode location or in the state of the preparation. Therefore, if the last and first record did not match, we discarded the whole set of data. We only used for further analysis the data obtained from a stable preparation.

Force field reconstruction. For a single stimulation site, the force vectors measured at the different force locations were considered as samples of a continuous force field. By definition, a force field is a function relating every workspace location to a corresponding force vector. We used the measured force vectors to estimate the force field in a large region of the ankle's workspace. To this end, we implemented the following piecewise linear interpolation procedure (see Fig. 2).

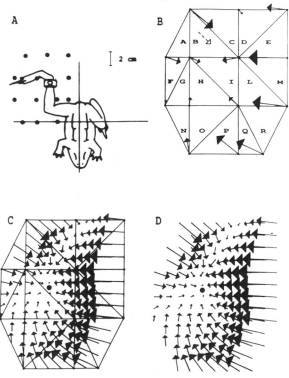

Figure 2. Force field analysis. (*A*) The tested locations of the workspace are shown in reference to the frog's body. (*B*) The tested workspace was partitioned into a set of nonoverlapping triangles (A,B,C,...). The vertices of each triangle were tested workspace locations. The force vectors measured at each location and at the same latency from the onset of the stimulus are displayed as solid arrows. The dashed arrow in triangle B was obtained by linearly interpolating the three force vectors at the vertices of B. (*C*) Interpolated field. The field's equilibrium point is indicated by a filled circle. (*D*) Same field as in *C* without the interpolating triangles. This is the graphic format used for the subsequent illustrations.

1. First, we partitioned the ankle's workspace into a set of nonoverlapping triangles (A,B,C,... in Fig. 2B). The vertices of each triangle were tested grid points. Initially, the triangles were chosen so as to have a small minimal edge length. More recently, we have implemented a Delaunay triangulation algorithm (Preparata and Shamos 1985), which partitions the workspace into triangles as close to equilateral as possible. The two methods gave compatible results with the regular grids that we used in our experiments.

2. Within each triangle, we applied a linear interpolation to the force vectors measured at the corners. Thus, within each interpolation triangle the force components were given as:

$$F_x = a_{1,1}x + a_{1,2}y + a_{1,3}$$
$$F_y = a_{2,1}x + a_{2,2}y + a_{2,3}$$

Note that the above expression has six parameters, $a_{i,j}$. Therefore, the interpolation problem with three data vectors (i.e., six data components) had a unique solution.

3. The above interpolation procedure was applied to the data vector collected at a given latency from the onset of the stimulus. Using data sets obtained at two subsequent latencies, we derived two estimates (or "frames") of the force field generated by a single spinal stimulation. The presence of one or more equilibria was tested for by searching within each interpolation triangle for a location (x_0, y_0) at which F_x and F_y were both zero.

RESULTS

EMG Responses

The EMG responses of 11 hindlimb muscles following the microstimulation of a single spinal cord locus are shown in Figure 3. In this instance, the stimulation of the gray matter induced a response in 6 muscles, while 5 muscles remained silent. The responses in the 6 activated muscles appeared with different latencies from the onset of the stimulus.

One of the main methodological features of our experiments involved placing the ankle in different workspace locations while stimulating the same spinal cord site. As shown in Figure 4, changing the leg's configuration only modestly affected the EMG response to the stimulation. However, we did observe some modulation of the EMG responses as the ankle was placed at different locations. In a few instances, we failed to observe EMG responses in some muscles, especially at locations corresponding to extreme limb flexion or extension. Possibly, these changes in EMG were influenced by different levels of reflex activity generated at different limb configurations.

Mechanical Responses at Single Leg Locations

The mechanical response to a stimulation of the spinal gray matter is shown in Figure 5. We obtained

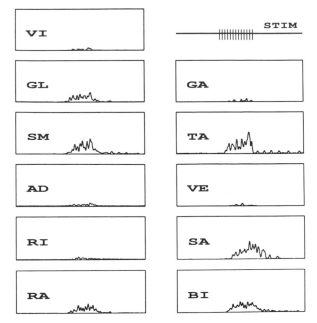

Figure 3. EMG responses to a microstimulation measured in 11 muscles. The trace in the top right corner shows the onset and the duration of the stimulus, which was a train of impulses lasting for 300 msec. The implanted muscles were gluteus (GL), vastus externus (VE), vastus internus (VI), rectus anticus (RA), rectus internus (RI), biceps (BI), semimembranosus (SM), gastrocnemius (GA), tibialis anticus (TA), sartorius (SA), and adductor magnus (AD).

this level of force response with the same stimulation that generated the EMG traces in Figure 3. The six force traces represent, respectively, the x, y, and z components of the force vector at the ankle and the x, y, and z components of the torque at the same point.

Before the onset of the stimulus, each force component was at a resting value that depended on the configuration of the limb. The mechanical response to the stimulation appeared as a change from this resting value after a latency of about 30–50 msec. The mechanical effect of the stimulation sometimes outlasted the duration of the electrical stimulus. After a variable period, the force components returned to their baseline level.

In our force field analysis, we have only considered the x and y components of the force vector. However, Figure 5 indicates that the stimulus elicited a mechanical response also in the other force and torque components.

Force Fields

Up to this point, we have presented our mechanical data as time-varying signals representing the components of a six-dimensional force/torque vector. Now, we restrict our attention to the x-y components of the force, and we introduce an alternative description. At any time, t, we regard our xy force data as a collection of samples of a force field, $\mathbf{F}(\mathbf{r}, t)$. These samples were taken by placing the frog's ankle at a set of xy locations in the horizontal plane. Then, for each sampling time,

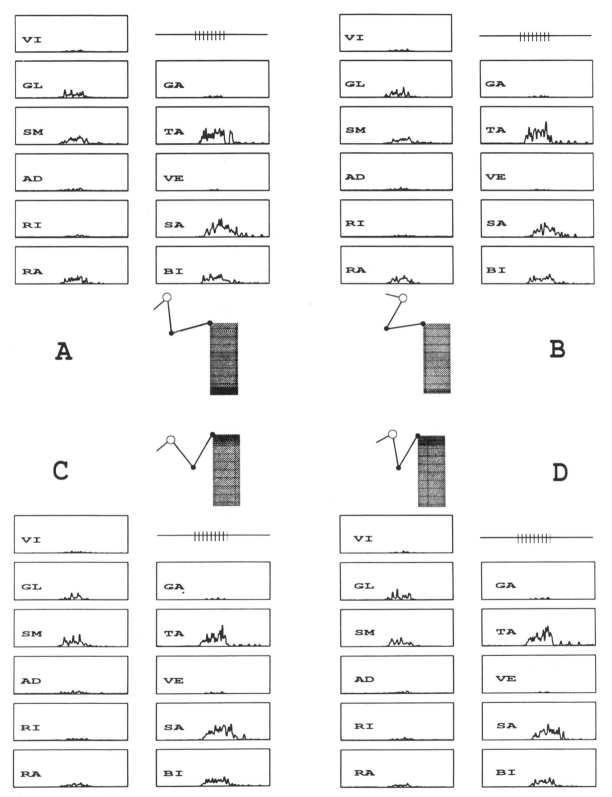

Figure 4. EMG responses with the leg in four different configurations. These responses were obtained with the electrode delivering the same stimulus at the same spinal site. In each panel are shown the same EMG channels and the stimulus as in Fig. 3. The configuration of the right leg with respect to the frog's body is schematically shown in each panel by a stick figure. The unfilled circle indicates the location of the ankle. The filled rectangle indicates the frog's body.

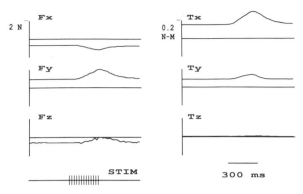

Figure 5. Force (*left*) and torque (*right*) signals measured by the force transducer before, during, and after a stimulation (STIM). Each signal represents a force or a torque component with respect to one of the coordinate axes. Scales are from −2.0 N to +2.0 N for forces, and from −0.2 NM to +0.2 NM for torques.

we applied to the data vectors the linear interpolation algorithm described in the Methods section. In this way, we obtained an estimate of the field within the whole convex polygonal region delimited by the sampling locations (Fig. 6).

Figure 6A shows the "resting" field as measured at an instant of time before the onset of the stimulus. The forces form a pattern that converges to a single location, the "resting equilibrium point." This location is

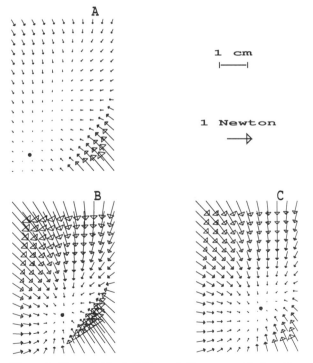

Figure 6. Force fields. (*A*) Force field measured before the onset of the stimulus (passive field). (*B*) Force field measured 460 msec after the onset of a stimulation lasting 300 msec. (*C*) The "active field" obtained by a vector subtraction of force in *A* from the corresponding force in *B*. The filled circle indicates the equilibrium point.

indicated by a filled circle. The force field after 460 msec from the onset of the stimulus is shown in Figure 6B. Here, the mechanical effect of the stimulation has reached its peak. The equilibrium position is now at a different location, and the stiffness about this location has also increased. We defined the "active field" as the difference at each location between the actual force and the resting force (i.e., the force before the stimulation). The active field corresponding to Figure 6B is shown in Figure 6C. The presence of an equilibrium point in this active field indicates that the joint torques induced by the stimulus at the hip and at the knee change from flexion to extension at different ankle locations. Thus, the structure of the total field (and in particular the presence of an equilibrium point) cannot be accounted for by the simple interaction of a constant torque coupled with a passive elastic element, since active torques change sign moving across the workspace.

Temporal Evolution of the Force Fields

After the delivery of a stimulation, each measured force component changed with time. Consequently, the force field as a whole changed with time. The dependency of the force field on time is graphically captured by a sequence of "frames" (Fig. 7). Each frame shows the force field measured at a given latency from the onset of the stimulus. In the first frame (latency = 0), we have the resting force field, that is, the field as it was before the stimulus had produced any effect. The subsequent frames are separated by intervals of 86 msec. They show the effect of the stimulus as a smooth change in the overall pattern of forces. In several instances, we have observed the following sequence of events (as indicated in Fig. 7):

1. After a brief delay from the onset of the stimulus (~50 msec), the pattern of forces began to change and the equilibrium position started to "move" in a given direction (Fig. 7, frames 1–3).
2. Then (Fig. 7, frame 4) the equilibrium position reached a point of maximum displacement within the workspace. This point was maintained for a time interval depending on the stimulation parameters (current, train duration, etc.). At the same time, the field forces reached a maximum amplitude around the equilibrium position, corresponding to a maximum in endpoint stiffness.
3. Finally (Fig. 7, frames 5 and 6), the field forces started to decrease in amplitude and rotate toward their original directions. At the same time, the equilibrium moved back to its resting location. Figure 8 displays a summary of the temporal evolution of the equilibrium point corresponding to the sequence of fields in Figure 7. This sequence of static equilibria is by definition an "equilibrium trajectory": As the neuromuscular activity changes gradually in time (as shown in Fig. 3), the equilibrium undergoes a gradual shift. Furthermore, after the EMG activities have returned to their resting

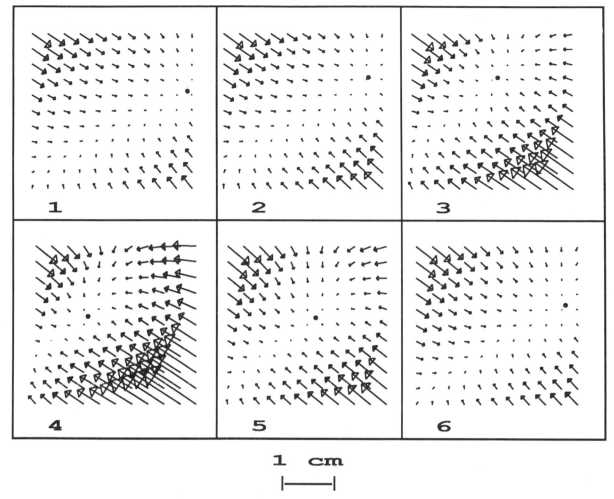

Figure 7. Temporal sequence of fields following the stimulation of a spinal site. The six frames are ordered by increasing latency from the stimulus and are separated by intervals of 86 msec. The filled circle indicates the equilibrium point.

value, the equilibrium returns to the resting location.

A significant feature of our data is the continuity of the equilibrium trajectory at the boundary between two interpolating triangles. This is a remarkable result, since the only pieces of information that enter into our algorithmic derivation of the equilibrium point are three force vectors: These vectors were measured at the vertices of the triangle that includes the equilibrium point. Therefore, when the equilibrium point moves from one triangle to the next, a data vector is suddenly replaced by a new one in the computation. If the sampled force data were not consistent with a smooth vector field, one might expect to observe a sudden jump of the equilibrium location in the transition between interpolating triangles. In contrast, the continuity of the equilibrium trajectory provides further evidence that our force samples truly reflect the structure of a continuous field with single, well-defined equilibrium.

DISCUSSION

Our results show that the stimulation of the premotor layers in the gray matter of the spinal cord produces a field of mechanical forces in the leg. We have measured the effect of these acting on the ankle. This force field has a single equilibrium point that is the point at which the ankle would rest at steady state when constrained to the horizontal plane. The stimulation of a spinal site was generally followed by the activation of a group of leg muscles. For some of the tested muscles, the amount of EMG activity elicited by a given stimulation depended on the position of the leg. However, the qualitative pattern of active and silent muscles was more a characteristic of the stimulation site than of the ankle location. For each ankle location, the force vector produced by a spinal stimulation changed in time. In most instances, this change followed a simple course: Starting from a resting amplitude and direction, the vector changed to a new value and then came back to the resting state. The smooth evolution of each mea-

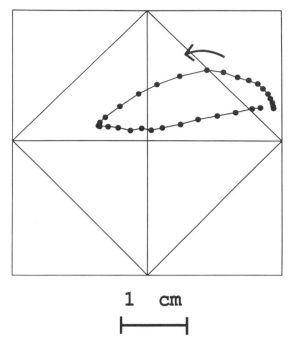

1   cm

Figure 8. Equilibrium-point trajectory following the stimulation of a spinal site. The trajectory corresponds to the sequence shown in Fig. 7. The equilibrium points have been plotted as filled circles every 14 msec. The tessellation triangles are shown. Note the smooth transition of the computed equilibrium over triangle boundaries.

sured force vector corresponded to a gradual transformation of the force field as a whole. In particular, the equilibrium point shifted gradually from the resting site to a new location and then back to the resting site.

Our results show a clear-cut relationship to the equilibrium-point hypothesis. This hypothesis was first proposed by Feldman (1974). The gist of this hypothesis is that the CNS generates movements as a shift of the limb's equilibrium posture—that posture at which the net torque generated by the muscles at the joints is zero. The equilibrium-point hypothesis is strongly rooted in the biomechanics of muscles and, in particular, in their tunable spring-like behavior (Rack and Westbury 1969; Hogan 1984): The isometric force generated by a muscle depends on the level of neuromuscular activity as well as on the length of the muscle. In other words, the state of activation of a muscle does not determine tension alone, but a whole length-tension curve. Experimental work on single-joint movements (Bizzi et al. 1984) has supported the idea that posture control is achieved by the CNS through the choice of agonist and antagonist length-tension curves. These curves determine the equilibrium position for the limb and the stiffness about the joints.

It is significant that this muscle behavior is in conflict with the traditional engineering notion of an "ideal actuator." According to this notion, the output of an ideal actuator—for example, the torque produced by a torque motor—is independent of the operating state (position and velocity). This requirement is analogous to the specification of an ideal voltage source in an

electrical circuit. We believe that there is a deep relationship between the characteristics of the actuators and the computational problems that have been central to the research in robotics. An example of such a problem is the computation of inverse dynamics: To make this computation, one finds the torque that must be applied to the joints to produce a desired motion when the inertial parameters of a manipulator are given. The formulation of this problem assumes implicitly that an ideal force generator is available for translating the output of the computation (a torque) into a control signal. From this perspective, the biological muscle would be a poor actuator.

The above argument can be reversed, however: Since the biological actuators are spring-like, the inverse-dynamics problem does not need to be solved. In fact, the equilibrium-point hypothesis asserts that the CNS can directly express the desired trajectory of a limb as a sequence of equilibrium positions. Then the muscles' spring-like properties transform the error between actual position and desired position of the limb into an elastic restoring force. This force is directed at all times toward the desired position. Such a process does not require any explicit computation of joint torques.

At low speeds and accelerations, viscous and inertial torques are modest and can be regarded as "perturbing torques" that make the arm deviate from the virtual trajectory by an acceptable amount (Flash 1987). As the speed of movement increases, limb inertia and viscosity would be expected to cause larger deviations from the equilibrium trajectory. These deviations may cease to be acceptable, and they can be prevented by increasing the stiffness and by modifying the equilibrium trajectory itself (McIntyre 1990).

The equilibrium-point hypothesis has important implications for the central representation of movement and posture. According to the views based on the explicit representation of inverse dynamics, posture and movements are separate issues: Complex computations are necessary for generating movements, whereas posture is a separate feedback control problem with practically no computational content. In contrast, according to the equilibrium-point hypothesis, the major task for a biological system is that of establishing a map between patterns of neuromuscular activities and limb postures. This map may be considered the primal form of motor coordination upon which rests the ability to generate limb movements.

The experiments described in this paper have demonstrated that the stimulation of a site in the spinal cord generates a particular pattern of EMG activities and a field of elastic forces with a single equilibrium point. The field of elastic forces is a complete characterization of limb posture: It specifies an equilibrium location together with the restoring forces generated by the muscles when the limb is away from the equilibrium. Stimulation of different spinal sites produced different EMG patterns as well as different displacements of the equilibrium point.

In summary, we have observed a clear correspondence between neuromuscular activations and limb postures. We have also observed that movements generated by spinal neural activation are accomplished by a gradual change of the equilibrium position and of the surrounding field of restoring forces. Therefore, we conclude that our experiments provide the first neurophysiological evidence for the equilibrium-point hypothesis in the generation of movement by the spinal cord.

ACKNOWLEDGMENTS

This work was supported by National Institutes of Health grants NS-09343 and AR-26710 and Office of Naval Research grant N-00014/88/K/0372.

REFERENCES

Bizzi, E., A. Polit, and P. Morasso. 1976. Mechanisms underlying achievement of final head position. *J. Neurophysiol.* **39:** 435.

Bizzi, E., N. Accornero, W. Chapple, and N. Hogan. 1984. Posture control and trajectory formation during arm movement. *J. Neurosci.* **4:** 2738.

Feldman, A.G. 1974. Change of muscle length due to shift of the equilibrium point of the muscle-load system. *Biofizika* **19:** 534.

Flash, T. 1987. The control of hand equilibrium trajectories in multi-joint arm movements. *Biol. Cybern.* **57:** 257.

Fukson, O.I., M.B. Berkinblitt, and A.G. Feldman. 1980. The spinal frog takes into account the scheme of its body during the wiping reflex. *Science* **209:** 1291.

Giszter, S.F., J. McIntyre, and E. Bizzi. 1989. Kinematic strategies and sensorimotor transformations in the wiping movements of frogs. *J. Neurophysiol.* **62:** 750.

Hogan, N. 1984. An organizing principle for a class of voluntary movements. *J. Neurosci.* **4:** 2745.

Hollerbach, J.M. and T. Flash. 1982. Dynamic interactions between limb segments during planar arm movement. *Biol. Cybern.* **44:** 67.

Kelso, J.A.S. 1977. Motor control mechanisms underlying human movement reproduction. *J. Exp. Psychol.* **3:** 529.

Kelso, J.A.S. and K.G. Holt. 1980. Exploring a vibratory system analysis of human movement production. *J. Neurophysiol.* **43:** 1183.

McIntyre, J. 1990. "Utilizing elastic system properties for the control of posture and movement." Ph.D. thesis, Massachusetts Institute of Technology, Cambridge.

Mussa-Ivaldi, F.A., N. Hogan, and E. Bizzi. 1985. Neural, mechanical and geometric factors subserving arm posture in humans. *J. Neurosci.* **5:** 2732.

Preparata, F.P. and M.I. Shamos. 1985. *Computational geometry. An introduction.* Springer-Verlag, Heidelberg.

Rack, P.M.H. and D.R. Westbury. 1969. The effects of length and stimulus rate on tension in the isometric cat soleus muscle. *J. Physiol.* **217:** 419.

Schotland J.L., W.A. Lee, and W.Z. Rymer. 1989. Wiping reflex and flexion withdrawal reflexes display different EMG patterns prior to movement onset in the spinalized frog. *Exp. Brain Res.* **78:** 649.

Roles of Proprioceptive Input in the Programming of Arm Trajectories

C. GHEZ,* J. GORDON,† M.F. GHILARDI,* C.N. CHRISTAKOS,* AND S.E. COOPER*

*Center for Neurobiology and Behavior, New York State Psychiatric Institute, †Program in Physical Therapy, College of Physicians & Surgeons, Columbia University, New York, New York 10032

It has been known for more than 100 years that loss or impairment of sensation in our limbs may produce severe disorders of movement and that sensory input plays a critical role in controlling movement. Indeed, the skin, muscles, and joints of our limbs are richly innervated by a variety of sensory receptors that convey proprioceptive information to all levels of the nervous system. What role this input plays in movement control has been a question of recurring interest but remains incompletely understood. In 1895, Mott and Sherrington demonstrated that surgical deafferentation of a monkey's limb produces severe disorders of movement and an unwillingness to use the limb in purposeful action. They therefore concluded that movement initiation requires the support of afferent information and proposed that coordinated movement results from the concatenation of reflex responses. Subsequently, however, it was established that deafferentation does not abolish the capacity to make purposeful movements and that motor performance may be substantially preserved when deafferentation is bilateral or when specific training procedures are used (Munk 1909; Knapp et al. 1963; Taub and Berman 1963; Polit and Bizzi 1979). This indicated that sensory input from the limbs is required neither to initiate movement nor to perform complex motor acts, as originally believed by Sherrington. Rather, the central nervous system makes use of motor programs to direct movements (Keele 1968). Nevertheless, the movements of deafferented monkeys have been repeatedly described as clumsy, inaccurate, and poorly coordinated (Munk 1909; Bossom 1974). Thus, although not necessary for the production of movement, sensory information, particularly from muscle receptors, clearly plays an important role in its control.

To examine the role of proprioceptive input in the control of limb movement, several investigators (Forget and Lamarre 1982, 1983, 1987; Rothwell et al. 1982; Sanes et al. 1985) have examined control of single-joint arm movements in patients with large-fiber sensory neuropathies. In this rare condition, there is degeneration of large afferent fibers, notably those conveying proprioceptive information, with little or no effect on motor fibers. These investigations have shown that such patients have major deficits in the feedback control of movement, i.e., in the ability to correct errors based on information from the moving limb. Thus, patients are neither able to maintain the limb in a fixed position nor to maintain their force at a constant level without visually monitoring the position of the limb or the force applied. They also cannot compensate for unexpected changes in loads encountered during the course of limb movements (Rothwell et al. 1982; Sanes et al. 1985). Errors are reduced, however, when patients are able to watch the limb during movement, so that visual feedback is apparently able to compensate, at least in part, for the loss of proprioceptive information. Lack of cutaneous feedback also readily explains the loss of dexterity in fine movements, such as buttoning clothes or grasping small objects, in which tactile cues are used to guide movement.

In contrast, the mechanisms involved in programming the trajectories of movements before they begin, a process referred to as feedforward control, have appeared largely normal in the deafferented patients of these studies. However, several considerations suggest that, in addition to deficits in feedback control, impairments of feedforward control might also contribute to the motor impairments that occur in these patients. First, Rothwell and colleagues (1982) reported that the learning of new and complex tasks, such as driving an unfamiliar automobile, was impaired in their deafferented patient. Second, the increased variability and lack of precision in the patterning of muscle contraction in isotonic (Forget and Lamarre 1983, 1987) and isometric tasks (Gordon et al. 1987) suggests an impairment in feedforward control. Third, the apparent absence of deficits in programming trajectories could have resulted from the relative simplicity of the processing required to specify the direction and extent of single-joint as opposed to multijoint movements (Flash 1987; Soechting 1989). The accurate performance of multijoint movements requires the nervous system to transform the spatial coordinates of the target, represented in extrinsic or retinotopic coordinates, into a complex set of commands specified in terms of an intrinsic coordinate system based on the controlled biomechanical variables of the limb (Atkeson 1989; Soechting 1989). In the case of even simple pointing and reaching movements, in which two or more limb segments must be rotated by multiple muscle groups acting in different ways, the task is biomechanically quite complicated. Therefore, it is reasonable to assume that specification of movement parameters requires precise information about the state of the limb prior to movement (Polit and Bizzi 1979; Hasan and Stuart 1988).

In the present studies, we used a multijoint reaching task in which subjects moved a hand-held cursor to different targets on a two-dimensional surface. Subjects did not view the cursor or the targets directly. Rather, target locations and cursor position were displayed on a computer monitor. This allowed us to control the visual information subjects obtained about the position of the arm and the results of their movements. In this paper, we first characterize the alterations in the trajectory of the hand that occur in the absence of proprioceptive input from the limb. We then present evidence that, without sensory input from the limbs, programs for reaching movements fail to compensate for anisotropies in the inertial properties of the arm. Finally, we examine how vision of the limb helps deafferented patients to improve their accuracy. We show that this improvement arises in large part by enabling a feedforward compensation for anisotropies in limb inertia. Some of the results have been reported previously in abstract form (Gordon et al. 1987; Ghez et al. 1988).

METHODS

Subjects. Subjects were four neurologically normal adults (three males and one female, aged 27–41) and three female patients (G.L., 39; M.A., 43; and M.B., 66). The patients had each developed severe large-fiber sensory neuropathies affecting both arms, the trunk, and, to a variable degree, both lower extremities. Onset was gradual, progressing over several months to 2 years. In the two younger patients, the etiology of the disease was unknown, and the disease had not progressed for several years. Both patients had complete loss of position sense in the hand and wrist and could only detect movements of the elbow and shoulders at the extremes of range. Temperature and pain sensation were preserved. Deep tendon reflexes were absent in all muscles of the upper extremities, but muscle strength was normal on clinical examination. The restriction of the neuropathy to large sensory fibers was confirmed by somatosensory evoked potentials, electromyography and nerve conduction studies, and, in one patient, by nerve and muscle biopsy. These two younger patients were intensively studied over a long series of testing sessions, and they became highly practiced in the tasks we asked them to perform. It should also be noted that, although muscle strength was normal, both patients were severely disabled and were unable to successfully perform many activities of daily living, such as dressing, drinking from a cup, or writing. One of the patients was confined to a wheelchair because of her difficulty in balancing. The other, although unsteady, was able to walk independently on a wide base. In the third, older patient we examined, the sensory neuropathy was secondary to a carcinoma of the lung. In this patient, sensory deficits were less severe at the shoulder and elbow. Nevertheless, this patient was also severely impaired in functional activities, and her deficits in our experiments were qual-

itatively similar to those of the other two. We were only able to examine this patient in one session.

Apparatus and tasks. Subjects were seated facing the screen of a computer (17 cm × 12 cm, Macintosh SE, Apple Computer) and moved a hand-held cursor on a digitizing tablet (42 cm × 30 cm, Numonics Corp.) with their dominant hand. The position of the cursor on the tablet (x and y coordinates) was sampled by the computer at 200 Hz and displayed on the computer screen as a cursor with the shape of a crosshair. The ratio of cursor movement on the tablet to cursor movement on the screen was approximately 2.4 to 1. In most experiments, the tablet was positioned at waist level, so that the upper arm was approximately vertical and the elbow was flexed at about 90°. In some experiments, to facilitate theoretical analysis and computer simulations, the tablet was positioned at shoulder level so that the entire arm moved in a horizontal plane. In this position, the subject's upper arm was supported by a sling and cable hanging from the ceiling. In all experiments described here, the tablet was directly in front of the subject, so that its center was aligned with the midsagittal plane of the subject.

In this paper, we present results from a reaching task, in which subjects were required to make a quick and accurate movement of the cursor from one point to another on the tablet without visual feedback. At the start of a trial, two small circles were displayed on the computer screen, a start circle and a target circle. During the initial alignment phase, subjects monitored their movements on the screen as movement of a crosshair cursor, and they used this feedback to position the cursor in the center of the start circle on the screen. After alignment was achieved, a "go" tone was presented; subjects were told to then move "when ready" and to make a "single, quick, and uncorrected movement" to attempt to reach the target circle. In most experiments, the screen cursor was blanked at the time of presentation of the tone, so that visual information could not be used to correct the movement trajectory. At the end of the movement, the trajectory was displayed to the subject to provide knowledge of results. Subjects were encouraged to try to be as accurate as possible and were provided with a running score of their performance. Targets were typically presented in a variety of locations (from 9 to 24 in different experiments), requiring movements in different directions and of different extents. The order of target presentation was varied in random fashion, and no target was presented twice in succession, to prevent subjects from progressively refining a stereotyped movement strategy for a specific target. In most experiments, vision of the hand and arm was blocked by the combination of a drape attached around the neck and a two-way mirror covering the hand. In some experiments, described below, vision of the hand was allowed either before trials or during trials, by illumination of the hand from underneath the mirror. In addition, in some experiments, subjects were allowed to visually monitor the screen cursor during movement. These manipulations allowed us to assess the roles of different types of visual information in achieving accurate control of movement trajectories.

RESULTS

Deafferented Patients Make Increased Errors in Trajectory and in End Position

In general, subjects with normal sensation and motor control had little difficulty in producing relatively accurate movements to different targets without visual feedback, and the trajectories of their movements were stereotyped in form. Figure 1 shows typical trajectories of one control subject to nine different targets (three directions and three amplitudes). Movements are straight and terminate close to the required target. The precision with which direction is specified is evident from the overlap of paths to targets in the same direction. Since the direction of movement is specified from the very beginning of the trajectory, it must be largely preplanned and thus controlled by a motor program. In addition, movements are terminated cleanly with a stable end position. As illustrated for one patient in Figure 1, however, movements made by deafferented subjects were highly variable and inaccurate. Trajectories in this figure can be seen to be curved and frequently misdirected at their onset. Terminal endpoints are also unstable: Secondary movements and drifts often occur at the termination of the movements. It should be noted that the patients were typically unaware of such drifts and believed that their hand had come to a stable resting position.

Movement accuracy was assessed by characterizing the spatial distributions of endpoints at each of the target locations, as shown in Figure 2A for the control subject and deafferented patient of Figure 1. Movement endpoints here were defined as the point at which velocity reached zero or at which the movement sharply changed direction; thus, terminal drifts were not included. In this figure, each endpoint distribution is surrounded by a contour whose shape was computed using principal-components analysis and a fitting procedure based on the quartiles in the principal and orthogonal axes of the two-dimensional distribution. The fitted contours closely surround most of the points in each distribution and allow assessment of the shapes and sizes of the distributions. In the control subject, endpoint distributions have a characteristic elliptical shape with the long axis aligned close to the average direction of movement (defined using the center of the distribution). Thus, errors in direction are considerably smaller than errors in extent. The deafferented patient, however, shows markedly larger endpoint dispersions, with distributions that are more circular in shape or whose long axis is unrelated to the average direction of movement. The other deafferented patients showed similar distributions. Thus, the variable errors are larger in the patients than in controls. Moreover, errors in direction appear increased disproportionately to errors in extent.

To assess this trend quantitatively across subjects, we measured separately the "on-axis" errors (deviation of each endpoint from the average endpoint along the axis of the average movement direction) and "off-axis" errors (deviation from average endpoint along an axis perpendicular to average movement direction). The ratio of off-axis to on-axis errors then provides a measure of the shape of the endpoint distributions. In control subjects, this ratio varied from 0.3 to 0.4, indicating that the lengths of the endpoint distributions were on average 2.5–3 times larger than the widths. In deafferented subjects, the ratios ranged from 0.6 to 1.2, indicating that their endpoint distributions were more circular. The overall size of the distributions was measured as the average deviation of each endpoint from the average endpoint. Deafferented subjects showed an average deviation that was 2.4 times larger than the average deviations of controls (mean deviation for controls = 1.18 cm, mean for patients = 2.83 cm).

Average velocity profiles for responses to the 30° targets are shown in Figure 2B (direction angle is defined as increasing counterclockwise with 0° at the 3

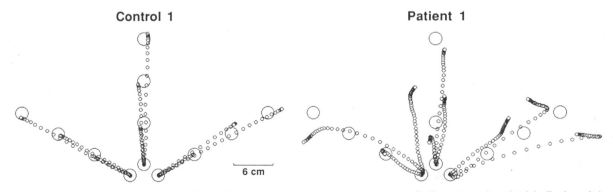

Figure 1. Selected movement paths to each of nine targets made by a control subject (*left*) and a patient (*right*). Each path is plotted with small circles that correspond to *x-y* coordinates in bins spaced 20 msec apart. The large circles indicate starting points and targets. The starting points for movements in each of the three directions are superimposed. Actual starting points for movements in the three directions had a different spatial relationship to each other than that shown.

A

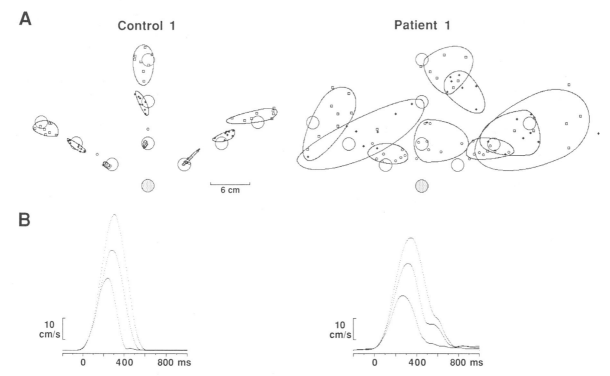

Figure 2. Endpoint distributions (*A*) and average tangential velocities (*B*) of movements made by a control subject (*left*) and a patient (*right*). (*A*) Endpoint distributions show terminations of movements made to nine different targets in three directions. Terminations are measured as locations where hand velocity reached zero or reversed in direction. Endpoints of movements to targets requiring smallest movement extent are designated by circles, medium extents as diamonds, and largest extents as squares. The distribution of endpoints to each target is surrounded by a contour whose orientation is computed by the method of principal components and whose size and shape are based on the interquartile range in each of the major axes. (*B*) Average tangential velocities of responses to the three targets in the 150° direction (requiring movements diagonally to the left). Each trace is the average of eight movements aligned on movement onset.

o'clock position). In general, both control subjects and deafferented patients showed bell-shaped velocity profiles, with increases in peak velocity and peak acceleration as greater distances are reached. These characteristically shaped velocity profiles are typically seen in relatively fast movements (Abend et al. 1982; Hollerbach and Flash 1982) and are taken to indicate that the extent of movement is programmed in advance (Brooks 1974; Ghez 1979).

In both the control subjects and the patients, peak velocities showed systematic differences for movements made in the three directions; responses made to the 30° target consistently reached higher peak velocities than the responses to the 90° and 150° targets (not shown). In parallel with these directional differences in trajectories, directionally dependent errors are evident in the endpoint distributions shown in Figure 2A. In both control subjects and patients, there are systematic errors in direction and extent that depend on the target direction: For example, movements made to the 30° target are typically hypermetric, whereas movements made to the 150° target are hypometric. Moreover, there are errors in direction that are consistent for each of the different target directions. This systematic dependence of extent and direction errors on target direction was observed consistently in all subjects. However,

although these errors were small in controls, they were frequently large in the patients.

Increased Systematic Errors in Deafferented Patients Result from Failure to Compensate for Mechanical Anisotropy

It is known from the work of Hogan and other investigators (Hogan 1985; Mussa-Ivaldi et al. 1985) that the inertial load at the hand differs for movements in different directions. With the arm oriented vertically, the 30° movement is largely carried out by rotating around the long axis of the humerus and thus involves principally the inertia of the forearm, whereas for movements in the 150° direction, the inertias of both upper arm and forearm resist movement. We therefore hypothesized that systematic differences between movements made in different directions could have resulted from a failure to program joint torques in accord with differences in inertia.

We analyzed the effect of the intended direction of movement on trajectory variables and on errors by presenting subjects with targets located in 24 different directions spaced 15° apart, all requiring a movement of the same extent (7.5 cm) from a central starting point. To simplify the mechanical conditions and the computations of the effects of inertia, the subject's arm was now placed in a horizontal plane (see Methods), restricting movement to 2 degrees of freedom (one at the shoulder and one at the elbow).

If subjects fail to compensate for direction-dependent variations in limb inertia, the initial acceleration of the movements should show a systematic dependence on direction. Figure 3 shows vector plots of the average peak accelerations and average movement extents for each of the 24 target directions. Responses of a control subject and of a patient are shown. Three important findings are illustrated in these plots. First, in both controls and patients, the magnitude of peak acceleration varies in an orderly way for movements in different directions. Peak accelerations are highest along an axis oriented at approximately 60°–240°, and they are lowest along the axis perpendicular to this (see dashed line in upper left of Fig. 3: Note that the axis of least inertia varies according to the exact position of the subject's arm). Second, in the patient, this systematic variation in acceleration is carried over into the final movement extents, which are greatest in the same axis in which peak accelerations are largest. The control subject, in contrast, shows only a slight residual effect of the acceleration anisotropy. Third, there are systematic directional biases that also depend on target direction.

The peak accelerations for movements in different directions thus appear to vary inversely with limb inertia. As pointed out by Hogan (1985), the variation in "apparent mass" of the hand takes the form of an ellipse, whose long axis is oriented very close to the long axis of the forearm. This is shown for the conditions of this experiment in Figure 4A: When the subject moves to a target in the 60°–240° axis, the movement is largely carried out by moving the forearm. Relatively little movement of the upper arm is required. This means that the inertial resistance to movement is relatively low in this direction compared to the orthogonal direction, in which the inertias of both upper arm and forearm resist movement.

To gain further insight into whether variations in peak acceleration derive from anisotropy in inertial resistance, we used standard equations for the apparent mass of a two-link manipulator (Hogan 1985; Mussa-Ivaldi et al. 1985) to compute the initial acceleration vectors that would result from a constant impulse of force applied in each of the 24 directions from the initial position of the subject's arm. The predicted peak acceleration vectors in the different directions form an ellipse whose long axis is approximately perpendicular to the long axis of the forearm (Fig. 4B). This vector plot is similar in shape and orientation to the acceleration vector plots of both the control and the patient shown in Figure 3. When these simulated peak accelerations are plotted as a function of initial movement

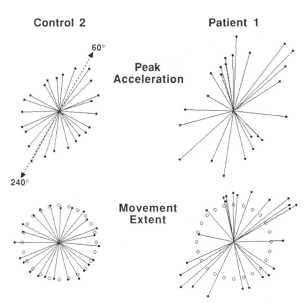

Figure 3. Vector plots of average peak acceleration (*top*) and average movement extent (*bottom*) of a control subject (*left*) and a patient (*right*). Each line represents the average of six trials aimed to a single target. Subjects were given 24 targets separated by 15° intervals (targets are shown as small circles in plots of movement extent). The acceleration vectors for each subject are scaled so that the average vector is the same length as the average extent vectors for that subject. The dashed line in the upper left plot indicates the approximate axis of least inertia.

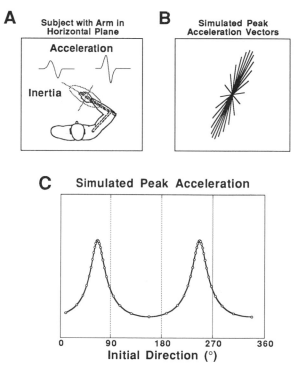

Figure 4. Anisotropy of the arm's inertial field. (*A*) Position of the subject in horizontal arm task. Superimposed ellipse shows calculated inertial field, which resists movements of the hand in different directions. Top part of figure shows average accelerations of a control subject for movements in the axis of highest inertia (*left*) and least inertia (*right*). (*B*) Calculated acceleration vectors for movements with a constant force applied at the hand in each of 24 equally spaced target directions. Compare to actual acceleration vectors in Fig. 3. (*C*) Calculated peak accelerations plotted as a function of initial movement direction. Compare to plots in Fig. 5.

direction (Fig. 4C), the plot shows two relatively sharp maxima and two broad minima. The peaks occur for directions in which inertia is minimal.

Figure 5 presents the measured peak accelerations by target direction and a line fitted to this distribution for the control subject and the patient whose responses were illustrated in Figure 3. As shown here, both control subjects and patients exhibit variations in peak acceleration that are quite similar in shape to the predicted values, with sharp maxima and broad minima close to those of the simulation. Therefore, peak acceleration varies inversely with the inertial resistance to

movement. This indicates that the initial net forces moving the hand, or, equivalently, the programmed joint torques, do not fully compensate for the inertial anisotropy of the limb.

Nevertheless, the control subjects largely compensated for the inertial anisotropy by the end of the movement by modulating movement time. The middle row of Figure 5 shows movement extent as a function of direction in a control subject and a patient, whereas the bottom row shows movement time, also as a function of direction. In the control subject, the plot of movement time is almost a mirror image of the peak acceleration

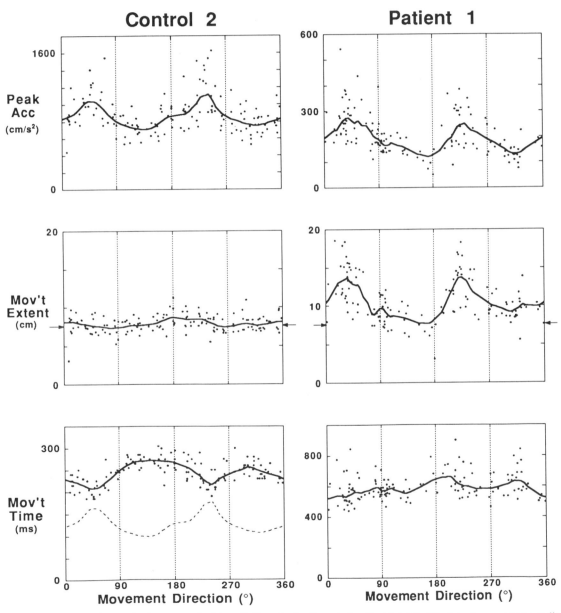

Figure 5. Directional anisotropies in a control subject (*left*) and a deafferented patient (*right*). All plots show movement direction on the horizontal axis. In top row, peak acceleration is plotted; in middle row, movement extent; and in bottom row, movement time is plotted. In all plots, a procedure called LOWESS (locally weighted scatterplot smoother) is used to fit a line to the scatterplots (Cleveland 1979). This procedure averages the data in local regions and gives less weight to outlying data points. The arrows on the sides of the movement extent plots in the middle row show target extent. The dashed line in the movement time plot for the control subject shows the best fitting line for peak acceleration (from the top row) to allow comparison.

plot. Thus, the control subject compensates for high peak accelerations by truncating movement time and for low accelerations by prolonging movement time. In contrast, the patient does not show this compensation, and there is relatively little variation in movement time as a function of direction. As a result, the variation in movement extent parallels the variation in peak acceleration.

In addition to variations in peak acceleration, the elliptical form of the arm's inertial field also results in a disparity between the direction of application of force

and the direction of the resulting acceleration. As can be seen in the simulated acceleration vector plot (Fig. 4B), even though unit forces are applied in 24 equally spaced directions, the directions of the accelerations are not distributed uniformly. There is a higher concentration of accelerations directed toward the long axis of the ellipse, that is, the direction in which inertia is least. Figure 6 shows that in the patient this mechanical anisotropy leads to marked nonuniformities in the distribution of the directions of movement paths. Whereas the control subject shows relatively evenly spread

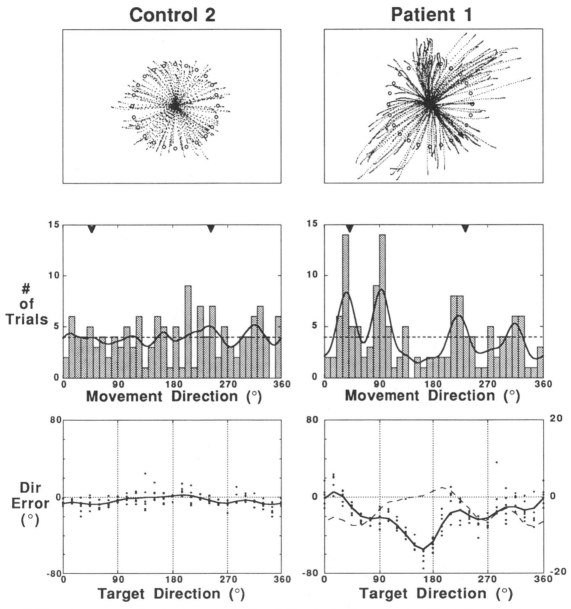

Figure 6. Biases in movement direction in a control subject (*left*) and a deafferented patient (*right*). Top plots show movement paths made to 24 targets spaced 15° apart (small circles indicate target locations). Each path is plotted as a series of dots; the dots represent locations of the hand every 5 msec. Drifts that occur after termination of movement are not shown. Middle plots show histograms of movement direction with local density superimposed. The dashed lines in these plots show expected density for a uniform distribution. Bottom plots show directional error plotted as a function of target direction. LOWESS is used to fit a line to the scatterplots (see Fig. 5). The dashed line in the directional error plot for the patient shows the best fitting line for the control subject (from the plot at left) displayed on a higher scale (see axis labels on right side of plot) to allow comparison.

paths, with only small gaps, the patient shows high densities of paths in some directions and large gaps in other directions. These nonuniformities become more apparent when movement directions are represented as histograms (with local density superimposed), as in the middle row of Figure 6. In this figure, it is apparent that the patient shows particularly high concentrations of movements in the directions in which peak acceleration is highest (indicated by triangles at top of histograms) as well as local concentrations in the directions approximately orthogonal to these. Both patients examined in this task showed qualitatively similar patterns of error. The bottom row of Figure 6 shows the directional errors that are associated with these nonuniformities in the distribution of movement directions. Although the patient makes much larger errors on average than the normal, these errors do not simply result from greater variability in response direction. Rather, the systematic error is much greater in the patient, whereas the variable error is only modestly increased. Therefore, the deafferented patients make exaggerated errors in both extent and direction that are consistent with anisotropies in the inertial field. This suggests that the patients do not adapt the amplitudes and directions of applied forces to the actual mechanical properties of their limbs.

Visual Monitoring of the Limb Reduces Error by Improving Feedforward Control

It is well known that deafferented patients are able to reach for objects a great deal more accurately if they can see their hands. One explanation is that vision provides deafferented patients with feedback information to correct errors that develop in the course of movement. Thus, the difference between the position of the hand and the target could serve as an error signal for the correction of movement trajectory. An alternative explanation (but one that need not exclude the first) is that vision of the arm might improve performance by providing feedforward information to improve the programming of movement itself. Perhaps by updating an internal model of the limb, such information could enable the patient to more accurately specify the commands needed to move his limbs with the appropriate direction and extent. In this section, we analyze the extent to which vision contributes to both feedback and feedforward control, by providing subjects with different forms of visual information.

We first analyzed the effect of two forms of visual information. In one condition (WithFB), subjects were allowed to monitor the cursor on the screen during the movement. In another condition (PreVision), subjects

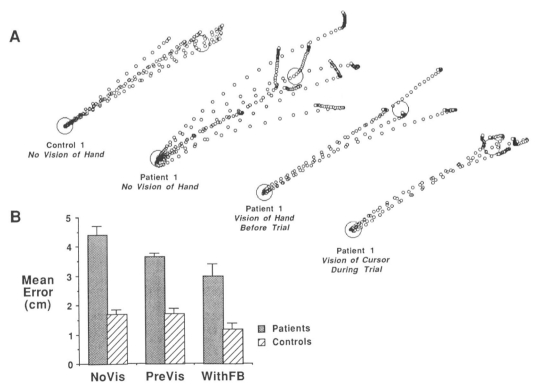

Figure 7. Effect of prior vision of the hand and vision of the cursor on errors in deafferented patients and controls. (*A*) Paths of all movements aimed to a single target are plotted for control subject with no vision (*n* = 8), deafferented patient with no vision (*n* = 8), patient with prior vision of hand (*n* = 4), and patient with vision of cursor on screen (*n* = 4). Each path is plotted as a series of small circles; the circles represent locations of the hand every 20 msec. The large circles show starting points and targets. (*B*) Mean error and standard error of the mean (distance from target to termination of movement) are shown by condition for patients (shaded bars, *n* = 3) and control subjects (hatched bars, *n* = 3).

were allowed to see their arms for a few seconds before each trial. We compared movements made under these two conditions with those in the standard condition of no vision of the arm or cursor (NoVision). For this experiment, we presented targets in three directions with three amplitudes in each direction. Figure 7A shows, as an example, movement paths to one target for a control subject in the NoVision condition and for a patient in all three conditions. PreVision substantially reduces error, primarily by decreasing the variability of the initial direction. Cursor feedback (WithFB) reduces error at both the initiation and the termination of movement. Figure 7B shows the average errors made by three control subjects and three patients in each of these conditions. In the control subjects, prior vision of the arm had little effect on accuracy, whereas cursor feedback produced modest but significant decreases in error. In the patients, on the other hand, both PreVision and cursor feedback led to significant decreases. In fact, in two of the three patients, PreVision was as potent in reducing error as cursor feedback.

These findings indicate that prior vision of the limb alone allows the deafferented patients to improve accuracy through a feedforward mechanism, that is, by improving the initial programming of the movement. This feedforward mechanism was further analyzed in two subjects by presenting them with 24 targets arranged, as before, in a circular array around a common origin. In addition to the blocks of no-vision trials, the subjects were now given blocks in which on alternate trials vision of the hand and arm was either allowed or prevented. In the trials with vision, the patients were able to see their arms in motion. However, since no two successive targets were the same, the visual information from these trials could not be directly used to program the following movements, which were made without vision. Any information gained on the trials with vision could only serve to improve the general rules used to plan subsequent movements or to calibrate an internal model of the limb on which such rules might be based.

The results of this experiment are shown for one patient in Figure 8. The three columns show perform-

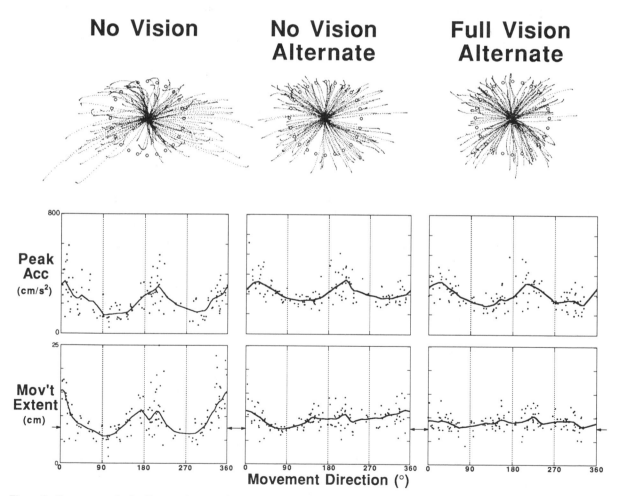

Figure 8. Responses of a deafferented patient (Patient 2) to 24 targets under three conditions: no vision (*left*), no vision alternate (*middle*), and full vision alternate (*right*). No-vision trials were run in separate blocks. No vision alternate and full vision alternate were run in the same blocks; trials with vision of the hand were followed by trials with no vision. Top row shows plots of movement paths (see Fig. 6 for explanation). Middle row shows plots of peak acceleration; bottom row shows plots of movement extent (see Fig. 6 for explanation).

ance in each of the three conditions: no vision, alternate no vision (trials with no vision that followed trials with vision of the arm), and alternate full vision (trials on which vision of the hand was allowed). The top row of plots shows the variation in acceleration as a function of movement direction. The middle row shows the variation in movement extent. The bottom row shows the movement paths to the 24 targets. The two groups of responses made without vision of the arm differ dramatically. In the blocks where the subject could never see her arm, there is again a failure of compensation for inertial anisotropy with fluctuations in movement extent that parallel the fluctuations in peak acceleration. In contrast, in the blocks of trials in which the subject had no vision of the arm but had previously viewed her arm during movement, the modulation in movement extent in different directions is considerably reduced. Finally, it can be seen that vision of the arm during movement provides only modest improvement over vision of the arm on the preceding movement. The other patient showed similar but less dramatic results. We therefore conclude that the major improvement in performance provided by vision during reaching is not, as might otherwise have been suspected, due to the availability of feedback signals. Instead, it results from improvement in the subject's ability to correctly program the forces needed to compensate for the variations in the inertia of the limb.

DISCUSSION

Our studies of reaching movements in normal and deafferented subjects lead to two main conclusions. First, information from the limb is necessary both to accurately program movement trajectory and to specify the patterns of muscle contraction necessary for the subsequent maintenance of posture. Because of the absence of proprioceptive input, deafferented patients are unable to compensate for the inherently non-uniform inertial properties of their limbs, as normals do, and they cannot maintain a steady position of the hand at the end position. Second, visual monitoring of the arm can partially substitute for deficient proprioceptive information. Although allowing for some feedback correction, vision of the limb acts principally by enabling patients to more accurately specify critical parameters of the motor programs to guide subsequent movements. This conclusion is based on the finding that prior vision of the limb, either in a static condition or while it is moving, is as effective as concurrent vision of the cursor in improving accuracy.

The fact that, under normal conditions, trajectories are straight and fairly accurate from their onset indicates that the direction of movement is planned to a substantial degree before the movement begins. Similarly, the normal scaling of initial acceleration to the distance to be traveled shows that movement distance is preprogrammed as well. The large errors in direction and extent of movement made by deafferented patients indicate that, contrary to conclusions derived from studies of single-joint movement, the programming of multijoint movement is critically dependent on proprioceptive information from the limb.

Although the large errors made by deafferented patients appear initially random, analysis of the initial kinematic features of movements shows that these errors are systematic and reflect anisotropy in the inertial field of the arm. A surprising finding of these studies was that anisotropy in limb inertia also influences the initial portions of the trajectories made by normal subjects. The systematic variations we find in peak acceleration with movement direction indicate that the motor program that specifies the trajectory of the limb does not take full account of the inertial anisotropy of the limb. A dramatic finding in the present study was that deafferented patients show severe directional biases that lead to gaps in the distributions of their movement paths. They appear as "motor scotomas," representing areas of the workspace that were rarely entered. Our preliminary evidence is that inertial anisotropy also contributes to these directional biases; however, their mechanism may be more complex.

Vision of the hand and arm at rest prior to movement or vision of the limb's motion in response to the subject's prior voluntary commands can substantially correct deficits in movement programming in deafferented patients. This intermittent information could only have acted through feedforward mechanisms, and not through feedback. These observations suggest that a fundamental role of proprioceptive information from the limb is to allow subjects to program the forces they exert in accord with the complex mechanical properties of their limbs. In deafferented subjects, knowledge of the current state and properties of the limb obtained through vision apparently can substitute for deficient somatosensory input and enable partial compensation for inertial anisotropy.

We propose that proprioceptive input is used by the central nervous system to update an internal representation, or model, of the mechanical properties of the limb. We hypothesize that such a model is used to specify both the general kinematic plan and the adjustments that are necessary to adapt this plan for movements in different directions. When somatosensory information is reduced or absent, as in our patients, the internal representation of the limbs is unstable and degrades with time, forcing patients to rely on visual input. This emphasizes the importance of precise and current information about the state of the limb in the control of movement. The sensory receptors in our muscles and joints, especially the spindles and tendon organs, appear well adapted to provide this information, for example, to enable the brain to take into account the varying inertial loads for movements in different directions. Finally, since the neural processes involved in using this state information to plan movements are distributed throughout many centers of the nervous system, it is likely that the deficits we have encountered in deafferented patients will have analogs in the deficits of patients with central lesions.

ACKNOWLEDGMENTS

Support for this research was provided by grant NS-22713 from the National Institutes of Health. We are indebted to Meenakshi Iyer and Dr. Roberto Bermejo who assisted during early experiments. Dr. Samuel Elias generously gave of his time and expertise in helping us to simulate limb mechanical properties. Dr. Yves Lamarre and Dr. Robert Forget graciously allowed us to study patient G.L., who has been the subject of several previous publications. Finally, we are deeply grateful to patient M.A., whose courage, commitment, and patience have been essential to the success of this project.

REFERENCES

Abend, W., E. Bizzi, and P. Morasso. 1982. Human arm trajectory formation. *Brain* **105**: 331.

Atkeson, C.G. 1989. Learning arm kinematics and dynamics. *Annu. Rev. Neurosci.* **12**: 157.

Bossom, J. 1974. Movement without proprioception. *Brain Res.* **71**: 285.

Brooks, V.B. 1974. Some examples of programmed limb movements. *Brain Res.* **71**: 299.

Cleveland, W.S. 1979. Robust locally weighted regression and smoothing scatterplots. *J. Am. Stat. Assoc.* **74**: 829.

Flash, T. 1987. The control of hand equilibrium trajectories in multi-joint arm movements. *Biol. Cybern.* **57**: 257.

Forget, R. and Y. Lamarre. 1982. Contribution of peripheral feedback to the control of a rapid flexion movement of the forearm in man. *Soc. Neurosci. Abstr.* **8**: 732.

———. 1983. Antagonist muscle activity during rapid flexion of the forearm in a functionally deafferented human subject. *Soc. Neurosci. Abstr.* **9**: 630.

———. 1987. Rapid elbow flexion in the absence of proprioceptive and cutaneous feedback. *Hum. Neurobiol.* **6**: 27.

Ghez, C. 1979. Contributions of central programs to rapid limb movements in the cat. In *Integration in the nervous system* (ed. H. Asanuma and V.J. Wilson), p. 305. Igaku-Shoin, Tokyo.

Ghez, C., R. Bermejo, and J. Gordon. 1988. Impairment in programming of response direction and amplitude in deafferented patients. *Soc. Neurosci. Abstr.* **14**: 953.

Gordon, J., M. Iyer, and C. Ghez. 1987. Impairment of motor programming and trajectory control in a deafferented patient. *Soc. Neurosci. Abstr.* **13**: 352.

Hasan, Z. and D.G. Stuart. 1988. Animal solutions to problems of movement control: The role of proprioceptors. *Annu. Rev. Neurosci.* **11**: 199.

Hogan, N. 1985. The mechanics of multi-joint posture and movement control. *Biol. Cybern.* **52**: 315.

Hollerbach, J.M. and T. Flash. 1982. Dynamic interactions between limb segments during planar arm movement. *Biol. Cybern.* **44**: 67.

Keele, S.W. 1968. Movement control in skilled motor performance. *Psychol. Bull.* **70**: 387.

Knapp, H.D., E. Taub, and A.J. Berman. 1963. Movements made in monkeys with deafferented forelimbs. *Exp. Neurol.* **7**: 305.

Mott, F.W. and C.S. Sherrington. 1895. Experiments upon the influence of sensory nerves upon movement and nutrition of the limbs. *Proc. R. Soc. Lond. B Biol. Sci.* **57**: 481.

Munk, H. 1909, ed. Über die Folgen des Sensibilitätsverlustes der Extremität für deren Motilität. Kap XIII. In *Über die Funktionen von Hirn und Rükenmark, Gessammelte Mitteilungen*, p. 247. Hirschwald, Berlin.

Mussa-Ivaldi, F.A., N. Hogan, and E. Bizzi. 1985. Neural, mechanical, and geometric factors subserving arm posture in humans. *J. Neurosci.* **5**: 2732.

Polit, A. and E. Bizzi. 1979. Characteristics of motor programs underlying arm movements in monkey. *J. Neurophysiol.* **42**: 183.

Rothwell, J.L., M.M. Traub, B.L. Day, J.A. Obeso, P.K. Thomas, and C.D. Marsden. 1982. Manual motor performance in a deafferented man. *Brain* **105**: 515.

Sanes, J.N., K.-H. Mauritz, M.C. Dalakas, and E.V. Evarts. 1985. Motor control in humans with large-fiber sensory neuropathy. *Hum. Neurobiol.* **4**: 101.

Soechting, J.F. 1989. Elements of coordinated arm movements in three-dimensional space. In *Perspectives on the coordination of movement* (ed. S.A. Wallace), p. 47. North-Holland, New York.

Taub, E. and A.J. Berman. 1963. Avoidance conditioning in the absence of relevant proprioceptive and exteroceptive feedback. *J. Comp. Physiol. Psychol.* **56**: 1012.

Neural Coding of the Direction of Reaching and a Comparison with Saccadic Eye Movements

A.P. GEORGOPOULOS

The Philip Bard Laboratories of Neurophysiology, Department of Neuroscience,
The Johns Hopkins University School of Medicine, Baltimore, Maryland 21205

The neural control of movement has captured the imagination for a long time. For example, Descartes (1664) attached a special role to the pineal gland in eye-hand coordination (Fig. 1). It is only recently that knowledge has accumulated concerning the control of arm and eye movements by the central nervous system (CNS). These movements share common characteristics reflected in the neural mechanisms that control them. First, they are vectors whose direction and amplitude need to be specified, and, second, they are implemented by concomitant engagement of several muscles.

The *specification problem* concerns the neural codes by which the direction and amplitude of the movement are generated in the brain. Recent studies have suggested that the specification of movement *direction* involves similar neural codes in both the arm and the eye movement systems: Information concerning the direction of the movement is distributed within a neuronal ensemble, and it is only at the level of the whole ensemble that the direction of movement is uniquely specified. In contrast, the neural mechanisms underlying the specification of movement *amplitude* are less well understood, especially for the arm motor system. This is partly due to the fact that changes in movement amplitude are associated with concomitant changes in other movement parameters, namely, duration and peak velocity (Keele 1981; Robinson 1981). These latter parameters can, in turn, be controlled independently of the amplitude of the movement. Because of these complexities, this review deals only with the CNS mechanisms underlying the specification of the direction of the movement. Moreover, it deals only with kinematics (i.e., the trajectory of the movement); the CNS implementation of arm movement dynamics (i.e., the generation of torques at the shoulder and elbow joints) is poorly understood.

The *implementation problem* concerns the neural mechanisms by which a specified direction and amplitude of an arm or eye movement is translated into patterns of activation of the corresponding muscles. Eye movements are produced by the action of 12 muscles (4 recti and 2 oblique muscles for each eye) which are very tightly coordinated at the brain stem level. In contrast, although reaching movements also involve tight coordination of the motion at elbow and shoulder joints (Soechting and Lacquaniti 1981), the neural substrate(s) of this organization at the spinal level has only

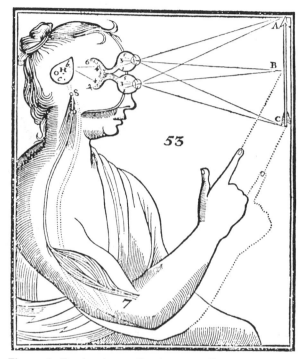

Figure 1. Eye-hand coordination according to Descartes (1664).

recently begun to be elucidated. Accordingly, the discussion of the implementation problem below will be focused on the arm motor system.

REACHING ARM MOVEMENTS

Representation of the Direction of Reaching in the Motor Cortex

Directional tuning of single cells. The activity of single cells in the motor cortex is broadly tuned with respect to the direction of reaching: Cell activity is most intense for reaching in a particular direction (the cell's "preferred direction") and decreases progressively for movements made farther away from this direction (Georgopoulos et al. 1982, 1986; Schwartz et al. 1988). The changes in cell activity relate to the direction and not the endpoint of the reaching movement (Georgopoulos et al. 1985). Quantitatively, the crucial variable on which cell activity depends is the angle formed between the direction of the movement and the cell's preferred direction: The intensity of cell activity is a linear function of the cosine of this angle (Georgopoulos et al. 1982, 1986; Schwartz et al. 1988). The directional tuning of motor cortical cells studied in two- and three-dimensional reaching tasks is illustrated in Figures 2 and 3, respectively. For movements of the same amplitude, the directional tuning equation is

$$d_i(\mathbf{M}) = b_i + k_i \cos\theta_{\mathrm{CiM}} \qquad (1)$$

where $d_i(\mathbf{M})$ is the discharge rate of the ith cell with movement in direction $\mathbf{M}$, b_i and k_i are regression coefficients, and the θ_{CiM} is the angle formed between the direction of movement $\mathbf{M}$ and the cell's preferred direction $\mathbf{C}_i$. Equation 1 holds both for two-dimensional reaching movements performed on a plane (Georgopoulos et al. 1982) and for free three-dimensional reaching movements (Georgopoulos et al. 1986; Schwartz et al. 1988). The preferred directions differ for different cells and are distributed in the whole three-dimensional directional continuum (Fig. 5, top panel).

The activity of a number of cells in motor cortex is also broadly tuned with respect to the direction of static loads (Kalaska et al. 1989); other cells show no tonic activity during load application. It is interesting that the load effect, when present, is statistically additive to that of the movement (Kalaska et al. 1989).

Neuronal population coding of the direction of reaching. The data discussed above indicate that a given cell participates in movements of various directions; from this, it follows that, conversely, a movement in a particular direction will involve the activation of a whole population of cells: How, then, is the direction of reaching represented in a unique fashion in a population of neurons each of which is directionally broadly tuned? To answer this question, it was hypothesized that the motor cortical command for the direction of reaching can be regarded as an ensemble of vectors (Georgopoulos et al. 1983, 1986, 1988). Each vector represents the contribution of a directionally tuned cell. A particular vector points in the cell's preferred direction and has length proportional to the change in cell activity associated with a particular movement direction: Then the vector sum of these weighted cell vectors (the "neuronal population vector") points at or near the direction of the movement (Georgopoulos et al. 1983, 1986, 1988). This is illustrated in Figure 4 for eight two-dimensional reaching movement directions

and in Figure 5 (middle panel) for one three-dimensional reaching direction. Using statistical bootstrapping techniques (Georgopoulos et al. 1988), 95% confidence intervals on the direction of the population vector can be generated; an example is illustrated in Figure 5, bottom panel. Some findings regarding the neuronal population vector are summarized below.

1. *The neuronal population vector predicts the direction of reaching during the reaction time.* Given that the changes in cell activity in the motor cortex precede the onset of movement by approximately 160–180 msec, on the average (Georgopoulos et al. 1982), it is an important finding that the population vector predicts the direction of the upcoming movement in that period during which the movement is being planned (Georgopoulos et al. 1984, 1988). This is illustrated in Figure 6.

2. *The neuronal population vector predicts the direction of reaching during an instructed delay period.* In these experiments, the monkeys were trained to withhold the movement for a period of time after the onset of a visual cue signal and to move later in response to a "go" signal. During this instructed delay period, the population vector in the motor cortex computed every 20 msec gave a reliable signal concerning the direction of the movement that was triggered later for execution (Georgopoulos et al. 1989a). However, it is noteworthy that the length of the population vector (i.e., the strength of the population signal) was smaller than that achieved following the go signal. This was due to two factors. First, during the instructed delay period, significant changes in cell activity were observed in about 50% of the cases, as compared to 85% in the nondelayed task. Second, the change in activity of the cells engaged during the delay was typically stronger following the go signal. These results establish the usefulness of the population vector as a sensitive probe into the directional tendency of the neuronal ensemble, but they also indicate that in the case of an instructed delay period, the signal is weak and is amplified after the go signal.

3. *The neuronal population vector predicts the direction of reaching for movements of different origin.* In these experiments, monkeys made movements that started from different points, were in the same direction, but described parallel trajectories in three-dimensional space. Under these conditions, the population vector in the motor cortex predicted well the direction of the reaching movement (Kettner et

Figure 2. Directional tuning of a cell recorded in the arm area of the motor cortex during two-dimensional reaching. (*Top*) Rasters are impulse activity during five trials of reaching in the directions indicated in the drawing at the center. Short vertical bars indicate the occurrence of an action potential. Rasters are aligned to the onset of movement (M). Longer vertical bars preceding the onset of movement indicate the onset of the target (T); those following the movement indicate, successively, the entrance to the target zone and the delivery of reward. (*Bottom*) Directional tuning curve of the cell illustrated at top. The average frequency of discharge (± S.E.M.) from the onset of the stimulus until the entry to the target window is plotted against the direction of movement. Continuous curve is a cosine function fitted to the data using multiple regression analysis. (Reprinted, with permission, from Georgopoulos et al. 1982; copyright by Society for Neuroscience.)

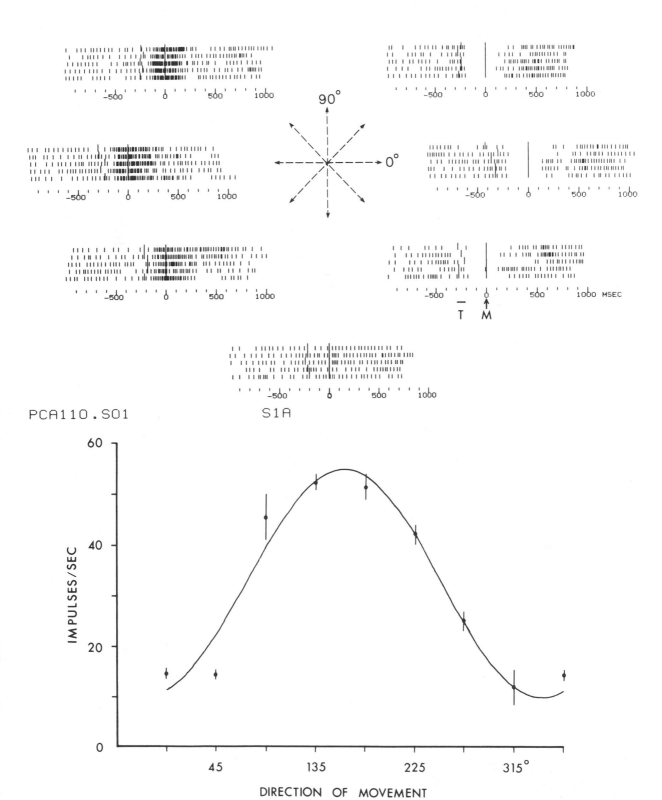

PCA110.S01   S1A

Figure 2. (*See facing page for legend.*)

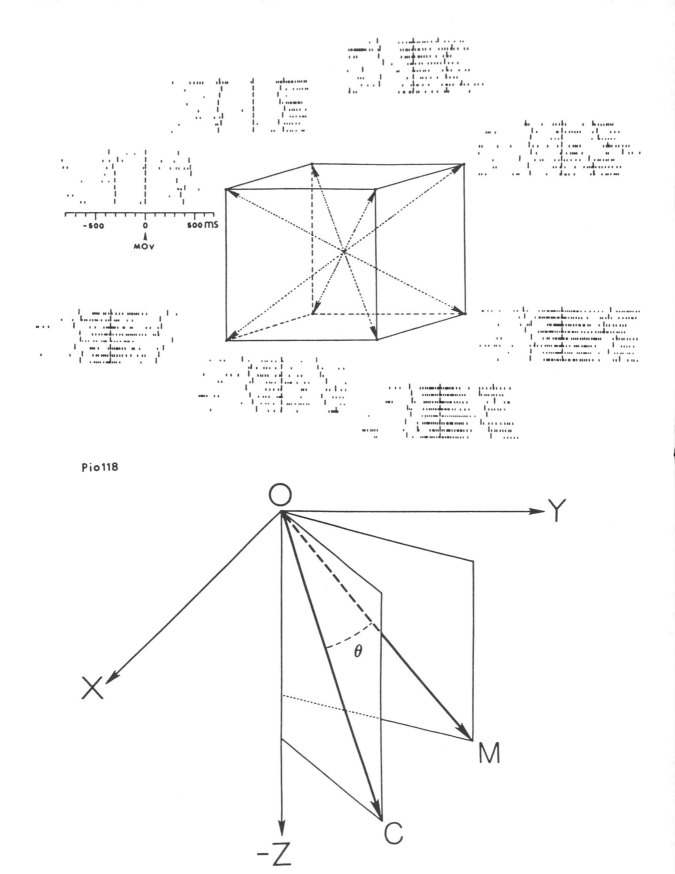

Pio118

Figure 3. Directional tuning of a cell recorded in the arm area of the motor cortex during three-dimensional reaching. (*Top*) Rasters are impulse activity during five trials of reaching in the directions indicated in the drawing at the center. Short vertical bars indicate the occurrence of an action potential. (*Bottom*) Diagram illustrating the general principle of directional tuning. The predicted frequency of cell discharge is a linear function of the cosine of the angle, θ, formed between the direction of movement, **M**, and the cell's preferred direction, **C**. (Reprinted, with permission, from Georgopoulos et al. 1986; copyright by the American Association for the Advancement of Science.)

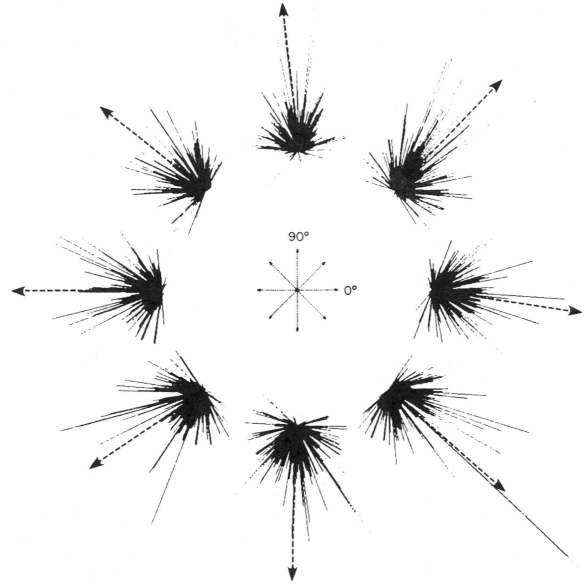

Figure 4. Neuronal population coding of the direction of reaching illustrated for a motor cortical population ($n = 241$ cells) and eight movement directions toward a two-dimensional working surface. Vectorial contributions of single cells (continuous lines) add to yield the population vector (interrupted line). Each cluster represents the same population; the movement directions are shown in the diagram at the center. The population vector points in or near the direction of the movement. (Reprinted, with permission, from Georgopoulos et al. 1983.)

al. 1988; Caminiti et al. 1990b), even if the preferred directions of individual cells shifted systematically in the horizontal plane with different movement origins (Caminiti et al. 1990a).

4. *The direction of reaching is predicted well by neuronal population vectors in the upper and lower cortical layers.* The average absolute angle between the population vector calculated from cells in the upper layers (II and III) and the direction of movement was $4.31° \pm 2.98°$ (mean $\pm$ s.d., $n = 8$ movement directions), compared to $2.32° \pm 2.06°$ for the lower layers (V and VI) (Georgopoulos 1990). This finding suggests that the ensemble operation of the population vector can be realized separately in the

upper and lower layers. This is important because that information can then be distributed to different structures according to the differential projections from the upper and lower layers (Jones and Wise 1977).

5. *The neuronal population vector predicts the movement trajectory in continuous, tracing movements* (Schwartz and Anderson 1989). In this experiment, monkeys were trained to trace smoothly with their index finger sinusoids displayed on a screen, from one end to the other. The direction of the population vectors, calculated every 20 msec along the trajectory, changed throughout the sinusoidal movement, closely matching the smoothly changing direc-

tion of the finger path. Moreover, a neural "image" of the sinusoidal trajectory of the movement was obtained by connecting successive population vectors tip-to-tail. This finding suggests that the length of the population vector carries information concerning the instantaneous velocity of the movement.

6. *The neuronal population coding of the direction of reaching is resistant to loss of cells.* The population coding described above is a distributed code and as such does not depend exclusively on any particular cell. This robustness was evaluated by calculating the population vector from progressively smaller samples of cells randomly selected from the original population (Georgopoulos et al. 1988). Indeed, the direction of the population vector can be reliably estimated from as few as 100–150 cells.

7. *The neuronal population vector transmits directional information comparable to that transmitted by the direction of movement.* The information transmitted by the direction of the population vector was calculated using an information-theoretical analysis and compared to the information transmitted by the direction of two-dimensional reaching movements (Georgopoulos and Massey 1988). It was found that both the neuronal population vector and the reaching movement transmitted comparable amounts of directional information at various levels of input information, but the information transmitted by the population vector was consistently higher than that transmitted by the movement by approximately 0.5 bits.

Implementation of Reaching Movement: Spinal Cord and Reaching

Reaching involves motion at the shoulder and elbow joints. Behaviorally, there is little doubt that these two joints are controlled as one functional unit (Soechting and Lacquaniti 1981) and that this control is separate from that of the wrist (Soechting 1984; Lacquaniti and Soechting 1982). Reaching movements are implemented by the concomitant activation and/or relaxation of a number of muscles acting on the forearm, the upper arm, and the shoulder girdle: Ultimately, movements are produced by the weighted action of these various muscles. Given that motions at the elbow and shoulder joints are tightly coupled in reaching, it is reasonable to suppose that the weighted activation of the muscles involved is "hard-wired" at a subcortical level. Indeed, the motor cortex could be regarded as controlling such a combinatorial arrangement (Georgopoulos 1988). The hard-wiring of these weighted muscle combinations could be achieved by specialized circuits in the spinal cord, such as the C3-C4 propriospinal system. Descending motor commands from the motor cortex and other brain areas influence the proximal arm motoneurons, i.e., those innervating muscles acting on the elbow and/or shoulder, through a set of interneurons located at the C3-C4 spinal segments, i.e.,

above the segments of the proximal motor nuclei. These interneurons ("C3-C4 propriospinal neurons" [Lundberg 1979]) have been studied extensively in the cat. They receive monosynaptic inputs from several supraspinal sources (Illert et al. 1978), including the pyramidal (i.e., corticospinal), and they distribute their axons to several proximal motoneuronal pools (Alstermark et al. 1987). Selective section of the output from these propriospinal neurons to their target motoneurons results in abnormal reaching with normal grasping, and similar effects are observed when the corticospinal input to the propriospinal neurons is removed (Alstermark et al. 1981). These results indicate that the C3-C4 propriospinal system is concerned with the neural integration of the reaching movement at the spinal level and that the motor cortex and other areas control reaching most probably through that system.

SACCADIC EYE MOVEMENTS

Pontine and Mesencephalic Reticular Formation

Neural systems controlling saccadic eye movements at the immediate premotoneuronal level control saccades made in a direction ipsilateral to the location of the system. Moreover, these systems are organized in Cartesian coordinates such that one system relates predominantly to the control of horizontal, and to a lesser degree vertical, saccades, whereas another system controls vertical saccades; the two systems have to work in tandem for the production of oblique saccades. Single cells in both the paramedian pontine reticular formation (PPRF) (Henn and Cohen 1976) and the mesencephalic reticular formation (MRF) (Büttner et al. 1977) are broadly tuned with respect to the direction of eye movement. In fact, for saccades of the same amplitude, the tuning function is a cosine function of the angle between the direction of the eye movement and the cell's preferred direction. However, the preferred directions of cells do not range throughout the directional continuum. In the PPRF, the preferred directions of most cells cluster at or near the horizontal plane (Henn and Cohen 1976; Hepp and Henn 1983); in the MRF, the preferred directions cluster at or near the vertical plane (Büttner et al. 1977). The presumed immediate premotoneuronal cells give a high-frequency burst that precedes the onset of the saccade by approximately 6–12 msec (medium-lead bursters). The axons of these cells are distributed to appropriate groups of eye motoneurons (Strassman et al. 1986).

Superior Colliculus

Electrical stimulation of the superior colliculus elicits saccadic eye movements toward the contralateral (to the stimulated colliculus) field (Robinson 1972). The direction and amplitude of the evoked saccades depend on the collicular locus stimulated. These results led to the hypothesis that saccades of specific direction and amplitude are generated by activating the appropriate

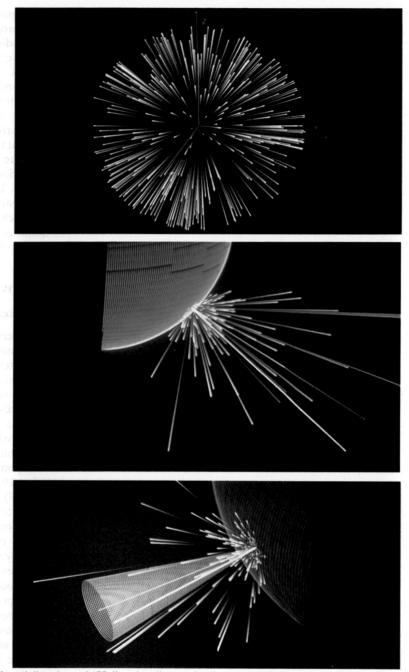

Figure 5. (*Top*) Preferred directions of 475 directionally tuned cells recorded during a three-dimensional reaching task. Lines are vectors of unit length. (Reprinted, with permission, from Schwartz et al. 1988; copyright by the Society for Neuroscience.) (*Middle*) Same population of cells (light blue lines) shaped for a movement in direction indicated by the yellow line. The preferred directions are the same as in top panel, but their length is proportional to the changes in cell activity associated with the particular movement direction illustrated. The direction of the population vector (orange) is close to that of the movement. (Reprinted, with permission, from Georgopoulos et al. 1988; copyright by the Society for Neuroscience.) (*Bottom*) 95% confidence cone for the direction of the population vector (line in the center of the cone); the movement direction (yellow line) is within the cone. (Reprinted, with permission, from Georgopoulos et al. 1988; copyright by the Society for Neuroscience.)

locus on the motor map. However, electrical microstimulation at a point in the colliculus can drive more than 50% of the tectal efferent neurons within an area 3 mm in diameter (McIlwain 1982), which suggests that the effects of microstimulation are brought about by the combined action of the population activated in that area.

The results of recording the activity of single cells pointed in the same direction. Thus, individual cells in the superior colliculus possess *movement fields*, i.e., they discharge in association with movements of certain directions and amplitudes (Schiller and Koerner 1971; Schiller and Stryker 1972; Wurtz and Goldberg 1972; Sparks et al. 1976). In general, the movement fields are

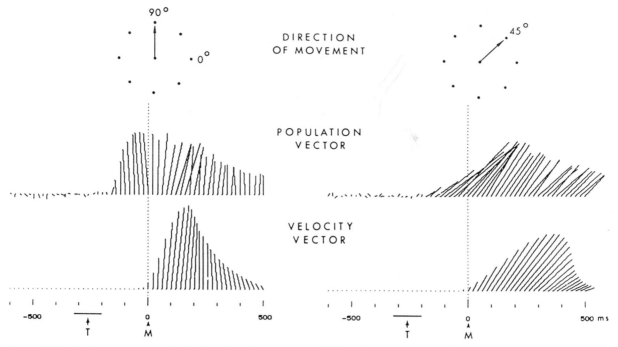

Figure 6. Population vector points in the direction of movement well before the movement begins. The results for two movement directions in the two-dimensional task are illustrated (*top*); the population vector was calculated every 20 msec (*middle*); the average instantaneous (20 msec bin) velocity of the movement is also shown (*bottom*). Before the target onset (T), the population vector is very small in length and its direction varies from moment to moment. Well before the onset of movement (M), it increases in length, and its direction points to the direction of the upcoming movement. This finding suggests that even the earliest inputs to the motor cortex are relevant to the direction of the upcoming movement. (Reprinted, with permission, from Georgopoulos et al. 1984.)

congruent with those observed using microstimulation. However, the changes in cell activity are not sharply tuned with respect to a specific direction and amplitude of a saccade; instead, a particular cell will discharge with various combinations of direction and amplitude (Sparks et al. 1976). Thus, the tuning is broad, and it is broader for cells with movement fields of larger movement amplitudes. It follows from the results above that the coding of the direction and amplitude of saccadic eye movements in the colliculus involves a large population of cells.

Early proposals for *population coding* ("weighted center of gravity") in the superior colliculus (Pitts and McCulloch 1947) were followed by a specific model for a weighted averaging of vectorial contributions to explain the finding that simultaneous stimulation of two points in the superior colliculus resulted in a saccade that was the vector average of the vectorial representation of movement in the two points stimulated, when the strength of electrical stimulation applied was used as the weight at each point (Robinson 1972). The implications of the distributed directional representation of saccadic eye movements in the superior colliculus were discussed (McIlwain 1975) and a weighted vectorial coding was considered (Sparks et al. 1976) in an attempt to explain how the activation of cells with widespread movement fields led to the production of a saccade with a specific direction and amplitude. Cells located in a particular point of the motor map could be

regarded as vectors with direction and amplitude those of the saccades elicited by electrical stimulation at the particular point of the motor map. Then, a particular saccade would be the outcome of vector averaging in this population. This was shown by selective inactivation of particular cell populations in the colliculus using localized injection of a local anesthetic (Lee et al. 1988). The vector-averaging model predicts saccades not only in the appropriate direction, but also of smaller or larger amplitudes, depending on the site inactivated by lidocaine. Indeed, this latter prediction was confirmed.

COMPARISON OF ARM AND EYE CENTRAL MOTOR STRUCTURES

Directional Tuning of Single Cells

Both arm and eye motor structures deal with the specification and control of movements implemented by the concomitant activation of several muscles. Although the muscle coupling is best understood for eye movements, the stereotypy of reaching movements and the tight link between the motions at the shoulder and elbow joints suggest that, under normal conditions, the coordination of arm muscles may also be tightly coupled. This basic similarity may underlie the similar functional properties of single cells (broad tuning) and of cell populations (population coding) in the arm and eye systems in the representation of the direction of movement. In structures related to the control of reaching movements, the directional tuning is best described by a cosine function. This is also the case for the immediate premotor eye movement structures (PPRF, MRF). The directional tuning in the superior colliculus is symmetric, but it does not follow a cosine function. Here, the broadness of tuning is a function of movement amplitude: The larger the amplitude, the broader the tuning.

A basic difference in the directional tuning of cells in arm and eye motor structures lies in the distribution of the cells' preferred directions. The preferred directions of cells in eye motor structures point toward the ipsilateral or contralateral field, depending on the structure. This was expected, since eye movement structures control ipsilateral (for example, PPRF) or contralateral (for example, superior colliculus) saccades. The preferred directions are distributed throughout the hemifield in the superior colliculus but cluster around the horizontal or vertical planes in the PPRF and the MRF, respectively. In contrast, the preferred directions of cells in the motor cortex are distributed throughout the directional continuum and without apparent clustering around particular directions.

Unfortunately, there are no studies of C3-C4 propriospinal neurons during reaching by behaving animals. Thus, important information concerning the transformation(s) of motor cortical output by this system is lacking. For example, it is important to know whether this or other subcortical premotor reaching systems are organized in Cartesian (horizontal/vertical) coordinates, as the PPRF/MRF systems. This problem remains to be investigated.

Neuronal Population Coding of Movement Direction in Motor Cortex and Superior Colliculus

The population coding of the direction of arm movements in motor cortex provides accurate information about the direction of movement and is based on the analysis of single-cell data; electrical stimulation of the motor cortex has not yielded a polar motor map, as it has in the superior colliculus. It appears that cells with the same preferred direction may be organized in cortical columns (Georgopoulos et al. 1984). Therefore, it seems that the neuronal population coding of reaching is an intercolumnar operation and is probably performed repeatedly, since cells with the same preferred directions are repeatedly represented in the cortex and are all active during reaching movements.

The neuronal population coding in the superior colliculus resembles but also differs from that in the motor cortex. In both structures, a large population of directionally heterogeneous cells is engaged preceding the initiation of the movement, and each cell is assumed to make a weighted vector contribution to the population operation. However, in the colliculus, unlike the motor cortex, single cells are tuned with respect to both the direction and the amplitude of the saccade, and the

proper vector operation seems to involve vector averaging.

CONCLUDING REMARKS

The purpose of this review was to compare the functional properties of arm and eye motor structures in the central nervous system with respect to the coding of the direction of reaching arm movements and saccadic eye movements. From this viewpoint, the two systems are quite similar, especially in the broad directional tuning of individual cells and the unique coding of this parameter by neuronal populations. Another general similarity between the two systems is that both code movements and neither specifies endpoints. Changes in cell activity recorded in the various motor structures relate to the upcoming movement, i.e., to the vector itself, not to its endpoint. The neural signal for desired final eye position is elusive (for a discussion of this issue, see Scudder 1988), as is the signal for the endpoint of the reaching movement (Georgopoulos et al. 1985; Godschalk et al. 1985; Wise et al. 1986).

A final aspect concerns the fact that the data reviewed above were interpreted mainly in the context of the output of a neural structure. However, at least the initial changes in cell activity must reflect the effects of inputs as well. In more central structures (e.g., motor cortex and frontal eye fields), this "motor intention" could be dissociated from the actual movement. In fact, the visualization of the directional motor intention in the motor cortex was identified in cases of delayed movement (see above).

The fact that the population vector calculated post hoc during the reaction time or during an instructed delay period points in the direction of the upcoming movement has important implications and potentially significant applications for tasks that require spatial transformations, because it provides an accurate and robust monitor of the directional motor intention of a neuronal ensemble as this tendency evolves and changes in time. This feature was utilized to gain an insight into the brain correlates of a mental transformation. The task required the making of two-dimensional reaching movements in a direction that was at an angle from a stimulus direction. Under these conditions, the reaction time of human subjects increases in a linear fashion with the angle (Georgopoulos and Massey 1987), suggesting that a mental rotation from the stimulus direction to the movement direction might underlie performance in this task. This hypothesis could be tested because the directions above could be visualized as the neuronal population vector. Indeed, recordings in the motor cortex of monkeys revealed that the neuronal population vector pointed first in the direction of the stimulus and then rotated gradually (like the hand of a clock) to point in the direction of the movement (Georgopoulos et al. 1989b) (Fig. 7). These findings provide evidence for the mental rotation hypothesis above and underscore the usefulness of the population analysis in general and the population vec-

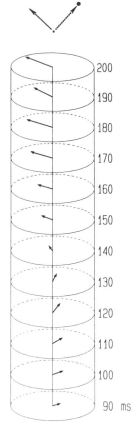

Figure 7. Rotation of the neuronal population vector during the reaction time in a task that required an angular transformation of movement direction. A monkey was trained to move a handle in a direction perpendicular and counterclockwise from a direction indicated by a stimulus. In the case illustrated here, the stimulus direction (around 2 o'clock) and the movement direction (around 10 o'clock) are indicated by the interrupted and continuous lines at the top. The population vector in the two-dimensional space is shown for successive time frames beginning 90 msec after stimulus onset. Notice its rotation counterclockwise from the direction of the stimulus to the direction of the movement. (Reprinted, with permission, from Georgopoulos et al. 1989b; copyright by the American Association for the Advancement of Science.)

tor in particular as meaningful tools for analysis and interpretation of brain events related to cognitive motor transformations.

ACKNOWLEDGMENTS

I thank Adonis Moschovakis for critical discussion of the manuscript. This work was supported by U.S. Public Health Service grant NS-17413 and Office of Naval Research contract N-00014-88-K-0751.

REFERENCES

Alstermark, B., H. Kümmel, M.J. Pinter, and B. Tantisira. 1987. Branching and termination of C3-C4 propriospinal neurons in the cervical spinal cord of the cat. *Neurosci. Lett.* **74:** 291.

Alstermark, B., S. Lindstrom, A. Lundberg, and E. Sybirska. 1981. Integration in descending motor pathways controlling the forelimb in the cat. 8. Ascending projection to the lateral reticular nucleus from C3-C4 propriospinal neurones also projecting to forelimb motoneurones. *Exp. Brain Res.* **42:** 282.

Büttner, U., J.A. Büttner-Ennever, and V. Henn. 1977. Vertical eye movement related unit activity in the rostral mesencephalic reticular formation of the alert monkey. *Brain Res.* **130:** 239.

Caminiti, R., P.B. Johnson, and A. Urbano. 1990a. Making of arm movements within different parts of space: Dynamic mechanisms in the primate motor cortex. *J. Neurosci.* **10:** 2039.

Caminiti, R., P.B. Johnson, C. Galli, S. Ferraina, Y. Burnod, and A. Urbano. 1990b. Premotor cortical representation of movement direction. *Soc. Neurosci. Abstr.* (in press).

Descartes, R. 1664. *L'Homme de René Descartes.* Charles Angot, Paris.

Georgopoulos, A.P. 1988. Neural integration of movement: Role of motor cortex in reaching. *FASEB J.* **2:** 2849.

————. 1990. Neurophysiology of reach. In *Attention and performance XIII* (ed. M. Jeannerod), p. 227. Erlbaum, Hillside, New Jersey.

Georgopoulos, A.P. and J.T. Massey. 1987. Cognitive spatial-motor processes. 1. The making of movements at various angles from a stimulus direction. *Exp. Brain Res.* **65:** 361.

————. 1988. Cognitive spatial-motor processes. 2. Information transmitted by the direction of two-dimensional arm movements and by neuronal populations in primate motor cortex and area 5. *Exp. Brain Res.* **69:** 315.

Georgopoulos, A.P., M.D. Crutcher, and A.B. Schwartz. 1989a. Cognitive spatial-motor processes. 3. Motor cortical prediction of movement direction during an instructed delay period. *Exp. Brain Res.* **75:** 183.

Georgopoulos, A.P., J.F. Kalaska, and R. Caminiti. 1985. Relations between two-dimensional arm movements and single cell discharge in motor cortex and area 5: Movement direction versus movement endpoint. *Exp. Brain Res. Suppl.* **10:** 176.

Georgopoulos, A.P., R.E. Kettner, and A.B. Schartz. 1988. Primate motor cortex and free arm movements to visual targets in three-dimensional space. II. Coding of the direction of movement by a neuronal population. *J. Neurosci.* **8:** 2928.

Georgopoulos, A.P., A.B. Schartz, and R.E. Kettner. 1986. Neuronal population coding of movement direction. *Science* **233:** 1416.

Georgopoulos, A.P., R. Caminiti, J.F. Kalaska, and J.T. Massey. 1983. Spatial coding of movement: A hypothesis concerning the coding of movement direction by motor cortical populations. *Exp. Brain Res. Suppl.* **7:** 327.

Georgopoulos, A.P., J.F. Kalaska, R. Caminiti, and J.T. Massey. 1982. On the relations between the direction of two-dimensional arm movements and cell discharge in primate motor cortex. *J. Neurosci.* **2:** 1527.

Georgopoulos, A.P., J.F. Kalaska, M.D. Crutcher, R. Caminiti, and J.T. Massey. 1984. The representation of movement direction in the motor cortex: Single cell and population studies. In *Dynamic aspects of neocortical function* (ed. G.M. Edelman et al.), p. 501. John Wiley, New York.

Georgopoulos, A.P., J. Lurito, M. Petrides, A.B. Schwartz, and J.T. Massey. 1989b. Mental rotation of the neuronal population vector. *Science* **243:** 234.

Godschalk, M., R.N. Lemon, H.G.J.M. Kuypers, and J. van der Steen. 1985. The involvement of monkey premotor cortex neurones in preparation of visually cued arm movements. *Behav. Brain Res.* **18:** 143.

Henn, V. and B. Cohen. 1976. Coding of information about rapid eye movements in the pontine reticular formation of alert monkeys. *Brain Res.* **108:** 307.

Hepp, K. and V. Henn. 1983. Spatio-temporal recording of rapid eye movement signals in the monkey paramedian pontine reticular formation (PPRF). *Exp. Brain Res.* **52:** 105.

Illert, M., A. Lundberg, Y. Padel, and R. Tanaka. 1978. Integration in descending motor pathways controlling the forelimb in the cat. 5. Properties of and monosynaptic excitatory convergence on C3-C4 propriospinal neurones. *Exp. Brain Res.* **33**: 101.

Jones, E.G. and S.P. Wise. 1977. Size, laminar and columnar distribution of efferent cells in the sensory-motor cortex of monkeys. *J. Comp. Neurol.* **175**: 391.

Kalaska, J.F., D.A.D. Cohen, M.L. Hyde, and M. Proud'-Homme. 1989. A comparison of movement direction-related versus load direction-related activity in primate motor cortex, using a two-dimensional reaching task. *J. Neurosci.* **9**: 2080.

Kelle, S.W. 1981. Behavioral analysis of movement. In *Handbook of physiology. The nervous system II* (ed. J.M. Brookhart and V.B. Mountcastle), p. 1391. American Physiological Society, Bethesda.

Kettner, R.E., A.B. Schwartz, and A.P. Georgopoulos. 1988. Primate motor cortex and free arm movements to visual targets in three-dimensional space. III. Positional gradients and population coding of movement direction from various movement origins. *J. Neurosci.* **8**: 2938.

Lacquaniti, F. and J.F. Soechting. 1982. Coordination of arm and wrist motion during a reaching task. *J. Neurosci.* **2**: 399.

Lee, C., W.H. Rohrer, and D.L. Sparks. 1988. Population coding of saccadic eye movements by neurons in the superior colliculus. *Nature* **332**: 357.

Lundberg, A. 1979. Integration in a propriospinal motor centre controlling the forelimb in the cat. In *Integration in the nervous system* (ed. H. Asanuma and V.J. Wilson), p. 47. Igaku-Shoin, Tokyo.

McIlwain, J.T. 1975. Visual receptive fields and their images in superior colliculus of the cat. *J. Neurophysiol.* **38**: 219.

———. 1982. Lateral spread of neural excitation during microstimulation in intermediate gray layer of cat's superior colliculus. *J. Neurophysiol.* **47**: 167.

Pitts, W. and W.S. McCulloch. 1947. How we know universals. The perception of auditory and visual forms. *Bull. Math. Biophys.* **9**: 127.

Robinson, D.A. 1972. Eye movements evoked by collicular stimulation in the alert monkey. *Vision Res.* **12**: 1795.

———. 1981. Control of eye movements. In *Handbook of physiology. The nervous system II* (ed. J.M. Brookhart and V.B. Mountcastle), p. 1274. American Physiological Society, Bethesda.

Schiller, P.H. and F. Koerner. 1971. Discharge characteristics of single units in superior colliculus of the alert rhesus monkey. *J. Neurophysiol.* **34**: 920.

Schiller, P.H. and M. Stryker. 1972. Single-unit recording and stimulation in superior colliculus of the alert rhesus monkey. *J. Neurophysiol.* **35**: 915.

Schwartz, A.B. and B.J. Anderson. 1989. Motor cortical images of sinusoidal trajectories. *Soc. Neurosci. Abstr.* **15**: 788.

Schwartz, A.B., R.E. Kettner, and A.P. Georgopoulos. 1988. Primate motor cortex and free arm movements to visual targets in three-dimensional space. I. Relations between single cell discharge and direction of movement. *J. Neurosci.* **8**: 2913.

Scudder, C.A. 1988. A new local feedback model of the saccadic burst generator. *J. Neurophysiol.* **59**: 1455.

Soechting, J.F. 1984. Effect of target size on spatial and temporal characteristics of a pointing movement in man. *Exp. Brain Res.* **54**: 121.

Soechting, J.F. and F. Lacquaniti. 1981. Invariant characteristics of a pointing movement in man. *J. Neurosci.* **1**: 710.

Sparks, D.L., R. Holland, and B.L. Guthrie. 1976. Size and distribution of movement fields in the monkey superior colliculus. *Brain Res.* **113**: 21.

Strassman, A., S.M. Highstein, and R.A. Crea. 1986. Anatomy and physiology of saccadic burst neurons in the alert squirrel monkey. I. Excitatory burst neurons. *J. Comp. Neurol.* **249**: 337.

Wise, S.P., M. Weinrich, and K.-H. Mauritz. 1986. Movement-related activity in the premotor cortex of rhesus macaques. *Prog. Brain Res.* **64**: 117.

Wurtz, R.H. and M.E. Goldberg. 1972. Activity of superior colliculus in behaving monkey. III. Cells discharging before eye movements. *J. Neurophysiol.* **35**: 575.

Cortical Neuronal Periodicities and Frequency Discrimination in the Sense of Flutter

V.B. Mountcastle, M.A. Steinmetz,* and R. Romo*
*The Philip Bard Laboratories of Neurophysiology, Department of Neuroscience,
The Johns Hopkins University School of Medicine, Baltimore, Maryland 21205*

Our objective in the present experiments was to determine what differences exist between the two sets of cortical neural activities evoked by two sensory stimuli between which primates can discriminate along some sensory continuum. Particularly, we sought to determine whether the temporal order in which cortical neurons discharge impulses, in response to sensory stimuli, provides signals critical for discriminations. The mechanoreceptive mode of somatic sensibility called flutter vibration, evoked by mechanical sinusoids of 2–500 Hz delivered to the skin, appeared suitable for these purposes, especially the low-frequency range of flutter (2–40 Hz). Monkeys and humans are known to have similar capacities for detecting and discriminating between such stimuli that differ in frequency or amplitude (Lattotte and Mountcastle 1975; Mountcastle et al. 1990). This sensory mode is suitable for the combined behavioral neurophysiological experiments we wished to make. The first-order afferent signals evoked in the range of flutter are known in detail: The frequency of the mechanical sinusoid is signaled by entrained sequences of nerve impulses in a set of large mechanoreceptive afferent fibers with intervals equal to the cycle lengths of the stimuli, over a wide range of stimulus amplitudes (Mountcastle et al. 1972). It is important for our purpose that sequential stimuli of discriminably different frequencies evoke, sequentially, different patterns of activity in the same set of primary afferent fibers, in the same set of linking neurons of the somatic afferent system, and in the same set of postcentral cortical neurons.

The Sense of Flutter Vibration

Humans sense as moving mechanical sinusoids delivered to the skin over a range from 2 Hz to about 500 Hz; higher frequencies are perceived as stationary. Low-frequency stimuli (2–40 Hz) evoke a local fluttering sensation on the skin that gives way at higher frequencies to the deep radiating hum of vibration. The human and monkey frequency-threshold functions are U-shaped and identical, with best frequencies at about 250 Hz. Local skin anesthesia produces a sensory dissociation, leaving the sense of vibration intact, eliminating the sense of flutter (Bing 1905; Cummings 1938; Talbot et al. 1968). Flutter and vibration are also dissociated by masking or adapting stimuli. Stimuli in the low-frequency range (e.g., 30 Hz) desensitize the flutter component, leaving the vibratory component intact, and vice versa (Gescheider 1976; Labs et al. 1978; Gescheider and Verrillo 1979; Gescheider et al. 1983). Masking remains when the stimuli are delivered to different locations on the same or opposite sides of the body (Gescheider and Verrillo 1982; Craig 1976). These observations suggest that masking depends on central mechanisms and that the two afferent channels remain to some degree separate in their central projections.

Peripheral Neural Mechanisms in Flutter Vibration

The glabrous skin of the primate hand is innervated by four classes of large afferent fibers linked to different mechanoreceptors. These are the quickly adapting Pacinian (PC) and Meissner (QA) and the slowly adapting Merkel (SA-I) and Ruffini (SA-II) classes. It is uncertain whether the latter exist in the monkey, and in the human, they are thought not to project to the cerebral cortex. The frequencies of mechanical stimuli delivered to the glabrous skin that primates detect are encoded in periodic sequences of nerve impulses, in the QA afferents with best frequencies at 20–30 Hz, and in the PCs with best frequencies at about 250 Hz (Mountcastle et al. 1972; Johansson and Vallbo 1983). Stimuli at absolute thresholds evoke afferent impulses at varying multiples of the stimulus cycle lengths, constrained to a restricted cycle phase. Increases of stimulus amplitude of 6–8 dB evoke perfectly tuned periodic afferent discharges of one impulse per stimulus cycle. The overlapping frequency ranges of tuning thresholds for the QA and PC afferents blanket the human and monkey frequency-detection functions (Mountcastle et al. 1972). The SA-I afferents are sensitive to low-frequency stimulation, but there are reasons to believe they contribute little to the sense of flutter vibration.

Central Neural Mechanisms in Flutter Vibration

Each of the four postcentral areas (3a, 3b, 1, and 2 from anterior to posterior) contains a somatotopic representation of the body form (Kaas et al. 1979; Nelson

* Present address: Departamento de Neurosciencias, Instituto de Fisiologia Celular, Universidad Nacional Autonoma de Mexico, Mexico, D.F., Mexico.

et al. 1980; Kaas 1983). These representations are thought to be maintained by dynamic mechanisms, for they can be altered by changing peripheral input (Merzenich et al. 1983, 1984, 1987; Jenkins et al. 1990). Areas 3b and 1 receive largely but not exclusively input relayed from cutaneous afferents, and areas 3a and 2 receive largely but not exclusively input from deep afferents. Area 2 also contains a representation of the glabrous skin of the contralateral hand (Iwamura et al. 1980; Darian-Smith 1984 et al.). Neurons within these glabrous skin areas have properties that suggest they are activated by afferent signals in one or another of the sets of first-order mechanoreceptive afferents (Powell and Mountcastle 1959; Mountcastle et al. 1969); we refer to these sets of cortical neurons as the QAs, SAs, and PCs, respectively. The SA and QA neurons of 3b and 1, and the deep neurons of area 2, are arranged in a columnar manner (Powell and Mountcastle 1959; Sur et al. 1980, 1984). There is a preponderance of SA columns in 3b and of QA columns in area 1, but this segregation is only partial. Columns of PC neurons are occasionally observed in areas 3b and 1 (Mountcastle and Powell 1959; Mountcastle et al. 1969).

Monkeys, after removal of the somatic areas of the postcentral gyrus, show initially a marked elevation of flutter thresholds, but with intense postoperative training, they achieve asymptotically thresholds 8–10 dB above normal. In contrast, these same monkeys never regain their preoperative capacity for frequency discriminations, even with prolonged training (LaMotte and Mountcastle 1979). The inference is that an animal with a lesion of the somatic sensory cortex may still learn to recognize an increment in neural activity in his lesioned somatic system, without postcentral cortical processing. However, such a monkey is never able again to differentiate between neural periodicities of different lengths. The latter requires a process that is uniquely intracortical.

In an earlier set of experiments, we examined the capacity of human subjects to make frequency discriminations in the sense of flutter and analyzed the results in the context of decision theory (Mountcastle et al. 1969). A parallel series of experiments employing single flutter stimuli was made in unanesthetized, neuro-muscularly blocked (denervated head) monkeys. It was found that the variance of the presumed sensory events from the first analysis changed in step with variances in the periodicities in the responses of postcentral neurons evoked by similar stimuli, delivered to the monkeys' hands. It was inferred from these covariations that the periodicities in the entrained postcentral activity adequately represent stimulus frequencies, that the periodicities depend on the serial order of impulse intervals, and that differences in the lengths of the periods in sets of evoked activity might serve as the neural discriminanda for frequency in the sense of flutter.

We tested this hypothesis directly in the present experiments by recording the activity of postcentral neurons evoked by mechanical sinusoids delivered to the glabrous skin of the hands of monkeys as they made frequency discriminations.

EXPERIMENTAL PROCEDURES

Primate psychophysics. The three human subjects were members of the laboratory staff. The four monkey subjects lived in $4' \times 4' \times 4'$ cages in a room housing 12–15 monkeys; all were tuberculin- and B-virus-negative. The monkeys sat in restraining chairs during daily 3-hour training-testing sessions and were then returned to living cages. Monkeys were deprived of water during training and testing periods; each earned or was given 30–35 ml water/kg body weight per day and allowed free access to water 1 day each week. Subjects were trained and tested in the discrimination task outlined in Figure 1. Humans sat facing a heavy metal table with left arms restrained in a half-cast arm and finger mold, palm upward. Monkeys sat in restraining chairs placed in a slot in the same table, for them air-suspended, arm and hand similarly placed. Stimuli were delivered to the distal pads of fingers 2, 3, or 4 with a noiseless Chubbuck linear motor stimulator bearing a rounded Lucite probe 1 or 2 mm in diameter. The trial sequence of the passive task of Figure 1 was initiated by the subject; he interrupted a light beam with his right hand when he perceived a step indentation of the skin of the left hand. Monkeys were rewarded for correct identification of the second stimulus as higher or lower in frequency than the first with a drop of liquid. Errors were signaled by an increase in the volume of a masking noise.

Two human subjects were trained and tested in the active form of the task of Figure 1. The subject initiated a trial upon appearance of a go signal by applying the distal pad of the left third finger to a flat circular manipulandum 6 cm in diameter. He was required to maintain force on the manipulandum within a preset range of 70–140 g while awaiting the two successive mechanical oscillations of the manipulandum to indicate the end of the second stimulus by releasing force and to choose the higher or lower frequency of the second stimulus by projecting his hand to one of two target switches. The programmed force windows and the force exerted by the subject were indicated visually with an LED board display.

The details of monkey training are given elsewhere (Mountcastle 1990); training to the liminal discrimination values required about 4 months.

Experimental control sets. The subjective intensity of a mechanical sinusoid delivered to the skin changes with stimulus frequency (Goff 1967; LaMotte and Mountcastle 1975). We determined equal subjective magnitude functions for the set of frequencies used in human subjects by psychophysical measures, and from the results, we constructed frequency-discrimination control sets, used for both human and monkey subjects, in which all stimuli of different frequencies were

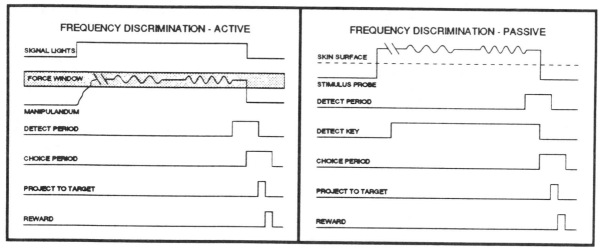

Figure 1. Schematic outlines of the active and passive modes of the frequency discrimination task. Descriptions of psychophysical experiments are made in the text. (Reprinted, with permission, from Mountcastle et al. 1990.)

equated for subjective magnitude. Control experiments described elsewhere (Mountcastle et al. 1990) indicated that our subjects were attending to and discriminating between the frequencies and not the intensities of the stimuli used.

The combined behavioral-neurophysiological experiment. We recorded the electrical signs of the impulse discharges of postcentral cortical neurons as monkeys worked in the passive frequency discrimination task of Figure 1. We adapted to the waking monkey the method of multiple microelectrode recording of Reitboeck (1983a,b) and constructed a matching multichannel data collection and processing system (for details, see Mountcastle et al. 1990; V.B. Mountcastle et al., in prep.). The method allows simultaneous trans-dural recording from seven independently movable microelectrodes that can be arranged in any x-y spatial arrangement desired, constrained by the 300-μm O.D. of the carrier tubes. The Reitboeck microelectrodes are quartz glass filaments 80 μm O.D., whose 30-μm central cores are filled with a tungsten-platinum alloy. The filaments are drawn in a high-temperature, helium-filled chamber, and then ground to the appropriate size, usually 1–2 μm tips with impedance of 3–4 megohms at 1000 Hz. Recordings were repeated in 6-hour daily sessions for many days. The 8-channel data collection system contains for each channel amplifiers, filters, discriminators, and impedance measuring devices, all under microprocessor control. Control of sequences in the behavioral task, data collection, and analysis are accomplished by a system of PDP 84 computers and Microvax workstations linked by Ethernet hardware and DecNet software.

Data analysis. Our initial survey of neural data included examination of impulse replica plots and of poststimulus time and cycle histograms, synchronized on stimulus events. These provided objective evidence

of the functional properties of each cortical neuron studied. Cyclic entrainment of neuronal responses was evaluated with expectation (autocorrelation) and renewal density functions were derived from impulse interval train data.

Fourier analysis was used to provide measures of the strength and periodicity of the rhythmic entrainment of cortical neuronal responses (Bloomfield 1976; Bracewell 1986). Unsmoothed frequency histograms were constructed from the neural discharges recorded during the 1-sec stimulus periods, using 1-msec bins averaged over repeated trials. Fast Fourier transforms of the frequency counts provided the periodogram ordinate values from 1 Hz through 500 Hz, in 1-Hz steps. The spectral density (power fraction) at individual frequencies was expressed as the ratio of the periodogram ordinate value at that frequency to the sum of all ordinate values. Statistical significance of individual power fractions was tested using Shimshoni's rank order modification of Fisher's significance test for harmonic analysis (Fisher 1929; Shimshoni 1971).

Psychometric functions were obtained for the human and monkey discriminations between vibratory stimuli of different frequency by plotting the percent of comparison stimuli called higher in frequency than the base stimuli as a function of the frequency of the comparison stimulus. Logistic functions of the form $f(x) = 100/(1 + e^{**}[x + b])$ were fitted to the data using an iterative method for least-squares solution (Draper and Smith 1981). All regressions were shown to be significant by analysis of variance ($p < 0.05$). Difference limens (DLs) were computed as one-half the difference between the stimulus frequency called higher than the standard on 75% of the trials and that called higher on 25% of the trials. These values were read directly from the fitted functions and expressed in terms of cycle lengths in milliseconds, and Weber fractions were calculated from them.

RESULTS

Primate Capacity for Frequency Discrimination in the Sense of Flutter

We first tested an experienced human subject, a male aged 34 years, in both the active and the passive modes of the discrimination task outlined in Figure 1. He achieved Weber fractions when working in the passive mode of 5.4% at 30 Hz base frequency, 6.5% at 40 Hz, 7% at 60 Hz, and 9.5% at 100 Hz. His Weber fractions when working in the active mode were 4% at 30 Hz, 4% at 40 Hz, 7% at 60 Hz, and 4% at 100 Hz. Although his performance was somewhat better in the active mode of the discrimination task, than in the passive mode, we chose to study other human subjects and our monkey subjects in the passive mode, for we had found great difficulty in earlier experiments on detection in flutter vibration in adapting the active mode of the task to the combined experiments we wished to execute.

The graphs to the left of Figure 2 show psychometric functions fitted to the pooled results obtained in study of three male subjects aged 25, 34, and 71 years, working in the passive form of the task, with 50 or more trials per point. The Weber fractions for the averages are 17% at 20 Hz, 7% at 30 Hz, and 7% at 40 Hz. We also tested these same subjects in the range of Pacinian vibration, where they achieved averaged Weber fractions of 10% at 60 Hz, 11% at 100 Hz, and 7% at 200 Hz. Thus, we found no decline in the discriminatory capacity with increases in the range of frequencies tested, as Goff (1967) did when working under different experimental circumstances.

The graphs to the right of Figure 2 show psychometric functions obtained from the performance of

monkey 109 as he worked in the passive task in the neurophysiological experiments described below. His Weber fractions were 15% at 20 Hz (180 trials per point), 12% at 30 Hz (100 trials per point), and 7.5% at 40 Hz (30 trials per point). His performance in the experimental situation was comparable to the average of our three human subjects. This same monkey performed somewhat better in the preexperimental testing period, with Weber fractions of 7%, 5.5%, and 4.3% at 20, 30, and 40 Hz, respectively. A second monkey, 108, performed as well in the preexperimental period, with Weber fractions of 7%, 5.5%, and 4.2% at 20, 30, and 40 Hz, respectively.

We conclude that humans and monkeys have virtually identical capacities for frequency discrimination in the frequency range of the sense of flutter and that the discriminatory capacity does not decline as the test frequencies are raised into the Pacinian range of vibration.

Neurophysiological Experiments

Data base. The neurophysiological results presented below were obtained in four monkeys, in experiments carried out using a variety of protocols for study of different aspects of somesthesis. We abstract from the data base of more than 900 postcentral cortical neurons those studied with frequency-discrimination stimulus control sets. As monkey 109 performed the passive discrimination task of Figure 1, 150 postcentral neurons were studied; 41 of these same cells were also studied while this alert animal performed no task. We define this latter as the irrelevant stimulus condition, for in it the stimuli do not control behavior. In addition,

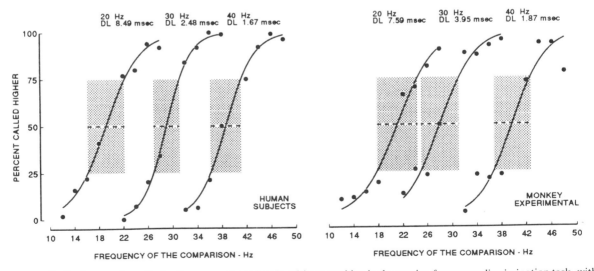

Figure 2. *(Left):* Averaged results for three experienced male subjects working in the passive-frequency discrimination task, with base frequencies of 20, 30, and 40 Hz. Data points (60 or 90 trials) indicate the percentage of trials in which the frequency of the comparison stimulus was judged higher than that of the base stimulus. The curves are logistic functions fitted to these data points. Difference limen (DL) is defined in the text. Stimuli are equated for equal subjective magnitude, and 10× thresholds. (Reprinted, with permission, from Mountcastle et al. 1990.) *(Right)* Results obtained in monkey 109 as he worked in similar frequency discrimination tests in the combined behavioral and neurophysiological experiments. Plots are as for *left;* further description is given in the text.

46 postcentral neurons were studied with frequency-discrimination control sets in monkeys 105, 106, and 107, in the irrelevant condition; these latter animals were not trained in frequency discrimination.

Neuron identification. It is generally accepted that postcentral neurons activated by gentle mechanical stimulation of the glabrous skin of the contralateral hand can be classified in terms of the functional properties of the sets of large mechanoreceptive afferent fibers innervating that skin. This specificity is thought to result from a limited cross-modal convergence between the linking neurons of the somatic system on which these sets of primary afferent fibers project, as well as by dynamic mechanisms such as the cross-modal inhibition we have occasionally observed. Cortical Pacinian neurons (PC, Pacinian afferents) are identified by their selective high-pass property, for they respond to low-amplitude, high-frequency (60–300 Hz) mechanical sinusoids delivered to the hand, and not to low frequencies. Their receptive fields are large and poorly defined. Cortical quickly adapting neurons (QA, Meissner afferents) and slowly adapting neurons (SA-I, Merkel afferents) both respond preferentially to low-frequency (5–40 Hz) and not to high-frequency mechanical sinusoids delivered to the glabrous skin, and both are related to small receptive fields in the glabrous skin of the contralateral hand. These two sets are differentiated by rapid versus slow rates of adaptation to step indentations of the skin.

Neuron location. Monkey 109 is still alive. The brains of the other three monkeys were perfused and sectioned serially at 25 μm; every section was stained and mounted (Mountcastle et al. 1990). Diligent search of these sections has not revealed the electrode tracks, due, we believe, to the atraumatic surface and constant shaft diameter of the Reitboeck microelectrode. The tracks of chronically implanted microelectrodes (2 hemispheres of monkey 105) and of guide tubes placed terminally in other brains allow us to define the location of recordings in those brains, but with some error in the x-y dimension of the cortex. We have therefore relied on physiological criteria to specify the cytoarchitectural area from which recordings have been made. Neurons were classified as being in area 2 if they subtended large, multifingered receptive fields and if similar fields were observed from cell to cell in cortical depth during a microelectrode penetration, a characteristic established for area 2 by Iwamura (1980) and Darian-Smith et al. (1984). We found a sharp transition in the posterior-to-anterior axis of the postcentral gyrus from neurons with multifingered receptive fields to those with single-fingered fields, as did those authors, and we have taken this transition in receptive field nature to mark the transition from area 2 posteriorly to area 1 anteriorly. We observed the equally sharp transition described by Kaas et al. (1979) and by Darian-Smith et al. (1984) to mark the transition from area 1 posteriorly to area 3b anteriorly; it is based on the reversal point in the progression and regression of receptive fields from

tip to base and from base to tip of the fingers. All neurons activated from single-fingered receptive fields and located more than 2000 μm below the top of activity in a microelectrode penetration of the postcentral gyrus were classed in area 3b. We found SA and QA neurons in both areas 1 and 3b. Our sample of postcentral PC neurons is small ($n = 28$) for definite conclusions, but we observed them in almost equal numbers in areas 3b and 1, and we have not identified any PC neurons in the glabrous skin hand region of area 2. The criteria we have used allow no statement concerning the laminar location of the neurons studied, but only the sequence in depth from the top of neural activity encountered in microelectrode penetrations. No conclusions of our study depend on laminar designations.

Cortical Neural Discriminandum for Frequency

An example of the observations made in the combined experiment is given in Figure 3. This 3b neuron was located 2508 μm below the top of neural activity in the postcentral gyrus and was related to a receptive field confined to the distal phalanx of the contralateral third digit. A tuning study revealed that the cell responded best to mechanical sinusoids at or near 20 Hz. The psychometric function to the right of Figure 3 plots the performance of the monkey in the discrimination task with base frequency of 20 Hz, a DL of 4.5 msec, and a Weber fraction of 9%. The replicas of the neural responses evoked in this same run are shown to the left: First those evoked by the base stimuli at 20 Hz, followed 1 second later by those evoked by the comparison stimuli of 12, 16, 18, 20, 22, 24, and 28 Hz, from above downward. Expectation density analyses of these records revealed that the neuron was strongly entrained in a periodic discharge at both base frequency and all comparison frequencies and that the lengths of the neuronal periods matched those of the stimulus cycles. Moreover, the rates of discharge evoked by base and comparison stimuli did not differ significantly (cf. Fig. 6).

The responses of a neuron of area 1 of monkey 107, studied in the irrelevant state, are shown in Figure 4. The first two columns at the left of Figure 4 are replicas of the impulse trains evoked by the base and comparison stimuli for selected classes of the control sets used. The third and fourth columns show the expectation density histograms constructed by analysis of the responses of columns 1 and 2. They reveal the periodic entrainment of the responses, and measurements showed that the period lengths in the neuronal discharges match precisely the cycle lengths of the stimuli evoking them. The renewal density histograms of column 5 show for the data of column 4 that a random shuffle of the sequential order of impulse intervals virtually destroyed the periodicities obvious in column 4. The inset impulse interval histograms of column 6, for the data of column 2, indicate that the periodicities are not due to the presence of large numbers of impulse

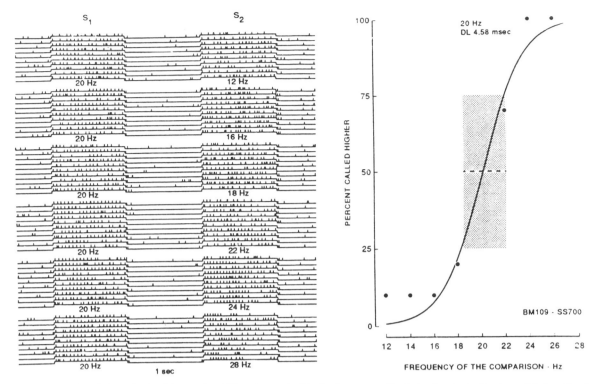

Figure 3. Examples of data obtained in monkey 109 as he worked in the frequency discrimination task. Psychometric function to the right shows his performance, plotted as for Fig. 2. Spike replicas to the left obtained simultaneously are of the discharges of a quickly adapting neuron of area 3b of the contralateral postcentral gyrus. Each line is a replica of a single trial; each small upstroke is the instant of impulse discharge. Steps indicate stimulus times. Further description is given in the text. (Reprinted, with permission, from Mountcastle et al. 1990.)

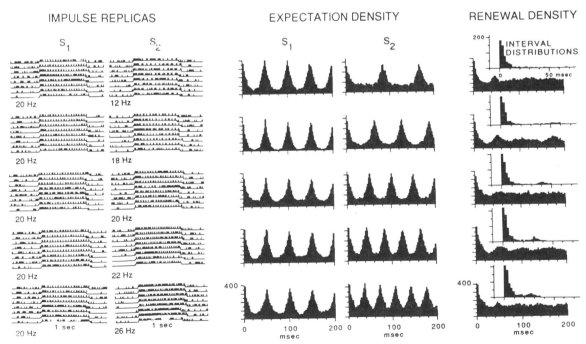

Figure 4. Results obtained in study of a postcentral neuron in an alert monkey, 107, not working in any task, the irrelevant state. Stimulus sequences are as for the passive task of Fig. 1. Neuron of the quickly adapting class is located in area 1 of the postcentral gyrus. The expectation density histograms of the activity replicated in columns 1 and 2 show the periodic entrainment of the cortical neuron by the base and the comparison stimuli. Full description is given in the text. (Reprinted, with permission, from Mountcastle et al. 1990.)

866

intervals at or near the stimulus cycle lengths. The periodicities of the responses of cortical neurons under drive by mechanical sinusoidal stimulation of the skin are produced by a sequential order coding of neuronal discharge.

We have carried out the experiment illustrated in Figures 3 and 4 for 73 neurons of areas 3b and 1 as monkey 109 worked in the discrimination task; 50 of these cells responded in the periodic manner observed. We have made a number of field studies, in which the stimulating probe was moved from run to run across the receptive field of the neuron under study. Reconstruction of the population of neurons evoked by these stimuli indicates that the strong periodic driving illustrated in Figures 3 and 5 is confined to the central core

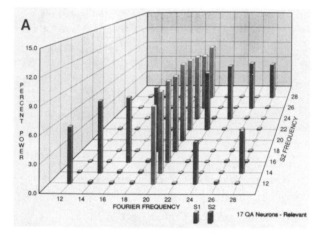

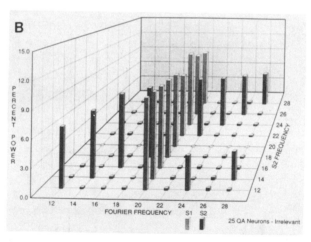

Figure 5. (*A*) Results of Fourier analysis of the averaged responses of 17 neurons of the quickly adapting class in the postcentral gyrus of monkey 109 as he worked in the passive task of Fig. 1, with base frequency of 20 Hz. Methods of analysis are described in the text. Gray columns indicate percent total spectral power evoked by the base stimuli, dark columns indicate that evoked by the comparison stimuli, from 12 to 28 Hz, in different rows. Thus, the same set of cortical neurons delivers, with a 1-sec interval, robust signals of the frequencies of the base and comparison stimuli presented for discrimination. (*B*) Results of a similar analysis for 25 postcentral neurons studied in monkey 107, alert but performing no task, the irrelevant state. (Reprinted, with permission, from Mountcastle et al. 1990.)

of the population and rapidly declines in intensity as the stimulus is moved away from the center toward the edge of the receptive field.

Harmonic analysis. We measured by Fourier analysis the strength and harmonic content of the periodic signals in the responses of neurons of areas 3b and 1. The results averaged for 17 QA neurons studied as monkey 109 worked in the discrimination task are given in Figure 5A. Analyses were made in 1-Hz steps over the range from 1 Hz to 500 Hz, but only the results at base and comparison frequencies are illustrated in Figure 5A. Power at all other frequencies was less than 0.5% of total power, except for the harmonics evoked in the responses of some neurons to low-stimulus frequencies. The data of Figure 5A show that this set of neurons responded to the base stimuli of 20 Hz with periodic signals whose harmonic content at 20 Hz was 8–10% of the total power in the signal. These same neurons responded after a 1-second delay with an equally powerful signal in which the harmonic content shifted dramatically to the frequency of the comparison stimuli; e.g., compare the 20 versus 22 Hz, or 20 versus 18 Hz sets of Figure 5A. The frequencies of the two stimuli compared in the discrimination task are represented in the responses of QA neurons of areas 3b and 1 as the lengths of the periodicities in the neural activity evoked by those stimuli. We conclude that these differences in the neuronal period lengths are the critical neural discriminanda underlying the primate capacity to make frequency discriminations in the sense of flutter and that they depend on serial order coding.

The Postcentral Neuronal Response Is Independent of Stimulus Relevance

The question arises of where in the neural processing stages leading to perception are the effects of attention and other central control states exerted. We have examined a number of neurons of areas 3b and 1 in both the relevant and irrelevant states and have not observed any significant difference in the evoked neural activity that depended on whether the stimuli guided behavior. In addition, we studied 46 neurons in alert monkeys not trained in the discrimination task (105, 106, 107), for whom the stimuli were irrelevant and did not control behavior. The result of harmonic analysis for 25 of these neurons is given in Figure 5B. They replicate almost exactly those studied in monkey 109 in the relevant state, shown in Figure 5A. Indeed, subtraction of one of these matrices from the other left remainders that fell into the range of "background," at 0.5% of total power, or less. We conclude that whether pairs of stimuli are relevant or irrelevant as guides in discriminatory performance makes no difference in the neural responses of QA neurons of areas 3b and 1 activated by those stimuli. We emphasize that the definitions of the relevant and irrelevant states make no inferences about where attention is allocated in the two states. However, our human subjects all reported that the frequency discrimination task requires intense attention to each of the pairs of stimuli.

Frequency Discrimination Cannot Be Based on a Neuronal Rate Code

The responses of the 17 QA neurons recorded as monkey 109 made discriminations, and analyzed by harmonic analysis for Figure 5, were also measured for frequency of discharge without concern for serial order. Population means and their standard errors are given in Figure 6. They show that the responses evoked by the base and comparison stimuli are virtually identical. We conclude that frequency discrimination cannot be based on differences in the overall frequencies of discharge of neurons of areas 3b and 1, evoked by the stimuli discriminated: A neuronal rate code will not suffice.

The Postcentral Neuronal Signal Provided by the Slowly Adapting System

The SA neurons of areas 3b and 1 have a selective low-pass frequency sensitivity almost identical to that of the QA neurons. This is illustrated in Figure 7, where the percentage of harmonic power evoked by the comparison stimuli over a wide frequency range is shown for a group of 12 SA neurons studied in the relevant state, compared with similar responses for populations of QA neurons. The responses of the two sets of neurons are similar both in overall frequencies and in harmonic content, over about the same range of

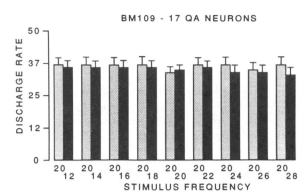

Figure 6. Results of rate analysis for the 17 QA neurons of Fig. 5A, studied in monkey 109 as he performed the frequency-discrimination task. Shaded columns indicate mean rates of responses to the base stimuli; solid columns indicate mean rates of the responses to the comparison stimuli. Vertical lines represent 1 S.E.M. This result shows that the capacity of monkeys to make frequency discriminations in the sense of flutter cannot be accounted for by a rate code. (Reprinted, with permission, from Mountcastle et al. 1990.)

test frequencies. We discuss below the reasons for our conclusion that the SA system is unlikely to contribute to frequency discrimination in the sense of flutter, despite its appropriate frequency-sensitivity range.

Observations on Neurons of Postcentral Area 2

It is known from the studies of several investigators that neurons of area 2 differ in their functional prop-

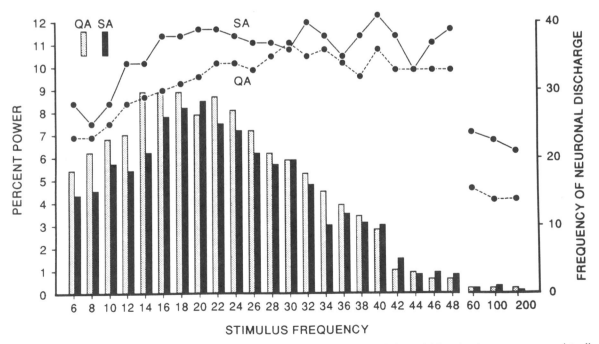

Figure 7. Illustration that the frequency bandwidths of the slowly adapting and the quickly adapting systems are virtually identical. Data obtained as monkey 109 worked in the passive discrimination task, and averaged here for 12 slowly adapting and 17 quickly adapting postcentral neurons. Vertical bars indicate the percent spectral power in the responses evoked in these populations by stimuli of different frequencies. They are not significantly different for the two sets. Similarly, the rates of discharge evoked in the two sets by stimuli of the same frequencies differ only slightly.

erties from neurons of areas 3b and 1 (Mountcastle et al. 1969; Whitsel et al. 1972; Constanzo and Gardner 1980; Iwamura et al. 1980; Darian-Smith et al. 1984). Indeed, we have used the fact that cells of area 2, but not those of areas 1 and 3, uniformly subtend multifingered receptive fields on the contralateral hand as a location marker. Area 2 neurons are exquisitely sensitive to lateral motion of stimuli across the skin, and a fraction are differentially sensitive to the direction of stimulus motion. We have identified both SA and QA types of neurons in area 2, and we have studied 77 area 2 cells in the relevant frequency-discrimination task in monkey 109. Only 10 of these 77 cells (13%) showed any degree of periodic entrainment by sinusoidal mechanical stimuli, which contrasts with the fact that 46 (72%) of the 64 neurons of areas 3b and 1 showed strong periodic entrainment under exactly the same experimental circumstances. The preliminary inference is that area 2 does not play a major role in the series of intracortical transformations of the neural activity evoked by peripheral stimuli discriminated for frequency, and which leads to perception, decision, and motor response.

DISCUSSION

Primate Capacity for Frequency Discrimination

Our observations confirm earlier ones that monkeys and humans have about the same capacity for frequency discrimination in the sense of flutter (LaMotte and Mountcastle 1975). Each makes such discriminations with Weber fractions in the range of 5-10%, and for humans, this fraction is invariant over the frequency range from 30 Hz to 200 Hz. Goff (1967) and Bekesy (1962) emphasized that vibratory pitch changes with stimulus amplitude. We therefore took care to construct stimulus sets in which stimuli of different frequencies were equated for subjective magnitude. Control experiments described elsewhere (Mountcastle et al. 1990) indicate that this was achieved and that our subjects discriminated between the frequencies and not the intensities of stimuli. The equal primate capacities for frequency discrimination lend some strength to our proposition that the neuronal activity observed in the postcentral gyrus of discriminating monkeys is generally similar to that occurring in the postcentral gyrus of humans under similar experimental circumstances.

Cortical Neuronal Discriminandum for Frequency

We conclude that frequency discrimination in the range of flutter depends on periodic neural signals evoked in postcentral neurons and that this periodicity is an example of a serial order neural code. Our conclusion is based on the following considerations: (1) The periods in the postcentral neural signals between which primates can discriminate are different and sharply defined, as shown by harmonic analysis. (2) Monkeys can never again make such frequency discriminations after

removal of the postcentral cortical areas. (3) The peripheral afferent and central neural signals evoked by the discriminated stimuli occur sequentially in the same sets of neural elements. Discrimination cannot be based on a place or a spatial code. (4) Discrimination cannot be based on differences in overall frequency of discharge, for stimuli easily discriminated evoke central neural responses indiscriminable for frequency, but which contain easily discriminated differences in neuronal period lengths.

Relevance or Irrelevance of Stimuli and the Direction of Attention

Many studies in humans made with the event-related-potential method indicate that the effects of attention on sensory performance are imposed at some point "central" to the initial representation of the physical characteristics of sensory stimuli in the primary sensory areas of the cerebral cortex. Our observations of the identity of response of neurons in areas 3b and 1 of the postcentral gyrus fit with this view, for the physical features of the stimuli discriminated in the relevant state are robustly represented in the activity of postcentral neurons whether or not the stimuli are used to guide behavior. We have no control of where attention is allocated in the irrelevant state. What is certain is that intense attention is required for optimal performance in making frequency discriminations.

Does the SA System Play a Role in Frequency Discrimination in Flutter?

Our findings suggest on first inspection that either the SA or the QA systems could provide cortical neuronal signals adequate for frequency discrimination in the sense of flutter. (1) Both SA and QA sets of postcentral neurons are entrained periodically by mechanical sinusoids delivered to their receptive fields in the glabrous skin of the hand, in the frequency range of flutter. (2) The strength and the narrow restriction of the harmonic power in the postcentral neuronal responses to stimulus frequencies are similar for the two systems. (3) The frequency bandwidths of the two are similar. However, observations in microneuronography experiments in human subjects suggest that the SA system does not evoke the sense of flutter (Torebjork and Ochoa 1980; Ochoa and Torebjork 1983; Torebjork et al. 1984, 1987; Vallbo et al. 1984; Vallbo and Johannson 1984). Electrical stimulation of single identified QA fibers innervating the glabrous skin of the human hand evokes a sense of flutter. Changes in the frequency of that stimulation evokes perceptions of flutter stimuli of different frequencies. On the other hand, electrical stimulation of similarly identified SA fibers evokes a sense of skin pressure, and changes in the frequency of that stimulation evoke changes in the perceived intensity of skin pressure.

The first implication of these findings is that what appears to be a neural signal of a sensory event, even at the cortical level, cannot be regarded as a neural code for that event unless it can be shown that the signal is used at the level of perception and behavioral response. Second, they imply that the SA and QA systems are kept separate from the initial postcentral representations to and through the neural levels of perceptual operations, and this fits with our observation of absence of convergence in areas 3b and 1 of SA and QA inputs, as judged by functional properties. Third, it implies that the perceptual operations set in motion by SA and QA input must themselves differ. That for the SA system must include an integrative operation that smooths input and leads to the perception of skin pressure and its variations in intensity. That for the QA system must specifically be free of such an integrative stage, and variations in the neuronal period lengths of different stimulus frequencies must lead to perceptions of differences in the cycle lengths of different stimulus frequencies.

Specificity and Isolation of Afferent Channels from the Skin of the Hand

An assumption in our present formulations concerning the central neural mechanisms in flutter vibration and for tactile sensibility in general is that each of the three sets of large, mechanoreceptive afferent fibers innervating the glabrous skin, known to project to the somatic sensory cortex (the PC, SA-I, and QA channels) is separate and has a separate and privileged access to perceptual processes. Each of these sets projects via linking neurons of the somatic system onto different sets of neurons in areas 3b and 1 of the postcentral gyrus. This specificity at the cortical level is thought to be produced by a restricted cross-channel divergence/convergence at each level of the system. Convergence/divergence is in the main restricted to homogeneous channels, setting receptive field sizes and surround inhibition. This restriction may also be maintained dynamically, for there is preliminary evidence that modality properties can be modified by changes in sensory experience (Recanzone et al. 1989; see also Merzenich et al., this volume). Modification by changes in sensory experience on a time scale of hours or days is thought to result from an increase in the efficacy of cross-linked but normally "silent" synapses between heterogeneous elements, produced by the activity evoked by intense sensory experiences driving activity in one particular channel. It is important to emphasize, however, that cross-channel convergences are necessary at some level to account for the more complex aspects of somesthesis, such as stereognosis.

Some Conjectures on the Higher-order Neuronal Mechanisms in Frequency Discrimination

We present in Figure 8 a simple flow diagram of the processes we surmise to play a role in frequency discrimination in the sense of flutter. The evidence presented above indicates that the frequencies of the two

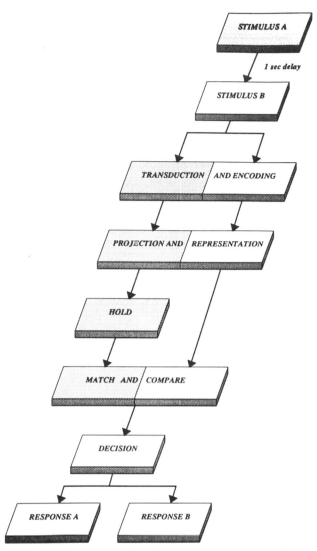

Figure 8. Schematic outline of processes thought to lead from the initial transduction and encoding of the periods of mechanical sinusoids delivered to the hand, and the final differentiated motor response that indicates frequency discrimination, indicated by responses A or B. For discussion, see the text. (Reprinted, with permission, from Mountcastle et al. 1990.)

stimuli discriminated are signaled (represented) by the lengths of the periods in the entrained sets of cortical neuronal activity evoked by the two stimuli. These must be compared sequentially in time, for they occur in the same sets of cortical elements. The comparison might be made if the period of the first stimulus is held in a short-term (sensory) memory, and compared directly with the period of the second set arriving one second later in the same set of elements. Alternatively, the period of the first might be identified and used to access a standard template for frequency in/from memory for comparison with the period of the second set of neuronal activity. Either alternative requires close attention to the frequency of each stimulus, as our human subjects report. Both monkey and human subjects have succeeded in making flutter discriminations when working with "mixed" stimulus sets that contain two or more different base stimuli and their associated comparison stimuli. Under these conditions, the base stimuli of different frequencies appear in random sequence, which suggests that each must be identified individually for successful discriminations, whichever of the two alternatives—or some other—is used.

We have not observed any sign of the "hold," "compare," or "decision" processes indicated in Figure 8 in the activity of neurons of the postcentral somatic sensory areas in animals working successfully in the discrimination task. We interpret this to mean that these higher-order operations must occur in more central nodes of the distributed somatic sensory networks of the homotypical cortex, perhaps in the parietal lobe.

ACKNOWLEDGMENT

The research described above was supported in part by grants 1 R01-NS-27776 and 5 P01-NS-20868 from the U.S. Public Health Service.

REFERENCES

Bekesy, G. 1962. Can we feel the nervous discharges of the end organs during vibratory stimulation of the skin. *J. Acoust. Soc. Am.* **34:** 850.

Bing, R. 1905. Die Knochensensibilitat und ihre Untersuchung durch die Stimmgabelmethode. *Med. Klin.* **1:** 332.

Bloomfield, P. 1976. *Fourier analysis of time series—An introduction.* Wiley, New York.

Bracewell, R.N. 1986. *The Fourier transform and its applications.* McGraw-Hill, New York.

Constanzo, R.M. and E.P. Gardner. 1980. A quantitative analysis of responses of direction-sensitive neurons in the somatosensory cortex of awake monkeys. *J. Neurophysiol.* **43:** 1319.

Craig, J.C. 1976. Attenuation of vibrotactile spatial summation. *Sens. Process.* **1:** 40.

Cummings, S.B., Jr. 1938. The effect of local anesthesia on tactile and vibratory thresholds. *J. Exp. Psychol.* **23:** 321.

Darian-Smith, I., A. Goodwin, M. Sugitani, and J. Heywood. 1984. The tangible features of textured surfaces: Their representation in the monkey's somatosensory cortex. In *Dynamic aspects of neocortical function* (ed. G.M. Edelman et al.), p. 475. Wiley, New York.

Draper, N. R. and H. Smith. 1981. *Applied regression analysis.* Wiley, New York.

Fisher, R.A. 1929. Test of significance in harmonic analysis. *Proc. R. Soc. Lond. A.* **125:** 54.

Gescheider, G.A. 1976. Evidence in support of the duplex theory of mechanoreception. *Sens. Process.* **1:** 68.

Gescheider, G.A. and R.T. Verrillo. 1979. Vibrotactile frequency characteristics as determined by adaptation and masking procedures. In *Sensory functions of the skin* (ed. D.R. Kenshalo), p. 183. Plenum Press, New York.

———. 1982. Contralateral enhancement and suppression of vibrotactile sensation. *Percept. Psychophys.* **32:** 69.

Gescheider, G.A., M.J. O'Malley, and R.T. Verrillo. 1983. Vibrotactile forward masking: Evidence for channel independence. *J. Acoust. Soc. Am.* **74:** 474.

Goff, G.D. 1967. Differential discrimination of frequency of cutaneous mechanical vibration. *J. Exp. Psychol.* **74:** 294.

Iwamura, Y., M. Tanaka, and O. Hikosaka. 1980. Overlapping representation of fingers in the somatosensory cortex (area 2) of the conscious monkey. *Brain Res.* **197:** 516.

Jenkins, W.M., M.M. Merzenich, M.T. Ochs, T. Allard, and E. Guic-Robles. 1990. Functional reorganization of primary somatosensory cortex in adult owl monkeys after behaviorly controlled tactile stimulation. *J. Neurophysiol.* **63:** 82.

Johansson, R.S. and A.B. Vallbo. 1983. Tactile sensory coding in the glabrous skin of the human hand. *Trends Neurosci.* **6:** 27.

Kaas, J.H. 1983. What, if anything, is SI? Organization of first somatosensory area of cortex. *Physiol. Rev.* **63:** 206.

Kaas, J.H., R.J. Nelson, M. Sur, C.S. Lin, and M.M. Merzenich. 1979. Multiple representations of the body within the primary somatosensory cortex of primates. *Science* **204:** 521-523.

Labs, S.M., G.A. Gescheider, R.R. Fay, and C.H. Lyons. 1978. Psychophysical tuning curves in vibrotaction. *Sens. Process.* **2:** 231.

LaMotte, R.H. and V.B. Mountcastle. 1975. The capacities of humans and monkeys to discriminate between vibratory stimuli of different frequency and amplitude; a correlation between neural events and psychophysical measurements. *J. Neurophysiol.* **38:** 539.

———. 1979. Disorders in somesthesis following lesions of parietal lobe. *J. Neurophysiol.* **42:** 400-419.

Merzenich, N.M., J.H. Kaas, J.T. Wall, M. Sur, R.J. Nelson, and D.J. Felleman. 1983. Progression of change following median nerve section in the cortical representation of the hand in areas 3b and 1 in adult owl and squirrel monkeys. *Neuroscience* **10:** 639.

Merzenich, M.M., R.J. Nelson, M.P. Stryker, M.S. Cynader, A. Schoppmann, and J.M. Zook. 1984. Somatosensory cortical map changes following digit amputation in adult monkeys. *J. Comp. Neurol.* **224:** 591.

Merzenich, M.M., R.J. Nelson, J.H. Kaas, M.P. Strycker, W.M. Jenkins, J.M. Zook, M.S. Cynader, and A. Schoppmann. 1987. Variability in hand surface representations in areas 3b and 1 in adult owl and squirrel monkeys. *J. Comp. Neurol.* **258:** 281.

Mountcastle, V.B. and T.P.S. Powell. 1959. Neural mechanisms subserving cutaneous sensibility, with special reference to the role of afferent inhibition in sensory perception and discrimination. *Bull. Johns Hopkins Hosp.* **105:** 201.

Mountcastle, V.B., R.H. LaMotte, and G. Carli. 1972. Detection thresholds for stimuli in humans and monkeys: Comparison with threshold events in mechanoreceptive afferent nerve fibers innervating the monkey hand. *J. Neurophysiol.* **35:** 122.

Mountcastle, V.B., M.A. Steinmetz, and R. Romo. 1990. Frequency discrimination in the sense of flutter: Psychophysical measurements correlated with postcentral events in behaving monkeys. *J. Neurosci.* (in press).

Mountcastle, V.B., W.H. Talbot, H. Sakata, and J. Hyvarinen. 1969. Cortical neuronal mechanisms in flutter vibration studied in unanesthetized monkeys. *J. Neurophysiol.* **32:** 453.

Nelson, R.J., M. Sur, D.J. Felleman, and J. H. Kaas. 1980. Representations of the body surface in the postcentral parietal cortex of *Macaca fascicularis. J. Comp. Neurol.* **192:** 611.

Ochoa, J. and E. Torebjork. 1983. Sensations evoked by intraneuronal microstimulation of single mechanoreceptive units innervating the human hand. *J. Physiol.* **342:** 633.

Powell, T.P.S. and V.B. Mountcastle. 1959. Some aspects of the functional organization of the cortex of the postcentral gyrus of the monkey: A correlation of findings obtained in a single unit analysis with cytoarchitecture. *Bull. Johns Hopkins Hosp.* **105:** 133.

Recanzone, G.H., W.M. Jenkins, G.T. Hrqadek, C.E. Schreiner, K.A. Grajski, and N.M. Merzenich. 1989. Frequency discrimination training alters topographical representations and distributed temporal response properties of neurons in SI cortex of adult owl monkeys. *Soc. Neurosci. Abstr.* **15:** 1223.

Reitboeck, H.J. 1983a. Fiber microelectrodes for electrophysiological recordings. *J. Neurosci. Methods* **8:** 249.

————. 1983b. A 19-channel matrix drive with individually controllable fiber microelectrodes for neurophysiological applications. *IEEE Trans. Syst. Man Cybernet.* **13**: 676.

Shimshoni, M. 1971. On Fisher's test of significance in harmonic analysis. *Geophys. J. R. Astro. Soc.* **23**: 373.

Sur, M., M.M. Merzenich, and J.H. Kaas. 1980. Magnification, receptive-field area, and "hypercolumn" size in areas 3b and 1 of somatosensory cortex in owl monkey. *J. Neurophysiol.* **44**: 395.

Sur, M., J.T. Wall, and J.H. Kaas. 1984. Modular distribution of neurons with slowly adapting and rapidly adapting responses in area 3b of somatosensory cortex in monkeys. *J. Neurophysiol.* **51**: 724.

Talbot, W.H., I. Darian-Smith, H.H. Kornhuber, and V.B. Mountcastle. 1968. The sense of flutter-vibration: Comparison of the human capacity with response patterns of mechanoreceptive afferents from the monkey's hand. *J. Neurophysiol.* **31**: 301.

Torebjork, H.E. and J.L. Ochoa. 1980. Specific sensations evoked by activity in single identified sensory units in man. *Acta. Physiol. Scand.* **110**: 445.

Torebjork, H.E., W. Schady, and J. Ochoa. 1984. Sensory correlates of somatic afferent fibre activation. *Hum. Neurobiol.* **3**: 15.

Torebjork, H.E., A.B. Vallbo, and J.L. Ochoa. 1987. Intraneural microstimulation in man. Its relation to specificity of tactile sensations. *Brain* **110**: 1509.

Vallbo, A.B., K.A. Olsson, K.G. Westberg, and F.J. Clark. 1984. Microstimulation of single tactile afferents from the human hand. Sensory attributes related to unit type and properties of receptive fields. *Brain* **107**: 727.

Whitsel, B.L., J.R. Roppolo, and G. Werner. 1972. Cortical information processing of stimulus motion on primate skin. *J. Neurophysiol.* **35**: 691.

Adaptive Mechanisms in Cortical Networks Underlying Cortical Contributions to Learning and Nondeclarative Memory

M.M. Merzenich, G.H. Recanzone, W.M. Jenkins, and K.A. Grajski*

Coleman Laboratory, Departments of Otolaryngology and Physiology, University of California, San Francisco, California 94143-0732

The purpose of this paper is to summarize our research progress in studies of the dynamic mechanisms of the cerebral cortex underlying its contributions to learning and nondeclarative memory in experiments conducted over the past five years. Five years ago, we and other workers (see below) had discovered that the details of cortical representations could be altered by peripheral lesions in adult primates. Furthermore, we argued that the cortical representational reorganization in somatosensory (SI) cortical fields following peripheral nerve injuries did not merely reflect the existence of aberrantly sprouted connections (see Merrill and Wall 1978), but must manifest normal dynamic cortical processes by which the selective, distributed responses of cortical neurons—cortical "maps"—are shaped by our experiences throughout life (Merzenich et al. 1983b, 1984a,b; Merzenich 1986). We set out to confirm and extend preliminary behavioral/physiological experiments in somatosensory cortical area 3b that supported this conclusion; to determine how such distributed representational plasticity applied to other neocortical areas; to define the "rules" of the processes underlying these experience-driven changes in distributed cortical responses; to define how such changes could specifically account for improvements in perceptual abilities with training; and to relate these changes to practical medical issues and especially to the possibility that a "representational recovery" could underlie the often remarkable functional recovery from brain injury.

All of these objectives have been at least partly achieved. We have demonstrated that the specific inputs effective for exciting cortical neurons—and considered in the distributed realm, cortical maps—can be altered by our experiences throughout life. We have defined the basic rules of this process and now understand much about underlying mechanisms. We have demonstrated how changes in cortical cell assemblies and in distributed network element responses might account for progressive improvements in discriminative abilities with training. We have successfully extended these studies to other functional cortical areas; considered with the work of other investigators (much of which preceded our own), these studies make it clear that the dynamic processes in our model systems are general for at least much of the neocortex. We have documented representational changes following stroke that are probably a major basis for functional recovery. We have documented major distributed neural network changes generated by direct motor and somatosensory cortical network microstimulation and clearly related to kindling and the genesis of epilepsy. We have studied changes following a variety of peripheral nerve and skin manipulations paralleling common plastic surgery procedures. We have developed realistic neural network models in an attempt to further understand the distributed cortical changes underlying the representational plasticity recorded experimentally. In addition, we have studied "natural" changes in cortical representations, e.g., by documenting normal variability in somatosensory, motor, and auditory cortical fields; by demonstrating that the motor representations of preferred hands are substantially more complex than are those of nonpreferred hands; by demonstrating that cortical representations can be easily distorted by enriching behavioral experiences; and by demonstrating that cortical areas of the rat ventrum are substantially altered by the onset and progression of nursing behaviors in adult female rats.

In this paper, some of the specific findings derived in these studies conducted over the past five years will be briefly summarized. Some general implications of these results will then be discussed.

SOME SPECIFIC FINDINGS

Cortical Representations—the Distributed, Specific Responses of Cortical Neurons—Are Remodeled by Our Experiences Throughout Life

This continuous remodeling manifests *the* basic adaptive processes underlying cortical contributions to learning and nondeclarative memory. Five years ago, we had concluded that the reorganization of the to-

*Present address: Ford Aerospace, 220 Henry Ford II Drive, San Jose, California 95161-9041.

pographies of representations of the skin in somato-sensory cortical fields induced by peripheral nerve lesions (Kalaska and Pomeranz 1979; Franck 1980; Merzenich et al. 1983a,b, 1984a; Wall and Cusick 1984) and by digit amputation (Rasmusson 1982; Kelehan and Deutsch 1984; Merzenich et al. 1984b) probably reflected a normal capacity for functional representational plasticity underlying cortical contributions to the acquisition of new behaviors (Merzenich et al. 1983b, 1984a,b). Recent studies have confirmed this hypothesis. Moreover, they have led to a much more complete understanding of the cortical network origins of experience-driven representational plasticity (for review, see Merzenich 1986, 1987; Merzenich et al. 1988, 1990, 1991a; Allard 1989; Recanzone and Merzenich 1991).

Many Basic Aspects of the Adaptive Responses of Cortical Networks to Specific Behaviorally Important Stimuli Are Now Understood

1. The discriminative abilities of monkeys (Recanzone 1990; G.H. Recanzone et al., in prep.), like those of humans (see, e.g., James 1890; Snoddy 1926; Gibson 1953; Anderson 1981), improve continuously and progressively with training. These training-dependent changes in discriminability and nondeclarative memory (Squire and Zola-Morgan 1987) are almost certainly accounted for by cortical representational remodeling.

2. Although training gains apply primarily to behaviorally engaged skin, some of the gains of discrimination training are "conferred" on nearby skin surrounding the trained hand location(s) (G.H. Recanzone et al., in prep.). Similarly, some of the gains of discrimination training on restricted skin surfaces in humans are conferred on nearby but not distant skin surfaces (see, e.g., Volkmann 1858; James 1890; Craig 1988; Singley and Anderson 1989).

3. Engagement of a restricted skin surface in a behavioral task in which the hand is either moving or held static results in an enlargement of the territory of representation of those skin surfaces in cortical area 3b (see Fig. 1) (Jenkins et al. 1990b; G.H. Recanzone et al., in prep.).

4. When behaviorally important stimuli move across the skin or are applied to an inconstant skin location, the spatially selective responses of cortical neurons in the directly engaged cortical region—their "receptive fields"—are *reduced* in size over time. This decline in receptive field size is roughly inversely proportional to the increase in cortical representational territory with training (see Fig. 2) (Jenkins et al. 1990b).

5. When the behaviorally stimulated skin site is highly restricted and the directly stimulated skin location is unchanging, cortical receptive fields commonly *enlarge* severalfold in extent (Fig. 2) (G.H. Recanzone et al., in prep.). Here, the normal distance/overlap rule of area 3b organization (Sur et al. 1981) is *not* maintained.

6. The areas of representation of the specific stimuli applied in tactile discrimination training increase greatly over time in directly behaviorally engaged cortical network sectors (Jenkins et al. 1990b; G.H. Recanzone et al., in prep.).

7. Responses to behaviorally important inputs can emerge over large cortical sectors that were formerly completely unresponsive to these stimuli (Jenkins et al. 1990b; G.H. Recanzone et al., in prep.).

8. With the emergence of newly effective excitatory inputs across new and enlarged cortical sectors, inputs formerly represented at those locations are no longer able to drive these cortical neurons to discharge, i.e., this reorganization is marked by widespread *substitutions* of effective inputs (Jenkins et al. 1990b; G.H. Recanzone et al., in prep.).

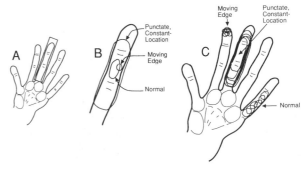

Figure 2. A principal finding of these behavioral/physiological experiments: Receptive fields are either reduced or enlarged severalfold in their areal extents when the animal is trained in a task in which stimuli move across a small skin region or in which stimuli are always applied to a small, constant skin location, respectively (*B*). Both behaviors result in a change in local cortical map topography (*C*), with the emergence of a substantial cortical sector over which receptive fields are all centered over the behaviorally stimulated skin surface (Jenkins et al. 1990b; G.H. Recanzone et al., in prep.).

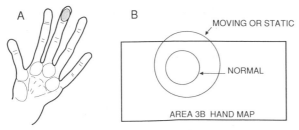

Figure 1. A principal finding of these behavioral/physiological experiments: The cortical territory of representation of a behaviorally engaged skin surface (e.g., as in *A*) enlarges in cortical area 3b (*B*) when the animal is trained in a task in which either static or moving stimuli are applied to this skin surface and in tasks in which the hand is either statically positioned while stimuli are applied to the skin or is actively maintaining contact with a stimulanda surface (Jenkins et al. 1990b; G.H. Recanzone et al., in prep.).

9. Systematic changes in cortical receptive fields and representational topographies were commonly recorded in the cortical representations of skin areas surrounding the directly behaviorally stimulated skin. These spatially conferred changes are an apparent consequence of cortical network effects that extend away from the excited cortical network region from which spike discharges are directly evoked (see Merzenich et al. 1984a, 1990; G.H. Recanzone et al., in prep.).

10. No changes are recorded in the hand area of contralateral cortical area 3b in animals in which dramatic representational changes are driven by training in the opposite-hemisphere representation (see Calford and Tweedale 1990; Jenkins et al. 1990b; G.H. Recanzone et al., in prep.).

11. The cortical area 3b hand representation commonly enlarges as a consequence of behavioral training to extend across its former functional boundaries into cortical area 3a and to encroach on the area 3b cortical zones of representation of the hand or face (Jenkins et al. 1990b).

12. Distributed responses of neurons over behaviorally "trained" cortical network sectors had shorter latencies and were more highly temporally synchronized (G.H. Recanzone et al., in prep.).

13. Changes in mean discharge rates to identical stimuli were very modestly, but statistically significantly, elevated by a period of intensive training engaging a restricted skin—and cortical network—sector (G.H. Recanzone et al., in prep.).

14. Temporal discrimination can improve in animals in which spatial topographic order is maintained as locally precise or in animals in which spatial topographic order is greatly degraded (G.H. Recanzone et al., in prep.). This suggests that cortical representational changes driven by temporal discrimination tasks may be at least partly independent of changes driven by spatial discrimination tasks.

Distributed Changes across the Cortical Network Representation of Behaviorally Important Stimuli Account for Progressive Gains in Frequency Discrimination Abilities with Training

As a consequence of such training, as noted above, the cortical zone of representation of the behaviorally engaged skin surface is substantially enlarged. At the same time, the responses across this far larger cortical network sector are more temporally coherent than are the distributed responses representing untrained skin surfaces. We hypothesize that this is partly due to changes in synaptic effectivenesses for stimuli applied to this behaviorally trained skin *and* to stronger and emergent positive coupling between excitatory neurons in this behaviorally engaged cortical network sector (Dinse et al. 1990; Recanzone and Merzenich 1991; G.H. Recanzone et al., in prep.). In any event, these

differences in distributed temporal responses are highly correlated (correlation coeff. >0.96; see Recanzone 1990; G.H. Recanzone et al., in prep.) with the monkeys' ability to discriminate frequency differences in the flutter-vibration range. Other experience-driven changes (e.g., changes in cortical areas of representation, changes in receptive field sizes, changes in response magnitudes, changes in response tuning, changes in vector strengths of responses) *cannot* account for these behavioral gains with training (G.H. Recanzone et al., in prep.).

When applied stimuli are moving or are introduced at inconstant locations, receptive fields decrease to a fraction of their normal sizes and the behaviorally engaged skin surface is thereby represented in much finer spatial grain (Jenkins et al. 1990b). This generation of a finer-grained cortical representation presumably contributes to gains in tactile spatial acuity achieved with practice with such stimuli—although in this case, behavioral performance changes have not yet been directly related to distributed representational changes.

Cortical Representational Remodeling Is Induced by a Variety of Surgically Induced Peripheral Input Manipulations in Adult Monkeys

Cortical network response remodeling has been studied following a variety of peripheral cutaneous lesions and skin transfers in an attempt to further understand principles of representational plasticity in adult primates and to model neurological consequences of these common human surgical procedures.

Cortical representations of the hand were studied in detail at different stages before and after digital amputation (Merzenich et al. 1984b; T. Allard et al., unpubl.). The cortical representation of the hand reorganized to occupy the cortical network sector formerly representing the now-missing digit, with topographically expanded representations of surrounding skin surfaces. These effects have been tracked with a chronic electrode array that sampled from neurons in the zone of representation of the amputated and adjacent digits and revealed that an early enlargement of receptive fields was followed by recreation of restricted, translocated fields, apparently thereby establishing a new, shifted representational topography (see also Calford and Tweedale 1988). These representational changes parallel (and probably account for) earlier-described perceptual changes over time for the sensibility of the skin on the stumps of amputees (Henderson and Smyth 1948; Teuber et al. 1949; Haber 1955, 1958; Merzenich et al. 1984b).

Cortical representations of the median nerve (Wall et al. 1986; and see Paul et al. 1972) and of digital cutaneous nerves (Allard et al. 1988 and in prep.) were studied in adult monkeys after these peripheral cutaneous nerves were transected and surgically repaired. These surgical procedures result in a shuffling of skin-to-central-nervous-system addresses because there are no bases for guiding the direction of axonal growth cone migration in these nerve-repair regions. That shuffling of addresses is demonstrated by studies of representational topographies within repaired nerves examined just proximal to the site of repair (Hallin et al. 1981; T.A. Allard et al., in prep.). After skin rein-nervation in these monkeys, there was a reestablish-ment of topographically ordered representations of af-fected skin surfaces in cortical areas 3b and 1. The highly ordered constructions that emerged in the cortex could not be explained by subcortical responses to these shuffled inputs; in the thalamus, representational topographies remained chaotic (Allard et al. 1988 and in prep.). In the case of digital cutaneous nerve repair, a virtually normal topography of representation could be reestablished after nerve regeneration. In parallel, human adults with small-nerve injuries commonly re-gain normal tactile acuity and image recognition abilities over the affected skin.

For larger skin field nerves like the median or ulnar nerves, reemergent cortical skin representations were highly ordered locally, but overall topographies re-mained disrupted and were marked by extensive over-laps of skin surfaces that were widely separated on the hand (Paul et al. 1972; Wall et al. 1986). These persis-tent representational overlaps probably account for the persistence of correctly located stimulation simulta-neously perceived with stimulus "ghosts" falsely local-ized to other skin field sites in adult patients with such large-nerve injuries. These false localization phenom-ena generate confusions that greatly impair recovery of the functional use of hands. We believe that they arise because the cortical network creates its topographies on temporal bases (see below) and cannot effectively sort inputs arising from distant skin surfaces, from which most inputs will be temporally unrelated (see Merzenich et al. 1987, 1990, 1991a; Grajski and Merze-nich 1990a,b).

Cortical representations of the hand were studied after fingers were fused by splitting the skin of adjacent digits along the midlateral line and resuturing dorsal and ventral surfaces. In these monkeys, normally separately and discontinuously represented digits came to be represented in cortical area 3b by a continuously overlapping representational topography (Clark et al. 1988; T.A. Allard et al., in prep.). This reorganization was central (and probably primarily cortical) in origin. These experiments further demonstrate that represen-tational discontinuities recorded in normal body sur-face representations (Merzenich et al. 1978; Kaas et al. 1981) are functional constructs created by the dynamic, adaptive cortical machinery and reflect normal pro-cesses by which cortical networks segregate inputs that are largely temporally independent (Grajski and Merzenich 1990a,b; Merzenich et al. 1991a).

Cortical representations of the hand were studied after transfer of innervated, vascularized skin islands to a new hand location (Clark et al. 1986; Merzenich et al. 1988, 1991a). They were dramatically reorganized by these innervated skin transfers, even though such trans-fers do not substantially modify the relationships be-tween skin innervation addresses and central nervous system addresses. By this cortical representational re-modeling, transferred skin islands came to be repre-sented in entirely new cortical regions, there in topo-graphic relationship to the skin of the recipient digit. Similar results were obtained in monkeys in which the skin of the hand was left intact, with single digital cutaneous nerves of adjacent fingers transected, then cross-connected (T.A. Allard et al., in prep.).

Cortical Reorganization Follows Induction of Restricted Cortical Lesions

Cortical reorganization has also been tracked follow-ing induction of restricted cortical lesions modeling small strokes (Jenkins and Merzenich 1987, 1991; Jen-kins et al. 1990a). In these studies, the hand representa-tion was reconstructed in detail in a sterile surgical procedure, then a small lesion was introduced to utterly destroy the representation of the surfaces of one or two or three digits. The cortical representation was again mapped immediately after lesion induction and/or mapped in detail later as a function of time after the cortical lesion. Lesions were later reconstructed his-tologically with reference to electrophysiological ex-periment landmarks. Among the many findings of this ongoing research, are the following:

1. Cortical representations respond passively to lesion induction by generating a functional lesion which is significantly smaller than that expected on the basis of prelesion maps and with a widespread inward shift of receptive field locations induced by the le-sion over a several-hundred-micron-wide zone sur-rounding it (C. Xerri et al., unpubl.).
2. Over the next several days, the representation shifts outward so that at 4 or 5 days after lesion induction, the functional representational losses can be *greater* than those estimated at the time of the lesion. The progression of changes resulting in this dramatic reversal of the trend of immediate postlesion effects is unknown (Jenkins et al. 1990a).
3. Over subsequent weeks, a representation of skin surfaces represented overtly only within the zone of the lesion at the time of its induction emerges in the cortical network sector around it (Jenkins and Merzenich 1987; Jenkins et al. 1990a).
4. In long-surviving animals with such lesions, recep-tive fields in this perilesion zone can remain large, with much cruder than normal representational to-pographies, or they can have almost normally selec-tive inputs and topographies.

Cortical Representational Remodeling by Natural Experiences and Behavioral Training in Adult Rats

We have also tracked changes in the SI cortical fields of rats (1) trained in vibrissal roughness discrimination tasks, (2) maintained in a tactually enriched environment with all but a few whiskers trimmed daily, or (3) with long whiskers glued to get rats to selectively attend to them (Yun et al. 1987; E. Guic-Robles et al., in prep.). We have also tracked changes in the representations of the female rat ventrum that occur with postnatal nursing behaviors (J. Stern et al., unpubl.).

In *all* of these experimental paradigms, two- to sevenfold changes in the territories of representation of the behaviorally engaged cutaneous inputs have been recorded. These regions of expanded representation have short-latency responses and must reflect changes in the distributed effectivenesses of mainline somatosensory system inputs. Inputs that coconcur in these behaviors are represented together with high probability in these behaviorally remodeled representations. As a consequence of training or experience directed toward rat vibrissae, receptive fields expanded to respond to behaviorally important inputs, or receptive fields representing behaviorally important inputs were substituted for those normally represented at those locations. Among many other implications, these studies challenge experiments conducted in rats which have claimed that recorded receptive field locations and extents of functional representations strictly correspond to predictions based on patterns of the "barrels" of the rat SI field (see, e.g., Killackey 1990).

Evidence That Cortical Self-organizing Mechanisms Recorded in Somatosensory Cortical Field 3b Are General in the Neocortex

An extensive series of experiments conducted in somatosensory cortical fields 1 and 3a and in the movement representations in cortical area 4 were designed to determine, among many other specific objectives, whether or not the dramatic functional self-organization of the somatosensory koniocortical field (area 3b in adult monkeys; SI in rats) applies generally across the neocortex.

Cortical area 1. In some experiments in several of the above-described series, changes in the area 1 representations of adult monkeys induced by these special behaviors were also recorded. Limited experiments completed to date have revealed the following: (1) Changes in area 1 are not predicted by distributed response changes in area 3b (Merzenich 1986; Merzenich et al. 1987, 1990). (2) In postbehavior maps, differentially stimulated digital surfaces in the rotating disk digit tip stimulation behavior (Jenkins et al. 1990b) lose their cortical zone of representation within area 1. (3) Preliminarily, in postbehavior maps, representations of stimulated digital surfaces in monkeys discriminating differences in flutter-vibration frequency undergo a severalfold enlargement.

These paradoxical findings are consistent with recent findings of Nelson and colleagues (Nelson 1987; Nelson

and Douglas 1989; see also Shin and Chapin 1989a,b), who found that inputs into area 1 in macaques were gated "on" for a positionally static hand and "off" during active hand exploration. In the rotating disk behavioral stimulation task, the monkey actively controlled the contact of fingertips with the stimulanda, and changes recorded in area 1 were consistent with the gated "off" condition. In the frequency discrimination task, the hand was placed onto a hand mold and was sitting passively when stimuli were delivered up onto it. Recorded changes were consistent with the gated "on" condition.

Although behaviorally driven changes in area 1 must be more completely documented, it is clear that (1) its representations, like those in area 3b, are remodeled by an animal's experiences; (2) presumably because of corticocortical gating or "reafference" influences, the behaviorally driven representational changes within cortical area 1 can be dependent on the motor context of the behavior; and (3) the changes driven in cortical area 1 can thereby be very different from those driven by the same behavior in cortical area 3b.

Cortical area 3a. We have also completed a study of the changes in distributed responses in cortical area 3a that emerge in a monkey performing a behavioral task involving a "go–no go" hand reach signaled by discriminated differences in light tactile stimuli (Recanzone 1990; G.H. Recanzone et al., in prep.). In a normal adult monkey, neurons in cortical field 3a are predominantly excited by inputs from receptors innervating muscles and joints (Phillips et al. 1971; Lucier et al. 1975; Heath et al. 1976; Friedman and Jones 1981; Lin et al. 1979; Ze-hui et al. 1986). In these behaviorally trained monkeys, roughly half of the hand representation in area 3a came to be driven most effectively by *cutaneous* inputs. Earlier investigators have shown that such inputs are delivered anatomically into this zone from cortical area 3b and possibly from the thalamus (see Cusick and Gould 1990) but are only occasionally effective in driving neurons within it. At the same time, electrical stimulation of purely cutaneous nerves has revealed that area 3a neurons have subthreshold inputs from the skin, as a rule (Zarzecki and Wiggin 1982; Zarzecki and Herman 1983).

In an owl monkey responding to tactile stimulation by moving his hand within reaction-time limits, cutaneous input comes to be *dominant* over a very large 3a sector (see also Nelson and Douglas 1989). This reorganization can be described as a "substitution" of effective inputs, in the sense that deep inputs from muscles and joints formerly dominating the excitatory response behavior of neurons in this region are no longer evident within large, emergent area 3a zones now driven by cutaneous inputs in these trained monkeys. It has been hypothesized that the inputs from cortical area 3a are one source of afferent inputs controlling or modulating movement initiation in motor cortex (see, e.g., Phillips et al. 1971; Lucier et al. 1975; Nelson and Douglas 1989). With this behavior, the hand is held stationary and can provide no kinesthetic inputs that can signal a reaction movement. As the monkey practices this behavior, these behavior-guiding skin inputs are the only inputs engaged in area 3a in the crucial premovement phase of the behavior. They are (we hypothesize) therefore progressively differentially strengthened (see G.H. Recanzone et al., in prep.).

All three SI cortical areas that we have studied (3b, 3a, 1) project with excitatory inputs to the principal somatosensory field of SII and are the principal sources of inputs to this field (see Pons et al. 1987; Burton et al. 1990; Garraghty et al. 1990). This SII field undergoes remarkable representational remodeling following ablation of the hand areas of SI (Pons et al. 1988). This raises the interesting question of how the very different use-driven changes recorded in different SI cortical fields in a monkey trained in one of these simple behaviors might be integrated in an experience-remodeled SII field.

Movement representations of cortical area 4. Highly detailed microstimulation movement maps were derived in adult squirrel monkeys before and after a period of training in a simple motor task (Merzenich et al. 1988, 1990; Jenkins et al. 1990a; R. Nudo et al., unpubl.). Monkeys were trained to retrieve food pellets from small food wells in a modified Kluver board. In their daily feeding sessions, monkeys rapidly and progressively improved their retrieval/attempt ratio. The motor cortical zones representing specific digital, hand, wrist, elbow, and shoulder movements were mapped in great detail after 10–15 hours of such training and compared to equally detailed maps derived earlier in a baseline period. Significant increases in the territories over which digit movements required for the task were evoked at threshold by intracortical microstimulation were recorded in all studied animals, with the greatest changes in anterior aspect of the area 4 movement representation. New movement relationships that were intrinsic to the behavior emerged in the map. For example, digit and wrist movements that were concurrent in the behavior more commonly overlapped or bordered each other in the postbehavior movement representation. A statistically significant change in the fractionation of evoked digit movements was also recorded in these monkeys. Thus, changes in movement representations were induced by a few hours of training at a simple motor skill, and the magnitudes of representational changes were on a scale equal to or greater than those recorded in somatosensory cortical field studies.

Taken together, and combined with studies conducted by other workers demonstrating neuronal response plasticity in many other neocortical areas (see, e.g., Olds et al. 1972; Woody and Engel 1972; Disterhoft and Stuart 1976; Buchhalter et al. 1978; Kitzes et al. 1978; Diamond and Weinberger 1986, 1989; Woody 1986; Delacour et al. 1987; Ichikawa et al. 1987; Sakamoto et al. 1987; Miyashita 1988; Miyashita and Chang 1988; Weinberger and Diamond 1988; Iriki et al. 1989; Robertson and Irvine 1989; Rolls et al. 1989; Kaas et al. 1990; Sanes et al. 1990; Weinberger et al. 1990), there would appear to be little question that these basic self-organizing processes are general in the neocortex (Merzenich 1987; Merzenich et al. 1988, 1990, 1991a).

Self-organizing Neocortical Processes Account for Cortical Contributions to Idiosyncratic Neurobehavioral Development in Animals and in Man

These studies indicate that use-dependent alteration of cortical representational detail is a major determinant of the idiosyncratic variability in cortical topographic representations, reflecting the behavioral specializations of every individual human or monkey. Thus, for example, we have documented the significant variability in "untrained" monkeys in somatosensory cutaneous cortical representations in areas 3b and 1 (Merzenich 1986; Merzenich et al. 1987), in the "deep" receptor representations of cortical area 3a (G.H. Recanzone et al., in prep.), in the movement representations of cortical area 4 (Nudo et al. 1988 and in prep. and see, e.g., Leyton and Sherrington 1917; Lashley 1923; Gould et al. 1986), and in the primary auditory cortical field in adult cats (Merzenich et al. 1975; Reale and Imig 1980; Schreiner and Mendelson 1990) and monkeys (Merzenich and Brugge 1973; Imig et al. 1977; Aitkin et al. 1986; Merzenich and Schreiner 1991; Merzenich et al. 1991b). In all these cortical zones, there are very substantial idiosyncratic differences in the details of the representations of the skin surface, of movements, and of sound stimulus parameters in different individual adult monkeys. Representations of hand movements are significantly more complicated for the hand preferentially used by the monkey for food retrieval and in which a strong hand preference was evident (Nudo et al. 1988 and in prep).

These idiosyncratic features of cortical representations have been largely ignored by cortical electrophysiologists. In fact, magnitudes of representational changes driven by different hand or auditory uses as well as cortical representational changes incurred by peripheral input losses in these monkeys, especially in the hearing domain (see Robertson and Irvine 1989), clearly account for much of the representational variability recorded in cortical mapping experiments (Merzenich 1986; Merzenich et al. 1987, 1988; Merzenich and Schreiner 1991). This shaping of these representations by experience must be a major contributor to idiosyncratic neurobehavioral development (Merzenich et al. 1991a).

One important implication of these findings is that the details of representations recorded in any given adult animal reflect what an animal has done and can do operationally in the perceptual/motor domain represented by the field(s) under study. Cortical experiments directed toward understanding the origins of behavior must *necessarily* be conducted with strict behavioral controls.

New Studies Contribute to Our Understanding of Basic Mechanisms Underlying This Cortical Representational Plasticity

The cortex is probably the site of greatest behaviorally induced changes, although the contributions of subcortical structures are still incompletely defined. We have begun deriving thalamic maps in animals from which cortical representations have been constructed. These studies have shown that (1) thalamic representational topographies are jumbled in monkeys recovered from peripheral nerve transections (Allard et al. 1988 and in prep.), whereas cortical representational topographies are highly ordered in these same monkeys; (2) the dramatic remodeling of cortical representations recorded after transferring islands of innervated skin across the hand (see above) cannot be accounted for by changes in thalamic representations; (3) representational remodeling can be induced rapidly by direct cortical stimulation, i.e., by stimulation that does not directly engage subcortical levels with excitatory inputs (see Fig. 3) (Recanzone and Merzenich 1988; Dinse et al. 1990; Nudo et al. 1990; G.H. Recanzone et al., in prep.).

Although subcortical lemniscal system contributions to representational remodeling following peripheral nerve injuries are undeniable (see Wall and Egger 1971; Dostrovsky et al. 1976; Millar et al. 1976; Merrill

and Wall 1978; Devor 1987), we have earlier pointed out that given the substantially greater divergence of the spreads of anatomical inputs at the cortical level, given great differences between the topographies of cortical representations that share common thalamic inputs, and given specific features of these cortical representations that differ from thalamic representations, whatever the subcortical reorganizational effects, the cortex must itself have a capacity for representational reorganization (Merzenich et al. 1983a, 1984a, 1988, 1990, 1991a; Merzenich 1987; Recanzone and Merzenich 1991; G.H. Recanzone et al., in prep.). Recent studies indicate that the spreads of inputs in the cortex are at least 5 or 6 times greater than are the spreads of inputs at subcortical levels (see, e.g., Rainey and Jones 1983; Hicks and Dykes 1984; Juliano and Whitsel 1985; Snow et al. 1988; Alloway et al. 1989; Florence et al. 1989; Garraghty et al. 1989, 1990; Raussel and Jones 1989; Recanzone et al. 1990). Moreover, plastic changes induced by training a monkey in a temporal discrimination task probably apply primarily to the cortical level, since most of the temporal degradation of responses across this projection system and hence most of the sharpening of responses to improve distinctions of temporal differences with training must apply to the cortical level (G.H. Recanzone et al., in prep.). This issue has been addressed directly in the auditory system, where the mainline lateral and dorsal parts of the medial geniculate body projecting to auditory cortical fields were found to be unaltered by behavioral training that induced major changes in neuronal responses at the cortical level (Ryugo and Weinberger 1978). The full extents of subcortical participation in cortically recorded representational plasticity in behaviorally trained animals will ultimately be fully resolved only by deriving detailed thalamic maps in behaviorally trained animals and by more directly determining possible thalamic contributions to cortical input selection processes.

Specific cortical neuron responses are time-based. Results of many different studies individually reveal (and collectively, overwhelmingly confirm) that cortical representations can be altered by changing the temporal distributions of inputs into the engaged cortical network sector (Clark et al. 1986, 1988; Allard et al. 1988, 1990, and in prep.; Merzenich et al. 1988, 1991a; Dinse et al. 1990; Jenkins et al. 1990b; Recanzone and Merzenich 1991; G.H. Recanzone et al., in prep.). Thus, for example, we find the following:

1. Representational discontinuities are destroyed by digital fusion that greatly reduces the quantities of temporally independent inputs originating on facing surfaces of adjacent fingers (Clark et al. 1988; Allard et al. 1990).
2. Representations are remodeled by transferring innervated skin sectors across the hand, and with the creation of a new representation of the transferred

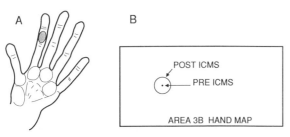

Figure 3. A principal finding of these behavioral/physiological experiments: Cortical representations are also rapidly altered by a brief period of very low level intracortical microstimulation. Prior to conditioning stimulation, a specific cutaneous receptive field (e.g., as in *A*) is recorded for neurons within a very small neuronal population usually comprising a few hundred cortical neurons extending over a horizontal cortical area not usually more than 40–100 μm across. After a period of very discrete conditioning stimulation, *all* neurons over a cortical zone several hundreds of microns across, and now including several thousand neurons, come to be driven by the specific receptive field initially recorded only at the pre-stimulation cortical network location (Recanzone and Merzenich 1991). With this dramatic substitution of the stimulation-site receptive field for the formerly effective inputs in this surrounding cortical zone, neurons across this region also come to be strongly positively coupled (Dinse et al. 1990).

skin, many receptive fields have component parts from across the new scar line, and that must reflect new receptive field formation based on temporal coselection (Clark et al. 1986; Merzenich et al. 1988, 1991a).

3. Temporally based coselection of inputs must underlie the reemergence of small receptive fields and local topographies following nearly random mixing of peripheral-to-central somatosensory connections by peripheral nerve transection and repair (Wall et al. 1986; Allard et al. 1988 and in prep.).

4. Changes in receptive fields and distributed changes in cortical maps driven by training monkeys in tasks that engage small skin regions (Jenkins et al. 1990b; G.H. Recanzone et al., in prep.) are specifically consistent with alterations in cortical responses based on temporally based input selection processes.

5. Movements that coconcur in learned motor skills are represented together with increased probability in the movement maps of trained monkeys (Merzenich et al. 1988, 1991a; R. Nudo et al., unpubl.).

6. Distributed, selectively effective responses in both areas 4 and 3b are rapidly altered by intracortical microstimulation that results in a highly localized, synchronous excitation of inputs and neurons at a highly restricted cortical location (Nudo and Merzenich 1987; Recanzone and Merzenich 1988; Dinse et al. 1990; Nudo et al. 1990; G.H. Recanzone et al., in prep.).

Taken together, these studies reveal that, considered in detail, cortical representations actually topographically represent *temporal* continua.

Both effective afferent inputs and the coupling between cortical neurons—functional cortical cell assemblies—are altered by use.   Such changes were first documented by defining non-stimulus-driven correlations between neurons across a sector of cortical network driven to change by intracortical microstimulation (see Fig. 3) (Dinse et al. 1990). Changes in the stimulus-engaged cortical network sector of behaviorally trained monkeys were later found to closely parallel changes recorded in these intracortical microstimulation network-perturbation studies (Recanzone and Merzenich 1991; G.H. Recanzone et al., in prep.). These experimental findings support long-standing conclusions by theorists that nearly coincident inputs delivered into the cortical network should result in the formation of positively coupled (cooperative) cortical cell assemblies (see, e.g., Edelman and Mountcastle 1978; Edelman and Finkel 1984; Pearson et al. 1987; Cowan and Sharp 1988; Edelman 1988; von der Malsburg and Singer 1988; Palm 1990; Singer 1990).

The cortical network responds in different ways when it is challenged by moving or stationary stimuli.   As noted earlier, spot-like or wave-edge stimuli generate small receptive fields when stimuli are moved across the skin or engage it in inconstant locations; equivalently spot-like stimulation results in the genesis of large receptive fields when a highly restricted and constant skin site is stimulated (Fig. 2). This intuitively surprising result is nonetheless completely consistent with predicted cortical network model behavior and is explained by differences in network competition attributable to effectively competitive correlated inputs from widely distributed skin locations in the moving stimulus case, as compared with competitively winning inputs from one small skin site in the static spot-stimulation case.

Anatomical spreads of inputs support the observed cortical representational changes.   Numerous studies (including several conducted by us) indicate that the spreads of anatomical inputs are sufficient to account for the representational substitutions and translocations recorded in these cortical plasticity studies. Thus, e.g., arbors of thalamocortical afferents projecting into somatosensory cortical areas spread over distances of many hundreds of microns, as is revealed by the filling of individual axons with tracers (see Landry and Deschenes 1981; Garraghty et al. 1989; Garraghty and Sur 1990), the tracer-labeling of isorepresentational thalamic columns (Raussel and Jones 1989), the definition of the extents of cortical arbors of individual thalamic neurons using an antidromic spike-collision mapping technique (Snow et al. 1988), or the recording of excitatory postsynaptic potentials (EPSPs) in a sample of cortical neurons (see, e.g., Zarzecki and Wiggin 1982; Zarzecki and Herman 1983). The wide spreads of activity generated by point stimulation on the skin in metabolic maps are also consistent with relatively wide input spread from any given skin location (see, e.g., Juliano and Whitsel 1985). Moreover, receptive fields can be shown to enlarge severalfold in extent by blocking GABA responses (Hicks and Dykes 1984; Alloway et al. 1989) or by conditioning a cortical sector by a period of peripheral nerve stimulation (Recanzone et al. 1990). Taken together, these studies indicate that inputs from any given skin surface site richly feed an area 3b cortical zone 1.5–2.5 mm in diameter, with even greater input divergences in other SI cortical fields. Considered conversely, any given cortical site receives input from a large skin region; neurons at that site ordinarily respond to only a very small fraction of its anatomically delivered input. *All the changes recorded in somatosensory plasticity studies described above are within the limits of this input-arbor divergence.*

It might be noted, again, that most of this input spread in the somatosensory lemniscal system occurs at the cortical level. In contrast, spreads of inputs at subcortical levels are much more highly topographically constrained (see, e.g., Rainey and Jones 1983; Florence et al. 1989).

Cortical representational remodeling involves closely linked processes of input strengthening and input weakening. Representational remodeling in most cortical plasticity studies is marked by widespread *substitutions* of effective inputs.

The capacity for reorganization of somatosensory cortical fields is greater in very young animals than in adults. The representations of the body surface were also mapped in cats that had incurred early postnatal spinal injuries, in a series prepared to study the functional recovery from early spinal injury, by Dr. Patricia McKinley. Among other results, these mapping experiments (see McKinley et al. 1987) revealed the following: (1) After spinal transection incurred within the first 3 weeks of postnatal life, cortical area 3b was dramatically reorganized, with the emergence of a large, roughly mirror-image representation of the forelimb in the cortical sector that normally represents the now-denervated posterior trunk and hindlimb. (2) These emergent topographic representations extended across almost the entire mediolateral extent of the deprived SI sector. (3) In older kittens, as in adults, representations of skin nearer the denervated skin expanded topographically over significant distances, but never occupied cortical zones far into the deprived cortex, as in early postnatal cases.

Changes are gated as a function of the behavioral state of the animal. These use-dependent cortical network changes are recorded *only* when inputs are delivered into this system in an attended behavior (see, e.g., Olds et al. 1972; Disterhoft and Stuart 1976; Diamond and Weinberger 1986; G.H. Recanzone et al., in prep.). We have recently completed studies which show that only very minor changes are recorded in animals that were stimulated daily but were attending to other sensory stimuli; however, application of the same stimuli in the same schedule in an attended behavior resulted in major distributed changes (G.H. Recanzone et al., in prep.; and see Jenkins et al. 1990b). Moreover, when the behavior is extinguished, behaviorally induced response changes are "reversed" or again approach baseline levels (Jenkins et al. 1990b; and see Olds et al. 1972; Woody and Engel 1972; Disterhoft and Stuart 1976; Diamond and Weinberger 1986; Weinberger and Diamond 1988).

Some Theoretical Implications

Changes in input effectivenesses recorded in these experiments are consistent with time-concurrent Hebbian effects (Hebb 1949) involving an induction of immediate short-term changes by behaviorally important stimuli—e.g., by protein phosphorylation through a second-messenger system—followed by a longer-term modification most probably (but not necessarily) involving morphological changes of the pre- and post-

synaptic elements themselves (for a review, see Byrne 1988; Merzenich et al. 1991a; Recanzone and Merzenich 1991; G.H. Recanzone et al., in prep.). The integration time for inducing changes is probably on the order of several tens of milliseconds. Evoked spike discharge activity in postsynaptic cells may not be required to induce changes in synaptic effectivenesses, as is indicated by the fact that strong discharge activity emerges from cortical network regions in which this same input is earlier totally ineffective in evoking action potentials. As noted above, changes are almost certainly not limited to afferent input effectivenesses, but extend farther to effect changes in the positive coupling of neurons across cortical networks. We have recently begun documenting the extents of anatomical spreads of pyramidal cell collaterals across local SI cortical networks (Goldreich and Merzenich 1990). In these studies, we have preliminarily found that the spreads of these intracortical pyramidal cell axonal arbors are as great or greater than the network domains over which we have altered the effective positive coupling of cortical neurons (Dinse et al. 1990).

To further understand these behaviorally induced changes in cortical representations, we have constructed three-layer (input, subcortical, cortical) Hebbian network models using assumptions based on known anatomical and functional features of the somatosensory lemniscal system and cortical area 3b. Eight different peripheral-lesion, central-lesion, and behavioral-training experiments have been simulated with these models, with model results matching experimental results in most, but not all, respects (Grajski and Merzenich 1990a,b; see also Pearson et al. 1987; Edelman 1988). Although our real cortical networks are not yet fully understood, these model results have taken much of the mystery out of our experiments by helping us understand the cortical network bases of these complex experimental phenomena. They emphasize to us that cortical network responses to behaviorally delivered inputs that drive performance changes are not mysterious or surprising.

As this work progresses, these models and our experimental result descriptions should progressively merge. The ultimate result should be a mathematically expressed, general theory of neocortical function.

DISCUSSION: SOME GENERAL CONCLUSIONS

Early behavioral and forebrain experimentalists understood that enduring changes in the effective complex circuits of the forebrain must be induced by our behaviors (see, e.g., James 1890; Graham Brown and Sherrington 1912; Lashley 1933, 1950; Hebb 1949). For those accepting the mind-brain assumption, the distributed consequences of all these enduring changes up to any given point in our lives must account for the sum of our behavioral abilities and memories up to that moment. Many experimentalists have sought to discover the form of these "traces" (James 1890) or "engrams" (Lashley 1950) (i.e., the stored representations) of our learned behaviors. Almost all the numerous investigators on this quest who have studied the plasticity of cortical neurons in a learning behavior have relatively easily driven neurons to change their responses in direct relationship with the learning and have tracked response changes back toward a baseline or control response status when the learning was extinguished. They have thereby had repeated small glimpses of the trace of the learning and nondeclarative memories driven by this training in the cortex. The high success with which these experiments have been conducted and the relatively high percentage of sampled neurons whose responses are altered by behavioral training reveal that the extents of distributed changes induced by learning in the cortex are often massive. Excepting the very complexly organized olfactory system (see Hasselmo et al., this volume), the distributed form of representation of training-induced changes have not been earlier constructed across the cortical networks that they engage.

If these distributed training-induced changes represent the cortical contributions to nondeclarative memories and learned behaviors, as we believe they must, then their genesis is probably not particularly complicated in origin or particularly difficult to understand at the level of the dynamic cortical circuit. Most features of our results can be modeled by plausible neural network models, with distributions of excitatory and inhibitory effects similar to those that have been applied in models of the refinement of connections in the superior colliculus (see Cowan and Sharp 1988; Constantine-Paton, this volume) and by the operation of Hebb-like synapses in cortical network models based on real network parameters (Grajski and Merzenich 1990a,b; and see Pearson et al. 1987; Stryker et al.; Edelman and Cunningham; both this volume).

As we have progressed in deriving this large body of experimental data documenting the phenomenology of cortical plasticity in our own experiments, and as we have constructed and manipulated theoretical models designed to evaluate possible origins of these responses, our thinking about the study of the basic adaptive mechanisms of the neocortex has changed in a number of ways. First, the documentation of distributed, training-induced changes in cortical responses and studies of changes in cortical responses across a cortical network sector induced by very discrete intracortical microstimulation have provided new insights into the nature of the basic cortical self-organizing machinery accounting for the remodeling of distributed, selective cortical neuronal responses by experience. Among other findings, they revealed to us that effectively coupled cortical neuron populations—the functional "mini-columns" or "neuronal groups" of the neocortex —are *themselves* altered by our experiences (see Dinse et al. 1990; Recanzone and Merzenich 1991; Merzenich

et al. 1991a; G.H. Recanzone et al., in prep.). This is hardly surprising; it only means that plastic changes in the cortex advance past the afferent input synapse into the network itself.

A strong implication is that any real understanding of cortical dynamics requires derivation of a simultaneous, distributed sample of cortical network element responses derived in an appropriate spatial grain across these functionally coupled assemblies of cortical neurons. Requirements for obtaining this kind of spatially detailed, distributed neuron response sample have also been demonstrated in behavioral/physiological experiments in which cortical network changes could account for gains in perceptual discrimination *only* from consideration of the representation of behaviorally relevant stimuli *all across* the distributed cortical network sector engaged by these stimuli in behavioral training (see G.H. Recanzone et al., in prep.). That is, the basis of making fine temporal distinctions between flutter-vibration stimuli is not explained by any spatial or temporal response change expressed by individual neurons, but rather by changes in the distributed temporal response coherence of the thousands or tens of thousands of neurons that were engaged by these behaviorally important stimuli.

Theorists have long understood that there is a network atop our sensory systems. They have correctly emphasized that the responses of cortical neurons have to be understood in terms of their memberships in coupled cell assemblies (see, e.g., Edelman and Finkel 1984; Cowan and Sharp 1988; von der Malsburg and Singer 1988; Palm 1990; and see Singer 1990; Singer et al.; Edelman and Cunningham; both this volume).

Second, theorists also routinely do something to their model networks that experimentalists relatively rarely do: They turn them on. A principal point of interest in forebrain neuroscience is to document how the distributed representations of the brain are altered as we acquire new motor or perceptual abilities, as we drive our cortical network model to "learn" or "recognize" or "remember." In real life, that requires that we sample responses of neurons across cortical networks *during the acquisition of new behavior*. Few experiments are directed toward studying the cortex in this crucial context, and fewer still do so while recording across cortical networks for learning-induced changes. This is surprising, because there lies the cortical engram.

Third, modeling studies have had a major impact on our research planning, in large part because they have provided a logical framework for them to which all later experiments shall be related. To study how these model cortical networks are altered by specific inputs, one systematically manipulates spatial, temporal, and intensive continua in an attempt to achieve a logically complete reconstruction of input-induced cortical network behaviors. It has become increasingly clear to us that this is just what we must do with *real* cortical networks, to most efficiently complete first-generation cortical plasticity studies. Thus, a current major focus of our research is directed toward systematically defining how these dynamic networks respond to stimuli altered across these most fundamental of parametric continua.

Fourth, these studies generate insights into the possible origins of a number of functional disabilities and illnesses and have provided further insights into the neurological bases of recovery from brain injury. Thus, we have the following examples:

1. Changes in representational recovery in the cortex parallel described sequelae of changes in recovery from stroke, although functional recovery in the short term and in the long term following brain injury have often been usually attributed (we believe incorrectly) primarily to other causes (see, e.g., Finger and Stein 1982; Wade et al. 1985). These studies reveal that the competitive cortical network processes that underlie adaptive changes in learning and memory also account for recovery following brain injury. These results therefore bear important implications for the positive utility (and possible negative consequences) of application of different rehabilitative training strategies.

2. Striking cortical network cell assembly changes induced by cortical microstimulation probably constitute the key change underlying the emergence of kindling phenomena modeling epilepsy genesis (see, e.g., Cain 1977, 1979; for review, see McNamara et al. 1980). Pharmacological manipulation of kindling is in every way consistent with our current understanding of mechanisms underlying the behaviorally contingent modulation of cortical cell assembly and distributed-response representational changes recorded in our experimental studies (McNamara et al. 1980).

3. Recent studies of patients with a wide variety of "occupational cramps" or "focal dystonias" (Sheehy and Marsden 1982; Panizza et al. 1990) indicate that many are probably attributable to use-driven changes that disrupt and degrade detailed cortical representational topographies, simply because behaviorally important inputs are driven into the network within the limits of its basic input-selecting integration time window. Such effects have been recorded in our mapping studies and in behavioral experiments conducted in the laboratory of Dr. James Craig in Indiana (J. Craig and M. Merzenich, in prep.).

4. These mechanisms account for cortical contributions to our idiosyncratic behavioral abilities (see Merzenich et al. 1991a) and, in extension, for the geniuses, the fools, and the idiot savants among us.

5. Finally, these dynamic cortical areas must be subject to extremes of hyperstabilization or destabilization, which may be related to the great functional illnesses of depression and madness that plague this machine.

ACKNOWLEDGMENTS

This research was supported by National Institutes of Health grant NS-10414, the Coleman Fund, and Hearing Research, Inc. Collaborators in these many studies include Dr. Terry Allard (now at the Office of Naval Research); Dr. Ralph Beitel (University of California at San Francisco [UCSF]); Dr. Sharon Clark (Stanford University/UCSF); Dr. Hubert Dinse (Bochum Universität); Mr. Daniel Goldreich (UCSF); Dr. Patricia McKinley (McGill University); Dr. Randall Nelson (University of Tennessee, Memphis); Dr. Randolph Nudo (University of Texas, Houston); Dr. Marleen Ochs (Vanderbilt University); Mr. Brett Petersen (University of California at Berkeley/UCSF); Dr. William Rivers (University of Virginia); Dr. Christoph Schreiner (UCSF); Dr. Peter Snow (University of Queensland); Dr. Michael Stryker (UCSF); Dr. Christian Xerri (Provence Universite/UCSF); Dr. Junti Yun (Capital City Hospital, Beijing); and Dr. John Zook (Ohio University).

REFERENCES

Aitkin, L.M., M.M. Merzenich, D.R.F. Irving, J.C. Clarey, and J.E. Nelson. 1986. Frequency representation in auditory cortex of the common marmoset (*Callithrix jacchus jacchus*). *J. Comp. Neurol.* **252:** 275.

Allard, T. 1989. Biological constraints in a dynamic network: The somatosensory system. In *Connectionist modeling and brain function* (eds. S.J. Hanson and C.R. Olson), p. 149. MIT Press, Cambridge, Massachusetts.

Allard, T., S.A. Clark, H.A. Grajski, and M.M. Merzenich. 1988. Plasticity in primary somatosensory cortex after digital nerve section and regeneration in adult owl monkey. *Soc. Neurosci. Abstr.* **14:** 844.

Allard, T.A., S.A. Clark, W.M. Jenkins, and M.M. Merzenich. 1990. Reorganization of somatosensory area 3b representation in adult owl monkeys following digital syndactyly. *J. Neurophysiol.* (in press).

Alloway, K.D., P. Rosenthal, and H. Burton. 1989. Quantitative measurements of receptive field changes during antagonism of GABAergic transmission in primary somatosensory cortex of cats. *Exp. Brain Res.* **78:** 514.

Anderson, J.R. 1981. *Cognitive skills and their acquisition.* Erlbaum, Hillsdale, New Jersey.

Buchhalter, J., J. Brons, and C. Woody. 1978. Changes in cortical neuronal excitability after representations of a compound auditory stimulus. *Brain Res.* **157:** 162.

Burton, H., K. Sathian, and S. Dian-Hua. 1990. Altered responses to cutaneous stimuli in the second somatosensory cortex following lesions of the postcentral gyrus in infant and juvenile macaques. *J. Comp. Neurol.* **291:** 395.

Byrne, J.H. 1988. Cellular analysis of associative learning. *Physiol. Rev.* **57:** 329.

Cain, D.P. 1977. Seizure development following repeated electrical stimulation of central olfactory structures. *Ann. N.Y. Acad. Sci.* **290:** 201.

———. 1979. Sensory kindling: Implications for development of sensory prostheses. *Neurology* **29:** 1595.

Calford, M.B. and R. Tweedale. 1988. Immediate and chronic changes in responses of somatosensory cortex in adult flying fox after digit amputation. *Nature* **332:** 446.

———. 1990. Interhemispheric transfer of plasticity in the cerebral cortex. *Science* **249:** 805.

Clark, S.A., T. Allard, W.M. Jenkins, and M.M. Merzenich. 1986. Cortical map reorganization following neurovascular island skin transfers on the hands of adult owl monkeys. *Soc. Neurosci. Abstr.* **12:** 391.

———. 1988. Syndactyly results in the emergence of double digit receptive fields in somatosensory cortex in adult owl monkeys. *Nature* **332:** 444.

Cowan, J.D. and D.H. Sharp. 1988. Neural networks. *Q. Rev. Biophys.* **21:** 365.

Craig, J.C. 1988. The role of experience in tactual pattern perception: A preliminary report. *Int. J. Rehabil. Res.* **11:** 167.

Cusick, C.G. and H.J. Gould. 1990. Connections between area 3b of the somatosensory cortex and subdivisions of the ventroposterior nuclear complex and the anterior pulvinar nucleus in squirrel monkeys. *J. Comp. Neurol.* **292:** 83.

Delacour, H., O. Houcine, and B. Talbi. 1987. "Learned" changes in the responses of the rat barrel field neurons. *Neuroscience* **23:** 63.

Devor, M. 1987. On mechanisms of somatotopic plasticity. In *Effect of injury on trigeminal and spinal somatosensory systems* (ed. L.M. Pubols and B.J. Sessle), p. 215. A.R. Liss, New York.

Diamond, D.M. and N.M. Weinberger. 1986. Classical-conditioning rapidly induces specific changes in frequency receptive fields of single neurons in secondary and ventral ectosylvian auditory cortical fields. *Brain Res.* **372:** 357.

———. 1989. Role of context in the expression of learning-induced plasticity of single neurons in auditory cortex. *Behav. Neurosci.* **103:** 471.

Dinse, H.R., G.H. Recanzone, and M.M. Merzenich. 1990. Direct observation of neural assemblies during neocortical representational reorganization. In *Parallel processing in neural systems and computers* (ed. R. Eckmitler et al.), p. 65. Elsevier, North Holland, Amsterdam.

Disterhoft, J.F. and D.K. Stuart. 1976. Trial sequence of changed unit activity in auditory system of alert rat during conditioned response acquisition and extinction. *J. Neurophysiol.* **39:** 266.

Dostrovsky, J.O., J. Millar, and P.D. Wall. 1976. The immediate shift of afferent drive of dorsal column nucleus cells following deafferentation: A comparison of acute and chronic deafferentation in gracile nucleus and spinal cord. *Exp. Neurol.* **52:** 480.

Edelman, G.M. 1988. *Neuronal Darwinism: The theory of neuronal group selection.* Basic Books, New York.

Edelman, G.M. and L.H. Finkel. 1984. Neuronal group selection in the cerebral cortex. In *Dynamic aspects of neocortical function* (ed. G.M. Edelman et al.), p. 653. Wiley, New York.

Edelman, G.M. and V.B. Mountcastle. 1978. *The mindful brain: Cortical organization and the group-selective theory of higher brain function.* MIT Press, Cambridge, Massachusetts.

Finger, S. and D.G. Stein. 1982. *Brain damage and recovery: Research and clinical perspectives.* Academic Press, New York.

Florence, S.L., J.T. Wall, and J.H. Kaas. 1989. Somatotopic organization of inputs from the hand to the spinal gray and cuneate nucleus of monkeys with observations on the cuneate nucleus of humans. *J. Comp. Neurol.* **286:** 48.

Franck, J.I. 1980. Functional reorganization of cat somatic sensory-motor cortex (SmI) after selective dorsal root rhizotomies. *Brain Res.* **186:** 458.

Friedman, D.P. and E.G. Jones. 1981. Thalamic input to areas 3a and 2 in monkeys. *J. Neurophysiol.* **45:** 59.

Garraghty, P.E. and M. Sur. 1990. Morphology of single intracellularly stained axons terminating in area 3b of macaque monkeys. *J. Comp. Neurol.* **294:** 583.

Garraghty, P.E., T.P. Pons, and J.H. Kaas. 1990. Ablations of area 3b (SI proper) and 3a of somatosensory cortex in marmosets deactivates the second and parietal ventral somatosensory areas. *Somatosens. Mot. Res.* **7:** 125.

Garraghty, P.E., T.P. Pons, M. Sur, and J.H. Kaas. 1989. The arbors of axon terminations in middle cortical layers of somatosensory area 3b in owl monkeys. *Somatosens. Mot. Res.* **6:** 401.

Gibson, E.J. 1953. Improvement in perceptual judgments as a function of controlled practice or training. *Psychol. Bull.* **50:** 401.

Goldreich, D. and M.M. Merzenich. 1990. Spreads of intracortical axonal collaterals and basal dendrites in the barrelfield cortex of rats. *Barrels* **2:** 22.

Gould, H.J., C.G. Cusick, T.P. Pons, and J.H. Kaas. 1986. The relationship of corpus callosum connections to electrical stimulation maps of motor, supplementary motor, and frontal eye fields in owl monkeys. *J. Comp. Neurol.* **247:** 297.

Graham Brown, T. and C.S. Sherrington. 1912. On the instability of a cortical point. *Proc. R. Soc. Lond. B Biol. Sci.* **85:** 250.

Grajski, K.A. and M.M. Merzenich. 1990a. Hebb-type dynamics is sufficient to account for the inverse magnification rule in cortical somatotopy. *Neural Computat.* **2:** 74.

———. 1990b. Neuronal network simulation of somatosensory representational plasticity. In *Neural information processing systems* (ed. D.L. Touretzky), vol. 2. Morgan Kaufman, San Mateo, California. (In press.)

Haber, W.B. 1955. Effects of loss on limb on sensory functions. *J. Psychol.* **40:** 115.

———. 1958. Reactions to loss of limb: Physiological and psychological aspects. *Ann. N.Y. Acad. Sci.* **75:** 14.

Hallin, R.G., Z. Wiesenfeld, and H. Lungnegard. 1981. Neurophysiological studies of peripheral nerve functions after neural regeneration following nerve suture in man. *Int. J. Rehabil. Res.* **3:** 187.

Heath, C.J., J. Hore, and C.G. Phillips. 1976. Inputs from low threshold muscle and cutaneous afferents of hand and forearm to areas 3a and 3b of baboon's cerebral cortex. *J. Physiol.* **257:** 199.

Hebb, D.O. 1949. *The organization of behavior: A neuropsychological theory.* Wiley, New York.

Henderson, W.R. and G.E. Smyth. 1948. Phantom limbs. *J. Neurol. Neurosurg. Psychiatry* **11:** 88.

Hicks, T.P. and R.O. Dykes. 1984. Receptive field size for certain neurons in primary somatosensory cortex is determined by GABA-mediated intracortical inhibition. *Brain Res.* **274:** 160.

Ichikawa, M., K. Arissian, and H. Asanuma. 1987. Reorganization of the projections from the sensory cortex to the motor cortex following elimination of the thalamic projection to the motor cortex in cats; Golgi, electron microscope and degeneration study. *Brain Res.* **437:** 131.

Imig, T.J., M.A. Ruggero, L.M. Kites, E. Javel, and J.F. Brugge. 1977. Organization of the auditory cortex in the owl monkey (*Aotus trivirgatus*). *J. Comp. Neurol.* **171:** 111.

Iriki, A., C. Pavlides, A. Keller, and H. Asanuma. 1989. Long-term potentiation in the motor cortex. *Science* **245:** 1385.

James, W. 1890. *The principles of psychology*, vol. 1. Dover, New York.

Jenkins, W.M. and M.M. Merzenich. 1987. Reorganization of neocortical representations after brain injury: A neurophysiological model of the bases of recovery from stroke. *Prog. Brain Res.* **71:** 249.

———. 1991. Cortical representational plasticity: Some implications for the bases of recovery from brain damage. In *Brain damage and rehabilitation. A neuropsychological approach* (ed. D. van Cramon et al.). Springer, Berlin. (In press.)

Jenkins, W.M., M.M. Merzenich, and G. Recanzone. 1990a. Neocortical representational dynamics in adult primates:

Implications for neuropsychology, *Neuropsychologia* **28:** 573.

Jenkins, W.M., M.M. Merzenich, M. Ochs, T. Allard, and E. Guic-Robles. 1990b. Functional reorganization of primary somatosensory cortex in adult owl monkeys after behaviorally controlled tactile stimulation. *J. Neurophysiol.* **63:** 82.

Juliano, S.L. and B.L. Whitsel. 1985. Metabolic labeling associated with index finger stimulation in monkey SI: between animal variability. *Brain Res.* **342:** 242.

Kaas, J.H., M. Sur, R.J. Nelson, and M.M. Merzenich. 1981. Multiple representations of the body. In *Multiple somatic areas* (ed. C. N. Woolsey). Humana Press, Clifton, New Jersey.

Kaas, J.H., L.A. Krubitzer, Y.M. Chino, A.L. Langston, E.H. Polley, and N. Blair. 1990. Reorganization of retinotopic cortical maps in adult mammals after lesions of the retina. *Science* **228:** 229.

Kalaska, J. and B. Pomeranz. 1979. Chronic paw denervation causes and age-dependent appearance of novel responses from forearm in "paw cortex" of kittens and adult cats. *J. Neurophysiol.* **42:** 618.

Kelehan, A.M. and G.S. Deutsch. 1984. Time-dependent changes in the functional organization of somatosensory cerebral cortex following digit amputation in adult raccoons. *Somatosens. Res.* **2:** 49.

Killackey, H.P. 1990. Static and dynamic aspects of cortical somatotopy: A critical evaluation. *J. Cognit. Neurosci.* **1:** 1.

Kitzes, L.M., G.R. Farley, and A. Starr. 1978. Modulation of auditory cortex unit activity during the performance of a conditioned response. *Exp. Neurol.* **62:** 678.

Landry, P. and M. Deschenes. 1981. Intracortical arborizations and receptive fields of identified ventrobasal thalamocortical afferents to the primary somatic sensory cortex in the cat. *J. Comp. Neurol.* **199:** 345.

Lashley, K. 1923. Temporal variation in the function of the gyrus precentralis in primates. *Am. J. Physiol.* **65:** 585.

―――. 1933. Integrative functions of the cerebral cortex. *Physiol. Rev.* **13:** 1.

―――. 1950. In search of the engram. *Symp. Soc. Exp. Biol.* **4:** 454.

Leyton, A.S.F. and C.S. Sherrington. 1917. Observations on the excitable cortex of the chimpanzee, orangutan, and gorilla. *Q. J. Exp. Physiol.* **11:** 135.

Lin, C.S., M.M. Merzenich, M. Sur, and J.H. Kaas. 1979. Connections of areas 3b and 1 of the parietal somatosensory strip with the ventroposterior nucleus in the owl monkey (*Aotus trivirgatus*). *J. Comp. Neurol.* **185(2):** 355.

Lucier, C.E., D.C. Ruegg, and M. Wiesendanger. 1975. Responses of neurones in motor cortex and in area 3a to controlled stretches of forelimb muscles in cebus monkeys. *J. Physiol.* **251:** 833.

McKinley, P.A., W.M. Jenkins, J.L. Smith, and M.M. Merzenich. 1987. Age-dependent capacity for somatosensory cortex reorganization in chronic spinal cats. *Dev. Brain Res.* **31:** 136.

McNamara, J.O., M.C. Byrne, R.M. Dasheiff, and J.G. Fitz. 1980. The kindling model of epilepsy: A review. *Prog. Neurobiol.* **15:** 139.

Merrill, E.G. and P.D. Wall. 1978. Plasticity of connection in the adult nervous system. In *Neuronal plasticity* (ed. C.W. Cotman), p. 94. Raven Press, New York.

Merzenich, M.M. 1986. Sources of intraspecies and interspecies cortical map variability in mammals: Conclusions and hypotheses. In *Comparative neurobiology: Modes of communication in the nervous system* (ed. M.J. Cohen and F. Strumwasser), p. 105. Wiley, New York.

―――. 1987. Dynamic neocortical processes and the origins of higher brain functions. In *The neural and molecular bases of learning* (ed. J.-P. Changeux and M. Konishi), p. 337. Wiley, London.

Merzenich, M.M. and J.F. Brugge. 1973. Representation of the cochlear partition on the superior temporal plane of the macaque monkey. *Brain Res.* **50:** 275.

Merzenich, M.M. and C.E. Schreiner. 1991. Mammalian auditory cortex; some comparative observations. In *Evolutionary biology of hearing* (ed. A. Popper et al.). Academic Press, New York. (In press.)

Merzenich, M.M., T. Allard, and W.M. Jenkins. 1991a. Neural ontogeny of higher brain function; implications of some recent neurophysiological findings. In *Information coding in the somatosensory system* (ed. O. Franzen and P. Westman). Oxford University Press, England. (In press.)

Merzenich, M.M., W.M. Jenkins, and J.C. Middlebrooks. 1984a. Observation and hypotheses on special organizational features of the central auditory nervous system. In *Dynamic aspects of neocortical function* (ed. G.M. Edelman et al.), p. 397. Wiley, New York.

Merzenich, M.M., P.L. Knight, and G.L. Roth. 1975. Representation of cochlea within primary auditory cortex in the cat. *J. Neurophysiol.* **38:** 231.

Merzenich, M.M., G.H. Recanzone, and W.M. Jenkins. 1990. How the brain functionally rewires itself. In *Natural and artificial parallel computations* (ed. M. Arbib and J.A. Robinson). MIT Press, New York.

Merzenich, M.M., J.H. Kaas, M. Sur, and C.-S. Lin. 1978. Double representation of the body surface within cytoarchitectonic areas 3b and 1 in "SI" in the owl monkey (*Aotus trivigatus*). *J. Comp. Neurol.* **181:** 41.

Merzenich, M.M., G.H. Recanzone, W.M. Jenkins, T. Allard, and R.J. Nudo. 1988. Cortical representational plasticity. In *Neurobiology of neocortex* (ed. P. Rakic and W. Singer), p. 41. Wiley, New York.

Merzenich, M.M., C.E. Schreiner, G.H. Recanzone, R.E. Beitel, and M.L. Sutter. 1991b. Topographic organization of cortical field A-I in the owl monkey (*Aotus nancymai*). *ARO Abstr.* **13:** 61.

Merzenich, M.M., J.H. Kaas, J.T. Wall, R.J. Nelson, M. Sur, and D.J. Felleman. 1983a. Topographic reorganization of somatosensory cortical areas 3b and 1 in adult monkeys following restricted deafferentation. *Neuroscience* **10:** 33.

Merzenich, M.M., J.H. Kaas, J.T. Wall, M. Sur, R.J. Nelson, and D.J. Felleman. 1983b. Progression of change following median nerve section in the cortical representation of the hand in areas 3b and 1 in adult owl and squirrel monkeys. *Neuroscience* **10:** 639.

Merzenich, M.M., R.J. Nelson, M.P. Stryker, M.S. Cynader, A. Schoppmann, and J.M. Zook. 1984b. Somatosensory cortical map changes following digit amputation in adult monkeys. *J. Comp. Neurol.* **224:** 591.

Merzenich, M.M., R.J. Nelson, J.H. Kaas, M.P. Stryker, W.M. Jenkins, J.M. Zook, M.S. Cynader, and A. Schoppmann. 1987. Variability in hand surface representations in areas 3b and 1 in adult owl and squirrel monkeys. *J. Comp. Neurol.* **258:** 281.

Millar, J., A.I. Basbaum, and P.D. Wall. 1976. Restructuring of the somatotopic map and appearance of abnormal neuronal activity in the gracile nucleus after partial deafferentation. *Exp. Neurol.* **50:** 658.

Miyashita, Y. 1988. Neural correlate of visual associative long-term memory in the primate temporal cortex. *Nature* **335:** 817.

Miyashita, Y. and H.S. Chang. 1988. Neural correlate of pictorial short term memory in the primate temporal cortex. *Nature* **331:** 68.

Nelson, R.J. 1987. Activity of monkey primary somatosensory cortical neurons changes prior to active movement. *Brain Res.* **406:** 402.

Nelson, R.J. and V.D. Douglas. 1989. Changes in premovement activity in primary somatosensory cortex differ when monkeys make hand movements in response to visual vs. vibratory cues. *Brain Res.* **484:** 43.

Nudo, R.J. and M.M. Merzenich. 1987. Repetitive intracortical microstimulation alters the area for representation of movements. *Soc. Neurosci. Abstr.* **13:** 1596.

Nudo, R.J., W.M. Jenkins, and M.M. Merzenich. 1988. Interhemispheric asymmetry in the area 4 representation of movements is correlated with hand preference. *Soc. Neurosci. Abstr.* **14:** 508.

———. 1990. Repetitive microstimulation alters the cortical representation of movements in adult rats. *Somatosens. Mot. Res.* **7:** 463.

Olds, J., J.F. Disterhoft, M. Segal, C.L. Kornblith, and R. Hirsh. 1972. Learning centers of rat brain mapped by measuring latencies of conditioned unit responses. *J. Neurophysiol.* **35:** 202.

Palm, G. 1990. Cell assemblies as a guideline for brain research. *Concepts Neurosci.* **1:** 133.

Panizza, M., S. Lelli, J. Nilsson, and M. Hallett. 1990. H-reflex recovery curve and reciprocal inhibition of H-reflex in different kinds of dystonia. *Neurology* **40:** 324.

Paul, R.L., H. Goodman, and M.M. Merzenich. 1972. Alterations in mechanoreceptor input to Brodmann's areas 1 and 3 of the postcentral hand area of *Macaca mulatta* after nerve section and regeneration. *Brain Res.* **39:** 1.

Pearson, J.C., L.H. Finkel, and G.M. Edelman. 1987. Plasticity organization of adult cerebral cortical maps: A computer simulation based on neuronal group selection. *J. Neurosci.* **7:** 4209.

Phillips, C.G., T.P.S. Powell, and M. Wiesendanger. 1971. Projection from low-threshold muscle afferents of hand and forearm to area 3a of baboon's cortex. *J. Physiol.* **217:** 419.

Pons, T.P., P.E. Garraghty, and M. Mishkin. 1988. Lesion-induced plasticity in the second somatosensory cortex of adult macaques. *Proc. Natl. Acad. Sci.* **85:** 5279.

Pons T.P., P.E. Garraghty, D.P. Friedman, and M. Mishkin. 1987. Physiological evidence for serial processing in somatosensory cortex. *Science* **237:** 417.

Rainey, W.T. and E.G. Jones. 1983. Spatial distribution of individual medial lemniscal axons in the thalamic ventrobasal complex of the cat. *Exp. Brain Res.* **49:** 229.

Rasmusson, D.D. 1982. Reorganization of raccoon somatosensory cortex following removal of the fifth digit. *J. Comp. Neurol.* **205:** 313.

Raussel, E. and E.G. Jones. 1989. Modular organization of the thalamus VPM nucleus in monkeys. *Soc. Neurosci. Abstr.* **15:** 311.

Reale, R. and T.J. Imig. 1980. Tonotopic organization in auditory cortex of the cat. *J. Comp. Neurol.* **192:** 265.

Recanzone, G.H. 1990. "Changes in the junctional organization of SI following tactile frequency discrimination training in adult owl monkey." Ph.D. thesis, University of California, San Francisco.

Recanzone, G.H. and M.M. Merzenich. 1988. Intracortical microstimulation in somatosensory cortex in adult rats and owl monkeys results in a large expansion of the cortical zone of representation of a specific cortical receptive field. *Soc. Neurosci. Abstr.* **14:** 223.

———. 1991. Alterations of the functional organization of primary somatosensory cortex following intracortical microstimulation or behavioral training. In *Memory: Organization and locus of change* (ed. L. Squire et al.). Oxford University Press, England. (In press.)

Recanzone, G., T. Allard, W.M. Jenkins, and M.M. Merzenich. 1990. Receptive field changes induced by peripheral nerve stimulation in S1 of adult cats. *J. Neurophysiol.* **63:** 1213.

Robertson, D. and D.R.F. Irvine. 1989. Plasticity of frequency organization in auditory cortex of guinea pigs with partial unilateral deafness. *J. Comp. Neurol.* **282:** 456.

Rolls, E.T., G.C. Bayles, M.E. Hasselmo, and V. Nalwa. 1989. The effect of learning on the face selective responses of neurons in the cortex in the superior temporal sulcus of the monkey. *Exp. Brain Res.* **76:** 153.

Ryugo, D.K. and D.M. Weinberger. 1978. Differential plasticity of morphologically distinct nerve populations in the medial geniculate body of the cat during classical conditioning. *Behav. Biol.* **22:** 275.

Sakamoto, T., L.L. Porter, and H. Asanuma. 1987. Long-lasting potentiation of synaptic potentials in the motor cortex produced by stimulation of the sensory cortex in the cat: A basis of motor learning. *Brain Res.* **413:** 360.

Sanes, J.N., S. Suner, and J.P. Donoghue. 1990. Dynamic organization of primary motor cortex output to target muscles in adult rats. I. Long-term patterns of reorganization following motor or mixed peripheral nerve lesions. *Exp. Brain Res.* **79:** 479.

Schreiner, C.E. and J.R. Mendelson. 1990. Functional topography of cat primary auditory cortex: Distribution of integrated excitation. *J. Neurophysiol.* **64:** 1442.

Sheehy, M.P. and C.D. Marsden. 1982. Writers' cramp—A focal dystonia. *Brain* **105:** 461.

Shin, H.C. and J.K. Chapin. 1989a. Mapping the effects of motor cortex stimulation on single neurons in the dorsal column nuclei in the rat: Direct responses and afferent modulation. *Brain Res. Bull.* **22:** 245.

———. 1989b. Mapping the effects of motor cortex stimulation on somatosensory relay neurons in the rat thalamus: Direct responses and afferent modulation. *Brain Res. Bull.* **24:** 257.

Singer, W. 1990. Search for coherence: A basic principle of cortical self-organization. *Concepts Neurosci.* **1:** 1.

Singley, M.K. and J.R. Anderson. 1989. *The transfer of cognitive skill.* Harvard University Press, Cambridge, Massachusetts.

Snow, P.J., R.J. Nudo, W. Rivers, W.M. Jenkins, and M.M. Merzenich. 1988. Somatotopically inappropriate projections from thalamocortical neurons to the S1 cortex in the cat. *J. Somatosens. Res.* **5:** 349.

Snoddy, G.S. 1926. Learning and stability. *J. Appl. Psychol.* **10:** 1.

Squire, L.R. and S. Zola-Morgan. 1987. Memory: Brain systems and behavior. *Trends Neurosci.* **11:** 170.

Sur, M., M.M. Merzenich, and J.H. Kaas. 1981. Magnification, receptive fields area, and "hypercolumn" size in areas 3b and 1 of somatosensory cortex in owl monkeys. *J. Neurophysiol.* **44:** 295.

Teuber, H.L., H.P. Krieger, and M.B. Bender. 1949. Reorganization of sensory function in amputation stumps: Two-point discrimination. *Fed. Proc.* **8:** 156.

Volkmann, A.W. 1858. Über den Einfluss der Übung. *Leipzig Berichte Math.-phys. Classe* **10:** 38.

von der Malsburg, C. and W. Singer. 1988. Principles of cortical network organization. In *Neurobiology of neocortex* (ed. T.P. Rakic and W. Singer), p. 69. Wiley, New York.

Wade, D.T., R.L. Hewer, C. Skilbeck, and R.M. David. 1985. *Stroke. A critical approach to diagnosis treatment and management*, p. 175. Year Book Medical, Chicago.

Wall, J.T. and C.G. Cusick. 1984. Cutaneous responsiveness in primary somatosensory (S-I) hindpaw cortex before and after partial hindpaw deafferentation in adult rats. *J. Neurosci.* **4:** 1499.

Wall, J.T., J.H. Kaas, M. Sur, R.J. Nelson, D.J. Felleman, and M.M. Merzenich. 1986. Functional reorganization in somatosensory cortical areas 3b and 1 of adult monkeys after median nerve repair: Possible relationships to sensory recovery in humans. *J. Neurosci.* **6:** 218.

Wall, P.D. and M.D. Egger. 1971. Formation of new connections in adult rat brains after partial deafferentation. *Nature* **232:** 542.

Weinberger, N.M. and D.M. Diamond. 1988. Dynamic modulation of the auditory system by associative learning. In *Auditory function: Neurobiological bases of hearing* (ed. G.M. Edelman et al.), p. 485. Wiley, New York.

Weinberger, N.M., J.H. Ashe, R. Metherate, T.M. McKenna, D.M. Diamond, and J. Bakin. 1990. Retuning auditory cortex by learning: A preliminary model of receptive field plasticity. *Concepts Neurosci.* **1:** 91.

Woody, C.D. 1986. Understanding the cellular basis of memory and learning. *Annu. Rev. Psychol.* **37:** 433.

Woody, C.D. and J. Engel. 1972. Changes in unit activity and thresholds to electrical microstimulation at coronal-pericruciate cortex of cat with classical conditioning of different facial movements. *J. Neurophysiol.* **36:** 230.

Yun, J.T., M.M. Merzenich, and T. Woodruff. 1987. Alteration of functional representations of vibrissae in the barrel field of adult rats. *Soc. Neurosci. Abstr.* **13:** 1596.

Zarzecki, P. and D. Herman. 1983. Convergence of sensory inputs upon projection neurons of somatosensory cortex: Vestibular, neck, head, and forelimb inputs. *Exp. Brain Res.* **50:** 408.

Zarzecki, P. and D.M. Wiggin. 1982. Convergence of sensory inputs upon projection neurons of somatosensory cortex. *Exp. Brain Res.* **48:** 28.

Ze-hui, Z., W. Chien-ping, and X. Ming-chu. 1986. Thalamic projection to motor area and area 3a of the cat cerebral cortex. *Brain. Res.* **380:** 389.

Three-dimensional Object Recognition

S. ULLMAN

Department of Brain and Cognitive Sciences, Massachusetts Institute of Technology, Cambridge, Massachusetts 02139

The task of visual object recognition is performed efficiently and effortlessly by humans, including young children. Simpler animals, such as the pigeon, also exhibit a remarkable capacity to classify and recognize objects. In contrast, the task has proved to be exceedingly difficult in artificial systems. This is an intriguing contrast: It suggests that a better understanding of the recognition problem, and, in particular, why the task is so natural for biological systems and so difficult to mimic in artificial systems, may give us insights regarding some fundamental principles of brain organization.

In approaching the recognition problem, it may appear initially that the problem could be overcome by using a sufficiently large and efficient associative memory system. In performing recognition, we are trying to determine whether an image we currently see corresponds to an object we have seen in the past. It might be possible, therefore, to approach object recognition by storing a sufficient number of different views associated with each object, and then comparing the image of the currently viewed object with all the views stored in memory (Abu-Mostafa and Psaltis 1987). Several mechanisms, known as associative memories, have been proposed for implementing this "direct" approach to recognition. These mechanisms, usually embodied in neuron-like networks, can store a large number of patterns (P_1, P_2, ..., P_n), and then, given an input pattern Q, they can retrieve the pattern P_i which is most similar to Q (Willshaw et al. 1969; Kohonen 1978; Hopfield 1982).

Have associative memories of this type solved the problem of object recognition? Discussions of associative memories sometimes suggest that they have. When the system has stored a representative view, or a few views, of each object, a new view would automatically retrieve the stored representation that most closely resembles it.

The problem with using an associative memory directly to recognize objects from their images is that the notion of similarity used in associative memories is a restricted one. The typical similarity measure used is the so-called "Hamming distance." (This measure is defined for two binary vectors. Suppose that **u** and **v** are two binary vectors, i.e., strings of 1s and 0s. The Hamming distance between **u** and **v** is simply the number of coordinates in which they differ.)

Such a simple similarity measure may be appropriate for some special applications and for certain nonvisual domains, such as olfaction (Freeman 1979). For the general problem of visual object recognition, this direct approach is implausible for two reasons. First, the space of all possible views of all the objects to be recognized is likely to be prohibitively large. The second, and more fundamental reason, is that the image to be recognized will often not be sufficiently similar to any image seen in the past. There are four main sources for this variability, and it seems to me that the success of any recognition scheme will depend on its ability to cope with these four problems.

The first source of variability comes from photometric effects, i.e., the positions and distributions of light sources in the scene (including effects of mutual illumination by other objects, the relative orientation of the object with respect to the light sources, etc.). Illumination effects of this type can change drastically the light intensity distribution in the image, but they usually do not affect our ability to recognize the objects in the image.

The second source is the effect of context. Objects are rarely seen in isolation: They are usually seen against some background, next to or partially occluded by, other objects. Even when the image contains a familiar object, if we compare the image as a whole with images we have seen in the past, it is unlikely to match closely any image of the same object seen in the past.

The third reason for the variability between new and old images has to do with the effect of viewing position. Three-dimensional objects can be viewed from a variety of viewing positions (directions and distances), and these different views can give rise to widely different projections. It is sometimes difficult to appreciate this effect of viewing direction. Two views of the same object separated by, say, 20–30° usually appear perceptually quite similar. When two two-dimensional projections are superimposed, it becomes apparent, however, how different they can become with even a modest change in viewing direction.

The fourth and final reason is the effect of changing shape. Many objects, such as the human body, can maintain their identity while changing their three-dimensional shape. To identify such objects correctly, the recognition scheme must be able to deal, therefore, with the effects induced by changes of shape.

In this paper, I deal with aspects of the second and third of these sources, the effects of context and of viewing position. Before doing this, I will comment briefly, however, about the first source, the photo-

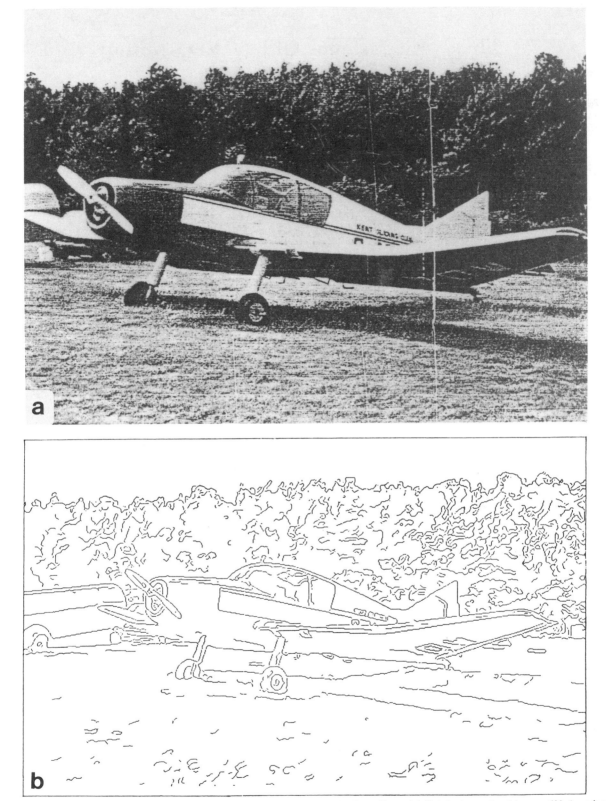

Figure 1. Edge images may be used to minimize variations due to illumination effects. (*a*) Original gray-level image. (*b*) An edge image of the original image.

metric effects. How can a recognition system deal with such changes in illumination conditions? The answer is not entirely known, but there has been primarily one

dominant approach to the problem, based on the notion of edge detection. The idea is to find in the light intensity distribution that forms the image, features that are affected as little as possible by changes in the illumination conditions. The best-known examples of such features are intensity edges, contours where the light intensity changes relatively abruptly from one level to another. Such edges are often associated with object boundaries and with material changes on an object's surface. When the illumination changes, the absolute light intensities change as well, but the locations of edges caused by physical surface discontinuities remain, on the whole, stable.

This process of edge detection is illustrated in Figure 1. Figure 1a is a gray-level image, and 1b is its edge-contour image. The edge image contains most of the relevant information in the original image. The advan-

tage, compared with the original image, is that this edge image, unlike the original one, will change only little when the illumination conditions change. This invariance is not complete, however: Some object edges might appear or disappear, some spurious edges will result from shadows and specularities, etc.

CONTEXT EFFECTS: SEGMENTATION AND SELECTION

The second source of variation listed above is the effect of varying context. The main approach that has been proposed to deal with this context problem is to precede the actual recognition and matching process by

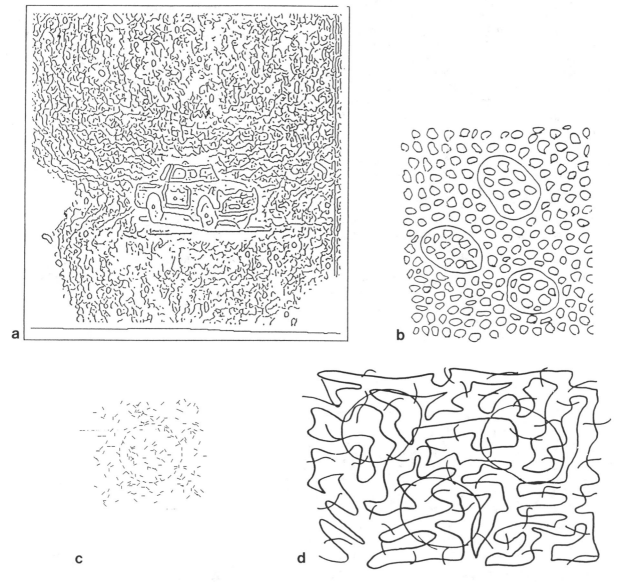

Figure 2. The perception of salient structures. The car in *a* attracts our attention; we can find it without scanning the image exhaustively. *b–d* do not contain recognizable objects, but certain structures in the image are more salient and figure-like than others. The saliency in *c* and *d* is global rather than local.

a stage called "segmentation" or "selection." The general idea is to select out of the image a region that contains an object to be recognized, and "hand it over" to the recognition process, which can then process selectively this region and ignore the rest of the image.

When we look at an image such as Figure 2a, it appears to us that our attention is somehow drawn immediately to the main object, which we then recognize as a car. For most observers, the car is found immediately, without the need to scan the image systematically, and without attempting to recognize first some structures in other parts of the image.

Structures that attract our attention need not be recognizable objects. In Figure 2b–d, for example, a number of round blobs are relatively easy to detect as the most salient, figure-like structures in these images.

In examining the processes that make such structures salient in our perception, it is useful to draw a distinction between local and global (or structural) saliency. Our attention is sometimes drawn to an item in the image because it is different in some local property from neighboring elements; for example, a green dot in an image of red dots, or a vertical line segment surrounded by horizontal ones. This phenomenon of local saliency has been investigated in a number of psychological studies (see, e.g., Treisman and Gelade 1980; Julesz 1981). In other cases (such as Fig. 2c,d), the salient structure has no conspicuous local part having a distinguishing local property such as color, orientation, contrast, or curvature. Although the elements comprising the structure are not individually salient, their arrangement makes the figure as a whole somehow globally conspicuous. In the more general case, the saliency of an image structure may be determined by the combination of both local and global aspects.

The section below describes a model that has been developed to extract certain classes of globally salient structures from images. This process on its own is not intended to provide a full solution to the selection problem, but, as discussed at the end of the section, it offers a useful first stage in solving the problem.

Detecting Globally Salient Image Structures

The model for extracting salient image structures proceeds by computing at each point in the image a measure of saliency. A successful model of this type will assign high saliency measure to image structures that are also salient in human perception, and should provide an efficient method for extracting from the image the conspicuous structures such as the car or the blobs in Figure 2, b–d.

For simplicity, the input image is assumed to be composed of contours. Such contours may be, for example, the lines and edges extracted from the image by line and edge detection processes. The saliency measure in the model increases with the contour's length, and decreases with its curvature or curvature variation. That is, the measure is designed to favor image contours that are long and smooth. I concentrate below on a somewhat simpler version that does not take into account curvature variation, and only increases with overall length and decreases with total curvature. The use of length and curvature parameters was motivated by psychophysical observations, and the exact form of saliency measure was determined by computational considerations that are discussed in more detail below.

In defining the mathematical form of the saliency measure, it is convenient to consider first a single contour Γ in the image, and ignore all others. Let p be a point on Γ, and $S_{\Gamma}(p)$ be the saliency measure at point p assuming that Γ is the only relevant curve. The saliency at p is then given by

$$S_{\Gamma}(p) = \sum_i w_i \sigma_i$$

In this expression, σ_i is the local saliency of the ith edge element along the curve (Fig. 3a). For now, σ_i can be thought of simply as having the value "1" for every edge element i, and "0" if the edge element is missing (i.e., there is a gap in the curve). More generally, the values of σ_i provide the link between local and global saliency. The idea is that the σ_i are determined by a

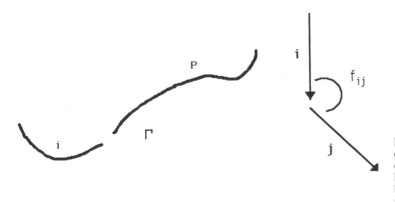

a   b

Figure 3. The saliency computation. (*a*) The contribution of element i to the saliency at p depends on the total curvature between the two locations. For details, see text. (*b*) Two neighboring line elements in the network for computing global saliency. The "coupling constant" $f_{i,j}$ between them decreases with the angle between the two elements.

local saliency measure; they increase, for example, for higher contrast, or when the ith edge element differs significantly from its neighbors in color or orientation, etc. The scheme can provide in this manner a measure of the global saliency based on length and curvature, while at the same time taking into account the local saliency of the individual components.

In the expression above, the overall saliency is obtained by a weighted sum of the local contributions σ_i along Γ. The weight w_i of the ith element is

$$e^{-c_i}$$

where c_i is the total curvature of the contour from p up to the ith element (a slight extension of this definition is introduced below).

The saliency measure defined so far depends on a particular curve Γ. The final saliency at p is given by

$$S(p) = max_\Gamma \, S_\Gamma(p)$$

The maximum is taken over all possible curves terminating at p. (This computes the contribution to p from one side of the curve; the contribution from the other side is determined in a similar way.) In practice, it is also convenient to use this definition limited to curves of length N

$$S_N(p) = max_{\Gamma_N} \, S_{\Gamma_N}(p)$$

where Γ_N stands for Γ restricted to length N. It is important to realize that the optimum is sought over all possible curves, including fragmented ones. In the case of the fragmented circle in Figure 2c, for example, the scheme will in effect consider all the possible curves running through any number of the individual line segments in the figure. This task appears quite demanding. To determine the salient figure, one must consider all possible curves through all the elements in the image, and integrate along each one the curvature-based saliency measure defined above. As it turns out, the saliency measure described above can in fact be computed by a surprisingly simple, locally connected network described below.

Computing Global Saliency by a Simple Local Network

To detect the globally salient structure in the image, the saliency measure $S(p)$ is computed at each image point p by a locally connected network of processing units. The processing elements can be thought of as "line detectors" that respond to the presence of lines or edges in the image. The entire image is covered by a grid of $n \times n$ points, where each point corresponds to a specific x, y location in the image. At each point p, there are k "orientation elements" coming into p from neighboring points, and the same number of orientation elements leaving p to nearby points. Each orientation element p_i (the ith orientation element at point p)

responds to an input image by signaling the presence of the corresponding line segment in the image. A lack of activity at p_i means that the corresponding line segment is not present in the image. The activity level of the element p_i, denoted by E_{p_i}, will eventually correspond to the saliency of this line element. The initial activity is determined by the local saliency of the element, denoted by σ_i. This local saliency is determined by comparing the element in question with surrounding elements along a number of dimensions. For example, if the ith element has high contrast, or if it is very different from the surrounding elements in color, orientation, or direction of motion, then its local saliency will be high. To account for global rather than local saliency, the activity $E(p_i)$ is then modified by interactions with the neighboring elements, so that eventually it also measures the length and the curvature of the contour passing through p_i.

The activity $E(p_i)$ is updated by the following simple local computation:

$$E_{p_i}^{(0)} = \sigma_i$$

$$E_{p_i}^{(n+1)} = \sigma_i + \rho_i \max_{p_j} E_{p_i}^{(n)} f_{i,j}$$

where p_j is one of k possible neighbors of p_i. In this formula, $f_{i,j}$ are "coupling constants" between neighboring line elements. Their values in this model are given by

$$f_{i,j} = e^{-2\alpha_{ij} \tan(\alpha_{ij}/2)/\Delta s}$$

where α_{ij} is the angle between the successive elements i and j (see Fig. 3b). The main property of these coupling constants is that they decrease with the angle between successive elements. The particular choice of the coupling constants above ensures that the computed saliency will depend directly on the total curvature along the contour. In terms of these constants, the discrete approximation to the total curvature measured along p_i, $...p_j$ is obtained by

$$e^{C_{i,j}} = \prod_{k=i}^{j-1} f_{k,k+1}$$

where $C_{i,j}$ is the total curvature (squared) between elements i and j. This quantity is equal to unity for a straight line and decays to zero as the curvature increases. The factors ρ_i are of secondary importance; they make the contributions of faraway locations smaller than that of nearby elements along the curve (for more detail, see Ullman and Shashua 1988).

The updating formula is in fact a very simple one, and the saliency computation as defined above is simple and local. At each step in the iteration at a given element, the element simply adds the maximal contribution of its k neighbors to its original local saliency σ_i.

The interesting point about this computation is that by using this simple updating formula, the quantity E_{p_i} computes at every point p the desired measure $S(p)$

defined above. It is remarkable that such a simple local computation is sufficient for this task. The saliency measure S at a point p in the image is in fact a rather elaborate measure. For each possible curve Γ passing through p, it must compute a measure S_Γ. Then, of all the curves passing through p, the best one (with highest S_Γ) must be selected. The computation achieves all of this without explicitly tracing and examining different curves. In addition, although the number of possible

curves of length N increases exponentially as the number N grows, the computation is only linear in the length N.

Figure 4 shows examples of the computation applied to three figures. The first is the car image in Figure 2a (only a portion of the image is shown). The left figure is a "saliency map" after 30 iterations of the computation. The wider, lighter contours are those with higher saliency $E(p)$. It can be seen that the activity at the

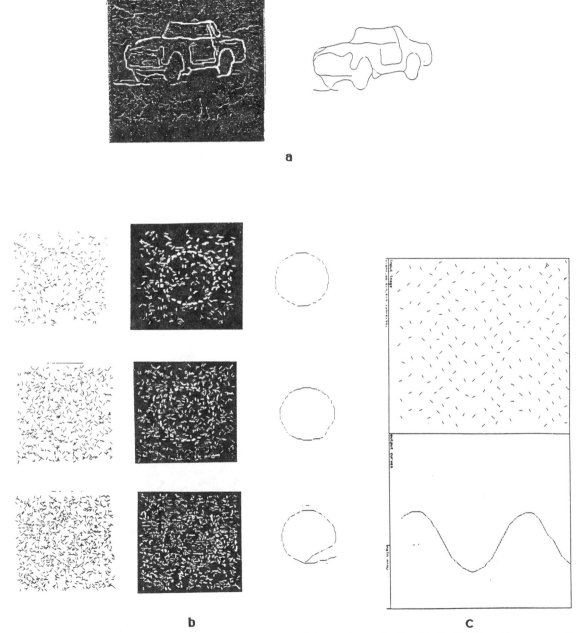

Figure 4. Results of the saliency computation. (*a*) A portion of the car image in Fig. 2d. (*Left*) The saliency map after 30 iterations. (*Right*) The five most active (salient) contours after 30 iterations. (*b*) A fragmented circle embedded in increasing amounts of noise. (*Left*) Original images. (*Center*) The saliency map after 10 iterations. (*Right*) The most salient contour following 10 iterations. (*c*) A sinusoidal curve in background noise. (*Top*) The input figure. (*Bottom*) The most salient contour in the input image.

background is reduced compared to the activity at the figure. The figure on the right shows the five most salient contours by the end of the 30 iterations.

Although the process successfully selects the main object in this image, it should be noted that, in general, the saliency computation described is not intended to model the entire process of selecting out a candidate object from the image. A more plausible view is that such a selection process is obtained in two stages. The first stage, which is applied uniformly and in parallel across the entire image, selects and "highlights" a small number of processes. A candidate object can be selected by processing these preferred contours further. This second stage can be more attentive and applied preferentially to the contours selected in the first stage, rather than to all the contours in the image.

Figure 4b shows a fragmented circle embedded in increasing amounts of noise. The left column illustrates the input figures. It can be noted that in the first two images the circle is immediately discernible by our perceptual system despite the gaps and the high noise level. The second column shows the saliency map after 10 iterations, and the right column shows the most active (salient) contour by the end of 10 iterations. The performance of the scheme appears to be comparable to human perception. It is also worth noting that the gaps in the original figure are filled in during the course of the computation.

Figure 4c was supplied to us by J. Beck from the University of Oregon. Beck has noted that the figure is a challenging one, but still perceivable by human observers. It is also interesting because it is not a simple closed compact figure. Schemes that are sensitive specifically to blob-like structures will not be able to extract such long curved structures. The scheme described above has some preference for closed figures, but, like human vision, can detect any smooth extended structure.

In summary of this part regarding the selection of salient image structures, a number of points are worth noting.

1. There are good reasons to believe, on the basis of psychophysical and computational considerations, that processes involved in segmenting the image and selecting structures for further processing are important in the early stages of visual information processing. The lower-level visual areas in the hierarchy of visual areas, such as V1 and V2, may be involved in this type of processing. The saliency map itself may also have a physiological counterpart, but not necessarily in V1 or V2.
2. Segmentation and selection probably involve a number of different processes, and they depend on both local (e.g., contrast, color, and motion) as well as global (e.g., length and overall curvature) properties.
3. The (global) saliency of a contour in the image increases when the contour is long and smooth.
4. The extraction of smooth long contours can be ob-

tained by a simple network of locally interacting line elements.

COMPENSATING FOR VIEWING DIRECTION

The problem of compensating for changes in the image induced by different orientations of objects in three-dimensional (3-D) space is a difficult one, and a number of schemes have been proposed over the years as possible models for how the visual system may overcome this problem. In this section, I present briefly a new scheme that differs from previous ones in that it uses collections of two-dimensional (2-D) images instead of storing 3-D object models. The scheme appears to be simpler and more direct than alternative schemes, and it is hoped, therefore, that it may correspond more closely to the processes used by biological visual systems in recognizing 3-D objects.

In most previous recognition theories, it has been assumed that the visual system somehow stores and manipulates 3-D object models. When confronted with a novel 2-D image of the object, the system must deduce whether it is a possible view of one of the already stored 3-D objects. For example, it may try to find a transformation in space (rotation, translation, and scaling) that will make a stored 3-D model compatible with the image. What we propose to do instead is to directly use small collections of 2-D images. The new approach has several advantages. First, there is no need in this scheme to explicitly recover and represent the 3-D structure of objects. Second, it handles all the rigid 3-D transformations, but it is not restricted to such transformations. Third, the processes involved are often simpler than in previous schemes. Fourth, it becomes easier to acquire new object models.

In our approach, a 3-D object is represented by the linear combination of 2-D images of the object. If $M = M_1, \ldots, M_k$ is the set of pictures representing a given object, and P is the 2-D image of an object to be recognized, then P is considered an instance of M if $P = \sum_{i=1}^{k} \alpha_i M_i$ for some constants α_i.

What I mean by a linear combination of views is the following. Suppose that (x_i, y_i), (x'_i, y'_i) (x''_i, y''_i) are the coordinates of corresponding points (i.e., points in the image that arise from the same point on the object) in three different views. Let X_1, X_2, X_3 be the vectors of x-coordinates of the points in the three views. Suppose that we are now confronted with a new image, and X' is the vector of the x-coordinates of the points in this new view. If X' arises from the same object represented by the original three views, then it will be possible to express X' as the linear combination of X_1, X_2, X_3. That is, $X' = a_1 X_1 + a_2 X_2 + a_3 X_3$ for some constants a_1, a_2, a_3. Similarly, for the y-coordinates, $Y' = b_1 Y_1 + b_2 Y_2 + b_3 Y_3$ for some constants b_1, b_2, b_3. This property is expressed by the following theorem: Note that, in general, different coefficients are required for the x and y components. In more pictorial terms, we can image that each of the three points x_i, x'_i, x''_i has a mass associated with it. The mass at x_i, x'_i, x''_i is a_1, a_2, a_3, respectively (the same weights are used for triplets). The linear combination of the points is now their center of mass.

Theorem: All possible views of a rigid object that can undergo rotation in space, translation, and scaling are spanned by the linear combinations of three views of the object.

The theorem assumes orthographic projection and objects with sharp bounding contours. For objects with smooth bounding contours, the number of views required is five rather than three. (Objects with smooth bounding contours, such as an egg or a football, are more complex because the object's silhouette is not generated by fixed contours on the object. The bounding contours generating the silhouette move on the object as the viewing position changes.) If the object is close to the camera and the perspective effects become large, the space spanned by all the object's views will

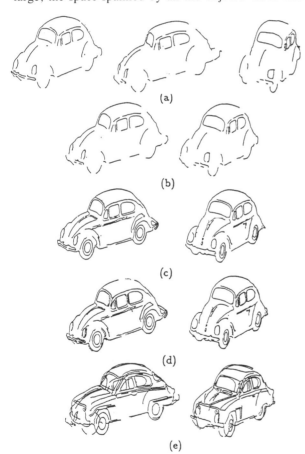

Figure 5. The linear combination of 2-D views. (*a*) Three views of a car (VW). Due to technical reasons, only some of the edges are illustrated. (*b*) Two new views of the VW. These new views were obtained by linear combinations of the views in *a*. (*c*) Two novel views of the VW. (*d*) Superposition of the images in *c* and the linear combinations in *b*. The new views are matched well by linear combinations of the original views. (*e*) The best matching linear combination to a similar, but different, car (a Saab). The match is less precise, illustrating that the linear combination can make fine distinctions between similar objects.

no longer be linear but will become slightly curved. Algorithms we develop (e.g., the RBF method below) can handle these cases and do not require strict linear combination. Finally, it should be noted that, due to self-occlusion, three views are insufficient for representing an object from all orientations. That is, a different set of views will be required to represent, e.g., the "front" and the "back" of the same object.

Figure 5 shows an example of using linear combinations of views to compensate for changes in viewing direction. Figure 5a shows three different views of a car (a Volkswagen [VW]). The figure shows only those edges that were extracted in all three views; as a result, some of the edges are missing. Figure 5b shows two new views of the VW car. These new images were not obtained from novel views of the car. They were generated instead using linear combinations of the first three views. Figure 5c shows two new views of the VW, obtained from new viewing positions. Figure 5d superimposes these new views and the linear combinations obtained in 5c. It can be seen that the novel views are matched well by linear combinations of the three original views. For comparison, Figure 5e shows the superposition of a different, but similar car (a Saab), with the best matching linear combinations of the VW images. As expected, the match is not as good. This illustrates that the linear combination method can be used to make fine distinctions between similar 3-D objects.

Using Combinations of Views for Recognition

The preceding section has stated and illustrated the fact that a novel view of a 3-D object can be matched by combinations of a small number of 2-D images. In this section, I consider briefly how this property may be used in a process for 3-D object recognition. There are several possible ways in which this can be accomplished. I briefly mention two possible methods. For a more complete discussion, see Ullman and Basri (1989).

The Use of a Linear Mapping

The linear combination property can be used to construct a linear operator that maps each view of a given object to a predefined vector, which identifies the object. We assume in this section that a correspondence has been established between the viewed object and the stored model. We then use a linear mapping to test whether the viewed object is a linear combination of the model views.

Suppose that a pattern of P is represented by a vector **p** of its coordinates, e.g., $(x_1, y_1, x_2, y_2, ..., x_n, y_n)$. Let P_1 and P_2 be two different patterns representing the same object. We can now construct a matrix L that maps both $\mathbf{p}_1$ and $\mathbf{p}_2$ to the same output vector **q**. That is, $L\mathbf{p}_1 = L\mathbf{p}_2 = \mathbf{q}$. Any linear combination $a\mathbf{p}_1 + b\mathbf{p}_2$ will then be mapped to the same output vector **q**, multiplied by the scalar $a + b$. We can choose, for example, $\mathbf{q} = \mathbf{p}_1$, in which case any view of the object will be mapped by L to a selected "canonical view" of it.

We have seen above that different views of the same object can be expressed as linear combinations $\Sigma a_i \mathbf{p}_i$ of a small number of representative views P_i. If the mapping matrix L is constructed in such a manner that $L\mathbf{p}_i = \mathbf{q}$ for all the views P_i in the same model, then any combined view $\hat{\mathbf{p}} = \Sigma a_i \mathbf{p}_i$ will be mapped by L to the same $\mathbf{q}$ (up to a scale), since $L\hat{\mathbf{p}} = (\Sigma a_i)\mathbf{q}$.

L can be constructed as follows. Let $\{\mathbf{p}_1, \ldots, \mathbf{p}_k\}$ be k linearly independent vectors representing the model pictures (we can assume that they are all linearly independent since a picture that is not is obviously redundant). Let $\{\mathbf{p}_{k+1}, \ldots, \mathbf{p}_n\}$ be a set of vectors such that $\{\mathbf{p}_1, \ldots, \mathbf{p}_n\}$ are all linearly independent. We define the following matrices:

$$P = (\mathbf{p}_1, \ldots, \mathbf{p}_k, \mathbf{p}_{k+1}, \ldots, \mathbf{p}_n)$$
$$Q = (\mathbf{q}, \ldots, \mathbf{q}, \mathbf{p}_{k+1}, \ldots, \mathbf{p}_n)$$

We require that

$$LP = Q$$

Therefore,

$$L = QP^{-1}$$

Note that since P is composed of n linearly independent vectors, the inverse matrix P^{-1} exists, therefore L can always be constructed.

By this definition, we obtain a matrix L that maps any linear combination of the set of vectors $\{\mathbf{p}_1, \ldots, \mathbf{p}_k\}$ to a scaled pattern $\alpha\mathbf{q}$. Furthermore, it maps any vector orthogonal to $\{\mathbf{p}_1, \ldots, \mathbf{p}_k\}$ to itself. Therefore, if $\hat{\mathbf{p}}$ is a linear combination of $\{\mathbf{p}_1, \ldots, \mathbf{p}_k\}$ with an additional orthogonal noise component, it would be mapped by L to $\mathbf{q}$ combined with the same amount of noise.

In our implementation, we have used $L\mathbf{p}_i = 0$ for all the view vectors $\mathbf{p}_i$ of a given object. The reason is that if a new view of the object $\hat{\mathbf{p}}$ is given by $\Sigma a_i \mathbf{p}_i$ with $\Sigma a_i = 0$, then $L\hat{\mathbf{p}} = 0$. This means that the linear mapping L may send a legal view to the zero vector, and it is therefore convenient to choose the zero vector as the common output for all the object's views. If it is desirable to obtain at the output level a canonical view of the object such as $\mathbf{p}_1$ rather than the zero vector, then one can use as the final output the vector $\mathbf{p}_1 - L\hat{\mathbf{p}}$.

The decision regarding whether or not $\hat{\mathbf{p}}$ is a view of the object represented by L can be based on comparing $\|L\hat{\mathbf{p}}\|$ with $\|\hat{\mathbf{p}}\|$. If $\hat{\mathbf{p}}$ is indeed a view of the object, then this ratio will be small (exactly 0 in the noise-free condition). If the view is "pure noise" (in the space orthogonal to the span of $[\mathbf{p}_1, \ldots, \mathbf{p}_k]$), then this ratio will be equal to 1.

The Use of Linear Receptive Fields

To use the above idea, it becomes necessary to establish a correspondence between the object in the image and a model in memory. There are several possible ways to approach this problem. Here we propose a simple method, motivated in part by considerations of biological plausibility, that is based on the notion of linear receptive fields.

A linear receptive field (LRF) can be thought of as an operator that takes a weighted contribution of the points falling within a given region, using a linear weighting function. We will assume here that the LRF response is simply the average contribution of the points falling inside its region. That is, given an image P, the response r is given by $\alpha\bar{x} + \beta\bar{y}$ (for some parameters α, β), where the average is taken over all the points of P falling within the receptive field.

Let us examine the response of an LRF of this type to the model and the viewed object. Let P_1 and P_2 be two pictures in the model set, $\hat{P}$ is the viewed object, and assume that $\hat{P} = aP_1 + bP_2$. Let r_1, r_2, and $\hat{r}$ be the responses of the LRF to P_1, P_2, and $\hat{P}$, respectively. For each pattern, the LRF "sees" only a subset of the points comprising the pattern. The other points fall outside the receptive field. If the points seen by the LRF in P_1, P_2, and $\hat{P}$ are corresponding points (even if the pointwise correspondence is unknown), then it is clear from the considerations above that $\hat{r} = ar_1 + br_2$. In practice, some of the points may not have counterparts inside the LRF, but the relation will hold approximately provided that the majority of points remain within the limits of the receptive field in P_1, P_2, and $\hat{P}$. To obtain this condition it is desirable to (1) use large receptive fields and (2) apply some rough alignment prior to the match. This rough alignment should compensate for large discrepancies in position, scale, and overall orientation in the image plane.

We can now proceed along the following line. Let $\mathbf{r} = (r_1, r_2, \ldots, r_m)$ be an ordered set of LRFs. We define a model to be the result of applying this set $\mathbf{r}$ to each of the model pictures. Given an image I, we first perform a process of rough alignment and denote the result by I'. We apply the set $\mathbf{r}$ to I', and then we check whether the result is a linear combination of the model pictures, that is, we look for a set $\{a_1, a_2, \ldots, a_k\}$ of coefficients such that for every $1 \leq i \leq m$ it holds that

$$r_i(I') = \sum_{j=1}^{k} a_j r_i(P_j)$$

This equality can be tested by using the linear mapping approach outlined earlier. This means that a matrix of connections is formed to map each of the vectors $\mathbf{r}(P_i)$ to a fixed canonical output vector. A preliminary stage of rough alignment is required in this scheme to bring each point in the image to lie close to a corresponding position in the model (one of the model pictures). Consequently, each linear receptive field will contain a relatively large proportion of corresponding points. As a result, the application of the set of LRFs to the image will yield approximately a linear combination of the results of applying the same set of LRFs to the model pictures.

The matching scheme has been outlined above in terms of abstract operations. In terms of an actual implementation within the visual system, it has the following meaning. First, a process of rough alignment is applied. This process will not be discussed here. Next, the image is passed through a set of linear receptive fields. The pattern of activity of these units is then mapped linearly onto a new set of units. The weights of this mapping embody the matrix L above. The output pattern is expected to be approximately invariant, even when the 3-D object changes its orientation in space. It appears premature to propose a more specific biological implementation. The above description is meant primarily to suggest that the use of 2-D images can be accomplished by rather straightforward and, from a biological standpoint, not implausible operations.

The use of LRFs serves in this scheme two distinct purposes. The first is to establish correspondence between subsets of image points, rather than individual points. The second is a conversion between two different types of representations. The linear mapping method assumes that the position of points is given by the numerical values of their x- and y-coordinates. The input image is given, however, in a different representation: a 2-D array of points. The LRF serves to translate the position of a point within the receptive field to a value representing the coordinate of the point. Other conversion schemes are possible, but the LRF is a simple one that also appears to be biologically plausible. It is interesting to note that cells with LRFs have been described in area 7a of macaque monkeys (Zipser and Andersen 1988). In Zipser and Andersen's model these cells also serve the role of converting position in the plane to a firing rate that represents x- or y-coordinate.

The Use of Radial Basis Function

An alternative scheme for combining 2-D views is the radial basis functions (RBF) method and its extensions described by T. Poggio (this volume). This method has the advantage that it is not limited to linear combinations of images; nonlinear combinations are also possible. To take full advantage of the results mentioned above (that the set of views of a given object spans a very low dimensional subspace in the space of possible views), the basic RBF method should be modified to allow the basis functions to be long and narrow rather than radial (and pointing in different directions in different parts of the space). Such an extended scheme may combine in an optimal manner the desired properties of the two methods, but it will not be considered here further.

The following points summarize the main conclusions of this part regarding the compensation for viewing direction.

1. In contrast with methods that use 3-D object models, the method outlined above uses directly small collections of 2-D images.
2. A particular view of a given 3-D object is represented in this scheme by the combined activity of units, where each unit is tuned in a broad manner to a particular 2-D view. This seems to be in general agreement with physiological findings regarding face-selective cells in the primate visual cortex (Perret et al. 1985). These cells usually respond best to a particular 2-D view of a face, but the response is broadly tuned and usually covers similar faces as well as the same face from a range of viewing directions.
3. The use of combinations of 2-D views in recognition appears more direct and straightforward compared with schemes that store and manipulate 3-D models, and may be more biologically plausible. The scheme is similar in certain respects to the direct use of an associative memory for 2-D patterns, but with a crucial difference. Given an input pattern, the system is not required to have an exact replica of the pattern already stored in memory. Instead, it is trying to establish whether the input pattern can be matched by combinations of small sets of stored patterns. As it turns out, such combinations are sufficient to compensate for the variations induced by changes in viewing direction.

ACKNOWLEDGMENTS

I thank my students and collaborators in this work, Amnon Shashua and Ronen Basri. S.U. and A.S. were supported in part by National Science Foundation grant IRI-8900207. A more expanded version of this material will appear in the Proceedings of the Conference on Attention and Performance, Ann Arbor, Michigan, 1990.

REFERENCES

Abu-Mostafa, Y.S. and D. Pslatis. 1987. Optical neural computing. *Sci. Am.* **256:** 66.
Freeman, W.J. 1979. EEG analysis gives model of neuronal template matching mechanism for sensory search with olfactory bulb. *Biol. Cybern.* **35:** 85.
Hopfield, J.J. 1982. Neural networks and physical systems with emergent collective computational abilities. *Proc. Natl. Acad. Sci.* **79:** 2554.
Julesz, B. 1981. Textons, the elements of texture perception, and their interactions. *Nature* **290:** 91.
Kohonen, T. 1978. *Associative memories: A system theoretic approach.* Springer-Verlag, Berlin.
Perret, D.I., P.A.J. Smith, D.D. Potter, A.J. Mistlin, A.S. Head, A.D. Milner, and M.A. Reeves. 1985. Visual cells in the temporal cortex sensitive to face view and gaze direction. *Proc. R. Soc. Lond. B Biol. Sci.* **223:** 293.
Treisman, A. and G. Gelade. 1980. A feature integration theory of attention. *Cognit. Psychol.* **12:** 97.
Ullman, S. and R. Basri. 1989. Recognition by linear combination of models. *M.I.T. A.I. Memo No. 1152.*
Ullman, S. and A. Shashua. 1988. Structural saliency: The detection of globally salient structures using a locally connected network. *M.I.T. A.I. Memo No. 1061.*
Willshaw, D.J., O.P. Buneman, and H.C. Longuet-Higgins. 1969. Non-holographic associative memory. *Nature* **222:** 960.
Zipser, D. and R.A. Andersen. 1988. A back-propagation programmed network that simulates response properties of a subset of posterior pariental neurons. *Nature* **331:** 679.

A Theory of How the Brain Might Work

T. POGGIO

I.R.S.T., Povo, 38100 Trento, Italy; Thinking Machines Co., Artificial Intelligence Laboratory, Cambridge, Massachusetts 02142; Center for Biological Information Processing, Massachusetts Institute of Technology, Cambridge, Massachusetts 02139

I wish to propose a quite speculative new version of the grandmother cell theory to explain how the brain, or parts of it, may work. In particular, I discuss how the visual system may learn to recognize three-dimensional objects. The model would apply directly to the cortical cells involved in visual face recognition. I also outline the relationship of our theory to existing models of the cerebellum and of motor control. Specific biophysical mechanisms can be readily suggested as part of a basic type of neural circuitry that can learn to approximate multidimensional input/output mappings from sets of examples and that is expected to be replicated in different regions of the brain and across modalities. The main points of the theory are:

1. The brain uses modules for multivariate function approximation as basic components of several of its information processing subsystems.
2. These modules are realized as HyperBF networks (Poggio and Girosi 1990a,b).
3. HyperBF networks can be implemented in terms of biologically plausible mechanisms and circuitry.

The theory predicts a specific type of population coding that represents an extension of schemes such as look-up tables. I conclude with some speculations about the trade-off between memory and computation and the evolution of intelligence.

I. THE GRANDMOTHER NEURON THEORY

A classic theme in the neurophysiological literature, at least since the work of Hubel and Wiesel (1962), is the idea of information processing in the brain as leading to "grandmother" neurons responding selectively to the precise combination of visual features that are associated with one's grandmother. Even when not explicitly stated, this notion seems to capture how many neuroscientists believe that the brain works. The grandmother neuron theory is of course not restricted to vision and applies as well to other sensory modalities and even to motor control under the form of cells corresponding to elemental movements. Why is this idea so attractive? The idea is attractive because of its simplicity: It replaces possibly complex information processing with the superficially simpler task of accessing a memory. The problem of recognition and motor control would be solved by simply accessing look-up tables containing appropriate descriptions of objects and of motor actions. The human brain can probably exploit a vast amount of memory with its 10^{14} or so synapses, making attractive any scheme that replaces computation with memory. In the case of vision, the apparent simplicity of this solution hides the difficult problems of an appropriate representation of an object and of how to extract it from complex images. Even assuming that these problems of representation, feature extraction, and segmentation could be solved by other mechanisms, a fundamental difficulty seems to be intrinsic to the grandmother cell idea. The difficulty consists of the combinatorial explosion in the number of cells that any scheme of the look-up table type would reasonably require for either vision or motor control. In the case of three-dimensional object recognition, for instance, there should be for each object as many entries in the look-up table as there are two-dimensional views of the object, in principle an infinite number!

The difficulty of a combinatorial explosion lies at the heart of theories of intelligence that attempt to replace information processing with look-up tables of precomputed results. In this paper, we suggest a scheme that avoids the combinatorial problem, while retaining the attractive features of the look-up table. The basic idea is to use only a few entries and interpolate or approximate among them. A mathematical theory based on this idea leads to a powerful scheme of learning from examples that is equivalent to a parallel network of simple processing elements. The scheme has an intriguingly simple implementation in terms of plausible biophysical mechanisms. We discuss in particular the case of three-dimensional object recognition but propose that the scheme is possibly used by the brain for several different information-processing tasks. Many information-processing problems can be represented as the composition of one or more multivariate functions that map an input signal into an output signal in a smooth way. These modules could be synthesized from a sufficient set of input/output pairs—the examples—by the scheme described here. Because of the power and general applicability of this mechanism, we speculate that a part of the machinery of the brain, including perhaps some of the cortical circuitry that is somewhat similar across the different modalities, may be dedicated to the task of function approximation.

II. HOW TO SYNTHESIZE THROUGH LEARNING THE BASIC APPROXIMATION MODULE: REGULARIZATION NETWORKS

This section describes a technique for synthesizing the approximation modules discussed above through learning from examples. I first explain how to rephrase the problem of learning from examples as a problem of approximating a multivariate function. The material in this section is from Poggio and Girosi (1989, 1990a,b), where more details can be found.

To illustrate the connection, let us draw an analogy between learning an input/output mapping and a standard approximation problem, two-dimensional surface reconstruction from sparse data points. *Learning* simply means collecting the *examples*, i.e., the input coordinates x_i, y_i, and the corresponding output values at those locations, the heights of the surface d_i. *Generalization* means estimating d at locations x, y where there are no examples, i.e., no data. This requires interpolating or, more generally, approximating the surface (i.e., the function) between the data points (interpolation is the limit of approximation when there is no noise in the data). In this sense, learning is a problem of *hypersurface reconstruction* (Omohundro 1987; Poggio et al. 1988, 1989).

From this point of view, learning a smooth mapping from examples is clearly ill-posed, in the sense that the information in the data is not sufficient to reconstruct uniquely the mapping at places where data are not available. In addition, the data are usually noisy. A priori assumptions about the mapping are needed to make the problem well-posed. One of the simplest assumptions is that the mapping is *smooth*: Small changes in the inputs cause a small change in the output. Techniques that exploit smoothness constraints in order to transform an ill-posed problem into a well-posed one are well known under the term of *regularization theory* and have interesting Bayesian interpretations (Tikhinov and Arsenin 1977; Poggio et al. 1985; Bertero et al. 1988). We have recently shown that the solution to the approximation problem given by regularization theory can be expressed in terms of a class of multilayer networks that we call regularization networks or Hyper Basis Functions (HyperBFs) (see Fig. 1). Our main result (Poggio and Girosi 1989) is that the regularization approach is equivalent to an expansion of the solution in terms of a certain class of functions:

$$f(\mathbf{x}) = \sum_{i=1}^{N} c_i G(\mathbf{x}; \xi_i) + p(\mathbf{x}) \qquad (1)$$

where $G(\mathbf{x})$ is one such function and the coefficients c_i satisfy a linear system of equations that depend on the N "examples," i.e., the data to be approximated. The term $p(\mathbf{x})$ is a polynomial that depends on the smoothness assumptions. In many cases, it is convenient to include up to the constant and linear terms. Under relatively broad assumptions, the Green's function G is radial and therefore the approximating function becomes

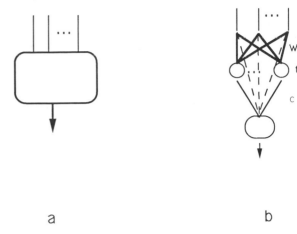

a   b

Figure 1. (*a*) The basic learning module that (we conjecture) is used by the brain for a number of tasks. The module learns to approximate a multivariate function from a set of examples (i.e., a set of input/output pairs). (*b*) A HyperBF network equivalent to a module for approximating a scalar function of three variables from sparse and noisy data. The data, a set of points where the value of the function is known, can be considered as examples to be used during learning. The hidden units evaluate the function $G(\mathbf{x}; \mathbf{t}_n)$, and a fixed, nonlinear, invertible function may be present after the summation. The units are in general fewer than the number of examples. The parameters that are determined during learning are the coefficients c_n, the centers $\mathbf{t}_n$ and the norm-weights $\mathbf{W}$. In the radial case $G = G(\|\mathbf{x} - \mathbf{t}_n\|_{\mathbf{W}}^2)$ and the hidden units simply compute the radial basis functions G at the "centers" $\mathbf{t}_n$. The radial basis functions may be regarded as matching the input vectors against the "templates" or "prototypes" that correspond to the centers (consider, for instance, a radial Gaussian around its center, which is a point in the n-dimensional space of inputs). There may be also connections computing the polynomial term of Fig. 1b: Constant and linear terms (the dotted lines in b) may be expected in most cases.

$$f(\mathbf{x}) = \sum_{i=1}^{N} c_i G(\|\mathbf{x} - \xi_i\|^2) + p(\mathbf{x}) \qquad (2)$$

which is a sum of radial functions, each with its *center* ξ_i on a distinct data point and of constant and linear terms (from the polynomial, when restricted to be of degree one). The number of radial functions, and corresponding centers, is the same as the number of examples.

Our derivation shows that the type of basis functions depends on the specific a priori assumption of smoothness. Depending on it, we obtain the Gaussian $G(r) = e^{-(r/c)^2}$, the well-known "thin plate spline" $G(r) = r^2 \ln r$, and other specific functions, radial and not. As observed by Broomhead and Lowe (1988) in the radial case, a superposition of functions like Equation 1 is equivalent to a network of the type shown in Figure 1b. The interpretation of Equation 2 is simple: in the two-dimensional case, for instance, the surface is approximated by the superposition of, say, several two-dimensional Gaussian distributions, each centered on one of the data points.

The network associated with Equation 2 can be made more general in terms of the following extension

$$f^*(\mathbf{x}) = \sum_{\alpha=1}^{n} c_\alpha G(\|(\mathbf{x} - \mathbf{t}_\alpha)\|_W^2) + p(\mathbf{x}) \qquad (3)$$

where the parameters $\mathbf{t}_\alpha$, which we call "centers," and the coefficients c_α are unknown, and are in general many fewer than the data points ($n \leqslant N$). The norm is a *weighted norm*

$$\|(\mathbf{x} - \mathbf{t}_\alpha)\|_W^2 = (\mathbf{x} - \mathbf{t}_\alpha)^T W^T W(\mathbf{x} - \mathbf{t}_\alpha) \qquad (4)$$

where W is an unknown square matrix and the superscript T indicates the transpose. In the simple case of diagonal W, the diagonal elements w_i assign a specific weight to each input coordinate, determining in fact the units of measure and the importance of each feature (the matrix W is especially important in cases in which the input features are of a different type and their relative importance is unknown). Equation 3 can be implemented by the network of Figure 1. Notice that a sigmoid function at the output may sometimes be useful without increasing the complexity of the system (see Poggio and Girosi 1989). Notice also that there could be more than one set of Green's functions, for instance, a set of multiquadrics and a set of Gaussians, each with its own $\mathbf{W}$. Notice that two or more sets of Gaussians, each with a diagonal $\mathbf{W}$, are equivalent to sets of Gaussians with their own σs.

Learning

Iterative methods can be used to find the optimal values of the various sets of parameters, the c_α, the w_i, and the $\mathbf{t}_\alpha$, that minimize an error functional on the set of examples. Steepest descent is *the* standard approach that requires calculations of derivatives. An even simpler method that does not require calculation of derivatives (suggested and found surprisingly efficient in preliminary work by B. Caprile and F. Girosi, pers. comm.) is to look for random changes (controlled in appropriate ways) in the parameter values that reduce the error. We define the error functional—also called energy—as

$$H[f^*] = H_{c,t,\mathbf{w}} = \sum_{i=1}^{N} (\Delta_i)^2$$

with

$$\Delta_i \equiv y_i - f^*(\mathbf{x}) = y_i - \sum_{\alpha=1}^{n} c_\alpha G(\|\mathbf{x}_i - \mathbf{t}_\alpha\|_{\mathbf{w}}^2)$$

In the first method, the values of c_α, $\mathbf{t}_\alpha$, and $\mathbf{W}$ that minimize $H[f^*]$ are regarded as the coordinates of the stable fixed point of the following dynamical system:

$$\dot{c}_\alpha = -\omega \frac{\partial H[f^*]}{\partial c_\alpha}, \qquad \alpha = 1, \ldots, n$$

$$\dot{\mathbf{t}}_\alpha = -\omega \frac{\partial H[f^*]}{\partial \mathbf{t}_\alpha}, \qquad \alpha = 1, \ldots, n$$

$$\dot{\mathbf{W}} = -\omega \frac{\partial H[f^*]}{\partial \mathbf{W}}$$

where ω is a parameter. The derivatives are rather complex (see Poggio and Girosi 1990a; and Notes section).

The second method is simpler: Random changes in the parameters are made and accepted if $H[f^*]$ decreases. Occasionally, changes that increase $H[f^*]$ may also be accepted (similarly to the Metropolis algorithm).

Interpretation of the Network

The interpretation of the network of Figure 1 is as follows. *After learning*, the centers of the basis functions are similar to prototypes, since they are points in the multidimensional input space. Each unit computes a (weighted) distance of the inputs from its center, that is, a measure of their similarity, and applies to it the radial function. In the case of the Gaussian, a unit will have maximum activity when the new input exactly matches its center. The output of the network is the linear superposition of the activities of all the basis functions in the network, plus direct, weighted connections from the inputs (the linear terms of $p[\mathbf{x}]$) and from a constant input (the constant term). Notice that in the limit case of the basis functions approximating delta functions, the system becomes equivalent to a look-up table. *During learning*, the weights c are found by minimizing a measure of the error between the network's prediction and each of the examples. At the same time, the centers of the radial functions and the weights in the norm are also updated during learning. Moving the centers is equivalent to modifying the corresponding prototypes and corresponds to task-dependent clustering. Finding the optimal weights $\mathbf{W}$ for the norm is equivalent to transforming appropriately, for instance scaling, the input coordinates and corresponds to task-dependent dimensionality reduction.

Regularization networks, of which HyperBFs are the most general and powerful version, represent a general framework for learning smooth mappings that rigorously connects approximation theory, generalized splines, and regularization with feedforward multilayer networks. They also contain as special cases the radial basis functions (RBF) technique (Micchelli 1986; Powell 1987; Broomhead and Lowe 1988) and several well-known algorithms, especially in the pattern recognition literature.

III. A PROPOSAL FOR A BIOLOGICAL IMPLEMENTATION

In this section, we point out some remarkable properties of Gaussian HyperBF, which may have implications for neurobiology.

Factorizable Radial Basis Functions

The synthesis of (weighted) RBFs in high dimensions may be easier if they are factorizable. It is easily seen that the *only RBF which is factorizable is the Gaussian (with diagonal* **W**). A multidimensional Gaussian function can be represented as the product of lower dimensional Gaussians. For instance, a two-dimensional Gaussian radial function centered in **t** can be written as

$$G(\|x - t\|^2_W) \equiv e^{-\|x-t\|^2_W} = e^{-(x-t_x)^2/2\sigma_x^2} \, e^{-(y-t_y)^2/2\sigma_y^2}$$

(5)

with $\sigma_x = 1/w_1$ and $\sigma_y = 1w_2$, where w_1 and w_2 are the elements of the matrix **W** assumed, in this section, to be diagonal.

This dimensionality factorization is especially attractive from the physiological point of view, since it is difficult to imagine how neurons could compute $G(\|x - t_\alpha\|^2)$. The scheme of Figure 2, on the other hand, is physiologically plausible. Gaussian radial functions in one, two, and possibly three dimensions can be implemented as *receptive fields* by weighted connections from the sensor arrays (or some retinotopic array

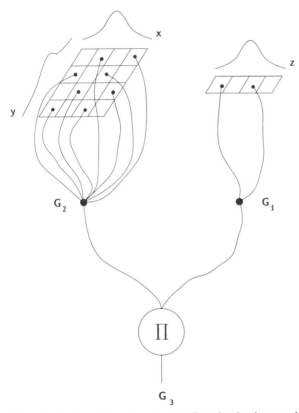

Figure 2. A three-dimensional radial Gaussian implemented by multiplying two-dimensional Gaussian and one-dimensional Gaussian receptive fields. The latter two functions are synthesized directly by appropriately weighted connections from the sensor arrays, as neural receptive fields are usually thought to arise. Notice that they transduce the implicit position of stimuli in the sensor array into a number (the activity of the unit). They thus serve the dual purpose of providing the required "number" representation from the activity of the sensor array and of computing a Gaussian function. Two-dimensional Gaussians acting on a retinotopic map can be regarded as representing two-dimensional "features," whereas the radial basis function represents the "template" resulting from the conjunction of those lower-dimensional features.

of units representing with their activity the position of features). Gaussians in higher dimensions can then be synthesized as products of one- and two-dimensional receptive fields.

This scheme has three additional interesting features:

1. The multidimensional radial functions are synthesized directly by appropriately weighted connections from the sensor arrays, without any need of an explicit computation of the norm and the exponential.
2. Two-dimensional Gaussians operating on the sensor array or on a retinotopic array of features extracted by some preprocessing transduce the implicit position of features in the array into a number (the activity of the unit).
3. Two-dimensional Gaussians acting on a retinotopic map can be regarded each as representing one two-dimensional "feature," i.e., a component of the input vector, whereas each center represents the "template," resulting from the conjunction of those lower-dimensional features. Notice that in this analogy the RBF is the AND of several features and could also include the negation of certain features, that is the AND NOT of them. **W** weights the importance of the different features.

Biophysical Mechanisms

The network. The multiplication operation required by the previous interpretation of Gaussian GRBFs to perform the "conjunction" of Gaussian receptive fields is not too implausible from a biophysical point of view. It could be performed by several biophysical mechanisms (see Koch and Poggio 1987). Here we mention three mechanisms:

1. Inhibition of the silent type and related circuitry (see Poggio and Torre 1978; Torre and Poggio 1978)
2. The AND-like mechanism of NMDA receptors
3. A logarithmic transformation, followed by summation, followed by exponentiation. The logarithmic and exponential characteristic could be implemented in appropriate ranges by the sigmoid-like pre-to-postsynaptic voltage transduction of many synapses.

If the first or the second mechanism is used, the product of Figure 3 can be performed directly on the dendritic tree of the neuron representing the corresponding radial function (alternatively, each dendritic tree may perform pairwise products only, in which case a logarithmic number of cells would be required). The scheme also requires a certain amount of memory per basis unit, in order to store the center vector. In the case of Gaussian receptive fields used to synthesize Gaussian RBFs, the center vector is effectively stored in the position of the two-dimensional (or one-dimensional) receptive fields and in their connections to the product unit(s). This is plausible physiologically.

The linear terms (the direct connections from the inputs to the output in Fig. 1) can be realized directly as

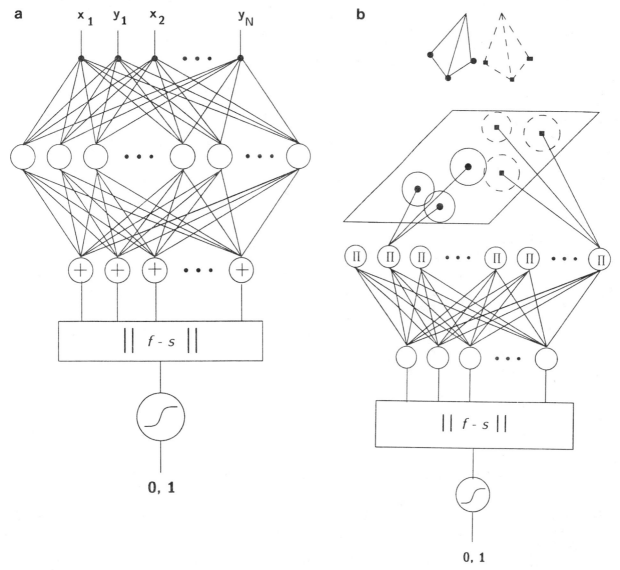

Figure 3. (*a*) The HyperBF network proposed for the recognition of a three-dimensional object from any of its perspective views (Poggio and Edelman 1990). The network attempts to map any view (as defined in the text) into a standard view, arbitrarily chosen. The norm of the difference between the output vector **f** and the standard view **s** is thresholded to yield a 0,1 answer. The $2N$ inputs accommodate the input vector **v** representing an arbitrary view. Each of the K radial basis functions is initially centered on one of a subset of the M views used to synthesize the system ($K < M$). During training, each of the M inputs in the training set is associated with the desired output, i.e., the standard view **s**. (*b*) A completely equivalent interpretation of *a* for the special case of Gaussian radial basis functions. Gaussian functions can be synthesized by multiplying the outputs of two-dimensional Gaussian receptive fields, that "look" at the retinotopic map of the object point features. The solid circles in the image plane represent the two-dimensional Gaussians associated with the first radial basis function, which represents the first view of the object. The dotted circles represent the two-dimensional receptive fields that synthesize the Gaussian radial function associated with another view. The two-dimensional Gaussian receptive fields transduce positions of features, represented implicitly as activity in a retinotopic array, and their product "computes" the radial function without the need of calculating norms and exponentials explicitly. (Reprinted, with permission, from Poggio and Girosi 1990b.)

inputs to the output neuron that summates linearly its synaptic inputs (an output nonlinearity is allowed and will not change the basic form of the model, see Poggio and Girosi 1989). They may also be realized through intermediate linear units.

Mechanisms for learning. Do the update schemes have a physiologically plausible implementation? Consider first the steepest descent methods, which require

derivatives. Equation 6 or a somewhat similar, quasi-Hebbian scheme is not too unlikely and may require only a small amount of neural circuitry. Equation 7 seems more difficult to implement for a network of real neurons.

Methods such as the random descent method, which do not require calculation of derivatives, are biologically much more plausible and seem to perform very well in preliminary experiments. In the Gaussian case, with basis functions synthesized through the product of Gaussian receptive fields, moving the centers means establishing or erasing connections to the product unit. A similar argument can be made also about the learning of the matrix **W**. Notice that in the diagonal Gaussian case, the parameters to be changed are exactly the σ of the Gaussians, i.e., the spread of the associated receptive fields. Notice also that the σ for all centers on one particular dimension is the same, suggesting that the learning of w_i may involve the modification of the scale factor in the input arrays rather than a change in the dendritic spread of the postsynaptic neurons. In all these schemes, the real problem consists in how to provide the "teacher" input (but see Fig. 5).

IV. VISUAL RECOGNITION OF THREE-DIMENSIONAL OBJECTS AND FACE-SENSITIVE NEURONS

We have recently suggested and demonstrated how to use a HyperBF network to learn to recognize a three-dimensional object. This section reviews very briefly this work (Poggio and Edelman 1990) and then suggests that the brain may use a similar strategy. Face-sensitive neurons are discussed as a specific instance.

HyperBF Networks for Recognizing Three-dimensional Objects

A three-dimensional object gives rise to an infinite variety of two-dimensional images or views, because of the infinite number of possible poses relative to the viewer, and because of arbitrarily different illumination conditions. Is it possible to synthesize a module that can recognize an object from any viewpoint, after it learns its three-dimensional structure from a small set of perspective views? We have recently shown (Poggio and Edelman 1990) that the HyperBF scheme may provide a solution to the problem provided that relatively stable and uniquely identifiable features (that we will call "labeled" features) can be extracted from the image.

In our scheme, a view is represented as a $2N$ vector $x_1, y_1, x_2, y_2, \ldots, x_N, y_N$ of the coordinates on the image plane of N labeled and visible feature points on the object. We assume that a view of an object is a vector of this type (instead of position in the image of feature points, we have also used angles between corners and length of segments or both), in general augmented by components that represent other properties of the object not necessarily related to its geometric shape, such as color or texture. We also assume that the function that maps the views into 0, 1 (0 if the view is of another object, 1 if the view is of the correct object) can be approximated by a smooth function (if this were false, one could approximate the mapping from the view to a "standard" view and then apply a radial function to the result, see Poggio and Edelman 1990).

The network used for this task is shown in Figure 3

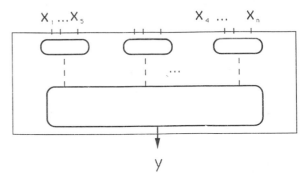

Figure 4. A hierarchical scheme in which HyperBF modules are inputs to another HyperBF module. As an example, a scheme of this type may be used for three-dimensional object recognition in the general case of spurious and missing features. Instead of encoding all n features, one encodes only subsets of dimensions d, where $d < n$. The input to each of the first row of modules is a different set of features of the object; the output is a value between 0,1 that indicates the degree of certainty that the input is the sought object. The last module is a decision module that integrates the various inputs. Notice that all modules could be synthesized by learning through independent sets of examples.

(see also Fig. 4). In the simplest version (fixed centers), the centers correspond to some of the examples, i.e., some views of the object. Updating the centers is equivalent to modifying the corresponding "prototypical views." Updating the weights of the matrix **W** corresponds to changing the relative importance of the various features that define the views of an object. This is important in the case in which these features are of a completely different type: A large w indicates a larger weight in the feature in the measure of similarity and is equivalent to a small σ in the Gaussian function. Features with a small role have a very large σ: Their exact position or value does not matter much.

An interesting conclusion of this work consists of the small number of views required to recognize an object from the infinite number of possible views. The results clearly show that the scheme avoids the main problem of look-up table schemes, the explosion in the number of entries. Furthermore, the performance of the HyperBF recognition scheme resembles human performance in a related task. As discussed in Poggio and Edelman (1990), the number of training views necessary to achieve an acceptable recognition rate on novel views, 80–100 for the full viewing sphere, is broadly compatible with the finding that people have trouble recognizing a novel wire-frame object previously seen from one viewpoint if it is rotated away from that viewpoint by about 30° (it takes 72 30° × 30° patches to cover the viewing sphere).

Recently, H. Buelthoff and S. Edelman (in prep.) have obtained interesting psychophysical results that support this model for human recognition of a certain class of three-dimensional objects against other possible models. In general, the experimental results fit closely the prediction of theories of the two-dimensional interpolation variety and appear to contradict theories that involve three-dimensional models.

Face-sensitive Neurons

The HyperBF recognition scheme we have outlined has suggestive similarities with some of the data about visual neurons responding to faces obtained by Perrett and co-workers recording from the temporal association cortex (see Perrett et al. 1987 and references therein; Poggio and Edelman 1990). Let us consider the network of Figure 3 as the skeleton for a model of the circuitry involved in the recognition of faces. One expects different modules, one for each different object of the type of the network of Figure 3. One also expects hierarchical organizations: For instance, a network of the HyperBF type may be used to recognize certain types of eyes and then may serve as input to another network involved in recognizing a certain class of faces, which may be itself one of the inputs to a network for a specific face. Different types of cells may then be expected. The overall output of a network for a specific face may be identified with the behavioral responses associated with recognition and may or may not coincide with an individual neuron. There should be cells or parts of cells corresponding to the centers, i.e., to the prototypes used by the networks. The response of these neurons should be a Gaussian function of the distance of the input to the template. These units would be somewhat similar to "grandmother" filters with a graded response, rather than binary detectors, each representing a prototype. They would be synthesized as the conjunction of, for instance, two-dimensional Gaussian receptive fields looking at a retinotopic map of features. During learning, the weights of the various prototypes in the network output are modified to find the optimal values that minimize the overall error. The prototypes themselves are slowly changed to find optimal prototypes for the task. The weights of the different input features are also modified to perform task-dependent dimensionality reduction.

Some of these expectations are consistent with the experimental findings of Perret et al. (1987). Some of the neurons described have several of the properties expected from the units of a HyperBF network with a center, i.e., a prototype that corresponds to a view of a specific face. Some of the main data (from Perret et al. 1987 and references therein) follow.

1. The majority of cells responsive to faces are sensitive to the general characteristics of the face, and they are somewhat invariant to its exact position and attitude.
2. Presenting parts of the face in isolation revealed that some of the cells responded to different subsets of features: Some cells are more sensitive to parts of the face such as eyes or mouth.
3. There are cells selective for a particular view of the head. Some cells were maximally sensitive to the front view of a face, and their response fell off as the head was rotated into the profile view, and others were sensitive to the profile view with no response to the front view of the face.
4. There are cells that are specific to the views of one individual. It seems that for each known person there would be a set of "face recognition units." Our model applies most directly to these neurons.

V. THEORIES OF THE CEREBELLUM AND OF MOTOR CONTROL

Cerebellum Models of Marr and Albus

The cerebellum is a part of the brain that is important in the coordination of complex muscle movements. The neural organization of the cerebellum is highly regular and well known (see Fig. 5). Marr (1969) and Albus (1971) modeled the cerebellum as a look-up table. The critical part of their theories is the assumption that the synapses between the parallel fibers and the Purkinje cells are modified as a function of the Purkinje cell activity *and* the climbing fibers input. I suggest (see Fig. 5) that the cerebellum is a HyperBF network or set of networks (one for each Purkinje cell). Instead of a simple look-up table, the cerebellum would be a *function approximation module* (in a sense, "an approximating look-up table"). In our conjecture, basket and Golgi cells would have different roles from the roles assumed in the Marr-Albus theory. In particular, the

Figure 5. (*a*) A sketch of the neurons of the cerebellum and their connections. In our conjecture, these would be the basic elements of a HyperBF network: The mossy fibers are the inputs, the granule cells correspond to the various centers and basis functions $G(x, x_i)$, the Purkinje cells correspond to the output units that summate the weighted activities of the basis units, whereas the climbing fibers carry the "teacher" signal y_i. The strength of the synapses between the parallel fibers and the Purkinje cells would correspond to the c_α. (*b*) The corresponding HyperBF network has two basis functions corresponding to the two granule cells in *a* and two output summation units corresponding to the two Purkinje cells in *a*.

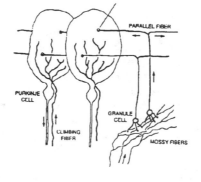

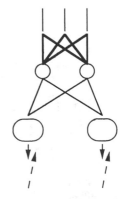

a

b

Golgi cells, which receive inputs from the parallel fibers and whose axons synapse on the granule cells/mossy fibers clusters, may be used to change the norm weights **W**.

Key assumptions include: (1) granule cells correspond to basis units (there may be as many as 200,000 granule cells per Purkinje cell) representing as many "examples"; (2) Purkinje cells are the outputs of the network; (3) climbing fibers are responsible for modifying synapses from granule cells to the Purkinje cell.

Theories of Motor Control

There are at least two aspects of motor control in which HyperBF modules could be used: (1) to compute smooth, time-dependent trajectories (for instance arm trajectories) given sparse points such as initial, final, and intermediate positions; (2) to associate to each position in the trajectory the appropriate field of muscle forces. These two problems may be solved by two modules that can be used in series, the first one providing the input to the second one (see Fig. 6a,b). I first consider the problem of computing appropriate smooth trajectories from sparse points in space-time. An interesting question is: Are HyperBFs a plausible implementation for Flash and Hogan's minimum jerk principle for the coordination of arm movements? Flash and Hogan (1985) found experimental evidence that arm trajectories minimize jerk, i.e., $C = \|x^{(3)}\|^2 + \|y^{(3)}\|^2$, where $x^{(3)}$ is the third temporal derivative of x. This suggests a regularization principle with a stabilizer corresponding to additive quintic splines. HyperBF could implement it using basis units recruited for the specific motion (as many as there are constrained points) with Gaussian-like or spline-like time-dependent activities (boundary conditions may have to be taken into account). The weights would be learned during training. As Morasso and Mussa-Ivaldi (1982) implied, approximation schemes of this type amount to composition of elemental movements. It is interesting to observe that jerk is automatically minimized by the linear superposition of the appropriate elemental movements, i.e., the appropriate Green's functions. Thus, a scheme of the Morasso-Mussa-Ivaldi type can be made to be perfectly equivalent to the Flash-Hogan minimization principle. The fact that the minimum jerk principle can be implemented directly by a HyperBF network is attractive from the point of view of a biological implementation, since biologically implausible direct minimization procedures are not required anymore. The minimization is implicit in the form of the elemental movements; weighted superposition of the elemental movements seems a much easier operation to implement in the motor system than explicit minimization.

The second problem requires a neural circuit that associates an equilibrium position to an appropriate activation. Bizzi (see, e.g., E. Bizzi et al., in prep.) suggests that a group of spinal cord interneurons specify the limb's final position and configuration

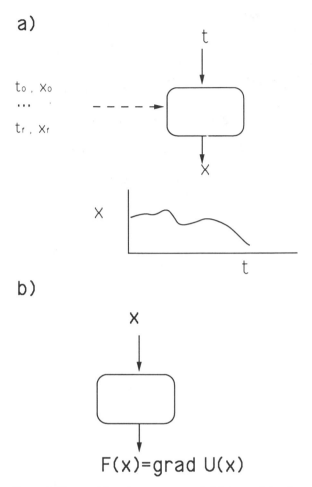

Figure 6. Two problems in motor control: (a) determining the trajectory x(t) from a small set of points (t_i, x_i) on the desired trajectory and (b) computing the field of muscle forces for each of the points on the trajectory. The figure suggests that two different HyperBF modules may be used to perform both tasks. In a, a HyperBF module approximates the trajectory from the sparse points by superimposing Gaussian distributions with the appropriate weights in such a way as to satisfy some minimum-jerk-like principle. In b, a module of the HyperBF type has been synthesized during development and continuously adapted to generate the appropriate field of forces for each equilibrium position x. It is similar to an approximating look-up table. A behavior of the look-up table type was suggested by Bizzi because of very recent experimental data (see E. Bizzi et al., in prep.).

through a field of muscle forces that have the appropriate equilibrium point. E. Bizzi et al. (in prep.) propose that the spinal cord contains aspects of motor behavior reminiscent of a look-up table. Their findings extend several results in the area of oculomotor research, where investigators have described neural structures whose activation brings the eyes or the head to a unique position. I suggest that the required look-up table behavior may be implemented through a HyperBF module that requires the storage of only a few equilibrium positions (or correspondingly, a few conservative-like fields, i.e., appropriate activation coefficients for the motoneurons) and can interpolate between them (see Fig. 6). Notice that the synthesis of a conservative field of muscle force could be achieved through the superposition (with arbitrary weights, over the index α) by the motor system of appropriate elementary motor fields of the form (see F. Mussa-Ivaldi and S. Giszter, in prep.)

$$\phi(\mathrm{x}, \alpha) = \frac{\mathrm{x} - \mathrm{x}_\alpha}{r_\alpha} \, G'(r_\alpha)$$

with $r_\alpha = \|\mathbf{x} - \mathbf{x}_\alpha\|$ and G is a radial basis function such as the Gaussian.

VI. SUMMARY: A PROPOSAL FOR HOW THE BRAIN WORKS

The theory proposed in this paper consists of three main points:

1. It assumes that the brain may use *modules that approximate multivariate functions and that can be synthesized from sparse examples* as basic components for several information-processing tasks.
2. It proposes that these modules are realized in terms of HyperBF networks, of which a rigorous theory is now available.
3. It shows how HyperBF networks can be implemented in terms of plausible biophysical mechanisms.

The theory is in a sense a modern version of the grandmother neurons idea, made computationally plausible by eliminating the combinatorial explosion in the number of required cells, which was the main problem in the old idea.

The proposal that much information processing in the brain is performed through modules that are similar to *enhanced look-up tables* is attractive for many reasons. It also promises to bring closer apparently orthogonal views, such as the *immediate perception* of Gibson and the *representational theory* of Marr, since almost iconic "snapshots" of the world may allow the synthesis of computational mechanisms completely equivalent to vision algorithms such as, say, structure-from-motion. The idea seems to change significantly the computational perspective on several vision tasks. As a simple example, consider the different specific tasks of hyperacuity, invented by the psychophysicists. The theory developed here would suggest that an appropriate module for the task, somewhat similar to a new "routine," may be synthesized by learning in the brain.

Notice that the theory makes two independent claims: The first is that the brain can be explained in part in terms of approximation modules, the second is that these modules are of the HyperBF type. The second claim implies that the modules are an extension of look-up tables. Notice that there are schemes other than HyperBF that could be used to extend look-up tables. Notice also that multilayer Perceptrons, typically used in conjunction with back-propagation, can also be considered as approximation schemes, albeit still without a convincing mathematical foundation. Unlike HyperBF networks, they cannot be interpreted as direct extensions of look-up tables (they are more similar to an extension of multidimensional Fourier series).

The theory suggests that population coding (broadly tuned neurons combined linearly) is a consequence of extending a look-up table scheme (corresponding to interval coding) to yield interpolation (or more precisely approximation, since the examples may be noisy), that is, generalization.

The theory suggests some possibly interesting ideas about the evolution of intelligence. It also makes a number of predictions for physiology and psychophysics. More work is needed to specify sufficiently the details and some of the basic assumptions of the theory in order to make it useful to biologists. The next sections deal with these last three points.

Evolution of Intelligence: From Memory to Computation

There is a duality between *computation* and *memory*. Given infinite resources, the two points of view are equivalent: For instance, I could play chess by precomputing winning moves for every possible state of the chessboard. More to the point, notice that basic logical operations can be defined in terms of *truth tables* and that all Boolean predicates can be represented in disjunctive normal form, i.e., as a look-up table.

Given that the brain probably has a prodigious amount of memory and given that one can build powerful approximating look-up tables using techniques such as HyperBF, is it possible that part of intelligence may be built from a set of souped-up look-up tables? One advantage of this point of view is to make it perhaps easier to understand how intelligence may have evolved from simple associative reflexes. In more than one sense (biophysical and computational), HyperBF-like networks are a natural and rather straightforward development of very simple systems of a few neurons showing basic learning phenomena such as classic conditioning.

Predictions and Remarks

General Predictions

1. Computation, as generalization from examples, emerges from the superposition of receptive fields in a multidimensional input space.
2. Computation is performed by *Gaussian receptive fields* and their combination (through some approximation to multiplication), rather than by threshold functions.
3. The theory predicts the existence of low-dimensional feature-like cells and multidimensional Gaussian-like receptive fields, somewhat similar to template-like cells, a fact that could be tested experimentally on cortical cells.
4. The HyperBF scheme is a general-purpose circuitry, used in the brain to synthesize module that can be regarded as approximating look-up tables. If this

point of view is correct, we expect the same basic kind of neural machinery to be replicated in different parts of the brain across different modalities (in particular in different cortical areas).

5. The "programming style" used by the brain in solving specific perceptual and motor problems is to synthesize appropriate architectures from modules of the type shown in Figure 1 (a very simple architecture built from the basic module of Fig. 1 is shown in Fig. 4).

Face Neurons

1. Some of the face cells correspond to basis functions with centers in a high-dimensional input space and are somewhat similar to prototypes or coarse "grandmother cells."

2. They could be synthesized as the conjunctions of features with Gaussian-like distance from the prototype.

3. Face cells are *not* detectors; often several may be active simultaneously. The output of the network is a combination of several prototypes.

4. From our preliminary experiments (Poggio and Edelman 1990), the number of basis cells that are required per object is about 40–80 for the full viewing sphere, but much less (10–20) for each aspect (e.g., frontal views). I conjecture that a similar estimate holds for faces.

5. Input to the face cells are features such as eye positions, mouth position, and hair color.

6. Eye features cells may be themselves the output of HyperBF networks specialized for eyes.

Cerebellum

1. The cerebellum is a set of approximation modules for learning to perform motor skills (both movements and posture).

2. Its neurons are elements of a HyperBF network: The mossy fibers are the inputs, the granule cells correspond to the basis functions $G(x, x_i)$, the Purkinje cells correspond to the output units that summate the weighted activities of the basis units, whereas the climbing fibers carry the "teacher" signal y_i.

3. The strength of the modifiable synapses between the parallel fibers and the Purkinje cells corresponds to the c_α.

4. Golgi cells may be involved in modifying during learning the center positions t_α and the norm weights $\mathbf{W}$.

Motor Control

The qualitative expectation is to find cells and circuits corresponding to the two stages shown in Figure 6. Spinal cord neurons, according to very recent data by E. Bizzi et al. (in prep.), specify the limb's final position and configuration.

Future

The proposal of this paper is just a rough sketch of a theory. Many details (some of them critical) need to be filled in. Some basic questions remain: For instance, how reasonable is the idea of supervised learning schemes? To say it in a different and perhaps more constructive way, what are the systems that can be synthesized from building blocks that are just function approximation modules? What types of tasks can be solved by systems of that type? On the biological side of the theory, the obvious next task is to develop detailed proposals for the circuitries underlying face recognition and motor control (including the circuitry of the cerebellum) that take into account up-to-date physiological and anatomical data.

Notes to Section I

1. Segmentation of an image in parts that are likely to correspond to separate objects is probably the most difficult problem in vision. Remember that already in the Perceptron book (Minsky and Papert 1969) recognition-in-context was shown to be significantly harder than recognition of isolated patterns. We assume here that this problem has been "solved," at least to a reasonable extent.

2. The same basic machinery in the brain may be used for synthesizing many different, "small" learning modules, as components of many different systems. This is very different from suggesting a single giant network that learns everything.

Notes to Section II

The relevant derivatives for optimization methods that need them are for the c_α

$$\frac{\partial H[f^*]}{\partial c_\alpha} = -2 \sum_{i=1}^N \Delta_i G(\|\mathbf{x}_i - \mathbf{t}_\alpha\|_{\mathbf{w}}^2) \qquad (6)$$

for the centers $\mathbf{t}_\alpha$

$$\frac{\partial H[f^*]}{\partial \mathbf{t}_\alpha} = 4 c_\alpha \sum_{i=1}^N \Delta_i G'(\|\mathbf{x}_i - \mathbf{t}_\alpha\|_{\mathbf{w}}^2) \mathbf{W}^T \mathbf{W}(x_i - \mathbf{t}_\alpha) \qquad (7)$$

and for $\mathbf{W}$

$$\frac{\partial H[f^*]}{\partial \mathbf{W}} = -4\mathbf{W} \sum_{\alpha=1}^n c_\alpha \sum_{i=1}^N \Delta_i G'(\|\mathbf{x}_i - \mathbf{t}_\alpha\|_{\mathbf{w}}^2) Q_{i,\alpha} \qquad (8)$$

where $Q_{i,\alpha} = (\mathbf{x}_i - \mathbf{t}_\alpha)^T$ *is a dyadic product and G' is the first derivative of G* (for details, see Poggio and Girosi 1990a).

Notes to Section III

1. There are many nonradial functions derived from our regularization formulation, such as tensor product splines, that are factorizable.

2. I have assumed here that all centers have the same **W**. It is possible to have sets of different Green's functions, each set with its own **W** (see Poggio and Girosi 1990a).

3. It is natural to imagine hierarchical architectures based on the HyperBF scheme: A multidimensional Gaussian "template" unit may be a "feature" input for another radial function (again because of the factorization property of the Gaussian). Of course, a whole HyperBF network may be one of the inputs to another HyperBF network.

4. I conjecture that Equation 8 could be approximated by a Hebbian-like rule for the elements of the diagonal **W** such as

$$w_k(t+1) = w_i(t) - \sum_{\alpha=1}^{n} c_\alpha \gamma(x_k(t) - (t_\alpha)_k)y_k(t) \tag{9}$$

where **y** is the output of the upper layer of Figure 1a, i.e., $\mathbf{y} = \mathbf{Wx}$ and γ is

$$\gamma = \Delta_i G'(\|\mathbf{x}_i - \mathbf{t}_\alpha\|_\mathbf{w}^2) \tag{10}$$

and i labels the ith example. Such a Hebbian rule requires back-connections from later stages in the network to the upper layer—where **W** is updated—in order to broadcast quantities such as the error of the overall network relative to the ith example and the derivative of G' of the activation units.

5. The mechanisms and especially the connections needed to implement the learning equations or some equivalent scheme are an open question, in terms of biological plausibility. More work is needed.

Notes to Section IV

1. The HyperBF scheme addresses only one part of the problem of shape-based object recognition, the variability of object appearance due to changing viewpoint. The key issue of how to detect and identify image features that are stable for different illuminations and viewpoints is outside the scope of the network.

2. Notice that the HyperBF approach to recognition does not require as inputs the x, y coordinates of image features: Other parameters of appropriate features can also be used.

3. In a similar vein, notice that the HyperBF network can provide, with the same centers (but different **c**), other parameters of the object, such as its pose, instead of simply a *yes*, *no* recognition signal.

4. Recognition of noisy and partially occluded objects, using realistic feature identification schemes, requires an extension of the scheme. A natural extension of the scheme is based on the use of multiple lower-dimensional centers, corresponding to different subsets of detected features, instead of one 2N-dimensional center for each view in the example set. This corresponds to a set of networks capable of

recognizing different parts of an object. It is equivalent to a set of networks each with a diagonal **W** with some zero entries in the diagonal, instead of one network with **W** with nonzero diagonal elements.

5. Not all features may be always labeled correctly. In general, one expects a significant "correspondence" problem. Possibly the easiest solution is to generate all reasonable sequence of labels for a given input vector and simply try them out on the network. This is, of course, equivalent to trying in parallel the given input on many networks each with a different labeling of its inputs.

6. An obvious use of these learning/approximation modules based on the HyperBF technique is based on a hierarchical composition of GRBF modules, in which the outputs of lower-level modules assigned to detect object parts and their relative disposition in space are combined to allow recognition of complex structured objects. Figure 4 is an example of this architecture.

Notes to Section V

Zipser and Andersen (1988) have presented intriguing simulations suggesting that a back-propagation network trained to solve the problem of converting visual stimuli in retinal coordinates to head-centered coordinates generates receptive fields similar to the ones experimentally found in cortical area 7 of the monkey. We conjecture that Andersen's data may be better accounted for by a HyperBF network. For simplicity, let us consider the one-dimensional version of the problem Zipser and Andersen propose is solved by neurons in area 7. The position of a spot of light on the retina is given as r; the eye position relative to the head is also known as e. The problem is to compute the position of the spot of light relative to the head, i.e., $h = r + e$. Stated in these terms, the problem is computationally trivial, and its solution simply requires the addition of the two inputs r and e. The situation is, however, more complicated due to the actual representation in which r and e are given. In the equation, r and e are represented as numbers. Zipser and Andersen assume, in accordance with physiology, a different representation: They assume that the position r of a spot of light is coded by the presence or absence of activity of one or more cells in a retinotopic array. From this point of view, the goal of the computation carried out by the network is to change representation from *array representation* to *number representation*.

The simplest solution to the problem of changing from an array representation to a number representation is the following. Assume that only one cell in the array $f(x)$ is excited at any given position, i.e., $f(x) = \delta(r - x)$. Simplifying somewhat the situation assumed by Zipser and Andersen, but not altering it in any significant way, let us assume that e is represented directly as a number or a firing rate. The problem then is to convert the *array representation* $f(x) = \delta(r - x)$ for the retinal position into a number *(or a firing rate)* representation. Consider a linear unit that summates linearly all inputs with the "receptive field" $w(x)$. The output l is given by $l = \int w(x)f(x)dx$. For $f(x) = \delta(x - r)$, the choice $w(x) = x$ yields $l = r$. Thus, a simple solution to our problem of converting an array representation into a number representation only needs receptive fields that increase linearly with eccentricity (notice that $w[x] = ax$ may also be acceptable; simply a monotonic dependence on x may be a sufficient approximation).

If a Gaussian HyperBF network with a polynomial term of degree one is used to approximate the relation of the equation from a set of input/output examples, some of the basis functions will be linear units such as the ones described above, and some will be the product of two-dimensional Gaussians representing the visual receptive fields and two-dimensional Gaussians representing the eye position. These latter cells would probably account for the multiplicative property of the area 7 cells found by Andersen. We conjecture that other features of the cells could be replicated in a HyperBF simulation.

ACKNOWLEDGMENTS

The ideas of this paper about the biological implications of new function approximation techniques can be found, to a good extent, in Poggio and Girosi (1989). They depend critically on the work done together with Federico Girosi, Shimon Edelman, and Bruno Caprile on the theory and the applications of regularization networks. It is very likely that, although plausible, the ideas are wrong—unlike the work on which they rest. Anya Hurlbert, Sandro Mussa-Ivaldi, and Robert Thau read the manuscript and suggested several good ways to improve it, which I managed to implement only in part. This paper describes research done in part within the Artificial Intelligence (A.I.) Laboratory and the Center for Biological Information Processing in the Department of Brain and Cognitive Sciences. Support for this research is provided by a grant from the ONR Cognitive and Neural Sciences Division, and by the NATO Scientific Affairs Division (0403/87). Support for the A.I. Laboratory's artificial intelligence research is provided by the Advanced Research Projects Agency of the Department of Defense under Army contract DACA-76-85-C-0010 and in part under ONR contract N-00014-85-K-0124. T.P. is supported by the Uncas and Ellen Whitaker chair.

REFERENCES

Albus, J.S. 1971. A theory of cerebellar functions. *Math. Biosci.* **10**: 25.

Bertero, M., T. Poggio, and V. Torre. 1988. Ill-posed problems in early vision. *Proc. IEEE* **76**: 869.

Broomhead, D.S. and D. Lowe. 1988. Multivariable functional interpolation and adaptive networks. *Complex Syst.* **2**: 321.

Flash, T. and N. Hogan. 1985. The coordination of arm movements: An experiment confirmed mathematical model. *J. Neurosci.* **5**: 1688.

Hubel, D.H. and T.N. Wiesel. 1962. Receptive fields, binocular interaction and functional architecture in the cat's visual cortex. *J. Physiol.* **160**: 106.

Koch, C. and T. Poggio. 1987. Biophysics of computational systems: Neurons, synapses, and membranes. In *Synaptic function* (ed. G.M. Edelman et al.), p. 637. Wiley, New York.

Marr, D. 1969. A theory of cerebellar cortex. *J. Physiol.* **202**: 437.

Micchelli, C.A. 1986. Interpolation of scattered data: Distance matrices and conditionally positive definite functions. *Constr. Approx.* **2**: 11.

Minsky, M.L. and S. Papert. 1969. *Perceptrons.* MIT Press, Cambridge, Massachusetts.

Morasso, P. and F.A. Mussa-Ivaldi. 1982. Trajectory formation and handwriting: A computational model. *Biol. Cybern.* **45**: 131.

Omohundro, S. 1987. Efficient algorithms with neural network behaviour. *Complex Syst.* **1**: 273.

Perrett, D.I., A.J. Mistlin, and A.J. Chitty. 1987. Visual neurones responsive to faces. *Trends Neurosci.* **10**: 358.

Poggio, T. and S. Edelman. 1990. A network that learns to recognize 3D objects. *Nature* **343**: 263.

Poggio, T. and F. Girosi. 1989. A theory of networks for approximation and learning. In *A.I. Memo No. 1140.* Artificial Intelligence Laboratory, Massachusetts Institute of Technology, Cambridge.

———. 1990a. Extension of a theory of networks for approximation and learning: Dimensionality reduction and clustering. In *A.I. Memo No. 1167.* Artificial Intelligence Laboratory, Massachusetts Institute of Technology, Cambridge.

———. 1990b. Theory of networks for learning. *Science* **247**: 978.

Poggio, T. and V. Torre. 1978. A theory of synaptic interactions. In *Theoretical approaches in neurobiology* (ed. W.E. Reichardt and T. Poggio), p. 28. MIT Press, Cambridge, Massachusetts.

Poggio, T., V. Torre, and C. Koch. 1985. Computational vision and regularization theory. *Nature* **317**: 314.

Poggio, T. and the staff. 1988. MIT progress in understanding images. In *Proceedings image understanding workshop,* Cambridge, Massachusetts, April 1988. Morgan Kaufmann, San Mateo, California.

Poggio, T. and the staff. 1989. MIT progress in understanding images. In *Proceedings image understanding workshop,* Palo Alto, California, May 1989, p. 56. Morgan Kaufmann, San Mateo, California.

Powell, M.J.D. 1987. Radial basis functions for multivariable interpolation: A review. In *Algorithms for approximation* (ed. J.C. Mason and M.G. Cox). Clarendon Press, Oxford.

Tikhonov, A.N. and V.Y. Arsenin. 1977. *Solutions of ill-posed problems,* Winston, Washington, D.C.

Torre, V. and T. Poggio. 1987. An application: A synaptic mechanism possibly underlying motion detection. In *Theoretical approaches in neurobiology* (ed. W.E. Reichardt and T. Poggio), p. 39. MIT Press, Cambridge, Massachusetts.

Zipser, D. and R.A. Andersen. 1988. A back-propagation programmed network that simulates response properties of a subset of posterior parietal neurons. *Nature* **331**: 679.

Toward a Neural Understanding of Visual Surface Representation

K. NAKAYAMA* AND S. SHIMOJO†

The Smith-Kettlewell Eye Research Institute, San Francisco, California 94115

Independent Visual Modules?

Owing to the exploitation of available techniques in modern neuroanatomy and neurophysiology, an increasingly detailed picture of the primate cortical visual system is emerging. First, a topographic map of the retina appears to be duplicated many times in the cerebral cortex (Hubel and Wiesel 1965; Zeki 1978), and more than a dozen separate cortical maps of the retina have been described (Maunsell and Newsome 1987). Second, there seems to be a set of parallel anatomical pathways mediating visual function. This segregation begins as early as the retina and appears to continue through many cortical areas. Segregation is manifested particularly in the responses of individual cells. Cells differ in their selectivity to various characteristics of the visual image: binocular disparity, line orientation, motion direction, size, color, etc. (for review, see Livingstone and Hubel 1987).

This diversity in the coding properties of neurons and their anatomical distribution has given credence to the idea of relatively independent modules emerging early for the processing of different attributes of visual images. Such notions underlie various models, including those encoding motion (Adelson and Bergen 1985), binocular disparity (Sperling 1970; Julesz 1971; Nelson 1975; Marr and Poggio 1976), and color (Land 1977). What characterizes each of these models is a distinct module, composed of simple within-module elements. Thus, color and contour are not influenced by depth, depth is not influenced by color, etc. The most explicit support for this notion came from Julesz's demonstration of "purely cyclopean" perception (Julesz 1971). The idea of modularity also gains credibility from studies examining the selective damage to visual structures in the monkey. Restricted lesions can selectively knock out the perception of motion (Newsome and Pare 1988), light spots as opposed to dark (Schiller et al. 1986), and color (Schiller et al. 1990).

The assumption of independence between modules in fact has had a certain heuristic value. Yet, the success of such an approach should not blind us to the rather primitive nature of our current understanding of vision and the need to ask new questions. If we do have such modules, how are their activities coordinated so that we

see as we do? Ordinarily, we see textured and colored surfaces bounded by contours. We do not see color and motion separately disembodied from objects and surfaces. The problem of how specific visual attributes or features are combined has been identified as the "feature-binding problem," and a number of hypotheses have been advanced to address this issue, often positing specific neural or cognitive processes to perform such tasks (Treisman and Gelade 1980; Crick 1984).

Our immediate approach to this seemingly difficult problem is to sidestep it, at least temporarily. Rather than attempting to build up perception from the outputs of these hypothetically independent neural modules, we think it perhaps more fruitful to look out into the world, to examine how the optical properties of the real world constrain the structure of images formed on our retina. Then we ask how such images might be best interpreted for the brain to "see" as it does. This approach rests heavily on an appreciation of ecological optics (Gibson 1950) and is broadly related to computational vision (Marr 1982). It also relies on phenomenological observations, often used by Gestalt psychologists (Koffka 1935).

Natural Constraints and Surface Representation

In contrast to the approach that seeks to build up perception from sets of atomic features, based on physiological and psychophysical experiments, we suggest that it is as important to evaluate how the visual system might go about encoding real-world scenes by looking at the natural-optical constraints of this world. Furthermore, to understand the interactive nature of early vision, as opposed to its modularity, we think it of great importance to understand the encoding of surfaces.

A look at surfaces in the real world immediately reveals one of the most important facts about vision: Closer surfaces occlude more distant surfaces. The amount of occlusion varies greatly, depending on seemingly arbitrary factors—the relative positions of the distant surface, the closer surface, and the viewing eye. Yet, various aspects of visual perception remain remarkably unimpaired. Because animals, including ourselves, seem to see so well under such conditions and since this fact of occlusion is always with us, it would seem that many problems associated with occlusion would have been solved by visual systems throughout the course of evolution.

Present addresses: *Department of Psychology, Harvard University, 33 Kirkland Street, Cambridge, Massachusetts 02138; †Department of Psychology, College of Arts and Sciences, University of Tokyo, Komaba, Meguro-ku, Tokyo 153, Japan.

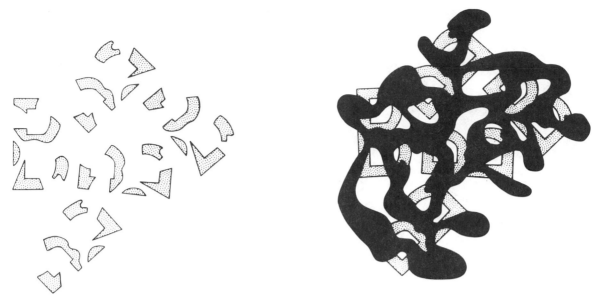

Figure 1. On the left are a series of letter fragments, made up of letter Bs that have been occluded by an invisible occluder. On the right are the exact same set of remaining fragments of the letter Bs, but here the black occluder is visible. Note that the letters can be recognized on the right but not on the left. (Reprinted, with permission, from Bregman 1981.)

We begin by thinking about the problem of object identification under occlusion. If we consider the image of several objects that have been occluded, some important things become apparent. Not only can an occluder conceal information from the viewer about the objects themselves, rendering them less visible for purposes of recognition, but it can also have two more effects which could be as damaging or more so. First, it could separate different parts of the same object from each other. Second, it could introduce spurious bounding contours around the object fragments themselves.

Perhaps these two points can be best appreciated by looking at the left portion of Figure 1 (from Bregman 1981). Here, we see a set of image fragments, remaining portions of letter Bs, scattered about. These Bs have been covered by an "invisible" occluder. Recognition is virtually impossible. Now examine the right portion of Figure 1, where the occluder is visible. Here, recognition becomes possible, almost easy. In each case, exactly the same fragments of the letters are visible, yet the difference is striking.

What accounts for this difference? To return to our points made earlier, it appears that without the visibility of the occluder, the separate fragments of each letter are not appropriately grouped. The invisible occluder divides the letters, and it is not possible to know which of the separate fragments go with which. With the visibility of the occluder, however, they are more correctly grouped.

Border Belongingness and Surface Continuation

To begin to understand what is going on, we would like to introduce some simple but useful concepts, similar in part to ideas outlined over 50 years ago by Koffka

(1935). First is the notion of border "belongingness" or "ownership." If there is a common border between two image regions, we argue that it is important for the visual system to make an early distinction as to which image region "owns" the common border. As an example of border ownership, consider the various borders in Figure 1. On the left, the contours surrounding the stippled letter fragments clearly belong to the fragments themselves. Each fragment appears as complete within itself. They do not group with other fragments. As a consequence, it is very difficult to make out the letters. It is very different, however, for the case shown on the right. Here, the contours that are common to the black region and the stippled region are seen as belonging to the black region and not to the stippled region. As such, the stippled region is phenomenally bounded only where it meets the white background, not where it meets the black region. At this boundary the stippled region appears to continue "amodally" (Michotte 1954; Kanizsa 1979) behind the black region. Now each fragment is no longer complete within itself because it is not entirely enclosed with its own bounding contour. We argue that this lack of "boundedness" enables it to link up with other similarly unbound image regions, thus forming larger units which are otherwise fragmented in the image.

Why does the boundary between the black and stippled region "belong" to the black region? Note that there is a T-junction where these two image regions meet. Ever since Helmholtz (1910), such junctions have been hypothesized to provide evidence for depth and occlusion, with the line forming the top of the T being the occluding contour (see Guzman 1984). Thus, the T-junction provides evidence that the black edge is an occluding contour. As such, it belongs to the black region and not to the stippled region.

We postulate that if a given image region is bounded by a contour that does not belong to it, the surface corresponding to this region is not bounded there. As such, it will be seen as continuing behind the bounding contour that belongs to its neighbor.

To summarize, contour ownership or belongingness is critical for depth and to surface continuation. Under most circumstances, if a surface is seen as nearer, the common boundary belongs to this nearer surface. This optical constraint of occlusion, in turn, ensures that the neighboring distal region is seen as continuing behind.

Something very similar can be seen in Figure 2, which should be first viewed monocularly, not as a stereogram. Here, it should be clear that one sees a large letter C, occluded by a gray patch in all three panels. Again, as a consequence of the T-junction, the gray patch is seen as in front, and it thus owns the common border. This means that the two letter fragments are effectively "unbounded" at this point and they are seen to continue behind the patch. This enables us to see the C as a single object.

What would happen, however, if we were to reverse the depth seen in this figure and to make the gray patch appear in back rather than in front? If our hypothesis regarding depth and contour belongingness is correct, this reversal should have a major effect. Under these conditions, the contour would no longer belong to the gray patch because it is no longer in front. The ownership would be transferred to the fragments of the letter. As a consequence of this ownership transfer, the fragments would be effectively bounded on all sides. As such they could not be linked to form a single letter.

Our strategy has been to use stereopsis because it can often overcome monocular depth cues, such as T-junctions. To see this, the reader should fuse the images shown in Figure 2 as stereograms. Supporting our hypothesis, it should be clear that there is a dramatic difference when the gray patch is seen as behind. The figure is seen as two image fragments, two U-shaped objects, separated. It can hardly be seen as a single object. If one views the stereogram in the reversed configuration, however, so that the gray patch pops out of the page, we then see the fragments linked and we are again aware of the unified C as expected.

The data presented so far are purely phenomenological. We argue that such observations provide important and valid evidence for an understanding of perception. Yet, we have also linked such observations to more objective measures of pattern recognition (Nakayama et al. 1989). In brief, we presented a set of human faces to naive experimental subjects, asking them to remember these faces for a recognition test to take place immediately thereafter. During the testing phase, the image of the face was incomplete, replaced in part by a set of horizontal "noise" strips. An example of such a stimulus can be seen in the stereograms in Figure 3. Two conditions with identical image information were presented in the stereograms. In one case, the strips of faces were seen in back, in the other case they were seen as in front, occasioned by a simple right-eye left-eye reversal of images. All subjects reported that the faces were more recognizable when seen in the back plane. The separate pieces of the face appeared to continue behind the occluders and recognition appeared much more certain in comparison to the case where the strips containing the face fragments were in front. These impressions were clearly confirmed in the performance accuracy in the recognition task. Recognition accuracy was significantly better if the horizontal pieces of the face were seen in back rather than in front. Note that the two depth conditions were identical in terms of pictorial information for face recognition, different only in the sign of disparity. This ensures that relative depth of surfaces is critical for

Figure 2. Note that the letter C is easily visible when not viewed as a stereogram. It is as if the hidden portions of the C continued behind the gray patch. If viewed as a stereogram such that the gray patch recedes in depth, the perception of the C disappears. One only sees two U- shaped objects, unconnected. If one views the reverse stereogram such that the gray patch pops out in depth, the C will be visible again. (Adapted from Nakayama et al. 1989.)

Note: To view this 3-section stereogram (as well as others in this paper) in its normal configuration, persons who cross their eyes should fuse the left and center images. Those who diverge to fuse should view the center and right images. To view the stereograms in the reversed configuration, do the opposite. Thus, cross-fusers should fuse the center and right images.

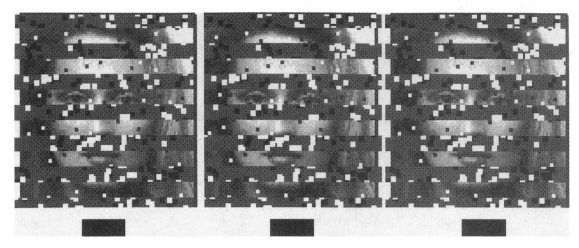

Figure 3. If one fuses these stereograms such that the faces are seen in the back plane, they are much easier to recognize than if they appear on the front disparity plane. Compare normal and reversed disparity case. (Adapted from Nakayama et al. 1989.)

image segmentation and grouping, which is a necessary stage of processing for object recognition.

Figure 4 summarizes our current understanding of how borders and surfaces are encoded. If the image patch labeled M is coded in front, contours C and C′ are owned by and belong to region M. As a consequence, surfaces corresponding to regions U and L

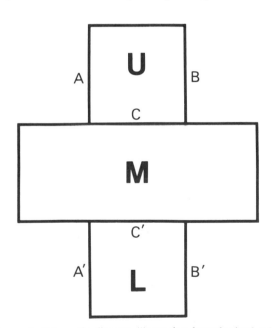

Figure 4. Schematic diagram illustrating hypothesized relationship between depth, contour ownership, and completion of image fragments behind occluders. If M in this diagram were to be encoded in front, M would own contours C and C′. As such, regions U and L would appear to continue behind M because they are effectively "unbounded" at C and C′. Then contours A and A′ as well as contours B and B′ would tend to be linked. If, however, M were to be encoded as behind, its common border with regions U and L would be owned and belong to U and L, respectively. As such, U and L would be effectively bounded and no perceptual linking between them would occur. (Reprinted, with permission, from Nakayama et al. 1989.)

are not bounded at C and C′. As such, they can have the opportunity to continue behind M. Contours A and A′ as well as B and B′ are then perceptually linked. Conversely, however, if region M is coded in back, then C and C′ belong to regions U and L, respectively, and A and A′ as well as B and B′ can no longer be linked.

Can we come up with a plausible neural mechanism to understand such large differences in perception? We can only speculate at this point. Yet, it is curious to note that frequently encountered cell types in striate and extrastriate cortex could combine their outputs to implement some of the seemingly "intelligent" distinctions mentioned above. For example, one of the most important decisions to be made in this context is whether a given line terminator in an image represents a real line termination in the three-dimensional world or whether it is more likely to continue behind another surface (see Shimojo et al. 1989).

Cells originally labeled "hypercomplex" by Hubel and Wiesel (1965) and now more recently designated as "end stopped" might indicate that a line ended in an image. Such cells respond less vigorously for long lines and fire more vigorously if the line stops in the image plane. However, such cells alone could not signal whether a real line might continue behind an occluder or whether it actually stops in the real world. Combining the output of these cells with cells sensitive to depth, however, could resolve the issue for the visual system. Consider a disparity-tuned, end-stopped cell with a receptive field coincident with contour B′ in Figure 4. It would fire vigorously because the line stops abruptly in the image. Suppose, however, that such a cell were to feed its output to higher order cells which also received input from cells that encoded the depth of region M. If M were coded as closer, then such higher order cells could indicate that the line continued behind. Conversely, if M were coded as further, such cells would provide information as to whether the line really did end in the three-dimensional world.

Up to now, we have only considered the possibility of surfaces that are opaque, showing how surfaces and contours might be seen as continuing behind occluders, depending on local depth signals. In addition, we suggested how plausible signals from different early mechanisms might interact to encode surface termination versus surface continuation.

Transparency and Color Spreading

Interaction between different putative early local mechanisms becomes even more apparent in our studies of surface formation. In these studies, we show that the perception of contour, depth, and color are closely coupled and are critically related to whether a given configuration is perceptually encoded as transparent or opaque.

Recently, in considering factors involved in space perception, there has been an implicit dichotomy between physiological versus cognitive cues to depth. These attitudes may have stemmed in part from the existence of neuronal units selective to binocular disparity (Barlow et al. 1967) and the lack of comparable evidence for pictorial cues. Such a bias toward stereopsis might lead one to assume that binocular disparity signals alone are sufficient to specify depth and that so-called cognitive occlusion cues were perhaps acquired later, built on early experience with stereopsis or perhaps motion parallax. If disparity did indeed play such a dominant role, it would seem to follow that if one reversed the disparity in a simple stereoscopic scene, the depth of elements in the scene should undergo a corresponding reversal. This is indeed the case for a large set of contrived stereograms. However, a closer examination of many types of other simple configurations indicates that local disparity alone is far from

sufficient to specify the depth values of points in many scenes. As such, the reversal of right and left eye views can have effects very different from an expected exchange of depth values.

Examine the cross, shown in Figure 5. Although appearing as a cross if viewed monocularly, it should be clear that there is a difference in relative disparity between the vertical and horizontal limbs of the cross if fused stereoscopically. In such an untextured figure, classical stereopsis makes no obvious prediction regarding the depth value of the untextured region at the very center of the cross. Will it take a value intermediate to the front and back region of the stereogram—i.e., some form of averaging? If so, might not one assume the average would be weighted more by the depth defined by the vertical limb of the cross? We mention this possible expectation, because disparity signals along the vertical line defining the vertical limb are certainly closer to the center than the short vertical lines far out on the horizontal limb. As such, they might be expected to contribute more, that is, if we assume simple local propagation of depth signals.

If the reader fuses the stereograms seen in Figure 5, it should be obvious that perception does not correspond to any of the expectations outlined above, and yet the answer is clear and unambiguous. The middle of the cross is seen in front even when the disparity of the closer vertical limb indicates that this region is in back.

More telling are the specific details of the perceived surface layout. If the ends of the horizontal portion of the cross are nearer, one sees a horizontal bar in front of a vertical bar. In the reversed case, the vertical bar is in front. Yet something new is also seen. Although each monocular cross is homogeneous, this homogeneity is now broken by an obvious contour when viewed stereoscopically. An illusory occluding contour "com-

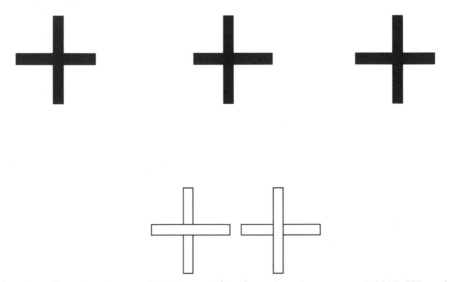

Figure 5. Top is a cross when viewed monocularly. Areas within the cross are homogeneously black. When viewed in its normal stereo configuration, however, one sees a black horizontal bar in front of a vertical bar. In the reversed stereo configuration (right-eye left-eye reversal), one sees a vertical bar in front of a horizontal bar. Bottom two figures portray what is seen in the fused stereograms, showing the subjective occluding contours.

pletes" the vertical or horizontal bar in front. A schematic description of these two perceptual outcomes can be seen in the bottom of Figure 5.

Although the perception of this stereogram reminds us that disparity is certainly important and can propagate when necessary, more importantly, it also tells us that local disparity alone is not sufficient to explain what is going on in this scene. No model based on local disparity signals can account for these results. It appears that when the visual system is confronted with this simple stereogram, it acts by "constructing" a set of depth values that correspond more to possible configurations in the world rather than performing an algebraic summation of local disparity signals. Thus, instead of providing a smoothed output profile of depth, as current neural models might suggest, the visual system comes up with a concise and seemingly intelligent answer: in this case, one surface occluding another.

This "problem solving" or "inferential" aspect of perception is perhaps even more dramatically supported in the next demonstration shown at the top of Figure 6. Here, the exact same cross is colored red and embedded in a white cross which itself has no "within" differences in disparity. As such, one might expect to see another version of what we have just described: a horizontal bar in front of a vertical bar, lying within a white cross.

The perception, however, is strikingly different. No longer does one see two bars, the horizontal in front of the vertical. Instead one sees a red transparent surface, sitting in front of a white cross. Furthermore, even though there is no red coloring in the black regions around the center of the disk, one sees a distinct reddening of this area, enclosed by a circular "subjective" contour bounding this disk. All of these descriptions are most succinctly summarized by saying that one sees a red filter in front of a white cross.

Reversing the disparity (by looking at the other pair of the three half-images) also leads to something unexpected from our previous discussion. Instead of seeing a vertical bar in front of a horizontal bar, one sees a flat circular red disk, lying behind, seen through a cruciform aperture. Note that the spreading of red color into the black region is essentially absent and that the surface color is matte rather than transparent. It is as if one sees a Japanese flag behind a window.

Another configuration that yields a very similar set of results can be seen by inspecting the stereogram seen at the bottom of Figure 6. In the normal configuration, one sees a transparent green square in front. Note the spread of color into the black background. In the reversed configuration, one only sees pieces of a green square viewed through four circular apertures. Here the green region is no longer transparent and it does not spread into the black background (for details, see Nakayama et al. 1990).

These very striking changes in perception with small changes in the display are puzzling if we think only about local "within-module" signal processing. How can such a small change in color and configuration lead

to such a very different global perception? In particular, how can just the addition of the outer limbs of the cross, combined with changing the color of the inner limbs, lead to such a dramatic change in appearance? A small change in the configuration leads to the creation and/or destruction of contours, depth, and color. Each of these seemingly primitive features appears as subordinate to the global interpretation of the scene as a set of surfaces.

Discontinuity Edges, Transparency, and Contrast Conditions

To extend this observation even further, we choose what is perhaps the simplest one-dimensional configuration (Fig. 7). The pattern consists of sets of horizontal bars, which if they were not divided into white and gray regions, would have no depth when viewed stereoscopically because the ends of these bars all have the same disparity. What makes these bars interesting is that the vertical dividing border between the gray and white regions has crossed disparity. As a consequence, it should be seen as in front. At issue is the perceived depth of the intermediate regions. Again, these portions of the image are untextured, and classic stereopsis has no explicit prediction as to their perceived depth. If one takes the now popular view, however, that the visual system is looking to maximize smoothness in terms of interpreting the image (Hildreth 1984; Poggio et al. 1985), one might expect some form of interpolation: either a set of tilted planes if continuity alone is maintained, or a bowed plane (similar to a spline fit) if both continuity and smoothness are preserved. These expected interpretations (labeled 1 and 2) are shown in Figure 8A.

Our perception is quite different from either of these expectations. Instead of the kink or bulge in a continuous surface as might be predicted from an interpolation of disparity-based depth signals, two distinct planes in depth emerge. We see a transparent surface in front of white regions in back. In the top stereogram of Figure 7, we see a transparent filter covering the central region as schematized in the bottom of Figure 8A (labeled "perceived"). We also see the spreading of color into the black regions as well as vertical subjective contours, appearing to contain the spreading color. If we examine the lower set of stereograms shown in Figure 7, something very different happens. Here we have exactly the same stereograms as shown in the top of Figure 7, except that the luminances have been exchanged. Regions that were gray are now white and vice versa.

Such a reversal of contrast has a dramatic perceptual effect. No longer is the center region transparent, but transparency has shifted to the outer gray regions. Also striking is the concomitant change of depth (see schematic drawing in Fig. 8B). In this demonstration, with exactly the same disparity, this central region is no longer seen in front, but in back; the outer regions are now in front. Thus, by the simple manipulation of luminance, we obtain a radically different perception of

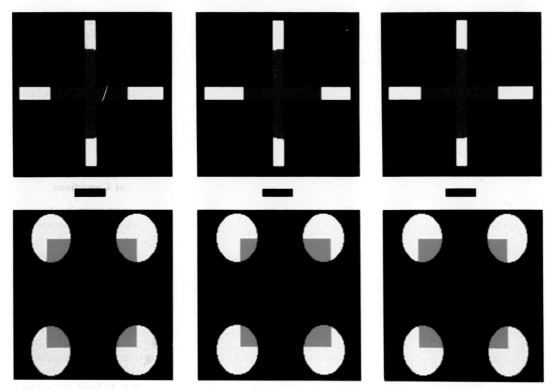

Figure 6. Top row shows the stereoscopic modification of a configuration introduced by Redies and Spillmann (1981). Inner red cross has the same disparity as the cross shown in Fig. 5, yet the perception is very different. Instead of seeing a horizontal bar in front of a vertical bar, one sees a transparent colored disk, covering the central cross. Thus, color spreads out into the dark regions nearby, confined by a circular "illusory" contour forming the outer perimeter of the transparent disk. When the stereograms are viewed in their reversed configuration, one perceives a more distant disk, seen through a cruciform aperture. Color is matte and no longer spreads. Bottom row shows the stereoscopic modification of the Varin (1971) configuration where transparency, opacity, and subjective contours are also determined by the sign of disparity. (Adapted from Nakayama et al. 1990.)

depth. These results support Metelli's (1974) observation that the region of intermediate luminance is seen as the transparent surface. They go further, however, in indicating that hand in hand with this switch in the region seen as transparent, there is a corresponding switch in depth. A region previously appearing opaque and in back now looks transparent and in front. Thus, a small change in luminance can have a profound influence on perceived depth. It is as if the visual system with exactly the same disparity signals makes a decision from various sorts of information (including luminance) to come up with a coherent interpretation of the scene.

This brief series of results indicates that we cannot consider depth, color, and contour as elemental primitives, acting within confined regions of the visual field according to within-module local rules. There is far too much interaction between these seemingly distinct primitives such that small changes in one can influence not only the surface interpretation, but also the same primitives themselves. Thus, changes in disparity can determine whether a surface is seen as transparent or opaque, and this in turn can determine whether subjective contours are visible and whether color is confined to a particular region or spreads elsewhere. In short, it seems that to understand surface perception we need to come to grips with terms like intelligence or inference.

It appears that our vision acts as if it were a detective, piecing together image data to come up with the most plausible interpretation of the scene. Such a view is not new. It was espoused forcefully by Helmholtz (1910) in his discussion of "unconscious inference" in perception, and this general view has had a number of contemporary adherents (Gregory 1970; Rock and Anson 1979; Hochberg 1981).

With the hope of delving more deeply into the specific nature of visual intelligence, let us again think about the striking changes in perception as we made the seemingly small modification from the stereogram in Figure 5 (the crossed bars) to the transparent surface seen in the top of Figure 6. How does such a small change in target configuration (with no changes in disparity) lead the visual system from seeing the inner cross as two crossed bars in one case (Fig. 5) to something that seems quite far-fetched, constructing in a seemingly unexpected way a transparent surface (as in Fig. 6)?

Generic View and Conditional Probabilities

Thinking in terms of the detective analogy, it would seem that the visual system would need to ask a number of questions. First, could a particular interpretation

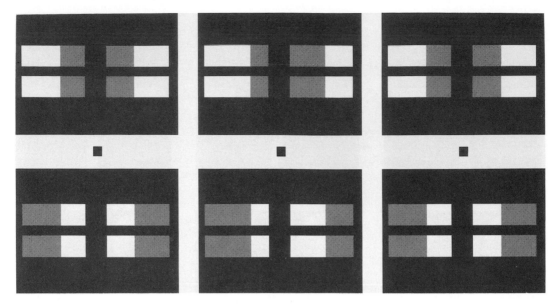

Figure 7. Top stereogram shows four horizontal bars whose right and left endings have the same disparity. These bars are each divided into two regions, the border of which has crossed disparity when viewed in the regular configuration. Thus, it should appear in front. What is perceived is a transparent gray figure covering the central region of the two bars; this colored region is bounded by "illusory" contours, oriented vertically. Bottom stereogram is the same except the gray and white have been exchanged. Despite the identical disparity, this simple switch in luminance leads to a very different perception. Now there is a closer surface on the outer edges of the figure; the closer surface in the inner region is gone. Note that this stereogram should be viewed only in its normal, not its reversed, configuration.

under consideration give rise to the facts at hand? Second, given the "reality" corresponding to a given interpretation, could it have plausibly given rise to these same facts?

The first question can be rephrased as follows. Does the perceived configuration correspond to the image data? The answer is yes for the perceived transparency configuration. One can (in retrospect) understand how the particular spatial pattern perceived (shown in the top of Fig. 6) could have given rise to the image data shown in the stereograms. The luminance and disparity relations conform to the underlying physics of such a scene. Yet, the answer to this question is not sufficient because there was at least one other interpretation; namely, the one we expected from an analysis of Figure 5 (two crossed red bars in front of a white cross). Why did the system choose the transparent disk rather than this second and seemingly reasonable interpretation?

The second question is perhaps more critical. Given a particular scene, how likely could it have given rise to the image data? Such conditional probabilities are dictated by the geometry and optics of scene viewing. In this context, we briefly introduce two interlinked concepts characterizing the totality of vantage points in space from which this scene could be viewed: the generic and the accidental views (see Richards et al. 1987; Koenderink 1990). By generic viewpoint, we mean those positions where, for arbitrarily small perturbations of this vantage point, there are no qualitative changes in the image. Conversely, by accidental viewpoint, we mean those very few vantage points in space where small perturbations will lead to qualitative

differences in the image. Our hypothesis is that, given a choice, the visual system will show a strong preference for a scene interpretation based on the generic rather than the accidental view.

As an illustration, consider the two figures seen in Figure 9. We see a square on the left and a cube on the right. Why do we only see a square on the left and not a cube? In terms of fitting the image data, it is certainly possible for a cube to be turned so that one just sees its face. Yet, if we appeal to the notion of the generic view, stated above, it is clear that if the object were a cube, the image on the left could only have arisen from a very small number of accidental viewpoints out of an infinite number of generic viewpoints. On the other hand, if it were a square, it could be seen from many (generic) viewpoints. We argue that the visual system has implicit knowledge of the conditional probabilities associated with these various views and hence rejects any interpretation based on an accidental view.

Now we use the same reasoning to explain why the visual system chooses the transparency interpretation seen in Figure 6 (top). Here, there are at least two physical interpretations, but only the transparent disk interpretation survives the generic view test. If the surface configuration in the real world was indeed a set of red crossed bars in front of a white cross, the binocular image seen in Figure 6 could have arisen only from a privileged or accidental view, such that the observer's position led to an exact alignment of image contours. It is obviously accidental because a small perturbation of viewing position leads to a very different image (note the top stereogram in Fig. 10 and compare it with the

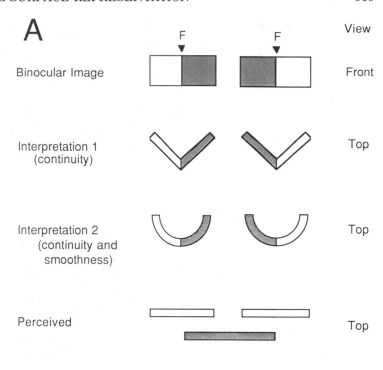

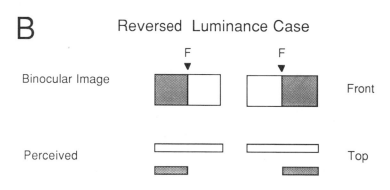

Figure 8. Schematic illustration of expected and actual perceived depth of single one-dimensional stereograms. In *A* we show the case for the top stereogram shown in Fig. 7, including the binocular image, the expected depths (from considerations of continuity and smoothness), and the central transparent surface perceived in front. F refers to the edge coded in front by binocular disparity. In *B* we show that the simple reversal of luminance leads to a dramatic reversal of depth. Now the transparent surface moves from the central region to the periphery.

top one in Fig. 6). If, on the other hand, the surface configuration was a transparent disk in front of a white cross, the image could have arisen from a generic view: Here for a similar change in vantage point, there is no qualitative change in image data. Note the invariant nature of the perception (aside from the color differ-

ence) as one compares the bottom stereogram in Figure 10 with that shown in the top of Figure 6.

Like a good detective, the visual system does not simply jump to conclusions but avoids a major pitfall. It does not base its "reasoning" on assumptions that are highly improbable. As such, it rejects any interpreta-

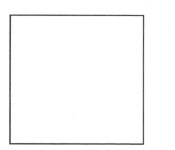 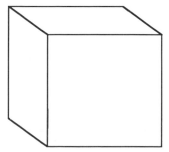

Figure 9. Accidental vs. generic view I. We hypothesize that we do not see a cube on the left because such a view can only arise from a small number of accidental vantage points (see text).

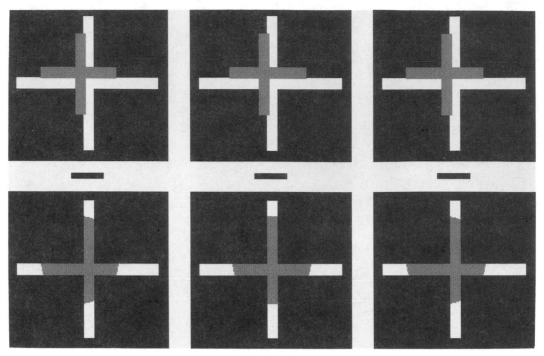

Figure 10. Accidental vs. generic view II. Binocular image of two possible surface configurations that could have given rise to the scene in Fig. 6 (top) under a perturbation of vantage point. Top stereogram shows the binocular image if the scene consisted of two crossed bars lying within a white cross. Bottom stereogram shows the binocular image of a transparent disk in front of a white cross. Note the large qualitative change in image for the first (crossed bars) but not the second (transparency) configuration.

tion based on the assumption of an accidental view.

Where in the brain might such "intelligence" reside? Is it in the visual system or is it higher up, part of some generalized cognitive function. as has been postulated by antiphysiological theorists (Gregory 1970; Rock and Anson 1979)? If we think of the word detective, we think of words like executive or agent "homunculus." If we look at the anatomy of the brain, it is not obvious from the structure of the system that there is an apparent "place" for this executive or agent, at least for vision. A more plausible alternative is that inference or intelligence must be distributed and that there needs to be no agent as such. Somehow, by the operation of many small distributed units, each showing some limited inferential capacities, the work of the apparent detective is done. Thus, there is no inherent reason why this process in vision cannot begin very early, possibly in areas now undergoing intensive neurophysiological investigation.

da Vinci Stereopsis and Possible Neural Mechanisms

To support this alternative way of thinking, we present our final set of demonstrations. Here, we make the case that at least one class of such inferences must begin very early in cortical information processing, possibly as early as primary visual cortex. To appreciate the logic of this argument, consider the case of surfaces viewed by the two eyes, not just one. Ever since Leonardo da Vinci, it has been known that a closer

surface occludes a background surface differentially in the two eyes (see Wheatstone 1838). Thus, there will be background points to the left of an occluding surface that are visible only to the left eye, and correspondingly, there will be background points to the right of an occluding surface that are visible only to the right eye. Thus, points P_L and P_R shown in Figure 11A are visible only to the left or right eye, respectively. It should be clear that such unmatched binocular points can hardly be avoided if we view real-world scenes. An interesting question is how the visual system might interpret the presence of such left-eye-only and right-eye-only points in a simple stereogram where there are no disparity-based depth cues and where the occluder is not physically present in the display. Would the visual system make the correct "unconscious inference" that such an occluding surface did still exist?

To see whether this is indeed the case, we created a stereogram with four unpaired image points, where two image points were seen only by the left eye and where the other two image points were seen only by the right eye. The positioning of such points is illustrated in Figure 11B. The only plausible scene in real life that could have given rise to this configuration of binocular and monocular points would be a surface in front (partially delineated by the dashed lines in Fig. 11C).

What is remarkable is that when most viewers examined such a scene in a stereoscope, it was reported that such a surface was indeed perceived (Nakayama and Shimojo 1990). A faint but distinct triangular-shaped surface bounded by illusory contours (posi-

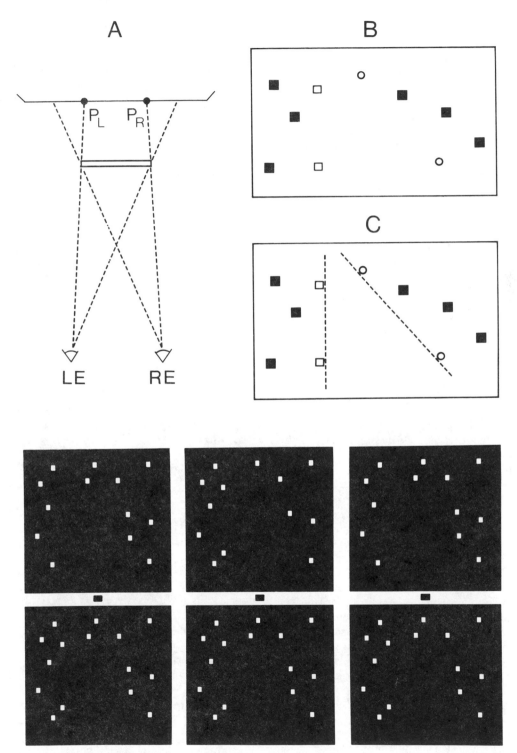

Figure 11. (*A*) Occlusion is different for the two viewing eyes. Because of the existence of an opaque surface, point P_L in the background is visible only to the left eye, and point P_R is visible only to the right eye. (*B*) Schematic of a stereogram where all filled circles represent points that are viewed binocularly and have zero disparity. Open squares and open circles identify points visible to the left eye only and right eye only, respectively. (*C*) Same as in *B*, except showing the boundaries of a surface that could have given rise to the monocular points. It also identifies where observers see subjective contours in the stereograms below. In the stereogram depicted in the next portion of the figure, the top portion has four unpaired points as illustrated in *B*. In the bottom portion, all points are paired.

tioned as the dashed lines in Fig. 11C) was seen to lie in front of the background dots. Thus, an illusory occluding contour was seen to the immediate right of the left-eye-only dots and to the immediate left of right-eye-only dots. Similar to the case of other surfaces bounded by illusory contours (see Petry and Meyer 1987), the surface was also seen as slightly darker than the dark background. The case just described is shown in the upper stereogram presented in Figure 11. A control case where all points are interocularly matched is seen in the lower stereogram. When presented in a stereoscope, it should be clear for most viewers (with normal stereoscopic vision) that an approximately triangular surface can be seen in the upper but not in the lower stereogram.

We think that this latest demonstration again makes the point. Perception is remarkably adaptive and intelligent. What makes this latest demonstration of added interest, however, is its very specific reliance on eye-of-origin information. In this demonstration as in others (see Shimojo et al. 1988; Nakayama and Shimojo 1990; Shimojo and Nakayama 1990), it is of importance for the visual system to know which eye was presented with the unpaired stimulus. The position of the illusory occluding contour had a very specific position in relation to whether the monocular dot came through the right or left eye. If it was presented to the left eye, the illusory occluding contour appeared to its immediate right. If it was presented to the right eye, the contour appeared to its immediate left. This is not surprising, given the nature of the real-world geometry described in Figure 11A. Putting this observation together with our current understanding of the properties of cells in striate and extrastriate cortex, however, leads us to propose an unexpectedly strong hypothesis; the inferential process responsible for the perception of the surface must begin very early in the cortical visual pathway, perhaps as early as striate cortex and at least as early as its immediate cortical projection zones.

The argument runs as follows. Eye-of-origin information is preserved in the ocular dominance structure of V1. Here, many cells respond preferentially to right-eye or left-eye stimulation. Beyond V1, however, this explicit coding of eye preference is essentially gone. Instead of finding cells that respond more to one eye than to the other, extrastriate cortex is characteristic in having cells that are equal in responsiveness to stimulation of either eye (Burkhalter and Van Essen 1986; Maunsell and Van Essen 1983; Hubel and Livingstone 1987). Thus, it would seem that the neural mechanism responsible for the illusory contours and the associated surface must have direct access to the signals from these monocular striate cells. At the very latest, therefore, cortical areas with such inputs from striate cortex comprise the possible candidates.

Cortical Organization and Surface Representation

Having provided some support for the view that the encoding of occlusion and surface formation can begin fairly early in cortical visual processing, we are in a position to return to the original problem presented in the introduction, namely, the feature-binding problem. How do separate features in an image get associated into unitary perceptual wholes?

Our approach to this problem has been to concentrate on the perception of surfaces, because it is here that one obtains clear evidence for differential linkage and visibility of features depending on global scene encoding. Depending on the final interpretation of the image data, the encoding of seemingly primitive processes such as contour, depth, and color can be radically altered. The perception of surfaces is influenced by primitives, and moreover, the final outcome can alter these same primitives. Obviously, the strong notion of modularity is inconsistent with this view. By the same token, this might be taken as evidence against any model based on a sequence or hierarchy of information processing. Yet, information obtained over the past 30 years indicates that cortex is highly organized and hierarchical, at least for vision (van Essen 1985).

To reconcile our perceptual results with the clear sequence and hierarchy seen in cortex, we briefly outline a speculative framework to consider the cortical analysis of surfaces. Figure 12 shows two levels of cortical organization, a hypothetical area V_m projecting to V_n (where index m < n). Thus, V_n represents an as yet unspecified extrastriate area (V2, V3, V4, etc.). In any given cortical area of interest, anatomical and physiological data support the view of vertical columns, patchy regions where function is more or less the same within a given vertical extent and differs more along a horizontal direction. Thus, one has thick, thin, and interstripes of V2. For the case of V2, color, contour, depth, and motion, for example, all have slightly differ-

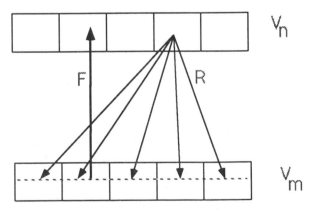

Figure 12. Hypothesized hierarchial relationship between two cortical visual areas, a lower level V_m projecting to a higher V_n showing its possible relation to visual surface formation. Primitive features segregated into different vertical columns of V_m project to V_n, where surface formation is hypothesized to occur. Forward connections (labeled F) between the regions are relatively local and tend to preserve segregation of pathways and topography. Reciprocal projections (labeled R), however, are not local but project widely and diffusely to a given lamina back in V_m (see text). Such backward connections enable different pathways to interact over wider retinotopic regions.

ent distributions with respect to these columnar subdivisions (Hubel and Livingstone 1987). As such, one might still consider these subregions as functional modules. In addition, these separate columns project forward to higher cortical regions in a reasonably local and discrete manner, roughly preserving segregation and hence modularity at each stage.

Of interest, however, is the fact that the backward projection (from V_n to V_m) appears to have a very different projection rule (Krubitzer and Kaas 1989; Zeki 1990). Instead of a given patch, say in V_n, projecting just to the patch from which it received its projection, the backward projection tends to be a laminar one (confined to particular horizontal layers), and it is much more diffuse, projecting across many columns in V_n. As such, a back projection has a much greater opportunity to operate across modules, as well as across larger retinotopic areas. This means that higher-order processing, say surface formation, could be influenced by and yet still influence the earlier processing of features.

Neurophysiological Implications

A number of hypotheses advanced in this paper may be directly testable in single unit experiments. We mention a few. First, regarding the possibility that eye-of-origin information participates in surface and depth perception, one could imagine a certain class of illusory contour cells (identified by von der Heydt et al. 1984; Peterhans and von der Heydt 1989; von der Heydt and Peterhans 1989) in which the responses of such cells would be stimulated by unpaired monocular regions, much in the way that such regions evoke illusory contours seen in Figure 11. Thus, one might predict that certain contour-specific cells would be more vigorously stimulated by unpaired rather than paired dots. In addition, one might also predict that the position of dots which would best stimulate such cells would correspond to the fact that contours appear to the right of left-eye-only and to the left of right-eye-only points.

Second, we think that our hypothesis regarding the close interdependence of contour, color, and depth might be explored by seeing whether color-specific cells might alter their firing rates in a predicted direction from a subtle manipulation of disparity. Thus, by simply reversing the disparity of figures like those seen in Figure 6, one might see changes in the response of color-specific cells whose receptive fields are in the "filled-in" region surrounded by physically colored regions. In addition, the removal of the outer limbs of the white cross from Figure 6 might be expected to stimulate illusory contour cells having horizontally oriented receptive fields, in accordance with the horizontal illusory contour seen in Figure 5.

CONCLUDING SUMMARY

In the course of attempting to understand the visual encoding of surfaces, we have made a number of points. First, we introduced the concept of contour belongingness or ownership and outlined its relationship to the linkage of image fragments. We demonstrated that if an image region is bounded by a contour that it does not own, linkage to other image regions becomes a possibility. Furthermore, we hypothesized that cell types encountered in visual cortex could begin to make the distinction between contours that actually ended in the three-dimensional world from those that continued behind occluding surfaces.

Second, we showed that the local pooling of disparity signals is insufficient to understand the perception of some very simple stereoscopic scenes. One must view the visual system as constructing a consistent interpretation of the scene rather than pooling local disparity signals.

Third, we argued from our studies of transparency that the visual system effectively avoids the assumption of the accidental view in interpreting scenes. These studies also show a strong two-way relationship between underlying features and surface formation. Thus, the triggering of transparency can lead to the destruction and creation of illusory contours, the spreading of color, and a radically different perception of depth.

Fourth, we showed that binocularly unpaired points can lead to the perception of a surface bounded by illusory contours. Because such eye-of-origin information is available only at the earliest stages of cortical processing, we suggested that the inferential process for surface formation must begin very early, as early as area V1 or its immediate cortical projection zones.

Fifth, we hypothesized a relationship between feature and surface representation that is derived from our perceptual observations and the known anatomy of extrastriate cortical areas.

ACKNOWLEDGMENTS

The current research is partially supported by Air Force Office of Scientific Research grant 83-0320. S.S. was supported by a fellowship from the Japanese Society for the Promotion of Science for Japanese Junior Scientists and by a Rachel C. Atkinson Fellowship.

REFERENCES

Adelson, E.H. and J.R. Bergen. 1985. Spatiotemporal energy models for the perception of motion. *J. Opt. Soc. Am.* **2:** 284.

Barlow, H.B., C. Blakemore, and J.D. Pettigrew. 1967. The neural mechanism of binocular depth discrimination. *J. Physiol.* **193:** 327.

Bregman, A.L. 1981. Asking the "what for" question in auditory perception. In *Perceptual organization* (ed. M. Kubovy and J.R. Pomerantz), p. 99. Lawrence Earlbaum, Hillsdale, New Jersey.

Burkhalter, A. and D.C. van Essen. 1986. Processing of color, form and disparity information in visual areas VP and V2 of ventral extrastriate cortex in the macaque monkey. *J. Neurosci.* **6:** 2327.

Crick, F. 1984. Function of the thalamic reticular complex: The searchlight hypothesis. *Proc. Natl. Acad. Sci.* **81:** 4586.

Gibson, J.J. 1950. *The perception of the visual world*. Houghton Mifflin, Boston.

Gregory, R.L. 1970. *The intelligent eye*. McGraw-Hill, New York.

Guzman, A. 1984. Decomposition of a visual scene into three dimensional borders: Fall Joint Conference 33. In *Information technology series*, volume VI. *Artificial intelligence* (ed. O. Fischein), p. 310. Reston, Virginia.

Helmholtz, H. 1910. *Treatise on physiological optics*. (Translated from the third German edition; reprinted in 1962) (ed. J.P.C. Southall), vol. 3. Dover, New York.

Hildreth, E. 1984. *The measurement of visual motion*. ACM Distinguished Dissertation Series. MIT Press, Cambridge.

Hochberg, J. 1981. Levels of perceptual organization. In *Perceptual organization* (ed. M. Kubovy and J.R. Pomerantz), p. 255. Lawrence Erlbaum, Hillsdale, New Jersey.

Hubel, D.H. and M.S. Livingstone. 1987. Segregation of form, color, and stereopsis in primate area 18. *J. Neurosci.* **7:** 3378.

Hubel, D.H. and T.N. Wiesel. 1965. Receptive fields and functional architecture in two non-striate visual areas (18 and 19) of the cat. *J. Neurophysiol.* **28:** 229.

Julesz, B. 1971. *Foundations of cyclopean perception*. University of Chicago Press, Illinois.

Kanizsa, G. 1979. *Organization in vision*. Praeger Publishers, New York.

Koenderink, J.J. 1990. *Solid shape*. MIT Press, Cambridge.

Koffka, K. 1935. *Principles of Gestalt psychology*, p. 107. Harcourt, Brace, and World, Cleveland.

Krubitzer, L.A. and J.H. Kaas. 1989. Cortical integration of parallel pathways in the visual system of primates. *Brain Res.* **478:** 161.

Land, E.H. 1977. The retinex theory of color vision. *Sci. Am.* **237:** 108.

Livingstone, M.S. and D.H. Hubel. 1987. Psychophysical evidence for separate channels for the perception of form, color, movement, and depth. *J. Neurosci.* **7:** 3416.

Marr, D. 1982. *Vision*. Freeman, San Francisco.

Marr, D. and T. Poggio. 1976. Cooperative computation of stereo disparity. *Science* **194:** 283.

Maunsell, J.H.R. and W.T. Newsome. 1987. Visual processing in monkey extrastriate cortex. *Annu. Rev. Neurosci.* **10:** 363.

Maunsell, J.H.R. and D.C. Van Essen. 1983. Functional properties of neurons in the middle temporal visual area (MT) of the macaque monkey. I. Selectivity for stimulus direction, speed and orientation. *J. Neurophysiol.* **49:** 1127.

Metelli, F. 1974. The perception of transparency. *Sci. Am.* **230:** 90.

Michotte, A. 1954. *La perception de la causalite*. Publications Universitaires de Louvain, France.

Nakayama, K. and S. Shimojo. 1990. daVinci Stereopsis: Depth and subjective occluding contours from unpaired image points. *Vision Res.* **30:** (in press).

Nakayama, K., S. Shimojo, and V.S. Ramachandran. 1990. Transparency: Relation to depth, subjective contours, luminance, and neon color spreading. *Perception* (in press).

Nakayama, K., S. Shimojo, and G.H. Silverman. 1989.

Stereoscopic depth: Its relation to image segmentation, grouping, and the recognition of occluded objects. *Perception* **18:** 55.

Nelson, J.I. 1975. Globality and stereoscopic fusion in binocular vision. *J. Theor. Biol.* **49:** 1.

Newsome, W.T. and E.B. Pare. 1988. A selective impairment of motion perception following lesions in the middle temporal visual area (MT). *J. Neurosci.* **8:** 2201.

Peterhans, E. and R. von der Heydt. 1989. Mechanisms of contour perception in monkey visual cortex. II. Contours bridging gaps. *J. Neurosci.* **9:** 1749.

Petry, S. and G.E. Meyer. 1987. *The perception of illusory contours*. Springer Verlag, New York.

Poggio, T., V. Torre, and C. Koch. 1985. Computational vision and regularization theory. *Nature* **317:** 314.

Redies, C. and L. Spillmann. 1981. The neon-color effect in the Ehrenstein illusion. *Perception* **10:** 667.

Richards, W., J.J. Koenderink, and D.D. Hoffman. 1987. Inferring three-dimensional shapes from two-dimensional silhouettes. *J. Opt. Soc. Am. A* **4:** 1168.

Rock, I. and R. Anson. 1979. Illusory contours as the solution to a problem. *Perception* **8:** 665.

Schiller, P.H., N.K. Logothetis, and E.R. Charles. 1990. Functions of the colour-opponent and broad-band channels of the visual system. *Nature* **343:** 68.

Schiller, P.H., J.H. Sandell, and J.H. Maunsell. 1986. Functions of the ON and OFF channels of the visual system. *Nature* **322:** 824.

Shimojo, S. and K. Nakayama. 1990. Real world occlusion constraints and binocular rivalry interaction. *Vision Res.* **30:** 69.

Shimojo, S., G.H. Silverman, and K. Nakayama. 1988. An occlusion-related mechanism of depth perception based on motion and interocular sequence. *Nature* **333:** 265.

———. 1989. Occlusion and the solution to the aperature problem for motion. *Vision Res.* **29:** 619.

Sperling, G. 1970. Binocular vision: A physical and neural theory. *Am. J. Psychol.* **83:** 461.

Treisman, A. and G. Gelade. 1980. A feature integration theory of attention. *Cognit. Psychol.* **12:** 97.

Van Essen, D.C. 1985. Functional organization of primate visual cortex. *Cereb. Cortex* **3:** 259.

Varin, D. 1971. Fenomini di contrasto e diffusione chromatica nell' organizzazione spaziale del campo percettivo. *Riv. Psicol.* **65:** 101.

von der Heydt, R. and E. Peterhans. 1989. Mechanisms of contour perception in monkey visual cortex. I. Lines of pattern discontinuity. *J. Neurosci.* **9:** 1731.

von der Heydt, R., E. Peterhans, and G. Baumgartner. 1984. Illusory contours and cortical neuron responses. *Science* **224:** 1260.

Wheatstone, C. 1838. On some remarkable, and hitherto unobserved, phenomena of binocular vision. *Philos. Trans. R. Soc. Lond. B* **128:** 371.

Zeki, S. 1978. Functional specialization in the visual cortex of the rhesus monkey. *Nature* **274:** 423.

———. 1990. The motion pathways of the visual cortex. In *Vision: Coding and efficiency* (ed. C. Blakemore), Cambridge University Press, United Kingdom. (In press.)

Haptic Illusions: Experiments on Human Manipulation and Perception of "Virtual Objects"

N. Hogan,* B.A. Kay,† E.D. Fasse,* and F.A. Mussa-Ivaldi†

*Department of Mechanical Engineering, †Department of Brain and Cognitive Sciences, Massachusetts Institute of Technology, Cambridge, Massachusetts 02139

The use of tools is one of the distinctive features of human behavior. Although other species make and use rudimentary tools, this behavior is most highly developed in humans. What is the nature of the underlying neural processes? What does the brain have to do to accomplish effective tool use?

To address this question, we have adopted an approach combining biological and robotic methods. One of the impediments to gaining a deeper understanding of motor behavior is that biological systems can be quite deceptive; superficial inspection (or introspection) rarely reveals the true complexity of what is going on. In biological systems, we see the solutions; the underlying problems are typically disguised. In contrast, attempts to accomplish comparable behavior in robotic systems quickly reveal the problems; however, solutions are often less obvious.

Control of Contact

Contact with objects is clearly a fundamental prerequisite for the use of tools, yet the apparently trivial problem of controlling the force exerted by a robot on a surface has proven surprisingly difficult. The "obvious" approach is to measure the force of contact and send that information to the controlling computer so that it may adjust or regulate the force exerted. Unfortunately, that approach has been plagued by a phenomenon that has been termed *contact instability*. Robotics researchers in numerous laboratories have reported that a robot which is capable of executing unrestrained motions stably and accurately will break into a pathologically uncontrollable chattering instability on contact with a rigid surface, bouncing off the surface and impacting it repeatedly. This problem has been listed as one of the prominent challenges of robotics (Paul 1987). Yet biological systems clearly have little difficulty contacting and manipulating objects. The manifest dexterity of humans provides an "existence proof" that this problem admits at least one excellent solution. To understand the nature of that solution, it is helpful to "look inside" the system, and that is perhaps more easily accomplished in a robot.

The necessary and sufficient condition for a manipulator to remain stable when coupled to any passive object has recently been derived mathematically and verified experimentally (Colgate 1988; Colgate and Hogan 1988; Hogan 1988b): The combination of ac-

tuators, feedback sensors, and control circuits must mimic the behavior of a passive object (e.g., a spring or a mass). It is a well-established fact (Matthews 1959; Gordon et al. 1966; Joyce et al. 1969; Rack and Westbury 1969; Crago et al. 1976; Houk 1979; Hoffer and Andreassen 1981; Loeb 1984) that muscles, both with and without their associated neural feedback networks, exhibit a spring-like behavior. Recent psychophysical experiments on human subjects have established that the entire multijoint upper limb mimics the behavior of a passive, multijoint spring (Mussa-Ivaldi et al. 1985), even though that requires finely balanced interjoint neural feedback (Hogan 1985). Spring-like behavior is consistent with the theoretical requirement for preserving stability on contact with objects. This provides one example of the synergy that can exist between biology and robotics.

Haptic Illusions

In an attempt to understand the neural basis of tool-using behavior, we have begun to investigate haptic perception: sensory exploration intimately linked with control of motor behavior. For example, when feeling an object, haptic perception (defined as the combination of touch and kinesthetic sense; see, e.g., Gibson 1966) provides information about the object's size, weight, compliance, etc. Movement is often required to extract these properties. In this paper, we describe psychophysical experiments conducted to examine the foundations of haptic perception.

Human visual perception is subject to many characteristic illusions or distortions such as the horizontal-vertical illusion, Mach bands, the Müller-Lyer illusion, and the Poggendorf illusion (Schiffman 1976). Investigating these illusions can provide insight into the underlying neural processes. For example, there is a clear relationship between the psychophysical observation of Mach bands and the center-surround receptive field of visual neurons and its implementation in lateral-inhibition networks (Schiffman 1976).

Human haptic perception, which requires intimate interaction between motor and sensory behavior, is also subject to characteristic illusions or distortions (Davidson 1972; Wong 1977; Kay et al. 1989a,b). These distortions may reveal much about the organization of human motor behavior and sensory perception. To use an object as a tool, it would appear that some form of internal model or representation of the limb and the object to be wielded is necessary. In fact, most proposed computational models of human motor control implicitly assume geometrically structured models of the body and the environment. Hypotheses about the existence of internal models have been criticized as being untestable. The experiments described here show that such hypotheses can be tested. We obtained information about our subjects' internal models by having them make psychophysical judgments about the properties of objects using whole-arm movements. That is, our primary datum takes the form of a transformation from the external world (i.e., the physical part of psychophysical) to the internal model (i.e., the psychopart of psychophysical). We show that this transformation is not a geometrically consistent one.

METHODS

Experimental apparatus. The experimental apparatus shown schematically in Figure 1 featured a unique computer-controlled manipulandum that was essentially a two-degree-of-freedom robot arm constrained to move in a horizontal plane. Seated subjects grasped a handle mounted on a force/torque transducer that was mounted, in turn, on the end of the manipulandum. Motion of the subjects' arms was also constrained to the horizontal plane, with motion allowed at the shoulder and elbow only. Two torque motors driven by current-controlled amplifiers were mounted on the links of the robot arm. Optical encoders measured the angular position of the links. The digitized output of analog tachometers mounted on the torque motors measured the angular speed of the links.

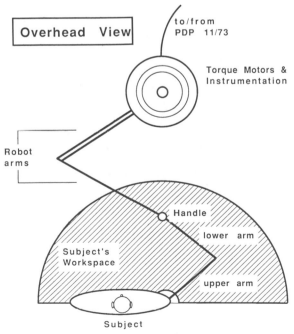

Figure 1. Schematic diagram of the experimental apparatus. The subject is depicted in a typical position relative to the apparatus.

Measured motions and forces at the human/machine interface were recorded at a sampling rate of 100 Hz by an LSI-11/73 digital computer.

The digital computer also controlled the voltages applied to the amplifiers. The control algorithm was designed to provide a programmable mechanical impedance that was varied as a function of the position of the handle. Mechanical impedance refers to the combination of apparent stiffness, viscosity, inertia, and other forces that impede attempted motion of the handle. In this way, the device simulated the presence of planar *virtual objects* in the workspace. Under computer control, we modified the *apparent* location, size, shape, and material properties (e.g., stiffness) of the simulated virtual objects that the human subjects felt.

Experiment 1: Judgment of length. In the first set of experiments, the apparatus simulated rectangular objects with different shapes. When the handle was outside the boundary of the rectangle, no force was exerted. When the handle crossed the boundary, an outward force was generated perpendicular to the boundary and proportional to the depth of penetration into the virtual object, thus providing a virtual stiffness at the boundary. Force proportional to velocity was also simulated, providing a virtual damping force that minimized any tendency of the handle to bounce on the surface of the virtual object. Values of stiffness and damping (0.8 N/mm and 15.0 N/mm/sec, respectively) were chosen to produce a compelling impression of a real object.

Two features of the rectangular objects were varied, the first being the ratio of the lengths of their sides. All simulated rectangular objects had the same area of 100 cm^2 and were placed with their centers at the same location in the center of the robot's workspace. The "Y" side of each rectangle was parallel to the subject's sagittal plane, and the "X" side was perpendicular to the "Y" side. Rectangles with 21 different aspects ratios of X:Y = 2.0, 1.9, ..., 1.1, 1.0 and Y:X = 1.1, 1.2, ..., 1.9, 2.0 were presented.

The second feature varied was the distance of the center of the simulated rectangles from the subject's shoulder. This was achieved by moving the subject back and forth with respect to the apparatus. In this way, we eliminated the possibility that any observed workspace-dependent effects could be attributed to variations in the control algorithm due to the kinematic configuration of the robot. Three distances from the shoulder were investigated: "proximal" at approximately 45%, "medial" at approximately 65%, and "distal" at approximately 85% of the subject's maximum reach.

One distance condition was tested in each of three experimental sessions. Subjects were instructed to close their eyes and feel the simulated rectangular object using only arm movements. Using a forced-choice paradigm, subjects were required to judge which side of the rectangle was longer, X or Y. They were allowed to feel the objects in any way and for as long as necessary in order to make their decision. Five blocks of trials were presented in each session, each block consisting of a randomized presentation of all of the aspect ratio conditions. A total of 12 subjects participated in the experiment.

Experiment 2: Judgment of stiffness. In a second set of experiments, the apparatus simulated objects of constant shape with sides of different stiffnesses. All simulated objects were square with the same area of 25 cm^2 and were placed with their centers at the same location in the center of the robot's workspace. The ratio of the stiffness of the X and Y sides, $K_X:K_Y$, was varied over 11 stimulus values. The ratio of the linear viscosity of the X and Y sides was covaried to preserve a constant damping ratio. Stiffnesses ranged from 0.4 to 0.8 N/mm and damping coefficients from 10.61 to 15.00 N/mm/sec.

The distance to the center of the simulated objects was varied as in the first experiment. One distance condition was tested in each of three experimental sessions. Subjects were instructed to close their eyes and feel the simulated object using only arm movements. Using a forced-choice paradigm, subjects were required to judge which side of the rectangle was stiffer, X or Y. Five blocks of trials were presented in each session, each block consisting of a randomized presentation of all of the stiffness ratio conditions. A total of six subjects participated in the experiment.

RESULTS

Judgment of Length

The judgment data for lengths were fitted to the standard psychometric function (Gescheider 1985), and the point of subjective equality (PSE) and the discrimination threshold (DT) were measured in terms of the aspect ratio X:Y. The PSE was defined as that aspect ratio for which 50% of a subject's judgments were that X was the longer side. Thus, a simulated rectangular object of this aspect ratio was perceived as square. The difference threshold was defined as the difference between the aspect ratios at which 25% and 75% of the subject's judgments were that X was the longer side. It provides a measure of the change in aspect ratio necessary to produce a just-noticeable difference in the simulated objects and indicates the resolution of the perceptual system in this task.

The measured X:Y ratios at the PSEs were always greater than one, by 29% on average. At all three workspace locations, a rectangular object with its X side longer than its Y side was perceived to be square. We also found a systematic trend for this perceptual illusion to become more pronounced with increasing distance from the shoulder. In contrast, the measured difference threshold did not show any trend. The average discriminable difference in the X:Y ratio was 0.078. The experimental results are summarized in Figure 2. A linear regression of the X:Y ratio at the point of

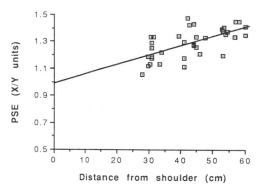

Figure 2. Plot of the ratio of lengths X:Y at the PSE for length judgment vs. distance from the shoulder in cm.

subjective equality onto the distance from the shoulder in centimeters was performed and is shown by the straight line in Figure 2. Curiously, if we extrapolate on the basis of this linear regression, the X:Y ratio at the PSE would equal unity at the shoulder. That is, the perceptual illusion would disappear if the object were felt at the shoulder.

Judgment of Stiffness

The judgment data for stiffness were fitted to the standard psychometric function, and the PSE and the DT were measured in terms of the aspect ratio $K_X:K_Y$. Unlike the judgments of length, the measured $K_X:K_Y$ ratios at the PSEs were typically *less* than one, by 15% on average. However, some of the PSE ratios were greater than one. The results are summarized in Figure 3. As with the judgments of length, we found a systematic trend for this perceptual illusion to become more pronounced with increasing distance from the shoulder, and no trend for the DT. The average discriminable difference in the $K_X:K_Y$ ratio was 0.15. A linear regression of the $K_X:K_Y$ ratio at the PSE onto the distance from the shoulder in centimeters was performed and is shown by the straight line in Figure 3. If we extrapolate on the basis of this linear regression, the

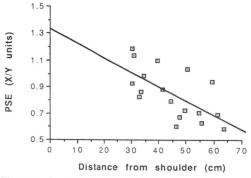

Figure 3. Plot of the ratio of stiffnesses $K_X:K_Y$ at the PSE for stiffness judgment vs. distance from the shoulder in cm.

$K_X:K_Y$ ratio at the PSE would equal unity at a point just inside "proximal" position.

DISCUSSION

A distortion of length perception similar to that reported here and by Kay et al. (1989a,b) was reported by Wong (1977), but to the authors' knowledge, the variation of this phenomenon with location in a subject's workspace has not been reported previously. It is similar to the horizontal-vertical visual illusion (Avery and Day 1969) and von Helmholtz's "horopter" illusion (Luneburg 1950). Likewise, to our knowledge, the distortion of stiffness perception and its variation with location in a subject's workspace has not been reported previously.

Metrically Consistent Internal Models

What are the implications of these observations for neural computation and the control of motor behavior? An implicit assumption underlying most proposed computational models of sensorimotor behavior is that they are founded on a consistent, geometrically structured model of the body and the environment—the typical robotics approach. The majority of robotic control schemes assume an internal geometric model of the robot, which is used for perception, planning, and control purposes. This internal model has a *metric structure* that is used to measure such quantities as velocity, force, and distance between points. A key feature of the model is that it is metrically consistent. By consistent we mean that given the position metric, the metric for force, angle, velocity, stiffness—all of the relevant geometric and mechanical quantities—can be determined.

Similar architectures have been proposed for biological motor control. One of the more controversial of these is the so-called tensor theory proposed by Pellionisz and Llinás (1978) and elaborated in a series of subsequent papers (see, e.g., Pellionisz and Llinás 1979, 1980, 1982). This theory proposes that certain prominent neural structures such as the cerebellum are the embodiment of the metric tensor of an internal geometric model.

A common criticism of the tensor theory of Pellionisz and Llinás (and of hypotheses about internal models in general) is that it is untestable. That is not the case for a consistent, metrically structured model. If a consistent metric underlies sensorimotor behavior, there should be a precise, mathematical relation between the distortion of haptic length perception and the distortion of haptic stiffness perception. Suppose a perceived position $\mathbf{x}_p$ is related to an actual position $\mathbf{x}$ by a known nonlinear function

$$\mathbf{x}_p = \mathbf{L}(\mathbf{x})$$

where the quantities $\mathbf{x}_p$ and $\mathbf{x}$ are arrays or vectors of the appropriate dimension. If this relation is smooth

enough to be differentiable, then the relation between infinitesimal displacements is

$$d\mathbf{x}_p = \mathbf{J}_p(\mathbf{x})d\mathbf{x}$$

where

$$\mathbf{J}_p(\mathbf{x}) = \partial \mathbf{L}(\mathbf{x})/\partial \mathbf{x}$$

If there is a consistent metric, infinitesimal work done is the same in both representations.

$$\mathbf{f}^t d\mathbf{x} = \mathbf{f}_p^t d\mathbf{x}_p$$

where superscript t denotes the transpose operator. Therefore, the relation between actual and perceived forces is

$$\mathbf{f} = \mathbf{J}_p^t(\mathbf{x})\mathbf{f}_p$$

The relation between perceived and actual stiffness may also be derived. Assume small displacements about an equilibrium point at zero force. Denote the perceived stiffness by

$$\mathbf{f}_p = \mathbf{K}_p d\mathbf{x}_p$$

Using the above relations between forces and displacements

$$\mathbf{f} = \mathbf{J}_p^t(\mathbf{x})\mathbf{K}_p\mathbf{J}_p(\mathbf{x})d\mathbf{x}$$

But, assuming small displacements about an equilibrium point at zero force, the actual stiffness is

$$\mathbf{f} = \mathbf{K}d\mathbf{x}$$

so the relation between perceived and actual stiffness is

$$\mathbf{K} = \mathbf{J}_p^t(\mathbf{x})\mathbf{K}_p\mathbf{J}_p(\mathbf{x})$$

Loosely speaking, if a consistent metric underlies sensorimotor behavior, the distortion of stiffness perception should be inversely proportional to the square of the length perception distortion.

Relation to Motor Control

Conscious comparison of lengths and stiffnesses requires a cognitive process that might be unrelated to the information processing associated with the production of motor behavior. However, the general trends in our experimental data are *qualitatively* similar to what would be expected if there were a distorted but consistent internal model of the external world. Comparing Figures 2 and 3, whereas the point of subjective equality for length is always greater than one, the point of subjective equality for stiffness is typically less than one, and the variations of these two measurements with location in the workspace are in the opposite senses, as indicated by the regression lines in Figures 2 and 3. If we compute the inverse square of the mean PSE for length at each position, we find that the mean point of subjective equality for stiffness at the same position is between one and two of the corresponding standard deviations for stiffness from that value. This approximate qualitative agreement with a metrically consistent internal model provides some evidence that the cognitive and perceptual processes involved in these experiments are, in fact, related to the processes of motor control.

Haptic Perception Is Not Metrically Consistent

If we examine the *quantitative* details of our experimental data, we find a significant departure from the predictions of a metrically consistent internal model. In the "proximal position," the mean PSE for length is a ratio of 1.2. To be metrically consistent, the PSE for stiffness should be about 0.69; in fact, it is 0.99. Conversely, our measurements indicate no significant distortion in the perception of stiffness in the proximal position. If the perceptions of length and stiffness were metrically consistent, we would expect no significant distortion of haptic length perception, but our measurements indicate otherwise. Figure 4 summarizes our results. Measured mean PSEs for length are shown by unfilled squares; the inverse squares of these measurements are shown by triangles; and the measured mean PSEs for stiffness are shown by filled squares. The PSEs for stiffness and the inverse squares of the PSEs for length are significantly different for all three distances ($t[16] = 4.72$, 2.99, and 4.02, proximal, medial, and distal, respectively; $p < 0.01$ for each) and overall ($t[52] = 5.56$, $p < 0.001$). The tensor theory of sensorimotor coordination of Pellionisz and Llinás cannot be reconciled with these observations.

It might be argued that the inconsistencies found between the perception of length and the perception of stiffness could be attributed to errors in the production

and perception of forces and do not conclusively disprove the existence of a metrically consistent internal model. However, a similar approach has been taken in a purely geometric context by comparing the distortion of length perception with the distortion of perception of angle. As before, if there is a metrically consistent internal representation of geometry, there is a rigorously quantifiable mathematical relation between these two perceptual illusions. Recent results (Fasse et al. 1990) again show that experimental observation is irreconcilable with a metrically consistent model.

Implications for Movement Production

Our findings do not preclude the existence of an internal model; they simply show that it is not metrically correct. These results may be compatible with the picture of motor planning and production that is beginning to emerge from recent studies. One key feature of the motor system is that in the absence of external loads, the effective mechanical behavior of groups of muscles and their associated neural feedback networks establishes a neurally modifiable equilibrium configuration for the limbs (see, e.g., Bizzi et al. 1976; Polit and Bizzi 1979). Because it may differ from the actual position of the limb (e.g., during movement or in the presence of an external load), the neurally defined equilibrium posture has been termed a virtual position and its time course a virtual trajectory (Hogan 1984). Movement may be generated by continuously modulating the neurally defined equilibrium posture. This proposal, originally made by Feldman (1966) in the context of single-joint movements, has since been elaborated to multijoint movements (see, e.g., Hogan 1985, 1988a; Flash 1987) and corroborated by a substantial body of neurophysiological (see, e.g., Bizzi et al. 1982; 1984), psychophysical (see, e.g., Cooke 1979; Kelso and Holt 1980; Schmidt and McGown 1980), and simulation (Flash 1987) studies.

One major implication of this hypothesis is that the computational complexity of Bernstein's (1967) problem—coordinating multimuscle, multijoint behavior—is dramatically simplified. The notoriously difficult "inverse dynamics" problem of robotics (Hollerbach 1982) is completely circumvented because the forces generated by the muscles and the torques exerted about the joints need not be explicitly computed. Even more compelling, the same control architecture that produces unrestrained motion can be used to control the force exerted on an object. It is only necessary to move the virtual position *inside* the object; force is exerted in relation to the distance between the actual position of the limb (which is confined to the surface of the object) and the neurally defined virtual position.

In the present context, an important implication of this motor control strategy is that forces need not be explicitly computed and may not be accurately represented in the central nervous system. Under normal circumstances, exertion of a force may be an implicit result of motor behavior rather than an explicit goal.

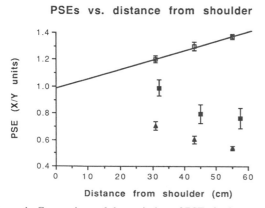

PSEs vs. distance from shoulder

Figure 4. Comparison of the variation of PSEs for length and stiffness judgment with distance from the shoulder in cm. (□) Measured mean points of subjective equality for length; (▲) inverse squares of these measurements; (■) measured mean PSEs for stiffness. Vertical bars denote one standard error.

Thus, the brain may not have encountered the need to develop mutually consistent perceptions of motion, force, and stiffness or any of the other quantities that are related in a metrically consistent model.

At this time, we cannot rule out the possibility that our results are due to the experimental context in which they were obtained. However, although the robotic apparatus used to generate virtual objects is novel and unusual, the tasks investigated are physiologically and psychologically relevant. In particular, the perception of stiffness (or, more generally, mechanical impedance) provides vital information about objects that cannot reliably be obtained by other means. We routinely assess the stiffness or impedance of objects; we commonly judge the ripeness of a fruit or the consistency of a cheese by squeezing it, and we do so because that information cannot be obtained by visual inspection alone. This may explain why our measurements show that near the center of the workspace (in the "proximal" position), haptic perception of stiffness is essentially undistorted, whereas in the same position, haptic perception of length (which could be corrected by comparison with visual perception) is substantially distorted. Clearly, further experimentation is required to establish the significance of these speculations.

ACKNOWLEDGMENTS

This research was supported in part by National Institutes of Health grants AR-40029 and NS-09343, National Science Foundation grant 8914032-BCS, Office of Naval Research grant N-00014-88-K-0372, Sloan Foundation grant 87-2-16, and The Fairchild Foundation. The authors are indebted to Dr. Gerald E. Loeb for his insightful comments.

REFERENCES

Avery, G.C. and R.H. Day. 1969. Basis of the horizontal-vertical illusion. *J. Exp. Psychol.* **81:** 376.

Bernstein, N.A. 1967. *The co-ordination and regulation of movements.* Pergamon Press, New York.

Bizzi, E., A. Polit, and P. Morasso. 1976. Mechanisms underlying achievement of final head position. *J. Neurophysiol.* **39:** 435.

Bizzi, E., N. Accornero, W. Chapple, and N. Hogan. 1982. Arm trajectory formation in monkeys. *Exp. Brain Res.* **46:** 139.

———. 1984. Posture control and trajectory formation during arm movement. *J. Neurosci.* **4:** 2738.

Colgate, J.E. 1988. "The control of dynamically interacting systems." Ph.D. thesis, Massachusetts Institute of Technology, Cambridge.

Colgate, J.E. and N. Hogan. 1988. Robust control of dynamically interacting systems. *Int. J. Control* **48:** 65.

Cooke, J.D. 1979. Dependence of human arm movements on limb mechanical properties. *Brain Res.* **165:** 366.

Crago, P.E., J.C. Houk, and Z. Hasan. 1976. Regulatory actions of the human stretch reflex. *J. Neurophysiol.* **39:** 925.

Davidson, P.W. 1972. Haptic judgements of curvature by blind and sighted humans. *J. Exp. Psychol.* **93:** 43.

Fasse, E.D., B.A. Kay and N. Hogan. 1990. Human haptic

illusions in virtual object manipulation. In *Proceedings of the 12th Annual Conference of the Institute of Electrical and Electronic Engineers.* Engineering in Medicine and Biology Society. (In press.)

Feldman, A.G. 1966. Functional tuning of the nervous system with control of movement or maintenance of a steady posture. III. Mechanographic analysis of the execution by man of the simplest motor tasks. *Biophysics* **11:** 766.

Flash, T. 1987. The control of hand equilibrium trajectories in multi-joint arm movements. *Biol. Cybern.* **57:** 257.

Gescheider, G.A. 1985. *Psychophysics: Method, theory and application,* 2nd edition. Erlbaum, Hillsdale, New Jersey.

Gibson, J.J. 1966. *The senses considered as perceptual systems.* Houghton-Mifflin, New York.

Gordon, A.M., A.F. Huxley, and F.J. Julian. 1966. The variation in isometric tension with sarcomere length in vertebrate muscle fibers. *J. Physiol.* **184:** 170.

Hoffer, J.A. and S. Andreassen. 1981. Regulation of soleus muscle stiffness in premammillary cats: Intrinsic and reflex components. *J. Neurophysiol.* **45:** 267.

Hogan, N. 1984. An organising principle for a class of voluntary movements. *J. Neurosci.* **4:** 2745.

———. 1985. The mechanics of multi-joint posture and movement control. *Biol. Cybern.* **52:** 315.

Hogan, N. 1988a. Planning and execution of multi-joint movements. *Can. J. Physiol. Pharmacol.* **66:** 508.

———. 1988b. On the stability of manipulators performing contact tasks. *IEEE J. Robotics Automation* **4:** 677.

Hollerbach, J.M. 1982. Computers, brains and the control of movement. *Trends Neurosci.* **6:** 189.

Houk, J.C. 1979. Regulation of stiffness by skeletomotor reflexes. *Annu. Rev. Physiol.* **41:** 99.

Joyce, G., P.M.H. Rack, and D.R. Westbury. 1969. The mechanical properties of cat soleus muscle during controlled lengthening and shortening movements. *J. Physiol.* **204:** 461.

Kay, B.A., N. Hogan, F.A. Mussa-Ivaldi, and E.D. Fasse. 1989a. Perceiving the properties of objects using arm movements: Workspace dependent effects. In *Proceedings of the 11th Annual Conference of the Institute of Electrical and Electronic Engineers,* vol. 11, part 5, p. 1522. Engineering in Medicine and Biology Society. IEEE, New York.

———. 1989b. Perceived properties of objects using kinesthetic sense depend on workspace location. *Soc. Neurosci. Abstr.* **15:** 173.

Kelso, J.A.S. and K.G. Holt. 1980. Exploring a vibratory system analysis of human movement production. *J. Neurophysiol.* **43:** 1183.

Loeb, G.E. 1984. The control and responses of mammalian muscle spindles during normally executed motor tasks. *Exercise Sport Sci. Rev.* **12:** 157.

Luneburg, R.K. 1950. The metric of binocular visual space. *J. Opt. Soc. Am.* **40:** 627.

Matthews, P.B.C. 1959. The dependence of tension upon extension in the stretch reflex of the soleus muscle of the decerebrate cat. *J. Physiol.* **147:** 521.

Mussa-Ivaldi, F.A, N. Hogan, and E. Bizzi. 1985. Neural, mechanical and geometric factors subserving arm posture in humans. *J. Neurosci.* **5:** 2732.

Paul, R.P. 1987. Problems and research issues associated with the hybrid control of force and displacement. In *Proceedings of the IEEE Conference on Robotics and Automation,* p. 1966. IEEE Computer Society Press, Washington, D.C.

Pellionisz, A. and R. Llinás. 1978. A formal theory for cerebellar function: The predictive distributed property of the cortico-nuclear cerebellar system as described by tensor network theory and computer simulation. *Soc. Neurosci. Abstr.* **4:** 68.

———. 1979. Brain modelling by tensor network theory and computer simulation. The cerebellum: Distributed processor for predictive coordination. *Neuroscience* **4:** 323.

————. 1980. Tensorial approach to the geometry of brain function: Cerebellar coordination via the metric tensor. *Neuroscience* **5:** 1125.

————. 1982. Space time representation in the brain. The cerebellum as a predictive space-time metric tensor. *Neuroscience* **7:** 2949.

Polit, A. and E. Bizzi. 1979. Characteristics of motor programs underlying arm movements in monkeys. *J. Neurophysiol.* **42:** 183.

Rack, P.M.H. and D.R. Westbury. 1969. The effects of length and stimulus rate on tension in the isometric cat soleus muscle. *J. Physiol.* **204:** 443.

Schiffman, H.R. 1976. *Sensation and perception: An integrated approach.* Wiley, New York.

Schmidt, R.A. and C. McGown. 1980. Terminal accuracy of unexpectedly loaded rapid movements: Evidence for a mass-spring mechanism in programming. *J. Mot. Behav.* **12:** 149.

Wong, T.S. 1977. Dynamic properties of radial and tangential movements as determinants of the horizontal-vertical illusion with an L figure. *J. Exp. Psychol. Hum. Percept. Perform.* **3:** 151.

Intrinsic Electrical Properties of Nerve Cells and Their Role in Network Oscillation

R. LLINÁS

*Department of Physiology and Biophysics, New York University Medical Center,
New York, New York 10016*

For almost a century now, it has been agreed that the functional properties of the nervous system are the result of interactions among its constituent neuronal elements. Fundamental to this perspective has been the realization that nerve cells are truly individual anatomical elements. Indeed, although brilliant turn-of-the-century morphologists described in elegant detail the variety of forms that nerve cells may manifest, their most salient contribution was the proposal of the neuron doctrine (cf. Ramon y Cajal 1911).

On the other hand, from a physiological point of view, the neuron doctrine was long believed to imply unity of excitability in which any variability of function among nerve cells was ascribable to differences in synaptic connectivity. Many neuroscientists still believe that central neurons are brought to electrical activity or to quiescence only by their synaptic inputs. Accordingly, central neurons are thought to serve as mere *relay elements* in a neuronal chain that allows the conductance of impulses along the different pathways in a rapid race to some unknown portion of the brain that "puts it all together." This view of the organization of the nervous system is, at best, incomplete.

Over the last 15 years, however, another issue regarding neuronal function has emerged—that of *the intrinsic electroresponsive properties of neurons*. This concept may be stated as "nerve cells are not functionally interchangeable." That is, a neuron of a given kind (e.g., a thalamic cell) cannot replace, functionally, a neuron of another type (e.g., an inferior olivary cell), even if their morphology, synaptic connectivity, neurotransmitters, and neuromodulators were to be precisely reproduced. The reason for this uniqueness is that the intrinsic electrophysiological properties of thalamic cells are different from those of inferior olivary neurons.

Recognition of the functional significance of the intrinsic electrophysiological properties of neurons implies de facto that the overall activity of the nervous system emerges from the interplay of synaptic activity and intrinsic electroresponsive properties. The latter are responsible for one of the most remarkable properties of central nervous system (CNS) neurons, that of the generation of the membrane potential oscillations. Because this property allows neurons to respond preferentially to given frequencies of synaptic input, intrin-

sic oscillations play an important role in the organization of nervous system function.

NEURONAL OSCILLATION IN THE MAMMALIAN CNS

One of the truly remarkable findings relating to the electrical activity of the brain was the discovery by Hans Berger (1929) that rhythmic electrical activity could be recorded from the surface of the human cranium. Equally remarkable was the discovery that different rhythms may be associated with given states of consciousness. Seventy years later, we continue to be amazed by the fact that sufficiently coherent neuronal activity may be recruited to generate macroscopic oscillatory states in a structure as complex and massive as the human brain.

More recently, the in vitro study of single-cell electrical activity in many areas of the mammalian CNS has provided significant information regarding the possible mechanisms underlying the membrane oscillations. Although due to the simplified nature of brain slices this research paradigm cannot yield a complete picture of the oscillatory properties of neuronal ensembles, it has afforded a first step toward understanding network rhythmic activity in the in vivo system. Below I review the oscillatory properties of four cell types and discuss the possible role of intrinsic electrical properties in the generation of global functional states.

Inferior Olivary Neuron Oscillations

Threshold oscillations. In vitro experiments using brain-stem slices demonstrated that inferior olivary (IO) neurons have a set of ionic conductances that allow them to act as single-cell oscillators (Benardo and Foster 1986; Llinás and Yarom 1981a, 1986). The firing of IO cells is characterized by an initial fast-rising action potential (a somatic sodium spike), which is prolonged to 10–15 msec by a powerful dendritic calcium-dependent after-depolarization (Fig. 1A). This broad plateau is followed by the activation of a calcium-dependent potassium conductance ($gK_{(Ca)}$), which hyperpolarizes the cell, shunts most synaptic input, and silences the spike-generating activity. The hyperpolarization is terminated by a sharp active rebound arising

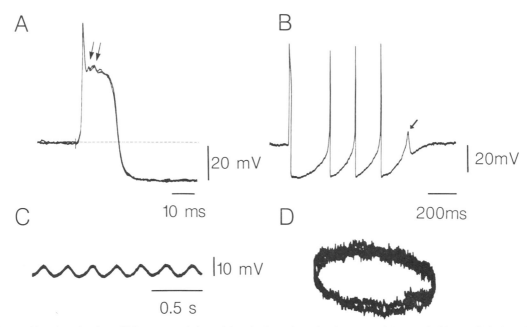

Figure 1. Antidromic activation of IO neurons. (*A*) Antidromically activated action potentials recorded intracellularly. Initial fast depolarization followed by an after-depolarization (arrows) and a prolonged after-hyperpolarization can be seen. (*B*) Oscillation of IO cell. The initial spike is followed by three action potentials and a subthreshold rebound (arrow). Note that the threshold for the rebound response is negative to the resting membrane potential. (*C*) Spontaneous oscillatory potentials in IO cells. Oscillatory potentials occurring at close to resting potential, having a peak-to-peak average of ~8 mV and a peak-to-peak frequency of ~5 Hz in vitro. (*D*) A Lissajous figure generated by utilizing a record similar to that in *C* in the vertical plane of the CRT while the horizontal was fed by a sinusoidal oscillator. (Modified from Llinás and Yarom 1981a, 1986).

from a membrane potential negative to the resting level. This rebound response, a "low-"threshold calcium spike (Fig. 1B, arrow), is due to the activation of a somatic voltage-gated calcium conductance that is inactivated at the resting membrane potential (about −65 mV) and is de-inactivated by the after-hyperpolarization described above (Llinás and Yarom 1981a,b). The rebound low-threshold spike serves to maintain the oscillatory firing of IO neurons at a frequency determined largely by the duration and amplitude of the after-hyperpolarization. In turn, as expected from activation of the $gK_{(Ca)}$, the amount of calcium entering the dendrites during the after-depolarization modulates the duration of the after-hyperpolarization. Thus, if the dendritic calcium action potential is small, the duration of the after-hyperpolarization is shorter, and the rebound response will have a low amplitude. (Fig. 1B). This point is central to understanding the oscillatory properties of IO cells, because it indicates that calcium entry determines the cycle time of this neuronal oscillator. Indeed, in Figure 1B, the first spike of the sequence has a broader after-depolarization (arrow) and a more prolonged after-hyperpolarization. The spikes that follow, arriving from a more negative membrane potential, produce a smaller after-depolarization, and their interspike integral becomes stabilized at close to 5 Hz in the in vitro slice. Note that the last rebound calcium spike failed to generate a full action potential.

Subthreshold oscillations. In addition to spike oscillations, subthreshold membrane-potential oscillations

may be recorded intracellularly in slices (Fig. 1C) and are an emerging property of the IO neuronal ensemble. These spontaneous oscillations are symmetrical and close to sinusoidal with a frequency that is independent of the electroresponsive state of any individual neuron, since direct activation of the recorded cell does not alter the oscillation frequency (Benardo and Foster 1986; Llinás and Yarom 1986). The regularity of these oscillations is illustrated in the Lissajous figure in Figure 1D.

The sequence of events that serves as the basis for this oscillation is similar to those described above for the threshold oscillations. It involves an inward Ca^{++} current that activates a $gK_{(Ca)}$, which in turn leads to a hyperpolarization followed by a calcium-dependent low-threshold spike. Indeed, if tetrodotoxin (TTX) is added to the bath at a sufficient concentration to block the sodium-dependent action potentials, the subthreshold oscillations are unaltered. However, if the calcium conductances are blocked by either Co^{++} or Cd^{++}, or Ca^{++} is replaced by Mn^{++}, the oscillatory rhythm disappears (Llinás and Yarom 1986).

The electrical properties outlined above provide olivary neurons with the ability to resonate at two distinct frequencies, one ranging from 3 Hz to 6 Hz, the other from 9 Hz to 12 Hz. These two frequencies reflect, respectively, the predominantly dendritic or predominantly somatic distribution of the calcium electroresponsiveness of these cells, as modulated by the resting membrane-potential level. In a slightly depolarized cell, the firing frequency will be dominated by the calcium entering during the dendritic spike, which, in turn, governs the size and duration of the after-hyperpolarization. At more hyperpolarized levels, however, active invasion of the dendrites is reduced (due to their rather high threshold), and the firing frequency is dominated by the de-inactivating rebound Ca^{++} conductance (Llinás and Yarom 1986). From a global point of view, other experiments indicate that intrinsic properties, such as those giving rise to membrane oscillations, are essential in the timing properties of motor execution that characterizes the cerebellar control of motor coordination (Llinás and Sasaki 1989).

Thalamic Neuron Oscillations

In contrast to the rather stereotypical membrane oscillations of IO cells, thalamic cells may fire in a tonic or repetitive fashion, resembling other CNS neurons where the frequency of firing is proportional to the level of membrane depolarization. Indeed, as shown in Figure 2A, a step depolarization can drive the cell to high-frequency tonic firing. This type of firing occurs because the thalamic dendritic calcium conductance is

not as powerful as that in the IO, making the after-hyperpolarization that follows each thalamic spike smaller than its olivary counterpart. However, when thalamic cells are hyperpolarized, a short and phasic burst of spikes is generated. This burst is activated by a low-threshold calcium spike similar to that in the IO (Fig. 2C) (Jahnsen and Llinás 1984). These two types of electrical behaviors allow thalamic cells to switch from a tonic to a phasic firing pattern by a simple modulation of the membrane potential.

In addition to being able to fire in two distinct modes, thalamic cells fire at one of two preferred frequencies: near 6 Hz or near 10 Hz. The ionic mechanisms underlying thalamic neuron oscillatory behavior are in some aspects quite similar to those encountered in IO cells. However, thalamic cells, in addition to having rather limited dendritic calcium-dependent excitability, display an early potassium conductance (A current) similar to that described in invertebrate neurons (Hagiwara et al. 1961; Connor and Stevens 1971) and a noninactivating sodium conductance similar to that seen in Purkinje cells (Llinás and Sugimori 1980). This particular set of conductances allows oscillatory single-cell responses near 6 Hz at negative membrane potentials.

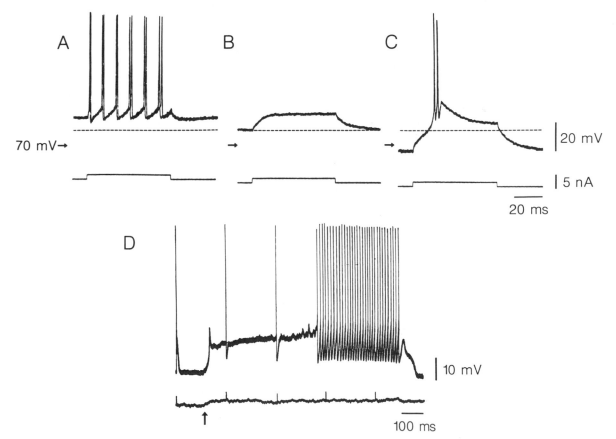

Figure 2. Stimulation of thalamic cell with a constant amplitude transmembrane current pulse at three different membrane potentials. (*A*) A depolarizing current pulse produces a train of action potentials if superimposed on a slightly depolarized membrane potential level. (*B*) The same current pulse produces a subthreshold depolarization, from resting membrane potential. (*C*) The cell was directly stimulated while being hyperpolarized by a constant current injection. The outward current pulse, which had the same amplitude as those in *A* and *B*, now triggers an all-or-none burst of spikes. (*D*) Injection of a minute constant current from resting membrane potential produced a ~ 12-mV depolarization generated by the persistent sodium current. At this level the cell fires in an oscillatory mode at close to 10 Hz. (Modified from Jahnsen and Llinás 1984.)

However, when depolarized, the activation of a persistent sodium conductance dominates neuronal excitability and triggers fast sodium-dependent spikes at close to 10 Hz (Fig. 2D). The point of interest here is that the switching of firing modes in thalamic neurons can trigger macroscopic changes in functional states as dramatic as the difference between somnolence and arousal (Steriade et al. 1990).

Entorhinal Stellate Cells of Layer II Subthreshold Oscillations and Theta Rhythmicity

Whereas oscillations in olivary and thalamic cells are dependent on the activation of calcium and potassium conductances, the subthreshold intrinsic oscillations in stellate cells of layer II in the entorhinal cortex (EC) are subserved by the activation of voltage-dependent sodium and potassium conductances. In these cells, in vitro membrane depolarization generates action potentials (Fig. 3A) and sustained sinusoidal-like membrane oscillations (Fig. 3B) with a dominant frequency near 8 Hz (Fig. 3B) (Alonso and Llinás 1989). These oscillations develop and reach a maximum amplitude at membrane potentials near -55 to -50 mV. Since the ionic mechanism of this oscillation involves voltage-gated sodium and potassium conductances, application of TTX to the bath totally blocks this activity (Fig. 3C). A similar result was found if extracellular sodium was replaced by choline, as well as after intracellular injection of QX314 (which blocks gNa from the inner surface of the plasmalemma). The advantage of having a slow sodium conductance—rather than the usual calcium conductance underlying these subthreshold oscillatory events—may be related to the ability to generate oscillations without triggering the biochemical cascades that accompany Ca^{++} entry (Greengard 1986). Of interest here, taking a broad perspective, is the fact that these cells are known to be the origin of the perforant path (Ramon y Cajal 1911) and to be intimately involved in the generation of the theta rhythm (Alonso and Llinás 1989).

Subthreshold Oscillation of Neocortical Interneurons at 40 Hz

Subthreshold oscillations at 30–45 Hz have been recorded from fourth-layer neocortical neurons (Fig. 4) (Llinás and Grace 1989). Intracellular staining revealed that these cells correspond anatomically to the sparsely spinous interneurons identified as being GABAergic and having axons that span from the third to the fifth cortical layers (Peters and Saint-Marie 1984). Unlike IO and thalamic neurons but similar to the entorhinal stellate cells, the ionic basis for the 40-Hz oscillation involves voltage-gated sodium and potassium conductances.

An intriguing possibility relating to the function of this oscillation in inhibitory cells is that their inhibitory potentials may induce oscillations in other cortical neurons, including pyramidal cells. Pyramidal cells, in turn, may transmit 40-Hz excitation to both the nucleus reticularis thalami, the intrinsic inhibitory neurons of the thalamus, and the projection thalamic neurons (cf. Steriade and Llináas 1988). This input would then establish a resonance state in the thalamocortical system via feedback through the fourth-layer interneurons. The combination of intrinsic oscillations and resonance in the cortico-thalamocortical circuit can thus form the basis of the 40-Hz rhythm recorded at the cortex (Llinás 1990). Although Gray et al. (1989) have not observed 40-Hz oscillation in the thalamus, Bouyer et al. (1987) have demonstrated such activity at thalamic sites. Furthermore, intracellular recordings from geniculate neurons have demonstrated that 40-Hz activity is triggered by light stimulation, although the authors, while showing the oscillations in one of their figures, failed to mention it in their paper (Fuster et al. 1965).

This 40-IIz oscillation in the thalamocortical system is intriguing in that it may serve as the nexus for the temporal correction of events that must be considered as a single motor or perceptual entity: the so-called "conjunction principle," or the "binding property" as described by Crick and Koch (this volume).

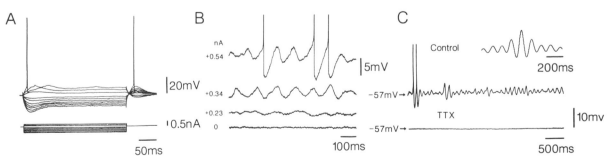

Figure 3. Electrophysiological properties of EC layer-II cells. (*A*) Intracellular current pulse injections demonstrate the presence of delayed and anomalous rectifications. Note that the membrane potential overshoots the resting potential (-64 mV) after the break of the inward current pulses. (*B*) Subthreshold voltage oscillations for three levels of constant current injection. The oscillatory activity became most apparent with current injection of $+0.34$ nA (mean membrane potential, -57 mV). (*C*) The autocorrelogram illustrates the rhythmic character of the voltage oscillation at a dominant frequency of 8 Hz. Note that this oscillatory activity was abolished by bath application of TTX (1 μM). (Modified from Alonso and Llinás 1989.)

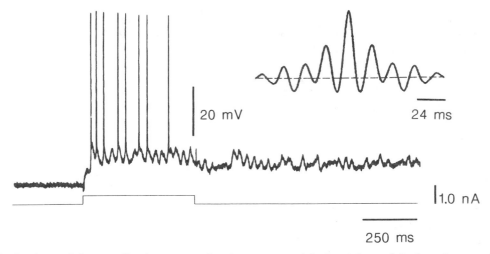

Figure 4. In vitro intracellular recording from a sparsely spinous neuron of the fourth layer of the frontal cortex of guinea pig. Shown is the characteristic response obtained in the cell following direct depolarization, consisting of a sustained subthreshold oscillatory activity on which single spikes can be observed. The intrinsic oscillatory frequency was 42 Hz, as demonstrated by the autocorrelogram shown (R. Llinás and A.A. Grace, unpubl.).

NEURONAL OSCILLATION AND SYNAPTIC PLASTICITY

So far, I have reviewed the ionic mechanisms responsible for neuronal oscillation and the possible role of this oscillation in network function. There is also the intriguing possibility that neuronal oscillation may be important in the plastic properties of neurons. Indeed, the neurons in layer II of the EC are of particular interest in this respect because they demonstrate long-

term potentiation (LTP) that seems to be controlled in a non-Hebbian manner by subthreshold oscillation.

It has been recently shown that LTP can be elicited in EC layer-II neurons by afferent stimulation as well as by direct subthreshold rhythmic depolarization (Alonso et al. 1990). Indeed, theta-pattern (Larson et al. 1986) afferent stimulation results in clear-cut LTP that is NMDA-dependent and of the Hebbian variety (Bliss and Lomo 1973).

Non-Hebbian LTP was also demonstrated in these

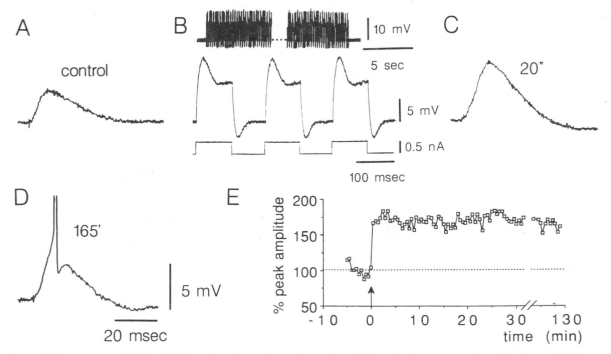

Figure 5. Time course of LTP of EPSPs induced by postsynaptic subthreshold rhythmic membrane depolarizations. (*A*) Control trace. (*B*) Postsynaptic stimulation applied at time 0. *C* and *D* were recorded at the times indicated. Note the rapid increase in the EPSP amplitude. (*E*) Peak EPSP amplitudes before and after the non-Hebbian potentiation as a function of time. (Modified from Alonso et al. 1990.)

neurons. Excitatory postsynaptic potentials (EPSPs) were evoked by white matter stimulation after intracellular conditioning stimulation (20-sec bursts of 100-msec subthreshold depolarizing current pulses delivered at 5 Hz). Intracellularly induced increases in synaptic strength, as determined by EPSP amplitude, developed within 30 seconds of the intracellular stimulation. Figure 5 illustrates this postsynaptically induced LTP. The control postsynaptic response to white matter afferent stimulation is illustrated in Figure 5A. Test white matter stimuli of the same amplitude as that eliciting the control response were delivered after the intracellular conditioning train demonstrated an enhanced EPSP amplitude (Fig. 5C) which reached firing threshold (Fig. 5D) and could be maintained for several hours (Fig. 5E). Administration of APV prior to extracellular or subthreshold direct stimulation prevented potentiation, indicating that the activation of NMDA receptors is necessary for the induction of both Hebbian and non-Hebbian LTP in the EC. Both types of LTP in EC layer-II neurons induced and expressed a selective increase in the NMDA-mediated component of the EPSP, suggesting that the enhancement of synaptic transmission during intracellular induced LTP seems to be due to purely postsynaptic factors (Alonso et al. 1990).

The finding that LTP in the EC occurs in Hebbian as well as non-Hebbian paradigms raises the question of the role of LTP in CNS function other than memory. Indeed, the fact that rhythmic conditioning stimuli induce Hebbian and non-Hebbian LTP in the same cell, utilizing the same ionic mechanisms, indicates that LTP may also serve to enhance resonance in rhythmically firing networks.

ACKNOWLEDGMENT

This research was supported by grant NS-13742 from the National Institute of Neurological and Communicative Disorders and Stroke.

REFERENCES

Alonso, A. and R. Llinás. 1989. Subthreshold Na-dependent theta-like rhythmicity in stellate cells of entorhinal cortex layer II. *Nature* 342: 175.

Alonso, A., M. deCurtis, and R. Llinás. 1990. Postsynaptic Hebbian and non-Hebbian long-term potentiation of synaptic efficacy in the entorhinal cortex in slices and in the isolated adult guinea pig brain. *Proc. Natl. Acad. Sci.* 87: 9280.

Benardo, L.S. and R.E. Foster. 1986. Oscillatory behavior in inferior olive neurons: Mechanism, modulation, cell aggregates. *Brain Res. Bull.* 17: 773.

Berger, H. 1929. Über das Elektrenkephalogramm des Menschen. *Arch. Psychiatr.* 87: 527.

Bliss, T.V. and T. Lomo. 1973. Long-lasting potentiation of synaptic transmission in the dentate area of the anesthetized rabbit following stimulation of the perforant path. *J. Physiol.* 232: 331.

Bouyer, J.J., F. Montaron, J.M. Vahneed, M.P. Albert, and A. Rougeul. 1987. Anatomical localization of cortical beta rhythms in cat. *Neuroscience* 22: 863.

Connor, J.A. and C.F. Stevens. 1971. Voltage-clamp studies of a transient outward membrane current in gastropod neural somata. *J. Physiol.* 213: 21.

Fuster, J.M., O.D. Creutzfelt, and M. Straschill. 1965. Intracellular recording of neuronal activity in the visual system. *Z. Vgl. Physiol.* 49: 605.

Gray, C.M., P. Konig, A.K. Engel, and W. Singer. 1989. Oscillatory responses in cat visual cortex exhibit intercolumnar synchronization which reflects global stimulus properties. *Nature* 338: 334.

Greengard, P. 1986. Protein phosphorylation and neuronal function. *Fidia Res. Found. Neurosci. Award Lect.* 1: 52.

Hagiwara, S., K. Kusano, and N. Saito. 1961. Membrane changes of *Onchidium* nerve cell in potassium-rich media. *J. Physiol.* 155: 470.

Jahnsen, H. and R. Llinás. 1984. Electrophysiological properties of guinea pig thalamic neurones: An *in vitro* study. *J. Physiol.* 349: 205.

Larson, J., D. Wong, and G. Lynch. 1986. Induction of synaptic potentiation in hippocampus by patterned stimulation involves two events. *Science* 232: 985.

Llinás, R. 1990. Intrinsic electrical properties of mammalian neurons and CNS function. *Fidia Res. Found. Neurosci. Award Lect.* 4: 173.

Llinás, R. and A.A. Grace. 1989. Intrinsic 40-Hz oscillatory properties of layer IV neurons in guinea pig cerebral cortex in vitro. *Soc. Neurosci. Abstr.* 15: 660.

Llinás and K. Sasaki. 1989. The functional organization of the olivocerebellar system as examined by multiple Purkinje cell recordings. *Eur. J. Neurosci.* 1: 587.

Llinás, R. and M. Sugimori. 1980. Electrophysiological properties of *in vitro* Purkinje cell somata in mammalian cerebellar slices. *J. Physiol.* 305: 171.

Llinás, R. and Y. Yarom. 1981a. Electrophysiology of mammalian inferior olivary neurones in vitro. Different types of voltage-dependent ionic conductances. *J. Physiol.* 315: 549.

———. 1981b. Properties and distribution of ionic conductances generating electroresponsiveness of mammalian inferior olivary neurones *in vitro. J. Physiol.* 315: 569.

———. 1986. Oscillatory properties of guinea pig inferior olivary neurones and their pharmacological modulation: An *in vitro* study. *J. Physiol.* 376: 163.

Peters, A. and R.L. Saint-Marie. 1984. Smooth and sparsely spinous nonpyramidal cells forming local axonal plexus. In *Cerebral cortex* (ed. A. Peters and E.G. Jones), vol. 1, p. 419. Plenum Press, New York.

Ramon y Cajal, S. 1911. *Histologie du systeme nerveux de l'homme et des vertebres*, tome 2, p. 993. Maloine, Paris.

Steriade, M. and R.R. Llinás. 1988. The functional states of the thalamus and the associated neuronal interplay. *Physiol. Rev.* 68: 649.

Steriade, M., E.G. Jones, and R.R. Llinás. 1990. *Thalamic oscillations and signalling.* Wiley, New York.

Formation of Cortical Cell Assemblies

W. SINGER, C. GRAY, A. ENGEL, P. KÖNIG, A. ARTOLA, AND S. BRÖCHER
Max Planck Institute for Brain Research, D-6000 Frankfurt/Main 71, Federal Republic of Germany

Scene Segmentation: An Early Visual Process

The retinal image of a visual scene consists of a two-dimensional, continuous distribution of gray levels. Before the visual system can identify particular figures or objects, it needs to determine which of the various luminance values belong to individual objects or to the embedding background. Some grouping has to be performed in order to associate these luminance distributions with contours, to associate particular contours with a single object, and to segregate objects with overlapping contours from each other and from the background.

Psychophysical evidence suggests as principal criteria for this grouping (1) the spatial contiguity of contours and (2) the coherence of pattern elements in particular feature domains (for review and examples, see Marr 1976, 1982; Julesz 1971; Bergen and Julesz 1983; Treisman 1980, 1986; Ramachandran 1988). The visual system interprets luminance gradients as originating from the same object or the same figure, if they are closely spaced, or continuous, or if they share similarities within particular feature domains. A particularly powerful criterion is coherence of motion. Spatially distributed contrast borders are interpreted as belonging to the same object if they move with the same speed in the same direction. The following psychophysical experiment exemplifies this. If one produces on a television display a cloud of dots of identical size and luminance that move with the same speed in randomized directions, and then suddenly makes a subset of dots move in the same direction, one perceives these dots as the outline of a figure that drifts through the cloud of randomly moving dots. Apparently, the visual system interprets dots that have a common fate, in this case the same movement vector, as belonging together and segregates the assembly of these coherently moving dots from the cloud of randomly moving dots.

To achieve this segregation, a neuronal mechanism is required which allows us (1) to compare responses of spatially distributed feature detectors and (2) to distinguish the responses to pattern elements that have certain features in common. One possibility is to have neurons that are spatially separate but prefer similar features interact with each other through selective excitatory connections. Such reciprocal connections have the effect of selectively enhancing the responses to pattern elements that have certain features in common (for further discussion of coding by cooperativity, see Julesz 1971; Marr 1982; Lehky et al., this volume).

If the cells of the assembly responding to coherent elements of a scene, however, are solely distinguished by the increased amplitudes of their responses, some ambiguities remain unresolved. Problems arise when the scene contains more than one coherent figure or when the background itself has some coherent properties, such as a regular texture. In this case, several assemblies of neurons with enhanced responses coexist, and it would become impossible to distinguish between the assemblies representing the various figures and the background. Individual figures would no longer be distinguishable. This problem has been addressed as the "superposition problem" by von der Malsburg and Schneider (1986). These authors have postulated that assemblies of neurons, representing particular relationships between the features of a figure, ought to be defined by the temporal correlation rather than by enhanced amplitudes of their responses. These authors have proposed that cell assemblies coding for different figures should be activated in alternating bursts, synchronization of the bursts being the key element in the segmentation process (see also Crick 1984; Crick and Koch, this volume). Recent simulation experiments have confirmed that this approach can in principle solve the superposition problem (von der Malsburg and Bienenstock 1986; Bienenstock and von der Malsburg 1987).

Experimental Evidence for Temporal Coding in Cell Assemblies

In recordings from the visual cortex of awake kittens, which had been implanted with multiple floating microelectrodes (Mioche and Singer 1988), we observed that neurons exhibited oscillatory responses to moving light stimuli. The rhythmic discharges were time-locked with the negative phase of an oscillatory field potential recorded simultaneously through the same electrodes. Correlation analysis revealed that these oscillations occurred in a frequency range of 40–60 Hz (Gray and Singer 1987a,b). Given the theoretical considerations summarized above, this suggested the possibility that oscillatory activity might play a role in structuring the activity of functionally coupled cell assemblies. Therefore, we sought to determine more quantitatively the stimulus dependence of this activity.

We found that even in anesthetized preparations, a large fraction of visual cortex neurons engage in oscillatory activity in a frequency range of 40–60 Hz when activated with light stimuli to which the neurons are tuned (Gray and Singer 1987a,b, 1989; Gray et al. 1990). This phenomenon is illustrated in Figure 1. Responses were recorded from an electrode capable of detecting the activity of a small cluster of neurons as well as the local extracellular field potential (LFP). When an appropriately oriented light bar passed through the receptive field, a vigorous response was recorded in both signals, which had a distinctly oscillatory character, the occurrence of spikes being phase-locked to the negative polarity of the LFP. The peak frequency of both signals, as revealed by the autocorrelogram of the spike train and the power spectrum of the LFP, could vary between trials and ranged from 35 to 45 Hz (see also Fig. 2).

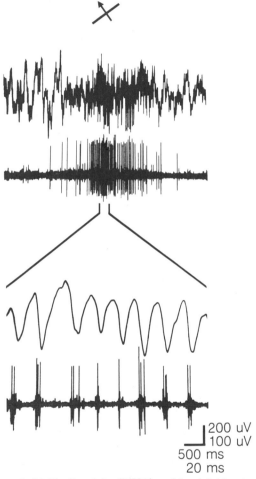

Figure 1. Multiunit activity (MUA) and local field potential (LFP) responses recorded from area 17 in an adult cat to the presentation of an optimally oriented light bar moving across the receptive field. Oscilloscope records of a single trial showing the response to the preferred direction of stimulus movement. In the upper two traces, at a slow time scale, the onset of the neuronal response is associated with an increase in high-frequency activity in the LFP. The lower two traces display the activity at the peak of the response at an expanded time scale. Note the presence of rhythmic oscillations in the LFP and MUA that are correlated in phase with the peak negativity of the LFP. Upper and lower voltage scales are for the LFP and MUA, respectively. (Reprinted, with permission, from Gray and Singer 1989.)

The large amplitude of the LFP and its close correlation with the activity of simultaneously recorded neurons suggest that a large number of closely spaced neurons are activated rhythmically and in synchrony. In many instances, the orientation tuning of the LFP was similar to that of the neurons recorded from the same electrode. This suggests that the local, synchronously active population of cells is limited roughly to the dimensions of a cortical orientation column (Gray and Singer 1989; Gray et al. 1990).

Three observations suggest that the oscillatory activity is not phase-locked to the stimulus and hence does not simply reflect the temporal structure of stimulus-driven afferent activity. First, onset latency, duration, frequency content, and amplitude of the oscillatory responses varied from trial to trial (Fig. 2). Thus, the oscillations do not reflect the temporal structure of stimulus-driven afferent activity. Second, cross-correlations of responses to identical but subsequently presented stimuli (shift predictor analysis) were flat, excluding stimulus-related phase relations. Third, there was no evidence from recordings in the lateral geniculate nucleus for stimulus-dependent oscillatory responses in the relevant frequency range (Gray and Singer 1989; Gray et al. 1990). These results indicate that the oscillatory activity is the result of dynamic interactions within the cortical network itself.

To identify the neurons participating in the generation of oscillatory responses, we recorded the activity of single units and analyzed their receptive fields. The results of these experiments revealed clear differences in the occurrence of oscillatory responses in the different classes of cortical cells (Gray et al. 1990). Roughly 40% of the complex cells showed evidence of oscillatory responses in the autocorrelograms, whereas only 10% of the simple cells exhibited rhythmic firing in the frequency range near 50 Hz. Within the complex category, the vast majority of cells having oscillatory responses were of the standard complex type, special complex cells showing little or no evidence of rhythmic firing (Gilbert 1977). The cells showing oscillatory responses were located primarily in upper (2 and 3) and lower (5 and 6) layers. These findings, however, do not exclude the likely possibility that the firing probability of nonoscillatory neurons is statistically related to the overtly oscillatory cells. In the olfactory bulb, for example, firing probability of single cells is closely related to the negativity of an oscillatory field potential, but autocorrelation of the spike trains usually fails to reveal this rhythmicity (Freeman 1975). Likely reasons for this are the brevity and the instationarity of the oscillatory responses. These make it difficult to extend autocorrelation analysis over intervals that are long enough to reveal the rhythmic changes in firing probability.

Although oscillatory responses were not phase-locked to the visual stimuli, some of their characteristics were found to be influenced by variations of stimulus parameters. The corresponding results are summarized by Gray et al. (1990). In general, those

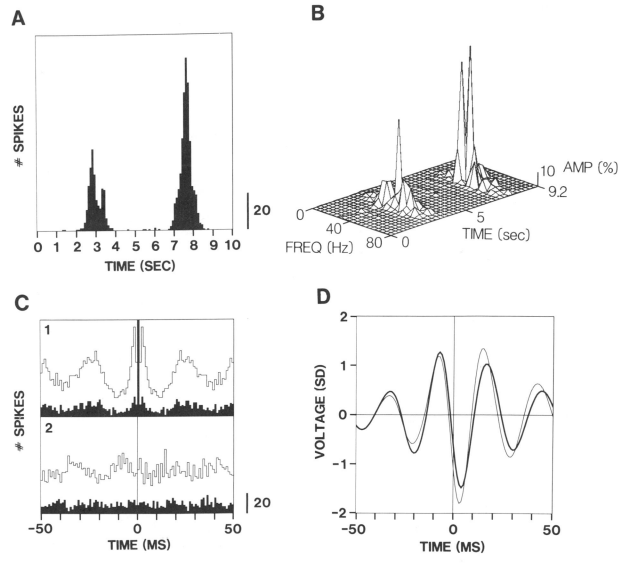

Figure 2. Temporal properties of the MUA and LFP responses recorded from area 17 in a 5-week-old kitten. (*A*) Poststimulus-time histogram of the MUA. (*B*) Distribution of the LFP amplitude vs. frequency and time on a single trial recorded from the same electrode in which the MUA was sampled. The frequency resolution is 4 Hz, and the temporal resolution is 256 msec. The amplitude scale is expressed as a fractional percentage of the peak amplitude. Examination of these plots across repeated trials revealed that the precise distribution of frequencies and amplitudes was never twice the same from one trial to the next. (*C1*) Autocorrelation functions (ACF) of the same MUA recorded in *A* displayed for both the forward (filled bars) and reverse (unfilled bars) direction of stimulus movement. Note the rhythmic firing pattern with a period length near 25 msec for both directions of stimulus movement. (*C2*) Recomputation of the ACF after shuffling the trial sequence by one stimulus period (i.e., shift predictor). This procedure demonstrated that the onset and phase of the oscillatory responses was not synchronized across trials. (*D*) Normalized spike-triggered average of the LFP for both the forward (thick line) and the reverse (thin line) directions of stimulus movement demonstrates a close correlation between the unit activity and the LFP. Results are expressed in units of standard deviation of the LFP voltage recorded during each direction of movement. (Reprinted, with permission, from Gray and Singer 1989.)

stimuli evoke optimal oscillatory responses that match best the response properties of the local group of neurons.

Intercolumnar Synchronization of Oscillatory Responses

Once it was established that oscillatory responses are a characteristic feature of stimulus-induced cortical activity, we sought to determine if there are any relation-

ships between oscillatory responses recorded from different locations within the striate cortex. As outlined above, such relationships are to be expected if the temporal structure of neuronal activity, in this case the phase of oscillatory responses, is used to establish relations between the responses of spatially distributed feature detectors. To address this problem, we recorded with arrays of 6–7 electrodes with interelectrode distances ranging from 0.4 mm to as much as 12 mm. Neurons that are separated in cortex by 0.4–2.0

942   SINGER ET AL.

mm have overlapping receptive fields and therefore can be activated together by a single moving light bar. Neurons separated by distances greater than 2.0 mm have spatially separate receptive fields and can be activated simultaneously by two independently controlled visual stimuli. We found that neurons with overlapping receptive fields, when activated by a single stimulus, synchronized their respective oscillatory responses with, on the average, no phase difference (Fig. 3). This synchronization was found to occur, with high prob-

ability, for all combinations of orientation preferences (Gray et al. 1989; Engel et al. 1990b).

We also found that oscillatory responses would synchronize across columns when the receptive fields of the recorded neurons were spatially nonoverlapping. These interactions extended to distances up to 7 mm in the cortex, and again synchronous responses showed, on the average, no phase difference. However, synchronization now depended on the spatial separation and the orientation preferences of the neurons. The

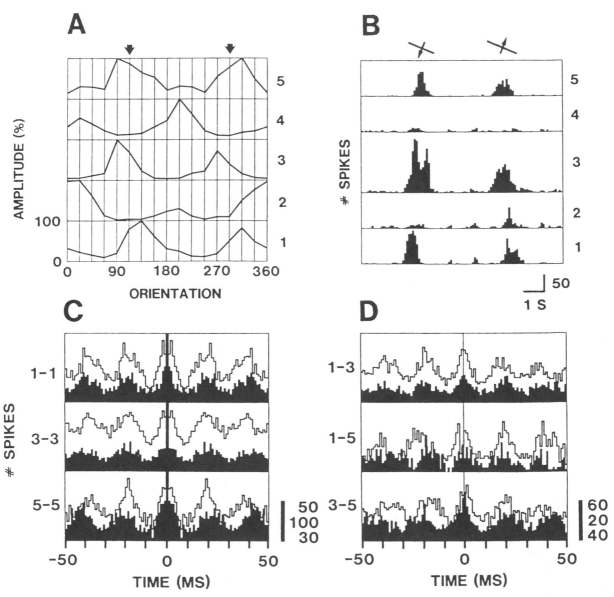

Figure 3. Orientation-specific intercolumnar synchronization of oscillatory neuronal responses in area 17 of an adult cat. (*A*) Normalized orientation tuning curves of the neuronal responses recorded from 5 electrodes spaced 400 μm apart and centered on the representation of the area centralis. Response amplitudes (ordinate) to stimuli of different orientations (abscissa) are expressed as a percentage of the maximum response for each electrode. The arrows indicate the stimulus orientation (112°) at which the responses were recorded in *B*, *C*, and *D*. (*B*) Poststimulus-time histograms recorded simultaneously from the same 5 electrodes at an orientation of 112°. Note the small difference in the latencies of the responses, indicating overlapping but slightly offset receptive field locations. (*C*) Autocorrelograms of the responses recorded at sites 1 (1-1), 3 (3-3), and 5 (5-5). (*D*) Cross-correlograms computed for the 3 possible combinations (1-3, 1-5, 3-5) between responses recorded on electrodes 1, 3, and 5. Correlograms computed for the first direction of stimulus movement are displayed with unfilled bars, with the exception of comparison 1-5 in *D*. (Reprinted, with permission, from Gray et al. 1989.)

probability of synchronization decreased with increasing distance and was higher for neurons with similar than with dissimilar orientation preference (Gray et al. 1989; Engel et al. 1990b). Moreover, synchronization of oscillatory responses tended to be more robust when the stimuli activating the respective neuron populations shared some common property. In the case of neuron groups with colinearly aligned receptive fields, the phase-locking of oscillatory responses was enhanced when contours of the same orientation were moved in the *same* direction, and it was maximal when a single, continuous contour stimulated both receptive fields simultaneously. No correlation was observed between the respective oscillatory responses when the two

groups of cells were activated with two bars moving in opposite directions over the two receptive fields (Fig. 4) (Gray et al. 1989). Thus, the degree of synchrony between the oscillatory responses reflects the coherence of the stimulus as it is perceived by a human observer. Two bars moving in counterphase are perceived as two independent stimuli; two coherently moving bars tend to be perceived as the interrupted outlines of a single moving figure; and the continuous bar is unambiguously perceived as a single figure. We consider this good correlation between the degree of synchrony of neuronal responses and perceptual coherence as compatible with the hypothesis that binding between spatially distributed features of an object may

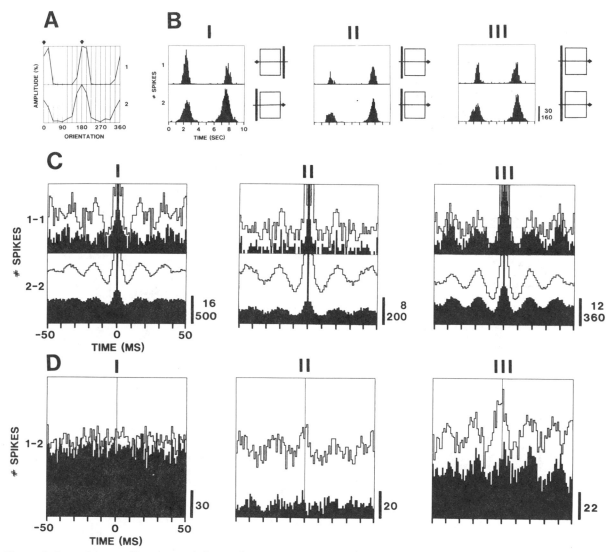

Figure 4. Long-range oscillatory correlations reflect global stimulus properties. (*A*) Orientation tuning curves of neuronal responses recorded from 2 electrodes (1,2) separated by 7 mm show a preference for vertical light bars (0 and 180°) at both recording sites. (*B*) Poststimulus-time histograms of the neuronal responses recorded at each site for each of three different stimulus conditions: (I) two light bars moved in opposite directions; (II) two light bars moved in the same direction; and (III) one long light bar moved across both receptive fields. A schematic diagram of the receptive field locations and the stimulus configuration used is displayed to the right of each poststimulus-time histogram. (*C,D*) Autocorrelograms (*C*, 1-1, 2-2) and cross-correlograms (*D*, 1-2) computed for the neuronal responses at both sites (1 and 2 in *A* and *B*) for each of the three stimulus conditions (I,II,III) displayed in *B*. For each pair of correlograms, except the two displayed in *C* (I, 1-1) and *D* (I), the second direction of stimulus movement is shown with unfilled bars. (Reprinted, with permission, from Gray et al. 1989.)

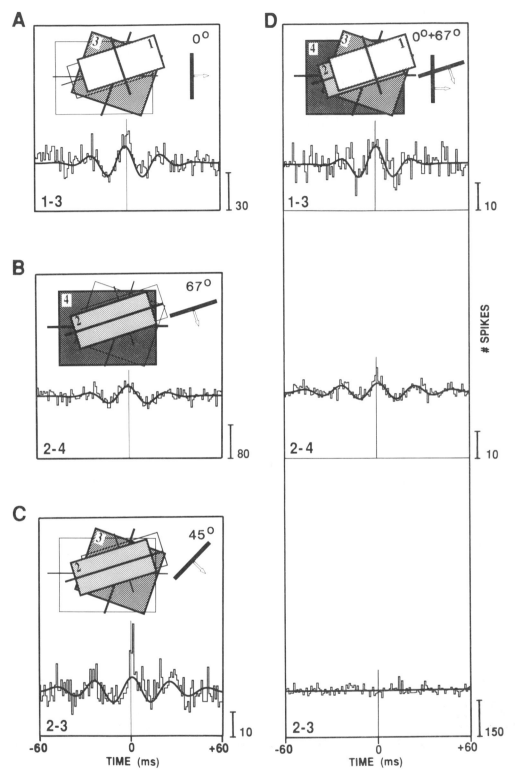

Figure 5. Effect of conflicting stimuli on the cross-columnar interaction. We recorded simultaneously from 4 different cell groups that were narrowly tuned to orientation preferences of 157° (site 1), 67° (2), 22° (3), and 90° (4), as indicated in D. The electrode separation was 400 μm. The figure compares responses to stimulation with single light bars of 0° (A), 67° (B), and 45° (C) orientation with responses to combined presentation of 0° and 67° light bars (D). For each stimulus condition, the shading of the receptive fields indicates the sites at which responses were elicited. The cross-correlation function (CCF) computed from the respective responses is shown with unfilled histogram bars. The thick continuous line represents the Gabor function, which was fitted to the correlogram. Note that the CCF of (2-3) in D does not show an oscillatory modulation, i.e., the Gabor function amplitude was not significantly different from 0. Scale bars indicate the number of spikes. (Reprinted, with permission, from Engel et al. 1990a.)

be achieved through phase-locking of oscillatory responses.

Further support for this interpretation comes from experiments in which four spatially separate clusters of cells with overlapping receptive fields were recorded simultaneously (Engel et al. 1990a). When single moving light bars were presented, those subsets became active whose orientation preferences were sufficiently similar to the orientation of the stimulus. As characteristic for cells with overlapping receptive fields, the oscillatory responses of these coactivated cells were always synchronous. When presented with two moving light bars of appropriately adjusted orientations, all four clusters could be activated simultaneously. However, in this case, response synchronization was no longer global but selective. Two synchronously oscillating cell assemblies emerged, each comprising two of the four clusters. Clusters 1 and 3 oscillated in phase and clusters 2 and 4 as well, but there was no constant phase relation between clusters 1 and 2 or 3 and 4. As indicated in Figure 5, clusters 1 and 3 had preferences that corresponded best to the vertically oriented first stimulus, whereas clusters 2 and 4 had preferences corresponding better to the second, oblique stimulus. Thus, the cell clusters had synchronized their oscillatory responses as a function of their respective affinities for either of the two stimuli. By evaluating the phase relations between the oscillatory responses of all four clusters, it is thus possible to infer that there were at least two figures; moreover, it is possible to identify the clusters associated with a particular figure. Such a coding mechanism could contribute to solving the superposition problem because it allows us to distinguish between responses originating from different but simultaneously present figures.

Interareal Synchronization

To evaluate the synchrony of neuronal responses related to a particular figure, a sampling process is required that is sensitive to temporal coincidence and capable of selecting those responses which are synchronous or coherent. Such a sampling device at higher processing levels could again consist of an assembly of distributed cells if these are able to generate oscillatory responses and to establish fixed phase relations with the oscillating assemblies at lower levels (Damasio 1989). These higher-order assemblies would thus serve as "detectors" of synchronously active lower-order assemblies. This hypothesis predicts, first, that oscillatory activity of similar frequency should occur also in other visual areas and, second, that synchronization should be possible between cells in different cortical areas.

Both predictions are supported by data. Oscillatory responses have been found in area 18 (Eckhorn et al. 1988; Gray and Singer 1989) and more recently also in the visual area of the posterior mediolateral suprasylvian sulcus (PMLS) (A. Engel et al., in prep.), a region probably specialized in the analysis of motion (Rauschecker et al. 1987). These oscillatory responses occur in the same frequency range as those in area 17 and show the same relationship between single unit activity and field potential. This suggests that the ability of local clusters of neurons to engage in rhythmic activity is a general property of cortical networks. Moreover, it was found that the oscillatory responses of neuron clusters can synchronize across different cortical areas if the clusters are activated by stimuli that have certain features in common, such as the same orientation or the same direction of motion. Such interareal synchronization has been demonstrated between areas 17 and 18 (Eckhorn et al. 1988), between area 17 and PMLS (A. Engel et al., in prep.), and even between the primary visual cortices of the two hemispheres (A. Engel et al., in prep.). Thus, available data are compatible with the view that synchronization of oscillatory responses may be used to establish relationships between responses of spatially distributed cell clusters and to distinguish functionally coherent cell assemblies by the temporal structure of their activity.

Substrate of Response Synchronization

The circuits responsible for synchronization have not been identified with certainty. The finding that synchronization occurs across the two hemispheres suggests corticocortical projections as a likely substrate. There are only a few subcortical projection systems that project bilaterally and could synchronize activity in the visual cortices of both hemispheres (Salin et al. 1989). However, most of these lack feature-selective visual input and innervate striate cortex in a rather diffuse manner (Foote and Morrison 1987). This makes it unlikely that they can mediate stimulus-specific synchronization of circumscribed cell populations. Thus, the corticocortical projections traveling through the corpus callosum appear as the most likely candidates for interhemispheric synchronization. They convey feature-selective visual responses and show topological specificity. Since the callosal projections are organized in a similar way as the ipsilateral corticocortical projections, it is conceivable that the latter also contribute to the long-range synchronization of oscillatory responses.

Another question is how synchronization is achieved. Two constraints have to be met by the synchronizing connections. First, they must not drive the cells in the target column, because, in that case, coupled cells would have multiple, spatially distributed receptive fields. Second, they have to allow for synchronization with zero phase lag and hence require a compensation mechanism for transmission delays. These problems are presently being investigated in simulation studies. Results compatible with experimental evidence have been obtained by implementing synchronizing connections that either drive inhibitory interneurons (König and Schillen 1990; Schillen 1990; Schillen and König 1990a,b) or possess nonlinear excitatory synapses that become efficient only when their respective target cells are active (Borisyuk et al. 1990).

Are Oscillatory Responses an Epiphenomenon?

The data reviewed above are compatible with the hypothesis that the synchronization of oscillatory responses is used by the nervous system to define functionally coherent cell assemblies and to encode coherence in feature space. However, it needs to be emphasized that there are other possibilities. Oscillatory responses and their synchronization could be epiphenomena of networks comprising feedback connections and could have no functional significance. Proof of the contrary will require the use of alert animals in which behavioral feedback can be utilized to examine the relationships between oscillatory activity and perceptual discrimination. However, if relevant, synchronization of oscillatory responses could also have other functions than those proposed above. Thus, it could serve to open pathways with high transmission thresholds that are only reached if large numbers of converging afferents are active simultaneously. Another possibility is that synchrony plays a role in use-dependent long-term modifications of synaptic efficacy. As discussed below, synaptic modifications have a high threshold and occur only if there is sufficient cooperativity between converging inputs. Thus, it can be predicted that synchronization of large cell assemblies is a particularly suitable condition for the induction of changes in synaptic transmission. Synchrony could therefore serve as a "now print" signal and define functional states that are sufficiently consistent to warrant storage. Moreover, because of their defined temporal structure, oscillatory responses could be important for processes relying on coincidence detection, such as Hebbian learning. If the activities that are to be compared are oscillatory, the temporal window of the Hebbian matching process is defined much more precisely than if activities lack a distinct temporal structure.

Finally, there is the possibility that oscillatory responses serve as a basis for dynamic processes in a more general sense. Coupled oscillators, even if their number is small, can engage in highly nonlinear dynamics that have a number of attractive properties (for review, see Basti and Perrone 1989; Skarda and Freeman 1987; Singer 1990b). Such nonlinear systems can assume a very large number of different quasi-stable states and are capable of very rapid state transitions. Both are considered to be important properties of neuronal networks subserving pattern recognition and pattern generation. Moreover, if cortical networks had such dynamic properties, attractive functions could be assigned to the modulatory systems that control cortical excitability (for review, see Singer 1979; Foote and Morrison 1987). In dynamic systems, the stability of individual states and the threshold for state changes do depend on the overall excitability of interacting neurons. Therefore, global modulation of excitability can serve to erase existing states, facilitate state changes, or stabilize a selected state. If one considers further that spatially and temporally structured sensory input determines the probability with which such a system stabilizes in a particular state, it becomes obvious that the dynamic properties of such a network exhibit many of the features postulated to be essential for cortical functions (see Edelman and Mountcastle 1978; Singer 1979; Crick 1984; Edelman and Finkel 1984).

Development of Selective Coupling

The results of the cross-correlation analysis have indicated that the probability of synchronization depends on the spatial separation of the neurons and on their feature selectivity. This implies that the connections responsible for synchronization need to be selective and raises the question how this selectivity is achieved during development.

To establish relationships between colinear contours, for example, selective connections must be implemented between neurons that have the same orientation preference and whose receptive fields are aligned colinearly. Because of the columnar organization of striate cortex, such neurons are distributed in spatially separate columns. Thus, it is not possible to simply connect nearest neighbors. Since the arrangement of iso-orientation domains in the striate cortex is not very regular, and in some species even shows marked anisotropies, it is also not possible to define a simple rule for these selective connections (see Fig. 6). The same holds true for connections between neurons that code for the same direction of motion or for the same color, etc. This raises the problem of how such selective connections can develop.

Selection according to functional criteria provides one solution. This is particularly attractive in the present case, since the feature detectors that must be selectively coupled can be identified with high probability on the basis of their responses. If, for example, an object moves across the visual field, movement detectors with similar preferences for speed and direction will become activated simultaneously by the moving contours of the object. The same holds true for the assembly of orientation detectors whose receptive fields are aligned colinearly if a straight contrast border is present. It would thus be sufficient to provide initially redundant sets of connections that link in an unselective way the various subpopulations of feature detectors and then to selectively stabilize connections between neurons that are often activated simultaneously. Such a process would be advantageous for two reasons. First, it would greatly economize on the genetic instructions. Second, it would assure that selective coupling is established preferentially between feature detectors whose combined properties are matched by actual and frequent feature constellations present in the physical environment.

In the following paragraph, developmental results are summarized that are compatible with the hypothesis that corticocortical connections attain some of their selectivity by a use-dependent pruning process.

One of the prominent features of cortical organization is the presence of an extremely dense network of

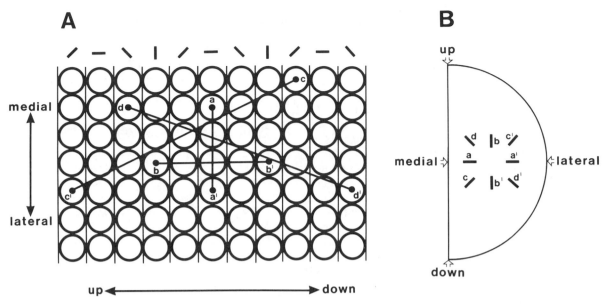

Figure 6. Schematic diagram showing the representation of retinal coordinates and iso-orientation domains in striate cortex. (*A*) Top view of the cortical sheet. Iso-orientation domains are assumed to be arranged in parallel stripes, which is an idealization of the conditions found in the cat visual cortex. (*B*) Representation of the contralateral visual field mapped onto the cortical sheet in *A*. The oriented contours *a–d* are assumed to activate the corresponding feature detectors at the appropriate locations as indicated in *A*. The connections in *A* link cell clusters activated by contours that have the same orientation and are aligned colinearly as indicated in *B*. Note that each of the combinations requires trajectories of connections of different length and direction. (Reprinted, with permission, from Singer 1990b.)

far-reaching connections that are tangential to the cortical lamination (Fisken et al. 1973; Szentagothai 1973). Electron microscopy (McGuire et al. 1985; LeVay 1988) and electrophysiological (Luhmann et al. 1990b) data indicate that these connections are excitatory, originate predominantly from pyramidal cells, and terminate on the apical dendrites of other pyramidal cells, as well as on inhibitory interneurons. These pathways are thus capable of mediating interactions between cortical neurons that are located in different columns. Furthermore, there are indications that these connections are selective (Rockland and Lund 1982; Gilbert and Wiesel 1983), linking in a reciprocal way neuron clusters that share certain functional properties, such as the same orientation preference and/or the same eye dominance (T'so et al. 1986; Gilbert and Wiesel 1989; Gray et al. 1989; but see also Matsubara et al. 1985).

Developmental studies in the cat have shown that these tangential connections essentially appear postnatally, pass through a phase of exuberant proliferation during which they are particularly numerous and far-reaching, and subsequently become pruned (Price and Blakemore 1985a,b; Callaway and Katz 1990; Luhmann et al. 1990a). This pruning occurs at a time when visual signals are readily available and appears to be influenced by retinal activity. If visual experience is unrestricted, subpopulations of these pathways are stabilized; if vision is prevented by dark-rearing or binocular deprivation, elimination of tangential connections is initially retarded (Callaway and Katz 1990) but subsequently enhanced so that eventually only a

rudimentary network of horizontal connections is maintained (Luhmann et al. 1986, 1990a).

The anatomical indications that excitatory tangential connections are initially exuberant and imprecise and assume their selectivity through pruning are supported by physiological data. In kitten visual cortex, excitatory interactions occur over much larger tangential distances, and the receptive fields of individual cortical neurons are significantly larger than in adult cats (Luhmann et al. 1990 b,c). Moreover, in kittens, about 20% of the cells have additional ectopic receptive fields, which are excitatory and can be located as far as 20° away from the center of the conventional receptive field. These ectopic fields occur mainly in cells located in supragranular layers where also tangential connections are densest and most far-reaching (Luhmann et al. 1990c; see also Singer and Tretter 1976). The laminar distribution and the numerical reduction of such cells with age correlate well with the organization and postnatal pruning of corticocortical projections, suggesting a causal relation. More direct evidence for this possibility comes from a study of kittens whose visual experience had been restricted to vertically oriented gratings of constant spatial frequency (Singer and Tretter 1976). These kittens developed neurons with ectopic receptive fields that matched precisely the orientation and spacing of the grating. Such a result is expected from selective stabilization of connections between columns that are often activated simultaneously by the regularly spaced bars of the grating.

The development of the network of intrinsic tangential connections thus resembles in a number of aspects that of the connections between the eyes and their target structures in the visual cortex (for review, see Miller et al. 1989; Singer 1990a). Both projections continue to develop postnatally and achieve topological selectivity through a pruning process. For the connections from the eyes to visual cortex, there is direct electrophysiological evidence that this pruning is guided by visual experience and leads to selective stabilization of connections conveying correlated activity. For the intracortical projection, this proof is still lacking, but there are indications that the use-dependent modifications of these pathways follow the same rules as the selection of binocular connections (see below). This predicts selective strengthening of interactions between neurons that are often activated together. Since responses of cortical neurons are feature-selective, the architecture of the selected intracortical connections is then expected to reflect the probability with which certain constellations of features have occurred during early development.

Selective stabilization of tangential intrinsic connections would thus generate a nontopographically organized map representing the coherent properties of "feature constellations" in physical reality. The principle is the same as for use-dependent pruning of binocular connections. The selective connections between the two eyes and common cortical target cells have the effect that the cortical cells become "detectors" of a particular interocular disparity. As an analogy, selective connections between distributed clusters of feature detectors with related preferences have the effect that the selectively coupled cells, as an assembly, become a detector of coherent constellations of features. Thus, by iteration of the very same processes of self-organization which, at peripheral levels of the visual system, increase the precision of topographic maps, it is possible to generate nontopographic maps that represent relations in feature space. Once such maps are established, they can be used to detect coherences among features of a visual scene and to segment the scene accordingly.

Use-dependent Modifications of Synaptic Gain in the Mature Visual Cortex

If selective interactions between spatially distributed cell groups in the visual cortex serve to establish neuronal representations of particular feature constellations, one is led to postulate that the connections responsible for these interactions preserve some malleability, even in the adult cortex. Otherwise, it would be impossible to modify through experience the criteria for the segmentation of patterns. Since growth and pruning of connections are probably restricted to development, changes of intercolumnar interactions in the adult need to involve modifications of synaptic efficacy of existing connections.

In accordance with this prediction, use-dependent long-term modifications of synaptic transmission have been observed in slices of the mature visual cortex (Artola and Singer 1987, 1990). Interestingly, the con-

ditions for the induction of synaptic modifications in the adult resemble in many respects those of the experience-dependent changes of cortical connectivity during development. In both cases, changes require the activation of NMDA-receptor-dependent conductances

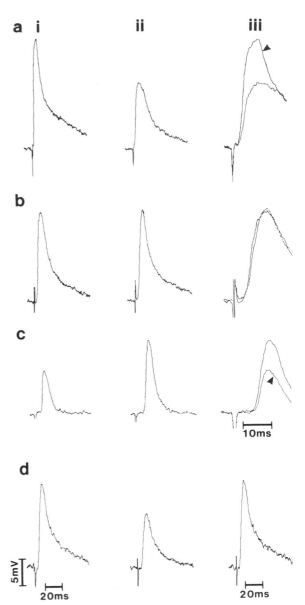

Figure 7. Effect of depolarizing and hyperpolarizing current pulses on the induction of LTD and LTP. (a–c) Averaged (n = 5, 0.03 Hz) responses to white matter stimulation recorded before (i) and 20 min after the tetanus (ii) from a cell receiving no current injection during the tetanus (a), in a cell hyperpolarized by −40 mV below V_{mr} (b), and in a cell depolarized by +20 mV above V_{mr} (c). Responses i and ii are superimposed at expanded time scale in iii. Arrows indicate the pretetanic response. d shows the induction and the reversal of LTD. First, a tetanus was applied without current injection and caused LTD (compare the control i with the posttetanic response ii). Then a second tetanus was applied in conjunction with a depolarizing current pulse, and this caused LTP of the previously depressed response resulting in a resetting of LTD (iii). V_m = −71 mV in a, −69 mV in b, −71 mV in c, and −73 mV in d. (Reprinted, with permission, from Artola et al. 1990.)

(Artola and Singer 1987, 1990; Kleinschmidt et al. 1987; Kimura et al. 1989), and modifications are facilitated by the neuromodulators noradrenaline and acetylcholine (Kasamatsu and Pettigrew 1979; Bear and Singer 1986; Greuel et al. 1988; Bröcher et al. 1989). Because in vitro the activation state of pre- and postsynaptic elements can be controlled, it has recently become possible to study directly how the synaptic gain changes depend on the activation state of pre- and postsynaptic elements. Examples of such modifications and the resulting modification rules are summarized in Figures 7 and 8. We found that there are two different

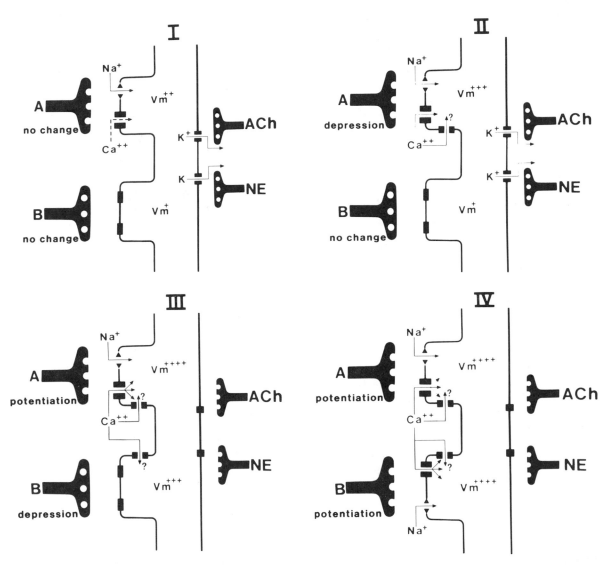

Figure 8. Schematic representation of processes likely to be involved in activity-dependent synaptic modifications in the developing and mature visual cortex. Inputs A and B correspond to two modifiable excitatory inputs. Inputs labeled ACh and NE correspond to cholinergic and noradrenergic afferents, respectively. (*I*) Input A is active while input B is inactive. Resulting depolarization is assumed to be neither sufficient to remove the Mg^{++} block of NMDA receptors at synapse A nor to reach the threshold of the homosynaptic depression mechanism. Consequently, postsynaptic activation also fails to reach the threshold for the heterosynaptic depression process. There is no change of synapses A and B. This occurs when permissive modulatory inputs are silent (Bear and Singer 1986). (*II*) Input A is active while input B is silent. Now, depolarization is assumed to be sufficient to reach the threshold for homosynaptic depression but still insufficient to cause substantial activation of NMDA-receptor-dependent Ca^{++} conductances. Consequently, the heterosynaptic depression threshold is not reached. Input A weakens while input B remains unchanged. In vivo this condition has been observed only after pharmacological manipulation of neuronal excitability. (*III*) Input A is active while input B is inactive. Now input A is assumed to cause a sufficiently strong depolarization of the membrane potential to lift the Mg^{++} block and to trigger substantial activation of the Ca^{++} conductance of the NMDA-receptor-gated channel. As a consequence, the threshold of the heterosynaptic depression mechanism is reached and synapse B weakens. The active synapse A is protected from depression because of the activation of NMDA-receptor-gated conductances at this synapse. Question marks indicate the possibility of additional activation of voltage-dependent Ca^{++} conductances. (*IV*) Afferents A and B are active simultaneously and in conjunction with permissive modulatory inputs. Inputs A and B are both assumed to cause sufficient depolarization to substantially activate the NMDA-receptor-gated conductances at their respective synapses. This protects both synapses from depression despite strong postsynaptic activation. The result is that the conjointly activated inputs A and B consolidate. (Reprinted, with permission, from Collingridge and Singer 1990.)

thresholds for synaptic modifications, both of which appear to depend on the activation state of the post-synaptic target cell. If an input fails to reach either threshold, there is no change in synaptic gain. If the first, lower threshold is reached by an active input, synaptic gain *decreases* at the activated synapses, but there is no change at other, inactive synapses. The threshold for this homosynaptic depression mechanism is lower than that of the activation threshold of NMDA-receptor-dependent conductances. Accordingly, depression occurs even if NMDA receptors are pharmacologically blocked at the active synapses. If activation increases further, a second threshold is reached, and the active input is no longer depressed but now becomes potentiated (Artola et al. 1990). This second threshold is related to NMDA-receptor-dependent conductances and cannot be reached if NMDA receptors are blocked. If this threshold is reached, however, the active input induces in addition to its own potentiation heterosynaptic depression of other inputs, i.e., other synapses on the same neuron become weakened if they are inactive. These inputs can in turn be protected from depression if they are also active and capable of activating NMDA-receptor-dependent conductances at their respective synapses. Thus, synapses capable of activating the NMDA-receptor mechanism have a double competitive advantage: First, they increase their gain and are protected against heterosynaptic depression and second, they are capable of repressing other synapses if these are not sufficiently active.

The synaptic modifications observed in the mature visual cortex have all the properties postulated for mechanisms subserving associative learning. They can mediate both Hebbian and anti-Hebbian modifications. This is compatible with recent theoretical arguments predicting use-dependent gain changes of connections between neurons in the striate cortex that follow Hebbian (von der Malsburg and Bienenstock 1986; von der Malsburg and Schneider 1986) and anti-Hebbian (Barlow and Földiák 1989) rules. At first sight, it may appear surprising that synaptic connections in a primary sensory area of adult animals remain susceptible to use-dependent changes of synaptic gain. However, if one considers the great similarities in the organization of different cortical areas, it would be equally surprising if synaptic plasticity, which is thought to be a constituent property of cortical networks, were restricted to "higher" cortical areas.

CONCLUSIONS

In conclusion, the data reviewed here are compatible with the following hypotheses:

1. It is one of the functions of primary visual cortex to evaluate relationships between spatially distributed features of a pattern.
2. These relationships are expressed by phase-locking of oscillatory responses, the ensemble of synchro-

nously oscillating cells serving as the neuronal representation of a particular constellation of features.
3. The criteria for the grouping of distributed features are set by the architecture of the synchronizing connections and by the gain of the respective synapses.
4. During development, this architecture is susceptible to experience-dependent modifications. Thus, through epigenetic shaping, the grouping criteria can be adapted to the actual requirements of the environment in which the organism happens to evolve.
5. Grouping criteria remain modifiable in the mature system but only within the constraints of the architecture of connections. These continuing modifications are realized through activity-dependent changes of synaptic gain.
6. The modification rules for changes in functional connectivity are similar in the developing and the mature system. In essence, these modifications strengthen connections between cell groups that are often active simultaneously, and they weaken interactions between cell groups that are only rarely coactivated.

In combination, these mechanisms lead to a network that is able to evaluate relationships between spatially distributed features and to create representations for particular, frequently occurring constellations of features. These representations in turn can be used for scene segmentation because they allow for the grouping that is necessary to assign signals from spatially distributed contours to particular objects, figures, and background.

ACKNOWLEDGMENTS

I thank Renate Ruhl for the artwork and Irmi Pipacs for editing the manuscript.

REFERENCES

Artola, A. and W. Singer. 1987. Long-term potentiation and NMDA receptors in rat visual cortex. *Nature* **330:** 649.
———. 1990. The involvement of N-methyl-D-aspartate receptors in induction and maintenance of long-term potentiation in rat visual cortex. *Eur. J. Neurosci.* **2:** 254.
Artola, A., S. Bröcher, and W. Singer. 1990. Different voltage-dependent thresholds for the induction of long-term depression and long-term potentiation in slices of the rat visual cortex. *Nature* (in press).
Barlow, H.B. and P. Földiák. 1989. Adaptation and decorrelation in the cortex. In *The computing neuron* (ed. C. Miall et al.), p. 54. Addison Weslay, Wokingham, England.
Basti, G. and A. Perrone. 1989. Neural networks, intentionality and some properties of non-linear dynamics. In *Proceedings of IEEE/IJCNN-89 International Joint Conference on Neural Networks.* Washington, D.C.
Bear, M.F. and W. Singer. 1986. Modulation of visual cortical plasticity by acetylcholine and noradrenaline. *Nature* **320:** 172.
Bergen, J.R. and B. Julesz. 1983. Parallel versus serial processing in rapid pattern discrimination. *Nature* **303:** 696.
Bienenstock, E. and C. von der Malsburg. 1987. A neural

network for invariant pattern recognition patterns. *Europhys. Lett.* **4:** 121.

Borisyuk, G.N., R.M. Borisyuk, and A.B. Kirillov. 1990. Modeling of oscillatory activity of neuron assemblies of the visual cortex. In *Proceedings of the IEEE/IJCNN-90 International Joint Conference on Neural Networks.* vol. 2, p. 431. (Abstr.) San Diego, California.

Bröcher, S., A. Artola, and W. Singer. 1989. Norepinephrine and acetylcholine act synergistically in facilitating LTP in the rat visual cortex. *Eur. Neurosci. Assoc. Abstr.* **21:** 18.

Callaway, E.M. and L.C. Katz. 1990. Emergence and refinement of clustered horizontal connections in cat striate cortex. *J. Neurosci.* **10:** 1134.

Collingridge, G. and W. Singer. 1990. Excitatory amino acid receptors and synaptic plasticity. *Trends Pharmcol. Sci.* **11:** 290.

Crick, F. 1984. Function of the thalamatic reticular complex: The searchlight hypothesis. *Proc. Natl. Acad. Sci.* **81:** 4586.

Damasio, A.R. 1989. The brain binds entities and events by multiregional activation from convergence zones. *Neural Computation* **1:** 123.

Eckhorn, R., R. Bauer, W. Jordan, M. Brosch, W. Kruse, M. Munk, and H.J. Reitböck. 1988. Coherent oscillations: A mechanism for feature linking in the visual cortex? *Biol. Cybern.* **60:** 121.

Edelman, G.M. and L.H. Finkel. 1984. Neuronal group selection in the cerebral cortex. In *Dynamic aspects of neocortical function.* (ed. G.M. Edelman et al.), p. 653. Wiley, New York.

Edelman, G.M. and V.B. Mountcastle. 1978. *The mindful brain: Cortical organization and the group selective theory of higher brain function.* MIT Press, Cambridge, Massachusetts.

Engel, A.K., P.König, C.M. Gray, and W. Singer. 1990a. Synchronization of oscillatory responses: A mechanism for stimulus-dependent assembly formation in cat visual cortex. In *Parallel processing in neural systems and computers* (ed. R. Eckmiller et al.), p.105. Elsevier, Amsterdam.

———. 1990b. Stimulus-dependent neuronal oscillations in cat visual cortex: Inter-columnar interaction as determined by cross-correlation analysis. *Eur. J. Neurosci.* **2:** 588.

Fisken, R.A., L.J. Garey, and T.P.S. Powell. 1973. Patterns of degeneration after intrinsic lesions of the visual cortex (area 17) of the monkey. *Brain Res.* **53:** 208.

Foote, S.L. and I.H. Morrison. 1987. Extrathalamic modulation of cortical function. *Annu. Rev. Neurosci.* **10:** 67.

Freeman, W.J. 1975. *Mass action in the nervous system.* Academic Press, New York.

Gilbert, C.D. 1977. Laminar differences in receptive field properties of cells in cat primary visual cortex. *J. Physiol.* **268:** 391.

Gilbert, C.D. and T.N. Wiesel. 1983. Clustered intrinsic connections in cat visual cortex. *J. Neurosci.* **3:** 1116.

———. 1989. Columnar specificity of intrinsic horizontal and corticocortical connections in cat visual cortex. *J. Neurosci.* **9:** 2432.

Gray, C.M. and W. Singer. 1987a. Stimulus-specific neuronal oscillations in the cat visual cortex: A cortical functional unit. *Soc. Neurosci. Abstr.* **13:** 404.3.

———. 1987b. Stimulus-dependent neuronal oscillations in the cat visual cortex area 17. *IBRO Abstr. Neurosci. Lett.* (suppl.) **22:** 1301P.

———. 1989. Stimulus-specific neuronal oscillations in orientation columns of cat visual cortex. *Proc. Natl. Acad. Sci.* **86:** 1698.

Gray, C.M., A.K. Engel, P. König, and W. Singer. 1990. Stimulus-dependent neuronal oscillations in cat visual cortex. Receptive field properties and feature dependence. *Eur. J. Neurosci.* **2:** 607.

Gray, C.M., P. König, A.K. Engel, and W. Singer. 1989. Oscillatory responses in cat visual cortex exhibit inter-

columnar synchronization which reflects global stimulus properties. *Nature* **338:** 334.

Greuel, J.M., H.J. Luhmann, and W. Singer. 1988. Pharmacological induction of use-dependent receptive field modifications in the visual cortex. *Science* **242:** 74.

Julesz, B. 1971. *Foundations of cyclopean perception.* The University of Chicago Press, Illinois.

Kasamatsu, T. and J.D. Pettigrew. 1979. Preservation of binocularity after monocular deprivation in the striate cortex of kittens treated with 6- hydroxydopamine. *J. Comp. Neurol.* **185:** 139.

Kimura, F., A. Nighigori, T. Shirokawa, and T. Tsumoto. 1989. Long-term potentiation and N-methyl-D-aspartate receptors in the visual cortex of young rats. *J. Physiol.* **414:** 125.

Kleinschmidt, A., M.F. Bear, and W. Singer. 1987. Blockade of "NMDA" receptors disrupts experience-dependent plasticity of kitten striate cortex. *Science* **238:** 355.

König, P. and T.B. Schillen. 1990. Segregation of oscillatory responses by conflicting stimuli—Desynchronizing connections in neural oscillator layers. In *Parallel processing in neural systems and computers* (ed. R. Eckmiller et al.), p.117. Elsevier, Amsterdam.

LeVay, S. 1988. Patchy intrinsic projections in visual cortex, area 18, of the cat: Morphological and immunocytochemical evidence for an excitatory function. *J. Comp. Neurol.* **269:** 265.

Luhmann, H.J., J.M. Greuel, and W. Singer. 1990a. Horizontal interactions in cat striate cortex: II. A current source-density analysis. *Eur. J. Neurosci.* **2:** 358.

———. 1990b. Horizontal interactions in cat striate cortex. III. Ectopic receptive fields and transient exuberancy of tangential connections. *Eur. J. Neurosci.* **2:** 369.

Luhmann, H.J., L. Martinez-Millan, and W. Singer. 1986. Development of horizontal intrinsic connections in cat striate cortex. *Exp. Brain Res.* **63:** 443.

Luhmann, H.J., W. Singer, and L. Martinez-Millan. 1990c. Horizontal interactions in cat striate cortex: I. Anatomical substrate and postnatal development. *Eur. J. Neurosci.* **2:** 344.

Marr, D. 1976. Early processing of visual information. *Philos. Trans. R. Soc. Lond. B Biol. Sci.* **275:** 483.

———. 1982. *Vision: A computational investigation into the human representation and processing of visual information.* Freeman, San Francisco.

Matsubara, J., M. Cynader, N.V. Swindale, and M.P. Stryker. 1985. Intrinsic projections within visual cortex: Evidence for orientation-specific local connections. *Proc. Natl. Acad. Sci.* **82:** 935.

McGuire, B.A., C.D. Gilbert, and T.N. Wiesel. 1985. Ultrastructural characterization of long-range clustered horizontal connections in monkey striate cortex. *Soc. Neurosci. Abstr.* **11:** 17.

Miller, K.D., J.B. Keller, and M.P. Stryker. 1989. Ocular dominance column development: Analysis and simulation. *Science* **245:** 605.

Mioche, L. and W. Singer. 1988. Long-term recordings and receptive field measurements from single units of the visual cortex of awake unrestrained kittens. *J. Neurosci. Methods* **26:** 83.

Price, D.J. and C. Blakemore. 1985a. The postnatal development of the association projection from visual cortical area 17 to area 18 in the cat. *J. Neurosci.* **5:** 2443.

———. 1985b. Regressive events in the postnatal development of association projections in the visual cortex. *Nature* **316:** 721.

Ramachandran, V.S. 1988. Perception of shape from shading. *Nature* **331:** 163.

Rauschecker, J.P., M.W. von Grünau, and C. Poulin. 1987. Centrifugal organization of direction preferences in the cat lateral suprasylvian visual cortex and its relation to flow field processing. *J. Neurosci.* **7:** 943.

Rockland, K.S. and J.S. Lund. 1982. Widespread periodic intrinsic connections in the tree shrew visual cortex. *Science* **215:** 1532.

Salin, P.A., J. Bullier, and H. Kennedy. 1989. Convergence and divergence in the afferent projections to cat area 17. *J. Comp. Neurol.* **283:** 486.

Schillen, T.B. 1990. Simulation of delayed oscillators with the *mens* general purpose modelling environment for network systems. In *Parallel processing in neural systems and computers* (ed. R. Eckmiller et al.). p. 135. Elsevier, Amsterdam.

Schillen, T.B. and P. König. 1990a. Coherency detection by coupled oscillatory responses—Synchronizing connections in neural oscillator layers. In *Parallel processing in neural systems and computers* (ed. R. Eckmiller et al.), p. 139. Elsevier, Amsterdam.

————. 1990b. Coherency detection and response segregation by synchronizing and desynchronizing delay connections in a neuronal oscillator model. In *Proceedings of the IEEE/IJCNN-90 International Joint Conference on Neural Networks*, vol. 2, p. 387. (Abstr.) San Diego, California.

Singer, W. 1979. Central-core control of visual cortex functions. In *The neurosciences, fourth study program* (ed. F.O. Schmitt and F.G. Worden), p. 1093. MIT Press, Cambridge, Massachusetts.

————. 1990a. Ontogenetic self-organization and learning. In *Brain organization and memory: Cells, systems and circuits*

(ed. J.L. McGaugh et al.), p. 211. Oxford University Press, New York.

————. 1990b. Search for coherence: A basic principle of cortical self-organization. *Concepts Neurosci.* **1:** 1.

Singer, W. and F. Tretter. 1976. Unusually large receptive fields in cats with restricted visual experience. *Exp. Brain Res.* **26:** 171.

Skarda, C. and W.J. Freeman. 1987. How brains make chaos in order to make sense of the world. *Behav. Brain Sci.* **10:** 161.

Szentagothai, J. 1973. Synaptology of the visual cortex. In *Handbook of sensory physiology* (ed. R. Jung), p. 269. Springer Verlag, Berlin.

Treisman, A.M. 1980. A feature-integration theory of attention. *Cognit. Psychol.* **12:** 97.

————. 1986. Properties, parts and objects. In *Handbook of perception and human performances* (ed. K. Boff et al.), p. 1. Wiley, New York.

Ts'o, D.Y., C.D. Gilbert, and T.N. Wiesel. 1986. Relationship between horizontal interactions and functional architecture in cat striate cortex as revealed by cross-correlation analysis. *J. Neurosci.* **6:** 1160.

von der Malsburg, C. and E. Bienenstock. 1986. A neural network for the retrieval of superimposed connection patterns. *Europhys. Lett.* **3:** 1243.

von der Malsburg, C. and W. Schneider. 1986. A neural cocktail-party processor. *Biol. Cybern.* **54:** 29.

Some Reflections on Visual Awareness

F. CRICK* AND C. KOCH†

*The Salk Institute, La Jolla, California 92037; †Computation and Neural Systems Program, 216-76,
California Institute of Technology, Pasadena, California 91125

We have recently published a paper entitled *Towards a Neurobiological Theory of Consciousness* (Crick and Koch 1990) that outlined a sketch of such a theory. Our aim was not to produce as complete a theory of consciousness as possible but to indicate promising lines of experimental work, mainly neurobiological, that might lead eventually toward a solution of the problem. We made the plausible assumption that all forms of consciousness (e.g., seeing, thinking, and pain) employ, at bottom, rather similar mechanisms and that if one form were understood, it would be much easier to tackle the others. We then made the personal choice of the mammalian visual system as the most promising one for an experimental attack.

This choice means that fascinating aspects of the subject, such as volition, intentionality, and self-consciousness, to say nothing of the problem of qualia, have had to be left on one side. We have also not dwelt on unusual psychological states, such as hypnosis, dreaming, lucid dreaming, and sleepwalking, to say nothing of meditative states, since we do not see any special advantage in studying them experimentally at this stage.

Our method is to combine what is known experimentally from both psychological and neurobiological experiments with plausible theoretical arguments of a general nature. We have not so far attempted detailed computer simulations, since it is unlikely that we understand the details of the system well enough for such modeling to provide decisive answers. In the long run, however, modeling is essential, and even at this stage, well-conceived computer simulations should suggest plausible general principles and thus guide the experimental attack on what is obviously a system of enormous complexity and subtlety.

In our previous paper (Crick and Koch 1990), we listed a number of topics and assumptions that we did not intend to discuss. This list will not be repeated here in toto except to say that we have assumed the higher mammals have a form of visual awareness fairly similar to ours, so that we can, with discretion, combine experimental results on humans with those from monkeys, cats, and so on.

THE THEORY IN OUTLINE

Our knowledge of the visual system of the macaque monkey, which is probably fairly similar to that of humans, suggests that there is no single place in the brain that corresponds to what we see. (For a detailed description of the macaque visual system, see Van Essen et al., this volume, and for the human visual system, see Zeki, this volume.) Thus, some mechanism must unite some of the neural activity in the many different visual areas to provide our global percept of the scene before us.

The problem of how to do this is sometimes referred to as the "binding problem." We distinguish three sorts of binding. The first is built in by genes acting on the developmental processes. The second is built up by experience, probably by strengthening existing but weak connections. An example might be neurons that respond to a familiar word. The third—the ad hoc binding problem—is what concerns us here. It is needed because the number of conceivable visual objects is so vast that there cannot be a special neuron (a "grandmother cell") for each one of them.

It is suggested that this binding is done mainly by the synchronized firing of the relevant neurons (as proposed by von der Malsburg and Schneider in 1986) and that such synchronized firing usually takes the form of semisynchronous oscillations in the 40–70-Hz range, sometimes called γ oscillations. (For a review of much of the recent experimental work on the "40 Hz" oscillations, see Singer et al., this volume.)

Psychological experiments show that we do not see everything in the visual scene at once. There appears to be a rapid, parallel process of handling the incoming visual information, followed by a further process that takes time and thus can be roughly described as "serial." This latter process is often referred to as "focal attention." It can happen to some extent without eye movements, as shown by Posner (1986), and is probably more rapid than eye movements, themselves another, slower, form of visual attention.

Whereas the initial, parallel, processing steps deal with the many "features" already encoded in the brain, we surmise that the steps involving focal attention serve temporarily to bind features that are not already coded there by fairly strong connections.

It has been suggested for many years that an essential feature of visual awareness is the temporary storage of what we have just seen in short-term memory (often called working memory) that decays within a few seconds. It is thought to have a somewhat limited capacity at any one moment, probably in the range of four to seven objects.

The deciphering by the brain of the visual scene before us is not an easy task, since in mathematical terms the problem is "ill-posed" (Poggio et al. 1985); that is, the information coming into our eyes is often ambiguous and can only be interpreted by using "constraints" built into the system by epigenetic processes and by previous experience. What needs to enter awareness is the result of these "computations," not the details of the computations themselves. We therefore suggest:

1. It is the result of these neural computations on an attended object that are expressed by phase-locked 40-Hz oscillations.
2. These phase-locked oscillations are the neural correlate of vivid visual awareness.
3. These oscillations then activate working memory.

These are our basic hypotheses. We also suggest very tentatively that there might be an even more transient form of awareness, linked to iconic memory, which we called "fleeting awareness." This is probably not associated with oscillatory firing patterns. Since this appears very difficult to study, we shall say no more about it here.

The reader is referred to our earlier paper (Crick and Koch 1990) both for a much fuller discussion of the rationale for these suggestions and for more extensive references. Our main object here is to build on that previous discussion in order to fill out some of these theoretical ideas. Our suggestions mostly concern ideas and phenomena that need to be studied, rather than being detailed proposals. We shall say little here about possible experimental tests, some of which are sketched in the earlier paper. We shall assume, without further discussion, that the 40-Hz oscillations are not an artifact and do indeed play the role we hypothesize for them. This assumption is far from being firmly established experimentally.

OSCILLATIONS

The Nature of Oscillations

The neurons involved do not strictly oscillate at 40 Hz. By "oscillate" we mean that when a neuron fires at 40 Hz, it does so at approximately 25-msec intervals. "Firing" here implies that the neuron produces an axonal spike, or sometimes two or three in very rapid succession. Sometimes a neuron may miss the opportunity to fire, but when it does fire it does so approximately "on the beat." The frequency at any one time is not especially regular. The mean frequency may vary somewhat with time and may vary also from neuron to neuron unless their phases have become locked together. At other times, such neurons may not oscillate but fire in a desynchronized manner. (For further details, see Singer et al., this volume.)

We shall assume, without further discussion, that certain neurons in the cerebral cortex (and perhaps elsewhere) have an inherent tendency to fire at about 40 Hz in the sense described above. This may be due to their intrinsic properties (as suggested by Llinás, this volume) or to circuit properties or, more likely, to both together. For example, a time delay of about 7–13 msec in the production of a short burst of inhibition might help to promote oscillations in the 40–70-Hz range.

The Number of Oscillations

How many distinct oscillations can exist in the brain at any one moment? This is a difficult question. It is unlikely to be only one, since there would then be little point in having oscillations. For instance, the activity leading to awareness need only be the "best" set of neurons, all firing very strongly together, say at 400 Hz, and no oscillations would be required. One of the advantages of having oscillations is that more than one coherent set of neurons can be active at any one moment without interfering too much with each other.

Moreover, it is an obvious advantage to maintain the representations of several objects simultaneously, since then further processing on this group of objects can proceed more rapidly and more efficaciously. This may be especially important for language, and for handling ideas in general.

Two different oscillations may have the same frequency but different phases. If these oscillations spread so that they overlap, they are likely either to cancel each other out in the overlap region or to coalesce to form one single set of oscillations of the same phase over the whole region. Oscillations of different frequencies may be able to interpenetrate more easily, but how much they will interfere with each other remains to be seen, since the system is probably highly nonlinear. It is by no means clear, on theoretical grounds, how many oscillations can exist together without significant interference. It may depend somewhat on whether they largely overlap in certain brain areas or whether, on the other hand, they dominate rather separate brain regions. An educated guess (meaning a guess with no sound theoretical foundations) might be four in the first case (heavy overlap) and up to seven or so in the second (little overlap).

It seems highly plausible that these restrictions on the maximum number of simultaneous oscillations are the main causes of the well-known limitations on the capacity, at any one moment, of the attentional or memory mechanism (for a somewhat different viewpoint, see Allport 1989).

It will thus be important, as more facts become known, to describe for a variety of cases the time of buildup of one set of oscillating neurons, the time between establishing one oscillatory set and establishing the next one, the length of time for which any one of them persists, and thus the number active at any particular moment. In interpreting the psychological data, it will be important to know whether an oscillatory set persists without interruption or whether it has lapsed but been recalled by a rapid readdressing system.

The Buildup of Oscillations

How easy is it for oscillations to build up and phase-lock? It is plausible to assume that for a simple, straightforward object, the time is likely to be shorter than for a more complex, ambiguous one. If there are several possible interpretations of the incoming information, it may take some time for the one particular interpretation to dominate its rivals and establish itself. In the case of "rivalry," when the percepts alternate, as in the well-known case of the Necker cube, we assume that the oscillations that first became established eventually habituate somewhat so that the other interpretation gets the upper hand by establishing the oscillations relevant to it and, in doing so, pushes down its rival. After a delay, it is then itself pushed down, and so on.

For complex objects, there is likely to be a constant struggle between rival sets of oscillations (strictly, between rival sets of neurons each trying to establish a coherent set of oscillations), except in very straightforward cases when one set of neurons is so dominant that it captures the oscillations without any significant challenge from other sets. The set of neurons that establishes strongly developed oscillations corresponds to those that embody the best interpretation of relevant parts of the visual scene, taking account of all the various mutual excitatory and inhibitory contacts already established by previous experience. We do not discuss at all any of the neural computations that underlie finding this best interpretation, that is, the visual algorithms computing the optical flow field, structure-from-motion, etc.

In all this, we have assumed that there will be competition between different sets of neurons, all attempting to set up coalitions to support each other's oscillations. Exactly how this is done is a very complicated matter that we shall not discuss here.

Oscillations and Awareness

It should not be assumed that all neurons showing some degree of 40-Hz oscillations in their autocorrelograms, or even sets of neurons showing some degree of phase-locking (see Singer et al., this volume), are the neural correlates of visual awareness. They may represent phases in the struggle to establish a coherent set of oscillations. This may be especially true in lightly anesthetized cats whose exact state of awareness we can only guess at.

What kind of oscillation corresponds, then, to full perceptual awareness? Two extreme views are possible. In the first view, visual awareness would require phase-locked sets of only very strong oscillations. (Strong here means that the peaks of the autocorrelation function are high and the troughs low.) Individual neurons of this type are occasionally seen among the oscillating neurons studied experimentally (Engel et al. 1990; Gray et al. 1990). In the second view, it could be argued that even for a fully established percept, the strengths of the oscillations needed are more distributed so that oscillations of various strengths contribute, since in this way more information might be conveyed. In both these cases, we lack any secure data on the fraction of cortical neurons, in one cortical region, that need to oscillate to produce full visual awareness. A different experimental approach suggests that the fraction of active neurons to lead to visual awareness may be quite small (see Newsome et al., this volume). Interpretation of the experimental results would be simpler if the first alternative were true, but the second sounds almost equally plausible.

The Importance of Short Chains

At what levels in the visual system do neurons interact to build up these phase-locked oscillations? We shall argue that a general principle may be involved. Rather simple simulations (Kammen et al. 1989) suggest that it is difficult to phase-lock oscillations quickly between two neurons or groups of neurons if they are not fairly directly connected but instead have many distinct neurons in the shortest chain connecting them. We believe that there has been intense evolutionary pressure for mechanisms that can build up coherent sets of oscillations as quickly as possible. Thus, as a general principle, we suggest that all pathways that help to synchronize oscillations will turn out to have as few intervening neurons as possible.

Since the coalitions that form are likely to involve interactions both locally and globally, we suggest that these synchronizing pathways will occur at many levels in the system. In particular, we expect such connections to occur within a cortical area, both at short distances (under 0.5 mm) and to some extent up to longer distances (a few mm) and also between different cortical areas, and especially between areas connected at adjacent levels in the hierarchy. This may well involve some of the so-called "back" pathways (see Van Essen et al., this volume). In addition, we think there will likely be pathways that help to synchronize whole sets of cortical areas. Obvious places to look for such pathways are the thalamus (Jones 1985) and the claustrum (Sherk 1986).

Because of our general principle, we suspect that more indirect pathways, for example, from cortical areas high in the Van Essen hierarchy to those much lower down, will be less useful for this purpose, unless there are fairly direct connections between them.

A general theoretical problem of considerable interest is the design of efficient systems that can quickly set up phase-locked oscillations. We strongly suspect that the design would be hierarchical, with feedback pathways that spread somewhat, together with some semi-global and global pathways. Although the detailed design would obviously depend on the problems any particular system has to solve, there may be theoretical arguments that favor certain styles of design. Whether this is true remains to be seen.

The Problem of Time Delays

In considering mechanisms for phase-locking, it is of the first importance to allow for the inevitable time delays in the pathways. Already simple simulations (Kammen et al. 1989; Sporns et al. 1989) have shown that delays in excitation of more than a quarter of a cycle make phase-locking difficult, although presumably delays of a full cycle will work. Of course, if a synchronizing pathway produces inhibition, time delays of about half a cycle between onset of excitation and onset of inhibition would be expected.

An interesting possibility is that the neurons with an inherent tendency to oscillate at about 40 Hz are mainly some of the inhibitory neurons, as indeed Llinás's results suggest (see Llinás, this volume). Inhibitory neurons in the cortex only project locally (i.e., within a single cortical area). Thus, if they sometimes oscillate in error, these errors will at first be fairly local. It may be that what mainly matters for perception is oscillations in sets of pyramidal cells (all of which are excitatory), since pyramidal cells usually project over long distances, both to other cortical areas and subcortically.

Delays in transmission down dendrites might in some cases produce unacceptably long delays for synchronization purposes. Most inhibitory neurons have many excitatory synapses on their somas, whereas excitatory neurons (such as pyramidal cells) have none, the synapses on their somas being almost entirely inhibitory (for review, see Crick and Asanuma 1986). Thus the circuit:

excitation → activation of → inhibition of a
                   inhibitory cell   pyramidal cell

can be a fast one, since it may not be subject to the delays of dendritic transmission.

For this reason, we expect that such "somatic" circuits will be used for fast processes, such as those needed to phase-lock 40-Hz oscillations. The main function of certain types of inhibitory cells (e.g., basket cells) may be to generate and phase-lock 40-Hz oscillations, even though the expression of these oscillations is mainly required in appropriate sets of pyramidal cells. This is, of course, quite distinct from the more traditional role of subtraction or vetoing assigned to them.

That inhibitory cells may be able to help the phase-locking of oscillations is suggested by the quite independent work of W.W. Lytton and T.J. Sejnowski (in prep.). By detailed modeling of the various ion currents, etc., they have shown how inhibitory cells, such as basket cells and chandelier cells, could help entrain an existing 40-Hz oscillation in a pyramidal cell, partly via a mechanism related to "anodal break excitation."

A set of coherent oscillations may not always build up in the same way, i.e., always starting in the same visual area. It seems more likely that in many cases, one cortical region will set up a strong coalition very rapidly and that the effects of this powerful alliance will then spread to other cortical areas where they can assist further coherent additions to the coalition. Sudden transitions from nonoscillating to oscillating behavior may sometimes be due to such effects.

Oscillations and Gestalt

The roles we are suggesting for the 40-Hz oscillations bring to mind some of the ideas of the Gestalt psychologists. What we have referred to as an object would be better termed a "gestalt." A transient coalition of neurons, all expressing the phase-locked oscillations, is probably built up by neuronal interactions that correspond somewhat to the "laws" of gestalt psychology, such as proximity, continuity of direction, common fate, good continuation, and even symmetry. What to a psychologist is a particular gestalt would, to the neuroscientist, be expressed by a particular set of phase-locked oscillating neurons. Today, these laws are interpreted within the current computational vision framework as constraints needed to arrive at a unique perceptual solution (Poggio et al. 1985).

A psychologist might complain that this reformulation does nothing more than define the problems confronting him in other terms, and moreover, in terms he is not certain how to manipulate. This is true, but this disadvantage is quite outweighed by the advantage of being able to tie cognitive ideas to neuronal behavior, so that several distinct types of experimental evidence can be brought to bear on the same problem. If the brain does in fact behave in the way we are suggesting, then explanations at the psychological level will have to be recast in terms that more closely correspond to the underlying neurobiological reality.

ATTENTION

The idea that attention and consciousness are closely connected dates back to the last century. It is impossible here to give a detailed review of all the current theories of visual attention, if only for limitations of space. Instead, we shall try to organize the various ideas into broad classes. Because of the complexity of the subject, both psychologically and neurobiologically, our discussion must be regarded as preliminary.

Almost all the psychologists involved have accepted that in vision there is an early, rapid, highly parallel process, followed by a slower one that usually takes longer and is often considered to be serial.

We shall deal only briefly with the early phase, often associated with iconic memory (Coltheart 1983). This memory is thought to have a large capacity but to be transient, with decay times in the range of a fraction of a second. All workers have considered it to contain visual "features," but some have emphasized simple features, such as orientation or color, whereas others have argued that it also contains more elaborate features, such as letters, numerals, and familiar words (see the discussion in the earlier parts of Allport 1989). In our terms, anything that has been already "built in" (and thus does not need the 40-Hz oscillations to relate its features) is likely to be processed in parallel, often rather rapidly, and to a high level in the system unless this early processing produces conflicts in interpretation. By a high level, we mean a level at which the neurons respond to such things as familiar words or faces.

This early phase is often called "preattentive." In some psychological models (Treisman 1988), an object can "pop out" into awareness by the parallel process alone. In others (Koch and Ullman 1985; Duncan and Humphreys 1989; Cave and Wolfe 1990), it needs the serial stage for this. Pop-out in these latter models is then the first, rapid step of the serial process.

Iconic memory may involve rapid synaptic modification (see Crick and Koch 1990); but whether it does or not, we believe that it will always involve the continued firing of the relevant neurons. How this firing is maintained is not yet understood. It may be due to processes inherent in the neurons themselves, but it seems likely that it will also involve reverbatory circuits of neurons of some sort or another.

Is There a Saliency Map?

The later, more serial stage has been explained by psychologists and theoreticians in several ways (Koch and Ullman 1985; Treisman 1988; Duncan and Humphreys 1989; Cave and Wolfe 1990; Van Essen and Anderson 1990). One of the main differences between these theories is whether a topographical saliency map exists or not. The basic idea of a saliency map (Koch and Ullman 1985) is that various visual areas send retinotopically mapped signals to a distinct area of the brain. This area does not code information on *what* it is that is salient but only *where* it is. Saliency is here meant to be understood in terms of simple operations, implemented by center-surround types of operations, e.g., a green object among many red ones or a moving stimulus among a stationary scene would both be very salient objects. In some versions, this area then selects, by some kind of winner-take-all mechanism (with or without noise in it), the most salient region in the visual field and directs attention to it. This attention can take the form either of boosting the firing of the neurons in that region of the visual field (for all retinotopically mapped areas) or of damping down the firing of regions outside the attentional spotlight, or both. There is neurophysiological evidence for both these effects in the region V4 of macaque monkeys (Moran and Desimone 1985; Spitzer et al. 1988).

From our point of view, we want the attentional mechanism to boost the appropriate 40-Hz oscillations in that region of the visual field. On the other hand, others (Duncan and Humphreys 1989) have argued that no saliency map is needed and that the struggle for saliency takes place in the cortical areas themselves. In our terminology, the struggle to establish the best set of

40-Hz oscillations would take place all over the visual cortex.

The Spotlight and the Oscillations

Let us consider three broad alternatives. In each case, there is first a highly parallel feature stage, either in the broad or the narrow sense of feature. We shall assume that in all three models, sets of 40-Hz oscillations compete with each other to some extent. In the models A and B, the spotlight promotes activity in the region of its beam and/or inhibits activity in the surroundings of the beam.

A. The 40-Hz oscillations only start in the neurons related to an object when some form of spotlight lights them up. When the oscillations are set up, they can continue (for a time) while the spotlight lights up the neurons representing the next most salient object. There is a saliency mechanism to control the spotlight.

B. The 40-Hz oscillations start up everywhere, as best they can. A spotlight (controlled by a crude saliency map) picks out the representations of the most salient item in several cortical areas and boosts them. When those oscillations are established they can continue, but the spotlight moves on to help the neurons corresponding to the next most salient item.

C. There is no saliency map, with its associated spotlight. The 40-Hz oscillations all start together, but the competition is such that the best set of oscillations wins, although it does not suppress the others entirely (they simply grow more slowly). After a time, this first one "fatigues" while others press forward to become the most favored one(s).

Thus, in model C, there is no separate attentional mechanism, but rather competition between sets of 40-Hz oscillations (P. Braam, pers. comm.).

It may not be easy to decide definitely, by psychophysical experiments alone, whether a separate saliency map exists or not. We are inclined to favor the view that it does, for the reason that it is difficult enough to establish quickly the oscillation of the best set of neurons for even a single object within the visual field (including solving the so-called figure-ground problem) without requiring this complex mechanism to cope by itself with competition between objects. Since the exact order of processing objects may only matter in extreme cases, it seems better to let the order in which objects are processed be decided by a much cruder and faster mechanism. At the moment, model B above seems the most attractive.

Where Is the Saliency Map?

A saliency map for eye movements is known to exist in the superior colliculus of mammals. It would not be surprising if it were used by the brain to help decide the saliency needed for the faster attentional system. Since the colliculus projects to the pulvinar, and since experimental evidence points to the thalamus, and the pulvinar in particular (see Desimone et al., this volume), as involved in attention, the pulvinar seems a promising place to look for saliency maps. The thalamic reticular nucleus may also be involved (Rafal and Posner 1987), although probably not exactly in the way previously suggested by one of us (Crick 1984), since that particular mechanism is now believed to occur only in slow-wave sleep (Steriade et al. 1990). There is also experimental evidence that the posterior parietal region is involved (Posner et al. 1987). Whatever its location, the attentional system must have access—in one way or another—to information from both cerebral hemispheres.

Since the thalamus has many distinct areas, including several visual ones, it would not be surprising if many of them were associated with one or another form of attention (see Allport 1989), so that even for vision, the single-map mechanism sketched above may well be too simple.

The Preattentive Stage

It is well established that the brain can process external stimuli, even to the point of initiating behavior, without consciously perceiving them. Such nonconscious, unconscious, or subconscious processes include blindsight, priming, implicit memory, subliminal perception, and automatic processes (Holender 1986; Kihlstrom 1987). For instance, patients with prosopagnosia, an inability to recognize familiar faces, show significant electrodermal skin conductance responses to pictures of persons they had previously known but were now unable to recognize, at the same time failing to show such an autonomic response to unfamiliar faces (Tranel and Damasio 1985).

We postulate that in these cases, the relevant stimuli give rise to strong firing responses in the associated cortical areas, without leading to phase-locked 40-Hz oscillations. Since it lacks the 40-Hz oscillations, this neuronal activity will not stimulate short-term memory and produce awareness. Nevertheless, this nonoscillatory (or weakly oscillatory) activity may be sufficient to leave a forward-reaching trace of the sort seen in priming and implicit memory (Tulving and Schacter 1990), perhaps partly by a non-Hebbian mechanism of synaptic modification. This possibly non-Hebbian mechanism is described more fully in our earlier paper (Crick and Koch 1990).

We can now suggest why some workers emphasize primitive features for the early visual stage, whereas others emphasize more complex features, such as familiar letters. The neurons that respond to the simpler features, being mapped retinotopically, may be the main ones that feed into the saliency map. Neuronal activity, as we have suggested, may very quickly reach the neurons in higher cortical areas that respond to more complex features, but because these features are probably not mapped retinotopically, their activity will not feed into the retinotopic saliency map. The activity of these complex feature-detectors will not reach awareness unless there is time and sufficient saliency for them to build up phase-locked 40-Hz oscillations.

NEUROPHYSIOLOGICAL EXPERIMENTS

Since the pioneer studies of Mountcastle et al. (1981), there have been a number of demonstrations that for an alert monkey the response of certain neurons depends on whether the monkey is attending or not. Some of these experiments are mentioned in the review by Wise and Desimone (1988). Here, we concentrate on a set of experiments by Moran and Desimone (1985), since these show that the idea of a simple spotlight of attention is inadequate. In their review Wise and Desimone state: (our italics)

Neurons in area V4 ... have receptive fields so large that many stimuli typically fall within them. One might expect that the responses of such cells would reflect the properties of *all* stimuli inside their receptive fields. However it has been found that when a monkey restricts its attention to *one* location within a V4 ... cell's receptive field, the response of the cell is determined primarily by the stimulus at the attended location, *almost as if the receptive field "shrinks" around the attended stimulus.* For example, consider a cell that responds strongly to red stimuli and not to green when only a single stimulus appears inside its receptive field [see Fig. 1]. If red and green stimuli appear simultaneously at different locations within the field, and the animal focuses its attention on only the red one, the cell will respond strongly [Fig. 1A]. If, however, the animal attends to only the green stimulus, the cell will respond weakly or not at all to the red stimulus [Fig. 1B], even though the red stimulus is still inside the receptive field and the retinal stimulation is identical to the previous condition.

So far, these results could be explained by a small spotlight of attention, surrounded by a larger suppressive penumbra at a lower level in the visual hierarchy, since this suppression could account for the V4 neuron's poor response in Figure 1B (other neurons in V4 are presumed to respond to the green stimulus).

The next experiment shows that this explanation is too simple. In the case illustrated in Figure 1C, Moran and Desimone (1985) kept the two stimuli the same distance apart, but placed the attended green one outside the receptive field, while the unattended red one remained in its place within the receptive field. The neuron's response was not reduced, as it was in Figure 1B, but remained strong as shown in Figure 1C (for a further description of these experiments, together with those on IT [inferotemporal] neurons, see Moran and Desimone [1985]).

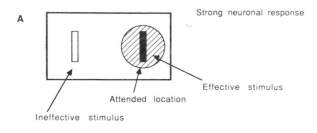

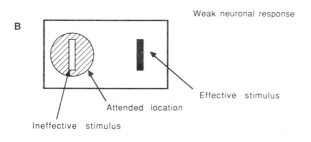

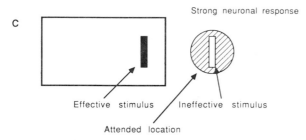

Figure 1. Simple diagrams to illustrate Moran and Desimone's (1985) results for one particular neuron in V4. The rectangle shows the receptive field of this neuron. The alert trained monkey fixated a point outside this field. This particular neuron responded only to red bars (shown black here) and not to green bars (shown open here). Thus, a red bar was an effective stimulus: a green bar an ineffective stimulus. For each trial the monkey was trained to pay attention (while maintaining fixation) to one particular place in the visual field, symbolized here by the circle, representing the hypothetical spotlight of attention. Note that the distance between the effective and the ineffective stimulus in C was the same as in A or B. The response of the neuron in each case is described to the right of each sketch. See text for a fuller discussion.

A simple spotlight, with a suppressive penumbra, will not explain this result, since the penumbra in the case of Figure 1C would have been expected to suppress the neuron and produce a poor response, whereas the observed response was strong. How is this very unexpected result to be explained?

A Possible Model

We suggest that there is indeed a spotlight of attention that, as implied in Figure 1, is smaller in area than a typical receptive field in V4. This spotlight provides some kind of boost or tag to certain of the neurons whose receptive fields are in that location in the visual field. These neurons are probably at a lower level in the visual hierarchy (e.g., in V2), where receptive fields are smaller than those in V4. In addition, we suggest a more elaborate mechanism. This will only be outlined here in an oversimplified form.

Suppose that in V4, there are many different stacks of neurons. Within each stack, the neurons have receptive fields all the same size and all in the same place in the visual field, some responding to blue, others to green, others to red, and so on. We consider two states of a single stack: without retinotopic attention (within that receptive field) and with attention. We postulate that the members of the stack do not compete when attention there is lacking but do compete strongly when attention is present. In other words, attention facilitates competition between the different neurons in the same stack but not between those in different stacks.

In our theory, this boosting or tagging would take the form of synchronized oscillations. Thus, neurons in a lower level—whose receptive field is smaller than those in V4—oscillate in response to the attended red object, expressing the neuronal correlate of attention. These neurons, feeding into the V4 neuron Moran and Desimone (1985) recorded from, will induce similar phase-locked oscillations in this cell but not in the other neurons in this stack responding to, say, green or blue. Neurons in this stack will then compete against each other, such that the oscillatory and phase-locked neurons will win out over the neurons with less synchronized or desynchronized firing. The response in Figure 1B is weak because the spotlight has activated competition between all the neurons in that stack and has also tagged the attended ("green") neurons at a lower level, so that in the resulting competition in V4 the "green" neurons there suppress the "red" ones. In Figure 1C, the spotlight of attention, while promoting competition in other stacks, fails to do so for the particular stack illustrated. Thus, lacking competition among nonoverlapping stacks, all neurons in the stack respond strongly to any incoming stimulus of the appropriate characters.

As the results show, an unattended stimulus (as in Fig. 1C) can sometimes give a fairly strong response. However, Moran and Desimone (1985) also studied neurons in visual region IT (inferotemporal). Here, the receptive fields are so large that they often fill much of the visual field. Thus, in the case of Figure 1C, the strong response of the neuron in V4 would be attenuated when it reached IT. There the roles of the two stimuli would be described by a figure that corresponded conceptually to Figure 1B, since in IT both stimuli would lie in the same receptive field and thus in the same stack, and so would compete with each other. The unattended red stimulus would therefore be suppressed somewhat in IT, as indeed Moran and Desimone found.

We can express the essence of our idea in more familiar words by using the concept of columns suggested by Mountcastle (Edelman and Mountcastle 1978).

In oversimplified terms, when a macrocolumn is not attended to, it can have several outputs. When it is attended to, it will have only one. This particular formulation is not to be taken too literally.

The above model has been simplified for didactic purposes. The idea of sets of stacks that do not overlap is far too simplistic. A more realistic model would have neurons whose receptive fields overlapped to varying degrees. Broadly speaking, for any two neurons, the greater the overlap of their receptive fields, the greater the competition the model would allow between them. This competition would, of course, depend on local activation by the spotlight in one way or another.

How might this "facilitation of competition" be done? We suggest by involving the 40-Hz oscillations, assuming competition between oscillations is fiercer than that between nonoscillatory activity, an idea that is not implausible. Moreover, the boost referred to above might be due, at least in part, to the resonances produced by 40-Hz oscillations. In other words, whenever a neuron is oscillating, it shuts down the nonoscillating neurons in that stack, or, more precisely, shuts down those neurons whose receptive fields heavily overlap with its own.

Unfortunately, it is not known whether 40-Hz oscillations occurred in Desimone's experiments. We would hope that the neuron in cases like that of Figure 1A would show strong 40-Hz oscillations, whereas for cases like Figure 1C, we would expect 40-Hz oscillations to be weak or absent. Whether this is true remains to be seen. We think that the idea that attention facilitates local competition may shed an entirely new light on mechanisms of attention and deserves further detailed study.

Top-down Effects

It would take us too far afield to consider top-down effects (see Julesz, this volume), except to say that they are undoubtedly important. It would not be too surprising if some of them originated in frontal cortex. Such top-down effects might act directly to bias the saliency map, or more indirectly by biasing some of the neurons in the various visual areas of the neocortex that project to the saliency map. There may also be top-down effects that adjust the size of the attentional spotlight. In addition, there must be mechanisms for remembering the task in a psychophysical experiment and for recognizing a target object when it springs into awareness. We shall discuss none of these subjects here.

WORKING MEMORY

It is difficult to say much about the neurological basis of working memory because there has been so little experimental work on it. We have to distinguish two broad possibilities. In the first, neural activity is maintained for some seconds by one mechanism or another (see Crick and Koch 1990), with or without transient synaptic modification. In the second, neuronal activity is not maintained, but only transient synaptic modifications take place. Both mechanisms may be used to some extent.

Let us first consider the activity taking place before working memory is activated. When a 40-Hz oscillation is both strongly active and phase-locked over many cortical areas, we expect this global activity to correspond to vivid visual awareness. There are likely to be certain regions that have easily formed this strong coalition (we call these the core of the activity) and have then spread their oscillations to other regions that we refer to as the periphery. These in their turn may activate further peripheral regions, but not necessarily to the extent of promoting phase-locked oscillations there. Some of these peripheral activities may correspond to what might be considered the "meaning" of the percept.

What will happen when, for one reason or another, this whole set of neurons ceases to oscillate in phase? In some case, the core regions may maintain mainly nonoscillatory activity, perhaps with the assistance of transient synaptic modifications. We suggest that this is the neural correlate of working memory. Because of the lack of global oscillations, their activity is not correlated with vivid awareness; however, should the attentional spotlight return to it (or should competition from other oscillatory sets greatly decrease), the core will quickly set up all or part of the previous phase-locked oscillatory set and thus enter awareness again in a very short time.

Recall that in some cases, it may have taken an appreciable time for a set of coherent oscillations to be set up in the first place. If this activity has produced some transient synaptic modification, there may be no need to repeat this prolonged setup time when the memory is evoked again.

A second possibility is that, after all oscillations have died away, all the neurons concerned lapse into firing at background rates. Even in such a case the memory may still be retrievable if sufficiently strong (transient) synaptic modifications have taken place. In this case, however, a fairly strong and specific cue, directed to the right place, will be needed to start up the oscillatory activity again.

In the first case discussed above, strong cueing should not be needed because the self-sustained (nonoscillatory) activity should be able itself to act as a sufficient cue under the right circumstances. If something more is required to reactivate the memory, it need only be a rather unspecific nudge. One form of recalling a previous item in working memory is often called rehearsal. Rehearsal may explain the rather large differences in the decay time of working memory reported by different workers. For example, in the case of Damasio's patient Boswell (Damasio et al. 1985), the time quoted is about 40 seconds (A.R. Damasio, pers. comm.). In those studies on normal people (Baddeley 1986) in which any form of rehearsal was discouraged, the decay times tended to be only a few seconds.

Although rehearsal may be obvious in some cases, it may sometimes escape introspection.

OTHER OSCILLATIONS

The main theoretical requirement for mechanisms that produce global activity among neurons is that they should promote correlated firing. Such in-phase firing of the incoming axons is likely to produce a larger effect at the soma than desynchronized firing at the same average rate, but this increase is likely, by itself, to be fairly small. A further advantage of oscillations as a form of coordinated firing is that they may be able to induce membrane-bound resonances if some neurons have a strong, but latent, tendency to fire at or near that particular frequency.

For the purpose of exposition, we have considered only γ oscillations (in the 40–80-Hz range), but no theoretical reason has been given so far why the brain should use these particular frequencies. On general grounds, one would expect the best oscillations to be as fast as possible, allowing for the unavoidable time delays in axonal, synaptic, and dendritic transmission. This argument is at the moment too imprecise to favor one frequency range over another.

The brain shows a whole range of oscillations, the most notable being the θ rhythm of the hippocampus and the α rhythm mainly associated with the neocortex. Exactly what these other rhythms are used for is unclear, but they should not be forgotten. The α rhythm tends to occur when the brain is awake but somewhat inactive. Duncan and Humphreys (1989) in their theory of attention propose a subsidiary mechanism that they call the "spreading suppression" of similar nontargets (the reader is referred to their paper for details). It is just conceivable that the α rhythm provides this hypothetical function. According to this view, the function of the α rhythm would be to hinder the establishment and spread of 40-Hz oscillations.

A major unanswered question concerns the interaction between different oscillations, either within a family or between families (e.g., between α rhythms and γ rhythms). Of course, even in a linear system, the interaction of two oscillations of different frequency will often produce "beats." The 40-Hz oscillations may perhaps be too irregular for such beats to be very prominent unless the oscillations become rather more regular when fully established. Nevertheless, it is conceivable that some mechanism based on beats tends to set a certain distance between the frequencies of two interacting sets of oscillations and, by this means, spaces simultaneous frequencies fairly uniformly over the allowed frequency range. The problem is complex and deserves more detailed theoretical study.

THE OVERALL PICTURE

Let us now try to describe the overall behavior of the neurons in the visual cortex of an alert animal. Whatever the details of the attentional mechanism, we expect that there will be several sets of phase-locked neurons oscillating at the same time and having somewhat different frequencies and/or phases. Some of these oscillations may be dying away while new ones may be struggling to grow. All this occurs against a large background of neurons firing in a more desynchronized or chaotic manner. Because we do not yet have a clear idea of the usual lifetime of one particular oscillation set, the time scale of all this transient activity is difficult to estimate precisely, but the changes are likely to be fairly fast, probably taking a small fraction of a second. For this reason, it may be difficult to study the oscillations in the brain of an alert monkey viewing a typical visual scene, since any particular set of neurons may oscillate in such a transient manner as to be difficult to pin down. An alert animal trained to fixate and looking at a straightforward rather uniform stimulus, such as a drifting grating, may be somewhat easier to study, but the results obtained may be so simple as to be misleading.

Eventually other devices may be needed. Perhaps the speed at the animal's attentional mechanism can be either slowed down or disabled, possibly by lesions to the parietal region (Posner et al. 1987). This slowing down may be one of the main effects of a state of light anesthesia. (It is also possible that an anesthetic reduces or prevents the effects of the oscillations on working memory, so that subjectively the subject is largely unconscious even though his brain may display oscillations to some extent.)

Radically new experimental methods may have to be invented if we are to understand what is going on. For example, it may be possible to follow many of the main features of the oscillations by recording multiunit activity (see Singer et al. or Bower; both this volume) in many places simultaneously. Perhaps an array of 10,000 "electrodes" could be placed on the exposed cortex of a monkey whose cortex had few convolutions, such as the owl monkey (or even on that of the humble, rather nonvisual rat; see Wilson and Bower, 1990). The results could be displayed on a television monitor, probably slowed down considerably, so that the dynamic features of the recording can be grasped more easily. Another possible technique that would allow monitoring of the 40-Hz oscillations simultaneously over large areas of cortex is that of voltage-sensitive dyes (Grinvald et al. 1988). It remains to be seen whether the time resolution and the signal-to-noise ratio can be brought to acceptable levels.

CONCLUSION

The object of this paper is not to put forward detailed theories but rather to outline a few of the ideas that have arisen rather naturally by assuming that the 40-Hz oscillations are doing what we are guessing they do. These considerations should alert neurobiologists both to ideas proposed by psychologists and to several rather complex dynamic activities in the brain that urgently need further study.

To psychologists, these ideas outline some neurobiological facts and possibilities that could provide new idioms with which to construct their models. For example, there may be two somewhat distinct forms of neural activity: (1) nonoscillatory or weakly oscillatory activity that does not produce awareness but can leave a forward-reaching trace of the sort seen in priming and (2) phase-locked oscillatory activity that does produce awareness and activates the working memory system.

To neural modelers, and to theorists in general, these ideas raise numerous theoretical problems, often very complex and difficult ones, although even simple models might give suggestive solutions of a general nature.

It is our personal view that none of these three approaches, by themselves, will provide definitive answers. On the other hand, we hope that a combined attack, with a constant interplay between theory and experiments of all types, may eventually lead to an understanding of what is clearly a highly complex nonlinear dynamic system whose behavior skips rapidly from one semistable state to another. Our suggestions should be regarded as a preliminary skirmish in such an attack.

ACKNOWLEDGMENTS

We thank Kyle Cave and Charles Gray for helpful comments on drafts of this manuscript. F.C. is supported by the J.W. Kieckhefer Foundation. C.K. is supported by the Air Force Office of Scientific Research, a Presidential Young Investigator Award from the National Science Foundation, and the James S. McDonnell Foundation.

REFERENCES

Allport, A. 1989. Visual attention. In *Foundations of cognitive science* (ed. M.I. Posner), p. 631. MIT Press, Cambridge.

Baddeley, A. 1986. *Working memory*. Oxford University Press, United Kingdom.

Cave, K.R. and J.M. Wolfe. 1990. Modeling the role of parallel processing in visual search. *Cognit. Psychol.* **22**: 225.

Coltheart, M. 1983. Iconic memory. *Philos. Trans. R. Soc. Lond. B* **302**: 283.

Crick, F.H.C. 1984. The function of the thalamic reticular complex: The searchlight hypothesis. *Proc. Natl. Acad. Sci.* **81**: 4586.

Crick, F. and C. Asanuma. 1986. Certain aspects of the anatomy and physiology of the cerebral cortex. In *Parallel distributing processing: Explorations in the microstructure of cognition* (eds. D. Rumelhart and J.L. McClelland), vol. 2, p. 333. MIT Press, Cambridge.

Crick, F. and C. Koch. 1990. Towards a neurobiological theory of consciousness. *Semin. Neurosci.* (in press).

Damasio, A.R., P.J. Eslinger, H. Damasio, G.H. Van Hoesen, and S. Cornell. 1985. Multimodal amnesic syndrome following bilateral temporal and basal forebrain damage. *Arch. Neurol.* **42**: 252.

Duncan, J. and G.W. Humphreys. 1989. Visual search and stimulus similarity. *Psychol. Rev.* **96**: 433.

Edelman, G. and V.B. Mountcastle. 1978. *The mindful brain: Cortical organization and the group selective theory of higher brain function*. MIT Press, Cambridge.

Engel, A.K., P. König, C.M. Gray, and W. Singer. 1990. Stimulus-dependent neuronal oscillations in cat visual cortex: II. Inter-columnar interaction as determined by cross correlation analysis. *Eur. J. Neurosci.* (in press).

Gray, C.M., A.K. Engel, P. Knig, and W. Singer. 1990. Stimulus-dependent neuronal oscillations in cat visual cortex: I. Receptive field properties and feature dependence. *Eur. J. Neurosci.* (in press).

Grinvald, A., R.D. Frostig, E. Lieke, and R. Hildesheim. 1988. Optical imaging of neuronal activity. *Physiol. Rev.* **68**: 1285.

Holender, D. 1986. Semantic activation without conscious identification in dochotic listening, parafoveal vision, and visual masking: A survey and appraisal. *Behav. Brain Sci.* **9**: 1.

Jones, E.G. 1985. *The thalamus*. Plenum Press, New York.

Kammen, D.M., P.J. Holmes, and C. Koch. 1989. Cortical architecture and oscillations in neuronal networks: Feedback versus local coupling. In *Models of brain function* (ed. R.M.J. Cotterill), p. 273. Cambridge University Press, United Kingdom.

Kihlstrom, J.F. 1987. The cognitive unconscious. *Science* **237**: 1445.

Koch, C. and S. Ullman. 1985. Shifts in selective visual attention: Towards the underlying neural circuitry. *Hum. Neurobiol.* **4**: 219.

Moran, J. and R. Desimone. 1985. Selective attention gates visual processing in the extrastriate cortex. *Science* **229**: 782.

Mountcastle, V.B., R.A. Andersen, and B.C. Motter. 1981. The influence of attentive fixation upon the excitability of the light-sensitive neurons of the posterior parietal cortex. *J. Neurosci.* **1**: 1218.

Poggio, T., V. Torre, and C. Koch. 1985. Computational vision and regularization theory. *Nature* **317**: 314.

Posner, M.I. 1986. *Chronometric explorations of mind*. Oxford University Press, United Kingdom.

Posner, M.I., J.A. Walker, F.A. Friedrich, and R.D. Rafal. 1987. How do the parietal lobes direct covert attention? *Neurophysiologia* **25**: 135.

Rafal, R.D. and M.I. Posner. 1987. Deficits in human visual spatial attention following thalamic lesions. *Proc. Natl. Acad. Sci.* **84**: 7349.

Sherk, H. 1986. The claustrum and the cerebral cortex. In *Cerebral cortex*, Volume 5: *Sensory-motor areas and aspects of cortical connectivity* (eds. E.G. Jones and A. Peters), p. 467. Plenum Press, New York.

Spitzer, H., R. Desimone, and J. Moran. 1988. Increased attention enhances both behavioral and neuronal performance. *Science* **240**: 338.

Sporns, O., J.A. Gally, G.N. Reeke, Jr., and G.M. Edelman. 1989. Reentrant signaling among simulated neuronal groups leads to coherency in their oscillatory activity. *Proc. Natl. Acad. Sci.* **86**: 7265.

Steriade, M., E.G. Jones, and R.R. Llinas. 1990. *Thalamic oscillations and signaling*. Wiley, New York.

Tranel, D. and A.R. Damasio. 1985. Knowledge without awareness: An autonomic index of facial recognition by prosopagnosics. *Science* **228**: 1453.

Treisman, A. 1988. Features and objects: The fourteenth Bartlett Memorial Lecture. *Q. J. Exp. Psychol.* **40A**: 201.

Tulving, E. and D.L. Schacter. 1990. Priming and human memory systems. *Science* **247**: 301.

Van Essen, D. and C.H. Anderson. 1990. Information processing strategies and pathways in the primate retina and visual cortex. In *An introduction to neural and electronic networks* (ed. S.F. Zornetzer et al.), p. 43. Academic Press, San Diego.

von der Malsburg, C. and W. Schneider. 1986. A neural cocktail-party processor. *Biol. Cybern.* **54**: 29.

Wilson, M. and J. Bower. 1990. Cortical oscillations and temporal interactions in a computer simulation of piriform cortex. *J. Neurophysiol.* (in press).

Wise, S.P. and R. Desimone. 1988. Behavioral neurophysiology: Insights into seeing and grasping. *Science* **242**: 736.

Attentional Control of Visual Perception: Cortical and Subcortical Mechanisms

R. Desimone,* M. Wessinger,* L. Thomas,* and W. Schneider,†
*Laboratory of Neuropsychology, National Institute of Mental Health, Bethesda, Maryland 20892;
†Learning Research and Development Center, University of Pittsburgh, Pittsburgh, Pennsylvania 15260

Given the properties of muscles (and the laws of physics), it is obviously not possible to direct the eyes or move an arm to more than one object at a time. What may not be so obvious is that neither is it possible to fully process or store in memory more than one or two visual stimuli in a single moment. In this sense, memory and muscles are very much alike. Thus, neurobiologists working in both sensory and motor systems must confront the problem of selective attention, i.e., how the brain selects which of the many images typically stimulating the retina will be the target for an eye movement or will have access to memory at a given moment. It is an interesting question whether these attentional mechanisms are the *same* mechanisms for both sensory and motor systems, and we address this later in this paper.

In our work, we have tried to understand the neural mechanisms of attention through recordings in the extrastriate cortex of macaque monkeys. The extrastriate cortex contains 20 or more areas with visual functions. Although there are a great many areas, and an even greater number of connections between them, they appear to form only two or three major processing systems, or "pathways." According to a model originally proposed by Ungerleider and Mishkin (1982), the striate, or primary visual, cortex is the source of two major information-processing pathways, both of which involve several prestriate visual areas. One of the pathways is directed ventrally into the temporal lobe and is crucial for object recognition. The other is directed dorsally into the parietal lobe and is crucial for spatial perception and visuomotor performance (for reviews, see Ungerleider and Mishkin 1982; Desimone et al. 1985; Van Essen 1985; Maunsell and Newsome 1987; Desimone and Ungerleider 1989). Recently, evidence has emerged for a third processing pathway within the cortex of the superior temporal sulcus of the macaque, and it has been speculated that this pathway mediates the perception of complex visual motion and/or integrates spatial and object vision (Boussaoud et al. 1990). The three major pathways are shown diagrammatically in Figure 1.

Because the occipitotemporal, or "ventral," pathway is known to be critical for the recognition of objects, it is in this pathway that we would expect that attention would influence the neural processing of visual information. This pathway begins with striate cortex and continues through areas V2, V3, V4, and areas TEO

and TE in inferior temporal (IT) cortex. As one proceeds from one area to the next along this pathway, neuronal properties change in two obvious ways. First, the complexity of neuronal processing increases. For example, whereas neurons in striate cortex are sensitive to local features of objects such as the orientation of contours at a specific retinal location, neurons in V2 have been shown to respond to "virtual" or illusory contours in certain figures (von der Heydt et al. 1984), and neurons in IT cortex are sensitive to global or overall object features, such as shape (Schwartz et al. 1983; Desimone et al. 1984). Second, the receptive

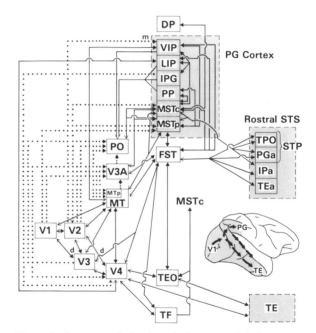

Figure 1. Summary of visual cortical areas and their connections in macaque monkeys. Solid lines indicate projections that originate from both central and peripheral field representations, and dotted lines indicate projections that arise exclusively from peripheral field representations. Solid arrowheads indicate "forward" connections, open arrowheads indicate "backward" connections, and lines connected with closed arrowheads at both ends indicate "intermediate" connections. The small *d*'s and *m*s indicate projections limited to the dorsal or medial portions of certain visual areas. The diagram shows a dorsal pathway directed into the parietal cortex (cytoarchitectonic area PG) that is specialized for spatial vision, a ventral pathway directed into the temporal cortex (cytoarchitectonic area TE) that is specialized for object vision, and a third pathway directed into the superior temporal sulcus (STS). (Adapted from Boussaoud et al. 1990.)

field size of individual neurons increases. Neurons in the central field representation of striate cortex often have receptive fields that are less than 0.1% in linear size (see, e.g., Dow et al. 1981). In contrast, neurons in the corresponding visual field representation in area V4 have receptive fields that are 1°–5° in size (Desimone and Schein 1987), and neurons in IT cortex, where receptive fields usually include the fovea, have a median receptive field size of 25° (Desimone and Gross 1979). As a result of these two trends, namely, increased complexity and larger receptive field size, neurons at the highest levels of the occipitotemporal pathway may provide a global description of object features that is invariant over changes in retinal location (Gross and Mishkin 1977). Furthermore, large receptive fields are an example of a "coarse coding" mechanism, which is very economical for coding large amounts of information by few neurons (see Hinton et al. 1986).

Attention and Large Receptive Fields

Although large receptive fields may be an economical coding mechanism and may also contribute to the ability to recognize an object regardless of where its image appears on the retina, they do not come without a cost. Large receptive fields allow for multiple independent objects to potentially stimulate the same neuron. Receptive fields of cells in IT cortex, for example, are large enough to encompass an entire scene. Likewise, in a page of text at normal reading distance, the receptive field of even a V4 neuron might contain the image of several words. Thus, an IT or V4 neuron's response will necessarily reflect the influence of all of the stimuli inside the field. Consider, for example, a color-coding scheme in which the color of a stimulus is determined by the relative activities of three cells coarsely tuned to red, green, or blue and with receptive fields at the same location. Such a scheme will work only if there is a single stimulus inside the joint field. If there are two or more differently colored stimuli each stimulating the three cells, the output of this three-neuron network will be completely ambiguous. This situation, sometimes termed the "binding problem" (Hinton et al. 1986), thwarts any coding efficiency obtained with large fields. Large receptive fields, then, bring us to just the problem that attentional mechanisms are supposed to solve, namely, how to limit the amount of information that is processed by the visual system in a single moment.

A possible solution to this problem was found in recordings from neurons in the occipitotemporal pathway in monkeys. In this study, monkeys were trained to attend to one or another of two stimuli within the receptive field of a V4 or IT neuron and it was found that the neuron's response was gated by the locus of the animal's attention within the receptive field (Moran and Desimone 1985).

First, the cell's receptive field was mapped with bars of various colors, orientations, and sizes while the animal fixated a small target. On the basis of the cell's responses, two sets of stimuli were selected, one set that was effective in eliciting a response from the cell and a second set that was ineffective. An effective stimulus was then presented at one location inside the receptive field and an ineffective stimulus at another. The monkey was trained on a task that required it to attend to the stimulus at one location and ignore the stimulus at another (the distractor). The monkey's attention was "covert," since eye movements were not permitted (fixation was monitored with the magnetic search coil technique). After a block of trials, the monkey was cued to switch its attention to the other location. Blocks of trials with attention directed toward one or the other location were alternated repeatedly. Because identical sensory conditions were maintained in the two types of blocks, any difference in the response of the cell could be attributed to the effects of attention.

The particular task used to focus the animal's attention was a matching-to-sample task. The animal was first cued by a special instructional trial at the start of the block which location in the visual field was relevant. At the relevant location, a sample stimulus was presented briefly and, after a short delay, was followed by a briefly presented test stimulus. The animal was required to indicate whether or not the test stimulus matched the sample. At another location in the visual field, irrelevant, or distracting, stimuli were paired with both the sample and test. If the animal mistakenly based his behavior on the distractors, its performance would be at chance levels. In the next block, the formerly distracting stimuli became the relevant sample and test.

The locus of the animal's attention within the receptive field of the recorded neuron had a large effect on the neuron's response. When both effective and ineffective sensory stimuli were presented within the receptive field, and the animal attended to the effective stimulus, the neuron responded well. When the animal attended to the ineffective stimulus, however, the neuron's response was greatly attenuated (a threefold reduction in response, on the average), even though the effective (but ignored) sensory stimulus was still present within the receptive field. The neuron responded as if the receptive field had contracted around the attended stimulus, so that the influence of distracting stimuli at other locations in the field was reduced or eliminated (Fig. 2). No effects of attention were found in either V1 or V2 in this paradigm, indicating that V4 is probably the first area in the occipitotemporal pathway where responses are gated by spatial attention.

One initially surprising finding was that the attentional effects observed in V4 depended on both the attended and ignored stimuli being located within the recorded neuron's receptive field. If one stimulus was located within the receptive field and one outside, it apparently made no difference (to the neuron) which stimulus the animal attended. That is, if the stimuli are sufficiently separated spatially, it apparently makes no

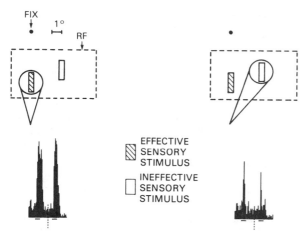

EFFECTIVE
SENSORY
STIMULUS

INEFFECTIVE
SENSORY
STIMULUS

Figure 2. Effect of selective attention on the responses of a neuron in extrastriate area V4. The neuronal responses shown are from when the monkey attended to one location inside the receptive field (RF) and ignored another. At the attended location (circled), two stimuli (sample and test) were presented sequentially, and the monkey responded differently depending on whether they were the same or different. Irrelevant stimuli were presented simultaneously with the sample and test but at a separate location in the receptive field. In the initial mapping of the field, the cell responded well to red bars but not at all to green bars. A horizontal or a vertical red bar (effective sensory stimuli) was then placed at one location in the field and a horizontal or a vertical green bar (ineffective sensory stimuli) at another. When the animal attended to the location of the red bar at the time of presentation of either the sample or test, the cell gave a good response (*left*), but when the animal attended to the location of the green bar, the cell gave only a small response (*right*), even though the two stimuli on the retina were identical in the two conditions. Thus, the responses of the cell were determined predominantly by the attended stimulus. The horizontal bars under the graphs indicate the 200-msec period when the sample and test stimuli were on. Because of the random delay between the sample and test presentations, the graphs were synchronized separately at the onsets of the sample and test stimuli (indicated by the vertical dashed lines). (Adapted from Moran and Desimone 1985.)

difference in V4 to which one the animal attends. This only makes sense if one considers that a major purpose of attentional mechanisms is to "disambiguate" a neuron's response when there are multiple stimuli inside the receptive field. If there is only a single stimulus inside the field, the neuron's response is determined solely by that stimulus and thus is already unambiguous.

Yet, there is still a puzzle, since we know from psychological studies that ignored stimuli often do not reach awareness no matter where they are located with respect to the attended stimulus. Somewhere along the occipitotemporal pathway we would expect to find an attentional mechanism that works over a larger spatial extent than in V4. Such a mechanism is found in IT cortex (see Fig. 1), where neurons have receptive fields so large as to include the entire central visual field. When there are two stimuli within an IT receptive field, IT neuronal responses are determined primarily by the attended stimulus, even when the attended and ignored stimuli are separated by a substantial distance. In fact,

the receptive fields in IT cortex were so large, and the attentional effects covered such a large spatial range, that it was not possible to test the effects of the animal attending outside the receptive field. These results suggest that the filtering of unwanted information is at least a two-stage process, with the first stage working over a small spatial range in V4, and a second stage working over a much larger spatial range in IT cortex.

These effects of attention in V4 and IT cortex presumably underlie the attenuated processing and the reduced awareness for unattended stimuli shown psychophysically in humans. Furthermore, the fact that neurons respond to an attended stimulus as if their receptive fields had contracted around it may allow for cells to communicate information with high spatial resolution despite their large receptive fields. Thus, the visual system achieves the advantages of large receptive fields without incurring the expected costs in spatial resolution, at least within the focus of attention. However, outside the focus of attention, large receptive fields may indeed incur a cost. Given that attention works over only a limited spatial range in V4, one might expect that spatial resolution outside the focus of attention to be poor, a possibility that is consistent with the results of a number of psychophysical studies. Julesz (1981), for example, has shown that focal attention is required to perceive the spatial arrangement of local line elements, and Triesman (1986, 1988) has found that the features of stimuli outside the focus of attention may be perceived in the wrong locations and consequently form "illusory conjunctions."

Increasing Resolution for Features

So far, all of these neurophysiological data fit a "suppressive" model of attention control, i.e., attention serves to suppress processing of unwanted stimuli. There is, however, recent neurophysiological evidence that increasing the *amount* of attention devoted to an attended stimulus enhances the processing of that stimulus within the occipitotemporal pathway (Spitzer et al. 1988). In this study, neurons were studied in the same matching-to-sample paradigm described above, except that there were no irrelevant stimuli within the visual field. Color and orientation tuning curves were compared when the animal was operating in either of two "modes," an easy one and a difficult one. In the easy mode, the sample and test stimuli in the task were either very different from each other (on nonmatching trials) or identical to each other (on matching trials). In the difficult mode, the same set of stimuli were paired in such a way that the sample and test stimulus were either very similar to one another (on nonmatching trials) or identical (on matching trials). For example, in the easy mode, the animal might be required to discriminate red versus aqua and blue versus orange, whereas in the difficult mode, the animal would have to discriminate red versus orange and blue versus aqua. It was reasoned that the difficult mode required more of the animal's attention than the easy mode.

Recordings from V4 neurons under these two conditions showed that neuronal responses in the difficult mode were stronger and more tightly tuned to the stimuli than were responses to the same stimuli in the easy mode. These effects, which were found for both color and orientation discriminations, are consistent with both psychophysical studies of attentional enhancement in humans (see, e.g., Bergen and Julesz 1983; Kahneman 1973; Treisman 1986; Posner and Presti 1987) and neurophysiological reports of attentional modulation of extrastriate neurons (see, e.g., Mountcastle et al. 1987; Richmond and Sato 1987; Spitzer and Richmond 1990).

Although these sharpening effects on V4 tuning curves might seem qualitatively different from the narrowing effects of spatial attention on V4 receptive fields, they actually share some similarities if a broad view of "receptive fields" is adopted. In the study of spatial attention in V4, cells responded as if their receptive fields contracted around the attended stimulus in order to exclude unwanted stimuli from the field, i.e., to enhance spatial resolution. If a cell's color or orientation tuning properties are regarded as a type of nonspatial receptive field, then it could be said that the color and orientation receptive fields of V4 neurons can also contract in order to exclude nonoptimal stimuli, i.e., to enhance "featural" resolution. It is not yet clear, however, whether these two phenomena could result from the same attentional mechanism.

A Pulvinar Source for the Attentional Modulation of V4 and IT Neurons?

Now that we know that attention modulates the responses of V4 and IT neurons, it is important to understand how these effects come about. The lateral pulvinar nucleus in the thalamus attracted our interest as a possible candidate for the source of these modulating inputs, for a number of reasons. First, the lateral pulvinar has reciprocal connections with all of the areas in the occipitotemporal pathway and thus is in a good anatomical position to influence cortical responses (Benevento and Davis 1974; Benevento and Rezak 1976; Ungerleider et al. 1983). Second, Crick (1984) has proposed a model of spatial attention based on interactions between the pulvinar and cortex. Third, studies of humans with thalamic lesions involving the pulvinar have shown impairments in the ability to engage attention (Rafal and Posner 1987), and PET studies in humans have shown activation of the pulvinar in attentional tasks (LaBerge and Buchsbaum 1990). Finally, and most importantly, Petersen et al. (1987) have reported that reversible chemical deactivation of the PDm portion of the pulvinar in monkeys (which can be regarded as the most medial and dorsal portion of the lateral pulvinar) causes an increased reaction time in switching attention from the ipsilesional to contralesional visual field. This impairment, which may be caused by an impairment in disengaging attention, resembles the attentional impairments found following

lesions of the posterior parietal cortex (Posner et al. 1984, 1987), with which this portion of the pulvinar is connected. Thus, we reasoned that perhaps the more lateral portion of the pulvinar, the portion connected with V4 and IT cortex, plays a role in gating V4 and IT responses to ignored stimuli, i.e., focusing attention.

Although our goal was to understand the gating of extrastriate cortical responses, we decided to pursue first a behavioral strategy. If a structure plays a critical role in gating out extrastriate responses to distracting stimuli, then deactivating that structure should impair the animal's ability to perceive or respond appropriately to an attended stimulus in the presence of a distractor but should not impair its ability to perceive or respond to a stimulus in the absence of any distractor. The first structure we tested in this way was the lateral pulvinar (Desimone et al. 1989).

The task we used was a color discrimination task with a spatial attentional cue. While the monkey maintained its gaze on a fixation spot (eye movements were prohibited throughout the trial), a small white spatial cue flashed briefly in the visual field. In the "distractor condition," the cue was followed by two briefly presented color bars, one of which was the target and one a distractor. The target was, by definition, the bar that was presented at the same location as the cue, and the animal had to indicate the color of the target with a lever press, ignoring the distractor. The animal moved the lever one direction if the target was red or yellow, and another direction if it was green or blue. The distractor was also a colored bar, but the color was either chosen randomly or consistently a different color from the target. As a control, we also ran the same task without a distractor.

The general strategy of the experiment was to test, on alternate days, the ability to perform the task with or without a distractor when the animal was normal, versus when its lateral pulvinar had been unilaterally deactivated. To reversibly deactivate the lateral pulvinar, we injected the GABA agonist muscimol through a cannula directly into the appropriate portion of the lateral pulvinar. Although the visual topography of the posterior portion of the lateral pulvinar, the portion connected with IT cortex and V4, is not yet clear, there is evidence for some degree of visual topography (Benevento and Rezak 1976; Benevento and Davis 1977; Bender 1981; Ungerleider et al. 1983, 1984). Thus, we attempted to deactivate all of the posterior lateral pulvinar in order to affect the complete contralateral field representation. Recordings following one of the injections showed that all neural activity in the lateral pulvinar was silenced. Behavioral data were collected from two monkeys.

Figure 3 shows the results from the "no distractor" condition when the animal was normal (baseline results) compared to when the lateral pulvinar of the left hemisphere was deactivated. The pulvinar deactivation caused, at most, a slight increase in errors when the target was located in either the left or right visual field. In contrast, when a distractor was present in the normal

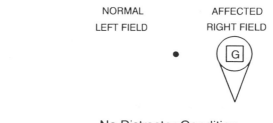

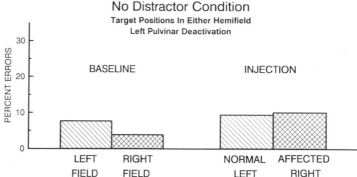

Figure 3. Effects of deactivation of the pulvinar in the left hemisphere on the discrimination of a target presented alone, in either the left or right visual field. Target locations were 3° from fixation.

left visual field and the target in the right visual field, the animal was severely impaired ($\sim 30\%$ errors), as shown in Figure 4. Performance on the opposite condition, when the target was located in the normal left visual field and the distractor was in the affected right field, actually appeared to be improved following the pulvinar deactivation.

The lateral pulvinar thus appears to play a critical role in attention only when attention is directed to a target in the presence of a distractor. When there are no competing stimuli in the opposite visual field, the absence of the lateral pulvinar does not affect an animal's ability to respond to a target appropriately. This is exactly the behavioral effect we expected from our previous neurophysiological results, given that we only

observed attentional gating in V4 and IT cortex when there was a distractor in the visual field. Specifically, the results suggest that the pulvinar deactivation interfered with the attentional gating of IT neuronal responses, since the placement of target and distractor in opposite visual fields was an appropriate stimulus configuration for IT but not V4 receptive fields.

What about a stimulus configuration more appropriate for V4 receptive fields, i.e., with a target and distractor both located in the field contralateral to the deactivated pulvinar? Surprisingly, we found very little effect of the pulvinar deactivation under this condition. Thus, the pulvinar cannot be a necessary source of the neural signals that gate V4 responses, nor even the necessary source of signals that gate IT responses when

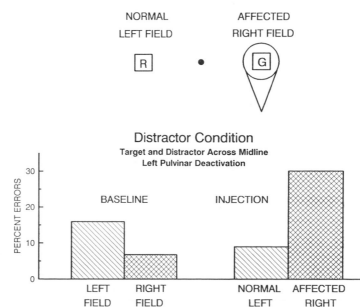

Figure 4. Effects of deactivation of the pulvinar in the left hemisphere on the discrimination of a target in the presence of a distractor in the opposite field. Target and distractor locations were 3° from fixation.

target and distractor are located within the same visual hemifield. This result was hard to understand until we recently obtained some preliminary results from deactivation of the superior colliculus in one monkey (Desimone et al. 1989).

A Possible Role for the Superior Colliculus

Unlike the case for the lateral pulvinar, it was not possible to test the effects of deactivating the entire contralateral field representation in the superior colliculus because such a large deactivation caused a severe nystagmus. We therefore recorded receptive fields in the colliculus and deactivated individual small zones corresponding to the recorded field. In contrast to the pulvinar results, this time we found impaired performance with a distractor located anywhere within the visual field, even in the same hemifield as the target, as long as the target was located at the receptive field location of the site we deactivated in the colliculus (Fig. 5). As was the case with pulvinar deactivation, there was little or no effect of the colliculus deactivation on target discrimination when there was no distractor present in the visual field. We should emphasize that all of these effects were obtained in the absence of eye movements.

It may seem surprising that we obtained attentional deficits in the absence of eye movements from deactivation of the superior colliculus, which is commonly thought to be an oculomotor structure. For example, cells in the intermediate layers of the superior colliculus give enhanced responses to visual stimuli when they will be the target for a saccadic eye movement but not when the stimuli elicit a different type of motor response, such as a bar release (for review, see Wurtz and Albano 1980). Furthermore, local deactivation of the superior colliculus impairs saccadic eye movements to targets located at the visual field location of the deacti-

vation site (Hikosaka and Wurtz 1986). Yet, other results have also suggested a role for the colliculus in attentional control in the absence of eye movements. Albano et al. (1982) have found that lesions of the superior colliculus cause an increase in reaction time to detect (with a lever release) a peripheral target, even when fixation is maintained on a central fixation spot. They suggested that the collicular lesions cause a visual neglect that is "related to but not necessarily limited to the generation of saccadic eye movements." In addition, Kertzman and Robinson (1988) have recently reported that local deactivation of the colliculus causes an increase in the time it takes to switch attention from the "ipsilesional" to "contralesional" hemifield, again in the absence of eye movements. Thus, some sort of attentional role of the colliculus is likely, although it is not yet clear how this role is expressed at the physiological level. Because the colliculus does not have direct projections to the cortex, any effect it has on cortical responses must arise from indirect anatomical connections.

Spatial Attention and Oculomotor Control

The close relationship between structures involved in the control of eye movements and spatial attention has been noted by several investigators (see, e.g., Matelli et al. 1983; Rizzolati 1983; Posner and Presti 1987), and Rizzolati (1983) has proposed a premotor theory of attentional control. Shifts of gaze typically follow shifts of attention, although, as we have seen, shifts of gaze are not imperative. Both gaze and attentional shifts require that a new target be selected. It would seem that the difference between oculomotor control and attentional control derives from whether or not neurons give the "go" signal for the eyes to actually move to the new target. In fact, whether or not the eyes actually move, the effects on visual processing in extrastriate

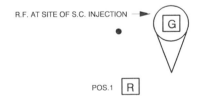

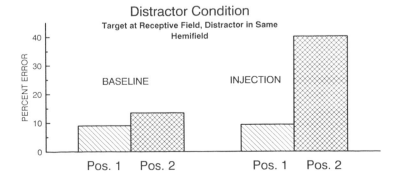

Figure 5. Effects of deactivation of a site in the superior colliculus on the discrimination of a target in the same hemifield. Target and distractor coordinates, in degrees, were (3, 0.25) and (1, −2.8), respectively.

cortex may be very similar. When the eyes fixate a new target, the visual system is dominated by new input because of the magnification of the foveal representation in cortical visual areas. Our work in V4 and IT cortex has shown that shifts in attention, without a concomitant eye movement, may also cause extrastriate visual processing to be dominated by new input.

It is probably not a coincidence that three of the structures presumed to play a major role in high-level oculomotor control, namely, the frontal eye field, the posterior parietal cortex, and the superior colliculus, have also been implicated in the control of spatial attention (for a recent review, see Goldberg and Colby 1989). Less is known about the role of the pulvinar in oculomotor control, but there is both behavioral and physiological evidence for such a role (Ungerleider and Christensen 1979; Petersen et al. 1985; Robinson et al. 1986).

One other common feature of the oculomotor and attentional control systems deserves comment. Because critical oculomotor functions appear to be carried out in parallel in more than one structure, a substantial degree of oculomotor control typically returns following lesions of any single "high-level" oculomotor structure. In monkeys, it requires a combined lesion of both the superior colliculus and frontal eye field to produce a lasting impairment in the ability to produce directed saccadic eye movements (Schiller et al. 1979). Likewise, permanent neglect is very uncommon following lesions in monkeys or man, except in the case of very large lesions or lesions that involve white matter. A distributed attentional control system (see, e.g., Posner and Presti 1987) may explain, in part, why we did not see an impairment in our pulvinar study when target and distractor were both located in the field contralateral to the pulvinar deactivation. If the attentional control system is a highly distributed one, then some other structure must be capable of controlling attention (and presumably modulating extrastriate responses) in the absence of the pulvinar. This is not a complete explanation, however, since it does not explain why we found an impairment from the pulvinar deactivation when target and distractor were located in opposite fields, nor does it account for our colliculus results.

A Model of Attention Control Based on Competition

Our own pulvinar and colliculus findings, as well the results of many other neuropsychological studies in humans and monkeys, are consistent with a model of attentional control based on competition within the attentional control system (Fig. 6). Within this system, every point in the visual field is in competition with every other point for control over attention. A stimulus will normally win the competition if it is particularly salient, if its location has been "precued," or if the subject has been instructed to attend to its location. Such "saliency maps" are an integral feature of the attention models of Koch and Ullman (1985) and Treisman and her colleagues (Treisman and Souther 1985;

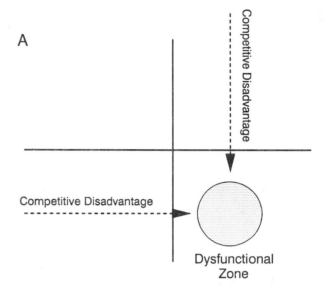

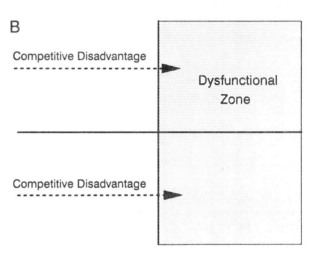

Figure 6. Competition within the attentional control system. (*A*) A dysfunction in one small portion of the visual field will put that point at a competitive disadvantage to all other points, within both hemifields. (*B*) A dysfunction that affects a complete visual hemifield will not put points within that hemifield at a disadvantage relative to one another. It will only put them at a disadvantage relative to points in the opposite hemifield.

Triesman 1986, 1988), among others. In fact, Koch and Ullman (1985) specifically propose that the saliency map contains a "winner-take-all" competitive network. Both the anatomical substrate of this map and the mechanism by which activity in the map affects sensory processing are at issue. Koch and Ullman (1985) speculate that the map may actually be located in the lateral geniculate nucleus, and Treisman (1988) has also recently speculated that the map may exist either before or after striate cortex.

On the basis of our work, we propose that there is no single saliency map in the attentional control system, but rather a series of maps (or possibly a distributed map), which are closely associated with the oculomotor system. Stimuli located at the point in space that is the winner of the competition within the attentional control system will be processed preferentially in extrastriate cortex. If a point is put at a competitive disadvantage to other points as a result of dysfunction (e.g., a lesion or deactivation) in one of the attention control structures, then that point will lose the competition to any other visually stimulated points (i.e., distractors) outside the dysfunctional zone. In our colliculus study, our local deactivation put a single point in the visual field at a competitive disadvantage to every other point, and thus we found impairments when a distractor was located anywhere within the field. However, according to the competition model, if there are no distractors, there is no competition, and the target will always win control over attention. This would explain why neither pulvinar nor colliculus lesions had much effect when the visual field was empty except for the target. In fact, our neurophysiological results in V4 and IT cortex raise the question of whether attention is even *required* when there is only a single target in the visual field.

Why did we find an impairment in the pulvinar study only when the target and distractor were located in opposite fields? According to the model, this came about because our pulvinar deactivation affected the complete contralateral visual field representation in the pulvinar, putting the entire contralateral hemifield at a competitive disadvantage to the ipsilateral hemifield within the remainder of the attentional control system. This would explain why distractors in the ipsilateral visual field were so disruptive. In contrast, no point within the contralateral field was at a competitive disadvantage to any other point in the contralateral field. Thus, when target and distractor both appeared within the contralateral field, the target was able to win the competition within the remainder of the attentional control system, explaining why we found little or no impairment following the pulvinar deactivation in this situation. The model predicts that we will find an impairment with a contralateral target and distractor if we confine our deactivation to a single small zone in the contralateral field representation, as we did in our colliculus study. This prediction remains to be tested in the pulvinar.

A competition model raises the obvious question of whether a lesion or dysfunction in any portion of the visual system might lead to an attentional impairment similar to that seen following lesions in the "attentional control" system. We do not have any results from local deactivation in visual cortex, but we have tested the effects of a local lesion in area V4 on an animal's ability to discriminate a target in the presence of a distractor. Although the animal was, as expected, impaired on both color and form discriminations when the discriminanda were confined to the visuotopic locus of the lesion (Desimone et al. 1990), we did not find any worsening of the deficit when there was a distractor in the visual field (R. Desimone et al., unpubl.). Although the results are not conclusive, since the animal might have recovered from an attentional impairment before we conducted our test, they are suggestive that

competition for spatially directed attention is confined to an attentional control system and does not extend to structures that are the *recipients* of attentional control.

Competition models provide a broad framework for understanding the results of neurophysiological and behavioral studies of attention. They do not specify the mechanism by which the responses of extrastriate neurons are modulated by attention. At present, it is still not even clear whether there is one or multiple proximal sources of attentional control signals to extrastriate cortex, or whether the pulvinar is, in fact, one of the proximal sources. Working out the wiring diagram for attention will be an interesting challenge.

ACKNOWLEDGMENTS

We gratefully acknowledge the advice and support of Mortimer Mishkin during all phases of the studies. Leslie Ungerleider made valuable comments on an earlier version of the manuscript, and Thelma Galkin helped in its preparation. This work was supported in part by Office of Naval Research contract N-00014-87K-0397 to W.S.

REFERENCES

Albano, J.E., M. Mishkin, L.E. Westbrook, and R.H. Wurtz. 1982. Visuomotor deficits following ablation of monkey superior colliculus. *J. Neurophysiol.* **48:** 338.

Bender, D.B. 1981. Retinotopic organization of macaque pulvinar. *J. Neurophysiol.* **46:** 672.

Benevento, L.A. and B. Davis. 1977. Topographical projections of the prestriate cortex to the pulvinar nuclei in the macaque monkey: An autoradiographic study. *Exp. Brain Res.* **30:** 405.

Benevento, L.A. and M. Rezak. 1976. The cortical projections of the inferior pulvinar and adjacent lateral pulvinar in the rhesus monkey (*Macaca mulatta*): An autoradiographic study. *Brain Res.* **108:** 1.

Bergen J.R. and B. Julesz. 1983. Rapid discrimination of visual patterns. *IEEE Trans. Sys. Man Cybernet.* **13:** 857.

Boussaoud, D., L.G. Ungerleider, and R. Desimone. 1990. Pathways for motion analysis: Cortical connections of the medial superior temporal and fundus of the superior temporal visual areas in the macaque. *J. Comp. Neurol.* **296:** 462.

Crick, F. 1984. The function of the thalamic reticular complex: The searchlight hypothesis. *Proc. Natl. Acad. Sci.* **81:** 4586.

Desimone R. and C.G. Gross. 1979. Visual areas in the temporal cortex of the macaque. *Brain Res.* **178:** 363.

Desimone, R. and S.J. Schein. 1987. Visual properties of neurons in area V4 of the macaque: Sensitivity to stimulus form. *J. Neurophysiol.* **57:** 835.

Desimone, R. and L.G. Ungerleider. 1989. Neural mechanisms of visual processing in monkeys. In *Handbook of neuropsychology* (ed. F. Boller and J. Grafman), vol. II, p. 267. Elsevier, Amsterdam.

Desimone, R., T.D. Albright, C.G. Gross, and C. Bruce. 1984. Stimulus selective properties of inferior temporal neurons in the macaque. *J. Neurosci.* **4:** 2051.

Desimone, R., S.J. Schein, J. Moran, and L.G. Ungerleider. 1985. Contour, color and shape analysis beyond the striate cortex. *Vision Res.* **25:** 441.

Desimone, R., M. Wessinger, L. Thomas, and W. Schneider. 1989. Effects of deactivation of lateral pulvinar or superior colliculus on the ability to selectively attend to a visual stimulus. *Soc. Neurosci. Abstr.* **15:** 162.

Desimone, R., L. Li, S. Lehky, L.G. Ungerleider, and M. Mishkin. 1990. Effects of V4 lesions on visual discrimination and on responses of neurons in inferior temporal cortex. *Soc. Neurosci. Abstr.* **16:** (in press).

Dow, B.M., A.Z. Snyder, R.G. Vautin, and R. Bauer. 1981. Magnification factor and receptive field size in foveal striate cortex of the monkey. *Exp. Brain Res.* **44:** 213.

Goldberg, M.E. and C.L. Colby. 1989. The neurophysiology of spatial vision. In *Handbook of neuropsychology* (ed. F. Boller and J. Grafman), vol. II, p. 267. Elsevier, Amsterdam.

Gross C.G. and M. Mishkin. 1977. The neural basis of stimulus equivalence across retinal translation. In *Lateralization in the nervous system* (ed. S. Harnad et al.), p. 109. Academic Press, New York.

Hikosaka, O. and R.H. Wurtz. 1986. Saccadic eye movements following injection of lidocaine into the superior colliculus. *Exp. Brain Res.* **61:** 531.

Hinton, G.E., J.L. McClelland, and D.E. Rumelhart. 1986. Distributed representations. In *Parallel distributed processing* (ed. D.E. Rumelhart et al.), p. 77. MIT Press, Cambridge, Massachusetts.

Julesz, B. 1981. Textons, the elements of texture perception, and their interactions. *Nature* **290:** 91.

Kahneman, D. 1973. *Attention and effort.* Prentice-Hall, Englewood Cliffs, New Jersey. Kertzman, C. and D.L. Robinson. 1988. Contributions of the superior colliculus of the monkey to visual spatial attention. *Soc. Neurosci. Abstr.* **14:** 831.

Koch, C. and S. Ullman. 1985. Shifts in selective visual attention: Towards the underlying neural circuitry. *Hum. Neurobiol.* **4:** 219.

LaBerge, D. and M.S. Buchsbaum. 1990. Positron emission tomographic measurements of pulvinar activity during an attention task. *J. Neurosci.* **10:** 613.

Matelli, M., M.F. Oliviere, A. Saccani, and G. Rizzolatti. 1983. Upper visual space neglect and motor deficits after section of the midbrain commissures in the cat. *Behav. Brain Res.* **10:** 263.

Maunsell, J.H.R. and W.T. Newsome. 1987. Visual processing in monkey extrastriate cortex. *Annu. Rev. Neurosci.* **10:** 363.

Moran, J. and R. Desimone. 1985. Selective attention gates visual processing in the extrastriate cortex. *Science* **229:** 782.

Mountcastle, V.B., B.C. Motter, M.A. Steinmetz, and A.K. Sestokas. 1987. Common and differential effects of attentive fixation on the excitability of parietal and prestriate (V4) cortical visual neurons in the macaque monkey. *J. Neurosci.* **7:** 2239.

Petersen, S.E., D.L. Robinson, and W. Keys. 1985. Pulvinar nuclei of the behaving rhesus monkey: Visual responses and their modulation. *J. Neurophysiol.* **54:** 867.

Petersen, S., D.L. Robinson, and J.D. Morris. 1987. Contributions of the pulvinar to visual spatial attention. *Neuropsychologia* **25:** 97.

Posner, M.I. and D.E. Presti. 1987. Selective attention and cognitive control. *Trends Neurosci.* **10:** 13.

Posner, M.I., J.A. Walker, F.J. Friedrich, and R.D. Rafal. 1984. Effects of parietal lobe injury on covert orienting of visual attention. *J. Neurosci.* **4:** 1863.

———. 1987. How do the parietal lobes direct covert attention? *Neuropsychologia* **25:** 135.

Rafal, R.D. and M.I. Posner. 1987. Deficits in human visual spatial attention following thalamic lesions. *Proc. Natl. Acad. Sci.* **84:** 7349.

Richmond, B.J. and T. Sato. 1987. Enhancement of inferior temporal neurons during visual discrimination. *J. Neurophysiol.* **6:** 1292.

Rizzolatti, G. 1983. Mechanisms of selective attention in mammals. In *Advances in vertebrate Neuroethology* (ed. J.-P. Ewert et al.), p. 261. Plenum Press, London.

Robinson, D.L., S.E. Petersen, and W. Keys. 1986. Saccade-related and visual activities in the pulvinar nuclei of the behaving rhesus monkey. *Exp. Brain Res.* **62:** 625.

Schiller, P.H., S.D. True, and J.L. Conway. 1979. Effects of frontal eye field and superior colliculus ablations on eye movements. *Science* **206:** 590.

Schwartz, E.L., R. Desimone, T.D. Albright, and C.G. Gross. 1983. Shape recognition and inferior temporal neurons. *Proc. Natl. Acad. Sci.* **80:** 5776.

Spitzer, H. and B.J. Richmond. 1990. Task difficulty: Ignoring, attending to, and discriminating a visual stimulus yield progressively more activity in inferior temporal neurons. *Exp. Brain Res.* (in press).

Spitzer, H., R. Desimone, and J. Moran. 1988. Increased attention enhances both behavioral and neuronal performance. *Science* **240:** 338.

Treisman, A. 1986. Features and objects in visual processing. *Sci. Am.* **225:** 114B.

———. 1988. Features and objects: The Fourteenth Bartlett Memorial Lecture. *Q. J. Exp. Psychol.* **40A:** 201.

Treisman, A. and J. Souther. 1985. Search asymmetry: A diagnostic for preattentive processing of separable features. *J. Exp. Psychol.* **114:** 285.

Ungerleider, L.G. and C.A. Christensen. 1979. Pulvinar lesions in monkeys produce abnormal scanning of a complex visual array. *Neuropsychologia* **17:** 493.

Ungerleider, L.G. and M. Mishkin. 1982. Two cortical visual systems. In *Analysis of visual behavior* (ed. D.J. Ingle et al.), p. 549. MIT Press, Cambridge, Massachusetts.

Ungerleider, L.G., T.W. Galkin, and M. Mishkin. 1983. Visuotopic organization of projections from striate cortex to inferior and lateral pulvinar in rhesus monkey. *J. Comp. Neurol.* **217:** 137.

Ungerleider, L.G., R. Desimone, T.W. Galkin, and M. Mishkin. 1984. Subcortical projections of area MT in the macaque. *J. Comp. Neurol.* **223:** 368.

Van Essen, D.C. 1985. Functional organization of primate visual cortex. In *Cerebral Cortex* (ed. E.G. Jones and A.A. Peters), vol. 3, p. 259. Plenum Press, New York.

von der Heydt, R., E. Peterhans, and G. Baumgartner. 1984. Illusory contours and cortical neuron responses. *Science* **224:** 1260.

Wurtz, R.H. and J.E. Albano. 1980. Visual-motor function of the primate superior colliculus. *Annu. Rev. Neurosci.* **3:** 189.

Early Vision Is Bottom-up, Except for Focal Attention

B. JULESZ

Laboratory of Vision Research, Psychology Department, Rutgers University, New Brunswick, New Jersey 08903
and Division of Biology, California Institute of Technology, Pasadena, California 91125

It is the 30-year anniversary of the introduction of computer-generated random-dot stereograms and cinematograms in psychology (Julesz 1960). These stimuli, together with texture pairs with identical second-order statistics (Julesz 1962), are devoid of all familiarity cues and are briefly presented (followed by a mask), yet yield vivid depth, motion, and preattentive texture discrimination, respectively. This demonstrates that these perceptual processes must operate at an early stage in the central nervous system (CNS). Only in recent years was it established by Gian Poggio (1984) that global stereopsis (of dynamic random-dot stereograms) is extracted as early as layer IVB in V1, i.e., at the very input of the monkey cortex. Therefore, what I called originally "cyclopean" vision, I am now calling "early" vision. Only recently did it also become apparent that these early visual processes are independent of top-down processes based on semantic memory. Some of these findings will be demonstrated and discussed, particularly depth from shading and asymmetry of texture discrimination, which until now were assumed to be based on semantics. The latter can be explained by perceptual closure of gaps due to subjective contours (Williams and Julesz 1990), and these subjective contours are extracted by special neural units in V2 as shown by von der Heydt et al. (1988). This independence from semantics makes some perceptual phenomena of early vision amenable to direct linkage to neurophysiological feature extractors, as revealed by single microelectrode recordings in V1, V2, V3, V4, and middle temporal (MT) areas. Whereas these "cognitively impenetrable modules" (an expression of Jerry Fodor [1983]) seem too limited to account for the rich phenomena of cognitive psychology, I will show that by evoking the mechanism of focal attention, it is possible to extend the scope of early vision. Indeed, with my collaborators and others, we were able to measure the aperture size and scanning rate of focal attention and determine some of the stimulus features that capture it, without having to study the enigmatic factors based on personal preferences and memory. Particularly important are the neurophysiological findings by Robert Desimone and his collaborators, who found receptive fields as early as V4 for which feature extraction properties change with the attentional state of the monkey. Since my criterion of "science" is to be able to derive phenomena at level i (psychology) by interactions at level (i-1) (neurophysiology), it is most encouraging that the study of early vision became a scientific en-

terprise. It is also promising that these processes of early vision are now intensively studied by mathematical model builders, thus linking psychology, neurophysiology, and neuroanatomy to the emerging field of machine vision.

Some of us who witnessed the miraculous growth of human psychology and monkey neurophysiology of visual perception in the last 30 years are still skeptical of the maturity of our field. It is most likely that brain research is still at the stage where physics was prior to Galileo or where monocular biology was prior to the discovery of the DNA double helix by Watson and Crick. Because of this, there is no consensus in brain research of what a real strategic problem might be, and my own views are probably as good as those of others, although each of us believes in his own paradigm.

My definition of *science*, particularly of a *scientific psychology*, is influenced by thermodynamics. There one is able to define phenomena, such as temperature, pressure, entropy, and enthalpy, that can be experienced at *level i* by interactions on a lower *level (i-1)* between molecules or atoms that merely collide with each other according to the well-known physical laws of mechanics. It is my belief that psychology (at level i) should be able to derive its mental phenomena, such as the percepts of depth, motion, and texture segregation, by the excitatory and inhibitory interactions of neurons, or pools of neurons, in the CNS, which I regard as a level (i-1) description. Of course, since the CNS of monkey and man are many orders of magnitude more complex than molecules, this quest cannot be strictly carried out at present.

Let me illustrate this by the oldest area of psychology: color perception. It started with George Palmer, who stated his trichromacy theory of color perception in 1777, which was later rediscovered by Thomas Young in 1802 (whose publications are reprinted in a historical collection by MacAdam 1970). The opponent-color theory of Hering (1878), the first perceptual model of how basic color channels interact, is also very old, even if only recently was the existence of these opponent-color channels hinted at by indirect neurophysiological evidence (Gouras 1970; DeValois 1973). Further linking between psychophysical color phenomena, including the retinex theory of Land (1986) and neurophysiological findings in V4 of the monkey cortex by Zeki (1980), illustrates an ever-increasing trend to explain mental phenomena by the activity of cortical neurons and their interactions. Most of this work on color perception does not study color per se, but rather conditions under which metameric color matches can be obtained, thus constituting a highly simplified subset of color perception.

Here I briefly discuss how this conceptual approach has been extended in the last three decades to link mental phenomena of stereoscopic depth (stereopsis) and preattentive texture discrimination to neurophysiological findings in V1, V2, V3, and V4. It started with the introduction of computer-generated random-dot stereograms (RDS) and random-dot cinematograms (RDC) into psychology (Julesz 1960), together with computer-generated texture pairs having controlled geometrical and statistical properties (Julesz 1962). Because motion perception cannot be demonstrated on the printed page, I will not discuss the great progress in trying to link motion perception with neurophysiological findings in the early cortical areas in the monkey, including MT.

In essence, computer-generated stimuli with controlled mathematical and statistical properties, but devoid of all cues except a few to be studied, simplify the study of perceptual phenomena and make it amenable for direct linking to neurophysiological phenomena. In my youth, I thought that artificial intelligence (AI) models would be the appropriate level (i-1) to account for perceptual findings; however, in the few cases when such models were proposed (particularly for stereopsis), these models were too robust and work well even though they were based on diametrically opposed principles. For example, David Marr and Tomy Poggio have had a cooperative and a noncooperative model of stereopsis published in brief succession (Marr and Poggio 1976, 1979), which can cope with RDS rather well. Grimson (1981) even wrote a monograph on the noncooperative model. However, it has been shown by Mayhew and Frisby (1979) and Mowforth et al. (1981), among others, that the noncooperative model of Marr and Poggio (based on convergence eye movements bringing into alignment spatial-frequency [SF]-tuned channels of ever increasing bandwidth) is not used in human stereopsis. These psychologists have shown that high SF RDS with low and medium SF filtered out can still elicit large disparity convergence eye movements and yield fusion when presented in a brief flash. Thus, only psychophysical experiments and neurophysiological facts can weed out the possible ones from among the many AI models.

GLOBAL STEREOPSIS

Above I alluded to the fact that there is no consensus of what might be a strategic question in psychobiology, and each researcher has his or her preferred problem. In my view, a basic problem of vision is how to reconstruct from two two-dimensional projections cast on the retinae the best three-dimensional percept of the environment. Can this be done in the absence of the enigmatic familiarity and Gestalt cues? The invention of the computer-generated RDS and RDC (Julesz

1960) answered the second question in the affirmative and transformed the first question into a simpler one: How are binocular images matched and false targets eliminated (as illustrated in Fig. 1)? Indeed, the false-target problem of stereopsis (Julesz 1971) initiated a hectic research activity. For a detailed review, see Julesz (1986) in the 25th Anniversary Issue of *Vision Research*.

Of the many models that try to eliminate false targets, I prefer the cooperative ones, the more so since with Jih Jie Chang, we showed that global stereopsis is a cooperative phenomenon exhibiting multiple stable states, disorder-order transitions, and hysteresis (Julesz and Chang 1976).

Space does not permit me to discuss these models. The main feature of all these models is based on some global process, similar to cross-correlation between left and right areas of similar binocular disparities. In essence, such correlation is much simpler than form recognition, which was believed to underlie binocular pattern matching prior to 1960. So, the main insight obtained by the fusion of RDS, particularly that they can be fused in 60 msec (Julesz and Chang 1976), is that stereopsis must occur at a rather early stage. My view of the CNS is schematically portrayed by Figure 2. Here, bottom-up and top-down processings are taking place simultaneously, and it appears that stereopsis would occur at an early bottom-up stage. Even so, it was a great event in my scientific life when Gian Poggio (1984) found units in layer IVB of V1 in the monkey cortex that fired for dynamic RDS. Since these stimuli consisted of stereo pairs uncorrelated in successive frames and presented at 100 frames/sec, there was no monocular luminance gradient between corresponding left and right image. It seems certain that these neurons extracted binocular disparities of correlated areas. That

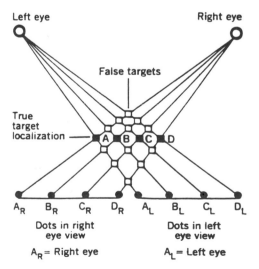

Figure 1. Binocular matching, or the problem of false-target elimination. Of the 4 identical targets (dots), there are 16 possible localizations, out of which only 4 are correct. Without monocular labeling, only some global constraints can eliminate the false matches. (Reprinted, with permission, from Julesz 1971.)

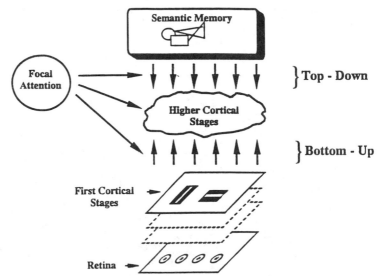

Figure 2. Bottom-up vs. top-down processes in the visual system, and focal attention. (Modified from Julesz 1990.)

global stereopsis can occur at the very input stage of the cortex was an unexpected confirmation of the psychophysical predictions of cyclopean perception research (using RDS). In recent years I renamed "cyclopean perception" as "global stereopsis of early vision."

THE LIMITED ROLE OF TOP-DOWN PROCESSES

The essence of the technique of RDS is to present dynamic noise devoid of the many semantic cues that are processed by top-down stages. Furthermore, these stimuli are presented briefly, followed by a mask, to assure that the top-down stream cannot reach the stimulus. Because of all these precautions, one might argue that research with RDS might study visual perception under unnatural conditions, and the higher cognitive processes might still have a role in more natural conditions.

Of course, many of our mental processes are so rich because of memory and symbolic logic, which together with focal attention, are intermeshed with the bottom-up processes. Nevertheless, I can demonstrate that most of the phenomena of stereopsis, motion perception, and texture discrimination are carried out by bottom-up processes, and the higher cognitive processes, except for focal attention, have limited roles, if any.

For instance, monocular depth from shading, such as seeing egg crates (and craters on the Moon) as either convex or concave, depending on whether the illumination is from above or below, might be construed as a top-down phenomenon interfering with bottom-up processes. Indeed, Ramachandran (1988) exploited this phenomenon in his study of apparent motion perception and suggested that this "shape from shading" process operates prior to motion perception. The motion perception Ramachandran studies is of the "long-range" kind that often disambiguates false matches by higher-order top-down processes, yet it is interesting

whether the bottom-up processes of "short-range" motion perception, and particularly stereopsis, are also influenced by shape-from-shading. After all, this egg-crate phenomenon must be of a high-level kind, based on the fact that Earth has only *one* sun that shines from *above*. If global stereopsis were to utilize such a complex top-down process, based on either some learned or genetically inherited information, we would have a counterexample of global stereopsis being based on early visual processing alone. To test this "counterexample" with Jih Jie Chang, we constructed a randomly speckled egg-crate pair portraying the convex (or concave) depth from shading phenomenon when monocularly viewed (see Fig. 3). However, 30% of the egg-crate pair is speckled by a RDS with crossed disparity (if reader views the stereogram binocularly with crossed eyes). Depending on whether the reader views these figures right-side-up or up-side-down, it becomes apparent that the convex shape portrayed by stereopsis will dominate depth-from-shading. Several variations of these experiments, including ambiguous RDS, demonstrate that the monocular cue of depth-from-shading is rather weak and does not influence global stereopsis (Chang and Julesz 1990).

In summary, it is most likely that global stereopsis is mediated by early visual processes without top-down influences. It is, in the usage of Jerry Fodor (1983), a "cognitively impenetrable module."

TEXTURE DISCRIMINATION AND FOCAL ATTENTION

In my youth, I posed a second paradigm: the preattentive texture discrimination of iso-second-order texture pairs (Julesz 1962). For an up-to-date review, see Julesz (1984). The essence of the findings is shown in Figure 4. The textures are composed of orthogonal line segments forming Ls, Ts, and Xs; however, only the Xs pop out from the aggregate of Ls, whereas the Ts among the Ls can be only found after an element-by-

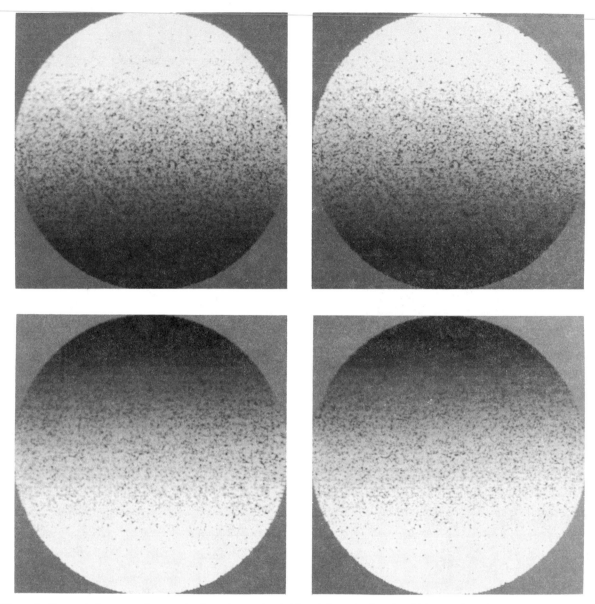

Figure 3. Monocularly convex (concave) sphere due to depth (shape) from shading, in which a random-dot stereogram (RDS) is mixed. When binocularly fused, depth from stereopsis dominates perceived depth. (*Top*) The RDS has crossed binocular disparity. (*Bottom*) The RDS has uncrossed binocular disparity. (Reprinted, with permission, from Chang and Julesz 1990.)

element scrutiny. I regard the effortless pop-out a parallel preattentive process that does not depend on the element size, whereas scrutiny is a serial time-consuming process that depends on the element size and requires focal attention.

This dichotomy of visual perception of preattentive/attentive processing is of great explanatory power, at least for texture segregation. As we have shown (Sagi and Julesz 1987), texture gradients pop out only if the element density is above a critical value. Even then, one can only tell the locations of the gradients in a brief flash (e.g., where are the horizontal or vertical line segments in diagonal ones), but identifying them (i.e., that they are actually horizontal or vertical) requires scrutiny by focal attention that depends on the number of the texture gradients (Sagi and Julesz 1985). We also determined the aperture of focal attention that increases with eccentricity (Sagi and Julesz 1986). Particularly interesting is the rate of speed with which focal attention can scan the items without eye movements. Although evidence is indirect, based on some models in which the experimental results are interpreted, the "searchlight of attention" scans rapidly about 30–60 msec/item (Treisman and Gelade 1980; Bergen and Julesz 1983; Weichselgartner and Sperling 1987). Obviously, this rate depends on the visibility of the texture gradients, and some parallel mechanism seems to facilitate serial search (Kröse and Julesz 1989). To find the neurophysiological mechanism of this "searchlight" and how this searchlight "glues together" in exact

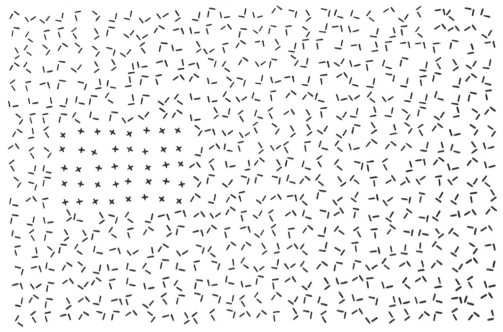

Figure 4. Preattentive (parallel) texture discrimination vs. serial scrutiny by focal attention. The Xs among the Ls pop out effortlessly, but finding the Ts among the Ls requires element-by-element search. (Reprinted, with permission, from Julesz and Bergen 1983.)

alignment various feature (texton) pools appears to me another strategic question of brain research.

Years ago, we showed (Julesz and Bergen 1983) how texture pairs with identical third-order statistics could be segregated by some linear spatial filter (Kuffler unit) followed by a nonlinear stage. That a nonlinear stage is essential can be easily demonstrated (Williams and Julesz 1990), as shown in Figure 5. As is apparent, adding to a strongly discriminable texture pair a homogeneous array of small Ls renders the sum indiscriminable, thus the law of superposition (a fundamental requirement for linearity) is flagrantly violated.

Despite the first successes of spatial filters to automatically segregate textures, until recently I was skeptical that such simple bottom-up processing could be adequate. My initial pessimism was based on the curious asymmetries of texture discrimination. For example, circles with a gap embedded into an array of intact circles pop out less than vice versa. This asymmetry seemed ominous, since it appeared that some complex figure-ground phenomenon might be at play. With Doug Williams, however, we found that the closure of gaps by subjective contours can account for such asymmetries (Williams and Julesz 1990). Since von der

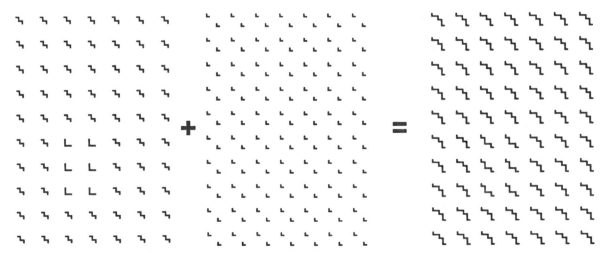

Figure 5. Demonstration of the nonlinearity of human texture discrimination. When to the highly discriminable texture pair (*left array*) a uniform, nondiscriminable array of small Ls (*middle array*) is added, a nondiscriminable texture pair (*right array*) is obtained. Thus, the law of superposition is violated. (Reprinted, with permission, from Williams and Julesz 1990.)

Heydt et al. (1988) found neural units in V2 of the monkey cortex that fire for subjective contours, I am now confident that many of the asymmetric texture discrimination phenomena can be explained by bottom-up processes. Indeed, recently Fogel and Sagi (1989) and Malik and Perona (1990), using Gabor filters followed by a nonlinear stage, have achieved machine segmentation in agreement with the psychophysical findings of Kröse (1987). The two models are not similar. The latter authors use lateral inhibition in their nonlinear stage, whereas the former authors have a second stage of spatial filters for segmentation after the nonlinear stage. More recently, Rubinstein and Sagi (1989) showed that their models exhibit segmentation asymmetries due to asymmetries in signal/noise characteristics of their filters and can explain the many asymmetrical texture discrimination findings of human observers obtained by Gurnsey and Browse (1987).

CONCLUSION

In this brief review, I have shown how successful the cyclopean perception paradigm was during 30 years and how it helped to link human perception of depth, motion, and texture discrimination with neurophysiological evidence obtained in the early stages of the monkey cortex. This joint field is now called *early vision*. I have also illustrated that early vision is essentially bottom-up and the enigmatic top-down processes have little influence. There is, however, an additional process that has to be evoked to understand visual perception: *focal attention*. Luckily, focal attention, although sharing several properties of consciousness, can now be studied experimentally by psychologists, and as the exciting studies of Robert Desimone and his collaborators (Moran and Desimone 1985), among others, show, can be successfully studied by the neurophysiologists.

REFERENCES

Bergen, J.R and B. Julesz. 1983. Parallel versus serial processing in rapid pattern discrimination. *Nature* **303:** 696.

Chang, J.J. and B. Julesz. 1990. Low-level processing of disparity-tuned binocular neurons takes precedence of shape from shading. *Invest. Ophthalmol. Visual Sci.* **31:** 525.

DeValois, R.L. 1973. Central mechanisms of color vision. In *Handbook of sensory physiology* (ed. R. Jung), vol. 7, p. 209. Springer, Berlin.

Fodor, J. 1983. *Modularity of mind.* MIT Press, Cambridge.

Fogel, I. and D. Sagi. 1989. Gabor filters as texture discriminators. *Biol. Cybern.* **61:** 103.

Gouras, P. 1970. Trichromatic mechanisms in single cortical neurons. *Science* **169:** 489.

Gurnsey, R. and R. Browse. 1987. Micropattern properties and presentation conditions influencing visual texture discrimination. *Percept. Psychophys.* **41:** 239.

Hering, E. 1878. *Zur Lehre vom Lichtsinn.* Gerold's Sohn, Vienna.

Julesz, B. 1960. Binocular depth perception of computer-generated patterns. *Bell Syst. Tech. J.* **39:** 1125.

———. 1962. Visual pattern discrimination. *IRE Trans. Info. Theory* **IT-8:** 84.

———. 1971. *Foundations of cyclopean perception.* University of Chicago Press, Illinois.

———. 1984. Toward an axiomatic theory of preattentive vision. In *Dynamic aspects of neocortical function* (ed. G.M. Edelman et al.), p. 585. Wiley, New York.

———. 1986. Stereoscopic vision. *Vision Res.* **26:** 1601.

———. 1990. Concepts in early vision. In *Synergetics in cognition* (ed. H. Haken and M. Stadler), p. 218. Springer Verlag, Berlin.

Julesz, B. and J.R. Bergen. 1983. Textons, the fundamental elements in preattentive vision and perception of textures. *Bell Syst. Tech. J.* **62:** 1619.

Julesz, B. and J.J. Chang. 1976. Interaction between pools of binocular disparity detectors tuned to different disparities. *Biol Cybern.* **22:** 107.

Kröse, B.J.A. 1987. Local structure analysers as determinants of preattentive pattern discrimination. *Biol. Cybern.* **55:** 289.

Kröse, B.J.A. and B. Julesz. 1989. The control and speed of shifts of attention. *Vision Res.* **29:** 1607.

Land, E.H. 1986. Recent advances in retinex theory. *Vision Res.* **26:** 7.

MacAdam, D.L. 1970. *Sources of color science.* MIT Press, Cambridge.

Malik, J. and P. Perona. 1990. Preattentive texture discrimination with early vision mechanisms. *J. Opt. Soc. Am.* **7:** 923.

Marr, D. and T. Poggio. 1976. Cooperative computation of stereo disparity. *Science* **194:** 283.

———. 1979. A theory of human stereopsis. *Proc. R. Soc. Lond. B.* **204:** 301.

Mayhew, J.E.W. and J.P. Frisby. 1979. Convergent disparity discriminations in narrow-band-filtered random-dot stereograms. *Vision Res.* **19:** 63.

Moran, T. and R. Desimone. 1985. Selective attention gates: Visual processing in the extrastriate cortex. *Science* **229:** 782.

Mowforth, P., J.E.W. Mayhew, and J.P. Frisby. 1981. Vergence eye movements made in response to spatial-frequency-filtered random-dot stereograms. *Perception* **10:** 299.

Poggio, G. 1984. Processing of stereoscopic information in primate visual cortex. In *Dynamic aspects of neocortical function* (ed. G.M. Edelman et al.), p. 613. Wiley, New York.

Ramachandran, V.S. 1988. Perception of shape from shading. *Nature* **331:** 163.

Rubinstein, B. and D. Sagi. 1989. Texture variability across the orientation spectrum can yield asymmetry in texture discrimination. *Perception* **18:** 517.

Sagi, D. and B. Julesz. 1985. "Where" and "what" in vision. *Science* **228:** 1217.

———. 1986. Enhanced detection in the aperture of focal attention during simple discrimination tasks. *Nature* **321:** 693.

———. 1987. Short-range limitation on detection of feature differences. *Spat. Vision* **2:** 39.

Treisman, A. and G. Gelade. 1980. A feature-integration theory of attention. *Cognit. Psychol.* **12:** 97.

von der Heydt, R., E. Peterhans, and G. Baumgartner. 1988. Illusory contours and cortical neuron responses. *Science* **224:** 1260.

Weichselgartner, E. and G. Sperling. 1987. Dynamics of automatic and controlled visual attention. *Science* **238:** 778.

Williams, D. and B. Julesz. 1990. On the asymmetries of preattentive texture discrimination. In *Neural networks for human and machine perception* (ed. H. Wechsler). Academic Press, Orlando, Florida.

Zeki, S.M. 1980. The representation of color in the cerebral cortex. *Nature* **284:** 412.

Cytochrome Oxidase and Functional Coding in Primate Striate Cortex: A Hypothesis

J. ALLMAN* AND S. ZUCKER†

*Division of Biology, California Institute of Technology, Pasadena, California 91125;
†Department of Electrical Engineering and the Canadian Institute for Advanced Research, McGill University,
Montreal, Quebec, Canada H3A 2A7

In 1978, Margaret Wong-Riley stained sections of squirrel monkey striate cortex for the activity of the mitochondrial enzyme, cytochrome oxidase, and noticed a periodic distribution of "puffs" of increased enzyme activity in layers 2 and 3 (letter to D. Hubel cited in Livingstone and Hubel [1984]). Her discovery anticipated a whole series of anatomical and physiological findings from many laboratories that correlated with the distribution of this enzyme in the striate cortex of primates, yet there has never been a satisfactory explanation as to why the distribution of this enzyme, crucial for aerobic energy metabolism, would be related to the functional organization of visual cortex (Martin 1988). The puffs have also been called blobs, spots, dots, and patches, with the term blob used most frequently.

When the striate cortex is viewed from above, the blobs form a periodic array intercalated within a lattice of lower cytochrome oxidase concentration. We propose that the distinction between the blobs and the lattice is related to two different modes for representing stimulus variables. We submit that *scalar* variables related to the *intensity* of the stimulus are represented in the blobs. Intensity information is encoded explicitly over a very broad dynamic range, in which activity is proportional to the intensity variable (e.g., contrast). This encoding strategy requires that neurons have the energetic capacity to sustain a broad range of activity levels, which in turn is related to the high concentration of cytochrome oxidase. The situation is analogous to red muscle, which also is rich in cytochrome oxidase and which is able to maintain a sustained level of contraction over time (Needham 1971).

We propose that in the surrounding lattice of lower cytochrome oxidase concentration, *geometric* variables are carried by neurons with orientation preferences and lead to different representational requirements. Each stimulus orientation is possible at every retinotopic location, and each is represented explicitly within an orientation hypercolumn. Activity varies with how well each individual orientation *matches* image structure at that location. However, there is rarely more than one orientation at any retinotopic location, so, on average, most oriented cells in each hypercolumn are quiet. The preference of these neurons for higher spatial frequencies (and possibly binocular disparities) further reduces the statistical probability that they will be active at any particular instant in time. The average level

of neural activity over time is thus much less in the lattice than in the blobs, which is consistent with the lower levels of cytochrome oxidase in the lattice. There is an analogy with white muscle, which contains less cytochrome oxidase and typically has short bouts of rapid contraction interspersed with longer resting periods.

We review the main empirical findings that have led us to this hypothesis. Tootell et al. (1988b) showed that the blobs were preferentially responsive to low spatial frequency gratings, whereas the lattice preferred higher spatial frequencies in experiments in which the functional activity of macaque monkey striate cortex was mapped with 2-deoxyglucose autoradiography. Silverman et al. (1989) found a strong negative correlation between cytochrome oxidase concentration and spatial frequency preference in electrophysiological recording experiments. Probably related to the spatial frequency organization of the blobs and the intervening lattice is the observation of Livingstone and Hubel (1984) that blob neurons tend to be much less sensitive to the orientation of elongated stimuli than are neurons in the lattice.

Livingstone and Hubel (1984) also noted that many neurons in the blobs were preferentially activated by stimulus color, and they found "double-opponent" color cells in the blobs. Tootell et al. (1988a) found that the blobs were more activated by colored stimuli than by gray stimuli of equal luminance. However, there are comparative data which suggest that the blobs have important functions that transcend color vision. Galagos, lorises, and owl monkeys, which are nocturnal primates[1] and therefore live in dim lighting conditions in which color vision is virtually impossible, nevertheless have well-developed cytochrome oxidase

---

[1]Galagos appear to be strictly nocturnal. They become active in the evening twilight at the time that human observers can no longer see color and cease to be active in the morning twilight when humans can just begin to discern color (Martin 1990). Owl monkeys are less strictly nocturnal. The activity cycle in owl monkeys varies in different parts of South America. In Peru, they are nocturnal; in Paraguay, they are active for several hours after sunrise and for several hours before sunset (Wright 1989). In the laboratory, owl monkeys are often active during the day, whereas galagos housed under the same conditions are active only at night (J. Allman, pers. obs.). Jacobs (1977) found that owl monkeys have a weakly developed capacity for color vision. Wikler and Rakic (1989) found that cones, identified immunocytochemically, are relatively abundant in galagos and owl monkeys. Possibly the cones in these nocturnal species serve to regulate daily activity cycles.

blobs (Horton and Hubel 1981; Horton 1984; Tootell et al. 1985; McGuinness et al. 1986; Condo et al. 1987; J. Allman and E. McGuinness, in prep.). There also are two diurnal primates, *Hapalemur griseus* and *Propithecus verrauxi*, that lack blobs, although the color vision capacities of these rare prosimians are unknown (McGuinness et al. 1986; J. Allman and E. McGuinness, in prep.). Blobs also are absent in a diurnal nonprimate with well-developed color vision, the tree shrew (Horton 1984; Jacobs and Neitz 1986; Wong-Riley and Norton 1988).

In macaque monkeys, the blobs are located in the centers of ocular dominance columns (Horton and Hubel 1981; Wong-Riley and Carroll 1984; Blasdel and Salama 1986) and are driven strongly by one eye (T'so and Gilbert 1988). The intervening lattice appears to have more complex binocular interactions. In this context, it is interesting to note that the lattice has higher concentrations of the calcium-binding protein, calbindin (Celio et al. 1986). Calbindin is abundant in neural structures in which precise timing of signals is important, such as the time-dependent pathways in electroreceptive fish (Maler et al. 1984) and the nuclei responsible for interaural time comparisons for sound localization in owls (Takahashi et al. 1987). There is a precise trade-off between spatial and temporal binocular disparity in stereopsis (Burr and Ross 1979); it is an intriguing possibility that the distribution of calbindin in the lattice is related to precise spatial-temporal binocular processing.

Maguire and Baizer (1982) investigated the responses of neurons in striate cortex of awake monkeys to different luminances against a constant background. They found that cells lacking orientation selectivity responded in a graded fashion to as much as 4 log units of variation in luminance from threshold to saturation.[2] At saturation, some of these nonoriented cells reached firing rates of 300 spikes per second, which is remarkably high for cortical neurons. The oriented cells usually responded to about 1 log unit of variation from threshold to saturation. These authors did not localize their recording sites to specific structures within striate cortex, but is it likely that their nonoriented cells were either in layer 4C or in the blobs, whereas their oriented cells were probably in the lattice.

The two styles of coding proposed in our hypothesis are classical, although the application to the blob-lattice system is novel. Intensity coding may be conceptually viewed as the more primitive form and is more commonly described in the brain stem oculomotor system, whereas coding in proportion to strength of match is more commonly described in the cortex (Marr 1970; Barlow 1972; Ballard 1986).

Although the above data indirectly support our hypothesis that cells containing high concentrations of cytochrome oxidase in the blobs are coding intensity variables, and the lattice cells are coding the match between geometric variables and the image, testable predictions do arise. The first series of predictions involve the coding of contrast, and the most direct of these is that, if contrast sensitivity were measured for blob cells, they would have the relationship to lattice cells illustrated in Figure 1. The contrast sensitivity curves that have been measured in striate cortex are for cells with an orientation preference (Sclar et al. 1989) and agree with the prediction for lattice cells; no direct measurements for blob cells have been made to our knowledge.

A second prediction of our hypothesis is that the blob system should exhibit relatively little contrast adaptation or gain control. This differs from the lattice system, which could use contrast adaptation to extend its operating range from dim to bright light. However, if the blob system were to adapt, then the baseline for calibrating contrasts would be lost. Blob cells would resemble lateral geniculate neurons in this regard (Derrington and Lennie 1984).

Third, if the blob system is coding contrast, then how can luminance values be recovered? One possibility is suggested by interpreting the circular surround receptive fields mathematically and then simply adding the responses together from cells spanning a range of receptive field sizes (Zucker and Hummel 1986). This suggests mapping the spatial properties of receptive fields for cells within blobs, and that a range of sizes will be found. The findings of Silverman et al. (1989) are consistent with this suggestion.

Surfaces can not only be covered with paint to give them contrast and color, but they can also be sprinkled with spots. Our next class of predictions are thus related to textures lacking orientation, such as salt-and-pepper patterns. Psychophysical evidence (Barlow 1979) indicates that density is a key property of such patterns, and it is another basic scalar intensity variable. Thus, we predict that the density of unoriented texture patterns is carried by the blob system. Furthermore, it follows that the smearing of textures outside of borders should be no more noticeable than the smear-

---

[2]These neurons might correspond in part to the "luxotonic" cells recorded from striate cortex of the squirrel monkey (Bartlett and Doty 1974) and the macaque (Kayama et al. 1979). The luxotonic cells were defined as having a maintained discharge to diffuse light and/or having a discharge that varied monotonically with change in light intensity over a range of at least 3 log units.

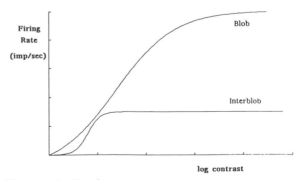

Figure 1. Predicted contrast sensitivity curves for blob and lattice neurons.

ing of color and contrast (for examples, see Livingstone and Hubel 1987). If there is no context provided by the geometric system, and if a class of blob cells represents the density of small spots, then there will be no geometric anchors to hold the dots in place. They would thus be free to drift in position and depth; perhaps this is the basis of the autokinetic effect.

The blobs are reduced following eye removal or tetrodotoxin injection into the linked eye (Wong-Riley and Carroll 1984; Wong-Riley et al. 1989). However, the blobs are not absolutely dependent on visual input. The blobs are present in newborn primates (Horton 1984) and even in monkeys that have had their eyes removed well before birth (Kuljis and Rakic 1990). One possible explanation for this is that a sizable portion of the neurons in the blobs may be very nonselective and respond simply to a graded input encoding contrast, whereas the lattice circuitry requires a precise coincidence of inputs. Thus, the surviving population of neurons in the lateral geniculate nucleus in monkeys with their eyes removed well before birth might be sufficient to provide a tonic drive to the blobs and thus engage their metabolic machinery.

The blob-lattice distinction is not an absolute dichotomy. There is a gradient in the concentration of cytochrome oxidase between the blobs and the lattice (Silverman et al. 1989). Similarly, the blob neurons are not uniform in cytochrome oxidase content (Wong-Riley et al. 1989). In particular, one class of blob neuron (type C) is much richer in cytochrome oxidase. Type C neurons constitute about one quarter of the blob population, and Wong-Riley and her collaborators have suggested that they correspond to the non-color-coded blob neurons that comprise a similar portion of the recording sample for blob neurons (Livingstone and Hubel 1984; T'so and Gilbert 1988). We hypothesize that this cytochrome-oxidase-rich population of blob neurons encodes contrast over a broad dynamic range and serves as the basis for a cortical brightness constancy system. We suspect that cytochrome-oxidase-rich neurons may constitute a larger portion of the blob population in nocturnal species. There is considerable evidence that primates evolved from nocturnal ancestors (Allman 1977), and the blobs may have developed originally as part of a cortical system for brightness constancy in highly visual animals living in a dimly illuminated environment. When primates became diurnal, they may have elaborated this system to encompass the color-specific lightnesses for determining color constancy.

In summary, the blob system is involved in color, contrast, and texture density; in short, in carrying scalar intensity variables. We are suggesting a difference in the interpretation of activity for neurons in the blobs and lattice: Firing rate encodes intensity in the blobs and "strength of match" in the lattice. Intuitively, we find this new view compelling: Otherwise, why would the visual system have evolved the blobs if it were simply "colorizing" the outlines provided by the lattice system?

ACKNOWLEDGMENTS

This work was supported by the Hixon Professorship at the California Institute of Technology, the Canadian Institute for Advanced Research, the Air Force Office of Scientific Research, and the Medical Research Council.

REFERENCES

Allman, J. 1977. Evolution of the visual system in the early primates. *Prog. Psychobiol. Physiol. Psychol.* **7**: 1.

Ballard, D. 1986. Cortical connections and parallel processing: Structure and function. *Behav. Brain Sci.* **9**: 67.

Barlow, H. 1972. Single units and sensation: A neural doctrine for perception. *Perception* **1**: 371.

———. 1979. The efficiency of detecting changes of density in random dot patterns. *Vision Res.* **18**: 637.

Bartlett, J. and R. Doty. 1974. Response of units in striate cortex of squirrel monkeys to visual and electrical stimuli. *J. Neurophysiol.* **37**: 621.

Blasdel, G. and G. Salama. 1986. Voltage-sensitive dyes reveal a modular organization in monkey striate cortex. *Nature* **321**: 579.

Burr, D. and J. Ross. 1979. How does binocular delay give information about depth. *Vision Res.* **19**: 523.

Celio, M., L. Scharer, J. Morrison, A. Norman, and F. Bloom. 1986. Calbindin immunoreactivity alternates with cytochrome c-oxidase-rich zones in some layers of the primate visual cortex. *Nature* **323**: 715.

Condo, G., S. Florence, and V. Casagrande. 1987. Development of laminar and columnar patterns of cytochrome oxidase activity in galago visual cortex. *Soc. Neurosci. Abstr.* **13**: 1025.

Derrington, A. and P. Lennie. 1984. Spatial and temporal contrast sensitivities of neurones in lateral geniculate nucleus of macaque. *J. Physiol.* **357**: 219.

Horton, J. 1984. Cytochrome oxidase patches: A new cytoarchitectonic feature of monkey cortex. *Philos. Trans. R. Soc. Lond. B Biol. Sci.* **304**: 199.

Horton, J. and D. Hubel. 1981. Regular patchy distribution of cytochrome oxidase staining in primate visual cortex of macaque monkey. *Nature* **292**: 762.

Jacobs, G. 1977. Visual capacities of the owl monkey (*Aotus trivirgatus*). 1. Spectral sensitivity and color vision. *Vision Res.* **17**: 811.

Jacobs, G. and J. Neitz. 1986. Spectral mechanisms and color vision in the tree shrew (*Tupaia belangeri*). *Vision Res.* **26**: 291.

Kayama, Y., R. Riso, J. Bartlett, and R. Doty. 1979. Luxotonic responses of units in macaque striate cortex. *J. Neurophysiol.* **42**: 1495.

Kuljis, R. and P. Rakic. 1990. Hypercolumns in primate visual cortex can develop in the absence of cues from photoreceptors. *Proc. Natl. Acad. Sci.* **87**: 5303.

Livingstone, M. and D. Hubel. 1984. Anatomy and physiology of a color system in primate visual cortex. *J. Neurosci.* **4**: 309.

———. 1987. Psychophysical evidence for separate channels for the perception of form, color, movement, and depth. *J. Neurosci.* **7**: 3416.

Maguire, W. and J. Baizer. 1982. Luminance coding of briefly presented stimuli in area 17 of the rhesus monkey. *J. Neurophysiol.* **47**: 128.

Maler, L., S. Jande, and D. Lawson. 1984. Localization of vitamin D-dependent calcium binding protein in the electrosensory and electromotor system of high frequency gymnotic fish. *Brain Res.* **301**: 166.

Marr, D. 1970. A theory for cerebral neocortex. *Proc. R. Soc. Lond. B Biol. Sci.* **176**: 161.

Martin, K. 1988. From enzymes to visual perception: A bridge too far? *Trends Neurosci.* **11:** 380.

Martin, R. 1990. *Primate origins and evolution.* Chapman and Hall, London.

McGuinness, E., C. MacDonald, M. Sereno, and J. Allman. 1986. Primates without blobs: The distribution of cytochrome oxidase activity in striate cortex of *Tarsius, Hapalemur* and *Cheirogaleus. Soc. Neurosci. Abstr.* **12:** 130.

Needham, D. 1971. *Machina carnis.* Cambridge University Press, England.

Sclar, G., P. Lennie, and D. DePriest. 1989. Contrast adaptation in striate cortex of macaque. *Vision Res.* **29:** 747.

Silverman, M., D. Grosof, R. DeValois, and S. Elfar. 1989. Spatial-frequency organization in primate striate cortex. *Proc. Natl. Acad. Sci.* **86:** 711.

Takahashi, T., C. Carr, N. Brecha, and M. Konishi. 1987. Calcium binding protein-like immunoreactivity labels the terminal field of nucleus laminaris of the barn owl. *J. Neurosci.* **7:** 1843.

Tootell, R., S. Hamilton, and M. Silverman. 1985. Topography of cytochrome oxidase activity in owl monkey cortex. *J. Neurosci.* **5:** 2786.

Tootell, R., M. Silverman, S. Hamilton, R. DeValois, and E. Switkes. 1988a. Functional anatomy of macaque striate cortex. III. Color. *J. Neurosci.* **8:** 1569.

Tootell, R., M. Silverman, S. Hamilton, E. Switkes, and R. DeValois. 1988b. Functional anatomy of macaque striate cortex. V. Spatial frequency. *J. Neurosci.* **8:** 1610.

T'so, D. and C. Gilbert. 1988. The organization of chromatic and spatial interactions in primate striate cortex. *J. Neurosci.* **8:** 1712.

Wikler, K. and P. Rakic. 1989. Immunocytochemical identification of cones in the retina of nocturnal and diurnal primates. *Soc. Neurosci. Abstr.* **15:** 1206.

Wong-Riley, M. and E. Carroll. 1984. The effect of impulse blockage on cytochrome oxidase activity in the monkey visual system. *Nature* **222:** 18.

Wong-Riley, M. and T. Norton. 1988. Histochemical localization of cytochrome oxidase activity in the visual system of the tree shrew: Normal patterns and the effects of retinal impulse blockage. *J. Comp. Neurol.* **272:** 562.

Wong-Riley, M., S. Tripathi, T. Trusk, and D. Hoppe. 1989. Effects of retinal impulse blockage on cytochrome oxidase-rich zones in the macaque striate cortex. I. Quantitative electron-microscopic (EM) analysis of neurons. *Vis. Neurosci.* **2:** 483.

Wright, P. 1989. The nocturnal primate niche in the new world. *J. Hum. Evol.* **18:** 635.

Zucker, S. and R. Hummel. 1986. Receptive fields and the representation of visual information. *Human Neurobiol.* **5:** 121.

Anatomical Explorations of Mind:
Studies with Modern Imaging Techniques

M.E. RAICHLE

Mallinckrodt Institute of Radiology, Department of Neurology and Neurological Surgery,
McDonnell Center for Studies of Higher Brain Function, Washington University School of Medicine,
St. Louis, Missouri 63110

Theories of how single words are processed by the normal human brain have been developed through studies of patients with various lesions affecting areas of the brain thought to be important in language processing (LaBerge and Samuels 1974; Damasio 1984; Coltheart 1985). From these studies, two general theories have emerged: a serial model that posits information flow in an obligatory, stepwise fashion from perception to speech, and a parallel model that posits a flexible modular organization governed by specific information processing requirements that can vary under particular circumstances. We have studied the processing of single words in normal adult humans using positron emission tomography (PET) to determine whether either of these theories best explains the manner in which single words are processed by the human brain. Results from our work indicate that the processing of single words is accomplished in a highly modular, parallel fashion that is flexibly determined by specific task requirements and the familiarity of the subject with the task (i.e., learning of an unfamiliar task leads to a complete rearrangement of the cortical areas involved in the execution of the task). This work not only provides important new information on theories of information processing in the human brain, but also demonstrates the important role to be played by modern imaging techniques used in conjunction with carefully designed experimental paradigms.

EXPERIMENTAL PROCEDURES

Emission tomography is a technique that produces an image of the distribution of a previously administered radionuclide in any desired section of the body. PET uses the unique properties of the annihilation radiation that is generated when positrons are absorbed in matter (Raichle 1983) to provide an image that is a highly faithful representation of the spatial distribution of the radionuclide at a selected plane through the tissue. Such an image is effectively equivalent to a *quantitative tissue autoradiogram* obtained with laboratory animals, but PET has the added advantage that it is noninvasive; hence, studies are possible in living animals, including humans. PET has been used in humans to measure brain blood flow, blood volume, metabolism of glucose and oxygen, acid-base balance, receptor pharmacol-

ogy, and transmitter metabolism (for an introduction to this literature, see Raichle 1986).

In this paper, I focus on the measurement of brain blood flow and its use in mapping the local functional activity within the normal human brain. Changes in neuronal activity are accompanied by rapid (< 1 sec) changes in local blood flow and metabolism in the brain (for review, Raichle 1987). PET accurately and rapidly measures changes in local blood flow (Raichle et al. 1983; Herscovitch et al. 1987). Assuming that all mental activity is accompanied by changes in local blood flow, PET is ideally suited to accomplish the task of relating changes in local neuronal activity to mental activity.

Our strategy for the functional mapping of neuronal activity in the human brain with PET measurements of local blood flow is composed of a number of important elements. These include the deliberate selection of blood flow measured with the PET adaptation of the Kety autoradiographic technique (Herscovitch et al. 1983, 1987; Raichle et al. 1983), or estimated from the radioactive counts accumulating in brain tissue during 40 seconds following the intravenous bolus administration of $H_2^{15}O$ (Fox et al. 1985), as the most accurate and flexible signal of changes in local neural activity that can be detected with PET (Fox et al. 1988b). Linearly scaled images of blood flow or radioactive counts in a control state are subtracted from images obtained during functional activation in each subject (i.e., paired image subtraction). The control state and the stimulated state are carefully chosen so as to isolate, as far as possible, a single mental operation (see, e.g., Petersen et al. 1988). By subtracting blood-flow measurements made in the control state from each task state, it is possible to identify those areas of the brain concerned with the mental operations unique to the task state. This extends to our work a strategy first introduced to psychology by Donders in 1868, in which reaction time was used to dissect out the components of mental operations (Donders 1969). In our work, we can now do so in terms of specific regions of the brain. These subtraction images form the basis of a data set that is composed of averaged responses across many individual subjects or across many runs in the same individual. Image averaging dramatically enhances the signal-to-noise properties of such data. This enables us to detect even low-level responses associated with mental activity with a spatial accuracy of a few millimeters (Fox et al. 1988a; Mintun et al. 1989).

RESULTS

For several years now, we have been examining the cortical anatomy of single-word processing (Petersen et al. 1988, 1989, 1990) as an initial step in the study of language. Because of the great complexity of language, restriction of our efforts to an understanding of the processing of individual words seemed warranted. Furthermore, the design of tasks appropriate for such studies with PET was greatly aided by extant knowledge in cognitive psychology, linguistics, and clinical neurology (see, e.g., LaBerge and Samuels 1974; Damasio 1984; Coltheart 1985).

In this project, we used four behavioral conditions in each subject to form a three-level subtractive hierarchy in which each task state was intended to add a small number of mental operations to those of its subordinate (control) state. In the *first level* comparison, the visual presentation of single words without a lexical task was compared to visual fixation on a small cross hairs on a television monitor without word presentation. Words were presented for 150 msec at the rate of once per second on a television screen during the 40-second measurement of blood flow. No motor output or volitional lexical processing was required in this task; rather, simple sensory input and involuntary word-form processing were targeted by this subtraction.

The areas of brain identified as active during the passive viewing of words appear to support two different computational levels, one of passive sensory processing in primary visual cortex and a second level of modality-specific word-form processing in extrastriate areas. The main regions activated (Fig. 1, triangles labeled PV) were in striate cortex bilaterally (Fig. 1, PV4 and PV5) and three extrastriate areas, one on the left (Fig. 1, PV1) and two on the right (Fig. 1, PV2 and PV3), extending to the temporal-occipital boundary on the right. The primary striate responses were similar to those produced by simple sensory stimuli such as the checkerboard annuli used in our earlier experiments (retinotopy experiments). The regions in extrastriate cortex became candidates for a network of cortical modules that code for visual word form. Subsequent experiments (Petersen et al. 1990) demonstrated that the area located at PV1 (Fig. 1) was activated by words and nonwords obeying rules of English and not by

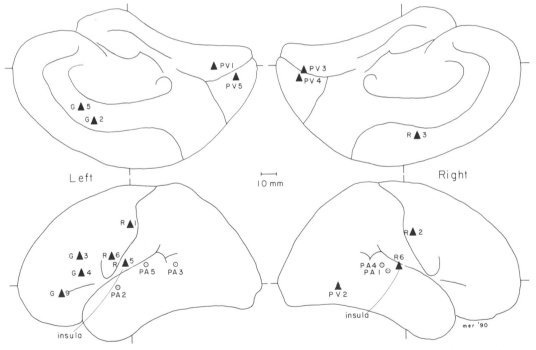

Figure 1. Location of averaged local blood-flow *changes* during the processing of single visual words in the cerebral cortex of normal adult subjects. (*Top*) Saggital views of the medial surfaces of the cerebral hemispheres; (*bottom*) the lateral surfaces. The medial views are oriented with dorsal down and the lateral views are oriented with dorsal up. Anterior is to the left for the left hemisphere and to the right for the right hemisphere. The cerebral hemisphere fiducial markers represent the zero planes for the Z (horizontal) and Y (vertical) axes of the Talairach stereotaxic system (Talairach et al. 1967). Three different *task states* were studied in each subject: passive presentation of visual or auditory words (PV and PA, respectively), repeating visual words (R), and generating a verb for a presented visual noun (G). The words, common English nouns, were presented on a television monitor at the rate of 1 Hz. The control state for the passive viewing of nouns was looking at a fixation point on the monitor. The control state for repeating nouns was the passive presentation of the same nouns. Finally, the control state for generating verbs was repeating nouns. The relative magnitude of each response within conditions is shown to the right of the symbol. These data are replotted from Petersen et al. (1988, 1989).

consonant letter strings or false fonts. Taken together, the several regions of striate and extrastriate cortex activated by passive visual words appear to combine, functionally, to analyze visual symbols that behave according to rules of the English language. As such, they must represent a learned response.

Words presented auditorily with subjects passively fixating on the visual cross hairs activated an entirely separate set of areas in temporal cortex bilaterally (Fig. 1, PA1–5). An area in left, posterior, temporal cortex (PA3, an appropriate candidate for Wernicke's area) was clearly seen with auditory presentation but was conspicuous by its absence during the presentation of words visually. Only when subjects were asked to judge whether pairs of *visual words rhymed* were responses seen in these areas (Petersen et al. 1988, 1989), emphasizing the functionally flexible nature of these modular relationships.

In the *second level* comparison, subjects were asked to repeat the words presented auditorily or visually. The control state for the PET blood-flow subtraction was the passive presentation of auditory or visual words. Areas related to motor output and articulatory coding were activated. In general, similar regions were activated for visual (responses labeled R, Fig. 1) and auditory presentation (not shown). Responses occurred in cerebellum (not shown), primary sensorimotor mouth cortex bilaterally (Fig. 1, R1,2), the supplementary motor area or SMA (Fig. 1, R3), premotor cortex (Fig. 1, R6), and insular cortex bilaterally (Fig. 1, R5,6). The left insular and premotor responses are near Broca's area, a region often viewed as specifically serving language output. But similar insular activation was also found when subjects were instructed to simply move their mouths and tongues (P.T. Fox et al., unpubl.), arguing against specialization of this region for speech output.

Finally, in the *third level* of comparison, subjects were asked to speak a verb for each noun presented, either auditorily or visually, again while monitoring a fixation point. Responses were identified in two areas of cerebral cortex as well as for both auditory (not shown) and visual word presentation (Fig. 1, G). A left inferior prefrontal area (Fig. 1, G9) was identified that participates in an undefined way in the process of semantic association. A second area in the anterior cingulate gyrus (Fig. 1, G2,5) is probably part of an anterior attentional system engaged in selection for action. This localization of function was suggested by the performance of converging experiments detailed elsewhere (Posner et al. 1988; Pardo et al. 1990).

Responses in the cerebellum (not shown), especially in the right lateral cerebellar hemisphere were also detected in this task. Because we had subtracted the motoric aspects of simply saying words, this result strongly suggests that the cerebellum plays an important role in high-level information processing involving a novel task that engages the left prefrontal cortex. This is the first direct evidence in support of the hypothesis that the cerebellum plays an important role

in high-level information processing in humans as suggested by other investigators (Berntson and Torello 1984; Bracke-Tolkmitt et al. 1989; Leiner et al. 1989).

One additional preliminary (M.E. Raichle et al., unpubl.) observation may be of importance in understanding the information processing role of the responses observed in this task. Specifically, the responses in left prefrontal cortex and anterior cingulate cortex were only present when subjects were first exposed to this task (i.e., when it was novel and required active attention). Practice generating verbs to a specific list of nouns resulted in disappearance of the left inferior prefrontal and anterior cingulate responses. These results suggest a role for these areas of cortex in the *acquisition* of a new skill, in this case linguistic.

DISCUSSION

What do such results suggest about the modular organization of the human brain for tasks associated with single-word processing? They suggest a *flexible* modular organization consisting of multiple routes. For example, there is no activation in any of our visual tasks near Wernicke's area or the angular gyrus in posterior temporal cortex unless a specific phonological judgment must be made (i.e., rhyme judgment). Visual information from occipital cortex appears to have access to output coding without undergoing phonological recoding in these areas in posterior temporal cortex. Furthermore, tasks calling for semantic processing of single words activate frontal cortices (i.e., left prefrontal and anterior cingulate) and the cerebellum, rather than posterior, temporal regions. Finally, sensory-specific information appears to have independent access to semantic and output codes; simple repetition of a presented word failed to activate the left-frontal semantic areas.

More generally, this brief review of our studies of single-word processing in the human brain was intended to demonstrate that a combination of cognitive and neurobiological approaches to the study of normal human subjects, aided by modern imaging techniques, can give us important new information about the flexible, distributed, modular organization of cognition in the human brain. Progress in our evolving understanding of the implementation of mental activities in the human brain will be dependent on an appreciation of the very distributed nature of this processing. Inferences drawn about the role of specific local neuronal ensembles, in particular mental activities, must be guided by the knowledge that an ensemble may be only a part of a very distributed network in which local areas of the brain contribute highly specialized component functions. Modern functional imaging studies of normal humans and awake behaving primates should play an important and unique role in defining these networks. Continued progress in this type of work should serve to enlighten us about the solution to the problem of mind-brain interaction that has intrigued us for so long. Finally, one must hope that the insights gained will provide a more rational basis for the understanding and treatment of some of the most devastating diseases of humans.

ACKNOWLEDGMENTS

This work was supported by National Institutes of Health grants NS-06833, HL-13851, AG-08377, and a grant from the MacArthur Foundation.

REFERENCES

Berntson, G.G. and M.W. Torello. 1984. The paleocerebellum and the integration of behavioral function. *Physiol. Psychol.* **10**: 2.

Bracke-Tolkmitt, R., A. Linden, A.G.M. Canavan, B. Rockstroh, E. Scholz, K. Wessel, and H.-C. Diener. 1989. The cerebellum contributes to mental skills. *Behav. Neurosci.* **103**: 442.

Coltheart, M. 1985. Cognitive neuropsychology and the study of reading. In *Attention and performance XI* (ed. M.I. Posner and O.S.M. Marlin), p. 3. Lawrence Erlbaum Associates, Hillsdale, New Jersey.

Damasio, A.R. 1984. The neural basis of language. *Annu. Rev. Neurosci* **7**: 127.

Donders, F.C. 1969. On the speed of mental processes. (Reprinted). *Acta Psychol.* **30**: 412.

Fox, P.T., J. Perlmutter, and M.E. Raichle. 1985. A stereotactic method of anatomical localization for positron emission tomography. *J. Comput. Assisted Tomogr.* **9**: 141.

Fox, P.T., M.A. Mintun, E.M. Reiman, and M.E. Raichle. 1988a. Enhanced detection of focal brain responses using intersubject averaging and distribution analysis of subtracted PET images. *J. Cereb. Blood Flow Metab.* **8**: 642.

Fox, P.T., M.E. Raichle, M.A. Mintun, and C. Dence. 1988b. Nonoxidative glucose consumption during focal physiologic neural activity. *Science* **241**: 462.

Herscovitch, P., J. Markham, and M.E. Raichle. 1983. Brain blood flow measured with intravenous $H_2^{15}O$. I. Theory and error analysis. *J. Nucl. Med.* **24**: 782.

Herscovitch, P., M.E. Raichle, M.R. Kilbourn, and M.J. Welch. 1987. Positron emission tomographic measurement of cerebral blood flow and permeability surface area product of water using ^{15}O-water and ^{11}C-butanol. *J. Cereb. Blood Flow. Metab.* **7**: 527.

LaBerge, D. and S.J. Samuels. 1974. Toward a theory of automatic information processing in reading. *Cognit. Psychol.* **6**: 293.

Leiner, H.C., A.I. Leiner, and R.S. Dow. 1989. Reappraising the cerebellum: What does the hindbrain contribute to the forebrain? *Behav. Neurosci.* **103**: 998.

Mintun, M.A., P.T. Fox, and M.E. Raichle. 1989. A highly accurate method of localizing regions of neuronal activation in the human brain with positron emission tomography. *J. Cereb. Blood Flow Metab.* **9**: 96.

Pardo, J.V., P.J. Pardo, K.W. Janer, and M.E. Raichle. 1990. The anterior cingulate cortex mendiates processing selection in the stoop attentional conflict paradigm. *Proc. Natl. Acad. Sci.* **87**: 256.

Petersen, S.E., P.T. Fox, A.Z. Snyder, and M.E. Raichle. 1990. Activation of extrastriate and frontal cortical areas by visual words and word-like stimuli. *Science* **249**: 1041.

Petersen, S.E., P.T. Fox, M.I. Posner, M.A. Mintun, and M.E. Raichle. 1988. Positron emission tomographic studies of the cortical anatomy of single word processing. *Nature* **331**: 585.

———. 1989. Positron emission tomographic studies of the processing of single words. *J. Cognit. Neurosci.* **1**: 153.

Posner, M.I., S.E. Petersen, P.T. Fox, and M.E. Raichle. 1988. Localization of cognitive functions in the human brain. *Science* **240**: 1627.

Raichle, M.E. 1983. Positron emission tomography. *Annu. Rev. Neurosci.* **6**: 249.

———. 1986. Neuroimaging. *Trends Neurosci.* **9**: 525.

———. 1987. Circulatory and metabolic correlates of brain function in normal humans. In *Handbook of physiology. The nervous system.* (ed. V.B. Mountcastle and F. Plum), vol. 5, p. 643. The American Physiological Society, Bethesda.

Raichle, M.E., W.R.W. Martin, P. Herscovitch, M. Mintun, and J. Markham. 1983. Brain blood flow measured with $H_2^{15}O$. II. Implementation and validation. *J. Nucl. Med.* **24**: 790.

Talairach, J., G. Sxikla, P. Tournoux, A. Prossalentis, M. Bordas-Ferrer, L. Covello, M. Iacob, and E. Mempel. 1967. *Atlas d'anatomie stereotaxique du telencephale.* Masson, Paris.

Frontal Lobes and Memory for the Temporal Order of Recent Events

B. MILNER, M.P. MCANDREWS, AND G. LEONARD

Montreal Neurological Institute and Department of Neurology and Neurosurgery,
McGill University, Montreal, Quebec, Canada, H3A 2B4

One of the earliest and most frequently replicated findings concerning the effects of frontal-lobe lesions in the monkey is the impairment in delayed response (Jacobsen 1935) and delayed alternation (Jacobsen and Nissen 1937) that follows bilateral removal of the prefrontal cortex. In these short-term memory tasks, the animal is confronted with two food wells with identical covers and must choose either the left- or the right-hand one on the basis of information received a few seconds before. In delayed response, the predelay cue is the sight of one food well being baited before both wells are screened from view; in delayed alternation, the cue is the location that was correct on the previous trial and must now be avoided. Because in both tasks the correct location varies from trial to trial, it is important to be able to suppress the potentially interfering memory of previous trials and respond on the basis of the most recent information.

The traditional delayed-response and delayed-alternation procedures are unsuitable for the study of human frontal-lobe function, because on these tasks even long time intervals can be bridged by verbal mediation. Instead, Prisko (1963 [reported in Milner 1964]) used the delayed-comparison method (Konorski 1959; Stepien and Sierpinski 1960) to elicit deficits in patients who had undergone a frontal cortical excision for the relief of epilepsy; this method also embodies an intratrial delay as an essential feature. In Prisko's experiment, two easily discriminable stimuli in the same sensory modality were presented in succession, 60 seconds apart, and the subject had to say whether the second stimulus was the same as, or different from, the first. Patients with frontal-lobe lesions, unlike those with temporal-lobe lesions, were impaired on those tasks in which a few stimuli recurred in different pairings throughout the test, but not on the one task in which new stimuli were used on each trial. This contrast was taken to indicate that patients with frontal-lobe lesions had a heightened susceptibility to proactive interference from the effects of preceding trials, rather than an inability to retain new information over a short time interval.

RECENCY JUDGMENTS

Prisko's findings led Milner (1968a) to suggest that the frontal lobes play a critical role in the temporal structuring of events in memory, so that, in a situation lacking strong contextual cues, patients with frontal-lobe lesions would be less able than normal subjects to distinguish a stimulus presented 60 seconds ago from one that had appeared earlier in the same series of trials. Yntema and Trask (1963) have proposed that items in memory normally carry time-tags that permit the discrimination of the more from the less recent, and it seemed that such a time-marking process might be disturbed by frontal-lobe injury, so that serial-order judgments would be impaired. Corsi (cited in Milner 1971) has since provided a direct test of the hypothesis that the frontal lobes play a role in the temporal ordering of events, by examining recency discrimination in patients with frontal- or temporal-lobe lesions and normal control subjects. For this purpose, he devised three formally similar tasks, embodying different kinds of stimulus material: concrete words, representational drawings, and abstract paintings.

In the verbal recency-discrimination task, the subject is given a deck of 184 cards, on each of which two high-imagery, spondaic words are inscribed (e.g., *peanut–ashtray*). The instruction is to read the words aloud and then turn to the next card; whenever a card appears bearing a question mark between the two words, the subject must indicate which word was read more recently. Usually both words on the test card will have appeared before (say, 8 items ago compared with 32), but in the limiting condition one of them will be new, in which case the task reduces to a simple test of item recognition. Inspection cards and test cards alternate after the first few inspection cards have been shown. A similar procedure is followed for the representational drawings, the subject being allowed 3 seconds to view each inspection card before being instructed to turn to the next card. Again, whenever a test card appears, the task is to indicate which of the two items has been seen more recently.

Figure 1 illustrates the stimulus material used in the abstract-paintings task. In this case, the inspection time for each card was extended to 6 seconds and the series was reduced to 92 cards, thus ensuring that the difficulty level for this more complex material would be roughly equivalent to that of the other two recency-discrimination tasks.

The results confirmed the important contribution of the frontal lobes to recency judgments, as well as revealing differential effects related to the side of the lesion. Patients with left frontal-lobe lesions showed a moder-

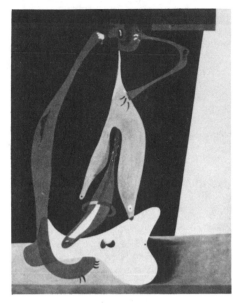 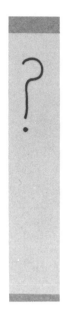 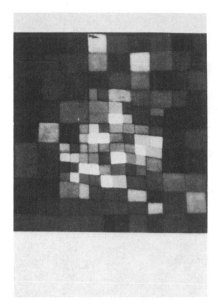

Figure 1. Sample test card from the abstract-paintings recency-discrimination task. Original in color. (Reprinted, with permission, from Milner 1974).

ate deficit when the stimuli to be ordered were verbal, but were unimpaired on the two pictorial tests. In contrast, patients with right frontal-lobe removals were totally unable to judge the relative recency of the abstract paintings and were significantly impaired on the representational drawings. In addition, their performance on the verbal task was only slightly better than that of the left frontal-lobe group. Thus, not only did the results vary as a function of the stimulus material, but there was also a suggestion that the right frontal lobe plays a more important role than the left in recency discrimination. It must, however, be borne in mind that the removals from the right tended to be a little larger than those from the left, because of the need to spare Broca's area in the language-dominant hemisphere.

Whereas neither frontal-lobe group in Corsi's study was impaired at simple item recognition, both the temporal-lobe groups showed mild, material-specific deficits in recognition memory, verbal for the left temporal-lobe group and pictorial for the right; the temporal-lobe groups did not, however, have any undue difficulty with recency discrimination as such. This contrasting pattern of results points to some separability of the processes mediating item recognition from those mediating temporal-order judgments (cf. Sagar et al. 1990).

Since the first brief reports of these findings (Milner 1971, 1974), we have added new patients to our frontal-lobe groups in order to test the hypothesis, based on behavioral and electrophysiological studies in the monkey (Fuster 1989; Goldman-Rakic 1987), that removals encroaching significantly on the midlateral frontal cortex (as sketched in Fig. 2) would prove particularly damaging to performance on recency-discrimination

tasks. This study, to be published in extenso elsewhere (B. Milner et al., in prep.), is summarized below.

Subjects

The subjects were 117 patients at the Montreal Neurological Hospital, each of whom had undergone a unilateral brain operation for the relief of focal cerebral seizures, and 20 normal control subjects, matched as closely as possible to the patient groups with respect to age, sex, and socioeconomic status. The total group ranged in age from 16 to 56 years, with a mean age of 28 years. Sixty patients were tested in the early postoperative period, from 14 to 20 days after surgery, and the remaining 57 were tested in follow-up study, from 1 to 20 years later. The various subgroups did not differ in the proportion tested early and the proportion

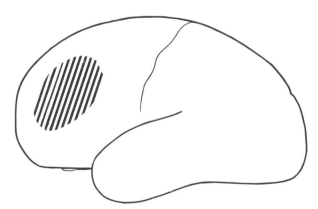

Figure 2. Brain map showing the approximate location in the lateral frontal cortex of an area hypothesized to be implicated in recency judgments.

tested late. All patients had received extensive neuro-psychological evaluation, and those with a full-scale Wechsler IQ rating below 75 were excluded, as were those with bilateral, or right-hemisphere, speech representation, as demonstrated by preoperative intracarotid sodium-amobarbital tests (Branch et al. 1964). The patient group included eight cases of indolent cerebral tumor, but otherwise the epileptogenic lesions were static and atrophic, typically dating from birth or early life.

Frontal-lobe and fronto-temporal groups. The 59 patients making up these groups included 36 subjects with cortical excisions limited to the frontal lobe (17 in the left hemisphere, 19 in the right), and 23 subjects whose removals involved both the frontal cortex and the anterior temporal region (13 in the left hemisphere, 10 in the right). The frontal-lobe removals always spared Broca's area (in the left hemisphere) and the primary motor cortex, as mapped out by electrical stimulation, but otherwise they varied considerably in locus and extent.

These patients were subdivided according to side of lesion and according to whether or not the removal (as drawn by the surgeon at the time of operation) encroached appreciably on the proposed critical area shown in Figure 2. The classification of the brain maps was made by an independent judge (M. Petrides, pers. comm.), who was unaware of how the patients had performed on the recency-discrimination tasks. This led to the formation of three left-hemisphere and three right-hemisphere groups, representative removals being shown in Figures 3 and 4, respectively. The left-hemisphere groups were defined as follows: (1) left

frontal removal invading (LFinv) proposed critical area (Fig. 3, Ch.Kn.); (2) left fronto-temporal removal invading (LFTinv) critical area (Fig. 3, Te.Al.); (3) left frontal removal sparing (LFsp) plus left fronto-temporal removal sparing (LFTsp) critical area (Fig. 3, Fr.Kl., Ro.Bl.). This composite group was formed because of the small number of patients in the LFsp and LFTsp categories.

The corresponding three right-hemisphere groups were defined in a similar way to the left, and representative removals are illustrated in Figure 4 (RFinv, Ma.Si.; RFTinv, Pe.De.; RFsp + RFTsp, Ly.Au., Ja.Be.).

Temporal-lobe groups. The 58 patients with removals limited to the temporal lobe were subdivided into left temporal-lobe (LT) and right temporal-lobe (RT) groups. Representative removals are shown in Figure 5. The cortical excisions ranged from 3.5 to 6.5 cm along the Sylvian fissure, and from 3.5 to 7.5 cm along the base of the brain. The removals always included the amygdala but varied in the amount of hippocampus and parahippocampal gyrus excised. All removals from the left hemisphere were anterior to the temporal speech area.

Results

Verbal recency task. Table 1 displays the results for the verbal task, for both word recognition and recency discrimination. Analysis of variance revealed no significant group differences in the ability to discriminate an item that had been presented before from one that was new, although the mean recognition score of the LT

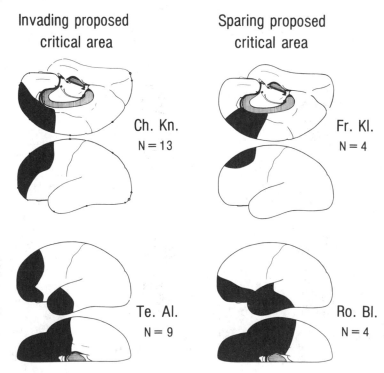

Invading proposed critical area

Sparing proposed critical area

Ch. Kn.
N = 13

Fr. Kl.
N = 4

Te. Al.
N = 9

Ro. Bl.
N = 4

Figure 3. Representative brain maps illustrating composition of the three groups with excisions from the left frontal lobe: Ch. Kn., left frontal-lobe removal invading proposed area (LFinv); Te. Al., left fronto-temporal removal invading proposed area (LFTinv); Fr. Kl. and Ro. Bl., left frontal and left fronto-temporal removals sparing proposed area (LFsp and LFTsp, respectively).

Invading proposed
critical area

Sparing proposed
critical area

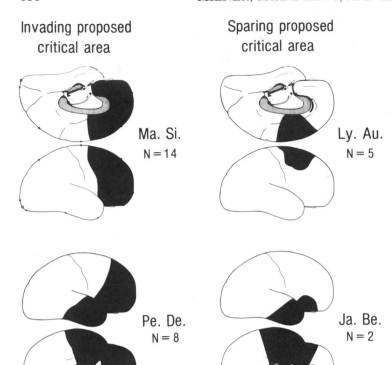

Ma. Si.
N = 14

Ly. Au.
N = 5

Pe. De.
N = 8

Ja. Be.
N = 2

Figure 4. Representative brain maps illustrating the composition of the three groups with excisions from the right frontal lobe: Ma. Si., RFinv; Pe. De., RFTinv; Ly. Au. and Ja. Be., RFsp and RFTsp, respectively.

group was a little lower than that of the other groups. On the more difficult task of recency discrimination, both the LFinv and the LFTinv groups were impaired, whereas the group of patients with left frontal or left fronto-temporal excisions that spared the midlateral area were not. In the right hemisphere, only the RFinv group differed significantly from the normal control group. Thus, the results of this verbal task provide some support for the hypothesis that frontal-lobe re-

Pa. St.   Ka. Fi.

Mi. Ep.   An. Co.

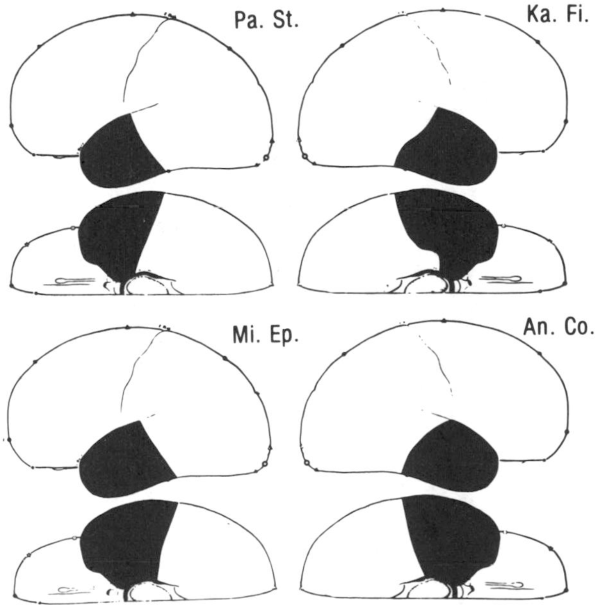

Figure 5. Representative left and right temporal lobectomies: Pa.St., Ka.Fi., small hippocampal removals; Mi.Ep., An.Co., large hippocampal removals.

movals that invade the midlateral frontal cortex are more likely to impair temporal-order judgments than those that do not.

Pictorial recency task A: Representational drawings. On this relatively easy task, the only significant finding was a mild impairment in recency discrimination in the RFinv group (but not in the RFTinv group).

Pictorial recency task B: Abstract paintings. The mean scores of the various groups for both picture recognition and recency judgments are shown in Table 2. The analysis disclosed significant impairments in item recognition for the RFTinv and the RT groups, as well as for the combined group of patients with RF or RFT lesions sparing the midlateral region, but no deficit in the RFinv group, nor in any of the left-hemisphere groups. This finding of a deficit in recognition memory for abstract paintings in all three groups involving patients with right temporal-lobe excisions (RT; RFTinv; RFsp + RFTsp) is consistent with the known detrimental effect of right temporal-lobe lesions on memory for complex visual patterns (Kimura 1963; Milner 1968b, 1990).

As shown in Table 2, the findings for picture recognition contrast markedly with those for recency judgments. In the latter case, the three groups of patients with removals invading the right frontal lobe were severely impaired, performing at, or near, the chance level, whereas the mean score of the RT group was within normal limits. There is, therefore, a double dissociation between the effects of right temporal- and right frontal-lobe excisions on picture recognition and recency discrimination, respectively. Again we note the

Table 1. Verbal Recency Task: Mean Percent Correct Responses (50 = chance performance)

Group	N	Item recognition	Recency discrimination
Normal control	20	94	71
Left frontal invading critical area	13	92	60**
Left fronto-temporal invading critical area	7	92	59**
Left frontal and fronto-temporal sparing critical area	8	92	64
Left temporal	26	87	68
Right frontal invading critical area	13	93	62*
Right fronto-temporal invading critical area	8	91	70
Right frontal and fronto-temporal sparing critical area	7	93	72
Right temporal	28	93	71

$*p < 0.05.$
$**p < 0.01.$

unimpaired performance of all the left-hemisphere groups on this nonverbal version of the recency-discrimination task. Taken together, these findings point to strong laterality effects but provide no evidence for a critical area within the right frontal lobe implicated in temporal-order judgments.

RECENCY DISCRIMINATION FOR MANIPULATED AND NONMANIPULATED OBJECTS

The results outlined above have confirmed and extended Corsi's demonstration of a major contribution from the frontal cortex to memory for temporal order. Similar findings have also been reported in cases of frontal-lobe epilepsy (Ladavas et al. 1979), as well as for other groups of patients with unilateral or bilateral frontal-lobe excisions (Shimamura et al. 1988). Yet thus far there have been few attempts to characterize more precisely the nature of the underlying disorder.

In the case of the monkey, Pribram has argued that deficits on delayed alternation after dorsolateral frontal-lobe lesions reflect a failure to "parse" or segment the ongoing stream of experience into discrete temporal moments (Pribram and Tubbs 1967; Pribram et al. 1977). This notion arose from the fact that monkeys with such lesions were unimpaired when the experimenter imposed external "temporal landmarks" by asymmetrically manipulating the duration of the delay period between trials (for a different interpretation, see Rosenkilde et al. 1981). If the frontal lobes do indeed parse and organize the temporal contexts of events, one outcome of such operations could be thought of as a direct encoding of temporal tags for events in memory, such as Yntema and Trask (1963) had postulated as forming the basis of human temporal-order judgments. According to this view, patients with frontal-lobe lesions do poorly on recency-discrimination tasks because this time-marking process is disrupted (Schacter 1987), and their performance should benefit if external temporal landmarks are provided.

Table 2. Abstract-Paintings Recency Task: Mean Percent Correct Responses (50 = chance performance)

Group	N	Item recognition	Recency discrimination
Normal control	20	92	77
Left frontal invading critical area	13	83	70
Left fronto-temporal invading critical area	9	85	69
Left frontal and fronto-temporal sparing critical area	8	88	65
Left temporal	28	92	79
Right frontal invading critical area	14	81	50**
Right fronto-temporal invading critical area	8	76**	56**
Right frontal and fronto-temporal sparing critical area	7	79*	54**
Right temporal	30	78**	66

$*p < 0.05.$
$**p < 0.01.$

If the impairment in temporal-order judgments shown by patients with frontal-lobe lesions stems, instead, from a failure to develop appropriate encoding and retrieval strategies for the reconstruction of temporal order, as some theories would imply (Underwood 1977), the use of a task that makes minimal demands on such strategies should lead to better performance. To test this notion, McAndrews and Milner (1991) constructed a new recency-discrimination task designed to bring the frontal-lobe groups up to the normal level. For this, they used series of toy objects and small real objects that were presented one at a time to the subject. For most items, a simple naming response was required, but for some of them, the subject was also instructed to carry out an action involving the object (e.g., "Squeeze the sponge" or "Blow the whistle"). Previous research has shown that memory for such subject-performed tasks (SPTs), or "action items," is superior to that for many other types of material. Recall is also relatively unaffected by variations in such subject characteristics as age and IQ, or in such presentation variables as level of semantic elaboration of the items, all of which are known to influence recall of other kinds of memoranda (Backman and Nilsson 1985; Cohen 1981, 1983; Nilsson and Cohen 1988).

McAndrews and Milner (1991) predicted that patients with frontal-lobe lesions would be unimpaired at judging which of a pair of action items had been presented more recently, but that they would show an impairment in recency discrimination for pairs of objects that they had merely named (Non-SPTs). In case they should do poorly on temporal-order judgments for both action and nonaction items, the experiment also incorporated a size-discrimination memory task as a control procedure. In this task, the names of two objects from the presentation series were spoken, and the subject had to say which was the larger (or smaller) of the two items as they had appeared in the series. To create pairs for the relative-size judgments, items were selected that were closest in shape and size to one another within the series, and which were such that the size judgment could rarely be based on the relative size of such objects in reality (e.g., by pairing a large button with a small bottle cap, or a plastic flower with a toy dinosaur).

Nine series were made up, using 198 objects. Each series consisted of 20 target items and 2 fillers, presented at the beginning and end of each series. Within each series, 12 objects (6 pairs) were designated as targets for the relative-recency judgments, and 8 objects (4 pairs) were used for judgments of relative size. Critical items within each pair were separated by three or four intervening items in the presentation sequence. Assignment of particular items to the different presentation conditions was counterbalanced across subjects, as was the order of items within each pair.

In addition, 44 new objects were used to create two homogeneous series, which were constructed in the same manner as the mixed series described above, except that they included no action items and no items designated for size discrimination. Thus, they provided a measure of recency discrimination for named objects uncontaminated by the presence of potentially more salient items or by changing task demands.

Each of the 11 series involved a presentation and a test phase. In the presentation phase, the 22 items were shown one at a time and then withdrawn behind a screen. For SPT items, the experimenter gave the instruction at the same time as the object was presented, whereupon the subject named the item and carried out the appropriate action. The rate of presentation was approximately 4 seconds per item, with a 2-second interstimulus interval. Immediately after presentation of the last item in each series, subjects carried out an intervening distractor task for 40 seconds before proceeding to the test phase, in which recency and size decisions were interspersed in predetermined random order. For the recency judgments, subjects were shown two objects from the series and had to decide which had been presented later in the series. Approximately 1–2 minutes of conversation preceded the presentation of each subsequent list. Across subjects, the order in which the 11 lists were given was randomly determined.

Subjects

This task was administered to 52 patients at the Montreal Neurological Hospital, each of whom had undergone either a frontal- or a temporal-lobe excision for the relief of focal epilepsy. The criteria for inclusion were the same as for the previous study, and the patients were drawn from a similar population. A normal control group of 20 subjects, matched as closely as possible to the patient groups with respect to age, sex, and socioeconomic status, was also tested.

The patient groups comprised 18 cases of frontal-lobe excision (8 left, 8 right) and 36 cases of anterior temporal lobectomy (16 left, 16 right). Except for one removal limited to the left inferior and orbital frontal cortex, all frontal-lobe excisions involved the dorsolateral cortex, and in some cases extended into the medial frontal region. Five patients in the right frontal-lobe group were tested within 3 months of surgery, and the remaining 13 frontal-lobe patients were seen in follow-up, from 6 months to 25 years postoperatively.

The temporal-lobe groups included 10 cases of extensive removal from the left hippocampus and parahippocampal gyrus, and 8 from the right (cf. Fig. 4). Fourteen patients (5 left temporal, 9 right temporal) were tested in the early postoperative period, and the remainder were tested in follow-up, one or more years later.

Results

Figure 6 displays the mean proportion of correct recency judgments (averaged across the 9 mixed lists), as related to subject group and presentation condition. Analysis of variance revealed a significant group by condition interaction; although there were no group

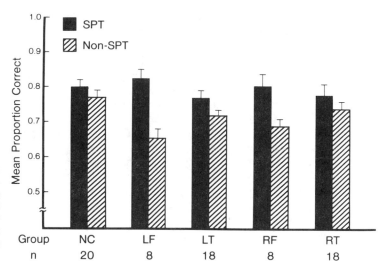

Figure 6. Objects recency-discrimination task: Histograms showing the mean proportion of correct temporal-order judgments for the various groups on the self-manipulated objects (SPT) and the objects (Non-SPT) that were merely named. NC, normal control; LF, left frontal; LT, left temporal; RF, right frontal; RT, right temporal.

differences on the action items (SPTs), both the left and right frontal-lobe groups were impaired in temporal-order judgments for the items that were only named (Non-SPTs). The normal control group and the two temporal-lobe groups performed equally well under the two presentation conditions. No group differences were seen on size discrimination, all groups having mean scores close to the 90% level.

A separate analysis was undertaken to determine whether performance on nonaction items was affected by the inclusion of enacted items in the series. No differences in overall level of performance were found between the homogeneous and the mixed lists, suggesting that the presence of action items was not detrimental to the encoding and retrieval of temporal information about nonenacted items within the same series. The results for the homogeneous lists replicated the findings of a deficit in recency discrimination for named objects in both frontal-lobe groups.

DISCUSSION

The results of this latest study confirm and extend our earlier finding of an impairment in recency discrimination after unilateral excisions from the frontal cortex. The present findings for the temporal ordering of named objects resemble most closely those obtained for the verbal recency-discrimination task (Table 1), in that an impairment was found after either left or right frontal-lobe lesions, but with some indication of a greater and more consistent effect of left-hemisphere removals than of right (Fig. 6). This contrasts with the outcome of the two pictorial tasks, where an impairment in recency discrimination was observed after right frontal-lobe excisions but not after left, thus emphasizing hemispheric specialization within the human frontal lobes.

The new finding reported here is that patients with frontal-lobe lesions are capable of normal recency discrimination when making temporal-order judgments

about objects that they have actively manipulated at the time of presentation. There are several reasons why such action items should be more salient than items that are merely named or viewed silently. In the first place, the actions bring in modalities other than vision, including tactile, kinesthetic, and, in some cases, auditory cues. This enriched sensory experience should increase the memorability of the event. Second, in this experiment, each action was distinct and meaningful, since it typically involved the demonstration of how a common object is habitually used. Thus, the richness and distinctiveness of the memory trace per se may have been the critical factor in enhancing the performance of the frontal-lobe groups when making temporal-order judgments for enacted items. It has in fact been shown, in normal subjects, that variations in materials and encoding instructions that are thought to influence elaboration and distinctiveness can also affect memory for temporal order (Michon and Jackson 1984).

This notion would not in itself be surprising, were it not for the fact that in the present study neither the normal control subjects nor the patients with temporal-lobe lesions benefited significantly from the opportunity to manipulate the objects in the recency-discrimination task. Yet their performance was not at ceiling in either presentation condition (Fig. 6). We interpret these findings as indicating that the objects themselves were sufficiently salient memoranda for normal subjects, and that to increase further the memorability of the items could not entirely compensate for the intrinsic difficulty of temporal-order judgments. If frontal-lobe lesions decrease the salience of remembered events from the recent past, then factors that enhance salience may facilitate the performance of patients with such lesions on recency-discrimination tasks.

It is of some interest that neither frontal-lobe group in the present study had any difficulty with the size-discrimination task, although this task required the subject to recall from memory the size of the specific objects that had been shown in the presentation series, because the inclusion of toy objects in the series prevented the use of prototypes as a basis for comparison. That frontal-lobe lesions did not impair performance on this task is consistent with the many studies showing normal performance on recognition and recall tasks after frontal lobectomy (Milner 1964, 1985).

A striking feature of the findings reported here has been the consistently normal performance of the temporal-lobe groups on all the recency-discrimination tasks; this was true irrespective of the extent of hippocampal removal in the unilateral temporal lobectomy. These results are in marked contrast to the well-established material-specific deficits in recognition memory and free recall that are associated with such lesions (Milner 1985) and which point to an impairment in the long-term storage of information.

ACKNOWLEDGMENTS

We thank Drs. W. Feindel, R. Leblanc, A. Olivier, T. Rasmussen, and J.-G. Villemure for the opportunity to study their patients and for providing detailed information concerning the surgical removals. Dr. M. Petrides classified the frontal-lobe removals. We also wish to thank the patients and normal control subjects who participated in these experiments. This work was supported by a postdoctoral fellowship to M.P. McAndrews from the Natural Sciences and Engineering Research Council of Canada, and by grant MT-2624 and a Career Investigatorship award to B. Milner from the Medical Research Council of Canada.

REFERENCES

Backman, L. and L.-G. Nilsson. 1985. Prerequisites for lack of age differences in memory performance. *Exp. Aging Res.* **11:** 67.

Branch, C., B. Milner, and T. Rasmussen. 1964. Intracarotid sodium Amytal for the lateralization of cerebral speech dominance. *J. Neurosurg.* **21:** 399.

Cohen, R.L. 1981. On the generality of some memory laws. *Scand. J. Psychol.* **22:** 267.

———. 1983. The effect of encoding variables in the free recall of words and action events. *Mem. Cognit.* **11:** 575.

Fuster, J.M. 1989. *The prefrontal cortex*, 2nd edition. Raven Press, New York.

Goldman-Rakic, P.S. 1987. Circuitry of primate prefrontal cortex and regulation of behavior by representational memory. In *Handbook of physiology: The nervous system* (ed. F. Plum), vol. 5, p. 373. American Physiological Society, Bethesda, Maryland.

Jacobsen, C.F. 1935. Functions of the frontal association area in primates. *Arch. Neurol. Psychiatry* **33:** 558.

Jacobsen, C.F. and H.W. Nissen. 1937. Studies of cerebral function in primates. IV. The effects of frontal lobe lesions on the delayed alternation habit in monkeys. *J. Comp. Physiol. Psychol.* **23:** 101.

Kimura, D. 1963. Right temporal-lobe damage. *Arch. Neurol.* **8:** 264.

Konorski, J. 1959. A new method of physiological investigation of recent memory in animals. *Bull. Acad. Pol. Sci.* **7:** 115.

Ladavas, E., C. Umilta, and L. Provinciali. 1979. Hemisphere-dependent cognitive performances in epileptic patients. *Epilepsia* **20:** 493.

McAndrews, M.P. and B. Milner. 1991. The frontal cortex and memory for temporal order. *Neuropsychologia* (in press).

Michon, J.A. and J.L. Jackson. 1984. Attentional effort and cognitive strategies in the processing of temporal information. *Ann. N.Y. Acad. Sci.* **423:** 298.

Milner, B. 1964. Some effects of frontal lobectomy in man. In *The frontal granular cortex and behavior* (ed. J.M. Warner and K. Akert), p. 313. McGraw-Hill, New York.

———. 1968a. Memory. In *Analysis of behavioural change* (ed. L. Weiskrantz), p. 328. Harper and Row, New York.

———. 1968b. Visual recognition and recall after right temporal-lobe excision in man. *Neuropsychologia* **6:** 191.

———. 1971. Interhemispheric differences in the localization of psychological processes in man. *Br. Med. Bull.* **27:** 272.

———. 1974. Hemispheric specialization: Scope and limits. In *The neurosciences: Third study program* (ed. F.O. Schmitt and F.G. Worden), p. 75. MIT Press, Cambridge, Massachusetts.

———. 1985. Memory and the human brain. In *How we know: Nobel Conference 20* (ed. M. Shafto), p. 31. Harper and Row, New York.

———. 1990. Right temporal-lobe contribution to visual perception and visual memory. In *Vision, memory and the temporal lobe* (ed. E. Iwai), p. 42. Elsevier, New York.

Nilsson, L.-G. and R.L. Cohen. 1988. Enrichment and generation in the recall of enacted and non-enacted instructions. In *Practical aspects of memory* (ed. M.M. Gruneberg et al.), vol. 1, p. 427. Wiley, London.

Pribram, K.H. and W.E. Tubbs. 1967. Short-term memory, parsing, and frontal cortex. *Science* **156:** 1765.

Pribram, K.H., H.C. Plotkin, R.M. Anderson, and D. Leong. 1977. Information sources in the delayed alternation task for normal and frontal monkeys. *Neuropsychologia* **15:** 329.

Prisko, L.-H. 1963. "Short-term memory in focal cerebral damage." Unpublished Ph.D. thesis, McGill University, Montreal, Canada.

Rosenkilde, C.E., H.E. Rosvold, and M. Mishkin. 1981. Time discrimination with positional responses after selective prefrontal lesions in monkeys. *Brain Res.* **210:** 129.

Sagar, H.J., J.D.E. Gabrieli, E.V. Sullivan, and S. Corkin. 1990. Recency and frequency discrimination in the amnesic patient H.M. *Brain* **113:** 581.

Schacter, D.L. 1987. Memory, amnesia and frontal-lobe dysfunction. *Psychobiology* **15:** 21.

Shimamura, A.P., J.S. Janowsky, and L.R. Squire. 1988. Memory for temporal order in patients with frontal-lobe lesions and patients with amnesia. *Soc. Neurosci. Abstr.* **14:** 1043.

Stepien, L. and S. Sierpinski. 1960. The effect of focal lesion of the brain upon auditory and visual recent memory in man. *J. Neurol. Neurosurg. Psychiatr.* **23:** 344.

Underwood, B.J. 1977. *Temporal codes for memories: Issues and problems.* Lawrence Erlbaum Associates, Hillsdale, New Jersey.

Yntema, D.B. and F.P. Trask. 1963. Recall as a search process. *J. Verb. Learn. Verb. Behav.* **2:** 65.

Theoretical and Neurophysiological Analysis of the Functions of the Primate Hippocampus in Memory

E.T. ROLLS

University of Oxford, Department of Experimental Psychology, Oxford OX1 3UD, England

The aims of this paper are to consider which spatial functions are performed by the primate hippocampus, how these are related to the memory functions performed by the hippocampus, and how the hippocampus performs these functions. In addition to the evidence that is available from anatomical connections, the effects of lesions to the system, and recordings of the activity of single neurons in the system, neuronal network models of hippocampal function will also be introduced, as they have the promise of enabling one to understand what and how the hippocampus computes, and thus the functions being performed by the hippocampus. Many of the studies described have been performed with macaque monkeys to provide information as relevant as possible to understanding amnesia in humans. Effects on memory are produced by damage to the hippocampus or to some of its connections, such as the fornix, and these structures are collectively referred to below as the hippocampal system.

Damage to the Hippocampal System and Spatial Function

Damage to the hippocampus or to some of its connections, such as the fornix, in monkeys produces deficits in simple left-right-discrimination learning in which, for example, food is hidden consistently on the right or the left under one of two identical objects, and the monkey must learn whether to displace the left or the right object in order to find food (Mahut 1972). Fornix lesions also impair conditional left-right-discrimination learning, in which the visual appearance of an object specifies whether a response is to be made to the left or the right (Gaffan et al. 1984; Rupniak and Gaffan 1987) (in humans, see Petrides 1985). (An example of such a conditional spatial response task is that if two objects shown are red, then the object on the left must be chosen to obtain a reward, and if the two objects shown are green, then the object on the right must be chosen to obtain a reward.) Two possible interpretations of these spatial learning impairments produced by fornix section are as follows.

First, it is possible that the learning system disrupted is only for the acquisition of map-like knowledge about the environment, such as that there is food in a certain place. This is not the case, because lesioned monkeys were impaired in learning to make a response to one side when one picture was shown and to the other side

when a different picture was shown (Rupniak and Gaffan 1987), i.e., in conditional spatial response learning as described above. The spatial environment was held constant, and thus damage to the hippocampal system does not impair only the ability to acquire map-like knowledge of the environment. The experiment does show, on the other hand, that there is an impairment when monkeys must learn to make spatial responses on the basis of nonspatial stimuli.

Second, it is possible that the hippocampal learning system is only for the control of spatially directed movements, such as go left and go right. This is not the case, for fornix-sectioned monkeys are impaired in learning on the basis of a spatial cue which object to choose (e.g., if two objects are on the left, choose object A, but if the two objects are on the right, choose object B) (Gaffan and Harrison 1989a). Thus, the deficit is not just in learning spatial responses, for in this task the response was not spatial. The spatial aspect of this task was in the spatial position of the stimuli.

These findings suggest that fornix damage can impair learning about both the places of objects and the places of responses. Gaffan and Harrison (1989b) have analyzed further what it is that characterizes the spatial learning deficit of monkeys with damage to the hippocampal system in experiments in which the monkey was moved to different positions in a room. Impairments were found when which of two or more objects the monkey had to choose depended on the position of the monkey in the room, provided that the same parts of the room were in view from both positions of the monkey, so that the relative positions of room cues had to be remembered in order to solve the task (Gaffan and Harrison 1989b, experiment 1). This requirement is referred to as "whole scene analysis." If the parts of the room visible from the monkey's testing positions were different, then there was no impairment in learning which object to choose (Gaffan and Harrison 1989b, experiment 2). However, if the monkey had to make a spatial response to one of two identical objects which depended on different environmental cues (whether room-based or local), then fornix-sectioned monkeys displayed a learning impairment (Gaffan and Harrison, 1989b, experiments 3 and 5). These experiments suggest that fornix-sectioned monkeys can predict which of two different objects is rewarded on the basis of a conjunction of background items in the environment and the object displaced. Accordingly, they can thus choose one of two (visually) different objects in a scene provided that the scene has different items visible in it, whether locally or distantly. However, a deficit is produced by fornix section when the monkey has to store the spatial relations of the background items and of identical objects in a scene. Accordingly, the fornix-sectioned monkeys are impaired in learning to select different objects depending on the spatial relations of items in the scene, or to make spatial responses to identical objects in a scene, as these involve storing the relative positions of places to which to respond (Gaffan and Harrison 1989b).

Another spatial task impaired by damage to the hippocampal system in monkeys (Gaffan and Saunders 1985; Parkinson et al. 1988) and humans (Smith and Milner 1981) is an object-place memory task. In this task, not only which objects have been seen before, but also where in space each object was located must be remembered. The task has been run with macaques by showing a picture in each of four positions on a screen twice (Rolls et al. 1989). The first time the monkey saw the picture in a particular position, he had to withhold a lick response (in order to avoid saline). The second time a picture appeared in a given position on the screen, the monkey could lick to obtain fruit juice. Each picture was shown in each position twice, once as novel and once as familiar for that position, and many different pictures were used in sequence. Thus, in order to perform the task, the monkey had to remember not only which pictures had been seen before, but also the position on the screen in which the picture had been seen. In humans, the object-place task was run by showing the subjects a tray containing a set of objects, and then asking later not only which objects had been seen before, but also where they were on the tray (Smith and Milner 1981). Such object-place tasks require a whole-scene or snapshot-like memory in which spatial relations in a scene must be remembered. It is not sufficient just to be able to remember the objects that have been seen before. The deficit in the object-place memory task is thus analogous to the deficit in the spatial tasks described above, in that the deficit is fully apparent when not just objects, but objects and their spatial relations to each other, must be remembered.

Nonspatial Aspects of the Function of the Hippocampus in Primates: Its Role in Memory

In addition to the spatial deficits described above that are produced by damage to the hippocampal system in primates, there are also deficits in nonspatial memory tasks. For example, the anterograde amnesia associated with damage to the hippocampus in humans is evident as a major deficit in learning to recognize new stimuli, and the recognition memory deficit encompasses nonspatial items (e.g., objects and people) as well as places (Scoville and Milner 1957; Milner 1972; Squire 1986; Squire and Zola-Morgan 1988). Recognition memory is also impaired in monkeys with damage to the hippocampal system (Gaffan 1974, 1977; Gaffan

and Weiskrantz 1980; Owen and Butler 1981; Zola-Morgan et al. 1986), although it is possible that severe deficits in recognition memory are only found when there is also damage to the amygdala (Mishkin 1978, 1982; Murray and Mishkin 1984). In a typical recognition memory task in the monkey, a stimulus is shown to the monkey, and when it is shown again later, the monkey can choose it to obtain a reward. If no other stimuli intervene between the first and second presentations of a given stimulus, then the task is described as a match-to-sample task. If other stimuli intervene between the first (novel) and second (familiar) presentations of a stimulus, then the task is described as a serial or running recognition task. A serial recognition task is often used when analyzing the role of the hippocampus in memory, because a memory task with intervening stimuli is more difficult than a delayed match-to-sample task and may therefore be a more sensitive indicator of an effect on memory (Gaffan 1974, 1977).

It is interesting that the impairment produced by damage to the hippocampal system in recognition memory tasks as usually implemented (e.g., choose or respond to objects seen before, that is delayed match-to-sample, perhaps with intervening stimuli) is much less clear if delayed nonmatch-to-sample is used (choose the novel stimulus) (Gaffan et al. 1984). The impairment is also much less severe if the monkeys are trained initially with the long (and therefore difficult) intervals between stimuli with which they are tested later (Gaffan et al. 1984). The implication of these findings is that the deficit produced by the fornix section is not simply due to an inability to distinguish novel from familiar stimuli, but is due perhaps just as much to a difficulty these lesioned animals have in altering their instrumental response strategies, e.g., so that they respond to familiar stimuli when the natural tendency is to respond to novel stimuli, and so that they start responding at long memory intervals when they have been trained previously to respond with short memory intervals (see Gaffan et al. 1984). However, although the deficit usually found in recognition memory tasks may not strictly be due to an inability to distinguish novel from familiar stimuli, there is nevertheless a nonspatial impairment apparent in recognition memory tasks. Another nonspatial impairment produced by fornix section in monkeys is a deficit in learning the unnatural instrumental response rule "Choose the object not previously paired with reward," sometimes called the win-shift rule (Gaffan et al. 1984). (Fornix section did not impair use of the natural instrumental rule "Choose the object previously associated with reward," sometimes called the win-stay rule [Gaffan et al. 1984].) Thus, in monkeys, hippocampal function is involved not only in some types of spatial learning, but also in some aspect of nonspatial learning, even if this latter may not be pure novelty versus familiarity learning, but is instead related in some way to organizing flexibly adaptive instrumental responses.

There is also evidence from humans that the hippocampus is involved in nonspatial (as well as spatial) memory, for e.g., in paired (word) associate learning, and in episodic memory, such as the memory of events that happened and people met on previous days (see Squire et al. 1989).

Relation between Spatial and Nonspatial Aspects of Hippocampal Function

One way of relating the impairment of spatial processing to other aspects of hippocampal function is to note that this spatial processing involves a snapshot type of memory, in which one whole scene must be remembered. This memory may then be a special case of episodic memory, which involves an arbitrary association of a set of events that describe a past episode. Furthermore, the nonspatial tasks impaired by damage to the hippocampal system may be impaired because they are tasks in which a memory of a particular episode rather than of a general rule is involved. Thus, the learning of tasks with nongeneral rules, such as choose the object not previously rewarded (i.e., win-shift, lose-stay), may be impaired because to solve them the particular pairing in the particular context (of performing with this special rule) must be remembered in order to choose the correct object later. (The natural rule, which will in the natural environment usually lead to reward, is to choose the object previously associated with reward.) Another example is that choosing familiar rather than novel objects in a recognition memory task may be particularly difficult for monkeys with damage to the hippocampal system because it involves a special rule, choose the familiar object in this task, rather than what may be a more general tendency, i.e., to choose the novel rather than the familiar object. The latter rule is what normally guides behavior, as this rule is more likely to lead to reward for objects without an explicit reward association already in the natural en-

vironment. Furthermore, recognition memory may be particularly impaired when this involves the memory of particular and arbitrary associations between parts of the image, especially when the same elements may occur in different combinations in other images. In addition, the deficit in paired associate learning in humans may be especially evident when this involves arbitrary associations between words, for example, window–lake. I suggest that the reason why the hippocampus is used for the spatial and nonspatial types of memory described above, and the reason that these two types of memory are so analogous, is that the hippocampus contains one stage, the CA3 stage, which acts as an autoassociation memory. (The structure, operation, and properties of autoassociation memories are described below.) It is suggested that an autoassociation memory implemented by the CA3 neurons equally enables whole (spatial) scenes or episodic memories to be formed, with a snapshot quality that depends on the arbitrary associations that can be made and the short temporal window that characterizes the synaptic modifiability in this system (see below and Rolls 1987, 1989a,b). The ways in which the architecture of the hippocampus appears to be specialized to perform these functions in spatial snapshot and episodic memory are described next, to lead toward a deeper understanding of hippocampal function in these types of learning.

Computational Significance of the Functional Architecture of the Hippocampus

The internal connections of the hippocampus and the learning rules implemented at its synapses are described first to delineate its functional architecture, which provides the basis for a computational theory of the hippocampus.

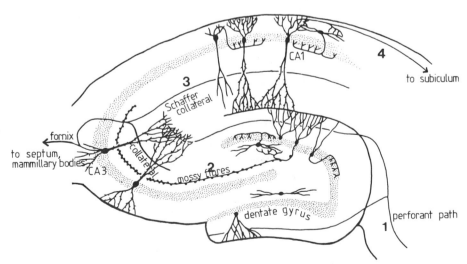

Figure 1. Representation of connections within the hippocampus. Inputs reach the hippocampus through the perforant path (1), which makes synapses with the dendrites of the dentate granule cells and also with the apical dendrites of the CA3 pyramidal cells. The dentate granule cells project via the mossy fibers (2) to the CA3 pyramidal cells. The well-developed recurrent collateral system of the CA3 cells is indicated. The CA3 pyramidal cells project via the Schaffer collaterals (3) to the CA1 pyramidal cells, which in turn have connections (4) to the subiculum.

Schematic diagrams of the connections of the hippocampus are shown in Figures 1 and 2. In primates, major input connections are from the association areas of the cerebral cortex, including the parietal cortex (which processes spatial information), the temporal lobe visual and auditory areas, and the frontal cortex. Within the hippocampus, there is a three-stage sequence of processing, consisting of the dentate granule cells (which receive from the entorhinal cortex via the perforant path), the CA3 pyramidal cells, and the CA1 pyramidal cells (see below). Outputs return from the hippocampus to the cerebral cortex via the subiculum, entorhinal cortex, and parahippocampal gyrus.

CA3 pyramidal cells. One major feature of hippocampal neuronal networks is the recurrent collateral system of the CA3 cells, formed by the output axons of the CA3 cells having a branch that returns to make synapses with the dendrites of the other CA3 cells, as shown in Figures 1 and 2. Given that the region of the CA3 cell dendrites on which the recurrent collaterals synapse is long (~ 12 mm), and that the total dendritic length is approximately 16 mm and has approximately 16,000 spines (Squire et al. 1989; Amaral et al. 1990), and that each spine receives one synapse, approximately 12,000 synapses per CA3 pyramidal cell could be devoted to recurrent collaterals, which with 304,000 CA3 neurons on each side of the brain in the (Sprague-Dawley) rat (Boss et al. 1987; Amaral et al. 1990) makes the probability of contact between the CA3 neurons 3.9%. (The quantitative values given here have been updated a little from those given by Rolls [1989a,b] in light of new estimates provided by Amaral et al. [1990].) It is remarkable that the contact probability is so high, and also that the CA3 recurrent collateral axons travel so widely in all directions that

they can potentially come close to almost all other CA3 neurons (Amaral and Witter 1989; Rolls 1989a,b; Squire et al. 1989; D.G. Amaral, pers. comm.). The connectivity of these CA3 cells is even more remarkable than this, for, in addition, there is a commissural system in which CA3 neurons on one side of the brain send axons to end primarily on the dendrites of the CA3 neurons of the other side of the brain. The terminals are made on the same stretch of the CA3 dendrites as the recurrent collaterals, so that the contact probability calculated above must be reduced (with the lower limit being perhaps 2.0%, representing 12,000 synapses shared among 608,000 CA3 neurons). The remarkable effect achieved by this is that the CA3 neurons provide one interconnected network of neurons for both sides of the brain, with a reasonably high probability that any CA3 neuron will be connected to any other CA3 neuron, irrespective of the side of the brain. Although connectivity across the midline is likely to be high in the rat, the two sides of the hippocampus are probably not fully interconnected in humans, as indicated by the evidence that damage to the right temporal lobe affects spatial tasks (such as conditional spatial response learning) more than nonspatial memory tasks, whereas damage to the left temporal lobe affects nonspatial tasks such as paired word associate learning more than nonspatial tasks (Milner 1982; Kolb and Whishaw 1985).

There is evidence from studies of long-term potentiation (Bliss and Lomo 1973; Kelso et al. 1986; Wigstrom et al. 1986; P.O. Andersen 1987; Brown et al. 1990; Collingridge and Singer 1990) that the synapses in this recurrent collateral system are Hebb-modifiable, i.e., that they become stronger when there is strong conjunctive postsynaptic and presynaptic activity (Miles 1988).

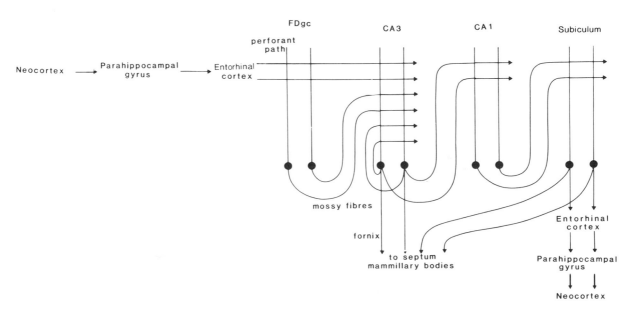

Figure 2. Schematic representation of the connections of the hippocampus, showing also that the cerebral cortex (neocortex) is connected to the hippocampus via the parahippocampal gyrus and entorhinal cortex, and that the hippocampus projects back to the neocortex via the subiculum, entorhinal cortex, and parahippocampal gyrus. (FDgc) Dentate granule cells.

Autoassociation memory implemented by the CA3 recurrent collateral system. This functional anatomy of the CA3 pyramidal cells immediately suggests that this is an autoassociation (or autocorrelation) matrix memory. The autoassociation arises because the outputs of the CA3 cells are fed back by the recurrent collateral axons to make Hebb-modifiable synapses with the dendrites of the other CA3 neurons. The result of implementation of the Hebb rule in this architecture is that any strongly activated cell or set of cells becomes linked by strengthened synapses with any other conjunctively strongly activated cell or set of cells. During learning, the matrix of synaptic weights that link the cells together (see Fig. 3) comes to reflect the correlations between the activities of the CA3 cells. Because the matrix of synaptic weights stores the correlations between the activities of the cells of the memory, this type of memory is called an autocorrelation or autoassociation matrix memory. During recall, presentation of even a part of the original pattern of activity of the CA3 cells, which might represent one part of or key to the memory, elicits the firing of the whole set of cells that were originally conjunctively activated. This important property of this type of memory is termed completion and is fundamental to any biological memory system. During recall, if a pattern similar to one learned by the system is presented, then insofar as some of the neurons active in the key stimulus were also part of a pattern stored previously in the memory, the previously stored pattern is recalled. This property, which is also fundamental to biological memory, is termed generalization. Another property of this type of memory is that it continues to function moderately well if it is partially damaged, or if, for example, not every

synapse in the matrix is present, either because of limitations of fan-in of individual neurons or because of limitations of the precision of development. This property is also important for a biological memory system and is termed graceful degradation or fault tolerance. More extensive descriptions of the properties of autoassociation matrix memories are given by Kohonen et al. (1981), Kohonen (1984), and Rolls (1987). The suggestion made here is that the output of the CA3 pyramidal cells is fed back along the horizontally running recurrent collateral axons that make Hebb-modifiable synapses with other CA3 dendrites so that the pattern of activity in the CA3 pyramidal cells is associated with itself.

For this autoassociation to work correctly, it is important that a depolarization produced by synaptic input on one part of the dendrite is effective on other parts of the dendrite, so that even distant active synapses experience the postsynaptic term required for the Hebb rule to be implemented. This condition does appear to be met, as shown by the short electrical length of the dendrites and by the cooperation which occurs between inputs that synapse on different parts of the dendrite in setting up the postsynaptic depolarization required for long-term potentiation (McNaughton 1984; P.O. Andersen 1987). This cooperativity between active synapses made at different positions along the postsynaptic membrane, so that active synapses onto a neuron alter their strength only when other synapses are active on the same dendrite and produce postsynaptic activation, enables associations to be formed on the basis of temporal conjunctions that occur between any set of conjunctively active afferents. In a sense, the large number of synapses of these CA3 cells devoted to the recurrent collaterals allows correlations of firing across a large information space to be detected. Consistent with this suggestion about the computational role of the CA3 system of the hippocampus, it is known that the probability of contact of the neurons in an autoassociation matrix memory must not be very low if it is to operate usefully (see Marr 1971; Gardner-Medwin 1976). The synaptic modifiability implemented in the CA3 recurrent collateral system may utilize NMDA receptors, which allow synaptic modifiability only when the postsynaptic membrane is strongly activated. This interesting nonlinearity of the learning rule means that only correlations between strongly activated CA3 pyramidal cells are stored, which help to maximize the storage capacity of the system and to minimize interference.

It is suggested below that the systems level function of this autoassociation memory is to enable events occurring conjunctively in quite different parts of the association areas of the cerebral cortex to be associated together to form a memory that could well be described as episodic. Each episode would be defined by a conjunction of a set of events, and each episodic memory would consist of the association of one set of events (such as where, with whom, and what one ate at lunch on the preceding day). It is suggested that the "snapshot, whole-scene" spatial memory in which the hip-

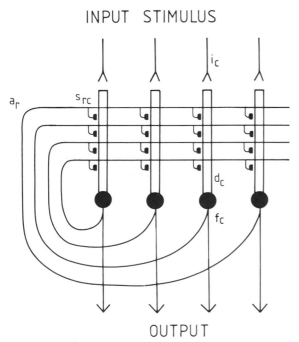

INPUT STIMULUS

OUTPUT

Figure 3. An autoassociation matrix memory. The dendrites, d_c, have recurrent collateral axons, a_r, which make Hebb-modifiable synapses, s_{rc}, with the other neurons in the population.

pocampus is implicated, as shown above, is what the hippocampus can achieve for spatial information processing by allowing all the parts of a whole scene to be associated together to provide a memory of the whole scene. The importance of the hippocampus in episodic memory and "whole-scene" memory may arise from the fact that in one part of it, the CA3 region, there is one autoassociation matrix memory with a relatively high contact probability that receives information originating in many different areas of the cerebral cortex, and from both sides of the brain. It is suggested that this ability to link information originating from different brain regions in a single autoassociation matrix in the CA3 regions is a key feature of hippocampal architecture, which is unlikely to be implemented in input regions such as the entorhinal cortex and dentate granule cells, which not only do not have the required system of recurrent collaterals over the whole population of cells, but also appear to maintain some segregation of inputs originating from different parts of the cerebral cortex (Insausti et al. 1987). One reason why there may not be more cells in the CA3 region is that it is important that the connectivity be kept relatively high so that any event represented by the firing of a sparse set of CA3 cells can be associated with any other event represented by a different set of CA3 cells firing. Because each CA3 pyramidal cell has a limited fan-in or number of synapses (perhaps 16,000, see above), the total number of cells in the autoassociation memory cannot be increased beyond the limit set by the fan-in and the connectivity. The advantages of sparse encoding and a well interconnected matrix are that a large number of different (episodic) memories can be stored in the CA3 system and that the advantageous emergent properties of a matrix memory, such as completion, generalization, and graceful degradation (see Kohonen et al. 1977, 1981; Kohonen 1984; Rolls 1987), are produced efficiently. Completion may operate particularly effectively here with a sparse representation, because it is under these conditions that the simple autocorrelation effect can reconstruct the whole of one pattern without interference, which would arise if too high a proportion of the input neurons was active.

Dentate granule cells and the CA1 pyramidal cells. The theory is developed elsewhere that the dentate granule cell stage of hippocampal processing that precedes the CA3 stage acts in two ways to produce the sparse yet efficient (i.e., nonredundant) representation in CA3 neurons that is required for the autoassociation to perform well (Rolls 1989a,b). The first way is that the perforant path/dentate granule cell system with its Hebb-like modifiability is suggested to act as a competitive learning matrix to remove redundancy from the inputs, producing a more orthogonal and categorized set of outputs. The second way arises because there is a very low (0.008% in the rat) contact probability in the mossy fiber/CA3 connections, which achieves by pattern separation relatively orthogonal representations (compared to those on the dentate granule cells, and within the limits set by the relative numbers of dentate

granule and CA3 cells; see Rolls 1989a), which are required if the autoassociation matrix memory formed by the CA3 cells is to operate with usefully large memory capacity and with minimal interference (see Kohonen et al. 1977, 1981; Rolls 1987). As the neurons have positive continuous firing rates, the only way in which relatively orthogonal representations can be formed is by making the number of neurons active for any one input stimulus relatively low (see, e.g., Jordan 1986), and this sparse representation is exactly what can be achieved by the low contact probability pattern separation effect of the mossy fibers (Rolls 1989a,b). The pattern separation effect refers to the point that input patterns which are correlated produce output patterns which are less correlated with each other.

The function of the CA1 stage that follows the CA3 cells (see Figs. 1 and 2) is also considered to be related to the CA3 autoassociation effect in which several arbitrary patterns of firing occur together on the CA3 neurons and become associated together to form an episodic or "whole-scene" memory. It is essential for this operation that several different sparse representations are present conjunctively in order to form the association. Moreover, when completion operates in the CA3 autoassociation system, all the neurons firing in the original conjunction can be brought into activity by only a part of the original set of conjunctive events. For these reasons, a memory in the CA3 cells consists of several different simultaneously active ensembles of activity. It is suggested that the CA1 cells, which receive these groups of simultaneously active ensembles, can detect the conjunctions of firing of the different ensembles that represent the episodic memory, and allocate by competitive learning a relatively few neurons to represent each episodic memory. The episodic memory would thus consist in the CA3 region of ensembles of active cells, each ensemble representing one of the subcomponents of the episodic memory (including context), whereas the whole episodic memory would be represented not by its parts, but as a single collection of active cells at the CA1 stage. It is suggested below that one role these economical (in terms of the number of activated fibers) and relatively orthogonal signals in the CA1 cells have is to guide information storage or consolidation in the cerebral cortex. To understand how the hippocampus may perform this function for the cerebral cortex, it is necessary to turn to a systems level analysis to show how the computations performed by the hippocampus fit into overall brain function. It may be noted that by forming associations of events derived from different parts of the cerebral cortex (the CA3 stage) and by building new economical (i.e., less redundant) representations of the conjunctions detected (the CA1 stage), the hippocampus provides an output that is suitable for directing the long-term storage of information.

Synaptic modification occurs with presynaptic firing rates in the physiological range in the hippocampus. The ideas introduced above on the operation of neuronal networks in the hippocampus during learning include the postulate that synapses in the hippocampus modify according to rules analyzed in studies of long-term potentiation. In studies of long-term potentiation, the presynaptic neurons are typically induced to fire synchronously at a high frequency by electrical stimulation. In a recent series of experiments (Cahusac and Rolls 1989), we investigated whether pairing of the normal firing of presynaptic neurons (i.e., at physiologically occurring firing rates and without the synchronous firing induced by electrical stimulation) could be effective when paired with postsynaptic activation in leading to synaptic enhancement.

Recordings were made extracellularly of action potentials from hippocampal neurons while macaques performed a task in which hippocampal neurons were known to be activated by visual stimuli (Miyashita et al. 1989). The task was a visual discrimination task in which the monkey could make lick or arm-reach responses when one visual stimulus was shown and had to avoid such responses when the other visual stimulus was shown in order to avoid the taste of saline. When a neuron was found that had some response to one or both of the visual stimuli, one of the stimuli was temporally paired with the ionophoretic application of L-glutamate (25–190 nA), which was switched on to cause firing for 350–950 msec while that stimulus was displayed. The visual stimuli were presented in random sequence until 30–50 pairings of one of the visual stimuli with firing of the postsynaptic neuron induced by glutamate had occurred.

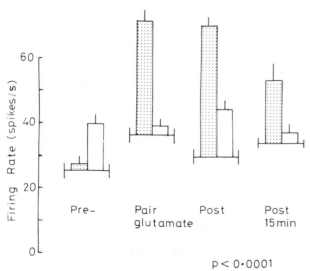

Figure 4. Evidence on synaptic modification in the primate hippocampus when the presynaptic firing is that induced by natural inputs to the hippocampus. (Pre-) The responses of the single neuron to two visual stimuli (dotted and open bars) in a visual discrimination task are shown (means ± S.E.M. shown above the spontaneous firing rate of the neuron). (Pair glutamate) One of the visual stimuli (dotted bars) was paired with ionophoretic application of glutamate, which produced fast firing of the neuron during the presentation of that stimulus. This pairing was repeated for many trials. (Post) After pairing with glutamate, the neuron responded more to the visual stimulus previously paired with glutamate. (Post 15 min) This effect lasted for at least 15 min.

Of 28 neurons studied, 6 showed potentiation of responses to the visual stimulus paired with the ionophoretic application of glutamate (as indicated by $p < 0.001$ in each case in an ANOVA) (see, e.g., Fig. 4). There was no potentiation to the unpaired visual stimulus. The modifications of responses lasted for at least 8–18 minutes. These experiments provide evidence that pairing of naturally induced firing of presynaptic neurons with postsynaptic activation in the primate hippocampus can lead to modifications of the neuronal responses elicited by the input paired with the postsynaptic activation. In terms of the network models described above, these experiments provide additional evidence that synaptic modification rules of the type incorporated in the models do operate in the hippocampus (for further details, see Rolls 1989c).

Systems Level Analysis of Hippocampal Function, Including Neuronal Activity in the Primate Hippocampus

We have just utilized the functional architecture (internal anatomy and physiology) of the hippocampus to suggest a computational theory of how it operates. To understand how these computations are used and how they contribute to the information processing being performed by other parts of the brain, we now turn to a systems level analysis in which we consider the connections of the hippocampus with the rest of the brain, and the activity of single neurons in the hippocampus when it is performing its normal function, as assessed by the effects of selective damage to the hippocampus as described above.

Systems level anatomy. The primate hippocampus receives inputs via the entorhinal cortex (area 28) and the parahippocampal gyrus from many areas of the cerebral association cortex, including the parietal cortex, which is concerned with spatial functions, the visual and auditory temporal association cortical areas, and the frontal cortex (Van Hoesen 1982; Amaral 1987; Rolls 1989a,b). In addition, the entorhinal cortex receives inputs from the amygdala. There are also subcortical inputs from, for example, the amygdala and septum. The hippocampus in turn projects back via the subiculum, entorhinal cortex, and parahippocampal gyrus (area TF-TH), to the cerebral cortical areas from which it receives inputs (Van Hoesen 1982), as well as to subcortical areas such as the mammillary bodies (see Figs. 1 and 2).

Systems level neurophysiology. The information processing being performed by the primate hippocampus while it is performing the functions for which lesion studies have shown it is needed has been investigated in studies in which the activity of single hippocampal neurons has been analyzed during the performance and learning of these (and related) spatial tasks. Watanabe and Niki (1985) analyzed hippocampal neuronal activity while monkeys performed a delayed spatial response task. In a delayed spatial response task, a stimulus is shown, for example, on the left; there is then a delay period, and after this the monkey can respond by touching the left stimulus position. They reported that 6.4% of hippocampal neurons responded differently while the monkey was remembering left as compared to right. The responses of these neurons could reflect preparation for the spatial response to be made, or they could reflect memory of the spatial position in which the stimulus was shown. To provide evidence on which was important, Cahusac et al. (1989) analyzed hippocampal activity in this task, and in an object-place memory task. In the object-place memory task, the monkey was shown a sample stimulus in one position on a video screen; there was a delay of two seconds, and then the same or a different stimulus was shown in the same or in a different position. The monkey remembered the sample and its position, and if both matched the delayed stimulus, he licked to obtain fruit juice. Of the 600 neurons analyzed in this task, 3.8% responded differently for the different spatial positions, with some of these responding differentially during the sample presentation, some in the delay period, and some in the match period. Thus, some hippocampal neurons (those differentially active in the sample or match periods) respond differently for stimuli shown in different positions in space, and some (those differentially active in the delay period) respond differently when the monkey is remembering different positions in space. In addition, some of the neurons responded to a combination of object and place information, in that they responded only to a novel object in a particular place. These neuronal responses were not due to any response being made or prepared by the monkey, because information about which behavioral response was required was not available until the match stimulus was shown. Cahusac et al. (1989) also found that the majority of the neurons that responded in the object-place memory task did not respond in the delayed spatial response task. Instead, a different population of neurons (5.7% of the total) responded in the delayed spatial response task, with differential left-right responses in the sample, delay, or match periods. Thus, this latter population of hippocampal neurons had activity that was related to the preparation for or initiation of a spatial response, which in the delayed response task could be encoded as soon as the sample stimulus was seen. These recordings showed that there are some neurons in the primate hippocampus with activity that is related to the spatial position of stimuli or to the memory of the spatial position of stimuli (as shown in the object-place memory task) and that there are other neurons in the hippocampus with activity that is related not to the stimulus or the memory of the stimulus, but instead to the spatial response that the monkey is preparing and remembering (as shown in the delayed spatial response task).

The responses of hippocampal neurons in primates with activity related to the place in which a stimulus is shown were further investigated using a serial multiple object-place memory task. The task required a memory for the position on a video monitor in which a given object had appeared previously (Rolls et al. 1989). This task was designed to allow a wider area of space to be tested than in the previous study and was chosen also because memory of where objects had been seen previously in space was known to be disrupted by hippocampal damage (Gaffan and Saunders 1985; Gaffan 1987). In the task, a visual image appeared in one of four or nine positions on a screen. If the stimulus had been seen in that position before, the monkey could lick to obtain fruit juice, but if the image had not appeared in that position before, the monkey had not to lick in order to avoid the taste of saline. Each image appeared in each position on the screen only twice, once as novel and once as familiar. The task thus required memory not only of which visual stimuli had been seen before, but of the positions in which they had been seen, and is an object-place memory task. It was found that 9% of neurons recorded in the hippocampus and parahippocampal gyrus had spatial fields in this and related tasks, in that they responded whenever there was a stimulus in some but not in other positions on the screen. Of the neurons, 2.4% responded to a combination of spatial information and information about the object seen, in that they responded more the first time a particular image was seen in any position. Six of these neurons were found that showed this combination even more clearly, because they, for example, responded only to some positions and only if it was the first time a particular stimulus had appeared there. Thus, not only is spatial information processed by the primate hippocampus, but it also can be combined, as shown by the responses of single neurons, with information about which stimuli have been seen before (Rolls et al. 1989).

The ability of the hippocampus to form such arbitrary associations of information probably originating from the parietal cortex about position in space with information originating from the temporal lobe about objects may be important for its role in memory. Moreover, these findings provide neurophysiological support for the computational theory described above, according to which such arbitrary associations should be formed onto single neurons in the hippocampus.

These "space" neurons (Cahusac et al. 1989; Rolls et al. 1989) may be compared with "place" cells recorded in the rat hippocampus (see McNaughton et al. 1983; O'Keefe 1984). The "place" cells described in the rat respond when the rat is in a particular place in the environment as specified by extra-maze cues, whereas the cells described here respond to particular positions in space, or at least when stimuli are shown in particular positions in space (for further details, see Feigenbaum and Rolls 1990).

These studies showed that some hippocampal neurons in primates have spatial fields. To investigate how space is represented in the hippocampus, Feigenbaum et al. (1987) and Feigenbaum and Rolls (1990) investigated whether the spatial fields use egocentric or some form of allocentric coordinates. This was investigated by finding a neuron with a space field and then moving the monitor screen and the monkey relative to each other and to different positions in the laboratory. For 10% of the spatial neurons, the responses remained in the same position relative to the monkey's body axis when the screen was moved or the monkey was rotated or moved to a different position in the laboratory. These neurons thus represented space in egocentric coordinates. For 46% of the spatial neurons analyzed, the responses remained in the same position on the screen or in the room when the monkey was rotated or moved to a different position in the laboratory. These neurons thus represented space in allocentric coordinates. Evidence for two types of allocentric encoding was found. In the first type, the field was defined by its position on the monitor screen independently of the position of the monitor relative to the monkey's body axis and independently of the position of the monkey and the screen in the laboratory. These neurons were called "frame of reference" allocentric, since their fields were defined by the local frame provided by the monitor screen. The majority of the allocentric neurons responded in this way. In the second type of allocentric encoding, the field was defined by its position in the room and was relatively independent of position relative to the monkey's body axis or to position on the monitor screen face. These neurons were called "absolute" allocentric, since their fields were defined by position in the room. These results provide evidence that in addition to neurons with egocentric spatial fields, which have also been found in other parts of the brain (Sakata 1985; R.A. Andersen 1987), there are neurons in the primate hippocampal formation that encode space in allocentric coordinates.

In another type of task for which the primate hippocampus is needed, conditional spatial response learning, in which the monkeys had to learn which spatial response to make to different stimuli, i.e., to acquire associations between visual stimuli and spatial responses, 14% of hippocampal neurons responded to particular combinations of stimuli and responses (Miyashita et al. 1989). The firing of these neurons could not be accounted for by the motor requirements of the task, nor wholly by the stimulus aspects of the task, as demonstrated by testing their firing in related visual discrimination tasks. These results showed that single hippocampal neurons respond to combinations of the visual stimuli and the spatial responses with which they must become associated in conditional response tasks and are consistent with the computational theory described above according to which part of the mechanism of this learning involves associations between visual stimuli and spatial responses learned by single hippocampal neurons. In a following study, it was found that during such conditional spatial response learning, 22% of this type of neuron analyzed in the hippocampus and parahippocampal gyrus altered their responses so that their activity, which was initially equal to the two new stimuli, became progressively differential to the two stimuli when the monkey learned to make different responses to the two stimuli (Rolls et al. 1990b). These changes occurred for different neurons

just before, at, or just after the time when the monkey learned the correct response to the stimuli. In addition to these neurons, which had differential responses that were sustained for as long as the recordings continued, another population of neurons (45% of this type of neuron analyzed) developed differential activity to the two stimuli, yet showed such differential responses transiently for only a small number of trials at about the time when the monkey learned. These findings are consistent with the hypothesis that some synapses on hippocampal neurons modify during this type of learning so that some neurons come to respond to particular stimulus/spatial response associations that are being learned. Furthermore, the finding that many hippocampal neurons started to reflect the new learning, but then stopped responding differentially (the transient neurons), is consistent with the hypothesis that the hippocampal neurons with large sustained changes in their activity inhibited the transient neurons, which then underwent reverse learning, thus providing a competitive mechanism by which not all neurons are allocated to any one learned association or event. These transient modifications are consistent with the computational theory outlined above and elsewhere (Rolls 1989a,b), since the return of the neuronal activity to nondifferential responsiveness is consistent with an implementation of competitive networks using reverse learning when the postsynaptic neuron is inhibited conjunctively with active afferents (see Rolls 1989c).

The activity of hippocampal neurons in nonhuman primates has also been analyzed during the performance of nonspatial tasks for which the hippocampus is needed, such as recognition memory tasks (Rolls et al. 1985, 1990a). It has been found that in the macaque hippocampus, some neurons do respond differently to novel and familiar stimuli in a serial recognition memory task, with those that did respond differentially typically responding more to novel than to familiar visual stimuli. It was notable that the proportion of hippocampal neurons that responded in this way was small, 2.3%, but that this is not inconsistent with the hypothesis that the hippocampus is involved in episodic memory. It might be of interest in future studies of recognition memory and hippocampal function to investigate whether there are hippocampal neurons tuned to respond to only rather few of a set of stimuli being remembered and whether the representation found is sparse, as would be useful if the CA3 neurons are to store many different stimuli using an autoassociation network. Brown et al. (1987) have also found context sensitivity of hippocampal neurons recorded during a delayed match-to-sample memory task (consistent with a role in episodic memory, in which context is important), but the task also included a conditional response component that may have contributed to the neuronal responses found.

Systems level theory. The effects of damage to the hippocampus indicate that the very long term storage of information is not in the hippocampus, at least in humans, because the retrograde amnesia produced by damage to the hippocampal system in humans is not always severe and because very old memories (e.g., for events which occurred 30 years previously) arc not destroyed (Squire 1986; Squire and Zola-Morgan 1988). On the other hand, the hippocampus does appear to be necessary for the storage of certain types of information (characterized by the description declarative, or knowing that, as contrasted with procedural, or knowing how, which is spared in amnesia). Declarative memory includes what can be declared or brought to mind as a proposition or an image. Declarative memory includes episodic memory, i.e., memory for particular episodes, and semantic memory, i.e., memory for facts (Squire and Zola-Morgan 1988; Squire et al. 1989).

These computational and systems level analyses suggest that the hippocampus is specialized to detect the best way in which to store information, and then by the return paths to the cerebral cortex to direct memory storage there. The hypothesis is that the CA3 autoassociation system is ideal for remembering particular episodes, for perhaps uniquely in the brain it provides a single autoassociation matrix that receives from many different areas of the cerebral association cortex. It is thus able to make almost any arbitrary association, including incorporation by association of the context in which a set of events occurred. This autoassociation type of memory is also required for paired-associate learning, in which arbitrary associations must be made between words, and an impairment of which is almost a defining test of anterograde amnesia. Impairment of this ability to remember episodes by using the CA3 autoassociation matrix memory may also underlie many of the memory deficits produced by damage to the hippocampal system. For example, conditional spatial response learning (see Miyashita et al. 1989) may be impaired by hippocampal damage because a monkey or human cannot make use of the memory of the episode of events on each particular trial (e.g., that a particular stimulus and a particular response were made, and reward was received). Similarly, object-place memory tasks, also impaired by hippocampal damage, require associations to be made between particular locations and particular objects—again a natural function for an autoassociation memory. Furthermore, the difficulty with memory for places produced by hippocampal damage (see Barnes 1988) may be because a place is normally defined by a conjunction of a number of features or environmental cues or stimuli, and this type of conjunction is normally made by the autoassociation memory capability of the hippocampus (see further, Rolls et al. 1989). Clearly, the hippocampus, with its large number of synapses on each neuron, its potentiation type of learning, and its CA3 autoassociation system, is able to detect when there is conjunctive activation of arbitrary sets of its input fibers and is able, as indicated both theoretically and by recordings made in the behaving monkey, to allocate neurons economically (i.e., with relatively few neurons active) to code for each complex input event (by the output or CA1

stage). Such output neurons could then represent an efficient way in which to store information, since complex memories with little redundancy would have been generated. It should be noted that this theory is not inconsistent with the possibility that the hippocampus provides a working memory, since in the present theory, the hippocampus sets up a representation using Hebbian learning, which is useful in determining how information can best be stored in the neocortex, and this representation could provide a useful working memory. Perhaps by understanding the operations performed by the hippocampus at the neuronal network level, it can be seen how the hippocampus could contribute to several functions that are not necessarily inconsistent.

The question of how the hippocampal output is used by the neocortex (i.e., cerebral cortex) is considered next. Given that the hippocampal output returns to the neocortex, a theory of back projections in the neocortex will be needed. This is developed elsewhere (Rolls 1989a,b). By way of introduction, it may be noted that which particular hippocampal neurons happen to represent a complex input event is not determined by any teacher or forcing (unconditioned) stimulus. Thus, the neocortex must be able to utilize the signal rather cleverly. One possibility is that any neocortical neuron with a number of afferents active at the same time as hippocampal return fibers in its vicinity are active modifies its responses so that it comes to respond better to those afferents the next time they occur. This learning by the cortex would involve a Hebb-like learning mechanism. It may be noted that one function served by what are thus in effect back projections from the hippocampus is some guidance for or supervision of neocortical learning. Unsupervised learning systems can detect local conjunctions efficiently, but these are not necessarily those of most use to the whole system. It is exactly this problem which it is proposed the hippocampus helps to solve by detecting useful conjunctions globally (i.e., over the whole of information space) and then directing storage locally at earlier stages of processing so that filters are built locally and provide representations of input stimuli useful for later processing. It is also suggested (Rolls 1989a,b) that the back projections are used for recall, for dynamic adjustment of the processing of earlier stages to facilitate the optimal satisfaction of multiple constraints, and for attention.

CONCLUSION

A computational theory of the hippocampus that has as a key feature the ability to implement an autoassociation memory using the CA3 pyramidal cells has been proposed. It is proposed that the hippocampus is involved in both spatial and episodic memory as a result of its ability to form arbitrary associations between input stimuli, so that whole spatial scenes or all the events that comprise a single episodic memory can be associated together. Recordings from single neurons in the primate hippocampus are consistent with the theory that inputs to the hippocampus originating from different parts of the cerebral cortex are brought together onto single neurons within the hippocampus and that synaptic modifications within the hippocampus implement the associations, although further work is needed to test the detailed predictions of the theory.

ACKNOWLEDGMENTS

The author has worked on some of the experiments and neuronal network modeling described here with A. Bennett, P.M.B. Cahusac, D. Cohen, J.D. Feigenbaum, R.P. Kesner, G. Littlewort, Y. Miyashita, H. Niki, R. Payne, and A. Treves, and their collaboration is sincerely acknowledged. Discussions with David G. Amaral of the Salk Institute, La Jolla, California, were also much appreciated. This research was supported by the Medical Research Council.

REFERENCES

Amaral, D.G. 1987. Memory: Anatomical organization of candidate brain regions. In *Handbook of neurophysiology. Section 1: The nervous system* (ed. V.B. Mountcastle), vol. V, part 1, p. 211. American Physiological Society, Washington, D.C.

Amaral, D.G. and M.P. Witter. 1989. The three-dimensional organization of the hippocampal formation: A review of anatomical data. *Neuroscience* 31: 571.

Amaral, D.G., N. Ishizuka, and B. Claiborne. 1990. Neurons, numbers and the hippocampal network. *Prog. Brain Res.* 83: 1.

Andersen, P.O. 1987. Properties of hippocampal synapses of importance for integration and memory. In *New insights into synaptic function* (ed. G.M. Edelman et al.), p. 403. Neuroscience Research Foundation/Wiley, New York.

Andersen, R.A. 1987. Inferior parietal lobule function in spatial perception and visuomotor integration. In *Handbook of physiology. Section 1: The nervous system. Higher functions of the brain* (ed. V.B. Mountcastle), vol. V, part 2, p. 483. American Physiological Society, Washington, D.C.

Barnes, C.A. 1988. Spatial learning and memory processes: The search for their neurobiological mechanisms in the rat. *Trends Neurosci.* 11: 163.

Bliss, T.V.P. and T. Lomo. 1973. Long-lasting potentiation of synaptic transmission in the dentate area of the anaesthetized rabbit following stimulation of the perforant path. *J. Physiol.* 232: 331.

Boss, B.D., K. Turlejski, B.B. Stanfield, and W.M. Cowan. 1987. On the numbers of neurons in fields CA1 and CA3 of the hippocampus of Sprague-Dawley and Wistar rats. *Brain Res.* 406: 280.

Brown, M.W., F.A.W. Wilson, and I.P. Riches. 1987. Neuronal evidence that inferomedial temporal cortex is more important than hippocampus in certain processes underlying recognition memory. *Brain Res.* 409: 159.

Brown, T.H., E.W. Kairiss, and C.L. Keenan. 1990. Hebbian synapses: Biophysical mechanisms and algorithms. *Annu. Rev. Neurosci.* 13: 475.

Cahusac, P.M.B. and E.T. Rolls. 1989. Modifications of neuronal responses to natural inputs paired with activation of the post-synaptic neurone by ionophoretic L-glutamate in the macaque hippocampus. *J. Physiol.* 420: 45P.

Cahusac, P.M.B., Y. Miyashita, and E.T. Rolls. 1989. Responses of hippocampal formation neurons in the monkey related to delayed spatial response and object-place memory tasks. *Behav. Brain Res.* 33: 229.

Collingridge, G.L. and W. Singer. 1990. Excitatory amino acid receptors and synaptic plasticity. *Trends Pharmacol. Sci.* 11: 290.

Feigenbaum, J.D. and E.T. Rolls. 1990. Allocentric and egocentric spatial information processing in the hippocampal formation of the behaving primate. *Psychobiology* (in press).

Feigenbaum, J., P.M.B. Cahusac, and E.T. Rolls. 1987. The coding of spatial information by neurons in the primate hippocampal formation. *Soc. Neurosci. Abstr.* 13: 608.

Gaffan, D. 1974. Recognition impaired and association intact in the memory of monkeys after transection of the fornix. *J. Comp. Physiol. Psychol.* 86: 1100.

———. 1977. Monkey's recognition memory for complex pictures and the effects of fornix transection. *Q. J. Exp. Psychol.* 29: 505.

———. 1987. Amnesia, personal memory and the hippocampus: Experimental neuropsychological studies in monkeys. In *Cognitive neurochemistry* (ed. S.M. Stahl et al.), p. 46. Oxford University Press, United Kingdom.

Gaffan, D. and S. Harrison. 1989a. A comparison of the effects of fornix section and sulcus principalis ablation upon spatial learning by monkeys. *Behav. Brain Res.* 31: 207.

———. 1989b. Place memory and scene memory: Effects of fornix transection in the monkey. *Exp. Brain Res.* 74: 202.

Gaffan, D. and R.C. Saunders. 1985. Running recognition of configural stimuli by fornix transected monkeys. *Q. J. Exp. Psychol.* 37B: 61.

Gaffan, D. and L. Weiskrantz. 1980. Recency effects and lesion effects in delayed non-matching to randomly baited samples by monkeys. *Brain Res.* 196: 373.

Gaffan, D., E.A. Gaffan, and S. Harrison. 1984. Effects of fornix transection on spontaneous and trained non-matching by monkeys. *Q. J. Exp. Psychol.* 36B: 285.

Gaffan, D., R.C. Saunders, E.A. Gaffan, S. Harrison, C. Shields, and M.J. Owen. 1984. Effects of fornix transection upon associative memory in monkeys: Role of the hippocampus in learned action. *Q. J. Exp. Psychol.* 26B: 173.

Gardner-Medwin, A.R. 1976. The recall of events through the learning of associations between their parts. *Proc. R. Soc. Lond. B.* 194: 375.

Insausti, R., D.G. Amaral, and W.M. Cowan. 1987. The entorhinal cortex of the monkey. II. Cortical afferents. *J. Comp. Neurol.* 264: 356.

Jordan, M.I. 1986. An introduction to linear algebra in parallel distributed processing. In *Parallel distributed processing. Foundations* (ed. D.E. Rumelhart and J.L. McClelland), vol. 1, p. 365. MIT Press, Cambridge.

Kelso, S.R., A.H. Ganong, and T.H. Brown. 1986. Hebbian synapses in the hippocampus. *Proc. Natl. Acad. Sci.* 83: 5326.

Kohonen, T. 1984. *Self-organization and associative memory.* Springer-Verlag, Berlin.

Kohonen, T., E. Oja, and P. Lehtio. 1981. Storage and processing of information in distributed associative memory systems. In *Parallel models of associative memory* (ed. G.E. Hinton and J.A. Anderson), p. 105. Erlbaum, New Jersey.

Kohonen, T., P. Lehtio, J. Rovamo, J. Hyvarinen, K. Bry, and L. Vainio. 1977. A principle of neural associative memory. *Neuroscience* 2: 1065.

Kolb, B. and I.Q. Whishaw. 1985. *Fundamentals of human neuropsychology*, 2nd edition. Freeman, New York.

Mahut, H. 1972. A selective spatial deficit in monkeys after transection of the fornix. *Neuropsychologia* 10: 65.

Marr, D. 1970. A thoery for cerebral cortex. *Proc. R. Soc. Lond. B* 176: 161.

———. 1971. Simple memory: A theory for archicortex. *Philos. Trans. R. Soc. Lond. B* 262: 23.

McNaughton, B.L. 1984. Activity dependent modulation of hippocampal synaptic efficacy: Some implications for memory processes. In *Neurobiology of the hippocampus* (ed. W. Seifert), p. 233. Academic Press, London.

McNaughton, B.L., C.A. Barnes, and J. O'Keefe. 1983. The contributions of position, direction, and velocity to single unit activity in the hippocampus of freely-moving rats. *Exp. Brain Res.* **52:** 41.

Miles, R. 1988. Plasticity of recurrent excitatory synapses between CA3 hippocampal pyramidal cells. *Soc. Neurosci. Abstr.* **14:** 19.

Milner, B. 1972. Disorders of learning and memory after temporal lobe lesions in man. *Clin. Neurosurg.* **19:** 421.

———. 1982. Some cognitive effects of frontal lobe lesions in man. *Philos. Trans. R. Soc. Lond. B* **298:** 211.

Mishkin, M. 1978. Memory severely impaired by combined but not separate removal of amygdala and hippocampus. *Nature* **273:** 297.

———. 1982. A memory system in the monkey. *Philos. Trans. R. Soc. Lond. B* **298:** 85.

Miyashita, Y., E.T. Rolls, P.M.B. Cahusac, H. Niki, and J.D. Feigenbaum. 1989. Activity of hippocampal neurons in the monkey related to a conditional spatial response task. *J. Neurophysiol.* **61:** 669.

Murray, E.A. and M. Mishkin. 1984. Severe tactual as well as visual memory deficits follow combined removal of the amygdala and hippocampus in monkeys. *J. Neurosci.* **4:** 2565.

O'Keefe, J. 1984. Spatial memory within and without the hippocampal system. In *Neurobiology of the hippocampus* (ed. W. Seifert), p. 375. Academic Press, London.

Owen, M.J. and S.R. Butler. 1981. Amnesia after transection of the fornix in monkeys: Long-term memory impaired, short-term memory intact. *Behav. Brain Res.* **3:** 115.

Parkinson, J.K., E.A. Murray, and M. Mishkin. 1988. A selective mnemonic role for the hippocampus in monkeys: Memory for the location of objects. *J. Neurosci.* **8:** 4059.

Petrides, M. 1985. Deficits on conditional associative-learning tasks after frontal- and temporal-lobe lesions in man. *Neuropsychologia* **23:** 601.

Rolls, E.T. 1987. Information representation, processing and storage in the brain: Analysis at the single neuron level. In *The Neural and molecular bases of learning* (ed. J.-P. Changeux and M. Konishi), p. 503. Wiley, Chichester.

———. 1989a. Functions of neuronal networks in the hippocampus and neocortex in memory. In *Neural models of plasticity: Experimental and theoretical approaches* (ed. J.H. Byrne and W.O. Berry), p. 240. Academic Press, San Diego.

———. 1989b. The representation and storage of information in neuronal networks in the primate cerebral cortex and hippocampus. In *The computing neuron* (ed. R. Durbin et al.), p. 125. Addison-Wesley, Wokingham.

———. 1989c. Functions of neuronal networks in the hippocampus and cerebral cortex in memory. In *Models of brain function* (ed. R.M.J. Cotterill), p. 15. Cambridge University Press, United Kingdom.

Rolls, E.T., P.M.B. Cahusac, J.D. Feigenbaum, and Y. Miyashita. 1990. Responses of single neurons in the hippocampus of the macaque related to recognition memory. *Exp. Brain Res.* (in press).

Rolls, E.T., Y. Miyashita, P. Cahusac, and R.P. Kesner. 1985. The responses of single neurons in the primate hippocampus related to the performance of memory tasks. *Soc. Neurosci. Abstr.* **11:** 525.

Rolls, E.T., Y. Miyashita, P.M.B. Cahusac, R.P. Kesner, H. Niki, J. Feigenbaum, and L. Bach. 1989. Hippocampal neurons in the monkey with activity related to the place in which a stimulus is shown. *J. Neurosci.* **9:** 1835.

Rupniak, N.M.J. and D. Gaffan. 1987. Monkey hippocampus and learning about spatially directed movements. *J. Neurosci.* **7:** 2331.

Sakata, H. 1985. The parietal association cortex: Neurophysiology. In *The scientific basis of clinical neurology* (ed. M. Swash and C. Kennard), p. 225. Churchill Livingstone, London.

Scoville, W.B. and B. Milner. 1957. Loss of recent memory after bilateral hippocampal lesions. *J. Neurol. Neurosurg. Psych.* **20:** 11.

Smith, M.L. and B. Milner. 1981. The role of the right hippocampus in the recall of spatial location. *Neuropsychologia* **19:** 781.

Squire, L. 1986. Mechanisms of memory. *Science* **232:** 1612.

Squire, L.R. and S. Zola-Morgan. 1988. Memory: Brain systems and behavior. *Trends Neurosci.* **11:** 170.

Squire, L.R., A.P. Shimamura, and D.G. Amaral. 1989. Memory and the hippocampus. In *Neural models of plasticity: Theoretical and empirical approaches* (ed. J. Byrne and W.O. Berry), p. 208. Academic Press, New York.

Van Hoesen, G.W. 1982. The parahippocampal gyrus. New observations regarding its cortical connections in the monkey. *Trends Neurosci.* **5:** 345.

Watanabe, T. and H. Niki. 1985. Hippocampal unit activity and delayed response in the monkey. *Brain Res.* **325:** 241.

Wigstrom, H., B. Gustaffson, Y.-Y. Huang, and W.C. Abraham. 1986. Hippocampal long-term potentiation is induced by pairing single afferent volleys with intracellularly injected depolarizing currents. *Acta Physiol. Scand.* **126:** 317.

Zola-Morgan, S., L.R. Squire, and D.G. Amaral. 1986. Human amnesia and the medial temporal region: Enduring memory impairment following a bilateral lesion limited to field CA1 of the hippocampus. *J. Neurosci.* **6:** 2950.

Memory: Organization of Brain Systems and Cognition

L.R. Squire,*† S. Zola-Morgan,*† C.B. Cave,* F. Haist,*‡
G. Musen,* and W.A. Suzuki*
*University of California, San Diego; †Veterans Affairs Medical Center, San Diego;
‡San Diego State University, San Diego, California 92161

Cognitive neuroscience is that part of the brain sciences concerned with the functional organization and neural substrates of higher cortical functions, e.g., perception, attention, language, memory, problem solving, and the organization of action. Among these diverse topics, the topic of memory has been a particularly fruitful target of experimental inquiry. Work on memory is currently benefiting from approaches at many levels of analysis, from studies of cellular and molecular mechanisms underlying synaptic plasticity to studies of brain systems and behavior. Cellular and molecular approaches address questions about how neurons exhibit history-dependent activity. Systems-level questions address a more global level of analysis: How is memory organized? Is there one kind of memory or many? Where are memories stored? What are the structures and connections involved in memory and what jobs do they do?

One useful strategy for asking systems-level questions about memory is to study instances of relatively selective memory impairment. In such cases, particularly in human patients, an analysis of the deficit can provide useful information about the normal function of the damaged system and about the organization of normal memory. In addition, study of animal models of human memory impairment, especially a recently developed model of amnesia in the monkey, can identify the anatomical structures and connections that comprise the damaged system.

The sections that follow summarize what has been learned from such an approach. First, we consider the nature of the primary deficit in human amnesia: impaired ability to learn new material. Second, we discuss what has been learned about memory from the analysis of retrograde amnesia, i.e., the loss of material acquired before the onset of memory impairment. Third, we review the scope and limits of human memory impairment, focusing on the important finding that even severely amnesic patients are entirely normal at some kinds of learning and memory. Finally, we consider recent work in monkeys, which has been successful during the past decade in establishing an animal model of human amnesia. With this animal model, it has been possible to identify the structures and connections that comprise the medial temporal lobe memory system.

ANTEROGRADE AMNESIA

Amnesia is a severe deficit in the ability to learn new facts and events (anterograde amnesia), which occurs against a background of intact intellectual ability (Fig. 1) (Milner 1972; Cermak 1982; Hirst 1982; Schacter 1985; Squire 1987; Weiskrantz 1987; Mayes 1988). The deficit extends to both verbal and nonverbal material and to material presented in any sensory modality. Memory for facts and events from the period prior to the onset of amnesia is also affected. Language, social skills, and personality can be intact, as well as memory for material acquired very early in life.

Patients with amnesia are also able to perform normally on memory tasks in which the material to be retained is within the capacity of immediate memory (usually on the order of 7 items). For example, the ability to repeat strings of digits is generally normal. The difficulty that amnesic patients have is in placing new information into *long-term memory*, which can be demonstrated with any number of standardized neuropsychological tests (Squire and Shimamura 1986). Figure 1 illustrates the performance of amnesic patients on three conventional measures of new learning ability.

In amnesia, the new learning of both events and facts is affected, i.e., both episodic and semantic memory (cf. Tulving 1983). Indeed, amnesic patients seem to have about as much difficulty acquiring new semantic knowledge (facts) as event-specific (episodic) knowledge. Nevertheless, some new semantic knowledge can usually be acquired through repeated exposures to factual material. Such an ability to acquire new information through repetition, albeit at an impaired rate, would be expected to exceed the ability to acquire episodic knowledge, because episodic knowledge is by definition unique to time and place and cannot be repeated. In other words, repeated material is always easier to learn than material that is not repeated (see Ostergaard and Squire 1990). The issue then is not that amnesic patients can accumulate some semantic knowledge over time without acquiring episodic knowledge (Tulving and Schacter 1990). The issue is whether their ability to acquire semantic knowledge is disproportionately spared, i.e., is it special in some way (e.g., outside the province of the structures and functions damaged in amnesia)? Or does it reflect simply the residual learning

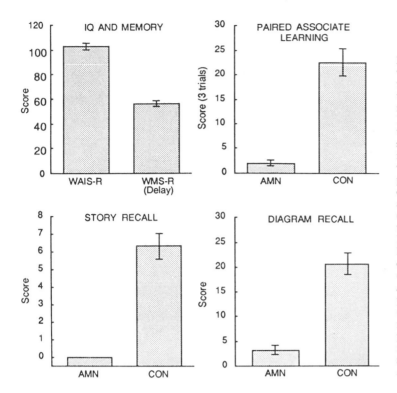

Figure 1. (*Upper left*) Performance of patients with amnesia ($n = 14$) on a standard intelligence test (Full Scale WAIS-R [Wechsler Adult Intelligence Scale-Revised]) and on a standard memory test (WMS-R [Wechsler Memory Scale-Revised] Delay Index). In the normal population, both tests yield average scores of 100 with a standard deviation of 15. The amnesic patients include 7 with alcoholic Korsakoff's syndrome, 6 with confirmed or suspected damage to the hippocampal formation, and 1 with a bilateral medial thalamic infarction. Also shown is performance of the same 14 patients with amnesia (AMN) and 8 control subjects (CON) on three tests of new learning ability. (*Upper right*) Paired-associate learning measures the ability to learn unrelated word pairs by reporting the second word in a pair when cued with the first word (10 pairs, 3 trials, maximum score = 30). (*Lower left*) Story recall measures retention of a short prose passage consisting of 21 meaning segments (maximum score = 21). (*Lower right*) Diagram recall measures the ability to reconstruct a complex line drawing (Rey Osterreith figure) from memory (maximum score = 36). Brackets show S.E.M. See Squire and Shimamura (1986) for additional description of these tests.

capacity of an incompletely damaged system? This important question has not yet been adequately addressed.

Recall and Recognition Memory in Amnesia

When amnesic patients are tested for their memory of recently presented material, they perform poorly whether they are requested to recall the material or to recognize it, i.e., choose the correct answers from among alternatives. An important question (one that is difficult to address experimentally) concerns whether recall and recognition are affected similarly. Free recall is usually considered more dependent on retrieval processes than is recognition. Accordingly, if recall were more impaired than recognition, one might suppose that amnesia is due to faulty retrieval processes. Alternatively, if recall and recognition were affected similarly, one would suppose that amnesia is due to an impairment in functions that are equally important for recall and recognition. The best way to compare recall and recognition performance is to test both recall and recognition at several times after learning and then to compare the forgetting functions produced by both normal subjects and amnesic patients (Haist et al. 1989).

Figure 2 shows the results of such an experiment. On each of 12 occasions, a different list of 20 common words was presented for learning. After a delay that ranged from 15 seconds to 8 weeks, retention was tested either by free recall or by recognition (6 different delays for recall and 6 delays for recognition). The free recall test required subjects to report as many of the words from the list as they could remember. The recognition test (2 alternative, forced choice) required subjects to choose which word they had seen before. Amnesic patients performed overall much worse than the normal subjects. However, recall and recognition were similarly affected. Specifically, the free recall scores obtained by the two subject groups (amnesic patients and control subjects) matched each other at exactly the same retention intervals at which the recognition scores matched. (Amnesic performance at delays from 15 sec to 10 min matched control performance at delays from 1 day to 8 weeks.) Thus, although recall and recognition tests differ in their sensitivity for detecting memory, the same difference in sensitivity was observed in amnesia that was observed in normal memory during the course of forgetting. These results provide strong evidence that recall and recognition memory are similarly dependent on the structures and functions damaged in amnesia. The findings are consistent with the idea that the structures damaged in amnesia are essential for establishing representations in long-term memory. An imperfectly or incompletely established representation should result in both poor recall and poor recognition.

It should be noted that Hirst and his colleagues (Hirst et al. 1986, 1988) have suggested, on the basis of work with a different group of memory-impaired patients and on the basis of tests done at single retention intervals, that free recall can be somewhat more impaired in amnesia than recognition memory.

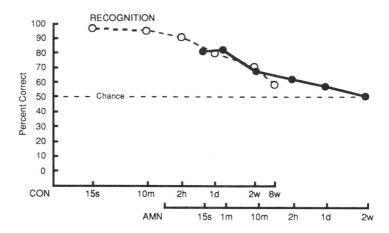

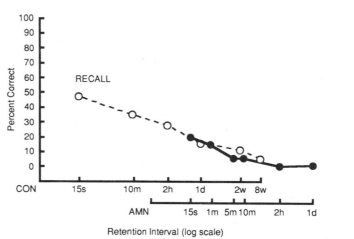

Figure 2. Performance of patients with amnesia (closed circles, $n = 12$) and control subjects (open circles, $n = 20$), who were tested for either recognition (2 alternative, forced choice) or free recall of different groups of 20 words at one of the indicated delays after learning. Control subjects were tested at relatively long intervals after learning so that their performance could be evaluated at a time when it was as poor as that of the amnesic patients. The performance of control subjects tested about 1 day after learning matched the performance of amnesic patients who were tested 15 sec after learning. The forgetting curves continued to match at longer delays following learning. The correspondence between control and amnesic performance was the same when memory was measured by recognition (*top*) as when memory was measured by recall (*bottom*). Accordingly, recall and recognition memory appear to be similarly affected in amnesia.

Associated and Dissociated Deficits: Identifying the Essential Components of Amnesia

Some deficits that occur commonly in memory-impaired patients are not essential to the memory impairment. As these deficits are identified, a more accurate picture develops about which deficits are inextricably a part of memory impairment and which ones are related only incidentally. One major strategy for identifying the essential nature of amnesia has been to carry out comparative studies of patients with alcoholic Korsakoff's syndrome, patients with confirmed or suspected damage to the hippocampal formation (non-Korsakoff amnesic patients), and patients with radiographically confirmed lesions restricted to the frontal lobes. These three groups have different lesions and different patterns of cognitive impairment. Amnesic patients with Korsakoff's syndrome have midline diencephalic lesions (which on their own are known to be sufficient to cause amnesia), and they also have frontal lobe damage, as demonstrated by quantitative analysis of computed tomography (CT) scans (Jacobson and Lishman 1987; Shimamura et al. 1988). The non-Korsakoff amnesic patients studied in this context have medial temporal lobe lesions, but do not have detectable frontal lobe lesions. Finally, the patients

with frontal lobe lesions have no known pathology outside the frontal lobes and are not amnesic (Janowsky et al. 1989b).

The logic of this approach is to suppose that deficits observed only in the two amnesic groups are reflections of memory impairment due to medial temporal lobe or diencephalic pathology, whereas deficits observed both in patients with Korsakoff's syndrome and frontal patients, but not in other amnesic patients, are due to frontal lobe dysfunction.

The comparisons summarized in Table 1 suggest that many deficits exhibited by patients with Korsakoff's syndrome are due to frontal lobe damage and are dissociable from amnesia. Consider, for example, the finding that patients with Korsakoff's syndrome are poor at making judgments and predictions about their own memory ability, i.e., they have impaired metamemory. In the absence of other information, one might suppose that impaired metamemory is an inextricable part of disordered memory. One might even suspect that an impairment in the ability to monitor and to be aware of one's own memory abilities could be a cause of disordered memory. However, impaired metamemory abilities are not observed in non-Korsakoff amnesic patients, even when the severity of their amnesia is similar to the severity of memory impairment in pa-

Table 1. Associated and Dissociated Deficits in Amnesia

Test	Amnesia	Korsakoff's syndrome	Frontal lobe damage
Delayed recall	+	+	−
Dementia rating scale: memory index	+	+	−
Dementia rating scale: initiation/perseveration index	−	+	+
Wisconsin card sort	−	+	+
Temporal order memory	+	+ +	+ +
Metamemory	−	+	+
Release from proactive interference	−	+	−

Constructed from data in Janowsky et al. (1989a,b); Shimamura et al. (1990); Shimamura and Squire (1986). Amnesia: Amnesic patients with confirmed or suspected damage to the hippocampal formation; Korsakoff's syndrome: amnesic patients with diencephalic lesions and confirmed frontal lobe atrophy; frontal lobe damage: patients with lesions restricted to the frontal lobes. (+) Deficit; (−) no deficit; (+ +) disproportionally impaired relative to item memory.

tients with Korsakoff's syndrome (Shimamura and Squire 1986). Moreover, patients with frontal lobe lesions exhibit metamemory deficits in the absence of amnesia (Janowsky et al. 1989a). These findings indicate that metamemory functions are separately organized from memory ability itself. Memory ability depends on the integrity of the medial temporal lobe and midline diencephalon. Metamemory functions depend importantly on the frontal lobe.

As Table 1 shows, patients with amnesia can have somewhat heterogeneous patterns of symptoms, which vary depending on what anatomical damage has occurred. Certain deficits are found in virtually all amnesic patients and likely reflect damage to the medial temporal lobe or midline diencephalon. These include difficulty in learning new facts and events, as measured by tests of both recall and recognition. Other deficits are sometimes present as well that are not obligatory to memory impairment. These include deficits in problem solving (Oscar-Berman 1980; Janowsky et al. 1989b), temporal order memory (Milner 1971; Squire 1982; Meudell et al. 1985; Shimamura et al. 1990), metamemory (Shimamura and Squire 1986), and sensitivity to proactive interference, i.e., failure to show the normal improvement in performance when attempting to learn words belonging to a new category after attempting several word lists from another category (Cermak et al. 1974; Squire 1982). These deficits are associated with frontal lobe dysfunction, which occurs in some cases of amnesia but not in others.

RETROGRADE AMNESIA

Retrograde amnesia refers to impaired memory for information that was acquired prior to the onset of amnesia. It has long been recognized that the status of retrograde amnesia has important implications for understanding both the organization of normal memory and the function of the damaged brain structures. In 1881, Theodule Ribot brought together a large number of clinical case reports indicating that recent memory is typically lost more readily than remote memory (Ribot 1882). These case reports formed the basis of his Law of Regression that in memory "the new perishes before the old," an idea that has been affirmed repeatedly by clinical observers during this century. Considering the limitations of informal observation, it is surprising that quantitative studies of retrograde amnesia were initiated only 20 years ago (Sanders and Warrington 1971). Since that time a great deal has been learned, despite the fact that most methods for assessing retrograde amnesia in humans are imperfect in a number of ways (Squire 1974; Squire and Cohen 1982). Indeed, the most decisive tests of Ribot's Law, which distinguish between alternative interpretations of his basic observation, have been carried out prospectively with experimental animals.

Useful descriptions of retrograde amnesia have come from formal studies of groups of amnesic patients (Fig. 3), including patients with Korsakoff's syndrome (Albert et al. 1979; Meudell et al. 1980; Cohen and Squire 1981; Squire et al. 1989a), patients with confirmed or suspected hippocampal damage (Squire et al. 1989a), and patients with transient global amnesia (TGA) (Kritchevsky and Squire 1989). For these patients, remote memory impairment is extensive and temporally graded, affecting the most recent decades more than remote decades. Indeed, very remote memory can be intact, even when the test items are so difficult that they can be answered by fewer than 20% of normal subjects (Squire et al. 1989a). The findings from the (non-Korsakoff) amnesic patients and the patients with TGA are particularly useful, because these patients, unlike patients with Korsakoff's syndrome, became amnesic on a known calendar day. In this circumstance, there can be no ambiguity about which test items measure retrograde amnesia.

Retrograde amnesia can be quite brief when damage is limited to the hippocampus and when anterograde amnesia is only moderately severe (e.g., patient R.B., who had bilateral lesions limited to the CA1 region of the hippocampus and retrograde amnesia of a few years

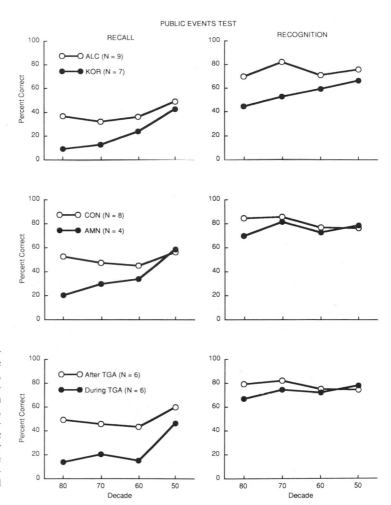

Figure 3. Remote memory performance of amnesic patients with Korsakoff's syndrome (KOR, $n = 7$), alcoholic control subjects (ALC, $n = 9$), amnesic patients with confirmed or suspected damage to the hippocampal formation (AMN, $n = 4$), healthy control subjects (CON, $n = 8$), and patients with transient global amnesia (TGA, $n = 6$). (*Left*) Recall of past public events that had occurred in one of the four decades from 1950 to 1985. (*Right*) Performance on a multiple-choice test (4 alternatives) involving the same public events (Kritchevsky and Squire 1989; Squire et al. 1989a).

at the most [Zola-Morgan et al. 1986]). Retrograde amnesia may be more extensive when anterograde amnesia is more severe, as was the case for the patients whose data appear in Figure 3: the Korsakoff patients, the (non-Korsakoff) amnesic patients, and the patients with TGA. Thus, retrograde amnesia may vary in its severity and extent as a function of the severity of anterograde amnesia. Moreover, both medial temporal lobe and diencephalic damage can produce similarly extensive and temporally graded retrograde amnesia. These ideas replace an earlier proposal that distinguished two different types of retrograde amnesia—a brief, temporally limited impairment and a more extensive impairment—depending on whether the locus of damage is medial temporal or diencephalic (Cohen and Squire 1981).

What accounts for the finding that the four (non-Korsakoff) amnesic cases in Figure 3, who became amnesic following an anoxic or ischemic event, have more severe anterograde and retrograde amnesia than R.B.? One would expect that their pathology is more extensive than was found in R.B., i.e., that it is not restricted to the CA1 region of the hippocampus. Two of these four patients have been examined recently with

an improved protocol for imaging the human hippocampus with magnetic resonance (Press et al. 1989). In both patients, the hippocampal formation was markedly reduced in size bilaterally, apparently affecting all the fields of the hippocampus including the CA1 region, together with the dentate gyrus and the subicular complex (Fig. 4).

It is important to note that some memory-impaired patients have extensive remote memory impairment covering many decades with no evidence of a temporal gradient (for discussion, see Squire et al. 1989a). It is not clear whether this extreme form of retrograde amnesia is always accompanied by a correspondingly more severe form of anterograde amnesia, i.e., an impairment that would be more severe than is found in the patients contributing to Figure 3. Although this is a possibility, an alternative is that severe, ungraded retrograde amnesia requires damage beyond the medial temporal lobe and midline diencephalic structures usually associated with circumscribed amnesia and that this damage impairs performance on remote memory tests without producing a proportional impairment of new learning. This possibility appears tenable because most of the clinical conditions in which severe, ungraded

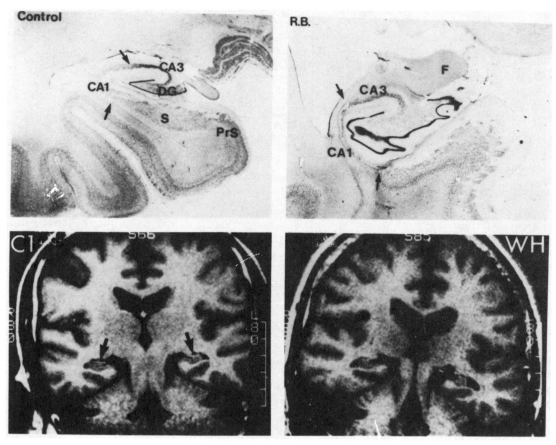

Figure 4. (*Top left panel*) Section through the hippocampus of a normal subject. (*Top right panel*) Section through the hippocampus of amnesic patient R.B., showing damage to the CA1 region. (*Bottom left panel*) Magnetic resonance scan of a normal subject (resolution = 0.625 mm). Several anatomical features of the hippocampal formation can be distinguished. (*Bottom right panel*) Magnetic resonance scan of amnesic patient W.H. using the same protocol. The hippocampal formation is markedly reduced in size. The calibration bars to the right represent 5 cm in 1-cm increments. (Top panels reprinted, with permission, from Squire 1986; bottom panels reprinted, with permission, from Press et al. 1989.)

retrograde amnesia is observed are conditions in which additional damage is known to occur, especially in neocortex, which is a likely repository of permanent memory (Mishkin 1982; Squire 1987).

In correspondence with their performance on tests of remote memory for factual material, amnesic patients also exhibit retrograde amnesia on tests that assess autobiographical memory for specific episodes (Butters and Cermak 1986; see also Beatty et al. 1987; Gabrieli et al. 1988; Kopelman 1989; MacKinnon and Squire 1989). Across individual patients, the severity of the impairment is similar for autobiographical memory and fact memory. The work reviewed to this point suggests that extensive, temporally graded retrograde amnesia for facts and personal events is a common feature of memory impairment. In addition, repeated testing across a period of years has shown that retrograde amnesia can be highly stable (Squire et al. 1989a).

Recently, a single-case report suggested that retrograde amnesia can be severe and extensive when assessed with standard tests, but that it is not observed at all when the same tests are redesigned as semantic memory tests, e.g., when one assesses simple familiari-

ty for famous names or name completion ability rather than associative memory (Warrington and McCarthy 1988). However, such tests could be too easy to discriminate between normal and impaired performance, i.e., retrograde amnesia might be obscured by a ceiling effect. To explore these issues further, we constructed similar tests of simple familiarity and name completion ability but made the tests more difficult. We tested two amnesic patients who have severe and extensive retrograde amnesia, as assessed by standard tests of remote memory (Boswell [Damasio et al. 1985] and W.I.). The first test asked subjects to select the famous name from a group of nonfamous names (e.g., Arthur Elliot, David Conner, Richard Daley). The second test asked subjects to complete a fragment to form a famous name (e.g., Adlai Stev_____). The famous names for both tests spanned the time period 1940–1985 and were taken from a standard famous faces test. On the new tests, both patients performed better than on more conventional remote memory tests. However, they still scored outside the range of control subjects for every decade and at every decade scored more than two standard deviations below the control mean (Fig. 5)

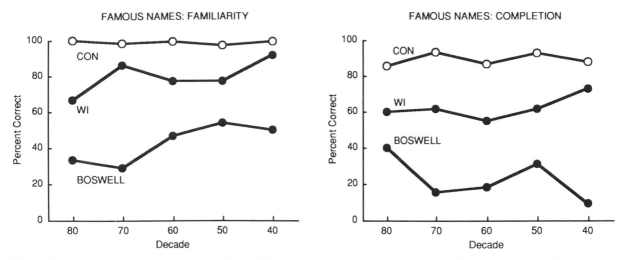

Figure 5. Performance of amnesic patients W.I. and Boswell on two tests of remote memory that were redesigned as semantic memory tests. In one case, subjects selected the famous names from two nonfamous names. In the other case, subjects attempt to complete the famous name when given the first name and a fragment of the last name. Performance of both amnesic patients was severely impaired. CON = 8 control subjects.

(Haist et al. 1990). Thus, there seems little basis for supposing that retrograde amnesia can be mitigated by simple changes in test procedure.

There are two ways to understand the important finding that amnesia affects recent memory for facts and events more than remote memory. One possibility is that the structures damaged in amnesia are necessary for the retrieval of components or features of memory that are ordinarily short-lasting. These memories will be abundant in recent memory and relatively uncommon in remote memory. By this scenario, amnesia will always affect recent memory more than remote memory. However, there is no transformation or consolidation of information across time, only differential attrition of memory by type. A second possibility is that information is reorganized or consolidated with the passage of time after learning. Memory initially depends on the integrity of the structures damaged in amnesia. As time passes after learning, memory is gradually reorganized and becomes independent of these structures.

These two alternatives can be distinguished by determining the precise shape of the performance curve in retrograde amnesia. The difficulty is that the precise shape of the temporal gradient of retrograde amnesia cannot be established with certainty on the basis of the available methods for testing remote memory retrospectively in humans. One can imagine two possibilities (Fig. 6A,B). The critical feature of the data illustrated in the right panel is that scores for more remote periods are actually better than scores for more recent periods. Only this pattern of data requires that active reorganization or consolidation occurs in memory (for discussion, see Zola-Morgan and Squire 1990b).

Findings from patients prescribed electroconvulsive therapy (ECT) (Squire et al. 1975), using a specially constructed test that permitted equivalent sampling of past time periods, and findings from mice given electro-

convulsive shock (ECS) (Squire and Spanis 1984), have shown unequivocally (in accordance with Fig. 6B) that a consolidation process must occur in very long-term memory. However, treatments like ECT and ECS cannot be usefully related to neuroanatomy. Accordingly, these gradients of retrograde amnesia do not reveal how the structures damaged in amnesia participate in the maintenance and consolidation of memory. The findings are useful primarily in showing that long-term memory retains considerable dynamism and that changes continue in memory storage for a long time after learning.

Recently, retrograde amnesia was assessed prospectively in monkeys with bilateral lesions of the hippocampal formation (Zola-Morgan and Squire 1990a). The key finding was that operated monkeys remembered object discriminations learned 12 weeks previously significantly better than object discriminations learned 2 weeks previously (Fig. 6C). These results provide unequivocal evidence for a gradual process of reorganization or consolidation in memory. Similar results were also reported recently for rats given hippocampal lesions, although the gradient of retrograde amnesia extended across a period of only 2–5 days (Winocur 1990). The hippocampal formation is essential for memory storage for a limited period of time. As time passes after learning, the contribution of the hippocampal formation gradually diminishes and a more permanent memory system develops, presumably in neocortex, which is independent of the hippocampal formation. A temporary memory in the hippocampal formation (a simple memory, a conjunction, or an index [Marr 1971; Teyler and Discenna 1986; Squire et al. 1989b]) is eventually replaced by a gradually developing, more permanent memory elsewhere.

Since quantitative studies of retrograde amnesia were undertaken beginning 20 years ago, a considerable amount has been learned about the organization of

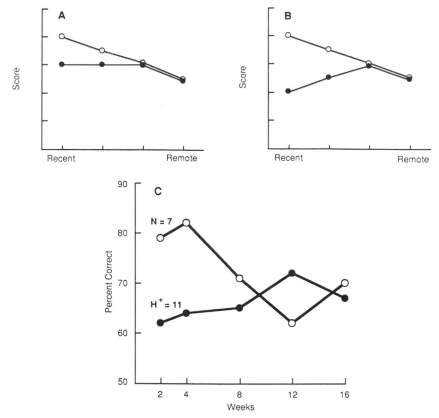

Figure 6. (*A, B*) Hypothetical retrograde amnesia data for normal subjects (○) and amnesic patients (●), assuming an optimal remote memory test, i.e., a test for which the information sampled from each time period is known to have been learned to the same level and forgotten at the same rate. Only the curves shown in *B* require the hypothesis that memory is actively reorganized or consolidated across time. (*C*) Temporally graded retrograde amnesia in monkeys with bilateral lesions of the hippocampal formation (H⁺). Monkeys were trained on 20 different object discrimination problems on each of five occasions, beginning 16, 12, 8, 4, and 2 weeks prior to surgery. Two weeks after surgery, retention for all 100 pairs was tested by presenting each object pair for a single trial. The results were similar to the hypothetical data in *B* (Zola-Morgan and Squire 1990b).

normal memory. Extensive and temporally graded amnesia can occur across a decade or more, even in patients with well-circumscribed amnesia. Very remote memory can be preserved. Similar findings are obtained for tests based on factual information and tests based on autobiographical, event-specific information. When damage is limited to the CA1 region of the human hippocampus, retrograde amnesia is limited to a period of only a few years at most. Retrograde amnesia is more extensive when the anatomical damage is more extensive, and it increases in severity as anterograde amnesia increases. The memory loss represents a loss of usable knowledge that cannot be mitigated in any known way by altering the manner in which remote memory questions are presented. Finally, a prospective study in monkeys has provided the first direct evidence in primates for the dynamic role of the hippocampal formation in memory storage. The hippocampal formation is initially essential for the storage and retrieval of memory, but its contribution diminishes and a more permanent memory develops elsewhere that is independent of the hippocampal formation. The hippocampal formation must interact with neocortex during a lengthy period of reorganization and consolidation,

if memory is to be established and then maintained in a usable form.

MULTIPLE FORMS OF MEMORY

The evidence from anterograde and retrograde amnesia indicates that the system damaged in amnesia is essential for establishing long-term memory at the time of learning and that it remains essential during a lengthy period of reorganization. Eventually, a more permanent memory develops that is independent of this system. The important finding to be considered in this section is that this sequence of events involves only one kind of memory. The kind of memory that is impaired in amnesia, which is dependent on the integrity of the damaged system, has been termed declarative (explicit) memory. Declarative memory refers to information about previously encountered facts and events, the kind of information that is ordinarily available as conscious recollections.

Although amnesic patients are gravely disabled by their disorder in declarative memory, performance on some learning tasks is entirely intact. The kinds of learning that are spared are a heterogeneous group of

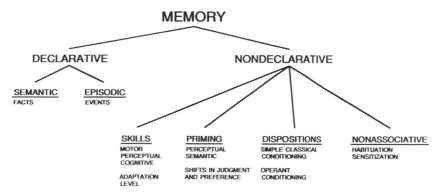

Figure 7. A tentative memory taxonomy. Declarative memory is available as conscious recollection. Nondeclarative memory refers to a large number of separable learning and memory abilities where performance changes but without affording access to the original experience or to any memory content.

abilities, collectively termed nondeclarative (implicit) memory (see Fig. 7). Examples of preserved learning include perceptuomotor skills (Milner 1962; Brooks and Baddeley 1976), perceptual and cognitive skills (Cohen and Squire 1980; Nissen and Bullemer 1987; Squire and Frambach 1990), and priming (Graf et al. 1984; Shimamura 1986; Tulving and Schacter 1990). Priming refers to an increased facility for identifying words or other perceptual objects, which is caused by their recent presentation. Amnesic patients also show normal shifts in preference after exposure to novel material (Johnson et al. 1985), normal adaptation-level effects (Benzing and Squire 1989), and a normal pattern of acquisition and extinction in simple classic conditioning (Weiskrantz and Warrington 1979; Daum et al. 1989). Taken together, these findings have provided the best evidence for the important idea that memory is not a unitary mental function, but a collection of different abilities.

Skill Learning

Early work showed that amnesic patients could learn perceptuomotor skills such as mirror drawing (Milner 1962) and could improve on a rotary pursuit tracking task (Corkin 1968; Brooks and Baddeley 1976). Subsequently, it became clear that perceptual skills and cognitive skills can also be learned normally, even when there is no motor component to the acquired skill. Thus, amnesic patients improved as rapidly as normal subjects at the skill of reading mirror-reversed words and exhibited normal retention after a 3-month interval (Cohen and Squire 1980). They were also normal during the early phase of learning a cognitive skill task, which required subjects to interact with a computer to maintain a specific target value across trials (Squire and Frambach 1990). In these cases, normal learning occurred, but the amnesic patients could not answer simple questions about the learning experience, even when the questions were presented in a multiple-choice test. One important feature of these tasks is that

memory is tested implicitly. That is, performance is based on speed or proficiency and does not depend on explicit reference to any previously presented information.

Acquired skills could potentially depend on generic information, which is acquired cumulatively across many study trials, or skills could depend on specific information that is based on the particular items that are encountered. For example, in the case of mirror reading, a skill could be general (i.e., a subject improves at reading any reversed letters or words) or a skill could be specific to the particular letters or words that were practiced. If item-specific information is retained, a further question is whether such information is nondeclarative, i.e., whether amnesic patients are entirely intact at acquiring item-specific information that is part of a skill.

One experimental approach to these questions has focused on reading skills for text. The phenomenon of interest is that, when subjects reread a passage of text, they tend to read it faster on the second reading than on the first. Studies of normal subjects have shown that this facilitation is specific to familiar passages and is not a nonspecific improvement in reading ability (Kolers 1975). To determine whether amnesic patients can acquire and retain text-specific reading skills, patients were asked to read a text passage aloud three times in succession and were then given a second text to read three times (Musen et al. 1990). The results were that reading speed improved at a similar rate in both amnesic patients and normal subjects and was specific to the text that was read (Fig. 8). After improving at reading the first passage, both groups read the second passage at the same slower speed with which they had initially read the first passage. In both groups, the facilitation persisted for about 10 minutes and disappeared within 2 hours. These results, and similar findings obtained in other studies (Moscovitch et al. 1986), show clearly that very specific skill-based information (e.g., information about the words and ideas presented in text) can be supported by nondeclarative (implicit) memory.

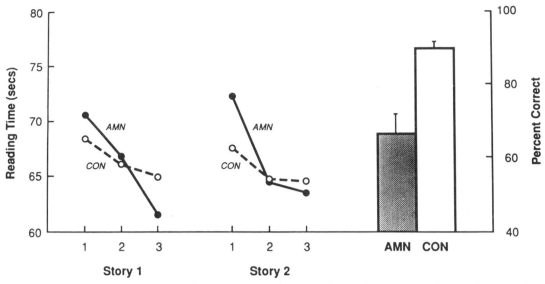

Figure 8. Time required to read aloud two different stories, each presented three times in succession (AMN, amnesic patients, $n = 8$; CON, control subjects, $n = 9$). The bars show the performance of each group on a test of story content given immediately after the final reading of the second story (chance = 33%). Brackets show S.E.M. (Reprinted, with permission, from Musen et al. 1990.)

Priming

Priming occurs when performance is facilitated or biased by recently encountered information (Shimamura 1986; Tulving and Schacter 1990). For example, in perceptual identification tasks, subjects try to identify words or pictures that are presented very briefly (for about 50 msec). Priming is indicated by more accurate identification or by faster response times for previously presented items compared to new items. In word-stem completion tasks, subjects are given word stems (e.g, MOT_____) and asked to form the first words that come to mind. Priming is indicated by an increased tendency to complete the stems to form recently presented words (e.g., MOTEL), compared with a condition when words were not presented first. Amnesic patients exhibit fully intact priming effects (Graf et al. 1984; Cermak et al. 1985; Schacter 1985). Some forms of priming are rather short-lived, disappearing within 2 hours. In these cases, the duration of priming is identical for normal subjects and amnesic patients (Graf et al. 1984; Shimamura and Squire 1984). Longer-lasting priming effects (e.g., days or weeks) have also been reported in normal subjects (see Tulving et al. 1982), but it is not yet clear when and if amnesic patients also show long-lasting effects (Moscovitch et al. 1986; McAndrews et al. 1987; Squire et al. 1987).

One way to understand priming is to suppose that preexisting representations are transiently activated, thereby influencing behavior for a period of time. The difficulty with this view is that in normal subjects priming-like effects have been found for novel stimuli, including pronounceable nonwords (Cermak et al. 1985; Smith and Oscar-Berman 1990) and novel patterns and objects (Gabrieli et al. 1990; Musen and Treisman 1990; Schacter et al. 1990). These observations suggest that priming may operate at early stages of perceptual processing, prior to the analysis of meaning. If so, priming of novel material may be supported entirely by nondeclarative memory and may be intact in amnesic patients. At the present time, the evidence for amnesic patients on this point is unclear (Cermak et al. 1985; Gabrieli and Keane 1988; Gordon 1988; Gabrieli et al. 1990).

One interesting possibility is that there are two forms of priming: perceptual and semantic (Gabrieli 1990; Schacter 1990; Tulving and Schacter 1990). Perceptual priming operates on early-stage perceptual systems (e.g., a presemantic word-form system), and semantic priming depends on access to word meanings. Perceptual priming is illustrated in word-identification or object-identification tasks that do not require access to meaning. Semantic priming is illustrated by the increased tendency of amnesic patients and normal subjects to produce presented words (e.g., BABY) when they are asked to "free associate" to semantically related words (e.g., CHILD [Shimamura and Squire 1984]).

This distinction between perceptual and semantic priming might illuminate the issue of whether the acquisition of entirely novel information can be supported by nondeclarative memory. Amnesic patients may be able to acquire novel information only when the information does not require access to or integration into meaning systems. For example, when normal subjects study WINDOW-REASON, they are later more likely to produce the word REASON when given WINDOW-REA than when given OFFICER-REA (Graf and Schacter 1985). This effect of context depends on forming a meaningful link between the two words at the time of study. Amnesic patients do not show this effect (Cermak et al. 1988; Shimamura and Squire 1989), perhaps because they lack the ability to join the two words into a unitized representation at the time the words are initially studied. Similarly, priming of pronounceable nonwords may occur in amnesic patients only when the task requires that items be read aloud, but not when items must be identified as words or nonwords. For example, in one study a lexical decision task was used in which subjects needed to decide rapidly whether a previously presented letter string was a real word or not (Smith and Oscar-Berman 1990). Normal subjects showed priming for both words and nonwords in this task, i.e., they made the lexical decision faster when either a word or nonword had been presented recently. Amnesic patients also showed priming of words, but they showed no priming of nonwords. In contrast, in another study, subjects were simply asked to read lists of repeated and unique words and nonwords as rapidly as possible. Amnesic patients and normal subjects showed similar increases in reading speed for repeated (as compared to unique) items. Importantly, amnesic patients improved their reading speed for repeated nonwords to the same extent as normal subjects (G. Musen and L.R. Squire, in prep.). Further study of priming and the perceptual-semantic distinction should be useful in order to clarify what kinds of new knowledge can be supported by nondeclarative memory.

Figure 7 illustrates a taxonomic organization of memory. Declarative memory is impaired in amnesia. It includes memory for both facts and events, which are represented such that learned information can be brought to mind as a conscious recollection. Declarative memory is flexible, available to multiple response systems, and is adapted for rapid, even one-trial learning. Nondeclarative memory includes a wide variety of examples where behavior changes with experience, but without conscious access to what has been learned. Information is embedded in specific procedures or stored as tunings, biases, or activations. The knowledge gained occurs as changes in particular perceptual systems, response systems, or as the development of specific production rules. The knowledge is inflexible and is best expressed through the same response systems within which it was acquired (Glisky et al. 1986; Eichenbaum et al. 1989; Saunders and Weiskrantz 1989).

Declarative memory depends on the integrity of the structures and connections damaged in amnesia. These structures provide a mechanism for forming new relationships rapidly in long-term memory, such as when a stimulus is associated to its spatial/temporal context (thus representing a new event) or when names and terms are associated to a semantic context (thus representing a new concept). Nondeclarative memory depends on anatomical structures and connections specific to what is being acquired. The striatum may be important for some kinds of nondeclarative memory, especially where a habit is acquired incrementally (Pack-

ard et al. 1989), but pathways in cerebellum (Thompson 1988) and amygdala (LeDoux et al. 1988) are also important, as, for example, in classic conditioning of skeletal musculature and in the conditioning of emotional responses. These and other observations are consistent with the idea that nondeclarative memory is heterogeneous (Squire 1987; Butters et al. 1990). For example, Heindel et al. (1989) found that word-completion priming was impaired in patients with Alzheimer's disease, but skill learning was intact. Patients with Huntington's disease showed the opposite pattern.

NEUROANATOMY OF MEMORY: RECENT FINDINGS FROM ANIMAL MODELS OF HUMAN AMNESIA

Careful neuropsychological descriptions of amnesic patients have contributed enormously to understanding how memory is organized in the brain. An important related issue is to identify the structures that when damaged produce amnesia. One promising approach to identifying these structures has taken advantage of an animal model of human amnesia in the nonhuman primate. The following sections describe a series of studies that used this approach to identify the components of the medial temporal lobe memory system.

Evaluating Memory Function in the Nonhuman Primate

Memory function in monkeys can be evaluated using a number of behavioral tasks that assess memory in a variety of ways (Zola-Morgan and Squire 1990a). Some of the tests are identical to ones failed by amnesic patients (delayed nonmatching to sample, delayed retention of object discriminations, and concurrent discrimination; Squire et al. 1988), and others are analogous to ones that amnesic patients do not fail (motor skill learning and pattern discrimination learning; Zola-Morgan and Squire 1984). These tasks, taken together, provide useful measures of the severity, the scope (impaired vs. spared memory functions), and the duration of memory deficit.

Contribution of the Medial Temporal Lobe to Memory Function

It is established in the monkey that large bilateral lesions of the medial temporal lobe, which include the structures thought to been removed in amnesic patient H.M. (Scoville and Milner 1957), produce severe memory impairment (Mishkin 1978; Mahut et al. 1982; Zola-Morgan and Squire 1985). In the monkey, this lesion involves the hippocampal formation (i.e., the dentate gyrus, the hippocampus proper, the subicular complex, and the entorhinal cortex), the amygdala, and the surrounding perirhinal and parahippocampal cortices. The lesion is termed the H^+A^+ lesion, where H refers to the hippocampus, A to the amygdala, and $^+$ to the respective, adjacent cortical regions (Zola-

Morgan and Squire 1985; Squire and Zola-Morgan 1988). The memory deficit in monkeys produced by the H^+A^+ lesion (Fig. 9A) parallels the deficit in human amnesia in several important ways (see Zola-Morgan and Squire 1990a): The deficit increases as the delay

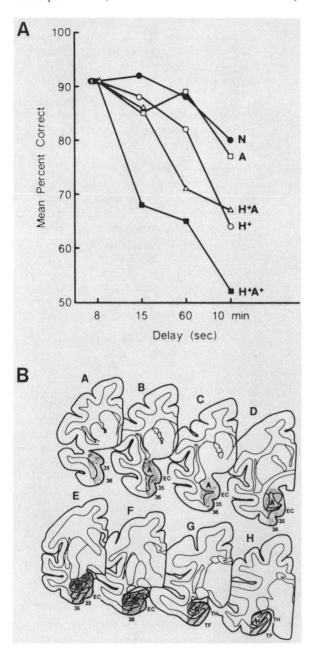

Figure 9. (*A*) Performance on the delayed nonmatching-to-sample task by normal monkeys (N), monkeys with lesions of the amygdala (A), monkeys with damage of the hippocampal formation (H^+), monkeys with conjoint lesions of the hippocampal formation and the amygdala (H^+A), and monkeys with large medial temporal lobe resections (H^+A^+). (*B*) Representative cross sections, rostral to caudal (A through H), through the brain of a monkey showing the regions damaged in the (H^+A^+) lesion (gray shading) and the (H^+) lesion (diagonal lines). Abbreviations: A, amygdala; H, hippocampus; EC, entorhinal cortex; 35 and 36, subdivisions of perirhinal cortex (Brodmann 1909); TH and TF, subdivisions of parahippocampal cortex (Bonin and Bailey 1947).

interval increases between acquisition and retention, it is severe and enduring, short-term memory is spared, it is modality general, and skill-based learning is spared. These parallels provide strong evidence that monkeys with the H^+A^+ lesion provide a good animal model of medial temporal lobe amnesia in humans. The work to be described next assesses the importance to memory functions of the components of the H^+A^+ lesion.

Hippocampal Formation and the Parahippocampal Cortex

As shown in Figure 9A, the H^+A^+ removal is not required to produce significant memory impairment. A substantial, though less severe memory deficit is observed in monkeys following a lesion limited to the hippocampal formation and parahippocampal cortex (referred to as the H^+ lesion; the anterior portion of the entorhinal cortex is spared in this lesion; Zola-Morgan et al. 1989a). This deficit is also enduring and appears to be similar qualitatively to the deficit associated with H^+A^+ lesions. (Importantly, only a transient impairment was observed following complete transection of the fornix, a major efferent projection of the hippocampal formation, or following complete destruction of the mammillary nuclei, a major subcortical target of this projection [Zola-Morgan et al. 1989a].) One possibility for the more severe memory deficit associated with the H^+A^+ lesion could be that the amygdala is included in the H^+A^+ lesion but not in the H^+ lesion (Fig. 9B).

Amygdaloid Complex

Recent findings suggest that amygdala damage does not contribute to the severe memory deficit exhibited by monkeys with H^+A^+ lesions. Lesions of the amygdaloid complex that spared the surrounding perirhinal and entorhinal cortex (the A lesion) produced no detectable memory impairment on any of four amnesia-sensitive tasks (Fig. 9A) (Zola-Morgan et al. 1989b). Moreover, adding an amygdala lesion to the H^+ lesion (H^+A lesion) did not exacerbate the level of memory deficit exhibited after the H^+ lesion alone (Fig. 9A).

Perirhinal and Parahippocampal Cortex

Recently, reevaluation of the extent of damage to the components of the original H^+A^+ lesion revealed that the perirhinal cortex (areas 35 and 36; Brodmann 1909) was more extensively damaged than previously appreciated (Zola-Morgan et al. 1989c). Neuroanatomical studies had already identified the perirhinal cortex and the closely associated parahippocampal cortex (areas TH and TF; Bonin and Bailey 1947) as important links between the polymodal and unimodal associational areas of neocortex and the hippocampal formation (Fig. 10A). Specifically, the perirhinal and parahippocampal cortex provide the major source of cortical input to the hippocampal formation, by way of

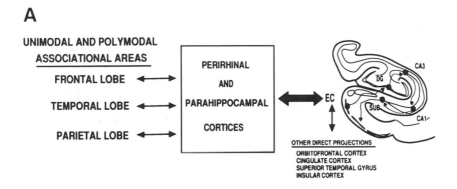

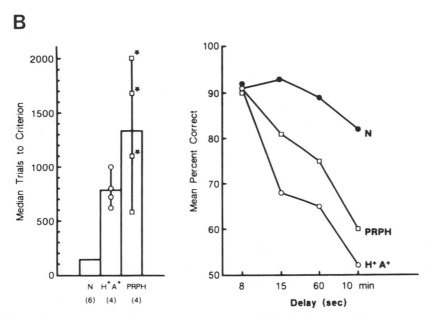

Figure 10. (*A*) Schematic representation of the connectivity of the perirhinal and the parahippocampal cortices in the monkey brain. The width of the arrows corresponds to the relative proportion of cortical inputs arising from the areas indicated. Abbreviations: EC, entorhinal cortex; DG, dentate gyrus; SUB, subicular complex; CA3 and CA1, fields of the hippocampus proper. (*B*) Performance on the delayed nonmatching-to-sample task by normal monkeys (N), monkeys with conjoint lesions of the perirhinal and parahippocampal cortices (PRPH), and monkeys with large medial temporal lobe resections (H$^+$A$^+$). (*Left*) Initial learning of this task with a delay of 8 sec. Symbols show trials required to reach learning criterion for individual animals. Asterisk indicates animals for which the task was made easier by providing two presentations of the sample object on each trial, instead of one (double-sample presentation). One monkey was performing at only 56% correct when testing was discontinued after 2000 trials. (*Right*) Performance across delays for the same groups. The curve for the PRPH animals underestimates the severity of impairment, because two of the three monkeys required double-sample presentation during this portion of the task. Indeed, when the single-sample procedure was used, performance of these two PRPH monkeys was considerably poorer than the performance of the H$^+$A$^+$ monkeys (8 sec: 70%; 15 sec: 60%; 60 sec: 55%).

the entorhinal cortex (Van Hoesen 1982; Insausti et al. 1987). These anatomical considerations suggest that lesions limited to the perirhinal and parahippocampal cortices, which spare the hippocampal formation and the amygdala (the PRPH lesion), should produce a severe memory deficit. Recently, monkeys with PRPH lesions were found to be severely impaired on three amnesia-sensitive tasks (Zola-Morgan et al. 1989c). On the delayed nonmatching-to-sample task, the PRPH group exhibited a more severe impairment than either the H$^+$ group or the H$^+$A$^+$ group (Fig. 10B). Neuroanatomical studies of the brains of the PRPH monkeys

showed that the PRPH lesion eliminated most of the cortical inputs to the entorhinal cortex that arise from structures other than perirhinal and parahippocampal cortex. In contrast, the cortical inputs to the amygdala were largely intact. The latter finding was consistent with the observation that monkeys with PRPH lesions showed none of the changes in emotionality that have invariably occurred following direct damage to the amygdala, even when damage to the amygdala is incomplete (Alvarez-Royo et al. 1988; Zola-Morgan et al. 1991).

Three conclusions can be reached from the findings

described to this point. First, damage to the amygdala does not appear to contribute to the memory deficit exhibited by monkeys with either H⁺A⁺ lesions or PRPH lesions. Second, the hippocampal formation and the anatomically related perirhinal and parahippocampal cortices are critical for normal memory function. Consistent with this view, in another operated group (the H⁺⁺ lesion), damage to the perirhinal cortex, sparing the amygdala, exacerbated the memory impairment associated with damage to the hippocampal formation (Clower et al. 1990). This finding contrasts sharply with the finding that amygdala damage did not increase the deficit associated with H⁺ lesions. Third, the PRPH lesion produced more severe impairment than the H⁺ lesion. One difference between the PRPH and H⁺ lesion was that the perirhinal cortex was included in the PRPH lesion but not in the H⁺ lesion. A second difference was that the PRPH lesion substantially deafferented the entorhinal cortex from cortical input, whereas the H⁺ lesion damaged only the posterior portion of entorhinal cortex. Accordingly, either of these two differences, either separately or in combination, could have contributed to the more severe impairment produced by the PRPH lesion, as compared to the H⁺ lesion. The important point is that the structures and connections damaged in the PRPH lesion, but not in the H⁺ lesion, must make a contribution to memory functions. Other studies will be needed to identify separate contributions to memory function of the perirhinal cortex, the entorhinal cortex, the parahippocampal cortex, and other cortical areas whose projections to entorhinal cortex were damaged by the PRPH lesion. In summary, the results strongly suggest that the severe memory impairment resulting from the H⁺A⁺ lesion depends not on conjoint damage to the hippocampus and the amygdala but on conjoint damage to the hippocampal formation and the surrounding perirhinal and parahippocampal cortices.

Hippocampus Proper

An additional issue is whether lesions limited to the hippocampus proper produce a significant memory deficit, or whether additional cortical damage is required. Valuable evidence pertaining to this point comes from patient R.B., who as the result of an ischemic episode sustained a lesion involving the entire CA1 field of the hippocampus bilaterally (Fig. 4). The perirhinal, entorhinal, and parahippocampal cortices were spared. R.B. exhibited a significant and enduring memory impairment (Zola-Morgan et al. 1986). This case showed that damage limited to the hippocampus proper is sufficient to cause a clinically significant and enduring memory deficit.

Monkeys that underwent a noninvasive procedure to produce cerebral ischemia (the ISC lesion) sustained substantial, bilateral loss of CA1 pyramidal cells in the hippocampus and were as impaired on the delayed non-matching-to-sample task as monkeys with H⁺ lesions (Fig. 11) (Zola-Morgan et al. 1989d). Moreover, the memory deficit exhibited by the ISC group was enduring. Across the three tasks that were given, the ISC group was less impaired than the H⁺ group, in keeping with the fact that the ISC lesion involved less damage to the hippocampal formation than the H⁺ lesion.

The findings from the ISC group make several points: First, the procedure used to produce global ischemia in the monkey consistently resulted in selective damage to the hippocampal formation sufficient to cause memory impairment. Second, lesions of either the hippocampal formation (H⁺) or incomplete hippocampal lesions (ISC) produced significant and long-lasting amnesia in the monkey. Third, the finding of significant and enduring memory impairment following even partial damage to the hippocampus (in the ISC group) contrasts with the lack of impairment that followed complete amygdala (A) damage.

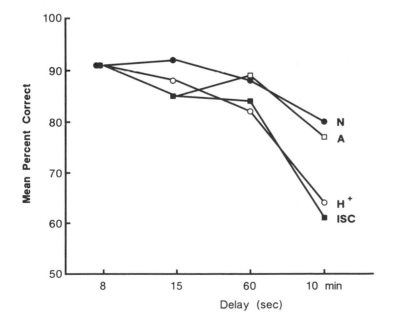

Figure 11. Performance on the delayed non-matching-to-sample task by normal monkeys (N), monkeys with lesions of the amygdala (A), monkeys with lesions of the hippocampal formation (H⁺), and monkeys with ischemic lesions of the hippocampus (ISC).

Medial Temporal Lobe Memory System

Cumulative and systematic work in monkeys has identified structures and connections important for memory function. The findings to date suggest that the hippocampal formation and the closely related perirhinal and parahippocampal cortices comprise the medial temporal lobe memory system. The amygdala does not appear to be an essential component of this memory system, although it has been implicated in other kinds of cognitive functions, e.g., ones that involve the association between a stimulus and its affective component (Mishkin and Aggleton 1981; Gaffan and Harrison 1987).

CONCLUSION

In this paper, we have reviewed recent progress in understanding the organization of memory and its neurological foundations. Parallel study of memory-impaired patients and an animal model of human memory impairment has illuminated the function of a medial temporal lobe/diencephalic system essential for the establishment of long-term memory. The role of this system is temporary, however, and it is eventually replaced by a gradually developing, more permanent memory elsewhere, probably in neocortex. Other work has led to the proposal that multiple forms of memory must be distinguished. The kind of memory that depends on the integrity of the medial temporal lobe/diencephalic system has been termed declarative (or explicit) memory. This kind of memory stores representations about facts and events and is accessible to conscious recollection. Nondeclarative (or implicit) memory is a heterogeneous collection of memory abilities, including the capacity for skill learning, priming, conditioning, and other instances in which memory is expressed through performance without access to prior encounters or to memory content. Nondeclarative memory depends on anatomical structures and connections that vary depending on what is being learned. Declarative memory depends on neocortex and on specific medial temporal lobe and diencephalic structures. On the basis of work with monkeys, the critical structures in the medial temporal lobe are the hippocampal formation and adjacent, anatomically related structures, especially the perirhinal and parahippocampal cortices.

ACKNOWLEDGMENTS

We thank Dr. Antonio Damasio for permission to test his patient, Boswell. This work was supported by the Medical Research Service of the Veterans Affairs, National Institute of Mental Health grant MH-24600, National Institutes of Health grant 19063, the Office of Naval Research, the McKnight Foundation, a Bioscience Grant for International Joint Research from NEDO, Japan, National Institute of Mental Health postdoctoral fellowship to G.M., and National Institute of Mental Health Research Service Award to C.B.C.

REFERENCES

Albert, M.S., N. Butters, and J. Levin. 1979. Temporal gradients in the retrograde amnesia of patients with alcoholic Korsakoff's disease. *Arch. Neurol.* **36:** 211.

Alvarez-Royo, P., M. Mesches, J. Allen, W. Saltzmann, L.R. Squire, and S. Zola-Morgan. 1988. Independence of memory functions and emotional behavior: Separate contributions of the hippocampal formation and the amygdala. *Soc. Neurosci. Abstr.* **14:** 1194.

Beatty, W.W., D.P. Salmon, N. Bernstein, and N. Butters. 1987. Remote memories in a patient with amnesia due to hypoxia. *Psychol. Med.* **17:** 657.

Benzing, W.C. and L.R. Squire. 1989. Preserved learning and memory in amnesia: Intact adaptation-level effects and learning of stereoscopic depth. *Behav. Neurosci.* **103:** 548.

Bonin, G. and P. Bailey. 1947. *The neocortex of Macaca mulatta.* University of Illinois Press, Urbana.

Brodmann, K. 1909. *Vergleichende Lokalizationslehre der Grosshirnrinde.* Barth, Leipzig.

Brooks, D. and A. Baddeley. 1976. What can amnesic patients learn? *Neuropsychologia* **14:** 111.

Butters, N. and L.S. Cermak. 1986. A case study of the forgetting of autobiographical knowledge: Implications for the study of retrograde amnesia. In *Autobiographical memory* (ed. D. Ruben), p. 253. Cambridge University Press, New York.

Butters, N., W.C. Heindel, and D.P. Salmon. 1990. Dissociation of implicit memory in dementia: Neurological implications. *Bull. Psychon. Soc.* **28:** 359.

Cermak, L.S., ed. 1982. *Human memory and amnesia.* Erlbaum, Hillsdale, New Jersey.

Cermak, L.S., R.P. Bleich, and S.P. Blackford. 1988. Deficits in implicit retention of new associates by alcoholic Korsakoff patients. *Brain Cog.* **1:** 145.

Cermak, L.R., N. Butters, and J. Moreines. 1974. Some analyses of the verbal encoding deficit of alcoholic Korsakoff patients. *Brain Lang.* **1:** 141.

Cermak, L.S., N. Talbot, K. Chandler, and L.R. Wolbarst. 1985. The perceptual priming phenomenon in amnesia. *Neuropsychologia* **23:** 615.

Clower, R.P., S. Zola-Morgan, and L.R. Squire. 1990. Lesions of perirhinal cortex, but not lesions of the amygdala, exacerbate memory impairment in monkeys following lesions of the hippocampal formation. *Soc. Neurosci. Abstr.* **16:** (in press).

Cohen, N.J. and L.R. Squire. 1980. Preserved learning and retention of pattern analyzing skill in amnesic patients: Dissociation of knowing how and knowing that. *Science* **210:** 207.

———. 1981. Retrograde amnesia and remote memory impairment. *Neuropsychologia* **19:** 337.

Corkin, S. 1968. Acquisition of motor skill after bilateral medial temporal lobe excision. *Neuropsychologia* **6:** 225.

Damasio, A.R., N.R. Graff-Radford, P.J. Eslinger, H. Damasio, and N. Kassell. 1985. Amnesia following basal forebrain lesions. *Arch. Neurol.* **42:** 263.

Daum, I., S. Channon, and A. Canavar. 1989. Classical conditioning in patients with severe memory problems. *J. Neurol. Neurosurg. Psychiatry* **52:** 47.

Eichenbaum, H., P. Matthews, and N.J. Cohen. 1989. Further studies of hippocampal representation during odor discrimination learning. *Behav. Neurosci.* **6:** 1207.

Gabrieli, J.D.E. 1990. Differential effects of aging and age-related neurological diseases on memory subsystems of the brain. In *The handbook of neuropsychology* (ed. F. Boller and J. Grafman). Elsevier, New York. (In press.)

Gabrieli, J.D.E. and M.M. Keane. 1988. Priming in the amnesic patient H.M.: New findings and a theory of impaired priming in patients with memory disorders. *Soc. Neurosci. Abstr.* **14:** 1290.

Gabrieli, J.D.E., N.J. Cohen, and S. Corkin. 1988. The impaired learning of semantic knowledge following medial temporal-lobe resection. *Brain Cog.* **7:** 157.

Gabrieli, J.D.E., W. Milberg, M.M. Keane, and S. Corkin. 1990. Intact priming of patterns despite impaired memory. *Neuropsychologia* **28:** 417.

Gaffan, D. and S. Harrison. 1987. Amygdalectomy and disconnection in visual learning for auditory secondary reinforcement by monkeys. *J. Neurosci.* **7:** 2285.

Glisky, E.L., D.L. Schacter, and E. Tulving. 1986. Computer learning by memory-impaired patients: Acquisition and retention of complex knowledge. *Neuropsychologia* **24:** 313.

Gordon, B. 1988. Preserved learning of novel information in amnesia: Evidence for multiple memory systems. *Brain Cog.* **7:** 257.

Graf, P. and D.L. Schacter. 1985. Implicit and explicit memory for new associations in normal and amnesic subjects. *J. Exp. Psychol. Learn. Mem. Cog.* **11:** 501.

Graf, P., L.R. Squire, and G. Mandler. 1984. The information that amnesic patients do not forget. *J. Exp. Psychol. Learn. Mem. Cog.* **10:** 164.

Haist, F., A.P. Shimamura, and L.R. Squire. 1989. The structures damaged in amnesia contribute similarity to recall and recognition memory. *Soc. Neurosci. Abstr.* **15:** 341.

Haist, F., L.R. Squire, and A.R. Damasio. 1990. Extensive retrograde amnesia on tests of familiarity and name completion ability. *Soc. Neurosci. Abstr.* (in press).

Heindel, W.C., D.P. Salmon, C.W. Shults, P.A. Walicks, and N. Butters. 1989. Neuropsychological evidence for multiple implicit memory systems: A comparison of Alzheimer's, Huntington's, and Parkinson's disease patients. *J. Neurosci.* **9:** 582.

Hirst, W. 1982. The amnesic syndrome: Descriptions and explanations. *Psychol. Bull.* **91:** 435.

Hirst, W., M.K. Johnson, E.A. Phelps, and B.T. Volpe. 1988. More on recognition and recall in amnesics. *J. Exp. Psychol. Learn. Mem. Cog.* **14:** 758.

Hirst, W., M. Johnson, J. Kim, E. Phelps, G. Risse, and B. Volpe. 1986. Recognition and recall in amnesics. *J. Exp. Psychol. Learn. Mem. Cog.* **12:** 4456.

Insausti, R., D.G. Amaral, and W.M. Cowan. 1987. The entorhinal cortex of the monkey: II. Cortical afferents. *J. Comp. Neurol.* **264:** 356.

Jacobson, R.R. and W.A. Lishman. 1987. Selective memory loss and global intellectual deficits in alcoholic Korsakoff's syndrome. *Psychol. Med.* **17:** 649.

Janowsky, J.S., A.P. Shimamura, and L.R. Squire. 1989a. Memory and metamemory: Comparison between patients with frontal lobe lesions and amnesic patients. *Psychobiology* **17:** 3.

Janowsky, J.S., A.P. Shimamura, M. Kritchevsky, and L.R. Squire. 1989b. Cognitive impairment following frontal lobe damage and its relevance to human amnesia. *Behav. Neurosci.* **103:** 548.

Johnson, M.J., J.K. Kim, and G. Risse. 1985. Do alcoholic Korsakoff's syndrome patients acquire affective reactions? *J. Exp. Psychol. Learn. Mem. Cog.* **11:** 22.

Kolers, P.A. 1975. Specificity of operations in sentence recognition. *Cog. Psychol.* **7:** 289.

Kopelman, M.D. 1989. Remote and autobiographical memory, temporal context memory and frontal atrophy of Korsakoff and Alzheimer patients. *Neuropsychologia* **27:** 437.

Kritchevsky, M. and L.R. Squire. 1989. Transient global amnesia: Evidence for extensive, temporally graded retrograde amnesia. *Neurology* **39:** 213.

LeDoux, J.E., J. Iwata, P. Cicchetti, and D.J. Reis. 1988. Different projections of the central amygdaloid nucleus mediate autonomic and behavioral correlates of conditioned fear. *J. Neurosci.* **7:** 2517.

MacKinnon, D.F. and L.R. Squire. 1989. Autobiographical memory and amnesia. *Psychobiology* **17:** 247.

Mahut, H., S. Zola-Morgan, and M. Moss. 1982. Hippocampal resections impair associative learning and recognition memory in the monkey. *J. Neurosci.* **2:** 1214.

Marr, D. 1971. Simple memory: A theory of archicortex. *Philos. Trans. R. Soc. Lond. B* **262:** 23.

Mayes, A.R. 1988. *Human organic memory disorders.* Cambridge University Press, England.

McAndrews, M.P., E.L. Glisky, and D.L. Schacter. 1987. When priming persists: Long-lasting implicit memory for a single episode in amnesic patients. *Neuropsychologia* **18:** 211.

Meudell, P.R., A.R. Mayes, A. Ostergaard, and A. Pickering. 1985. Recency and frequency judgements in alcoholic amnesics and normal people with poor memory. *Cortex* **21:** 487.

Meudell, P.R., B. Northern, J.S. Snowden, and D. Neary. 1980. Long-term memory for famous voices in amnesia and normal subjects. *Neuropsychologia* **18:** 133.

Milner, B. 1962. Les troubles de la memoire accompagnant des lesions hippocampiques bilaterales [Memory impairment accompanying bilateral hippocampal lesions]. In *Physiologia de l'hippocampe.* Centre National de la Recherche Scientifique, Paris.

———. 1971. Interhemispheric differences in the localization of psychological processes in man. *Br. Med. Bull.* **127:** 272.

———. 1972. Disorders of memory after temporal lobe lesions in man. *Clin. Neurosurg.* **19:** 421.

Mishkin, M. 1978. Memory in monkeys severely impaired by combined but not by separate removal of amygdala and hippocampus. *Nature* **273:** 297.

———. 1982. A memory system in the monkey. *Philos. Trans. R. Soc. Lond. B.* **298:** 85.

Mishkin, M. and J.P. Aggleton. 1981. Multiple functional contributions of the amygdala in the monkey. In *The amygdaloid complex* (ed. Y. Ben-Ari). Elsevier, Amsterdam.

Moscovitch, M., G. Winocur, and D. McLachlan. 1986. Memory as assessed by recognition and reading time in normal and memory-impaired people with Alzheimer's disease and other neurological disorders. *J. Exp. Psychol. Gen.* **115:** 331.

Musen, G. and A. Treisman. 1990. Implicit and explicit memory for visual patterns. *J. Exp. Psychol. Learn. Mem. Cog.* **16:** 127.

Musen, G., A.P. Shimamura, and L.R. Squire. 1990. Intact text-specific reading skill in amnesia. *J. Exp. Psychol. Learn. Mem. Cog.* (in press).

Nissen, M.M. and P. Bullemer. 1987. Attentional requirements of learning: Evidence from performance measures. *Cog. Psychol.* **19:** 1.

Oscar-Berman, M. 1980. The neuropsychological consequences of long-term chronic alcoholism. *Am. Sci.* **68:** 410.

Ostergaard, A.L. and L.R. Squire. 1990. Childhood amnesia and distinctions between form of memory. A comment on Wood, Brown and Felton. *Brain Cog.* (in press).

Packard, M.G., R. Hirsch, and N.M. White. 1989. Differential effects of fornix and caudate nucleus lesions on two radial maze tasks: Evidence for multiple memory system. *J. Neurosci.* **9:** 1465.

Press, G., D.G. Amaral, and L.R. Squire. 1989. Hippocampal abnormalities in amnesic patients revealed by high-resolution magnetic resonance imaging. *Nature* **341:** 54.

Ribot, T. 1882. *Diseases of memory* (translated by W.H. Smith). Appleton-Century-Crofts, New York. (Original work published 1881.)

Sanders, H.I. and E.K. Warrington. 1971. Memory for remote events in amnesic patients. *Brain* **94:** 661.

Saunders, R.C. and L. Weiskrantz. 1989. The effects of fornix transection and combined fornix transection, mammillary body lesions and hippocampal ablations on object-pair association in rhesus monkey. *Behav. Brain Res.* **2**: 85.

Schacter, D.L. 1985. Multiple forms of memory in humans and animals. In *Memory systems of the brain: Animal and human cognitive processes* (ed. N. Weinberger et al.), p. 351. Guilford Press, New York.

———. 1990. Perceptual representation systems and implicit memory: Toward a resolution of the multiple memory systems debate. *Ann. N.Y. Acad. Sci.* (in press).

Schacter, D.L., L.A. Cooper, and S.M. Delaney. 1990. Implicit memory for unfamiliar objects depends on access to structural descriptions. *J. Exp. Psychol. Gen.* **119**: 5.

Scoville, W.B. and B. Milner. 1957. Loss of recent memory after bilateral hippocampal lesions. *J. Neurol. Neurosurg. Psychiatry* **20**: 11.

Shimamura, A.P. 1986. Priming effects in amnesia: Evidence for a dissociable memory function. *Q. J. Exp. Psychol.* **38A**: 619.

Shimamura, A.P. and L.R. Squire. 1984. Paired-associate learning and priming effects in amnesia: A neuropsychological study. *J. Exp. Psychol. Gen.* **113**: 556.

———. 1986. Memory and metamemory: A study of the feeling-of-knowing phenomenon in amnesic patients. *J. Exp. Psychol. Learn. Mem. Cog.* **12**: 452.

———. 1989. Impaired priming of new associations in amnesia. *J. Exp. Psychol. Learn. Mem. Cog.* **15**: 721.

Shimamura, A.P., J.S. Janowsky, and L.R. Squire. 1990. Memory for the temporal order of events in patients with frontal lobe lesions and amnesic patients. *Neuropsychologia* (in press).

Shimamura, A.P., T.L. Jernigan, and L.R. Squire. 1988. Korsakoff's syndrome: Radiological (CT) findings and neuropsychological correlates. *J. Neurosci.* **8**: 4400.

Smith, M.E. and M. Oscar-Berman. 1990. Activation and the repetition priming of words and pseudowords in normal memory and amnesia. *J. Exp. Psychol. Learn. Mem. Cog.* (in press).

Squire, L.R. 1974. A stable impairment in remote memory following electroconvulsive therapy. *Neuropsychologia* **13**: 51.

———. 1982. Comparisons between forms of amnesia: Some deficits are unique to Korsakoff's syndrome. *J. Exp. Psychol. Learn. Mem. Cog.* **8**: 560.

———. 1987. *Memory and brain.* Oxford University Press, New York.

Squire, L.R. and N.J. Cohen. 1982. Remote memory, retrograde amnesia, and the neuropsychology of memory. In *Human memory and amnesia* (ed. L. Cermak), p. 275. Erlbaum, Hillsdale, New Jersey.

Squire, L.R. and M. Frambach. 1990. Cognitive skill learning in amnesia. *Psychobiology* **18**: 109.

Squire, L.R. and A.P. Shimamura. 1986. Characterizing amnesic patients for neurobehavioral study. *Behav. Neurosci.* **100**: 866.

Squire, L.R. and C.W. Spanis. 1984. Long gradient of retrograde amnesia in mice: Continuity with the findings in humans. *Behav. Neurosci.* **98**: 345.

Squire, L.R. and S. Zola-Morgan. 1988. Memory: Brain systems and behavior. *Trends Neurosci.* **11**: 170.

Squire, L.R., F. Haist, and A.P. Shimamura. 1989a. The neurology of memory: Quantitative assessment of retrograde amnesia in two groups of amnesic patients. *J. Neurosci.* **9**: 828.

Squire, L.R., A.P. Shimamura, and D.G. Amaral. 1989b. Memory and the hippocampus. In *Neural models of plasticity* (ed. J. Byrne and W. Berry), p. 208. Academic Press, New York.

Squire, L.R., A.P. Shimamura, and P. Graf. 1987. Strength and duration of priming effects in normal subjects and amnesic patients. *Neuropsychologia* **25**: 1195.

Squire, L.R., P.C. Slater, and P.M. Chace. 1975. Retrograde amnesia: Temporal gradient in very long-term memory following electroconvulsive therapy. *Science* **187**: 77.

Squire, L.R., S. Zola-Morgan, and K. Chen. 1988. Human amnesia and animal models of amnesia: Performance of amnesic patients on tests designed for the monkey. *Behav. Neurosci.* **102**: 210.

Teyler, T.J. and P. DiScenna. 1986. The hippocampal memory indexing theory. *Behav. Neurosci.* **100**: 147.

Thompson, R.F. 1988. The neural basis of basic associative learning of discrete behavioral responses. *Trends Neurosci.* **4**: 152.

Tulving, E. 1983. *Elements of episodic memory.* Oxford University Press, New York.

Tulving, E. and D.L. Schacter. 1990. Priming and human memory systems. *Science* **247**: 385.

Tulving, E., D. Schacter, and H.A. Stark. 1982. Priming effects in word-fragment completion are independent of recognition memory. *J. Exp. Psychol. Learn. Mem. Cog.* **8**: 352.

Van Hoesen, G. 1982. The parahippocampal gyrus. *Trends. Neurosci.* **5**: 345.

Warrington, E.K. and P.A. McCarthy. 1988. The fractionation of retrograde amnesia. *Brain Cog.* **7**: 184.

Weiskrantz, L. 1987. Neuroanatomy of memory and amnesia: A case for multiple memory systems. *Hum. Neurobiol.* **6**: 93.

Weiskrantz, L. and E.K. Warrington. 1979. Conditioning in amnesic patients. *Neuropsychologia* **17**: 187.

Winocur, G. 1990. Anterograde and retrograde amnesia in rats with dorsal hippocampal or dorsomedial thalamic lesions. *Behav. Brain Res.* **38**: 145.

Zola-Morgan, S. and L.R. Squire. 1984. Preserved learning in monkeys with medial temporal lesions: Sparing of motor and cognitive skills. *J. Neurosci.* **4**: 1072.

———. 1985. Medial temporal lesions in monkeys impair memory on a variety of tasks sensitive to human amnesia. *Behav. Neurosci.* **99**: 22.

Zola-Morgan, S. and L.R. Squire. 1990a. Neuropsychological investigations of memory and amnesia: Findings from humans and nonhuman primates. In *The development and neural bases of higher cognitive functions* (ed. A. Diamond). MIT Bradford Press, Cambridge. (In press.)

———. 1990b. The primate hippocampal formation: Evidence for a time-limited role in memory storage. *Science* (in press).

Zola-Morgan, S., L.R. Squire, and D.G. Amaral. 1986. Human amnesia and the medial temporal region: Enduring memory impairment following a bilateral lesion limited to field CA1 of the hippocampus. *J. Neurosci.* **6**: 2950.

———. 1989a. Lesions of the hippocampal formation but not lesions of the fornix or the mammillary nuclei produce long-lasting memory impairments in monkeys. *J. Neurosci.* **9**: 898.

———. 1989b. Lesions of the amygdala that spare adjacent cortical regions do not impair memory or exacerbate the impairment following lesions of the hippocampal formation. *J. Neurosci.* **9**: 1922.

Zola-Morgan, S., L.R. Squire, P. Alvarez-Royo, and R.P. Clower. 1991. Independence of memory functions and emotional behavior: Separate contributions of the hippocampal formation and the amygdala. *Hippocampus* (in press).

Zola-Morgan, S., L.R. Squire, D.G. Amaral, and W.A. Suzuki. 1989c. Lesions of the perirhinal and parahippocampal formation produce severe memory impairment. *J. Neurosci.* **9**: 4355.

Zola-Morgan, S., L.R. Squire, D.G. Amaral, G. Fleischer, M.S. Scheller, and M.H. Zornow. 1989d. An animal model of global ischemia in the monkey: Neuropathological and behavioral findings. *Soc. Neurosci. Abstr.* **15**: 341.

Neocortical Memory Circuits

P.S. Goldman-Rakic, S. Funahashi, and C.J. Bruce

Section of Neuroanatomy, Yale University School of Medicine, New Haven, Connecticut 06510

For many decades, the hippocampus and associated limbic areas of the mammalian central nervous system have been the structures most closely associated with memory (Scoville and Miner 1957; Mishkin 1982; Amaral et al. 1987). Indeed, the hippocampus is essential for acquiring and consolidating new knowledge about events, people, and places. In the unusual circumstance that both medial temporal lobes are damaged, as in the famous case of H.M., memory is reduced to that acquired before the injury (Scoville and Milner 1957); after suffering this type of injury, an individual is unable to remember most events for even a few minutes.

Other areas of the central nervous system are also important for memory processes. Among these, the prefrontal cortex has been consistently implicated in mnemonic functions (see, e.g., Warrington and Weiskrantz 1982; Fuster 1985; Kesner 1985; Milner et al. 1985), although the precise nature of these functions has been difficult to define. The question naturally arises as to the character of the prefrontal contribution compared to that of other areas and whether and how it differs from these other areas. In this paper, we review our recent studies on the physiological properties of prefrontal neurons engaged in oculomotor memory tasks (Funahashi et al. 1989, 1990, 1991). An understanding of the prefrontal contribution to memory should allow more precise comparisons with that of the hippocampus and other brain regions.

Delayed Response: Basic Probe of Short-term Memory

Evidence that the prefrontal cortex is involved in memory processes comes from the well-established, and often repeated, finding that monkeys with bilateral prefrontal lesions, primarily of the dorsolateral principal sulcus (PS) region of the frontal lobe, are severely impaired on delayed-response tasks (for review, see Goldman-Rakic 1987a; Fuster 1989). As their name implies, these tasks employ a temporal delay to separate the process of *encoding* a stimulus from the *execution of a response* to that stimulus. The simple expedient of introducing a time delay forces the monkey to guide its response on the basis of an *internal representation*, or memory, of the reward location. In the classic version of the task, after the monkey watches a reward being hidden under the cover of one of two food wells, an opaque screen is lowered to prevent the animal from reaching the hidden reward immediately. Following a

1–5-second delay, the screen is raised and selection of one of the locations is then allowed. Since the placement of the concealed item is randomly varied from trial to trial, the animal has to continually update his memory; accordingly, what is relevant on trial *n* becomes irrelevant on trial *n* + 1. Distinct from associative memory, this transient memory process is analogous to the process that cognitive psychologists refer to as "working memory" (Just and Carpenter 1985; Baddeley 1986).

Neuronal Elements of Short-term Memory

In a remarkable set of studies, in which monkeys performed the delayed-response task while activity was recorded from individual prefrontal neurons, neurophysiologists have observed neuronal activity in precise registration with the cue, the delay, or response periods of this task, suggesting that separate and distinct neuronal populations encode the input, hold, and output functions required in delayed-response tasks (Kubota and Niki 1971; Fuster 1973; Niki 1974c). These results confirm, at a neuronal level, what could be analytically derived; namely, that performance on a delayed-response task involves several levels of information processing: sensory encoding, temporary storage of information, and response execution. It has been hypothesized that the prefrontal cortex contains multiple working memory "centers," each dedicated to a different information-processing domain, and that within these centers, specific classes of neurons are specialized for carrying out the subfunctions necessary to accomplish an integrated memory-driven act (Goldman-Rakic 1987a, 1988).

Issues in the Study of Short-term Memory

Although the basic neuronal elements for construction of a cortical memory circuit have been identified, some of them are complex, and their role in behavior is not well understood. Fuster (1973) identified at least five types of prefrontal activity in monkeys performing a manual delayed-response task. Subsequently, additional neuronal profiles have been described as investigators have employed a variety of behavioral paradigms and/or variations of delayed-response tasks, including spatial delayed-alternation tasks (Kubota and Niki 1971; Niki 1974a,b), nonspatial delay tasks (Kubota et al. 1980; Rosenkilde et al. 1981; Fuster et al. 1982; Quintana et al. 1988; Yajeya et al. 1988), and oculomotor paradigms (Joseph and Barone 1987; Barone and Joseph 1989; Funahashi et al. 1989).

In this paper, we review the basic neuronal profiles in prefrontal cortex and address the question of their interdependence. Our studies have exploited an oculomotor paradigm which, as will be described below, controls the monkey's sensory input and performance requirements to an unprecedented degree. Our goal is to understand the role played by the prefrontal cortex vis-a-vis other cortical and subcortical structures in the memory systems of the brain.

EXPERIMENTAL CONTEXT

Behavioral Requirements

Rhesus monkeys served as subjects in the experiments to be described. They were trained to perform an oculomotor delayed-response task (ODR) (Fig. 1). Details of the training procedure and how eye position is monitored may be found in Funahashi et al. (1989). Briefly, in the ODR, the monkey was seated in a primate chair and trained to fixate a central spot on a cathode ray tube, monitored by a magnetic search coil technique (Robinson 1963). As soon as the monkey maintained fixation for 0.75 second, the *cue period* began with presentation of a visual target (a $0.7° \times 0.7°$ square) for 0.5 second at one of four or eight peripheral locations. As in the classic delayed-response task, the location of the stimulus is randomized over trials so that the monkey cannot predict where the cue will appear on any given trial. An important feature of the task is that the monkey is required to maintain fixation when the peripheral target appears and throughout the subsequent 3–5-second *delay period* as well. At the end of the delay, the extinction of the fixation spot signaled the *response period* in which the monkey is expected to make a saccade within the next 0.5 second to the position where the cue *had been* presented just seconds before. If the saccade fell within a predetermined diameter of the cue, the monkey was rewarded with a drop (0.2 ml) of lightly sweetened water or juice. Training the monkey to perform all steps in the ODR task at a high level of accuracy and consistency generally required several months. In the ODR, as in the classic delayed-response tasks, the monkey's response is memory-guided, i.e., the directional cue is presented only briefly and, importantly, is not available at the time of response. Unlike the traditional tests, however, the requirement of fixation throughout a trial ensures compliance with the memory requirements of the task, since it prevents anticipatory responses during the delay, as well as experimental control over the input (retinal coordinates of the stimulus to be remembered).

Single neuron activity was recorded with Parylene-coated tungsten microelectrodes (2–5 MΩ at 1 kHz, Micro Probe Inc.) or glass-coated elgiloy microelectrodes (0.5–1.0 MΩ at 1 kHz). The latter are ideal for making a small iron deposit at the recording site (Suzuki and Azuma 1977). Electric current (20 µA for

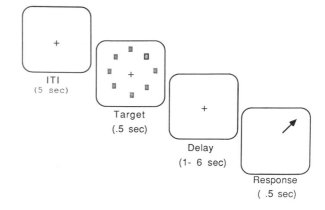

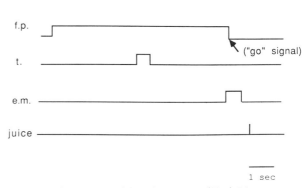

Figure 1. Oculomotor delayed response. (*Top*) Diagram representing the cathode ray monitor and temporal parameters of the response trials. From left to right: the intertrial interval (ITI), the cue period (target), the delay period, and the response period. The arrow indicates for the reader the correct direction of responding at the end of the delay; it is not a signal for the monkey. (*Bottom*) Temporal relationship of events in the oculomotor task. (f.p.) Fixation point; (t) target; (e.m.) eye movement.

10–15 sec) was passed at some electrode sites to mark the location of selected functionally characterized neurons.

For data analysis, an on-line computer system, in addition to carrying out the behavioral paradigms, sampled neuronal and ocular signals and stored the data in relation to task events on magnetic media. Event buffer files contain the time of appearance and disappearance of visual cues and also the time, duration, direction, and amplitude of each saccade. Using these files, we constructed rasters and histograms of neuronal activity for each position of the visuospatial cue. The rasters and histograms were made with different alignment points, including the start of the delay period, the start of the response period, the offset of the fixation point, and the initiation and completion of saccadic eye movement. Thus, not only were we able to track and record precisely the beginning and the end of saccadic eye movements and determine their latency and velocity, but we were also able to discriminate neuronal activity as pre- or postsaccadic (Funahashi et al. 1991).

To obtain a comprehensive view of neuronal activity, composite histograms were constructed that sum activity across defined classes of neurons, e.g., those neurons with delay-period activation. In addition, tuning curves were constructed for each neuron to determine directional specificity; tuning specificity was evaluated by fitting a neuron's activity at each of eight cue locations to a Gaussian function, using the method of least squares with the neuron's spontaneous rate and its rate and direction of best responses as constants.

RESULTS

Data Base

This review is based on a detailed examination of 434 fully analyzed neurons from the PS in six hemispheres of four rhesus monkeys performing the ODR task. A considerable percentage, 60%, or 261 neurons, were related to task parameters; i.e., they showed excitatory or inhibitory responses in relation to one or more events (cue, delay, and/or response period) of the ODR task. A breakdown of the 261 PS neurons with task-related activity, without regard to the sign of the response, revealed seven basic functional categories as follows: cue ($n = 21$), delay ($n = 73$), or response-related ($n = 62$) activity; cue and delay ($n = 20$); cue and response ($n = 10$); delay and response ($n = 52$); and cue, delay, and response activity ($n = 23$). Thus, overall, neurons showed a variety of responses: simple responses in that they related to only one event in the task (as shown in Fig. 2), but also complex responses, i.e., involving two or more task-related events. We have examined the temporal and spatial distribution of these major categories of neuronal activation and, for convenience, these are presented in functional groups below.

Cue Period Activity

One class of neuron recorded in and around the PS responded to the presentation of the cue in the ODR task (Fig. 3). Most neurons of this class gave a phasic excitatory response following cue onset, with a median latency of 116 msec; a small percentage (less than 10%) were inhibited by the cue. Additionally, the directional selectivity of these neurons reflects primarily their visual receptive fields (for details, see Funahashi et al. 1990). Whereas similar neurons have been recorded previously in manual delayed-response tasks (see, e.g., Fuster 1973), the use of visual perimetry (i.e., presenting the visual cue in a number of positions throughout the visual field) enabled us to show that over 95% of these cells are directionally selective; i.e., they increased their firing rate only for one or a few positions of the cue in the ODR task (Fig. 3). Furthermore, most neurons had their "best directions" (the target to which the neuron responded most strongly) in the visual field contralateral to the recording (Fig. 4, upper). The median tuning value of these responses was 37°. Thus, a

class of prefrontal neuron in and near the PS accesses specific information about the spatial coordinates of objects in the visual world, and all polar directions within the peripheral visual fields are represented (see Fig. 4).

Neurons that exhibited cue-related activity *only* were encountered relatively infrequently in our population of task-related neurons (~7% of the total). On the other hand, many more neurons showed identical phasic responses to a particular cue, or subset of cues, while *also* exhibiting delay-period activity or response-related activation (e.g., Fig. 5). When cells coded multiple events, it was generally the case that the tuning of these multiple "activities" was highly correlated; for example, a neuron that discharged preferentially to a target presented at the 90° position also responded best to that same direction during the delay or response periods of the ODR task.

Delay-period Activity

The largest class of task-related neurons in our entire sample (~50%) are those that increased or decreased their discharge in a directionally selective pattern during the delay period (Figs. 2 and 5). Such neurons discharged most vigorously (or were inhibited) when the to-be-remembered stimulus disappeared from view and during the period that motor action was deferred, thus making them particularly relevant to the memory process. Indeed, a given neuron was consistently activated *during the delay period* for only one or a few locations in space, and different neurons coded different locations. The neuron shown in Figure 5 was activated during the delay only when the monkey had to remember the target at the 270° location. The same neuron's activity was suppressed at the 90° location and did not differ significantly from baseline firing when the target was presented at all other locations. We have termed the neuron's activation to a specific best direction its "memory field" in analogy with the receptive fields of sensory cortical neurons (Funahashi et al. 1989). When we plotted the best directions for the entire sample of neurons with directional memory fields in polar coordinates, we discovered that different neurons coded different locations preferentially and that there was a bias for representing the contralateral visual field in memory (Fig. 4, lower) (see also Funahashi et al. 1989).

A number of additional findings support a mnemonic role for delay-period activity. The neuron shown in Figure 6 was tested with four target locations and two different delays. When the delay period was prolonged, the delay period activity expanded; when the delay was shortened, the neuronal activity contracted correspondingly. Although the upper limits for a sustained response are not known, sustained activation for as long as 16 seconds has been observed (S. Funahashi et al., unpubl.). Finally, delay-period activation seems to be necessary for correct responding. Figure 7 is a composite histogram of the delay-period activity for the

1. Cue period activity

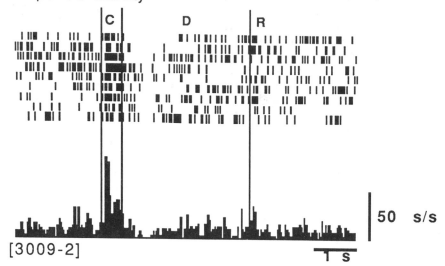

[3009-2]

50 s/s

1 s

2. Delay period activity

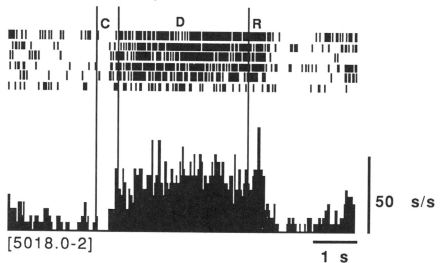

[5018.0-2]

50 s/s

1 s

3. Response period activity

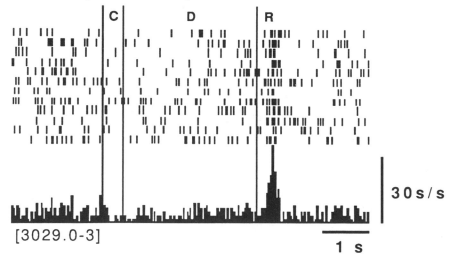

[3029.0-3]

30 s/s

1 s

Figure 2. Three elemental patterns of activity, recorded from different neurons in and around the PS. (C) Cue period; (D) delay period; (R) response period.

A. ODR task

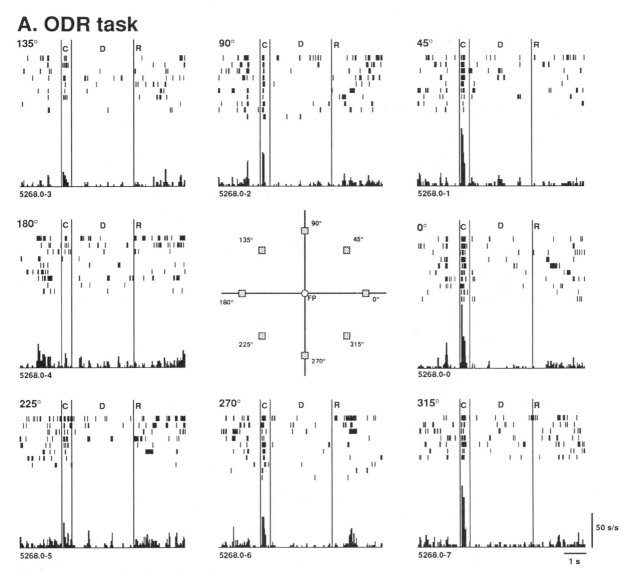

B. cue period activity

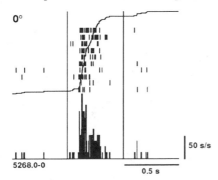

Figure 3. (*A*) Directional cue period activity of a PS neuron recorded while the monkey performed the oculomotor delayed-response task. This neuron had a strong phasic excitatory response to the onset of cues in the right visual field, with its best direction of response at 0°. Visual cues were randomly presented at one of the eight locations indicated in the central diagram. All cue eccentricities were 13°, and all delay periods were 3 sec. The histogram bin width is 40 msec. (*B*) Cue period activity on the 0° trials is shown with the time scale expanded and a cumulative histogram, in addition to the rasters and conventional histogram. The visual response at the 0° location occurred with a latency of 94 msec, as judged by the inflection of the cumulative histogram. The histogram bin width is 15 msec. (Reprinted, with permission, from Funahashi et al. 1990.)

A. Cue period activity (n=84)

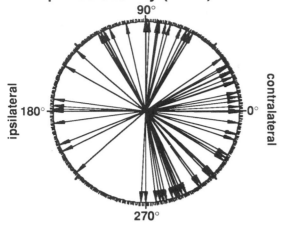

B. Delay period activity (n=171)

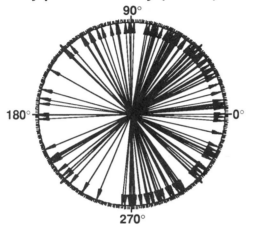

Figure 4. (*A*) Polar plots of the best directions of cue period activity for 84 PS neurons that displayed directionally specific responses in the ODR task. (*B*) Polar plots of the best directions of delay-period activity for 171 cells in and around the PS with directionally specific responses in the ODR task. The best directions were determined as described by Funahashi et al. (1989) and presented as if all neurons were recorded from the left hemisphere. A contralateral bias is evident.

best directions of nine prefrontal neurons whcn the animal performed correctly and the corresponding activity of the same neurons on trials in which the monkey made errors. The neurons exhibited enhanced activity during the delay on correct trials whereas the composite activity during the error trials did not differ from baseline, indicating that delay-period activity represents directional information that is used by the animal to guide correct responses. The difference in delay-period activity between the correct and incorrect trials was highly significant (paired $t = 2.76$, $df = 8$, $p < 0.025$).

As in the case of cue-related activity described above, delay-period activity can exist as the only activity of a neuron (e.g., Fig. 2) or it can be part of a compound neuronal response related to more than one event in the ODR task (e.g., Fig. 5). Many neurons

with delay-period activity also responded in relation to the cue ($n = 20$; 7%), to the response ($n = 52$; 20%), or to both cue and response ($n = 23$; 9%). Several of these compound responses are described in the next section.

Oculomotor Activity

Almost one-fourth of task-related neurons were related to the motor response, with latencies ranging from -192 to 460 msec relative to initiation of the saccadic responses required in the ODR task. About one fourth of the oculomotor responses were presaccadic, but the majority were postsaccadic, i.e., they increased firing after the initiation of the eye movement. Both presaccadic and postsaccadic responses, like delay-period and cue-period activity, were directionally specific, again favoring contralateral fields.

Saccade-related activity was registered in neurons unaccompanied by cue- and delay-period activity, again indicating that separate neurons code different events in the task. An example is shown in Figure 8, where the same neuron shows postsaccadic excitation for the 180°, 135°, and 225° stimulus directions and not for any other direction. However, it was not uncommon for oculomotor responses to be associated with cue-period activity, delay-period activity, or both. In a number of cells with mixed responses, we found an interesting functional dichotomy: In Figure 9, the excitatory delay-period activity at the 90° location was followed by phasic *presaccadic* activity; whereas inhibitory delay-period activity following presentation of the target at 0° was followed by phasic *postsaccadic* activity (see also Fig. 5).

Our ability to measure precisely the onset of the saccadic response and the latency of neuronal activation in relation to that response enabled us to detect strong temporal relationships between neurons. The postsaccadic responses observed in our experiments began about 50–100 msec after the completion of the saccadic eye movement. The peak of postsaccadic activation in one set of neurons turned out to coincide precisely with the termination and return to baseline of excitatory (and inhibitory) delay-period activity in independent neurons (Fig. 10). We have tentatively interpreted the postsaccadic activation in prefrontal neurons as a feedback signal that serves to inform the animal that the appropriate response has been executed, and delay-period activity (on-line memory) is no longer required. Definitive information is lacking on whether this feedback signal is a form of efference copy but, regardless, the erasure of the delay-period activity sets the stage for the next bit of information to come "on line" to guide the next response.

GENERAL DISCUSSION

Working memory is the term applied by cognitive psychologists to the type of memory that is active and relevant only for a brief segment of time, usually on the

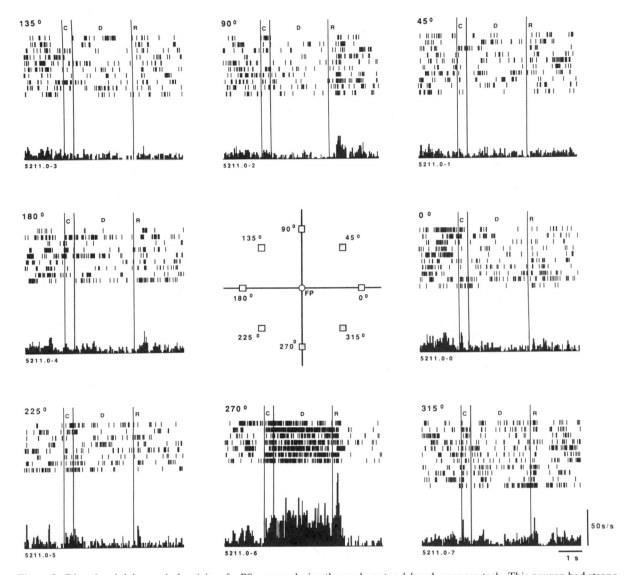

Figure 5. Directional delay-period activity of a PS neuron during the oculomotor delayed-response task. This neuron had strong directional delay-period activity ($F = 48.35$; $df = 7, 68$; $p < 0.001$), responding only when the cue had been presented at the bottom (270°) location. It was suppressed during the delay when the cue was presented in the upper visual field and, in all three cases, delay-period activity was significantly below the ITI rate (45°, $t = 2.350$, $df = 84$, $p < 0.025$; 90°, $t = 3.451$, $df = 85$, $p < 0.001$; 135°, $t = 2.607$, $df = 84$, $p = 0.025$). Visual cues were randomly presented at one of the eight locations indicated in the center diagram. All cue eccentricities were 13°, and all delay periods were 3 sec. (Reprinted, with permission, from Funahashi et al. 1989.)

scale of seconds (Just and Carpenter 1985; Baddeley 1986). A common but trivial example of working memory is keeping in mind a newly read phone number until it is dialed and immediately forgotten. Other still simple operations requiring working memory are "mental" arithmetic, planning chess moves, and "mental" rotation. The criterion—useful or relevant only transiently—distinguishes working memory from the very different processes of reference memory (Olton and Papas 1979), episodic memory (Tulving 1972), and procedural memory (Cohen and Squire 1980); all of which have in common that they are acquired by repetitive association of events and/or are long-lasting. However, the products of associative learning usually com-

prise the contents of working memory, indicating that the two types of mnemonic process are interdependent. In the classic terminology of memory research, associative memory deals with acquisition and consolidation, whereas working memory deals with retrieval of acquired knowledge.

We have argued that the classic and contemporary versions of delayed-response tasks depend on a working memory process in nonhuman primates. The ability of a monkey to keep a location or feature of an object "in mind" is not unlike the ability of humans to keep a phone number or the name of a person in mind. As reviewed here, a variety of neuronal responses can be recorded from the prefrontal cortex during perfor-

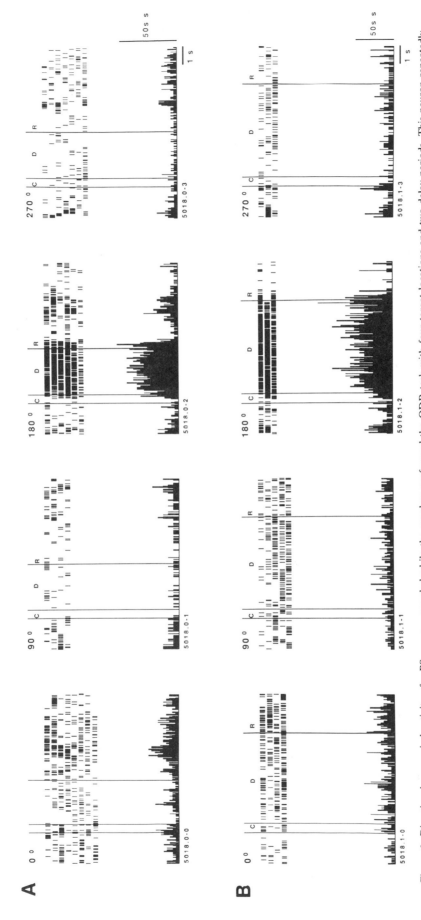

Figure 6. Directional cue period activity of a PS neuron recorded while the monkey performed the ODR task with four target locations and two delay periods. This neuron repeatedly responded with a strong tonic excitatory response in the delay period after cues presented in the 180° location. All cue eccentricities were 13° and all delay periods were 3 sec. The histogram bin width is 40 msec. (Reprinted, with permission, from Funahashi et al. 1989.)

A. Correct trials

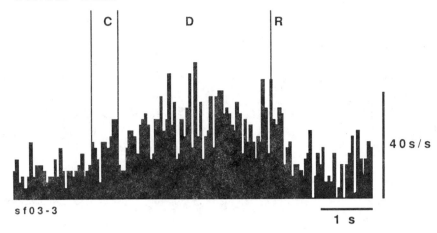

sf03-3

40 s/s

1 s

B. Error trials

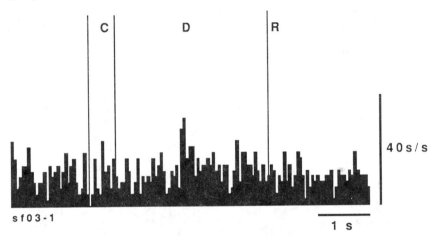

sf03-1

40 s/s

1 s

Figure 7. Comparison of delay-period activity for correct trials with activity for error trials. The first correct trial and the first error trial were taken from each of nine principal sulcus neurons that had excitatory delay-period activity. The error was made on a trial in the neuron's preferred direction. The comparison shows that the delay-period activation present on the correct trials (*top*) was absent on the error trials (*bottom*). (Reprinted, with permission, from Funahashi et al. 1989).

mance of the oculomotor delayed-response task, and there is every reason to believe that similar neurons play some role in the integrated process that underlies comprehension, thought, and problem solving in humans. Because a similar variety of neuronal responses has been recorded from the *same* regions of the prefrontal cortex for the manual version of the task (for review, see Fuster 1989), it would appear that the memory mechanisms could influence a number of effector systems conjointly or independently.

Working Memory or Motor Set

The present study provides insight into the types of, and timing relationships among, prefrontal neurons and their functional interaction. A central issue is whether the prefrontal neurons recorded do, indeed, provide the cellular substrates for memory-guided behavior. It could be argued, for example, that enhanced

neuronal discharge during the delay of a delayed-response trial does not represent substantive information to be remembered, but is instead the "motor set" of the animal to respond in a particular direction. The act of preparing to respond could invoke postural mechanisms, both peripheral and central, and not necessarily require processing of stored information. However, the prefrontal neurons with delay-period activity exhibit increased discharge only for targets in specific directions, even though the animal is set to respond, and does respond, correctly at the end of the delay period on every trial, regardless of target direction. Furthermore, the requirement that the animal maintain fixation in the delay period negates anticipatory saccades and rehearsal much as distractor tasks, such as counting backwards, control conscious rehearsal in human cognitive testing (see, e.g., Baddeley 1986). An important finding is that errors are committed on trials when delay-period activity is truncated

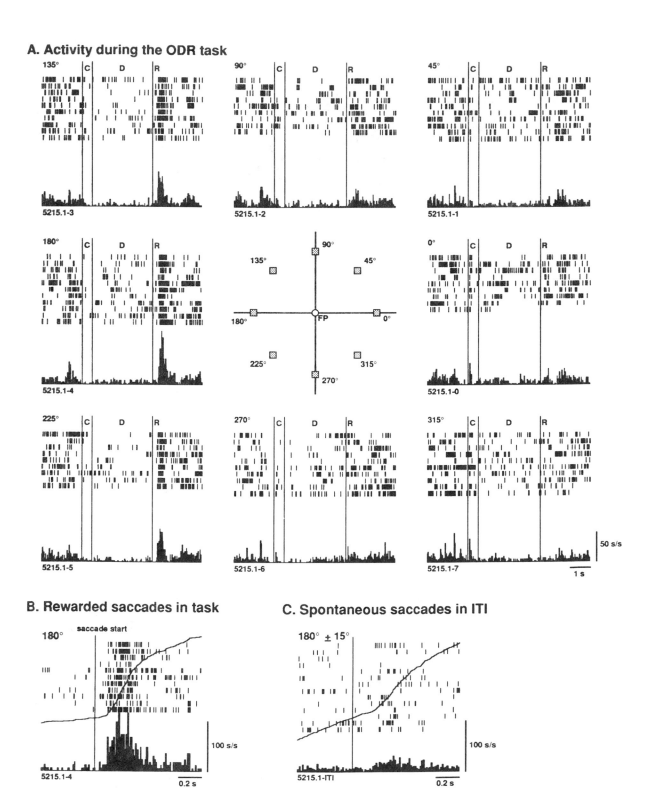

A. Activity during the ODR task

Figure 8. (*A*) Directional postsaccadic activation of a PS neuron during the oculomotor task. This neuron exhibited a strong phasic postsaccadic response when the monkey made saccades to the left visual field (135°, 180°, and 225°) but was not responsive in any other direction examined. (*B*) Oculomotor activity aligned at the initiation of saccades in the response period of the 180° trials. The latency of the oculomotor response was 110 msec. (*C*) Much reduced activity in conjunction with spontaneous saccades made during intertrial interval having the same direction (180° ± 15°) as those in *B*. (Reprinted, with permission, from Funahashi et al. 1991.)

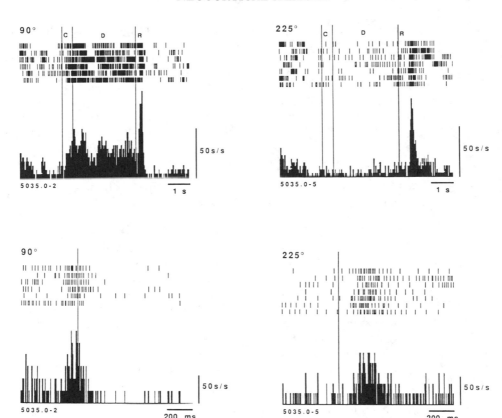

Figure 9. The neuron displayed showed directional delay-period excitatory activity for the 90° location (*top left*), but was inhibited during the delay for the opposite 225° location (*top right*). The neuron activity aligned at the initiation of the saccade reveals that the same neuron has a phasic discharge before the saccade at the 90° location (*lower left*) and a phasic response after the saccade is initiated for the opponent direction (*lower right*). Note that excitatory activity is associated with presaccadic activation, and inhibitory activity is associated with postsaccadic responses. (Modified from Funahashi et al. 1989.)

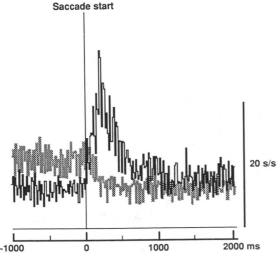

Figure 10. Composite histograms representing best-direction excitatory delay-period activity of 65 neurons (patterned line) and best-direction postsaccadic activity of 42 neurons (solid line). Both histograms are aligned at the initiation of the saccadic response. Note that the start of postsaccadic activation coincides with the termination of delay-period activity. Bin width is 15 msec. (Reprinted, with permission, from Funahashi et al. 1991.)

(Funahashi et al. 1989); also, the activity of prefrontal cells in the delay period expands and contracts as the delay is increased or foreshortened (see also Kojima and Goldman-Rakic 1982; Funahashi et al. 1989), as would be expected of a mnemonic process. Finally, a memory interpretation of prefrontal function is supported by recent studies of prefrontal neuronal responses in an antisaccade task. In this task, the monkey is required to direct his responses at the end of the delay to the location *opposite* that in which the cue was presented. Under this condition, the direction of the cue and direction of response are dissociable, and we can compare the activity of a neuron to the same set of targets in both conventional and antisaccade trials. Indeed, two-thirds of the prefrontal neurons that increased their discharge for a particular direction of target in the conventional paradigm also discharged for the same target direction in the antisaccade task, even though the eye movements were made to the opposite direction (Funahashi and Goldman-Rakic 1990). Thus, a substantial fraction of prefrontal neurons code the direction of the stimulus (rather than the response), in support of the idea that a subset of prefrontal neurons both carry information in the absence of the external cues that are represented and constitute a mental representation of the spatial coordinates of those cues.

Neuronal Properties and Local Circuits

A challenging issue is to explain the generation of the neuronal activity in prefrontal neurons. The present study provides evidence of both independence and interdependence among functionally related neurons located within the local territory of the caudal PS. As reported above, distinct populations of neurons registered the sensory information at the time it was presented or maintained that information "on-line," and still other neurons responded phasically immediately before or just after the response. In all categories, different neurons coded different target locations, but collectively they represented information from all polar directions within the visual field, although coding of contralateral targets predominated. At the same time, many neurons showed phasic or tonic responses that were time-locked to more than one phase of the delayed-response trial. Still other prefrontal cells registered directional afferent input, directional delay-period activity, *and* pre- and postsaccadic activation (for opposite directions).

A number of findings in the present study suggest that the compound response profiles in many neurons may be constructed from the separate inputs of neurons that register only the cue, the delay, or oculomotor events. For example, the cue-, delay-, or oculomotor-period activities in neurons that had more than one response were indistinguishable in terms of latency and response profile from the same responses in neurons that exhibited only one of these responses. In addition, the finding that excitatory (or inhibitory) delay-period activity expressed in one group of neurons terminated abruptly at the moment of onset of postsaccadic activity in another group of neurons is indicative of communication between these functionally distinct cells.

The extrinsic and intrinsic connections underlying the basic and compound functional properties of prefrontal neurons are under investigation, and the relationship between the circuitry and physiology is merely conjectural at present. We might hypothesize that prefrontal neurons with presaccadic responses lie in layer V, wherein reside the corticotectal, corticostriatal, and some corticocortical neurons that project to eye and/or hand movement centers directly or via premotor relays (for review, see Goldman-Rakic 1987b). The apical dendrites of such a cell passing through layers IV and III would be a primary target of mediodorsal and medial pulvinar thalamic afferents (Giguere and Goldman-Rakic 1988) and, as they reached into layers I and II, the recipient of sensory afferents from the posterior parietal cortex (Cavada and Goldman-Rakic 1989b) and contralateral prefrontal cortex (Goldman-Rakic and Schwartz 1982). In this way, they would receive an input from the striatonigrothalamocortical loop circuitry that is ideally situated to provide feedback information about the status of the motor action

and turn off the delay-period activity initiated by corticocortical afferents carrying visuospatial data from the areas that represent spatial vision.

The finding that tonic excitatory delay-period activity tends to be coupled with phasic presaccadic activity, whereas inhibitory delay-period activity is invariably followed by phasic postsaccadic activity in the opponent direction, provides the interesting possibility that the same neuron that participates in selection and initiation of motor programs in one direction may at the same time suppress inappropriate responses, i.e., responses that are not selected and are not appropriate at the moment. Formerly, it has been common to attribute the impulsive disinhibitory symptoms of frontal lobe patients to damage in orbital areas of the prefrontal cortex (see, e.g., Eslinger and Damasio 1985; Fuster 1989) and cognitive symptoms to dorsolateral prefrontal damage. The presence of both inhibitory and excitatory oculomotor responses in the *same* neuron suggests a cellular basis for the paradoxical positive and negative effects of prefrontal injury. The excitatory presaccadic activation, occurring as early as 192 seconds before the response, firmly supports the idea that prefrontal neurons can issue a motor command and/or influence the direction of movement in a direct and *prospective* manner. On the other hand, the large proportion of postsaccadic responses in neurons with inhibitory delay period activity may have a disinhibitory influence and thus a major role in suppression of unwanted responses. Thus, it is not surprising that the failure to inhibit inappropriate behavior is a cardinal symptom of prefrontal cortical damage (Luria 1973; Milner 1982; Milner et al. 1985; Stuss and Benson 1986). Loss of neuronal populations with opponent oculomotor responses may explain this long-standing puzzle.

Distributed Working Memory Network

Response features that at first seemed characteristic only of prefrontal neurons, such as enhanced activity during the delay period, have now been observed in a number of other structures, including the frontal eye field (Bruce and Goldberg 1985), the posterior parietal cortex (Gnadt and Andersen 1988), the basal ganglia (Hikosaka and Wurtz 1983; Hikosaka et al. 1989), the premotor and motor cortex (Tanji et al. 1980; Tanji and Kurata 1985), and the hippocampus (Watanabe and Niki 1985). Because each of these areas is connected with the dorsolateral prefrontal center whose neurons we have described in the present report (Selemon and Goldman-Rakic 1989; Cavada and Goldman-Rakic 1990a,b), the cooperation of a large number of areas in a function as complex as working memory could have been predicted, and it is possible to speculate on the contribution made by each of the components of this distributed network (see, e.g., Goldman-Rakic 1988). For illustrative purposes, in this last section, we consider how the studies of prefrontal function relate to the role of the hippocampal formation in memory functions of the brain. This issue is particularly challenging, because the two structures have often been considered as serving quite different functions in primates, although they are strongly interconnected (Goldman-Rakic et al. 1984). Our view, based on the limited physiological and behavioral evidence available, is that the hippocampus and prefrontal cortex are in a cooperative relationship with respect to working memory. Lesions of the prefrontal cortex disrupt performance on delayed-response and delayed nonmatching-to-sample tasks when the delays are brief or long (Goldman et al. 1971), but monkeys with hippocampal lesions are impaired on delayed-response tasks when delay periods are longer than about 10 seconds (Zola-Morgan et al. 1989). Congruent with the lesion results, studies in our laboratory have recently shown, in intact monkeys, that metabolic activity in the granule cell layer of the dentate gyrus and the molecular layers of CA1 and CA3 are elevated significantly when monkeys perform the traditional delayed-response task with 12-second delays; similar activation does not occur when they perform other tasks, such as visual pattern discriminations (Friedman and Goldman-Rakic 1988). These data are beginning to indicate that the prefrontal cortex and hippocampal formation are part of a common circuit which share common cognitive domains but subserve different subfunctions in the overall cognitive operation. The prefrontal contribution may be preeminent when information has to be rapidly processed, whereas the hippocampal contribution becomes more important when information needs to be associated

with other data in long-term memory or moved into longer-term stores. This latter process may occur with longer delays that allow time for and perhaps induce mental rehearsal and/or associative processing. It may be relevant that recent studies in monkeys show that the perirhinal cortices, including the parahippocampal gyrus, may be the critical foci for memory loss following medial temporal lesions. These medial temporal cortices are directly connected with the principal sulcus in the prefrontal cortex (Fig. 11) (Goldman-Rakic et al. 1984).

Similar conclusions with respect to cooperativity in the cortical network underlying spatial cognition are emerging in our preliminary analysis of neuronal activity in the posterior parietal cortex of monkeys performing the oculomotor delayed-response task (Chaffee et al. 1989). The parietal cortex is considered the brain's center for spatial vision, and our recordings there show that this region makes an important yet unique contribution to ODR performance (Chaffee et al. 1989). Thus, the regulation of behavior by mental representations requires the collaboration of a large set of cortical and subcortical structures, which together constitute the brain's machinery for spatial cognition, and much work remains before the secrets of this collaborative effort are uncovered. We believe these studies establish a framework for analysis of complex functions carried out by cortical networks.

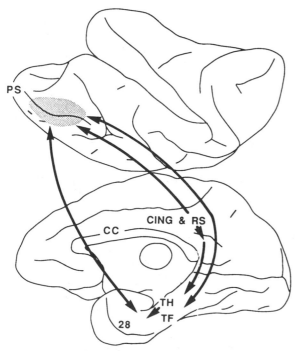

Figure 11. Principal sulcus (PS) connections with the cingulate (CING) and retrosplenal (RS) cortices, parahippocampal gyrus (areas TH and TF), entorhinal cortex (area 28), presubiculum (PSUB), and caudomedial lobule (CML). (Adapted from Goldman-Rakic 1987a.)

REFERENCES

Amaral, D.G., R. Insausti, and W.M. Cowan. 1987. The entorhinal cortex of the monkey. I. Cytoarchitectonic organization. *J. Comp. Neurol.* **264:** 326.

Baddeley, A.D. 1986. *Working memory.* Oxford University Press, London.

Barone, P. and J.-P. Joseph. 1989. Prefrontal cortex and spatial sequencing in macaque monkeys. *Exp. Brain Res.* **78:** 447.

Bruce, C.J. and M.E. Goldberg. 1985. Primate frontal eye fields. I. Single neurons discharging before saccades. *J. Neurophysiol.* **53:** 606.

Cavada, C. and P.S. Goldman-Rakic. 1989a. Posterior parietal cortex in rhesus monkey. I. Parcellation of areas based on distinctive limbic and sensory cortico-cortical connections. *J. Comp. Neurol.* **286:** 393.

———. 1989b. Posterior parietal cortex in rhesus monkey. II. Evidence for networks linking limbic and sensory areas to the frontal lobe. *J. Comp. Neurol.* **286:** 422.

Chafee, M., S. Funahashi, and P.S. Goldman-Rakic. 1989. Unit activity in the primate posterior parietal cortex during an oculomotor delayed response task. *Soc. Neurosci. Abstr.* **15:** 786.

Cohen, N.J. and L.R. Squire. 1980. Preserved learning and retention of pattern analyzing skill in amnesia: Dissociation of knowing how and knowing that. *Science* **210:** 207.

Eslinger, P.J. and A.R. Damasio. 1985. Severe disturbance of higher cognition after bilateral frontal lobe ablation: Patient EVR. *Neurology* **35:** 1731.

Friedman, H.R. and P.S. Goldman-Rakic. 1988. Activation of the hippocampus and dentate gyrus by working-memory: A 2-deoxyglucose study of behaving rhesus monkeys. *J. Neurosci.* **8:** 4693.

Funahashi, S. and P. Goldman-Rakic. 1990. Delay-period activity of pre-frontal neurons in delayed saccade and anti-saccade tasks. *Soc. Neurosci. Abstr.* **16:** 1223.

Funahashi, S., C.J. Bruce, and P.S. Goldman-Rakic. 1989. Mnemonic coding of visual space in the primate dorsolateral prefrontal cortex. *J. Neurophysiol.* **61:** 331.

———. 1990. Visuospatial coding in primate prefrontal neurons revealed by oculomotor paradigms. *J. Neurophysiol.* **63:** 814.

———. 1991. Neuronal activity related to saccadic eye movements in the monkey's dorsolateral prefrontal cortex. *J. Neurophysiol.* (in press).

Fuster, J.M. 1973. Unit activity in prefrontal cortex during delayed-response performance: neuronal correlates of transient memory. *J. Neurophysiol.* **36:** 61.

———. 1985. The prefrontal cortex and temporal integration. In *Cerebral cortex* (ed. E.G. Jones and A. Peters), p. 151. Plenum Press, New York.

———. 1989. *The prefrontal cortex*, 2nd edition, p. 255. Raven Press, New York.

Fuster, J.M., R.H. Bauer, and J.P. Jervey. 1982. Cellular discharge in the dorsolateral prefrontal cortex of the monkey in cognitive tasks. *Exp. Neurol.* **77:** 679.

Giguere, M. and P.S. Goldman-Rakic. 1988. The mediodorsal nucleus: Areal, laminar, and tangential distribution of afferents and efferents in the frontal lobe of rhesus monkey. *J. Comp. Neurol.* **277:** 195.

Gnadt, J.W. and R.A. Andersen. 1988. Memory related motor planning activity in posterior parietal cortex of macaque. *Exp. Brain Res.* **70:** 216.

Goldman, P.S., H.E. Rosvold, V. Vest, and T.W. Galkin. 1971. Analysis of the delayed-alternation deficit produced by dorsolateral prefrontal lesions in the rhesus monkey. *J. Comp. Physiol. Psychol.* **77:** 212.

Goldman-Rakic, P.S. 1987a. Circuitry of primate prefrontal cortex and regulation of behavior by representational memory. In *Handbook of physiology. The nervous system: Higher functions of the brain* (ed. F. Plum), vol. 5, p. 373. American Physiology Association, Bethesda, Maryland.

———. 1987b. Motor control function of the prefrontal cortex. In *Motor areas of the cerebral cortex* (ed. G. Bock et al.), p. 187. Wiley, Chichester, England.

———. 1988. Topography of cognition: Parallel distributed networks in primate association cortex. *Annu. Rev. Neurosci.* **11:** 137.

Goldman-Rakic, P.S. and M. Schwartz. 1982. Interdigitation of contralateral and ipsilateral columnar projections to frontal association cortex in primates. *Science* **216:** 755.

Goldman-Rakic, P.S., L.D. Selemon, and M.L. Schwartz. 1984. Dual pathways connecting the dorsolateral prefrontal cortex with the hippocampal formation and parahippocampal cortex in the rhesus monkey. *Neuroscience* **12:** 719.

Hikosaka, O. and R.H. Wurtz. 1983. Visual oculomotor functions of monkey substantia nigra pars reticulata. III. Memory-contingent visual and saccade responses. *J. Neurophysiol.* **49:** 1268.

Hikosaka, O., M. Sakamoto, and S. Usui. 1989. Functional properties of monkey caudate neurons. III. Activities related to expectation of target and reward. *J. Neurophysiol.* **61:** 814.

Joseph, J.P. and P. Barone. 1987. Prefrontal unit activity during a delayed oculomotor task in the monkey. *Exp. Brain Res.* **67:** 460.

Just, M.A. and P.A. Carpenter. 1985. Cognitive coordinate systems: Accounts of mental rotation and individual differences in spatial ability. *Psychol. Rev.* **92:** 137.

Kesner, R.P. 1985. Correspondence between humans and animals in coding of temporal attributes: Role of hippocampus and prefrontal cortex. *Ann. N.Y. Acad. Sci.* **444:** 122.

Kojima, S. and P.S. Goldman-Rakic. 1982. Delay-related activity of prefrontal cortical neurons in rhesus monkeys performing delayed response. *Brain Res.* **248:** 43.

Kubota, K. and H. Niki. 1971. Prefrontal cortical unit activity and delayed alternation performance in monkeys. *J. Neurophysiol.* **34:** 337.

Kubota, K., M. Tonoike, and A. Mikami. 1980. Neuronal activity in the monkey dorsolateral prefrontal cortex during a discrimination task with delay. *Brain Res.* **183:** 29.

Luria, A.R. 1973. The frontal lobes and the regulation of behavior. In *Psychophysiology of the frontal lobes* (ed. K.H. Pribam and A.R. Luria), p. 3. Academic Press, New York.

Milner, B. 1982. Some cognitive effects of frontal lobe lesions in man. *Philos. Trans. R. Soc. Lond. B Biol. Sci.* **298:** 211.

Milner, B., M. Petrides, and M.L. Smith. 1985. Frontal lobes and the temporal organization of memory. *Hum. Neurobiol.* **4:** 137.

Mishkin, M. 1982. A memory system in the monkey. *Philos. Trans. R. Soc. Lond. B Biol. Sci.* **298:** 85.

Niki, H. 1974a. Prefrontal unit activity during delayed alternation in the monkey. I. Relation to direction of response. *Brain Res.* **68:** 185.

———. 1974b. Prefrontal unit activity during delayed alternation in the monkey. II. Relation to absolute versus relative direction of response. *Brain Res.* **68:** 197.

———. 1974c. Differential activity of prefrontal units during right and left delayed response trials. *Brain Res.* **70:** 346.

Olton, D.S. and B.C. Papas. 1979. Spatial memory and hippocampal function. *Neuropsychologia* **17:** 667.

Quintana, J., J. Yajeya, and J.M. Fuster. 1988. Prefrontal representation of stimulus attributes during delay tasks. I. Unit activity in cross-temporal integration of sensory and sensory-motor information. *Brain Res.* **474:** 211.

Robinson, D.A. 1963. A method of measuring eye movement using a scleral search coil in a magnetic field. *IEEE Trans. Biomed. Elect.* **10:** 137.

Rosenkilde, C.E., R.H. Bauer, and J.M. Fuster. 1981. Single cell activity in ventral prefrontal cortex of behaving monkeys. *Brain Res.* **209:** 275.

Scoville, W.B. and B. Milner. 1957. Loss of recent memory after bilateral hippocampal lesions. *J. Neurol. Neurosurg. Psychiatry* **20:** 11.

Selemon, L.D. and P.S. Goldman-Rakic. 1990. Topographic intermingling of striatonigral and striatopallidal neurons in the rhesus monkey. *J. Comp. Neurol.* **297:** 359.

Stuss, D.T. and D.F. Benson. 1986. *The frontal lobes.* Raven Press, New York.

Suzuki, H. and M. Azuma. 1977. Prefrontal neuronal activity during gazing at a light spot in the monkey. *Brain Res.* **126:** 497.

Tanji, J. and K. Kurata. 1985. Contrasting neuronal activity in supplementary and precentral motor cortex of monkeys. I. Responses to instruction determining motor responses to forthcoming signals of different modalities. *J. Neurophysiol.* **53:** 8.

Tanji, J., K. Tanuguchi, and T. Saga. 1980. Supplementary motor area: Neuronal response to motor instructions. *J. Neurophysiol.* **43:** 60.

Tulving, E. 1972. Episodic and semantic memory. In *Organization of memory*, p. 381. Academic Press, New York.

Warrington, E.K. and L. Weiskrantz. 1982. Amnesia: A disconnection syndrome? *Neuropsychologia* **20:** 233.

Watanabe, T. and H. Niki. 1985. Hippocampal unit activity and delayed response in the monkey. *Brain Res.* **325:** 241.

Yajeya, J., J. Quintana, and J.M. Fuster. 1988. Prefrontal representation of stimulus attributes during delay tasks. II. The role of behavioral significance. *Brain Res.* **474:** 222.

Zola-Morgan, S., L.R. Squire, and D. Amaral. 1989. Lesions of the hippocampal formation but not lesions of the fornix or the mammillary nuclei produce long-lasting memory impairment in monkeys. *J. Neurosci.* **9:** 898.

Neural Regionalization of Knowledge Access: Preliminary Evidence

A.R. Damasio, H. Damasio, D. Tranel, and J.P. Brandt
*Department of Neurology, Division of Behavioral Neurology and Cognitive Neuroscience,
University of Iowa College of Medicine, Iowa City, Iowa 52242*

We have previously noted that some patients with bilateral damage in occipitotemporal cortices fail to recognize visually a large number of natural entities (Damasio et al. 1982, 1990; Damasio, 1990). An example is patient EH-034, who, in addition to not recognizing the unique identity of faces, buildings, animals, and objects, also did not recognize many of those entities as members of a category. Confronted with the picture of a fox or a lion, the patient said it was "an animal," but the specific category eluded her. Shown a robin, she said it was a "bird." She was unable to indicate the approximate size, habitat, or typical behavior of the unrecognized species. As we have pointed out elsewhere, the failure did not cover entire conceptual categories (*all* animals, or *all* living things). For instance, some animals were readily recognized, e.g., elephant and giraffe, suggesting that less prototypical animals with either global or local "outlier" shapes fared better than those which, despite belonging to a distinctive species, had a greater similarity of shapes and thus formed a visually "ambiguous" grouping. In contrast, man-made entities were for the most part readily recognized, e.g., tools and utensils posed no problem. Even among those, however, there were exceptions. For instance, several musical instruments, which are as man-made and manipulable as any garden tool or kitchen utensil, were not recognized through the visual route, beyond their supraordinate assignment as musical instruments. This stood in contrast to their specific and rapid recognition from sound.

Work from other laboratories has revealed virtually identical findings in patients whom we presume to have damage in comparable neural systems (Warrington and Shallice 1984; Warrington and McCarthy 1987; Young et al. 1989), but the interpretation of those findings has not been identical. For instance, Warrington has suggested that the evidence favors the existence of systems dedicated to conceptual categories (e.g., living/nonliving and animate/inanimate), which would be duplicated for each sensory modality. As noted below, we account for the findings in a different way (even if our explanations coincide in the importance accorded to the sensory characteristics of entities).

To us, the data available so far have suggested that the process of evoking the concept behind an entity is based on different neural systems, depending on the nature of each entity and the history of learning and interaction relative to that entity (Damasio 1990).

Damage within a given neural system impairs access to the concepts behind some entities, but leaves intact access to concepts for other entities. In patients with damage to the same system, the breakdown line between entities whose recognition is impaired or intact does *not* appear to respect the boundary of intuitive conceptual categories. Instead, impaired and intact entities appear to be grouped according to a variety of factors on the basis of which several subcategories can be formed, e.g., a combination of similar shapes and operations. On occasion, those subcategories overlap with traditional conceptual categories, but they are not necessarily coextensive.

Elsewhere, we have proposed a number of factors leading to such subcategorization and, in turn, to the differential neural mapping of various entities (Damasio 1989a,b,c, 1990). They include (1) physical structure (local and global shapes, configuration, color, texture); (2) operation (range of interactions, motion, displacement, outcome of interactions); (3) sensory modality engaged in perceiver and involvement required of perceiver; and (4) frequency in the environment and value to perceiver. In addition, we have noted that the size of the class formed by entities sharing similar physical structures is a probable factor in the learning and retrieval of knowledge related to them, e.g., for most individuals, the size of the class formed by animals with variants of the wolf shape is larger than that formed by elephant-like animals. (Sharing of physical structures determines what we have termed ambiguity [Damasio et al. 1982]. As will be discussed below, ambiguity per se may well account for some of the variance in recognition performance and must be distinguished from conflated and virtually meaningless factors such as "difficulty" or "complexity.") We believe that the weighted combination of some of these factors determines the system or systems in which a given entity is mapped. In individuals who have suffered focal damage to one of those neural systems, the differential mapping probably determines the ease of access to pertinent knowledge under constrained stimulus presentation (e.g., strictly visual presentation without concomitant somatosensory or auditory input).

The evidence discussed above has not specified in anatomical detail the systems underlying knowledge of different kinds or their access devices. From our early observations in patients EH-034 and Boswell, it appeared that bilateral damage to the occipitotemporal region was necessary for defects in visual recognition to appear, but the possibility remained open that unilateral damage to the left or right components of this broad region might cause the defect. Furthermore, the sector of occipitotemporal cortices responsible for the defect remained uncharacterized. For instance, might damage in anterior temporal structures alone cause the defect? Also not addressed was the relationship between concepts and names denoting those concepts. When patients fail to recognize an entity, i.e., access the concept, they also fail to name, i.e., retrieve the specific lexical item. But the converse is not true: Failure to *name* does not predict failure to *know*. Are the systems that permit lexical access, then, separable from those that permit concept access?

The study described below provides preliminary evidence on the neural correlates of these defects using visual recognition and visual naming tasks for which control data had been obtained in non-brain-damaged individuals of different ages, gender, and education. It was aimed at exploring the following hypotheses.

1. The neural systems that support conceptual nonverbal knowledge for nonunique entities and the access devices for this knowledge are separate from the neural systems that support verbal lexical knowledge and its access. It is postulated that the former systems are based on bilateral occipitotemporal and parietal cortices, whereas the latter are based on left temporal cortices.
2. The neural systems that support knowledge of entities learned and transacted predominantly by the visual modality are separate from the neural systems that support knowledge about entities learned and transacted through the visual *and* somatosensory modalities.
3. In general, the physical structure of entities determines further segregation in the systems that support knowledge and its access. For instance, the local and global physical structure of an entity, and the size of a class of entities formed on the basis of physical structure, determine the system, or the level within a system, at which recognition can occur. Specifically, entities with prototypical global shapes and lacking atypical local features require a different neural system from that required by entities with aprototypical global shapes and/or aprototypical local features.

METHODS

Experimental tasks. The experimental tasks called for subjects to recognize or to name, as members of a conceptual category, entities that were presented visually. The distinction between recognition and naming is important and should be clearly understood. In our task, naming calls for the assignment of a specific verbal tag to a particular entity, and the level of specificity corresponds to what Rosch et al. (1976) define as the "basic object level." A response is scored as correct only when the specific name is offered. Thus, a squirrel must be named as "squirrel," and not as "animal."

Accurate naming indicates normal recognition, i.e., when a subject names a particular entity correctly at basic object level, it can be assumed that the subject also recognizes the entity. The reverse is not true. When a subject fails to name an entity, the subject may nevertheless know the entity and thus be able to recognize it. Evidence for the evocation of the appropriate concept (even when the name is missing), at basic object level, can be obtained from (1) unequivocal definition of the concept, which the subject may offer spontaneously or produce in response to the prompt, "Tell me what this is"; or (2) satisfactory responses upon probing systematically for defining traits of the entity, e.g., color, texture, size, operation, function, and habitat. In both cases, the subject's responses are audiotaped and transcribed, and the scoring is made against the definition of the entity available in Webster's dictionary. An accurate response is that which can evoke the appropriate concept in an independent observer who is not seeing the stimulus.

Stimuli. The visual stimuli were developed by combining the 260 line drawings from Snodgrass and Vanderwart (1980) with 300 photographs of actual objects. This set was then pruned to eliminate excessive redundancy and pictures that featured items in highly noncanonical positions, and further culled to accomplish the objectives of (1) including stimuli that would also be amenable to presentation in auditory and tactile formats and (2) covering a broad range of variation along several key stimulus dimensions, which were enumerated above as important factors in object recognition and naming. The battery was constructed so as to probe the conceptual-lexical "categories" of animals, fruits/vegetables, tools, utensils, musical instruments, vehicles, body parts, clothing, personal effects, furniture, and buildings. The first four of these were given special emphasis, and a large number of items were maintained in each of these categories (specific numbers ranged between 15 and 60).

The final visual battery comprised 320 stimuli. The stimuli were prepared as black and white slides, and on each slide, all background material was masked, so that the target item was featured exclusively. The slides depicted stimuli in singular (e.g., horse), except in cases where plural presentation is more canonical (e.g., grapes).

Standardization studies: Procedure and data quantification. The visual stimuli were administered to two groups of normal control subjects:

Elderly controls. Twenty-four older persons (mean age, 69) completed the battery. The group included 14 women and 10 men, with educational backgrounds that varied from 8 to 16 years. These subjects are part of a normal elderly group in our community that has participated in a variety of neuropsychological norming studies. The subjects have all been screened for cognitive defects and positive neurological history, and their participation was voluntary. The subjects were tested in small groups (~3–5 per group). The stimuli were shown on a white screen, one at a time, and the subjects were required to write the name of each item on a response sheet. Subjects were instructed that if they could not remember the specific name for an item but recognized what the object was, they should write down information that would indicate such knowledge, e.g., the function or operation, or distinguishing features. Strict time limits were not enforced, but in general, most stimuli were presented for about 10 seconds, and response latencies rarely exceeded 20 seconds.

For each subject and for each conceptual-lexical category, two scores were calculated: (1) *Naming*: This refers to the number of items for which the correct name was produced; (2) *Recognition*: Items for which the subject produced correct and unequivocal descriptors (e.g., "This animal is black with a white stripe, and makes a terrible odor if you get too close" [skunk]), but not the name, were scored as correct recognitions. These were added to the naming score (as pointed out above, items correctly named are assumed to be correctly recognized) to obtain a recognition score. Recognition responses were rated by two raters and were scored correct only when the raters agreed that the response was unequivocal. The naming and recognition scores were divided by the number of items in each category and multiplied by 100, so that final scores were expressed in terms of percent correct.

Young controls. This was a group of 7 normal young adults (4 women, 3 men; mean age, 23.3). Subjects were recruited via ads in local news bulletins, screened for positive neurologic history and learning disability, and paid for their participation. Individual testing sessions were conducted. For each subject, the visual stimuli were presented one stimulus at a time on the internal screen of a Caramate 4000 slide projector. Subjects were asked to name the item pictured. If the name was not produced, or if the response was overly general or nonspecific (e.g., "animal"), the subject was prompted to provide additional information regarding particulars of the object, such as its function, operation, or identifying features. Responses were audiotaped. Typewritten transcriptions of the response protocols were used to score the young controls' performances, using the same procedure as described above for the elderly controls.

Selection of target subjects. The experimental "target" subjects for these experiments were drawn from our registry of patients with focal lesions of the telencephalon. The choice of subjects was dictated by our stated hypotheses and performed by an investigator who was not involved in the administration or scoring of the experimental tasks, according to the following procedure.

Preliminary evidence available from our laboratory indicated that damage to frontal association cortices and to superior occipitoparietal cortices does not compromise performance in the experimental tasks. Accordingly, subjects with damage in a variety of fields of temporal, inferior occipital, and lower parietal cortices were selected. In the current study, we included subjects with either bilateral ($n = 4$), left-sided ($n = 11$), or right-sided ($n = 8$) damage in these structures.

The anatomical localization of damage to neural systems was performed with a standard method (Damasio and Damasio 1989), based on magnetic resonance images. One purpose of the analysis was to determine whether inferotemporal cortex (IT) formed by fields 20, 21, and 37 was involved, unilaterally or bilaterally, entirely or partially. (The human IT is formed by fields 20, 21, and 37, as outlined in Figure 1. The lateral limit is the superior temporal sulcus; the mesial limit is the collateral sulcus; the anterior border is area 38; and the posterior border is area 19.) We also wanted to determine the presence or absence of damage in areas surrounding IT, e.g., anteriormost temporal (area 38), superior temporal (area 22), and "early" visual association cortices (areas 18, 19).

Procedure. Target subjects were administered the visual tasks as part of a comprehensive neuropsychological evaluation conducted in connection with their voluntary participation in our program project. Subjects were tested individually, and the tasks were administered by an investigator blind to the neuroanatomical and general neuropsychological status of the subject. Testing sessions were audiotaped, and typewritten transcriptions of these audiotapes were used to score the protocols. The stimuli were administered one at a time on the internal screen of a Caramate 4000 slide projector, in free field. The subject was

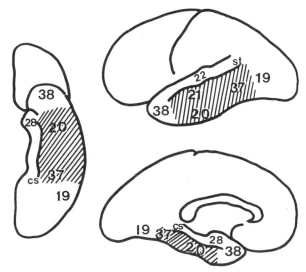

Figure 1. The human inferotemporal region (IT) is constituted by the Brodmann fields 21, 20, and 37. The superior temporal sulcus (ST) and the collateral sulcus (CS) are the natural boundaries, laterally and mesially. The anterior and posterior boundaries are defined by cytoarchitectonic fields 38 and 19, respectively. Note that area 37 is far larger in the human than in the monkey, where it probably corresponds to TF.

simply asked to tell the investigator what each stimulus was. If naming did not occur, or was too general, or if an incorrect name was offered, a standard semi-structured questioning procedure followed to probe the subject's *recognition* of the stimulus. The questioning procedure explored progressively more detailed and specific levels of knowledge: e.g., "Is this an animal?"; "What is the body covering like?" Size, color, weight, and typical actions, habitats, and functions were also explored. The objective of this questioning was to establish as comprehensively as possible whether or not the subject recognized the stimulus. The procedure was standard but flexible, so that each follow-up question was determined in part by the quality and detail of information provided to the previous question. The subject was not under a time limit, and stimuli were displayed on the screen for the duration of the questioning process.

Data quantification. For the visual tasks, two outcomes from the control subjects were important influences on the eventual data quantification format for the experimental subjects. First, the controls showed extremely little difference between naming and recognition. Since the naming score was always the same or slightly lower than the recognition score, we chose to be conservative and to utilize the control naming score as the control standard for each stimulus category. Second, scores in most categories were quite high for both young and elderly controls and showed little variation. In fact, in all categories except musical instruments, control scores were well over the 90% level, and standard deviations were in the range of only 2–5 percentage points. With these outcomes in mind, we utilized the following procedure to formulate a control score for each category: The average performances of the young controls and of the elderly controls were added together and divided by 2. Thus, for each category, the control score was the average of the average elderly score and the average young score.

For each subject, the naming and recognition performances were quantified as follows: (1) *Naming*: The subject's percent correct naming score in each category was subtracted from the control score for that category. (2) *Recognition*: The subject's percent correct recognition score in each category was subtracted from the control score for that category. These difference scores were graphed for separate categories. On the graphs, the ordinate ranges from −20 to +80 and is expressed in units of percentage points. The zero-line denotes the level at which the performance of the subject matches the control score, i.e., the subject is performing at the same level as control subjects. Positive values indicate increasing levels of deficiency on the part of the subject, whereas negative values indicate that the subject actually performed above the control average.

RESULTS

The main results are presented in Figures 2–7. The figures contain the difference scores for each target subject reported here, on two distinctive categories of stimuli: animals and tools/utensils. These two categories were chosen to illustrate the results because (1) the former includes entities that were learned through the visual modality alone and that do not generally engage the perceiver through any other modality; in particular, the entities are not manipulable; and (2) the latter category is learned and regularly transacted through both the visual *and* somatosensory modalities, i.e., the entities are all manipulable. (The figures do not describe the performances in other categories, which were nonetheless available for comparative qualitative and quantitative analyses. Those analyses are not reported in this paper.) The figures also contain the summary of the neuroanatomical analysis for each target subject. The findings can be summarized as follows:

1. Patients with bilateral (Fig. 2) or unilateral (Fig. 3) damage involving the inferotemporal region (areas 20, 21, and 37) had defects in the recognition of animals but not tools/utensils. The defect was most severe in the bilateral cases and less so in the left unilateral cases. In all the affected individuals, the

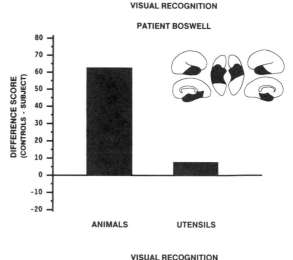

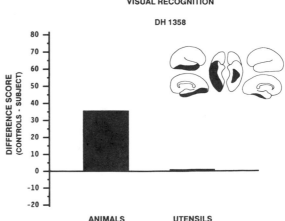

Figure 2. Severe defect for the recognition of animals, and normal performance in the tools group, in patients with bilateral damage involving IT.

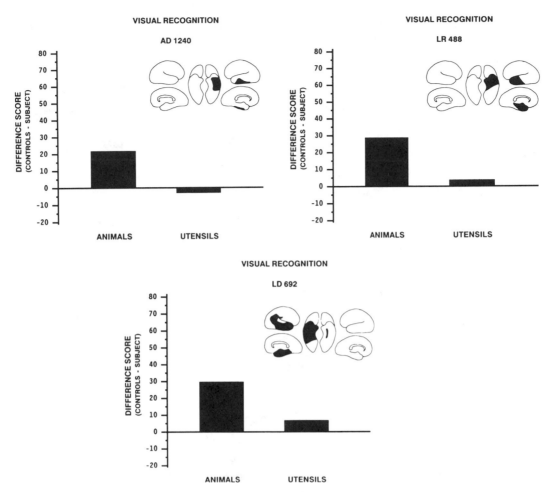

Figure 3. Unilateral damage involving IT in either left (AD1240 and LR488) or right (LD692) hemisphere. The dissociation is the same noted in the bilateral cases, but the magnitude of the defect is smaller.

defects were not subtle, since the subjects performed several standard deviations below the normal controls.

2. A patient with bilateral damage involving the hippocampus alone did not have any recognition defect (Fig. 4).

3. Patients with unilateral damage in the left (Fig. 5) or right (Fig. 6) hemisphere performed normally in the recognition task, provided the inferotemporal region was spared. Specifically, involvement of the anterior or superior sectors of each temporal lobe did not affect performance on the task.

4. Involvement in the *left* (but not right) anterior temporal region affected naming of entities, but not recognition, i.e., the former performance was impaired, but the latter was intact (Fig. 7).

In every individual, the defect did not cover *all* entities in the animal group, just as it did not spare *all* entities in the tool/utensil group. In short, the defect did not respect the boundaries of broad conceptual categories, e.g., natural/manmade, animate/inanimate, and living/nonliving, nor did it observe the boundary of traditional taxonomies. A preliminary qualitative analysis of errors in these data (not reported

here) supports the hypothesis that prototypicality of global and local shapes (or lack thereof) is a significant factor in the failure or success of recognition for each item. This finding is strengthened further by analysis of stimuli for other categories in which other prototypical,

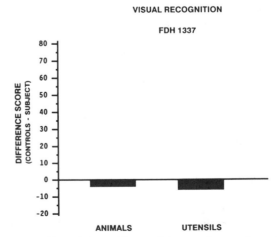

Figure 4. Normal recognition performance in a patient with bilateral damage to the hippocampal system due to an anoxic/ischemic episode, resulting in severe anterograde amnesia.

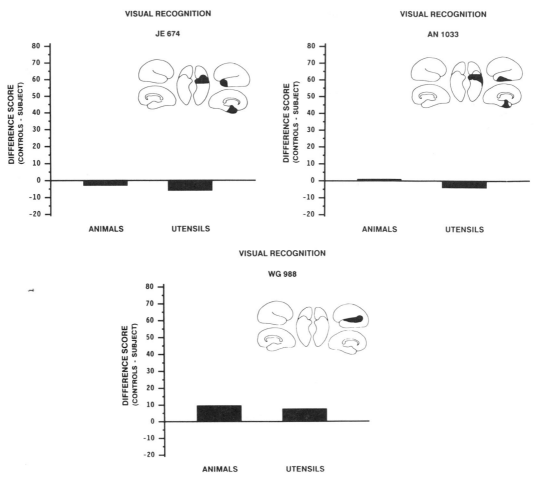

Figure 5. Unilateral damage to left temporal cortices sparing IT does not affect recognition in our tasks.

visually ambiguous entities are also recognized defectively.

In short, the evidence supports the first two hypotheses (that the systems that support conceptual nonverbal knowledge and those that support verbal tags are separate; that the systems that support knowledge for "visual" entities are separate from those that support "visual/somatosensory" entities). The evidence also offers preliminary support for the hypothesis that the physical structure of entities helps to determine the systems in which their representations are inscribed.

COMMENT

The first conclusion from this study is that when selective damage impairs visual recognition, it does not do so uniformly for all kinds of stimuli. Only certain kinds are sensitive, a strong suggestion that the mapping of knowledge about the world may be constrained by the nature of the stimuli, the biological properties of the system, and the interaction between stimuli and perceiver. The data indicate that the visual recognition of certain entities is resistant to virtually all combinations of damage beyond the extrastriate visual region contained in the human cortices of areas 18 and 19. The

characteristics of the "protected" entities include (1) having been learned and predominantly transacted through *both* visual and somatosensory modalities (most such entities happen to be manmade, manipulable, and have a clearly assigned operation/function) or (2) having outlier local or global shapes, regardless of having been learned and transacted exclusively through the visual channel (such entities may be either natural or manmade). In contrast, some entities are sensitive to damage in selected sectors of the higher-order cortices. They are characterized by (1) having been learned and predominantly transacted through the visual modality and (2) having a marked sharing of physical structure with entities that belong to other subcategories, i.e., belonging to a sizable group of visually ambiguous entities. Most entities, although not all, with such characteristics are natural, and animals from certain species are the most frequent examples. We will refer to them as "visual-ambiguous."

The recognition defect for the visual-ambiguous kinds is related to specific neural systems. The data indicate the following:

1. Bilateral damage to human inferotemporal region (IT) leads to a marked defect in the recognition of

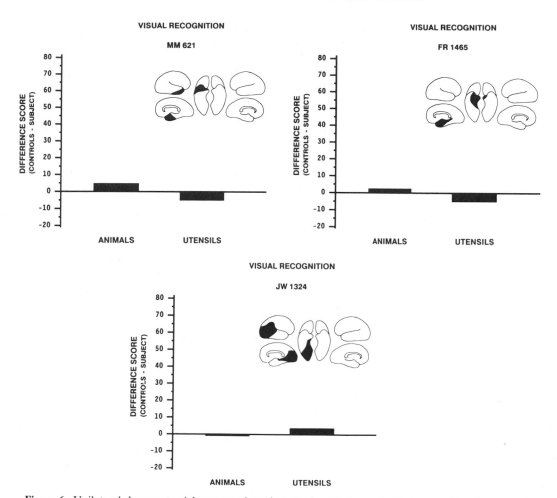

Figure 6. Unilateral damage to right temporal cortices sparing IT does not affect recognition in our tasks.

visual-ambiguous entities; unilateral damage to the same region in the right hemisphere causes the same defect, qualitatively, but to a lesser degree; unilateral damage to the left also causes the defect but the magnitude is even smaller.

2. Damage to superior temporal gyrus (area 22) has no effect on performance of these tasks.

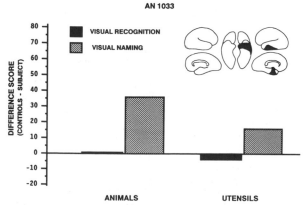

Figure 7. Damage to the anterior sector of the left IT severely compromises access to the names of entities, but leaves their recognition intact, as noted in Fig. 5.

3. Damage to hippocampus, even when it is bilateral, has no effect on the performance of these tasks.
4. Damage to left or right anteriormost temporal cortex (area 38) does not affect visual recognition.
5. Damage to virtually all right hemisphere visual areas other than IT fails to alter performance of these tasks; a comparable statement is not yet possible for the equivalent left hemisphere areas.

The current study leaves numerous questions unanswered. For instance, we have some evidence that nonambiguous, nonexclusively visual entities can be resolved in early visual association cortices in the left hemisphere alone, but further evidence is necessary to verify this impression. Should this impression prove to be true, we will need to determine whether the system that resolves such entities is parallel to the one that preferentially processes visual-ambiguous entities or is, instead, part of a sequential progression of processing from V1 toward IT cortices. Yet another unanswered question relates to the different role that each IT cortex is likely to play and to the cooperation between them in the normal recognition process.

The second conclusion from this study is that the neural systems based on the human IT cortices play a critical role in the retrieval of knowledge necessary to recognize visual-ambiguous entities but do not appear necessary to retrieve knowledge for visual nonambiguous entities. Our interpretation is that these systems permit the linkage between the record for an ambiguous visual shape and information that pertains uniquely to that shape and is based on other neural systems. Drawing on our model of neural architecture for cognition proposed elsewhere (Damasio 1989a,b), we believe that the record of an entity exists as an abstract set of parameters that defined the object as it was seen in the past, rather than as a permanently stored "image" or "template." That set of parameters can be used to visualize the object (as an internal representation in the perceiver's "mind's eye"), something that we believe can be achieved by synchronous feedback activation of earlier visual cortices (see model cited above). However, it should be clear that an internal revisualization of the object is *not* necessary for recognition. Recognition occurs when records are activated in IT systems by the renewed percept of the object. Those records exist in convergence zones that can activate, in turn, neurally distributed records that pertain uniquely to the entity and define, as a set, the concept of its category (Damasio 1989c). In short, IT contains records of parameters that define how things were seen, rather than iconic representations of percepts. The IT records serve two purposes: (1) They can be a conduit to the activation of other records, not necessarily visual, or (2) they can be operated in reverse to produce a degraded image of the entity in recall. It should be clear from this statement that we see IT as part of a memory system, rather than as part of a perceptual system, despite the obvious fact that IT utilizes perceptual data.

Finally, damage to only the anterior half of the left IT sector causes a marked defect in the access to names of entities but leaves intact the recognition of those entities. The anatomical correlates of the name retrieval defect can be circumscribed further, because damage to the anteriormost sector of the temporal region (area 38) on the left is accompanied by a defect in the retrieval of proper names (proper nouns), but leaves intact the access to names of entities at categorical level (common nouns); similar damage on the right appears to have no discernible effect on any of these tasks.

The third conclusion, then, is that access to names depends on a part of the anterior sector of the left IT region. Additional data not reported here suggest that this sector can be subdivided further. The more posterior and lateral aspect is probably related to access of names that denote nonambiguous entities; the more anterior sector is related to visual-ambiguous entities.

The evidence does not support the notion that there are systems solely dedicated to the knowledge of conceptual categories and, in particular, that there are systems linked to natural and living things versus manmade and inanimate things. The differences in the recognition of natural versus man-made entities can be accounted for by a combination of factors, including (1) physical structure, (2) sensorimotor route of learn-

ing and prevailing interaction with the perceiver, and (3) frequency of encounter (familiarity) and value to perceiver. Factor 1 can be decomposed into many other subfactors and largely conditions factor 2.

In the perspective of the "where" and "what" visual processing streams proposed by Ungerleider and Mishkin (1982) based on work in the monkey, our findings suggest that the "what" stream is not a single system or pathway. Rather, it can be subdivided in relation to the kind of entities it processes. Furthermore, the subsystems may well be asymmetric. The right IT may be critically involved in recording minimal differences among global configurations, whereas the left may be specialized for recording differences among local components of entities, as well as relationships among such components. The systems that feed into IT, and which, on the face of current evidence, appear capable of resolving the recognition of the tool/utensil type of stimulus, may also be asymmetric and biased toward the left.

Finally, the findings on lexical retrieval suggest that the left anterior temporal cortices contain a large number of functional regions that are language-related. This is especially important to note because the typical aphasia-producing lesions do not involve this region, and the lesion work on language had not established these cortices as part of a language network. The exceptions to this can be found in other preliminary reports from our laboratory (Tranel et al. 1988; Graff-Radford et al. 1990). In addition, our findings are in full agreement with the data reported by Ojemann and Creutzfeldt (1987) regarding electrical stimulation of left anterolateral temporal regions in humans undergoing surgery for treatment of seizures.

ACKNOWLEDGMENT

This work was supported by the National Institute for Neurological Diseases and Stroke Program Project grant NS-19632.

REFERENCES

Damasio, A.R. 1989a. The brain binds entities and events by multiregional activation from convergence zones. *Neural Computat.* **1:** 123.

———. 1989b. Time-locked multiregional retroactivation: A systems-level proposal for the neural substrates of recall and recognition. *Cognition* **33:** 25.

———. 1989c. Concepts in the brain. *Mind Lang.* **4:** 24.

———. 1990. Category-related recognition defects as a clue to the neural substrates of knowledge. *Trends Neurosci.* **13:** 95.

Damasio, A.R., H. Damasio, and D. Tranel. 1990. Impairments of visual recognition as clues to the processes of memory. In *Signal and sense: Local and global order in perceptual maps* (ed. G.M. Edelman et al.). Wiley-Liss, New York. (In press.)

Damasio, A.R., H. Damasio, and G.W. Van Hoesen. 1982. Prosopagnosia: Anatomic basis and behavioral mechanisms. *Neurology* **32:** 331.

Damasio, H. and A.R. Damasio. 1989. *Lesion analysis in neuropsychology.* Oxford University Press, New York.

Graff-Radford, N.R., A.R. Damasio, B.T. Hyman, M.N. Hart, D. Tranel, H. Damasio, G.W. Van Hoesen, and K. Resai. 1990. Progressive aphasia in a patient with Pick's disease: A neuropsychological, radiologic, and anatomic study. *Neurology* **40:** 620.

Ojemann, G.A. and O.D. Creutzfeldt. 1987. Language in humans and animals: Contribution of brain stimulation and recording. In *The nervous system: Higher functions of the brain* (ed. V.B. Mountcastle et al.), sect. 1, part 2. *Handb. Physiol.* **5:** 675.

Rosch, E., C.B. Mervis, W.D. Gray, D.M. Johnson, and P. Boyes-Braem. 1976. Basic objects in natural categories. *Cognit. Psychol.* **8:** 382.

Snodgrass, J.G. and M. Vanderwart. 1980. A standardized set of 260 pictures: Norms for name agreement, image agreement, familiarity, and visual complexity. *J. Exp. Psychol. Hum. Learn. Mem.* **6:** 174.

Tranel, D., H. Damasio, and A.R. Damasio. 1988. Dissociated verbal and nonverbal retrieval and learning following left anterotemporal damage. *Neurology* (suppl. 1) **38:** 322.

Ungerleider, L.G. and M. Mishkin. 1982. Two cortical visual systems. In *The analysis of visual behavior* (ed. D.J. Ingle et al.), p. 549. MIT Press, Cambridge, Massachusetts.

Warrington, E.K. and R.A. McCarthy. 1987. Categories of knowledge: Further fractionations and an attempted integration. *Brain* **110:** 1273.

Warrington, E.K. and T. Shallice. 1984. Category specific semantic impairments. *Brain* **107:** 829.

Young, A.W., F. Newcombe, D. Hellawell, and E. de Haan. 1989. Implicit access to semantic information. *Brain Cognit.* **11:** 186.

Summary: The Brain in 1990

M.P. STRYKER

Department of Physiology and Neuroscience Graduate Program,
University of California, San Francisco, California 94143-0444

The decreasing intervals between Cold Spring Harbor Symposia on neurobiology (The Neuron, 1952; Sensory Receptors, 1965; The Synapse, 1975; Molecular Neurobiology, 1983) provide an indication not only of the increasing rate of progress in neuroscience, but also of the increasingly wide appreciation of the unity of biology. Neuroscientists no longer immerse themselves in arcana impenetrable to anyone without a medical degree and a fondness for the history of psychology, psychiatry, and the neurological sciences, and few biologists outside neuroscience continue to dismiss it as too complex to merit productive thought. Many of the talks presented at the Symposium were the fruit of a productive interaction between neuroscience and the rest of biology.

"The Brain" is the most comprehensive and ambitious of the Cold Spring Harbor Symposium neuroscience topics. To what extent is the ambition evident in this title justified? Is biology ready to take on the brain? Although even philosophical difficulties remain in the study of the mind, these difficulties have not prevented the study of the mind's organ, the brain, and its component machinery. Even aspects of brain structure and function subserving consciousness, awareness, and the will are now receiving serious, if still speculative, attention, and new experimental approaches are appearing to address these most difficult questions. As one example, the link between perceptions and the activities of specific neurons in the brain has become very strong in the past several years.

Pervasive themes of the Symposium were (1) the dramatic demonstrations of the unity of biology at the molecular and cellular levels, and the rapid progress on the brain made possible as a result of discoveries in other species and other nonneural cells; (2) the overall progress of neuroscience from an abstract and more general level to the concrete and fundamental, so that we can now deal productively with neurons and neural circuits directly at the level at which they operate; (3) the newly serious manner in which we can discuss neural networks in both models and brains that are capable of organizing themselves and learning to do interesting things, such as memory and discrimination; (4) the increasing appreciation of a new cognitive science as an essential element in the understanding of the brain, both in animals and in humans; and (5) the enormous range of technological advances, from patch-clamping to PCR to PET, that have put us in a position to address the concrete questions that we can now pose about the brain.

NEW TOOLS

What are some of the tools and techniques that have allowed neurobiology to flourish so recently? At a molecular level, a variety of techniques have made it possible, and in many cases almost routine, to identify genes of interest, clone them, and make good guesses as to their function and mechanism of action. In *Drosophila*, for example, P-element mutagenesis and the polymerase chain reaction (PCR) make it possible to go from a mutant fly today to the sequence of the gene next week, if not tomorrow. Cloning of biophysically important molecules in mammalian neurons such as channels and receptors can now be done on the basis of the expression of the biophysical properties of interest in *Xenopus* oocytes (Hollmann et al.). When the genes are sequenced, computer data bases allow rapid searches for homologies that in many cases suggest common mechanisms of action in cells of widely different lineage and function (Edelman and Cunningham; Vaessin et al.). A variety of other molecular genetic technologies allow one to test hypotheses about structure-function relationships by making specific mutations and inserting the transgenes into cells or animals that will express them.

Neurophysiology has been revolutionized through the use of tight-seal patch electrodes (Sakmann and Neher 1983), which can be used in a variety of modes either to record single-channel currents or to establish a low-noise, low-resistance pathway into isolated neurons. Patch electrodes have now been applied to neurons in mammalian brain slices, allowing the clear resolution of miniature synaptic potentials in functional neuronal circuits (Busch and Sakmann). Advances in neurophysiology have been synergistic with those in the molecular biology of neurons, as illustrated, for example, in the studies of the GABA receptor (Seeburg et al.).

Neuroanatomy as well has profited from the molecular revolution, in large part through the more or less routine use of molecular probes on sections of neural tissue (Jones et al.). The neuroanatomy of early development in particular has also been revolutionized through the use of new postmortem dyes like DiI that can allow one to trace neuronal connections in fixed tissue (Shatz et al.; O'Leary et al.).

New imaging techniques have had impacts at many levels, from the monitoring of intracellular ion concentrations (Tsien 1989) to the display of the functional architecture of primate cortex (Grinvald et al. 1988) to the mapping of functional areas involved in particular tasks in human cortex (Raichle). Advances in the theory and practice of neural networks, together with the widespread availability of fast computers, have made it feasible to use network models as a way of posing and exploring hypotheses (Lehky et al.). Computers are now routinely used for behavioral and stimulus control and for the recording of neuronal responses (Newsome et al.).

MOLECULAR MECHANISMS OF NEURAL SIGNALING

Ion Channels and Receptors

Fifteen years ago, at the time of "The Synapse" Symposium, the nicotinic acetylcholine receptor molecule had been isolated by virtue of its binding to certain snake toxins and partially characterized. By the time of the "Molecular Neurobiology" Symposium 7 years ago, this receptor had been cloned by several groups, but we still knew little about the structures of the sodium, potassium, and calcium channels or about the receptors and associated channels for the most common neurotransmitters in the brain: glutamate for excitation and GABA for inhibition. Thus, most of the important players in our picture of the neuron, the transmembrane molecules responsible for its electrical, signaling, and integrative behavior, were, if not anonymous, known only through their electrical and pharmacological properties. It remained an article of faith that "the X channel," drawn as a variable resistor on one's picture of the neuron after electrical and pharmacological characterization, was a single molecule.

This situation has now changed completely. The sodium channel has been cloned (for review, see Numa and Noda 1986), along with the potassium channel (Isacoff et al.), a calcium channel (which appears also to function as the voltage sensor for excitation-contraction coupling in skeletal muscle; Numa et al.), the serotonin receptor (Julius et al. 1988), the $GABA_A$ receptor and channel (Seeburg et al.), and at least some of the glutamate receptors and channels (Hollmann et al.). The molecular clones have permitted structure-function analyses that in many cases point clearly toward parts of these molecules responsible for different features of their physiological functions, such as ligand binding, voltage gating, or inactivation (Aldrich et al.; Isacoff et al.; Numa et al.).

For the student of the brain, what has emerged to date from these studies is both appealing in its general unity and simplicity and appalling in its diversity. The appealing simplicity is that the ion channels and neurotransmitter receptors appear generally to fall into one of three types. The voltage-gated potassium and type-L calcium channels bear many similarities of overall structure to the sodium channel that was the first of these to be cloned and sequenced, and they all can be thought of as an extended family homologous to this voltage-gated sodium channel. The ligand-gated ion channels, such as $GABA_A$ and glutamate receptors, have structural similarities to the nicotinic acetylcholine receptor, and the whole group of ligand-gated ion channels can be thought of as another extended family. In addition, there is a large class of receptors that are coupled to G proteins, some of which, like the $GABA_B$ or muscarinic acetylcholine receptor, are activated by the same ligand that also gates an ion channel (for discussion, see Schofield et al. 1990). The similarities among the channels of each family that we had understood from physiology and pharmacology thus appear also to be evident in their molecular structures.

The appalling note is that most of these channels are not single molecules; instead, the channels of one type comprise a remarkably diverse set of molecules produced by the mixing and matching of different subunits or functional domains. It thus does not make sense, for example, to speak of a unique rat brain $GABA_A$ receptor (Seeburg et al.) or a *Drosophila* potassium channel (Isacoff et al.), since there are a large number of closely or more distantly related versions of each, even within a single species. The variant channels can differ greatly in their gating and kinetic properties, and we still do not know the full extent of this diversity. In situ hybridization studies indicate that a number, and perhaps all, of these variants are used in the brain (Seeburg et al.; Hollmann et al.). Single neurons may well express a large fraction of this variety. Although one may imagine that channels with different properties are localized to different parts of a cell or that a change in the mix of channels plays an important part in the long-term modulation of neuronal integrative properties, these hypotheses remain speculative for the time being. What is clear is that the richness and heterogeneity of the physiology of ion channels and receptors, even for a single neurotransmitter in a single cell (Hestrin et al.), are matched or perhaps exceeded by a rich molecular diversity.

Such molecular diversity allows, at least in principle, the possibility of a new molecular pharmacology, whose goal would be to generate reagents specifically targeted toward populations of cells or regions of cells that expressed a particular subtype of ion channel or receptor. In addition, we may expect, but do not yet know, that the neurons that can be considered to be a class on morphological, physiological, or other grounds will be similar in their expression of receptor and channel subtypes. This variety of molecules may well allow us to label functional classes of cells in order to study their properties further.

We are left with greater complexity than we might have hoped for or had dreamed of. If these channels are the major players in a neuron, the stadium vendors' refrain, "Get your scorecard; you can't tell the players without a scorecard," will remain in effect for the foreseeable future. On the other hand, the molecular biology does or will give us the scorecard. As the molecular biology of channels and receptors continues to flourish, we may finally get to the bottom of the roster and begin to exploit our new knowledge to intervene in the functioning nervous system with a degree of specificity hitherto unimaginable.

Synaptic Mechanisms and Plasticity

Until recently, our model for the microphysiology of the synapse in its natural state was the vertebrate neuromuscular junction, supplemented by many interesting findings from invertebrates and from cultured neurons or neuron-like cells. At the neuromuscular junction, synaptic transmission takes place by the rapid release of packets or quanta consisting of 10,000–20,000 molecules of acetylcholine, which diffuse quickly across the synaptic cleft and bind to a matching number of nicotinic acetylcholine receptors, causing the associated channels to open and producing a large transient transmembrane current. High-quality intracellular recordings capable of resolving these currents have been routine for more than 20 years. Similar events were not adequately resolved by penetrating microelectrodes in the small noisy cells of the central nervous system.

Whole-cell recordings. The introduction of gigohm-seal whole-cell recording to slice preparations from the mammalian forebrain has made it possible to study central nervous system synaptic mechanisms at a level of resolution previously unattainable (Busch and Sakmann). Strong evidence that both excitatory and inhibitory synaptic transmission in the mammalian forebrain are quantal has begun to emerge from such an analysis of miniature synaptic potentials and currents (Jack et al.; Busch and Sakmann; P. Andersen et al.; Tsien and Malinow). Several peculiarities of central nervous system synapses have emerged, however. One is that probabilities of release appear to fluctuate over minutes to tens of minutes and often to be near zero for many synapses (Jack et al.). A second peculiarity is that, at least in many cases, the central nervous system quanta are remarkably small, with only about 30 $GABA_A$ channels activated per quantum in inhibitory synapses onto hippocampal granule cells (Busch and Sakmann). In some excitatory synapses as well, quanta appear to be very much smaller than the number of transmitter molecules likely to be released (Jack et al.). These findings, if general, could provide a mechanism for stability in quantal size in the face of fluctuating numbers of transmitter molecules released. They would, however, rule out, or at least severely limit, the capacity for modulation of synaptic strength to be produced by a presynaptic mechanism, since the available postsynaptic receptors would be more than saturated by the amount of transmitter that is released. Although our mental cartoon of central nervous system synaptic physiology derived from the neuromuscular junction still appears to stand, unique features are beginning to be apparent. The next few years, in which these new techniques will be fully exploited in a variety of brain synapses, promise exciting advances in our understanding of synaptic mechanisms.

The use of whole-cell recordings in the slice preparation has also affected profoundly our understanding of how neurons integrate information from multiple synaptic inputs. In such recordings, many neurons have input resistances tenfold greater than they were thought to have from measurements with penetrating microelectrodes, so that a given synaptic current now gives rise to a tenfold bigger voltage change in the postsynaptic cell. P. Andersen et al. analyzed the consequences of this effect on synaptic integration in recordings from hippocampal pyramidal cells. They found that as few as ten of the many thousands of synaptic inputs present on a cell would suffice to fire the cell and that only a few inputs were necessary if they fired in brief bursts. Computationally, this turns the neuron from something more like an AND-gate, in which all of the inputs must be active to fire the cell, into something much closer to an OR-gate, in which the cell fires when any one of its many inputs is active. It will be important in the next few years to determine whether we have drastically to revise downward our notions of the numbers of active synaptic inputs necessary to fire neurons in many parts of the brain.

Molecular bases of synaptic plasticity. The structural and biochemical components of the synapse have also been revealed in much greater detail. The localization and regulatory capacities of several molecules make them prime candidates for the biochemical substrates of synaptic plasticity. Such a biochemical capacity for plasticity appears to be present both pre- and postsynaptically.

The type II calcium-calmodulin-dependent protein kinase (CaM-kinase II) has been established as a major constituent of the postsynaptic density that lies directly under the neurotransmitter receptors (Kennedy et al.). This protein occurs as a stable multimer. Its ability to phosphorylate a variety of substrates depends on both calcium levels and the protein's own state of phosphorylation. When the CaM-kinase II multimer is adequately phosphorylated, its autocatalytic activity appears to be sufficient to keep it phosphorylated for some time without neural activity or elevated calcium, even in the presence of endogenous phosphatases. CaM-kinase II thus appears to be able to act as a molecular switch, capable of persistently storing information about the recent history of postsynaptic activity in its state of phosphorylation. By its ability to phosphorylate other substrates, CaM-kinase II appears to be in a position to regulate a variety of postsynaptic events, including those responsible for synaptic plasticity.

The synapsins have been established as important components of the synaptic vesicles in the presynaptic terminal, and P. Greengard (meeting participant) presented current hypotheses and a large body of evidence regarding their role in the mobilization of synaptic vesicles for release and the possible regulation of that role by phosphorylation. Greengard reviewed physiological experiments that have demonstrated a powerful reduction of transmitter release by the injection of dephosphorylated synapsin I, and the reversal of this effect by the injection of CaM-kinase II. A molecular genetic analysis of presynaptic proteins from purified synaptic vesicles has revealed genes encoding at least two forms of a vesicle-associated membrane protein called VAMP (homologous to bovine synaptobrevin and to a *Drosophila* protein) along with synaptophysin (also known as p38), and protein studies have shown that synaptic vesicles contain several low-molecular-weight GTP-binding proteins (Ngsee et al.). The location of these three molecules in the synaptic vesicle membrane is consistent with their playing regulatory roles in synaptic release, but these roles remain to be established in physiological experiments. Insulin-like peptides may also play a role as neuromodulators (Schwartz et al.).

Long-term potentiation. Physiological studies of synaptic plasticity have taken great advantage of molecular reagents that act specifically on some of the components of the synapse identified above. Four papers reviewed experiments on long-term potentiation (LTP) in mammalian hippocampus. LTP is a long-lasting (hours to weeks) increase in the efficacy of synaptic transmission produced by activation of a presynaptic input in association with the depolarization of the postsynaptic cell. From the point of view of the postsynaptic cell, at least, LTP is specific to the synapse at which it was produced, in that other inputs to the same postsynaptic cell that were not active in association with the postsynaptic depolarization are not potentiated. These properties result in a form of synaptic plasticity that is both cooperative and associative. The induction of LTP in the CA1 region of the hippocampus depends on the presence of two general types of glutamate receptors on the postsynaptic cell: the *N*-methyl-D-aspartate (NMDA) receptor and the kainate/quisqualate or AMPA (non-NMDA) receptors. Each of these two general receptor types may consist of several different molecules (Hollmann et al.). The non-NMDA receptors have conventional properties of ligand-gated transmembrane channels reminiscent of those of the nicotinic acetylcholine receptor on muscle; they produce fast EPSPs as a result of permeability to univalent cations. Current through the NMDA receptor channels is unconventional, in that it depends on the membrane voltage and on the concentration of a modulator, glycine, as well as on the neurotransmitter, glutamate (for review, see Bekkers and Stevens); almost no current flows through this receptor unless the postsynaptic membrane is substantially depolarized, because the channel is blocked in the resting membrane by magnesium ions when they are present at physiological concentrations. NMDA-mediated EPSPs are also relatively slow and prolonged (for review, see Hestrin et al.). Finally, unlike all other ligand-gated channels at

these synapses, the NMDA receptor channels are highly permeable to calcium, as well as to other alkali metal cations. The computational properties of NMDA receptor channels are discussed by Bekkers and Stevens.

The explanation offered for LTP, then, is that when the postsynaptic cell is depolarized (artificially by an experimenter or by spatial or temporal summation of other synaptic inputs in the natural situation), active presynaptic inputs produce influxes of calcium at the synapse through NMDA receptors, and that the increase in postsynaptic calcium triggers a series of reactions that result in the specific strengthening of the active synapse without a strengthening of inactive synapses onto the same cell (for review, see Tsien and Malinow). The calcium influx appears to act through two calcium-dependent protein kinases, CaM-kinase II and protein kinase C, since specifically blocking either kinase by intracellular application of reagents generated from knowledge of the molecular biology of these kinases blocks LTP (for review, see Tsien and Malinow). The results of manipulations of calcium, membrane voltage, and specific blockade of NMDA and non-NMDA receptors in the hippocampus are all consistent with this explanation. There is now almost universal consensus on these facts of and explanations for the induction of LTP in the CA1 region of the hippocampus (for review, see Morris; Bliss et al.). Hippocampal LTP appears likely to be a mechanism that operates in normal life, and not merely to be the neurophysiologist's toy, since Morris has shown that the learning, but not the retrieval, of some behaviors thought to depend on the hippocampus has a pharmacology quantitatively and qualitatively identical to that of the induction of LTP in hippocampal slices.

The controversies over LTP relate not so much to its induction as to its expression (for review, see Tsien and Malinow). Is the persistent increase in synaptic efficacy that is induced as described above a result of a change in postsynaptic sensitivity to a constant presynaptic release of glutamate or is the increase in efficacy a result of an increased presynaptic release of neurotransmitter? If there is increased presynaptic release of transmitter, is this an increase in the probability of release at many synapses that previously failed to release transmitter or is it an increase in the amount of transmitter released at synapses that previously did release transmitter? If the expression of LTP is due to presynaptic changes, how is the instruction to increase synaptic efficacy communicated from the postsynaptic side of the synapse, which is responsible for the induction of LTP, specifically to its presynaptic terminal? Some perspective on these controversies is afforded by the realization that if the mechanisms responsible for LTP are also to participate in the long-term changes in synaptic efficacy that accompany the growth and rearrangement of synapses in development, as reviewed by Constantine-Paton, then the sizes and strengths of the pre- and postsynaptic components of the synapse must ultimately be regulated together, since one does not see a tremendous mismatch between the sizes of postsynaptic structures and their presynaptic terminals. This realization does not, however, answer the question of the locus of the changes in the few hours after the induction of LTP.

Kauer et al. (1988) and Muller and Lynch (1988) presented evidence that the expression of LTP consisted of an increase in the synaptic currents through non-NMDA receptor channels without a proportional increase through NMDA receptor channels; these findings suggested a postsynaptic locus. Tsien and Malinow present evidence from a quantal analysis of miniature PSPs using whole-cell patch electrode recordings that presynaptic neurotransmitter release is dramatically enhanced after LTP. In their experiments, potentiation was powerful, was accompanied by a prompt reduction in the number of response failures after stimulation of single presynaptic cells, and was accompanied by changes in the coefficient of variation of the single-fiber responses, which is a statistical sign consistent with a change in presynaptic release. Bliss et al. have interpreted increases in stimulus-evoked glutamate release seen after LTP using push-pull cannulae as evidence that LTP is expressed on the presynaptic side; their finding of enhanced release of arachidonic acid in association with LTP suggests that arachidonic acid could be the retrograde messenger responsible for informing the presynaptic terminal that its release should be enhanced.

If LTP is expressed presynaptically, how far does it spread? Although many experiments have shown that LTP is specific from the point of view of the postsynaptic cell, these experiments have not for the most part looked for changes in the efficacy of synapses made by a potentiated presynaptic axon onto other postsynaptic cells with which its activity was not paired. Bonhoeffer et al. have examined this question by making both intracellular recordings from hippocampal slice cultures and optical records of the spread of activation in a visual cortex slice as monitored by voltage-sensitive dyes; the results are consistent with their interpretation that synapses from input fibers that are potentiated onto one cell by being paired with depolarization also become potentiated onto other control cells that were not depolarized during the period of presynaptic activity. If it is confirmed that the subsynaptic membrane of the unpaired control cells was not inadvertently depolarized during the pairing, this finding would suggest that a retrograde messenger might spread over some tens or hundreds of microns to affect recently active presynaptic terminals, or else that the consequences of a synapse-specific retrograde messenger might spread to other terminals within the presynaptic fiber over a similar distance.

At the present time, it is difficult to reconcile or to dismiss many of the results favoring either a pre- or postsynaptic locus for the expression of LTP (for discussion, see Tsien and Malinow). Further work, including molecular characterization of the possible heterogeneity of glutamate receptors before and after LTP, further quantal analysis, statistical exploration of the

implications of possible postsynaptic heterogeneity for the interpretation of quantal analysis, and firm identification of the hypothesized retrograde messenger may all be necessary for a secure understanding. If progress in the next few years continues at the present rate, all of these goals and more may soon be at hand.

Molecular Mechanisms of Learning and Memory

At some level, mechanisms of synaptic plasticity like those discussed above appear likely to be used in learning and memory. Memory is, however, long-lasting, and changes lasting days or weeks are difficult to follow in the mammalian brain slice preparations that have been so productive in the analysis of LTP.

Students of memory have traditionally divided their topic into two or more stages, most simply into short-term memory and long-term memory. Short-term memory is thought to require ongoing patterns of activity in the brain, and it appears somehow to be transformed or fixed into long-term memory over time. Operationally, short-term memory is distinguished from long-term memory on the basis of its greater susceptibility to disruption by seizures, trauma, inhibition of protein synthesis, and other manipulations. In humans, such manipulations can produce a period of retrograde amnesia for events taking place previously, and thought to be stored only in short-term and not yet in long-term memory, as well as a period of post-traumatic amnesia for subsequent events.

How might long-term memory be encoded in the brain? Two issues emerge in an attempt to answer this question. The first historically was the locus of these changes: Where in the brain is the representation of the remembered event, referred to as the *engram*, stored? Our present understanding of distributed computation (see below) makes it clear why a systematic search for the locus of the engram using focal lesions might fail (Lashley 1950). The second issue that arises is the nature of the engram: What sort of change in the brain might be responsible for memory? Again, our present understanding of distributed computation reveals that the engram could consist of a set of long-lasting or permanent changes in the efficacy of many synapses distributed over a network. Because of the requirement of protein synthesis for memorizing and the inability of many manipulations to disrupt long-term memory, it was thought that the persistent changes in synaptic efficacy that constitute the engram must result from structural changes in synapses. Over the years, a number of attempts to study such structural changes have been made in the mammalian nervous system (for discussion, see P. Andersen et al.). Structural changes in synapses, however, take place most prominently during the growth and development of the nervous system. A unified view of the regulation of synaptic structure and efficacy might therefore encompass both growth and development, on the one hand, and learning and memory, on the other. The molecular machinery involved in the regulation of synaptic structure and efficacy may well be common to the two domains.

Much of our understanding of learning and memory in molecular terms is emerging from studies of invertebrates, from flies to molluscs to crustaceans. In the molluscs in particular, a combination of behavioral, neurophysiological, molecular genetic, and biochemical approaches has allowed the analysis of simple neural circuits that exhibit sophisticated forms of learning and memory. Models of these circuits reveal which of their properties are likely to be responsible for such behavioral phenomena as second-order conditioning, blocking, and operant conditioning (Byrne et al.). Schacher et al. have discussed the remarkable similarities between the processes responsible for the induction of short-term memory and long-term memory in the sensitization of a simple sensory-motor reflex in *Aplysia*. Both involve an increase in synaptic strength brought about by an increase in transmitter release as a result of a decrease in a presynaptic potassium current. Both use serotonin as a sensitizing presynaptic neurotransmitter and are mediated by increases in cAMP in the presynaptic terminal. Only the long-term process requires transcription and protein synthesis and is accompanied by growth of both pre- and postsynaptic structures. Phosphorylation patterns that are transient in the short-term process become persistent in the long-term process, apparently by the autonomous activation of the catalytic subunit of a protein kinase that is normally dependent on cAMP; this activation appears to involve a transcription factor and several regulatory steps. Two-dimensional gels reveal ten proteins whose expression is enhanced and five proteins whose expression is decreased within half an hour following stimuli that produce long-term sensitization; most of these changes in expression persist only for 2–3 hours. Four of the proteins whose expression is decreased cross-react to antibodies that recognize neural cell-adhesion molecules of the immunoglobulin superfamily. These four proteins are expressed at high levels at stable synapses in cell cultures and are down-regulated at times of growth and synaptic rearrangement. These molecules at least, and perhaps others as well, appear then to work in common in development and in long-term memory (Schacher et al.). Although many aspects of the regulatory cascade involved in this long-term sensitization model of learning remain to be worked out, the overall picture, involving kinases, transcription factors, apparent homologs of cellular immediate-early genes, pre- and postsynaptic growth, and homologs of cell adhesion molecules, provides a model for future studies of long-term memory in the mammalian nervous system.

Tully et al.; W. Quinn (meeting participant), and S. Benzer (meeting participant) discussed the promise of the fruit fly for studies of learning and memory. The remarkable similarity of cAMP-dependent protein kinase defects in several known fly mutants affecting learning to some of the presumed biochemical substrates of synaptic plasticity in molluscs and mammals suggests that the neural machinery of learning is likely to be phylogenetically ancient. The development of new training procedures that will allow flies to exhibit more robust learning, in combination with techniques like P-element mutagenesis that now allow a gene to be cloned within a few weeks of the observation of a mutant phenotype, hold out hope for rapid progress in the genetic dissection of the stages of learning and memory in this species.

NEURAL DEVELOPMENT

The study of neural development is one of the topics most revolutionized by recent progress in molecular genetics and by advances in dyes and molecular probes. As Jack McMahan remarked in an aside, at the time of the 1975 Symposium, we mainly discussed the *principles* of neural development. Although this may at times seem preferable to looking at the thousandth gel or nucleotide sequence of the day, we now have many of the tools to study neural development at the level at which it actually operates. The much more concrete level of the current discussions is a sign of progress, rather than a fascination with detail for detail's sake. We may well come to regard the broad developmental principles of yesteryear with the fondness reserved for other generalizations about the behavior of complex systems, like those of economics. Nevertheless, in this summary, nearly all of the detail will be ignored in an effort to highlight new directions and make generalizations.

The events in neural development that must be accounted for are many: the production of appropriate numbers of neuronal precursors and their acquisition of particular neuronal cell identities, either by lineage or by some cell-cell or cell-substrate interaction; their differentiation into distinct neuronal types; the adhesive and recognition events involved in growth cone extension, pathway finding, and target recognition; the establishment of synaptic connections and the macroscopic organization of local neural circuits; the further regulation of cell number by selective cell death; and the activity-dependent or other final remodeling of synaptic connections. As the previous section suggests, the mechanisms of synaptic plasticity, learning, and memory may be the same as those of some of the later stages of development, so that there may be no time at which one can assert that development is over.

Acquisition of Cell Identity

The early stages in the acquisition of neuronal cell identity are worked out most thoroughly in *Drosophila*, as reviewed by Vaessin et al. In this species, about half of the genome has to date been screened for the genes whose deletion prevents the normal development of a particular population of peripheral neurons, and it appears possible to screen the entire genome and identify all of the genes required in this process. The genes important in the acquisition of neuronal cell identity appear to fall into several groups responsible for different stages of the process. After the basic dorsal-ventral and anterior-posterior axes of the embryo are set up by so-called "prepattern" genes, the selection of a neural rather than an epidermal fate is governed by a set of "proneural" genes, among them *daughterless* (*da*) and the genes of the *achaete-scute complex* (*AS-C*). In the next stage of development, interactions among developing neuroblasts regulate the numbers of neuronal precursors by a process of lateral inhibition governed by the "neurogenic" genes, such as *Notch*, *big brain*, and *Enhancer of split*. Additional specificity is produced by later-acting "neuronal precursor-type selector" genes. Vaessin et al. present evidence that at least ten of the proneural and neurogenic gene products contain helix-loop-helix (HLH) domains, which regulate transcription by binding to specific DNA sequences as homo- or heterodimers. These HLH domains appear likely to participate in a complex regulatory network for transcription, with redundancy and feedback. Although such complexity demands great ingenuity on the part of the experimenter who attempts to understand it, it also affords the richness that may be needed to account for the specification of neuronal cell identity. HLH proteins are present and likely to play a similar role in vertebrates.

In the vertebrate peripheral nervous system, Mori et al. have studied the factors that control the differentiation of the sympathoadrenal precursor cells of the neural crest into either sympathetic neurons or adrenal chromaffin cells. Exposure to a sequence of polypeptide factors such as fibroblast growth factor (FGF) and nerve growth factor (NGF) is required for full neuronal differentiation, whereas exposure to glucocorticoids is required for chromaffin differentiation. Some of the genes that regulate these differentiation events are under study. Remarking on the enormous variety of neuronal phenotypes, in which different classic neurotransmitters are combined in particular types of neurons with different levels of some of the many neuropeptides, Nawa et al. have pointed out the similarity of neuronal differentiation to that of the hematopoietic cells. In both cell types, a variety of factors can have different but overlapping effects on differentiation. Strikingly, one of the most important factors responsible for inducing and maintaining cholinergic differentiation of autonomic neurons is identical to the leukemia inhibitory factor known to affect hematopoietic differentiation.

Much of the speculation in past years about the acquisition of neuronal cell identity and the regulation of neuron number depended on the existence of additional neurotrophic factors that would act like NGF but be secreted from different targets and cause responses in different neurons. Until very recently, for over 40 years, no other such molecule had been isolated. Those who held out hope for additional neurotrophic factors have now been rewarded. Yancopoulos et al. review recent findings of the molecular cloning of two new neurotrophic factors in the NGF or neurotrophin family: brain-derived neurotrophic factor (BNDF) and neurotrophin-3 (NT-3). They also note the cloning of a fourth, unrelated ciliary neurotrophic factor (CNTF). Both BNDF and NT-3 molecules are extraordinarily highly conserved, with identical amino acid sequences in every mammal in which they have been investigated. The three neurotrophins have distinct patterns of expression, and changes in their expression mirror other important developmental changes. Yancopoulos et al. also describe a procedure for isolating cells that have receptors for particular neurotrophic factors. Neurotrophic factors may well exist in sufficient profusion to account for all of the decades of speculation that has surrounded them.

The acquisition of neuronal cell identity in the vertebrate central nervous system is to date less clear than in the periphery, where clear precedents or counterparts in vivo have been demonstrated for the effects of factors and cocultures shown in vitro (Nawa et al.). McKay et al. have identified an intermediate filament protein which they call nestin that is expressed by embryonic neuronal-glial precursor cells in the vertebrate central nervous system. They have immortalized lines of nestin-positive cells in vitro by the insertion of a temperature-sensitive oncogene and have shown that the cells will differentiate to resemble neurons in culture in response to defined growth factors or in coculture with other cell types. Most promising for future studies is the possibility of further genetic manipulation of the cells in vitro followed by transplantation of the cells back into the developing brain, where they will no longer proliferate because the elevated temperature inactivates the product of the temperature-sensitive oncogene. In the differentiation of different types of glial cells in optic nerve cultures, soluble factors, factors associated with the extracellular matrix, and timing all can play a role (Raff et al.). It is not yet clear whether these factors play the same role in vivo. Whether cell lineage is responsible for the identity of neocortical neurons as members of a particular functional column has been investigated using replication-incompetent retrovirus vectors; although a number of cells in a column did commonly share a lineage, there were a sufficient number of exceptions to exclude a powerful role for lineage in this aspect of neuronal identity (Cepko et al.).

Neuronal Cell Adhesion, Pathway Selection, and Target Recognition

Molecular bases of cell and process adhesion. Edelman and Cunningham discuss the role of the regulation of adhesion in the differentiation of tissues. They note that there are adhesive interactions between cells mediated by cell adhesion molecules (CAMs), further adhesive interactions between cell and substrate mediated by different molecules, and still further adhesive interactions between cells and junctions. They propose that morphological differentiation is brought about by the interactions of these adhesive forces, which generate mechanical and chemical changes that feed back upon the expression of adhesion molecules. The domains of the CAMs involved in these interactions are under investigation.

Reichardt et al. have analyzed some of the major classes of molecules that regulate axon outgrowth and growth-cone movement. In addition to the CAMs, these include glycoproteins of the extracellular matrix (ECM) and the integrins, a class of transmembrane heterodimers responsible for most of the interactions with ECM glycoproteins. The large variety of CAMs and integrins appears to allow for specific interactions that either promote or retard growth along particular pathways.

A third major class of molecule involved in neural development is the cadherins, a group of calcium-dependent cell-cell adhesion molecules that homophilically bind to similar cadherins on other cells. Reduced or ectopic expression of N-cadherin dramatically alters the development of *Xenopus* embryos (Takeichi et al.). Grenningloh et al. report that N-CAM-like molecules are also present and appear to play a role in the developing insect nervous system.

The growth cone in the recognition of pathway and target. Kater and Guthrie have focused attention on the neuronal growth cone as the integrator of multiple environmental and endogenous stimuli that inform the growing neurite which pathway to follow, when to grow straight, when to turn, and when to stop growing. Growth cones of different identified neurons in the snail *Helisoma* differ in their responses to the same stimuli, whereas the same identified neuron from different individual snails, or different individual neurons of the same class in mammals, exhibits highly stereotyped behavior. Many, but not all, of these phenomena appear to be mediated by their effects on calcium levels within the growth cone.

In vivo, axonal growth is directed along appropriate pathways to appropriate targets. It has long been attractive to suppose that pathways need not be marked explicitly but that diffusible factors secreted from the target might establish a gradient of increasing concentration that the growth cone can follow to the target. Placzek et al. provide evidence from studies in vitro and in vivo that the growth cones of developing spinal axons are guided by a diffusible chemoattractant secreted by cells of the floor plate of the spinal cord. The molecular identity of this putative diffusible chemoattractant is not yet known.

O'Leary et al. provide similar evidence for a factor secreted by the pontine nuclei to which corticospinal axons are sensitive. The O'Leary et al. experiments, however, cast considerable doubt on the hypothesized unique sensitivity of the growth cone to chemoattractant or target recognition factors. In their system, the growth cones of corticospinal axons in vivo ordinarily grow past the pontine nuclei; several days later, the naked axons sprout interstitially at the point at which they pass closest to either normal or ectopically located pontine nuclei. These experiments suggest strongly that axons are sensitive to at least some target-derived factors all along their course and not merely at specialized endings.

In many cases, when growth cones reach a target, they not only must recognize it, but must also participate in a topographic map within the target structure. In the most recent of a long series of studies of a model of this process in vitro, Stahl et al. have devised assays that reveal a preference for axons from the nasal retina of the chick to grow on stripes of membrane prepared from posterior tectum. This preferential growth mirrors the arrangement in vivo and complements the specificity previously demonstrated by temporal retinal axons for anterior tectum. With the further biochemical characterization of the repellent substance responsible for the preference of temporal retinal axons in this assay, Stahl et al. discuss how it may guide axonal growth through its influence on the growth cone. This and similar systems promise soon to take the hypothesis that chemospecific gradients are responsible for topographic specificity from the realm of theoretical speculation to concrete fact.

Molecular specificity of the neuromuscular synapse. Just as we know more about the synaptic physiology of the neuromuscular junction than we do about any other synapse, so too do we have our most concrete appreciation of the molecules involved in the specificity of development and regeneration at this synapse (for review, see Sanes et al.). Falls et al. review progress toward the isolation and molecular cloning of a factor called *aria*, for its action on cultured muscle cells of mimicking the activity of nerve terminals in the induction of new acetylcholine receptor expression and clustering. Changeux et al. consider the molecular mechanisms by which the expression of the acetylcholine receptor gene comes to be enhanced in and restricted to the particular nuclei of the multinucleate muscle fibers that lie under the end plate. McMahan describes the characterization and molecular cloning of agrin, which (1) is released by motoneurons at the end plate, (2) persists in the synaptic basal lamina for long periods of time even in the absence of nerve or muscle cells, and (3) may be responsible for the reestablishment of regenerating synapses at the specific sites of previous synapses.

Sanes et al. review evidence that a very large number of molecules participate in the specificity of neuromuscular reinnervation (see Fig. 2 in Sanes et al.). These molecules appear to be of four classes, including soluble factors that might attract axonal ingrowth from a distance, such as insulin-like growth factors 1 and 2; extrasynaptic adhesive factors that might signal denervation such as N-CAM and N-cadherin; perisynaptic adhesive molecules such as tenascin and fibronectin; and synapse-specific factors such as acetylcholinesterase, agrin, and particularly a synapse-specific form of laminin called s-laminin. Sanes et al. suggest that basal laminae may differ enormously from place to place in the combinations of their numerous molecular components that are expressed and that these differences may be the molecular substrates of recognition.

Central Nervous System Development In Vivo and In Vitro

Recent studies of central nervous system development have taken great advantage of new optical techniques such as confocal microscopy, new stains such as the postmortem dye DiI, new labels for specific molecular components of the central nervous system, and new approaches to cell culture such as "organotypic" slice culture or collagen matrix cultures. Most of the experiments described below would not have been possible without the technical advances of the past few years, and work in this area appears likely to be revolutionized again in the next few years by further advances in technology.

The initial aim of many of these studies is at least to outline a sort of *Peyton Place* of neural development, a narrative about developing axons and dendrites that reveals who does what to whom, and how often. With such a narrative in hand, describing developmental events at or near the level at which they actually take place, we may hope to advance from the present level of description and explanation, usually posed in terms of principles of development, such as "competition" versus "disuse" and "trophic" effects versus "activity" effects, closer to a mechanistic understanding.

Neural circuitry in many regions of the central nervous system is organized into macroscopic patches, columns, or clusters. The glomeruli of the olfactory bulb constitute one such macroscopic arrangement of neural and glial circuitry. Purves and LaMantia took advantage of recent advances in optics and dye technology to examine the mode of growth of these macroscopic structures by repeatedly imaging the arrangement of glomeruli in individual animals. They found that new glomeruli are added in the spaces between existing glomeruli, which appear to be essentially permanent, with little hint of fission, turnover, or other forms of gradual reorganization.

The early development of neocortex and its inputs and outputs is a major topic of study. P. Rakic (meeting participant) focused on the roles of intrinsic cortical cell properties versus thalamocortical inputs in the specification of cortical areas. By removing the eyes sufficiently early in the development of fetal monkeys, he reduced the size of the major thalamic recipient of input from the eyes, the lateral geniculate nucleus (LGN), to approximately one third of normal. This reduction in the size of the LGN was accompanied by a similar reduction in the size of V1 or area 17, the primary visual cortex and recipient of input from the LGN. After these animals grew up, histochemical analysis revealed that reduced area 17 was essentially normal; the normally neighboring cortical region, area 18, however, no longer extended to the border of area 17. Much or all of the cortex that would have become part

of area 17 in normal development took on entirely novel characteristics, appropriate for no area of normal cortex. These results make it likely that both thalamocortical inputs and intrinsic cortical cell properties play a role in the specification of cortical areas. A contrasting view emerged from the experiments of Blakemore and Molnar, who studied the innervation cocultures of LGN and cortex. Although these cocultures produced mutual stimulation of axonal outgrowth, the outgrowth and innervation under these conditions showed no sign of positional or areal specificity, perhaps because these experiments were conducted at a different developmental stage than those of Rakic. Although many features of the early development of different cortical areas are in common, as O'Leary et al. showed for the collaterals of the descending axons cortical layer V cells, differences among the areas are ultimately clearly asserted.

Shatz et al. have found that prior to the development of the cortical plate, neurons within the subplate send and receive synaptic inputs and pioneer many axonal pathways, including those between thalamus and cortex. In many species including the one that these authors have principally studied, the cat, most of these subplate cells die before maturity. Evidence that these transient cells may play an important role in the production of the mature nervous system comes from experiments in which the subplate cells are destroyed before the normal time of thalamocortical innervation, causing the thalamic fibers to fail to enter the apparently intact cortical plate above the damaged subplate. Shatz et al. hypothesize that this system constitutes a neural scaffold, possibly allowing thalamocortical afferents to become organized appropriately before growing into the cortical plate.

Role of neural activity. Patterns of neural activity can also play an important role in development. In several systems, synaptic connections appear to rearrange under the influence of neural activity in normal development (for review, see Stryker et al.). Constantine-Paton exploited the experimentally induced reorganization of inputs produced when two eyes innervate a single tectum in amphibians. She revealed an activity-dependent segregation of inputs from the two eyes that is strikingly similar to the cortical ocular dominance columns in higher mammals. Agents that block or stimulate the NMDA subtype of glutamate receptor disrupt or enhance this segregation. Explanations of this phenomenon have much in common with those above for LTP. Stryker et al. presented evidence that cortical orientation columns, like all of the other known features of organization of carnivore visual cortex, are paralleled by a specific organization of the thalamocortical afferent input. Mathematical models are reviewed which demonstrate that a variety of mechanisms, including ones like LTP, can account for the development of this and the other known fine-scale specificities of thalamocortical innervation.

Patterns of neural activity can have important consequences for the expression of specific molecules in both the developing nervous system and the mature nervous system. Certain neuronal proteoglycans are expressed at high levels in the extracellular matrix (ECM) surrounding stable, mature synapses. Hock-field et al. show that the expression of one of these, Cat-301, is regulated by neural activity and reflects neuronal maturation. Jones et al. have shown an amazing variety of prompt (2–4 days) molecular changes in the visual cortex of the adult monkey following unilateral eye removal or activity blockade. Dramatic changes were evident in the GABA system, in the expression of certain peptide neurotransmitters, and in the expression of CaM kinase II (see above). Similar but smaller and much slower changes were seen in the weeks following monocular visual occlusion.

A number of "cellular immediate-early" genes involved in transcriptional regulation are also induced by various patterns of activity in the mammalian central nervous system. Curran et al. have induced the proto-oncogenes c-*fos* and c-*jun* in rat cortex by creating seizures, and they discuss attempts to understand the transcriptional targets of these gene products and the potentially mutually regulatory relationships among the variety of transcriptional regulators that can be induced to transient high levels of expression. Worley et al. present evidence that physiological levels of visual stimulation powerfully modulate the level of expression of *zif/268*, another transcription factor, that is also developmentally regulated and induced under circumstances that produce LTP. Future work promises to disclose the precise roles that these genes play in development and in long-term synaptic plasticity.

SENSORY AND MOTOR SYSTEMS OF THE BRAIN

The past 15 years have witnessed major advances in our understanding of sensory and motor systems. Most of these advances have, however, been evolutionary rather than revolutionary. The appreciation of multiple parallel channels or streams of central processing within a single modality is not new, for example, but it has now become the dominant view even in areas of research and among researchers that had previously favored a more nearly serial, hierarchical view of sensory organization.

Although few experimental approaches or questions are entirely new, several have recently received much more widespread appreciation at the forefront of current research. Most prominent among these is a renewed concern for parallel psychophysical and neurophysiological investigations. This psychophysiological parallelism is pursued at two levels, one in which the general organization of a sensory system, for example, is explored with an eye to the general organization of perceptual representations as we understand them, and a second level that has the goal of explaining particular aspects of perception or movement in terms of the activities of particular central neurons.

A second change in approach is the new or renewed engagement of experimental neurobiologists with formal models. Fifteen years ago, modeling at any level but the most fundamentally cellular and biophysical was widely thought among experimentalists to be counterproductive or, at best, a harmless vice to be pursued in secret for one's own amusement. Now the formulation and testing of models are more than respectable; they are a major industry in many laboratories.

A third advance is that many neural systems are conceived of and described in terms of parallel distributed processing networks, and the computational power of such networks is now better appreciated. Although such an approach has yet fully to bear fruit, it is now widely regarded as promising.

A fourth change from the predominant practice of 15 years ago, largely as a result of the proliferation of inexpensive, powerful laboratory computers, is that central nervous system neuroscience has gradually become more quantitative, and many more aspects of central nervous system structure and function are now measured and not just described. Although premature quantitation can not only be tedious, but also misleading, as is evident, for example, from much of the visual cortex literature prior to 1960, the peculiarities of neuronal responses can make qualitative categorization a fragile and subjective enterprise.

A fifth important new development, not fully represented at the Symposium, is the ability to monitor neural activity optically (Grinvald et al. 1988). Powerful new findings from the application of these techniques to the study of cortical organization are now beginning to appear.

We may look forward to several promising new approaches as well. The use of specific molecular reagents for the isolation of functional cell types in the brain and in perception may well bear great fruit. If different functional classes of central neurons within one area of the brain turn out to use distinct ion channels or receptors, for example, it should be possible to stimulate or block their activity selectively. Pharmacological experiments along these lines have been successful (Schiller et al. 1986). Higher-resolution brain-imaging studies in humans and animals of metabolism, transmitters, or blood flow, perhaps in combination with extremely high-resolution magnetic resonance anatomical studies of the same individual brains, also promise great advances in the understanding of which brain areas are involved in which tasks (Raichle).

Sensory Transduction

Studies of sensory transduction have profited most directly from recent advances in molecular biology and genetics. Bargmann et al. have begun the analysis of chemosensation in the nematode *Caenorhabditis elegans* through a combination of lesions and genetics. Berg has used a genetic analysis of bacterial sensory-motor function in combination with biophysical techniques to work out many aspects of bacterial "chemotaxis."

Jacobs and Hudspeth have devised preparative conditions under which they can photograph filaments that connect adjacent stereocilia of the auditory hair cell along its axis of polarization. These filaments or tip-links are reminiscent of the "springs" that were hypothesized to transduce the shearing motion between neighboring stereocilia that is thought to be the basis of hair-cell mechanosensitivity by opening channels to which the springs were connected. If these tip-links play the role hypothesized, their identification may lead to a way of identifying the transduction channels, which are elusive in part because they appear to be so few in number. Such an eventuality would also be remarkable in the extent to which biological reality would mimic the cartoon model of hair-cell transduction devised purely on biophysical grounds.

With the cloning and sequencing of the genes for rhodopsin and the cone photopigments (Nathans), the study of color vision and its anomalies at the level of the photoreceptors has changed over the past 5 years from the construction of Stiles plots of spectral sensitivity and exercises in the interpretation of family trees to biochemistry. Few other areas of neuroscience have experienced such a rapid reduction from the abstract and inferential to the concrete. The most speculative issue now surrounding the genetics of photopigments is their evolution. Nathans is using site-directed mutagenesis to investigate the biochemistry responsible for the precise spectral sensitivities of the different cones. By making recordings of the photocurrent from single cones, Kraft et al. found excellent agreement between cone spectral sensitivities and the sensitivity of human color vision. These studies suggest strongly that the different cone pigments are essentially pure, since the presence of as little as 1 molecule in 100,000 of the blue cone pigment could have been detected in the red and green cones if it were present. Although the central representation of color remains puzzling in many respects (Hubel and Livingstone), transduction is now a question of biochemical mechanisms rather than inference from psychophysics.

Psychophysiological Explanations: What Does That Neuron Do for You?

The explanation of psychophysical thresholds, the limits of human or animal performance, in terms of the transduction and encoding capacities of sensory receptors and peripheral neurons has been a long-standing program of sensory physiology, the many successes of which are well known (Kraft et al.). In some fields of study, such as somatic sensation (Mountcastle et al.) and neuroethology (Konishi; Suga et al.), this pursuit has been followed into the central nervous system with success, and behavioral capacities for the analysis of stimulus qualities not directly represented in the discharge rates of peripheral neurons have been explained in terms of successive stages of neural computation evident in the receptive field properties of sometimes complex central neurons. In other areas of sensory physiology, these concerns have lain dormant for many years while other goals were pursued.

In the mammalian central visual system, for example, the major endeavor has been for many years to follow the transformation of visual information from lower- to higher-order stations. These investigations have disclosed many features of organization, but they have not revealed the functions of these features. Although we have known of the center-surround receptive fields of retinal ganglion cells for nearly 40 years, only in the past 5 years do we have clear evidence that the on-center receptive fields are actually used for detecting brightening or for stimuli brighter than the background and the off-center fields for darkening or for stimuli darker than the background (Schiller et al. 1986). In the visual cortex, we have known of orientation columns for nearly 30 years and of ocular dominance columns for more than 25 years. Although it was once in some circles (but is no longer) fashionable to speak of visual cortical neurons as "orientation detectors," the fact remains that we have no clear indication of the function or behavioral role of the particular receptive-field properties of these neurons or of their arrangements in columns, stripes, or patches.

Much of the excitement in current research comes from a renewed investigation of the neurophysiological basis of sensory and motor psychophysics. Examples from several areas of the central nervous system show that the psychophysically relevant information is present in simple patterns of activity distributed over populations of neurons. In cases in which this has been investigated, the neurons may be arranged in maps according to the psychophysically relevant parameter.

Neuroethology. Suga et al. have analyzed the sonar system of the mustache bat. This animal hunts flying insects by emitting pulses of sound that have a long constant frequency (CF) component with significant energy at 4 harmonics, followed by a brief frequency-modulated (FM) component. From the echoes of these pulses reflected back from a target, the bat determines the direction, range, velocity, movement, and something about the surface properties of the target. The analyses of these different qualities are carried out in different computational maps that define different auditory cortical areas. The neural machinery for the computation of target range is described, and Suga et al. review the evidence for a similar degree of auditory cortical specialization in other species, including humans.

Konishi recommends a similar "top-down" approach, in which one starts with the information known on psychophysical grounds to be encoded in high-level neurons and then looks for the input connections and neural circuitry responsible for this encoding. His examples of this approach are the processing of information in parallel pathways for the computation of the direction of auditory stimuli in the barn owl and for the electrosensory system of the weakly electric fish, *Eignemannia*. Similar computational algorithms or procedures involving amplitude and phase encodings are required and are used in the two systems, but the neural implementations of these procedures are completely different.

Somatic sensation. Mountcastle et al. present human and monkey psychophysical studies of the discrimination of different frequencies of sinusoidally vibratory light tactile stimuli. They compare the responses of peripheral, subcortical, and cortical neurons to stimuli that are just barely discriminable in an effort to determine what features of the neural response are used for making the discrimination. For the range of frequencies investigated, the period of the oscillating neuronal response appeared to be the only feature available for making the discrimination, requiring that the brain somehow store the period evoked by one stimulus and compare it with that evoked by a later stimulus. No sign of these storage and comparison operations was evident in the primary cortical areas investigated. A further surprising finding was that cortical responses to a particular stimulus were not affected by the relevance of the stimulus to the behavioral discrimination task in which the monkey was engaged.

Merzenich et al. present evidence that the representations of tactile stimuli that are made behaviorally relevant in an experiment increase in size and that the total response to such newly relevant stimuli, distributed over the reorganized network, increases sufficiently to account for the improvements in discrimination that take place over weeks and months. They show that a variety of other manipulations also produce dramatic reorganizations of cortical sensory representations within limits set by an apparently fixed anatomical convergence and divergence of input. The plasticity of cortical representation is viewed as the substrate for the improvement in behavioral capacity.

Vision. Newsome et al. investigated whether motion-sensitive neurons in the middle temporal cortical visual area (MT or V5) are responsible for the monkey's ability to discriminate the direction of movement. First, the threshold responses of MT neurons were compared with the animal's psychophysical thresholds for the detection of correlated movement in a field of otherwise randomly moving dots and were found to be similar. Then, taking advantage of the fact that MT neurons sensitive to the same direction of motion are clustered in columns or patches, Newsome et al. stimulated electrically in one patch of MT neurons while the animal was performing a discrimination for movement either in the direction preferred by the neurons near the stimulating electrode or in the opposite direction. In nearly all cases, the animal was more likely with the stimulation than without to respond as if the stimulus were moving in the neurons' preferred direction. If the stimulating electrode could be considered to activate only the neurons near its tip, this experiment would provide strong evidence that the activity of these MT

neurons underlies the capacity for the discrimination of the direction of motion.

Movement. Sparks et al. probed the encoding of the size and direction of eye movements in the monkey superior colliculus. Colliculus neurons discharge optimally in association with saccadic eye movements of a particular size and direction, but they discharge well over a broad range of eye movements. The hypothesis tested was that the activities of the entire population of eye-movement cells in the colliculus are used to guide eye movements, i.e., that each neuron contributes to the eye-motor control system the equivalent of a command to move along a vector of the neuron's optimal size and direction weighted by the rate of discharge of the neuron. The hypothesized population code is therefore the weighted sum of all these eye-movement vectors. Pharmacologically enhancing or reducing the discharge of part of this population caused the eye movements to deviate as predicted. These powerful experiments establish beyond doubt that saccadic eye-movement commands are issued through the superior colliculus. Along with previous work on this system, these experiments provide a model of the sorts of evidence needed to establish the existence of a proposed distributed coding in the nervous system.

Georgoupolos compared the population coding of eye movements in the superior colliculus, now firmly established, with the code that may be present for the direction of arm movements in the motor cortex. If one accepts that the neurons in motor cortex do produce arm movements (rather than merely reflecting their production elsewhere), then, as few as 150 neurons could encode the direction of arm movement with an accuracy similar to that of the animal. The suggestion that the direction of arm movement encoded by the population of motor cortex neurons rotates continuously under circumstances that would be thought to induce the monkey to rotate mentally the direction of his reach provides further support for such a population coding.

Movshon et al. compared the motion signals evident in the responses of MT neurons to the features of visual motion that appear to be responsible for smooth pursuit eye movements. The match is surprisingly good. Although such evidence is to date merely correlative, it suggests that the limitations of the pursuit eye movement system may be fundamentally sensory rather than motor.

Parallel Channels in Vision

Parallel channels in the visual system have their origin in the retina. At the level of the lateral geniculate nucleus (LGN), there are channels for the two eyes and for lightness and darkness (corresponding to ON- and OFF-center inputs). There are also two major channels for different classes of retinal inputs: one, in the magnocellular layers of the LGN and referred to as the magno channel, receives input from the largest, most rapidly conducting retinal ganglion cells and has broad-band spectral sensitivity and high contrast sensitivity, and the other channel, in the parvocellular layers of the LGN, receives input from more slowly conducting retinal ganglion cells and typically has smaller, color-opponent receptive fields and lower contrast sensitivity.

Hubel and Livingstone, Zeki, and Van Essen et al. have followed these channels from the LGN through modular subdivisions of the primary visual cortex (V1) and onto many other cortical areas using a combination of anatomical tracing, metabolic staining, physiological study of visual response properties, and psychophysics. Within and V1 and V2, three functional streams, one magno and two parvo, are segregated into different layers or modules. Beyond V2, these streams lead on to different cortical areas, including MT for the magno stream, and different modules of V4 and of the posterior inferotemporal cortex for the two parvo streams. Because of the different spectral and spatial contrast sensitivities of the different streams, it is possible to devise psychophysical stimuli that should activate one of the streams well and the others minimally. Using such stimuli, Hubel and Livingstone have inferred the cortical loci at which several different perceptual tasks are performed. Zeki has combined these stimuli with positron emission tomographic measurements of cerebral blood flow in human volunteers and patients with visual defects to infer the existence of similar functional streams in visual areas of the human cortex. Allman and Zucker propose a hypothesis that assigns the encoding of geometrical and intensity differences to different modules in V1.

Although the different functional streams may remain largely segregated in separate modules and laminae within V1 and V2, horizontal interactions over distances that span at least several modules are also prominent in the experiments of Gilbert et al. Some of these interactions were highly specific for stimulus orientation, but others showed a convergence of influences from different orientations. Following peripheral lesions, much of the recovery in the responsiveness of cortex originally denervated by the lesion appeared to be mediated by widespread horizontal interactions within cortex. One must conclude that the cortical modules can make both selective and nonselective connections with one another.

Multiple cortical areas. Van Essen et al. and Zeki have arranged the many cortical visual areas into a rough hierarchy. It has been conventional to suppose that these different cortical areas are specialized in terms of the cues or sensory qualities that modulate the discharge of neurons in each area. Accordingly, one would expect to find some areas sensitive only to motion, others only to color, and still others only to binocular disparity, the cue to the stereoscopic perception of depth. Quantitative experimental findings rarely show such qualitative distinctions, and studies of all or nearly all cortical visual areas reveal more than an insignificant fraction of neurons whose responses are graded along each of the stimulus dimensions. Van Essen et al. have therefore raised the alternative possibility that these cortical visual areas may be specialized in terms of the perceptual features represented by their outputs, rather than by the particular stimulus cues to which the neurons respond. The position of objects in three-dimensional space might be represented in one visual area, for example, and neurons there might respond to the many different cues that contribute to this perception, including stereopsis, occlusion, motion parallax, and the direction of shadows. Nakayama and Shimojo show psychophysically that each of the stimulus qualities like color, depth, or motion that is thought to be processed in its own stream or module can profoundly influence the perception of stimuli thought to be processed in a different stream or module, a finding incompatible with a strict separation of the streams according to stimulus cues. These psychophysical findings may well be compatible with this alternative view of functional specialization.

Westheimer pointed to difficulties for distributed representations in multiple cortical areas posed by the tremendously high resolution of human vision (about 10 times better than the grain of the photoreceptor mosaic) in tasks involving relative spatial localization. Such hyperacuity, which is evident not only in stereoscopic vision, but also in vernier and other localization tasks, is little affected by blurring or image motion up to 2.5°/sec. It is difficult to imagine that hyperacuity could be attained by comparison of the spatial signs present in different cortical areas. Accordingly, it appears necessary to suppose that some cortical areas contain within themselves special machinery for the representation of differences in position, with receptive fields that are individually sensitive to the stimulus properties that allow hyperacuity. Psychophysically, Westheimer sees no sign of discontinuities in the cortical representation that might be thought to result from ocular dominance columns, on a fine scale, or multiple cortical representations, on the larger scale.

Visual motion. R. Andersen et al. have compared the motion-selective responses of neurons in V1, MT, and MST. Confirming the hierarchical arrangement of these areas, the responses of V1 neurons were the most simple and spatially confined, those of MT intermediate and more strongly influenced by surrounding stimulation, and those of MST quite complex in that their selective responses to certain small patterns were unaffected by varying the position of the pattern in the visual field. Comparison of the responses of neurons in MT and different parts of MST by Wurtz et al. also confirms the general hierarchical organization among higher cortical visual areas. Responses of neurons in MST suggest strongly that, unlike its immediate predecessor area, MT, MST is not homogeneous. Instead, different regions of MST appear to be specialized for different aspects of visual motion, such as the maintenance of pursuit eye movements in the lateral portion of MST.

Stereopsis. G. Poggio studied neurons in alert monkeys in V1 and V2 that are sensitive to the binocular disparity of visual stimuli. Similar types of responses were found at three successive stages of the proposed hierarchy of visual areas, in V1, V2, and V3a, but the proportion of disparity-selective cells increased from stage to stage. Disparity-selective responses were usually of one of three types, broadly tuned cells responding to objects nearer than the plane of fixation (called "near" or crossed-disparity cells); similarly broadly tuned cells selective for objects behind the plane of fixation ("far" or uncrossed-disparity cells), or tuned excitatory or inhibitory cells, whose optimal responses were usually to stimuli almost exactly on the plane of fixation. Many cells responded with identical tuning to light or dark bars as to random-dot stereograms (Julesz), a pure disparity stimulus in which no figure can be seen except by the correlations between the patterns of dots presented to the two eyes.

The finding of three pools of broadly disparity-selective cells rather than a series of disparity filters, each of which is tightly tuned to a different particular disparity, is reminiscent of color vision, in which the broad overlapping spectral sensitivities of the three types of cone photoreceptors allow excellent color discrimination by a comparison of the relative responses of two classes of cones using a population code. Lehky et al. have made models of human stereoacuity incorporating such a broadly distributed representation of near and far disparity pools and compared such a population code to models of other forms of encoding of binocular depth information. The population code was the most successful model at accounting for a number of features of the psychophysics. Calculations and simulations indicated that fewer than 20 such disparity neurons would be required to attain human levels of performance.

Distributed Representations in Motor Control

The motor control system appears at first sight to be needlessly complicated, with multiple feedback loops through many anatomical pathways. Just working out the basic framework of the circuitry is daunting and, in some respects, is still far from complete. The complexity becomes more comprehensible if one realizes that the system has not only to move, but to learn to improve its performance and to stabilize its performance in the face of loads, muscle weakness, or injury.

Mussa-Ivaldi et al. propose a simplifying notion that they examined in a simple vertebrate preparation, the spinalized frog. Their equilibrium-point hypothesis presupposes that each posture of the limb corresponds to a certain balance tension among the muscles (which act like opposing springs), corresponding to a certain pattern of motoneuronal activity. Movement is conceived of as a shift in this equilibrium point, so that the central nervous system would have the opportunity to represent different equilibrium points in different premotor interneurons by their projection patterns to the motoneurons. Consistent with their hypothesis, electri-cal stimulation in the interneuronal pools of the spinal cord gray matter produced force fields corresponding to new equilibrium points within the limb's work space.

Hogan et al. point out benefits of studying biological motor control in parallel with robotics: The complexity of apparently simple control problems is revealed by the difficulty in making robots perform smoothly when programmed with the principles thought to be present in the biological system. Features of biological motor control widely believed to be messy, inconvenient, or inessential may have profound importance. For example, recent robotics research has revealed mathematically and experimentally that a manipulator must have or must mimic the properties of a passive mechanical object (i.e., springs, masses, etc.) if it is to make stable contact with a rigid surface. The spring-like properties of muscles and limbs are now seen to be essential. Explorations in human subjects of the haptic sense, which allows one to infer the shape and surface properties of an object by manipulating it, reveal systematic distortions and illusions that cannot quantitatively be reconciled with the geometry of space. This suggests that the human motor control system does not need a self-consistent representation of objects.

Ghez et al. examined the role of proprioceptive input in the programming of movement by human patients whose limbs hand become deafferented. They show that the lack of proprioception prevents the patients from compensating for the complex and changing inertia presented by the limb in its different postures. This finding suggests that the complex biomechanics of limb movement is neither entirely precomputed by the motor control system nor entirely dependent on proprioceptive feedback. The feedback appears instead to fine-tune an existing program.

Lisberger et al. have systematically investigated the pathways responsible for motor learning in the vestibulo-ocular reflex (VOR), the simple reflex that stabilizes eye position in space by rotating the eyes by an amount equal and opposite to head movements. This reflex is actively adapted to a state of near perfection, and its strength can be experimentally controlled over a few days by fitting animals with magnifying or minifying spectacles. The reflex is produced through several parallel pathways leading from the sensor, the vestibular organ, that sum together on the effector, the motoneurons of the eye muscles. Using electrical rather than mechanical stimulation of the vestibular apparatus in order to improve the time resolution of responses, they find no sign of motor learning in the early part of the reflex mediated by the most rapid and direct pathways. Motor learning was evident only in the indirect pathways that affected eye movements with a protracted time course. These findings suggest that one function of parallel pathways in the nervous system may be to add sufficient flexibility for calibration and control without either delaying the onset of the signal in the recipient structure or introducing an additional stage of synaptic processing in more than the minimal fraction of the pathway needed for plasticity.

Models in Neurobiology

Models, formal and informal, have been an essential part of biophysical approaches to neurobiology. Informal modeling, as a kind of rough guide for a research program, is more widespread than one would suspect from reading the literature. For example, in the investigation of the mechanism of inactivation using variants of the *Shaker* potassium channels, Aldrich et al. discussed a "ball-and-chain" model, in which a hydrophilic ball at the amino terminus of the channel molecule was thought to dangle from a chain of amino acids until it landed in the channel and blocked the passage of current. Comparing three channels identical except at their amino-terminal regions, they found, consistent with the ball-and-chain model, that the channel with the longest and most hydrophilic amino-terminal region had the fastest inactivation rate, with the other two channels progressively slower to inactivate, shorter, and less hydrophilic. Interestingly, their chapter, unlike the oral presentation, makes no mention of this valuable informal model.

One of the early triumphs of formal mathematical modeling was Hodgkin and Huxley's (1952) simulation of the action potential in the squid axon. Torre et al. have modeled the light response and adaptation in photoreceptors with even greater biophysical and biochemical realism. Such formal models are not mere exercises in curve-fitting. Because the elements of the formal model of Torre et al. correspond to genuine biophysical and biochemical entities, the model *embod*ies our understanding of the biological system. Comparing the understanding presented in Torre et al. with the understanding of photoreceptors at the time of the "Molecular Neurobiology" Symposium in 1983, one will appreciate how rapid progress has been in this field. We can test this understanding, whose mathematical expression is the system of coupled differential equations written by Torre et al., to see where it breaks down or fails in principle. Each of these equations is fundamental, in the sense that the relationship it describes is a consequence of physical and chemical laws, rather than a matter of empirical observation. We can determine what the values of the model parameters must be for it to mimic the behavior that we find in the photoreceptors, and we can measure experimentally the values of the biological entities that the parameters represent. If the model cannot be made to work with values of its parameters consistent with experimental measurements, then our understanding of the processes taking place in the photoreceptor must simply be wrong.

Simulations using compartmental models of neurons connected in realistic circuits, like the model of lamprey locomotion presented by Grillner et al., can establish whether the known features of the neurons and the circuitry are capable of generating the range of behaviors observed experimentally. They can also assist in the interpretation of the sometimes complex effects of pharmacological treatments on such distributed systems. It is not possible simply to intuit the behavior of complexly connected systems containing feedback. If one takes the system apart to the extent that it becomes intuitively comprehensible, then the behaviors of interest may be lost. Modeling can thus be essential for understanding. It is important to note that the major elements of such a model do correspond directly to real features of the system being modeled. In the case of Grillner et al., in contrast to that of Torre et al. above, those elements are synapses and circuits rather than enzyme molecules. Although enzyme molecules underlie, for example, the effects of serotonin application that are reproduced in the lamprey model, the neurotransmitter effects are described at a higher level, in terms of time courses of conductances rather than levels of phosphodiesterase. The model of Lisberger et al., whose elements are even more abstract—firing rates and "gains" rather than conductances and synapses—plays a similar role in supplementing intuition and quantitatively testing the effects of experimental manipulations.

Except for biophysics and compartmental and circuit models like those described above, many biologically inclined neuroscientists have considered modeling to be a form of hand waving, an inexpensive and easy substitute for the often difficult work of finding out what is really going on. Computer modeling, which with modern graphics produces pictures that can mislead by their resemblance to biology, may be even worse; perhaps computers just permit the modeler to wave his hands 100,000 times as fast? For the reasons described above, models like that of Torre et al. are not susceptible to the old MIT criticism, "Give me 5 free parameters, and I'll make you an elephant. Give me a sixth, and I'll make him wag his tail." This criticism, however, may apply to models in fields such as economics as well as to many models in developmental neurobiology, central nervous system processing, and psychology. In these topics, the equations that modelers write usually do not embody fundamental laws; they are frequently just summaries of past behavior. The elements in such equations commonly do not correspond to anything that is really present at the level at which things actually operate in the system being modeled. Stryker et al. and Stryker (1991) review further features that make models useful.

Another goal of many current models is to answer the question, What arrangement of neural circuitry could accomplish a particular task? So-called "neural net" models are made to solve a problem, given a set of neural inputs and desired neural outputs, using learning algorithms that have no relation to the rules responsible for the development of the biological circuitry. The point of these models is merely to get a good or even an optimal solution by whatever means. The modeler may then compare the receptive fields and circuitry of the model neurons with those of the biological nervous system. This approach has the promise and pitfalls of the "ideal receiver" approach to sensory transduction. One assumes that the biological system will have evolved something like ideal performance, subject to various constraints. If the biological system performs much worse than the model, modelers ask whether they have to understand the task or the biological constraints correctly. Loeb et al. have applied this approach to sensorimotor feedback; Arnold and Robinson, to the oculomotor control system; and Bankman et al., to somatosensory cortical processing. In every case, they see a surprising similarity between the model neurons and the real ones, giving one confidence that the sometimes counterintuitive receptive field properties of central neurons can be important to the solution of the problem in which the neuronal circuit under study is engaged.

MEMORY, ATTENTION, AND HUMAN NEUROSCIENCE

In a sense, the topics discussed above have all to do with the neural machinery necessary to make neurons function as cells, form circuits, and make the body move and react to stimuli. The topics discussed in this section may eventually be regarded in this light as well, but they also must at least skirt issues that are at present much more difficult to think of in mechanistic terms, issues closer to the mind. Some of these issues are raised clearly by phenomena that are peculiarly difficult to investigate, like language, which exists only in humans, or like conscious awareness, which we have trouble knowing how to think about at all. For other issues, like perception and memory, it is an article of faith that they have clear animal counterparts, but their investigation in humans and our own introspection reveal aspects we would never have dreamed of from animal studies (although, once we take account of them, we may see their operation clearly in animals).

Neural Nets and Memory

There appears to be a great gulf between biological studies of memory—in the immune system, in flies and molluscs, and in hippocampal slices—and what is meant when a person says he remembers something. In part, that gulf is apparent because of the difficulty in comprehending how changes in neural circuitry could be used to "remember" anything the least bit interesting. It is easy to comprehend how a reflex that already exists could become stronger or weaker, but how could we make an arbitrary association? Although the difficulty in principle is alleviated by the (perhaps apocryphal) truism that no neuron is more than five to ten synapses away from any other neuron in the brain, that realization is little help in practice. How could we construct neural circuitry for memorizing arbitrary connections between things?

Studies of so-called "neural net" algorithms and the "parallel distributed processing" (PDP; Rumelhardt and McClelland 1986; not a brand of computer, as most neurophysiologists had thought) movement in cogni-

tive science have provided new insight into this problem during the past 15 years. A variety of "neural" networks (from now on in this section, I will stop using the quotation marks, but most of the unfortunate jargon of this field is expropriated from biology, making a discussion like the present one needlessly confusing) and learning rules can encode and store a fantastic amount of arbitrary information in an architecture reminiscent of the organization of a simple nervous system. The simplest powerful form of these networks consists of three layers of neural units (analogous to Herrick's sensory neurons, interneurons, and motor neurons). Each unit in one layer makes connections to all of the units in the next higher layer, and recipient units add up the total of the excitations of their inputs, weighted by the strength of each input connection. The recipient units then pass on some function of the excitation that they receive to their output connections onto the units in the next higher layer. Networks like these, if they are sufficiently large, have been proved mathematically to be capable of transforming any limited set of patterns given at their inputs into any arbitrary set of patterns at their outputs. Much of the excitement of the past 10 years in this field has resulted from the rediscovery of learning rules that allow one to adjust the strengths of the connections between the units in order to make the network behave as desired. In some learning-rule algorithms, the adjustment of strength is made solely on the basis of information available at the synapse, i.e., on the basis of the activities of presynaptic and postsynaptic units. A gradient-descent procedure called the back-propagation algorithm is commonly used to teach (i.e., to adjust the strengths of the connections in) a network so that, starting from a random state, with a set of examples of input activity patterns and desired output activity patterns, the network will come closer and closer to giving the right outputs for the right inputs.

This still may not sound much like interesting memory, but it is. Suppose the task is to start with a set of sample spellings and pronunciations and from them to learn and memorize the rules of phonics, and their exceptions, to allow a network to come up with the correct pronunciation of words written in English. Sejnowski and Rosenberg (1987) have used a back-propagation learning rule to train a three-layer network like the one described above to do a good job of producing the correct phonemes at the output from written English text. The particular learning process used may not be biologically realistic, but the network's computational and memory-storage abilities once it has learned provide a biologically plausible model of how an interesting memory could be encoded as a pattern of synaptic strengths in neuron-like circuitry. Lehky et al. provide other examples of such networks.

The architecture and unit properties of computational neural networks can be made to conform to those of actual, more complex networks. Hasselmo et al. have analyzed the ability of a more realistic neural network, modeled after the olfactory cortex, to do problems of categorization. Such a network might take as input the neural responses from a huge number of olfactory tract axons, each with its idiosyncratic response to the chemicals presented at the olfactory mucosa. The network could then generate outputs characteristic of its response to the smell of a rose, even if some of the inputs were absent or were different from those produced by the archetypal rose. Hasselmo et al. also show that the network will mimic some pharmacological effects of the biological olfactory cortex.

A major issue that must be considered in dealing with memory and with neural networks is representation. What is represented by the activities of the input units and output units is the most crucial choice in the design of neural networks. The representation in the brain of what it is that we remember is also perhaps the most difficult problem in grappling with human memory. Rolls addresses this problem in the hippocampus, reviewing theoretical work and neurophysiological findings consistent with the theory.

Goldman-Rakic et al. have explored memory in monkeys using a combination of behavioral memory tasks that are disrupted by particular brain lesions and anatomical, physiological, and pharmacological studies of the inputs, outputs, and patterns of neural activity of brain regions found behaviorally to be important for memory. When they trained monkeys to remember the position of a stimulus for a period of time before responding to it, Goldman-Rakic et al. showed that particular neurons in the dorsolateral prefrontal cortex maintain high rates of discharge for many seconds during the time between the disappearance of a stimulus in a particular part of the visual field and the time the monkey is allowed to respond to it. This neuronal activity could be interpreted as the neural representation of the remembered location of the stimulus. When a lesion was made in the region of these neurons, the monkeys could no longer do the memory task in that specific region of the visual field, even though they were perfectly capable of responding to a stimulus that was present there. These and other experiments suggest that neurobiology has located many of the brain regions important for memory in the performance of at least certain tasks. Ongoing studies promise to reveal much more of the neurobiology of these memory circuits.

Milner et al. reviewed evidence that memory is not unitary, but is dissociable into at least two forms: an associative or nondeclarative memory for habits, skills, and the like that is built up with practice, and a cognitive or declarative memory of thoughts and experiences. She describes the effects of different limbic and cortical lesions in human patients on a variety of memory tasks. These findings support the notion that different brain regions are specialized for different forms of memory. Squire et al. discussed cases of retrograde amnesia in human patients and its experimental production in animals. His work supports the dissocia-

tion of memory referred to above and the particular importance of limbic structures in the brain for memory and recall.

Artificial Intelligence

The area of study called artificial intelligence has made important theoretical contributions to neuroscience by separating conceptually the tasks that the brain needs to do from the algorithms or procedures by which the brain does them and from the neural circuitry or "hardware" that implements these algorithms. Few biological neuroscientists except in neuroethology (Konishi; Suga et al.) actually use an artificial intelligence approach in their experimental work, but this approach can provide powerful insights into the nature of perceptual and motor problems.

Ullman reviewed the problem of the visual recognition of familiar three-dimensional objects in the presence of distracting backgrounds. This is a task at which neuroanatomists in particular excel, but even pigeons are pretty good at it. Part of the difficulty of this problem is separating the object from the background without recognizing it or knowing what it is in the first place. Another part of the difficulty is that the view of the object changes depending on the position from which it is viewed. Ullman demonstrated that computationally simple algorithms can do a surprisingly good job of solving these problems. The algorithms have a structure that would be natural to construct out of elements like neurons.

T. Poggio demonstrated that there is a trade-off between the amount of computation needed to do a perceptual task and the amount of memory devoted to it. For example, we could either remember our multiplication tables or add up the multiplicand the number of times given by the multiplier. He outlined a mathematical approach that makes this trade-off explicit and suggested that the brain might use a memory-intensive approach to tasks involved in perception and movement.

Regional Specialization of the Human Brain

Damasio et al. have studied a large variety of perceptual, linguistic, and cognitive tasks in patients with a variety of brain lesions, the locations of which were independently determined with good resolution by magnetic resonance imaging. Their work provides powerful evidence that there are many highly specialized cortical areas that serve these higher functions. One is left with the impression that the 20–30 visual cortical areas may be few compared to the number of areas that deal with the more complex aspects of behavior.

Raichle reviews the range of imaging techniques available for studying the human brain and the role these techniques can play in disclosing regional specializations of structure and function. He describes experiments on language that attempt to separate production of language from its comprehension.

Experimental Studies of Attention and a Proposed Substrate of Awareness

The understanding of consciousness, the will, or awareness appears initially not to be susceptible to experimental investigation by neuroscientists. It seems to be the sort of problem best left for philosophers. But the phenomenon of attention, which may be conceived of as the direction of consciousness or awareness toward a particular object, has prominent neurophysiological consequences. Investigating attention may be one possible approach to the ultimate investigation of awareness.

In practice, if one sees an effect of attention in the nervous system, such as the enhancement of a response to the presentation of a visual stimulus when that stimulus is made important to an animal, it is always hard to distinguish from a possible effect of movement, since humans and animals will ordinarily move or orient themselves, if only very subtly, toward the objects to which they attend. Such movement can be blocked peripherally, of course, and more than 100 years ago, Helmhotz described the effects of an eye movement that was so prevented—a perceived shifting of the world in the direction of the intended eye movement (which makes sense because such a shift in the position of the world would leave the retinal image unchanged if eyes had actually succeeded in moving; see Stevens et al. 1976). For this reason, it is necessary to study the substrates of attention in awake, behaving animals so that one can hope to dissociate effects of attention from those of movement.

Goldberg et al. studied neurons in the parietal lobe that were active during the performance of a complex visual and eye-movement task. Like neurons previously studied in the frontal lobe, these neurons showed evidence of participation in the system that transforms the representation of visual stimuli from the coordinate system of the eyes to that of the animal's head or body. Unlike the frontal neurons, in the parietal lobe, the neuronal responses were not invariably coupled to the monkey's eye movements, suggesting that the parietal neurons are participating in a shifting of visual attention that ordinarily (but need not) precedes an eye movement.

Desimone et al. study visual responses in the extrastriate visual cortex and superior colliculus of monkeys under conditions in which the same stimulus is sometimes a signal for a task in which the monkey is engaged and on other trials is irrelevant to the task. Profound differences in visual responses were evident in some neurons, and it seems reasonable to attribute these differences to the attention that the monkey paid to the stimulus in the former case. Working backward from these effects of attention to the neural circuitry responsible for it may reveal something of the substrates and control of attention in the brain.

Julesz reviews his psychophysical studies of early cortical visual processing. He points out the tremendous similarity between many aspects of the central representations of visual stimuli deduced from psychophysical experiments and the receptive fields of cortical neurons. Several of his "textons," or basic elements of early visual perception, resemble nothing so much as cells in the visual cortex. However, his experiments also disclose the operation of a serial search mechanism, an internal shift of attention, that can focus on only a limited area of the visual stimulus field at one time but that can do complex discriminations. One cannot understand even quite simple aspects of human visual perception without considering attention.

Crick and Koch proposed that the study of visual awareness, which encompasses attention and the binding together in consciousness of all the many aspects of a stimulus that are thought to be represented in many separate visual areas (Van Essen et al.; Zeki), may become a productive enterprise. They suggested that the coherent oscillations of neuronal discharge and extracellular field potentials that have been observed between distant sites in the visual cortex responding to a single stimulus (Singer et al.) may be the substrate of this awareness. These oscillations were proposed to be the "glue" that binds the different representations of a single object together and constitute it as an object in consciousness. Llinás discussed the intrinsic membrane properties responsible for oscillatory activity in many cells and suggested that intrinsic properties of neurons and their circuits contribute to many features of neuronal activity and plasticity. The hypothesis put forth by Crick and Koch would represent an important step forward if the phenomena that it predicts are confirmed in alert-animal studies designed to test it as rigorously as, for example, Sparks ct al. have tested the role of the superior colliculus in the control of saccadic eye movements. Such an outcome would represent further progress, as we try as scientists to take yet another topic away from the philosophers.

CONCLUDING REMARKS

Progress in the field of neuroscience depends on interactions across an amazingly diverse intellectual landscape, stretching at the far right from physics and mathematics, which set our standards for theoretical work; through a core area of biophysics, biochemistry, and molecular, cell, and developmental biology; through a second core of neuroanatomy and neurophysiology; through a third core of studies of perception, ethology, attention, language, and memory; and onto the philosophy of mind on the far left. Theorists, engineers who try to build devices capable of doing some of the things that animals and people do, and physicians whose patients illuminate neuroscience or benefit from the insight it may yield burrow in and contribute to this landscape at many points. No one person is capable of seeing the whole landscape at once, at least at any distance close enough to be useful.

But for those with the energy to take it in, this Symposium offered the closest view available of the excitement of current research in its central 90%. Many did have that energy and will remember as well the pleasure of companionship and late night discussions over beer in Blackford Hall.

Nearly all who work in neuroscience, regardless of where they work on its landscape, do so at least in part because they believe that understanding the mind would be the most exciting accomplishment of human culture. Although this is a distant prospect, and we are far even from understanding the mind's organ, the brain, progress in many areas of neuroscience has been much more rapid than anyone would have imagined 20 years ago. In large part, this rapid progress has resulted from the open attitudes among most neuroscientists and their generous sharing of ideas about experiments dreamed of, planned, or in progress. It could also not have happened in the same way without a few people, like Steve Kuffler and Hans-Lukas Teuber, who first saw the expanse of neuroscience and who helped to unify it, and a few institutions, like the Cold Spring Harbor Laboratory, that have fostered it with summer courses that brought many talented people into the field and have helped to make its whole expanse respectable among biologists.

ACKNOWLEDGMENT

The author is grateful to the staff of the Meetings and Publications Departments of Cold Spring Harbor Laboratory, who organized the meeting and the book, respectively, with remarkable grace and efficiency, and to the members of the Long Island Biological Society, for hospitality that made our brief time away from neuroscience such a pleasure.

REFERENCES

Grinvald, A., R.D. Frostig, E. Lieke, and R. Hildesheim. 1988. Optical imaging of neuronal activity. *Physiol. Rev.* **68:** 1285.

Hodgkin, A. and H. Huxley. 1952. A quantitative description of membrane current and its application to conduction and excitation in nerve. *J. Physiol.* **117:** 500.

Julius, D., A.B. McDermott, R. Axel, and T.M. Jessell. 1988. Molecular characterization of a functional cDNA encoding the serotonin 1c receptor. *Science* **241:** 558.

Kauer, J.A., R.C. Malenka, and R.A. Nicoll. 1988. A persistent postsynaptic modification mediates long-term potentiation in the hippocampus. *Neuron* **1:** 911.

Lashley, K. 1950. In search of the engram. *Symp. Soc. Exp. Biol.* **4:** 454.

Muller, D. and G. Lynch. 1988. Long-term potentiation differentially affects two components of synaptic responses in hippocampus. *Proc. Natl. Acad. Sci.* **85:** 9346.

Numa, S. and M. Noda. 1986. Molecular structure of sodium channels. *Ann. N.Y. Acad. Sci.* **479:** 338.

Rumelhardt, D.E. and J.L. McClelland, eds. 1986. *Parallel distributed processing: Explorations in the microstructure of cognition*, vols. 1 and 2. MIT Press, Cambridge, Massachusetts.

Sakmann, B. and E. Neher. 1983. *Single-channel recording.* Plenum Press, New York.

Schiller, P.H., J.H. Sandell, and J.H. Maunsell. 1986. Functions of the ON and OFF channels of the visual system. *Nature* **322:** 824.

Schofield, P.R., B.D. Shivers, and P.H. Seeburg. 1990. The role of receptor subtype diversity in the CNS. *Trends Neurosci.* **13:** 8.

Sejnowski, T.J. and C.R. Rosenberg. 1987. Parallel networks that learn to pronounce English text. *Complex Systems* **1:** 145.

Stevens, J.K., R.C. Emerson, G.L. Gerstein, T. Kallos, G.R. Neufeld, C.W. Nichols, and A. C. Rosenquist. 1976. Paralysis of the awake human: Visual perceptions. *Vision Res.* **16:** 93.

Stryker, M.P. 1991. Activity-dependent reorganization of afferents in the developing mammalian visual system. In *Development of the visual system* (ed. D.M.K. Lam and C.J. Shatz), p. 267. MIT Press, Cambridge, Massachusetts.

Tsien, R.Y. 1989. Fluorescent probes of cell signaling. *Annu. Rev. Neurosci.* **12:** 227.

For the reader's (and the author's) convenience, all references insofar as possible are to chapters in this volume and are cited without dates. Although this practice does not respect the priority of scientific discovery, only a small number of reviews or primary papers are cited in connection with topics not covered in the chapters.

Author Index

Subject Index